MEDICAL MICROBIOLOGY

NOTE TO INSTRUCTORS:
Contact your Elsevier Sales Representative for teaching resources, including slides and image banks, for *Medical Microbiology*, 8e, or request these supporting materials at: http://[illegible].elsevier.com/Murray/microbiology/

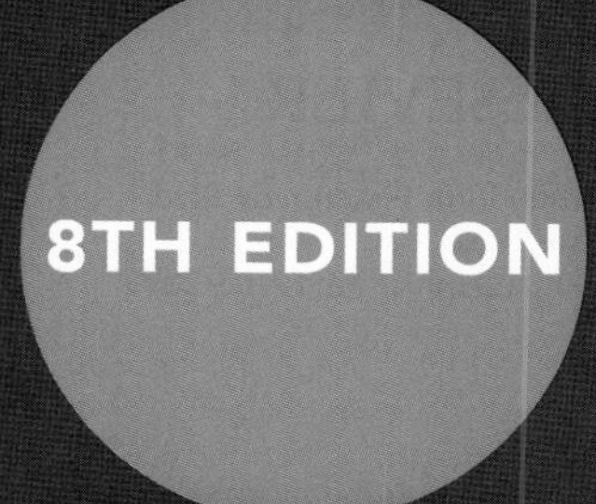

MEDICAL MICROBIOLOGY

PATRICK R. MURRAY, PhD
Senior Worldwide Director, Scientific Affairs
BD Diagnostics Systems
Sparks, Maryland;
Adjunct Professor, Department of Pathology
University of Maryland School of Medicine
Baltimore, Maryland

KEN S. ROSENTHAL, PhD
Professor of Biomedical Sciences
Director of Microbiology and Immunology
Roseman University of Health Sciences College of Medicine
Las Vegas, Nevada;
Emeritus Professor
Northeastern Ohio Medical University
Rootstown, Ohio

MICHAEL A. PFALLER, MD
Chief Medical Officer
T2 Biosystems
Lexington, Massachusetts;
Professor Emeritus
University of Iowa College of Medicine and College of Public Health
Iowa City, Iowa

ELSEVIER

ELSEVIER

1600 John F. Kennedy Blvd.
Ste 1800
Philadelphia, PA 19103-2899

MEDICAL MICROBIOLOGY, EIGHTH EDITION ISBN: 978-0-323-29956-5

Notices

Knowledge and best practice in this field are constantly changing. As new research and experience broaden our understanding, changes in research methods, professional practices, or medical treatment may become necessary.

Practitioners and researchers must always rely on their own experience and knowledge in evaluating and using any information, methods, compounds, or experiments described herein. In using such information or methods they should be mindful of their own safety and the safety of others, including parties for whom they have a professional responsibility.

With respect to any drug or pharmaceutical products identified, readers are advised to check the most current information provided (i) on procedures featured or (ii) by the manufacturer of each product to be administered, to verify the recommended dose or formula, the method and duration of administration, and contraindications. It is the responsibility of practitioners, relying on their own experience and knowledge of their patients, to make diagnoses, to determine dosages and the best treatment for each individual patient, and to take all appropriate safety precautions.

To the fullest extent of the law, neither the Publisher nor the authors, contributors, or editors assume any liability for any injury and/or damage to persons or property as a matter of products liability, negligence or otherwise, or from any use or operation of any methods, products, instructions, or ideas contained in the material herein.

Library of Congress Cataloging-in-Publication Data

Murray, Patrick R., author.
Medical microbiology / Patrick R. Murray, Ken S. Rosenthal, Michael A. Pfaller ; consultant, JMI Laboratories.—8th edition.
p. ; cm.
Includes bibliographical references and index.
ISBN 978-0-323-29956-5 (pbk. : alk. paper)
I. Rosenthal, Ken S., author. II. Pfaller, Michael A., author. III. Title.
[DNLM: 1. Microbiology. 2. Microbiological Techniques. 3. Parasitology. QW 4]
QR46
616.9′041—dc23

2015030867

Senior Content Strategist: James Merritt
Content Development Manager: Kathryn DeFrancesco
Publishing Services Manager: Catherine Jackson
Project Manager: Rhoda Howell
Design Direction: Brian Salisbury

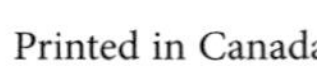

Printed in Canada

Last digit is the print number: 9 8 7 6 5 4 3 2 1

- *To all who use this textbook, that they may benefit from its use as much as we did in its preparation*

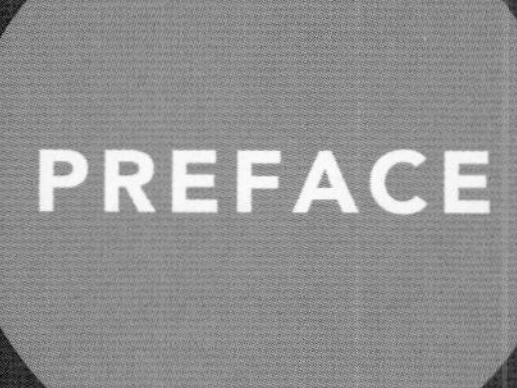

PREFACE

Our knowledge about microbiology and immunology is constantly growing, and by building a good foundation of understanding in the beginning, it will be much easier to understand the advances of the future.

Medical microbiology can be a bewildering field for the novice. We are faced with many questions when learning microbiology: How do I learn all the names? Which infectious agents cause which diseases? Why? When? Who is at risk? Is there a treatment? However, all these concerns can be reduced to one essential question: **What information do I need to know that will help me understand how to diagnose and treat an infected patient?**

Certainly, there are a number of theories about what a student needs to know and how to teach it, which supposedly validates the plethora of microbiology textbooks that have flooded the bookstores in recent years. Although we do not claim to have the one right approach to teaching medical microbiology (there is truly no one perfect approach to medical education), we have founded the revisions of this textbook on our experience gained through years of teaching medical students, residents, and infectious disease fellows, as well as on the work devoted to the seven previous editions. We have tried to present the basic concepts of medical microbiology clearly and succinctly in a manner that addresses different types of learners. The text is written in a straightforward manner with, it is hoped, uncomplicated explanations of difficult concepts. In this edition, we challenged ourselves to improve the learning experience even more. We are using the new technology on StudentConsult.com (e-version) to enhance access to the material. New to this edition, **chapter summaries** and learning aids are placed at the beginning of each of the microbe chapters, and on the e-version these are keyed to the appropriate sections in the chapter. In addition, many of the **figures** are enhanced to assist learning. **Details** are summarized in tabular format rather than in lengthy text, and there are colorful illustrations for the visual learner. **Clinical Cases** provide the relevance that puts reality into the basic science. **Important points** are emphasized in **boxes** to aid students, especially in their review, and the **study questions,** including Clinical Cases, address relevant aspects of each chapter. Each section (bacteria, viruses, fungi, parasites) begins with a chapter that summarizes microbial diseases, and this also provides **review material.**

Our understanding of microbiology and immunology is rapidly expanding, with new and exciting discoveries in all areas. We used our experience as authors and teachers to choose the most important information and explanations for inclusion in this textbook. Each chapter has been carefully updated and expanded to include new, medically relevant discoveries. In each of these chapters, we have attempted to present the material that we believe will help the student gain an interest in as well as a clear understanding of the significance of the individual microbes and their diseases.

With each edition of *Medical Microbiology* we refine and update our presentation. There are many changes to the eighth edition, both in the print and e-versions of the book. The book starts with a general introduction to microbiology and new chapters on the human microbiome and epidemiology of infectious diseases. The human microbiome (that is, the normal population of organisms that populate our bodies) can now be considered as another organ system with 10 times as many cells as human cells. This microbiota educates the immune response, helps digest our food, and protects us against more harmful microbes. Additional chapters in the introductory section introduce the techniques used by microbiologists and immunologists and are followed by chapters on the functional immune system. The immune cells and tissues are introduced, followed by an enhanced chapter on innate immunity and updated chapters on antigen-specific immunity, antimicrobial immunity, and vaccines. The sections on bacteria, viruses, fungi, and parasites have also been reorganized. Each section is introduced by the relevant basic science chapters and then the specific microbial disease summary chapter before proceeding into descriptions of the individual microbes, "the bug parade." Each chapter on the specific microbes begins with a summary (including trigger words), which is keyed to the appropriate part of the chapter in the e-version. As in previous editions, there are many summary boxes, tables, clinical photographs, and original clinical cases. **Clinical Cases** are included because we believe students will find them particularly interesting and instructive, and they are a very efficient way to present this complex subject. Each chapter in the "bug parade" is introduced by relevant questions to excite students and orient them as they explore the chapter. Finally, students are provided with access to the new Student Consult website, which provides links to additional reference materials, clinical photographs, animations (including new animations), and answers to the introductory and summary questions of each chapter. Many of the figures are presented in step-by-step manner to facilitate learning. A very important feature on the website is access to more than 200 **practice exam questions** that will help students assess their mastery of the subject matter and prepare for their course and licensure exams. In essence, this edition provides an understandable text, details, questions, examples, and a review book all in one.

• To Our Future Colleagues: The Students

On first impression, success in medical microbiology would appear to depend on memorization. Microbiology may seem to consist of only innumerable facts, but there is also a logic to microbiology and immunology. Like a medical detective, the first step is to know your villain. Microbes establish a niche in our bodies; some are beneficial and help us to digest our food and educate our immune system, while others may cause disease. Their ability to cause disease, and the disease that may result, depend on how the microbe interacts with the host and the innate and immune protective responses that ensue.

There are many ways to approach learning microbiology and immunology, but ultimately the more you interact with the material using multiple senses, the better you will build memory and learn. A **fun** and **effective** approach to learning is to **think like a physician and treat each microbe and its diseases as if it were an infection in your patient. Create a patient for each microbial infection, and compare and contrast the different patients.** Perform role-playing and ask the seven basic questions as you approach this material: Who? Where? When? Why? Which? What? and How? For example: Who is at risk for disease? Where does this organism cause infections (both body site and geographic area)? When is isolation of this organism important? Why is this organism able to cause disease? Which species and genera are medically important? What diagnostic tests should be performed? How is this infection managed? Each organism that is encountered can be systematically examined. Use the following acronym to create a clinical case and learn the essential information for each microbe: **DIVIRDEPT.** How does the microbial *d*isease present in the patient and the differential diagnosis? How would you confirm the diagnosis and *i*dentify the microbial cause of disease? What are the *v*irulence properties of the organism that cause the disease? What are the helpful and harmful aspects of the *i*nnate and *i*mmune response to the infection? What are the specific conditions or mechanisms for *r*eplicating the microbe? What are all the *d*isease characteristics and consequences? What is the *e*pidemiology of infection? How can you *p*revent its disease? What is its *t*reatment? Answering the DIVIRDEPT questions will require that you jump around in the chapter to find the information, but this will help you learn the material. For each of the microbes, learn three to five words or phrases that are associated with the microbe—words that will stimulate your memory (**trigger words,** provided in the new chapter summary) and organize the diverse facts into a logical picture. Develop **alternative associations.** For example, this textbook presents organisms in the systematic taxonomic structure (frequently called a "bug parade," but which the authors think is the easiest way to introduce the organisms). Take a given virulence property (e.g., toxin production) or type of disease (e.g., meningitis) and list the organisms that share this property. Pretend that an imaginary patient is infected with a specific agent and create the case history. Explain the diagnosis to your imaginary patient and also to your future professional colleagues. In other words, do not simply attempt to memorize page after page of facts; rather, use techniques that stimulate your mind and challenge your understanding of the facts presented throughout the text and **it will be more fun.** Use the summary chapter at the beginning of each organism section to **review** and help refine your "differential diagnosis" and classify organisms into logical "boxes." Get familiar with the textbook and its bonus materials and you will not only learn the material but also have a review book to work from in the future.

No textbook of this magnitude would be successful without the contributions of numerous individuals. We are grateful for the valuable professional help and support provided by the staff at Elsevier, particularly Jim Merritt, Katie DeFrancesco, and Rhoda Howell. We also want to thank the many students and professional colleagues who have offered their advice and constructive criticism throughout the development of this eighth edition of *Medical Microbiology*.

Patrick R. Murray, PhD; Ken S. Rosenthal, PhD; and Michael A. Pfaller, MD

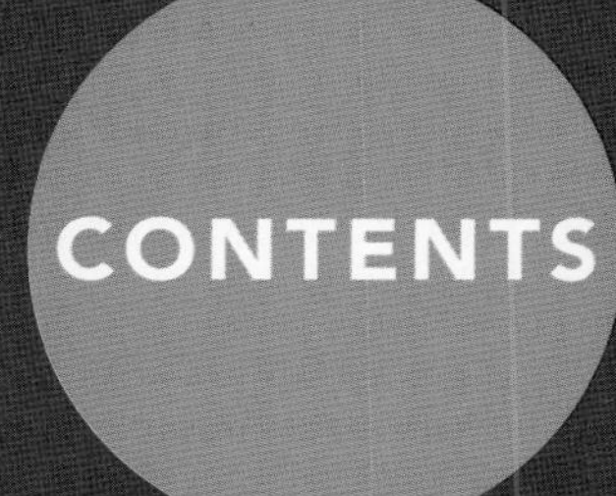

CONTENTS

SECTION 6
Mycology

SECTION 7
Parasitology

SECTION

1

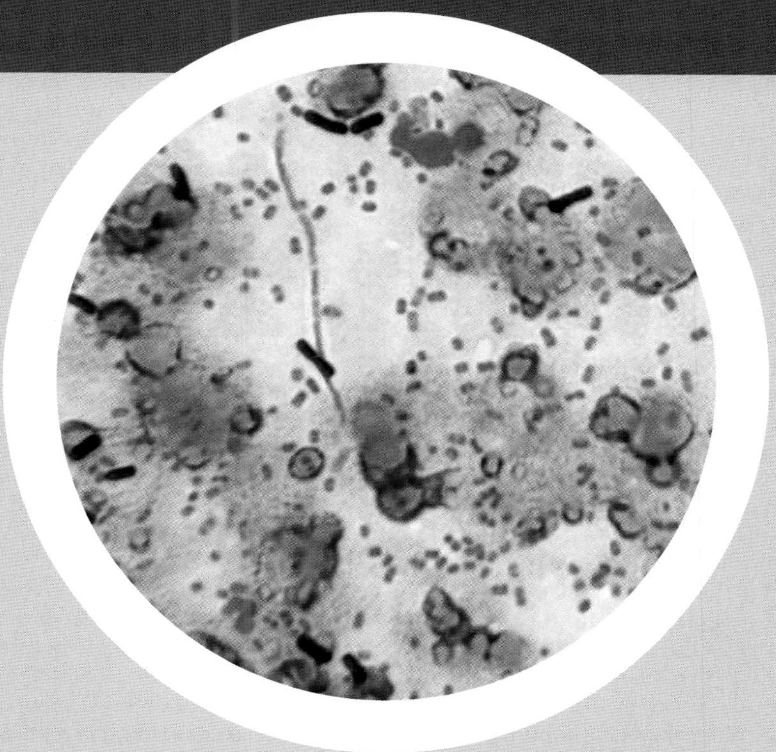

INTRODUCTION

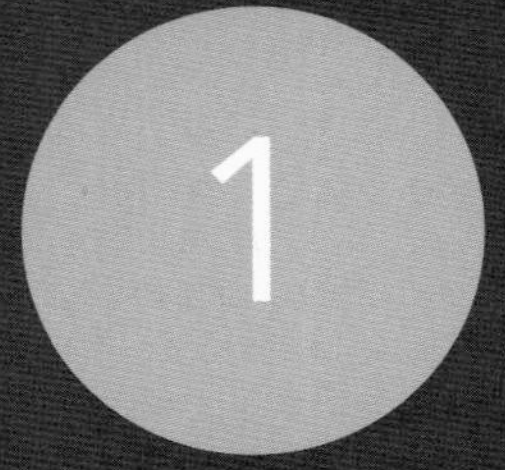

CHAPTER 1

INTRODUCTION TO MEDICAL MICROBIOLOGY

Imagine the excitement felt by the Dutch biologist Anton van Leeuwenhoek in 1674 as he peered through his carefully ground microscopic lenses at a drop of water and discovered a world of millions of tiny "animalcules." Almost 100 years later, the Danish biologist Otto Müller extended van Leeuwenhoek's studies and organized bacteria into genera and species according to the classification methods of Carolus Linnaeus. This was the beginning of the taxonomic classification of microbes. In 1840, the German pathologist Friedrich Henle proposed criteria for proving that microorganisms were responsible for causing human disease (the "germ theory" of disease). Robert Koch and Louis Pasteur confirmed this theory in the 1870s and 1880s with a series of elegant experiments proving that microorganisms were responsible for causing anthrax, rabies, plague, cholera, and tuberculosis. Other brilliant scientists went on to prove that a diverse collection of microbes was responsible for causing human disease. The era of chemotherapy began in 1910, when the German chemist Paul Ehrlich discovered the first antibacterial agent, a compound effective against the spirochete that causes syphilis. This was followed by Alexander Fleming's discovery of penicillin in 1928, Gerhard Domagk's discovery of sulfanilamide in 1935, and Selman Waksman's discovery of streptomycin in 1943. In 1946, the American microbiologist John Enders was the first to cultivate viruses in cell cultures, leading the way to the large-scale production of virus cultures for vaccine development. Thousands of scientists have followed these pioneers, each building on the foundation established by his or her predecessors, and each adding an observation that expanded our understanding of microbes and their role in disease.

Our knowledge of microbiology is now undergoing a remarkable transformation founded in the rapid technologic advances in genome analysis. The Human Genome Project was a multinational program that concluded in 2005 with the comprehensive sequencing of the human genome. The techniques developed for this program have rapidly moved into the research and clinical laboratories, leading to microbial sequencing and revealing previously unappreciated insights about pathogenic properties of organisms, taxonomic relationships, and functional attributes of the endogenous microbial population. Clearly, we are at the early stages of novel approaches to diagnostics and therapeutics based on the monitoring and manipulations of this population (the microbiome).

The world that van Leeuwenhoek discovered was complex, consisting of protozoa and bacteria of all shapes and sizes. However, the complexity of medical microbiology we know today rivals the limits of the imagination. We now know that there are thousands of different types of microbes that live in, on, and around us—and hundreds that cause serious human diseases. To understand this information and organize it in a useful manner, it is important to understand some of the basic aspects of medical microbiology. To start, the microbes can be subdivided into the following four general groups: viruses, bacteria, fungi, and parasites, each having its own level of complexity.

• Viruses

Viruses are the smallest infectious particles, ranging in diameter from 18 to 600 nanometers (most viruses are < 200 nm and cannot be seen with a light microscope). Viruses typically contain either deoxyribonucleic acid (DNA) or ribonucleic acid (RNA) but not both; however, some viral-like particles do not contain any detectable nucleic acids (e.g., prions), whereas the recently discovered Mimivirus contains both RNA and DNA. The viral nucleic acids required for replication are enclosed in a protein shell with or without a lipid membrane coat. Viruses are true parasites, requiring host cells for replication. The cells they infect and the host response to the infection dictate the nature of the clinical manifestation. More than 2000 species of viruses have been described, with approximately 650 infecting humans and animals. Infection can lead either to rapid replication and destruction of the cell or to a long-term chronic relationship with possible integration of the viral genetic information into the host genome. The factors that determine which of these takes place are only partially understood. For example, infection with the human immunodeficiency virus, the etiologic agent of the acquired immunodeficiency syndrome (AIDS), can result in the latent infection of CD4 lymphocytes or the active replication and destruction of these immunologically important cells. Likewise, infection can spread to other susceptible cells, such as the microglial cells of the brain, resulting in the neurologic manifestations of AIDS. The virus determines the disease and can range from the common cold to gastroenteritis to fatal catastrophes such as rabies, Ebola, smallpox, or AIDS.

• Bacteria

Bacteria are relatively simple in structure. They are **prokaryotic** organisms—simple unicellular organisms with no nuclear membrane, mitochondria, Golgi bodies, or endoplasmic reticulum—that reproduce by asexual division. The bacterial cell wall is complex, consisting of one of two basic forms: a gram-positive cell wall with a thick peptidoglycan layer, and a gram-negative cell wall with a thin peptidoglycan layer and an overlying outer membrane. Some bacteria lack this cell wall structure and compensate by surviving only inside host cells or in a hypertonic environment. The size (1 to 20 μm or larger), shape (spheres, rods, spirals), and spacial arrangement (single cells, chains, clusters) of the cells are used for the preliminary classification of bacteria, and the phenotypic and genotypic properties of the bacteria form the basis for the definitive classification. The human body is inhabited by thousands of different bacterial species—some living transiently, others in a permanent parasitic relationship. Likewise, the environment that surrounds us, including the air we breathe, water we drink, and food we eat, is populated with bacteria, many of which are relatively avirulent and some of which are capable of producing life-threatening disease. Disease can result from the toxic effects of bacterial products (e.g., toxins) or when bacteria invade normally sterile body tissues and fluids.

• Fungi

In contrast to bacteria, the cellular structure of fungi is more complex. These are **eukaryotic** organisms that contain a well-defined nucleus, mitochondria, Golgi bodies, and endoplasmic reticulum. Fungi can exist either in a unicellular form **(yeast)** that can replicate asexually or in a filamentous form **(mold)** that can replicate asexually and sexually. Most fungi exist as either yeasts or molds; however, some fungi can assume either morphology. These are known as **dimorphic** fungi and include such organisms as *Histoplasma, Blastomyces,* and *Coccidioides.*

• Parasites

Parasites are the most complex microbes. Although all parasites are classified as eukaryotic, some are unicellular and others are multicellular. They range in size from tiny protozoa as small as 4 to 5 μm in diameter (the size of some bacteria) to tapeworms that can measure up to 10 meters in length and arthropods (bugs). Indeed, considering the size of some of these parasites, it is hard to imagine how these organisms came to be classified as microbes. Their life cycles are equally complex, with some parasites establishing a permanent relationship with humans and others going through a series of developmental stages in a progression of animal hosts. One of the difficulties confronting students is not only an understanding of the spectrum of diseases caused by parasites but also an appreciation of the epidemiology of these infections, which is vital for developing a differential diagnosis and an approach to the control and prevention of parasitic infections.

• Immunology

It is difficult to discuss human microbiology without also discussing the innate and immune responses to the microbes. Our innate and immune responses evolved to protect us from infection. At the same time, the microbes that live in our bodies as normal flora or disease-causing organisms must be able to withstand or evade these host protections sufficiently long to be able to establish their niche within our bodies or spread to new hosts. The peripheral damage that occurs during the war between the host protections and microbial invaders contributes to or may be the cause of the symptoms of the disease. Ultimately, the innate and immune responses are the best prevention and cure for microbial disease.

• Microbial Disease

One of the most important reasons for studying microbes is to understand the diseases they cause and the ways to control them. Unfortunately, the relationship between many organisms and their diseases is not simple. Specifically, most organisms do not cause a single well-defined disease, although there are certainly ones that do (e.g., *Clostridium tetani* [tetanus], Ebola virus [Ebola], *Plasmodium* species [malaria]). Instead, it is more common for a particular organism to produce many manifestations of disease (e.g., *Staphylococcus aureus*—endocarditis, pneumonia, wound infections, food poisoning) or for many organisms to produce the same disease (e.g., meningitis caused by viruses, bacteria, fungi, and parasites). In addition, relatively few organisms can be classified as always pathogenic, although some do belong in this category (e.g., rabies virus, *Bacillus anthracis, Sporothrix schenckii, Plasmodium* species). Instead, most organisms are able to establish disease only under well-defined circumstances (e.g., introduction of an organism with a potential for causing disease into a normally sterile site such as the brain, lungs, and peritoneal cavity). Some diseases arise when a person is exposed to organisms from external sources. These are known as **exogenous infections,** and examples include diseases caused by influenza virus, *C. tetani, Neisseria gonorrhoeae, Coccidioides immitis,* and *Entamoeba histolytica.* Most human diseases, however, are produced by organisms in the person's own microbial flora that spread to normally sterile body sites where disease can ensue **(endogenous infections).**

The interaction between an organism and the human host is complex. The interaction can result in transient colonization, a long-term symbiotic relationship, or disease. The virulence of the organism, the site of exposure, and the host's ability to respond to the organism determine the outcome of this interaction. Thus the manifestations of disease can range from mild symptoms to organ failure and death. The role of microbial virulence and the host's immunologic response is discussed in depth in subsequent chapters.

The human body is remarkably adapted to controlling exposure to pathogenic microbes. Physical barriers prevent invasion by the microbe; innate responses recognize molecular patterns on the microbial components and activate local defenses and specific adapted immune responses that target the microbe for elimination. Unfortunately, the immune response is often too late or too slow. To improve the human body's ability to prevent infection, the immune system can be augmented either through the passive transfer of antibodies present in immune globulin preparations or through active immunization with components of the microbes (vaccines). Infections can also be controlled with a variety of chemotherapeutic agents. Unfortunately, microbes can mutate and share genetic information, and those that cannot be recognized by the immune response because of **antigenic variation** or those that are resistant to antibiotics will be selected and will endure. Thus the battle for control between microbe and host continues, with neither side yet able to claim victory (although the microbes have demonstrated remarkable ingenuity). There clearly is no "magic bullet" that has eradicated infectious diseases.

• Diagnostic Microbiology

The clinical microbiology laboratory plays an important role in the diagnosis and control of infectious diseases. However, the ability of the laboratory to perform these functions is limited by the quality of the specimen collected from the patient, the means by which it is transported from the patient to the laboratory, and the techniques used to demonstrate the microbe in the sample. Because most diagnostic tests are based on the ability of the organism to grow, transport conditions must ensure the viability of the pathogen. In addition, the most sophisticated testing protocols are of little value if the collected specimen is not representative of the site of infection. This seems obvious, but many specimens sent to laboratories for analysis are contaminated during collection with the organisms that colonize mucosal surfaces. It is virtually impossible to interpret the testing results with contaminated specimens, because most infections are caused by endogenous organisms.

The laboratory is also able to determine the antimicrobial activity of selected chemotherapeutic agents, although the value of these tests is limited. The laboratory must test only organisms capable of producing disease and only medically relevant antimicrobials. To test all isolated organisms or an indiscriminate empirical selection of drugs can yield misleading results with potentially dangerous consequences. Not only can a patient be treated inappropriately with unnecessary antibiotics, but also the true pathogenic organism may not be recognized among the plethora of organisms isolated and tested. Finally, the in vitro determination of an organism's susceptibility to a variety of antibiotics is only one aspect of a complex picture. The virulence of the organism, site of infection, and patient's ability to respond to the infection influence the host-parasite interaction and must also be considered when planning treatment.

• Summary

It is important to realize that our knowledge of the microbial world is evolving continually. Just as the early microbiologists built their discoveries on the foundations established by their predecessors, we and future generations will continue to discover new microbes, new diseases, and new therapies. The following chapters are intended as a foundation of knowledge that can be used to build your understanding of microbes and their diseases.

CHAPTER

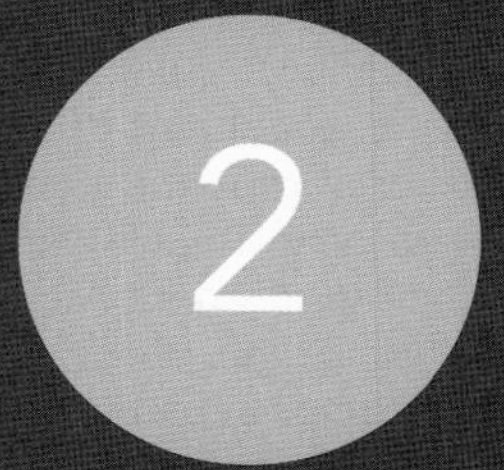

HUMAN MICROBIOME IN HEALTH AND DISEASE

Up until the time of birth, the human fetus lives in a remarkably protected and for the most part sterile environment; however, this rapidly changes as the infant is exposed to bacteria, archaea, fungi, and viruses from the mother, other close contacts, and the environment. Over the next few years, communities of organisms (**microbiota** or **normal flora** [Table 2-1]) form on the surfaces of the skin, nares, oral cavity, intestines, and genitourinary tract. The focus of this chapter is to gain an understanding of the role these communities play in the metabolic and immunologic functions of healthy individuals, factors regulating the composition of these communities, and how disruption of these communities can result in disease states.

• Human Microbiome Project

Our current knowledge of the **microbiome** is rooted in the successful completion of the Human Genome Project, a 13-year international effort initiated in 1990 that determined the sequences of the approximately 3 billion nucleotides that make up the 23,000 protein-encoding genes in human DNA. Much like efforts to send a man to the moon, the greatest legacy of this work was the development of technologies and informatic solutions that allow the generation and analysis of tremendous amounts of DNA and messenger RNA sequencing data.

The Human Microbiome Project was a 5-year multinational study to analyze the genetic composition (**microbiome**) of the microbial populations that live in and on healthy adults. To put the complexity of this program into perspective, it is estimated that bacterial cells outnumber human cells in the host by 10 : 1, and the bacterial population contributes at least 300-fold more protein genes.

The Human Microbiome Project was launched in 2007 with the collection of samples from the nose, mouth, skin, gut, and vagina from healthy adult volunteers. The microbes were identified by sequencing targeted regions of the 16S ribosomal RNA gene, and information about the gene content of the entire population was determined by sequencing the whole genome of a subset of specimens. These analyses showed that there is substantial variation in the species and gene composition for individuals and at different body sites. For example, bacteria colonizing the gut are different from those in the mouth, skin, and other body sites. The body site with the greatest taxonomic and genetic diversity was the intestine, and the vagina was the least complex. Microenvironments such as different regions of the mouth, gut, skin surface, and vagina also had their own unique microbiome (Figure 2-1).

• Core Microbiome

Most individuals share a **core microbiome,** arbitrarily defined as the species that are present at a specific site in 95% or more of individuals. The greatest numbers of shared species are present in the mouth, followed by the nose, intestine, and skin, and the fewest shared species are found in the vagina. Additionally, the small numbers of species that comprise the core microbiome are the most numerous, representing the majority of the total population, whereas the remaining portion of the population **(secondary microbiome)** consists of small numbers of many species that may not be widely shared by individuals. This would imply that the members of the core microbiome are critically important, providing essential functions that must be retained for normal metabolic and immunologic activities, and the functions provided by the secondary microbiome are also critically important but can be provided by a variety of organisms. In other words, although there is tremendous variation of species among individuals, there is less variation in the genetic composition at each site. The **taxonomic diversity** of a population is great, but the functional properties are highly conserved **(functional redundancy)** in microbiomes associated with health. This is not surprising if we consider that the microbiome is a community that exists in a symbiotic relationship with its host, providing needed metabolic functions, stimulating innate immunity, and preventing colonization with unwanted pathogens. Thus interpersonal variations of the microbiome can exist in healthy individuals as long as the needed functions are satisfied.

• Evolution of the Microbiome and Normal Flora

The **normal flora** of a particular site of the body consists of a unique community of core and secondary microbiota that evolved through a symbiotic relationship with the host and a competitive relationship with other species. The host provides a place to colonize, nutrients, and some protection from unwanted species (innate immune responses). The microbes provide needed metabolic functions, stimulate innate and regulatory immunity, and prevent colonization with unwanted pathogens (Figure 2-2). The ability to tolerate

Table 2-1 Glossary of Terms

Term	Definition
Microbiota	Community of microbes that live in and on an individual; can vary substantially between environmental sites and host niches in health and disease
Normal flora	Microbiota
Microbiome	Aggregate collection of microbial genomes in the microbiota
Core microbiome	Commonly shared microbial species among individuals at specific body sites; although typically represented by a limited number of species, these comprise the largest proportion of the microbial population
Secondary microbiome	Microbial species that contribute to the unique diversity of individuals at specific body sites; typically present in proportionately small numbers
Functional redundancy	Required functions (e.g., metabolism of nutrients, regulation of the immune response) that are provided by the diverse members of the microbiota
Taxonomic diversity	The diverse number of species that comprise the microbiota
Prebiotic	Food ingredient that supports the growth of one or more members of the microbiota
Probiotic	Live organism that when ingested is believed to provide benefit to the host

the amount of oxygen or lack thereof (redox state) and the pH and salt concentration, as well as to scavenge essential minerals and harvest and metabolize the available nutrients, determines the numbers and nature of the species that populate a site of the body. Anaerobic or facultative anaerobic bacteria colonize most of the sites of the body because of the lack of oxygen in sites such as the mouth, intestine, and genitourinary tract.

The composition of the microbiota is influenced by personal hygiene (e.g., use of soap, deodorants, mouthwash, skin peels, enemas, vaginal douches), diet, water source, medicines (especially antibiotics), and exposure to environmental toxins. Drinking well water versus chlorinated city water or a diet consisting of more or less fiber, sugar, or fats can select for different intestinal bacteria based on their ability to utilize the essential minerals (e.g., iron) and nutrients. Alteration of the environment with foods or medicines can also alter the microbiota (Figure 2-3). These changes can be acceptable if the core microbiome and critical functional properties of the microbiome are maintained but can result in disease if these functions are lost. Historically, the greatest concern with the use of broad-spectrum antibiotics was the selection of resistant bacteria; however, a greater concern should be the disruption of the microbiome and loss of essential functions.

Of the approximately 200 unique species of bacteria that colonize the gut, most are members of the Actinobacteria (e.g., *Bifidobacterium*), Bacteroidetes (e.g., *Bacteroides*), and Firmicutes (e.g., *Eubacterium, Ruminococcus, Faecalibacterium, Blautia*). Interestingly, the importance of many of these bacteria was not appreciated before gene sequencing was used to identify and quantitate the gut microbiota. Within the colon, some bacteria wage interspecies warfare to establish their niche with bacteriocins (e.g., colicins produced by *Escherichia coli*), other antibacterial proteins, and metabolites that deter other species from growing. These molecules also benefit the host by eliminating invading bacteria including *Salmonella, Shigella, Clostridium difficile, Bacillus cereus,* and other pathogens. The bacteria must also resist antimicrobial peptides and immunoglobulin (Ig)A produced by the host and released into the bowel.

Metabolism of nutrients plays a major role in the symbiotic relationship between the human host and microbe. Bacteria in the human gut are responsible for metabolizing complex carbohydrates (including cellulose) to provide small-chain fatty acids such as acetate, propionate, and butyrate that can be readily transported and used by the cells of our body. These acids also limit the growth of undesirable bacteria. Other bacteria graze on the carbohydrates, the mucins that line the epithelium, or the oils released in our sweat. Bacteroidetes and Firmicutes are more efficient than others at breaking down complex carbohydrates, including plant cell wall compounds (cellulose, pectin, xylan) as well as host-derived carbohydrates, including those attached to the mucins or chondroitin sulfates of the protective mucous layer of the intestine. Increases in the ratio of these bacteria in the gut microbiome can lead to a higher efficiency in storage of the metabolic byproducts. This can be a benefit for malnourished populations or patients with debilitating diseases such as cancer, or can lead to obesity in well-nourished populations.

Role of the Microbiome in Disease

If the normal microbiome characterizes health, alterations in the microbiome can signify disease, a relationship we are only beginning to understand. In 1884 Robert Koch and Friedrich Loeffler defined the relationship between an organism and infection. The **Koch postulates** were based on the concept of one organism: one disease. Microbiome research has introduced a new concept—disease caused by a community of organisms rather than a single species of bacteria, and the influence extends beyond traditional "infectious" diseases to include immunologic and metabolic disorders such as inflammatory bowel disease, obesity, type 2 diabetes, and celiac disease. We are now at the forefront of a new era of defining infectious diseases.

Disruption of the normal microflora (commonly referred to as **dysbiosis**) can lead to disease by the elimination of needed organisms or allowing the growth of inappropriate bacteria. For example, following exposure to antibiotics and suppression of the intestinal normal flora, *C. difficile* is able to proliferate and express enterotoxins, leading to inflammation of the colon **(antibiotic-associated colitis).** Another disease of the colon, **ulcerative colitis,** is associated with an increased level of bacteria producing mucin-degrading sulfatases, leading to degradation of the protective mucosal lining of the intestinal wall and stimulation of inflammatory immune responses. Individuals with an intestinal microbiota that is more efficient at breaking down complex carbohydrates internalize rather than void these nutrients and are therefore susceptible to **obesity** and a predisposition to metabolic syndromes such as **type 2 diabetes.** Not all patients genetically predisposed to **celiac disease,** an

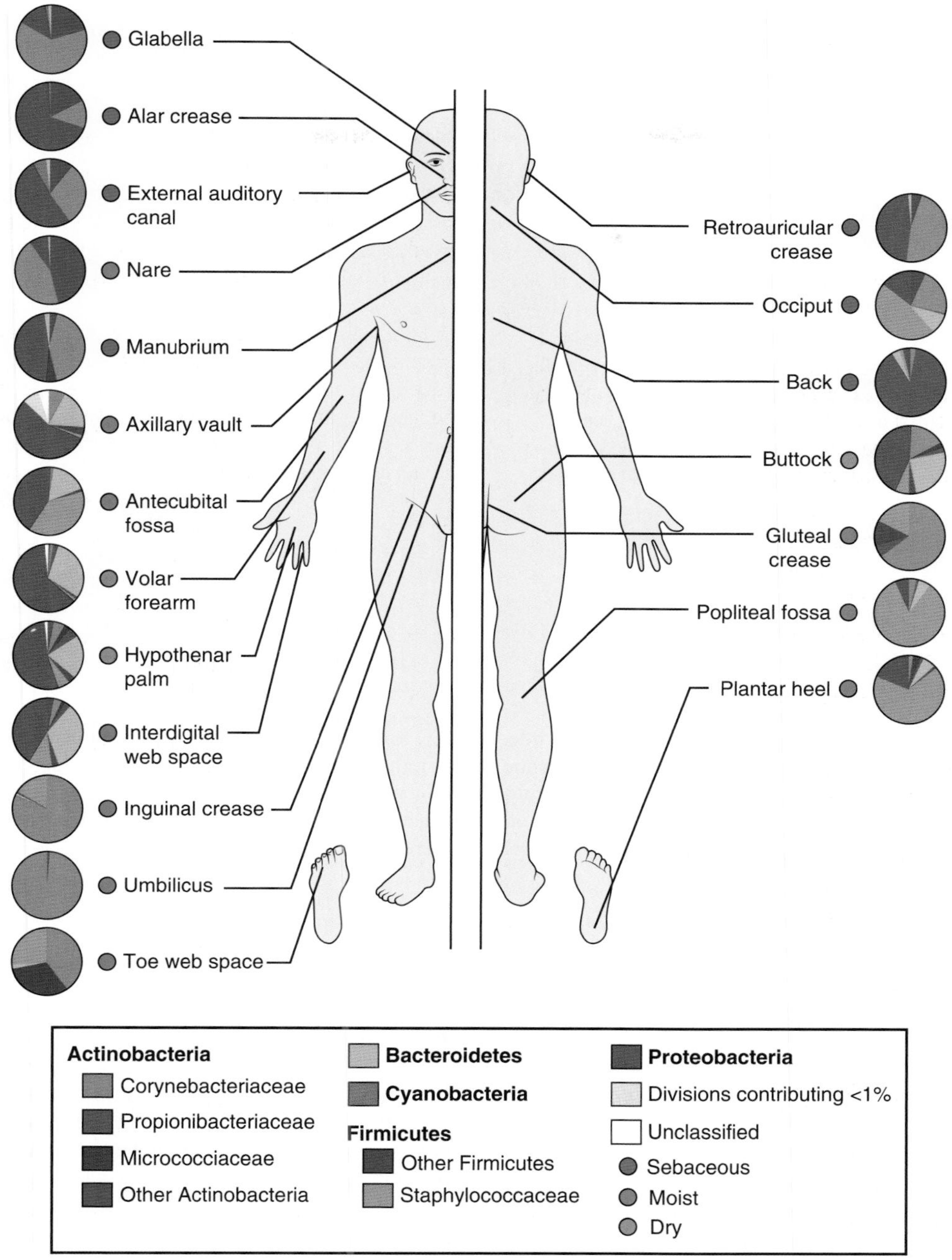

FIGURE 2-1 Topographical distribution of bacteria on skin sites. As at other body sites, the distribution of the skin microbiome is dependent on the microenvironment of the sampled site, such as sebaceous or oily *(blue circles),* moist *(green circles),* and dry, flat surfaces *(red circles).* (From Grice E, Segre J: The skin microbiome, *Nat Rev Microbiol* 9:244–253, 2011.)

immune-mediated enteropathology precipitated by exposure to gluten proteins, are symptomatic. The intestinal microbiota of most individuals is composed of bacteria capable of digesting glutens, which may be sufficient to protect these genetically predisposed individuals. In the absence of these bacteria, disease may occur. Shifts in the skin microbiome are associated with progression to **chronic wound infections** and episodic exacerbations of **atopic dermatitis.** Alteration in the vaginal microbiome from relatively few predominant organisms to a heterogeneous mixed population is associated with the progression to **vaginitis.**

Diagnostics and Therapeutics

An understanding of the influence of dysbiosis on disease pathology can lead to both advanced diagnostic tests and paths for therapeutic intervention. Just as the presence of *Salmonella* or *Shigella* signifies disease, changes in the diversity and composition of the fecal microflora can also indicate susceptibility to or onset of disease. The most obvious example is *C. difficile* disease—clinical disease is preceded by a depletion of the normal flora owing to antibiotic use. Interestingly, patients with chronic relapsing *C. difficile* infections

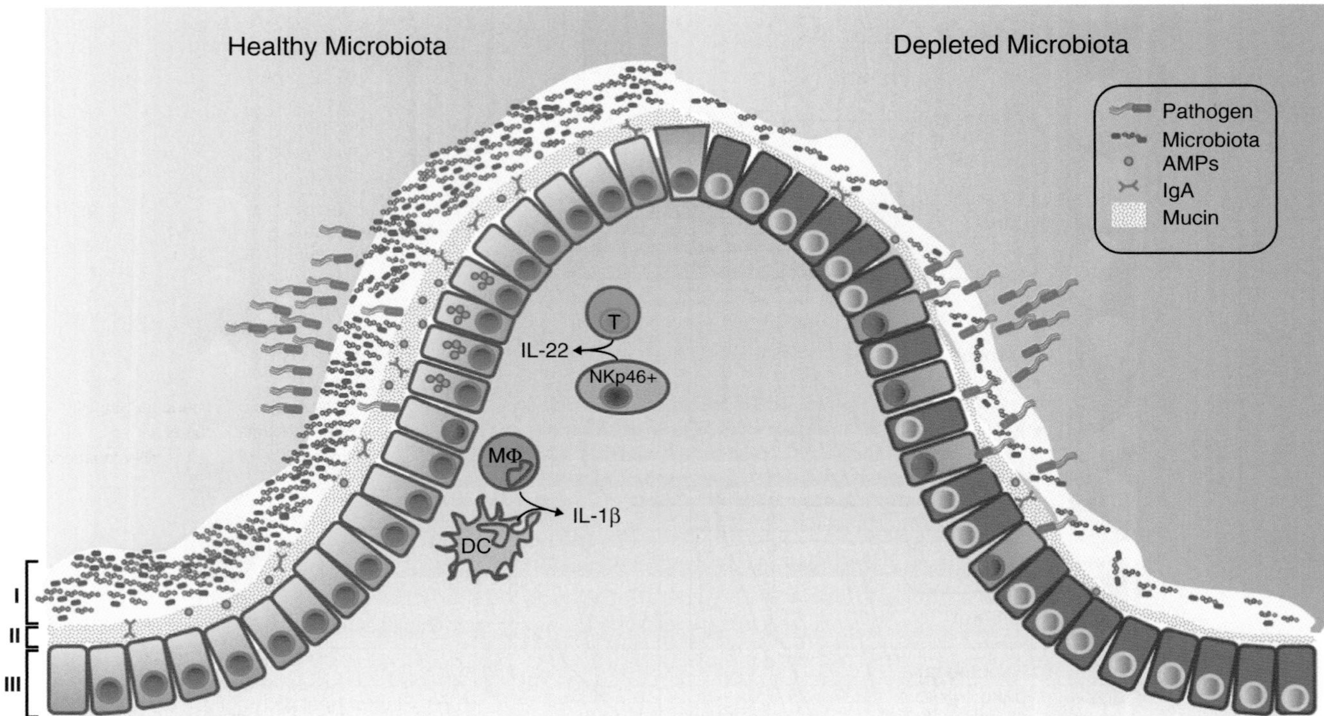

FIGURE 2-2 Intestinal microbiota protection against enteric infections. (I) Saturation of colonization sites and consumption of nutrients limit pathogen access to host tissues; (II) the microbiota prime innate immunity by stimulating mucin production, immunoglobulin *(Ig)*A, and antimicrobial peptides *(AMPs);* and (III) the microbiota stimulate interleukin *(IL)*-22 expression, which increases epithelial resistance, and IL-1β production, which promotes recruitment of inflammatory cells. (From Khosravi A, Mazmanian S: Disruption of the gut microbiome as a risk factor for microbial infections, *Curr Opin Microbiol* 16:221–227, 2013.)

are treated successfully by repopulating (some say **"repoopulating"**) the intestines with stool transplants from a healthy spouse or close relative, or with artificially created stool specimens consisting of a complex mixture of aerobic and anaerobic fecal organisms.

More subtle alterations in the gut microbiome may predict development of diseases such as **necrotizing enterocolitis (NEC),** inflammatory bowel disease, and a predilection for obesity. NEC is a devastating intestinal disease that afflicts preterm infants. Prospectively collected stool samples from infants younger than 29 weeks' gestational age who develop NEC demonstrate a distinct dysbiosis prior to the development of disease. Infants with early-onset disease have a dominance of Firmicutes (predominantly *Staphylococcus*), whereas infants with late-onset NEC have a dominance of Enterobacteriaceae.

The effects of microbiome alterations have also been described for the pathogenesis of inflammatory bowel disease and colorectal cancer. Proliferation of bacteria such as *Akkermansia muciniphila* that produce mucin-degrading sulfatases is responsible for degradation of the intestinal wall lining. Additionally, an increase in members of the anaerobic family Prevotellaceae leads to up-regulation of chemokine-mediated inflammation. Enterotoxigenic *Bacteroides fragilis* can also induce T helper cell–mediated inflammatory responses that are associated with colitis and are a precursor to colonic hyperplasia and colorectal tumors. Finally, *Methanobrevibacter smithii,* a minor member of the gut microbiome, enhances digestion of dietary glycans by *Bacteroides thetaiotaomicron* and other core intestinal bacteria, leading to accumulation of fat.

• Probiotics

Probiotics are mixtures of bacteria or yeast that upon ingestion colonize and proliferate, even temporarily, the intestine. Consumers of probiotics believe they act by rebalancing the microbiome and its functions, such as enhancing digestion of food and modulating the individual's innate and immune response. The most common reason people use over-the-counter probiotics is to promote and maintain regular bowel function and improve tolerance to lactose. Probiotics are commonly gram-positive bacteria (e.g., *Bifidobacterium, Lactobacillus*) and yeasts (e.g., *Saccharomyces*). Many of these microbes are found in ingestible capsules and as food supplements (e.g., yogurt, kefir). Probiotics have been used to treat *C. difficile*–associated diarrhea and inflammatory bowel disease, to provide protection from *Salmonella* and *Helicobacter pylori* disease, as therapy for pediatric atopic dermatitis and autoimmune diseases, and even for reduction in dental caries, although the value of probiotics for many of these conditions is unproven. Although probiotics are safe dietary supplements, not all probiotics are effective and for all people. The species, mixture of species, and dose and viability of the probiotic organisms within a probiotic formulation influence its potency, efficacy, and therapeutic potential. What is clear is that much like the use of complex artificial mixtures of

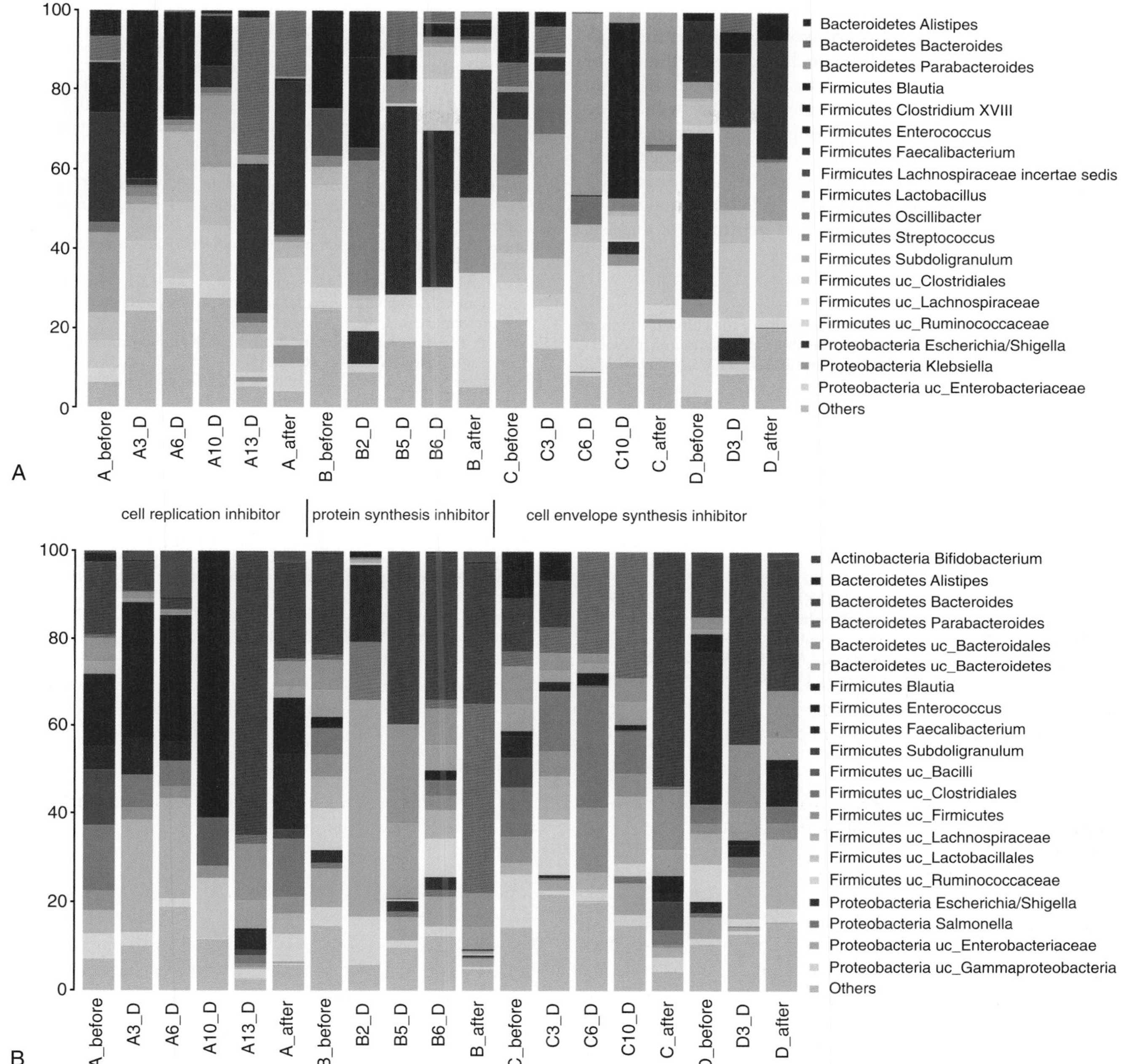

FIGURE 2-3 Effect of antibiotics on the gut microbiota. Fecal samples were collected from four patients treated with antibiotics: patient A, moxifloxacin; patient B, penicillin + clindamycin; patient C, cefazolin followed by ampicillin/sulbactam; patient D, amoxicillin. Fecal samples collected before, during (e.g., 3_D is day 3 of therapy), and after therapy were used to assess the total microbiota. Changes are noted both during therapy and after therapy is discontinued. **A,** Total microbiota (16S rRNA gene). **B,** Metabolically active microbiota (16S rRNA transcripts). (From Perez-Cobas AE, Artacho A, Knecht H, et al: Differential effects of antibiotic therapy on the structure and function of human gut microbiota, *PLoS One* 8:e80201, 2013.)

organisms to treat recurrent *C. difficile* disease, carefully designed "smart probiotics" will likely be an important adjunct to medical therapy in the future.

• Perspective

In the near future, with faster and cheaper DNA sequencing procedures, analysis of a person's microbiome may become a routine diagnostic test for predicting and treating a wide range of diseases. However, a number of questions remain to be resolved, including: can we predict disease in an individual by monitoring changes in the microbiome; which changes are most important—taxonomic or genetic function; can we prevent disease or treat disease by reestablishing a healthy microbiome; can this be done by prescribing specific replacement microbes (e.g., fecal transplant) or with a universal mixture (probiotic); can the use of metabolic supplements (**prebiotics**) promote a healthy microbiota; and will use of antibiotics be replaced by use of "smart microbiome" therapies? Other questions include: what is the role of the host genome, environmental factors, and our hygienic practices in shaping the microbiome; and what will be the informatic requirements for guiding diagnostics or therapeutics? Regardless of the answers to these and other questions, it is certain that we are witnessing the beginning of a new era of microbiology that can radically change our approach to prediction, diagnosis, and treatment of disease.

Bibliography

Caminero A, Herran AR, Nistal E, et al: Diversity of the cultivable human gut microbiome involved in gluten metabolism: isolation of microorganisms with potential interest for celiac disease, *FEMS Microbiol Ecol* 88:309–319, 2014.

Cho I, Blaser MJ: The human microbiome: at the interface of health and disease, *Nat Rev Genet* 13:260–270, 2012.

Damman CJ, Miller SI, Surawicz CM, et al: The microbiome and inflammatory bowel disease: is there a therapeutic role for fecal microbiota transplantation? *Am J Gastroenterol* 107:1452–1459, 2012.

David LA, Maurice CF, Carmody RN, et al: Diet rapidly and reproducibly alters the human gut microbiome, *Nature* 505:559–563, 2014.

Deweerdt S: A complicated relationship status, *Nature* 508:S62–S63, 2014.

Faith JJ, Guruge JL, Charbonneau M, et al: The long-term stability of the human gut microbiota, *Science* 341:1237439, 2013.

Gevers D, Knight R, Petrosino JF, et al: The Human Microbiome Project: a community resource for the healthy human microbiome, *PLoS Biol* 10:e1001377, 2012.

Grice E, Segre J: The skin microbiome, *Nat Rev Microbiol* 9:244–253, 2011.

Hajishengallis G, Darveau R, Curtis M: The keystone-pathogen hypothesis, *Nat Rev Microbiol* 10:717–725, 2012.

Human Microbiome Project Consortium: A framework for human microbiome research, *Nature* 486:215–221, 2012.

Human Microbiome Project Consortium: Structure, function and diversity of the healthy human microbiome, *Nature* 486:207–214, 2012.

Khosravi A, Mazmanian S: Disruption of the gut microbiome as a risk factor for microbial infections, *Curr Opin Microbiol* 16:221–227, 2013.

Landers ES, Linton LM, Birren B, et al: Initial sequencing and analysis of the human genome, *Nature* 409:860–921, 2001.

Li K, Bihan M, Methé BA: Analyses of the stability and core taxonomic memberships of the human microbiome, *PLoS ONE* 8:e63139, 2013.

McDermott AJ, Huffnagle GB: The microbiome and regulation of mucosal immunity, *Immunology* 142:24–31, 2014.

Morgan XC, Segata N, Huttenhower C: Biodiversity and functional genomics in the human microbiome, *Trends Genet* 29:51–58, 2013.

Morrow AL, Lagomarcino AJ, Schibler KR, et al: Early microbial and metabolomics signatures predict later onset of necrotizing enterocolitis in preterm infants, *Microbiome* 1:13, 2013.

Murray P: The Human Microbiome Project: the beginning and future status, *Ann Clin Microbiol* 16:162–167, 2013.

Perez-Cobas AE, Artacho A, Knecht H, et al: Differential effects of antibiotic therapy on the structure and function of human gut microbiota, *PLoS ONE* 8:e80201, 2013.

Petrof EO, Claud EC, Gloor GB, et al: Microbial ecosystems therapeutics: a new paradigm in medicine? *Benef Microbes* 4:53–65, 2013.

Petschow B, Dore J, Hibberd P, et al: Probiotics, prebiotics, and the host microbiome: the science of translation, *Ann N Y Acad Sci* 1306:1–17, 2013.

Srinivasan S, Hoffman NG, Morgan MT, et al: Bacterial communities in women with bacterial vaginosis: high resolution phylogenetic analysis reveal relationships of microbiota to clinical criteria, *PLoS ONE* 7:e37818, 2012.

Venter JC, Adams MD, Myers EW, et al: The sequence of the human genome, *Science* 291:1304–1351, 2001.

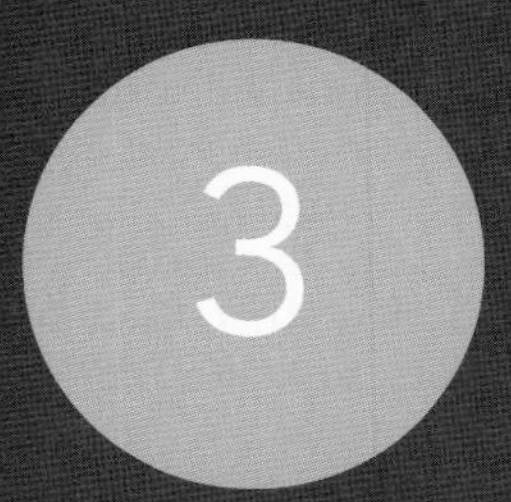

CHAPTER 3

STERILIZATION, DISINFECTION, AND ANTISEPSIS

An important aspect of the control of infections is an understanding of the principles of sterilization, disinfection, and antisepsis (Box 3-1).

• Sterilization

Sterilization is the total destruction of all microbes, including the more resilient forms such as bacterial spores, mycobacteria, nonenveloped (non-lipid) viruses, and fungi. This can be accomplished using physical, gas vapor, or chemical sterilants (Table 3-1).

Saturated steam under pressure is a widely used, inexpensive, nontoxic, and reliable method of sterilization. Three parameters are critical: the time of exposure to steam, temperature, and amount of moisture. The most commonly used sterilization cycle is use of saturated steam heated at 121° C for 15 minutes. Maintaining the proper temperature is critical because a drop of 1.7° C increases the needed exposure time by 48%. If no moisture is present, then the temperature must reach 160° C. Dry heat sterilization requires prolonged exposure times and damages many instruments, so it is not currently recommended.

Ethylene oxide gas is used to sterilize temperature- or pressure-sensitive items. Treatment is generally for 4 hours, and sterilized items must be aerated for an additional 12 hours to eliminate the toxic gas before the items are used. Although ethylene oxide is highly efficient, strict regulations limit its use, because it is flammable, explosive, and carcinogenic to laboratory animals. For these reasons, ethylene oxide sterilization is avoided if acceptable alternatives are available.

Hydrogen peroxide vapors are effective sterilants because of the oxidizing nature of the gas. This sterilant is used for the sterilization of instruments. A variation is **plasma gas sterilization,** in which hydrogen peroxide is vaporized, and then reactive free radicals are produced with either microwave-frequency or radio-frequency energy. Because this is an efficient sterilizing method that does not produce toxic byproducts, plasma gas sterilization has replaced many of the applications for ethylene oxide. However, it cannot be used with materials that absorb hydrogen peroxide or react with it.

Two **chemical sterilants** have also been used: **peracetic acid** and **glutaraldehyde.** Peracetic acid, an oxidizing agent, has excellent activity, and the end products (i.e., acetic acid and oxygen) are nontoxic. In contrast, safety is a concern with glutaraldehyde, and care must be used when handling this chemical.

• Disinfection

Microbes are also destroyed by disinfection procedures, although more resilient organisms can survive. Unfortunately, the terms *disinfection* and *sterilization* are casually interchanged and can result in some confusion. This occurs because disinfection processes have been categorized as high level, intermediate level, and low level. High-level disinfection can generally approach sterilization in effectiveness, whereas spore forms can survive intermediate-level disinfection, and many microbes can remain viable when exposed to low-level disinfection.

Even the classification of disinfectants (Table 3-2) by their level of activity is misleading. The effectiveness of these procedures is influenced by the nature of the item to be disinfected, number and resilience of the contaminating organisms, amount of organic material present (which can inactivate the disinfectant), type and concentration of disinfectant, and duration and temperature of exposure.

High-level disinfectants are used for items involved with invasive procedures that cannot withstand sterilization procedures (e.g., certain types of endoscopes and surgical instruments with plastic or other components that cannot be autoclaved). Disinfection of these and other items is most effective if cleaning the surface to remove organic matter precedes treatment. Examples of high-level disinfectants include treatment with moist heat and use of liquids such as glutaraldehyde, hydrogen peroxide, peracetic acid, and chlorine compounds.

Intermediate-level disinfectants (i.e., alcohols, iodophor compounds, phenolic compounds) are used to clean surfaces or instruments where contamination with bacterial spores and other highly resilient organisms is unlikely. These have been referred to as semicritical instruments and devices and include flexible fiberoptic endoscopes, laryngoscopes, vaginal specula, anesthesia breathing circuits, and other items.

Low-level disinfectants (i.e., quaternary ammonium compounds) are used to treat noncritical instruments and devices, such as blood pressure cuffs, electrocardiogram electrodes, and stethoscopes. Although these items come into contact with patients, they do not penetrate through mucosal surfaces or into sterile tissues.

Box 3-1 Definitions

Antisepsis: Use of chemical agents on skin or other living tissue to inhibit or eliminate microbes; no sporicidal action is implied

Disinfection: Use of physical procedures or chemical agents to destroy most microbial forms; bacterial spores and other relatively resistant organisms (e.g., mycobacteria, viruses, fungi) may remain viable; disinfectants are subdivided into high-, intermediate-, and low-level agents

Germicide: Chemical agent capable of killing microbes; includes virucide, bactericide, sporicide, tuberculocide, and fungicide

High-level disinfectant: A germicide that kills all microbial pathogens except large numbers of bacterial spores

Intermediate-level disinfectant: A germicide that kills all microbial pathogens except bacterial endospores

Low-level disinfectant: A germicide that kills most vegetative bacteria and lipid-enveloped and medium-size viruses

Sterilization: Use of physical procedures or chemical agents to destroy all microbial forms, including bacterial spores

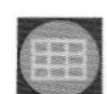

Table 3-1 Methods of Sterilization

Method	Concentration or Level
Physical Sterilants	
Steam under pressure	121° C or 132° C for various time intervals
Filtration	0.22- to 0.45-μm pore size; HEPA filters
Ultraviolet radiation	Variable exposure to 254-nm wavelength
Ionizing radiation	Variable exposure to microwave or gamma radiation
Gas Vapor Sterilants	
Ethylene oxide	450-1200 mg/L at 29° C to 65° C for 2-5 hr
Hydrogen peroxide vapor	30% at 55° C to 60° C
Plasma gas	Highly ionized hydrogen peroxide gas
Chemical Sterilants	
Peracetic acid	0.2%
Glutaraldehyde	2%

HEPA, High-efficiency particulate air.

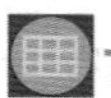

Table 3-2 Methods of Disinfection

Method	Concentration (Level of Activity)
Heat	
Moist heat	75° C to 100° C for 30 min (high)
Liquid	
Glutaraldehyde	2%-3.2% (high)
Hydrogen peroxide	3%-25% (high)
Chlorine compounds	100-1000 ppm of free chlorine (high)
Alcohol (ethyl, isopropyl)	70%-95% (intermediate)
Phenolic compounds	0.4%-5.0% (intermediate/low)
Iodophor compounds	30-50 ppm of free iodine/L (intermediate)
Quaternary ammonium compounds	0.4%-1.6% (low)

The level of disinfectants used for environmental surfaces is determined by the relative risk these surfaces pose as a reservoir for pathogenic organisms. For example, a higher level of disinfectant should be used to clean the surface of instruments contaminated with blood than that used to clean surfaces that are "dirty," such as floors, sinks, and countertops. The exception to this rule is if a particular surface has been implicated in a nosocomial infection, such as a bathroom contaminated with *Clostridium difficile* (spore-forming anaerobic bacterium) or a sink contaminated with *Pseudomonas aeruginosa*. In these cases, a disinfectant with appropriate activity against the implicated pathogen should be selected.

• Antisepsis

Antiseptic agents (Table 3-3) are used to reduce the number of microbes on skin surfaces. These compounds are selected for their safety and efficacy. A summary of their germicidal properties is presented in Table 3-4. **Alcohols** have excellent activity against all groups of organisms except spores and are nontoxic, although they tend to dry the skin surface because they remove lipids. They also do not have residual activity and are inactivated by organic matter. Thus the surface of the skin should be cleaned before alcohol is applied. **Iodophors** are also excellent skin antiseptic agents, having a range of activity similar to that of alcohols. They are slightly more toxic to the skin than is alcohol, have limited residual activity, and are inactivated by organic matter. Iodophors and iodine preparations are frequently used with alcohols for disinfecting the skin surface. **Chlorhexidine** has broad antimicrobial activity, although it kills organisms at a much slower rate than alcohol. Its activity persists, although organic material and high pH levels decrease its effectiveness. The activity of **parachlorometaxylenol (PCMX)** is limited primarily to gram-positive bacteria. Because it is nontoxic and has residual activity, it has been used in hand washing products. **Triclosan** is active against bacteria but not against many other organisms. It is a common antiseptic agent in deodorant soaps and some toothpaste products.

• Mechanisms of Action

The following section briefly reviews the mechanisms by which the most common sterilants, disinfectants, and antiseptics work.

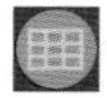

Table 3-3 Antiseptic Agents

Antiseptic Agent	Concentration
Alcohol (ethyl, isopropyl)	70%-90%
Iodophors	1-2 mg of free iodine/L; 1%-2% available iodine
Chlorhexidine	0.5%-4.0%
Parachlorometaxylenol	0.50%-3.75%
Triclosan	0.3%-2.0%

Table 3-4 Germicidal Properties of Disinfectants and Antiseptic Agents

Agents	Bacteria	Mycobacteria	Bacterial Spores	Fungi	Viruses
Disinfectants					
Alcohol	+	+	–	+	+/–
Hydrogen peroxide	+	+	+/–	+	+
Phenolics	+	+	–	+	+/–
Chlorine	+	+	+/–	+	+
Iodophors	+	+/–	–	+	+
Glutaraldehyde	+	+	+	+	+
Quaternary ammonium compounds	+/–	–	–	+/–	+/–
Antiseptic Agents					
Alcohol	+	+	–	+	+
Iodophors	+	+	–	+	+
Chlorhexidine	+	+	–	+	+
Parachlorometaxylenol	+/–	+/–	–	+	+/–
Triclosan	+	+/–	–	+/–	+

Moist Heat

Attempts to sterilize items using boiling water are inefficient because only a relatively low temperature (100° C) can be maintained. Indeed, spore formation by a bacterium is commonly demonstrated by boiling a solution of organisms and then subculturing the solution. Boiling vegetative organisms kills them, but the spores remain viable. In contrast, steam under pressure in an autoclave is a very effective form of sterilization; the higher temperature causes denaturation of microbial proteins. The rate of killing organisms during the autoclave process is rapid but is influenced by the temperature and duration of autoclaving, size of the autoclave, flow rate of the steam, density and size of the load, and placement of the load in the chamber. Care must be taken to avoid creating air pockets, which inhibit penetration of the steam into the load. In general, most autoclaves are operated at 121° C to 132° C for 15 minutes or longer. Including commercial preparations of *Bacillus stearothermophilus,* spores can help monitor the effectiveness of sterilization. An ampule of these spores is placed in the center of the load, removed at the end of the autoclave process, and incubated at 37° C. If the sterilization process is successful, the spores are killed and the organisms fail to grow.

Ethylene Oxide

Ethylene oxide is a colorless gas (soluble in water and common organic solvents) that is used to sterilize heat-sensitive items. The sterilization process is relatively slow and is influenced by the concentration of gas, relative humidity and moisture content of the item to be sterilized, exposure time, and temperature. The exposure time is reduced by 50% for each doubling of ethylene oxide concentration. Likewise, the activity of ethylene oxide approximately doubles with each temperature increase of 10° C. Sterilization with ethylene oxide is optimal in a relative humidity of approximately 30%, with decreased activity at higher or lower humidity. This is particularly problematic if the contaminated organisms are dried onto a surface or lyophilized. Ethylene oxide exerts its sporicidal activity through the alkylation of terminal hydroxyl, carboxyl, amino, and sulfhydryl groups. This process blocks the reactive groups required for many essential metabolic processes. Examples of other strong alkylating gases used as sterilants are formaldehyde and β-propiolactone. Because ethylene oxide can damage viable tissues, the gas must be dissipated before the item can be used. This aeration period is generally 16 hours or longer. The effectiveness of sterilization is monitored with the *Bacillus subtilis* spore test.

Aldehydes

As with ethylene oxide, aldehydes exert their effect through alkylation. The two best-known aldehydes are **formaldehyde** and **glutaraldehyde,** both of which can be used as sterilants or high-level disinfectants. Formaldehyde gas can be dissolved in water, creating a solution called formalin. Low concentrations of formalin are bacteriostatic (i.e., they inhibit but do not kill organisms), whereas higher concentrations (e.g., 20%) can kill all organisms. Combining formaldehyde with alcohol can enhance this microbicidal activity. Exposure of skin or mucous membranes to formaldehyde can be toxic, and vapors may be carcinogenic. For these reasons, formaldehyde is now rarely used in health care settings. Glutaraldehyde is less toxic for viable tissues, but it can still cause burns on the skin or mucous membranes. Glutaraldehyde is more active at alkaline pH levels ("activated" by sodium hydroxide) but is less stable. Glutaraldehyde is also inactivated by organic material, so items to be treated must first be cleaned.

Oxidizing Agents

Examples of oxidants include ozone, peracetic acid, and hydrogen peroxide, with the last used most commonly. **Hydrogen peroxide** effectively kills most bacteria at a concentration of 3% to 6% and kills all organisms, including spores, at higher concentrations (10% to 25%). The active oxidant form is not hydrogen peroxide but rather the free hydroxyl radical formed by the decomposition of hydrogen peroxide. Hydrogen peroxide is used to disinfect plastic implants, contact lenses, and surgical prostheses.

Halogens

Halogens, such as compounds containing iodine or chlorine, are used extensively as disinfectants. **Iodine compounds** are the most effective halogens available for disinfection. Iodine is a highly reactive element that precipitates proteins and oxidizes essential enzymes. It is microbicidal against virtually all organisms, including spore-forming bacteria and mycobacteria. Neither the concentration nor the pH of the iodine solution affects the microbicidal activity, although the efficiency of iodine solutions is increased in acid solutions because more free iodine is liberated. Iodine acts more rapidly than do other halogen compounds or quaternary ammonium compounds. However, the activity of iodine can be reduced in the presence of some organic and inorganic compounds, including serum, feces, ascitic fluid, sputum, urine, sodium thiosulfate, and ammonia. Elemental iodine can be dissolved in aqueous potassium iodide or alcohol, or it can be complexed with a carrier. The latter compound is referred to as an *iodophor* (iodo, "iodine"; phor, "carrier"). Povidone iodine (iodine complexed with polyvinylpyrrolidone) is used most commonly and is relatively stable and nontoxic to tissues and metal surfaces, but it is expensive compared with other iodine solutions.

Chlorine compounds are also used extensively as disinfectants. Aqueous solutions of chlorine are rapidly bactericidal, although their mechanisms of action are not defined. Three forms of chlorine may be present in water: elemental chlorine (Cl_2), which is a very strong oxidizing agent; hypochlorous acid (HOCl); and hypochlorite ion (OCl_2). Chlorine also combines with ammonia and other nitrogenous compounds to form chloramines, or *N*-chloro compounds. Chlorine can exert its effect by the irreversible oxidation of sulfhydryl (SH) groups of essential enzymes. Hypochlorites are believed to interact with cytoplasmic components to form toxic *N*-chloro compounds, which interfere with cellular metabolism. The efficacy of chlorine is inversely proportional to the pH, with greater activity observed at acid pH levels. This is consistent with greater activity associated with hypochlorous acid rather than with hypochlorite ion concentration. The activity of chlorine compounds also increases with concentration (e.g., a twofold increase in concentration results in a 30% decrease in time required for killing) and temperature (e.g., a 50% to 65% reduction in killing time with a 10° C increase in temperature). Organic matter and alkaline detergents can reduce the effectiveness of chlorine compounds. These compounds demonstrate good germicidal activity, although spore-forming organisms are 10- to 1000-fold more resistant to chlorine than are vegetative bacteria.

Phenolic Compounds

Phenolic compounds (germicides) are rarely used as disinfectants. However, they are of historical interest because they were used as a comparative standard for assessing the activity of other germicidal compounds. The ratio of germicidal activity by a test compound to that by a specified concentration of phenol yielded the phenol coefficient. A value of 1 indicated equivalent activity, greater than 1 indicated activity less than phenol, and less than 1 indicated activity greater than phenol. These tests are limited because phenol is not sporicidal at room temperature (but is sporicidal at temperatures approaching 100° C), and it has poor activity against non–lipid-containing viruses. This is understandable because phenol is believed to act by disrupting lipid-containing membranes, resulting in leakage of cellular contents. Phenolic compounds are active against the normally resilient mycobacteria because the cell wall of these organisms has a very high concentration of lipids. Exposure of phenolics to alkaline compounds significantly reduces their activity, whereas halogenation of the phenolics enhances their activity. The introduction of aliphatic or aromatic groups into the nucleus of halogen phenols also increases their activity. Bisphenols are two phenol compounds linked together. The activity of these compounds can also be potentiated by halogenation. One example of a halogenated bisphenol is **hexachlorophene,** an antiseptic with activity against gram-positive bacteria.

Quaternary Ammonium Compounds

Quaternary ammonium compounds consist of four organic groups covalently linked to nitrogen. The germicidal activity of these cationic compounds is determined by the nature of the organic groups, with the greatest activity observed with compounds having 8- to 18-carbon-long groups. Examples of quaternary ammonium compounds include **benzalkonium chloride** and **cetylpyridinium chloride.** These compounds act by denaturing cell membranes to release the intracellular components. Quaternary ammonium compounds are bacteriostatic at low concentrations and bactericidal at high concentrations; however, organisms such as *Pseudomonas, Mycobacterium,* and the fungus *Trichophyton* are resistant to these compounds. Indeed, some *Pseudomonas* strains can grow in quaternary ammonium solutions. Many viruses and all bacterial spores are also resistant. Ionic detergents, organic matter, and dilution neutralize quaternary ammonium compounds.

Alcohols

The germicidal activity of alcohols increases with increasing chain length (maximum of five to eight carbons). The two most commonly used alcohols are **ethanol** and **isopropanol.** These alcohols are rapidly bactericidal against vegetative bacteria, mycobacteria, some fungi, and lipid-containing viruses. Unfortunately, alcohols have no activity against bacterial spores and have poor activity against some fungi and non–lipid-containing viruses. Activity is greater in the presence of water. Thus 70% alcohol is more active than 95% alcohol. Alcohol is a common disinfectant for skin surfaces and, when followed by treatment with an iodophor, is extremely effective for this purpose. Alcohols are also used to disinfect items such as thermometers.

Bibliography

Block SS: *Disinfection, sterilization, and preservation,* ed 2, Philadelphia, 1977, Lea & Febiger.

Brody TM, Larner J, Minneman KP: *Human pharmacology: molecular to clinical,* ed 3, St Louis, 1998, Mosby.

Widmer A, Frei R: Decontamination, disinfection, and sterilization. In Versalovic J, et al, editors: *Manual of clinical microbiology,* ed 10, Washington, DC, 2011, American Society for Microbiology.

SECTION

2

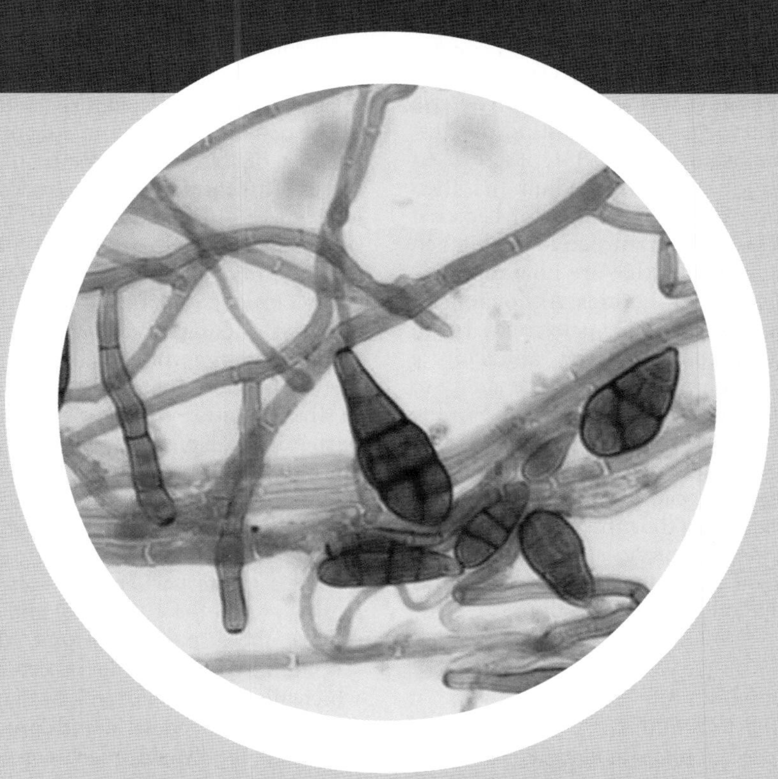

GENERAL PRINCIPLES OF LABORATORY DIAGNOSIS

CHAPTER

4 MICROSCOPY AND IN VITRO CULTURE

The foundation of microbiology was established in 1676 when Anton van Leeuwenhoek, using one of his early microscopes, observed bacteria in water. It was not until almost 200 years later that Pasteur was able to grow bacteria in the laboratory in a culture medium consisting of yeast extract, sugar, and ammonium salts. In 1881, Hesse used agar from his wife's kitchen to solidify the medium that then permitted the growth of macroscopic colonies of bacteria. Over the years, microbiologists have returned to the kitchen to create hundreds of culture media that are now routinely used in all clinical microbiology laboratories. Although tests that rapidly detect microbial antigens and nucleic acid–based molecular assays have replaced microscopy and culture methods for the detection of many organisms, the ability to observe microbes by microscopy and grow microbes in the laboratory remains an important procedure in clinical laboratories. For many diseases, these techniques remain the definitive methods to identify the cause of an infection. This chapter will provide an overview of the most commonly used techniques for microscopy and culture, and more specific details will be presented in the chapters devoted to laboratory diagnosis in the individual organism sections.

• Microscopy

In general, microscopy is used in microbiology for two basic purposes: the initial detection of microbes and the preliminary or definitive identification of microbes. The microscopic examination of clinical specimens is used to detect bacterial cells, fungal elements, parasites (eggs, larvae, or adult forms), and viral inclusions present in infected cells. Characteristic morphologic properties can be used for the preliminary identification of most bacteria and are used for the definitive identification of many fungi and parasites. The microscopic detection of organisms stained with antibodies labeled with fluorescent dyes or other markers has proved to be very useful for the specific identification of many organisms. Five general microscopic methods are used (Box 4-1).

Microscopic Methods

Brightfield (Light) Microscopy

The basic components of light microscopes consist of a light source used to illuminate the specimen positioned on a stage, a condenser used to focus the light on the specimen, and two lens systems **(objective lens** and **ocular lens)** used to magnify the image of the specimen. In brightfield microscopy the specimen is visualized by transillumination, with light passing up through the condenser to the specimen. The image is then magnified, first by the objective lens and then by the ocular lens. The total magnification of the image is the product of the magnifications of the objective and ocular lenses. Three different objective lenses are commonly used: low power (10-fold magnification), which can be used to scan a specimen; high dry (40-fold), which is used to look for large microbes such as parasites and filamentous fungi; and oil immersion (100-fold), which is used to observe bacteria, yeasts (single-cell stage of fungi), and the morphologic details of larger organisms and cells. Ocular lenses can further magnify the image (generally 10-fold to 15-fold).

The limitation of brightfield microscopy is the resolution of the image (i.e., the ability to distinguish that two objects are separate and not one). The **resolving power** of a microscope is determined by the wavelength of light used to illuminate the subject and the angle of light entering the objective lens (referred to as the **numerical aperture**). The resolving power is greatest when oil is placed between the objective lens (typically the 100× lens) and the specimen, because oil reduces the dispersion of light. The best brightfield microscopes have a resolving power of approximately 0.2 μm, which allows most bacteria, but not viruses, to be visualized. Although most bacteria and larger microorganisms can be seen with brightfield microscopy, the **refractive indices** of the organisms and background are similar. Thus organisms must be stained with a dye so they can be observed, or an alternative microscopic method must be used.

Darkfield Microscopy

The same objective and ocular lenses used in brightfield microscopes are used in darkfield microscopes; however, a special **condenser** is used that prevents transmitted light from directly illuminating the specimen. Only oblique scattered light reaches the specimen and passes into the lens systems, which causes the specimen to be brightly illuminated against a black background. The advantage of this method is that the resolving power of darkfield microscopy is significantly improved compared with that of brightfield microscopy (i.e., 0.02 μm versus 0.2 μm) and makes it possible to detect extremely thin bacteria such as *Treponema pallidum* (etiologic agent of syphilis) and *Leptospira* spp. (leptospirosis). The disadvantage of this method is that light passes around rather than through organisms, making it difficult to study their internal structure.

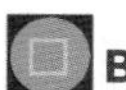 **Box 4-1 Microscopic Methods**

Brightfield (light) microscopy
Darkfield microscopy
Phase-contrast microscopy
Fluorescent microscopy
Electron microscopy

Phase-Contrast Microscopy

Phase-contrast microscopy enables the internal details of microbes to be examined. In this form of microscopy, as parallel beams of light are passed through objects of different densities, the wavelength of one beam moves out of "phase" relative to the other beam of light (i.e., the beam moving through the more dense material is retarded more than the other beam). Through the use of **annular rings** in the condenser and the objective lens, the differences in phase are amplified so that in-phase light appears brighter than out-of-phase light. This creates a three-dimensional image of the organism or specimen and permits more detailed analysis of the internal structures.

Fluorescent Microscopy

Some compounds called **fluorochromes** can absorb short-wavelength ultraviolet or ultrablue light and emit energy at a higher visible wavelength. Although some microorganisms show natural fluorescence **(autofluorescence),** fluorescent microscopy typically involves staining organisms with fluorescent dyes and then examining them with a specially designed fluorescent microscope. The microscope uses a high-pressure mercury, halogen, or xenon vapor lamp that emits a shorter wavelength of light than that emitted by traditional brightfield microscopes. A series of filters are used to block the heat generated from the lamp, eliminate infrared light, and select the appropriate wavelength for exciting the fluorochrome. The light emitted from the fluorochrome is then magnified through traditional objective and ocular lenses. Organisms and specimens stained with fluorochromes appear brightly illuminated against a dark background, although the colors vary depending on the fluorochrome selected. The contrast between the organism and background is great enough that the specimen can be screened rapidly under low magnification, and then the material is examined under higher magnification once fluorescence is detected.

Electron Microscopy

Unlike other forms of microscopy, **magnetic coils** (rather than lenses) are used in electron microscopes to direct a beam of electrons from a tungsten filament through a specimen and onto a screen. Because a much shorter wavelength of light is used, magnification and resolution are improved dramatically. Individual viral particles (as opposed to viral inclusion bodies) can be seen with electron microscopy. Samples are usually stained or coated with metal ions to create contrast. There are two types of electron microscopes: **transmission electron microscopes,** in which electrons such as light pass directly through the specimen, and **scanning electron microscopes,** in which electrons bounce off the surface of the specimen at an angle and a three-dimensional picture is produced. Today, electron microscopy is used more as a research tool than a diagnostic aid, with highly sensitive and specific nucleic acid amplification assays the primary diagnostic test in current use.

Examination Methods

Clinical specimens or suspensions of microorganisms can be placed on a glass slide and examined under the microscope (i.e., direct examination of a wet mount). Although large organisms (e.g., fungal elements, parasites) and cellular material can be seen using this method, analysis of the internal detail is often difficult. Phase-contrast microscopy can overcome some of these problems; alternatively, the specimen or organism can be stained by a variety of methods (Table 4-1).

Direct Examination

Direct examination methods are the simplest for preparing samples for microscopic examination. The sample can be suspended in water or saline **(wet mount),** mixed with alkali to dissolve background material **(potassium hydroxide [KOH] method),** or mixed with a combination of alkali and a contrasting dye (e.g., **lactophenol cotton blue, iodine**). The dyes nonspecifically stain the cellular material, increasing the contrast with the background, and permit examination of the detailed structures. A variation is the **India ink method,** in which the ink darkens the background rather than the cell. This method is used to detect capsules surrounding organisms, such as the yeast *Cryptococcus* (the dye is excluded by the capsule, creating a clear halo around the yeast cell) and encapsulated *Bacillus anthracis.*

Differential Stains

A variety of differential stains are used to stain specific organisms or components of cellular material. The **Gram stain** is the best known and most widely used stain and forms the basis for the phenotypic classification of bacteria. Yeasts can also be stained with this method (yeasts are gram-positive). The **iron hematoxylin** and **trichrome** stains are invaluable for identifying protozoan parasites, and the **Wright-Giemsa** stain is used to identify blood parasites and other selected organisms. Stains such as methenamine silver and toluidine blue O have largely been replaced by more sensitive or technically easier differential or fluorescent stains.

Acid-Fast Stains

At least three different acid-fast stains are used, each exploiting the fact that some organisms retain a primary stain even when exposed to strong decolorizing agents such as mixtures of acids and alcohols. The **Ziehl-Neelsen** is the oldest method used but requires heating the specimen during the staining procedure. Many laboratories have replaced this method with either the cold acid-fast stain **(Kinyoun method)** or the fluorochrome stain **(auramine-rhodamine method).** The fluorochrome method is the stain of choice because a large area of the specimen can be examined rapidly by simply searching for fluorescing organisms against a black background. Some organisms are "partially acid-fast," retaining the primary stain only when they are decolorized with a weakly acidic solution. This property is characteristic of only a few organisms (see Table 4-1), making it quite valuable for their preliminary identification.

 **Table 4-1 Microscopic Preparations and Stains Used in the Clinical Microbiology Laboratory**

Staining Method	Principle and Applications
Direct Examination	
Wet mount	Unstained preparation is examined by brightfield, darkfield, or phase-contrast microscopy.
10% KOH	KOH is used to dissolve proteinaceous material and facilitate detection of fungal elements that are not affected by strong alkali solution. Dyes such as lactophenol cotton blue can be added to increase contrast between fungal elements and background.
India ink	Modification of KOH procedure in which ink is added as contrast material. Dye primarily used to detect *Cryptococcus* spp. in cerebrospinal fluid and other body fluids. Polysaccharide capsule of *Cryptococcus* spp. excludes ink, creating halo around yeast cell.
Lugol iodine	Iodine is added to wet preparations of parasitology specimens to enhance contrast of internal structures. This facilitates differentiation of amebae and host white blood cells.
Differential Stains	
Gram stain	Most commonly used stain in microbiology laboratory, forming basis for separating major groups of bacteria (e.g., gram-positive, gram-negative). After fixation of specimen to glass slide (by heating or alcohol treatment), specimen is exposed to crystal violet and then iodine is added to form complex with primary dye. During decolorization with alcohol or acetone, complex is retained in gram-positive bacteria but lost in gram-negative organisms; counterstain safranin is retained by gram-negative organisms (hence their red color). The degree to which organism retains stain is function of organism, culture conditions, and staining skills of the microscopist.
Iron hematoxylin stain	Used for detection and identification of fecal protozoa. Helminth eggs and larvae retain too much stain and are more easily identified with wet-mount preparation.
Methenamine silver	In general, performed in histology laboratories rather than in microbiology laboratories. Used primarily for stain detection of fungal elements in tissue, although other organisms (e.g., bacteria) can be detected. Silver staining requires skill because nonspecific staining can render slides unable to be interpreted.
Toluidine blue O stain	Used primarily for detection of *Pneumocystis* organisms in respiratory specimens. Cysts stain reddish-blue to dark purple on light blue background. Background staining is removed by sulfation reagent. Yeast cells stain and are difficult to distinguish from *Pneumocystis* cells. Trophozoites do not stain. Many laboratories have replaced this stain with specific fluorescent stains.
Trichrome stain	Alternative to iron hematoxylin for staining protozoa. Protozoa have bluish-green to purple cytoplasms with red or purplish-red nuclei and inclusion bodies; specimen background is green.
Wright-Giemsa stain	Used to detect blood parasites, viral and chlamydial inclusion bodies, and *Borrelia, Toxoplasma, Pneumocystis,* and *Rickettsia* spp. This is a polychromatic stain that contains a mixture of methylene blue, azure B, and eosin Y. Giemsa stain combines methylene blue and eosin. Eosin ions are negatively charged and stain basic components of cells orange to pink, whereas other dyes stain acidic cell structures various shades of blue to purple. Protozoan trophozoites have a red nucleus and grayish-blue cytoplasm; intracellular yeasts and inclusion bodies typically stain blue; rickettsiae, chlamydiae, and *Pneumocystis* spp. stain purple.
Acid-Fast Stains	
Ziehl-Neelsen stain	Used to stain mycobacteria and other acid-fast organisms. Organisms are stained with basic carbolfuchsin and resist decolorization with acid-alkali solutions. Background is counterstained with methylene blue. Organisms appear red against light blue background. Uptake of carbolfuchsin requires heating specimen (hot acid-fast stain).
Kinyoun stain	Cold acid-fast stain (does not require heating). Same principle as Ziehl-Neelsen stain.
Auramine-rhodamine	Same principle as other acid-fast stains, except that fluorescent dyes (auramine and rhodamine) are used for primary stain, and potassium permanganate (strong oxidizing agent) is the counterstain and inactivates unbound fluorochrome dyes. Organisms fluoresce yellowish-green against a black background.
Modified acid-fast stain	Weak decolorizing agent is used with any of three acid-fast stains listed. Whereas mycobacteria are strongly acid-fast, other organisms stain weaker (e.g., *Nocardia, Rhodococcus, Tsukamurella, Gordonia, Cryptosporidium, Isospora, Sarcocystis,* and *Cyclospora*). These organisms can be stained more efficiently by using a weak decolorizing agent. Organisms that retain this stain are referred to as partially acid-fast.
Fluorescent Stains	
Acridine orange stain	Used for detection of bacteria and fungi in clinical specimens. Dye intercalates into nucleic acid (native and denatured). At neutral pH, bacteria, fungi, and cellular material stain reddish-orange. At acid pH (4.0), bacteria and fungi remain reddish-orange, but background material stains greenish-yellow.
Auramine-rhodamine stain	Same as acid-fast stains.
Calcofluor white stain	Used to detect fungal elements and *Pneumocystis* spp. Stain binds to cellulose and chitin in cell walls; microscopist can mix dye with KOH. (Many laboratories have replaced traditional KOH stain with this stain.)

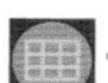 Table 4-1 **Microscopic Preparations and Stains Used in the Clinical Microbiology Laboratory—cont'd**

Staining Method	Principle and Applications
Direct fluorescent antibody stain	Antibodies (monoclonal or polyclonal) are complexed with fluorescent molecules. Specific binding to an organism is detected by presence of microbial fluorescence. Technique has proved useful for detecting or identifying many organisms (e.g., *Streptococcus pyogenes, Bordetella, Francisella, Legionella, Chlamydia, Pneumocystis, Cryptosporidium, Giardia,* influenza virus, herpes simplex virus). Sensitivity and specificity of test are determined by number of organisms present in test sample and quality of antibodies used in reagents.

KOH, Potassium hydroxide.

Fluorescent Stains

The auramine-rhodamine acid-fast stain is a specific example of a fluorescent stain. Numerous other fluorescent dyes have also been used to stain specimens. For example, the **acridine orange stain** can be used to stain bacteria and fungi, and **calcofluor white** stains the chitin in fungal cell walls. Although the acridine orange stain is rather limited in its applications, the calcofluor white stain has replaced the potassium hydroxide stains. Another procedure is the examination of specimens with specific antibodies labeled with fluorescent dyes **(fluorescent antibody stains).** The presence of fluorescing organisms is a rapid method for both detection and identification of the organism.

• In Vitro Culture

The success of culture methods is defined by the biology of the organism, the site of the infection, the patient's immune response to the infection, and the quality of the culture media. The bacterium *Legionella* is an important respiratory pathogen; however, it was never grown in culture until it was recognized that recovery of the organism required using media supplemented with iron and L-cysteine. *Campylobacter,* an important enteric pathogen, was not recovered in stool specimens until highly selective media were incubated at 42° C in a microaerophilic atmosphere. *Chlamydia,* an important bacterium responsible for sexually transmitted diseases, is an obligate intracellular pathogen that must be grown in living cells. *Staphylococcus aureus,* the cause of staphylococcal toxic shock syndrome, produces disease by release of a toxin into the circulatory system. Culture of blood will almost always be negative, but culture of the site where the organism is growing will detect the organism. In many infections (e.g., gastroenteritis, pharyngitis, urethritis), the organism responsible for the infection will be present among many other organisms that are part of the normal microbial population at the site of infection. Many media have been developed that suppress the normally present microbes and allow easier detection of clinically important organisms. The patient's innate and adaptive immunity may suppress the pathogen, so highly sensitive culture techniques are frequently required. Likewise, some infections are characterized by the presence of relatively few organisms. For example, most septic patients have less than one organism per milliliter of blood, so recovery of these organisms in a traditional blood culture requires inoculation of a large volume of blood into enrichment broths. Finally, the quality of the media must be carefully monitored to demonstrate it will perform as designed.

Relatively few laboratories prepare their own media today. Most media are produced by large commercial companies with expertise in media production. Although this has obvious advantages, it also means that media are not "freshly produced." Although this is generally not a problem, it can impact the recovery of some fastidious organisms (e.g., *Bordetella pertussis*). Thus laboratories that perform sophisticated testing frequently have the ability to make a limited amount of specialized media. Dehydrated formulations of most media are available, so this can be accomplished with minimal difficulty. Please refer to the references in the Bibliography for additional information about the preparation and quality control of media.

Types of Culture Media

Culture media can be subdivided into four general categories: (1) enriched nonselective media, (2) selective media, (3) differential media, and (4) specialized media (Table 4-2). Some examples of these media are summarized below.

Enriched Nonselective Media

These media are designed to support the growth of most organisms without fastidious growth requirements. The following are some of the more commonly used media:

Blood agar. Many types of blood agar media are used in clinical laboratories. The media contain two primary components—a basal medium (e.g., tryptic soy, brain heart infusion, *Brucella* base) and blood (e.g., sheep, horse, rabbit). Various other supplements can also be added to extend the range of organisms that can grow on the media.

Chocolate agar. This is a modified blood agar medium. When blood or hemoglobin is added to the heated basal media, it turns brown (hence the name). This medium supports the growth of most bacteria, including some that do not grow on blood agar (i.e., *Haemophilus,* some pathogenic *Neisseria* strains).

Mueller-Hinton agar. This is the recommended medium for routine antibiotic susceptibility testing of bacteria. It has a well-defined composition of beef and casein extracts, salts, divalent cations, and soluble starch that is necessary for reproducible test results.

Thioglycolate broth. This is one of a variety of enrichment broths used to recover low numbers of aerobic and anaerobic bacteria. Various formulations are used, but most include casein digest, glucose, yeast extract, cysteine, and sodium thioglycolate. Supplementation with hemin and vitamin K will enhance the recovery of anaerobic bacteria.

Table 4-2 Types of Culture Media

Type	Media (examples)	Purpose
Nonselective	Blood agar	Recovery of bacteria and fungi
	Chocolate agar	Recovery of bacteria including *Haemophilus* and *Neisseria gonorrhoeae*
	Mueller-Hinton agar	Bacterial susceptibility test medium
	Thioglycolate broth	Enrichment broth for anaerobic bacteria
	Sabouraud dextrose agar	Recovery of fungi
Selective, differential	MacConkey agar	Selective for gram-negative bacteria; differential for lactose-fermenting species
	Mannitol salt agar	Selective for staphylococci; differential for *Staphylococcus aureus*
	Xylose lysine deoxycholate agar	Selective, differential agar for *Salmonella* and *Shigella* in enteric cultures
	Lowenstein-Jensen medium	Selective for mycobacteria
	Middlebrook agar	Selective for mycobacteria
	CHROMagar	Selective, differential for selected bacteria and yeasts
	Inhibitory mold agar	Selective for molds
Specialized	Buffered charcoal yeast extract (BCYE) agar	Recovery of *Legionella* and *Nocardia*
	Cystine-tellurite agar	Recovery of *Corynebacterium diphtheriae*
	Lim broth	Recovery of *Streptococcus agalactiae*
	MacConkey sorbitol agar	Recovery of *Escherichia coli* 0157
	Regan Lowe agar	Recovery of *Bordetella pertussis*
	Thiosulfate citrate bile salts sucrose (TCBS) agar	Recovery of *Vibrio* species

Sabouraud dextrose agar. This is an enriched medium consisting of digests of casein and animal tissue supplemented with glucose that is used for the isolation of fungi. A variety of formulations have been developed, but most mycologists use the formulation with a low concentration of glucose and neutral pH. By reducing the pH and adding antibiotics to inhibit bacteria, this medium can be made selective for fungi.

Selective Media and Differential Media

Selective media are designed for the recovery of specific organisms that may be present in a mixture of other organisms (e.g., an enteric pathogen in stool). The media are supplemented with inhibitors that suppress the growth of unwanted organisms. These media can be made differential by adding specific ingredients that allow identification of an organism in a mixture (e.g., addition of lactose and a pH indicator to detect lactose fermenting organisms). The following are some examples of selective and differential media:

MacConkey agar. This is a selective agar for gram-negative bacteria and differential for differentiation of lactose-fermenting and lactose-nonfermenting bacteria. The medium consists of digests of peptones, bile salts, lactose, neutral red, and crystal violet. The bile salts and crystal violet inhibit gram-positive bacteria. Bacteria that ferment lactose produce acid that precipitates the bile salts and causes a red color in the neutral red indicator.

Mannitol salt agar. This is a selective medium used for the isolation of staphylococci. The medium consists of digests of casein and animal tissue, beef extract, mannitol, salts, and phenol red. Staphylococci can grow in the presence of a high salt concentration, and *S. aureus* can ferment mannitol, producing yellow-colored colonies on this agar.

Xylose-lysine deoxycholate (XLD) agar. This is a selective agar used for detection of *Salmonella* and *Shigella* in enteric cultures. This is an example of a very clever approach to detecting important bacteria in a complex mixture of insignificant bacteria. The medium consists of yeast extract with xylose, lysine, lactose, sucrose, sodium deoxycholate, sodium thiosulfate, ferric ammonium citrate, and phenol red. Sodium deoxycholate inhibits the growth of the majority of nonpathogenic bacteria. Those that do grow typically ferment lactose, sucrose, or xylose, producing yellow colonies. *Shigella* does not ferment these carbohydrates, so the colonies appear red. *Salmonella* ferments xylose but also decarboxylates lysine, producing the alkaline diamine product cadaverine. This neutralizes the acid fermentation products, thus the colonies appear red. Because most *Salmonella* produce hydrogen sulfide from sodium thiosulfate, the colonies will turn black in the presence of ferric ammonium citrate, thus differentiating *Salmonella* from *Shigella*.

Lowenstein-Jensen (LJ) medium. This medium, used for the isolation of mycobacteria, contains glycerol, potato flour, salts, and coagulated whole eggs (to solidify the medium). Malachite green is added to inhibit gram-positive bacteria.

Middlebrook agar. This agar medium is also used for the isolation of mycobacteria. It contains nutrients required for the growth of mycobacteria (i.e., salts, vitamins, oleic acid, albumin, catalase, glycerol, glucose) and malachite green for the inhibition of gram-positive bacteria. In contrast with LJ medium, it is solidified with agar.

CHROMagar. These selective differential agars are used for the isolation and identification of a variety of bacteria (e.g., *Staphylococcus aureus,* enteric bacteria) and yeasts. An example of design of these media is the one developed for *Candida* species. This medium has chloramphenicol to inhibit bacteria and a mixture of proprietary chromogenic substrates. The different species of *Candida* have enzymes that can use one or more of the substrates, releasing the color compound and producing colored colonies. Thus *Candida albicans* forms green colonies, *Candida tropicalis* forms purple colonies, and *Candida krusei* forms pink colonies.

Inhibitory mold agar. This medium is an enriched selective formulation used for the isolation of pathogenic fungi other than dermatophytes. Chloramphenicol is added to suppress the growth of contaminating bacteria.

Specialized Media

A large variety of specialized media have been created for the detection of specific organisms that may be fastidious or typically present in large mixtures of organisms. The more commonly used media are described in the specific organism chapters in this textbook.

Cell Culture

Some bacteria and all viruses are **strict intracellular microbes;** that is, they can only grow in living cells. In 1949, John Franklin Enders described a technique for cultivating mammalian cells for the isolation of poliovirus. This technique has been expanded for the growth of most strict intracellular organisms. The cell cultures can either be cells that grow and divide on a surface (i.e., **cell monolayer**) or grow suspended in broth. Some cell cultures are well established and can be maintained indefinitely. These cultures are commonly commercially available. Other cell cultures must be prepared immediately before they are infected with the bacteria or viruses and cannot be maintained in the laboratory for more than a few cycles of division **(primary cell cultures).** Entry into cells is frequently regulated by the presence of specific receptors, so the differential ability to infect specific cell lines can be used to predict the identity of the bacterium or virus. Additional information about the use of cell cultures is described in the following chapters.

Bibliography

Chapin K: Principles of stains and media. In Murray P, et al, editors: *Manual of clinical microbiology*, ed 9, Washington, DC, 2007, American Society for Microbiology Press.

Murray P, Shea Y: *ASM pocket guide to clinical microbiology*, ed 3, Washington, DC, 2004, American Society for Microbiology Press.

Snyder J, Atlas R: *Handbook of media for clinical microbiology*, ed 2, Boca Raton, Fla, 2006, CRC Press.

Wiedbrauk D: Microscopy. In Versalovic J, et al, editors: *Manual of clinical microbiology*, ed 10, Washington, DC, 2011, American Society for Microbiology.

Zimbro M, Power D: *Difco and BBL manual: manual of microbiological culture media*, Sparks, Md, 2003, Becton Dickinson and Company.

CHAPTER

5 MOLECULAR DIAGNOSIS

Like the evidence left at the scene of a crime, the DNA (deoxyribonucleic acid), RNA (ribonucleic acid), or proteins of an infectious agent in a clinical sample can be used to help identify the agent. In many cases, the agent can be detected and identified in this way even if it cannot be isolated or detected by immunologic means. New techniques and adaptations of older techniques are being developed for the analysis of infectious agents.

The advantages of molecular techniques are their sensitivity, specificity, and safety. From the standpoint of safety, these techniques do not require isolation of the infectious agent and can be performed on chemically fixed (inactivated) samples or extracts. Because of their sensitivity, very dilute samples of microbial DNA or RNA can be detected in a tissue even if the agent is not replicating or producing other evidence of infection. These techniques can distinguish related strains on the basis of differences in their genotype (i.e., mutants). This is especially useful for distinguishing antiviral drug–resistant strains, which may differ by a single nucleotide.

• Detection of Microbial Genetic Material

Electrophoretic Analysis of DNA and Restriction Fragment Length Polymorphism

The genome structure and genetic sequence are major distinguishing characteristics of the family, type, and strain of microorganism. Specific strains of microorganisms can be distinguished on the basis of their DNA or RNA or by the DNA fragments produced when the DNA is cleaved by specific restriction endonucleases **(restriction enzymes)** or selectively amplified (see later). Restriction enzymes recognize specific DNA sequences that have a palindromic structure; an example follows:

GAATTC EcoR 1 recognition
CTTAAG sequence and cleavage

The DNA sites recognized by different restriction endonucleases differ in their sequence, length, and frequency of occurrence. As a result, different restriction endonucleases cleave the DNA of a sample in different places, yielding fragments of different lengths. The cleavage of different DNA samples with one restriction endonuclease can also yield fragments of many different lengths. The differences in the length of the DNA fragments among the different strains of a specific organism produced on cleavage with one or more restriction endonucleases is termed **restriction fragment length polymorphism (RFLP).**

DNA or RNA fragments of different sizes or structures can be distinguished by their electrophoretic mobility in an agarose or polyacrylamide gel. Different forms of the same DNA sequence and different lengths of DNA move through the mazelike structure of an agarose gel at different speeds, allowing their separation. The DNA can be visualized by staining with ethidium bromide. Smaller fragments (<20,000 base pairs), such as those from bacterial plasmids or viruses, can be separated and distinguished by normal electrophoretic methods. Larger fragments, such as those from whole bacteria, can be separated by using a special electrophoretic technique called *pulsed-field gel electrophoresis.*

RFLP is useful, for example, for distinguishing different strains of herpes simplex virus (HSV). Comparison of the restriction endonuclease cleavage patterns of DNA from different isolates can identify a pattern of virus transmission from one person to another or distinguish HSV-1 from HSV-2. RFLP has also been used to show the spread of a strain of *Streptococcus* causing necrotizing fasciitis from one patient to other patients, an emergency medical technician, and the emergency department and attending physicians (Figure 5-1). Often, comparison of the 16S ribosomal RNA is used to identify different bacteria.

Nucleic Acid Detection, Amplification, and Sequencing

DNA probes can be used like antibodies as sensitive and specific tools to detect, locate, and quantitate specific nucleic acid sequences in clinical specimens (Figure 5-2). Because of the specificity and sensitivity of DNA probe techniques, individual species or strains of an infectious agent can be detected even if they are not growing or replicating.

DNA probes are chemically synthesized or obtained by cloning specific genomic fragments or an entire viral genome into bacterial vectors (plasmids, cosmids). DNA copies of RNA viruses are made with the retrovirus reverse transcriptase and then cloned into these vectors. After chemical or heat treatments melt (separate) the DNA strands in the sample, the DNA probe is added and allowed to **hybridize** (bind) with the identical or nearly identical sequence in the sample. The **stringency** (the requirement for an exact sequence match) of the interaction can be varied so that related sequences can be detected or different strains (mutants) can be distinguished. The DNA probes are labeled with radioactive or chemically modified nucleotides (e.g.,

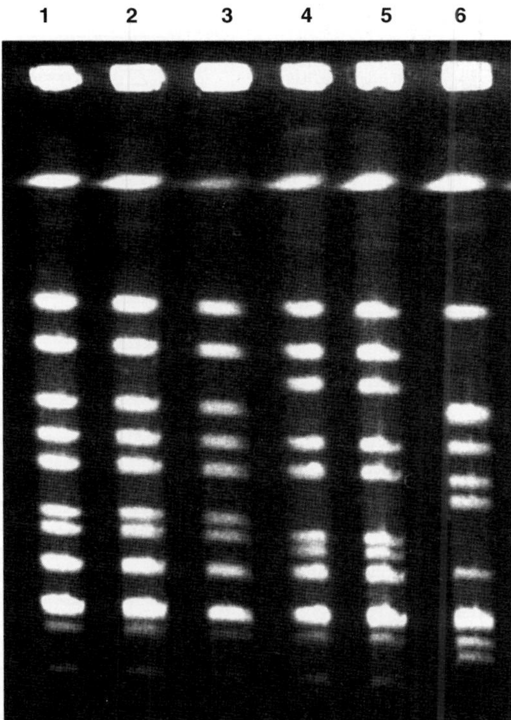

FIGURE 5-1 Restriction fragment length polymorphism distinction of DNA from bacterial strains separated by pulsed-field gel electrophoresis. Lanes 1 to 3 show Sma 1 restriction endonuclease-digested DNA from bacteria from two family members with necrotizing fasciitis and from their physician (pharyngitis). Lanes 4 to 6 are from unrelated *Streptococcus pyogenes* strains. (Courtesy Dr. Joe DiPersio, Akron, Ohio.)

biotinylated uridine) so that they can be detected and quantitated. The use of a biotin-labeled DNA probe allows the use of a fluorescent or enzyme-labeled avidin or streptavidin (proteins that bind tightly to biotin) molecule to detect viral nucleic acids in a cell in a way similar to how indirect immunofluorescence or an enzyme immunoassay localizes an antigen.

The DNA probes can detect specific genetic sequences in fixed permeabilized tissue biopsy specimens by **in situ hybridization.** When fluorescent detection is used, it is called **FISH: fluorescent in situ hybridization.** The localization of cytomegalovirus (CMV)-infected (Figure 5-3) or papillomavirus-infected cells by in situ hybridization is preferable to an immunologic means of doing so and is the only commercially available means of localizing papillomavirus. There are now many commercially available microbial probes and kits for detecting viruses, bacteria, and other microbes.

Specific nucleic acid sequences in extracts from a clinical sample can be detected by applying a small volume of the extract to a nitrocellulose filter **(dot blot)** and then probing the filter with labeled, specific viral DNA. Alternatively, the electrophoretically separated restriction endonuclease cleavage pattern can be transferred onto a nitrocellulose filter (**Southern blot**—DNA:DNA probe hybridization), and then the specific sequence can be identified by hybridization with a specific genetic probe and by its characteristic electrophoretic mobility. Electrophoretically separated RNA

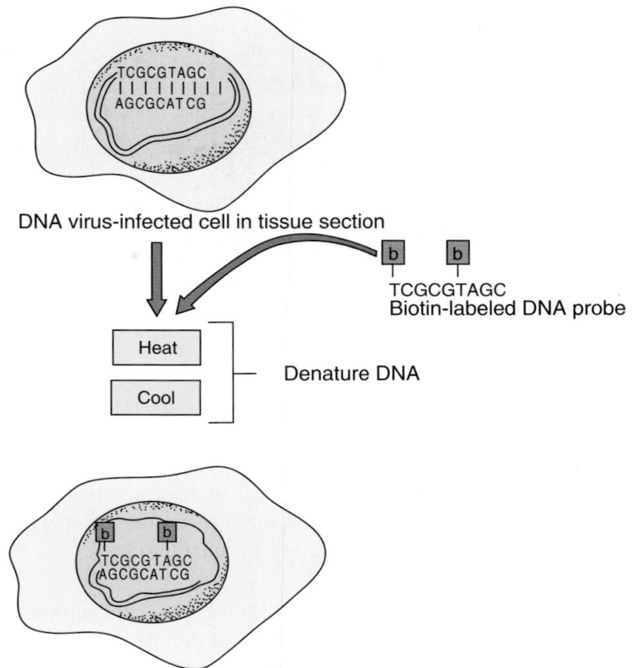

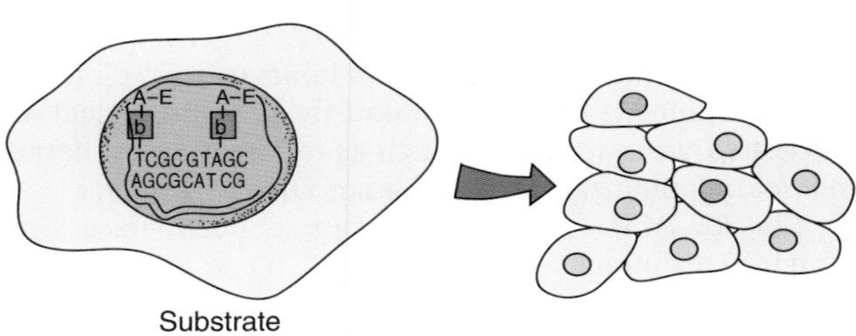

FIGURE 5-2 DNA probe analysis of virus-infected cells. Such cells can be localized in histologically prepared tissue sections using DNA probes consisting of as few as nine nucleotides or bacterial plasmids containing the viral genome. A tagged DNA probe is added to the sample. In this case, the DNA probe is labeled with biotin-modified thymidine, but radioactive agents can also be used. The sample is heated to denature the DNA and cooled to allow the probe to hybridize to the complementary sequence. Horseradish peroxidase–labeled avidin is added to bind to the biotin on the probe. The appropriate substrate is added to color the nuclei of virally infected cells. *A,* Adenine; *b,* biotin; *C,* cytosine; *G,* guanine; *T,* thymine.

(**Northern blot**—RNA:DNA probe hybridization) blotted onto a nitrocellulose filter can be detected in a similar manner.

The **polymerase chain reaction (PCR)** amplifies single copies of viral DNA millions of times over and is one of the most useful genetic analysis techniques (Figure 5-4). In this technique, a sample is incubated with two short DNA oligomers, termed **primers,** that are complementary to the ends of a known genetic sequence within the total DNA, a heat-stable DNA polymerase (Taq or other polymerase obtained from thermophilic bacteria), nucleotides, and buffers. The oligomers hybridize to the appropriate sequence of DNA and

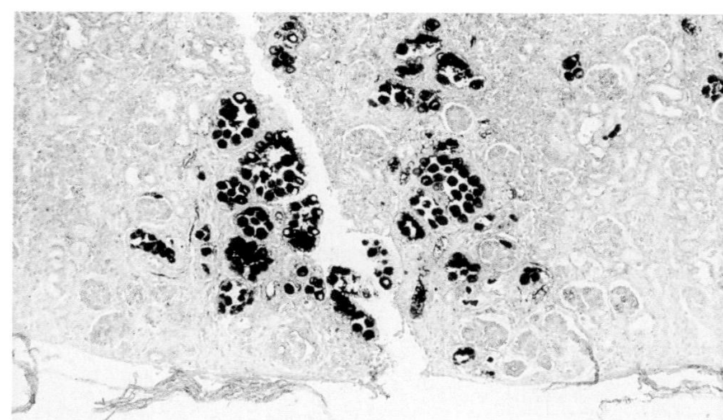

FIGURE 5-3 In situ localization of cytomegalovirus (CMV) infection using a genetic probe. CMV infection of the renal tubules of a kidney is localized with a biotin-labeled CMV-specific DNA probe and is visualized by means of the horseradish peroxidase–conjugated avidin conversion of substrate, in a manner similar to enzyme immunoassay. (Courtesy Donna Zabel, Akron, Ohio.)

act as primers for the polymerase, which copies that segment of the DNA. The sample is then heated to denature the DNA (separating the strands of the double helix) and cooled to allow hybridization of the primers to the new DNA. Each copy of DNA becomes a new template. The process is repeated many (20 to 40) times to amplify the original DNA sequence in an exponential manner. A target sequence can be amplified 1,000,000-fold in a few hours using this method. This technique is especially useful for detecting latent and integrated virus sequences, such as in retroviruses, herpesviruses, papillomaviruses, and other DNA viruses.

The **RT-PCR** (reverse transcriptase polymerase chain reaction) technique is a variation of PCR and involves use of the reverse transcriptase of retroviruses to convert viral RNA or messenger RNA to DNA before PCR amplification. In 1993, hantavirus sequences were used as primers for RT-PCR to identify the agent causing an outbreak of hemorrhagic pulmonary disease in the Four Corners area of New Mexico. It showed the infectious agent to be a hantavirus.

Real-time PCR can be used to quantitate the amount of DNA or RNA in a sample after it is converted to DNA by reverse transcriptase. Simply put, the more DNA in the sample, the faster new DNA is made in a PCR reaction, and the reaction kinetics are proportional to the amount of DNA. The production of double-stranded DNA is measured by the increase in fluorescence of a molecule bound to the amplified double-strand DNA molecule or by other means. This procedure is useful for quantitating the number of human immunodeficiency virus (HIV) genomes in a patient's blood to evaluate the course of the disease and antiviral drug efficacy.

The **branched-chain DNA assay** is a hybridization technique that is an alternative to PCR and RT-PCR for detecting small amounts of specific RNA or DNA sequences. This technique is especially useful for quantitating plasma levels of HIV RNA (plasma viral load). In this case, plasma is incubated in a special tube lined with a short complementary DNA (cDNA) sequence to capture the viral RNA. Another cDNA sequence is added to bind to the sample, but this DNA is attached to an artificially branched chain of DNA. On development, each branch is capable of initiating a detectable signal. This amplifies the signal from the original sample. The **antibody capture solution hybridization assay** detects and quantitates RNA:DNA hybrids using an antibody specific for the complex in a technique similar to an ELISA (enzyme-linked immunosorbent assay) (see Chapter 6).

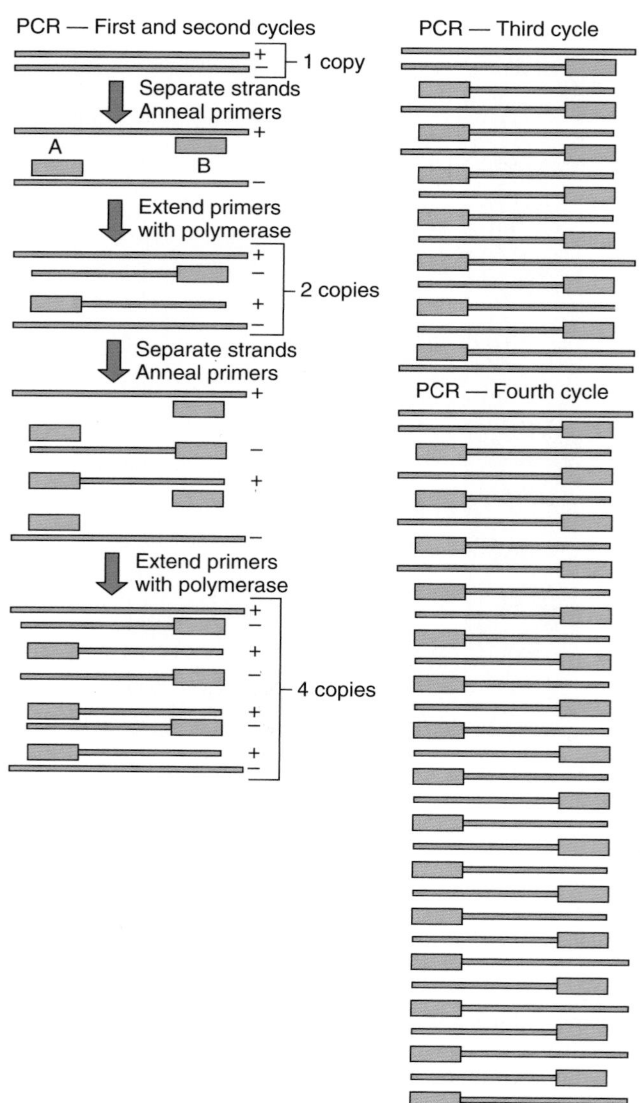

FIGURE 5-4 Polymerase chain reaction *(PCR)*. This technique is a rapid means of amplifying a known sequence of DNA. A sample is mixed with a heat-stable DNA polymerase, excess deoxyribonucleotide triphosphates, and two DNA oligomers **(primers),** which complement the ends of the target sequence to be amplified. The mixture is heated to denature the DNA and then cooled to allow binding of the primers to the target DNA and extension of the primers by the polymerase. The cycle is repeated 20 to 40 times. After the first cycle, only the sequence bracketed by the primers is amplified. In the **reverse transcriptase PCR** technique, RNA can also be amplified after its conversion to DNA by reverse transcriptase. Labels *A* and *B,* DNA oligomers used as primers; + and –, DNA strands. (Modified from Blair GE, Zajdel MEB: The polymerase chain-reaction—already an established technique. *Biochem Educ* 20:87–91, 1992.)

Table 5-1 Molecular Techniques

Technique	Purpose	Clinical Examples
RFLP	Comparison of DNA	Molecular epidemiology, HSV-1 strains
DNA electrophoresis	Comparison of DNA	Viral strain differences (up to 20,000 bases)
Pulsed-field gel electrophoresis	Comparison of DNA (large pieces of DNA)	Streptococcal strain comparisons
In situ hybridization	Detection and localization of DNA sequences in tissue	Detection of nonreplicating DNA virus (e.g., cytomegalovirus, human papillomavirus)
Dot blot	Detection of DNA sequences in solution	Detection of viral DNA
Southern blot	Detection and characterization of DNA sequences by size	Identification of specific viral strains
Northern blot	Detection and characterization of RNA sequences by size	Identification of specific viral strains
PCR	Amplification of very dilute DNA samples	Detection of DNA viruses
RT-PCR	Amplification of very dilute RNA samples	Detection of RNA viruses
Real-time PCR	Quantification of very dilute DNA and RNA samples	Quantitation of HIV genome: virus load
Branched-chain DNA	Amplification of very dilute DNA or RNA samples	Quantitation of DNA and RNA viruses
Antibody capture solution hybridization DNA assay	Amplification of very dilute DNA or RNA samples	Quantitation of DNA and RNA viruses
MALDI-TOF mass spectrometry	Rapid, sensitive analysis of DNA, RNA, and protein samples	Sequence analysis, microbial identification
SDS-PAGE	Separation of proteins by molecular weight	Molecular epidemiology of HSV

DNA, Deoxyribonucleic acid; *HIV,* human immunodeficiency virus; *HSV-1,* herpes simplex virus-1; *MALDI-TOF,* matrix-assisted laser desorption/ionization time-of-flight; *PCR,* polymerase chain reaction; *RFLP,* restriction fragment length polymorphism; *RNA,* ribonucleic acid; *RT-PCR,* reverse transcriptase polymerase chain reaction; *SDS-PAGE,* sodium dodecyl sulfate–polyacrylamide gel electrophoresis.

Assay kits that use variations on the aforementioned techniques to detect, identify, and quantitate different microbes are commercially available.

DNA sequencing has become sufficiently fast and inexpensive to allow laboratory determination of microbial sequences for identification of microbes. Sequencing of the 16S ribosomal subunit can be used to identify specific bacteria. Sequencing of viruses can be used to identify the virus and distinguish different strains (e.g., specific influenza strains).

Matrix-assisted laser desorption/ionization time-of-flight (MALDI-TOF) mass spectrometry is a powerful new rapid approach to determine RNA, DNA, and protein sequences. The DNA or RNA is inserted into the instrument, ionized, and fragmented, the fragments are separated based on their charge-to-mass ratio, and the nucleotide sequence is determined by analyzing the mass of the ionized fragments. Comparison of specific genes (e.g., 16S RNA) or PCR amplified sequences to a bank of gene sequences can allow rapid microbial detection and identification of bacteria and viruses and discrimination of specific strains of microbes.

• Detection of Proteins

In some cases, viruses and other infectious agents can be detected on the basis of finding certain characteristic enzymes or specific proteins. For example, the detection of reverse transcriptase enzyme activity in serum or cell culture indicates the presence of a retrovirus. The pattern of proteins from a virus or another agent after sodium dodecyl sulfate–polyacrylamide gel electrophoresis (SDS-PAGE) can also be used to identify and distinguish different strains of viruses or bacteria. In the SDS-PAGE technique, SDS binds to the backbone of the protein to generate a uniform peptide structure and peptide length-to-charge ratio such that the mobility of the protein in the gel is inversely related to the logarithm of its molecular weight. For example, the patterns of electrophoretically separated HSV proteins can be used to distinguish different types and strains of HSV-1 and HSV-2. MALDI-TOF mass spectrometry also uses molecular weight to distinguish different proteins. Antibody can be used to identify specific proteins separated by SDS-PAGE using a Western blot technique (see Figure 6-6). The molecular techniques used to identify infectious agents are summarized in Table 5-1.

Bibliography

DiPersio JR, File TM Jr, Stevens DL, et al: Spread of serious disease-producing M3 clones of group A *Streptococcus* among family members and health care workers, *Clin Infect Dis* 22:490–495, 1996.

Forbes BA, Sahm DF, Weissfeld AS: *Bailey and Scott's diagnostic microbiology*, ed 12, St Louis, 2007, Mosby.

Fredericks DN, Relman DA: Application of polymerase chain reaction to the diagnosis of infectious diseases, *Clin Infect Dis* 29:475–486, 1999.

Millar BC, Xu J, Moore JE: Molecular diagnostics of medically important bacterial infections, *Curr Issues Mol Biol* 9:21–40, 2007.

Murray PR: *ASM pocket guide to clinical microbiology*, ed 3, Washington, DC, 2004, American Society for Microbiology Press.

Persing DH, Tenover FC, Tang Y-W, et al: *Molecular microbiology, diagnostic principles and practice*, ed 2, Washington, DC, 2011, American Society for Microbiology Press.

Specter S, Hodinka RL, Young SA: *Clinical virology manual*, ed 3, Washington, DC, 2000, American Society for Microbiology Press.

Strauss JM, Strauss EG: *Viruses and human disease*, ed 2, San Diego, 2007, Academic.

Versalovic J, Carroll KC, Funke G, et al: *Manual of clinical microbiology*, ed 10, Washington, DC, 2011, American Society for Microbiology Press.

CHAPTER

6 SEROLOGIC DIAGNOSIS

Immunologic techniques are used to detect, identify, and quantitate antigen in clinical samples, as well as to evaluate the antibody response to infection and a person's history of exposure to infectious agents. The specificity of the antibody-antigen interaction and the sensitivity of many of the immunologic techniques make them powerful laboratory tools (Table 6-1). *In most cases, the same technique can be adapted to evaluate antigen and antibody.* Because many serologic assays are designed to give a positive or negative result, quantitation of the antibody strength is obtained as a titer. The **titer** of an antibody is defined as the greatest dilution of the sample that retains a detectable activity.

• Antibodies

Antibodies can be used as sensitive and specific tools to detect, identify, and quantitate the antigens from a virus, bacterium, fungus, or parasite. Specific antibodies may be obtained from convalescent patients (e.g., antiviral antibodies) or prepared in animals. These antibodies are **polyclonal;** that is, they are heterogeneous antibody preparations that can recognize many epitopes on a single antigen. **Monoclonal** antibodies recognize individual epitopes on an antigen. Monoclonal antibodies for many antigens are commercially available, especially for lymphocyte cell surface antigens.

The development of monoclonal antibody technology revolutionized the science of immunology. For example, because of the specificity of these antibodies, lymphocyte subsets (e.g., CD4 and CD8 T cells) and lymphocyte cell surface antigens were identified. Monoclonal antibodies are the products of hybrid cells generated by the fusion and cloning of a spleen cell from an immunized mouse and a myeloma cell, which produces a hybridoma. The myeloma provides immortalization to the antibody-producing B cells of the spleen. *Each hybridoma clone is a factory for one antibody molecule, yielding a monoclonal antibody that recognizes only one epitope.* Monoclonal antibodies can also be prepared and manipulated through genetic engineering and "humanized" for therapeutic usage.

The advantages of monoclonal antibodies are (1) that their specificity can be confined to a single epitope on an antigen and (2) that they can be prepared in "industrial-sized" tissue culture preparations. A major disadvantage of monoclonal antibodies is that they are often too specific, such that a monoclonal antibody specific for one epitope on a viral antigen of one strain may not be able to detect different strains of the same virus.

• Methods of Detection

Antibody-antigen complexes can be detected directly, by precipitation techniques, or by labeling the antibody with a radioactive, fluorescent, or enzyme probe, or they can be detected indirectly through measurement of an antibody-directed reaction, such as complement fixation.

Precipitation and Immunodiffusion Techniques

Specific antigen-antibody complexes and cross-reactivity can be distinguished by immunoprecipitation techniques. Within a limited concentration range for both antigen and antibody, termed the **equivalence zone,** the antibody cross-links the antigen into a complex that is too large to stay in solution and therefore precipitates. This technique is based on the multivalent nature of antibody molecules (e.g., immunoglobulin [Ig]G has two antigen-binding domains). The antigen-antibody complexes are soluble at concentration ratios of antigen to antibody that are above and below the equivalence concentration.

Various immunodiffusion techniques make use of the equivalence concept to determine the identity of an antigen or the presence of antibody. **Single radial immunodiffusion** can be used to detect and quantify an antigen. In this technique, antigen is placed into a well and allowed to diffuse into antibody-containing agar. The higher the concentration of antigen, the farther it diffuses before it reaches equivalence with the antibody in the agar and precipitates as a ring around the well.

The **Ouchterlony immuno–double-diffusion** technique is used to determine the relatedness of different antigens, as shown in Figure 6-1. In this technique, solutions of antibody and antigen are placed in separate wells cut into agar, and the antigen and antibody are allowed to diffuse toward each other to establish concentration gradients of each substance. A visible precipitin line occurs where the concentrations of antigen and antibody reach equivalence. On the basis of the pattern of the precipitin lines, this technique can also be used to determine whether samples are identical, share some but not all epitopes (partial identity), or are distinct. This technique is used to detect antibody and fungal antigens (e.g., *Histoplasma* species, *Blastomyces* species, and coccidioidomycoses).

In other immunodiffusion techniques, the antigen may be separated by electrophoresis in agar and then reacted with antibody (immunoelectrophoresis); it may be pushed into agar that contains antibody by means

Table 6-1 Selected Immunologic Techniques

Technique	Purpose	Clinical Examples
Ouchterlony immuno–double-diffusion	Detect and compare antigen and antibody	Fungal antigen and antibody
Immunofluorescence	Detection and localization of antigen	Viral antigen in biopsy (e.g., rabies, herpes simplex virus)
Enzyme immunoassay (EIA)	Same as immunofluorescence	Same as immunofluorescence
Immunofluorescence flow cytometry	Population analysis of antigen-positive cells	Immunophenotyping
ELISA	Quantitation of antigen or antibody	Viral antigen (rotavirus); viral antibody (anti-HIV)
Western blot	Detection of antigen-specific antibody or antigen	Confirmation of anti-HIV seropositivity (antibody)
Radioimmunoassay (RIA)	Same as ELISA	Same as for ELISA
Complement fixation	Quantitate specific antibody titer	Fungal, viral antibody
Hemagglutination inhibition	Antiviral antibody titer; serotype of virus strain	Seroconversion to current influenza strain; identification of influenza
Latex agglutination	Quantitation and detection of antigen and antibody	Rheumatoid factor; fungal antigens; streptococcal antigens

ELISA, Enzyme-linked immunosorbent assay; *HIV,* human immunodeficiency virus.

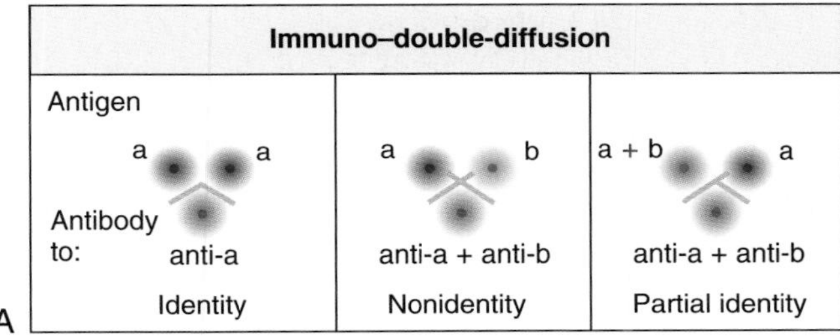

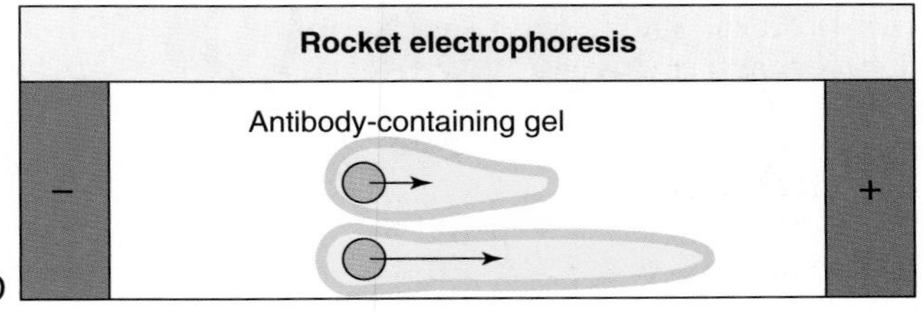

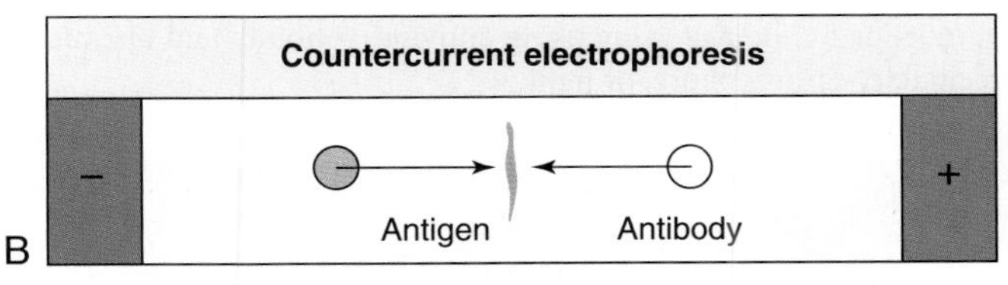

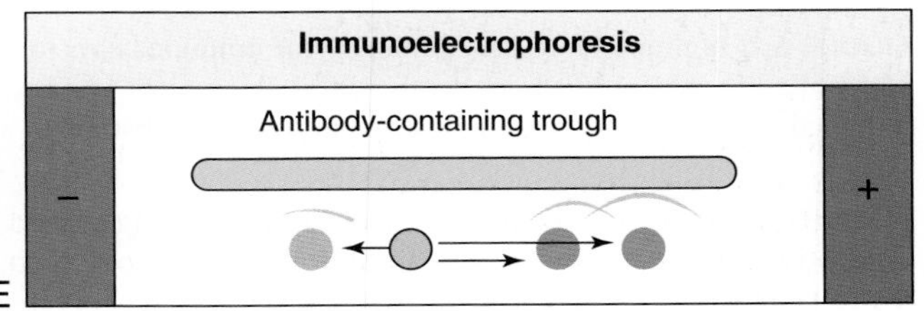

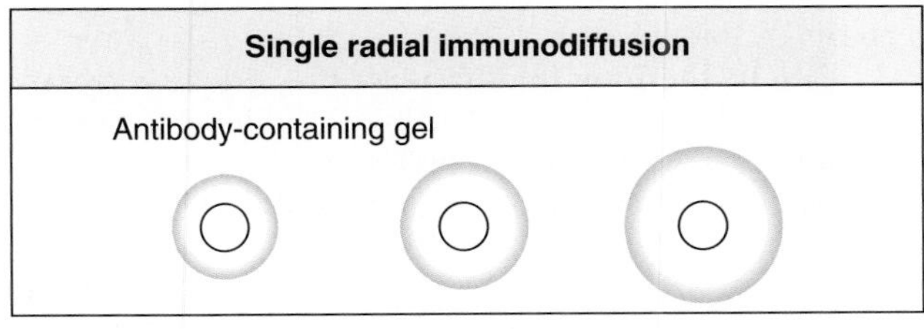

FIGURE 6-1 Analysis of antigens and antibodies by immunoprecipitation. The precipitation of protein occurs at the equivalence point, at which multivalent antibody forms large complexes with antigen. **A,** Ouchterlony immuno–double-diffusion. Antigen and antibody diffuse from wells, meet, and form a precipitin line. If identical antigens are placed in adjacent wells, the concentration of antigen between them is doubled, and precipitation does not occur in this region. If different antigens are used, two different precipitin lines are produced. If one sample shares antigen but is not identical, then a single spur results for the complete antigen. **B,** Countercurrent electrophoresis. This technique is similar to the Ouchterlony method, but antigen movement is facilitated by electrophoresis. **C,** Single radial immunodiffusion. This technique involves the diffusion of antigen into an antibody-containing gel. Precipitin rings indicate an immune reaction, and the area of the ring is proportional to the concentration of antigen. **D,** Rocket electrophoresis. Antigens are separated by electrophoresis into an agar gel that contains antibody. The length of the "rocket" indicates concentration of antigen. **E,** Immunoelectrophoresis. Antigen is placed in a well and separated by electrophoresis. Antibody is then placed in the trough, and precipitin lines form as antigen and antibody diffuse toward each other.

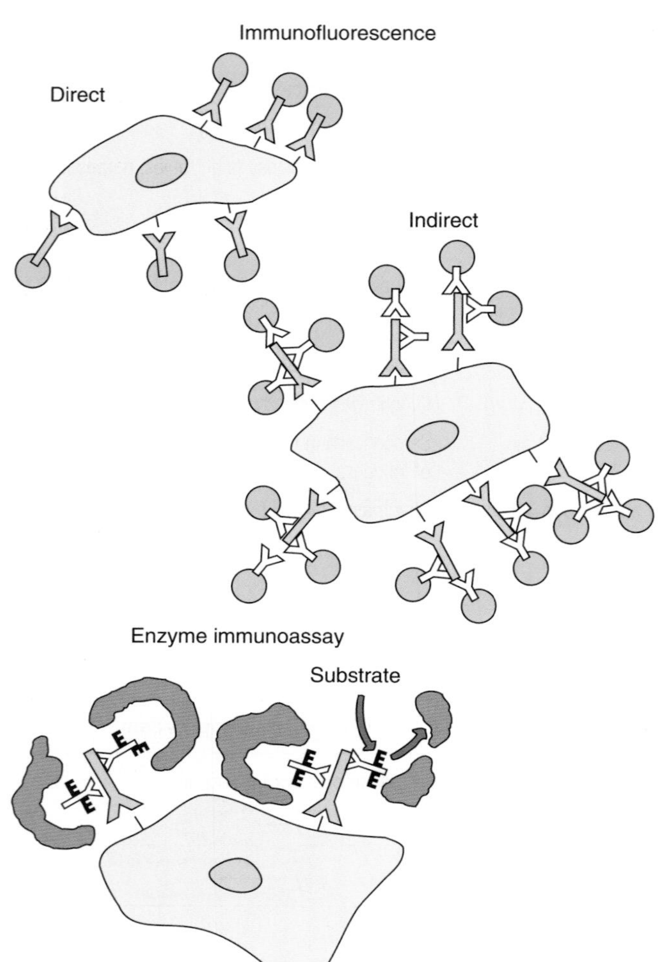

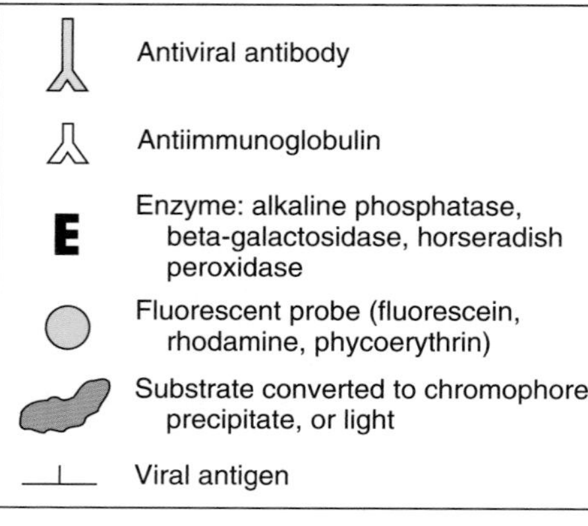

FIGURE 6-2 Immunofluorescence and enzyme immunoassays for antigen localization in cells. Antigen can be detected by *direct* assay with antiviral antibody modified covalently with a fluorescent or enzyme probe, or by *indirect* assay using antiviral antibody and chemically modified antiimmunoglobulin. The enzyme converts substrate to a precipitate, chromophore, or light.

of electrophoresis (rocket electrophoresis), or antigen and antibody may be placed in separate wells and allowed to move electrophoretically toward each other (countercurrent immunoelectrophoresis).

• Immunoassays for Cell-Associated Antigen (Immunohistology)

Antigens on the cell surface or within the cell can be detected by **immunofluorescence** and **enzyme immunoassay (EIA).** In **direct immunofluorescence,** a fluorescent molecule is covalently attached to the antibody (e.g., fluorescein-isothiocyanate [FITC]-labeled rabbit antiviral antibody). In **indirect immunofluorescence,** a second fluorescent antibody specific for the primary antibody (e.g., FITC-labeled goat anti-rabbit antibody) is used to detect the primary antiviral antibody and locate the antigen (Figures 6-2 and 6-3). In EIA, an enzyme such as horseradish peroxidase or alkaline phosphatase is conjugated to the antibody and converts a substrate into a chromophore to mark the antigen. Alternatively, an antibody modified by the attachment of a **biotin** (the vitamin) molecule can be localized by the very high-affinity binding of avidin or streptavidin molecules. A fluorescent molecule or an enzyme attached to the avidin and streptavidin allows detection. These techniques are useful for the analysis of tissue biopsy specimens, blood cells, and tissue culture cells.

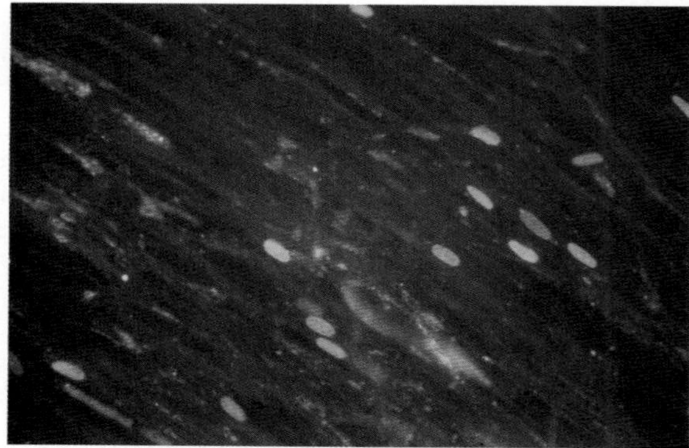

FIGURE 6-3 Immunofluorescence localization of herpes simplex virus–infected nerve cells in a brain section from a patient with herpes encephalitis. (Modified from Male D, Cooke A, Owen M, et al: *Advanced immunology,* ed 3, St Louis, 1996, Mosby.)

The **flow cytometer** can be used to analyze the immunofluorescence of cells in suspension and is especially useful for identifying and quantitating lymphocytes (immunophenotyping). A laser is used in the flow cytometer to excite the fluorescent antibody attached to the cell and to determine the size and the granularity of the cell by means of light-scattering measurements. The cells flow past the laser at rates of more than 5000 cells per second, and analysis is performed electronically. The **fluorescence-activated cell sorter (FACS)** is a flow cytometer that can also isolate specific subpopulations of cells for tissue culture growth on the basis of their size and immunofluorescence.

The data obtained from a flow cytometer are usually presented in the form of a histogram, with the fluorescence intensity on the x-axis and the number of cells on the y-axis, or in the form of a dot plot, in which more than one parameter is compared for each cell. The flow cytometer can perform a differential analysis of white blood cells and determine the numbers and compare other parameters of CD4 and CD8 T-cell populations simultaneously (Figure 6-4). Flow cytometry is also useful for analyzing cell growth after the fluorescent labeling of deoxyribonucleic acid (DNA) and other fluorescent applications.

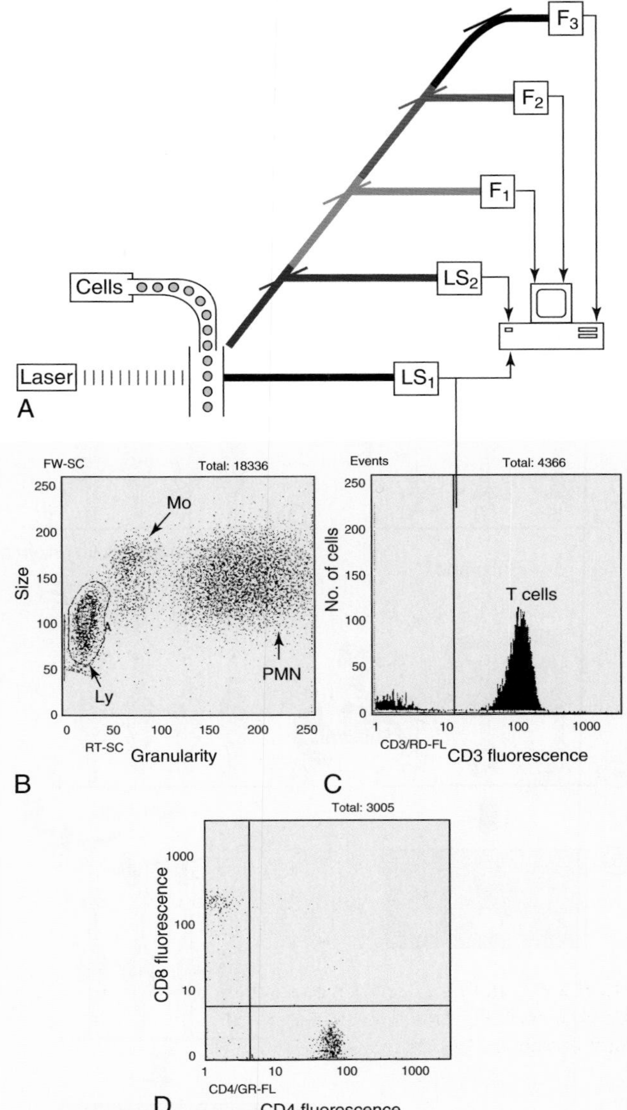

FIGURE 6-4 Flow cytometry. **A,** The flow cytometer evaluates individual cell parameters as the cells flow past a laser beam at rates of more than 5000 per second. Cell size and granularity are determined by light scattering *(LS)*, and antigen expression is evaluated by immunofluorescence *(F)*, using antibodies labeled with different fluorescent probes. Graphs **B** to **D** depict T-cell analysis of a normal patient. **B,** Light-scatter analysis was used to define the lymphocytes *(Ly)*, monocytes *(Mo)*, and polymorphonuclear (neutrophil) leukocytes *(PMN)*. **C,** The lymphocytes were analyzed for CD3 expression to identify T cells (presented in a histogram). **D,** CD4 and CD8 T cells were identified. Each dot represents one T cell. (Data courtesy Dr. Tom Alexander, Akron, Ohio.)

• Immunoassays for Antibody and Soluble Antigen

The **enzyme-linked immunosorbent assay (ELISA)** uses antigen immobilized on a plastic surface, bead, or filter to capture and separate the specific antibody from other antibodies in a patient's serum (Figure 6-5). An antihuman antibody with a covalently linked enzyme (e.g., horseradish peroxidase, alkaline phosphatase, β-galactosidase) then detects the affixed patient antibody. It is quantitated spectrophotometrically according to the optical density of the color produced in response to the enzyme conversion of an appropriate substrate. The actual concentration of specific antibody can be determined by comparison with the reactivity of standard human antibody solutions. The many variations of ELISAs differ in the way in which they capture or detect antibody or antigen.

ELISAs can also be used to quantitate the soluble antigen in a patient's sample. In these assays, soluble antigen is captured and concentrated by an immobilized antibody and then detected with a different antibody labeled with the enzyme. An example of a commonly used ELISA is the home pregnancy test for the human chorionic gonadotropin hormone.

Western blot analysis is a variation of ELISA. In this technique, viral proteins separated by electrophoresis according to their molecular weight or charge are transferred (blotted) onto a filter paper (e.g., nitrocellulose, nylon). When exposed to a patient's serum, the immobilized proteins capture virus-specific antibody and are visualized with an enzyme-conjugated antihuman antibody. This technique shows the proteins recognized by the patient's serum. Western blot analysis is used to confirm ELISA results in patients suspected to be infected with the human immunodeficiency virus (HIV) (Figure 6-6; also see Figure 39-7).

In **radioimmunoassay (RIA),** radiolabeled (e.g., with iodine-125) antibody or antigen is used to quantitate antigen-antibody complexes. RIA can be performed as a capture assay, as described previously for ELISA, or as a competition assay. In a competition assay, antibody in a patient's serum is quantitated according to its ability to compete with and replace a laboratory-prepared radiolabeled antibody from antigen-antibody complexes. The antigen-antibody complexes are precipitated and separated from free antibody, and the radioactivity is measured for both fractions. The amount

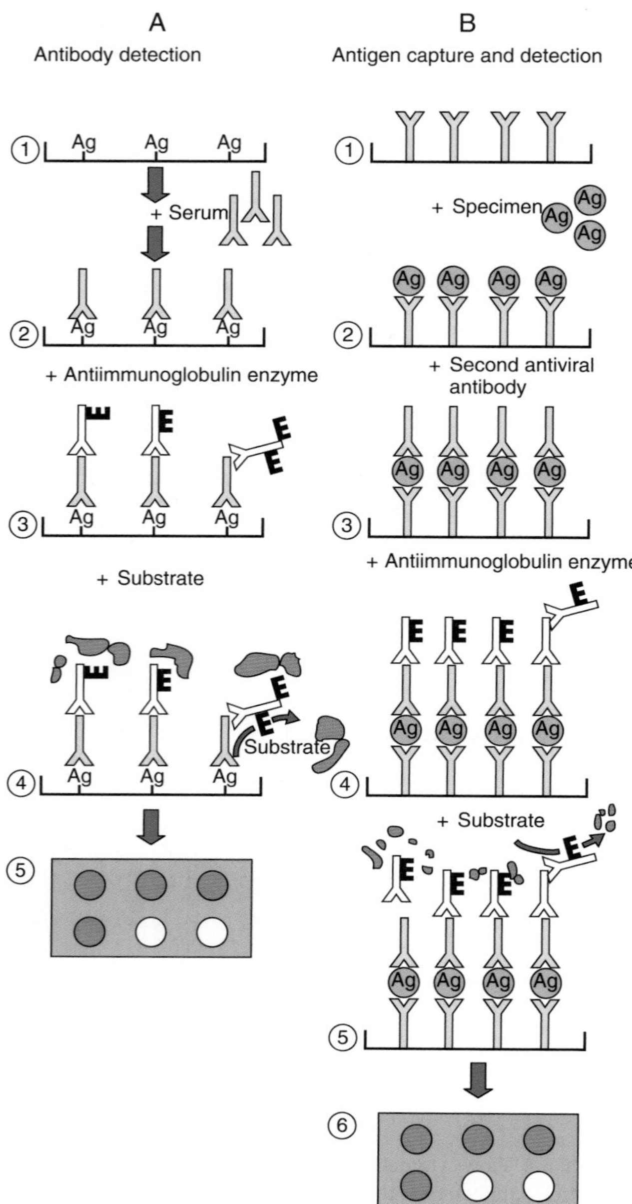

FIGURE 6-5 Enzyme immunoassays for quantitation of antibody or antigen. **A,** Antibody detection. *1,* Viral antigen *(Ag)* obtained from infected cells, virions, or genetic engineering is affixed to a surface. *2,* Patient serum is added and allowed to bind to the antigen. Unbound antibody is washed away. *3,* Enzyme-conjugated antihuman antibody *(E)* is added, and unbound antibody is washed away. *4,* Substrate is added and converted *(5)* into chromophore, precipitate, or light. **B,** Antigen capture and detection. *1,* Antiviral antibody is affixed to a surface. *2,* A specimen that contains antigen is added, and unbound antigen is washed away. *3,* A second antiviral antibody is added to detect the captured antigen. *4,* Enzyme-conjugated anti-antibody is added, washed, and followed by substrate *(5),* which is converted *(6)* into a chromophore, precipitate, or light.

of the patient's antibody is then quantitated from standard curves prepared with use of known quantities of competing antibody. The radioallergosorbent assay is a variation of an RIA capture assay in which radiolabeled anti-IgE is used to detect allergen-specific responses.

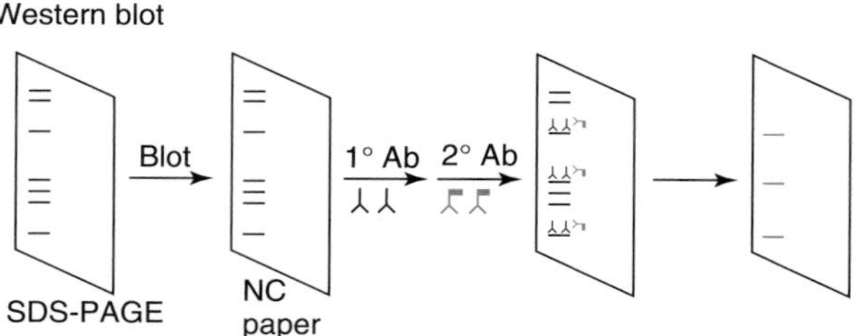

FIGURE 6-6 Western blot analysis. Proteins are separated by sodium dodecyl sulfate–polyacrylamide gel electrophoresis *(SDS-PAGE),* electroblotted onto nitrocellulose *(NC)* paper, and incubated with antigen-specific or patient's antisera *(1° Ab)* and then enzyme-conjugated antihuman serum *(2° Ab).* Enzyme conversion of substrate identifies the antigen.

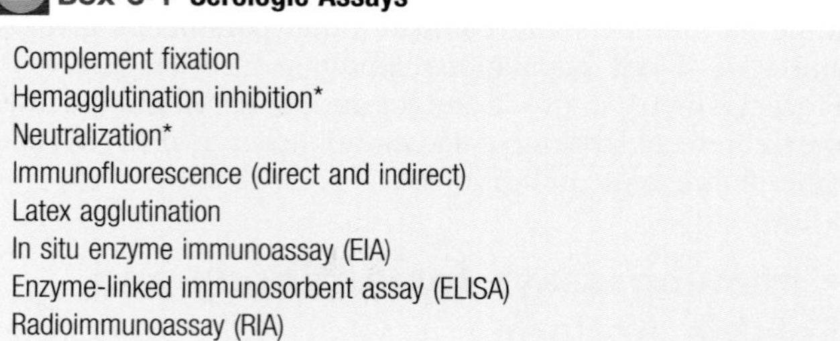

Box 6-1 Serologic Assays

Complement fixation
Hemagglutination inhibition*
Neutralization*
Immunofluorescence (direct and indirect)
Latex agglutination
In situ enzyme immunoassay (EIA)
Enzyme-linked immunosorbent assay (ELISA)
Radioimmunoassay (RIA)

*For detection of antibody or serotyping of virus.

Complement fixation is a standard but technically difficult serologic test (Box 6-1). In this test, the patient's serum sample is reacted with laboratory-derived antigen and extra complement. Antibody-antigen complexes bind, activate, and fix (use up) the complement. The residual complement is then assayed through the lysis of red blood cells coated with antibody. Antibodies measured by this system generally develop slightly later in an illness than those measured by other techniques. A variation of this test can also be used to identify genetic deficiencies in complement components.

Antibody inhibition assays make use of the specificity of an antibody to prevent infection **(neutralization)** or other activity **(hemagglutination inhibition)** to identify the strain of the infecting agent, usually a virus, or to quantitate antibody responses to a specific strain of virus. For example, hemagglutination inhibition is used to distinguish different strains of influenza A and the potency of antibody developed by new vaccines for influenza. These tests are discussed further in Chapter 49.

Latex agglutination is a rapid, technically simple assay for detecting antibody or soluble antigen. Virus-specific antibody causes latex particles coated with viral antigens to clump. Conversely, antibody-coated latex particles are used to detect soluble viral antigen. In passive hemagglutination, antigen-modified erythrocytes are used as indicators instead of latex particles.

• Serology

The humoral immune response provides a history of a patient's infections. Serology can be used to identify the

Box 6-2 Viruses Diagnosed by Serology*

Epstein-Barr virus
Rubella virus
Hepatitis A, B, C, D, and E viruses
Human immunodeficiency virus
Human T-cell leukemia virus
Arboviruses (encephalitis viruses)

*Serologic testing is also used to determine a person's immune status with regard to other viruses.

infecting agent, evaluate the course of an infection, or determine the nature of the infection—whether it is a primary infection or a reinfection, and whether it is acute or chronic. The antibody type and titer and the identity of the antigenic targets provide serologic data about an infection. Serologic testing is used to identify viruses and other agents that are difficult to isolate and grow in the laboratory or that cause diseases that progress slowly (Box 6-2).

The relative antibody concentration is reported as a titer. A **titer** is the inverse of the greatest dilution (lowest concentration [e.g., dilution of 1:64 = titer of 64]) of a patient's serum that retains activity in one of the immunoassays just described. The amount of IgM, IgG, IgA, or IgE reactive with antigen can also be evaluated through the use of a labeled second antihuman antibody that is specific for the antibody isotype.

Serology is used to determine the time course of an infection. **Seroconversion** occurs when antibody is produced in response to a primary infection. *Specific IgM antibody found during the first 2 to 3 weeks of a primary infection is a good indicator of a recent primary infection.* Reinfection or recurrence later in life causes an **anamnestic** (secondary or booster) response. Antibody titers may remain high, however, in patients whose disease recurs frequently (e.g., herpesviruses). Seroconversion or reinfection is indicated by the finding *of at least a fourfold increase in the antibody titer between serum obtained during the acute phase of disease and that obtained at least 2 to 3 weeks later during the convalescent phase.* A twofold serial dilution will not distinguish between samples with 512 and 1023 units of antibody, both of which would give a reaction on a 512-fold dilution but not on a 1024-fold dilution, and both results would be reported as titers of 512. On the other hand, samples with 1020 and 1030 units are not significantly different but would be reported as titers of 512 and 1024, respectively.

Serology can also be used to determine the stage of a slower or chronic infection (e.g., hepatitis B or infectious mononucleosis caused by Epstein-Barr virus), based on the presence of antibody to specific microbial antigens. The first antibodies to be detected are those directed against antigens most available to the immune system (e.g., on the surface of the virion, on infected cells, or secreted). Later in the infection, when cells have been lysed by the infecting virus or the cellular immune response, antibodies directed against the intracellular proteins and enzymes are detected.

Bibliography

Forbes BA, Sahm DF, Weissfeld AS: *Bailey and Scott's diagnostic microbiology*, ed 12, St Louis, 2007, Mosby.

Murray PR: *ASM pocket guide to clinical microbiology*, ed 3, Washington, DC, 2004, American Society for Microbiology Press.

Murray PR, Baron EJ, Jorgensen JH, et al: *Manual of clinical microbiology*, ed 9, Washington, DC, 2007, American Society for Microbiology Press.

Rosenthal KS, Wilkinson JG: Flow cytometry and immunospeak, *Infect Dis Clin Pract* 15:183–191, 2007.

Specter S, Hodinka RL, Young SA: *Clinical virology manual*, ed 3, Washington, DC, 2000, American Society for Microbiology Press.

Strauss JM, Strauss EG: *Viruses and human disease*, ed 2, San Diego, 2007, Academic.

SECTION

3

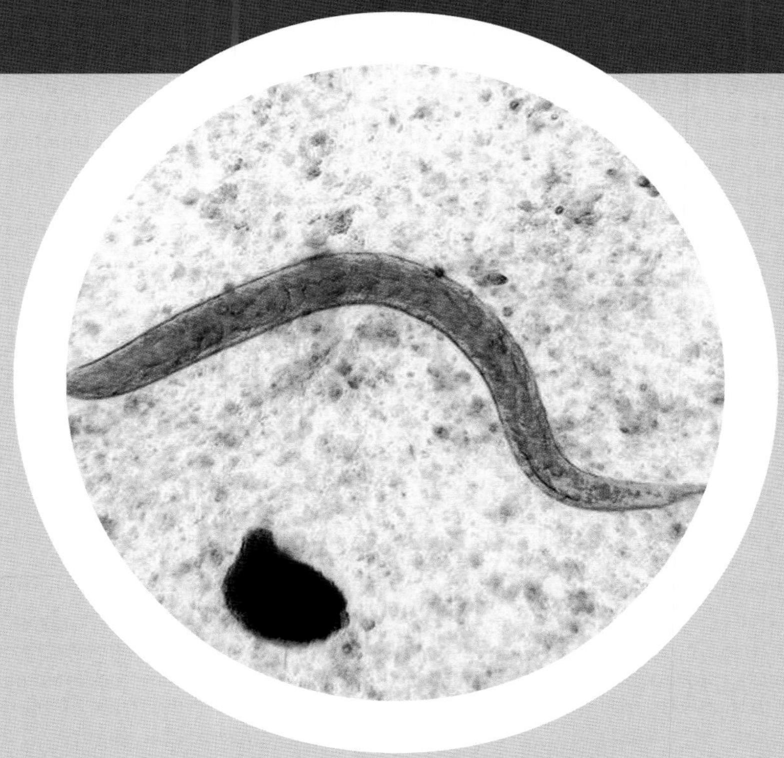

BASIC CONCEPTS IN THE IMMUNE RESPONSE

CHAPTER

ELEMENTS OF HOST PROTECTIVE RESPONSES

We live in a microbial world, and a microbial world lives on and within us. Our bodies are constantly being exposed to bacteria, fungi, parasites, and viruses (Box 7-1) and must restrict the normal flora from entering into sterile tissue sites, discriminate between friend and foe, and defend against invading microbes. Our bodies' defenses are similar to a military defense. The initial defense mechanisms are **barriers** such as the skin, acid and bile of the gastrointestinal tract, and mucus that inactivate and prevent entry of the foreign agents. If these barriers are compromised or the agent gains entry in another way, the local militia of **innate responses** must quickly rally to the challenge and prevent expansion of the invasion. Initially, toxic molecules (defensins and other peptides, complement) are thrown at the microbe while other molecules make them sticky (complement, lectins, and antibodies), facilitating the ingestion and destruction of the microbe by neutrophils and macrophages. Once activated, these responses also send an alarm (complement, cytokines, and chemokines) to other cells and open the vasculature (complement, cytokines) to provide access to the site. If these steps are not effective, the innate responses activate a major campaign specifically directed against the invader by **antigen-specific immune responses** (B cells, antibody, and T cells) at whatever cost (immunopathogenesis). Finally, the infected tissue must be repaired and the system returned to the status quo and a normal regulated balance. Knowledge of the characteristics of the enemy (antigens) through prior exposure or vaccination enables the body to mount a faster, more effective response (activation of memory B and T cells) on rechallenge.

The different elements of the immune system interact and communicate using soluble molecules and by direct cell-to-cell interaction. These interactions provide the mechanisms for activation and control of the protective responses. Unfortunately, the protective responses to some infectious agents are insufficient or too slow; in other cases, the response to the challenge is excessive and causes peripheral damage. In either case, disease occurs.

• Soluble Activators and Stimulators of Innate and Immune Functions

Innate and immune cells communicate by cell-cell interactions and with soluble molecules, including complement cleavage products, cytokines, interferons, and chemokines. **Cytokines** are hormone-like proteins that act on cells to activate and regulate the innate and immune response (Table 7-1 and Box 7-2). **Interferons** are also cytokines that are produced in response to viral and other infections (interferon [IFN]-α and IFN-β) or on activation of the immune response (IFN-γ); they promote antiviral and antitumor responses and stimulate immune responses (see Chapter 8). **Chemokines** are small proteins (≈8000 Da) that attract specific cells to sites of inflammation and other immunologically important sites. Neutrophils, basophils, natural killer (NK) cells, monocytes, and T cells express receptors and can be activated by specific chemokines. The chemokines and other proteins (e.g., the C3a and C5a products of the complement cascade) are chemotactic factors that establish a chemical path to attract phagocytic and inflammatory cells to the site of infection. The triggers that stimulate the production of these molecules and the consequences of the interactions with their receptors on specific cells determine the nature of the innate and immune response. *Useful mnemonics to help learn cytokines are:* ***STAT****—****s****ource (cell),* ***t****rigger,* ***a****ction,* ***t****arget (receptor and cell); and for the response,* ***TICTOC****—****t****rigger,* ***i****nducer,* ***c****ells (producer and responder),* ***t****imecourse,* ***o****utcome,* ***c****ytokines.*

• Cells of the Immune Response

Immune responses are mediated by specific cells with defined functions. Characteristics of these cells and their appearances are presented in Figure 7-1 and in Tables 7-2 and 7-3. *For each of the cells know the* ***CARP****:* ***c****ell surface markers (e.g., CD4, TCR, etc.),* ***a****ctions (kill, suppress, activate, etc.),* ***r****ole (type of response),* ***p****roducts (cytokines, antibody, etc.).* The white blood cells can be distinguished on the basis of (1) morphology, (2) histologic staining, (3) immunologic functions, and (4) intracellular and cell surface markers. B and T lymphocytes can be distinguished by expression of antigen receptors on their surfaces, immunoglobulin for B cells and T-cell receptors for T cells. Other cell surface proteins distinguish subsets of these and other types of cells. These marker proteins are identified with monoclonal antibodies. They are defined within clusters of differentiation (as determined by all of the monoclonal antibodies that recognize the same molecule [e.g., CD4]) or group of molecules (e.g., CD3) and the markers indicated by **"CD"** (cluster of differentiation) numbers (Table 7-4). In addition, **all nucleated cells express class I MHC (MHC I) antigens** (human: HLA-A, HLA-B, HLA-C).

A special class of cells that are **antigen-presenting cells (APCs) express class II major histocompatibility complex**

Box 7-1 Overview of the Immune Response

- There is a natural balance in the body between repair and debris removal and inflammation and attack; this balance is regulated by components of the innate and antigen-specific immune responses.
- The immune system is trained to ignore its own proteins and tolerate normal flora that stays in its normal habitat.
- Tissue damage and infection trigger host responses, each of which provides molecules (damage-associated molecular patterns [DAMP] and pathogen-associated molecular patterns [PAMP]) recognized by host receptors on immune and other cells that activate innate and inflammatory responses.
- Soluble effectors are released or activated in response to tissue damage or infection before phagocytes or immune cells become involved (soluble before cellular).
- The host response progresses from innate to antigen specific.
- The immune response facilitates, enhances, and regulates the innate responses.

(MHC) antigens (HLA-DR, HLA-DP, HLA-DQ). Cells that present antigenic peptides to T cells include dendritic cells, macrophage family cells, B lymphocytes, and a limited number of other cell types.

Hematopoietic Cell Differentiation

Differentiation of a common progenitor cell, termed the **pluripotent stem cell,** gives rise to all blood cells. Differentiation of these cells begins during development of the fetus and continues throughout life. The pluripotent stem cell differentiates into stem cells (sometimes referred to as colony-forming units) for different lineages of blood cells, including the lymphoid (T and B cells), myeloid, erythrocytic, and megakaryoblastic (source of platelets) lineages (see Figure 7-1). The stem cells reside primarily in the bone marrow but can also be isolated from the fetal blood in umbilical cords and as rare cells in adult blood. Differentiation of stem cells into the functional blood cells is triggered by specific cell surface interactions with the stromal cells of the marrow and specific cytokines produced by these and other cells.

The bone marrow and thymus are considered **primary lymphoid organs** (Figure 7-2 and Box 7-3). These sites of initial lymphocyte differentiation are essential to the development of the immune system. The thymus is essential at birth for T-cell development but shrinks with aging, and other tissues adopt its function later in life. **Secondary lymphoid organs** include the **lymph nodes, spleen, skin**, and **mucosa-associated lymphoid tissue (MALT);** the latter also includes gut-associated lymphoid tissue (GALT) (e.g., Peyer patches) and bronchus-associated lymphoid tissue (BALT) (e.g., lung). These sites are where dendritic cells and B and T lymphocytes reside and respond to antigenic challenges. The cells of the primary and secondary lymphoid organs produce chemokines and express cell surface adhesion molecules **(addressins)** that interact with homing receptors **(cell adhesion molecules)** expressed on B and T cells.

The spleen and lymph nodes are encapsulated organs in which the macrophages and B and T cells reside in defined regions. Their location facilitates interactions that promote immune responses to antigen (Figure 7-3). Proliferation of the lymphocytes in response to infectious challenge causes these tissues to swell (i.e., "swollen glands").

The **lymph nodes** are kidney-shaped organs, 2 to 10 mm in diameter, that filter the fluid that passes from intercellular spaces into the lymphatic system, almost like a sewage processing plant. The lymph node is constructed to optimize the meeting of the innate (dendritic cells and macrophages) and the immune response (B and T) cells to initiate and expand specific immune responses. A lymph node consists of three layers:

1. The cortex, the outer layer that contains mainly B cells, follicular dendritic cells, and macrophages arranged in structures called *follicles* and, if activated, in germinal centers
2. The paracortex, which contains T cells and dendritic cells, which present antigens to the T cells to initiate immune responses
3. The medulla, which contains B and T cells and antibody-producing plasma cells, as well as channels for the lymph fluid

The **spleen** is a large organ that acts like a lymph node and also filters antigens, encapsulated bacteria, and viruses from blood and removes aged blood cells and platelets (Figure 7-4). The spleen consists of two types of tissue, the white pulp and the red pulp. The white pulp consists of arterioles surrounded by lymphoid cells (periarteriolar lymphoid sheath) in which the **T cells** surround the central arteriole. **B cells** are organized into primary unstimulated or secondary stimulated follicles that have a germinal center. The germinal center contains memory cells, macrophages, and follicular dendritic cells. The red pulp is a storage site for blood cells and the site of turnover of aged platelets and erythrocytes. *A hint for remembering this is: There is no T in follicle or germinal center but there are Ts in paracortex and periarteriolar lymphoid sheet.*

The **epidermis of skin** contains Langerhans cells, and the **dermis** contains dendritic cells, B and T lymphocytes, macrophages, and mast cells. Large numbers of memory T cells continuously circulate into these layers of the skin. Keratinocytes in the epidermis are part of the innate antimicrobial defense system.

MALT contains less structured aggregates of lymphoid cells (Figure 7-5). For example, the **Peyer patches** along the intestinal wall have special cells in the epithelium (M cells) that deliver antigens from the lumen into a mini–lymph node–like structure containing dendritic cells and lymphocytes in defined regions (T [interfollicular] and B [germinal]). Dendritic cells, T cells, and B cells also reside in the lamina propria layer just under the epithelium. Once thought to be expendable, the **tonsils** are an important part of the MALT. These lymphoepithelial organs sample the microbes in the oral and nasal area. The tonsils contain a large number of mature and memory B cells (50% to 90% of the lymphocytes) that use their antibodies to sense specific pathogens and, with dendritic cells and T cells, can initiate immune responses. Swelling of the tonsils may be caused by infection or a response to infection.

Polymorphonuclear Leukocytes

Polymorphonuclear leukocytes (neutrophils) are short-lived cells that constitute 50% to 70% of circulating white blood cells (see Figure 7-1) and are a primary **phagocytic defense** against bacterial infection and major component of

Table 7-1 Cytokines and Chemokines

Factor	Source	Major Target	Function
Innate and Acute-Phase Responses			
IFN-α, IFN-β	Leukocytes, pDCs, fibroblasts, and other cells	Virally infected cells, tumor cells, NK cells	Induction of antiviral state; activation of NK cells, enhancement of cell-mediated immunity
IL-1α, IL-1β	Macrophages, DCs, fibroblasts, epithelial cells, endothelial cells	T cells, B cells, PMNs, tissue, central nervous system, liver, etc.	Many actions: promotion of inflammatory and acute-phase responses, fever, activation of T cells and macrophages
TNF-α (cachectin)	Similar to IL-1	Macrophages, T cells, NK cells, epithelial and many other cells	Similar to IL-1, and also antitumor, wasting (cachexia, weight loss) functions, sepsis, endothelial activation
IL-6	DCs, macrophages, T and B cells, fibroblasts, epithelial cells, endothelial cells	T and B cells, hepatocytes	Stimulation of acute-phase and inflammatory responses, T- and B-cell growth and development
IL-12, IL-23	DC, macrophage	NK cells, CD4 TH1, TH17 cells	Activation of T-cell–mediated and inflammatory responses, IFN-γ or IL-17 production
Growth and Differentiation			
Colony-stimulating factors (e.g., GM-CSF)	T cells, stromal cells	Stem cells	Growth and differentiation of specific cell types, hematopoiesis
IL-3	CD4 T cells, keratinocytes	Stem cells	Hematopoiesis
IL-7	Bone marrow, stroma	Precursor cells and stem cells	Growth of pre–B cell, thymocyte, T cell, and cytotoxic lymphocyte
TH1 and TH17 Responses			
IL-2	CD4 T cells (TH0, TH1)	T cells, B cells, NK cells	T- and B-cell growth, NK activation
IFN-γ	CD4 TH1 cells, NK cells	Macrophages,* DCs, T cells, B cells	Activation of macrophage, promotion of IgG class switch, inflammation and TH1 but inhibition of TH2 responses
TNF-β	CD4 TH1 cells	PMN, tumors	Lymphotoxin: tumor killing, activation of PMN, endothelial activation
IL-17	CD4 TH17 cells	Epithelial, endothelial, and fibroblast cells, neutrophils	Activate tissue to promote inflammation even in the presence of TGF-β.
TH2 Responses			
IL-4	CD4 T cells (TH0, TH2)	B and T cells	T- and B-cell growth; IgG, IgA, and IgE production; TH2 responses
IL-5	CD4 TH2 cells	B cells, eosinophils	B-cell growth and differentiation; IgG, IgA, and IgE production; eosinophil production; allergic responses
IL-10	CD4 TH2 and Treg cells	B cells, CD4 TH1 cells	B-cell growth, inhibition of TH1 response
Regulatory Response			
TGF-β (also IL-10)	CD4 Treg cells	B cells, T cells, macrophages	Immunosuppression of B, T, and NK cells and macrophages; promotion of oral tolerance, wound healing, IgA production
Chemokines			
α-Chemokines: CXC chemokines—two cysteines separated by one amino acid (IL-8; IP-10; GRO-α, GRO-β, GRO-γ)	Many cells	Neutrophils, T cells, macrophages	Chemotaxis, activation
β-Chemokines: CC chemokines—two adjacent cysteines (MCP-1; MIP-α; MIP-β; RANTES)	Many cells	T cells, macrophages, basophils	Chemotaxis, activation

CD, Cluster of differentiation; *DCs,* dendritic cells; *GM-CSF,* granulocyte-macrophage colony-stimulating factor; *GRO-γ,* growth-related oncogene-γ; *IFN-α, -β, -γ,* interferon-α, -β, -γ; *Ig,* immunoglobulin; *IL,* interleukin; *IP,* interferon-α protein; *MCP,* monocyte chemoattractant protein; *MIP,* macrophage inflammatory protein; *NK,* natural killer; *pDCs,* plasmacytoid dendritic cells, *PMN,* polymorphonuclear leukocyte; *RANTES,* regulated on activation, normal T expressed and secreted; *TGF-β,* transforming growth factor-β; *TH,* T helper (cell); *TNF-α,* tumor necrosis factor-α.

*Applies to one or more cell types of the monocyte-macrophage lineage.

the **inflammatory response. Neutrophils** are 9 to 14 μm in diameter, lack mitochondria, have a granulated cytoplasm in which granules stain with both acidic and basic stains, and have a multilobed nucleus. Neutrophils leave the blood and concentrate at the site of infection in response to chemotactic factors. During infection, the neutrophils in the blood increase in number and include precursor forms. These precursors are termed **band forms,** in contrast to the terminally differentiated and **segmented neutrophils.** The finding of such an increase and change in neutrophils by a blood count is sometimes termed *a left shift with an increase in bands versus segs.* Neutrophils ingest bacteria by phagocytosis and expose the bacteria to antibacterial substances and enzymes contained in **primary (azurophilic)** and **secondary (specific) granules.** Azurophilic granules are reservoirs for enzymes such as myeloperoxidase, β-glucuronidase, elastase, and cathepsin G. Specific granules serve as reservoirs for lysozyme and lactoferrin. Dead neutrophils release a sticky antimicrobial net of DNA and other fibers, termed **neutrophil extracellular trap (net)**, and dead neutrophils are the major component of **pus.**

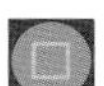

Box 7-2 Major Cytokine-Producing Cells

Innate (Acute-Phase Responses)

Dendritic cells, macrophages, other: IL-1, TNF-α, IL-6, IL-12, IL-18, IL-23, GM-CSF, chemokines, IFN-α, IFN-β

Immune: T Cells (CD4 and CD8)

TH1 cells: IL-2, IFN-γ, TNF-α, TNF-β, IL-3, GM-CSF

TH2 cells: IL-4, IL-5, IL-6, IL-10, IL-3, IL-9, IL-13, GM-CSF, TNF-α

TH17 cells: IL-17, TNF-α

Treg cells: TGF-β and IL-10

GM-CSF, Granulocyte-macrophage colony-stimulating factor; *IFN-α, -β, -γ,* interferon-α, -β, -γ; *IL,* interleukin; *TGF-β,* transforming growth factor-β; *TNF-α,* tumor necrosis factor-α.

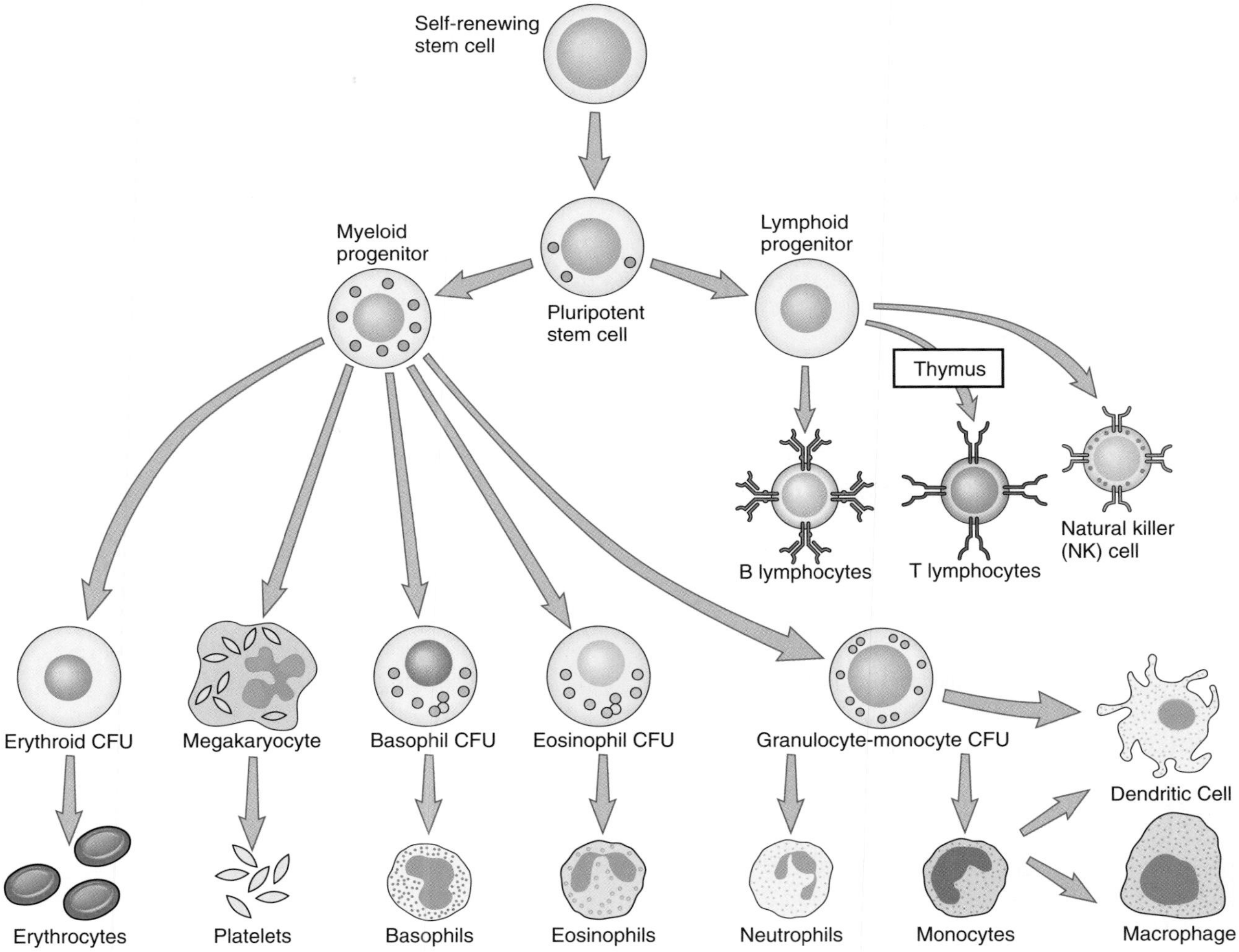

Eosinophils are heavily granulated cells (11 to 15 μm in diameter) with a bilobed nucleus that stains with the acid dye eosin Y. They are also phagocytic, motile, and granulated. The granules contain acid phosphatase, peroxidase, and eosinophilic basic proteins. Eosinophils play a role in the defense against **parasitic infections.** The eosinophilic basic proteins are toxic to many parasites. **Mast cells** and **basophils** are non-phagocytic granulocytes that release the

FIGURE 7-1 Morphology and lineage of cells involved in the immune response. Pluripotent stem cells and colony-forming units *(CFUs)* are long-lived cells capable of replenishing the more differentiated functional and terminally differentiated cells. (Modified from Abbas AK, Lichtman AH, Pillai S, et al: *Cellular and molecular immunology,* ed 8, Philadelphia, 2015, Elsevier.)

 Table 7-2 **Cells of the Immune Response**

Cells	Characteristics and Functions
Innate Lymphoid Cells (ILCs)	Produce cytokines
NK cells	Large, granular lymphocytes
	Markers: Fc receptors for antibody, KIR
	Kill antibody-decorated cells and virus-infected or tumor cell (no MHC restriction)
Phagocytic Cells	
Neutrophils	Granulocytes with short life span, multilobed nucleus and granules, segmented band forms (more immature)
	Phagocytose and **kill bacteria** (polymorphonuclear leukocytes)
Eosinophils	Bilobed nucleus, heavily granulated cytoplasm, stains with eosin
	Involved in parasite defense and allergic response
Antigen-Presenting Phagocytic Cells (APCs)	Marker: Class II MHC-expressing cells
	Process and present antigen to CD4 T cells
Monocytes*	Horseshoe-shaped nucleus, lysosomes, granules
	Precursors to macrophage-lineage and dendritic cells, cytokine release
Immature dendritic cells	Blood and tissue
	Cytokine response to infection, process antigen
Dendritic cells*	Lymph nodes, tissue
	Most potent APC; initiates and determines nature of T-cell response
Langerhans cells*	**Present in skin**
	Same as immature dendritic cell
Macrophages*	Possible residence in tissue, spleen, lymph nodes, and other organs; activated by IFN-γ and TNF
	Markers: large, granular cells; Fc and C3b receptors
	(M2) Remove debris, maintain normal tissue function, and facilitate repair, APC (M1) Activated cells initiate inflammatory and acute-phase response; **activated cells are antibacterial, APC**
Antigen-Responsive T Cells	
T cells (all)	Mature in thymus; large nucleus, small cytoplasm
	Markers: CD2, CD3, T-cell receptor (TCR)
α/β TCR CD4 T cells	Helper/DTH cells; **activation** by APCs through **class II MHC antigen presentation**
	Produce cytokines; stimulate T- and B-cell growth; promote B-cell differentiation (class switching, antibody production)
	TH1 subtype (IL-2, IFN-γ, LT production): promote antibody and cell-mediated defenses (local and systemic), including DTH, CD8 T killer cells
	TH2 subtype (IL-4, IL-5, IL-6, IL-10 production): promote humoral (antibody) responses (systemic)
	TH17 subtype (IL-17, TNF-α, IL-6): stimulate epithelial cells and neutrophils and inflammation
	T regulator (Treg) cells (TGF-β, IL-10): control CD4 and CD8 T-cell activation and other cells; important for immunotolerance
α/β TCR CD8 T-killer cells	**Recognition** of antigen presented by **class I MHC antigens**
	Kill viral, tumor, nonself (transplant) cells; secrete cytokines
γ/δ TCR T cells	Markers: CD2, CD3, γ/δ T-cell receptor
	Early sensor of some bacterial infections in tissue and blood
NKT cells	Express NK cell receptors, TCR, and CD3
	Rapid response to infection, cytokine release

Table 7-2 Cells of the Immune Response—cont'd

Cells	Characteristics and Functions
Antibody-Producing Cells	
B cells	Mature in bone marrow (bursal equivalent), Peyer patches
	Large nucleus, small cytoplasm; activation by antigens and T-cell factors
	Markers: surface antibody, **class II MHC antigens**
	Produce antibody and present antigen
Plasma cells	Small nucleus, large cytoplasm
	Terminally differentiated, antibody factories
Other Cells	
Basophils/mast cells	Granulocytic
	Marker: Fc receptors for IgE
	Release histamine, provide allergic response, are antiparasitic
Platelets	Release clotting factors, antimicrobial peptides, chemokines and cytokines upon activation

CNS, central nervous system; *DTH,* delayed-type hypersensitivity; *IFN-γ,* interferon-γ; *Ig,* immunoglobulin; *IL,* interleukin; *KIR,* killer cell immunoglobulin-like receptors; *LT,* lymphotoxin; *MHC,* major histocompatibility complex; *NK,* natural killer; *TCR,* T-cell receptor; *TGF-β,* transforming growth factor-β; *TH,* T helper (cell); *TNF-α,* tumor necrosis factor-α.

*Monocyte/macrophage lineage.

Table 7-3 Normal Blood Cell Counts

Cell Type	Mean Number per Microliter	Normal Range
White blood cells (leukocytes)	7400	4500-11,000
Neutrophils	4400	1800-7700
Eosinophils	200	0-450
Basophils	40	0-200
Lymphocytes	2500	1000-4800
Monocytes	300	0-800

Modified from Abbas AK, Lichtman AH, Pillai S, et al: *Cellular and molecular immunology,* ed 8, Philadelphia, 2015, Elsevier.

contents of their granules in response to inflammatory triggers and during allergic responses (type 1 hypersensitivity).

Mononuclear Phagocyte System

The **mononuclear phagocyte system** has myeloid cells and consists of monocytes (see Figure 7-1) in the blood, **macrophages,** and **dendritic cells. Monocytes** are 10 to 18 μm in diameter, with a single-lobed, kidney bean–shaped nucleus. They represent 3% to 8% of peripheral blood leukocytes. Monocytes follow neutrophils into tissue as an early cellular component of inflammation.

Macrophages are long-lived cells that are phagocytic, contain lysosomes, and unlike neutrophils, have mitochondria. Macrophages have the following basic functions: (1) phagocytosis of debris and microbes, (2) antigen presentation to T cells to expand specific immune responses, and (3) secretion of cytokines to either maintain normal tissue function and repair (M2 macrophages) or be antimicrobial and promote inflammation (M1 macrophages) (Figure 7-6; also see Figure 8-3). Macrophages express cell surface receptors for the Fc portion of immunoglobulin (Ig)G **(Fc-γ RI, Fc-γ RII, Fc-γ RIII)** and for the C3b product of the complement cascade **(CR1, CR3).** These receptors facilitate the phagocytosis of antigen, bacteria, or viruses coated with these proteins. **Toll-like and other pattern-recognition receptors** recognize pathogen-associated molecular patterns and activate protective responses. Macrophages also express the **class II MHC antigen,** which allows these cells to present antigen to CD4 helper T cells to expand the immune response. Macrophages secrete **interleukin (IL)-1, IL-6, tumor necrosis factor (TNF)-α, IL-12,** and other molecules upon sensing bacteria, which stimulates immune and inflammatory responses, including fever. A T-cell–derived cytokine, **IFN-γ,** activates inflammatory functions in macrophages. **Activated macrophages** (M1) have enhanced phagocytic, killing, and antigen-presenting capabilities.

Blood, alveolar, and serosal (e.g., peritoneal) macrophages are examples of "wandering" macrophages derived from bone marrow precursor cells. Tissue resident macrophages include: *alveolar macrophages in the lungs, Kupffer cells in the liver, intraglomerular mesangial cells in the kidney, histiocytes in connective tissue, osteoclasts, synovial cells, and microglial cells in the brain.* These macrophages are descended from cells of the yolk sac and are primarily involved in tissue maintenance and repair functions (M2 macrophages). The mature forms of these cells have different morphologies corresponding to their ultimate tissue location and function and may express a subset of macrophage activities or cell surface markers.

Dendritic Cells

Most **dendritic cells** have octopus-like tendrils and are professional antigen-presenting cells (APCs) that can also produce cytokines. Different types of immature and mature dendritic cells are found in tissue and blood; they include

Table 7-4 Selected CD Markers of Importance

CD Markers	Identity and Function	Cell
CD1 (a-d)	MHC I–like, glycolipid antigen presentation	DC, macrophage
CD2 (LFA-3R)	Erythrocyte receptor	T cells
CD3	TCR subunit (γ, δ, ε, ζ, η); activation	T cells
CD4	Class II MHC receptor	T-cell subset, monocytes, some DCs
CD8	Class I MHC receptor	T-cell subset
CD11b (CR3)	C3b complement receptor 3 (α chain)	NK, myeloid cells
CD14	LPS-binding protein receptor	Myeloid cells (monocytes, macrophages)
CD16 (Fc-γ RIII)	Phagocytosis and ADCC	NK-cell marker, macrophages, neutrophils
CD21 (CR2)	C3d complement receptor, EBV receptor, B-cell activation	B cells
CD25	IL-2 receptor (α chain), early activation marker, marker for regulatory cells	Activated T and B cells, regulatory T cells
CD28	Receptor for B7 co-stimulation: activation	T cells
CD40	Stimulation of B cell, DC, and macrophage	B cell, macrophage
CD40 L	Ligand for CD40	T cell
CD45RO	Isoform (on memory cells)	T cell, B cell
CD56 (NKH1)	Adhesion molecule	NK cell
CD69	Marker of cell activation	Activated T, B, NK cells and macrophages
CD80 (B7-1)	Co-stimulation of T cells	DC, macrophages, B cell
CD86 (B7-2)	Co-stimulation of T cells	DC, macrophages, B cell
CD95 (Fas)	Apoptosis inducer	Many cells
CD152 (CTLA-4)	Receptor for B7; tolerance	T cell
CD178 (FasL)	Fas ligand: apoptosis inducer	Killer T and NK cells
Adhesion Molecules		
CD11a	LFA-1 (α chain)	
CD29	VLA (β chain)	
VLA-1, VLA-2, VLA-3	α Integrins	T cells
VLA-4	α_4-Integrin homing receptor	T cell, B cell, monocyte
CD50	ICAM-3	Lymphocytes and leukocytes
CD54	ICAM-1	
CD58	LFA-3	

Modified from Male D, Cooke A, Owen M, et al: *Advanced immunology,* ed 3, St Louis, 1996, Mosby.

ADCC, Antibody-dependent cellular cytotoxicity; *APCs,* antigen-presenting cells; *CD,* cluster of differentiation; *CTLA-4,* cytotoxic T-lymphocyte–associated protein-4; *DC,* dendritic cell; *EBV,* Epstein-Barr virus; *ICAM-1, -3,* intercellular adhesion molecule-1, -3; *Ig,* immunoglobulin; *IL,* interleukin; *LFA-1, -3R,* leukocyte function–associated antigen-1, -3R; *LPS,* lipopolysaccharide; *MHC,* major histocompatibility complex; *NK,* natural killer; *TCR,* T-cell antigen receptor; *VLA,* very late activation (antigen).

Langerhans cells in the skin, **dermal interstitial cells, splenic marginal dendritic** cells, and dendritic cells in the **liver, thymus, germinal centers of the lymph nodes,** and **blood. Plasmacytoid dendritic cells** have a plasma cell–like appearance, are present in blood, and produce large amounts of IFN-α and cytokines in response to viral and other infections. Dendritic cells may be derived from stem cells or monocytes. **Immature dendritic cells** capture and phagocytose antigen efficiently and release cytokines to activate and steer the subsequent immune response. Upon maturation, dendritic cells move to lymph node regions rich in T cells to present antigen on class I and class II MHC antigens. *Dendritic cells are the only antigen-presenting cells that can initiate an immune response with a naïve T lymphocyte,* and they also determine the type of response (TH1, TH2, TH17, Treg). **Follicular dendritic cells** localize to B-cell regions of lymph nodes and spleen, are not hematopoietic in origin, and do not process antigen but have tendrils (dendrites) and a "sticky" surface to concentrate and display antigens to B cells.

Lymphocytes

The lymphocytes are 6 to 10 μm in diameter, which is smaller than leukocytes. There are three classes of lymphocytes: **T**

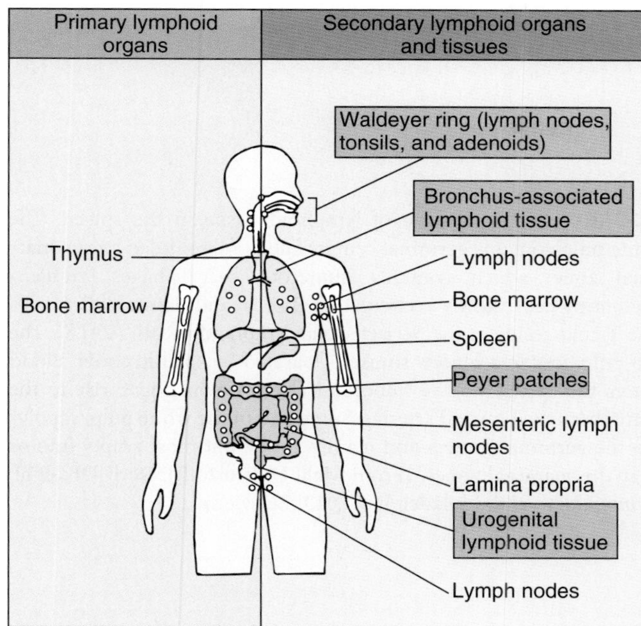

FIGURE 7-2 Organs of the immune system. Thymus and bone marrow are primary lymphoid organs. They are sites of maturation for T and B cells, respectively. Cellular and humoral immune responses develop in the secondary (peripheral) lymphoid organs and tissues; effector and memory cells are generated in these organs. The spleen responds predominantly to blood-borne antigens. Lymph nodes mount immune responses to antigens in intercellular fluid and in the lymph, absorbed either through the skin (superficial nodes) or from internal viscera (deep nodes). Tonsils, Peyer patches, and other mucosa-associated lymphoid tissues *(blue boxes)* respond to antigens that have penetrated the surface mucosal barriers. (From Male D, Brostoff J, Roth DB, et al: *Immunology,* ed 8, Philadelphia, 2013, Elsevier.)

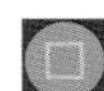
Box 7-3 Immune Organs

Thymus

Required at birth for T-cell development

Site of T-cell maturation and development of central tolerance

Bone Marrow

Source of stem cells

B-cell maturation and development of central tolerance

Lymph Node

Follicle: B-cell zone

Germinal center: site of B-cell proliferation, plasma and memory cell development

Paracortex: T-cell zone

Spleen

White pulp

Follicles: B-cell zone

Periarteriolar lymphoid sheath (PALS); T-cell zone

Red pulp

Macrophage-rich region for filtering blood, removal of damaged cells and microbes

Mucosa-Associated Lymphoid Tissue

Skin

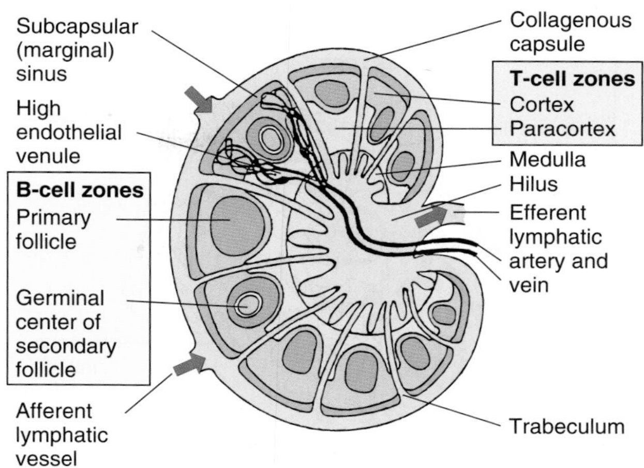

FIGURE 7-3 Organization of the lymph node. Beneath the collagenous capsule is the subcapsular sinus, which is lined with phagocytic cells. Lymphocytes and antigens from surrounding tissue spaces or adjacent nodes pass into the sinus via the afferent lymphatic system. The cortex contains B cells grouped in primary follicles and stimulated B cells in secondary follicles (germinal centers). The paracortex contains mainly T cells and dendritic cells (antigen-presenting cells). Each lymph node has its own arterial and venous supplies. Lymphocytes enter the node from the circulation through the specialized high endothelial venules in the paracortex. The medulla contains both T and B cells, as well as most of the lymph node plasma cells organized into cords of lymphoid tissue. Lymphocytes can leave the node only through the efferent lymphatic vessel. (From Male D, Brostoff J, Roth DB, et al: *Immunology,* ed 8, Philadelphia, 2013, Elsevier.)

cells, B cells, and innate lymphoid cells. These cells have a large nucleus and smaller, agranular cytoplasm. Although B and T cells are indistinguishable by their morphologic features, they can be distinguished on the basis of function and surface markers (Table 7-5). Lymphoid cells that are not B or T cells are termed **innate lymphoid cells (ILCs)** and include the **NK cells.**

T cells acquired their name because they develop in the *t*hymus. T cells have the following two major functions in response to foreign antigen:

1. Regulate, suppress (when necessary), and activate immune and inflammatory responses by cell-to-cell interactions and by releasing cytokines
2. Directly kill virally infected cells, foreign cells (e.g., tissue grafts), and tumors by promoting apoptosis

T cells make up 60% to 80% of peripheral blood lymphocytes. T cells were initially distinguished from B cells on the basis of their ability to bind and surround themselves (forming rosettes) with sheep erythrocytes through the CD2 molecule. All T cells express an antigen-binding **T-cell receptor (TCR),** which resembles but differs from antibody, and **CD2**- and **CD3-associated** proteins on their cell surface (Figure 7-7). T cells are divided into three major groups on the basis of the type of TCR and also by the cell surface expression of two proteins, CD4 and CD8. Most lymphocytes express the α/β **TCR. CD4-expressing T cells** are primarily cytokine-producing cells that help initiate, direct, and regulate innate and immune responses. The CD4 T cells can

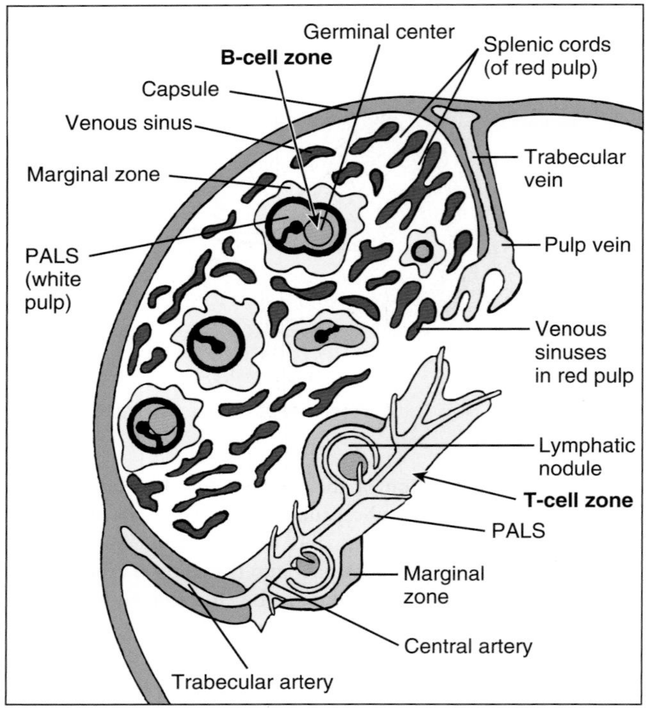

FIGURE 7-4 Organization of lymphoid tissue in the spleen. The white pulp contains germinal centers and is surrounded by the marginal zone, which contains numerous macrophages, antigen-presenting cells, slowly recirculating B cells, and natural killer cells. The T cells reside in the periarteriolar lymphoid sheath *(PALS)*. The red pulp contains venous sinuses separated by splenic cords. Blood enters the tissues via the trabecular arteries, which give rise to the many-branched central arteries. Some end in the white pulp, supplying the germinal centers and mantle zones, but most empty into or near the marginal zones. (From Male D, Brostoff J, Roth DB, et al: *Immunology,* ed 8, Philadelphia, 2013, Elsevier.)

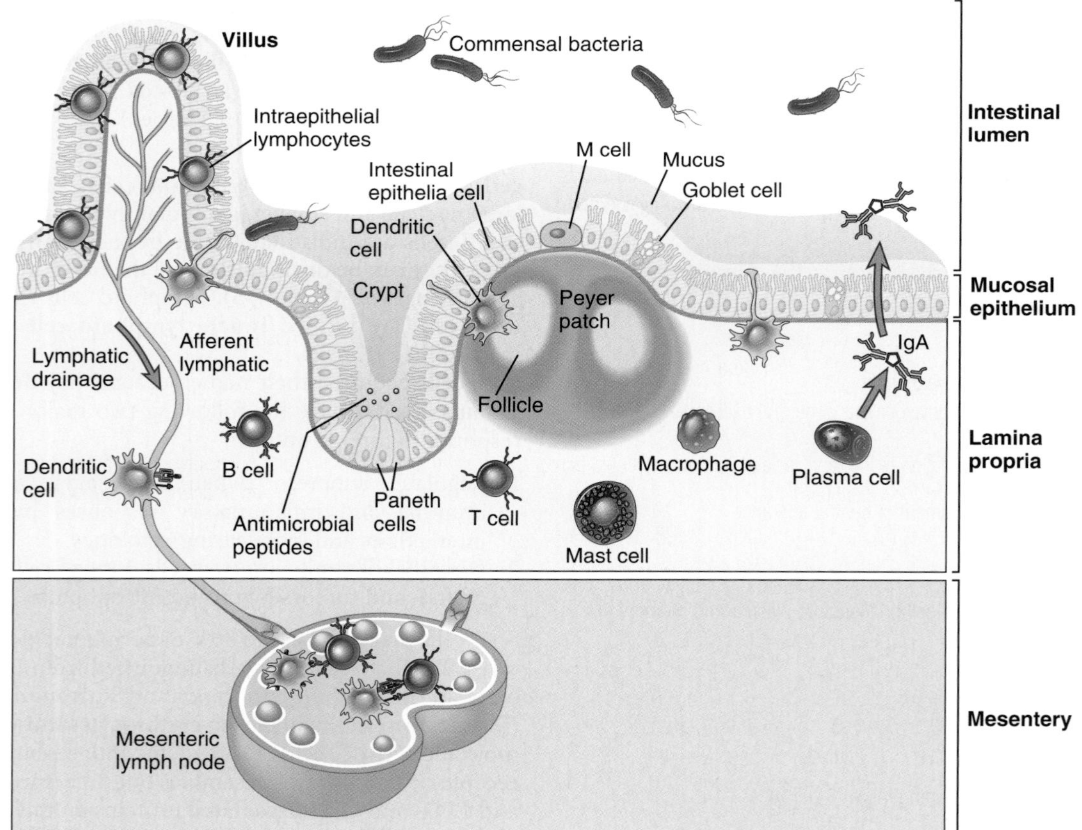

FIGURE 7-5 Lymphoid cells stimulated with antigen in Peyer patches (or lungs or another mucosal site) migrate via the regional lymph nodes and thoracic duct into the bloodstream and then to the lamina propria of the gut and probably other mucosal surfaces. Thus lymphocytes stimulated at one mucosal surface may become distributed throughout the MALT (mucosa-associated lymphoid tissue) system. *IgA,* Immunoglobulin A. (Modified from Abbas AK, Lichtman AH, Pillai S, et al: *Cellular and molecular immunology,* ed 8, Philadelphia, 2015, Elsevier.)

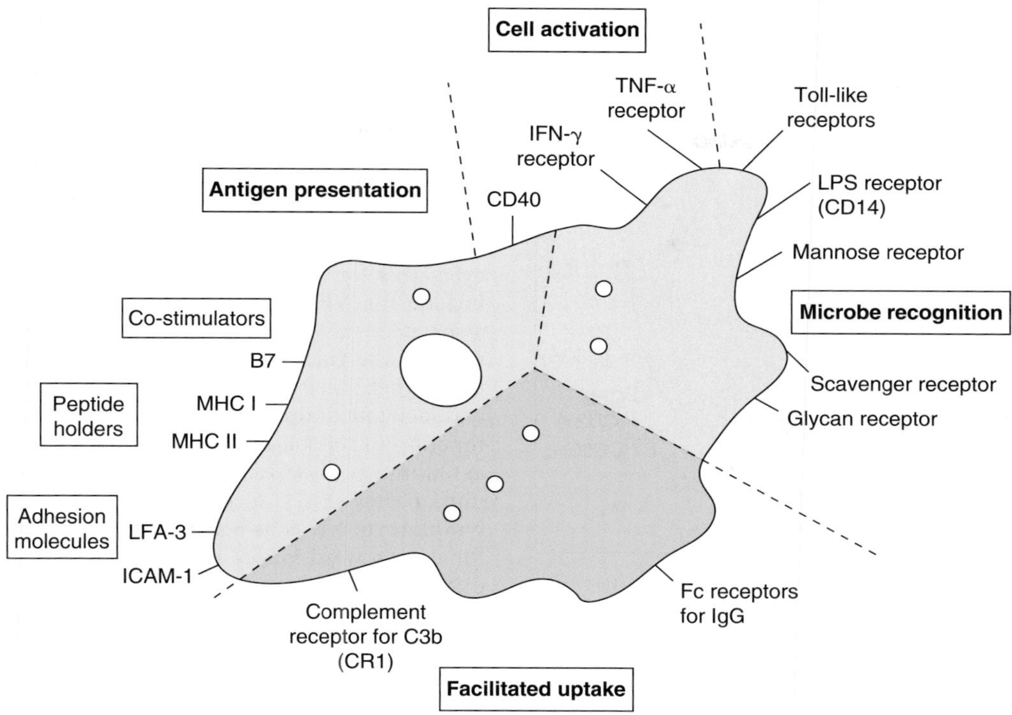

FIGURE 7-6 Macrophage surface structures mediate cell function. Receptors for bacterial components, antibody, and complement (for opsonization) promote activation and phagocytosis of antigen; other receptors promote antigen presentation and activation of T cells. The dendritic cell shares many of these characteristics. *ICAM-1,* Intercellular adhesion molecule-1; *IFN-γ,* interferon-γ; *Ig,* immunoglobulin; *LFA-3,* leukocyte function–associated antigen-3; *LPS,* lipopolysaccharide; *MHC,* major histocompatibility antigen I or II; *TNF-α,* tumor necrosis factor-α.

Table 7-5 Comparison of B and T Cells

Property	T Cells	B Cells
Origin	Bone marrow	Bone marrow
Maturation	Thymus	Bursal equivalent: bone marrow, Peyer patches
Functions	CD4: helper class II MHC-restricted **cytokine production** for initiation and promotion of immune response CD8: CTL class I MHC-restricted **cytolysis** NKT and γ/δ T: rapid response to infection Treg: control and suppress T-cell and other responses	**Antibody production** Antigen presentation to T cells
Protective response	Resolution of intracellular and fungal infections, enhance and control innate and immune responses	Antibody protects against rechallenge; blocks spread of agent in blood, opsonize, etc.
Products*	Cytokines, IFN-γ, growth factors, cytolytic substances (perforin, granzymes)	IgM, IgD, IgG, IgA, or IgE
Distinguishing surface markers	CD2 (sheep red blood cell receptor), TCR, CD3	Surface antibody, complement receptors, class II MHC antigens
Subsets	CD4 TH0: helper precursor CD4 TH1: activates B-, T-, and NK-cell growth; activates macrophages, CTLs, DTH responses, and IgG production CD4 TH2: activates B- and T-cell growth; promotes IgG, IgE, and IgA production CD4 TH17: inflammation CD4 CD25 Treg: suppression CD8: cytotoxic T cells (CTL) NKT, γ/δ T: rapid response to infection Memory cells: long-lived, anamnestic response	B cells (IgM, IgD): antibody, antigen presentation B cells (IgG or IgE or IgA): antibody, antigen presentation Plasma cell: terminally differentiated antibody factories Memory cells: long-lived, anamnestic response

CD, Cluster of differentiation; *CTL,* cytotoxic lymphocyte; *DTH,* delayed-type hypersensitivity; *IFN,* interferon; *Ig,* immunoglobulin; *MHC,* major histocompatibility complex; *NKT,* natural killer T (cell); *TCR,* T-cell receptor; *TH,* T helper (cell).

*Depending on subset.

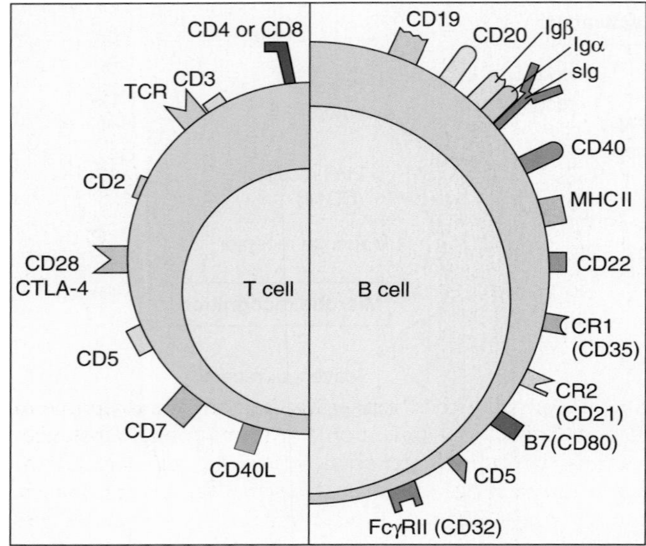

FIGURE 7-7 Surface markers of human B and T cells.

be further divided into TH0, TH1, TH2, TH17, Treg, and other subgroups according to the spectrum of cytokines they secrete and the type of immune response they promote. TH1 cells promote local antibody and cellular inflammatory responses, whereas TH2 cells promote antibody production. TH17 cells activate epithelial cell and neutrophil-driven inflammation and other responses, and Treg cells regulate the immune response to maintain balance and tolerance of self. The **CD8 T cells** also release cytokines but are better known for their ability to recognize and kill (through apoptosis) virally infected cells, foreign tissue transplants (nonself-grafts), and tumor cells as cytotoxic T cells. T cells also produce **memory cells** that express CD45RO. A variable number of T cells express the **γ/δ TCR** but do not express CD4 or CD8. These cells generally reside in skin and mucosa and are important for innate immunity. **NKT** cells are T cells that share characteristics with NK cells.

The primary function of **B cells** is to **make antibody,** but they also internalize antigen, process the antigen, and present the antigen to T cells to request T cell help and expand the immune response. B cells can be identified by the presence of immunoglobulins, class II MHC molecules, and receptors for the C3b and C3d products of the complement cascade (CR1, CR2) on their cell surfaces (see Figure 7-7). The B-cell name is derived from its site of differentiation, the ***b***ursa of Fabricius in birds and the ***b***one marrow of mammals. Activated B cells either apoptose, develop into **memory cells,** which express the CD45RO cell surface marker and circulate until activated by specific antigen, or terminally differentiate into plasma cells. **Plasma cells** have small nuclei and a large cytoplasm for their job as producers of antibody.

Innate lymphoid cells (ILCs) are non-B, non-T lymphocytes that resemble T cells in some characteristics and include the **NK cells.** Cytokine-producing ILCs are found associated with epithelial cells in the thymus and in the intestines. In the gut, these cells produce cytokines that regulate the epithelial cell and T-cell response to the intestinal flora and facilitate antiparasitic worm protection. Errors in their function are associated with immunopathology, including autoimmune diseases. ILCs are also involved in regulating immune responses during pregnancy. The **large, granular lymphocyte NK cells** resemble the CD8 T cells in cytolytic function toward virally infected and tumor cells, but they differ in the mechanism for identifying the target cell. NK cells are also capable of antibody-dependent killing and hence are also called **antibody-dependent cellular cytotoxicity (ADCC or K) cells.** The cytoplasmic granules contain cytolytic proteins to mediate the killing.

Bibliography

Abbas AK, Lichtman AH, Pillai S, et al: *Cellular and molecular immunology*, ed 7, Philadelphia, 2011, WB Saunders.

DeFranco AL, Locksley RM, Robertson M: *Immunity: the immune response in infectious and inflammatory disease*, Sunderland, Mass, 2007, Sinauer Associates.

Janeway CA, Travers P, Walport M, et al: *Immunobiology: the immune system in health and disease*, ed 6, New York, 2004, Garland Science.

Kindt TJ, Goldsby RA, Osborne BA: *Kuby immunology*, ed 7, New York, 2011, WH Freeman.

Kumar V, Abbas AK, Fausto N: *Robbins and Cotran pathologic basis of disease*, ed 7, Philadelphia, 2005, Elsevier.

Rosenthal KS: Are microbial symptoms "self-inflicted"? The consequences of immunopathology, *Infect Dis Clin Pract* 13:306–310, 2005.

Rosenthal KS: Vaccines make good immune theater: immunization as described in a three-act play, *Infect Dis Clin Pract* 14:35–45, 2006.

Rosenthal KS, Wilkinson JG: Flow cytometry and immunospeak, *Infect Dis Clin Pract* 15:183–191, 2007.

Sompayrac L: *How the immune system works*, ed 2, Malden, Mass, 2003, Blackwell Scientific.

Spits H, DiSanto JP: The expanding family of innate lymphoid cells: regulators and effectors of immunity and tissue remodeling, *Nat Immunol* 12:21–27, 2011.

Trends Immunol: Issues contain understandable reviews on current topics in immunology.

CHAPTER

▶ Animations for this chapter are available on StudentConsult.com.

8 INNATE HOST RESPONSES

Innate host responses are continuously working to keep the normal flora in their appropriate places and rapidly react to invading and inappropriate microbes and cells. The body protects itself from microbial invasion in ways that are similar to those used to protect a country from invasion. Barriers such as skin, mucosal surfaces, and the acid of the stomach restrict bacteria to the outer surfaces and the lumen of the gastrointestinal tract and prevent invasion by most microbes. The microbes capable of passing these barriers are bombarded with soluble antimicrobial molecules such as defensins, complement components, and lectins. As the infection expands, troops of cells of the innate response, including neutrophils, monocyte-macrophage lineage cells, immature dendritic cells (iDCs), Langerhans cells, dendritic cells (DCs), and natural killer (NK) cells, are called to action with instructions from cytokines and chemokines. Often these innate responses are sufficient to control the infection. Later, more sophisticated antigen-specific responses support, enhance, and control the cell-mediated innate responses (Box 8-1).

Innate protections are activated by direct contact with repetitive structures of the microbial surface or genome termed *pathogen-associated molecular patterns* (PAMPs) and by molecules released upon cell damage termed *damage-associated molecular patterns* (DAMPS). In contrast, the antigen-specific responses sense and are activated by small structures termed *epitopes*.

• Barriers to Infection

The **skin** and **mucous membranes** serve as barriers to most infectious agents (Figure 8-1), with few exceptions (e.g., papillomavirus, dermatophytes ["skin-loving" fungi]). Free fatty acids produced in sebaceous glands and by organisms on the skin surface, lactic acid in perspiration, and the low pH and relatively dry environment of the skin all form unfavorable conditions for the survival of most organisms.

The mucosal epithelium covering the orifices of the body is protected by mucus secretions and cilia. In the upper respiratory tract, large airborne particles get caught in the mucus, which is continuously transported toward the mouth by ciliated epithelial cells. Small particles (0.05 to 3 μm, the size of viruses or bacteria) that reach the alveoli are phagocytosed by macrophages and transported out of the airspaces. Some bacteria and viruses (e.g., *Bordetella pertussis*, influenza virus), cigarette smoke, or other pollutants can interfere with this clearance mechanism by damaging the ciliated epithelial cells, rendering the patient susceptible to secondary bacterial pneumonia. Antimicrobial substances (cationic peptides **[defensins]**, lysozyme, and lactoferrin) found in secretions at mucosal surfaces (e.g., tears, mucus, and saliva) also provide protection. Lysozyme induces lysis of bacteria by cleaving the polysaccharide backbone of the peptidoglycan of gram-positive bacteria. Lactoferrin, an iron-binding protein, deprives microbes of the free iron they need for growth (Table 8-1).

The **acidic environment** of the stomach, bladder, and kidneys and the **bile** of the intestines inactivate many viruses and bacteria. **Urinary flow** also limits the establishment of infection.

Body temperature, especially **fever,** limits or prevents the growth of many microbes, especially viruses. In addition, the immune response is more efficient at elevated temperatures.

• Soluble Components of Innate Responses

Antimicrobial Peptides and Chelators

Defensins and cathelicidins are peptides produced by neutrophils, epithelial cells, and other cells that are toxic to many microbes. **Defensins** are small (≈30 amino acids) cationic peptides that can disrupt membranes, kill bacteria and fungi, and inactivate viruses. When secreted by Paneth cells in the bowel, they limit and regulate the bacteria living in the lumen. Production of defensins may be constitutive or stimulated by microbial products or cytokines, including interleukin (IL)-17. Cathelicidins are cleaved to produce microbicidal peptides.

Metal ion–binding proteins that bind iron (e.g., lactoferrin, transferrin, ferritin, siderocalin) or bind zinc (e.g., calprotectin) sequester these essential ions to prevent growth of bacteria and yeast. Unfortunately, many pathogens have developed alternate means for acquiring these ions.

Complement

The complement system is an alarm and a weapon against infection, and is especially important against bacterial infections. The complement system is activated directly by bacteria and bacterial products **(alternate or properdin pathway),** by lectin binding to sugars on the bacterial or fungal cell surface **(mannose-binding protein),** or by complexes of antibody and antigen **(classical pathway)** (Figure 8-2; Animation 8-1). The three activation pathways of complement

Box 8-1 Innate Host Responses

Constitutive
Barriers: skin, stomach acid, bile, mucus
Body temperature
Antimicrobial peptides: defensins, cathelicidins
Enzymes: lysozyme
Lactoferrin, transferrin, hepcidin
Complement
Epithelial cell responses

Recruitment
Complement C3a, C5a
Chemokines from epithelium and macrophages

Pathogen-Responsive Cells
Neutrophils
Macrophages
Langerhans/dendritic cells
γ/δ T cells
NK, NKT cells

Acute-Phase/Inflammatory Cytokines
IL-1: fever, diapedesis, inflammation
Tumor necrosis factor-α: fever, diapedesis, inflammation, vascular permeability, tissue remodeling, metabolism, maintenance of macrophage activation, cachexia
IL-6: acute-phase protein synthesis by liver, lymphocyte activation

Other Cytokines and Activators
IL-12: promotes TH1 response and activates NK cells
IL-23: promotes TH17 response from memory cells
Type 1 interferons: antiviral effect, fever, promotes CD8 T-cell response
Interferon-γ (from NK, NKT cells): activation of macrophages and dendritic cells
Lipid mediators (prostaglandins and leukotrienes)

Acute-Phase Proteins from the Liver
C-reactive protein, mannose-binding protein, fibrinogen, complement

IL, Interleukin; *NK,* natural killer.

coalesce at a common junction point, the activation of the C3 component. Activation by either pathway initiates a cascade of proteolytic events that cleave the proteins into **"a"**, **"b"** and other subunits. *The **a** subunits (C3a, C5a) attract (chemotactic factors) phagocytic and inflammatory cells to the site, allow access to soluble molecules and cells by increasing vascular permeability (anaphylactic C3a, C4a, C5a), and activate responses. The **b** subunits are bigger and bind to the agent to promote their phagocytosis **(opsonization)** and elimination, and build a molecular drill that can directly kill the infecting agent.*

Alternate Pathway

The alternate pathway can be activated before the establishment of an immune response to the infecting bacteria because it does not depend on antibody and does not involve the early complement components (C1, C2, and C4). The C3 is spontaneously cleaved in serum and can covalently bind to bacterial surfaces. *Properdin factor B* binds to the C3b and *properdin factor D* splits *factor B* in the complex to yield the *Bb active fragment* that remains linked to *C3b (activation unit)*. The complement cascade then continues in a manner analogous to the classical pathway.

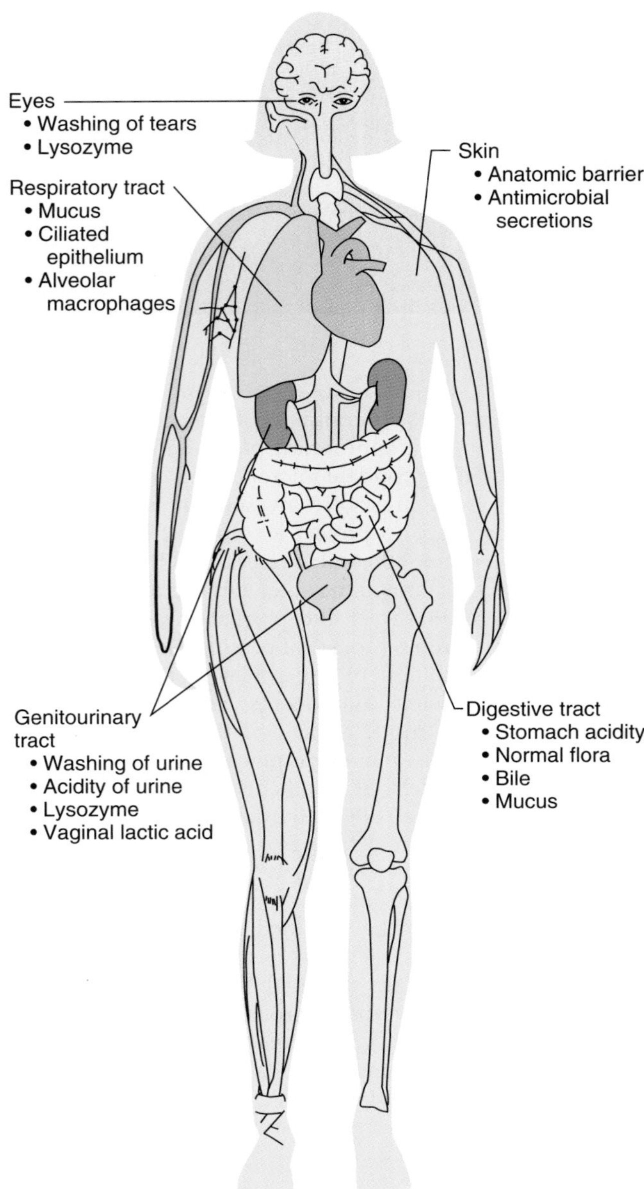

FIGURE 8-1 Barrier defenses of the human body.

Lectin Pathway

The lectin pathway is a bacterial and fungal defense mechanism independent of antibody. **Mannose-binding protein** is a large serum protein that binds to nonreduced mannose, fucose, and glucosamine on bacterial, fungal, and other cell surfaces. Mannose-binding protein resembles and replaces the C1q component of the classical pathways and, on binding to bacterial surfaces, activates the cleavage of the mannose binding protein–associated serine protease. Mannose binding protein–associated serine protease cleaves the C4 and C2 components to produce the C3 convertase, the junction point of the complement cascade.

Classical Pathway

The classical complement cascade is initiated by the binding of the first component, C1, to the Fc portion of antibody

Table 8-1 Soluble Innate Defense Mediators

Factor	Function	Source
Lysozyme	Catalyzes hydrolysis of bacterial peptidoglycan	Tears, saliva, nasal secretions, body fluids, lysosomal granules
Lactoferrin, transferrin	Bind iron and compete with microorganisms for it	Specific granules of PMNs
Lactoperoxidase	May be inhibitory to many microorganisms	Milk and saliva
β-Lysin	Is effective mainly against gram-positive bacteria	Thrombocytes, normal serum
Chemotactic factors	Induce directed migration of PMNs, monocytes, and other cells	Complement and chemokines
Properdin	Promotes complement activation in the absence of antibody-antigen complex	Normal plasma
Lectins	Bind to carbohydrates to promote microbial phagocytosis	Normal plasma
Cationic peptides	Disrupt membranes, block cell transport activities	Polymorphonuclear granules, epithelial cells, etc. (defensins, etc.)

PMNs, Polymorphonuclear neutrophils (leukocytes).

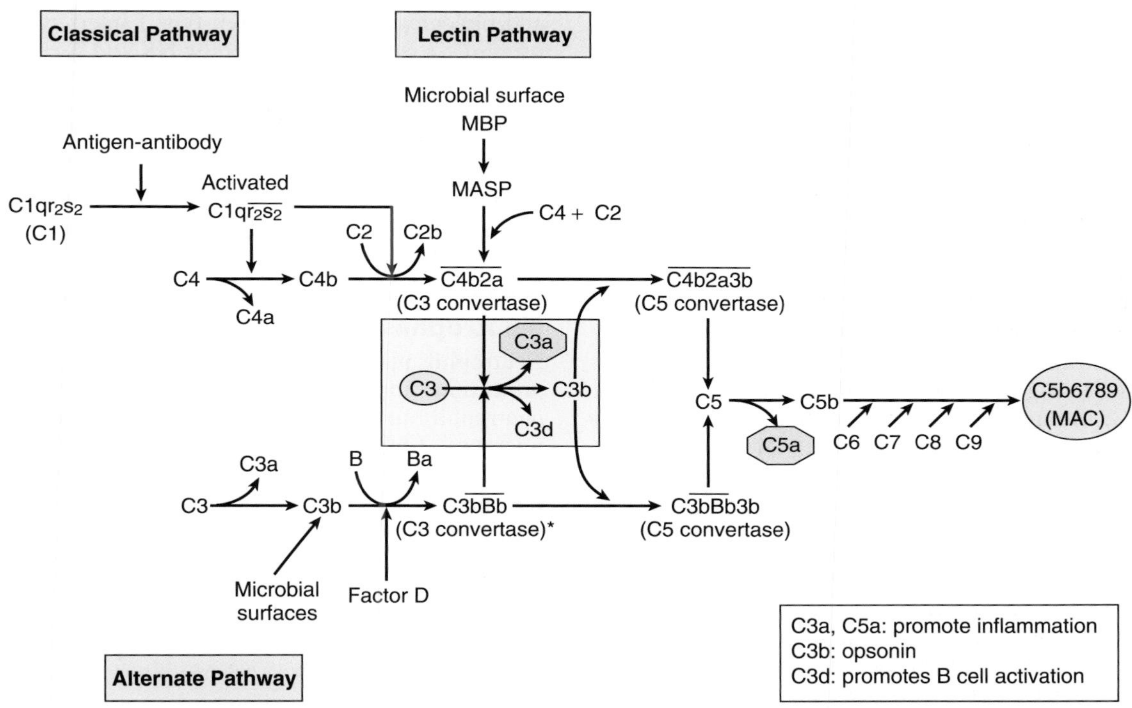

FIGURE 8-2 The classical, lectin, and alternate complement pathways. Despite different activators, all three pathways converge toward the cleavage of C3 and C5 to provide chemoattractants and anaphylotoxins *(C3a, C5a),* an opsonin *(C3b)* that adheres to membranes, and a B-cell activator *(C3d)* and to initiate the membrane attack complex *(MAC)* to kill cells. C9 resembles perforin (natural killer cells and cytotoxic T cells) to promote apoptosis in the target cell. *MASP,* MBP-associated serine protease; *MBP,* mannose-binding protein. (Redrawn from Rosenthal KS, Tan M: *Rapid review microbiology and immunology,* ed 3, St Louis, 2010, Mosby.)

(immunoglobulin [Ig]G or IgM, not IgA or IgE) that is bound to cell surface antigens or to an immune complex with soluble antigens. C1 consists of a complex of three separate proteins designated C1q, C1r, and C1s (see Figure 8-2). C1q binds to the Fc protein, leading to activation of the proteolytic activities of C1r and C1s. C1s then cleaves C4 to C4a and C4b, and C2 to C2a and C2b. The union of C4b and C2a produces **C4b2a,** which is known as **C3 convertase.** This complex binds to the cell membrane and cleaves C3 into C3a and C3b fragments. The C3b protein has a unique thioester bond that will covalently attach C3b to a cell surface or be hydrolyzed. The C3 convertase amplifies the response by splitting many C3 molecules. The interaction of C3b with C4b2a bound to the cell membrane produces **C4b3b2a,**

which is termed **C5 convertase.** This activation unit splits C5 into C5a and C5b fragments and represents yet another amplification step.

Biological Activities of Complement Components

The products of cleavage of the C3 and C5 components are essential for antibacterial responses, enhance clearance of the infectious agent, and promote inflammation. Complement fragments **C3a, C4a,** and **C5a** serve as powerful **anaphylatoxins** that stimulate mast cells to release histamine and tumor necrosis factor (TNF)-α, which enhances vascular permeability and smooth muscle contraction. **C3a** and **C5a** also act as attractants **(chemotactic factors)** for neutrophils and macrophages, facilitating their exit from the capillary near the infection. These proteins are powerful promoters of inflammatory reactions. C3b is an opsonin that promotes clearance of microbes by binding directly to the cell to make the cell more recognizable to phagocytic cells, such as neutrophils and macrophages, which have receptors for C3b. C3b can be cleaved further to generate C3d, which is an activator of B lymphocytes. For gram-positive and most other bacterial infections, these responses provide the major antimicrobial function of the complement system.

The complement system also interacts with the clotting cascade. Activated coagulation factors can cleave C5a, and a protease of the lectin pathway can cleave prothrombin to result in production of fibrin and activation of the clotting cascade.

Membrane Attack Complex

The terminal stage of the classical pathway involves creation of the **membrane attack complex (MAC),** also called the **lytic unit** (see Figure 8-2).The five terminal complement proteins (C5 through C9) assemble into a MAC on target cell membranes to mediate injury. Initiation of the MAC assembly begins with C5 cleavage into C5a and C5b fragments. A $(C5b,6,7,8)_1(C9)_n$ complex forms and drills a hole in the membrane, leading to apoptosis or the hypotonic lysis of cells. *Neisseria* bacteria are very sensitive to this manner of killing, whereas gram-positive bacteria are relatively insensitive. The peptidoglycan of gram-positive bacteria limits access of the complement components to the plasma membrane target unless disrupted by lysozyme. Unlike other gram-negative bacteria, the outer membrane of *Neisseria* bacteria contains lipooligosaccharide, which lacks O-antigenic side chains, and like stubble, it allows access of complement to the membrane surface. The C9 component is similar to perforin, which is produced by cytolytic T cells and NK cells.

Regulation of Complement Activation

Humans have several mechanisms for preventing generation of the C3 convertase to protect against inappropriate complement activation. These include C1 inhibitor, C4 binding protein, factor H, factor I, and the cell surface proteins decay-accelerating factor (DAF) and membrane cofactor protein. In addition, CD59 (protectin) prevents formation of the MAC. Most infectious agents lack these protective mechanisms and remain susceptible to complement. A genetic deficiency in these protection systems can result in disease.

Interferons

Interferons are small, cytokine-like proteins that can interfere with virus replication but also have systemic effects (described in more detail in Chapter 10). The type I interferons include α and β but not γ, which is a type II interferon. The type I interferons are primarily a very early antiviral response triggered by the double-stranded RNA intermediates of virus replication and other structures that bind to Toll-like receptors (TLRs), RIG-1 (retinoic acid–inducible gene 1), and other PAMP receptors (PAMPRs). Plasmacytoid DCs produce large amounts of IFN-α in response to viral infection, especially during viremia, but other cells can also make IFN-α. IFN-β is made primarily by fibroblasts. The type I interferons promote transcription of antiviral proteins in cells that become activated by viral infection. They also activate systemic responses, including fever, and enhance T-cell activation. Type I interferons will be discussed further with respect to the response to viral infections.

IFN-γ is a type II interferon and differs in biochemical and biological properties from type I interferons. IFN-γ is primarily a cytokine produced by NK and T cells as part of TH1 immune responses and activates macrophages and myeloid cells. IFN-γ will be discussed further with respect to T-cell responses.

• Cellular Components of Innate Responses

Neutrophils

Neutrophils play a major role in antibacterial and antifungal protections and a lesser role for antiviral protections. The neutrophil surface is decorated with receptors that bind microbes, such as lectins and scavenger receptors, and opsonin receptors for the Fc portion of immunoglobulin or C3b, bound to the microbial surface. These receptors promote phagocytosis of the microbe and their subsequent killing, as described later. Neutrophils have many granules that contain antimicrobial proteins and substances. These cells are terminally differentiated, spend less than 3 days in the blood, rapidly die in tissue, and **become pus** at the site of infection.

Mast Cells, Basophils, Eosinophils

Mast cells, basophils, and eosinophils have cytoplasmic granules containing antimicrobial substances and mediators of inflammation. Mast cells are present in skin, mucoepithelial tissue, and the lining of small blood vessels and nerves. Basophils are like mast cells but circulate in the blood, and their granules stain with basic dyes. Mast cells and basophils bind IgE, complement, and microbial products and release histamine and cytokines as part of allergic and inflammatory responses. Eosinophils circulate in the blood, their granules stain with acidic dyes (e.g., eosin), and they are important in antiparasitic responses.

Cells of the Monocyte-Macrophage Lineage

Macrophages may originate from bone marrow–derived monocytes or from embryonic yolk sac. The latter reside in tissue, such as the Kupffer cells in the liver. Like neutrophils,

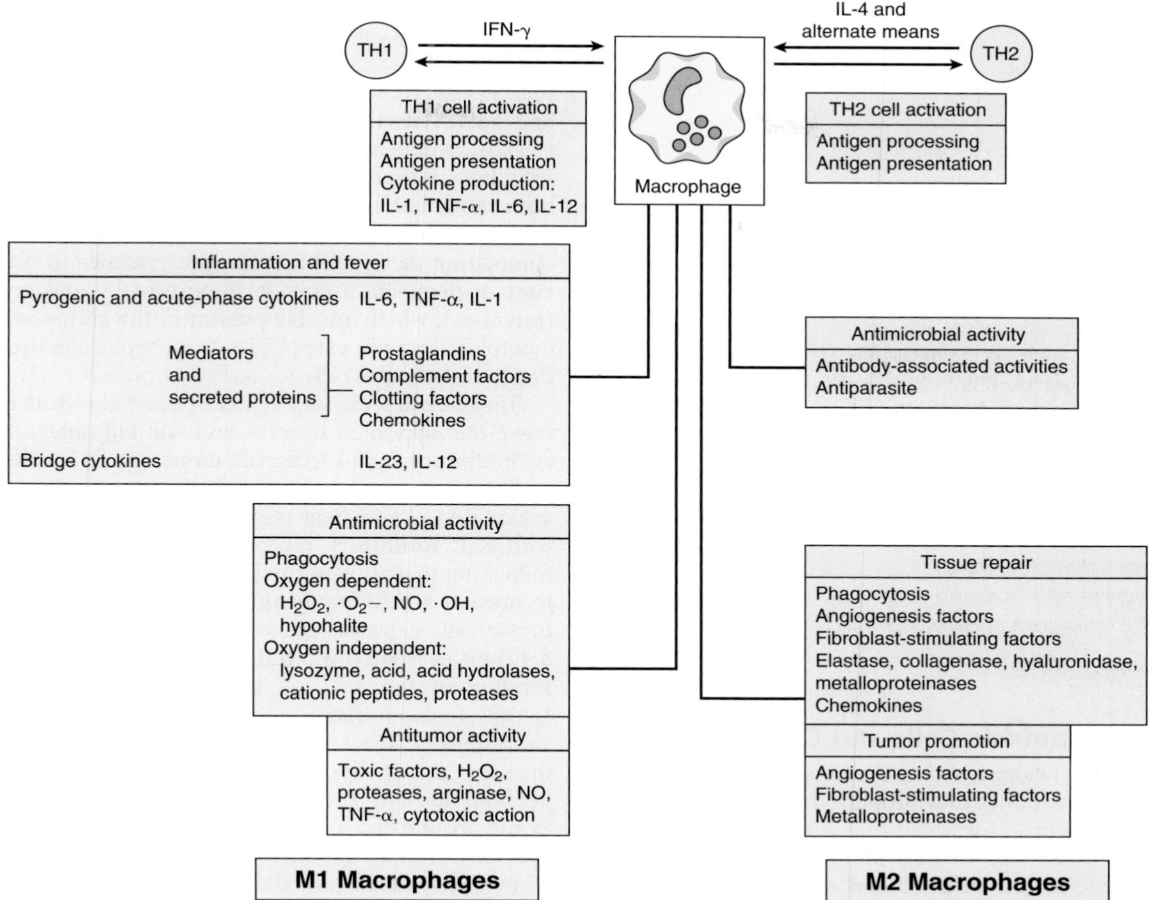

FIGURE 8-3 The many functions of macrophages and members of the macrophage family. M2 macrophages maintain the status quo and facilitate wound healing by removal of debris and promoting angiogenesis and tissue repair. M1 macrophages promote antimicrobial killing and inflammation. *H_2O_2,* Hydrogen peroxide; *IFN-γ,* interferon-γ; *IL,* interleukin; *NO,* nitric oxide; *O^-,* oxygen radical; *OH,* hydroxyl radical; *TH,* T helper (cell); *TNF-α,* tumor necrosis factor-α.

macrophages are phagocytes, but unlike neutrophils, they are long lived, can divide, present antigenic peptides to CD4 T cells on MHC II molecules, and must be activated to efficiently kill the phagocytosed bacteria.

The primary role of tissue macrophages is to remove debris and promote tissue repair and remodeling **(M2 macrophages).** Sometimes called alternatively activated macrophages, these cells can be further activated by the TH2-related cytokines, IL-4 and IL-13, to support antiparasitic responses. M2 macrophages are also present in tumors and reinforce the growth of tumor cells and promote angiogenesis (Figure 8-3).

In order to promote inflammatory responses and be able to kill phagocytosed bacteria, macrophages are activated by IFN-γ (classical activation) produced by NK cells and CD4 and CD8 T cells as part of the TH1 response **(M1 macrophages).** Activated M1 macrophages produce enzymes and other molecules to promote antimicrobial function (Box 8-2) and reinforce local inflammatory reactions by producing chemokines to attract neutrophils, iDCs, NK cells, and activated T cells and acute-phase cytokines (IL-1, TNF-α, IL-6) to promote the response. Macrophages get help by presenting antigen to T cells, which produce IFN-γ as long as the antigen is present. In the case of an unresolved mycobacterial infection, continuous (chronic) stimulation of macrophages by T cells promotes fusion of the macrophages into **multinucleated giant cells** and large macrophages called **epithelioid cells** that surround the infection and form a **granuloma.**

 **Box 8-2 The Many Functions of Macrophages**

Status Quo (Peacetime): M2 Macrophages

Phagocytosis and degradation of debris
Production of enzymes and factors for tissue growth and repair
Production of angiogenesis factors

During Infection and Inflammation (At War): M1 Macrophages (Activated by PAMPs, TNF-α, and IFN-γ)

Phagocytosis and oxygen-dependent and -independent antimicrobials
Acute-phase cytokines: IL-6, TNF-α, and IL-1 (endogenous pyrogens)
Other cytokines: IL-12, GM-CSF, G-CSF, M-CSF, IFN-α
Arachidonic acid metabolites
  Prostaglandin, thromboxane, leukotrienes
Enzymes, complement components, coagulation factors

G-CSF, Granulocyte colony-stimulating factor; *GM-CSF,* granulocyte-macrophage colony-stimulating factor; *IFN-α,* interferon-α; *IL,* interleukin; *M-CSF,* macrophage colony-stimulating factor; *TNF-α,* tumor necrosis factor-α.

 **Box 8-3 Dendritic Cells (DCs)**

Myeloid and Lymphoid
Morphology: octopus-like with tendrils
Activities
- **Immature DCs**
  - In blood and tissue
  - Danger sensors, phagocytosis, cytokine production, antigen processing
- **Mature DCs**
  - Only cell that can initiate a new T-cell response
  - Process antigenic proteins into peptides
  - Increased expression of molecules for antigen presentation
    - MHC I-peptide: CD8 T cells
    - CD1-glycolipids: CD8 T cells
    - MHC II-peptide: CD4 T cells
    - B7-1 and B7-2 co-receptors
  - Produce cytokines to initiate and direct T-helper response

Follicular DCs
In B-cell areas of lymphoid tissues
Express sticky receptors to display antigen to B cells (Fc and CR1, CR2, and CR3 complement receptors, lack MHC II)

MHC, Major histocompatibility complex.

Immature Dendritic Cells and Dendritic Cells

DCs provide the bridge between the innate and the immune responses. The cytokines they produce determine the nature of the T-cell response *(dendritic cells direct the T cells as to what to tell other cells to do).* Monocytes and precursor myeloid DCs circulate in the blood and then differentiate into iDCs in tissue and lymphoid organs. **iDCs** are phagocytic, and upon activation by danger signals, they release an early cytokine-mediated warning and then mature into DCs. These cells express different combinations of danger sensors that can detect tissue trauma (adenosine triphosphate [ATP], adenosine, reactive oxygen species [ROS], heat shock proteins) and infection, including **Toll-like receptors** and other receptors (see later). **Mature DCs** are the ultimate antigen-presenting cells, the only antigen-presenting cells that can initiate an antigen-specific T-cell response (Box 8-3). **Langerhans cells** are a type of iDC that remains in the epidermis of the skin until activated and then becomes a mature DC.

Natural Killer Cells, γ/δ T Cells, and NKT Cells

NK cells are **innate lymphoid cells (ILCs)** that provide an early cellular response to a viral infection, have antitumor activity, and amplify inflammatory reactions after bacterial infection. NK cells are also responsible for **antibody-dependent cellular cytotoxicity (ADCC),** in which they bind and kill antibody-coated cells. NK cells are large granular lymphocytes (LGLs) that share many characteristics with T cells, except the mechanism for target cell recognition. NK cells do not express a T-cell receptor (TCR) or CD3 and cannot make IL-2. They neither recognize a specific antigen nor require presentation of antigen by MHC molecules. The NK system does not involve memory or require sensitization and cannot be enhanced by specific immunization.

NK cells are activated by (1) IFN-α and IFN-β (produced early in response to viral and other infections), (2) TNF-α, (3) IL-12, IL-15, and IL-18 (produced by pre-DCs and activated macrophages), and (4) IL-2 (produced by CD4 TH1 cells). The NK cells express many of the same cell surface markers as T cells (e.g., CD2, CD7, IL-2 receptor [IL-2R], and **FasL [Fas ligand]**) but also the **Fc receptor for IgG (CD16),** complement receptors for ADCC, and NK-specific inhibitory receptors and activating receptors (including NK immunoglobulin-like receptors **[KIR]**). Activated NK cells produce IFN-γ, IL-1, and granulocyte-macrophage colony-stimulating factor (GM-CSF). The granules in an NK cell contain **perforin,** a pore-forming protein, and **granzymes** (esterases), which are also present in the granules of a CD8 cytotoxic T lymphocyte (CTL). These molecules promote the death of the target cell.

The NK cell sees every cell as a potential victim, especially those that appear in distress, and will kill unless it receives an inhibitory signal from the target cell. NK cells bind to carbohydrates and surface proteins on a distressed cell. Interaction of sufficient numbers of class I MHC molecules with KIR **inhibitory receptors** acts as a secret password, indicating that all is normal, to activate an inhibitory signal to prevent NK killing of the target cell. Virus-infected and tumor cells express "stress-related receptors" and are often deficient in MHC I molecules and become NK-cell targets. Binding of the NK cell to antibody-coated target cells (ADCCs) also initiates killing, but this is not controlled by an inhibitory signal. The **killing mechanisms** are similar to those of CD8 cytotoxic T cells. A synapse (pocket) is formed between the NK and target cell, and **perforin and granzymes** are released to disrupt the target cell and induce apoptosis. In addition, the interaction of the **FasL** on the NK cell with **Fas** protein on the target cell can also induce apoptosis.

Other **ILCs** resemble CD4 T cells and produce cytokines to regulate epithelial and lymphocyte responses. ILCs line the inside of the intestinal epithelium and produce cytokines to regulate their production of defensins as well as T-cell responses to the gut microbial flora and facilitate antiparasitic worm protections. Errors in their function are associated with inflammatory bowel diseases.

NKT cells and **γ/δ T cells** reside in tissue and in the blood and differ from other T cells because they have a limited repertoire of T-cell receptors. Unlike other T cells, NKT and γ/δ T cells can sense nonpeptide antigens, including bacterial glycolipids (mycobacteria) and phosphorylated amine metabolites from some bacteria (*Escherichia coli,* mycobacteria) but not others (streptococci, staphylococci). These T cells and NK cells produce IFN-γ, which activates macrophages and DCs to enforce a protective TH1 cycle of cytokines and local cellular inflammatory reactions. NKT cells also express NK-cell receptors.

• Activation of Innate Cellular Responses

The cells of the innate response are activated by cytokines, chemokines, and direct interaction with microbes and microbial components. These cells express different combinations of danger and damage sensors for microbes and cell trauma, including the **TLR** family of proteins, as well as other receptors. The TLRs include at least 10 different cell surface and

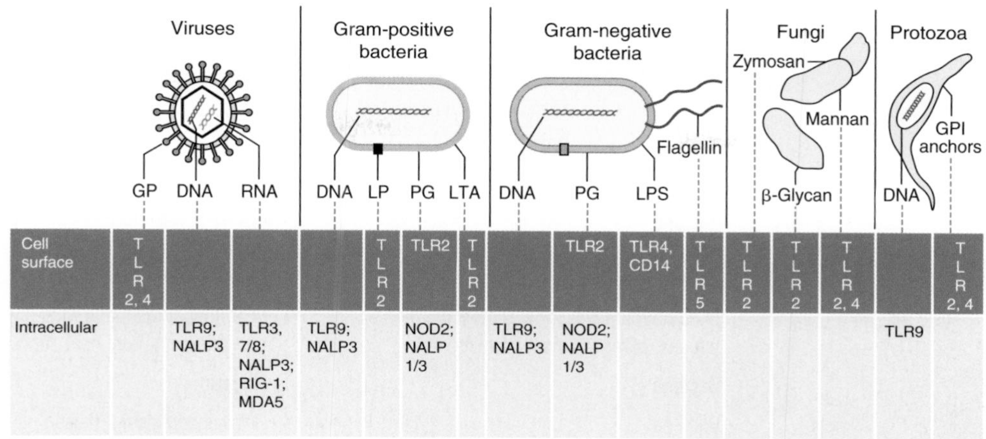

FIGURE 8-4 Recognition of pathogen-associated molecular patterns. Microbial structures, RNA, and DNA bind to specific receptors on the cell surface, in vesicles, or in the cytoplasm to activate innate responses. *FL,* Flagellin; *GP,* glycoproteins; *GPI,* phosphatidylinositol glycan–anchored proteins; *LP,* lipoproteins; *LPS,* lipopolysaccharide; *LTA,* lipoteichoic acid; *MDA5,* melanoma differentiation–associated gene 5; *NALP3,* Nacht, leucine-rich repeat, and pyrin domain–containing protein 1/3; *NOD2,* nucleotide-binding oligomerization domain protein 2; *PG,* peptidoglycan; *RIG-1,* retinoic acid-inducible gene protein-1; *TLR9,* Toll-like receptor 9. (Modified from Mogensen TH: Pathogen recognition and inflammatory signaling in innate immune defenses, *Clin Microbiol Rev* 22:240–273, 2009.)

intracellular proteins that bind repetitive structures that form **pathogen-associated molecular patterns (PAMPs)** (Figure 8-4 and Table 8-2). These patterns are present within the endotoxin component of lipopolysaccharide (LPS) and in lipoteichoic acid, fungal glycans, unmethylated cytosine-guanosine units of DNA (CpG oligodeoxynucleotides [ODNs]) commonly found in bacteria, double-stranded RNA produced during the replication of some viruses, and other molecules. Cytoplasmic sensors of bacterial peptidoglycan include nucleotide-binding oligomerization domain protein 1 (NOD1), NOD2, and cryopyrin and, for nucleic acids, RIG-1, melanoma differentiation–associated gene 5 (MDA5), etc. Binding of PAMPs to TLRs and other PAMPRs activates adaptor proteins that trigger cascades of protein kinases and other responses that result in the activation of the cell and production of specific cytokines. These cytokines can include IL-1 and TNF-α, IL-6, IFN-α and -β, and various chemokines.

In response to PAMPs and other stimuli, epithelial cells, DCs, macrophages, and other cells can assemble an **inflammasome** (Figure 8-5). This multiprotein complex is activated by several of the adaptor proteins induced in response to PAMPRs or tissue damage. Proteases released upon uric acid crystal (gout) or asbestos puncture of phagosomes and lysosomes can also activate inflammasome formation. The inflammasome activates the caspase 1 protease, which then cleaves, activates, and promotes the release of IL-1β and IL-18. These activated cytokines promote local inflammation. The activated inflammasome can also initiate an apoptosis-like cell death for cells bearing intracellular bacterial infections.

Chemotaxis and Leukocyte Migration

Chemotactic factors produced in response to infection and inflammatory responses, such as complement components (C3a, C5a), bacterial products (e.g., formyl-methionyl-leucyl-phenylalanine [f-met-leu-phe]), and chemokines, are powerful chemoattractants for neutrophils, macrophages, and later in the response, lymphocytes. **Chemokines** are small cytokine-like proteins that direct the migration of white blood cells to the site of infection or inflammation or to different tissue locations. Most chemokines are either CC (adjacent cysteines) or CXC (cysteines separated by one amino acid) chemokines and bind to specific G protein–coupled receptors. The chemokines establish a chemically lighted "runway" to guide these cells to the site of an infection and also activate them. Combined with TNF-α, the chemokines cause the endothelial cells lining the capillaries (near the inflammation) and the leukocytes passing by to express complementary adhesion molecules (molecular "Velcro"). The leukocytes slow, roll, attach to the lining, and then extravasate across (i.e., pass through) the capillary wall to the site of inflammation, a process called *diapedesis* (Figure 8-6).

Phagocytic Responses

Polymorphonuclear neutrophils (PMNs) are the first cells to arrive at the site in response to infection; they are followed later by monocytes and macrophages. **Neutrophils** provide the major antibacterial and antifungal response and contribution to inflammation. An increased number of neutrophils in the blood, body fluids (e.g., cerebrospinal fluid), or tissue usually indicates a bacterial infection. The infection recruits the release of immature **band forms** from the bone marrow described as a "left shift," (*left* refers to the beginning of a chart of neutrophil development).

Phagocytosis of bacteria or a fungus by macrophages and neutrophils involves three steps: attachment, internalization, and digestion. **Attachment** is mediated by receptors for cell surface carbohydrates (**lectins** [specific sugar-binding proteins]), fibronectin receptors (especially for *Staphylococcus aureus*), and **receptors for opsonins,** including complement (C3b), mannose-binding protein, and the Fc portion of antibody. After attachment, a section of plasma membrane surrounds the particle to form a **phagocytic vacuole** around the microbe. This vacuole fuses with the **primary lysosomes**

 Table 8-2 **Pathogen Pattern Receptors**

Receptor*	Microbial Activators	Ligand
Cell Surface		
TLR1	Bacteria, mycobacteria *Neisseria meningitidis*	Lipopeptides Soluble factors
TLR2	Bacteria Fungi Cells	LTA, LPS, PG, etc. Zymosan Necrotic cells
TLR4	Bacteria, parasites, host proteins Viruses, parasites, host proteins	**LPS,** fungal mannans, viral glycoproteins, parasitic phospholipids, host heat shock proteins, LDL
TLR5	Bacteria	Flagellin
TLR6	Bacteria Fungi	LTA, lipopeptides, zymosan
Lectins	Bacteria, fungi, viruses	Specific carbohydrates (e.g., mannose)
N-Formyl methionine receptor	Bacteria	Bacterial proteins
Endosome		
TLR3	Viruses	Double-stranded RNA
TLR7	Viruses	Single-stranded RNA Imidazoquinolines
TLR8	Viruses	Single-stranded RNA Imidazoquinolines
TLR9	Bacteria Viruses	Unmethylated DNA (CpG)
Cytoplasm		
NOD1, NOD2, NALP3	Bacteria	Peptidoglycan
Cryopyrin	Bacteria	Peptidoglycan
RIG-1	Viruses	RNA
MDA5	Viruses	RNA
DAI	Viruses, cytoplasmic DNA	DNA

Activators: *DAI,* DNA-dependent activator of interferon regulatory factors; *DNA,* deoxyribonucleic acid; *dsRNA,* double-stranded RNA; *LDL,* minimally modified low-density lipoprotein; *LPS,* lipopolysaccharide; *LTA,* lipoteichoic acid; *MDA5,* melanoma differentiation–associated gene 5; *NALP3,* Nacht, leucine-rich repeat and pyrin domain–containing protein 3; *NOD,* nucleotide-binding oligomerization domain; *PG,* peptidoglycan; *RIG-1,* retinoic acid–inducible gene-1; *TLR,* Toll-like receptor.

*Information about Toll-like receptors from Takeda A, Kaisho T, Akira S: Toll-like receptors, *Annu Rev Immunol* 21:335–376, 2003; and Akira S, Takeda K: Toll-like receptor signalling, *Nat Rev Immunol* 4:499–511, 2003.

(macrophages) or **granules** (PMNs) to allow inactivation and digestion of the vacuole contents.

Phagocytic killing may be oxygen dependent or oxygen independent (Figure 8-7). Neutrophils do not need special activation to kill internalized microbes, but their response is reinforced by IL-17 and TNF-α. Activation of macrophages is promoted by IFN-γ (best) and GM-CSF, which are produced early in the infection by NK and NKT cells or later by CD4 and CD8 T cells, and sustained by TNF-α and lymphotoxin (TNF-β). Activation of macrophages is required for macrophages to efficiently kill internalized microbes.

Oxygen-dependent killing is mediated by reactive oxygen species (ROS), hypochlorous ions, and nitric oxide (Box 8-4). In the neutrophil, but not the macrophage, hydrogen peroxide with **myeloperoxidase** (released by primary granules during fusion to the phagolysosome) transforms chloride ions into hypochlorous ions (chlorine bleach). **Nitric oxide** produced by neutrophils and activated macrophages has antimicrobial activity and is also a major second messenger molecule that enhances the inflammatory and other responses.

The **neutrophil** can also mediate **oxygen-independent killing** upon fusion of the phagosome with azurophilic granules containing cationic proteins (e.g., cathepsin G) and specific granules containing lysozyme and lactoferrin. These proteins kill gram-negative bacteria by disrupting their cell membrane integrity, but they are far less effective against gram-positive bacteria and fungi, which are killed principally through the oxygen-dependent mechanism.

The neutrophils also promote inflammation. Prostaglandins and leukotrienes, which increase vascular permeability, are released, causing swelling (edema) and stimulating pain receptors. In addition, during phagocytosis, the granules may leak their contents to cause tissue damage. The neutrophils have short lives; upon death at the site of infection, they release their DNA and granule contents to form a sticky net

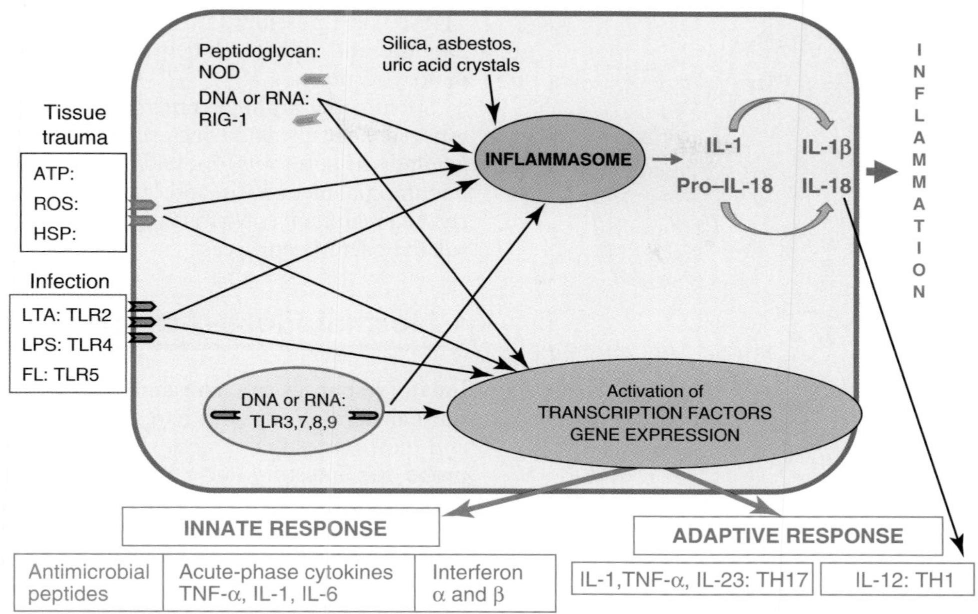

FIGURE 8-5 Induction of inflammatory responses. Receptors for pathogen-associated molecular patterns and damage-associated molecular pattern receptors at the cell surface, in vesicles, and in the cytoplasm (1) activate signal cascades that (2) produce adaptor proteins that (3) activate local inflammatory responses. The adaptor proteins initiate the assembly of the inflammasome and also trigger the transcription of cytokines. Cytokines activate innate and promote antigen-specific responses. In addition, crystalline materials lyse lysosomes, releasing proteases that cleave precursors to initiate assembly and activation of the inflammasome and promote inflammation. *ATP,* Adenosine triphosphate; *FL,* flagellin; *HSP,* heat shock protein; *IL,* interleukin; *LPS,* lipopolysaccharide; *LTA,* lipoteichoic acid; *NOD,* nucleotide-binding oligomerization domain protein; *RIG-1,* retinoic acid-inducible gene protein 1; *ROS,* reactive oxygen species; *TLR,* Toll-like receptor; *TNF-α,* tumor necrosis factor-α.

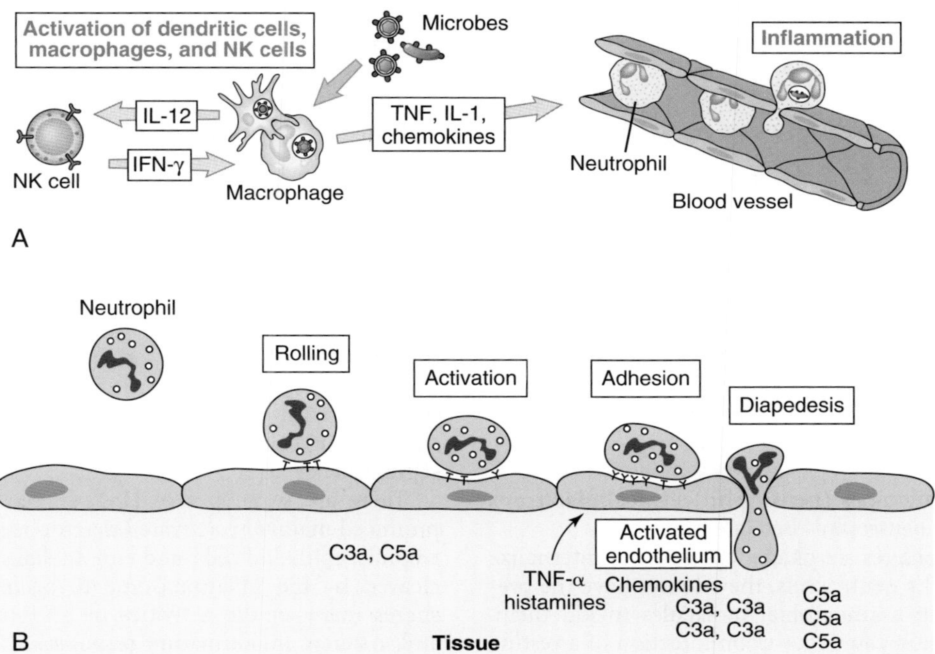

FIGURE 8-6 **A** and **B,** Neutrophil diapedesis in response to inflammatory signals. Tumor necrosis factor *(TNF)*-α and chemokines activate the expression of selectins and intercellular adhesion molecules on the endothelium near the inflammation and their ligands on the neutrophil: integrins, L-selectin, and leukocyte function–associated antigen-1 (LFA-1). The neutrophil binds progressively tighter to the endothelium until it finds its way through the endothelium. Epithelial cells, Langerhans cells, and macrophages activated by microbes and interferon *(IFN)*-γ make TNF-α and other cytokines and chemokines to enhance diapedesis. *IL,* Interleukin; *NK,* natural killer. (**A,** From Abbas AK, Lichtman AH: *Basic immunology: functions and disorders of the immune system,* ed 4, Philadelphia, 2012, WB Saunders.)

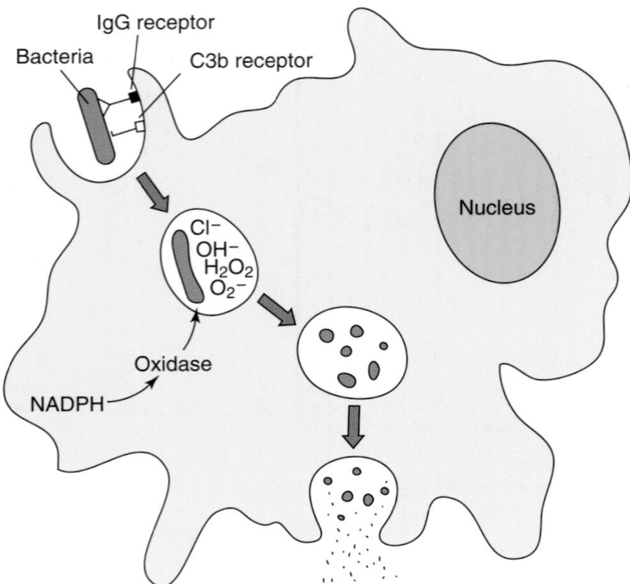

FIGURE 8-7 Phagocytosis and killing of bacteria. Bacteria are bound directly or are opsonized by mannose-binding protein, immunoglobulin *(Ig)*G, and/or C3b receptors, promoting their adherence and uptake by phagocytes. Within the phagosome, oxygen-dependent and oxygen-independent mechanisms kill and degrade the bacteria. *NADPH,* Nicotinamide adenine dinucleotide phosphate reduced.

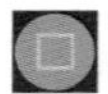 **Box 8-4 Antibacterial Compounds of the Phagolysosome**

Oxygen-Dependent Compounds
Hydrogen peroxide: NADPH oxidase and NADH oxidase
Superoxide
Hydroxyl radicals (·OH⁻)
Activated halides (Cl⁻, I⁻, Br⁻): myeloperoxidase (neutrophil)
Nitrous oxide

Oxygen-Independent Compounds
Acids
Lysosome (degrades bacterial peptidoglycan)
Lactoferrin (chelates iron)
Defensins and other cationic proteins (damage membranes)

Proteases: Elastase, Cathepsin G

NADH, Nicotinamide adenine dinucleotide reduced; *NADPH,* nicotinamide adenine dinucleotide phosphate reduced.

to catch and kill microbes **(neutrophil extracellular traps [NETs])** and dead neutrophils become **pus.**

Resting **macrophages** are phagocytic and will internalize microbes, but unlike neutrophils, they do not have the preformed granules of antimicrobial molecules to kill them. Intracellular infection can occur upon infection of a resting macrophage or if the microbe can counteract the antimicrobial activities of an activated macrophage. **Activation of the macrophage by IFN-γ,** making the macrophages "angry," promotes production of inducible nitric oxide synthase (iNOS) and nitric oxide, other ROS, and antimicrobial enzymes to kill internalized microbes. Activated macrophages also make acute-phase cytokines (IL-1, IL-6, and TNF-α) and possibly IL-23 or IL-12. Macrophages have a long life, and with T-cell help they can maintain the inflammatory response.

Splenic macrophages are important for clearing bacteria, especially encapsulated bacteria, from blood. Asplenic (congenitally or surgically) individuals are highly susceptible to pneumonia, meningitis, and other manifestations of *Streptococcus pneumoniae, Neisseria meningitidis,* and other encapsulated bacteria and yeast.

• Normal Flora–Associated Responses

Innate responses are constantly being stimulated by the normal flora of the skin, nares, oral region, and urogenital and gastrointestinal tracts. Dendritic cells continuously probe the intestine and sense the LPS, lipoteichoic acid (LTA), flagella, and other components of the bacteria within the lumen. An equilibrium is maintained between inflammatory and immune regulatory responses to microbial stimuli. Disruption of the equilibrium can result in gastroenteritis, inflammatory bowel disease, or autoimmune diseases.

• Inflammation

Proinflammatory Cytokines

The proinflammatory cytokines, sometimes referred to as *acute-phase cytokines,* are IL-1, TNF-α, and IL-6 (Figure 8-8 and Table 8-3). These cytokines are produced by activated macrophages and other cells. IL-1 and TNF-α share properties. Both of these cytokines are **endogenous pyrogens** capable of stimulating fever, promoting local inflammatory reactions and synthesis of acute-phase proteins.

TNF-α is the ultimate mediator of inflammation and the systemic effects of infection. TNF-α stimulates endothelial cells to express adhesion molecules and chemokines to attract leukocytes to the site of infection, loosens the epithelial tight junctions to allow diapedesis, activates mast cells lining the vasculature to release histamine to promote seepage of fluid, activates neutrophils and macrophages, and promotes apoptosis of certain cell types. Systemically, TNF acts on the hypothalamus to induce fever, can cause systemic metabolic changes, weight loss (cachexia), and loss of appetite, enhances production of IL-1, IL-6, and chemokines, and promotes acute-phase protein synthesis by the liver. At high concentrations, TNF-α elicits all of the functions leading to septic shock.

There are two types of **IL-1,** IL-1α and IL-1β. IL-1 is produced mainly by activated macrophages but also by neutrophils, epithelial cells, and endothelial cells. IL-1β must be cleaved by the inflammasome to become activated. IL-1 shares many of the activities of TNF-α to promote local and systemic inflammatory responses. Unlike TNF-α, IL-1 is a growth factor, cannot induce apoptosis, and will enhance but is not sufficient to cause septic shock.

IL-6 is produced by many cell types, promotes the synthesis of acute-phase proteins in the liver, production of neutrophils in bone marrow, and activation of T and B lymphocytes. **IL-23** and **IL-12** are cytokines that bridge the innate and immune responses. Both cytokines have two

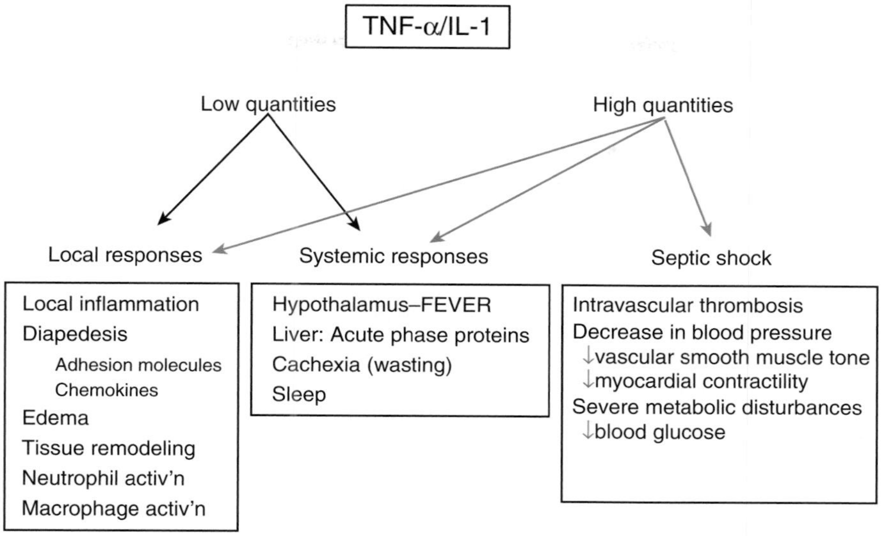

FIGURE 8-8 The good, the bad, and the ugly effects of tumor necrosis factor *(TNF)*-α and interleukin *(IL)*-1. Low concentrations activate local inflammation (promote movement of fluid, proteins, and cells from the blood to the site of infection) and supportive responses. High concentrations activate systemic inflammation and shock.

Table 8-3 Cytokines of Innate Immunity (STAT)*

Cytokine[†]	Source	Trigger	Action	Target
TNF-α	Macrophages, T cells	PAMP, inflammation	Acute-phase responses, promotes inflammation, fever, symptoms of sepsis, cachexia, vascular permeability, altered muscle tone, apoptosis (some cells)	Endothelial cells, neutrophils, macrophages, hypothalamus, liver, muscle, mast cells, other cells
IL-1 (α, β cleaved)	Macrophages, keratinocytes, endothelial and some epithelial cells	PAMP, inflammation	Acute-phase responses, promotes inflammation, fever, supports symptoms of sepsis, synthesis of acute-phase proteins	Endothelial cells, hypothalamus, liver, and other cells
IL-6	Macrophages, endothelial cells, T cells	PAMP, inflammation	Acute-phase responses, reinforces acute-phase responses, stimulation of T and B cells	Macrophages, endothelial cells, T cells
Type 1 IFNs (α, β)	Most cells, plasmacytoid dendritic cells	Viral infection (especially RNA viruses)	Inhibit virus replication, activate NK cells, enhance immune response	Virus-infected cells, NK cells, T cells
Chemokines	Macrophages, dendritic cells, many other cells	PAMP, inflammation, C5a, TNF-α	Chemotaxis, targeting of cells to infection/inflammation	Leukocytes, lymphocytes, endothelial cells, and other cells
IL-12 (p70)	Dendritic cells, macrophages	PAMP	Promotes TH1 immune response, activates NK cell	NK cells, T cells
IL-23	Dendritic cells, macrophages	PAMP	Promotes TH17 response	T cells
IL-18 (cleaved)	Macrophages/inflammasome	PAMP, inflammation	Promotes IFN-γ production	NK cells, T cells
Type II IFN (γ)	NK cells, T cells	IL-18, IL-12 (TH1 responses)	Activates antimicrobial activity, production of inducible nitric oxide synthetase, other	Macrophages, dendritic cells, B cells, etc.

IFN, Interferon; *IL,* interleukin; *NK,* natural killer; *PAMP,* pathogen-associated molecular pattern; *TH,* T helper (cell); *TNF,* tumor necrosis factor.
*STAT: acronym for essential information for each cytokine: *S*ource, *T*rigger, *A*ction, *T*arget.
[†]Table is not all-inclusive for cell sources, stimuli, activities, or targets.

subunits, a p40 subunit and a p35 subunit for IL-12 and a p19 subunit for IL-23. IL-23 promotes TH17 responses from memory T cells, which enhance neutrophil action. IL-12 promotes NK-cell function and is required to promote a TH1 immune response, which enhances macrophages and other myeloid cells functions. These cytokines will be discussed in Chapter 9 regarding their actions on T cells. **IL-18** is produced by macrophages, must be cleaved by the inflammasome to an active form, and promotes NK- and T-cell function.

Acute Inflammation

Acute inflammation is an early defense mechanism to contain the infection, prevent its spread from the initial focus, and activate subsequent immune responses. Initially, inflammation can be triggered by the response to danger signals resulting from infection and tissue damage. Mast cells respond by releasing histamines, TNF-α, and prostaglandins that can trigger increases in permeability of capillaries. With chemokines, IL-1, and complement, these agents can promote acute inflammation.

The three major events in acute inflammation are (1) expansion of capillaries to increase blood flow (causing redness or a rash and releasing heat); (2) increase in permeability of the microvasculature structure to allow escape of fluid, plasma proteins, and leukocytes from the circulation (swelling or edema); and (3) recruitment of neutrophils and their accumulation and response to infection at the site of injury. Inflammatory responses are beneficial but are associated with pain, redness, heat, and swelling and can also cause tissue damage. The mediators of inflammation are listed in Table 8-4.

Tissue damage is caused to some extent by complement and macrophages but mostly by neutrophils and their products. Dead neutrophils are a major component of **pus.** Kinins and clotting factors induced by tissue damage (e.g., factor XII [Hageman factor], bradykinin, fibrinopeptides) are also involved in inflammation. These factors increase vascular permeability and are chemotactic for leukocytes. Products of arachidonic acid metabolism also affect inflammation. Cyclooxygenase-2 (COX-2) and 5-lipooxygenase convert arachidonic acid to **prostaglandins** and **leukotrienes,** respectively, which can mediate essentially every aspect of acute inflammation. The course of inflammation can be followed by rapid increases in acute-phase proteins, especially C-reactive protein (which can increase 1000-fold within 24 to 48 hours) and serum amyloid A.

Table 8-4 Mediators of Acute and Chronic Inflammation

Action	Mediators
Acute Inflammation	
Increased vascular permeability	Histamine, bradykinin, C3a, C5a, leukotrienes, PAF, substance P
Vasodilation	Histamine, prostaglandins, PAF, nitric oxide (NO)
Pain	Bradykinin, prostaglandins
Leukocyte adhesion	Leukotriene B4, IL-1, TNF-α, C5a
Leukocyte chemotaxis	C5a, C3a, IL-8, chemokines, PAF, leukotriene B4
Acute-phase response	IL-1, IL-6, TNF-α
Tissue damage	Proteases, free radicals, NO, neutrophil granule contents
Fever	IL-1, TNF, prostaglandins
Chronic Inflammation	
Activation of T cells and macrophages, and acute-phase processes	T cells (TNF, IL-17, IFN-γ), macrophages (IL-1, TNF-α, IL-23, IL-12), cytokines

From Novak R: *Crash course immunology,* Philadelphia, 2006, Mosby.

IFN-γ, Interferon-γ; *IL,* interleukin; *PAF,* platelet activating factor; *TNF,* tumor necrosis factor.

Acute-Phase Response

The **acute-phase response** is triggered by infection, tissue injury, prostaglandin E_2, interferons associated with viral infection, acute-phase cytokines (IL-1, IL-6, TNF-α), and inflammation (Box 8-5). The acute-phase response promotes changes that support host defenses and include fever, anorexia, sleepiness, metabolic changes, and production of proteins. Acute-phase proteins that are produced and

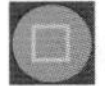

Box 8-5 Acute-Phase Proteins

α_1-Antitrypsin
α_1-Glycoprotein
Amyloids A and P
Antithrombin III
C-reactive protein
C1 esterase inhibitor
Complement C2, C3, C4, C5, C9
Ceruloplasmin
Fibrinogen
Haptoglobin
Orosomucoid
Plasminogen
Transferrin
Lipopolysaccharide-binding protein
Mannose-binding protein

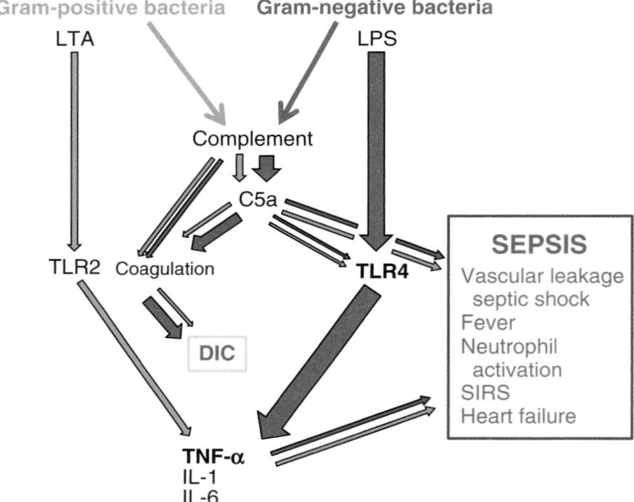

FIGURE 8-9 Gram-positive and gram-negative bacteria induce sepsis by shared and separate pathways. Bacterial surface lipopolysaccharides *(LPS)* activate complement, producing C5a, which promotes inflammation and activates coagulation. LPS, lipoteichoic acid *(LTA),* and other pathogen-associated molecular patterns interact with Toll-like receptors *(TLRs)* and other pathogen pattern receptors to activate inflammation and proinflammatory cytokine production. These add up to sepsis. The thickness of the arrow indicates the strength of the response. Red is for gram-negative and blue is for gram-positive bacteria. *DIC,* Disseminated intravascular coagulation; *IL,* interleukin; *SIRS,* systemic inflammatory response syndrome; *TNF-α,* tumor necrosis factor-α. (Modified from Rittirsch D, Flierl MA, Ward PA: Harmful molecular mechanisms in sepsis, *Nat Rev Immunol* 8:776–787, 2008.)

released into the serum include C-reactive protein, complement components, coagulation proteins, LPS-binding proteins, transport proteins, protease inhibitors, and adherence proteins. **C-reactive protein** binds to the polysaccharides of numerous bacteria and fungi and activates the complement pathway, facilitating removal of these organisms from the body by enhancing phagocytosis. **Hepcidin** inhibits iron uptake by the gut and macrophages, and this reduces availability to microbes. The acute-phase proteins reinforce the innate defenses against infection, but their excessive production during sepsis (induced by endotoxin or bacteremia) can cause serious problems such as shock.

Sepsis and Cytokine Storms

Cytokine storms are generated by an overwhelming release of cytokines in response to bacterial cell wall components (especially LPS), toxic shock toxins, and certain viral infections. Strong innate responses are triggered by the presence of microbes in the blood during bacteremia and viremia. During bacteremia, large amounts of complement C5a and cytokines are produced and distributed throughout the body (Figure 8-9). C5a and TNF-α promote vascular leakage, neutrophil activation, and activation of the coagulation pathway. Plasmacytoid DCs in the blood produce large amounts of inflammatory cytokines and IL-12 in response to bacterial PAMPs. Endotoxin is an especially potent activator of cells and inducer of cytokine production and sepsis (see Figure 14-4). Cytokine storms can also occur upon the abnormal stimulation of T cells and antigen-presenting cells (DCs, macrophages, and B cells) by superantigens produced by *S. aureus* or *Streptococcus pyogenes* (see Figure 14-3). During viremia, large amounts of IFN-α and other cytokines are produced by plasmacytoid DCs and T cells.

Although beneficial on a limited and local basis, excess cytokines in the blood induce life-threatening inflammatory trauma throughout the entire body. Most significantly, increases in vascular permeability can result in leakage of fluids from the bloodstream into tissue and cause shock. Septic shock is a consequence of cytokine storm and can be attributed to the systemic action of large quantities of C5a and TNF-α.

• Bridge to Antigen-Specific Immune Responses

The innate response is often sufficient to control an infection but also initiates antigen-specific immunity. DCs (and Langerhans cells if in the skin) provide the bridge between the innate and immune responses. They become activated at the site of infection, deliver and process antigenic proteins to the T cells in the lymph node, and make appropriate cytokines to elicit the necessary T-cell response (Figure 8-10).

iDCs, intestinal DCs, and Langerhans cells in the skin are constantly acquiring antigenic material by macropinocytosis, pinocytosis, or phagocytosis of apoptotic cells, debris,

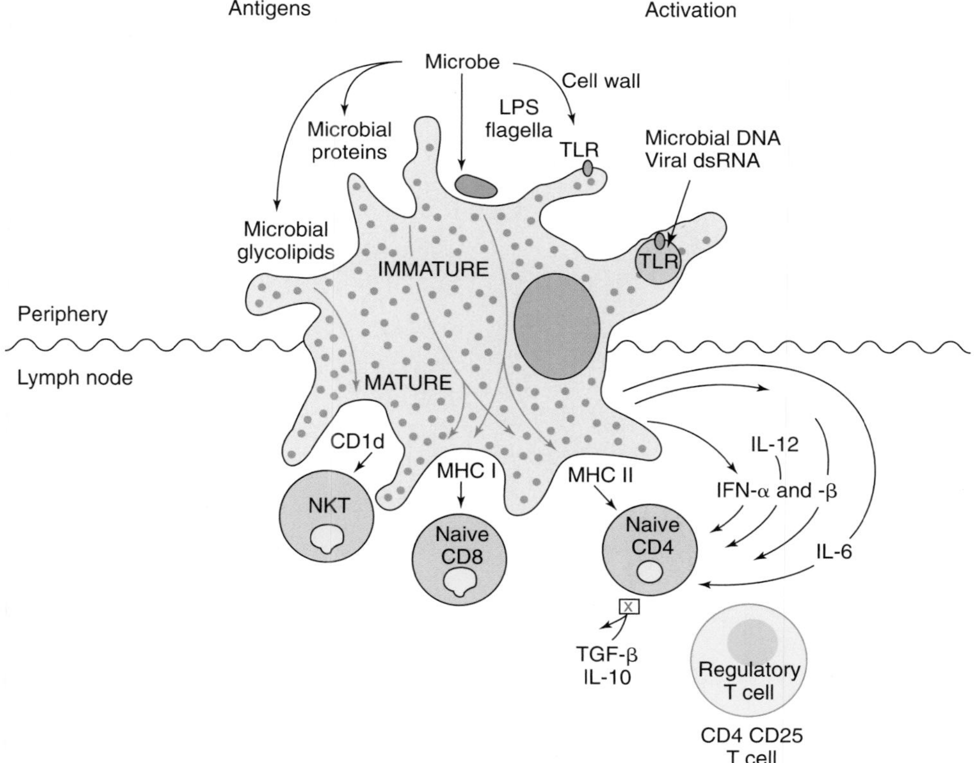

FIGURE 8-10 Dendritic cells (DCs) initiate and direct immune responses. Immature DCs constantly internalize and process proteins, debris, and microbes, when present. Binding of microbial components to Toll-like receptors *(TLRs)* activates the maturation of the DC so that it ceases to internalize any new material; moves to the lymph node and up-regulates major histocompatibility complex *(MHC)* II and co-receptors B7 and B7-1 molecules for antigen presentation; and produces cytokines to activate T cells. Cell surface interactions and cytokines activate the T cells and direct the nature of the subsequent response. *IFN,* Interferon; *LPS,* lipopolysaccharide.

and proteins in normal tissue and at the site of infection or tumor. Upon activation by a combination of damage and pathogen-associated signals, acute-phase cytokines (IL-1, IL-6, and TNF-α) are released, the iDC matures into a DC, and its role changes. The DC loses its ability to phagocytize, preventing it from acquiring irrelevant antigenic material other than the microbial debris, and it progresses to the lymph node. *By analogy, the iDC is like a clam, constantly surveying its environment by filter feeding the cellular and microbial debris (if present), but when triggered by a PAMPR signal, indicating that microbes are present, it releases a local cytokine alarm, closes its shell, and moves to the lymph node to trigger a response to the challenge. Having experienced the challenge, the DC directs the appropriate response in the T cells.* The mature DC moves to T-cell areas of lymph nodes and up-regulates its cell surface molecules for optimal antigen presentation (class II MHC and B7-1 and B7-2 [co-stimulatory] molecules). Microbe-activated mature DCs release cytokines (e.g., IL-12, IL23), which activate responses to reinforce local host defenses (TH1, TH17 responses). DCs present antigenic material attached to MHC class I and CD1 molecules to CD8 T and NKT cells, and on MHC class II molecules to CD4 T cells. DCs are so effective at presenting antigen that 10 cells loaded with antigen are sufficient to initiate protective immunity to a lethal bacterial challenge in a mouse. T-cell responses will be described in the next chapter.

Bibliography

Abbas AK, Lichtman AH, Pillai S, et al: *Cellular and molecular immunology*, ed 7, Philadelphia, 2011, WB Saunders.

Akira S, Takeda K: Toll-like receptor signaling, *Nat Rev Immunol* 4:499–511, 2004.

DeFranco AL, Locksley RM, Robertson M: *Immunity: the immune response in infectious and inflammatory disease*, Sunderland, Mass, 2007, Sinauer Associates.

Janeway CA, Travers P, Walport M, et al: *Immunobiology: the immune system in health and disease*, ed 6, New York, 2004, Garland Science.

Kindt TJ, Goldsby RA, Osborne BA: *Kuby immunology*, ed 7, New York, 2011, WH Freeman.

Kumar V, Abbas AK, Fausto N: *Robbins and Cotran pathologic basis of disease*, ed 7, Philadelphia, 2005, Elsevier.

Lamkanfi M: Emerging inflammasome effector mechanisms, *Nat Rev Immunol* 11:213–220, 2011.

Netea MG, van der Meer JW: Immunodeficiency and genetic defects of pattern-recognition receptors, *N Engl J Med* 364:60–70, 2011.

Rittirsch D, Flierl MA, Ward PA: Harmful molecular mechanisms in sepsis, *Nat Rev Immunol* 8:776–787, 2008.

Sompayrac L: *How the immune system works*, ed 2, Malden, Mass, 2003, Blackwell Scientific.

Takeda K, Kaisho T, Akira S: Toll-like receptors, *Annu Rev Immunol* 21:335–376, 2003.

Trends Immunol: Issues contain understandable reviews on current topics in immunology.

CHAPTER

Animations for this chapter are available on StudentConsult.com.

9 ANTIGEN-SPECIFIC IMMUNE RESPONSES

Antigen-specific immune responses provided by T and B cells and antibody expand the host protections provided by innate responses. Almost any molecule has the potential to initiate an immune response, and yet the system does not normally respond to its own molecules. The antigen-specific immune system is a randomly generated, coordinately regulated, inducible, and activatable system that ignores self-proteins but specifically responds to and protects against infection. When not working properly, the immune response can be unregulated, overstimulated, uncontrolled, reactive to self-proteins, unresponsive or poorly responsive to infections, and become the cause of pathogenesis and disease. Once specifically activated by exposure to a new antigen, the immune response rapidly expands in strength, cell number, and specificity. For proteins, immune memory develops to allow more rapid recall upon rechallenge.

Antibody and the antibody-like **T-cell receptor (TCR)** molecules recognize antigens and act as receptors to activate the growth and functions of those cells that can elicit the antigen-specific response. The soluble forms of antibody in the blood, body fluids, or secreted across membranes protect the body by inactivating and promoting the elimination of toxins and microbes, especially when they are in the blood (bacteremia, viremia). T cells are important for activating and regulating innate and immune responses and for direct killing of cells expressing inappropriate antigens.

Although some molecules elicit only a limited antibody response (carbohydrates and lipids), proteins and protein-conjugated molecules (including carbohydrates) elicit a more complete immune response that includes T cells. Activation of a complete immune response is highly controlled because it uses a large amount of energy, and once initiated, it develops memory and remains for most of a lifetime. Development of an antigen-specific immune response progresses from the innate responses through ***d***endritic cells (DCs), which ***d***irect the ***T*** cells to ***t***ell other T cells, B cells, and other cells to grow and activate the necessary responses. Cell-receptor and cytokine-receptor interactions provide the necessary signals to activate cell growth and respond to the challenge. ***T*** cells ***t***ell the B cell which type of antibody to produce (immunoglobulin [Ig]G, IgE, IgA) and promote memory cell development. T cells continuously regulate the entire system, maintaining a balance that normally minimizes inflammation but still allows protection from normal and pathogenic microbes.

Immunogens, Antigens, and Epitopes

Almost all proteins and carbohydrates associated with an infectious agent—whether a bacterium, fungus, virus, or parasite—are considered foreign to the human host and have the potential to induce an immune response. A protein or carbohydrate that is recognized and sufficient to initiate an immune response is called an **immunogen** (Box 9-1). Immunogens may contain more than one antigen (e.g., bacteria). An **antigen** is a molecule that is recognized by specific antibodies or the TCR on T cells. An **epitope (antigenic determinant)** is the actual molecular structure that interacts with a single antibody molecule or TCR. Within a protein, an epitope may be formed by a specific sequence **(linear epitope)** or a three-dimensional structure **(conformational epitope).** *The TCR can recognize only linear peptide epitopes.* Antigens and immunogens usually contain several epitopes, each capable of binding to a different antibody molecule or TCR. As described later in this chapter, a **monoclonal antibody** recognizes a single epitope.

Not all molecules are immunogens. In general, *proteins are the best immunogens, carbohydrates are weaker immunogens, and lipids and nucleic acids are poor immunogens.* **Haptens (incomplete immunogens)** are often too small to immunize (i.e., initiate a response) an individual but can be recognized by antibody. Haptens can be made immunogenic by attachment to a **carrier molecule,** such as a protein. For example, conjugation of penicillin to serum albumin converts it to an immunogen.

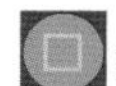

Box 9-1 Definitions

Adjuvant: substance that promotes immune response to immunogen
Antigen: substance recognized by immune response
Carrier: protein modified by hapten to elicit response
Epitope: minimal molecular structure recognized by immune response
Hapten: incomplete immunogen that cannot initiate response but can be recognized by antibody
Immunogen: substance capable of eliciting an immune response
T-dependent antigens: antigens that must be presented to T and B cells for antibody production
T-independent antigens: antigens with large, repetitive structures (e.g., bacteria, flagellin, lipopolysaccharide, polysaccharide)

During artificial immunization (e.g., vaccines), an adjuvant is often used to enhance the response to antigen. **Adjuvants** usually prolong the presence of antigen in the tissue, promote uptake of the immunogen, or activate DCs, macrophages, and lymphocytes. Some adjuvants mimic the activators of innate responses (e.g., microbial ligands for Toll-like receptors) present in a natural immunization.

Some molecules will not elicit an immune response in an individual. During growth of the fetus, the body develops **central immune tolerance** toward self-antigens and any foreign antigens that may be introduced before maturation of the immune system (Animation 9-1). Later in life, **peripheral tolerance** develops to other proteins to prevent uncontrolled or autoimmune responses. For example, our immune response is tolerant of the food we eat; alternatively, eating steak would induce an antimuscle response.

The type of immune response initiated by an immunogen depends on its molecular structure. A primitive but rapid antibody response can be initiated toward *bacterial polysaccharides (capsule), peptidoglycan, or flagellin.* Termed **T-independent antigens,** these molecules have a large repetitive structure that is sufficient to activate B cells directly to make antibody without the participation of T-cell help. In these cases, the response is limited to production of **IgM** antibody, memory cells are not generated, and **anamnestic (booster) responses** cannot occur. The transition from an IgM response to an IgG, IgE, or IgA response results from a big change in the B cell and is equivalent to differentiation of the cell. This requires help provided by T-cell interactions and cytokines. Portions of the antigen (likely to be different) must be recognized and stimulate T and B cells. **T-dependent antigens** are proteins; they generate all five classes of immunoglobulins and can elicit memory and an anamnestic response.

The structure of the antigen, the amount, route of administration, and other factors influence the type of immune response, including the types of antibody produced. For example, oral or nasal administration of a vaccine across mucosal membranes promotes production of a secretory form of **IgA** (sIgA) that would not be produced on intramuscular administration.

• T Cells

The thymus is essential for T-cell production. T cells were initially distinguished from B cells on the basis of their ability to bind sheep red blood cells through the CD2 molecule and form rosettes. These cells communicate through direct cell-to-cell interactions and with cytokines. T cells are defined through the use of antibodies that distinguish their cell surface molecules. The T-cell surface proteins include (1) the **TCR,** (2) the CD4 and CD8 co-receptors, (3) CD3 and accessory proteins that promote recognition, regulation, and activation, (4) cytokine receptors, and (5) adhesion proteins. T cells can be distinguished by the type of T-cell antigen receptor, either consisting of γ and δ chains or α and β chains, and for α/β T cells, the presence of CD4 or CD8 co-receptors. T cells can be further distinguished by the response that they initiate with the cytokines that they produce.

The helper T cells **(CD4)** activate and control immune and inflammatory responses by specific cell-to-cell interactions and by releasing cytokines. Helper T cells interact with peptide antigens presented on class II major histocompatibility complex (MHC) molecules expressed on antigen-presenting cells (APCs) (DCs, macrophages, and B cells). The repertoire of cytokines secreted by a specific CD4 T cell in response to antigenic challenge defines the type of CD4 T cell. CD4 T cells can also kill target cells with their Fas ligand surface protein.

CD8 T cells are categorized as cytolytic T cells but can also make cytokines similar to CD4 cells. Activated CD8 T cells "patrol" the body for virus-infected or tumor cells, which are identified by antigenic peptides presented by class I MHC molecules. Class I MHC molecules are found on all nucleated cells.

• Cell Surface Receptors of T Cells

The **TCR complex** is a combination of the antigen recognition structure (TCR) and cell-activation machinery **(CD3)** (Figure 9-1). T cells expressing the **γ/δ TCR** are present in blood, mucosal epithelium, and other tissue locations and are important for stimulating innate and mucosal immunity. These cells make up 5% of circulating lymphocytes but expand to between 20% and 60% of T cells during certain bacterial and other types of infections. The γ/δ TCR senses unusual microbial metabolites and initiates cytokine-mediated immune responses.

The **α/β TCR** is expressed on most T cells, and these cells are primarily responsible for antigen-activated immune responses. T cells with the α/β TCR are distinguished further by expression of either a CD4 or a CD8 molecule.

The specificity of the TCR determines the antigenic response of the T cell. Each TCR molecule is made up of two different polypeptide chains. As with antibody, each TCR chain has a constant region and a variable region. The repertoire of TCRs is very large and can identify a tremendous number of antigenic specificities (estimated to be able to recognize 10^{15} separate epitopes). The genetic mechanisms for the development of this diversity are also similar to those for antibody (Figure 9-2). The TCR gene is made up of multiple V ($V_1V_2V_3 \ldots V_n$), D, and J segments. In the early stages of T-cell development, a particular V segment genetically recombines with one or more D segments, deleting intervening V and D segments, and then recombines with a J segment to form a unique TCR gene. Like antibody, random insertion of nucleotides at the recombination junctions increases the potential for diversity and the possibility of producing inactive TCRs. Unlike antibody, somatic mutation does not occur for TCR genes. Only cells with functional TCRs will survive. Each T-cell and its progeny express a unique TCR.

Unlike antibody molecules, most TCRs can only recognize a linear peptide epitope held within a cleft on the surface of either the MHC I or MHC II molecules (see Figure 9-1). Presentation of the antigenic peptide requires specialized proteolytic processing of the protein (see later) and attachment to MHC II molecules by the antigen-presenting cell or to MHC I molecules by all nucleated cells.

The **CD3 complex** is found on all T cells and consists of the γ-, δ-, ε-, and ζ-polypeptide chains. The CD3 complex is the **signal transduction unit** for the TCR. **Tyrosine protein kinases** (ZAP-70, Lck) associate with the CD3 complex when antigen is bound to the TCR complex, promote a cascade of protein phosphorylations, activation of phospholipase C

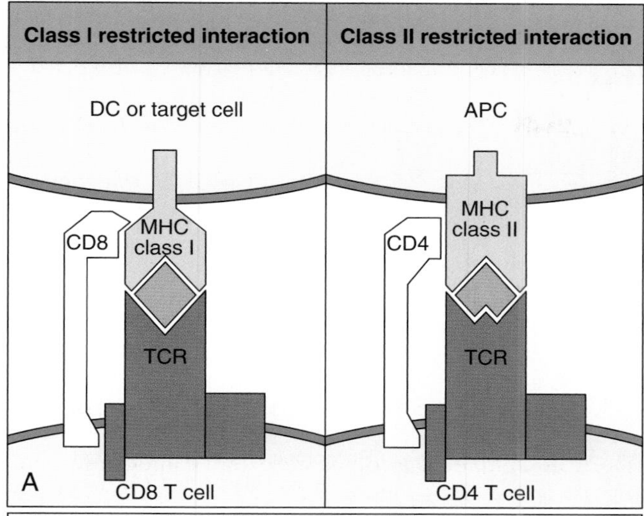

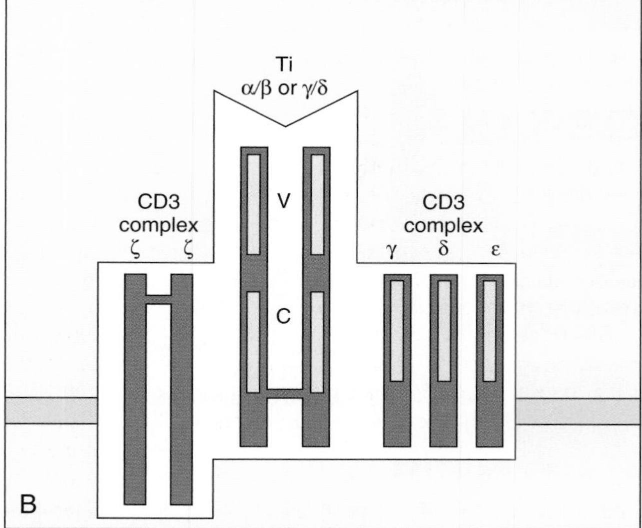

FIGURE 9-1 Major histocompatibility complex *(MHC)* restriction and antigen presentation to T cells. **A,** *Left,* Antigenic peptides bound to class I MHC molecules are presented to the T-cell receptor *(TCR)* on CD8 T-killer/suppressor cells. *Right,* Antigenic peptides bound to class II MHC molecules on the antigen-presenting cell *(APC)* (B cell, dendritic cell *[DC],* or macrophage) are presented to CD4 T-helper cells. **B,** T-cell receptor. The TCR consists of different subunits. Antigen recognition occurs through the α/β or γ/δ subunits. The CD3 complex of γ, δ, ε, and ζ subunits promotes T-cell activation. *C,* Constant region; *V,* variable region.

(PLC), and other events. The products of cleavage of inositol triphosphate by PLC cause the release of calcium and activate protein kinase C and **calcineurin,** a protein phosphatase. Calcineurin is a target for the immunosuppressive drugs cyclosporine and tacrolimus. Activation of membrane G-proteins, such as Ras, and the consequences of the previously described cascades result in the activation of specific transcription factors in the nucleus, activation of the T cell, and production of interleukin (IL)-2 and its receptor, IL-2R. These steps are depicted in Figure 9-3.

The **CD4 and CD8 proteins** are co-receptors for the TCR (see Figure 9-1) because they facilitate the interaction of the

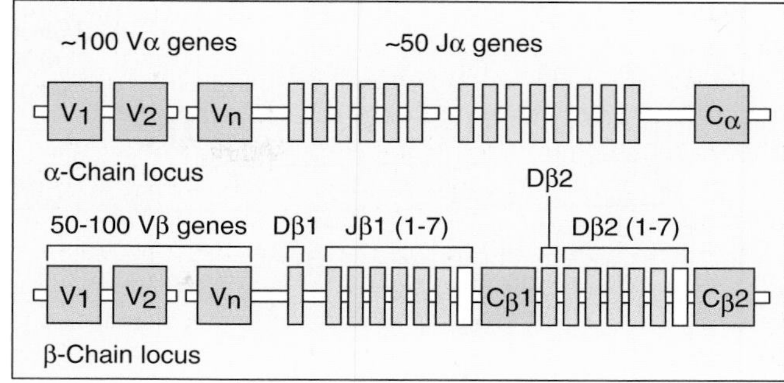

FIGURE 9-2 Structure of the embryonic T-cell receptor gene. Note the similarity in structure to the immunoglobulin genes. Recombination of these segments also generates a diverse recognition repertoire. *C,* Connecting sequences; *J* and *D,* segments; *V,* variable segments.

TCR with the antigen-presenting MHC molecule and can enhance the activation response. CD4 binds to class II MHC molecules on the surface of APCs. CD8 binds to class I MHC molecules on the surface of APCs and target cells. Class I MHC molecules are expressed on all nucleated cells (see more on MHC later in this chapter). The cytoplasmic tails of CD4 and CD8 associate with a protein tyrosine kinase (Lck), which enhances the TCR-induced activation of the cell on binding to the APC or target cell. CD4 or CD8 is found on α/β T cells but not on γ/δ T cells.

Accessory molecules expressed on the T cell include several protein receptors on the cell surface that interact with proteins on APCs and target cells, leading to activation of the T cell, promotion of tighter interactions between the cells, or facilitation of the killing of the target cell. These accessory molecules are as follows:

1. **CD45RA (native T cells)** or **CD45RO (memory T cells),** a transmembrane protein tyrosine phosphatase (PTP)
2. **CD28** or cytotoxic T-lymphocyte–associated protein 4 **(CTLA-4)** that binds to the B7 protein on APCs to deliver a co-stimulation or an inhibitory signal to the T cell
3. **CD154 (CD40L),** which is present on activated T cells and binds to CD40 on DCs, macrophages, and B cells to promote their activation
4. **FasL,** which initiates apoptosis in a target cell that expresses **Fas** on its cell surface.

Adhesion molecules tighten the interaction of the T cell with the APC or target cell and may also promote activation. Adhesion molecules include **leukocyte function–associated antigen-1 (LFA-1),** which interacts with the **intercellular adhesion molecules (ICAM-1, ICAM-2, and ICAM-3)** on the target cell. **CD2** was originally identified by its ability to bind to sheep red blood cells **(erythrocyte receptors).** CD2 binds to LFA-3 on the target cell and promotes cell-to-cell adhesion and T-cell activation. **Very late antigens (VLA-4 and VLA-5)** are expressed on activated cells later in the response and bind to fibronectin on target cells to enhance the interaction.

T cells express receptors for many cytokines that activate and regulate T-cell function (Table 9-1). Binding of the cytokine to the **cytokine receptor** activates protein kinase and other activation cascades that deliver their signal to the nucleus. **The IL-2 receptor (IL-2R)** is composed of three

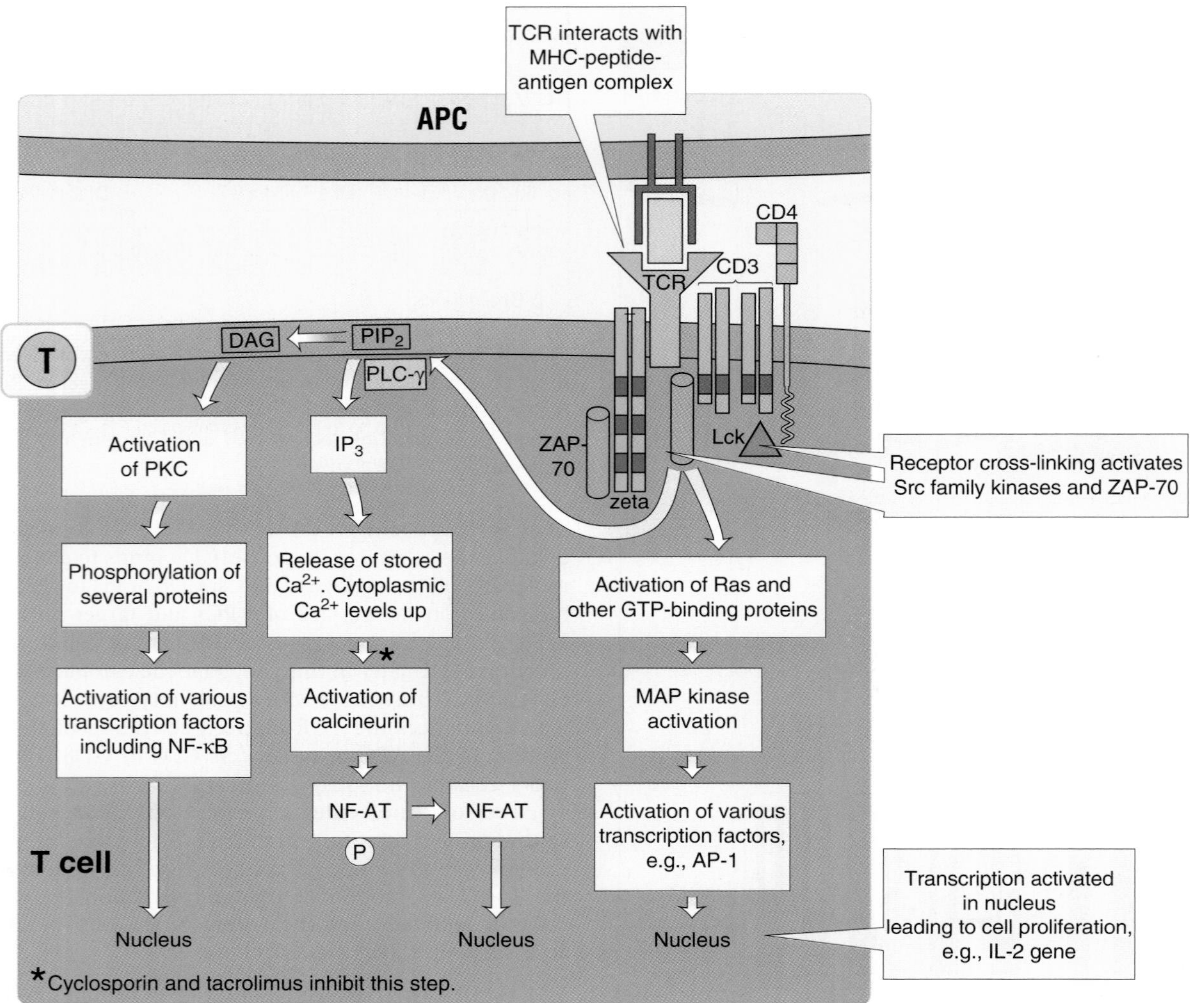

FIGURE 9-3 Activation pathways for T cells. Binding of major histocompatibility complex *(MHC)* II-peptide to CD4 and the T-cell receptor *(TCR)* activate kinase cascades and phospholipase C to activate the nuclear factor of activated T cells *(NF-AT),* nuclear factor-kappa B *(NF-κβ),* activation protein 1 *(AP-1),* and other transcription factors. *APC,* Antigen-presenting cell; *DAG,* diacylglycerol; *GTP,* guanosine triphosphate; *IL-2,* interleukin-2; *IP_3,* inositol 1,4,5-triphosphate; *Lck,* lymphocyte-specific tyrosine protein kinase; *MAP kinase,* mitogen-activated protein kinase; *PIP_2,* phosphatidylinositol 4,5-bisphosphate; *PKC,* protein kinase C; *PLC-γ,* phospholipase C-γ; *ZAP,* zeta-associated protein. (Modified from Nairn R, Helbert M: *Immunology for medical students,* ed 2, Philadelphia, 2007, Mosby.)

subunits. The β/γ subunits are on most T cells (also natural killer [NK] cells) and have intermediate affinity for IL-2. The α subunit **(CD25)** is induced by cell activation to form a high-affinity α/β/γ IL-2R. Binding of IL-2 to the IL-2R initiates a growth-stimulating signal to the T cell, which also promotes the production of more IL-2 and IL-2R. CD25 is expressed on activated, growing cells, including the Treg subset of CD4 T cells ($CD4^+CD25^+$). **Chemokine receptors** distinguish different T cells and guide the cell to where it will reside in the body.

• Development of T Cells

T-cell precursors are continuously developing into T cells in the thymus (Figure 9-4; Animation 9-2). Contact with the thymic epithelium and hormones such as thymosin, thymulin, and thymopoietin II in the thymus promote extensive proliferation and differentiation of the individual's T-cell population during fetal development. Individuals who congenitally lack a thymus (DiGeorge syndrome) lack T cells. While the T-cell precursors are in the thymus, each cell undergoes recombination of sequences within its TCR genes to generate a TCR unique to that cell. T cells without TCRs, bearing nonfunctional TCRs, TCRs that cannot interact with MHC molecules, or those that react too strongly with self-protein peptides (self-reactive) are forced into committing suicide (apoptosis). The epithelial cells in the thymus have a unique capacity to express most of the proteins of the human genome so that the developing T cells can be exposed to the normal repertoire of human proteins. In the thymic medullary epithelial cells, the autoimmune regulator (AIRE) protein is a transcription factor that promotes expression of most of the body's proteins. These proteins are processed and presented to the T cells so they can promote elimination of T cells that recognize self-antigens. The surviving CD4 T

 Table 9-1 **Cytokines That Modulate T-Cell Function**

Type of Response	Acute Phase*	TH1	TH17	TH2	Treg/Sup
Inducers	PAMPs	IL-12	IL-6 + TGF-β	IL-6	??
			IL-23 (memory cells)		
Mediators	IL-1	IL-2	IL-17	IL-4	I-10
	TNF-α	LT (TNF-β)	TNF-α	IL-5	TGF-β
	IL-6	IFN-γ	IL-22	IL-10	
	IFN-α IFN-β				
	IL-12, IL-23				

IFN, Interferon; *IL,* interleukin; *LT,* lymphotoxin; *PAMPs,* pathogen-associated molecular patterns; *Sup,* suppressor; *TGF-β,* transforming growth factor-β; *TH,* T helper (cell).

*Acute-phase responses influence but are not T-cell responses.

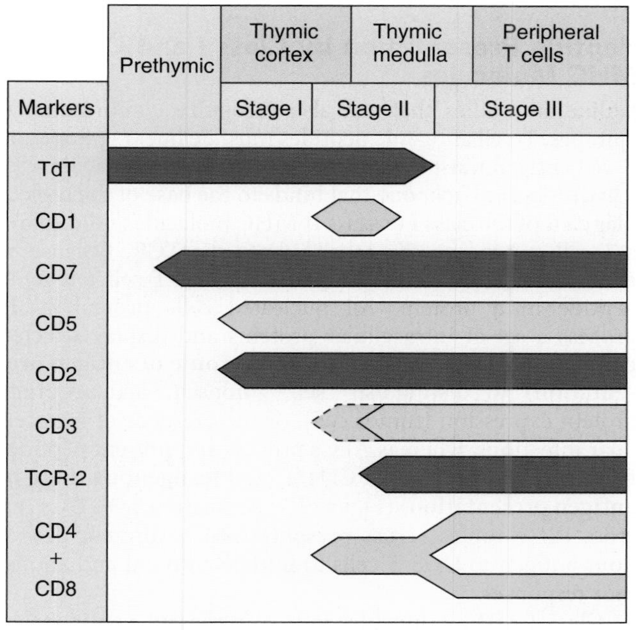

FIGURE 9-4 Human T-cell development. T-cell markers are useful for the identification of the differentiation stages of the T cell and for characterizing T-cell leukemias and lymphomas. *TCR,* T-cell receptor; *TdT,* cytoplasmic terminal deoxynucleotidyl transferase.

cells differentiate into the CD4 or CD8 subpopulations of T cells (Box 9-2). The T cells enter the blood and travel to lymph nodes, spleen, and other sites.

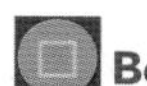 Box 9-2 **T Cells**

γ/δ T Cells

γ/δ TCR reactive to microbial metabolites
Local responses: resident in blood and tissue
Quicker responses than α/β T cells
Produce interferon-γ; activate dendritic cells and macrophages

α/β T Cells

CD4: α/β TCR reactive with peptides on MHC II on antigen-presenting cell
Cytokines activate and direct immune response (TH1, TH2, TH17)
Also, cytotoxic through Fas–Fas ligand interactions

CD4 CD25 Treg cells: control and limit expansion of immune response; promote tolerance and memory cell development

CD8: α/β TCR reactive with peptides presented on MHC I
Cytotoxic through perforin and granzymes and Fas–Fas ligand induction of apoptosis
Also, produce similar cytokines as CD4 cells

NKT cells: α/β TCR reactive with glycolipids (mycobacteria) on CD1d molecules
Kill tumor and viral-infected cells, similar to NK cells
Provide early cytokine support to antibacterial responses

MHC, Major histocompatibility complex; *NK,* natural killer; *TCR,* T-cell receptor.

 Box 9-3 **Activation of T-Cell Responses**

Only a dendritic cell (DC) can initiate a response from a naïve CD4 or CD8 T cell.

CD4:

Antigen-presenting cells present 11-13 amino acid peptide on MHC II.
Co-receptor (B7.1 or B7.2) interacts with CD28 to activate or CTLA4 to suppress response.
Cytokines activate and determine the nature of the response.
CD40L expression and binding to CD40 on APC is necessary for APC activation.
Activation of cell changes chemokine receptors and adhesion proteins, and it enters blood and cycles through skin, tissue, and B-cell zones of lymph node.

CD8:

DC activates CD8 T cell with help from CD4 T cell.
CD8 T cell enters blood and cycles through skin and tissue.
Target cell presents 8-9 amino acid peptide on MHC I.
Adhesion proteins create immune synapse.
Perforin and granzyme are secreted into immune synapse.
Target cell commits apoptosis.

• Initiation of T-Cell Responses

Antigen Presentation to T Cells

Activation of an antigen-specific T-cell response requires a combination of cytokine and cell-to-cell receptor interactions (Box 9-3) initiated by the interaction of the α/β TCR with MHC-bearing antigenic peptides. **Class I** and **II MHC** molecules provide a molecular cradle for the peptide. As such, these T cells only respond to protein epitopes. The **CD8** molecule on T cells binds to and promotes the interaction with class I MHC molecules on target cells (see Figure 9-1A). The **CD4** molecule on T cells binds to and promotes interactions with class II MHC molecules on APCs. The MHC molecules are encoded within the MHC gene locus (Figure 9-5). The MHC contains a cluster of genes important to the immune response.

Class I MHC molecules are found on all nucleated cells and are the major determinant of "self." The class I MHC

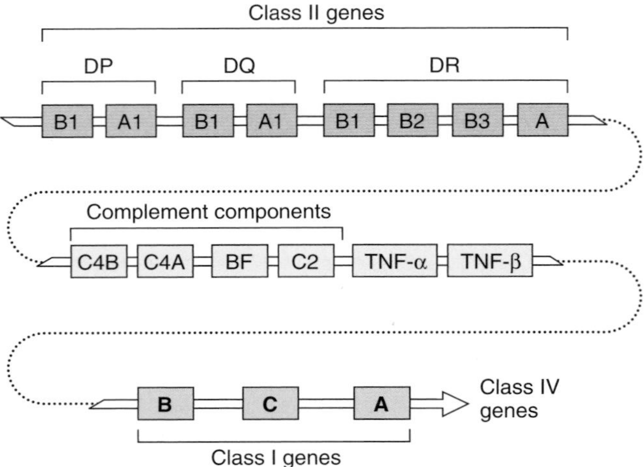

FIGURE 9-5 Genetic map of the major histocompatibility complex (MHC). Genes for class I and class II molecules, as well as complement components and tumor necrosis factor *(TNF),* are within the MHC gene complex.

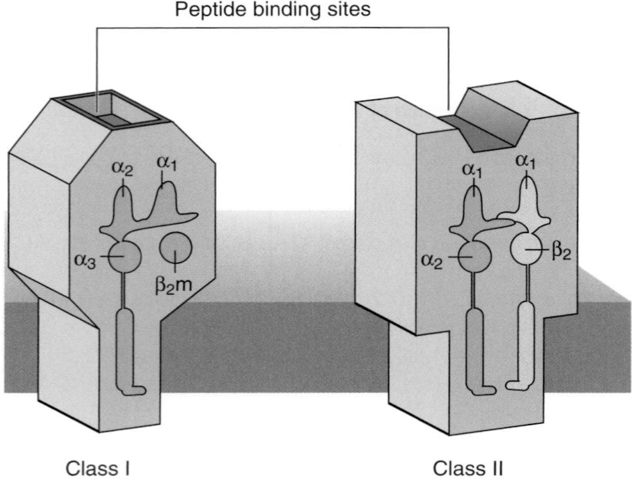

FIGURE 9-6 Structure of class I and class II major histocompatibility complex (MHC) molecules. The class I MHC molecules consist of two subunits, the heavy chain, and β_2-microglobulin. The binding pocket is closed at each end and can only hold peptides of 8 to 9 amino acids. Class II MHC molecules consist of two subunits, α and β, and hold peptides of 11 or more amino acids.

molecule, also known as **HLA** for human and H-2 for mouse, consists of two chains, a **variable heavy chain** and a **light chain (β_2-microglobulin)** (Figure 9-6). Differences in the heavy chain of the HLA molecule between individuals (*allotypic differences*) elicit the T-cell response that prevents graft (tissue) transplantation. There are three major HLA genes **(HLA-A, HLA-B,** and **HLA-C)** and other minor HLA genes. Each cell expresses a pair of different HLA-A, HLA-B, and HLA-C proteins, one from each parent, providing six different clefts to capture a repertoire of antigenic peptides. *The heavy chain of the class I MHC molecule forms a closed-ended cleft, like a pita bread pocket, that holds a peptide of eight to nine amino acids.* The class I MHC molecule presents antigenic peptides, most of which are from within the cell **(endogenous)**, to CD8-expressing T cells. Up-regulation of class I MHC molecules makes the cell a better target for T-cell action. Some cells (brain) and some virus infections (herpes simplex virus, cytomegalovirus) down-regulate the expression of MHC I molecules to reduce their potential as targets for T cells.

Class II MHC molecules are normally expressed on antigen-presenting cells, cells that interact with CD4 T cells (e.g., macrophages, DCs, B cells). The class II MHC molecules are encoded by the **DP, DQ,** and **DR** loci and, like MHC I, are also co-dominantly expressed to produce six different molecules. The class II MHC molecules are a dimer of **α and β subunits** (see Figure 9-6). *The chains of the class II MHC molecule form an open-ended peptide-binding cleft that resembles a hotdog bun and holds a peptide of 11 to 12 amino acids.* The class II MHC molecule presents ingested **(exogenous)** antigenic peptides to CD4-expressing T cells.

CD1 MHC molecules resemble MHC I molecules and have a heavy chain and a light chain (β_2-microglobulin) but bind glycolipids rather than peptides. CD1 molecules are primarily expressed on DCs and present antigen to a specialized invariant TCR on NKT ($CD4^-CD8^-$) cells. CD1 molecules are especially important for defense against mycobacterial infections.

Peptide Presentation by Class I and Class II MHC Molecules

Unlike antibodies that can also recognize conformational epitopes, T-cell antigenic peptides must be linear epitopes. A T-cell antigen must be a peptide of 8 to 12 amino acids with a hydrophobic backbone that binds to the base of the molecular cleft of the class I or class II MHC molecule and displays a T-cell epitope on the other side to the TCR. Because of these constraints, there may be only one T-cell antigenic peptide in a protein. All nucleated cells proteolytically process a set of intracellular proteins and display selected peptides to CD8 T cells **(endogenous route of antigen presentation)** to distinguish "self," "nonself," inappropriate protein expression (tumor cell), or the presence of intracellular infections, whereas APCs process and present peptides from ingested proteins to CD4 T cells **(exogenous route of antigen presentation)** (Figure 9-7; Animation 9-3). DCs can cross these routes **(cross-presentation)** to present exogenous antigen to CD8 T cells to initiate antiviral and antitumor responses.

Class I MHC molecules bind and present peptides that are degraded from cellular proteins by the **proteasome** (a protease machine) in the cytoplasm. These peptides are shuttled into the endoplasmic reticulum (ER) through the **transporter associated with antigen processing (TAP).** Most of these peptides come from misfolded or excess proteins (trash) marked by attachment of the **ubiquitin** protein. The antigenic peptide binds to the heavy chain of the class I MHC molecule. Then the MHC heavy chain can assemble properly with β_2-microglobulin, exit the ER, and proceed to the cell membrane.

During a **viral infection,** large quantities of viral proteins are produced and degraded into peptides and become the predominant source of peptides occupying the class I MHC molecules to be presented to CD8 T cells. **Transplanted cells (grafts)** express peptides on their MHC molecules, which differ from those of the host and therefore may be recognized as foreign. **Tumor cells** often express peptides derived

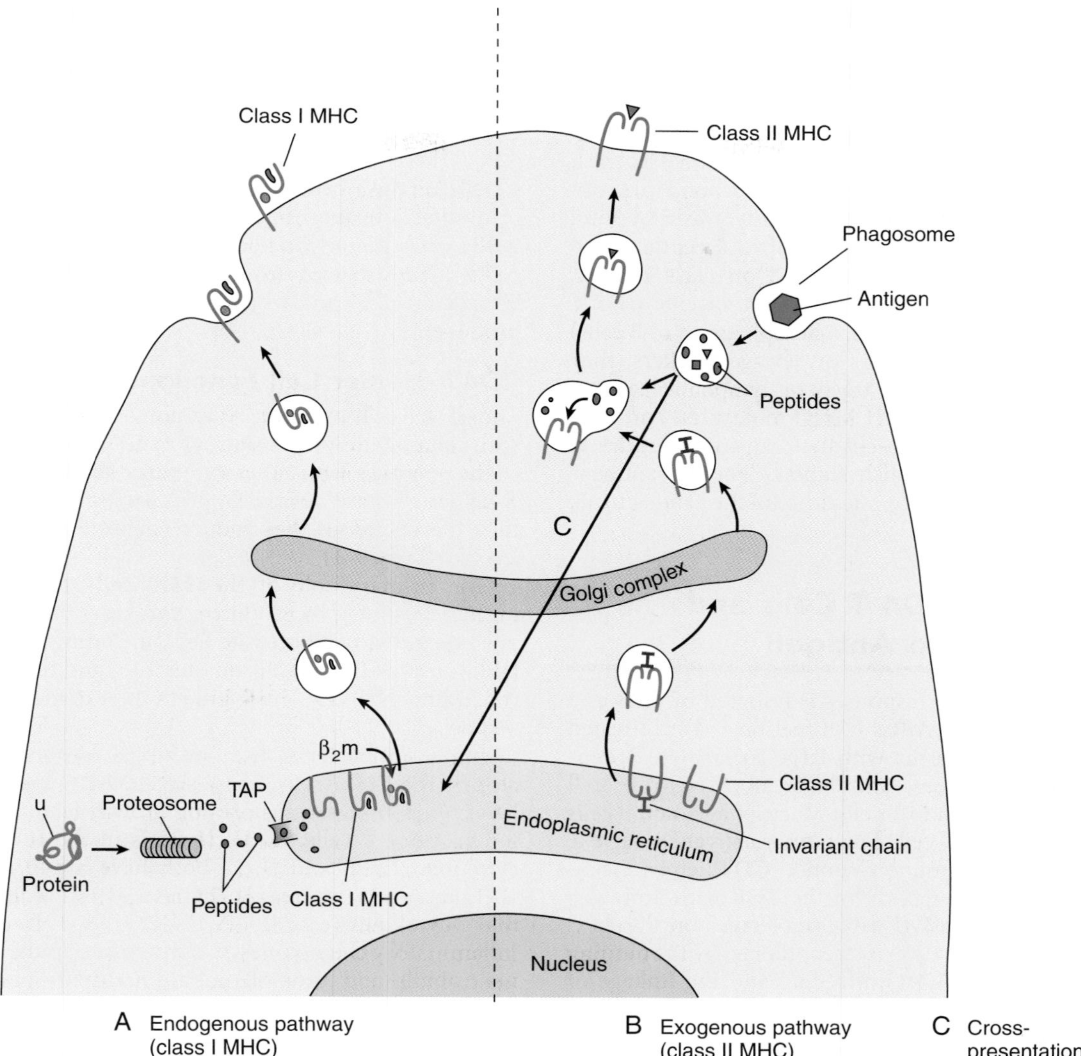

FIGURE 9-7 Antigen presentation. **A, Endogenous:** Endogenous antigen (produced by the cell and analogous to cell trash) is targeted by attachment of ubiquitin *(u)* for digestion in the proteasome. Peptides of eight to nine amino acids are transported through the transporter associated with antigen processing *(TAP)* into the endoplasmic reticulum *(ER)*. The peptide binds to a groove in the heavy chain of the class I major histocompatibility complex *(MHC)* molecule, and the β_2-microglobulin *(β_2m)* binds to the heavy chain. The complex is processed through the Golgi apparatus and delivered to the cell surface for presentation to CD8 T cells. **B, Exogenous:** class II MHC molecules assemble in the ER with an invariant chain protein to prevent acquisition of a peptide in the ER. They are transported in a vesicle through the Golgi apparatus. Exogenous antigen (phagocytosed) is degraded in lysosomes, which then fuse with a vesicle containing the class II MHC molecules. The invariant chain is degraded and displaced by peptides of 11 to 13 amino acids, which bind to the class II MHC molecule. The complex is then delivered to the cell surface for presentation to CD4 T cells. **C, Cross-presentation:** Exogenous antigen enters the ER of dendritic cells and is presented on MHC I molecules to CD8 T cells.

from abnormal or embryonic proteins, which may elicit responses in the adult because the adult was not tolerized to these proteins. Expression of these "foreign" peptides on MHC I at the cell surface allows the T cell to "see" what is going on within the cell.

Class II MHC molecules present peptides from exogenous proteins that were acquired by macropinocytosis, pinocytosis, or phagocytosis and then degraded in lysosomes by APCs. The class II MHC protein is also synthesized in the ER, but unlike MHC I, the invariant chain associates with MHC II to block the peptide-binding cleft and prevent acquisition of a peptide. MHC II acquires its antigenic peptide as a result of a merging of the vesicular transport pathway (carrying newly synthesized class II MHC molecules) and the lysosomal degradation pathway (carrying phagocytosed and proteolyzed proteins). The invariant chain is cleaved and antigenic peptides displace it and associate with the cleft formed in the class II MHC protein; the complex is then delivered to the cell surface.

Cross-presentation of antigen is used mostly by dendritic cells to present antigen to naïve CD8 T cells to initiate the response to viruses and tumor cells. After picking up antigen (including debris from apoptotic cells) in the periphery, the protein is degraded and its peptides enter the cytoplasm and are then shuttled through the transporter associated with processing (TAP) into the ER to bind to MHC I molecules.

The following analogy might aid in the understanding of antigen presentation: All cells degrade their protein "trash" and then display it on the cell surface on class I MHC trash cans. CD8 T cells "policing" the neighborhood are not alarmed by the normal, everyday peptide trash. A viral intruder would produce large amounts of viral peptide trash (e.g., beer cans, pizza boxes) displayed on class I MHC molecular garbage cans, which would alert specific CD8 T cells initiated by DCs. APCs (DCs, macrophages, and B cells) are similar to garbage collectors or sewage workers; they gobble up the neighborhood trash or lymphatic sewage, degrade it, display it on class II MHC molecules, and then move to a lymph node to present the antigenic peptides to the CD4 T cells in the "police station." Foreign antigens would alert the CD4 T cells to release cytokines and activate an immune response.

• Activation of CD4 T Cells and Their Response to Antigen

Activation of naïve T-cell responses is initiated by DCs and then expanded by other APCs (Animation 9-4). Activated DCs have octopus-like arms with large surface area (dendrites), produce cytokines, and have an MHC-rich cell surface to present antigen to T cells. Macrophages and B cells can present antigen to T cells but cannot activate a naïve T cell to initiate a new immune response. CD4 helper T cells are activated by the interaction of the TCR with antigenic peptide presented by class II MHC molecules on the APC (Figure 9-8A). The interaction is strengthened by the binding of CD4 to the class II MHC molecule and the linkage of adhesion proteins on the T cell and the APC. A **co-stimulatory signal** mediated by binding of B7 molecules on the macrophage, dendritic, or B-cell APC to CD28 molecules on the T cell is required to induce growth of the T cell as a fail-safe mechanism to ensure legitimate activation. B7 also interacts with CTLA4, which delivers an inhibitory signal. Activated APCs express sufficient B7 to fill up all the CTLA4 and then bind to the CD28. Cytokine signals (e.g., IL-1, IL-2, IL-6) are also required to initiate growth and overcome regulatory suppression of the cell. Proper activation of the helper T cell promotes production of IL-2 and increases expression of IL-2Rs on the cell surface, enhancing the cell's own ability to bind and maintain activation by IL-2 (Figure 9-9). Once activated, the IL-2 sustains the growth of the cell, and other cytokines influence the subsequent helper T-cell response (see following section). Effector and **memory T cells** are generated as the T cells divide (see Figure 9-9B).

Partial activation (TCR interaction with MHC peptide) of a CD4 T cell without co-stimulation leads to **anergy** (unresponsiveness) or apoptotic death (cell suicide). This is also a mechanism for (1) eliminating self-reactive T cells in the thymus and (2) promoting the development of **tolerance** to self-proteins. Anergy can also result from binding of B7 to CTLA-4 instead of CD28.

The activated, growing CD4 T cells express different adhesion proteins and new chemokine receptors, exit the T-cell sites of the lymph node, and enter the blood or move to B-cell zones of the lymph nodes and spleen. Many of the activated T cells cycle through the skin and mucoepithelium. Cells that present antigen recognized by the TCR initiate close interactions between the T cell and APC that allow the CD28 molecules on the T cell to bind B7 molecules on the APC. These interactions then stimulate the expression of CD40L on the T cell, which interacts with the APC, resulting in mutual activation of the T cell and the APC (see Figure 9-8B). This interaction and the cytokines produced by the T cell will activate and determine the function of the macrophages and DCs and which immunoglobulin the B cell will produce.

CD4 T-Helper Cell Functions

The CD4 T cells promote expansion of the immune response with cell growth–promoting cytokines and define the nature of the response with other cytokines. The different types of T-helper cells are defined by the cytokines they secrete and thus the responses they induce (Figure 9-10 and Box 9-4; also see Table 9-1).

The primary role of the **TH0 cells** is to expand the immune response by producing cytokines that promote lymphocyte growth and activate DCs, including IL-2, interferon (IFN)-γ, and IL-4. **IL-2** promotes T, B, and innate lymphoid (including NK cells) cell growth to expand the immune response.

Initial antibacterial and antifungal responses are mediated by the **TH17** cells. These are CD4 T-helper cells stimulated by IL-6 plus transforming growth factor (TGF)-β or, for memory T cells, IL-23. IL-23 is in the IL-12 family of cytokines. IL-23 and IL-12 both have a p40 subunit, but IL-12 has a p35, whereas IL-23 has a p19 subunit. TH17 cells make cytokines (e.g., IL-17, IL-22, IL-6, TNF-α) and pro-inflammatory chemokines, which activate epithelial cells and neutrophils and promote inflammatory responses. TH17 responses provide protection in immunoprivileged sites such as the eye, where there is an abundance of TGF-β. TH17 responses are associated with cell-mediated autoimmune inflammatory diseases such as rheumatoid arthritis.

The **TH1 response (1 meaning *early*)** *usually occurs early in response to an infection and activates both cellular and antibody responses* (Animation 9-5). Activation of **TH1** responses requires **IL-12** produced by DCs and macrophages. TH1 cells are characterized by secretion of **IL-2, IFN-γ,** and **TNF-β (lymphotoxin [LT]). IFN-γ,** also known as **macrophage activation factor,** reinforces TH1 responses by promoting more IL-12 production, creating a self-sustaining cycle. IFN-γ also promotes production of IgG and inhibits TH2 responses. **TNF-β** can activate neutrophils. TH1 cells are inhibited by IL-4 and IL-10, which is produced by TH2 cells. Activated TH1 cells also express the **FasL** ligand, which can interact with the **Fas** protein on target cells to promote apoptosis (killing) of the target cell and the CCR5 chemokine receptor that promotes relocation to sites of infection. Human immunodeficiency virus (HIV) uses the CCR5 chemokine receptor as a co-receptor with CD4 to initiate infection of an individual.

The TH1 responses amplify local inflammatory reactions and delayed-type hypersensitivity (DTH) reactions by activating macrophages, NK cells, and CD8 cytotoxic T cells and also expand the immune response by stimulating growth of B and T cells with IL-2. These responses are important for

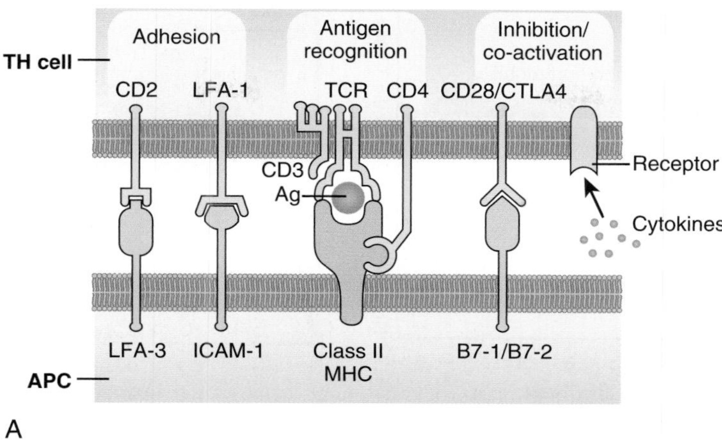

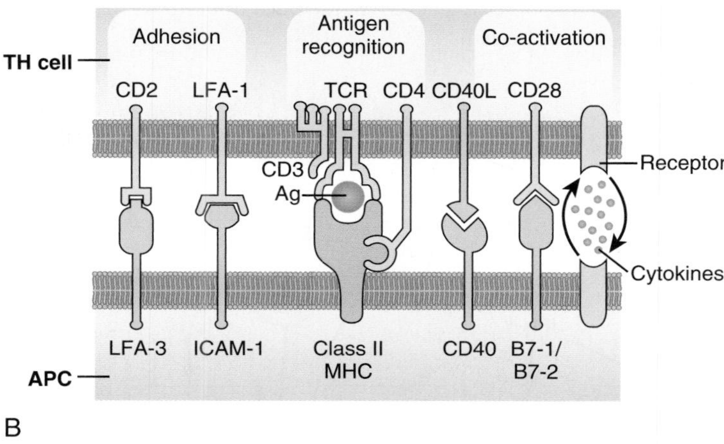

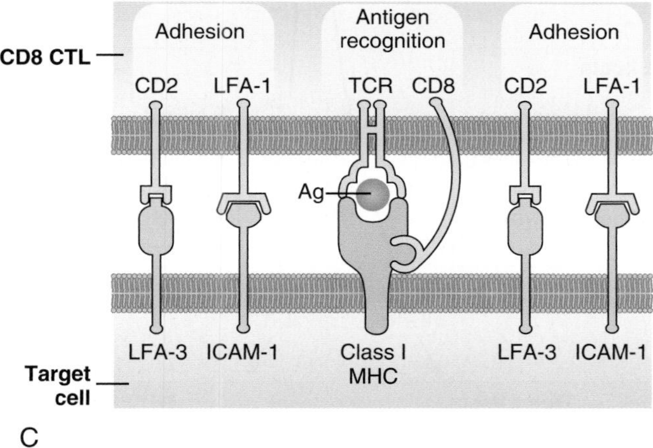

FIGURE 9-8 The molecules involved in the interaction between T cells and antigen-presenting cells *(APCs)*. **A,** Initiation of a CD4 T-cell response. Initiation of a CD8 T-cell response is similar, but CD8 and the T-cell receptor *(TCR)* interact with peptide major histocompatibility complex *(MHC)* I and the peptide it holds. **B,** CD4 T-cell helper binding to a B cell, dendritic cell, or macrophage. **C,** CD8 T cell binding to target cell creates an immunosynapse into which perforin and granzymes are secreted. Cell surface receptor-ligand interactions and cytokines are indicated with the direction of their action. *Ag,* Antigen; *CTLA4,* cytotoxic T lymphocyte A4; *ICAM-1,* intercellular adhesion molecule-1; *LFA-1,* leukocyte function–associated antigen-1. (From Rosenthal KS, Tan M: *Rapid reviews in microbiology and immunology,* ed 3, Philadelphia, 2010, Elsevier.)

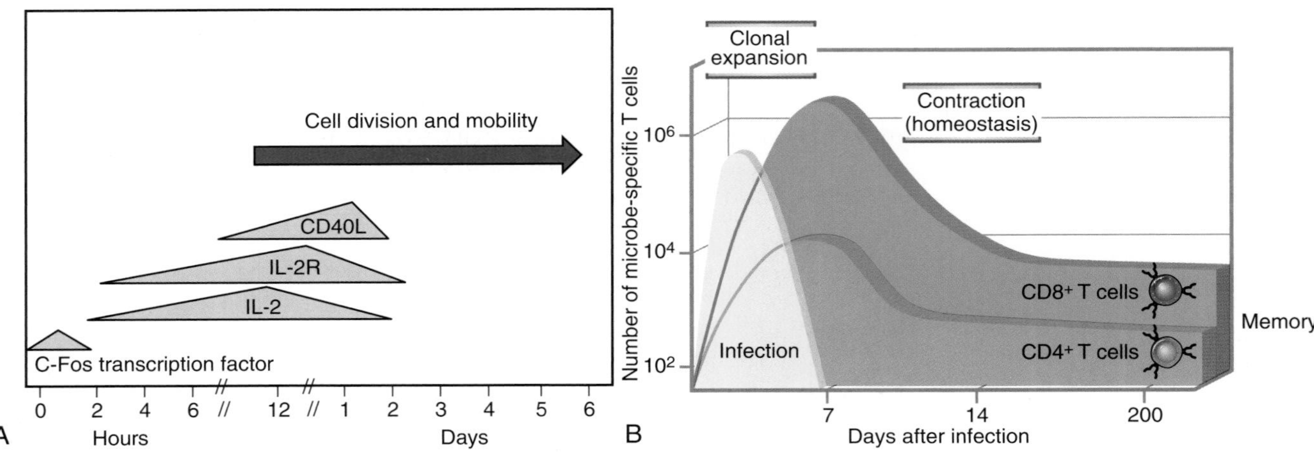

FIGURE 9-9 Progression of naïve T-cell activation and response. **A,** Interaction with antigen and co-receptors from the antigen-presenting cell (APC) activates expression of new transcription factors *(c-Fos),* interleukin *(IL)*-2 and the IL-2R to promote growth and CD40L to activate the APC. **B,** CD4 or CD8 T-cell numbers rise rapidly in response to infection, after which the activated T cells will apoptose, leaving memory T cells. Activation of memory T-cell responses is quicker. (**B,** Modified from Abbas AK, Lichtman AH, Pillai S, et al: *Cellular and molecular immunology,* ed 8, Philadelphia, 2015, Elsevier.)

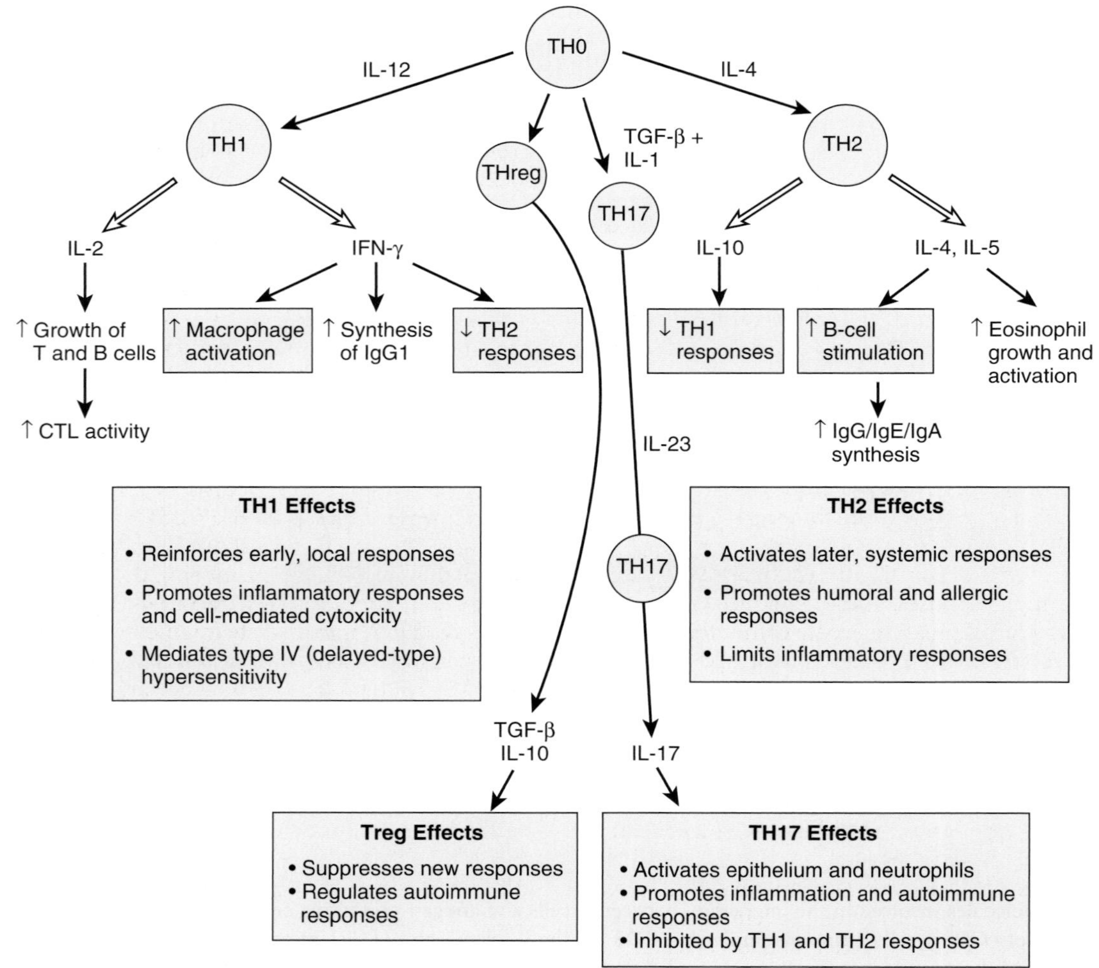

FIGURE 9-10 T-cell responses are determined by cytokines. Dendritic cells initiate and determine the type of CD4 T-cell responses by the cytokines they produce. Similarly, T cells tell other cells what to do with other cytokines. The response-defining cytokines are indicated. ↑, Increase; ↓, decrease; *CTL,* cytotoxic T lymphocyte; *IFN-γ,* interferon-γ; *IgG/IgE/IgA,* immunoglobulin G/E/A; *IL,* interleukin; *TGF-β,* transforming growth factor-β; *TH,* T helper (cell). (From Rosenthal KS, Tan M: *Rapid reviews in microbiology and immunology,* ed 3, Philadelphia, 2010, Elsevier.)

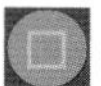 **Box 9-4 T-Helper Responses and Their Cytokines**

Activated TH cells express CD40L to activate B cells, macrophages, and DCs.
TH cells produce growth-stimulating and response-defining cytokines.
Growth-stimulating cytokines: GM-CSF, IL-3
TH1: requires induction with IL-12
IFN-γ: activates M1 (inflammatory) macrophages; promotes B-cell production of IgG; inhibits TH2
IL-2: promotes T, B, and NK cell growth
TNF-α and TNF-β: promote inflammation and cytotoxicity
TH2: induced by IL-4
IL-4: T-cell growth factor, stimulates immunoglobulin class switch (IgG, IgE), activation of mast cells, M2 (alternative) macrophage
IL-5: B-cell and eosinophil growth factor, stimulates immunoglobulin class switch (IgG, IgA)
IL-10: B-cell growth factor and inhibitor of TH1 and inflammatory responses
TH17: induced by TGF-β + IL-1; memory T cells by IL-23
IL-17: activates neutrophils, monocytes
IL-22: stimulates epithelium to produce antimicrobial peptides
TFH: influenced by TH1 or TH2 cytokines
IL-21: germinal center development, plasma cell and memory B-cell development
IFN-γ or IL-4: see above
Treg: requires IL-2
TGF-β: inhibits naïve T-cell and other T-cell activation, inhibits inflammation
IL-10: see above

DCs, Dendritic cells; *GM-CSF,* granulocyte-macrophage colony-stimulating factor; *IFN,* interferon; *Ig,* immunoglobulin; *IL,* interleukin; *TGF,* transforming growth factor; *TNF,* tumor necrosis factor.

eliminating intracellular infections (e.g., viruses, bacteria, parasites) and fungi and for antitumor responses but are also associated with cell-mediated autoimmune inflammatory diseases (e.g., multiple sclerosis, Crohn disease).

The **TH2 response (2 meaning second)** is the default T-cell response. It occurs later in response to infection and acts systemically through antibody-mediated responses. The TH2 response promotes antibody production to antigenic debris in the lymphatic system, which occurs in the absence of an IL-12/IFN-γ signal from innate responses. TH2 cells release IL-4, IL-5, IL-6, and IL-10 cytokines that promote humoral (systemic) responses. These cytokines stimulate the B cell to undergo recombination events within the immunoglobulin gene to switch from production of IgM and IgD to production of specific types and subtypes of IgG, IgE, or IgA. TH2 responses are associated with production of IgE, which is useful for antihelminthic responses but mediates allergies. TH2 responses can exacerbate an intracellular infection (e.g., *Mycobacterium leprae, Leishmania*) by prematurely shutting off protective TH1 responses. TH2 cell development is inhibited by IFN-γ.

Follicular helper T cells (TFH) reside in the follicles of the lymph node, the B cell zones of the lymph node. They relay the cytokine responses, whether TH1 or TH2, to the B cells to promote production of the appropriate antibody. They also promote development of germinal centers, which are foci of specific memory cell, plasma cell, and antibody production.

Treg cells expressing $CD4^+CD25^+$ are antigen-specific suppressor cells. These cells prevent development of autoimmune and overzealous responses by producing TGF-β and IL-10, help to keep T-cell responses under control, and promote memory cell development. Treg cells are especially important to regulate responses to normal flora on the skin and in the gastrointestinal tract. Other TH responses (e.g., TH9 and TH22) have been described, and their names refer to the primary cytokine they produce or the functions promoted by the cytokine.

• CD8 T Cells

CD8 T cells include cytotoxic T lymphocytes **(CTLs),** but they can also produce cytokines and influence immune responses. CTLs are part of the TH1 response and are important for eliminating virally infected cells and tumor cells. They release proteins that convince the target cell to commit apoptosis.

The CTL response is initiated when naïve CD8 T cells in the lymph node are activated by antigen-presenting DCs and cytokines produced by TH1 CD4 T cells, including IL-2 (similar to activation of CD4 T cells but with MHC I interacting with CD8, as in Figure 9-8A). The DC may have acquired the antigen as a result of a viral infection or by cross-presentation of an antigen acquired at the site of infection or tumor prior to maturation. The activated CD8 T cells divide and differentiate into mature CTLs which disseminate through the blood. During a viral challenge, the numbers of specific CTLs will increase up to 100,000 times. When the activated CTL finds a target cell, it binds tightly through interactions of the TCR with antigen-bearing class I MHC proteins and adhesion molecules on both cells (similar to the closing of a zipper). **Granules** containing toxic molecules, **granzymes (esterases),** and a pore-forming protein **(perforin)** move to the site of interaction and release their contents into the pocket **(immune synapse)** formed between the T cell and target cell. **Perforin** generates holes in the target cell membrane to allow the granule contents to enter and induce **apoptosis (programmed cell death)** in the target cell. CD8 T cells can also initiate apoptosis in target cells through the interaction of the **FasL on the T cell with the Fas protein on the target cell surface.** FasL is a member of the TNF family of proteins, and Fas is a member of the TNF receptor family of proteins. Apoptosis is characterized by degradation of the target cell DNA into discrete fragments of approximately 200 base pairs and disruption of internal membranes. The cells shrink into apoptotic bodies, which are readily phagocytosed by macrophages and DCs. Apoptosis is a clean method of cell death, unlike necrosis, which signals neutrophil action and further tissue damage. TH1 CD4 T cells and NK cells also express FasL and can initiate apoptosis in target cells.

Suppressor T cells provide antigen-specific regulation of helper T-cell function through inhibitory cytokines and other means. Like CTLs, suppressor T cells interact with class I MHC molecules.

• NKT Cells

NKT cells are like a hybrid between NK cells and T cells. They express an NK cell marker, NK1.1, and an **α/β** TCR. Unlike other T cells, the TCR repertoire is very limited. They may express CD4, but most lack CD4 and CD8 molecules ($CD4^-CD8^-$). The TCR of most NKT cells reacts with CD1 molecules, which present microbial glycolipids and glycopeptides. Upon activation, NKT cells release large amounts of IL-4 and IFN-γ. NKT cells help in the initial responses to infection and are very important for defense against mycobacterial infections.

• B Cells and Humoral Immunity

The primary molecular component of the humoral immune response is antibody produced by B cells and plasma cells. Antibodies provide protection from rechallenge by an infectious agent, block spread of the agent in the blood, neutralize virulence factors, and facilitate elimination of the infectious agent. To accomplish these tasks, an incredibly large repertoire of antibody molecules must be available to recognize the tremendous number of infectious agents and molecules that challenge our bodies. In addition to interacting specifically with foreign structures, the antibody molecules must also interact with host systems and cells (e.g., complement, macrophages) to promote clearance of antigen and activation of subsequent immune responses (Box 9-5). Antibody molecules also serve as the cell surface receptors that stimulate the appropriate B-cell antibody factories to grow and produce more antibody in response to antigenic challenge.

Box 9-5 Antimicrobial Actions of Antibodies

Are opsonins: promote ingestion and killing by phagocytic cells (immunoglobulin [Ig]G)
Neutralize (block attachment of) bacteria, toxins, and viruses
Agglutinate bacteria: may aid in clearing
Render motile organisms nonmotile
Combine with antigens on the microbial surface and activate the complement cascade, thus inducing an inflammatory response, bringing fresh phagocytes and serum antibodies into the site
Combine with antigens on the microbial surface, activate the complement cascade, and anchor the membrane attack complex involving C5b to C9

• Immunoglobulin Types and Structures

Immunoglobulins are composed of at least two heavy chains and two light chains, a dimer of dimers. They are subdivided into classes and subclasses based on the structure and antigenic distinction of their heavy chains. IgG, IgM, and IgA are the major antibody forms, whereas IgD and IgE make up less than 1% of the total immunoglobulins. The IgA and IgG classes of immunoglobulin are divided further into subclasses based on differences in the Fc portion. There are four subclasses of IgG, designated as IgG1 through IgG4, and two IgA subclasses (IgA1 and IgA2) (Figure 9-11).

Antibody molecules are Y-shaped molecules with two major structural regions that mediate the two major functions of the molecule (Table 9-2; also see Figure 9-11). The **variable-region/antigen-combining site** must be able to identify and specifically interact with an epitope on an antigen. A large number of different antibody molecules, each with a different variable region, are produced in every individual to recognize the seemingly infinite number of different antigens in nature. The **Fc portion** (stem of the antibody Y) interacts with host systems and cells to promote clearance of antigen and activation of subsequent immune responses. The Fc portion is responsible for fixation of complement and binding of the molecule to cell surface immunoglobulin receptors **(FcR)** on macrophages, NK cells, T cells, and other cells. For IgG and IgA, the Fc portion interacts with other proteins to promote transfer across the placenta and the mucosa, respectively (Table 9-3). In addition, each of the different types of antibody can be synthesized

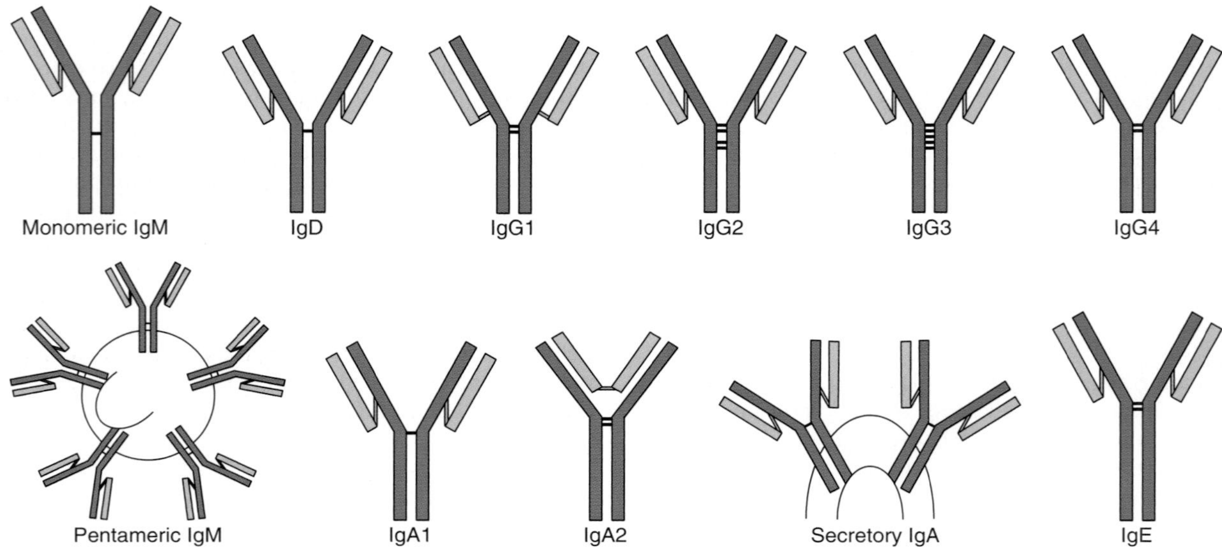

FIGURE 9-11 Comparative structures of the immunoglobulin classes and subclasses in humans. IgA and IgM are held together in multimers by the J chain. IgA can acquire the secretory component for the traversal of epithelial cells.

Table 9-2 Properties and Functions of Immunoglobulins

Properties and Functions	IgM	IgD	IgG	IgE	IgA
Heavy-chain	μ	δ	γ	ε	α
Subclasses			$\gamma_1, \gamma_2, \gamma_3, \gamma_4$		α_1, α_2
Molecular weight (kDa)	900	185	154	190	160
% Serum immunoglobulin	5-10	<1	75-85	<1	5-15
Half-life (days)	5	2-3	23	2-3	6
T-cell requirement	Independent	Independent	Dependent	Dependent	Dependent
Time/memory	Early, primary	Early, primary	Later, memory	Later, memory	Later, memory
Complement	++	–	++	–	–
Opsonization	*	–	++	–	–
ADCC	++	–	++	–	–
Crosses placenta	–	–	++	–	–
Protects mucosa	+	–	+†	–	+++
Activates mast cell	–	–	–	+++	–

ADCC, Antibody-dependent cellular cytotoxicity.
*Opsonizes by fixing complement.
†Transported by neonatal Fc receptor.

Table 9-3 Fc Interactions with Immune Components

Immune Component	Interaction	Function
Fc receptor	Macrophages	Opsonization
	Polymorphonuclear neutrophils	Opsonization
	T cells	Activation
	Natural killer cells (antibody-dependent cellular cytotoxicity)	Killing
	Mast cells for immunoglobulin (Ig)E	Allergic reactions, antiparasitic
	Neonatal IgG receptor	Transport across capillary membranes
Complement	Complement system	Opsonization, killing (especially bacteria), activation of inflammation

with a **membrane-spanning portion** to make it a cell surface antigen receptor.

IgG and IgA have a flexible **hinge region** rich in proline and susceptible to cleavage by proteolytic enzymes. Digestion of IgG molecules with **papain** yields two **Fab** fragments and one **Fc** fragment (Figure 9-12). Each Fab fragment has one antigen-binding site. **Pepsin** cleaves the molecule, producing an **F(ab′)$_2$** fragment with two antigen-binding sites and a **pFc′** fragment.

The different types and parts of immunoglobulin can also be distinguished using antibodies directed against different portions of the molecule. **Isotypes (IgM, IgD, IgG, IgA, IgE)** are determined by antibodies directed against the Fc portion of the molecule (*iso-* meaning the same for all people.) **Allotypic** differences occur for antibody molecules with the same isotype but contain protein sequences that differ from one person to another (in addition to the antigen-binding region). *(All ["allo"] of us have differences.)* The **idiotype** refers to the protein sequences in the variable region that comprise the large number of antigen-binding regions. *(There are many different idiots in the world.)*

On a molecular basis, each antibody molecule is made up of heavy and light chains encoded by separate genes. The basic immunoglobulin unit consists of **two heavy (H)** and **two light (L) chains.** IgM and IgA consist of multimers of this basic structure. The heavy and light chains of immunoglobulin are fastened together by **interchain disulfide bonds.** Two types of light chains—**κ** and **λ**—are present in all five immunoglobulin classes, although only one type is present in an individual molecule. Approximately 60% of human immunoglobulin molecules have κ light chains, and 40% have λ light chains. There are **five types of heavy chains,** one for each isotype of antibody **(IgM, μ; IgG, γ; IgD, δ; IgA, α; and IgE, ε)**. Intrachain disulfide bonds define molecular domains within each chain. Light chains have a variable and a constant domain. The heavy chains have a variable and three (IgG, IgA) or four (IgM, IgE) constant domains. The variable domains on the heavy and light chains interact to form the antigen-binding site. The constant domains from each chain make up the Fc portion, provide the molecular structure to the immunoglobulin, and define the interaction of the antibody molecule with host systems, hence its

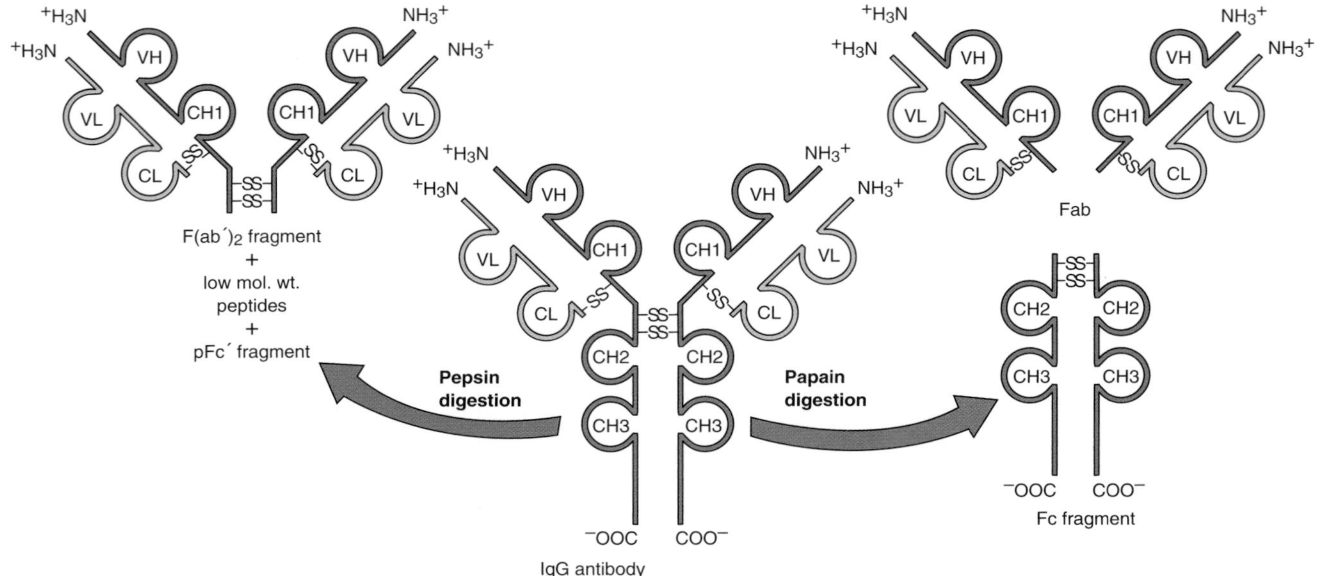

FIGURE 9-12 Proteolytic digestion of immunoglobulin *(Ig)*G. Pepsin treatment produces a dimeric $F(ab')_2$ fragment. Papain treatment produces monovalent Fab fragments and an Fc fragment. The $F(ab')_2$ and the Fab fragments bind antigen but lack a functional Fc region. The heavy chain is depicted in *blue;* the light chain in *orange. mol. wt.,* Molecular weight.

ultimate function. The heavy chain of the different antibody molecules can also be synthesized with a membrane-spanning region to make the antibody an antigen-specific cell surface receptor for the B cell.

Immunoglobulin D

IgD, which has a molecular mass of 185 kDa, accounts for less than 1% of serum immunoglobulins. IgD exists primarily as membrane IgD, which serves with IgM as an antigen receptor on early B-cell membranes to help initiate antibody responses by activating B-cell growth. IgD and IgM are the only isotypes that can be expressed together by the same cell.

Immunoglobulin M

IgM is the first antibody produced in response to antigenic challenge and can be produced in a T cell–independent manner. IgM makes up 5% to 10% of the total immunoglobulins in adults and has a half-life of 5 days. It is a **pentameric molecule** with five immunoglobulin units joined by the **J chain,** with a total molecular mass of 900 kDa. Theoretically, this immunoglobulin has 10 antigen-binding sites. IgM is the most efficient immunoglobulin for fixing (binding) complement. A single IgM pentamer can activate the classical complement pathway. Monomeric IgM is found with IgD on the B-cell surface, where it serves as the receptor for antigen. Because IgM is relatively large, it remains in the blood and spreads inefficiently from the blood into tissue. IgM is particularly important for immunity against polysaccharide antigens on the exterior of pathogenic microorganisms. It also promotes phagocytosis and promotes bacteriolysis by activating complement through its Fc portion. IgM is also a major component of rheumatoid factors (autoantibodies).

Immunoglobulin G

IgG comprises approximately 85% of the immunoglobulins in adults. It has a molecular mass of 154 kDa, based on two L chains of 22,000 Da each and two H chains of 55,000 Da each. The four subclasses of IgG differ in structure (see Figure 9-11), relative concentration, and function. Production of IgG requires T-cell help. IgG, as a class of antibody molecules, has the longest half-life (23 days) of the five immunoglobulin classes, binds the neonatal Fc receptor and is transported across the placenta and certain other membranes, and is the principal antibody in the **anamnestic (booster) response.** IgG shows high avidity (binding capacity) for antigens, fixes complement, stimulates chemotaxis, and acts as an opsonin to facilitate phagocytosis.

Immunoglobulin A

IgA comprises 5% to 15% of the serum immunoglobulins and has a half-life of 6 days. It has a molecular mass of 160 kDa and a basic four-chain monomeric structure. However, it can occur as monomers, dimers, trimers, and multimers combined by the J chain (similar to IgM). In addition to serum IgA, a **secretory IgA** appears in body secretions. IgA production requires specialized T-cell help and mucosal stimulation. The J chain of IgA binds to a **poly-Ig receptor** on epithelial cells for transport across the cell. The poly-Ig receptor remains bound to IgA and is then cleaved to become the **secretory component** when secretory IgA is secreted from the cell. An adult secretes approximately 2 g of IgA per day. Secretory IgA appears in colostrum, intestinal and respiratory secretions, saliva, tears, stool, and other secretions. IgA-deficient individuals have an increased incidence of respiratory tract infections.

Immunoglobulin E

IgE accounts for less than 1% of the total immunoglobulins and has a half-life of approximately 2.5 days. Most IgE is bound to Fc receptors on **mast cells,** on which it serves as a receptor for allergens and parasite antigens. When sufficient antigen binds to the IgE on the mast cell, the mast cell releases histamine, prostaglandin, platelet-activating factor,

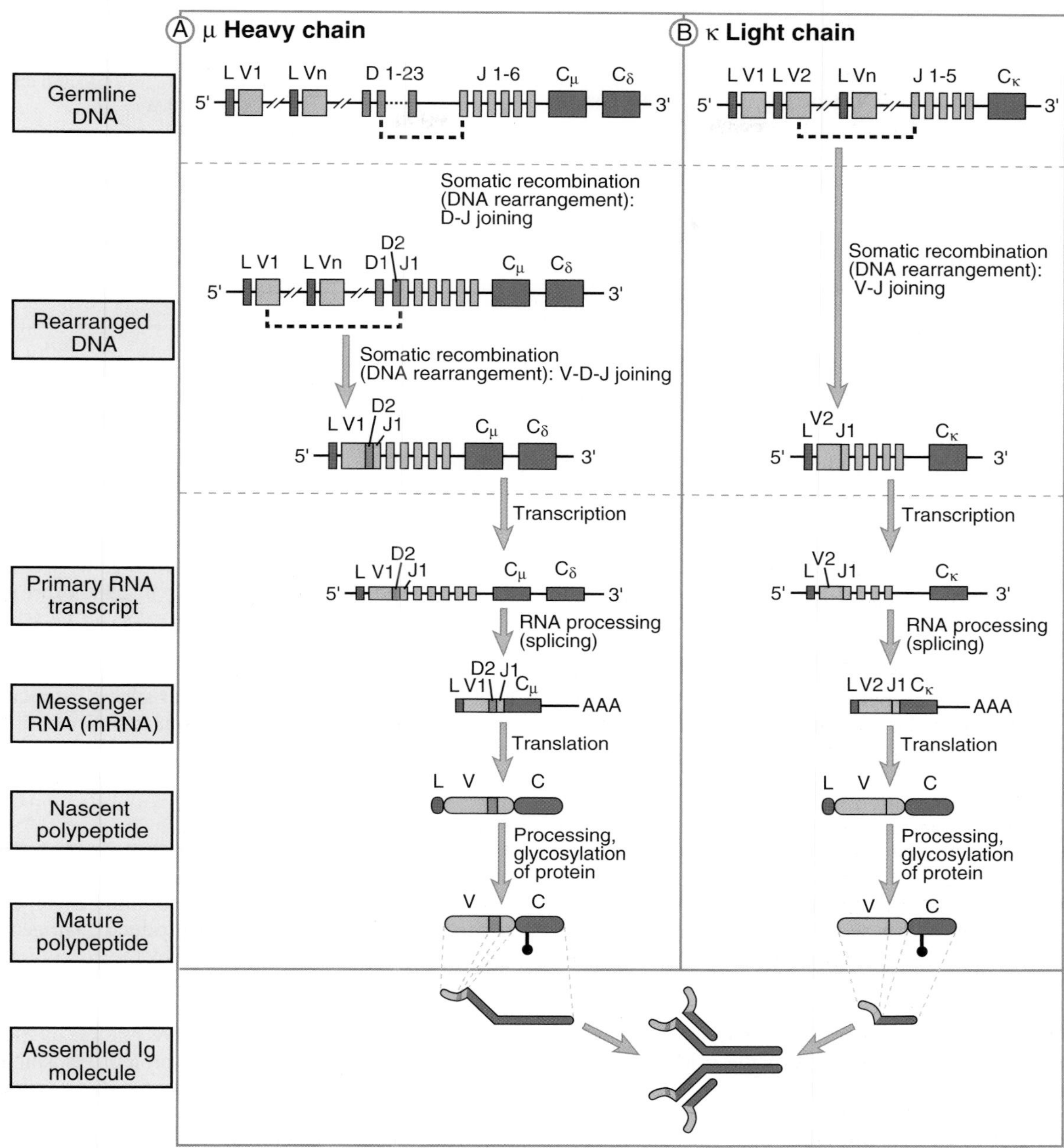

FIGURE 9-13 Immunoglobulin gene rearrangement to produce IgM (**A,** heavy-chain sequences and **B,** light-chain sequences). The germline immunoglobulin gene contains multiple V, D, and J genes that recombine and delete intervening sequences and juxtaposes the variable region sequences to the μ-δ heavy-chain sequences during the development of the B cell in the bone marrow. T-cell help induces differentiation of the B cell and promotes genetic recombination and immunoglobulin class switching. Switch regions in front of the constant-region genes (including IgG subclasses) allow attachment of the preformed VDJ region with other heavy-chain constant-region genes, genetically removing the μ, δ, and other intervening genes. This produces an immunoglobulin gene with the same VDJ region (except for somatic mutation) but different heavy-chain genes. Splicing of messenger RNA (mRNA) produces the final IgM and IgD mRNA.

and cytokines. IgE is important for protection against parasitic infection and is responsible for **anaphylactic hypersensitivity** (type 1) (rapid allergic reactions).

• Immunogenetics

The antibody response can recognize at least 10^8 structures but can still specifically amplify and focus a response directed to a specific challenge. The mechanisms for generating this antibody repertoire and the different immunoglobulin subclasses are tied to random genetic events that accompany the development (differentiation) of the B cell (Figure 9-13).

Human chromosomes 2, 22, and 14 contain immunoglobulin genes for κ, λ, and H chains, respectively. The **germline** forms of these genes consist of different and separate sets of genetic building blocks for the light **(V and J gene segments)** and heavy chains **(V, D, and J gene segments)**, which are genetically recombined to produce the immunoglobulin variable regions. These variable regions are then connected to the constant-region C gene segments. For the κ light chain, there are 300 V gene segments, 5 J gene segments, and only one C gene segment. The number of λ gene segments for V and J is more limited. For the heavy chain, there are 300 to 1000 V genes, 12 D genes, and 6 (heavy-chain) J genes but only 9 C genes (one for each class and subclass of antibody [**μ; δ; γ_3, γ_1, γ_2, and γ_4; ε; α_1 and α_2**]). In addition, gene segments for membrane-spanning peptides can be attached to the heavy-chain genes to allow the antibody molecule to insert into the B-cell membrane as an antigen-activation receptor.

Production of the antibody molecule in the pre-B cell occurs in the bone marrow. Genetic recombination at the deoxyribonucleic acid (DNA) level and posttranscriptional processing at the ribonucleic acid (RNA) level assemble the immunoglobulin gene and produce the functional messenger RNA (mRNA) (see Figure 9-13). Each of the V, D, and J segments is surrounded by DNA sequences that promote **directional recombination and loss of the intervening DNA sequences.** The enzyme produced by the **RAG gene** is essential for recombination of these segments. Randomly inserted nucleotides at the junction sites connect the two strands, which can enhance the diversity of sequences or inactivate the gene if it disrupts the reading frame for the subsequent mRNA. The light-chain gene segment is produced by juxtaposition of randomly chosen κ or λ V and J gene segments, and the variable region of the heavy-chain segment is produced by juxtaposition of its V, D, and J genes. These recombination reactions are analogous to matching and sewing together similar patterns from a long swatch of cloth and then cutting out the intervening loops of extra cloth.

The complete heavy-chain gene is produced by attachment of the variable-region sequences (VDJ) by recombination to the μ; δ; γ_3, γ_1, γ_2, and γ_4; ε; or α_1 and α_2 sequences of the constant region (C) gene segments. In the pre-B and immature B cells, mRNAs are produced that contain the variable-region gene segments connected to the C gene sequences for μ and δ. Processing of the mRNA removes either the μ or δ, as if it were an intron, to produce the final immunoglobulin mRNA. The pre-B cell expresses cytoplasmic IgM, whereas the B cell expresses cytoplasmic and cell surface IgM and cell surface IgD. IgM and IgD are the only pair of isotypes that can be expressed on the same cell.

Class switching (IgM to IgG, IgE, or IgA) occurs in mature B cells in response to different cytokines produced by TH1 or TH2 CD4 helper T cells (Figure 9-14). Each of the C gene segments, except δ, is preceded by a DNA sequence called the **switch site.** After the appropriate cytokine signal, the switch in front of the μ sequence recombines with the switch in front of the γ_3, γ_1, γ_2, or γ_4; ε; or α_1 or α_2 sequences, creating a DNA loop that is subsequently removed. Processing of the RNA transcript yields the final mRNA for the immunoglobulin heavy-chain protein. For example, IgG1 production would result from excision of DNA containing the C gene segments C_μ, C_δ, and $C_{\gamma3}$ to attach the variable region to the γ_1 C gene segment. **Class switching changes the function of the antibody molecule (Fc region) but does not change its specificity (variable region).**

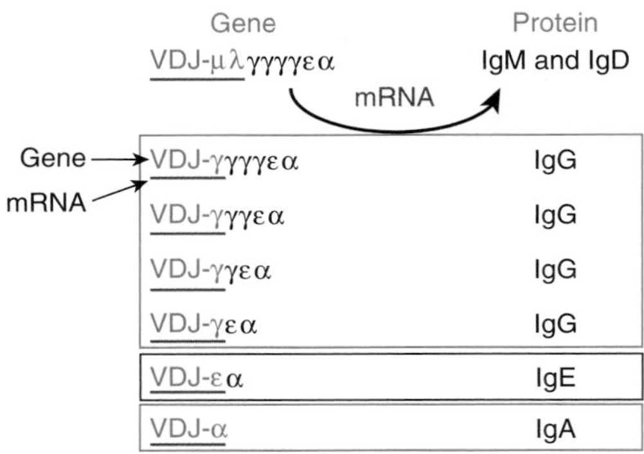

FIGURE 9-14 Immunoglobulin class switching. The VDJ portion recombines with different heavy-chain genes, deleting the intervening sequences to produce a gene for an antibody of the desired antigen specificity but with different Fc-determined functions.

The final steps in B-cell differentiation to memory cells or plasma cells do not change the antibody gene. **Memory cells** are long-lived, antigen-responsive B cells expressing the CD45RO surface marker. Memory cells can be activated in response to antigen later in life to divide and then produce its specific antibody. **Plasma cells** are terminally differentiated B cells with a small nucleus but a large cytoplasm filled with endoplasmic reticulum. Plasma cells are antibody factories with a finite lifetime.

• Antibody Response

The B cells that best recognize the different epitopes of the antigen are selected to increase in number in a process termed **clonal expansion.** B cells producing antigen-specific antibody are selected and activated by the binding of antigen to surface immunoglobulin. The cell surface antibody acts as an antigen receptor to trigger activation of the B cell through its associated signal transduction receptors, Ig-α (CD79a) and Ig-β (CD79b). A cascade of protein tyrosine kinases, phospholipase C, and calcium fluxes activate transcription and cell growth to mediate the activation signal. Other surface molecules, including the CR2 (CD21) complement (C3d) receptor, amplify the activation signal. The combination of these signals triggers growth and increases the number of cells making antibodies to that antigen (Animation 9-6).

T-independent antigens, such as flagellin and capsular polysaccharide, have repetitive structures that can cross-link sufficient numbers of surface antibody to stimulate growth of the antigen-specific IgM- and IgD-producing B cells. Binding of the C3d component of complement to its receptor (CR2, CD21) facilitates activation of the antibody response. In contrast, production of antibody to **T-dependent antigens** uses follicular dendritic cells as bulletin boards to display multiple units of the antigen to the surface antibody and requires help from CD4 T cells through binding of CD40L (T cell) to CD40 (on the B cell) and the action of cytokines. Different combinations of cytokines induce immunoglobulin class switching. *TH1-helper responses (IFN-γ) promote production of IgG. TH2-helper responses (IL-4,*

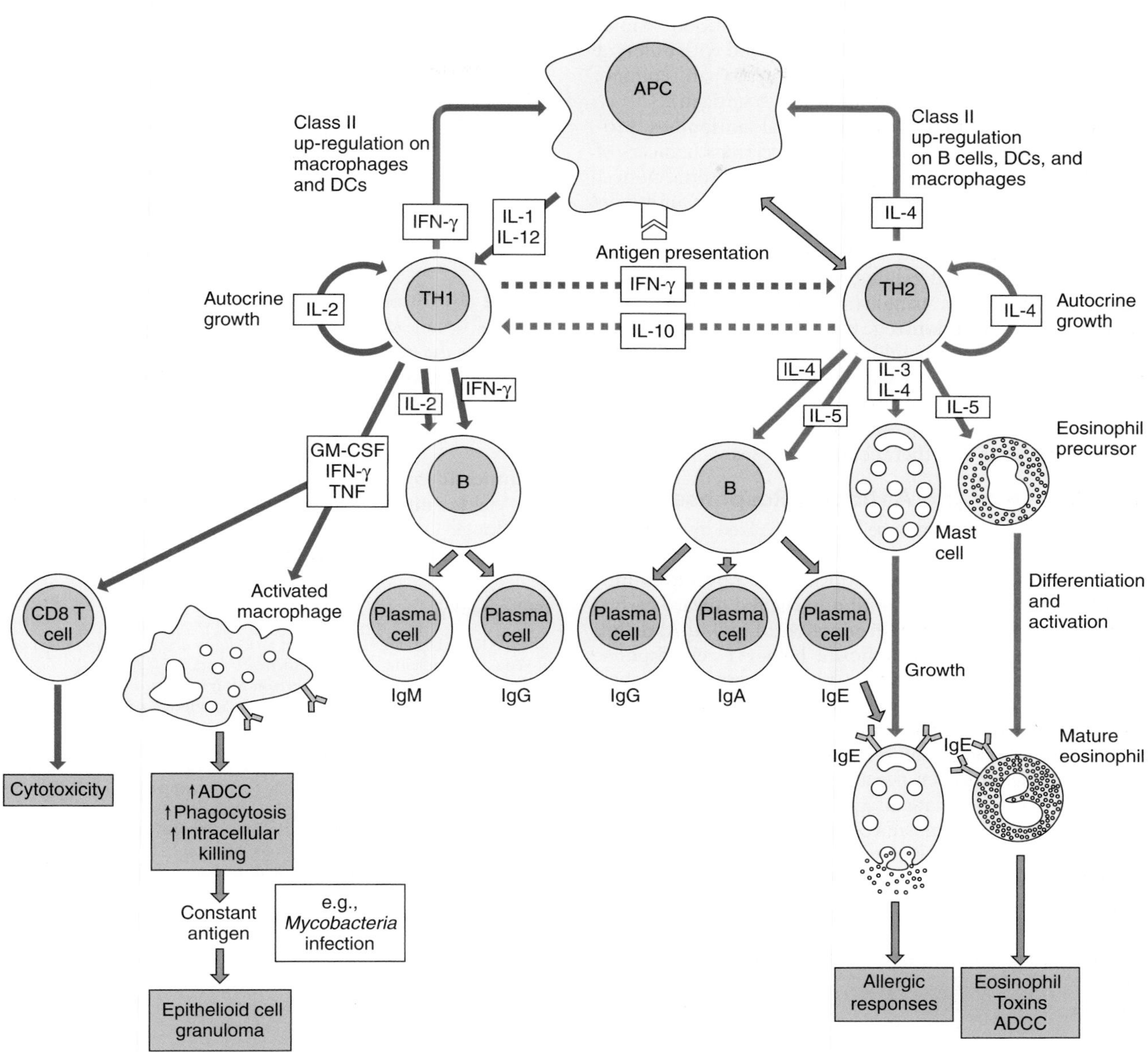

FIGURE 9-15 T-cell help determines the nature of the immune response. Receptor-ligand interactions between T cells and B cells and cytokines associated with TH1 or TH2 determine the subsequent response. TH1 responses are initiated by interleukin *(IL)*-12 and delivered by interferon-γ *(IFN-γ)* and IL-2 to promote cell-mediated and immunoglobulin *(Ig)*G production *(solid blue lines)* and inhibit TH2 responses *(dotted blue lines)*. IL-4 and IL-5 from TH2 cells promote humoral responses *(solid red lines),* and IL-4 and IL-10 inhibit TH1 responses *(dotted red lines)*. Mucosal epithelium promotes secretory IgA production. Colored boxes denote end results. ↑, Increase; ↓, decrease; *ADCC,* antibody-dependent cellular cytotoxicity; *APC,* antigen-presenting cell; *CTL,* cytotoxic T lymphocyte; *DCs,* dendritic cells; *DTH,* delayed-type hypersensitivity; *GM-CSF,* granulocyte-macrophage colony-stimulating factor; *TNF,* tumor necrosis factor.

IL-5) promote production of IgG, IgE, and IgA. IgA production is especially promoted by IL-5 and TGF-β (Figure 9-15).

Clonal expansion of the antigen-specific activated B cells occurs in the germinal centers with help from follicular helper T cells (Animation 9-7). Stimulation of B cell growth also promotes ***somatic mutation*** *of the variable region, increasing the diversity of antibody molecules* directed at the specific antigen. The B-cell clones that express antibody with the strongest antigen binding are preferentially stimulated. This selects a better antibody response. Ultimately, the process generates memory B cells and the ultimate antibody factory, the plasma cell.

With an increase in the number of antibody factories making the relevant antibody, the strength and specificity of the antibody response is thus increased. During an immune response, antibodies are made against different epitopes of the foreign object, protein, or infectious agent. *Specific antibody is a mixture of many different immunoglobulin molecules made by many different B cells* **(polyclonal antibody),** each immunoglobulin molecule differing in the epitope it recognizes and the strength of the interaction. Antibody molecules that recognize the same antigen may bind with different strengths (**affinity,** monovalent binding to an epitope; **avidity,** multivalent binding of antibody to antigen).

Monoclonal antibodies are identical antibodies produced by a single clone of cells or by myelomas (cancers of plasma cells) or hybridomas. Hybridomas are cloned, laboratory-derived cells obtained by the fusion of antibody-producing spleen cells and a myeloma cell. In 1975, Kohler and Millstein developed the technique for producing monoclonal antibodies from B-cell hybridomas. The hybridoma is immortal and produces a single (monoclonal) antibody. This technique has revolutionized the study of immunology because it allows selection (cloning) of individual antibody-producing cells and their development into cellular factories for production of large quantities of that antibody. Monoclonal antibodies have been commercially produced for both diagnostic reagents and therapeutic purposes.

Time Course of the Antibody Response

The primary antibody response is characterized by the initial production of IgM. IgM antibodies appear in the blood within 3 days to 2 weeks after exposure to a novel immunogen. This is the only type of antibody elicited toward carbohydrates (bacterial capsule). Production of IgG, IgA, or IgE requires development of a sufficient helper T-cell response to promote the class switch and requires approximately 8 days. The predominant serum antibody will be IgG antibodies (Figure 9-16). The first antibodies produced react with residual antigen and therefore are rapidly cleared. After the initial lag phase, however, the antibody titer increases logarithmically to reach a plateau. IgG has a half-life in blood of 23 days, and long-lived plasma cells may continue to produce the antibody for years, depending upon the strength and nature of the challenge.

Reexposure to an immunogen, a **secondary response,** induces a heightened antibody response (also termed **anamnestic response**). Activation of preformed memory cells yields a much more rapid production of antibody, which lasts longer and reaches a higher titer. The antibodies in a secondary response are principally of the IgG class.

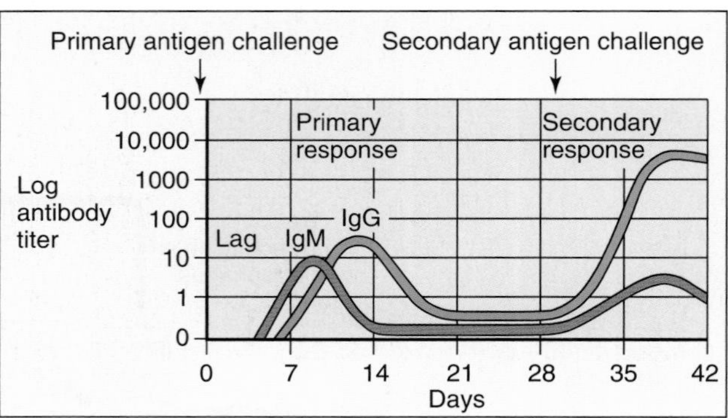

FIGURE 9-16 Time course of immune responses. The primary response occurs after a lag period. The immunoglobulin *(Ig)*M response is the earliest response. The secondary immune response (anamnestic response) reaches a higher titer, lasts longer, and consists predominantly of IgG.

Bibliography

Abbas AK, Lichtman AH, Pillai S, et al: *Cellular and molecular immunology*, ed 6, Philadelphia, 2007, Saunders.

DeFranco AL, Locksley RM, Robertson M: *Immunity: the immune response in infectious and inflammatory disease*, Sunderland, Mass, 2007, Sinauer Associates.

Janeway CA, Travers P, Walport M, et al: *Immunobiology: the immune system in health and disease*, ed 6, New York, 2004, Garland Science.

Kindt TJ, Goldsby RA, Osborne BA: *Kuby immunology*, ed 6, New York, 2007, WH Freeman.

Kumar V, Abbas AK, Fausto N: *Robbins and Cotran pathologic basis of disease*, ed 7, Philadelphia, 2005, Saunders.

Sompayrac L: *How the immune system works*, ed 2, Malden, Mass, 2003, Blackwell Scientific.

Trends Immunol: Issues contain understandable reviews on current topics in immunology.

CHAPTER

Animations for this chapter are available on StudentConsult.com.

IMMUNE RESPONSES TO INFECTIOUS AGENTS

The previous chapters in this section introduced the different immunologic actors and their characteristics. This chapter describes the different roles they play in host protection from infection, their interactions, and the immunopathogenic consequences that may arise as a result of the response (Box 10-1). Most infections are controlled by innate responses before immune responses can be initiated, but immune responses are necessary to resolve the more troublesome infections. Innate and immune responses are also important for restricting normal flora to their niche in the body and restricting virulent species. The importance of each of the components of the host response differs for different types of infectious agents (Table 10-1), and their importance becomes obvious when it is genetically deficient or diminished by chemotherapy, disease, or infection (e.g., acquired immunodeficiency syndrome [AIDS]).

Human beings have three basic lines of protection against inappropriate microbial infection:

1. **Natural barriers** such as skin, mucus, ciliated epithelium, gastric acid, and bile restrict entry of the agent.
2. **Innate antigen-nonspecific immune defenses** such as fever, antimicrobial peptides, interferon, complement, neutrophils, macrophages, dendritic cells (DCs), and natural killer (NK) cells provide rapid local responses to act at the infection site to restrict the growth and spread of the agent.
3. **Adaptive antigen-specific immune responses** such as antibody and T cells reinforce the innate protections and specifically target, attack, and eliminate the invaders that succeed in passing the first two defenses.

Symptoms and disease occur when barrier functions and innate responses are insufficient to keep normal flora within its niche or control other infections. Infections can grow, spread, and cause disease during the time period required to initiate a new antigen-specific immune response. Immune memory elicited by prior infection or vaccination can be activated quickly enough to control most infections before symptoms occur.

• Antibacterial Responses

Figure 10-1 illustrates the progression of protective responses to a bacterial challenge. Protection is initiated by activation of local innate and inflammatory responses and progresses to system-wide acute-phase and antigen-specific responses. A new response progresses from soluble antibacterial factors (peptides and complement) to cellular responses and then soluble antibody responses. *The most important antibacterial host responses are phagocytic killing by neutrophils and macrophages and antitoxin antibody.* Complement and antibody facilitate the uptake of microbes by phagocytes and TH17, and TH1 CD4 T-cell responses enhance and regulate their function. A summary of antibacterial responses is presented in Box 10-2.

Initiation of the Response

Once past the barriers, bacterial cell surfaces activate the alternative or lectin pathways of complement that are present in interstitial fluids and serum. The **complement system** (see Chapter 8) is a very early and important antibacterial defense. The **alternative complement pathway (properdin)** is activated by cleavage and binding of C3 to bacterial surfaces. Binding of the **mannose-binding protein** to polysaccharides activates the **lectin complement pathway.** Later, when immunoglobulin (Ig)M or IgG is present, the **classical complement pathway** is activated. All three pathways converge to cleave C3 into C3a, C3b, and C3d and generate the C5 convertase to produce C5a. The membrane attack complex (MAC) can directly kill gram-negative bacteria and, to a much lesser extent, gram-positive bacteria (the thick peptidoglycan of gram-positive bacteria shields them from the components). *Neisseria* are especially sensitive to complement lysis owing to the truncated structure of lipooligosaccharide in the outer membrane. Complement facilitates elimination of all bacteria by producing:

1. **Chemotactic factors (C3a and C5a)** to attract neutrophils and macrophages to the site of infection
2. **Anaphylotoxins (C5a, C3a, and to a lesser extent, C4a)** to stimulate mast cell release of histamine and thereby increase vascular permeability, allowing access to the infection site
3. **Opsonins (C3b),** which bind to bacteria and promote their phagocytosis
4. **B-cell activator (C3d)** to enhance antibody production

Bacterial cell wall molecules (teichoic acid, lipoteichoic acid, and peptidoglycan fragments of gram-positive bacteria and lipid A of lipopolysaccharide [LPS] of gram-negative bacteria) bind and activate **pathogen-associated molecular pattern (PAMP) receptors** (see Table 8-2 and Figure 8-4). **Lipid A (endotoxin)** binds to TLR4 and other PAMP receptors and is a very strong activator of DCs, macrophages, B cells, and selected other cells (e.g., epithelial and endothelial cells). Binding of these PAMPs to receptors on epithelial

 **Box 10-1 Summary of the Immune Response**

The drama of the host response to infection unfolds in several acts after an infectious challenge, with certain differences depending upon the microbial villain. The actors include cells of the innate response, including neutrophils; monocyte-macrophage lineage cells, immature dendritic cells (iDCs), and dendritic cells (DCs); natural killer (NK) cells; the T and B lymphocytes of the antigen-specific response; and other cells. These cells are distinguished by their outer structures, their costumes, which also define their roles in the immune response. Act 1 starts at the site of infection and involves innate responses. Activation of complement releases the "a" fragments, C3a, C4a, and C5a, which attract the actors to the site of infection. Neutrophils and, later, activated macrophages act directly on bacteria and infection. Type I interferons limit virus replication, activate NK cells, and also facilitate the development of subsequent T-cell responses. The NK cells provide early responses to infection and kill virally infected and tumor cells. The NK cells return in Act 2 to kill cells decorated with antibody (antibody-dependent cellular cytotoxicity [ADCC]). DCs bridge the gap between the innate and the antigen-specific protective responses, first by producing cytokines to enhance the action and then by taking their phagocytosed and pinocytosed cargo to the lymph node as the only antigen-presenting cell (APC) that can **initiate** an immune response. Act 2 commences in the lymph node, where the mature DCs present antigen to the T lymphocytes. The plot of this story may proceed to reinforce local-site inflammatory responses (TH17, TH1) or initiate systemic humoral responses (TH2), depending on the cytokine dialogue of the DC and the T cell. The T cells play a central role in activating and controlling (helping) immune and inflammatory responses through the release of cytokines. In Act 3, the T cells and B cells increase in number and terminally differentiate into effector and plasma cells to deliver antigen-specific cellular and antibody immune responses. Macrophages, DCs, and B cells refine and strengthen the direction of the response as APCs. Certain members of the B- and T-cell cast maintain a low profile and become memory cells to be able to replay the drama more quickly and efficiently in the future. Specific cellular actors, the receptor-ligand interactions between the actors, and the cytokine dialogue determine the drama that unfolds during the immune response.

cells, macrophages, Langerhans cells, and DCs leads to activation of the inflammasome and promotes cytokine production (including the **acute-phase cytokines interleukin [IL]-1, IL-6, and tumor necrosis factor [TNF]-α**), protective responses, and maturation of DCs. The inflammasome promotes the cleavage of IL-1β and IL-18 to reinforce local inflammation (see Figure 8-5). NK cells, NKT cells, and γ/δ T cells residing in tissue also respond, produce cytokines, and reinforce cellular responses.

IL-1 and TNF-α enhance the inflammatory response by locally stimulating changes in the tissue, promoting diapedesis of neutrophils and macrophages to the site, activating these cells, and activating systemic responses. IL-1 and TNF-α are endogenous pyrogens, inducing fever, and also induce the **acute-phase response.** The acute-phase response can also be triggered by inflammation, tissue injury, prostaglandin E_2, and interferons generated during infection. The acute-phase response promotes changes that support host defenses and include fever, anorexia, sleepiness, metabolic changes, and production of proteins. Acute-phase proteins that are produced and released into the serum include C-reactive protein, complement components, coagulation

 **Table 10-1 Importance of Antimicrobial Defenses for Infectious Agents**

Host Defense	Bacteria	Intracellular Bacteria	Viruses	Fungi	Parasites
Complement	+++	–	–	–	+
Interferon-α/β	–	–	++++	–	–
Neutrophils	++++	–	+	+++	++
Macrophages	+++	+++*	++	++	+
Natural killer cells	–	–	+++	–	–
CD4 TH1	+	++	+++	++	+
TH17	++	++	++	++++	+
CD8 cytotoxic T lymphocytes	–	++	++++	–	–
Antibody	+++	+	++	++	++ (IgE)†

*Activated M1 macrophages.
†Immunoglobulin E and mast cells are especially important for worm infections.

proteins, LPS-binding proteins, transport proteins, protease inhibitors, and adherence proteins. **C-reactive protein** complexes with the polysaccharides of numerous bacteria and fungi and activates the complement pathway, facilitating removal of these organisms from the body through greater phagocytosis. The acute-phase proteins reinforce the innate defenses against infection.

Antimicrobial peptides, including defensins, are released by activated epithelial cells, neutrophils, and other cells to protect skin and mucoepithelial surfaces. Their release is reinforced by TH17 responses. Antimicrobial peptides are very important for regulating the species of bacteria in the gastrointestinal tract. In addition, chelating peptides are released as part of the inflammatory response to sequester essential metal ions, such as iron and zinc, to limit microbial growth.

Immature DCs (iDCs), macrophages, and other cells of the macrophage lineage will produce IL-23 and IL-12 in addition to the acute-phase cytokines. IL-12 activates NK cells at the site of infection, which can produce interferon (IFN)-γ to further activate macrophages and DCs. IL-12 and IL-23 activate TH1 and TH17 immune responses, respectively, to reinforce macrophages and neutrophil function. Epithelial cells also respond to PAMPs and release cytokines to promote natural protections.

These actions initiate **local acute inflammation**. Expansion of capillaries and increased blood flow brings more antimicrobial agents to the site. Increase in permeability and alteration of surface molecules of the microvasculature structure attracts and facilitates leukocyte entry and provides access for fluid and plasma proteins into the site of infection. Kinins and clotting factors induced by tissue damage (e.g., factor XII [Hageman factor], bradykinin, fibrinopeptides) are also involved in inflammation. These factors increase vascular permeability and are chemotactic for leukocytes. Products of arachidonic acid metabolism also affect inflammation. Cyclooxygenase-2 (COX-2) and 5-lipooxygenase convert

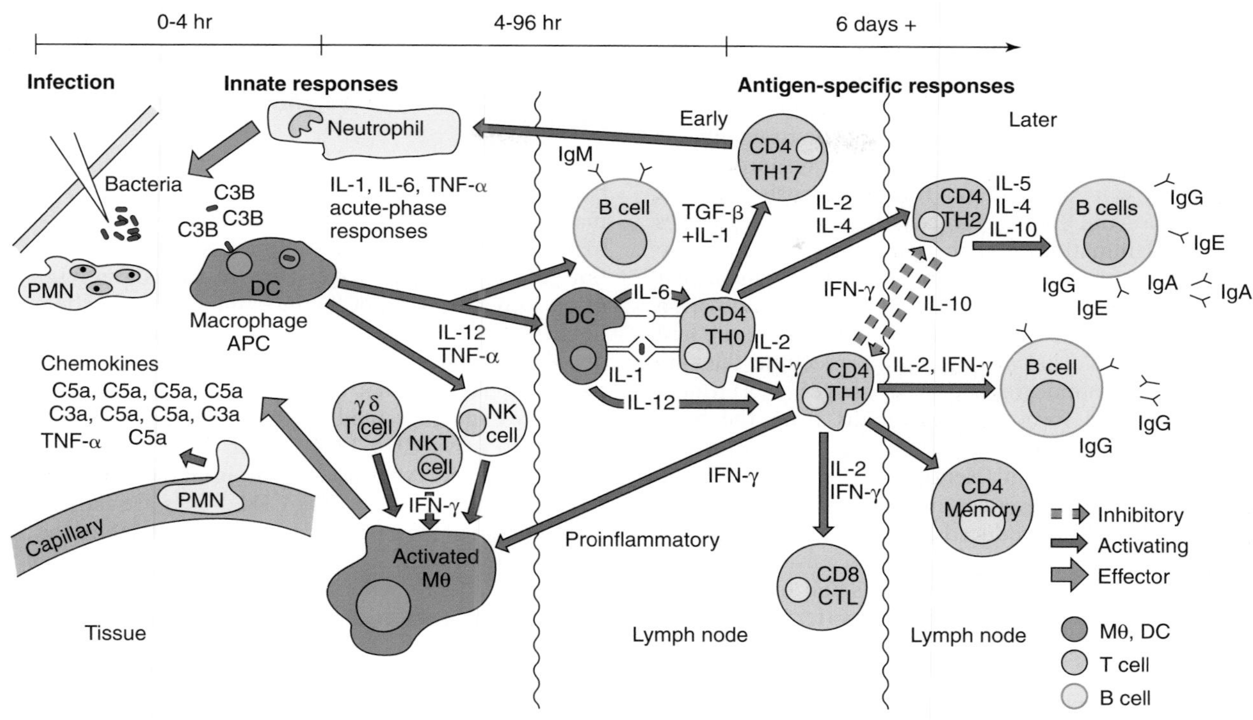

FIGURE 10-1 Antibacterial responses. First, innate antigen-nonspecific responses attract and promote polymorphonuclear neutrophil *(PMN)* and macrophage *(Mθ)* responses. Dendritic cells *(DCs)* and antigen reach the lymph node to activate early immune responses *(TH17, TH1, IgM,* and *IgG).* Later, TH2 systemic antibody responses and memory cells are developed. **The time course of events is indicated at the top of the figure.** *APC,* Antigen-presenting cell; *CTL,* cytotoxic T lymphocyte; *IFN-γ,* interferon-γ; *IL,* interleukin; *TGF-β,* transforming growth factor-β; *TH,* T helper (cell); *TNF-α,* tumor necrosis factor-α.

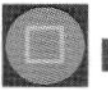 **Box 10-2 Summary of Antibacterial Responses**

Antimicrobial Peptides and Proteins
Defensins and other peptides disrupt membranes
Transferrin, lactoferrin, and other proteins sequester iron and other essential ions

Complement
Production of chemotactic and anaphylatoxic proteins (C3a, C5a)
Opsonization of bacteria (C3b)
Promotion of killing of gram-negative bacteria
Activation of B cells (C3d)

Neutrophils
Important antibacterial phagocytic cells
Killing by oxygen-dependent and oxygen-independent mechanisms

Activated Macrophages (M1)
Important antibacterial phagocytic cells
Killing by oxygen-dependent and oxygen-independent mechanisms
Production of TNF-α, IL-1, IL-6, IL-23, IL-12
Activation of acute-phase and inflammatory responses
Presentation of antigen to CD4 T cell

Dendritic Cells
Production of acute phase cytokines (TNF-α, IL-6, IL-1); IL-23; IL-12; IFN-α
Presentation of antigen to CD4 and CD8 T cells
Initiation of immune responses in naïve T cells

T Cells
γ/δ T-cell response to bacterial metabolites
Natural killer T (NKT) cell response to CD1 presentation of mycobacterial glycolipids
TH17 CD4 response activates neutrophils
TH1 CD4 responses important for bacterial, especially intracellular, infections
TH2 CD4 response important for antibody protections

Antibody
Binding to surface structures of bacteria (fimbriae, lipoteichoic acid, capsule)
Blocking of attachment
Opsonization of bacteria for phagocytosis
Promotion of complement action
Promotion of clearance of bacteria
Neutralization of toxins and toxic enzymes

IFN-α, Interferon-α; *IL,* interleukin; *TNF-α,* tumor necrosis factor-α.

arachidonic acid to **prostaglandins and leukotrienes,** respectively, which can mediate essentially every aspect of acute inflammation. The course of inflammation can be followed by rapid increases in serum levels of acute-phase proteins, especially C-reactive protein (which can increase 1000-fold within 24 to 48 hours) and serum amyloid A. Although these processes are beneficial, inflammation also causes **pain, redness, heat, and swelling and promotes tissue damage.** Inflammatory damage is caused to some extent by complement and macrophages but mostly by neutrophils.

Phagocytic Responses

C3a, C5a, bacterial products (e.g., formyl-methionyl-leucyl-phenylalanine [f-met-leu-phe]), and chemokines produced by epithelial cells, Langerhans cells, and other cells in skin and mucous epithelium are powerful chemoattractants for neutrophils, macrophages, and later in the response, lymphocytes. The chemokines and **tumor necrosis factor-α (TNF-α)** cause the endothelial cells lining the capillaries (near the inflammation) and the leukocytes passing by to express complementary adhesion molecules (molecular "Velcro") to promote diapedesis (see Figure 8-6; Animation 10-1). Polymorphonuclear neutrophils (PMNs) are the first cells to arrive at the site in response to infection; they are followed later by monocytes and macrophages. Recruitment of immature band forms of neutrophils from the bone marrow during infection is indicated by a "left shift" in the complete blood cell count. Neutrophils are recruited and activated by the TH17 response and macrophages, and DCs are activated by IFN-γ produced by NK and NKT cells and the TH1 response.

Bacteria are bound to the neutrophils and macrophages with receptors for bacterial carbohydrates (**lectins** [specific sugar-binding proteins]), fibronectin receptors (especially for *Staphylococcus aureus*), and **receptors for opsonins,** including complement (C3b), C-reactive protein, mannose-binding protein, and the Fc portion of antibody. The microbes are internalized in a **phagocytic vacuole** that fuses with **primary lysosomes** (macrophages) or **granules** (PMNs) to allow inactivation and digestion of the vacuole contents (see Figure 8-7 and Box 8-4).

The neutrophil kills the phagocytosed microbes by **oxygen-dependent killing** with hydrogen peroxide, superoxide ion, and hypochlorous ions and with **oxygen-independent killing** upon fusion of the phagosome with azurophilic granules containing cationic proteins (e.g., cathepsin G) and specific granules containing lysozyme and lactoferrin. These proteins kill gram-negative bacteria by disrupting their cell membrane integrity, but they are far less effective against gram-positive bacteria, which are killed principally through the oxygen-dependent mechanism. **Nitric oxide** produced by neutrophils and activated macrophages has antimicrobial activity and is also a major second messenger molecule that enhances the inflammatory and other responses.

Neutrophils contribute to the inflammation in several ways. Prostaglandins and leukotrienes are released and increase vascular permeability, cause swelling (edema), and stimulate pain receptors. During phagocytosis, the granules may leak their contents to cause tissue damage. The neutrophils have short lives, and upon death, neutrophils release a sticky DNA net (neutrophil extracellular trap) and become **pus.**

In contrast to neutrophils, macrophages have long lives, but the cells must be activated (made angry) with IFN-γ (best) in order to kill phagocytized microbes. Granulocyte-macrophage colony-stimulating factor (GM-CSF), TNF-α, and lymphotoxin (TNF-β) maintain the antimicrobial action (keep them aggravated). Early in the infection, IFN-γ is produced by NK and NKT cells and later by CD4 T cells. **Splenic macrophages** are important for clearing bacteria, especially encapsulated bacteria, from blood. Asplenic (congenitally or surgically) individuals are highly susceptible to pneumonia, meningitis, and other manifestations of *Streptococcus pneumoniae, Neisseria meningitidis,* and other encapsulated bacteria and yeast.

Antigen-Specific Response to Bacterial Challenge

On ingestion of bacteria and after stimulation of TLRs by bacterial components, Langerhans cells and iDCs become mature, cease to phagocytize, and move to the lymph nodes to process and deliver their internalized antigen for presentation to T cells (Figure 10-2). Dendritic cells also insert dendrites into the lumen of the intestine to "check" the normal flora. Antigenic peptides (having > 11 amino acids) produced from phagocytosed proteins (exogenous route) are bound to class II major histocompatibility complex (MHC) molecules and presented by these antigen-presenting cells (APCs) to naïve **CD4 TH0 T cells.** TH0 provides the first stage, a generic expansion of the immune cells needed to respond to the infection. The CD4 T cells are activated by a combination of (1) antigenic peptide in the cleft of the MHC II molecule with the T-cell antigen receptor (TCR) and with CD4, (2) co-stimulatory signals provided by sufficient numbers of interactions of B7 molecules on the DC with CD28 molecules on the T cells, and (3) IL-6 and other cytokines produced by the DCs. The TH0 cells produce IL-2, IFN-γ, and IL-4. Simultaneously, bacterial molecules with repetitive structures (e.g., capsular polysaccharide) interact with B cells expressing surface IgM and IgD specific for the antigen and activate the cell to grow and produce IgM. LPS and also the C3d component of complement activate B cells and promote the specific IgM antibody responses. Swollen lymph nodes are an indication of lymphocyte growth in response to antigenic challenge.

Early responses are also provided by γ/δ T cells, NKT cells, and innate lymphoid cells (including NK cells). **γ/δ T cells** in tissue and blood sense phosphorylated amine metabolites from some bacteria (*Escherichia coli*, mycobacteria) but not others (streptococci, staphylococci). DCs can present bacterial glycolipids to activate **NKT** cells. These T cells and **innate lymphoid cells** produce IFN-γ, which activates macrophages and DCs to enforce local cellular inflammatory reactions.

The conversion of TH0 cells to TH17 and TH1 cells initiates expansion of the host response. Acute-phase cytokines IL-1 and TNF-α together with the omnipresent transforming growth factor (TGF)-β promote the development of **CD4 TH17 T cells** (see Animation 9-5). *The acute phase cytokines provide a cry for help despite the calming influence of TGF-β to elicit a quick inflammatory cytokine yell by the CD4 TH17 T cells to the epithelial cells and neutrophils to activate inflammatory responses.* Memory TH17 cells are activated by IL-23. TH17 cells produce IL-17 and TNF-α to activate epithelial cells and neutrophils and also promote production of antimicrobial peptides. *TH17 responses are important for early antibacterial responses and antimycobacterial responses.* A balance of TH17 and Treg responses are also important to regulate the populations of intestinal flora.

DCs producing IL-12 promote TH1 responses. **CD4 TH1 T cells** (1) promote and reinforce inflammatory responses (e.g., IFN-γ activation of macrophage) and growth of T and B cells (IL-2) to expand the immune response, and (2) promote B cells to produce complement-binding antibodies (IgM and then IgG upon class switching) and mature into

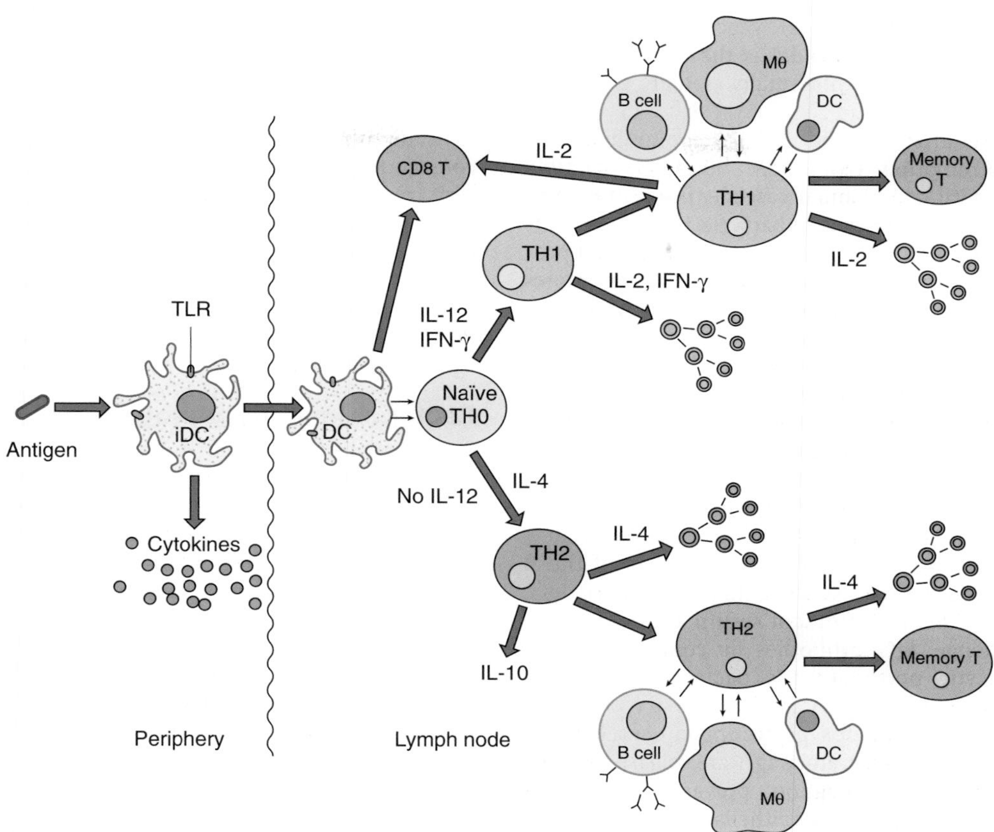

FIGURE 10-2 Initiation and expansion of specific immune responses. Immature dendritic cells *(iDCs)* at the site of infection acquire microbial debris, Toll-like receptors *(TLRs) and other pathogen pattern receptors bind their ligands and activate* dendritic cells *(DCs)* that produce cytokines, mature, and move to the lymph node. DCs present antigen to naïve T cells to initiate the antigen-specific and cytokine-directed response. During a secondary or memory response, B cells, macrophages, and DCs can present antigen to initiate the response. *IL*, Interleukin; *IFN-γ*, interferon-γ; *Mθ*, macrophage; *TH*, T helper (cell).

plasma cells and memory cells. These responses are important for the early phases of an antibacterial defense. TH1 responses are also essential for combating intracellular bacterial infections, including mycobacteria, which are hidden from antibody. IFN-γ activates macrophage to kill phagocytized microbes. Upon chronic stimulation by macrophages expressing microbial (e.g., mycobacterial or histoplasma) antigen, CD4 TH1 T cells will produce IFN-γ and TNF-α and cause transformation of other macrophages into epithelioid cells and giant cells, which can surround the infection and produce a granuloma. Granulomas wall off intracellular infections arising either because the microbe can evade antimicrobial responses (e.g., *Mycobacterium tuberculosis*), the macrophages are not activated and cannot kill them (normal alveolar macrophages), or a genetic defect prevents generation of antimicrobial reactive oxygen substances, as in chronic granulomatous disease. *CD8 T cells facilitate clearance of intracellular infections by producing cytokines but are not essential for antibacterial immunity.*

CD4 TH2 T-cell responses occur in the absence of IL-12 at more distant lymph nodes. These responses are also initiated by DCs and are sustained by the B-cell presentation of antigen. TH2 responses can occur at the same time as TH1 responses when antigen is delivered in lymph fluid to lymph nodes other than the draining lymph node. The DCs act as sewage inspectors who promote a response to clear out excess and damaged protein. This is the same type of response that occurs to injection of a bolus of antigen for an inactivated vaccine. Binding of antigen to the cell surface antibody on B cells activates the B cells and also promotes uptake, processing of the antigen, and presentation of antigenic peptides on class II MHC molecules to the CD4 TH2 cell. The TH2 cell produces IL-4, IL-5, IL-6, IL-10, and IL-13, which enhance IgG production and, depending on other factors, the production of IgE or IgA. **CD4TFH** cells are a conduit for the TH1 or TH2 responses to promote memory cell production and terminal differentiation of B cells to plasma-cell antibody factories.

$CD4^+CD25^+$ regulatory T cells (Treg) prevent spurious activation of naïve T cells, curtail both TH1 and TH2 responses, and promote development of some of the antigen-specific cells into memory T cells. Only DCs can override the Treg block to activate naïve T cells.

Antibodies are the primary protection against extracellular bacteria and toxins and promote the clearance and prevent the spread of bacteria in the blood (bacteremia). Antibody promotes complement activation, opsonizes bacteria for phagocytosis, blocks bacterial adhesion, and neutralizes (inactivates) exotoxins (e.g., tetanospasmin, botulinum toxin) and other cytotoxic proteins produced by bacteria (e.g., degradative enzymes). Vaccine immunization with inactivated exotoxins (toxoids) is the primary means of protection against the potentially lethal effects of exotoxins.

IgM antibodies are produced early in the antibacterial response (see Animation 10-1). IgM bound to bacteria activates the classical complement cascade, promoting both the direct killing of gram-negative bacteria and the inflammatory responses. IgM is usually the only antibody produced against capsular polysaccharides and promotes opsonization of the bacteria with complement. Splenic macrophages depend upon IgM bound to capsular polysaccharides to activate complement and opsonize the encapsulated bacteria so they can be recognized, phagocytized, and eliminated. The large size and limited transport mechanisms for IgM limits its ability to spread into tissue. IgM produced in response to polysaccharide vaccines (as for *Streptococcus pneumonia*) can prevent bacteremia but not infection of the interstitium of the lung. Approximately a week later, T-cell help promotes differentiation of the B cell and immunoglobulin class switching to produce IgG. **IgG** antibodies are the predominant serum antibody, especially on rechallenge. IgG antibodies fix complement and promote phagocytic uptake of the bacteria through Fc receptors on macrophages. **IgA** is the primary secretory antibody and is important for protecting mucosal membranes. Large amounts of secretory IgA are released to regulate the normal flora population, prevent adhesion of bacteria, and neutralize toxins at epithelial cell surfaces.

A primary antigen-specific response to bacterial infection takes at least 5 to 7 days. Movement of the DC to the lymph node may take 1 to 3 days, followed by activation, expansion, and maturation of the response. On rechallenge to infection, long-lived plasma cells may still be producing antibody. Memory T cells can respond quickly to antigen presentation by DCs, macrophages, or B cells, not just DCs; memory B cells are present to respond quickly to antigen, and the secondary antibody response occurs within 2 to 3 days.

Skin, Intestinal, and Mucosal Immunity

The skin, intestine, and mucous membranes are populated with bacteria upon traversing the birth canal and soon thereafter. The immune response matures, and a balance develops between regulatory and inflammatory cells in response to this normal flora.

The intestinal flora is constantly interacting with and being regulated by the innate and immune systems of the gut-associated lymphoid tissue (see Figure 7-5). Similarly, the immune response is shaped by its interaction with intestinal flora as regulatory cells limit the development of autoimmune responses and inflammation. DCs, innate lymphoid cells, Treg, TH17, TH1, and other T cells and B cells in the lamina propria, Peyer patches, and intestinal lymphoid follicles monitor and control the bacteria within the gut. These cells and epithelial and other cells lining the gut produce antimicrobial peptides, and plasma cells secrete IgA into the gut to maintain a healthy mixture of bacteria. At the same time, regulatory cells prevent the development of detrimental or excessive immune responses to the contents of the gut. Alterations in the microbial flora and its interaction with the innate and immune cells can disrupt the system and result in inflammatory bowel diseases. For example, absence or a mutation in the IL-23 receptor or NOD2 receptor for peptidoglycan enhances chances for certain types of Crohn disease.

In the skin, Langerhans cells are sentinel DCs responsive to trauma and infection. Memory CD4 and CD8 T cells constantly cycle into the skin from the blood. In the respiratory tract, antimicrobial peptides and secreted IgA control bacteria, mucus traps, and cilia move the mucus and bacteria out of the lungs. Inflammatory responses are controlled by alveolar macrophages (M2 macrophages) to prevent tissue damage to normal flora. Like in the gastrointestinal tract, DCs monitor the epithelium for normal and abnormal microbes.

Bacterial Immunopathogenesis

Activation of the inflammatory and acute-phase responses can initiate significant tissue and systemic damage. Activation of macrophages and DCs in the liver, spleen, and blood by endotoxin can promote release of acute-phase cytokines into the blood, causing many of the symptoms of **sepsis,** including hemodynamic failure, shock, and death (see Cytokine Storm section and Chapter 14). Although IL-1, IL-6, and TNF-α promote protective responses to a local infection, these same responses can be life threatening when activated by systemic infection. Increased blood flow and fluid leakage can lead to shock when it occurs throughout the body. Antibodies produced against bacterial antigens that share determinants with human proteins can initiate autoimmune tissue destruction (e.g., antibodies produced in poststreptococcal rheumatic fever). Nonspecific activation of CD4 T cells by **superantigens** (e.g., toxic shock syndrome toxin of *S. aureus*) promotes production of large amounts of cytokines and, eventually, the death of large numbers of T cells. The sudden massive release of cytokines ("cytokine storm") can cause shock and severe tissue damage (e.g., toxic shock syndrome) (see Cytokine Storm section and Chapter 14).

Bacterial Evasion of Protective Responses

The mechanisms used by bacteria to evade host-protective responses are discussed in Chapter 14 as virulence factors. These mechanisms include (1) inhibition of phagocytosis and intracellular killing in the phagocyte, (2) inactivation of complement function, (3) binding of the Fc portion of IgG and cleavage of IgA, (4) intracellular growth (avoidance of antibody), and (5) change in bacterial antigenic appearance. Some microorganisms, including but not limited to mycobacteria (also *Listeria* and *Brucella* species), survive and multiply within macrophages and use the macrophages as a protective reservoir or transport system to help spread the organisms throughout the body. However, cytokine-activated macrophages can often kill the intracellular pathogens.

• Antiviral Responses

Host Defenses against Viral Infection

The immune response is the best and, in most cases, the only means of controlling a viral infection (Figure 10-3 and Box 10-3). Unfortunately, it is also the source of pathogenesis for many viral diseases. Both humoral and cellular immune responses are important for antiviral immunity. **The**

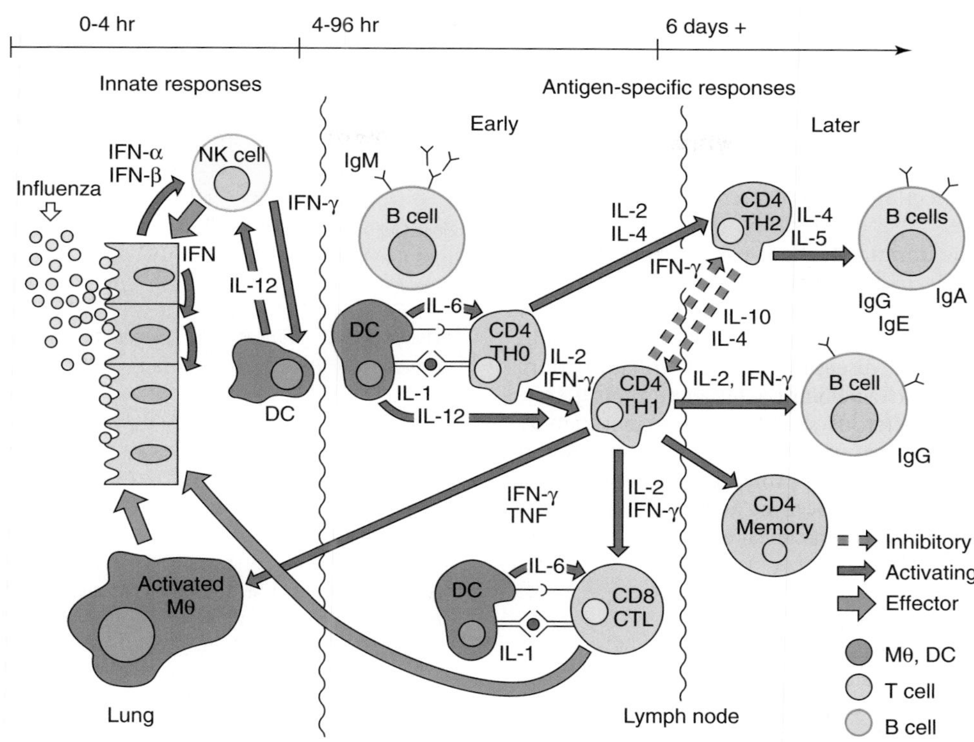

FIGURE 10-3 Antiviral responses. The response to a virus (e.g., influenza virus) initiates with interferon production and action and natural killer *(NK)* cells. Activation of antigen-specific immunity resembles the antibacterial response, except that CD8 cytotoxic T lymphocytes *(CTLs)* are important antiviral responses. **The time course of events is indicated at the top of the figure.** *IFN,* Interferon, *IL,* interleukin; *Mθ,* macrophage; *TH,* T helper (cell); *TNF,* tumor necrosis factor.

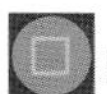 **Box 10-3 Summary of Antiviral Responses**

Interferon

Interferon is induced by double-stranded RNA, inhibition of cellular protein synthesis, or enveloped virus

Interferon initiates the antiviral state in surrounding cells

Antiviral state blocks viral replication

Interferon activates NK cells and systemic antiviral responses

NK Cells

NK cells are activated by IFN-α and interleukin-12, which activate macrophages with IFN-γ

NK cells target and kill virus-infected cells (especially enveloped viruses)

Macrophages and DCs

Macrophages filter viral particles from blood

Macrophages inactivate opsonized virus particles

Immature and plasmacytoid DCs produce IFN-α and other cytokines

DCs initiate and determine the nature of the CD4 and CD8 T-cell response

DCs and macrophages present antigen to CD4 T cells

T Cells

T cells are essential for controlling enveloped and noncytolytic viral infections

T cells recognize viral peptides presented by MHC molecules on cell surfaces

Antigenic viral peptides (linear epitopes) can come from any viral protein (e.g., glycoproteins, nucleoproteins)

CD8 cytotoxic T cells respond to viral peptide: class I MHC protein complexes on the infected cell surface

CD4 TH2 responses may be detrimental if they prematurely limit the TH1 inflammatory and cytolytic responses

Antibody

Antibody neutralizes extracellular virus:

It blocks viral attachment proteins (e.g., glycoproteins, capsid proteins)

It destabilizes viral structure

Antibody opsonizes virus for phagocytosis

Antibody promotes killing of target cell by the complement cascade and antibody-dependent cellular cytotoxicity

Antibody resolves lytic viral infections

Antibody blocks viremic spread to target tissue

IgM is an indicator of recent or current infection

IgG is a more effective antiviral than IgM

Secretory IgA is important for protecting mucosal surfaces

Resolution requires elimination of free virus (antibody) and the virus-producing cell (viral or immune cell–mediated lysis)

DC, Dendritic cell; *IFN,* interferon; *Ig,* immunoglobulin; *MHC,* major histocompatibility complex; *NK,* natural killer.

ultimate goal of the immune response in a viral infection is to eliminate both the virus and the host cells harboring or replicating the virus. Failure to resolve the infection may lead to persistent or chronic infection or death.

Interferons, NK cells, CD4 TH1 responses, and CD8 cytotoxic killer T cells are more important for viral infections than for bacterial infections. Complement has a limited role in antiviral defense.

The course of the immune response and the nature of the immunopathogenesis of bacterial and viral infections are different. For bacteria, complement and the recruitment of neutrophils and macrophages are the initial response, and they rapidly drive the disease-associated inflammation. Antibody can control extracellular bacteria and their toxins. For viruses, type I interferons and other cytokines initiate the response, prodrome symptoms are driven by interferon and cytokines, but protection, inflammatory responses and disease often wait until T cells become activated. As a result, the time course and nature of bacterial and viral disease are very different.

Innate Defenses

Body temperature, fever, interferons, other cytokines, the mononuclear phagocyte system, and NK cells provide a local rapid response to viral infection and also activate the specific immune defenses. Often the nonspecific defenses are sufficient to control a viral infection, thus preventing the occurrence of symptoms.

Body temperature and fever can limit replication or destabilize some viruses. Many viruses are less stable (e.g., herpes simplex virus) or cannot replicate (rhinoviruses) at 37° C or higher. The live influenza vaccine is attenuated because it cannot replicate above 25° C.

Viral infection can induce the release of cytokines (e.g., TNF, IL-1) and interferon from infected cells, iDCs, and macrophages. Viral RNA (especially dsRNA), DNA, and some viral glycoproteins are potent activators of TLRs and other pathogen pattern receptors to initiate these interferon and cytokine responses. Interferons and other cytokines trigger early local and systemic responses. Induction of fever and stimulation of the immune system are two of these systemic effects.

Cells of the **dendritic and mononuclear phagocyte system** phagocytose the viral and cell debris from virally infected cells. Macrophages in the liver (Kupffer cells) and spleen rapidly filter many viruses from the blood. Antibody and complement bound to a virus facilitate its uptake and clearance by macrophages (opsonization). DCs and macrophages also present antigen to T cells and release IL-1, IL-12, and IFN-α to expand the innate and initiate the antigen-specific immune responses. Plasmacytoid DCs in the blood produce large amounts of IFN-α and other cytokines in response to a viremia.

NK cells are activated by IFN-α, IFN-β, and IL-12 to kill virally infected cells. Viral infection may reduce the expression of MHC antigens to remove inhibitory signals or may alter the carbohydrates on cell surface proteins to provide cytolytic signals to the NK cell.

Interferon

Interferon was first described by Isaacs and Lindemann as a very potent factor that "interferes with" the replication of many different viruses. Interferon is the body's first active defense against a viral infection, an "early warning system." In addition to activating a target-cell antiviral defense to block viral replication, interferons activate the immune response and enhance T-cell recognition of the infected cell. Interferon is a very important defense against infection, but it is also a cause of the systemic symptoms associated with many viral infections, such as malaise, myalgia, chills, and fever (nonspecific flulike symptoms), especially during viremia. Type I interferon is also a factor in causing systemic lupus erythematosus.

Table 10-2 Basic Properties of Human Interferons (IFNs)

Property	IFN-α	IFN-β	IFN-γ
Previous designations	Leukocyte IFN type I	Fibroblast IFN type I	Immune IFN type II
Genes	>20	1	1
Molecular mass (Da)*	16,000-23,000	23,000	20,000-25,000
Acid stability	Stable†	Stable	Labile
Primary activator	Viruses	Viruses	Immune response
Principal source	Epithelium, leukocytes	Fibroblast	NK or T cell
Homology with human IFN-α	100%	30%-50%	<10%

Data from White DO: *Antiviral chemotherapy, interferons and vaccines,* Basel, Switzerland, 1984, Karger; and Samuel CE: Antiviral actions of interferon. Interferon-regulated cellular proteins and their surprisingly selective antiviral activities, *Virology* 183:1–11, 1991.

*Molecular mass of monomeric form.

†Most subtypes but not all.

Interferons comprise a family of proteins that can be subdivided according to several properties, including size, stability, cell of origin, and mode of action (Table 10-2). **IFN-α** and **IFN-β** are type I interferons that share many properties, including structural homology and mode of action. B cells, epithelial cells, monocytes, macrophages, and iDCs make **IFN-α.** Plasmacytoid DCs in blood produce large amounts in response to viremia. Fibroblasts and other cells make **IFN-β** in response to viral infection and other stimuli. **IFN-λ** (interferon lambda) is a type III interferon with activity similar to **IFN-α** and is important for anti-influenza responses. **IFN-γ** is a type II interferon, a cytokine produced by activated T and NK cells that occurs later in the infection. Although IFN-γ inhibits viral replication, its structure and mode of action differ from those of the other interferons. IFN-γ is also known as **macrophage activation factor** and is the defining component of the TH1 response.

The best inducer of IFN-α and IFN-β production is **dsRNA,** *produced as the replicative intermediates of RNA viruses* or from the interaction of sense/antisense messenger RNAs (mRNAs) for some DNA viruses (Box 10-4). One dsRNA molecule per cell is sufficient to induce production of interferon. Interaction of some enveloped viruses (e.g., herpes simplex virus and human immunodeficiency virus [HIV])

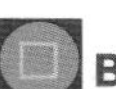

Box 10-4 Type I Interferons

Induction

Double-stranded ribonucleic acid (during virus replication)
Viral inhibition of cellular protein synthesis
Enveloped virus interaction with plasmacytoid dendritic cell

Mechanism of Action

Initial infected cell or plasmacytoid dendritic cell releases interferon
Interferon binds to a specific cell surface receptor on another cell
Interferon induces the "antiviral state":
 Synthesis of protein kinase R (PKR), 2′,5′-oligoadenylate synthetase, and ribonuclease L
Viral infection of the cell activates these enzymes
Protein synthesis inhibited to block viral replication
 Degradation of mRNA (2′,5′-oligoadenylate synthase and RNAase L)
 Inhibition of ribosome assembly (PKR)
Activation of innate and immune antiviral responses
Induction of flulike symptoms

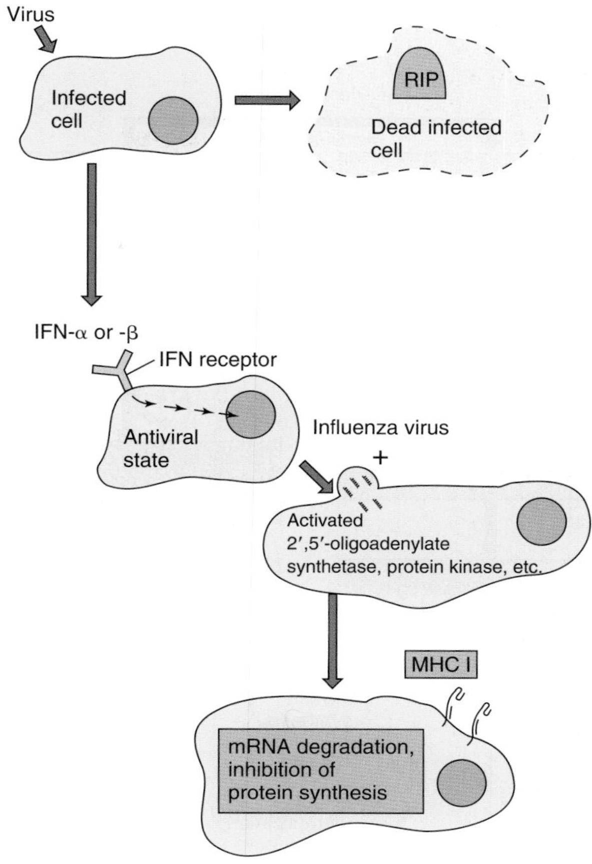

FIGURE 10-4 Induction of the antiviral state by interferon *(IFN)*-α or IFN-β. Interferon is produced in response to viral infection but does not protect the initially infected cell. The interferon binds to a cell surface receptor on other cells and induces production of antiviral enzymes (antiviral state). The infection and production of double-stranded RNA activates the antiviral activity. *MHC I,* Major histocompatibility antigen type I.

with plasmacytoid DCs can promote production of IFN-α. Alternatively, inhibition of protein synthesis in a virally infected cell can decrease production of a repressor protein of the interferon gene, allowing production of interferon. Nonviral interferon inducers include:

1. Intracellular microorganisms (e.g., mycobacteria, fungi, protozoa)
2. Activators of certain TLRs or mitogens (e.g., endotoxins, phytohemagglutinin)
3. Double-stranded polynucleotides (e.g., poly I:C, poly dA:dT)
4. Synthetic polyanion polymers (e.g., polysulfates, polyphosphates, pyran)
5. Antibiotics (e.g., kanamycin, cycloheximide)
6. Low-molecular-weight synthetic compounds (e.g., tilorone, acridine dyes)

IFN-α, IFN-β, and IFN-λ can be induced and released within hours of infection (Figure 10-4). The interferon binds to specific receptors on the neighboring cells and induces the production of antiviral proteins—**the antiviral state.** However, these antiviral proteins are not activated until they bind dsRNA. The major antiviral effects of interferon are produced by two enzymes, **2′,5′-oligoadenylate synthetase** (an unusual polymerase) and **protein kinase R (PKR)** (Figure 10-5), and for influenza, the **mx protein** is also important. Viral infection of the cell and production of dsRNA activate these enzymes and trigger a cascade of biochemical events that leads to (1) the inhibition of protein synthesis by PKR phosphorylation of an important ribosomal initiation factor (elongation initiation factor 2-α [eIF-2α]) and (2) the degradation of mRNA (preferentially, viral mRNA) by ribonuclease L, activated by 2′,5′-oligoadenosine. PKR and ribonuclease L bind to double-stranded RNA or 2′,5′-oligoadenosine, respectively, like beads on a string, and then bind to each other to form multimers to become activated. This process essentially puts the cellular protein synthesis factory "on strike" and prevents viral replication. It must be stressed that interferon does not directly block viral replication. The antiviral state lasts for 2 to 3 days, which may be sufficient for the cell to degrade and eliminate the virus without being killed.

Interferons stimulate cell-mediated immunity by activating effector cells and enhancing recognition of the virally infected target cell. Type I interferons activate NK cells and assist in activation of CD8 T cells. *IFN and activated NK cells provide an early, local, natural defense against viral infection.* IFN-α and IFN-β increase the expression of class I MHC antigens, enhancing the cell's ability to present antigen and making the cell a better target for cytotoxic T cells (CTLs). Activation of macrophages by IFN-γ promotes production of more IFN-α and IFN-β, secretion of other biological response modifiers, phagocytosis, production of reactive oxygen and nitrogen species, recruitment, and inflammatory responses. IFN-γ increases expression of class II MHC antigens on the macrophage to help promote antigen presentation to T cells. Interferon also has widespread regulatory effects on cell growth, protein synthesis, and the immune response. All three interferon types block cell proliferation at appropriate doses.

Genetically engineered recombinant interferon is being used as an antiviral therapy for some viral infections (e.g.,

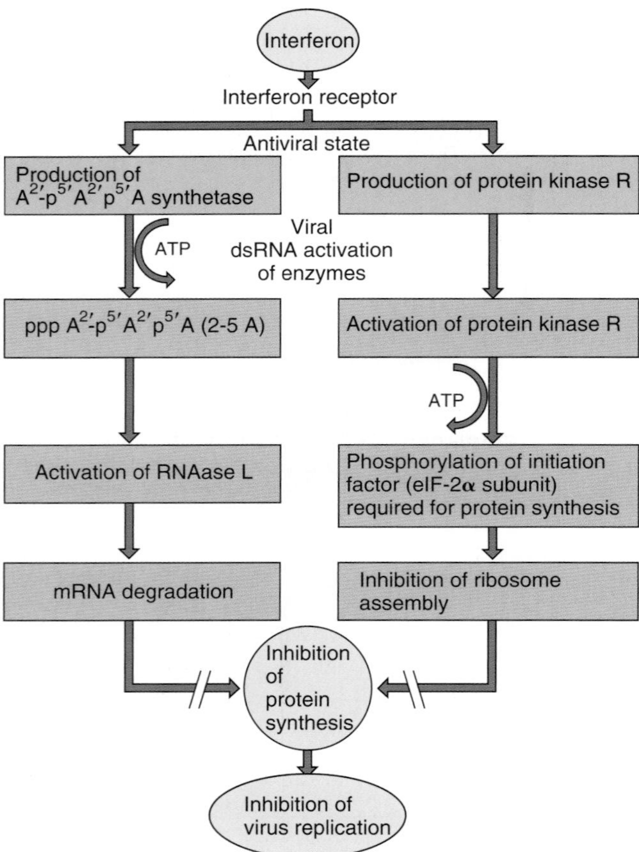

FIGURE 10-5 The two major routes for interferon inhibition of viral protein synthesis. One mechanism involves induction of an unusual polymerase (2′,5′-oligoadenylate synthetase [2-5A]) that is activated by double-stranded RNA *(dsRNA)*. The activated enzyme synthesizes an unusual adenine chain with a 2′,5′-phosphodiester linkage. The oligomer activates RNAase L that degrades messenger RNA *(mRNA)*. The other mechanism involves induction of protein kinase R (PKR), which prevents assembly of the ribosome by phosphorylation of the elongation initiation factor (eIF-2α) to prevent initiation of protein synthesis from capped mRNAs. *ATP,* Adenosine triphosphate.

human papilloma and hepatitis C viruses). Effective treatment requires the use of the correct interferon subtype(s) and its prompt delivery at the appropriate concentration. IFN-β is used for treatment of multiple sclerosis. Interferons have also been used in clinical trials for the treatment of certain cancers. However, *interferon treatment causes flulike side effects such as chills, fever, and fatigue.*

Antigen-Specific Immunity

The goal of antigen-specific immunity is to eliminate free virus and virus-producing cells, but sometimes it can only control a chronic infection. Humoral immunity and cell-mediated immunity play different roles in resolving viral infections (i.e., eliminating the virus from the body). Humoral immunity (antibody) acts mainly on extracellular virions, whereas cell-mediated immunity (T cells) is directed at the virus-producing cell.

Humoral Immunity

Practically all viral proteins are foreign to the host and are immunogenic (i.e., capable of eliciting an antibody response). However, not all immunogens elicit protective immunity.

Antibody blocks the progression of disease through the **neutralization and opsonization** of cell-free virus. Protective antibody responses are generated toward the viral capsid proteins of naked viruses and the glycoproteins of enveloped viruses that interact with cell surface receptors (viral attachment proteins). These antibodies can neutralize the virus by preventing viral interaction with target cells or by destabilizing the virus, thus initiating its degradation. Binding of antibody to these proteins also opsonizes the virus, promoting its uptake and clearance by macrophages. Antibody recognition of infected cells can also promote antibody-dependent cellular cytotoxicity (ADCC) by NK cells. Antibodies to other viral antigens may be useful for serologic analysis of the viral infection.

The major antiviral role of antibody is to prevent the spread of extracellular virus to other cells. Antibody is especially important in limiting the spread of the virus by **viremia,** preventing the virus from reaching the target tissue for disease production. Antibody is most effective at resolving cytolytic infections. *For cytolytic infections, resolution occurs because the virus kills the cell factory and the antibody eliminates the extracellular virus.*

T-Cell Immunity

T cell–mediated immunity promotes antibody and inflammatory responses (CD4 helper T cells) and kills infected cells (cytotoxic T cells [primarily CD8 T cells]). The **CD4 TH1** response is generally more important than TH2 responses for controlling a viral infection, especially noncytolytic and enveloped viruses. **CD8** killer T cells promote apoptosis in infected cells after their T-cell receptor binds to a viral peptide presented by a class I MHC protein. The peptides expressed on class I MHC antigens are obtained from viral proteins synthesized within the infected cell (endogenous route). *The viral protein from which these peptides are derived may not elicit protective antibody* (e.g., intracellular or internal virion proteins, nuclear proteins, improperly folded or processed proteins [cell trash]). For example, the matrix and nucleoproteins (cytoplasmic) of the influenza virus and the infected cell protein 4 (ICP4) (nuclear) of herpes simplex virus are targets for CTLs but do not elicit protective antibody. An **immune synapse** formed by interactions of the TCR and MHC I and adhesion molecules creates a space into which **perforin,** a complement-like membrane pore former, and granzymes (degradative enzymes) are released to induce apoptosis in the target cell. Interaction of the Fas ligand protein on CD4 or CD8 T cells with the Fas protein on the target cell can also promote apoptosis. *CTLs kill infected cells and, as a result, eliminate the source of new virus.*

The CD8 T-cell response probably evolved as a defense against viral infection. Cell-mediated immunity is especially important for resolving infections by syncytia-forming viruses (e.g., measles, herpes simplex virus, varicella-zoster virus, HIV), which can spread from cell to cell without exposure to antibody, and by noncytolytic viruses (e.g., hepatitis A and measles viruses). CD8 T cells also interact with neurons to control, without killing, the recurrence of latent

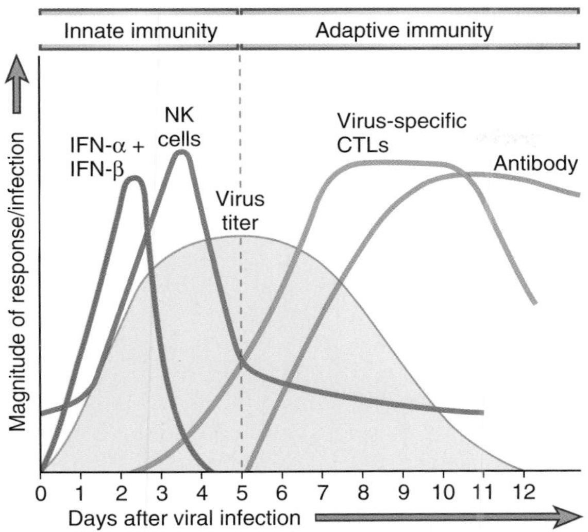

FIGURE 10-6 Time course of antiviral immune responses. (Modified from Abbas AK, Lichtman AH, Pillai S, et al: *Cellular and molecular immunology,* ed 8, Philadelphia, 2015, Elsevier.)

viruses (herpes simplex virus, varicella-zoster virus, and JC papillomaviruses).

Immune Response to Viral Challenge

Primary Viral Challenge

The innate host responses are the earliest responses to viral challenge and are often sufficient to limit viral spread (Figure 10-6; also see Figure 10-3). The **type I interferons** produced in response to most viral infections initiate the protection of adjacent cells, enhance antigen presentation by increasing the expression of MHC antigens, and initiate the clearance of infected cells by activating NK cells and antigen-specific responses. Virus and viral components released from the infected cells are phagocytosed by and activate **iDCs** to produce cytokines and then move to the lymph nodes. Macrophages in the liver and spleen are especially important for clearing virus from the bloodstream (filters). These phagocytic cells degrade and process the viral antigens. DCs present the appropriate peptide fragments bound to class II MHC antigens to CD4 T cells and can also cross-present these antigens on MHC I molecules to CD8 T cells to initiate the response. The APCs also release IL-1, IL-6, and TNF-α and, with IL-12, promote activation of helper T cells and specific cytokine production (TH1 response). The type I interferons and these cytokines induce the prodromal flulike symptoms of many viral infections. The activated T cells move to the site of infection and also B-cell areas of the lymph node, and macrophages and B cells present antigen and become stimulated by the T cells.

Antiviral antigen-specific responses are similar to antibacterial antigen-specific responses, except that the CD8 T cell plays a more important role. **IgM** is produced first, and its production indicates a primary infection. **IgG** and **IgA** are produced after 7 to 10 days. Secretory IgA is made in response to a viral challenge of mucosal surfaces at the natural openings of the body (i.e., eyes, mouth, and respiratory and gastrointestinal systems). Activated **CD4** and **CD8** T cells are present at approximately the same time as serum IgG. During infection, the number of CD8 T cells specific for antigen may increase 100,000-fold. The antigen-specific CD8 T cells move to the site of infection and kill virally infected cells. Recognition and binding to class I MHC viral-peptide complexes promotes apoptotic killing of the target cells, either through the release of perforin and granzymes (to disrupt the cell membrane) or through the binding of the Fas ligand with Fas on the target cell. Resolution of the infection occurs later, when sufficient antibody is available to neutralize all virus progeny or when cellular immunity has been able to reach and eliminate the infected cells. *For the resolution of most enveloped and noncytolytic viral infections, TH1-mediated responses are required to kill the viral factory in addition to antibody neutralization of free virus.*

Viral infections of the brain and the eye can cause serious damage because these tissues cannot repair tissue damage and are **immunologically privileged sites** of the body. TH1 responses are normally suppressed to prevent the serious tissue destruction that accompanies extended inflammation. TH17 responses and special neutrophils are initiated against herpes simplex virus and other virus infections of the eye.

Cell-mediated and IgG immune responses do not arise until 6 to 8 days after an initial viral challenge. For many viral infections, this is after innate responses have controlled viral replication. However, for other viral infections, this period allows the virus to expand the infection, spread through the body and infect the target tissue, and cause disease (e.g., brain, encephalitis; liver, hepatitis). Resolution of the expanded infection may require a larger and more intense immune response, which often includes the immunopathogenesis and tissue damage that cause disease symptoms.

Secondary Viral Challenge

In any war, it is easier to eliminate an enemy if its identity and origin are known and if establishment of its foothold can be prevented. Similarly in the human body, prior immunity established by prior infection or vaccination allows rapid, specific mobilization of defenses to prevent disease symptoms, promote rapid clearance of the virus, and block viremic spread from the primary site of infection to the target tissue to prevent disease. As a result, most secondary viral challenges are asymptomatic. Antibody and memory B and T cells are present in an immune host to generate a more rapid and extensive anamnestic (booster) response to the virus. Secretory antiviral IgA is produced quickly to provide an important defense to reinfection through the natural openings of the body, but it is produced only transiently.

Host, viral, and other factors determine the outcome of the immune response to a viral infection. Host factors include genetic background, immune status, age, and the general health of the individual. Viral factors include viral strain, infectious dose, and route of entry. The time required to initiate immune protection, the extent of the response, the level of control of the infection, and the potential for immunopathology (see Chapter 37) resulting from the infection differ after a primary infection and a rechallenge.

Viral Mechanisms for Escaping the Immune Response

A major factor in the virulence of a virus is its ability to escape immune resolution. Viruses may escape immune resolution by evading detection, preventing activation, or blocking delivery of the immune response. Specific examples

Table 10-3 Examples of Viral Evasion of Immune Responses

Mechanism	Viral Examples	Action
Humoral Response		
Hidden from antibody	Herpesviruses, retroviruses	Latent infection
	Herpes simplex virus, varicella-zoster virus, paramyxoviruses, HIV	Cell-to-cell infection (syncytia formation)
Antigenic variation	Lentiviruses (HIV)	Genetic change after infection
	Influenza virus	Annual genetic changes (drift) Pandemic changes (shift)
Secretion of blocking antigen	Hepatitis B virus	Hepatitis B surface antigen
Interferon		
Block production	Hepatitis B virus	Inhibition of IFN transcription
	Epstein-Barr virus	IL-10 analog (BCRF-1) blocks IFN-γ production
Block action	Adenovirus	Inhibits up-regulation of MHC expression; VA1 blocks double-stranded RNA activation of interferon-induced protein kinase (PKR)
	Herpes simplex virus	Inactivates PKR and activates phosphatase (PP1) to reverse inactivation of initiation factor for protein synthesis
Immune Cell Function		
Impairment of DC function	Measles, hepatitis C	Induction of IFN-β, which limits DC function
Impairment of lymphocyte function	Herpes simplex virus	Prevention of CD8 T-cell killing
	HIV	Kills CD4 T cells and alters macrophages
	Measles virus	Suppression of NK, T, and B cells
Immunosuppressive factors	Epstein-Barr virus	BCRF-1 (similar to IL-10) suppression of CD4 TH1 helper T-cell responses
Decreased Antigen Presentation		
Reduced class I MHC expression	Adenovirus 12	Inhibition of class I MHC transcription; 19-kDa protein (E3 gene) binds class I MHC heavy chain, blocking translocation to surface
	Cytomegalovirus	H301 protein blocks surface expression of β_2-microglobulin and class I MHC molecules
	Herpes simplex virus	ICP47 blocks TAP, preventing peptide entry into ER and binding to class I MHC molecules
Inhibition of Inflammation		
	Poxvirus, adenovirus	Blocking of action of IL-1 or tumor necrosis factor

DC, Dendritic cell; *ER,* endoplasmic reticulum; *HIV,* human immunodeficiency virus; *ICP47,* infected cell protein 47; *IFN,* interferon; *IL,* interleukin; *MHC I,* major histocompatibility complex, antigen type 1; *NK,* natural killer; *PMN,* polymorphonuclear neutrophil; *TAP,* transporter associated with antigen production.

are presented in Table 10-3. Some viruses even encode special proteins that suppress the immune response.

Viral Immunopathogenesis

The symptoms of many viral diseases are the consequence of cytokine action or overzealous immune responses. The flulike symptoms of influenza and any virus that establishes a viremia (e.g., arboviruses) are a result of the interferon and other cytokine responses induced by the virus. Antibody interactions with large amounts of viral antigen in blood, such as occurs with hepatitis B virus infection, can lead to immune complex diseases. The measles rash, the extensive tissue damage to the brain associated with herpes simplex virus encephalitis (*-itis* means "inflammation"), and the tissue damage and symptoms of hepatitis are a result of cell-mediated immune and inflammatory responses. The more aggressive NK-cell and T-cell responses of adults exacerbate some diseases that are benign in children, such as varicella-zoster virus, Epstein-Barr virus infectious mononucleosis, and hepatitis B infection. Yet, the lack of such a response in children makes them prone to chronic hepatitis B infection because the response is insufficient to kill the infected cells and resolve the infection. Viral infections may also provide the initial activation trigger that allows the immune system to respond to self-antigens and cause autoimmune diseases.

Autoimmune diseases may result from an override of the peripheral tolerance mediated by Treg cells following a cytokine storm produced in response to a virus infection, like influenza. In a person who is genetically predisposed to an autoimmune disease (MHC type), this can allow initiation of an anti-self CD4 T cell, antibody, or CD8 T-cell response.

 Box 10-5 **Summary of Antifungal Responses**

Antimicrobial peptides produced by epithelial cells, neutrophils, macrophages and other cells are a primary defense.
Neutrophils are very important. They release reactive oxygen species and antifungal compounds and phagocytize fungi.
Macrophages are also important.
TH17 responses reinforce antifungal neutrophil and epithelial cell function and antimicrobial peptide production but promote inflammation.
TH1 responses reinforce macrophage functions but promote inflammation.
Granuloma formation is important for intracellular infections *(Histoplasma).*
TH2 responses, through immunoglobulin (Ig)G and IgA, can block attachment of fungi and toxin action, but IgE can promote allergy and asthma.

• Specific Immune Responses to Fungi

The primary protective responses to fungal infection are initiated by fungal cell wall carbohydrates binding to TLRs and the dectin-1 lectin and are provided by **neutrophils, macrophages, and antimicrobial peptides** (Box 10-5). CD4 T-cell **TH17 and TH1 responses** stimulate the neutrophil and macrophage responses. Patients deficient in neutrophils or these CD4 T cell–mediated responses (e.g., patients with AIDS) are most susceptible to fungal (opportunistic) infections. Fungal infections can be held in check, undetectable for decades, by effective T cell–induced immune and neutrophil responses, only to awaken upon neutrophil or T-cell deficiency and become lethal. Defensins and other cationic peptides may be important for some fungal infections (e.g., mucormycosis, aspergillosis), and nitric oxide may be important against *Cryptococcus* and other fungi. Respiratory infection with *Histoplasma* causes intracellular infection of macrophages eliciting immune responses similar to *M. tuberculosis*. Antibody, as an opsonin, may facilitate clearance of the fungi but may also elicit disease-causing hypersensitivity reactions. Fungi and fungal spores are a common allergen and inducer of asthma and allergic alveolitis.

• Specific Immune Responses to Parasites

It is difficult to generalize about the mechanisms of antiparasitic immunity, because there are many different parasites that have different forms and reside in different tissue locations during their life cycles (Box 10-6 and Table 10-4). Stimulation of *CD4 TH1, TH17, CD8 T-cell, and macrophage responses are important for intracellular infections, and neutrophils, macrophages, and TH2 antibody responses are important for extracellular parasites in blood and fluids.* **IgE, eosinophil,** and **mast cell** action are triggered by and are especially important for eliminating worm (cestode and nematode) infections. The efficiency of control of the infection may depend on which response is initiated in the host. Dominance of a TH2 response against *Leishmania* infections results in the inhibition of TH1 activation of macrophages, inability to clear intracellular parasites, and a poor outcome. This observation provided the basis for the discovery that

 Box 10-6 **Summary of Antiparasitic Responses**

Different immune responses are necessary depending upon the nature of the parasite and the replicative stage.
Many parasites have multiple tricks to evade immune responses.
TH2 responses, through immunoglobulin (Ig)G and IgA, are important for preventing parasite binding to tissue, to block binding and entry into cells, to activate complement, and as an opsonin.
IgE bound to mast cells and eosinophils binds parasite and parasite antigen, and releases histamine and toxic substances to promote expulsion.
TH2 responses activate mucus secretion into colon to promote expulsion.
TH1 responses are especially important for intracellular infections *(Leishmania)* but promote inflammation.
Granuloma formation is important for intracellular infections *(Schistosoma).*
TH17 responses reinforce epithelial and neutrophil action for extracellular parasites.

TH1 and TH2 responses are separate and antagonistic. Parasites have developed sophisticated mechanisms for avoiding immune clearance and often establish chronic infections.

Extracellular parasites such as *Trypanosoma cruzi, Toxoplasma gondii,* and *Leishmania* species are phagocytosed by **macrophage. Antibody** may facilitate the uptake of (opsonize) the parasites. Killing of the parasites follows activation of the macrophage by IFN-γ (produced by NK, γ/δ T, or CD4 TH1 cells) or TNF-α (produced by other macrophages) and induction of **oxygen-dependent killing mechanisms** (peroxide, superoxide, nitric oxide). The parasites may replicate in the macrophage and hide from subsequent immune detection unless the macrophage is activated by TH1 responses.

TH1 production of IFN-γ and activation of macrophages are also essential for defense against intracellular protozoa and for the development of **granulomas** around *Schistosoma mansoni* eggs and worms in the liver. The granuloma, formed by layers of inflammatory cells, protects the liver from toxins produced by the eggs. However, the granuloma also causes fibrosis that interrupts the venous blood supply to the liver, leading to hypertension and cirrhosis.

Neutrophils phagocytize and kill extracellular parasites through both oxygen-dependent and oxygen-independent mechanisms. **Eosinophils** localize near parasites, bind to IgG or IgE on the surface of larvae or worms (e.g., helminths, *S. mansoni,* and *Trichinella spiralis*), degranulate by fusing their intracellular granules with the plasma membrane, and release the **major basic protein** into the intercellular space. The major basic protein is toxic to the parasite.

For parasitic worm infections, IL-4 and other cytokines produced by epithelial cells, innate lymphoid cells, and CD4 TH2 T cells are very important for stimulating production of IgE and activating mast cells (Figure 10-7). IgE bound to Fc receptors on mast cells targets the cells to antigens of the infecting parasite. In the lumen of the intestine, antigen binding and cross-linking of the IgE on the mast cell surface stimulate the release of histamine and substances toxic to the parasite. TH2 responses also promote mucus secretion to coat and promote expulsion of the worm.

Table 10-4 Examples of Antiparasitic Immune Responses

Parasite	Habitat	Main Host Effector Mechanism*	Method of Avoidance
Trypanosoma brucei	Bloodstream	Antibody + complement	Antigenic variation
Plasmodium species	Hepatocyte, erythrocyte	Antibody, cytokines, TH1 for hepatocyte	Intracellular growth, erythrocyte infection, antigenic variation
Toxoplasma gondii	Macrophage	O_2 metabolites, NO, lysosomal enzymes (TH1)	Inhibition of fusion with lysosomes
Trypanosoma cruzi	Many cells	O_2 metabolites, NO, lysosomal enzymes (TH1)	Escape into cytoplasm, thus avoiding digestion in lysosome
Leishmania species	Macrophage	O_2 metabolites, NO, lysosomal enzymes (TH1)	Impairment of O_2 burst and scavenging of products; avoidance of digestion
Trichinella spiralis	Gut, blood, muscle	Myeloid cells, antibody + complement (TH2)	Encystment in muscle
Schistosoma mansoni	Skin, blood, lungs, portal vein	Myeloid cells, antibody + complement (TH2)	Acquisition of host antigens, blockade by antibody; soluble antigens and immune complexes; antioxidants
Wuchereria bancrofti	Lymphatic system	Myeloid cells, antibody + complement (TH2)	Thick, extracellular cuticle; antioxidants
Helminths	Gut	IgE	Extracellular cuticle

Adapted from Roitt I, Brostoff J, Male D, et al: *Immunology,* ed 4, St Louis, 1996, Mosby.

IgE, Immunoglobulin E; *NO,* nitric oxide; *TH,* T helper (cell).

*Antibody is most important for extracellular pathogens. Cell-mediated immunity (TH1 response) is most important for intracellular pathogens.

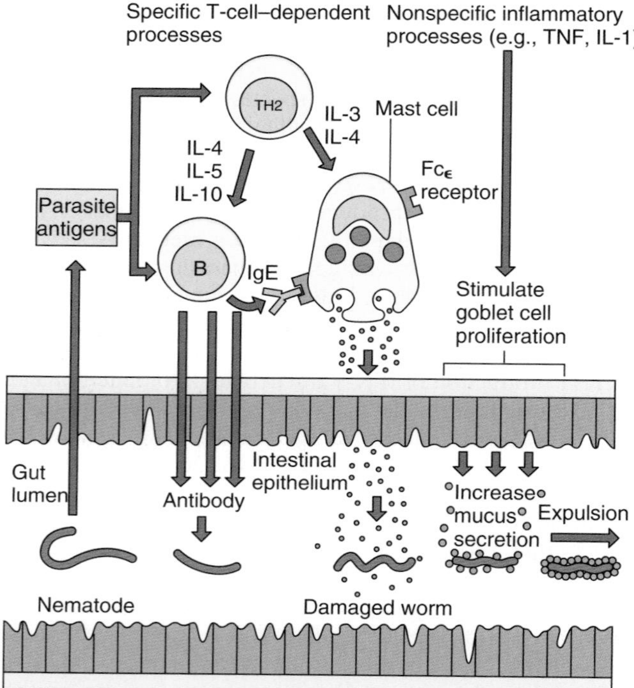

FIGURE 10-7 Elimination of nematodes from the gut. TH2 responses are important for stimulating the production of antibody. Antibody can damage the worm. Immunoglobulin E *(IgE)* is associated with mast cells, release of histamine, and toxic substances. Increased mucus secretion also promotes expulsion. *IL,* Interleukin; *TNF,* tumor necrosis factor. (From Roitt I, Brostoff J, Male D, et al: *Immunology,* ed 4, St Louis, 1996, Mosby.)

IgG antibody also plays an important role in antiparasitic immunity, as an opsonin and by activating complement on the surface of the parasite.

Malaria poses an interesting challenge for the immune response. Protective antibodies are made toward attachment and other surface proteins, but these differ for each of the stages of the parasite's development. TH1 responses and CTLs may be important during liver phases of infection. While in the erythrocyte, the parasite is hidden from antibody, unrecognizable by CTLs, but can stimulate NK- and NKT-cell responses. Cytokines, especially TNF-α, produced by these cells promote protection but also immunopathogenesis. Immune complexes containing malarial components and cell debris released upon erythrocyte lysis can clog small capillaries and activate type II hypersensitivity reactions (see later) and promote inflammatory tissue damage.

Evasion of Immune Mechanisms by Parasites

Animal parasites have developed remarkable mechanisms for establishing chronic infections in the vertebrate host (see Table 10-4). These mechanisms include intracellular growth, inactivation of phagocytic killing, release of blocking antigen (e.g., *Trypanosoma brucei, Plasmodium falciparum*), and development of cysts (e.g., protozoa: *Entamoeba histolytica;* helminths: *T. spiralis*) to limit access by the immune response. The African trypanosomes can reengineer the genes for their surface antigen (variable surface glycoprotein) and therefore change their antigenic appearance. Schistosomes can coat themselves with host antigens, including MHC molecules.

• Other Immune Responses

Antitumor responses and **rejection of tissue transplants** are primarily mediated by the TH1 immune response (Animation 10-2). CD8 cytolytic T cells recognize and kill tumors expressing peptides from embryologic proteins, mutated proteins, or other proteins on class I MHC molecules (endogenous route of peptide presentation). These proteins may be expressed inappropriately by the tumor cell, and the host immune response may not be tolerized to them. Most tumors activate wound healing responses (tissue remodeling and angiogenesis) from M2 macrophage and promote immunosuppression of T cells.

T-cell rejection of **allografts** used for tissue transplants is triggered by recognition of foreign peptides expressed on foreign class I MHC antigens. Antibody to foreign antigens can also cause rejection by activating complement and antibody-dependent cellular cytotoxicity killing of the graft. In addition to host rejection of the transplanted tissue, cells from the donor of a blood transfusion or a tissue transplant can initiate a response or react against the new host in a **graft-versus-host (GVH) response.** An in vitro test of T-cell activation and growth in a GVH-like response is the **mixed lymphocyte reaction.** Activation is usually measured as T-cell DNA synthesis.

• Immunopathogenesis

Hypersensitivity Responses

Once activated, the immune response is sometimes difficult to control and causes tissue damage. Hypersensitivity reactions are responsible for many of the symptoms associated with microbial infections. Hypersensitivity reactions occur to people who have already established immunity to the antigen. *The mediator and the time course* primarily distinguish the four types of hypersensitivity responses (Table 10-5).

Type I hypersensitivity is caused by **IgE** and is associated with **allergic, atopic,** and **anaphylactic reactions** (Figure 10-8; Animation 10-3). IgE allergic reactions are rapid-onset reactions. IgE binds to Fc receptors on mast cells and becomes the cell surface receptor for antigens **(allergens).** Cross-linking of several cell surface IgE molecules by an allergen (e.g., pollen) triggers degranulation, releasing **chemoattractants** (chemokines, leukotrienes) to attract eosinophils, neutrophils, and mononuclear cells; **activators** (histamine, platelet-activating factor, tryptase, kininogenase, cytokines) to promote vasodilation and edema; and **spasmogens** (histamine, prostaglandin D_2, leukotrienes) to directly affect bronchial smooth muscle and promote mucus secretion. Desensitization (allergy shots) produces IgG to bind the allergen and prevent allergen binding to IgE. After 8 to 12

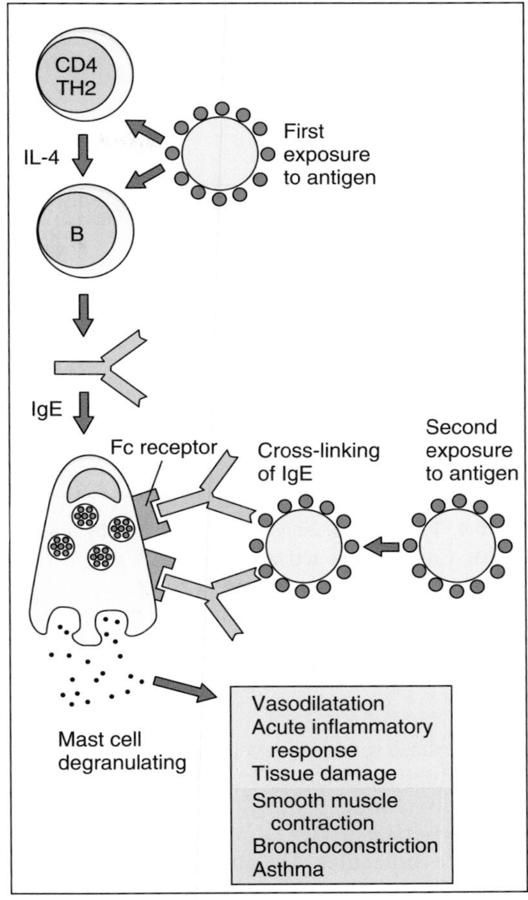

FIGURE 10-8 Type I hypersensitivity: immunoglobulin E *(IgE)*–mediated atopic and anaphylactic reactions. IgE produced in response to the initial challenge binds to Fc receptors on mast cells and basophils. Allergen binding and cross-linking of the cell surface IgE promotes release of histamine and prostaglandins from granules to produce symptoms. Examples are hay fever, asthma, penicillin allergy, and reaction to bee stings. *IL,* Interleukin; *TH,* T helper (cell).

Table 10-5 Hypersensitivity Reactions

Reaction Type	Onset Time	Key Features	Beneficial Effects	Pathologic Effects
Type I	<30 min	Soluble antigen-triggered, IgE-dependent release of vasoactive mediators followed by late-phase reaction	Antiparasitic responses and toxin neutralization	Localized allergies (e.g., hay fever, asthma) Systemic anaphylaxis
Type II	<8 hr	Cell-bound antibody promoting C′-mediated cytotoxicity; binding and modulation of receptor function	Direct lysis and phagocytosis of extracellular bacteria and other susceptible microbes	Destruction of red blood cells (e.g., transfusion reactions, Rh disease) Organ-specific tissue damage in some autoimmune diseases (e.g., Goodpasture syndrome)
Type III	<8 hr	Soluble antigen-antibody complexes activate C′	Acute inflammatory reaction at site of extracellular microbes and their clearance	Arthus reaction (localized) Serum sickness and drug reactions (generalized) Systemic autoimmune diseases
Type IV	24-72 hr (acute); >1 week (chronic)	Phagocytized soluble antigen presented to CD4 T cells activates macrophages and inflammation	Protection against infection by fungi, intracellular bacteria, and viruses	Acute: contact dermatitis, tuberculosis skin test Chronic: granuloma formation

ADCC, Antibody-dependent cellular cytotoxicity; *MHC,* major histocompatibility complex; *TH,* T helper (cell).

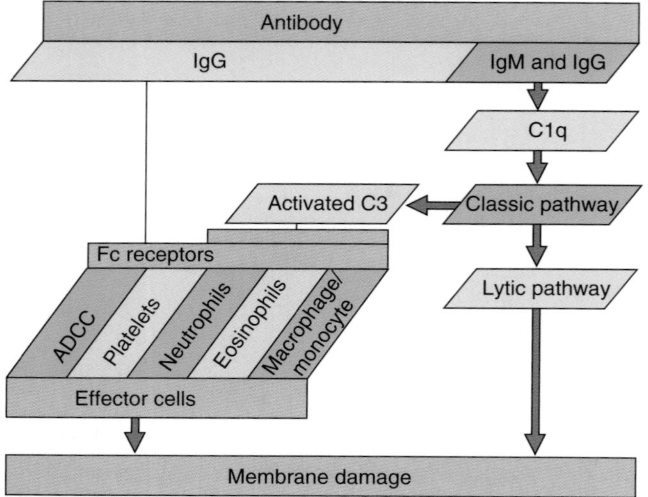

FIGURE 10-9 Type II hypersensitivity: mediated by antibody and complement. Complement activation promotes direct cell damage through the complement cascade and by the activation of effector cells. Examples are Goodpasture syndrome, the response to Rh factor in newborns, and autoimmune endocrinopathies. *ADCC,* Antibody-dependent cellular cytotoxicity; *Ig,* immunoglobulin.

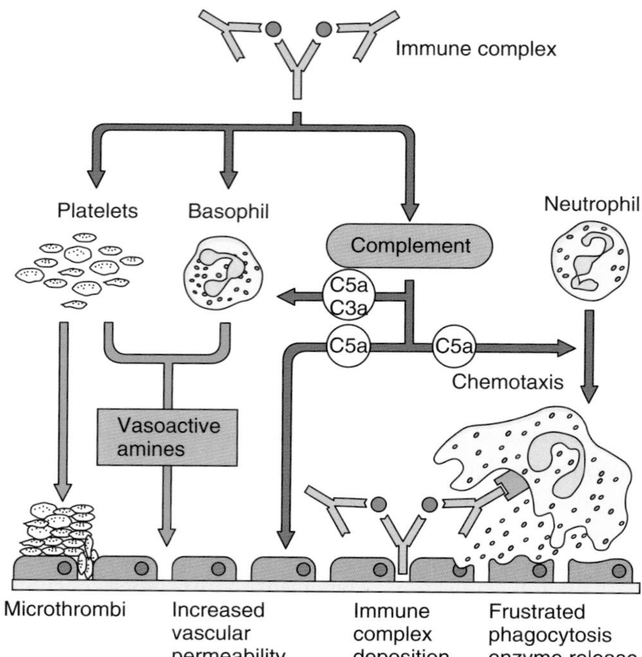

FIGURE 10-10 Type III hypersensitivity: immune complex deposition. Immune complexes can be trapped in the kidney and elsewhere in the body and can activate complement to promote inflammation. Examples are serum sickness, nephritis associated with chronic hepatitis B infection, and Arthus reaction.

hours, a late-phase reaction develops because of the infiltration of eosinophils and CD4 T cells and cytokine reinforcement of inflammation.

Type II hypersensitivity is caused by **antibody binding to cell surface molecules.** The antibody may promote cytolytic responses by the **classic complement cascade** or antibody-dependent cellular cytotoxicity (Figure 10-9). These reactions occur as early as 8 hours following a tissue or blood transplant or as part of a chronic disease. Examples of these reactions are autoimmune hemolytic anemia and Goodpasture syndrome (lung and kidney basement membrane damage). Another example is hemolytic disease of newborns (blue babies), which results when maternal IgG antibody, generated during the first pregnancy to an incompatible Rh factor on fetal erythrocytes, crosses the placenta and harms a second baby (Rh incompatibility).

Antireceptor antibody activation or inhibition of effector functions is also considered a type II response. Myasthenia gravis is due to antibodies to acetylcholine receptors on neurons, Graves disease results from antibody stimulation of the thyroid-stimulating hormone (TSH) receptor, and some forms of diabetes can result from antibodies blocking the insulin receptor.

Type III hypersensitivity responses result from activation of **complement** by **immune complexes** (Figure 10-10). In the presence of an abundance of soluble antigen in the bloodstream, large antigen-antibody complexes form, become trapped in capillaries (especially in the kidney), and then initiate the classical complement cascade. Activation of the complement cascade initiates inflammatory reactions. Immune complex disease may be caused by infections (e.g., hepatitis B, malaria, staphylococcal infective endocarditis, group A streptococcal–associated glomerulonephritis), autoimmunity (e.g., rheumatoid arthritis, systemic lupus erythematosus), or persistent inhalation of antigen (e.g., mold, plant, or animal antigens). For example, hepatitis B infection produces large amounts of hepatitis B surface antigen that may promote formation of immune complexes that lead to glomerulonephritis. Type III hypersensitivity reactions can be induced in presensitized people by the intradermal injection of antigen to cause an **Arthus reaction,** a skin reaction characterized by redness and swelling. Annual booster immunizations to influenza may elicit an Arthus reaction at the site of the immunization owing to the presence of antibody from the previous year's immunization. Serum sickness, extrinsic allergic alveolitis (a reaction to inhaled fungal antigen), and glomerulonephritis result from type III hypersensitivity reactions. Serum sickness can result after receiving animal immunoglobulin (e.g., anti-snake venom) on multiple occasions.

Type IV hypersensitivity responses are **TH1-mediated delayed-type hypersensitivity (DTH)** inflammatory responses (Figure 10-11 and Table 10-6). It usually takes 24 to 48 hours for antigen to be presented to **circulating CD4 T cells,** for them to move to the site, and then to **activate macrophages** to induce inflammation. DTH is responsible for **contact dermatitis** (e.g., cosmetics, nickel) and the response to poison ivy. Intradermal injection of **tuberculin antigen** (purified protein derivative) elicits firm swelling that is maximal 48 to 72 hours after injection and indicative of prior exposure to *M. tuberculosis* (Figure 10-12). Granulomatous hypersensitivity occurs with tuberculosis, leprosy, schistosomiasis, sarcoidosis, and Crohn disease. **Granulomas** form in response to continued stimulation by the intracellular growth of *M. tuberculosis.* These structures consist of epithelioid cells created from chronically activated macrophages, fused epithelioid cells (multinucleated giant cells) surrounded by lymphocytes, and

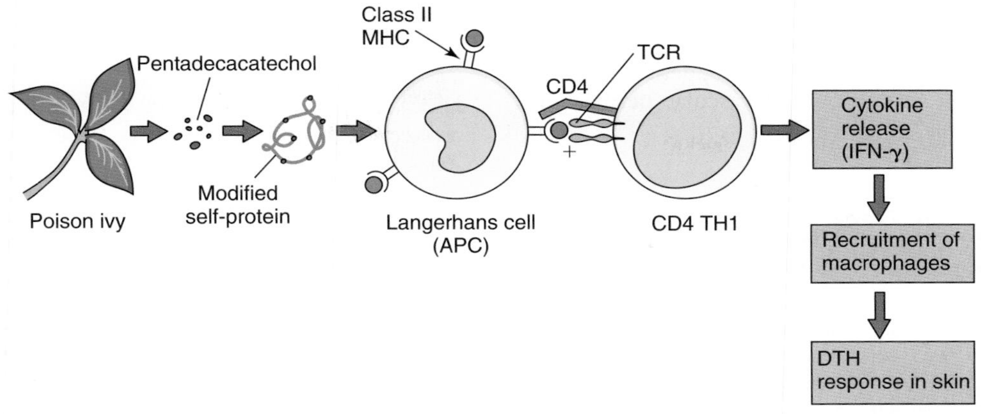

FIGURE 10-11 Type IV hypersensitivity: delayed-type hypersensitivity *(DTH)* mediated by CD4 T cells *(TH1)*. In this case, chemically modified self-proteins are processed, and peptides are presented to CD4 memory T cells cycling through the skin, which release cytokines (including interferon-γ *[IFN-γ]*) that promote inflammation. Other examples of DTH are the tuberculin response (purified protein derivative test) and reaction to metals such as nickel. *APC,* Antigen-presenting cell; *TCR,* T-cell receptor.

Table 10-6 Important Characteristics of Four Types of Delayed-Type Hypersensitivity Reactions

Type	Reaction Time	Clinical Appearance	Histologic Appearance	Antigen
Jones-Mote	24-48 hr	Skin swelling	Basophils, lymphocytes, mononuclear cells	Intradermal antigen: reaction to PPD or other protein antigen
Tuberculin	48 hr	Local induration and swelling with or without fever	Mononuclear cells, lymphocytes and monocytes, reduced macrophages	Dermal: tuberculin (PPD), mycobacterial, leishmanial
Contact	48 hr	Eczema	Mononuclear cells, edema, raised epidermis	Epidermal: nickel, rubber, poison ivy
Granulomatous	4 wk	Skin induration	Epithelioid cell granuloma, giant cells, macrophages, fibrosis with or without necrosis	Persistent antigen or antigen-antibody complexes in macrophages or "nonimmunologic" (e.g., talcum powder)

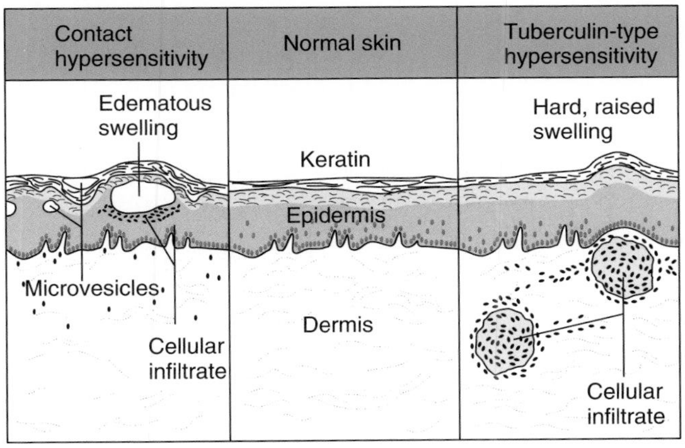

FIGURE 10-12 Contact and tuberculin hypersensitivity responses. These type IV responses are cell mediated but differ in the site of cell infiltration and in the symptoms. Contact hypersensitivity occurs in the epidermis and leads to the formation of blisters; tuberculin-type hypersensitivity occurs in the dermis and is characterized by swelling.

fibrosis caused by the deposition of collagen from fibroblasts. The granulomas restrict the spread of *M. tuberculosis* as long as CD4 T cells can provide IFN-γ.

Cytokine Storm

Sepsis, toxin-mediated shock syndrome (e.g., induced by *Staphylococcus* toxic shock syndrome toxin), some viral infections (e.g., severe acute respiratory syndrome [SARS]) and influenza, and graft-versus-host disease induce an overwhelming stimulation of innate and/or immune responses, producing excessive amounts of cytokines that disrupt the physiology of the body. The consequences are multisystem dysregulation, rash, fever, and shock. Superantigens clamp together TCRs with the MHC II molecules on antigen-presenting cells to activate up to 20% of T cells. This triggers uncontrolled release of excess T cell– and macrophage-produced cytokines until the T cell dies of apoptosis. Bacteria, endotoxin, or viruses in blood can promote production of large amounts of acute-phase cytokines and type I interferons by plasmacytoid DCs, and certain viruses are very potent activators of interferon and cytokine production. Large amounts of TNF-α are produced during cytokine storms. TNF-α can promote inflammatory processes such as enhanced vascular leakage and activation of neutrophils that can be beneficial on a local level, but on a systemic level will lead to fever, chills, aches, stimulation of coagulation pathways, elevated liver enzymes, loss of appetite, enhanced metabolism, weight loss, increased vascular permeability, and potentially shock.

• Autoimmune Responses

Normally a person is tolerized to self-antigens during the development of T cells and B cells and by Treg cells. Autoimmunity can be induced by any or all of the following: overriding Treg-induced tolerance by excessive cytokine production (e.g., cytokine storm, systemic lupus erythematosus), cross-reactivity with microbial antigens (e.g., group A streptococcal infection, rheumatic fever), polyclonal activation of lymphocytes induced by tumors or infection (e.g., malaria, Epstein-Barr virus infection), a genetic predisposition toward expression of self-antigenic peptides (MHC association), or lack of tolerization to specific antigens.

Autoimmune diseases result from the presence of autoantibodies, activated T cells, and hypersensitivity reactions. People with certain MHC antigens are at higher risk for autoimmune responses (e.g., HLA-B27: juvenile rheumatoid arthritis, ankylosing spondylitis). Once initiated, a cycle is established between antigen-presenting cells and T cells, which produce cytokines to promote inflammation and tissue damage and more self-antigen. TH17 and TH1 responses are responsible for rheumatoid arthritis and other diseases.

• Immunodeficiency

Immunodeficiency may result from genetic deficiencies, starvation, drug-induced immunosuppression (e.g., steroid treatment, cancer chemotherapy, chemotherapeutic suppression of tissue graft rejection), cancer (especially of immune cells), or disease (e.g., AIDS) and naturally occurs in neonates and pregnant women. Deficiencies in specific protective responses put a patient at high risk for serious disease caused by infectious agents that should be controlled by that response (Table 10-7). These "natural experiments" illustrate the importance of specific responses in controlling specific infections.

Immunosuppression

Immunosuppressive therapy is important for reducing excessive inflammatory or immune responses or for preventing the rejection of tissue transplants by T cells. The therapy addresses the symptoms, the activator, or the mediator of the response. Aspirin and nonsteroidal antiinflammatory drugs (NSAIDs) target the cyclooxygenases that generate inflammatory prostaglandins (e.g., PGD_2) and pain. Other **antiinflammatory treatments** target the production and action of TNF-α, IL-12, and IL-1. Corticosteroids prevent their production by macrophages and may be toxic to T cells. Soluble forms of the TNF-α receptor and antibody to TNF-α can be used to block the binding of TNF-α and prevent its action. Antibodies to other cytokines, adhesion proteins on T cells or antigen-presenting cells, and antagonists of CD28 can block T-cell activation of inflammatory and other responses.

Table 10-7 Infections Associated with Defects in Immune Responses

Defect	Pathogen
Induction by physical means (e.g., burns, trauma)	*Pseudomonas aeruginosa*
	Staphylococcus aureus
	Staphylococcus epidermidis
	Streptococcus pyogenes
	Aspergillus species
	Candida species
Splenectomy	Encapsulated bacteria and fungi
Granulocyte and monocyte defects in movement, phagocytosis, or killing or decreased number of cells (neutropenia)	*S. aureus*
	S. pyogenes
	Haemophilus influenzae
	Gram-negative bacilli
	Escherichia coli
	Klebsiella species
	P. aeruginosa
	Nocardia species
	Aspergillus species
	Candida species
Individual components of complement system	*S. aureus*
	Streptococcus pneumoniae
	Pseudomonas species
	Proteus species
	Neisseria species
T cells	Cytomegalovirus
	Herpes simplex virus
	Herpes zoster virus
	Human herpesvirus 8
	Listeria monocytogenes
	Mycobacterium species
	Nocardia species
	Aspergillus species
	Candida species
	Cryptococcus neoformans
	Histoplasma capsulatum
	Pneumocystis jirovecii
	Strongyloides stercoralis
B cells	Enteroviruses
	S. aureus
	Streptococcus species
	H. influenzae
	Neisseria meningitidis
	E. coli
	Giardia lamblia
	P. jirovecii
Combined immunodeficiency	See pathogens listed for T cells and B cells

Immunosuppressive therapy for transplantation generally inhibits the action or causes the lysis of T cells. Cyclosporine, tacrolimus (FK-506), and rapamycin prevent the activation of T cells (see Figure 9-3). Anti–CD40 ligand and anti–IL-2 prevent activation of T cells, whereas anti-CD3 promotes complement lysis of T cells to suppress T-cell responses. Anti–TNF-α and other ablative therapies increase risk of *M. tuberculosis* disease and anti–α4 integrin cell adhesion molecule increases the risk of JC virus reactivation disease (progressive multifocal leukoencephalopathy).

Hereditary Complement Deficiencies and Microbial Infection

Inherited **deficiencies of C1q, C1r, C1s, C4,** and **C2** components are associated with defects in activation of the classic complement pathway that lead to greater susceptibility to pyogenic (pus-producing) staphylococcal and streptococcal infections (Figure 10-13). These bacteria are not controlled by γ/δ T cell–induced responses. A **deficiency of C3** leads to a defect in activation of both the classical and the alternative pathways, which also results in a higher incidence of pyogenic infections. **Defects of the properdin factors** impair activation of the alternative pathway, which also results in an increased susceptibility to pyogenic infections. Finally, **deficiencies of C5 through C9** are associated with defective cell killing, which raises the susceptibility to disseminated infections by *Neisseria* species.

Defects in Phagocyte Action

People with defective phagocytes are more susceptible to bacterial infections but not to viral or protozoal infections (Figure 10-14). The clinical relevance of oxygen-dependent killing is illustrated by **chronic granulomatous disease** in children who lack the enzymes (e.g., NADPH oxidase) to produce superoxide anions. Although phagocytosis is normal, these children have an impaired ability to oxidize NADPH and destroy bacteria or fungi through the oxidative pathway. In patients with **Chédiak-Higashi syndrome,** the neutrophil granules fuse when the cells are immature in the bone marrow. Thus neutrophils from these patients can phagocytose bacteria but have greatly diminished ability to kill them. Granulomas are formed around the infected phagocyte to control the infection. **Asplenic individuals** are at risk for infection with encapsulated organisms, because such people lack the filtration mechanism of spleen macrophages. Other deficiencies are shown in Figure 10-14.

Deficiencies in Antigen-Specific Immune Responses

People deficient in **T-cell function** are susceptible to **opportunistic infections** by (1) viruses, especially enveloped and noncytolytic viruses and recurrences of viruses that establish latent infections, (2) intracellular bacteria, (3) fungi, and (4) some parasites. T-cell deficiencies can also prevent the

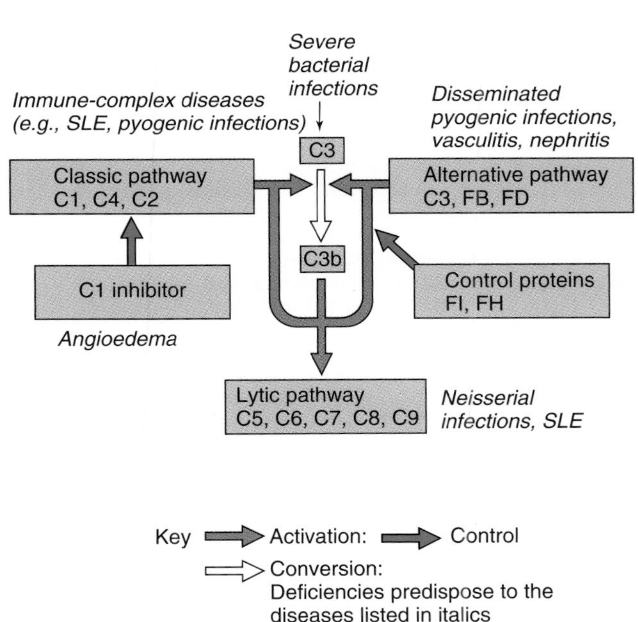

FIGURE 10-13 Consequences of deficiencies in the complement pathways. A deficiency in the activation or control of complement can lead to disease. The phagocytic response to bacterial infections is compromised when C3a and C5a are deficient. Factor B binds to C3b on cell surfaces, and the plasma serine protease D cleaves and activates B-C3b as part of the alternative pathway. Factors FI and FH limit inappropriate activation of complement. FH binds to C3b and prevents activation and is a cofactor for FI. FI is a serine protease that cleaves C3b and C4b. *SLE,* Systemic lupus erythematosus.

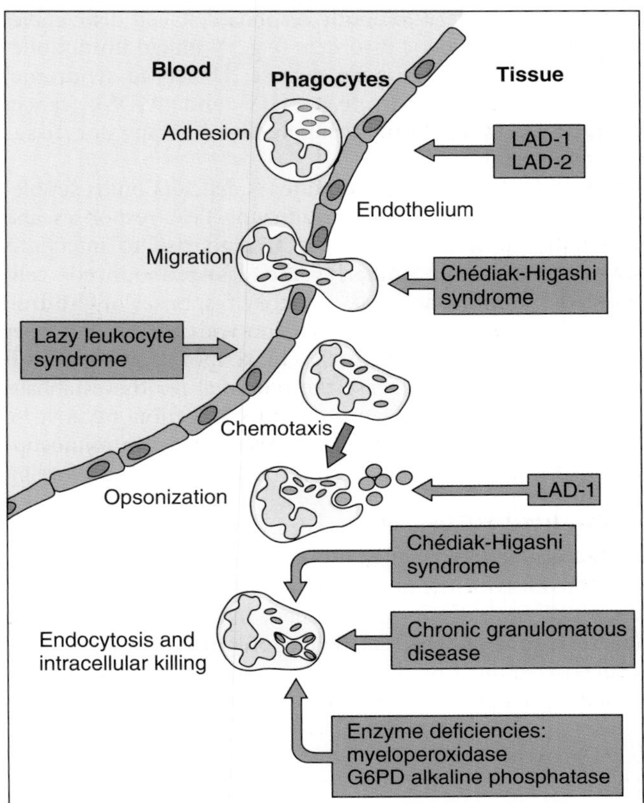

FIGURE 10-14 Consequences of phagocyte dysfunction. Inability to sense or access an infection or to bind, internalize, or kill internalized bacteria increases susceptibility to serious bacterial disease. *G6PD,* Glucose-6-phosphate dehydrogenase; *LAD-1,* leukocyte adhesion deficiency-1.

Table 10-8 Immunodeficiencies of Lymphocytes

Condition	T Cell No.	T-Cell Function	B Cell No.	Serum Antibodies	Incidence*
XLA, Bruton syndrome	✓	✓	↓↓	↓	Rare
RAG1 or RAG2 deficiency	↓↓	↓↓	↓↓	None	Rare
X-SCID	↓↓	↓	✓	↓	Rare
XLP, Duncan syndrome	✓	↓	✓	✓ or ↓	Rare
X-hyper IgM (CD40 or CD40L mutation)	✓	↓	✓	IgM↑↑ No IgG, IgE, or IgA	Rare
Wiskott-Aldrich syndrome	✓	↓	✓	↓	Rare
SCID: ADA or PNP deficiency	↓↓	↓↓	↓	↓	Very rare
HLA deficiency	↓	↓	✓	Poor Ag response	Very rare
Ataxia telangiectasia	↓	↓	✓	IgE↓, IgA↓, IgG2↓	Uncommon
DiGeorge syndrome	↓↓	↓	✓	IgG↓, IgE↓, IgA↓	Very rare
IgA deficiency	✓	✓	✓	IgA↓	Common

Modified from Brostoff J, Male DK: *Clinical immunology: an illustrated outline,* St Louis, 1994, Mosby.

✓, Normal; ↑, increased; ↓, decreased or defective; *ADA,* adenosine deaminase; *Ag,* antigen; *HLA,* human leukocyte antigen; *Ig,* immunoglobulin; *PNP,* purine nucleoside phosphorylase; *RAG,* recombination-activating gene; *XLA,* X-linked agammaglobulinemia; *XLP,* X-linked lymphoproliferative (syndrome); *X-SCID,* X-linked severe, combined immunodeficiency disease.

*Approximate incidence: very rare = $<10^{-6}$; rare = 10^{-5} to 10^{-6}; common = 10^{-2} to 10^{-3}.

maturation of B-cell antibody responses. T-cell deficiencies can arise from genetic disorders (e.g., X-linked immunodeficiency syndrome, Duncan disease, DiGeorge syndrome) (Table 10-8), infection (e.g., HIV and AIDS), cancer chemotherapy, or immunosuppressive therapy for tissue transplantation.

The T-cell response of **neonates** is deficient but is supplemented by maternal IgG. Insufficient TH1 responses and deficiency in IFN-γ puts them at high risk to infections by herpesviruses. Similarly, the less-pronounced cell-mediated immune and inflammatory responses of **children** decrease the severity (in comparison with adults) of herpes (e.g., infectious mononucleosis, chickenpox) and hepatitis B infections but also increase the potential for the establishment of a chronic hepatitis B virus infection because of incomplete resolution. Pregnancy also induces immunosuppressive measures to prevent rejection of the fetus (a foreign tissue).

B-cell deficiencies may result in a complete lack of antibody production (hypogammaglobulinemia), inability to undergo class switching, or inability to produce specific subclasses of antibody. People deficient in antibody production are very susceptible to **bacterial infection.** IgA deficiency, which occurs in 1 of 700 whites, results in a greater susceptibility to **respiratory infections.**

Bibliography

Abbas AK, Lichtman AH, Pillai S, et al: *Cellular and molecular immunology*, ed 6, Philadelphia, 2007, WB Saunders.

Alcami A, Koszinowski UH: Viral mechanisms of immune evasion, *Trends Microbiol* 8:410–418, 2000.

DeFranco AL, Locksley RM, Robertson M: *Immunity: the immune response in infectious and inflammatory disease*, Sunderland, Mass, 2007, Sinauer Associates.

Janeway CA, Travers P, Walport M, et al: *Immunobiology: the immune system in health and disease*, ed 6, New York, 2004, Garland Science.

Kindt TJ, Goldsby RA, Osborne BA: *Kuby immunology*, ed 6, New York, 2007, WH Freeman.

Kumar V, Abbas AK, Fausto N: *Robbins and Cotran pathologic basis of disease*, ed 7, Philadelphia, 2005, Elsevier.

Male D: *Immunology*, ed 4, London, 2004, Elsevier.

Mims C, Dockrell HM, Goering RV, et al: *Medical microbiology*, ed 3, London, 2004, Elsevier.

Novak R: *Crash course immunology*, Philadelphia, 2006, Mosby.

Rosenthal KS: Are microbial symptoms "self-inflicted"? The consequences of immunopathology, *Infect Dis Clin Pract* 13:306–310, 2005.

Rosenthal KS: Vaccines make good immune theater: immunization as described in a three-act play, *Infect Dis Clin Pract* 14:35–45, 2006.

Rosenthal KS, Wilkinson JG: Flow cytometry and immunospeak, *Infect Dis Clin Pract* 15:183–191, 2007.

Sompayrac L: *How the immune system works*, ed 2, Malden, Mass, 2003, Blackwell Scientific.

Trends Immunol: Issues contain understandable reviews on current topics in immunology.

CHAPTER

11 ANTIMICROBIAL VACCINES

Immunity, whether generated in reaction to infection or immunization or administered as therapy, can prevent or lessen the serious symptoms of disease. The memory immune responses activated upon challenge of an immunized individual are faster and stronger than for an unimmunized individual. The immunization of a population, like personal immunity, stops the spread of the infectious agent by reducing the number of susceptible hosts **(herd immunity).** Immunization programs on national and international levels have achieved the following goals:

1. Protection of population groups from the symptoms of pertussis, diphtheria, tetanus, and rabies
2. Protection and control of the spread of measles, mumps, rubella, varicella-zoster virus, influenza, rotavirus, and *Haemophilus influenzae* type B (Hib)
3. Elimination of wild-type poliomyelitis in most of the world and smallpox worldwide

In conjunction with immunization programs, measures can be taken to prevent disease by limiting the exposure of healthy people to infected people **(quarantine)** and by eliminating the source (e.g., water purification) or means of spread (e.g., mosquito eradication) of the infectious agent. As of 1977, natural smallpox was eliminated through a successful World Health Organization (WHO) program that combined vaccination and quarantine. Polio and measles have also been targeted for elimination.

Vaccine-preventable diseases still occur, however, where immunization is unavailable or too expensive (developing countries) or misinformation, personal beliefs, or complacency deter use. For example, measles outbreaks, which cause 2 million deaths annually worldwide, continue to occur in the United States for all of these reasons.

• Types of Immunizations

The injection of purified antibody, antibody-containing serum, or immune cells to provide rapid temporary protection or treatment of a person is termed **passive immunization.** Newborns receive natural passive immunity from maternal immunoglobulin that crosses the placenta or is present in the mother's milk. Therapeutic antibodies that block autoimmune responses and personalized T-cell or dendritic-cell antitumor therapy are also forms of passive immunity.

Active immunization occurs when an immune response is stimulated because of challenge with an immunogen, such as exposure to an infectious agent **(natural immunization)** or through exposure to microbes or their antigens in **vaccines.** On subsequent challenge with the virulent agent, a secondary immune response is activated that is faster and more effective at protecting the individual, or antibody is present to block the spread or virulence of the agent.

Passive Immunization

Passive immunization may be used as follows:

1. To prevent disease after a known exposure (e.g., needlestick injury with blood that is contaminated with hepatitis B virus [HBV])
2. To ameliorate the symptoms of an ongoing disease
3. To protect immunodeficient individuals
4. To block the action of bacterial toxins or venoms and prevent the diseases they cause (i.e., as therapy)

Immune serum globulin preparations derived from seropositive humans or animals (e.g., horses) are available as prophylaxis for several bacterial and viral diseases (Table 11-1). Human serum globulin is prepared from pooled plasma and contains the normal repertoire of antibodies for an adult. Special high-titer immune globulin preparations are available for hepatitis B virus (HBIg), varicella-zoster virus (VZIg), rabies (RIg), and tetanus (TIg). Human immunoglobulin is preferable to animal immunoglobulin because there is little risk of a hypersensitivity reaction (serum sickness).

Monoclonal antibody preparations are being developed for protection against various agents and diseases. In addition to infectious diseases, monoclonal antibodies are being used as therapy to block the overzealous cytokine and cellular responses in autoimmune diseases, to initiate antitumor responses, and for other therapies. Autologous activated dendritic cells loaded with tumor antigens and activated antitumor T cells can be prepared in the laboratory from the patient's own cells and injected back into the cancer patient as immunotherapy.

Active Immunization

The term *vaccine* is derived from vaccinia virus, a less virulent member of the poxvirus family that is used to immunize people against smallpox. Classical vaccines can be subdivided into two groups on the basis of whether they elicit an immune response on infection (**live vaccines** such as vaccinia) or not **(inactivated–subunit-killed vaccines)** (Figure 11-1). **Deoxyribonucleic acid (DNA) vaccines** represent a new means of immunization. In this approach, plasmid DNA is injected into muscle or skin and then taken up by dendritic, muscle, or macrophage cells, which express the gene for the immunogen as if for a natural infection. DNA

Table 11-1 Immune Globulins for Passive Immunity*

Disease	Source
Hepatitis A	Human
Hepatitis B	Human
Measles	Human
Rabies	Human†
Chickenpox, varicella-zoster	Human†
Cytomegalovirus	Human
Tetanus	Human,† equine
Botulism	Equine
Diphtheria	Equine
Respiratory syncytial virus	Monoclonal

*Immune globulins to other agents may also be available.
†Specific high-titer antibody is available and is the preferred therapy.

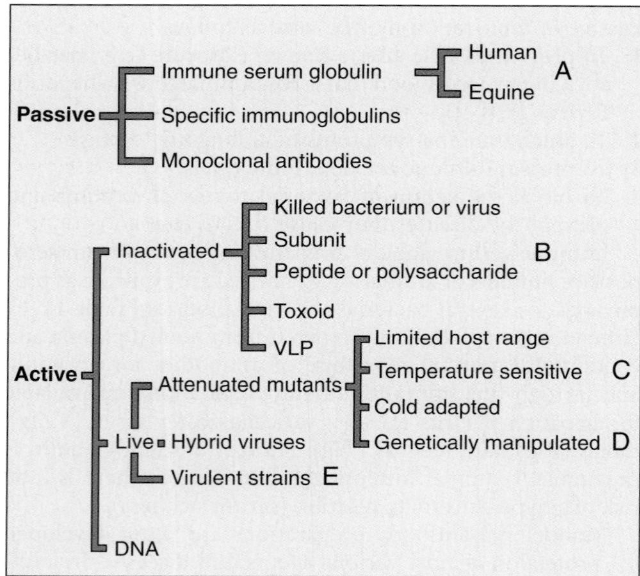

FIGURE 11-1 Types of immunizations. Antibodies (passive immunization) can be provided to block the action of an infectious agent, or an immune response can be elicited (active immunization) by natural infection or vaccination. The different forms of passive and active immunization are indicated. **A,** Equine antibodies can be used if human antibody is not available. **B,** Vaccine can consist of components purified from the infectious agent or can be developed through genetic engineering (virus-like particle *[VLP]*). **C,** Vaccine selected by passage at low or high temperature in animals, embryonated eggs, or tissue culture cells. **D,** Deletion, insertion, reassortment, and other laboratory-derived mutants. **E,** Vaccine composed of a virus from a different species that has a common antigen with the human virus.

vaccination stimulates T-cell immune responses, which can be boosted with antigen to elicit mature antibody responses.

Inactivated Vaccines

Inactivated vaccines use a large amount of antigen to produce a protective antibody response but without the risk of infection by the agent. Inactivated vaccines can be produced by chemical (e.g., formalin), irradiation, or heat inactivation of bacteria, bacterial toxins, or viruses, or by purification or synthesis of the components or subunits of the infectious agents. Inactivated vaccines usually generate antibody (TH2 responses) rather than cell-mediated immune responses.

These vaccines are usually administered with an **adjuvant** that boosts their immunogenicity by enhancing uptake by or stimulating dendritic cells (DCs) and macrophages. **Alum** (aluminum hydroxide or aluminum phosphate) is the most common and approved adjuvant. Many protein vaccines are precipitated onto alum to form particles and promote their uptake by DCs and macrophages. Other adjuvants may stimulate Toll-like receptors or activate the inflammasome in these antigen-presenting cells. MF59 (squalene microfluidized in an oil and water emulsion) and monophosphoryl lipid A (MPL) are adjuvants used in some newer vaccines. Experimental adjuvants include emulsions, virus-like particles, liposomes (defined lipid complexes), bacterial cell wall components, molecular cages for antigen, polymeric surfactants, and attenuated forms of cholera toxin and *Escherichia coli* lymphotoxin. These latter molecules are potent adjuvants for secretory antibody (immunoglobulin [Ig]A) after intranasal or oral immunization.

Table 11-2 Advantages and Disadvantages of Live versus Inactivated Vaccines

Property	Live	Inactivated
Route of administration	Natural* or injection	Injection
Dose of antigen	Low	High
Number of doses, amount	Single,† low	Multiple, high
Need for adjuvant	No	Yes
Duration of immunity	Long-term	Short-term
Antibody response	IgG, IgA‡	IgM, IgG
Cell-mediated immune response	Good	Poor
Potential lability	Yes	More stable
Side effects	Occasional mild symptoms	Occasional sore arm
Reversion to virulence	Rarely	None

Adapted from White DO, Fenner FJ: *Medical virology,* ed 3, New York, 1986, Academic.
Ig, Immunoglobulin.
*Oral or respiratory, in certain cases.
†A single booster may be required (yellow fever, measles, rubella) after 6 to 10 years.
‡IgA if delivered via the oral or respiratory route.

Inactivated, rather than live, vaccines are used to confer protection against toxins, most bacteria, and viruses that cannot be attenuated, may cause recurrent infection, or have oncogenic potential. Inactivated vaccines are generally safe except in people who have allergic reactions to vaccine components. The disadvantages of inactivated vaccines are listed below and compared to live vaccines in Table 11-2.

1. Immunity is not usually lifelong.
2. Immunity may be only humoral (TH2) and not cell mediated.

3. The vaccine does not elicit a local IgA response.
4. Booster shots are required.
5. Larger doses must be used.

There are three major types of inactivated bacterial vaccines: **toxoid** (inactivated toxins), **inactivated (killed)** bacteria, and surface components of the bacteria, such as **capsule or protein subunits.** The bacterial vaccines currently available are listed in Table 11-3. Most antibacterial vaccines protect against the pathogenic action of toxins.

Inactivated viral vaccines are available for **polio, hepatitis A, influenza, and rabies,** among other viruses. The Salk polio vaccine **(inactivated poliomyelitis vaccine [IPV])** is prepared through formaldehyde inactivation of virions. A rabies vaccine is prepared through the chemical inactivation of virions grown in human diploid tissue culture cells. Because of the slow course of rabies, the vaccine can be administered immediately after a person is exposed to the virus and still elicit a protective antibody response.

A **subunit vaccine** consists of the bacterial or viral components that elicit a protective immune response. Surface structures of bacteria and the viral attachment proteins (capsid or glycoproteins) elicit protective antibodies. T-cell antigens may also be included in a subunit vaccine. The immunogenic component can be isolated from the bacterium, virus, or virally infected cells by biochemical means, or the vaccine can be prepared through genetic engineering by the expression of cloned viral genes in bacteria or eukaryotic cells. For example, the HBV subunit vaccine was initially prepared from surface antigen obtained from human sera of chronic carriers of the virus. Today HBV vaccine is obtained from yeast bearing the HBsAg gene. The antigen is purified, chemically treated, and absorbed onto alum to be used as a vaccine. The subunit proteins used in the HBV and the human papillomavirus (HPV) vaccines form **virus-like particles (VLPs),** which are more immunogenic than individual proteins.

Most of the inactivated annual influenza vaccines consist of a mixture of the hemagglutinin and neuraminidase proteins obtained from embryonated eggs or tissue culture cells infected with different strains of influenza A and B or from genetically engineered protein. The vaccine mixture is formulated annually to elicit protection from the virus strains predicted to threaten the population in the coming year.

Vaccines against *H. influenzae* B, *Neisseria meningitidis, Salmonella typhi,* and *Streptococcus pneumoniae* (23 strains) are prepared from capsular polysaccharides. Unfortunately, polysaccharides are generally poor immunogens (T-independent antigens). The meningococcal vaccine contains the polysaccharides of four major serotypes (A, C, Y, and W-135). The pneumococcal vaccine contains polysaccharides from 23 serotypes. The immunogenicity of a polysaccharide can be enhanced by making it into a T-dependent antigen by chemical linkage to a protein carrier **(conjugate vaccine)** (e.g., diphtheria toxoid or *N. meningitidis* outer membrane protein) (Figure 11-2). The *H. influenzae* B (Hib) polysaccharide-diphtheria toxoid complex is approved for administration to infants and children. An *S. pneumoniae* "pneumococcal" conjugate vaccine has been developed in which polysaccharide from the 13 most prevalent strains in the United States is attached to a nontoxic form of the

Table 11-3 Bacterial Vaccines*†

Bacteria (Disease)	Vaccine Components	Who Should Receive Vaccinations
Corynebacterium diphtheriae (diphtheria)	Toxoid	Children and adults
Clostridium tetani (tetanus)	Toxoid	Children and adults
Bordetella pertussis (pertussis)	Acellular	Children and teens
Haemophilus influenzae B (Hib)	Capsule polysaccharide-protein conjugate	Children
Neisseria meningitidis A, C, Y, W135 (meningococcal disease) *N. meningitidis* B (protein vaccine)	Capsule polysaccharide-protein conjugate, capsule polysaccharide	People at high risk (e.g., those with asplenia), travelers to epidemic areas (e.g., military personnel), children
Streptococcus pneumoniae (pneumococcal disease; meningitis)	Capsule polysaccharides; capsule polysaccharide-protein conjugate	Children, people at high risk (e.g., those with asplenia), the elderly
Vibrio cholerae (cholera)	Killed cell	Travelers at risk to exposure
Salmonella typhi (typhoid)	Killed cell; polysaccharide	Travelers at risk to exposure, household contacts, sewage workers
Bacillus anthracis (anthrax)	Killed cell	Handlers of imported fur, military personnel
Yersinia pestis (plague)	Killed cell	Veterinarians, animal handlers
Francisella tularensis (tularemia)	Live attenuated	Animal handlers in endemic areas
Coxiella burnetii (Q fever)	Inactivated	Sheep handlers, laboratory personnel working with *C. burnetii*
Mycobacterium tuberculosis (tuberculosis)	Live attenuated bacillus Calmette-Guérin *Mycobacterium bovis*	Not recommended in United States

*Listed in order of frequency of use.

†A more complete list can be found at www.fda.gov/BiologicsBloodVaccines/Vaccines/ApprovedProducts/ucm093833.htm.

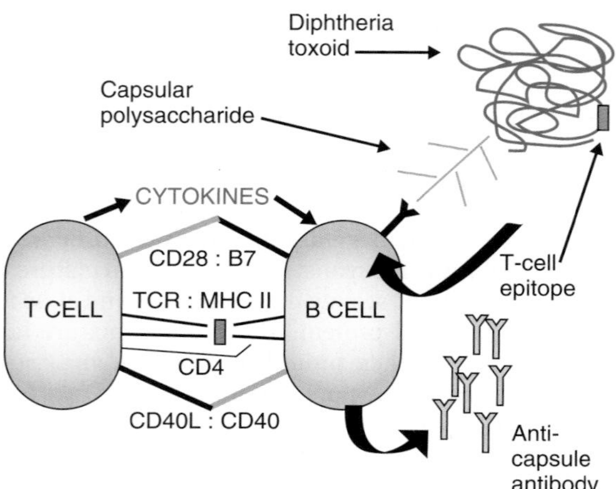

FIGURE 11-2 Capsular polysaccharide conjugate vaccines. Capsular polysaccharides are poor immunogens, do not elicit T-cell help, and only elicit immunoglobulin (Ig)M without memory. Capsule polysaccharide conjugated to a protein (e.g., diphtheria toxoid) binds to surface antipolysaccharide IgM on the B cell, the complex is internalized and processed, and then a peptide is presented on major histocompatibility complex II *(MHC II)* to CD4 T cells. The T cells become activated, produce cytokines, and promote immunoglobulin class switching for the polysaccharide-specific B cell. The B cell can become activated and make IgG, and memory cells will develop. *TCR,* T-cell receptor.

diphtheria toxoid. This vaccine is available for use in infants and young children. The other polysaccharide vaccines are less immunogenic and are administered to individuals older than 2 years.

Live Vaccines

Live vaccines are prepared with microbes limited in their ability to cause disease (e.g., **avirulent** or **attenuated** microbes). Live vaccines are especially useful for protection against infections caused by enveloped viruses, which require T-cell immune responses for resolution of the infection. Immunization with a live vaccine resembles the natural infection in that the immune response progresses through the natural innate and antigen-specific immune responses so that humoral, cellular, and memory immune responses are developed. Immunity is generally long lived and, depending on the route of administration, can mimic the normal immune response to the infecting agent. However, the following list includes three problems with live vaccines:

1. The vaccine virus may still be dangerous for immunosuppressed people or pregnant women, who do not have the immunologic resources to resolve even a weakened virus infection.
2. The vaccine may revert to a virulent viral form.
3. The viability of the vaccine must be maintained.

Live bacterial vaccines include the orally administered live, attenuated *S. typhi* strain (Ty2la) vaccine for typhoid; the bacillus Calmette-Guérin (BCG) vaccine for tuberculosis, which consists of an attenuated strain of *Mycobacterium bovis;* and an attenuated tularemia vaccine. A combination of antibody and cell-mediated immune responses elicited by a live vaccine may be required against intracellularly growing bacteria. The BCG vaccine is not used in the United States because immunization is not always protective and people vaccinated with it show a false-positive skin reaction to the purified protein derivative (PPD) test, which is the screening test used to control tuberculosis in the United States.

Live virus vaccines consist of less virulent mutants **(attenuated)** of the wild-type virus, viruses from other species that share antigenic determinants (vaccinia for smallpox, bovine rotavirus), or genetically engineered viruses lacking virulence properties (see Figure 11-1). Wild-type viruses are attenuated by growth in embryonated eggs or tissue culture cells at nonphysiologic temperatures (25° C to 34° C) and away from the selective pressures of the host immune response. These conditions **select** for or allow the growth of viral strains (mutants) that (1) are less virulent because they grow poorly at 37° C (**temperature-sensitive strains** [e.g., measles vaccine] and cold-adapted strains [influenza vaccine]), (2) do not replicate well in any human cell **(host-range mutants),** (3) cannot escape immune control, or (4) can replicate at a benign site but do not disseminate, bind, or replicate in the target tissue characteristically affected by the disease (e.g., polio vaccine replicates in the gastrointestinal tract but does not reach or infect neurons). Table 11-4 lists examples of attenuated live virus vaccines currently in use.

The first vaccine—that for smallpox—was developed by Edward Jenner. The idea for the vaccine came to him when he noted that cowpox (vaccinia), a virulent virus from another species that shares antigenic determinants with smallpox, caused benign infections in humans but conferred protective immunity against smallpox. Similarly, a mixture of genetic reassortant human and bovine rotaviruses are the basis for one of the current vaccines administered to protect infants against human rotavirus.

Albert Sabin developed the first live **oral polio vaccine (OPV)** in the 1950s. The attenuated virus vaccine was obtained by multiple passages of the three types of poliovirus through monkey kidney tissue culture cells. At least 57 mutations accumulated in the polio type 1 vaccine strain. When this vaccine is administered orally, IgA is secreted in the gut and IgG in the serum, providing protection along the normal route of infection by the wild-type virus. This vaccine is inexpensive, easy to administer, and relatively stable and can spread to contacts of the immunized individual. Effective immunization programs have led to the elimination of wild-type polio in most of the world. The IPV is used in most of the world for routine well-baby immunizations because of the risk of vaccine-virus–induced polio disease by the OPV (see Figure 11-2). Although the immune response elicited by the IPV can prevent spread of the virus to the central nervous system and muscles to protect the individual from disease, it does not prevent production of virus in the gastrointestinal tract and transmission to others in stool, as does the OPV.

The HBV and HPV vaccines are genetically engineered and grown in yeast cells. The viral attachment proteins from HBV (HBsAg) and HPV (L protein) form viral-like particles that are better immunogens than individual proteins. By limiting the spread of these viruses, these vaccines are also preventing their associated cancers (cervical carcinoma: HPV; primary hepatocellular carcinoma: HBV).

Table 11-4 **Viral Vaccines***†

Virus	Vaccine Components	Who Should Receive Vaccinations
Polio, inactivated	Trivalent (Salk vaccine)	Children
Attenuated polio	Live (oral polio vaccine, Sabin vaccine)	Children in epidemic areas
Measles	Attenuated	Children
Mumps	Attenuated	Children
Rubella	Attenuated	Children
Varicella-zoster	Attenuated Larger dose	Children Adults (>60) years
Rotavirus	Human-bovine hybrids Attenuated	Infants
Human papillomavirus	VLP	Girls and boys ages 9-26 yr
Influenza	Inactivated	Children, adults, especially medical personnel and the elderly
	Attenuated (nasal spray)	Ages 2-50 yr
Hepatitis B	Subunit (VLP)	Newborns, health care workers, high-risk groups (e.g., sexually promiscuous, intravenous drug users)
Hepatitis A	Inactivated	Children, child care workers, travelers to endemic areas, Native Americans, and Alaskans
Adenovirus	Attenuated	Military personnel
Yellow fever	Attenuated	Travelers at risk to exposure, military personnel
Rabies	Inactivated	Anyone exposed to virus Preexposure: veterinarians, animal handlers
Smallpox	Live vaccinia virus	People seeking protection from bioterrorism, military
Japanese encephalitis	Inactivated	Travelers at risk to exposure

VLP, Virus-like particle.

*Listed in order of frequency of use.

†A complete list can be found at www.fda.gov/BiologicsBloodVaccines/Vaccines/ApprovedProducts/ucm093833.htm.

Live vaccines for measles, mumps, and rubella (administered together as the MMR vaccine), **varicella-zoster,** and now **influenza** have been developed. Protection against these infections requires a potent cellular immune response. To elicit a mature T-cell response, the vaccine must be administered after 1 year of age, when there will be no interference by maternal antibodies and cell-mediated immunity is sufficiently mature. A killed measles vaccine proved to be a failure because it conferred an incomplete immunity that induced more serious symptoms (atypical measles) on challenge with wild-type measles virus than the symptoms associated with the natural infection.

The initial live measles vaccine consisted of the Edmonston B strain, which was developed by Enders and colleagues. This virus underwent extensive passage at 35° C through primary human kidney cells, human amnion cells, and chicken embryo cells. The currently used Moraten (United States) and Schwarz (other countries) vaccine strains of measles were obtained by further passage of the Edmonston B strain in chick embryos at 32° C.

The mumps vaccine (Jeryl Lynn strain) and rubella vaccine (Wistar RA 27/3) viruses were also attenuated by extensive passage of the virus in cell culture. The varicella-zoster vaccine uses the Oka strain, an attenuated virus. The varicella-zoster vaccine is administered along with the MMR vaccine, or a stronger version is administered to adults to prevent zoster (shingles).

The live tri- and tetravalent influenza vaccines are administered nasally within a mist and is cold adapted to 25° C. Unlike the inactivated vaccine, T- and B-cell responses and mucosal immunity are elicited by this vaccine. This vaccine can only be administered to individuals between ages 2 and 49 years.

Future Directions for Vaccination

Molecular biology techniques are being used to develop new vaccines. New live vaccines can be created by genetic engineering mutations that inactivate or delete a virulence gene instead of through random attenuation of the virus by passage through tissue culture. Genes from infectious agents that cannot be properly attenuated can be inserted into safe viruses (e.g., vaccinia, canarypox, attenuated adenovirus) to form **hybrid virus vaccines.** This approach holds the promise of allowing the development of a polyvalent vaccine to many agents in a single, safe, inexpensive, and relatively stable vector. On infection, the hybrid virus vaccine need not complete a replication cycle but simply promote expression of the inserted gene to initiate an immune response to the antigens. The vaccinia, canarypox, and adenovirus vector systems have been used in several experimental hybrid vaccines. A canarypox human immunodeficiency virus (HIV) vaccine followed by two booster immunizations with recombinant HIV glycoprotein 120 showed modest but promising results. A vaccinia-based vaccine is used to immunize forest animals against rabies. Other viruses have also been considered as vectors.

Genetically engineered **subunit vaccines** are being developed through cloning of genes that encode immunogenic proteins into bacterial and eukaryotic vectors. The greatest difficulties in the development of such vaccines are (1) identifying the appropriate subunit or peptide immunogen that can elicit protective antibody and, ideally, T-cell responses and (2) presenting the antigen in the correct conformation. Once identified, the gene can be isolated, cloned, and expressed in bacteria or yeast cells, and then large quantities of these proteins can be produced. The envelope protein gp120 of HIV, the hemagglutinin and neuraminidase of influenza, the G antigen of rabies, and the glycoprotein D of herpes simplex virus have been cloned, and their proteins have been generated in bacteria or eukaryotic cells for use (or potential use) as subunit vaccines.

Peptide subunit vaccines contain *specific epitopes* of microbial proteins that elicit neutralizing antibody or desired T-cell responses. To generate such a response, the peptide must contain sequences that bind to MHC I or MHC II (class I or class II major histocompatibility complex) proteins on DCs for presentation and recognition by T cells to initiate an immune response. The immunogenicity of the peptide can be enhanced by its covalent attachment to a carrier protein (e.g., tetanus or diphtheria toxoid or keyhole limpet hemocyanin [KLH]), a ligand for a Toll-like receptor (e.g., flagellin) or an immunologic peptide that can specifically present the epitope to the appropriate immune response. Better vaccines are being developed as the mechanisms of antigen presentation and T-cell receptor-specific antigens are better understood.

Adjuvants in addition to alum are being developed to enhance the immunogenicity and direct the response of vaccines to a TH1- or TH2-type response. These include activators of Toll-like receptors, such as oligodeoxynucleotides of CpG, derivatives of lipid A from lipopolysaccharide, cytokines, liposomes, nanoparticles, and others. Use of MF59 in a new influenza vaccine (not available in the United States) allows reduction in the amount of antigen required to elicit protective immunity.

DNA vaccines offer great potential for immunization against infectious agents and for tumor immunotherapy that require T-cell responses. For these vaccines, the gene for a protein that elicits protective responses is cloned into a plasmid that allows the protein to be expressed in eukaryotic cells. The naked DNA is injected into the muscle or skin of the vaccine recipient, where the DNA is taken up by cells, the gene is expressed, and the protein is produced, presented to, and activates T-cell responses. DNA vaccines usually require a boost with antigenic protein to produce antibody.

A new approach, termed *reverse vaccinology,* was used to develop a vaccine for *N. meningitidis* B. Based on protein properties predicted from the gene sequence, thousands of proteins were tested for their ability to confer protection against infection to identify protein candidates. With the advent of this and other new technology, it should be possible to develop vaccines against infectious agents such as *Streptococcus mutans* (to prevent tooth decay), the herpesviruses, HIV, and parasites such as *Plasmodium falciparum* (malaria) and *Leishmania.* In fact, it should be possible to produce a vaccine to almost any infectious agent once the appropriate protective immunogen is identified and its gene isolated.

• Immunization Programs

An effective vaccine program can save millions of dollars in health care costs. Such a program not only protects each vaccinated person against infection and disease but also reduces the number of susceptible people in the population, thereby preventing the spread of the infectious agent within the population. Although immunization may be the best means of protecting people against infection, vaccines cannot be developed for all infectious agents. One reason is that it is very time consuming and costly to develop vaccines. Box 11-1 lists the considerations that are weighed in the choice of a candidate for a vaccine program.

Box 11-1 Properties of Ideal Candidate for Vaccine Development

Microbe causes significant illness
Microbe exists as only one serotype
Antibody blocks infection or systemic spread
Vaccine is heat stable so that it can be transported to endemic areas
Immunization protects recipient and population

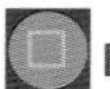

Box 11-2 Problems with Vaccines

Live vaccine can occasionally revert to virulent forms.
Vaccinating an immunocompromised person with a live vaccine can be life threatening.
Side effects to vaccination can occur; these include hypersensitivity and allergic reactions to the antigen, to nonmicrobial material in the vaccine, and to contaminants (e.g., eggs).
Vaccine development is high risk and very expensive.
Misinformation about safety causes underutilization of important vaccines.
Microbes with many serotypes are difficult to control with vaccination.

Natural smallpox was eliminated by means of an effective vaccine program because it was a good candidate for such a program; the virus existed in only one serotype, symptoms were always present in infected people, and the vaccine was relatively benign and stable. However, its elimination came about only as the result of a concerted cooperative effort on the part of the WHO and local health agencies worldwide. Rhinovirus is an example of a poor candidate for vaccine development, because the viral disease is not serious and there are too many serotypes for vaccination to be successful. Practical aspects of and problems with vaccine development are listed in Box 11-2.

From the standpoint of the individual, the ideal vaccine should elicit dependable lifelong immunity to infection, without serious side effects. Factors that influence the success of an immunization program include not only the composition of the vaccine but also the timing, site, and conditions of its administration. Misinformation regarding safety issues with vaccines has deterred some individuals or their children from being vaccinated, putting them at risk for disease.

Recommended schedules of vaccinations for children are given in Figure 11-3. Tables of recommended schedules for vaccination of children, teens, adults, and special cases are provided annually by the Advisory Committee on Immunization Practices (ACIP) of the Centers for Disease Control and Prevention. **Booster immunizations** of inactivated vaccines and the live measles vaccine are required later in life. Men and women younger than age 26 should receive the HPV vaccine, and college students should receive the meningococcal vaccine or a booster. Adults should be immunized with vaccines for *S. pneumoniae* (pneumococcus), influenza, rabies, varicella-zoster, HBV, and other diseases, depending on their age, jobs, the type of traveling they do, and other risk factors that may make them particularly susceptible to specific infectious agents. Further discussion of each of the vaccines is presented in later chapters with the disease they prevent.

Vaccine ▼ / Age ▶	Birth	1 month	2 months	4 months	6 months	12 months	15 months	18 months	19-23 months	2-3 years	4-6 years	12-26 years
Hepatitis B	HepB	HepB			HepB							
Rotavirus			Rota	Rota	Rota							
Diphtheria, tetanus, pertussis			DTaP	DTaP	DTaP		DTaP				DTaP	Tdap
Haemophilus influenzae type B			Hib	Hib	Hib	Hib						
Pneumococcal conjugate			PCV	PCV	PCV	PCV				PPV		
Inactivated poliovirus			IPV	IPV	IPV						IPV	
Influenza					Influenza (yearly)							
Measles, mumps, rubella						MMR					MMR	
Varicella						Varicella					Varicella	
Hepatitis A						HepA (2 doses)				HepA series		
Meningococcal					MCV4							
Human papillomavirus												HPV

Range of recommended ages — Certain high-risk groups

FIGURE 11-3 Recommended childhood immunization schedule from the Centers for Disease Control and Prevention. Vaccines are listed at the ages routinely recommended for their administration. Bars indicate the range of acceptable ages for vaccination. *DTaP,* Diphtheria, tetanus, and acellular pertussis; *HepA,* hepatitis A; *HepB,* hepatitis B; *Hib, Haemophilus influenzae* type B; *IPV,* inactivated poliovirus; *MCV4,* quadrivalent conjugated meningococcal; *MMR,* measles, mumps, rubella; *PCV,* pneumococcal conjugate; *PPV,* pneumococcal polysaccharide; *Rota,* rotavirus. (From the Centers for Disease Control and Prevention Advisory Committee on Immunization Practices: *Recommended immunization schedule for persons aged 0 through 6 years—United States, 2015* (PDF). www.cdc.gov/vaccines/recs/schedules/downloads/child/0-6yrs-schedule-pr.pdf. Accessed March 10, 2015.)

Bibliography

Centers for Disease Control and Prevention, Atkinson W, Wolfe S, Hamborsky J, editors: *Epidemiology and prevention of vaccine-preventable diseases (the pink book)*, ed 12, Washington, DC, 2011, Public Health Foundation.

Plotkin SA, Orenstein WA: *Vaccines*, ed 5, Philadelphia, 2005, WB Saunders.

Rosenthal KS: Vaccines make good immune theater: immunization as described in a three-act play, *Infect Dis Clin Pract* 14:35–45, 2006.

Rosenthal KS, Zimmerman DH: Vaccines: all things considered, *Clin Vaccine Immunol* 13:821–829, 2006.

Websites

Advisory Committee on Immunization Practices: Statements. www.cdc.gov/vaccines/recs/acip/default.htm. Accessed August 5, 2015.

American Academy of Pediatrics: Status of recently submitted, licensed, and recommended vaccines & biologics. http://redbook.solutions.aap.org/vaccine-status.aspx?gbosid=167073. Accessed April 6, 2015.

Centers for Disease Control and Prevention: Manual for the surveillance of vaccine-preventable diseases, ed 4, 2008–2009; ed 5, 2011. www.cdc.gov/vaccines/pubs/surv-manual/index.html. Accessed August 5, 2015.

Centers for Disease Control and Prevention: Vaccines & immunizations. www.cdc.gov/vaccines/default.htm. Accessed August 5, 2015.

Immunization Action Coalition: Vaccination information statements. www.immunize.org/vis. Accessed August 5, 2015.

Immunization Action Coalition: Vaccine information for the public and health professionals: vaccine-preventable disease photos. www.vaccineinformation.org/photos/index.asp. Accessed August 5, 2015.

National Foundation for Infectious Diseases: Fact sheets. www.nfid.org/publications/factsheets. Accessed August 5, 2015.

National Institute of Allergy and Infectious Diseases: Vaccines. www.niaid.nih.gov/topics/vaccines/Pages/Default.aspx. Accessed August 5, 2015.

World Health Organization: Immunization service delivery. www.who.int/vaccines-diseases/index.html. Accessed August 5, 2015.

SECTION

4

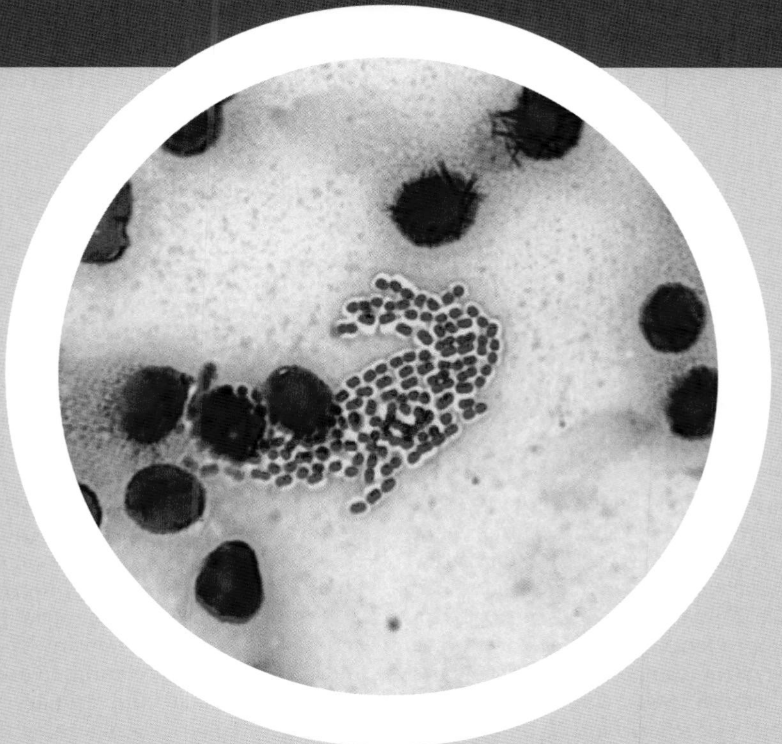

BACTERIOLOGY

CHAPTER

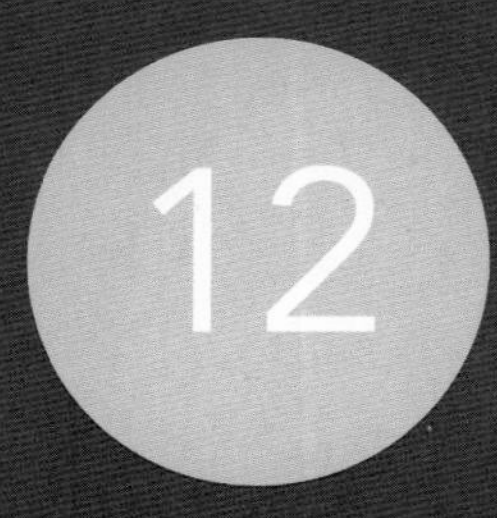

BACTERIAL CLASSIFICATION, STRUCTURE, AND REPLICATION

The smallest bacteria *(Chlamydia* and *Rickettsia)* are just 0.1 to 0.2 μm in diameter, whereas larger bacteria may be many microns in length. A newly described species is hundreds of times larger than the average bacterial cell and is visible to the naked eye. Most species, however, are approximately 1 μm in diameter and are therefore visible with the use of the light microscope, which has a resolution of 0.2 μm. In comparison, animal and plant cells are much larger, ranging from 7 μm (the diameter of a red blood cell) to several feet (the length of certain nerve cells).

Differences between Eukaryotes and Prokaryotes

Cells from animals, plants, and fungi are **eukaryotes** (Greek for "true nucleus"), whereas bacteria, **archae,** and blue-green algae belong to the **prokaryotes** (Greek for "primitive nucleus"). The archae (archaebacteria) resemble bacteria in most ways but represent a domain unique from bacteria and eukaryotes. In addition to lacking a nucleus and other organelles, the bacterial chromosome differs from the human chromosome in several ways. The chromosome of a typical bacterium, such as *Escherichia coli,* is a single, double-stranded, circular molecule of deoxyribonucleic acid (DNA) containing approximately 5 million base pairs, an approximate length of 1.3 mm (i.e., nearly 1000 times the diameter of the cell). The smallest bacterial chromosomes (from mycoplasmas) are approximately one fourth of this size. In comparison, humans have two copies of 23 chromosomes, which represent 2.9×10^9 base pairs 990 mm in length. Bacteria use a smaller ribosome, the 70S ribosome, and in most bacteria, a meshlike peptidoglycan cell wall surrounds the membranes to protect them against the environment. Bacteria can survive, and in some cases grow, in hostile environments in which the osmotic pressure outside the cell is so low that most eukaryotic cells would lyse, at temperature extremes (both hot and cold), with dryness, and with very dilute and diverse energy sources. Bacteria have evolved their structures and functions to adapt to these conditions. These and other distinguishing features are depicted in Figure 12-1 and outlined in Table 12-1. Several of these distinctions provide the basis for antimicrobial action.

Bacterial Classification

Bacteria can be classified by their macroscopic and microscopic appearance, by characteristic growth and metabolic properties, by their antigenicity, and finally by their genotype.

Macroscopic and Microscopic Distinction

The initial distinction between bacteria can be made by growth characteristics on different nutrient and selective media. Bacteria grow in colonies; each colony is like a city of as many as a million or more organisms. The sum of their characteristics provides the colony with distinguishing characteristics such as color, size, shape, and smell. The bacteria's ability to resist certain antibiotics, ferment specific sugars (e.g., lactose, to distinguish *Escherichia coli* from *Salmonella*), to lyse erythrocytes (streptococcal hemolytic properties), or to hydrolyze lipids (e.g., clostridial lipase) can also be determined using the appropriate growth media.

The microscopic appearance, including size, shape, and configuration of the organisms (cocci, rods, curved, or spiral) and their ability to retain the Gram stain (gram-positive or gram-negative) are the primary means for distinguishing bacteria. A spherical bacterium such as *Staphylococcus* is a coccus, a rod-shaped bacterium such as *E. coli* is a bacillus, and the snakelike treponeme is a spirillum. In addition, *Nocardia* and *Actinomyces* species have branched filamentous appearances similar to those of fungi. Some bacteria form aggregates, such as the grapelike clusters of *Staphylococcus aureus* or the diplococcus (two cells together) observed in *Streptococcus* or *Neisseria* species.

Gram stain is a rapid, powerful, easy test that allows clinicians to distinguish between the two major classes of bacteria, develop an initial diagnosis, and initiate therapy based on inherent differences in the bacteria (Figure 12-2). Bacteria are heat fixed or otherwise dried onto a slide, stained with **crystal violet** (Figure 12-3), a stain that is precipitated with **iodine,** and then the unbound and excess stain is removed by washing with the acetone-based **decolorizer** and water. A red counterstain, **safranin,** is added to stain any decolorized cells. This process takes less than 10 minutes.

For **gram-positive bacteria,** which turn **purple,** the stain gets trapped in a thick, cross-linked, meshlike structure, the peptidoglycan layer, which surrounds the cell.

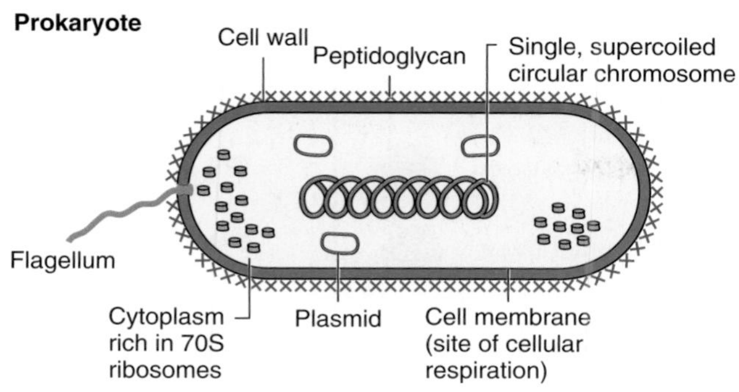

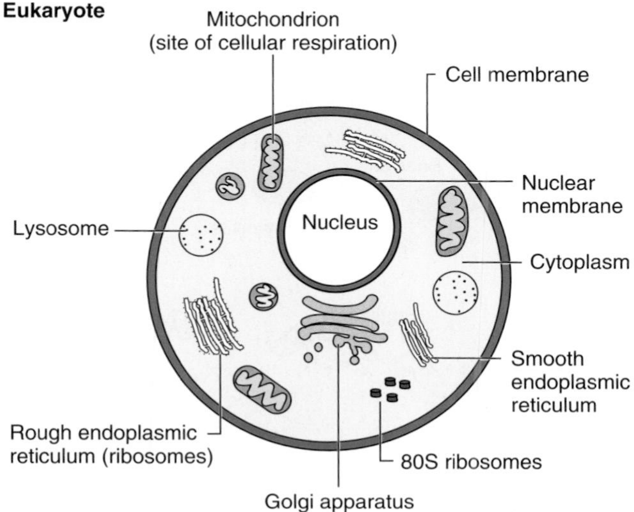

FIGURE 12-1 Major features of prokaryotes and eukaryotes.

Gram-negative bacteria have a thin peptidoglycan layer that does not retain the crystal violet stain, so the cells must be counterstained with safranin and turned red (Figure 12-4). A mnemonic device that may help is **"P-PURPLE-POSITIVE."**

Gram staining loses dependability for bacteria that are starved (e.g., old or stationary-phase cultures) or treated with antibiotics, owing to degradation of the peptoglycan. Bacteria that cannot be classified by Gram staining include mycobacteria, which have a waxy outer shell and are distinguished with the acid-fast stain, and mycoplasmas, which have no peptidoglycan.

Metabolic, Antigenic, and Genetic Distinction

The next level of classification is based on the metabolic signature of the bacteria, including requirement for anaerobic or aerobic environments, requirement for specific nutrients (e.g., ability to ferment specific carbohydrates or use different compounds as a source of carbon for growth), and production of characteristic metabolic products (acid, alcohols) and specific enzymes (e.g., staphylococcal catalase). Automated procedures for distinguishing enteric and other bacteria have been developed; they analyze the growth in different media and their microbial products and provide a numerical biotype for each of the bacteria.

A particular strain of bacteria can be distinguished using antibodies to detect characteristic antigens on the bacteria **(serotyping).** These serologic tests can also be used to identify organisms that are difficult (*Treponema pallidum,* the organism responsible for syphilis) or too dangerous (e.g., *Francisella,* the organism that causes tularemia), do not grow in the laboratory, are associated with specific disease syndromes (e.g., *E. coli* serotype O157:H7, responsible for hemorrhagic colitis), or need to be identified rapidly (e.g.,

Table 12-1 Major Characteristics of Eukaryotes and Prokaryotes

Characteristic	Eukaryote	Prokaryote
Major groups	Algae, fungi, protozoa, plants, animals	Bacteria
Size (approximate)	>5 μm	0.5-3.0 μm
Nuclear Structures		
Nucleus	Classic membrane	No nuclear membrane
Chromosomes	Strands of DNA diploid genome	Single, circular DNA haploid genome
Cytoplasmic Structures		
Mitochondria	Present	Absent
Golgi bodies	Present	Absent
Endoplasmic reticulum	Present	Absent
Ribosomes (sedimentation coefficient)	80S (60S + 40S)	70S (50S + 30S)
Cytoplasmic membrane	Contains sterols	Does not contain sterols (except mycoplasma)
Cell wall	Present for fungi; otherwise absent	Is a complex structure containing protein, lipids, and peptidoglycans
Reproduction	Sexual and asexual	Asexual (binary fission)
Movement	Complex flagellum, if present	Simple flagellum, if present
Respiration	Via mitochondria	Via cytoplasmic membrane

Modified from Holt S. In Slots J, Taubman M, editors: *Contemporary oral microbiology and immunology,* St Louis, 1992, Mosby.

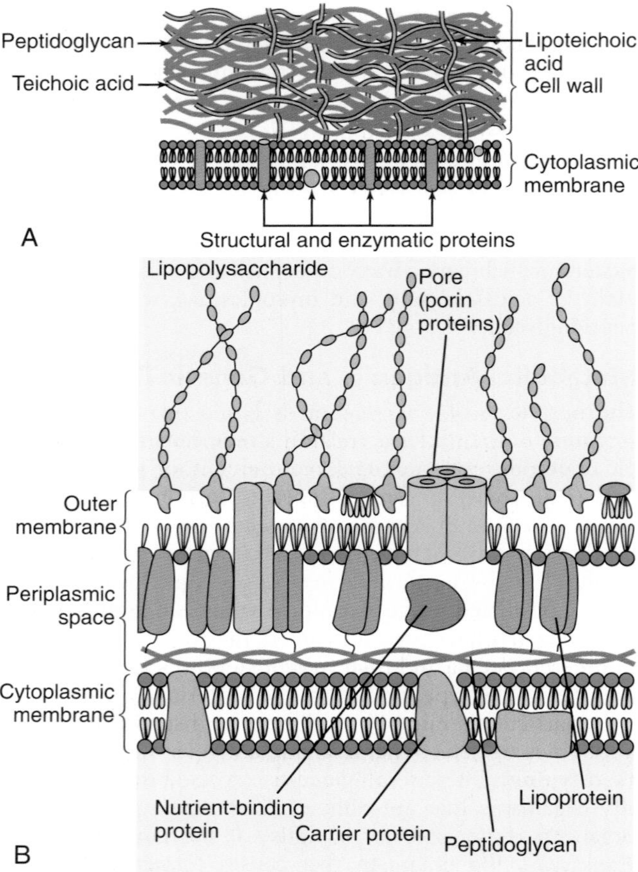

FIGURE 12-2 Comparison of gram-positive and gram-negative bacterial cell walls. **A,** A gram-positive bacterium has a thick peptidoglycan layer that contains teichoic and lipoteichoic acids. **B,** A gram-negative bacterium has a thin peptidoglycan layer and an outer membrane that contains lipopolysaccharide, phospholipids, and proteins. The periplasmic space between the cytoplasmic and outer membranes contains transport, degradative, and cell wall synthetic proteins. The outer membrane is joined to the cytoplasmic membrane at adhesion points and is attached to the peptidoglycan by lipoprotein links.

Streptococcus pyogenes, responsible for streptococcal pharyngitis). Serotyping is also used to subdivide bacteria below the species level for epidemiologic purposes.

The most precise method for classifying bacteria is by analysis of their genetic material. New methods distinguish bacteria by detection of specific characteristic DNA sequences. These techniques include **DNA hybridization, polymerase chain reaction (PCR) amplification, DNA sequencing,** and related techniques described in Chapter 5. These genetic techniques do not require living or growing bacteria and can be used for rapid detection and identification of slow-growing organisms (e.g., mycobacteria, fungi) or analysis of pathology samples of even very virulent bacteria. The technology is now available for rapid analysis of the nucleic acid sequence of specific segments or the entire bacterial chromosome. The most common application of this technique is analysis of sequences of ribosomal DNA to detect the highly conserved sequences that identify a family

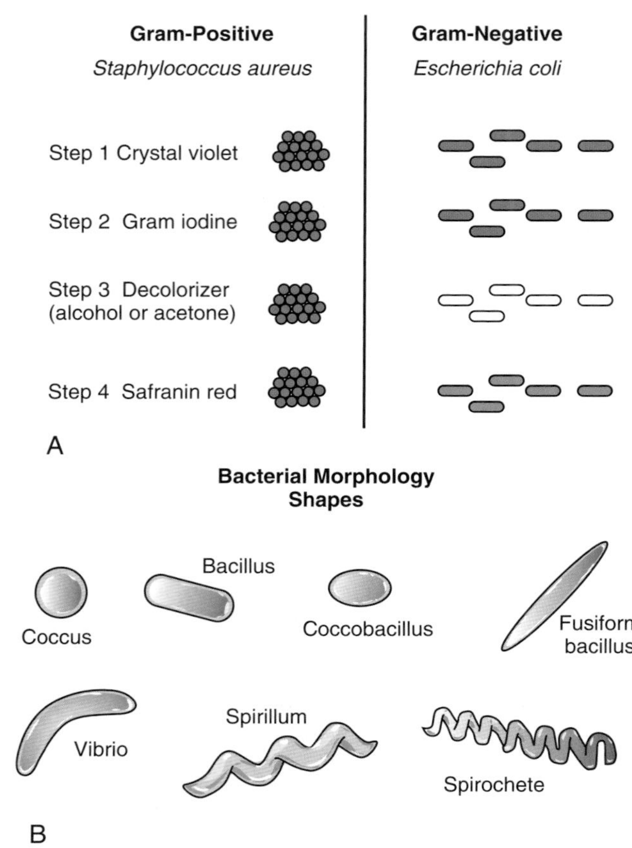

FIGURE 12-3 Gram-stain morphology of bacteria. **A,** The crystal violet of Gram stain is precipitated by Gram iodine and is trapped in the thick peptidoglycan layer in gram-positive bacteria. The decolorizer disperses the gram-negative outer membrane and washes the crystal violet from the thin layer of peptidoglycan. Gram-negative bacteria are visualized by the red counterstain. **B,** Bacterial morphologies.

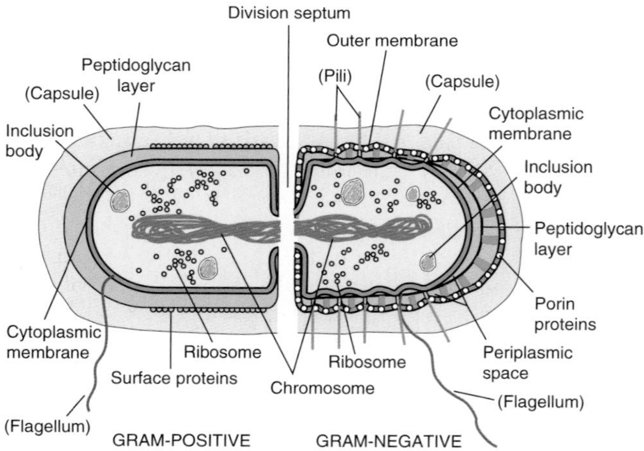

FIGURE 12-4 Gram-positive and gram-negative bacteria. A gram-positive bacterium has a thick layer of peptidoglycan (filling the purple space) *(left)*. A gram-negative bacterium has a thin peptidoglycan layer *(single black line)* and an outer membrane *(right)*. Structures in parentheses are not found in all bacteria. Upon cell division, the membrane and peptidoglycan grow toward each other to form a division septum to separate the daughter cells.

or genus and the highly variable sequences that distinguish a species or subspecies. It has also been used to define the evolutionary relationship among organisms and to identify organisms that are difficult or impossible to grow. Various other methods that have been used primarily to classify organisms at the subspecies level for epidemiologic investigations include: **plasmid analysis, ribotyping,** and **analysis of chromosomal DNA fragments.** In recent years the technical aspects of these methods have been simplified to the point that most clinical laboratories use variations of these methods in their day-to-day practice.

Bacterial Structure

Cytoplasmic Structures

The cytoplasm of the bacterial cell contains the DNA chromosome, messenger RNA (mRNA), ribosomes, proteins, and metabolites (see Figure 12-4). Unlike eukaryotes, most **bacterial chromosomes** are a single, double-stranded circle that is contained not in a nucleus but in a discrete area known as the **nucleoid.** Some bacteria may have two or three circular chromosomes or even a single linear chromosome. Histones are not present to maintain the conformation of the DNA, and the DNA does not form nucleosomes. **Plasmids,** which are smaller, circular, extrachromosomal DNAs, may also be present. Plasmids, although not usually essential for cellular survival, often provide a selective advantage: many confer resistance to one or more antibiotics.

The lack of a nuclear membrane simplifies the requirements and control mechanisms for the synthesis of proteins. Without a nuclear membrane, transcription and translation are coupled; in other words, ribosomes can bind to the mRNA, and protein can be made as the mRNA is being synthesized and still attached to the DNA.

The **bacterial ribosome** consists of 30S + 50S subunits, forming a **70S ribosome.** This is unlike the eukaryotic 80S (40S + 60S) ribosome. The proteins and RNA of the bacterial ribosome are significantly different from those of eukaryotic ribosomes and are major targets for antibacterial drugs.

The **cytoplasmic membrane** has a lipid bilayer structure similar to the structure of the eukaryotic membranes, but it contains no steroids (e.g., cholesterol); mycoplasmas are the exception to this rule. The cytoplasmic membrane is responsible for many of the functions attributable to organelles in eukaryotes. These tasks include electron transport and energy production, which are normally achieved in the mitochondria. In addition, the membrane contains transport proteins that allow uptake of metabolites and release of other substances, ion pumps to maintain a membrane potential, and enzymes. The inside of the membrane is lined with actin-like protein filaments that help determine the shape of the bacteria and the site of septum formation for cell division. These filaments determine the spiral shape of treponemes.

Cell Wall

The structure (Table 12-2), components, and functions (Table 12-3) of the cell wall distinguish gram-positive from gram-negative bacteria. Cell wall components are also unique to bacteria, and their repetitive structures bind to pathogen pattern receptors on human cells to elicit innate protective responses. The important differences in membrane characteristics are outlined in Table 12-4. Rigid **peptidoglycan (murein)** layers surround the cytoplasmic membranes of most prokaryotes. The exceptions are *Archaea* organisms (which contain pseudoglycans or pseudomureins related to peptidoglycan) and mycoplasmas (which have no peptidoglycan). Because the peptidoglycan provides rigidity, it also helps determine the shape of the particular bacterial cell. Gram-negative bacteria are also surrounded by outer membranes.

Gram-Positive Bacteria

A gram-positive bacterium has a *thick, multilayered cell wall consisting mainly of peptidoglycan* (150 to 500 Å) surrounding the cytoplasmic membrane (Figure 12-5). The peptidoglycan is a meshlike exoskeleton similar in function to the exoskeleton of an insect. Unlike the exoskeleton of the insect, however, the peptidoglycan of the cell is sufficiently porous to allow diffusion of metabolites to the plasma membrane. A new model for peptidoglycan suggests that the glycan extends out from the plasma membrane like bristles that are cross-linked with short peptide chains. The **peptidoglycan is essential** for structure, replication, and survival in the normally hostile conditions in which bacteria grow.

The peptidoglycan can be degraded by **lysozyme.** Lysozyme is an enzyme in human tears and mucus but is also produced by bacteria and other organisms. Lysozyme cleaves the glycan backbone of the peptidoglycan. Without the peptidoglycan, the bacteria succumb to the large osmotic pressure differences across the cytoplasmic membrane and lyse. Removal of the cell wall produces a **protoplast** that lyses unless it is osmotically stabilized.

The gram-positive cell wall may also include other components such as proteins, teichoic and lipoteichoic acids, and complex polysaccharides (usually called **C polysaccharides**). The M protein of streptococci and protein A of *S. aureus* are covalently bound to the peptidoglycan. **Teichoic acids** are water-soluble anionic polymers of polyol phosphates that are covalently linked to the peptidoglycan and essential to cell viability. **Lipoteichoic acids** have a fatty acid and are anchored in the cytoplasmic membrane. These molecules are common surface antigens that distinguish bacterial serotypes and promote attachment to other bacteria and to specific receptors on mammalian cell surfaces (adherence). Teichoic acids are important factors in virulence. Lipoteichoic acids are shed into the media and the host, and although weaker, they bind to pathogen pattern receptors and initiate innate protective host responses similar to endotoxin.

Gram-Negative Bacteria

Gram-negative cell walls are more complex than gram-positive cell walls, both structurally and chemically (see Figure 12-2). Structurally, a gram-negative cell wall contains two layers external to the cytoplasmic membrane. Immediately external to the cytoplasmic membrane is a *thin peptidoglycan layer* that accounts for only 5% to 10% of the gram-negative cell wall by weight. There are *no teichoic or lipoteichoic acids* in the gram-negative cell wall. External to the peptidoglycan layer is the **outer membrane,** which is unique to gram-negative bacteria. The area between the external surface of the cytoplasmic membrane and the internal surface of the outer membrane is referred to as the

 Table 12-2 **Bacterial Membrane Structures**

Structure	Chemical Constituents	Functions
Plasma membrane	Phospholipids, proteins, and enzymes	Containment, generation of energy, membrane potential, and transport
Cell Wall		
Gram-Positive Bacteria		
Peptidoglycan	Glycan chains of GlcNAc and MurNAc cross-linked by peptide bridge	Cell shape and structure; protection from environment and complement killing
Teichoic acid	Polyribitol phosphate or glycerol phosphate cross-linked to peptidoglycan	Strengthens cell wall; calcium ion sequestration
Lipoteichoic acid	Lipid-linked teichoic acid	Activator of innate host protections
Proteins	Covalently or binding to peptidoglycan or teichoic acid	Immune evasion, attachment, etc.
Gram-Negative Bacteria		
Peptidoglycan	Thinner version of that found in gram-positive bacteria	Cell shape and structure
Periplasmic space		Enzymes involved in transport, degradation, and synthesis
Outer membrane		Cell structure; protection from host environment
Proteins	Porin channel	Permeation of small hydrophilic molecules; restricts some antibiotics
	Secretory devices (types I, II, III, IV)	Penetrates and delivers proteins across membranes, including virulence factors
	Lipoprotein	Outer membrane link to peptidoglycan
LPS	Lipid A, core polysaccharide, O antigen	Outer membrane structure; potent activator of innate host responses
Phospholipids	With saturated fatty acids	
Other Structures		
Capsule	Polysaccharides or polypeptides (anthrax)	Antiphagocytic
Biofilm	Polysaccharides	Protection of colony from environment, antimicrobials, and host response
Pili	Pilin, adhesins	Adherence, sex pili
Flagellum	Motor proteins, flagellin	Movement, chemotaxis
Proteins	M protein of streptococci (for example)	Various

GlcNAc, N-Acetylglucosamine; *LPS,* lipopolysaccharide; *MurNAc, N*-acetylmuramic acid.

periplasmic space. This space is actually a compartment containing components of transport systems for iron, proteins, sugars and other metabolites, and a variety of hydrolytic enzymes that are important to the cell for the breakdown of large macromolecules for metabolism. These enzymes typically include proteases, phosphatases, lipases, nucleases, and carbohydrate-degrading enzymes. In the case of pathogenic gram-negative species, many of the virulence factors, such as collagenases, hyaluronidases, proteases, and β-lactamase, are in the periplasmic space.

The gram-negative cell wall is also traversed by different transport systems, including the **type I, II, III, IV, and V secretion devices.** Transport systems provide mechanisms for the uptake and release of different metabolites and other compounds. Production of the secretion devices may be induced during infection and contribute to the virulence of the microbe by transporting molecules that facilitate bacterial adhesion or intracellular growth. The type III secretion device is a major virulence factor for some bacteria, with a complex structure that traverses both the inner and outer membranes and can act as a syringe to inject proteins into other cells.

As mentioned previously, outer membranes (see Figure 12-2) are unique to gram-negative bacteria. The outer membrane is like a stiff canvas sack around the bacteria. *The outer membrane maintains the bacterial structure and is a permeability barrier to large molecules* (e.g., proteins such as lysozyme) *and hydrophobic molecules* (e.g., some antimicrobials). It also provides protection from adverse environmental conditions, such as the digestive system of the host (important for Enterobacteriaceae organisms). The outer membrane has an asymmetric bilayer structure that differs from any other biological membrane in the structure of the outer leaflet of the membrane. The inner leaflet contains phospholipids normally found in bacterial membranes. However, the outer leaflet is composed primarily of **lipopolysaccharide (LPS).**

Table 12-3 Functions of the Bacterial Envelope

Function	Component
Structure	
Rigidity	All
Packaging of internal contents	All
Bacterial Functions	
Permeability barrier	Outer membrane or plasma membrane
Metabolite uptake	Membranes and periplasmic transport proteins, porins, permeases
Energy production	Plasma membrane
Motility	Flagella
Mating	Pili
Host Interaction	
Adhesion to host cells	Pili, proteins, teichoic acid
Immune recognition by host	All outer structures and peptidoglycan
Escape from host immune protections	
Antibody	Protein A
Phagocytosis	Capsule, M protein
Complement	Gram-positive peptidoglycan
Medical Relevance	
Antibiotic targets	Peptidoglycan synthesis, outer membrane
Antibiotic resistance	Outer membrane barrier

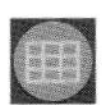

Table 12-4 Membrane Characteristics of Gram-Positive and Gram-Negative Bacteria

Characteristic	Gram-Positive	Gram-Negative
Outer membrane	–	+
Cell wall	Thick	Thin
Lipopolysaccharide	–	+
Endotoxin	–	+
Teichoic acid	Often present	–
Sporulation	Some strains	–
Capsule	Sometimes present	Sometimes present
Lysozyme	Sensitive	Resistant
Antibacterial activity of penicillin	More susceptible	More resistant
Exotoxin production	Some strains	Some strains

Except for those LPS molecules in the process of synthesis, the outer leaflet of the outer membrane is the only location where LPS molecules are found.

LPS is also called **endotoxin,** a powerful stimulator of innate and immune responses. LPS is shed from the bacteria into the host. LPS binds to pathogen pattern receptors and activates B cells and induces macrophage, dendritic, and other cells to release interleukin (IL)-1, IL-6, tumor necrosis factor (TNF), and other factors. LPS induces fever and can cause shock. The **Shwartzman reaction** (disseminated intravascular coagulation) follows the release of large amounts of endotoxin into the bloodstream. *Neisseria* bacteria shed large amounts of a related molecule, **lipooligosaccharide (LOS),** resulting in fever and severe symptoms.

The variety of proteins found in gram-negative outer membranes is limited, but several of the proteins are present in high concentration, resulting in a higher total protein content than that of the cytoplasmic membrane. Many of the proteins traverse the entire lipid bilayer and are thus transmembrane proteins. A group of these proteins is known as **porins** because they form pores **that allow diffusion of hydrophilic molecules less than 700 Da in mass through the membrane.** *The porin channel allows passage of metabolites and small hydrophilic antimicrobials.* The outer membrane also contains structural proteins, receptor molecules for bacteriophages, and other ligands and components of transport and secretory systems.

The outer membrane is connected to the cytoplasmic membrane at adhesion sites and is tied to the peptidoglycan by **lipoprotein.** The lipoprotein is covalently attached to the peptidoglycan and is anchored in the outer membrane. The adhesion sites provide a membranous route for the delivery of newly synthesized outer membrane components to the outer membrane.

The outer membrane is held together by divalent cation (Mg^{+2} and Ca^{+2}) linkages between phosphates on LPS molecules and hydrophobic interactions between the LPS and proteins. These interactions produce a stiff, strong membrane that can be disrupted by antibiotics (e.g., polymyxin) or by the removal of Mg and Ca ions (chelation with ethylenediaminetetraacetic acid [EDTA] or tetracycline). Disruption of the outer membrane weakens the bacteria and allows the permeability of large hydrophobic molecules. Disruption of the outer membrane can provide entry of lysozyme to produce **spheroplasts,** which, like protoplasts, are osmotically sensitive.

External Structures

Some bacteria (gram-positive or gram-negative) are closely surrounded by loose polysaccharide or protein layers called **capsules,** sometimes referred to as a **slime layer** or a **glycocalyx.** *Bacillus anthracis,* the exception to this rule, produces a polypeptide capsule. The capsule is hard to see in a microscope, but its space can be visualized by the exclusion of India ink particles.

Capsules are unnecessary for the growth of bacteria but are very important for survival in the host. *The capsule is poorly antigenic and antiphagocytic and is a major virulence factor* (e.g., *Streptococcus pneumoniae*). The capsule can also act as a barrier to toxic hydrophobic molecules, such as detergents, and can promote **adherence** to other bacteria or host tissue surfaces. For *Streptococcus mutans,* the dextran and levan capsules are the means by which the bacteria attach and stick to the tooth enamel. Bacterial strains lacking a capsule may arise during growth under laboratory conditions, away from the selective pressures of the host, and are therefore less virulent. Some bacteria (e.g., *Pseudomonas aeruginosa, S. aureus*) will produce a polysaccharide **biofilm**

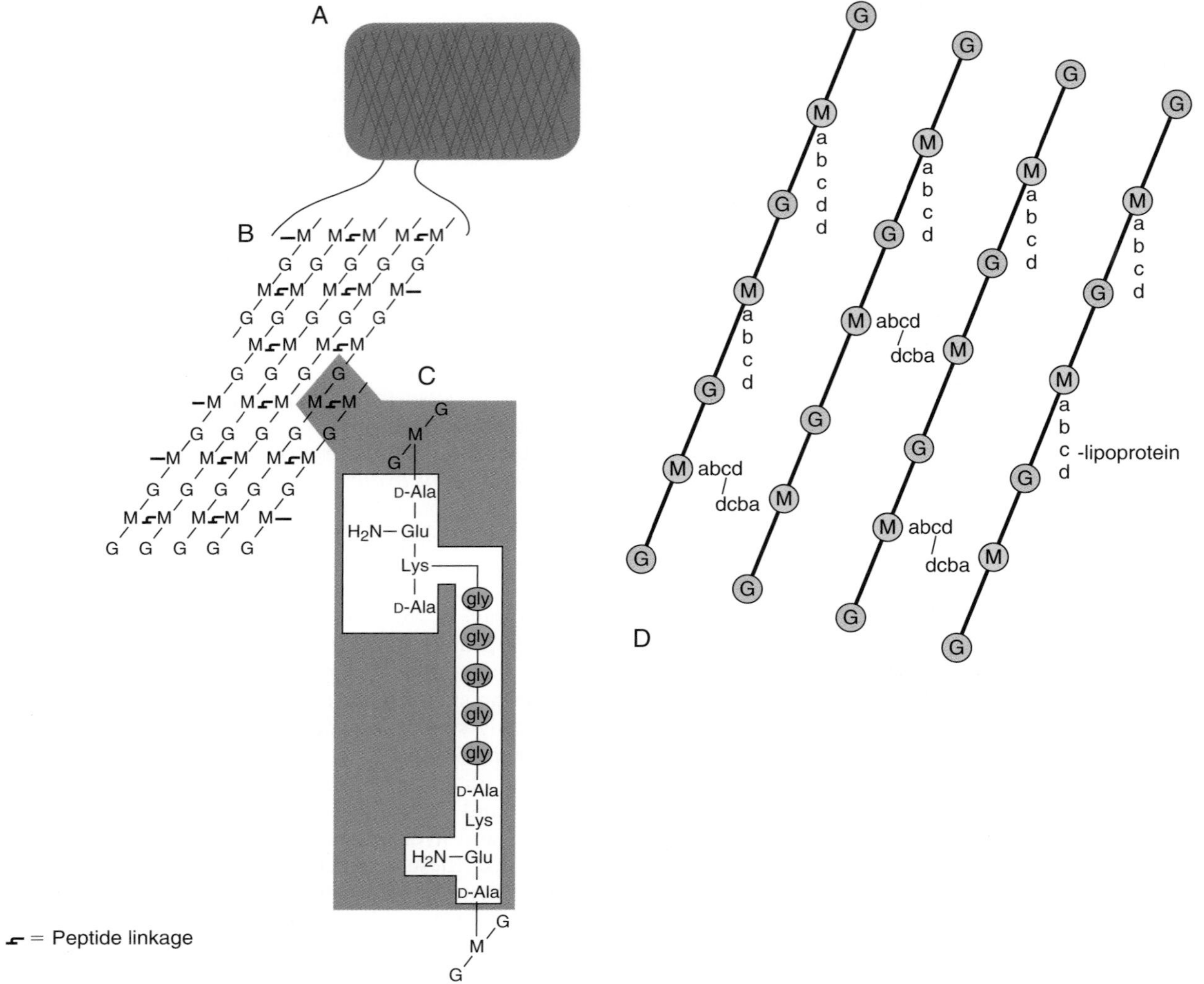

FIGURE 12-5 General structure of the peptidoglycan component of the cell wall. **A,** The peptidoglycan forms a meshlike layer around the cell. **B,** The peptidoglycan mesh consists of a polysaccharide polymer that is cross-linked by peptide bonds. **C,** Peptides are cross-linked through a peptide bond between the terminal D-alanine *(D-Ala)* from one chain and a lysine *(Lys)* (or another diamino amino acid) from the other chain. A pentaglycine bridge (gly_5) expands the cross-link in *Staphylococcus aureus* (as shown). **D,** Representation of the *Escherichia coli* peptidoglycan structure. Diaminopimelic acid, the diamino amino acid in the third position of the peptide, is *directly linked* to the terminal alanine of another chain to cross-link the peptidoglycan. Lipoprotein anchors the outer membrane to the peptidoglycan. *G, N*-Acetylglucosamine; *Glu,* D-glutamic acid; *gly,* glycine; *M, N*-acetylmuramic acid. (**A** to **C,** Modified from Talaro K, Talaro A: *Foundations in microbiology,* ed 2, Dubuque, Iowa, 1996, William C Brown. **D,** Modified from Joklik WK, Willett HP, Amos DB, et al: *Zinsser microbiology,* Norwalk, Conn, 1988, Appleton & Lange.)

when sufficient numbers (quorum) are present and under conditions that support growth. The biofilm contains and protects the bacterial community from antibiotics and host defenses. Another example of a biofilm is tooth plaque produced by *S. mutans.*

Flagella are ropelike propellers composed of helically coiled protein subunits **(flagellin)** that are anchored in the bacterial membranes through hook and basal body structures and are driven by membrane potential. Bacterial species may have one or several flagella on their surfaces, and they may be anchored at different parts of the cell. The membrane potential powers the protein motor, which spins a whiplike propeller made of multiple subunits of **flagellin.** Flagella provide motility for bacteria, allowing the cell to swim **(chemotaxis)** toward food and away from poisons. Bacteria approach food by swimming straight and then tumbling in a new direction. The swimming period becomes longer as the concentration of chemoattractant increases. The direction of flagellar spinning determines whether the bacteria swim or tumble. Flagella express antigenic and strain determinants and are a ligand for a pathogen pattern receptor to activate innate host protections.

Fimbriae (pili) (Latin for "fringe") are hairlike structures on the outside of bacteria; they are composed of protein subunits **(pilin).** Fimbriae can be morphologically distinguished from flagella because they are smaller in diameter (3 to 8 nm versus 15 to 20 nm) and usually are not coiled in structure. In general, several hundred fimbriae are arranged peritrichously (uniformly) over the entire surface of the bacterial cell. They may be as long as 15 to 20 μm or many times the length of the cell.

Fimbriae promote adherence to other bacteria or to the host (alternative names are *adhesins, lectins, evasins,* and *aggressins*). The tips of the fimbriae may contain proteins (lectins) that bind to specific sugars (e.g., mannose). As an adherence factor **(adhesin),** fimbriae are an important virulence factor for colonization and infection of the urinary tract by *E. coli, Neisseria gonorrhoeae,* and other bacteria. **F pili (sex pili)** bind to other bacteria and are a tube for transfer of large segments of bacterial chromosomes between bacteria. These pili are encoded by a plasmid (F).

Bacteria with Alternative Cell Wall Structures

Mycobacteria have a peptidoglycan layer (slightly different structure) that is intertwined with and covalently attached to an arabinogalactan polymer and surrounded by a **waxlike lipid coat** of mycolic acid (large α-branched β-hydroxy fatty acids), cord factor (glycolipid of trehalose and two mycolic acids), wax D (glycolipid of 15 to 20 mycolic acids and sugar), and sulfolipids (see Figure 22-1). These bacteria are described as **staining acid-fast.** The coat is responsible for virulence and is antiphagocytic. *Corynebacterium* and *Nocardia* organisms also produce mycolic acid lipids. **Mycoplasmas** have no peptidoglycan cell wall and incorporate steroids from the host into their membranes.

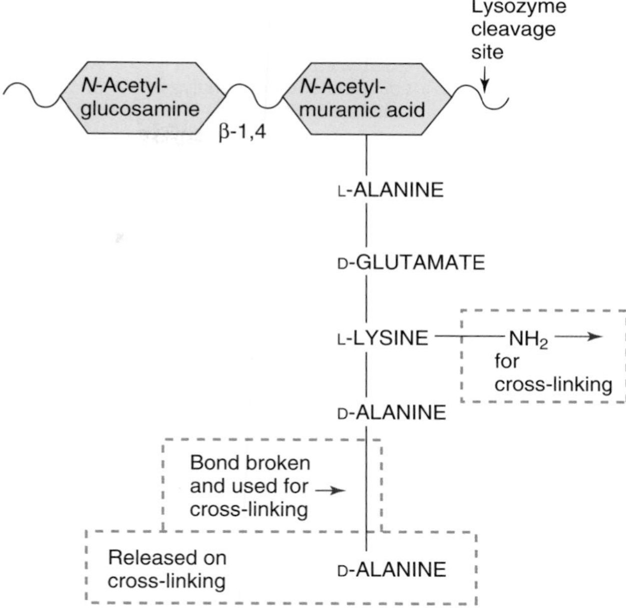

FIGURE 12-6 Precursor of peptidoglycan. The peptidoglycan is built from prefabricated units that contain a pentapeptide attached to the *N*-acetylmuramic acid. The pentapeptide contains a terminal D-alanine-D-alanine unit. This dipeptide is required for cross-linking the peptidoglycan and is the basis for the action of β-lactam and vancomycin antibiotics. The β-1,4 disaccharide link cleaved by lysozyme is indicated.

Structure and Biosynthesis of the Major Components of the Bacterial Cell Wall

The cell wall components are large structures made up of polymers of subunits. This type of structure facilitates their synthesis. Like astronauts building a space station, bacteria face problems assembling their cell walls. Synthesis of the peptidoglycan, LPS, teichoic acid, and capsule occurs on the outside of the bacteria, away from the synthetic machinery and energy sources of the cytoplasm and in an inhospitable environment. For both the space station and the bacteria, prefabricated precursors and subunits of the final structure are assembled in a factory-like setting on the inside, attached to a structure similar to a conveyor belt, brought to the surface, and then attached to the preexisting structure. For bacteria, the molecular conveyor belt–like structure is a large hydrophobic phospholipid called **bactoprenol (undecaprenol [C_{55} isoprenoid]).** The prefabricated precursors must also be activated with high-energy bonds (e.g., phosphates) or other means to power the attachment reactions occurring outside the cell. For gram-negative bacteria, the outer membrane components are delivered through adhesion sites.

Peptidoglycan (Mucopeptide, Murein)

The peptidoglycan is a rigid mesh made up of bristle-like linear polysaccharide chains cross-linked by peptides. The polysaccharide is made up of repeating disaccharides of ***N*-acetylglucosamine (GlcNAc, NAG, G)** and ***N*-acetylmuramic acid (MurNAc, NAM, M)** (Figure 12-6; see Figure 12-5).

A tetrapeptide is attached to the MurNAc. The peptide is unusual because it contains both D and L amino acids (D amino acids are not normally used in nature) and the peptide is produced enzymatically rather than by a ribosome. The first two amino acids attached to the MurNAc may vary for different organisms.

The diamino amino acids in the third position are essential for the cross-linking of the peptidoglycan chain. Examples of diamino amino acids include lysine and diaminopimelic and diaminobutyric acids. The peptide cross-link is formed between the free amine of the diamino amino acid and the D-alanine in the fourth position of another chain. *S. aureus* and other gram-positive bacteria use an amino acid bridge (e.g., a $glycine_5$ peptide) between these amino acids to lengthen the cross-link. The precursor form of the peptide has an extra D-alanine, which is released during the cross-linking step.

The peptidoglycan in gram-positive bacteria forms multiple layers and is often cross-linked in three dimensions, providing a very strong, rigid cell wall. In contrast, the peptidoglycan in gram-negative cell walls is usually only one molecule (layer) thick. The number of cross-links and the length of the cross-link determine the rigidity of the peptidoglycan mesh. The site where **lysozyme** cleaves the glycan of the peptidoglycan is shown in Figure 12-6.

Peptidoglycan Synthesis

Peptidoglycan synthesis occurs in four phases (Figure 12-7). First, the precursors are synthesized and activated inside the cell. Glucosamine is enzymatically converted into MurNAc

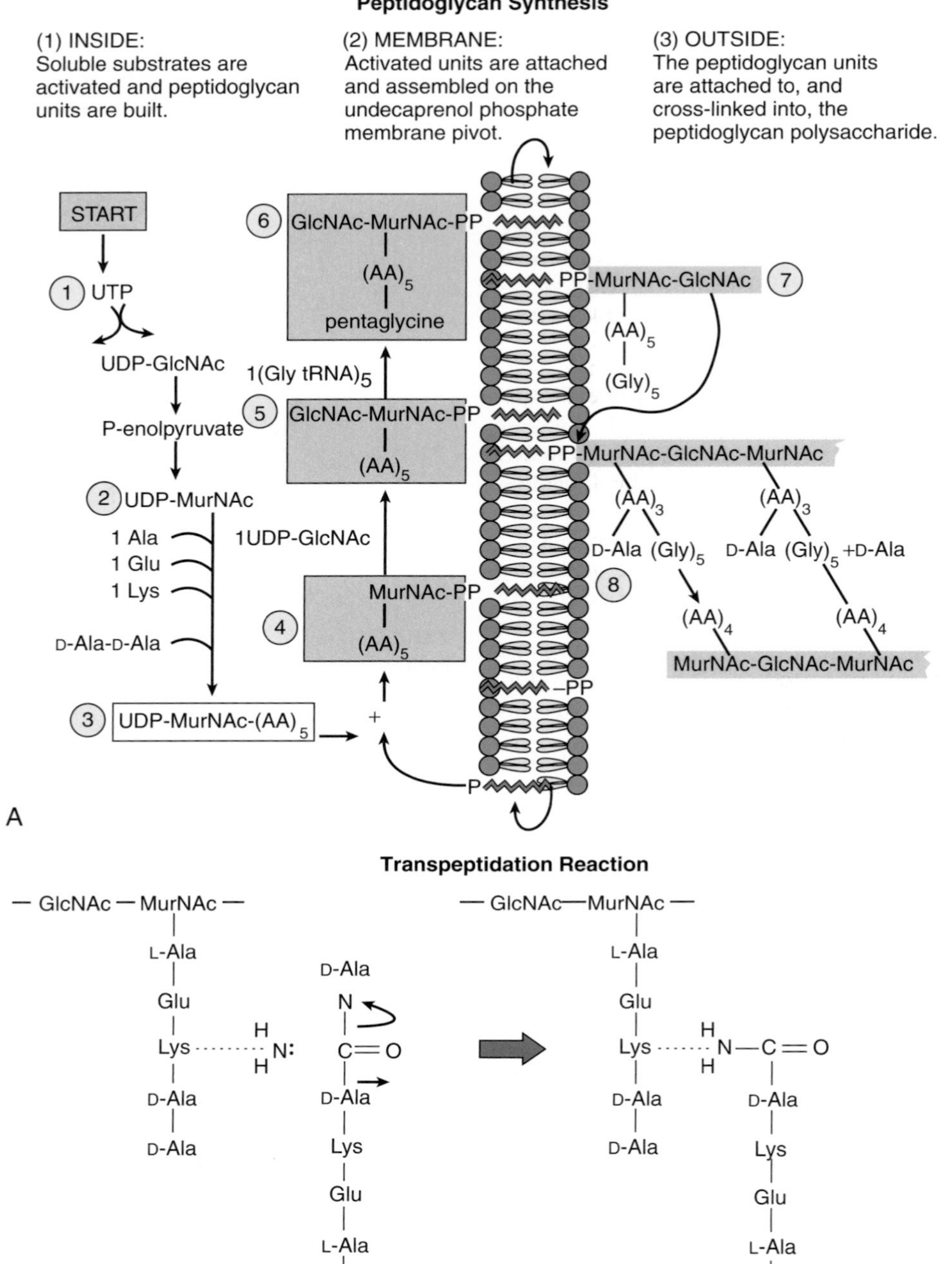

FIGURE 12-7 Peptidoglycan synthesis. **A,** Peptidoglycan synthesis occurs in the following four phases: (1) Peptidoglycan is synthesized from prefabricated units constructed and activated for assembly and transport inside the cell. (2) At the membrane the units are assembled onto the undecaprenol phosphate conveyor belt, and fabrication is completed. (3) The unit is translocated to the outside of the cell and (4) the unit is attached to the polysaccharide chain, and the peptide is cross-linked to finish the construction. *Staphylococcus aureus* utilizes a pentaglycine bridge in the cross-link. Such a construction can be compared with the assembly of a space station of prefabricated units. **B,** The cross-linking reaction is a transpeptidation. *Escherichia coli* uses a direct cross-link between D-alanine and lysine. One peptide bond (produced inside the cell) is traded for another (outside the cell) with the release of D-alanine. The enzymes that catalyze the reaction are called *D-alanine, D-alanine transpeptidase, or carboxypeptidases.* These enzymes are the targets of β-lactam antibiotics and are called penicillin-binding proteins. *AA_5,* pentapeptide with D-alanine-D-alanine; *AA_4,* tetrapeptide with terminal D-alanine; *AA_3,* tripeptide; *Glu,* glutamate; *Gly_5,* glycine pentapeptide; *Lys,* lysine; *MurNAc-PP, N*-acetylmuramic acid diphosphate; *tRNA,* transfer ribonucleic acid; *UDP-GlcNAc,* uridine diphosphate *N*-acetylglucosamine; *UDP-MurNAc,* uridine diphosphate-*N*-acetylmuramic acid; *UTP,* uridine triphosphate.

and then energetically activated by a reaction with uridine triphosphate (UTP) to produce uridine diphosphate-*N*-acetylmuramic acid (UDP-MurNAc). Next, the UDP-MurNAc-pentapeptide precursor is assembled in a series of enzymatic steps.

In the second phase, the UDP-MurNAc pentapeptide is attached to the **bactoprenol** "conveyor belt" in the cytoplasmic membrane through a pyrophosphate link, with the release of uridine monophosphate (UMP). GlcNAc is added to make the disaccharide building block of the peptidoglycan. Some bacteria (e.g., *S. aureus*) add a pentaglycine or another chain to the diamino amino acid at the third position of the peptide chain to lengthen the cross-link.

In the third phase, the bactoprenol molecule translocates the disaccharide:peptide precursor to the outside of the cell.

In the last phase, the peptidoglycan is extended at the outside surface of the plasma membrane. The GlcNAc-MurNAc disaccharide is attached to a peptidoglycan chain, using the pyrophosphate link between itself and the bactoprenol as energy to drive the reaction by enzymes called **transglycosylases.** The pyrophosphobactoprenol is converted back to a phosphobactoprenol and recycled. **Bacitracin** blocks the recycling. The peptide chains from adjacent glycan chains are cross-linked to each other by a peptide bond exchange **(transpeptidation)** between the free amine of the amino acid in the third position of the pentapeptide (e.g., lysine), or the N-terminus of the attached pentaglycine chain, and the D-alanine at the fourth position of the other peptide chain, releasing the terminal D-alanine of the precursor. This step requires no additional energy because peptide bonds are "traded."

The cross-linking reaction is catalyzed by membrane-bound **transpeptidases.** Related enzymes, **D-carboxypeptidases,** remove unreacted terminal D-alanines to limit the extent of cross-linking. The transpeptidases and carboxypeptidases are called **penicillin-binding proteins (PBPs)** because they are targets for penicillin and other β-lactam antibiotics. *Penicillin* and related **β-lactam antibiotics** resemble the "transition state" conformation of the D-Ala-D-Ala substrate when bound to these enzymes. **Vancomycin** binds to the D-Ala-D-Ala structure to block these reactions. Different PBPs are used for extending the peptidoglycan, creating a septum for cell division and curving the peptidoglycan mesh (cell shape). Peptidoglycan extension and cross-linking is necessary for cell growth and division.

The peptidoglycan is constantly being synthesized and degraded. **Autolysins,** such as lysozyme, are important for determining bacterial shape. Inhibition of synthesis or the cross-linking of the peptidoglycan does not stop the autolysins, and their action weakens the mesh and leads to cell lysis and death. New peptidoglycan synthesis does not occur during starvation, which leads to a weakening of the peptidoglycan and a loss in the dependability of the Gram stain.

An understanding of the biosynthesis of peptidoglycan is essential in medicine because these reactions are unique to bacterial cells and hence can be inhibited with little or no adverse effect on host (human) cells. As indicated earlier, a number of antibacterials target one or more steps in this pathway (see Chapter 17).

A
Ribitol Teichoic Acid
(*Staphylococcus*)

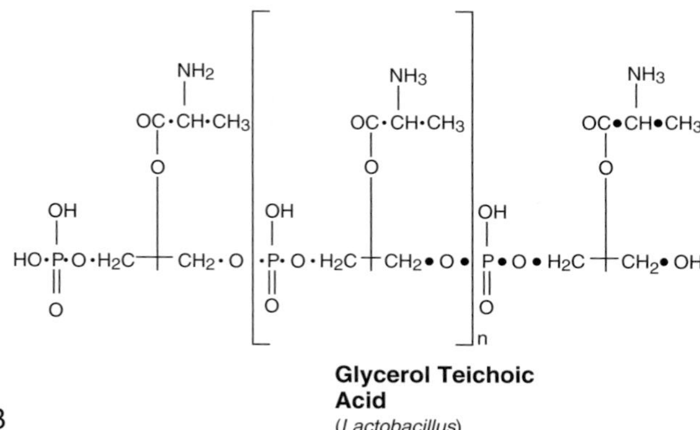

FIGURE 12-8 Teichoic acid. Teichoic acid is a polymer of chemically modified ribitol **(A)** or glycerol phosphate **(B).** The nature of the modification (e.g., sugars, amino acids) can define the serotype of the bacteria. Teichoic acid is covalently attached to the peptidoglycan. Lipoteichoic acid is anchored in the cytoplasmic membrane by a covalently attached fatty acid.

Teichoic Acid

Teichoic and **lipoteichoic acid** are polymers of chemically modified ribose or glycerol connected by phosphates (Figure 12-8). Sugars, choline, or D-alanine may be attached to the hydroxyls of the ribose or glycerol, providing antigenic determinants. These can be distinguished by antibodies and may determine the bacterial serotype. Lipoteichoic acid has a fatty acid and is anchored in the membrane. Teichoic acid is synthesized from building blocks using the bactoprenol in a manner similar to that of peptidoglycan. Teichoic acid is enzymatically attached to the N-terminus of the peptide of peptidoglycan and also secreted from the cells.

Lipopolysaccharide

LPS (endotoxin) consists of three structural sections: lipid A, core polysaccharide (rough core), and O antigen (Figure 12-9). Lipid A is a basic component of LPS and is essential for bacterial viability. Lipid A is responsible for the endotoxin activity of LPS. It has a phosphorylated glucosamine disaccharide backbone with fatty acids attached to anchor the structure in the outer membrane. The phosphates connect LPS units into aggregates. One carbohydrate chain is attached to each disaccharide backbone and extends away from the bacteria. The core polysaccharide is a branched polysaccharide of 9 to 12 sugars. Most of the core region is also

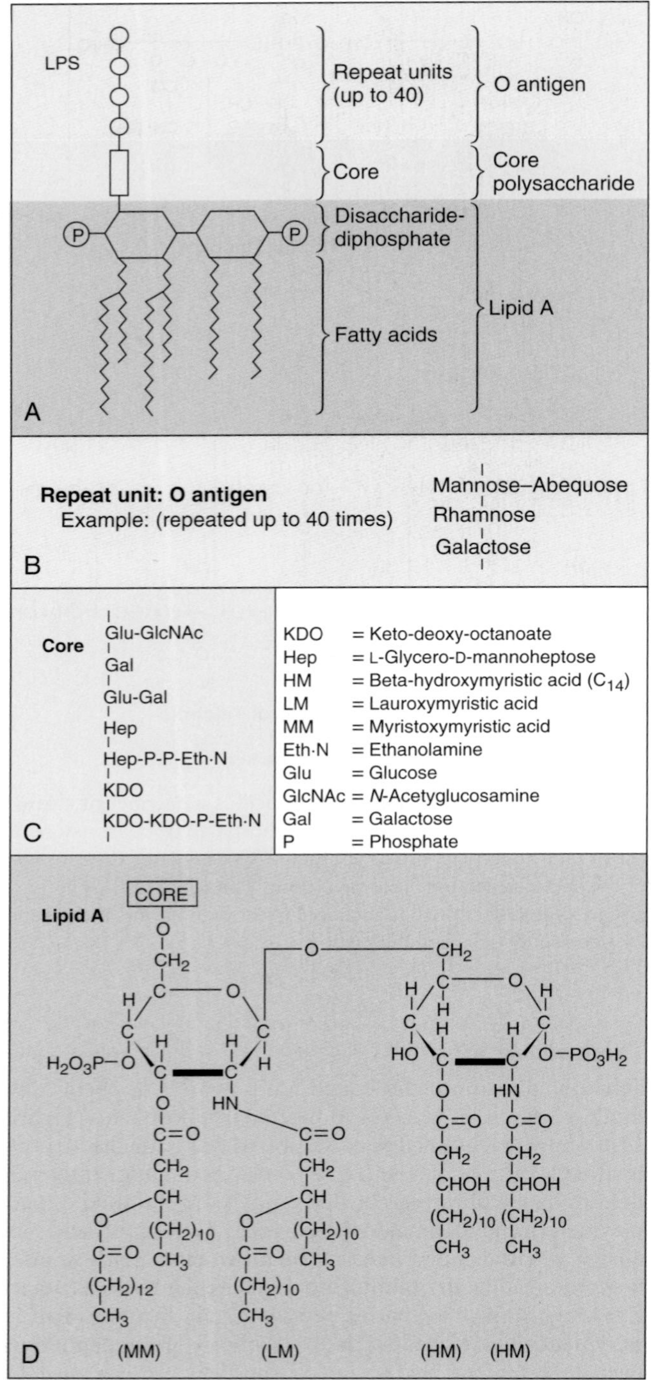

FIGURE 12-9 The lipopolysaccharide *(LPS)* of the gram-negative cell envelope. **A,** Segment of the molecule showing the arrangements of the major constituents. Each LPS molecule has one lipid A and one polysaccharide core unit but many repeats of O antigen. **B,** Typical O-antigen repeat unit *(Salmonella typhimurium).* **C,** Polysaccharide core. **D,** Structure of lipid A of *S. typhimurium.* (Modified from Brooks GF, Butel JS, Ornston LN: *Jawetz, Melnick, and Aldenberg's medical microbiology,* ed 19, Norwalk, Conn, 1991, Appleton & Lange.)

essential for LPS structure and bacterial viability. The core region contains an unusual sugar, 2-keto-3-deoxy-octanoate (KDO), and is phosphorylated. Divalent cations link the phosphates of the LPS and core to strengthen the outer membrane. The O antigen is attached to the core and extends away from the bacteria. It is a long, linear polysaccharide consisting of 50 to 100 repeating saccharide units of 4 to 7 sugars per unit. **Lipooligosaccharide (LOS),** which is present in *Neisseria* species, lacks the O-antigen portion of LPS and is readily shed from the bacteria. The shorter O antigen makes *Neisseria* more susceptible to host-mediated complement lysis.

LPS structure is used to classify bacteria. The basic structure of lipid A is identical for related bacteria and is similar for all gram-negative Enterobacteriaceae. The core region is the same for a species of bacteria. The O antigen distinguishes serotypes (strains) of a bacterial species. For example, the O157:H7 (O antigen : flagellin) serotype identifies the *E. coli* agent of hemolytic-uremic syndrome.

The lipid A and core portions are enzymatically synthesized in a sequential manner on the inside surface of the cytoplasmic membrane. The repeat units of the O antigen are assembled on a bactoprenol molecule and then transferred to a growing O-antigen chain. The finished O-antigen chain is transferred to the core lipid A structure. The LPS molecule is translocated through adhesion sites to the outer surface of the outer membrane.

Cell Division

Replication of the bacterial chromosome also triggers initiation of cell division (Figure 12-10). The production of two daughter bacteria requires growth and extension of the cell wall components, followed by production of a septum (cross wall) to divide the daughter bacteria into two cells. The septum consists of two membranes separated by two layers of peptidoglycan. Septum formation is initiated at midcell, at a site defined by protein complexes affixed to a protein filament ring that lines the inside of the cytoplasmic membrane. The septum grows from opposite sides toward the center of the cell, causing cleavage of the daughter cells. This process requires special transpeptidases (PBPs) and other enzymes. For streptococci, the growth zone is located at 180 degrees from each other, producing linear chains of bacteria. In contrast, the growth zone of staphylococci is at 90 degrees. Incomplete cleavage of the septum can cause the bacteria to remain linked, forming chains (e.g., streptococci) or clusters (e.g., staphylococci).

Spores

Some gram-positive—but never gram-negative—bacteria, such as members of the genera *Bacillus* (e.g., *Bacillus anthracis*) and *Clostridium* (e.g., *Clostridium tetani* or *botulinum*) (soil bacteria), are spore formers. Under harsh environmental conditions, such as loss of a nutritional requirement, these bacteria can convert from a **vegetative state** to a **dormant state,** or **spore.** The location of the spore within a cell is a characteristic of the bacteria and can assist in identification of the bacterium.

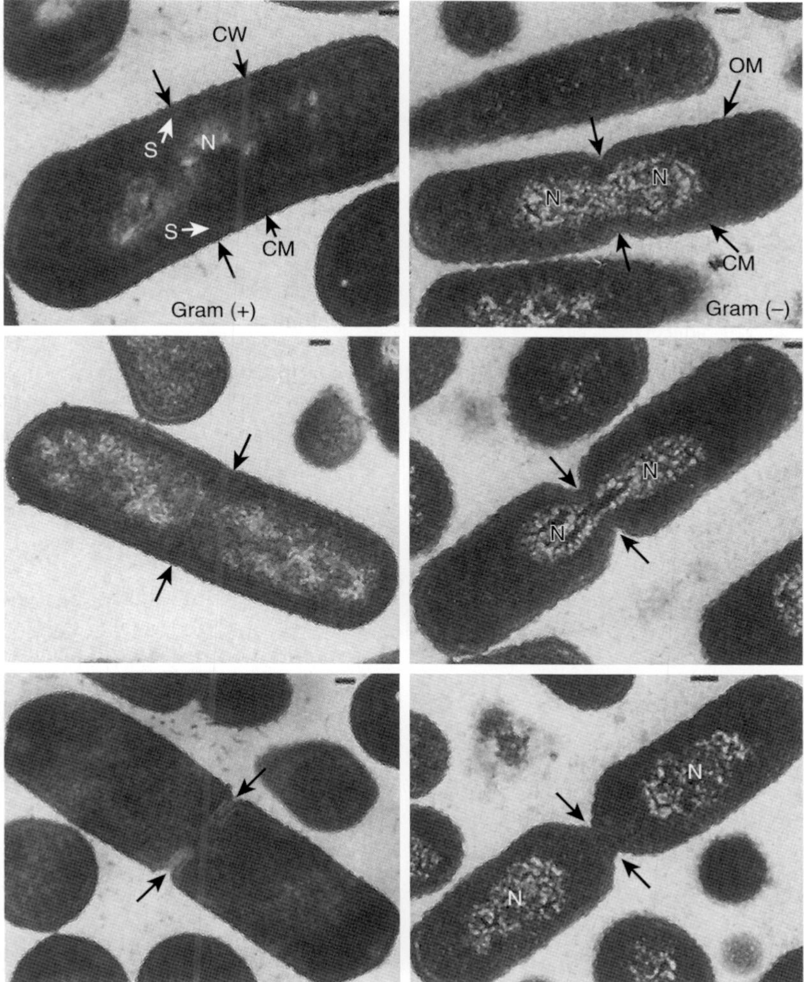

FIGURE 12-10 Electron photomicrographs of gram-positive *(Bacillus subtilis)* cell division *(left)* and gram-negative *(Escherichia coli)* cell division *(right)*. Progression in cell division from top to bottom. *CM,* Cytoplasmic membrane; *CW,* cell wall; *N,* nucleoid; *OM,* outer membrane; *S,* septum. Bar = 0.2 μm. (From Slots J, Taubman MA: *Contemporary oral biology and immunology,* St Louis, 1992, Mosby.)

The spore is a dehydrated multishelled structure that protects and allows the bacteria to exist in "suspended animation" (Figure 12-11). It contains a complete copy of the chromosome, the bare minimum concentrations of essential proteins and ribosomes, and a high concentration of **calcium bound to dipicolinic acid.** The spore has an inner membrane, two peptidoglycan layers, and an outer keratin-like protein coat. The spore looks refractile (bright) in the microscope. The structure of the spore protects the genomic DNA from intense heat, radiation, and attack by most enzymes and chemical agents. In fact, bacterial spores are so resistant to environmental factors that they can exist for centuries as viable spores. Spores are also difficult to decontaminate with standard disinfectants or autoclaving conditions.

Depletion of specific nutrients (e.g., alanine) from the growth medium triggers a cascade of genetic events (comparable to differentiation) leading to the production of a spore. Spore mRNAs are transcribed, and other mRNAs are turned off. Dipicolinic acid is produced, and antibiotics and toxins are often excreted. After duplication of the chromosome, one copy of the DNA and cytoplasmic contents **(core)** are surrounded by the cytoplasmic membrane, the peptidoglycan, and the membrane of the septum. This wraps the DNA in the two layers of membrane and peptidoglycan that would normally divide the cell. These two layers are surrounded by the **cortex,** which is made up of a thin inner layer of tightly cross-linked peptidoglycan surrounding a membrane (which used to be the cytoplasmic membrane) and a loose outer peptidoglycan layer. The cortex is surrounded by the tough **keratin-like protein coat** that protects the spore. The process requires 6 to 8 hours for completion.

Germination of spores into the vegetative state is stimulated by disruption of the outer coat by mechanical stress, pH, heat, or another stressor and requires water and a triggering nutrient (e.g., alanine). The process takes approximately 90 minutes. After the germination process begins, the spore will take up water, swell, shed its coats, and produce one new vegetative cell identical to the original vegetative cell, thus completing the entire cycle. Once germination has begun and the spore coat has been compromised, the spore is weakened and vulnerable and can be inactivated like other bacteria.

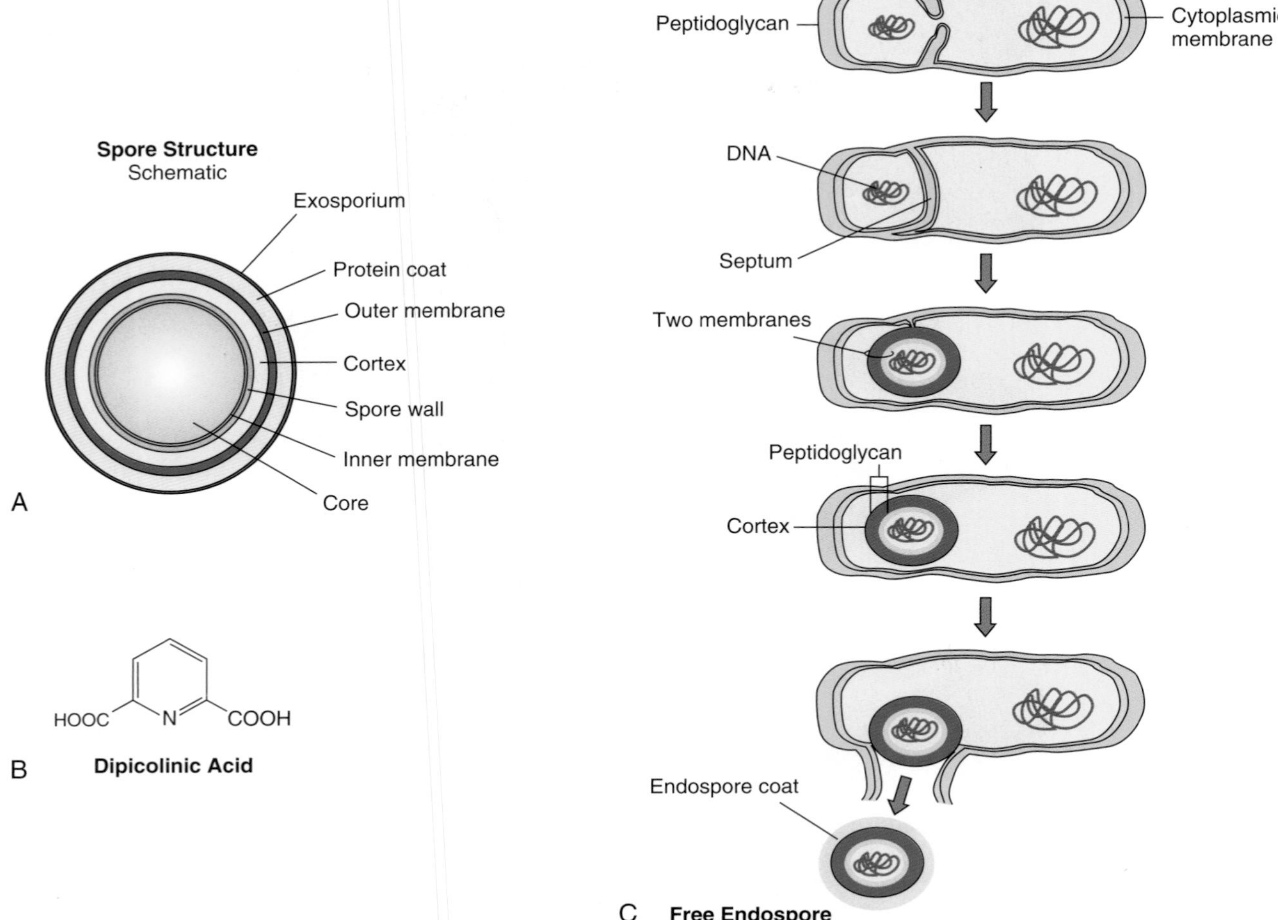

FIGURE 12-11 **A,** Structure of a spore. **B,** High concentrations of dipicolinic acid in the spore bind calcium and stabilize the contents. **C,** Sporogenesis, the process of endospore formation.

Bibliography

Bower S, Rosenthal KS: Bacterial cell walls: the armor, artillery and Achilles heel, *Infect Dis Clin Pract* 14:309–317, 2006.

Daniel RA, Errington J: Control of cell morphogenesis in bacteria: two distinct ways to make a rod-shaped cell, *Cell* 113:767–776, 2003.

Lutkenhaus J: The regulation of bacterial cell division: a time and place for it, *Curr Opin Microbiol* 1:210–215, 1998.

Meroueh SO, Bencze KZ, Hesek D, et al: Three-dimensional structure of the bacterial cell wall peptidoglycan, *Proc Natl Acad Sci U S A* 103:4404–4409, 2006.

Nanninga N: Morphogenesis of *Escherichia coli*, *Microbiol Mol Biol Rev* 62:110–129, 1998.

Staley JT, Gunsalus RP, Lory S, et al: *Microbial life*, ed 2, Sunderland, Mass, 2007, Sinauer.

Talaro K: *Foundations in microbiology*, ed 6, New York, 2008, McGraw-Hill.

Willey J, Sherwood L, Woolverton C: *Prescott/Harley/Klein's microbiology*, ed 7, New York, 2007, McGraw-Hill.

CHAPTER 13 BACTERIAL METABOLISM AND GENETICS

Bacterial Metabolism

Metabolic Requirements

Bacterial growth requires a source of energy and the raw materials to build the proteins, structures, and membranes that make up and power the cell. Bacteria must obtain or synthesize the amino acids, carbohydrates, and lipids used as building blocks of the cell.

The minimum requirements for growth are a source of carbon and nitrogen, an energy source, water, and various ions. The essential elements include the components of proteins, lipids, and nucleic acids (C, O, H, N, S, P), important ions (K, Na, Mg, Ca, Cl), and components of enzymes (Fe, Zn, Mn, Mo, Se, Co, Cu, Ni). **Iron** is so important that many bacteria secrete special proteins (siderophores) to concentrate iron from dilute solutions, and our bodies will sequester iron to reduce its availability as a means of protection.

Oxygen (O_2 gas), although essential for the human host, is actually a poison for many bacteria. Some organisms (e.g., *Clostridium perfringens*, which causes gas gangrene) cannot grow in the presence of oxygen. Such bacteria are referred to as **obligate anaerobes.** Other organisms (e.g., *Mycobacterium tuberculosis*, which causes tuberculosis) require the presence of molecular oxygen for metabolism and growth and are therefore referred to as **obligate aerobes.** Most bacteria, however, grow in either the presence or the absence of oxygen. These bacteria are referred to as **facultative anaerobes.** Aerobic bacteria produce superoxide dismutase and catalase enzymes, which can detoxify hydrogen peroxide and superoxide radicals that are the toxic byproducts of aerobic metabolism.

Growth requirements and metabolic byproducts may be used as a convenient means of classifying different bacteria. Some bacteria, such as certain strains of *Escherichia coli* (a member of the intestinal flora), can synthesize all the amino acids, nucleotides, lipids, and carbohydrates necessary for growth and division, whereas the growth requirements of the causative agent of syphilis, *Treponema pallidum,* are so complex that a defined laboratory medium capable of supporting its growth has yet to be developed. Bacteria that can rely entirely on inorganic chemicals for their energy and source of carbon (carbon dioxide [CO_2]) are referred to as autotrophs (lithotrophs), whereas many bacteria and animal cells that require organic carbon sources are known as heterotrophs (organotrophs). Clinical microbiology laboratories distinguish bacteria by their ability to grow on specific carbon sources (e.g., lactose) and the end products of metabolism (e.g., ethanol, lactic acid, succinic acid).

The metabolism of normal flora bacteria is optimized for the pH, ion concentration, and types of food present in their environment within the body. As in the rumen of a cow, the bacteria of the gastrointestinal (GI) tract break down complex carbohydrates into simpler compounds and produce short-chain fatty acids (e.g., butyrate, propionate, lactate, acetate) as byproducts of **fermentation.** The lactic acid and short-chain fatty acids that are produced can decrease luminal pH and are absorbed and metabolized more readily. Changes in diet, water, or health, antibiotics, and certain drugs can change the environment and influence the metabolism and composition of microbes in the GI tract. Probiotics are bacteria that can improve the function of the normal flora (Box 13-1).

Metabolism, Energy, and Biosynthesis

All cells require a constant supply of energy to survive. This energy is derived from the controlled breakdown of various organic substrates (carbohydrates, lipids, and proteins). This process of substrate breakdown and conversion into usable energy is known as **catabolism.** The energy produced may then be used in the synthesis of cellular constituents (cell walls, proteins, fatty acids, nucleic acids), a process known as **anabolism.** Together these two processes, which are interrelated and tightly integrated, are referred to as **intermediary metabolism.**

The metabolic process generally begins with hydrolysis of large macromolecules in the external cellular environment by specific enzymes (Figure 13-1). The smaller molecules that are produced (e.g., monosaccharides, short peptides, fatty acids) are transported across the cell membranes into the cytoplasm by active or passive transport mechanisms specific for the metabolite. These mechanisms may use specific carrier or membrane transport proteins to help concentrate metabolites from the medium. The metabolites are converted via one or more pathways to one common universal intermediate, **pyruvic acid.** From pyruvic acid, the carbons may be channeled toward energy production or the synthesis of new carbohydrates, amino acids, lipids, and nucleic acids.

Instead of releasing all of glucose's energy as heat (as for burning), the bacteria break down glucose in discrete steps and capture the energy in usable chemical and electrochemical forms. Chemical energy is typically in the form of a

Box 13-1 Metabolism of Probiotic and Gastrointestinal Microbes

Probiotic microbes are primarily gram-positive bacteria and include *Lactobacillus* spp., *Bifidobacterium* spp., and the yeast *Saccharomyces boulardii* (Stone S, Edmonds R, Rosenthal KS: Probiotics: helping out the normal flora, *Infect Dis Clin Pract* 21:305–311, 2013; Saad N, Delattre C, Urdaci M, et al: An overview of the last advances in probiotic and prebiotic field, *Food Sci Technol* 50:1–16, 2013). *Bifidobacterium infantis* is one of the bacteria acquired by newborns and then selected by the complex carbohydrates in mother's milk. Probiotics consist of microbes that can be ingested, facilitate the development and maintenance of a healthy gut flora, and influence the cells of the immune system. Many of these probiotic bacteria are present in yogurt and are capable of metabolizing complex carbohydrates, including those in milk. These bacteria break down complex carbohydrates into simpler compounds and produce short-chain fatty acids (e.g., butyrate, propionate, lactate, acetate) as byproducts of **fermentation.** The lactic acid and short-chain fatty acids produced can decrease luminal pH and are absorbed and metabolized more readily. Acidification of the colon can select for and promote the growth of beneficial lactate-producing endogenous bacteria. Short-chain fatty acids are taken up by the bowel and metabolized more efficiently by the body, enhance cell growth, and improve barrier function of the epithelial cells lining the gastrointestinal tract, as well as support the growth of T-regulator (Treg) cells to limit inflammatory and autoimmune responses (Smith PM, Howitt MR, Panikov N, et al: The microbial metabolites, short-chain fatty acids, regulate colonic Treg cell homeostasis, *Science* 341:569–573, 2013).

Some normal flora bacteria, such as *Bacteroidetes* and *Firmicutes,* are more efficient than others at breaking down complex carbohydrates, including plant cell wall compounds (cellulose, pectin, xylan) and mucins or chondroitin sulfates of the protective mucous layer of the intestine. Increases in the ratio of these bacteria in the gut microbiome can lead to obesity (Vijay-Kumar M, Aitken JD, Carvalho FA, et al: Metabolic syndrome and altered gut microbiota in mice lacking Toll-like receptor 5, *Science* 328:228–231, 2010).

high-energy phosphate bond in **adenosine triphosphate (ATP)** or guanosine triphosphate (GTP), whereas electrochemical energy is stored by reduction (adding electrons to) of **nicotinamide adenine dinucleotide (NAD) to NADH** or flavin adenine dinucleotide (FAD) to $FADH_2$. **The NADH** can be converted by a series of oxidation-reduction reactions into chemical (pH) and **electrical potential gradients (Eh)** across the cytoplasmic membrane. The electrochemical energy can be used by **ATP synthase** to drive the phosphorylation of ADP to ATP and also to drive the spinning of flagella and the transport of molecules across the membrane.

Bacteria can produce energy from glucose by—in order of increasing efficiency—fermentation, anaerobic respiration (both of which occur in the absence of oxygen), or aerobic respiration. Aerobic respiration can completely convert the six carbons of glucose to CO_2 and water (H_2O) plus energy, whereas two- and three-carbon compounds are the end products of fermentation. For a more complete discussion of metabolism, please refer to a textbook on biochemistry.

Glycolysis and Fermentation

The most common glycolytic pathway, the Embden-Meyerhof-Parnas (EMP) pathway, occurs under both aerobic

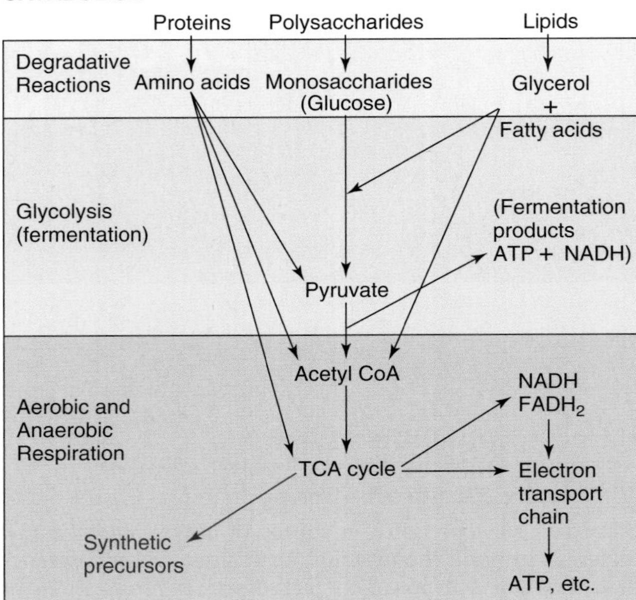

FIGURE 13-1 Catabolism of proteins, polysaccharides, and lipids produces glucose, pyruvate, or intermediates of the tricarboxylic acid *(TCA)* cycle and, ultimately, energy in the form of adenosine triphosphate *(ATP)* or the reduced form of nicotinamide adenine dinucleotide *(NADH). CoA,* Coenzyme A.

and anaerobic conditions. This pathway yields two ATP molecules per molecule of glucose, two molecules of reduced nicotinamide adenine dinucleotide (NADH) and two pyruvate molecules.

Fermentation occurs without oxygen, and the pyruvic acid produced from glycolysis is converted to various end products, depending on the bacterial species. Many bacteria are identified on the basis of their fermentative end products (Figure 13-2). These organic molecules, rather than oxygen, are used as electron acceptors to recycle the NADH to NAD. In yeast, fermentative metabolism results in the conversion of pyruvate to ethanol plus CO_2. Alcoholic fermentation is uncommon in bacteria, which most commonly use the one-step conversion of pyruvic acid to lactic acid. This process is responsible for making milk into yogurt and cabbage into sauerkraut. Other bacteria use more complex fermentative pathways, producing various acids, alcohols, and often gases (many of which have vile odors). These products lend flavors to various cheeses and wines and odors to wound and other infections.

Aerobic Respiration

In the presence of oxygen, the pyruvic acid produced from glycolysis and from the metabolism of other substrates may be completely oxidized (controlled burning) to H_2O and CO_2 using the tricarboxylic acid (TCA) cycle, which results in production of additional energy. The process begins with production of acetyl coenzyme A (acetyl CoA) and release of CO_2 and also produces two NADH molecules from pyruvate. The two remaining carbons derived from pyruvate in the acetyl CoA then enter the TCA by attachment to oxaloacetate to form the six-carbon citrate molecule. In a stepwise

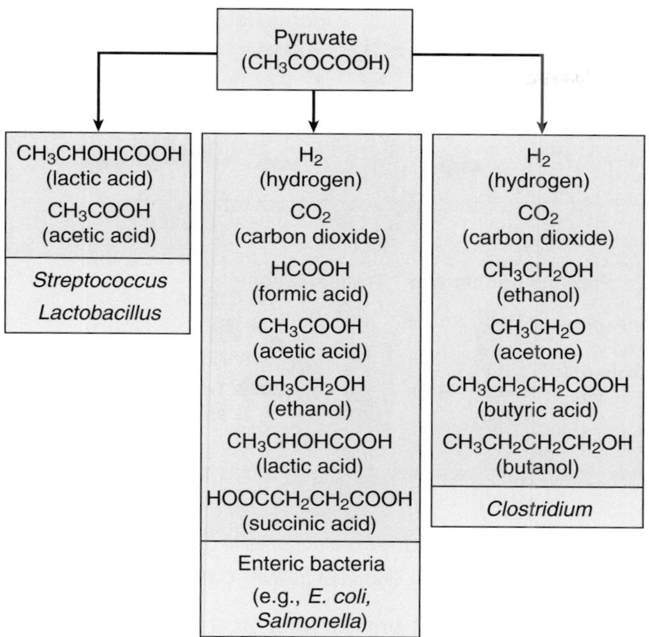

FIGURE 13-2 Fermentation of pyruvate by different microorganisms results in different end products. The clinical laboratory uses these pathways and end products as a means of distinguishing different bacteria.

series of oxidative reactions, the citrate is converted back to oxaloacetate (the cycle). The theoretical yield from each pyruvate is 2 moles of CO_2, 3 moles of NADH, 1 mole of flavin adenine dinucleotide ($FADH_2$), and 1 mole of guanosine triphosphate (GTP).

The TCA cycle allows the organism to generate substantially more energy per mole of glucose than is possible from glycolysis alone. In addition to the GTP (an ATP equivalent) produced by substrate-level phosphorylation, conversion of the NADH and $FADH_2$ back to NAD and FAD contributes electrons to the electron transport chain to produce ATP. In this chain the electrons are passed in a stepwise fashion through a series of donor-acceptor pairs (e.g., cytochromes) and ultimately to oxygen **(aerobic respiration)** to produce 3 ATP molecules for each NADH molecule and 2 ATP for each $FADH_2$. *Whereas fermentation produces only 2 ATP molecules per glucose, aerobic metabolism with electron transport and a complete TCA cycle can generate as much as 19 times more energy (38 ATP molecules) from the same starting material (and it is much less smelly).*

In addition to efficient generation of ATP from glucose (and other carbohydrates), the TCA cycle provides a means by which carbons derived from **lipids** (in the form of acetyl CoA) may be shunted toward either energy production or the generation of biosynthetic precursors. Similarly, the cycle includes several points at which **deaminated amino acids** may enter. For example, deamination of glutamic acid yields α-ketoglutarate, whereas deamination of aspartic acid yields oxaloacetate, both of which are TCA cycle intermediates. The TCA cycle therefore serves the following functions:

1. It is the most efficient mechanism for the generation of ATP.
2. It serves as the final common pathway for the complete oxidation of amino acids, fatty acids, and carbohydrates.
3. It supplies key intermediates (i.e., α-ketoglutarate, pyruvate, oxaloacetate) for the ultimate synthesis of amino acids, lipids, purines, and pyrimidines.

The last two functions make the TCA cycle a so-called **amphibolic cycle** (i.e., it may function to break down and synthesize molecules).

Anaerobic Respiration

During anaerobic respiration, other terminal electron acceptors are used instead of oxygen. Nitrate may be converted to NH_4, sulfate or molecular sulfur to H_2S, CO_2 to methane, ferric ion to ferrous ion, and fumarate to succinate. Less ATP is produced for each NADH than during aerobic respiration, because the reduction-oxidation potential is less for these reactions. These reactions are used by facultative anaerobic bacteria in the GI tract and other anaerobic environments.

Pentose Phosphate Pathway

The final pathway of glucose metabolism considered here is known as the **pentose phosphate pathway,** or the **hexose monophosphate shunt.** The function of this pathway is to provide nucleic acid precursors and reducing power in the form of nicotinamide adenine dinucleotide phosphate (reduced form) **(NADPH)** for use in biosynthesis.

Bacterial Genes and Expression

The bacterial genome is the total collection of genes carried by a bacterium, both on its chromosome and on its extrachromosomal genetic elements, if any. Bacteria usually have only one copy of their chromosomes (they are therefore **haploid**), whereas eukaryotes usually have two distinct copies of each chromosome (they are therefore diploid). With only one chromosome, alteration of a bacterial gene (mutation) will have a more obvious effect on the cell. In addition, the structure of the bacterial chromosome is maintained by polyamines, such as spermine and spermidine, rather than by histones.

In addition to protein-structural genes (**cistrons,** which are coding genes), the bacterial chromosome contains genes for ribosomal and transfer ribonucleic acid (RNA). Bacterial genes are often grouped into **operons** or islands (e.g., **pathogenicity islands**) that share function or to coordinate their control. Operons with many structural genes are **polycistronic.**

Bacteria may also contain **extrachromosomal genetic elements** such as **plasmids** or **bacteriophages** (bacterial viruses). These elements are independent of the bacterial chromosome and in most cases can be transmitted from one cell to another.

Transcription

The information carried in the genetic memory of the deoxyribonucleic acid (DNA) is transcribed into a **messenger RNA (mRNA)** for subsequent translation into protein. RNA synthesis is performed by a **DNA-dependent RNA polymerase.** The process begins when the **sigma factor** recognizes a particular sequence of nucleotides in the DNA (the promoter) and binds tightly to this site. **Promoter sequences** occur just before the start of the DNA that actually encodes a protein. **Sigma factors** bind to these promoters to provide a docking site for the RNA polymerase. Some bacteria encode several sigma factors to coordinate transcription of a group of genes under special conditions such as heat shock, starvation, special nitrogen metabolism, or sporulation.

Once the polymerase has bound to the appropriate site on the DNA, RNA synthesis proceeds with the sequential addition of ribonucleotides complementary to the sequence in the DNA. Once an entire gene or group of genes (operon) has been transcribed, the RNA polymerase dissociates from the DNA, a process mediated by signals within the DNA. The bacterial DNA-dependent RNA polymerase is inhibited by rifampin, an antibiotic often used in the treatment of tuberculosis.

Translation

Translation is the process by which the language of the **genetic code,** in the form of mRNA, is converted (translated) into a sequence of amino acids, the protein product. Each amino acid word and the punctuation of the genetic code is written as sets of three nucleotides known as **codons.** There are 64 different codon combinations encoding the 20 amino acids, plus start and termination codons. Some of the amino acids are encoded by more than one triplet codon. This feature is known as the *degeneracy of the genetic code* and may function in protecting the cell from the effects of minor mutations in the DNA or mRNA. Each tRNA molecule contains a three-nucleotide sequence complementary to one of the codon sequences. This tRNA sequence is known as the **anticodon;** it allows base pairing and binds to the codon sequence on the mRNA. Attached to the opposite end of the tRNA is the amino acid that corresponds to the particular codon-anticodon pair.

Bacterial protein synthesis (Figure 13-3) begins with the binding of the 30S ribosomal subunit and a special initiator tRNA for formyl methionine (fMet) at the methionine codon (AUG) start codon to form the **initiation complex.** The 50S ribosomal subunit binds to the complex to initiate mRNA synthesis. The ribosome contains two tRNA binding sites, the **A (aminoacyl) site** and the **P (peptidyl) site,** each of which allows base pairing between the bound tRNA and the codon sequence in the mRNA. The tRNA corresponding to the second codon occupies the A site. The amino group of the amino acid attached to the A site forms a peptide bond with the carboxyl group of the amino acid in the P site in a reaction known as **transpeptidation,** and the empty tRNA in the P site (uncharged tRNA) is released from the ribosome. The ribosome then moves down the mRNA exactly three nucleotides, thereby transferring the tRNA with attached nascent peptide to the P site and bringing the next codon into the A site. The appropriate charged tRNA is brought into the A site, and the process is then repeated. Translation continues until the new codon in the A site is one of the three termination codons, for which there is no corresponding tRNA. At that point the new protein is released to the cytoplasm and the translation complex may be disassembled, or the ribosome shuffles to the next start codon and initiates a new protein. The ability to shuffle along the mRNA to start a new protein is a characteristic of the 70S bacterial but not of the 80S eukaryotic ribosome. The

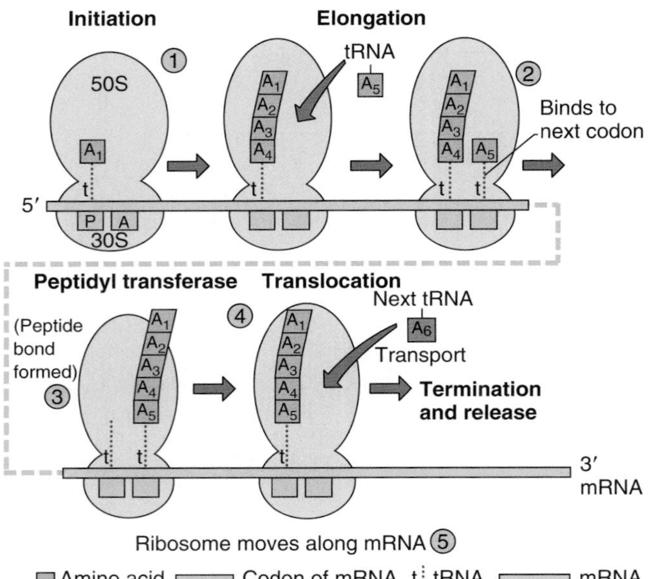

FIGURE 13-3 Bacterial protein synthesis. *1,* Binding of the 30S subunit to the messenger RNA *(mRNA)* with the formyl methionine transfer RNA (fMet-tRNA) at the AUG start codon allows assembly of the 70S ribosome. The fMet-tRNA binds to the peptidyl site *(P). 2,* The next *tRNA* binds to its codon at the *A* site and "accepts" the growing peptide chain. *3* and *4,* Before translocation to the peptidyl site. *5,* The process is repeated until a stop codon and the protein are released.

eukaryotic constraint has implications for the synthesis of proteins for some viruses.

The process of protein synthesis by the 70S ribosome represents an important target of antimicrobial action. The aminoglycosides (e.g., streptomycin and gentamicin) and the tetracyclines act by binding to the small ribosomal subunit and inhibiting normal ribosomal function. Similarly, the macrolide (e.g., erythromycin) and lincosamide (e.g., clindamycin) groups of antibiotics act by binding to the large ribosomal subunit. Also, formyl methionine peptides (e.g., fMet-Leu-Phe) are unique to bacteria, are chemotactic, and attract neutrophils to the site of an infection.

Control of Gene Expression

Bacteria have developed mechanisms to adapt quickly and efficiently to changes and triggers from the environment. This allows them to coordinate and regulate the expression of genes for multicomponent structures or the enzymes of one or more metabolic pathways. For example, temperature change could signify entry into the human host and indicate the need for a global change in metabolism and up-regulation of genes important for parasitism or virulence. Many bacterial genes are controlled at multiple levels and by multiple methods.

Promoters and operators are DNA sequences at the beginning of a gene or operon that are recognized by sigma factors, activator and repressor proteins that control expression of a gene or an operon. Thus all the genes coding for the enzymes of a particular pathway can be coordinately regulated.

Coordination of a large number of processes on a global level can also be mediated by small molecular activators, such as cyclic adenosine monophosphate (cAMP). Increased cAMP levels indicate low glucose levels and the need to use alternative metabolic pathways. Similarly, in a process called **quorum sensing,** each bacterium produces a specific small molecule, and when a sufficient number of bacteria are present, the concentration of the molecule will be sufficient to coordinate the expression of genes to support the colony rather than the individual bacterium. The trigger for biofilm production by *Pseudomonas* spp. is triggered by a critical concentration of *N*-acyl homoserine lactone (AHL) produced when sufficient numbers of bacteria (quorum) are present. Activation of biofilm, toxin production, and more virulent behavior by *Staphylococcus aureus* accompanies the increase in concentration of a cyclic peptide.

The genes for some virulence mechanisms are organized into a **pathogenicity island** under the control of a single promoter to coordinate their expression and ensure that all the proteins necessary for a structure or process are produced when needed. The many components of the type III secretion devices of *E. coli, Salmonella,* or *Yersinia* are grouped together within pathogenicity islands.

Transcription can also be regulated by the translation process. Unlike eukaryotes, the absence of a nuclear membrane in prokaryotes allows the ribosome to bind to the mRNA as it is being transcribed from the DNA. The position and speed of ribosomal movement along the mRNA can determine whether loops form in the mRNA, influencing the ability of the polymerase to continue transcription of new mRNA. This allows control of gene expression at both the transcriptional and translational levels.

Initiation of transcription may be under positive or negative control. Genes under **negative control** are expressed unless they are switched off by a **repressor protein.** This repressor protein prevents gene expression by binding to a specific DNA sequence within the operator, blocking the RNA polymerase from initiating transcription at the promoter sequence. Inversely, genes whose expression is under **positive control** are not transcribed unless an active regulator protein, called an **apoinducer,** is present. The apoinducer binds to a specific DNA sequence and assists the RNA polymerase in the initiation steps by an unknown mechanism.

Operons can be **inducible or repressible.** Introduction of a substrate **(inducer)** into the growth medium may induce an operon to increase the expression of the enzymes necessary for its metabolism. An abundance of the end products **(co-repressors)** of a pathway may signal that a pathway should be shut down or repressed by reducing the synthesis of its enzymes.

The *E. coli lac* operon includes all the genes necessary for lactose metabolism, as well as the control mechanisms for turning off (in the presence of glucose) or turning on (in the presence of galactose or an inducer) these genes only when they are needed. The *lac* operon includes a repressor sequence, a promoter sequence, and structural genes for the β-galactosidase enzyme, a permease, and an acetylase (Figure 13-4). Normally the bacteria use glucose, not lactose. In the absence of lactose, the operon is repressed by the binding of the repressor protein to the operator sequence, thus impeding the RNA polymerase function. In the absence of glucose, however, the addition of lactose reverses this repression. Full expression of the *lac* operon also requires a protein-mediated positive-control mechanism. In *E. coli,* when glucose decreases in the cell, cAMP increases to promote usage of other sugars for metabolism. Binding of cAMP to a protein called the **catabolite gene-activator protein (CAP)** allows it to bind to a specific DNA sequence present in the promoter. The CAP-cAMP complex enhances binding of the RNA polymerase to the promoter, thus allowing an increase in the frequency of transcription initiation.

The tryptophan operon **(*trp* operon)** contains the structural genes necessary for tryptophan biosynthesis and is under dual transcriptional control mechanisms (Figure 13-5). Although tryptophan is essential for protein synthesis, too much tryptophan in the cell can be toxic; therefore its synthesis must be regulated. At the DNA level, the repressor protein is activated by an increased intracellular concentration of tryptophan to prevent transcription. At the protein synthesis level, rapid translation of a "test peptide" at the beginning of the mRNA in the presence of tryptophan allows formation of a double-stranded loop in the RNA, which terminates transcription. The same loop is formed if no protein synthesis is occurring, a situation in which tryptophan synthesis would similarly not be required. This regulates tryptophan synthesis at the mRNA level in a process termed **attenuation,** in which mRNA synthesis is prematurely terminated.

Expression of the components of virulence mechanisms are also coordinately regulated from an operon. Simple triggers (e.g., temperature, osmolarity, pH, nutrient availability) or the concentration of specific small molecules (e.g., oxygen, iron) can turn on or turn off the transcription of a single gene or a group of genes. *Salmonella* invasion genes within a pathogenicity island are turned on by high osmolarity and low oxygen, conditions present in the GI tract or an endosomal vesicle within a macrophage. *E. coli* senses its exit from the gut of a host by a drop in temperature and inactivates its adherence genes. Low iron levels can activate expression of hemolysin in *E. coli* or diphtheria toxin from *Corynebacterium diphtheriae,* potentially to kill cells and provide iron. Quorum sensing for virulence factors and biofilm production by *S. aureus* and *Pseudomonas* spp. were discussed earlier. An example of coordinated control of virulence genes for *S. aureus* based on the growth rate, availability of metabolites, and the presence of a quorum is presented in Figure 13-6.

Replication of DNA

Replication of the bacterial genome is triggered by a cascade of events linked to the growth rate of the cell. Replication of bacterial DNA is initiated at a specific sequence in the chromosome called *oriC.* The replication process requires many enzymes, including an enzyme **(helicase)** to unwind the DNA at the origin to expose the DNA, an enzyme **(primase)** to synthesize primers to start the process, and the enzyme or enzymes **(DNA-dependent DNA polymerases)** that synthesize a copy of the DNA, but only if there is a **primer sequence** to add onto and only in the **5′ to 3′ direction.**

New DNA is synthesized **semiconservatively,** using both strands of the parental DNA as templates. New DNA synthesis occurs at **growing forks** and proceeds **bidirectionally.** One strand (the leading strand) is copied continuously in the 5′ to 3′ direction, whereas the other strand (the lagging

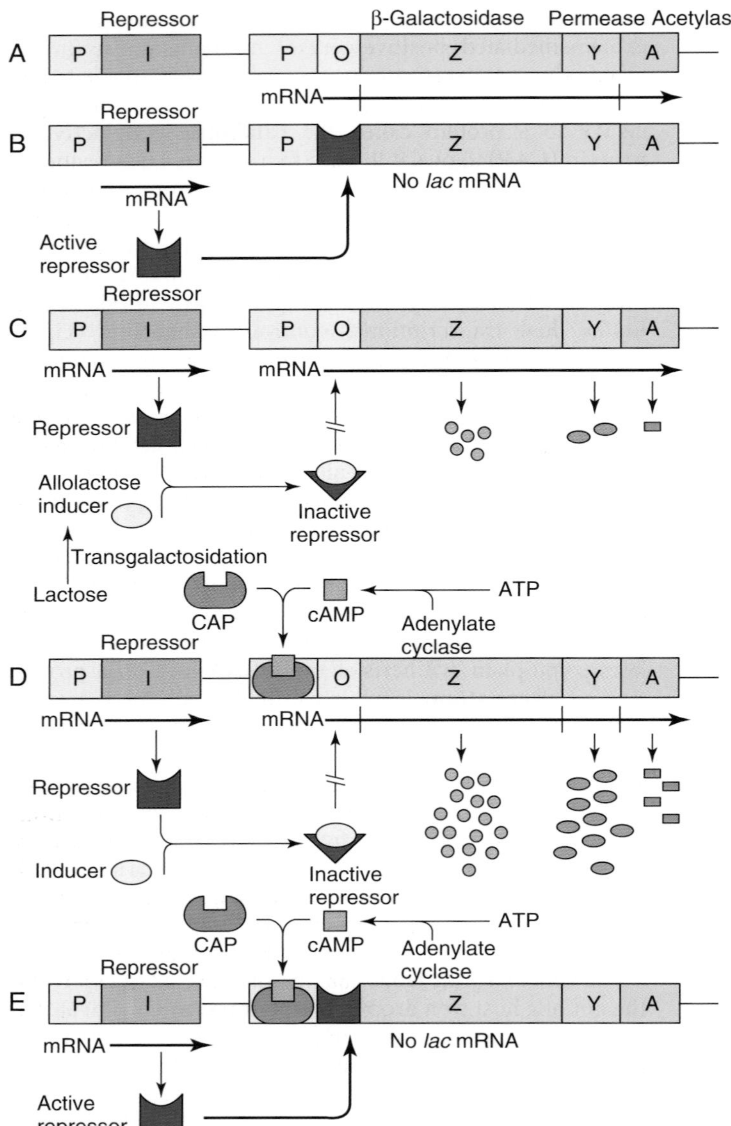

FIGURE 13-4 **A,** The lactose *(lac)* operon is transcribed as a polycistronic messenger RNA *(mRNA)* from the promoter *(P)* and translated into three proteins: β-galactosidase *(Z),* permease *(Y),* and acetylase *(A).* The *(I)* gene encodes the repressor protein. **B,** The lactose operon is not transcribed in the absence of an allolactose inducer, because the repressor competes with the RNA polymerase at the operator site *(O).* **C,** The repressor, complexed with the inducer, does not recognize the operator because of a conformation change in the repressor. The *lac* operon is thus transcribed at a low level. **D,** *Escherichia coli* is grown in a poor medium in the presence of lactose as the carbon source. Both the inducer and the CAP-cAMP complex are bound to the promoter, which is fully "turned on," and a high level of *lac* mRNA is transcribed and translated. **E,** Growth of *E. coli* in a poor medium without lactose results in the binding of the CAP-cAMP complex to the promoter region and binding of the active repressor to the operator sequence because no inducer is available. The result will be that the *lac* operon will not be transcribed. *ATP,* Adenosine triphosphate; *cAMP,* cyclic adenosine monophosphate; *CAP,* catabolite gene-activator protein.

strand) must be synthesized as many pieces of DNA using RNA primers (Okazaki fragments). The lagging-strand DNA must be extended in the 5′ to 3′ direction as its template becomes available. Then the pieces are ligated together by the enzyme DNA ligase (Figure 13-7). To maintain the high degree of accuracy required for replication, the DNA polymerases possess "proofreading" functions that allow the enzyme to confirm that the appropriate nucleotide was inserted and to correct any errors that were made. During log-phase growth in rich medium, many initiations of chromosomal replication may occur before cell division. This process produces a series of nested bubbles of new daughter chromosomes, each with its pair of growth forks of new DNA synthesis. The polymerase moves down the DNA strand, incorporating the appropriate (complementary) nucleotide at each position. Replication is complete when the two replication forks meet 180 degrees from the origin. The process of DNA replication puts great torsional strain on the chromosomal circle of DNA; this strain is relieved by **topoisomerases** (e.g., gyrase), which supercoil the DNA. Topoisomerases are essential to the bacteria and are targets for the fluoroquinolone antibiotics.

Bacterial Growth

Bacterial replication is a coordinated process in which two equivalent daughter cells are produced. For growth to occur, there must be sufficient metabolites to support synthesis of the bacterial components and especially the nucleotides for DNA synthesis. A cascade of regulatory events (synthesis of key proteins and RNA), much like a countdown at the Kennedy Space Center, must occur on schedule to initiate a replication cycle. *However, once it is initiated, DNA synthesis must run to completion even if all nutrients have been removed from the medium.*

Chromosome replication is initiated at the membrane, and each daughter chromosome is anchored to a different

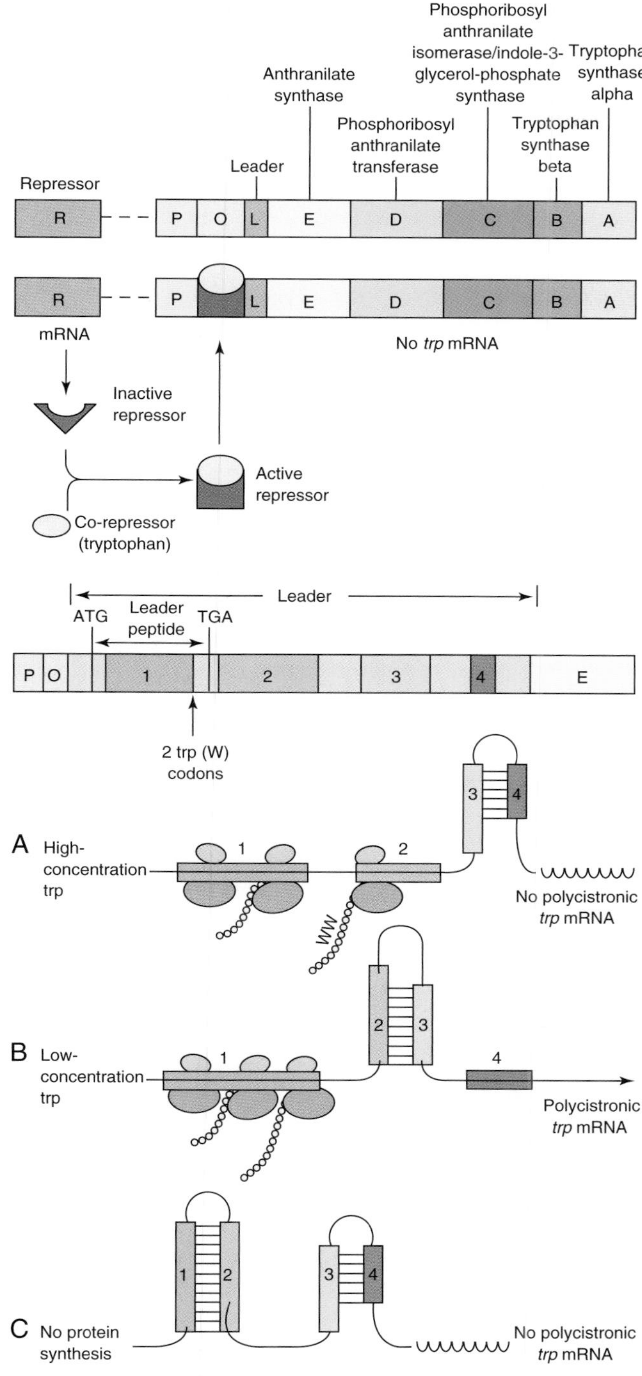

FIGURE 13-5 Regulation of the tryptophan *(trp)* operon. **A,** The *trp* operon encodes the five enzymes necessary for tryptophan biosynthesis. This *trp* operon is under dual control. **B,** The conformation of the inactive repressor protein is changed after its binding by the co-repressor tryptophan. The resulting active repressor *(R)* binds to the operator *(O),* blocking any transcription of the *trp* mRNA by the RNA polymerase. **C,** The *trp* operon is also under the control of an attenuation-antitermination mechanism. Upstream of the structural genes are the promoter *(P),* the operator, and a leader *(L),* which can be transcribed into a short peptide containing two tryptophans *(W),* near its distal end. The leader mRNA possesses four repeats (1, 2, 3, and 4), which can pair differently according to the tryptophan availability, leading to an early termination of transcription of the *trp* operon or its full transcription. In the presence of a high concentration of tryptophan, regions 3 and 4 of the leader mRNA can pair, forming a terminator hairpin, and no transcription of the *trp* operon occurs. However, in the presence of little or no tryptophan the ribosomes stall in region 1 when translating the leader peptide because of the tandem of tryptophan codons. Then regions 2 and 3 can pair, forming the antiterminator hairpin and leading to transcription of the *trp* genes. Finally, the regions 1 : 2 and 3 : 4 of the free leader mRNA can pair, also leading to cessation of transcription before the first structural gene *trpE. A,* Adenine; *G,* guanine; *T,* thymidine.

portion of membrane. *Bacterial membrane, peptidoglycan synthesis, and cell division are linked together such that inhibition of peptidoglycan synthesis will also inhibit cell division.* As the bacterial membrane grows, the daughter chromosomes are pulled apart. Commencement of chromosome replication also initiates the process of cell division, which can be visualized by the start of septum formation between the two daughter cells (Figure 13-8; see also Chapter 12). New initiation events may occur even before completion of chromosome replication and cell division.

Depletion of metabolites (starvation) or a buildup of toxic byproducts (e.g., ethanol) triggers production of chemical **alarmones,** which cause protein and other synthesis to stop, but degradative processes continue. DNA synthesis continues until all initiated chromosomes are completed, despite the detrimental effect on the cell. Ribosomes are cannibalized for deoxyribonucleotide precursors, peptidoglycan and proteins are degraded for metabolites, and the cell shrinks. Septum formation may be initiated, but cell division may not occur. Many cells die. Similar signals may initiate **sporulation** in species capable of this process (see Chapter 12). For some bacterial species, starvation promotes uptake of foreign DNA (transformation) that may encode the means to survive the challenge.

Population Dynamics

When bacteria are added to a new medium, they require time to adapt to the new environment before they begin dividing (Figure 13-9). This hiatus is known as the **lag phase** of growth. During the **logarithmic (log) or exponential phase,** the bacteria will grow and divide with a **doubling time** characteristic of the strain and determined by the conditions. The number of bacteria will increase to 2^n, in which n is the number of generations (doublings). The culture eventually runs out of metabolites, or a toxic substance builds up in the medium; the bacteria then stop growing and enter the **stationary phase,** followed by the **death phase.** During the death phase, some bacteria stop dividing but remain viable and are often insensitive to antibiotics.

• Bacterial Genetics

Mutation, Repair, and Recombination

Accurate replication of DNA is important to the survival of the bacteria, but mistakes and accidental damage to the DNA occur. The bacteria have efficient DNA repair systems, but

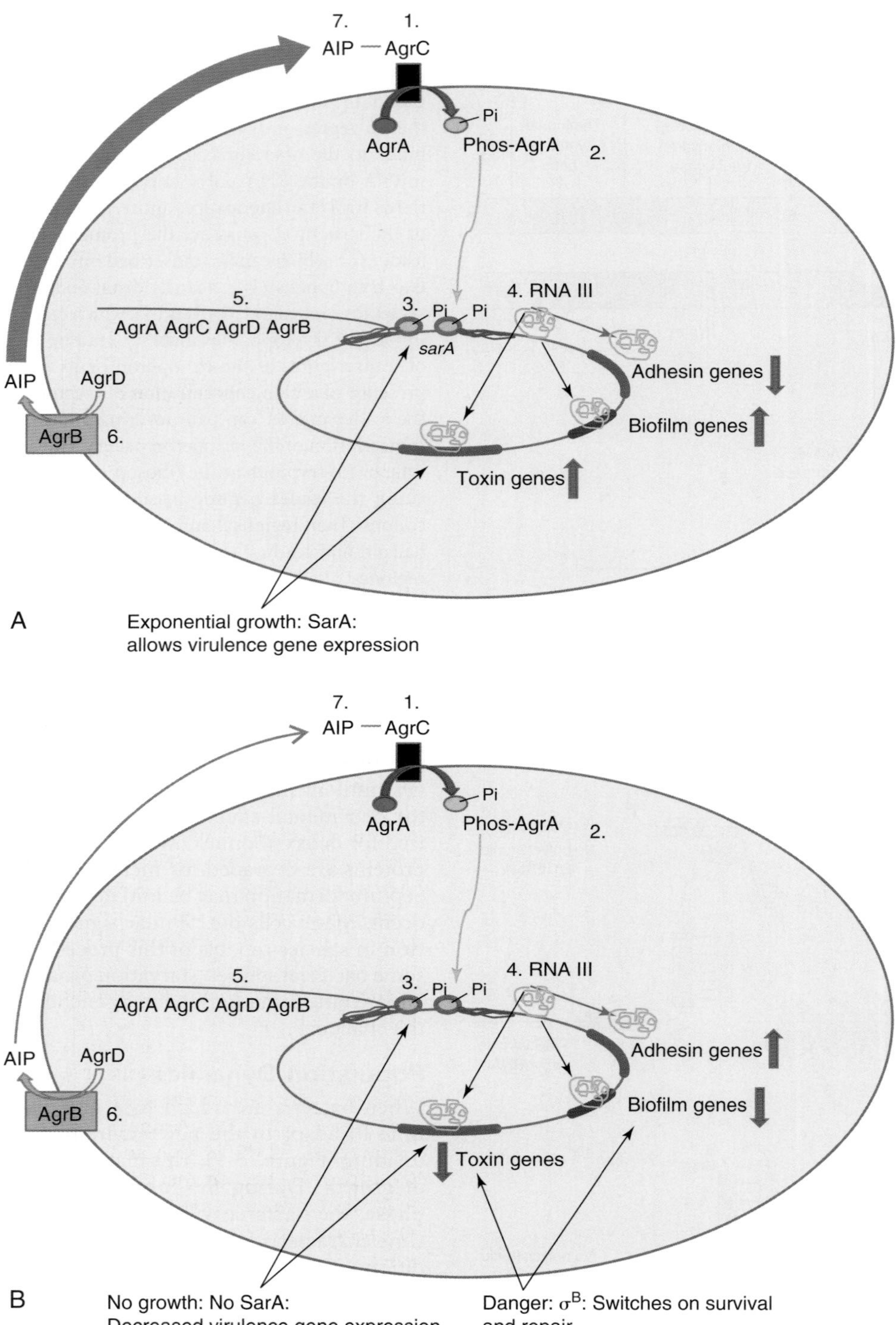

FIGURE 13-6 Control of virulence genes in *Staphylococcus aureus. S. aureus* switches on virulence factors when in exponential growth and when their numbers increase to a quorum. Toxin and protease are produced to kill host cells and supply the colony with food, and the colony produces a biofilm for protection. Cell wall thickness and adhesion factors are less important within the colony and are repressed. Quorum sensing is mediated and autoinduced by the **Agr (A-D)** proteins. **A,** *1.* The autoinducing peptide **(AIP)** binds to AgrC. *2,* **AgrC** is a receptor that phosphorylates **AgrA.** *3,* **Phosphorylated AgrA** activates the promoter for the *agr* operon and the promoter for a regulatory RNA called **RNA III.** *4,* RNA III contains the 26–amino acid δ-hemolysin RNA sequence. In addition, RNA III activates toxin and other virulence genes while decreasing expression of adhesion and cell wall synthesis genes. *5,* **AgrD** interacts with **AgrB,** in the membrane, to be converted into the AIP. As long as the bacteria are in exponential phase growth, they produce **SarA,** which also binds and activates the promoters for the *agr* and *RNAIII* genes. **B,** Upon metabolic problems and danger, SarA production is decreased and a new sigma factor, $\boldsymbol{\sigma}^B$, is produced to decrease production of these virulence factors, and σ^B turns on DNA and cellular repair mechanisms. *Large red arrows* indicate increases or decreases in expression.

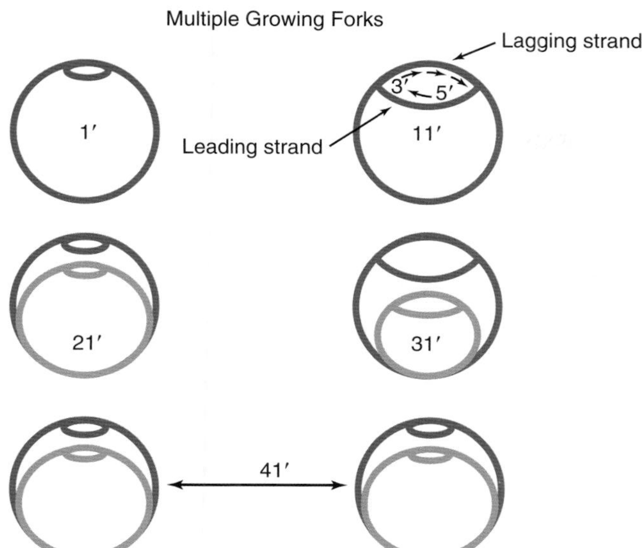

FIGURE 13-7 Bacterial DNA replication. New DNA synthesis occurs at growing forks and proceeds bidirectionally. DNA synthesis progresses in the 5′ to 3′ direction continuously (leading strand) or in pieces (lagging strand). Assuming it takes 40 minutes to complete one round of replication, and assuming new initiation every 20 minutes, initiation of DNA synthesis precedes cell division. Multiple growing forks may be initiated in a cell before complete septum formation and cell division. The daughter cells are "born pregnant."

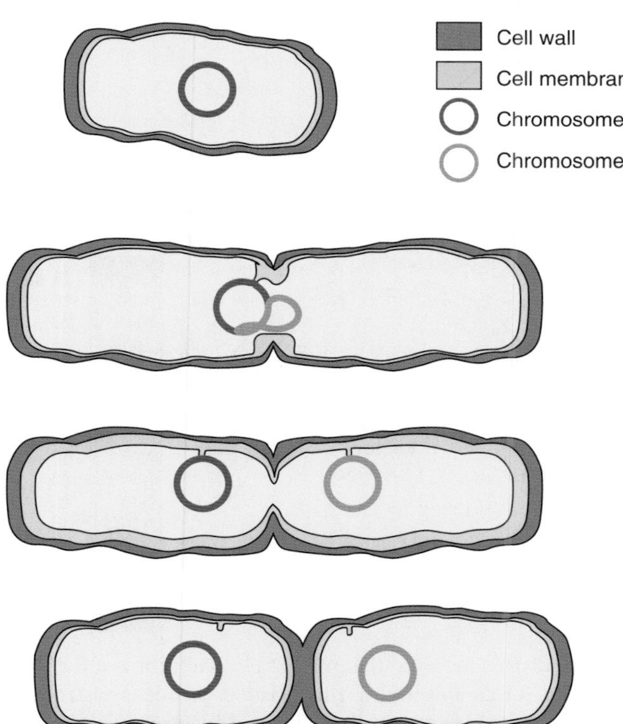

FIGURE 13-8 Bacterial cell division. Replication requires extension of the cell wall and replication of the chromosome and septum formation. Membrane attachment of the DNA pulls each daughter strand into a new cell.

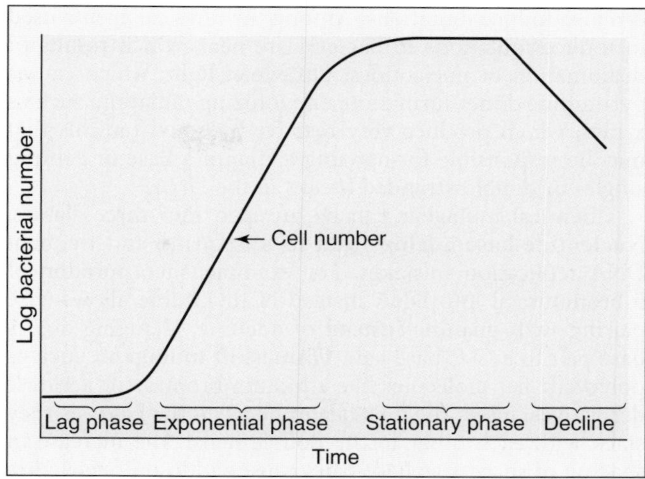

FIGURE 13-9 Phases of bacterial growth, starting with an inoculum of stationary-phase cells.

mutations and alterations to the DNA still occur. Most of these mutations have little effect on the bacteria or are detrimental, but some mutations may provide a selective advantage for survival of the bacteria when challenged by the environment, the host, or antibiotic therapy.

Mutations and Their Consequences

A mutation is any change in the base sequence of the DNA. A single base change can result in a **transition** in which one purine is replaced by another purine or in which a pyrimidine is replaced by another pyrimidine. A **transversion** in which, for example, a purine is replaced by a pyrimidine and vice versa may also result. A **silent mutation** is a change at the DNA level that does not result in any change of amino acid in the encoded protein. This type of mutation occurs because more than one codon may encode an amino acid. A **missense mutation** results in a different amino acid being inserted in the protein, but this may be a **conservative mutation** if the new amino acid has similar properties (e.g., valine replacing alanine). A **nonsense mutation** changes a codon encoding an amino acid to a stop codon (e.g., TAG [thymidine-adenine-guanine]), which will cause the ribosome to fall off the mRNA and end the protein prematurely. **Conditional mutations,** such as **temperature-sensitive mutations,** may result from a conservative mutation that changes the structure or function of an important protein at elevated temperatures.

More drastic changes can occur when numerous bases are involved. A small deletion or insertion that *is not in multiples of three* produces a **frameshift mutation.** This results in a change in the reading frame, usually leading to a useless peptide and premature truncation of the protein. **Null mutations,** which completely destroy gene function, arise when there is an extensive insertion, deletion, or gross rearrangement of the chromosome structure. Insertion of long sequences of DNA (many thousands of base pairs) by recombination, by transposition, or during genetic engineering can produce null mutations by separating the parts of a gene and inactivating the gene.

Many mutations occur spontaneously in nature (e.g., by polymerase mistakes); however, physical or chemical agents can also induce mutations. Among the physical agents used to induce mutations in bacteria are heat, which results in deamination of nucleotides; ultraviolet light, which causes pyrimidine dimer formation; and ionizing radiation, such as x-rays, which produce very reactive hydroxyl radicals that may be responsible for opening a ring of a base or causing single- or double-stranded breaks in the DNA.

Chemical mutagens can be grouped into three classes. **Nucleotide-base analogs** lead to mispairing and frequent DNA replication mistakes. For example, incorporation of 5-bromouracil into DNA instead of thymidine allows base pairing with guanine instead of adenine, changing a T-A base pair to a G-C base pair. **Frameshift mutagens,** such as polycyclic flat molecules like ethidium bromide or acridine derivatives, insert (or intercalate) between the bases as they stack with each other in the double helix. The increase in spacing of successive base pairs causes addition or deletion of a single base and leads to frequent mistakes during DNA replication. **DNA-reactive chemicals** act directly on the DNA to change the chemical structure of the base. These include nitrous acid (HNO_2) and alkylating agents, including nitrosoguanidine and ethyl methane sulfonate, which are known to add methyl or ethyl groups to the rings of the DNA bases. The modified bases may pair abnormally or not at all. The damage may also cause removal of the base from the DNA backbone.

Repair Mechanisms of DNA

A number of repair mechanisms have evolved in bacteria. These repair mechanisms can be divided into the following five groups:

1. **Direct DNA repair** is the enzymatic removal of damage, such as pyrimidine dimers and alkylated bases.
2. **Excision repair** is the removal of a DNA segment containing the damage, followed by synthesis of a new DNA strand. Two types of excision-repair mechanisms, generalized and specialized, exist.
3. **Recombinational** or **postreplication repair** replaces a missing or damaged section of DNA with the same or similar sequences that may be present during replication or on extrachromosomal DNA.
4. The **SOS response** is the induction of many genes (≈15) after DNA damage or interruption of DNA replication to promote recombination or error-prone repair.
5. **Error-prone repair** is the last resort of a bacterial cell before it dies. It is used to fill in gaps with a random sequence when a DNA template is not available for directing an accurate repair.

Gene Exchange in Prokaryotic Cells

Many bacteria, especially many pathogenic bacterial species, are promiscuous with their DNA. The exchange of DNA between cells allows exchange of genes and characteristics between cells, thus producing new strains of bacteria. This exchange may be advantageous for the recipient, especially if the exchanged DNA encodes antibiotic resistance. The transferred DNA can be integrated into the recipient chromosome or stably maintained as an extrachromosomal element **(plasmid)** or a bacterial virus **(bacteriophage)** and passed on to daughter bacteria as an autonomously replicating unit.

Plasmids are small genetic elements that replicate independently of the bacterial chromosome. Most plasmids are circular double-stranded DNA molecules varying from 1500 to 400,000 base pairs. However, *Borrelia burgdorferi,* the causative agent of Lyme disease, and the related *Borrelia hermsii* are unique among all eubacteria because they possess linear genomes and plasmids. Like the bacterial chromosomal DNA, plasmids can autonomously replicate and as such are referred to as **replicons.** Some plasmids, such as the *E. coli* F plasmid, are **episomes,** which means they can integrate into the host chromosome.

Plasmids carry genetic information that may not be essential but can provide a selective advantage to the bacteria. For example, plasmids may encode the production of antibiotic resistance mechanisms, bacteriocins, toxins, virulence determinants, and other genes that may provide the bacteria with a unique growth advantage over other microbes or within the host (Figure 13-10). The number of copies of plasmid produced by a cell is determined by the particular plasmid. The **copy number** is the ratio of copies of the

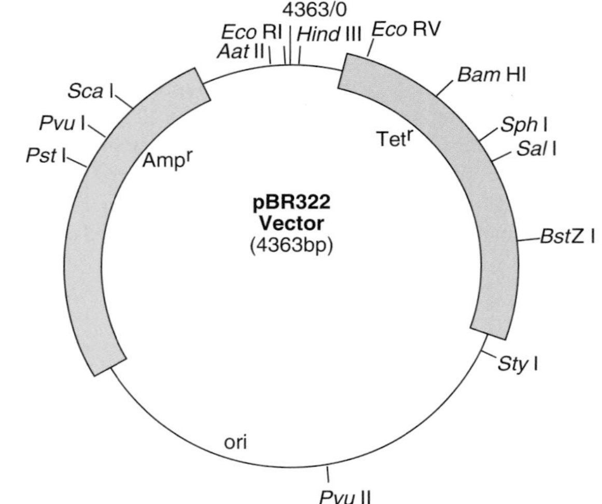

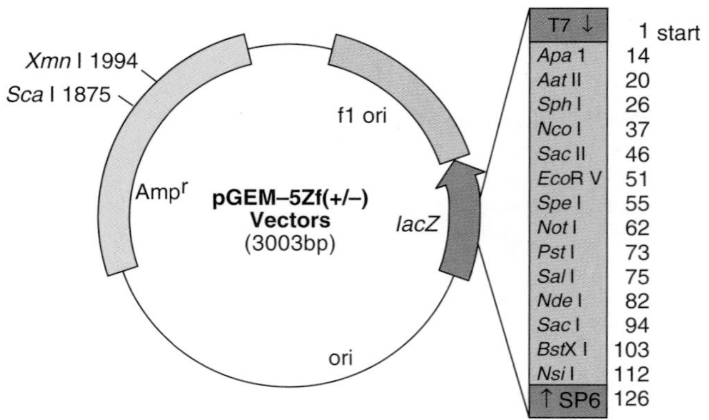

FIGURE 13-10 Plasmids. The pBR322 plasmid is one of the plasmids used for cloning DNA. This plasmid encodes resistance to ampicillin *(Amp)* and tetracycline *(Tet)* and an origin of replication *(ori)*. The multiple cloning site in the pGEM-5Zf(+/–) plasmid provides different restriction enzyme cleavage sites for insertion of DNA within the β-galactosidase gene *(lacZ)*. The insert is flanked by bacteriophage promoters to allow directional messenger RNA expression of the cloned sequence.

plasmid to the number of copies of the chromosome. This may be as few as one in the case of large plasmids or as many as 50 in smaller plasmids.

Large plasmids (20 to 120 kb), such as the **fertility factor F** found in *E. coli* or the resistance transfer factor (80 kb), can often mediate their own transfer from one cell to another by a process called **conjugation** (see the section on conjugation later in this chapter). These conjugative plasmids encode all the necessary factors for their transfer. Other plasmids can be transferred into a bacterial cell by means other than conjugation, such as transformation or transduction. These terms are also discussed later in the chapter.

Bacteriophages are bacterial viruses with a DNA or RNA genome usually protected by a membrane or protein shell. These extrachromosomal genetic elements can survive outside of a host cell and be transmitted from one cell to another. Bacteriophages infect bacterial cells and either replicate to large numbers and cause the cell to lyse **(lytic infection)** or, in some cases, **integrate** into the host genome without killing the host (the **lysogenic state**), such as the *E. coli* bacteriophage lambda. Some lysogenic bacteriophages carry toxin genes (e.g., corynephage beta carries the gene for the diphtheria toxin). Bacteriophage lambda remains lysogenic as long as a repressor protein is synthesized and prevents the phage genome from becoming unintegrated in order to replicate and exit the cell. Damage to the host cell DNA by radiation or by another means or inability to produce the repressor protein is a signal that the host cell is unhealthy and is no longer a good place for "freeloading."

Transposons (jumping genes) are mobile genetic elements (Figure 13-11) that can transfer DNA within a cell, from one position to another in the genome, or between different molecules of DNA (e.g., plasmid to plasmid or plasmid to chromosome). Transposons are present in prokaryotes and eukaryotes. The simplest transposons are called *insertion sequences* and range in length from 150 to 1500 base pairs, with inverted repeats of 15 to 40 base pairs at their ends and the minimal genetic information necessary for their own transfer (i.e., the gene coding for the transposase). Complex transposons carry other genes, such as genes that provide resistance against antibiotics. Transposons sometimes insert into genes and inactivate those genes. If insertion and inactivation occur in a gene that encodes an essential protein, the cell dies.

Some pathogenic bacteria use a transposon-like mechanism to coordinate expression of a system of virulence factors. The genes for the activity may be grouped together in a **pathogenicity or virulence island** surrounded by transposon-like mobile elements, allowing them to move within the chromosome and to other bacteria. The entire genetic unit can be triggered by an environmental stimulus (e.g., pH, heat, contact with the host cell surface) as a way to coordinate expression of a complex process. For example, the SPI-1 island of *Salmonella* is activated by environmental signals (e.g., pH) to express the 25 genes for a type III secretion device that allows the bacteria to enter nonphagocytic cells.

Mechanisms of Genetic Transfer between Cells

The exchange of genetic material between bacterial cells may occur by one of three mechanisms (Figure 13-12): (1) **transformation,** which is an active uptake and incorporation of exogenous or foreign DNA, (2) **conjugation,** which is the mating or quasi-sexual exchange of genetic information from one bacterium (the donor) to another bacterium (the recipient), or (3) **transduction,** which is the transfer of genetic information from one bacterium to another by a bacteriophage. Once inside a cell, a **transposon** can jump between different DNA molecules (e.g., plasmid to plasmid or plasmid to chromosome). Several of these mechanisms contributed to the generation of vancomycin-resistant *Staphylococcus aureus* (Figure 13-13 and Box 13-2).

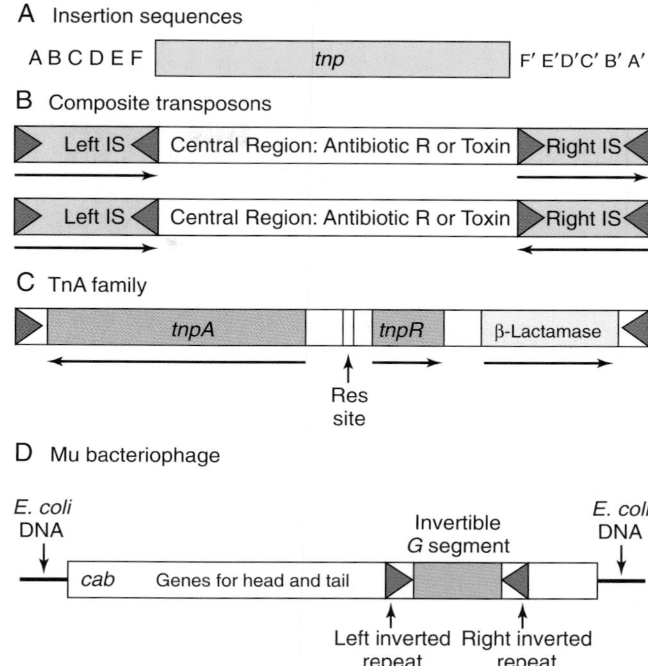

FIGURE 13-11 Transposons. **A,** The insertion sequences code only for a transposase *(tnp)* and possess inverted repeats (15 to 40 base pairs) at each end. **B,** The composite transposons contain a central region coding for antibiotic resistances or toxins flanked by two insertion sequences *(IS),* which can be either directly repeated or reversed. **C,** Tn*3*, a member of the Tn*A* transposon family. The central region encodes three genes—a transposase *(tnpA),* a resolvase *(tnpR),* and a β-lactamase—conferring resistance to ampicillin. A resolution site *(Res site)* is used during the replicative transposition process. This central region is flanked on both ends by direct repeats of 38 base pairs. **D,** Phage-associated transposon is exemplified by the bacteriophage mu.

Transformation

Transformation is the process by which bacteria take up fragments of naked DNA and incorporate them into their genomes. Transformation was the first mechanism of genetic transfer to be discovered in bacteria. In 1928, Griffith observed that pneumococcal virulence was related to the presence of a polysaccharide capsule and that extracts of encapsulated bacteria producing smooth colonies could transmit this trait to nonencapsulated bacteria, normally appearing as rough colonies. Griffith's studies led to Avery, MacLeod, and McCarty's identification of DNA as the transforming principle some 15 years later.

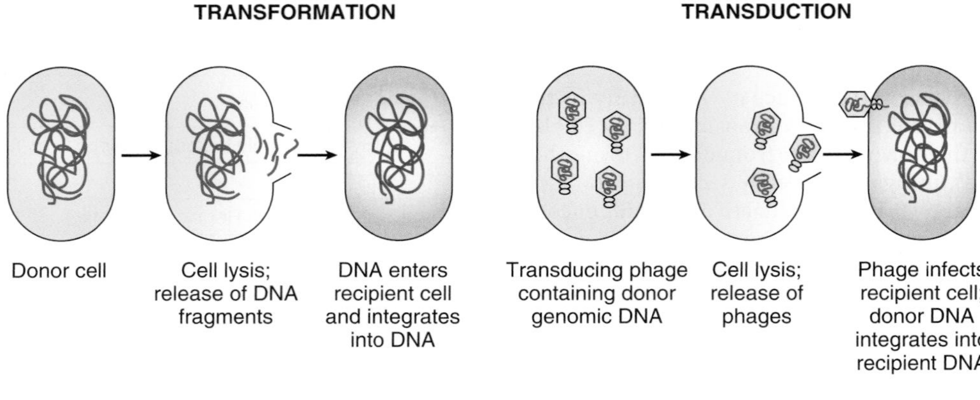

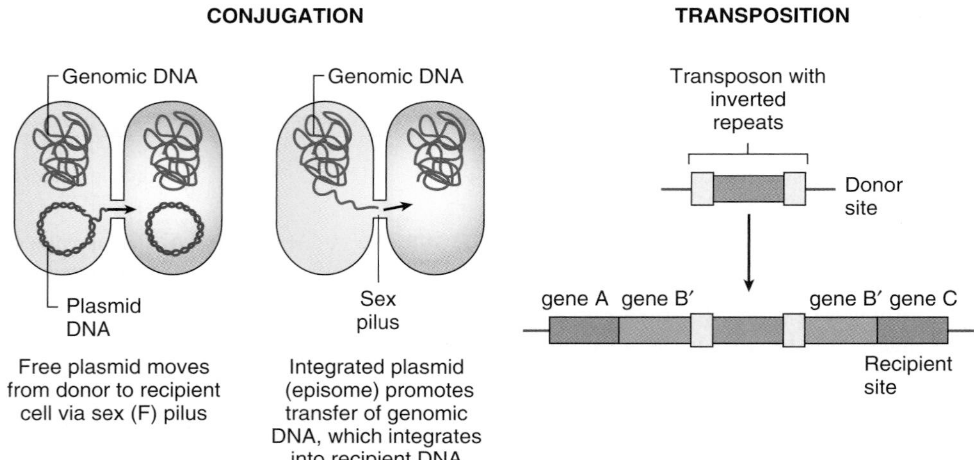

FIGURE 13-12 Mechanisms of bacterial gene transfer. (From Rosenthal KS, Tan J: *Rapid reviews microbiology and immunology,* St Louis, 2002, Mosby.)

Certain species are naturally capable of taking up exogenous DNA (such species are then said to be competent), including *Haemophilus influenzae, Streptococcus pneumoniae, Bacillus* spp., and *Neisseria* spp. Competence develops toward the end of logarithmic growth. *E. coli* and most other bacteria lack the natural ability for DNA uptake, and competence must be induced by chemical methods or electroporation (use of high-voltage pulses) to facilitate uptake of plasmid and other DNA.

Conjugation

Conjugation results in one-way transfer of DNA from a donor (or male) cell to a recipient (or female) cell through the **sex pilus.** Conjugation occurs with most, if not all, eubacteria, usually between members of the same or related species, but it has also been demonstrated to occur between prokaryotes and cells from plants, animals, and fungi.

The mating type (sex) of the cell depends on the presence (male) or absence (female) of a conjugative plasmid, such as the **F plasmid** of *E. coli.* The F plasmid is defined as conjugative because it carries all the genes necessary for its own transfer, including the ability to make sex pili and to initiate DNA synthesis at the transfer origin *(oriT)* of the plasmid. The sex pilus is a specialized type IV secretion device. Upon transfer of the F plasmid, the recipients become F^+ male cells. If a fragment of chromosomal DNA has been incorporated into the plasmid, it is designated an F prime (F′) plasmid. When it transfers into the recipient cell, it carries that fragment with it and converts it into an F′ male. If the F plasmid sequence is integrated into the bacterial chromosome, the cell is designated an Hfr (high-frequency recombination) cell.

The DNA that is transferred by conjugation is not a double helix but a single-stranded molecule. Mobilization begins when a plasmid-encoded protein makes a single-stranded site-specific cleavage at the oriT. The nick initiates rolling circle replication, and the displaced linear strand is directed to the recipient cell. The transferred single-stranded DNA is recircularized and its complementary strand synthesized. Conjugation results in transfer of a part of the plasmid sequence and some portion of the bacterial chromosomal DNA. Because of the fragile connection between the mating pairs, the transfer is usually aborted before being completed, such that only the chromosomal sequences adjacent to the integrated F are transferred. Artificial interruption of a mating between an Hfr and an F^- pair has been helpful in constructing a consistent map of the *E. coli* chromosomal DNA. In such maps, the position of each gene is given in minutes (based on 100 minutes for complete transfer at 37° C), according to its time of entry into a recipient cell in relation to a fixed origin.

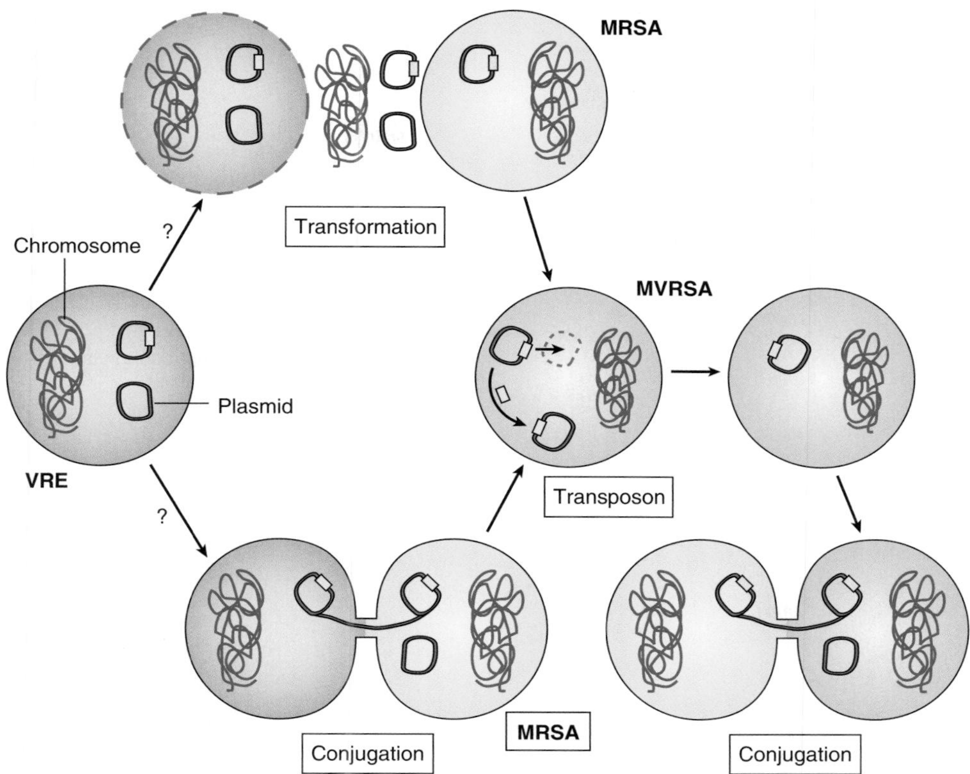

FIGURE 13-13 Genetic mechanisms of evolution of methicillin- and vancomycin-resistant *Staphylococcus aureus (MRSA* and *MVRSA)*. Vancomycin-resistant enterococcus *(VRE) (in blue)* contains plasmids with multiple antibiotic resistance and virulence factors. During co-infection, a MRSA *(in pink)* may have acquired the enterococcal resistance plasmid (e-plasmid) *(in purple)* by transformation (after lysis of the enterococcal cell and release of its DNA) or, more likely, by conjugation. A transposon in the e-plasmid containing the vancomycin resistance gene jumped out and inserted into the multiple antibiotic resistance plasmid of the MRSA. The new plasmid is readily spread to other *S. aureus* bacteria by conjugation.

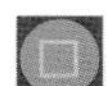

Box 13-2 Generation of Vancomycin-Resistant *Staphylococcus aureus* by Multiple Genetic Manipulations

Until recently, vancomycin was the last-resort drug for *Staphylococcus aureus* strains resistant to β-lactam (penicillin-related) antibiotics (e.g., methicillin-resistant *S. aureus* [MRSA]). Isolates of *S. aureus* acquired the vancomycin resistance gene during a mixed infection with *Enterococcus faecalis* (see Figure 13-13). The gene for vancomycin resistance was contained within a **transposon** (Tn*1546*) on a multiresistance conjugative plasmid. The plasmid was probably transferred by **conjugation** between *E. faecalis* and *S. aureus*. Alternatively, after lysis of the *E. faecalis, S. aureus* acquired the DNA by **transduction** and became **transformed** by the new DNA. The transposon then jumped from the *E. faecalis* plasmid, **recombined,** and **integrated** into the *S. aureus* multiresistance plasmid, and the *E. faecalis* DNA was degraded. The resulting *S. aureus* plasmid encodes resistance to β-lactams, vancomycin, trimethoprim, and gentamycin/kanamycin/tobramycin antibiotics and to quaternary ammonium disinfectants and can transfer to other *S. aureus* strains by **conjugation.** (For more information, refer to Weigel in the Bibliography at the end of the chapter.)

Transduction

Genetic transfer by transduction is mediated by bacterial viruses (bacteriophages) that pick up fragments of DNA and package them into bacteriophage particles. The DNA is delivered to infected cells and becomes incorporated into the bacterial genomes. Transduction can be classified as **specialized** if the phages in question transfer particular genes (usually those adjacent to their integration sites in the genome) or **generalized** if incorporation of DNA sequences is random because of accidental packaging of host DNA into the phage capsid. For example, a nuclease from the P1 phage degrades the host *E. coli* chromosomal DNA, and some of the DNA fragments are packaged into phage particles. The encapsulated DNA, instead of phage DNA, is injected into a new host cell, where it can recombine with the homologous host DNA. Generalized transducing particles are valuable in the **genetic mapping** of bacterial chromosomes. The closer two genes are within the bacterial chromosome, the more likely it is that they will be co-transduced in the same fragment of DNA.

Recombination

Incorporation of extrachromosomal (foreign) DNA into the chromosome occurs by recombination. There are two types of recombination: homologous and nonhomologous.

 **Table 13-1 Common Restriction Enzymes Used in Molecular Biology**

Microorganism	Enzyme	Recognition Site
Acinetobacter calcoaceticus	*Acc* I	5′ G T|(A/C) (G/T) A C C A (T/G) (C/A)|T G
Bacillus amyloliquefaciens H	*Bam* HI	5′ G|G A T C C C C T A G|G
Escherichia coli RY13	*Eco* RI	5′ G|A A T T C C T T A A|G
Haemophilus influenzae Rd	*Hind* III	5′ A|A G C T T T T C G A|A
H. influenzae serotype c, 1160	*Hinc* II	5′ G T (C/T)|(G/A) A C C A (G/A)|(C/T) T G
Providencia stuartii 164	*Pst* I	5′ G T G C A|G G|A C G T C
Serratia marcescens	*Sma* I	5′ C C C|G G G G G G|C C C
Staphylococcus aureus 3A	*Sau* 3AI	5′|G A T C C T A G|
Xanthomonas malvacearum	*Xma* I	5′ C|C C G G G G G G C C|C

Homologous (legitimate) recombination occurs between closely related DNA sequences and generally substitutes one sequence for another. The process requires a set of enzymes produced (in *E. coli*) by the *rec* genes. **Nonhomologous (illegitimate) recombination** occurs between dissimilar DNA sequences and generally produces insertions or deletions or both. This process usually requires specialized (sometimes site-specific) recombination enzymes, such as those produced by many transposons and lysogenic bacteriophages.

Genetic Engineering

Genetic engineering, also known as recombinant DNA technology, uses the techniques and tools developed by the bacterial geneticists to purify, amplify, modify, and express specific gene sequences. The use of genetic engineering and "cloning" has revolutionized biology and medicine. The basic components of genetic engineering are (1) **cloning and expression vectors,** which can be used to deliver the DNA sequences into receptive bacteria and amplify the desired sequence, (2) the **DNA sequence** to be amplified and expressed, (3) **enzymes,** such as **restriction enzymes,** which are used to cleave DNA reproducibly at defined sequences (Table 13-1), and (4) **DNA ligase,** the enzyme that links the fragment to the cloning vector.

Cloning and expression vectors must allow foreign DNA to be inserted into them but still must be able to replicate normally in a bacterial or eukaryotic host. Many types of vectors are currently used. Plasmid vectors, such as pUC, pBR322, and pGEM (Figure 13-14), are used for DNA fragments up to 20 kb. Bacteriophages, such as lambda, are used for larger fragments up to 25 kb, and **cosmid** vectors have combined some of the advantages of plasmids and phages for fragments up to 45 kb.

Most **cloning vectors** have been "engineered" to have a site for insertion of foreign DNA, a means of selection of the bacteria that have incorporated any plasmid (e.g., antibiotic resistance), and a means of distinguishing the bacteria that

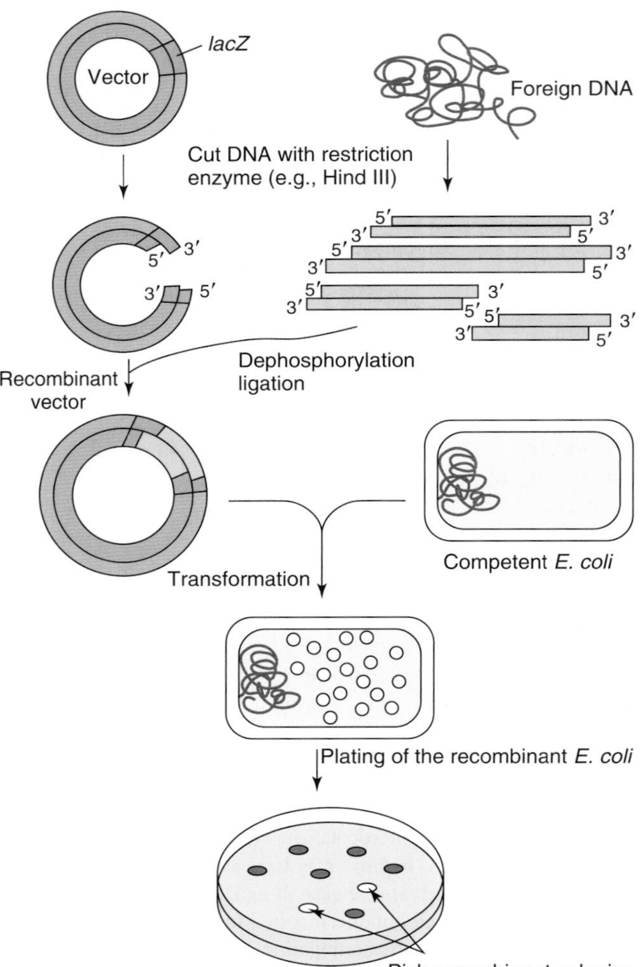

FIGURE 13-14 Cloning of foreign DNA in vectors. The vector and the foreign DNA are first digested by a restriction enzyme. Insertion of foreign DNA into the *lacZ* gene inactivates the β-galactosidase gene, allowing subsequent selection. The vector is then ligated to the foreign DNA, using bacteriophage T4 DNA ligase. The recombinant vectors are transformed into competent *Escherichia coli* cells. The recombinant *E. coli* cells are plated onto agar containing antibiotic, an inducer of the *lac* operon, and a chromophoric substrate that turns blue in cells having a plasmid but not an insert; those cells with a plasmid containing the insert remain white.

have incorporated those plasmids that contain inserted DNA. **Expression vectors** have DNA sequences to facilitate their replication in bacteria and eukaryotic cells and also the transcription of the gene into mRNA.

The DNA to be cloned can be obtained by purification of chromosomal DNA from cells, viruses, or other plasmids or by selective amplification of DNA sequences by a technique known as *polymerase chain reaction* (PCR) (PCR is explained further in Chapter 5). Both the vector and the foreign DNA are cleaved with restriction enzymes (see Figure 13-14). Restriction enzymes recognize a specific palindromic sequence and make a staggered cut that generates sticky ends or a blunt cut that generates blunt ends (see Table 13-1). Most cloning vectors have a sequence called the **multiple**

cloning site that can be cleaved by many restriction enzymes. Ligation of the vector with the DNA fragments generates a molecule called **recombinant DNA,** which is capable of replicating the inserted sequence. The total number of recombinant vectors obtained when cloning all the fragments that result from cleavage of chromosomal DNA is known as a **genomic library** because there should be at least one representative of each gene in the library. An alternative approach to cloning the gene for a protein is to use a retrovirus enzyme called *reverse transcriptase* (RNA-dependent DNA polymerase) to convert the mRNA in the cell into a complementary DNA (cDNA). A **cDNA library** represents the genes that are expressed as mRNA in a particular cell.

The recombinant DNA is then transformed into a bacterial host, usually *E. coli,* and the plasmid-containing bacteria are selected for antibiotic resistance (e.g., ampicillin resistance). The library can then be screened to find an *E. coli* clone possessing the desired DNA fragment. Various screening techniques can be used to identify the bacteria containing the appropriate recombinant DNA. The multiple cloning site used for inserting the foreign DNA is often part of the *lacZ* gene of the *lac* operon. Insertion of the foreign DNA into the *lacZ* gene inactivates the gene (acting almost like a transposon) and prevents the plasmid-directed synthesis of β-galactosidase in the recipient cell, which results in white bacterial colonies instead of blue colonies if β-galactosidase was produced and able to cleave an appropriate chromophore.

Genetic engineering has been used to isolate and express the genes for useful proteins such as insulin, interferon, growth hormones, and interleukin in bacteria, yeast, or even insect cells. Similarly, large amounts of pure immunogen for a vaccine can be prepared without the need to work with the intact disease organisms.

The vaccine against hepatitis B virus represents the first successful use of recombinant DNA technology to make a vaccine approved for human use by the U.S. Food and Drug Administration. The hepatitis B surface antigen is produced by the yeast *Saccharomyces cerevisiae.* Alternatively, the plasmid DNA capable of promoting expression of the desired immunogen (DNA vaccine) can be injected into an individual to let the host cells express the immunogen and generate an immune response. Recombinant DNA technology has also become essential to laboratory diagnosis, forensic science, agriculture, and many other disciplines.

Bibliography

Alberts B: *Molecular biology of the cell,* ed 4, New York, 2002, Garland Science.

Berg JM, Tymoczko JL, Stryer L: *Biochemistry,* ed 6, New York, 2006, WH Freeman.

Cotter PA, Miller JF: In vivo and ex vivo regulation of bacterial virulence gene expression, *Curr Opin Microbiol* 1:17–26, 1998.

Lewin B: *Genes IX,* Sudbury, Mass, 2007, Jones and Bartlett.

Lodish H, Berk A, Kaiser CA, et al: *Molecular cell biology,* ed 6, New York, 2007, WH Freeman.

Nelson DL, Cox M: *Lehninger principles of biochemistry,* ed 4, New York, 2004, Worth.

Novick RP, Geisinger E: Quorum sensing in staphylococci, *Ann Rev Genet* 42:541–546, 2008.

Patel SS, Rosenthal KS: Microbial adaptation: putting the best team on the field, *Infect Dis Clin Pract* 15:330–334, 2007.

Rutherford ST, Bassler BL: Bacterial quorum sensing: its role in virulence and possibilities for its control, *Cold Spring Harb Perspect Med* 2:pii: a012427, 2012. Available at www.perspectivesinmedicine.net/content/2/11/a012427.short.

Watson JD, Hopkins NH, Roberts JW, et al: *Molecular biology of the gene,* ed 4, Menlo Park, Calif, 1987, Benjamin-Cummings.

Weigel LM, Clewell DB, Gill SR, et al: Genetic analysis of a high-level vancomycin-resistant isolate of *Staphylococcus aureus, Science* 302:1569–1571, 2003.

Articles on Probiotics

Saad N, Delattre C, Urdaci M, et al: An overview of the last advances in probiotic and prebiotic field, *Food Sci Technol* 50:1–16, 2013.

Smith PM, Howitt MR, Panikov N, et al: The microbial metabolites, short-chain fatty acids, regulate colonic Treg cell homeostasis, *Science* 341:569–573, 2013.

Stone S, Edmonds R, Rosenthal KS: Probiotics: helping out the normal flora, *Infect Dis Clin Pract* 21:305–311, 2013.

Vijay-Kumar M, Aitken JD, Carvalho FA, et al: Metabolic syndrome and altered gut microbiota in mice lacking Toll-like receptor 5, *Science* 328:228–231, 2010.

CHAPTER 14

MECHANISMS OF BACTERIAL PATHOGENESIS

To a bacterium, the human body is a collection of environmental niches that provide the warmth, moisture, and food necessary for growth. Bacteria have traits that enable them to enter (invade) the environment, remain in a niche (adhere or colonize), gain access to food sources (degradative enzymes), sequester ions (e.g., iron), and escape clearance by host immune and nonimmune protective responses (e.g., **capsule**). When sufficient numbers of bacteria are present **(quorum),** they turn on functions to support the colony, including production of a biofilm. Unfortunately, many of the mechanisms bacteria use to maintain their niche and the byproducts of bacterial growth (e.g., acids, gas) can cause damage and problems for the human host. Many of these traits are **virulence factors** that enhance the ability of bacteria to cause disease. Although many bacteria cause disease by directly destroying tissue, some release toxins, which are then disseminated by the blood to cause system-wide pathogenesis (Box 14-1). The surface structures of bacteria are powerful stimulators of host responses (acute phase: interleukin [IL]-1, IL-6, tumor necrosis factor [TNF]-α) that can be protective but are often major contributors to the disease symptoms (e.g., sepsis). Production of disease results from the combination of damage caused by the bacteria and the consequences of the innate and immune (inflammation) responses to the infection (Box 14-2).

Not all bacteria or bacterial infections cause disease; however, some always cause disease. The human body is colonized with numerous microbes **(normal flora),** many of which serve important functions for their hosts. Normal flora bacteria aid in the digestion of food, produce vitamins (e.g., vitamin K), protect the host from colonization with pathogenic microbes, and activate appropriate host innate and immune responses. These endogenous bacteria normally reside in locations such as the gastrointestinal (GI) tract, mouth, skin, and upper respiratory tract, which can be considered to be outside the body (Figure 14-1). The composition of the normal flora can be disrupted by antibiotic treatment, diet, stress, and changes in the host response to the flora. The loss of the normal GI bacteria with broad-spectrum antibiotic treatment often allows the outgrowth of *Clostridium difficile,* which causes pseudomembranous colitis. An altered normal flora can lead to inappropriate immune responses, causing inflammatory bowel diseases.

Normal flora bacteria cause disease if they enter normally sterile sites of the body. **Virulent bacteria** have mechanisms that promote their growth in the host at the expense of the host's tissue or organ function. **Opportunistic bacteria** take advantage of preexisting conditions, such as immunosuppression, to grow and cause serious disease. For example, burn victims and the lungs of patients with cystic fibrosis are at higher risk of *Pseudomonas aeruginosa* infection, and patients with acquired immunodeficiency syndrome (AIDS) are very susceptible to infection by intracellularly growing bacteria, such as the mycobacteria.

Disease results from the damage or loss of tissue or organ function due to the infection or the host inflammatory responses. The **signs and symptoms of a disease** are determined by the change to the affected tissue. **Systemic responses** are produced by toxins and the cytokines produced in response to the infection. The **seriousness** of the disease depends on the importance of the affected organ and the extent of the damage caused by the infection. Infections of the central nervous system are especially serious. The **bacterial strain** and **inoculum size** are also major factors in determining whether disease occurs; however, the threshold for disease production is different for different bacteria (e.g., <200 *Shigella* are required for shigellosis, but 10^8 *Vibrio cholerae* or *Campylobacter* organisms are required for disease of the GI tract). Host factors can also play a role. For example, although a million or more *Salmonella* organisms are necessary for gastroenteritis to become established in a healthy person, only a few thousand organisms are necessary in a person whose gastric pH has been neutralized with antacids or other means. Congenital defects, immunodeficiency states (see Chapter 10), and other disease-related conditions might also increase a person's susceptibility to infection. *The longer a bacterium remains in the body, the greater its numbers, its ability to spread, and its potential to cause tissue damage and disease, and the larger the host response.*

Many of the virulence factors consist of complex structures or activities that are only expressed under special conditions (see Figure 13-6). The components for these structures are often encoded together in a **pathogenicity island.** Pathogenicity islands are large genetic regions in the chromosome or on plasmids that contain sets of genes encoding numerous virulence factors that may require coordinated expression. These genes may be turned on by a single stimulus (e.g., temperature of the gut, pH of a lysosome). A pathogenicity island is usually within a transposon and can be transferred as a unit to different sites within a chromosome or to other bacteria. For example, the SPI-2 pathogenicity island of *Salmonella* is activated by the acidic pH of a phagocytic vesicle within a macrophage. This promotes expression of approximately 25 proteins that assemble into a syringe-like molecular device (type III secretion device) that injects proteins into

 **Box 14-1 Bacterial Virulence Mechanisms**

Adherence
Invasion
Byproducts of growth (gas, acid)
Toxins
Degradative enzymes
Cytotoxic proteins
Endotoxin
Superantigen
Induction of excess inflammation
Evasion of phagocytic and immune clearance
Capsule
Resistance to antibiotics
Intracellular growth

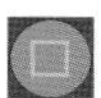 **Box 14-2 Bacterial Disease Production**

1. Disease is caused by damage produced by the bacteria plus the consequences of innate and immune responses to the infection.
2. The signs and symptoms of a disease are determined by the function and importance of the affected tissue.
3. The length of the incubation period is the time required for the bacteria and/or the host response to cause sufficient damage to initiate discomfort or interfere with essential functions.

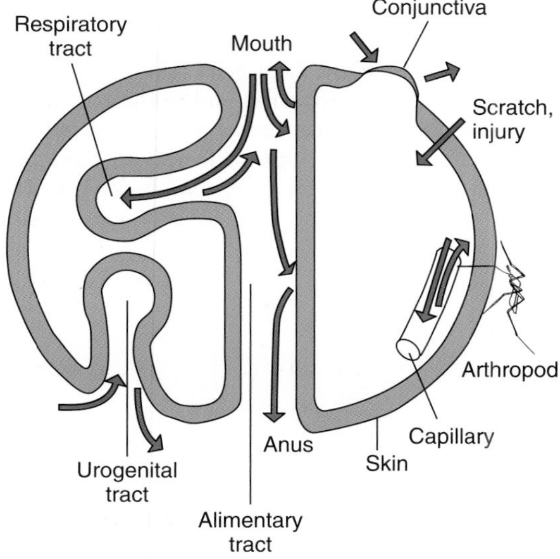

FIGURE 14-1 Body surfaces as sites of microbial infection and shedding. *Red arrows* indicate infection; *purple arrows* indicate shedding. (Modified from Goering RV, Dockrell HM, Zuckerman M, et al: *Mims' medical microbiology,* ed 5, Philadelphia, 2013, Elsevier.)

the host cell to facilitate the bacteria's intracellular survival and growth. Similarly, the biofilm produced by *Pseudomonas* is triggered when there are sufficient bacteria (a quorum) producing sufficient amounts of *N*-acyl homoserine lactone (AHL) to trigger expression of the genes for polysaccharide production.

 **Table 14-1 Bacterial Port of Entry**

Route	Examples
Ingestion	*Salmonella* spp., *Shigella* spp., *Yersinia enterocolitica*, enterotoxigenic *Escherichia coli*, *Vibrio* spp., *Campylobacter* spp., *Clostridium botulinum*, *Bacillus cereus*, *Listeria* spp., *Brucella* spp.
Inhalation	*Mycobacterium* spp., *Nocardia* spp., *Mycoplasma pneumoniae*, *Legionella* spp., *Bordetella*, *Chlamydophila psittaci*, *Chlamydophila pneumoniae*, *Streptococcus* spp.
Trauma	*Clostridium tetani*, *Staphylococcus aureus*
Needlestick	*Staphylococcus aureus*, *Pseudomonas* spp.
Arthropod bite	*Rickettsia*, *Ehrlichia*, *Coxiella*, *Francisella*, *Borrelia* spp., *Yersinia pestis*
Sexual transmission	*Neisseria gonorrhoeae*, *Chlamydia trachomatis*, *Treponema pallidum*

Entry into the Human Body

For infection to become established, bacteria must first gain entry into the body (Table 14-1; see Figure 14-1). Natural defense mechanisms and barriers (e.g., skin, mucus, ciliated epithelium) and secretions containing antibacterial substances (e.g., lysozyme, defensins) make it difficult for bacteria to gain entry into the body. However, these barriers are sometimes broken (e.g., a tear in the skin, a tumor or ulcer in the bowel), providing a portal of entry for the bacteria, or the bacteria may have the means to compromise the barrier and invade the body. On invasion, the bacteria can travel in the bloodstream to other sites in the body.

The **skin** has a thick, horny layer of dead cells that protects the body from infection. However, cuts in the skin, produced accidentally or surgically or kept open with catheters or other surgical appliances, provide a means for the bacteria to gain access to the susceptible tissue underneath. For example, *Staphylococcus aureus* and *Staphylococcus epidermidis,* which are a part of the normal flora on skin, can enter the body through breaks in the skin and pose a major problem for people with indwelling catheters and intravenous lines.

The mouth, nose, respiratory tract, ears, eyes, urogenital tract, and anus are sites through which bacteria can enter the body. These natural openings in the skin and their associated body cavities are protected by natural defenses such as the mucus and ciliated epithelium that line the upper respiratory tract, the lysozyme and other antibacterial secretions in tears and mucus, and the acid and bile in the GI tract, as well as secretory immunoglobulin (Ig)A. However, many bacteria are unaffected or have the means to evade these defenses. For example, the outer membrane of the gram-negative bacteria makes these bacteria more resistant to lysozyme, acid, and bile. The enterobacteria are thus enabled to colonize the GI tract. A break in the normal barrier can allow entry of these endogenous bacteria to normally sterile sites of the body, such as the peritoneum and the bloodstream, to cause disease. An example of this is the patient whose colon tumor was diagnosed after detection of a septicemia (blood-borne infection) caused by enteric bacteria.

Colonization, Adhesion, and Invasion

Different bacteria colonize different parts of the body. This may be closest to the point of entry or due to the presence of optimal growth conditions at the site. For example, *Legionella* is inhaled and grows in the lungs but does not readily spread because it cannot tolerate high temperatures (e.g., 35° C). Colonization of sites that are normally sterile implies the existence of a defect in a natural defense mechanism or a new portal of entry. Patients with cystic fibrosis have such defects because of the reduction in their ciliary mucoepithelial function and altered mucosal secretions; as a result, their lungs are colonized by *S. aureus* and *P. aeruginosa*. In some cases, colonization requires special structures and functions to remain at the site, survive, and obtain food.

Bacteria may use specific mechanisms to adhere to and colonize different body surfaces (Table 14-2). If the bacteria can adhere to epithelial or endothelial cell linings of the bladder, intestine, and blood vessels, they cannot be washed away, and this adherence allows them to colonize the tissue. For example, natural bladder function eliminates any bacteria not affixed to the bladder wall. *Escherichia coli* and other bacteria have **adhesins** that bind to specific receptors on the tissue surface and keep the organisms from being washed away. Many of these adhesin proteins are present at the tips of **fimbriae (pili)** and bind tightly to specific sugars on the target tissue; this sugar-binding activity defines these proteins as **lectins.** For example, most *E. coli* strains that cause pyelonephritis produce a fimbrial adhesin termed the *P fimbriae.* This adhesin can bind to α-D-galactosyl-β-D-galactoside (Gal-Gal), which is part of the P blood group antigen structure on human erythrocytes and uroepithelial cells. *Neisseria gonorrhoeae* pili are also important virulence factors; they bind to oligosaccharide receptors on epithelial cells. *Yersinia* organisms, *Bordetella pertussis,* and *Mycoplasma pneumoniae* express adhesin proteins that are not on fimbriae. *Streptococci, S. aureus, and other bacteria secrete proteins that bind components of the extracellular matrix of epithelial cells such as fibronectin, collagen, or laminin, termed* **MSCRAMMs** *(microbial surface components recognizing adhesive matrix molecules).*

A special bacterial adaptation that facilitates colonization, especially of surgical appliances such as artificial valves or indwelling catheters, is a **biofilm.** Bacteria in biofilms are bound within a sticky web of polysaccharide that binds the cells together and to the surface. Production of a biofilm requires sufficient numbers of bacteria (quorum). When *P. aeruginosa* determine that the colony size is large enough (quorum sensing) they produce a biofilm. Dental plaque is another example of a biofilm. The biofilm matrix can also protect the bacteria from host defenses and antibiotics.

Although bacteria do not have mechanisms that enable them to cross intact skin, several bacteria can cross mucosal membranes and other tissue barriers to enter normally sterile sites and more susceptible tissue. These invasive bacteria either destroy the barrier, induce inflammation to permeabilize the barrier, or penetrate into the cells of the barrier. *Salmonella* and *Yersinia* organisms are enteric bacteria that use fimbriae to bind to M (microfold) cells of the colon and then inject proteins into the M cell that stimulate the cell membrane to surround and take in the bacteria. These bacteria produce a type III secretion device that resembles a molecular syringe that injects pore-forming factors and effector molecules into the host cells. The effector proteins can facilitate uptake and invasion and promote intracellular survival and replication of the bacteria or the apoptotic death of the host cell. Enteropathogenic *E. coli* secretes proteins into the host cell that create a portable docking system for

Table 14-2 Examples of Bacterial Adherence Mechanisms

Microbe	Adhesin	Receptor
Staphylococcus aureus	Clumping factor A	Fibrinogen
Staphylococcus spp.	MSCRAMM	Extracellular matrix components (fibronectin, laminin, collagen, etc.)
Streptococcus, group A	LTA–M protein complex F protein, MSCRAMM	Extracellular matrix components (fibronectin, laminin, collagen, etc.)
Streptococcus pneumoniae	Adhesins and other proteins	*N*-Acetylhexosamine-galactose
Escherichia coli	Type 1 fimbriae	D-Mannose
	Colonization factor antigen fimbriae	GM ganglioside 1
	P fimbriae	P blood group glycolipid
Neisseria gonorrhoeae	Fimbriae	GD_1 ganglioside
Treponema pallidum	P_1, P_2, P_3	Fibronectin
Chlamydia trachomatis	Cell surface lectin	*N*-Acetylglucosamine
Mycoplasma pneumoniae	Protein P1	Sialic acid
Vibrio cholerae	Type 4 pili	Fucose and mannose

LTA, Lipoteichoic acid; *MSCRAMM,* microbial surface components recognizing adhesive matrix molecules.

itself, and *Salmonella* uses the device to promote its uptake into a vesicle and live intracellularly within the macrophage (see animations developed by the Howard Hughes Medical Institute [websites follow]). Many of the proteins injected into these cells by the type III secretion device promote actin polymerization. For *Salmonella,* this promotes phagocytic uptake; for *Shigella* and *Listeria monocytogenes,* movement within the cell and to other cells. Excellent videos of these processes can be seen at www.hhmi.org/biointeractive/disease/ecoli.html and www.hhmi.org/biointeractive/disease/salmonella.html. In addition, salmonella and other bacteria promote invasion of the GI tract by weakening the tight junctions between mucoepithelial cells with bacterial proteins or by inducing inflammation.

Pathogenic Actions of Bacteria

Tissue Destruction

Byproducts of bacterial growth, especially fermentation, include acids, gas, and other substances that are toxic to tissue. In addition, *many bacteria release degradative enzymes* to break down tissue, thereby providing food for the organisms' growth and also promoting bacterial spread. For example, *Clostridium perfringens* organisms are part of the normal flora of the GI tract but are also opportunistic pathogens that can establish infection in oxygen-depleted tissues and cause gas gangrene. These anaerobic bacteria produce enzymes (e.g., phospholipase C, collagenase, protease, hyaluronidase), several toxins, and acid and gas from bacterial metabolism, which destroy the tissue. Staphylococci produce many different enzymes that modify the tissue environment. These enzymes include hyaluronidase, fibrinolysin, and lipases. Streptococci also produce enzymes, including streptolysins S and O, hyaluronidase, DNAases, and streptokinases.

Toxins

Toxins are bacterial products that directly harm tissue or trigger destructive biological activities. Toxins and toxin-like activities are degradative enzymes that cause lysis of cells or specific receptor-binding proteins that initiate toxic reactions in a specific target tissue. In addition, endotoxin (lipid A portion of lipopolysaccharide) and superantigen proteins promote excessive or inappropriate stimulation of innate or immune responses.

In many cases, the toxin is completely responsible for causing the characteristic symptoms of the disease. For example, the **preformed toxin** present in food mediates the food poisoning caused by *S. aureus* and *Bacillus cereus* and the botulism caused by *Clostridium botulinum.* The symptoms caused by preformed toxin occur much sooner than for other forms of gastroenteritis because the effect is like eating a poison and the bacteria do not need to grow for the symptoms to occur. Because a toxin can be spread systemically through the bloodstream, symptoms may arise at a site distant from the site of infection, such as occurs in tetanus, which is caused by *Clostridium tetani.*

Exotoxins

Exotoxins are proteins that can be produced by gram-positive or gram-negative bacteria and include cytolytic enzymes and receptor-binding proteins that alter a function or kill the cell. In many cases, the toxin gene is encoded on a plasmid (tetanus toxin of *C. tetani,* heat-labile [LT] and heat-stabile [ST] toxins of enterotoxigenic *E. coli*) or a lysogenic phage (*Corynebacterium diphtheriae* and *C. botulinum*).

Cytolytic toxins include membrane-disrupting enzymes such as the α-toxin (phospholipase C) produced by *C. perfringens,* which breaks down sphingomyelin and other membrane phospholipids. Hemolysins insert into and disrupt erythrocyte and other cell membranes. Pore-forming toxins, including streptolysin O, can promote leakage of ions and water from the cell and disrupt cellular functions or cell lysis.

Many toxins are dimeric, with A and B subunits **(A-B toxins).** The **B** portion of the A-B toxins binds to a specific cell surface receptor, and then the A subunit is transferred into the interior of the cell, where it acts to promote cell injury *(B for binding, A for action).* The tissues targeted by these toxins are very defined and limited (Figure 14-2 and Table 14-3). The biochemical targets of A-B toxins include ribosomes, transport mechanisms, and intracellular signaling (cyclic adenosine monophosphate [cAMP] production, G-protein function), with effects ranging from diarrhea to loss of neuronal function to death. The functional properties of cytolytic and other exotoxins are discussed in greater detail in the chapters dealing with the specific diseases involved.

Superantigens are a special group of toxins (Figure 14-3). These molecules activate T cells by binding simultaneously to a T-cell receptor and a major histocompatibility complex class II (MHC II) molecule on an antigen-presenting cell without requiring antigen. *Superantigens activate large numbers of T cells to release large amounts (cytokine storm) of interleukins (including IL-1, IL-2, IL-6),* TNF-α, interferon (IFN)-γ, and various chemokines, causing *life-threatening fever, shock, rash, and autoimmune-like responses.* This superantigen stimulation of T cells can also lead to death of the activated T cells, resulting in the loss of specific T-cell clones and loss of their immune responses. Superantigens include the toxic shock syndrome toxin of *S. aureus,* staphylococcal enterotoxins, and the erythrogenic toxin A or C of *S. pyogenes.*

Endotoxin and Other Cell Wall Components

The presence of bacterial cell wall components acts as a signal of infection that provides a powerful multialarm warning to the body to activate the host's protective systems. The molecular patterns in these structures **(pathogen-associated molecular patterns [PAMPs])** bind to Toll-like receptors (TLRs) and other molecules and stimulate the production of cytokines (see Chapters 8 and 10). In some cases, the host response is excessive and may even be life threatening. The **lipid A portion of lipopolysaccharide (LPS)** produced by gram-negative bacteria is a powerful activator of acute-phase and inflammatory reactions and is termed **endotoxin.** It is important to appreciate that endotoxin is not the same as exotoxin and that *only gram-negative bacteria make endotoxin.* Weaker, endotoxin-like responses may occur to gram-positive bacterial structures, including **lipoteichoic acids.**

Gram-negative bacteria release endotoxin during infection. Endotoxin binds to specific receptors (CD14 and TLR4)

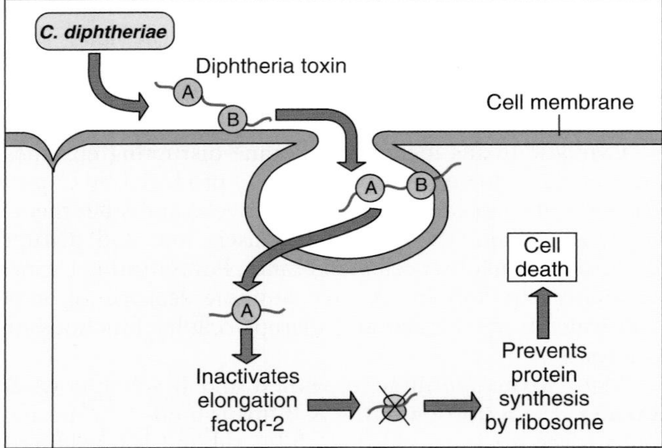

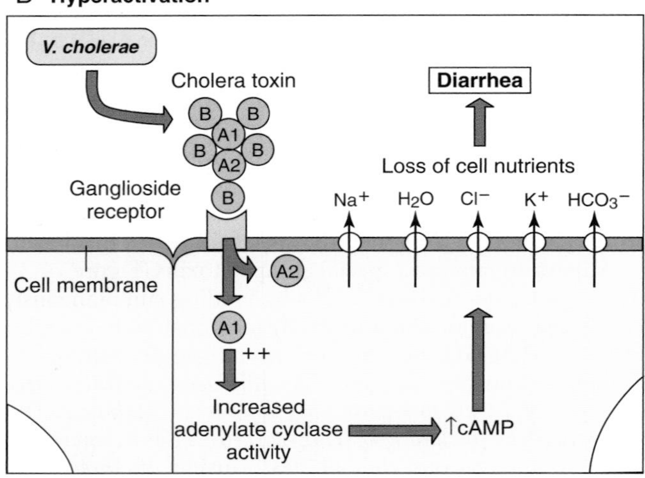

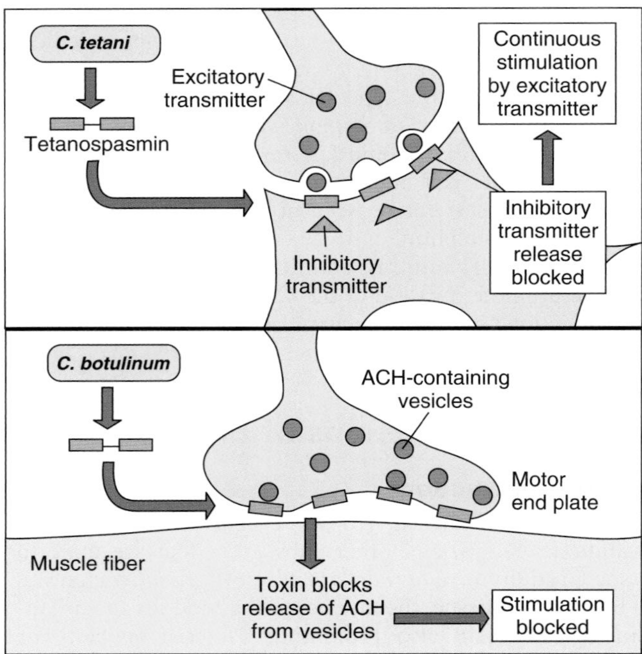

FIGURE 14-2 A-C, The mode of action of dimeric A-B exotoxins. The bacterial A-B toxins often consist of a two-chain molecule. The B chain binds and promotes entry of the A chain into cells, and the A chain has inhibitory activity against some vital function. *ACH,* Acetylcholine; *cAMP,* cyclic adenosine monophosphate; *C. botulinum, Clostridium botulinum; C. diphtheriae, Corynebacterium diphtheriae; C. tetani, Clostridium tetani; V. cholerae, Vibrio cholerae.* (Modified from Goering RV, Dockrell HM, Zuckerman M, et al: *Mims' medical microbiology,* ed 5, Philadelphia, 2013, Elsevier.)

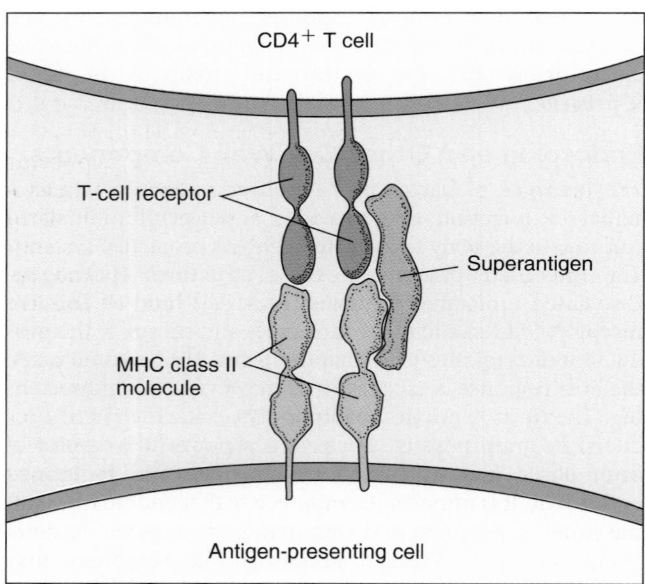

FIGURE 14-3 Superantigen binding to the external regions of the T-cell receptor and the major histocompatibility complex *(MHC)* class II molecules.

on macrophages, B cells, and other cells and stimulates production and release of **acute-phase cytokines,** such as IL-1, TNF-α, IL-6, and prostaglandins (Figure 14-4). Endotoxin also stimulates the growth (mitogenic) of B cells.

At low concentrations, endotoxin stimulates the development of protective responses such as fever, vasodilation, and activation of immune and inflammatory responses (Box 14-3). However, the endotoxin levels in the blood of patients with **gram-negative bacterial sepsis** (bacteria in the blood) can be very high, and the systemic response to these can be overpowering, resulting in shock and possibly death. High concentrations of endotoxin can also activate the alternative pathway of complement and production of anaphylatoxins (C3a, C5a), contributing to systemic vasodilation and capillary leakage. In combination with TNF-α and IL-1, this can lead to **hypotension** and **shock. Disseminated intravascular coagulation (DIC)** can also result from the activation of blood coagulation pathways. The high fever, petechiae (skin lesions resulting from capillary leakage), and potential symptoms of shock (resulting from increased vascular permeability) associated with *Neisseria meningitidis* infection can be related to the large amounts of endotoxin released during infection.

Table 14-3 Properties of A-B–Type Bacterial Toxins

Toxin	Organism	Gene Location	Subunit Structure	Target Cell Receptor	Biological Effects
Anthrax toxins	*Bacillus anthracis*	Plasmid	Three separate proteins (EF, LF, PA)	Tumor endothelial marker-8 (TEM-8); capillary morphogenesis protein 2 (CMG2)	EF + PA: increase in target cell cAMP level, localized edema; LF + PA: death of target cells and experimental animals
Bordetella	*Bordetella* spp.	Chromosomal	A-B	Unknown, probably glycolipid	Adenylate cyclase toxin. Increase in target cell cAMP level, modified cell function, or cell death
Botulinum toxin	*Clostridium botulinum*	Phage	A-B	Polysialogangliosides plus synaptotagmin (co-receptors)	Decrease in peripheral presynaptic acetylcholine release, flaccid paralysis
Cholera toxin	*Vibrio cholerae*	Chromosomal	A-B_5	Ganglioside (GM_1)	Activation of adenylate cyclase, increase in cAMP level, secretory diarrhea
Diphtheria toxin	*Corynebacterium diphtheriae*	Phage	A-B	Growth factor receptor precursor	Inhibition of protein synthesis, cell death
Heat-labile enterotoxins	*Escherichia coli*	Plasmid	Similar or identical to cholera toxin		
Pertussis toxin	*Bordetella pertussis*	Chromosomal	A-B_5	Surface glycoproteins with terminal sialic acid residues	Block of signal transduction mediated by target G proteins
Pseudomonas exotoxin A	*Pseudomonas aeruginosa*	Chromosomal	A-B	α_2-Macroglobulin receptor (α_2-MR)	Similar or identical to diphtheria toxin
Shiga toxin	*Shigella dysenteriae*	Chromosomal	A-B_5	Globotriaosylceramide (Gb3)	Inhibition of protein synthesis, cell death
Shiga-like toxins	*Shigella* spp., *E. coli*	Phage	Similar or identical to Shiga toxin		
Tetanus toxin	*Clostridium tetani*	Plasmid	A-B	Polysialogangliosides plus 15-kDa glycoprotein (co-receptors)	Decrease in neurotransmitter release from inhibitory neurons, spastic paralysis

Modified from Mandell G, Douglas G, Bennett J: *Principles and practice of infectious disease,* ed 3, New York, 1990, Churchill Livingstone.
cAMP, Cyclic adenosine monophosphate; *EF,* edema factor; *LF,* lethal factor; *PA,* protective antigen.

Box 14-3 Endotoxin-Mediated Toxicity

Fever
Leukopenia followed by leukocytosis
Activation of complement
Thrombocytopenia
Disseminated intravascular coagulation
Decreased peripheral circulation and perfusion to major organs
Shock
Death

• Immunopathogenesis

In many cases, the symptoms of a bacterial infection are produced by excessive innate, immune, and inflammatory responses triggered by the infection. When limited and controlled, the acute-phase response to cell wall components is a protective antibacterial response. However, these responses also cause fever and malaise, and when systemic and out of control, the acute-phase response and inflammation can cause life-threatening symptoms associated with sepsis and meningitis (see Figure 14-4). Activated neutrophils, macrophages, and complement can cause damage at the site of the infection. Activation of complement can also cause release of anaphylatoxins that initiate vascular permeability and capillary breakage. Cytokine storms generated by superantigens and endotoxin can cause shock and disruption of body function. Granuloma formation induced by CD4 T cells and macrophages in response to *Mycobacterium tuberculosis* can also lead to tissue destruction. Autoimmune responses can be triggered by some bacterial proteins, such as the M protein of *S. pyogenes,* which antigenically mimics heart tissue. The anti-M protein antibodies cross-react with and can initiate damage to the heart to cause rheumatic fever. Immune complexes deposited in the glomeruli of the kidney cause poststreptococcal glomerulonephritis. For *Chlamydia, Treponema* (syphilis), *Borrelia* (Lyme disease), and other bacteria, the host immune response is the principal cause of disease symptoms in patients.

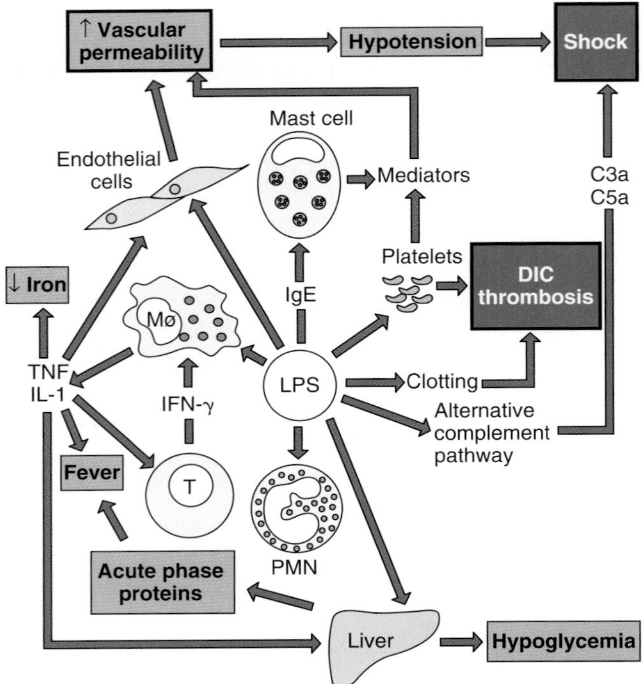

FIGURE 14-4 The many activities of lipopolysaccharide *(LPS)*. This bacterial endotoxin activates almost every immune mechanism, as well as the clotting pathway, which together make LPS one of the most powerful immune stimuli known. *DIC,* Disseminated intravascular coagulation; *IFN-γ,* interferon-γ; *IgE,* immunoglobulin E; *IL-1,* interleukin-1; *PMN,* polymorphonuclear (neutrophil) leukocytes; *TNF,* tumor necrosis factor. (Modified from Goering RV, Dockrell HM, Zuckerman M, et al: *Mims' medical microbiology,* ed 5, Philadelphia, 2013, Elsevier.)

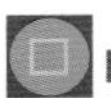
Box 14-4 Microbial Defenses against Host Immunologic Clearance

Encapsulation
Antigenic mimicry
Antigenic masking
Antigenic shift
Production of antiimmunoglobulin proteases
Destruction of phagocyte
Inhibition of chemotaxis
Inhibition of phagocytosis
Inhibition of phagolysosome fusion
Resistance to lysosomal enzymes
Intracellular replication

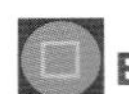
Box 14-5 Examples of Encapsulated Microorganisms

Staphylococcus aureus
Streptococcus pneumoniae
Streptococcus pyogenes (group A)
Streptococcus agalactiae (group B)
Bacillus anthracis
Bacillus subtilis
Neisseria gonorrhoeae
Neisseria meningitidis
Haemophilus influenzae
Escherichia coli
Klebsiella pneumoniae
Salmonella spp.
Yersinia pestis
Campylobacter fetus
Pseudomonas aeruginosa
Bacteroides fragilis
Cryptococcus neoformans (yeast)

Mechanisms for Escaping Host Defenses

Bacteria are parasites, and evasion of host protective responses is a selective advantage. Logically, the longer a bacterial infection remains in a host, the more time the bacteria have to grow and cause damage. Therefore bacteria that can evade or incapacitate the host defenses have a greater potential for causing disease. Bacteria evade recognition and killing by phagocytic cells, inactivate or evade the complement system and antibody, and even grow inside cells to hide from host responses (Box 14-4).

The capsule is one of the most important virulence factors (Box 14-5). These slime layers function by shielding the bacteria from immune and phagocytic responses. Capsules are typically made of polysaccharides, which are poor immunogens. The *S. pyogenes* capsule, for example, is made of hyaluronic acid, which mimics human connective tissue, thereby masking the bacteria and keeping them from being recognized by the immune system. The capsule also acts like a slimy football jersey, in that it is hard to grasp and tears away when grabbed by a phagocyte. The capsule also protects a bacterium from destruction within the phagolysosome of a macrophage or leukocyte. All of these properties can extend the time bacteria spend in blood (bacteremia) before being eliminated by host responses. Mutants of normally encapsulated bacteria that lose the ability to make a capsule also lose their virulence; examples of such bacteria are *Streptococcus pneumoniae* and *N. meningitidis.* A **biofilm,** which is made from capsular material, can prevent antibody and complement from getting to the bacteria.

Bacteria can evade antibody responses by **antigenic variation,** by **inactivation of antibody,** or **by intracellular growth.** *N. gonorrhoeae* can vary the structure of surface antigens to evade antibody responses and also produces a protease that degrades IgA. *S. aureus* makes an IgG-binding protein, protein A, which prevents antibody from activating complement or being an opsonin and masks the bacteria from detection. Bacteria that grow intracellularly include mycobacteria, francisellae, brucellae, chlamydiae, and rickettsiae (Box 14-6). Unlike most bacteria, control of these infections requires T-helper cell immune responses to activate macrophages to kill or create a wall (granuloma) around the infected cells (as for *M. tuberculosis*).

Bacteria evade complement action by preventing access of the components to the membrane, masking themselves, and inhibiting activation of the cascade. The thick peptidoglycan of gram-positive bacteria and the long O antigen of

Box 14-6 Examples of Intracellular Pathogens

Mycobacterium spp.
Brucella spp.
Francisella spp.
Rickettsia spp.
Chlamydia spp.
Listeria monocytogenes
Salmonella typhi
Shigella dysenteriae
Yersinia pestis
Legionella pneumophila

LPS of most gram-negative bacteria (not *Neisseria* spp.) limit access to complement and protect the bacterial membrane from being damaged. By degrading the C5a component of complement, *S. pyogenes* can limit the chemotaxis of leukocytes to the site of infection. To compensate for the lack of O antigen, *N. gonorrhoeae* attaches sialic acid to its lipooligosaccharide (LOS) to inhibit complement activation.

Phagocytes (neutrophils, macrophages) are the most important antibacterial defense, but many bacteria can circumvent phagocytic killing in various ways or kill the phagocyte. They can produce enzymes capable of lysing phagocytic cells (e.g., the streptolysin produced by *S. pyogenes* or the α-toxin produced by *C. perfringens*). They can inhibit phagocytosis (e.g., the effects of the **capsule** and the **M protein** produced by *S. pyogenes*) or block intracellular killing. Bacterial mechanisms for protection from intracellular killing include blocking fusion of the lysosome with the phagosome to prevent contact with its bactericidal contents (*Mycobacterium* spp.), capsule-mediated or enzymatic resistance to the bactericidal lysosomal enzymes or substances, and the ability to exit the phagosome into the host cytoplasm before being exposed to lysosomal enzymes (Figure 14-5 and Table 14-4). Production of catalase by staphylococci can break down the hydrogen peroxide produced by the myeloperoxidase system. Many of the bacteria that are internalized but survive phagocytosis can use the cell as a place to grow and hide from immune responses and as a means of being disseminated throughout the body.

S. aureus can also escape host defenses by walling off the site of infection. *S. aureus* can produce coagulase, an enzyme that promotes the conversion of fibrin to fibrinogen to produce a clotlike barrier; this feature distinguishes *S. aureus* from *S. epidermidis*. *S. aureus* and *S. pyogenes* and other bacteria are pyogenic (pus formers), and pus formation upon the death of neutrophils limits antibody or antibiotic access to the bacteria. *M. tuberculosis* is able to survive in a host by promoting the development of a granuloma, within which viable bacteria may reside for the life of the infected person. The bacteria may resume growth if there is a decline in the immune status of the person.

Summary

The primary virulence factors of bacteria are the capsule, adhesins, invasins, degradative enzymes, toxins, and mechanisms for escaping elimination by host defenses. Bacteria

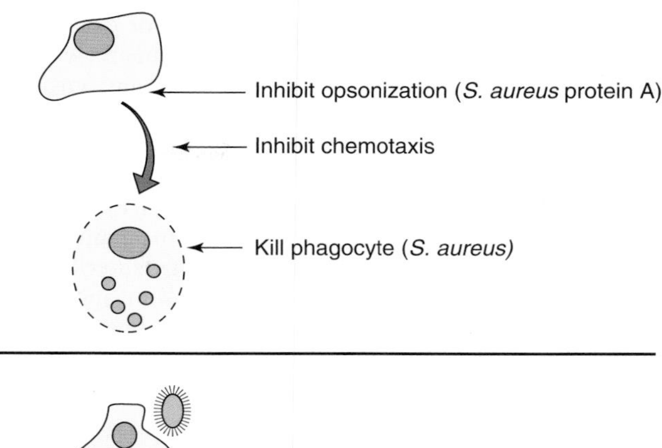

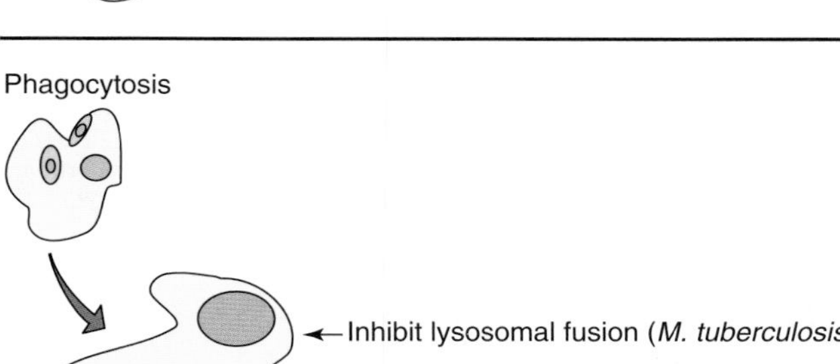

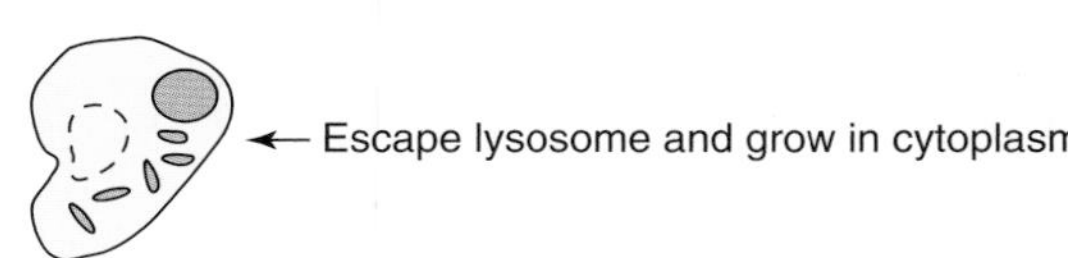

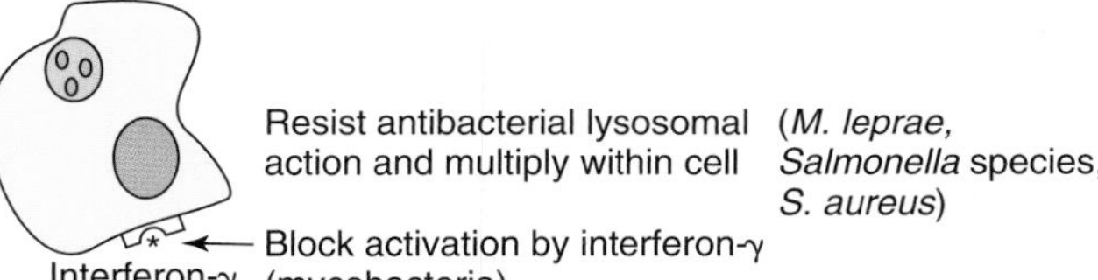

FIGURE 14-5 Bacterial mechanisms for escaping phagocytic clearance. Selected examples of bacteria that use the indicated antiphagocytic mechanisms are given. *M. leprae, Mycobacterium leprae; M. tuberculosis, Mycobacterium tuberculosis; S. aureus, Staphylococcus aureus.*

Table 14-4 Methods That Circumvent Phagocytic Killing

Method	Example
Inhibition of phagolysosome fusion	*Legionella* spp., *Mycobacterium tuberculosis, Chlamydia* spp.
Resistance to lysosomal enzymes	*Salmonella typhimurium, Coxiella* spp., *Ehrlichia* spp., *Mycobacterium leprae, Leishmania* spp.
Adaptation to cytoplasmic replication	*Listeria, Francisella,* and *Rickettsia* spp.

may only have one virulence mechanism. For example, *C. diphtheriae* has only one virulence mechanism, which is diphtheria toxin. Other bacteria express many virulence factors. *S. aureus* is an example of such a bacterium; it expresses adhesins, degradative enzymes, toxins, catalase, and coagulase, which are responsible for producing a spectrum of diseases. In addition, different strains within a bacterial species may express different virulence mechanisms. For example, the symptoms and sequelae of gastroenteritis (diarrhea) caused by *E. coli* may include invasion and bloody stools, cholera-like watery stools, and even severe hemorrhagic disease, depending on the specific infecting strain.

Bibliography

Behnsen J, Jellbauer S, Wong CP, et al: The cytokine IL-22 promotes pathogen colonization by suppressing related commensal bacteria, *Immunity* 40:262–273, 2014.

Bisno AL, Brito MO, Collins CM: Molecular basis of group A streptococcal virulence, *Lancet Infect Dis* 3:191–200, 2003.

Bower S, Rosenthal KS: Bacterial cell walls: the armor, artillery and Achilles heel, *Infect Dis Clin Pract* 14:309–317, 2006.

Brodell LA, Rosenthal KS: Skin structure and function: the body's primary defense against infection, *Infect Dis Clin Pract* 16:113–117, 2008.

Chagnot C, Listrat A, Astruc T, et al: Bacterial adhesion to animal tissues: protein determinants for recognition of extracellular matrix components, *Cell Microbiol* 14:1687–1696, 2012.

Cohen J, Powderly WC: *Infectious diseases*, ed 2, London, 2004, Mosby.

Desvaux M, Hebraud M, Henderson IR, et al: Type III secretion: what's in a name? *Trends Microbiol* 14:157–160, 2006.

Finlay BB, Falkow S: Common themes in microbial pathogenicity revisited, *Microbiol Mol Biol Rev* 61:136–169, 1997.

Groisman EA, Ochman H: How *Salmonella* became a pathogen, *Trends Microbiol* 5:343–349, 1997.

Lee CA: Pathogenicity islands and the evolution of bacterial pathogens, *Infect Agents Dis* 5:1–7, 1996.

Mandell GL, Bennet JE, Dolin R, editors: *Principles and practice of infectious diseases*, ed 6, Philadelphia, 2005, Churchill Livingstone.

McClane BA, Mietzner TA: *Microbial pathogenesis: a principles-oriented approach*, Madison, Conn, 1999, Fence Creek.

Papageorgiou AC, Acharya KR: Microbial superantigens: from structure to function, *Trends Microbiol* 8:369–375, 2000.

Reading N, Sperandio V: Quorum sensing: the many languages of bacteria, *FEMS Microbiol Lett* 254:1–11, 2006.

Rosenthal KS: Are microbial symptoms "self-inflicted"? The consequences of immunopathology, *Infect Dis Clin Pract* 13:306–310, 2005.

Excellent videos, prepared by the Howard Hughes Medical Institute, of the action of *E. coli* and *Salmonella* type III secretion devices promoting adhesion and intracellular growth can be seen at www.hhmi.org/biointeractive/disease/ecoli.html and www.hhmi.org/biointeractive/disease/salmonella.html. A video of *Salmonella* virulence mechanisms: www.youtube.com/watch?v=j5GvvQJVD_Y.

CHAPTER

15 ROLE OF BACTERIA IN DISEASE

This chapter summarizes material presented in Chapters 18 to 35, chapters that focus on individual organisms and the diseases they cause. We believe this is an important process in understanding how individual organisms produce disease; however, when a patient develops an infection, a physician approaches diagnosis by assessing the clinical presentation and constructing a list of organisms that are most likely to cause the disease. The etiology of some diseases can be attributed to a single organism (e.g., tetanus—*Clostridium tetani*). More commonly, however, multiple organisms can produce a similar clinical picture (e.g., sepsis, pneumonia, gastroenteritis, meningitis). The clinical management of infections is predicated on the ability to develop an accurate differential diagnosis; that is, it is critical to know which organisms are most commonly associated with a particular infectious process.

The development of an infection depends on the complex interactions of (1) the host's susceptibility to infection, (2) the organism's virulence potential, and (3) the opportunity for interaction between host and organism. It is impossible to summarize in a single chapter the complex interactions that lead to the development of disease in each organ system. That is the domain of comprehensive texts in infectious disease. Rather, this chapter is intended to serve as a very broad overview of the bacteria commonly associated with infections at specific body sites and with specific clinical manifestations (Tables 15-1 to 15-5). Because many factors influence the relative frequency with which specific organisms cause disease (e.g., age, underlying disease, epidemiologic factors, host immunity), no attempt is made to define all the factors associated with disease caused by specific organisms. That material is provided, in part, in the chapters that follow and in infectious disease texts. Furthermore, the roles of fungi, viruses, and parasites are not considered here but rather in the later sections of this book.

Tables 15-1 and 15-2 illustrate the complexity of summarizing the role of bacteria in infectious diseases. Simply stated, Table 15-1 is a list of bacteria and the diseases they cause and Table 15-2 is a list of diseases and the bacteria associated with the diseases. Unfortunately, neither list is comprehensive; more diseases are associated with many of the bacteria, and the list of bacteria responsible for most of the diseases is not complete. These two tables represent different approaches to understanding the role of bacteria in infectious disease. The overall approach taken in this book is to study the organisms, learning their biology in the context of their ability to cause disease. We have taken this traditional approach because we feel this provides a foundation for the student to understand the disease process. However, we recognize that the patient presents with a disease syndrome, and the student must remember which organisms can be responsible. For this reason, Table 15-2 is presented. In this edition of *Medical Microbiology,* we are using these summary chapters to introduce the discussions of bacteria, viruses, fungi, and parasites. We recognize that discussions of a large collection of organisms may be confusing for many students when they are introduced to microbiology. We hope that using these chapters as an introduction may provide students with a useful framework for cataloging the variety of organisms responsible for similar diseases.

Table 15-1 Overview of Selected Bacterial Pathogens

Organism	Clinical Features	Epidemiologic Features	Treatment
Aerobic and Facultatively Anaerobic Gram-Positive Cocci			
Enterococcus faecalis and *Enterococcus faecium*	Urinary tract infections, peritonitis, bacteremia, endocarditis	Elderly patients and patients who have been hospitalized for extended periods receiving broad-spectrum antibiotics	Penicillin/ampicillin or vancomycin; combined with gentamicin for endocarditis or severe infections; linezolid, daptomycin, tigecycline, or quinupristin/dalfopristin

Continued

 Table 15-1 **Overview of Selected Bacterial Pathogens—cont'd**

Organism	Clinical Features	Epidemiologic Features	Treatment
Staphylococcus aureus	Suppurative infections: impetigo, folliculitis, furuncles, carbuncles, wounds Disseminated infections: bacteremia, endocarditis, pneumonia, empyema, osteomyelitis, septic arthritis Toxin-mediated infections: toxic shock syndrome, scalded skin syndrome, food poisoning	Colonize human skin and mucosal surfaces; survive on environmental surfaces; able to grow at temperature extremes and in high salt concentrations	Localized infections: trimethoprim/sulfamethoxazole, doxycycline, clindamycin or linezolid Systemic infections: oxacillin (if susceptible) or vancomycin; daptomycin, tigecycline, or linezolid
Staphylococcus, coagulase-negative	Wound infections, urinary tract infections, catheter and shunt infections, prosthetic device infections	Colonize human skin and mucosal surfaces; survive on environmental surfaces; able to grow at temperature extremes	As with *S. aureus*
Streptococcus pyogenes (group A)	Suppurative infections: pharyngitis, scarlet fever, sinusitis, skin and soft-tissue infection (impetigo, erysipelas, cellulitis, necrotizing fasciitis), toxic shock–like syndrome; bacteremia Nonsuppurative infections: rheumatic fever, glomerulonephritis	Diverse populations	Penicillin V, amoxicillin; macrolides, cephalosporins, clindamycin, vancomycin; surgical debridement for necrotizing fasciitis
Streptococcus agalactiae (group B)	Neonatal disease (early onset, late onset): bacteremia, pneumonia, meningitis; postpartum endometritis, wound infection, skin and soft-tissue infection, urinary tract infections, pneumonia	Neonates; pregnant women; patients with diabetes, cancer, or alcoholism	Penicillin; cephalosporins or vancomycin
Viridans streptococci	Abscess formation; septicemia in neutropenic patients; subacute endocarditis; odontogenic infections; dental caries	Patients with abnormal heart valves; neutropenic patients	Penicillin; penicillin plus aminoglycoside; broad-spectrum cephalosporin, vancomycin
Streptococcus pneumoniae	Pneumonia, sinusitis, otitis media, meningitis, bacteremia, endocarditis, spontaneous bacterial peritonitis, septic arthritis	Diverse: neonates, children, adults with chronic diseases, elderly persons	Penicillin; levofloxacin, cephalosporins, clindamycin; broad-spectrum cephalosporins, vancomycin
Aerobic or Facultatively-Anaerobic Gram-Positive Rods			
Bacillus anthracis	Anthrax: cutaneous, GI, inhalation	Animal workers; microbiological accidents; bioterrorism	Cutaneous anthrax: amoxicillin Inhalation anthrax: ciprofloxacin or doxycycline plus rifampin, vancomycin, penicillin, imipenem, clindamycin or clarithromycin
Bacillus cereus	Food poisoning; ocular infections; bacteremia; pneumonia	Contaminated food; traumatic eye injury with introduction of contaminated soil; injection drug use	Food poisoning: symptomatic treatment Other infections: fluoroquinolones or vancomycin, clindamycin, gentamicin
Corynebacterium diphtheriae	Diphtheria: respiratory, cutaneous	Spread by respiratory droplets to unimmunized individuals	Penicillin or erythromycin to eliminate organism and terminate toxin production; immunize with diphtheria toxoid
Corynebacterium jeikeium	Opportunistic infections; bacteremia	Immunocompromised patients at increased risk	Vancomycin
Corynebacterium urealyticum	Urinary tract infections, including pyelonephritis with calculi; bacteremia	Risk factors include immunosuppression, underlying genitourinary disorders, antecedent urologic procedures, prior antibiotic therapy	Vancomycin

 Table 15-1 **Overview of Selected Bacterial Pathogens—cont'd**

Organism	Clinical Features	Epidemiologic Features	Treatment
Erysipelothrix rhusiophathiae	Erysipeloid (localized skin lesion); generalized cutaneous infection; septicemia	Occupational disease of butchers, meat processors, farmers, poultry workers, fish handlers, and veterinarians	Localized infection: penicillin, ciprofloxacin, clindamycin Disseminated infection: ceftriaxone, imipenem
Listeria monocytogenes	Early onset neonatal disease: granulomatosis infantiseptica Late-onset neonatal disease: meningitis with septicemia; flulike illness in adults; bacteremia or disseminated disease in pregnant women or patients with cell-mediated immune defect; meningitis	Immunocompromised hosts, elderly persons, neonates, pregnant women; ingestion of contaminated food	Gentamicin plus penicillin or ampicillin
Acid-Fast Bacteria			
Mycobacterium avium complex	Localized pulmonary disease; disseminated disease with multiorgan involvement	Localized disease in patients with chronic pulmonary disease; disseminated disease in AIDS and other immunocompromised patients	Clarithromycin or azithromycin combined with rifabutin or ethambutol
Mycobacterium leprae	Leprosy: range from tuberculoid form to lepromatous form	Close contact with infected individual most likely responsible for spread	Dapsone and rifampicin for tuberculoid form; add clofazimine for lepromatous form
Mycobacterium tuberculosis complex	Tuberculosis: pulmonary, extrapulmonary	All ages with HIV-infected patients at greatest risk for active disease	Multidrug therapy with isoniazid (INH), rifampin, ethambutol, and pyrazinamide, followed by INH plus rifampin; multidrug-resistant strains
Nocardia	Bronchopulmonary disease; brain abscess; primary or secondary cutaneous infections: mycetoma, lymphocutaneous infections, cellulitis, subcutaneous abscess	Opportunistic pathogen in immunocompetent patients with chronic pulmonary disease or immunocompromised patients with T-cell deficiencies	Trimethoprim/sulfamethoxazole for cutaneous infections in immunocompetent patients; add amikacin, imipenem, or broad-spectrum cephalosporin for disseminated infection or infection in immunocompromised patient
Rhodococcus equi	Bronchopulmonary disease; opportunistic infections in immunocompetent patients	Pathogen most commonly found in immunocompromised patients (e.g., AIDS patients, transplant recipients)	Combination therapy with vancomycin, carbapenems, aminoglycosides, ciprofloxacin, rifampin
Aerobic Gram-Negative Cocci			
Neisseria gonorrhoeae	Gonorrhea, septic arthritis; pelvic inflammatory disease; perihepatitis; septicemia	Sexual transmission, asymptomatic carriage	Ceftriaxone plus azithromycin or doxycycline
Neisseria meningitidis	Meningitis, septicemia (meningococcemia); pneumonia, arthritis, urethritis	Carrier state, aerosol transmission, most common in children and young adults	Ceftriaxone or cefotaxime
Aerobic and Facultatively Anaerobic Gram-Negative Rods			
Acinetobacter	Opportunistic infections: pneumonia, septicemia, urinary tract infections, wound infections	Nosocomial infections	Imipenem or ceftazidime combined with aminoglycosides for serious infections; multidrug resistance increasingly common
Aeromonas	Wound infections, gastroenteritis	Healthy and immunocompromised patients	Ciprofloxacin; trimethoprim/sulfamethoxazole, gentamicin, or amikacin as alternative therapy
Bartonella bacilliformis	Carrión disease (Oroya fever) + "Peruvian wart"	Bite of infected sandfly	Chloramphenicol + penicillin
Bartonella henselae	Bacillary angiomatosis (BA), subacute endocarditis, cat-scratch disease (CSD)	Healthy (endocarditis, CSD) and immunocompromised patients (BA)	Azithromycin; erythromycin or doxycycline

Continued

 Table 15-1 **Overview of Selected Bacterial Pathogens—cont'd**

Organism	Clinical Features	Epidemiologic Features	Treatment
Bartonella quintana	Trench fever (TF), BA, subacute endocarditis	Healthy (TF, endocarditis) or immunocompromised patients (BA)	Azithromycin; erythromycin or doxycycline
Bordetella pertussis, B. parapertussis	Pertussis (whooping cough)	Aerosol transmission; severe diseases in infants, milder in adults	Supportive therapy, erythromycin (or other macrolide) to decrease infectivity; azithromycin for contact prophylaxis
Brucella	Brucellosis	Exposure to infected goats, sheep, cattle, or other animals; bioterrorism	Doxycycline plus rifampin; trimethoprim/sulfamethoxazole
Burkholderia cepacia complex	Pulmonary infections, opportunistic infections	Compromised individuals, especially cystic fibrosis and chronic granulomatous disease patients	Trimethoprim/sulfamethoxazole; piperacillin, ceftazidime, or ciprofloxacin as alternative therapy if trimethoprim/sulfamethoxazole resistant
Burkholderia pseudomallei	Melioidosis (asymptomatic to severe pulmonary disease)	Opportunistic pathogen	Trimethoprim/sulfamethoxazole + ceftazidime
Campylobacter jejuni, C. coli, C. upsaliensis	Gastroenteritis	Zoonotic infection following ingestion of contaminated food, milk, or water	Self-limited; severe infections treated with azithromycin; tetracycline or fluoroquinolones used as alternative therapy
Campylobacter fetus	Septicemia, meningitis, gastroenteritis, spontaneous abortion	Infects elderly, immunocompromised patients	Aminoglycosides, carbapenems, chloramphenicol
Cardiobacterium hominis	Subacute endocarditis	Opportunistic pathogen in patients with previously damaged heart valve	Penicillin or ampicillin
Eikenella corrodens	Subacute endocarditis, wound infections	Human bite wounds; opportunistic pathogen in patients with previously damaged heart valve	Penicillin, cephalosporins, tetracycline, or fluoroquinolones
Escherichia coli: enteropathogenic (EPEC)	Watery diarrhea and vomiting	Infants in developing countries	Unknown
E. coli: Shiga toxin–producing (STEC)	Watery diarrhea, hemorrhagic colitis, hemolytic uremic syndrome	Foodborne, waterborne outbreaks in developed countries	Antibiotics contraindicated
E. coli: enterotoxigenic (ETEC)	Watery diarrhea	Childhood diarrhea in developing countries; travelers' diarrhea	Ciprofloxacin shortens course (high level of resistance)
E. coli: enteroaggregative (EAEC)	Diarrhea with mucus	Childhood diarrhea	Fluoroquinolones used in AIDS patients
E. coli: enteroinvasive (EIEC)	Watery diarrhea, hemorrhagic colitis	Childhood diarrhea in developing countries	Antibiotics reduce duration of disease and infectivity
E. coli: uropathogenic	Cystitis, pyelonephritis	Sexually active women	Trimethoprim/sulfamethoxazole, fluoroquinolones
E. coli: meningitis associated	Acute meningitis	Neonates	Extended-spectrum cephalosporins
Francisella tularensis	Tularemia: ulceroglandular, oculoglandular, pneumonic	Tick bites, exposure to infected rabbits, bioterrorism	Doxycycline or ciprofloxacin for mild infections; add gentamicin for serious infections
Haemophilus influenzae	Encapsulated type b strains: meningitis, septicemia, cellulitis, epiglottitis Unencapsulated strains: otitis media, sinusitis, bronchitis, pneumonia	Aerosol transmission in young unimmunized children; spread from upper respiratory tract in elderly patients with chronic respiratory disease	Broad-spectrum cephalosporin, azithromycin, or fluoroquinolone; many strains resistant to ampicillin
Helicobacter pylori	Gastritis, peptic and duodenal ulcers; gastric adenocarcinoma	Infections particularly common in people in low socioeconomic class or in developing countries	Multidrug therapy: omeprazole + amoxicillin + clarithromycin

Table 15-1 Overview of Selected Bacterial Pathogens—cont'd

Organism	Clinical Features	Epidemiologic Features	Treatment
Kingella kingae	Subacute endocarditis	Opportunistic pathogen in patients with previously damaged heart valve	β-Lactam with β-lactamase inhibitor, cephalosporins, macrolides, tetracycline, fluoroquinolone
Klebsiella pneumoniae	Pneumonia, urinary tract infections	Nosocomial infection; alcoholism	Cephalosporins, fluoroquinolones
Legionella pneumophila	Legionnaires' disease (pneumonia), Pontiac fever (flulike illness)	Waterborne; elderly and immunocompromised patients	Macrolides (erythromycin, azithromycin, clarithromycin); fluoroquinolones as alternative therapy
Moraxella catarrhalis	Bronchopneumonia, ear or eye infections	Children, patients with compromised pulmonary system	Cephalosporins, amoxicillin/clavulanic acid
Proteus mirabilis	Urinary tract infections, wound infections	Structural abnormality in urinary tract	Amoxicillin, trimethoprim/sulfamethoxazole, cephalosporins, fluoroquinolones
Pseudomonas aeruginosa	Pulmonary; primary skin and soft-tissue infection: burn wounds, folliculitis, osteochondritis; urinary tract infections; ear or eye infections; bacteremia; endocarditis	Nosocomial infections	Combination therapy generally required (e.g., aminoglycoside with extended-spectrum cephalosporins, piperacillin-tazobactam, or carbapenem)
Salmonella enterica	Diarrhea; enteric fever (serovar Typhi)	Contaminated food; immunocompromised patients at higher risk for bacteremia	May prolong carrier state in simple diarrhea treatment; fluoroquinolones for enteric fever
Serratia, Enterobacter	Pneumonia, urinary tract infections, wound infections	Nosocomial infections	Carbapenems, piperacillin-tazobactam
Shigella	Bacillary dysentery	Contaminated food or water; person-to-person spread	Ampicillin, trimethoprim/sulfamethoxazole, fluoroquinolones
Stenotrophomonas maltophilia	Wide variety of local and systemic infections	Nosocomial infections	Trimethoprim/sulfamethoxazole; doxycycline or ceftazidime as alternative
Streptobacillus moniliformis	Rat-bite fever; Haverhill fever	Bite of rat or other small rodent; ingestion of contaminated food or water	Penicillin, tetracycline
Vibrio cholerae	Severe watery diarrhea, septicemia	Children and adults in developing countries	Rehydration; azithromycin, doxycycline, or ciprofloxacin as alternative
Vibrio parahaemolyticus	Water diarrhea, wound infection	Seafood-borne outbreaks	Rehydration for diarrhea; doxycycline + ceftriaxone for wound infection
Vibrio vulnificus	Wound infections, primary septicemia	Compromised individuals with preexisting hepatic or chronic diseases	Minocycline or doxycycline + ceftriaxone or cefotaxime
Anaerobes			
Actinomyces	Actinomycosis: cervicofacial, thoracic, abdominal, pelvic, central nervous system	Colonizes human mucosal surface (oropharynx, intestine, vagina)	Surgical debridement; penicillin; carbapenems, macrolides, or clindamycin as alternative drugs
Bacteroides fragilis	Polymicrobial infections of abdomen, female genital tract, cutaneous and soft tissues	Normal inhabitant of the GI tract	Metronidazole; carbapenems; piperacillin/tazobactam
Clostridium botulinum	Botulism: foodborne, infant, wound	Found in environment (e.g., soil, water, sewage) and GI tract of animals and humans	Ventilatory support + metronidazole or penicillin + trivalent botulinum antitoxin
Clostridium difficile	Antibiotic-associated diarrhea; pseudomembranous colitis	Colonized human GI tract and female genital tract; contaminates hospital environment; prior antibiotic use	Discontinue implicated antibiotics; metronidazole or vancomycin

Continued

Table 15-1 Overview of Selected Bacterial Pathogens—cont'd

Organism	Clinical Features	Epidemiologic Features	Treatment
Clostridium perfringens	Soft-tissue infections: cellulitis, myositis, myonecrosis; food poisoning; enteritis necroticans; septicemia	Found in environment (e.g., soil, water, sewage) and GI tract of animals and humans	Surgical debridement + penicillin
Clostridium tetani	Tetanus: generalized, localized, neonatal	Found in environment (e.g., soil, water, sewage) and GI tract of animals and humans	Wound debridement + penicillin or metronidazole + vaccination with tetanus toxoid + passive immunization
Propionibacterium acnes	Acne; opportunistic infections (e.g., of catheters, shunts, and other prosthetic devices)	Colonizes human skin and mucosal surfaces	Acne treated with benzoyl peroxide + clindamycin or erythromycin
Anaplasma, Ehrlichia, Rickettsia, Coxiella, Chlamydia,* and *Chlamydophila			
Anaplasma phagocytophilum	Anaplasmosis (granulocytic ehrlichiosis)	Transmission by tick bite *(Ixodes)*	Doxycycline; rifampin as alternative therapy
Chlamydia trachomatis	Trachoma; neonatal conjunctivitis and pneumonia; urethritis; cervicitis; proctitis; salpingitis; lymphogranuloma venereum	Trachoma in developing countries; exposure to infected secretions during birth or sexual contact	Doxycycline, erythromycin, or azithromycin; fluoroquinolones
Chlamydophila pneumoniae	Pneumonia; cardiovascular disease (?)	Children, young adults	Macrolides; doxycycline, levofloxacin
Chlamydophila psittaci	Pneumonia	Exposure to birds and their secretions	Doxycycline or macrolides
Coxiella burnetii	Q fever: acute (fever, headache, chills, myalgias, granulomatous hepatitis) or chronic (endocarditis, hepatic dysfunction)	Persons exposed to infected livestock; primarily acquired by inhalation; relatively uncommon in United States	Acute disease: doxycycline Chronic disease: doxycycline + hydroxychloroquine; fluoroquinolones used as alternative to doxycycline
Ehrlichia chaffeensis	Monocytic ehrlichiosis	Transmission by tick bite *(Amblyomma)*	Doxycycline; rifampin used as alternative therapy
Mycoplasma pneumoniae	Tracheobronchitis; pharyngitis; atypical pneumonia	Symptomatic disease more common in children than adults; severe disease in patients with hypogammaglobulinemia	Erythromycin, doxycycline, fluoroquinolones
Rickettsia rickettsii	Rocky Mountain spotted fever	Most prevalent in hikers and other individuals who spend a lot of time outdoors; transmission by tick bite (*Dermacentor* in United States)	Doxycycline; fluoroquinolones used as alternative therapy
Spirochetes			
Borrelia burgdorferi, B. garinii, B. afzelii	Lyme disease: erythema migrans; cardiac, neurologic, or rheumatologic abnormalities	Transmission by ticks *(Ixodes)*	Early: amoxicillin, doxycycline, cefuroxime; late: ceftriaxone, cefotaxime, or penicillin G
Borrelia recurrentis	Epidemic relapsing fever	Transmission by human body louse; no animal host	Tetracyclines; penicillins
Borrelia species	Endemic relapsing fever	Transmission by tick bite *(Ornithodoros)*; rodent and small mammal reservoir	Tetracyclines; penicillins
Leptospira interrogans	Leptospirosis: mild, viral-like illness to severe multiorgan illness (Weil disease)	Transmission by exposure to infected urine or tissues of rodents, dogs, farm animals, wild animals	Penicillin; doxycycline
Treponema pallidum	Syphilis: primary, secondary, tertiary, congenital	Transmission congenitally or through sexual contact	Penicillins; doxycycline or azithromycin as alternative therapy

AAF, Aggregative adhesion fimbria; *AIDS,* acquired immunodeficiency syndrome; *EAEC,* enteroaggregative *E. coli; STEC,* Shiga toxin–producing *E. coli; EIEC,* enteroinvasive *E. coli; EPEC,* enteropathogenic *E. coli; ETEC,* enterotoxigenic *E. coli; GI,* gastrointestinal; *HIV,* human immunodeficiency virus.

 Table 15-2 **Summary of Bacterial Diseases**

System Affected	Pathogens
Upper Respiratory Infections	
Pharyngitis	***Streptococcus pyogenes,*** *Neisseria gonorrhoeae,* group C *Streptococcus, Arcanobacterium haemolyticum, Chlamydophila pneumoniae, Corynebacterium diphtheriae, Corynebacterium ulcerans, Mycoplasma pneumoniae, Francisella tularensis*
Sinusitis	***Streptococcus pneumoniae, Haemophilus influenzae, Moraxella catarrhalis,*** **mixed anaerobes and aerobes,** *Staphylococcus aureus,* group A *Streptococcus, Chlamydophila pneumoniae, Pseudomonas aeruginosa* and other gram-negative rods
Epiglottitis	*Haemophilus influenzae, Streptococcus pneumoniae, Staphylococcus aureus*
Ear Infections	
Otitis externa	***Pseudomonas aeruginosa, Staphylococcus aureus,*** group A *Streptococcus*
Otitis media	***Streptococcus pneumoniae, Haemophilus influenzae, Moraxella catarrhalis,*** *Staphylococcus aureus,* group A *Streptococcus,* mixed anaerobes and aerobes
Eye Infections	
Conjunctivitis	***Staphylococcus aureus, Streptococcus pneumoniae, Haemophilus aegyptius,*** *Neisseria gonorrhoeae, Pseudomonas aeruginosa, Francisella tularensis, Chlamydia trachomatis*
Keratitis	***Staphylococcus aureus, Streptococcus pneumoniae, Pseudomonas aeruginosa,*** group A *Streptococcus, Proteus mirabilis* and other Enterobacteriaceae, *Bacillus* species, *Neisseria gonorrhoeae*
Endophthalmitis	***Bacillus cereus, Staphylococcus aureus, Pseudomonas aeruginosa,*** coagulase-negative *Staphylococcus, Propionibacterium* species, *Corynebacterium* species
Pleuropulmonary and Bronchial Infections	
Bronchitis	***Moraxella catarrhalis, Haemophilus influenzae, Streptococcus pneumoniae,*** *Bordetella pertussis, Mycoplasma pneumoniae, Chlamydophila pneumoniae*
Empyema	***Staphylococcus aureus, Streptococcus pneumoniae,*** **group A *Streptococcus,*** *Bacteroides fragilis, Klebsiella pneumoniae* and other Enterobacteriaceae, *Actinomyces* species, *Nocardia* species, *Mycobacterium tuberculosis* and other species
Pneumonia	***Streptococcus pneumoniae, Staphylococcus aureus, Klebsiella pneumoniae,*** **other Enterobacteriaceae,** *Moraxella catarrhalis, Haemophilus influenzae, Neisseria meningitidis, Mycoplasma pneumoniae, Chlamydia trachomatis, Chlamydophila pneumoniae, Chlamydophila psittaci, Pseudomonas aeruginosa, Burkholderia* species, *Legionella* species, *Francisella tularensis, Bacteroides fragilis, Nocardia* species, *Rhodococcus equi, Mycobacterium tuberculosis* and other species, *Coxiella burnetii, Rickettsia rickettsii,* many other bacteria
Urinary Tract Infections	
Cystitis and pyelonephritis	***Escherichia coli, Proteus mirabilis,*** **other Enterobacteriaceae,** *Pseudomonas aeruginosa, Staphylococcus saprophyticus, Staphylococcus aureus, Staphylococcus epidermidis,* group B *Streptococcus, Enterococcus* species, *Aerococcus urinae, Mycobacterium tuberculosis*
Renal calculi	***Proteus mirabilis,*** *Morganella morganii, Klebsiella pneumoniae, Corynebacterium urealyticum, Staphylococcus saprophyticus, Ureaplasma urealyticum*
Renal abscess	***Staphylococcus aureus,*** mixed anaerobes and aerobes, *Mycobacterium tuberculosis*
Prostatitis	***Escherichia coli,*** *Klebsiella pneumoniae,* other Enterobacteriaceae, *Enterococcus* species, *Neisseria gonorrhoeae, Mycobacterium tuberculosis* and other species
Intraabdominal Infections	
Peritonitis	***Escherichia coli, Bacteroides fragilis*** and other species, ***Enterococcus* species,** *Klebsiella pneumoniae,* other Enterobacteriaceae, *Pseudomonas aeruginosa, Streptococcus pneumoniae, Staphylococcus aureus, Fusobacterium* species, *Clostridium* species, *Peptostreptococcus* species, *Neisseria gonorrhoeae, Chlamydia trachomatis, Mycobacterium tuberculosis*
Dialysis-associated peritonitis	**Coagulase-negative *Staphylococcus,*** *Staphylococcus aureus, Streptococcus* species, *Corynebacterium* species, *Propionibacterium* species, *Escherichia coli* and other Enterobacteriaceae, *Pseudomonas aeruginosa, Acinetobacter* species
Cardiovascular Infections	
Endocarditis	**Viridans *Streptococcus,* coagulase-negative *Staphylococcus,*** *Staphylococcus aureus, Aggregatibacter* species, *Cardiobacter hominis, Eikenella corrodens, Kingella kingii, Streptococcus pneumoniae, Abiotrophia* species, *Rothia mucilaginosa, Enterococcus* species, *Bartonella* species, *Coxiella burnetii, Brucella* species, *Erysipelothrix rhusiopathiae,* Enterobacteriaceae, *Pseudomonas aeruginosa, Corynebacterium* species, *Propionibacterium* species

Continued

Table 15-2 **Summary of Bacterial Diseases—cont'd**

System Affected	Pathogens
Myocarditis	***Staphylococcus aureus,*** *Corynebacterium diphtheriae, Clostridium perfringens,* group A *Streptococcus, Borrelia burgdorferi, Neisseria meningitidis, Mycoplasma pneumoniae, Chlamydophila pneumoniae, Chlamydophila psittaci, Rickettsia rickettsii, Orientia tsutsugamushi*
Pericarditis	***Staphylococcus aureus,*** *Streptococcus pneumoniae, Neisseria gonorrhoeae, Neisseria meningitidis, Mycoplasma pneumoniae, Mycobacterium tuberculosis* and other species
Sepsis	
General sepsis	***Staphylococcus aureus,* coagulase-negative *Staphylococcus, Escherichia coli,*** *Klebsiella* species, *Enterobacter* species, *Proteus mirabilis,* other Enterobacteriaceae, *Streptococcus pneumoniae* and other species, *Enterococcus* species, *Pseudomonas aeruginosa,* many other bacteria
Transfusion-associated sepsis	**Coagulase-negative *Staphylococcus,*** *Staphylococcus aureus, Yersinia enterocolitica, Pseudomonas fluorescens* group, *Salmonella* species, other Enterobacteriaceae, *Campylobacter jejuni* and other species, *Bacillus cereus* and other species
Septic thrombophlebitis	***Staphylococcus aureus, Bacteroides fragilis,*** *Klebsiella* species, *Enterobacter* species, *Pseudomonas aeruginosa, Fusobacterium* species, *Campylobacter fetus*
Central Nervous System Infections	
Meningitis	**Group B *Streptococcus, Streptococcus pneumoniae, Neisseria meningitidis, Listeria monocytogenes, Haemophilus influenzae,*** *Escherichia coli,* other Enterobacteriaceae, *Staphylococcus aureus,* coagulase-negative *Staphylococcus, Propionibacterium* species, *Nocardia* species, *Mycobacterium tuberculosis* and other species, *Borrelia burgdorferi, Leptospira* species, *Treponema pallidum, Brucella* species
Encephalitis	*Listeria monocytogenes, Treponema pallidum, Leptospira* species, *Actinomyces* species, *Nocardia* species, *Borrelia* species, *Rickettsia rickettsii, Coxiella burnetii, Mycoplasma pneumoniae, Mycobacterium tuberculosis* and other species
Brain abscess	***Staphylococcus aureus, Fusobacterium* species, *Peptostreptococcus* species, other anaerobic cocci,** Enterobacteriaceae, *Pseudomonas aeruginosa,* viridans *Streptococcus, Bacteroides* species, *Prevotella* species, *Porphyromonas* species, *Actinomyces* species, *Clostridium perfringens, Listeria monocytogenes, Nocardia* species, *Rhodococcus equi, Mycobacterium tuberculosis* and other species
Subdural empyema	***Staphylococcus aureus, Streptococcus pneumoniae,*** group B *Streptococcus, Neisseria meningitidis,* mixed anaerobes and aerobes
Skin and Soft-Tissue Infections	
Impetigo	**Group A *Streptococcus, Staphylococcus aureus***
Folliculitis	***Staphylococcus aureus, Pseudomonas aeruginosa***
Furuncles and carbuncles	***Staphylococcus aureus***
Paronychia	***Staphylococcus aureus,* group A *Streptococcus,*** *Pseudomonas aeruginosa*
Erysipelas	**Group A *Streptococcus***
Cellulitis	**Group A *Streptococcus, Staphylococcus aureus,*** *Haemophilus influenzae,* many other bacteria
Necrotizing cellulitis and fasciitis	**Group A *Streptococcus, Clostridium perfringens*** and other species, *Bacteroides fragilis,* other anaerobes, Enterobacteriaceae, *Pseudomonas aeruginosa*
Bacillary angiomatosis	***Bartonella henselae, Bartonella quintana***
Infections of burns	***Pseudomonas aeruginosa,*** *Enterobacter* species, *Enterococcus* species, *Staphylococcus aureus,* group A *Streptococcus,* many other bacteria
Bite wounds	***Eikenella corrodens, Pasteurella multocida,*** *Pasteurella canis, Staphylococcus aureus,* group A *Streptococcus,* mixed anaerobes and aerobes, many gram-negative rods
Surgical wounds	***Staphylococcus aureus,*** coagulase-negative *Staphylococcus,* groups A and B streptococci, *Clostridium perfringens, Corynebacterium* species, many other bacteria
Traumatic wounds	***Bacillus* species, *Staphylococcus aureus,*** group A *Streptococcus,* many gram-negative rods, rapidly growing mycobacteria
Gastrointestinal Infections	
Gastritis	***Helicobacter pylori***
Gastroenteritis	***Salmonella* species, *Shigella* species, *Campylobacter jejuni* and *coli, Escherichia coli* (STEC, EIEC, EHEC, EPEC, EAggEC), *Vibrio cholerae, Vibrio parahaemolyticus, Bacillus cereus,*** *Yersinia enterocolitica, Edwardsiella tarda, Pseudomonas aeruginosa, Aeromonas* species, *Plesiomonas shigelloides, Bacteroides fragilis, Clostridium botulinum, Clostridium perfringens, Clostridium difficile*

 Table 15-2 Summary of Bacterial Diseases—cont'd

System Affected	Pathogens
Food intoxication	***Staphylococcus aureus, Bacillus cereus,*** *Clostridium botulinum, Clostridium perfringens*
Proctitis	***Neisseria gonorrhoeae,*** *Chlamydia trachomatis, Treponema pallidum*
Bone and Joint Infections	
Osteomyelitis	***Staphylococcus aureus,*** *Salmonella* species, *Mycobacterium tuberculosis* and other species, β-hemolytic *Streptococcus, Streptococcus pneumoniae, Escherichia coli,* and other Enterobacteriaceae, *Pseudomonas aeruginosa,* many less common bacteria
Arthritis	***Staphylococcus aureus, Neisseria gonorrhoeae,*** *Streptococcus pneumoniae, Salmonella* species, *Pasteurella multocida, Mycobacterium* species
Prosthetic-associated infections	***Staphylococcus aureus,*** **coagulase-negative *Staphylococcus,*** group A *Streptococcus,* viridans *Streptococcus, Corynebacterium* species, *Propionibacterium* species, *Peptostreptococcus* species, other anaerobic cocci
Genital Infections	
Genital ulcers	***Treponema pallidum, Haemophilus ducreyi,*** *Chlamydia trachomatis, Francisella tularensis, Klebsiella granulomatis, Mycobacterium tuberculosis*
Urethritis	***Neisseria gonorrhoeae, Chlamydia trachomatis, Mycoplasma genitalium,*** *Ureaplasma urealyticum*
Vaginitis	***Mycoplasma hominis, Mobiluncus* species, other anaerobic species,** *Gardnerella vaginalis*
Cervicitis	***Neisseria gonorrhoeae, Chlamydia trachomatis, Mycoplasma genitalium,*** *Neisseria meningitidis,* group B *Streptococcus, Mycobacterium tuberculosis, Actinomyces* species
Granulomatous Infections	
General	***Mycobacterium tuberculosis* and other species, *Nocardia* species, *Treponema pallidum,*** *Brucella* species, *Francisella tularensis, Listeria monocytogenes, Burkholderia pseudomallei, Actinomyces* species, *Bartonella henselae, Tropheryma whippelii, Chlamydia trachomatis, Coxiella burnetii*

Organisms in boldface are the most common pathogens.

EIEC, Enteroinvasive *E. coli; EPEC,* enteropathogenic *E. coli; ETEC,* enterotoxigenic *E. coli; EAggEC,* enteroaggregative *E. coli; STEC,* Shiga toxin–producing (enterohemorrhagic) *E. coli.*

 Table 15-3 Selected Bacteria Associated with Foodborne Diseases

Organism	Implicated Food(s)
Aeromonas species	Meats, produce, dairy products
Bacillus cereus	Fried rice, meats, vegetables
***Brucella* species**	Unpasteurized dairy products, meat
***Campylobacter* species**	Poultry, unpasteurized dairy products
Clostridium botulinum	Vegetables, fruits, fish, honey
Clostridium perfringens	Beef, poultry, pork, gravy
Escherichia coli	Beef, unpasteurized milk, fruits and juices, vegetables, lettuce
Francisella tularensis	Rabbit meat
Listeria monocytogenes	Unpasteurized dairy products, coleslaw, poultry, cold-cut meats
Plesiomonas shigelloides	Seafood
***Salmonella* species**	Poultry, unpasteurized dairy products
Shigella species	Eggs, lettuce
Staphylococcus aureus	Ham, poultry, egg dishes, pastries
Streptococcus, group A	Egg dishes
***Vibrio* species**	Shellfish
Yersinia enterocolitica	Unpasteurized dairy products, pork

Organisms in boldface are the most common foodborne pathogens.

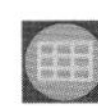 Table 15-4 Selected Bacteria Associated with Waterborne Diseases

Organism	Disease
Aeromonas species	Gastroenteritis, wound infections, septicemia
Campylobacter species	Gastroenteritis
Escherichia coli	Gastroenteritis
Francisella tularensis	Tularemia
***Legionella* species**	Respiratory disease
***Leptospira* species**	Systemic disease
Mycobacterium marinum	Cutaneous infection
Plesiomonas shigelloides	Gastroenteritis
***Pseudomonas* species**	Dermatitis
Salmonella species	Gastroenteritis
Shigella species	Gastroenteritis
***Vibrio* species**	Gastroenteritis, wound infection, septicemia
Yersinia enterocolitica	Gastroenteritis

Organisms in boldface are the most common waterborne pathogens.

Table 15-5 Arthropod-Associated Disease

Arthropod	Organism	Disease
Tick	*Anaplasma phagocytophilum*	Human anaplasmosis (formerly called human granulocytic ehrlichiosis)
	Borrelia afzelii	Lyme disease
	Borrelia burgdorferi	Lyme disease
	Borrelia garinii	Lyme disease
	Borrelia, other species	Endemic relapsing fever
	Coxiella burnetii	Q fever
	Ehrlichia chaffeensis	Human monocytic ehrlichiosis
	Ehrlichia ewingii	Canine (human) granulocytic ehrlichiosis
	Francisella tularensis	Tularemia
	Rickettsia rickettsii	Rocky Mountain spotted fever
Flea	*Rickettsia prowazekii*	Sporadic typhus
	Rickettsia typhi	Murine typhus
	Yersinia pestis	Plague
Lice	*Bartonella quintana*	Trench fever
	Borrelia recurrentis	Epidemic relapsing fever
	Rickettsia prowazekii	Epidemic typhus
Mite	*Orientia tsutsugamushi*	Scrub typhus
	Rickettsia akari	Rickettsialpox
Sandfly	*Bartonella bacilliformis*	Bartonellosis (Carrión disease)

Bibliography

Borriello P, Murray P, Funke G: *Topley & Wilson's microbiology and microbial infections: bacteriology*, ed 10, London, 2005, Hodder.

Longo DL, Fauci AS, Kasper DL, et al: *Harrison's principles of internal medicine*, ed 18, New York, 2011, McGraw-Hill.

Mandell GL, Bennett JE, Dolin R: *Principles and practice of infectious diseases*, ed 7, New York, 2009, Churchill Livingstone.

Murray P, Shea Y: *Pocket guide to clinical microbiology*, ed 3, Washington, DC, 2004, American Society for Microbiology Press.

Versalovic J, Carroll KC, Funke G, et al: *Manual of clinical microbiology*, ed 10, Washington, DC, 2011, American Society for Microbiology Press.

CHAPTER

16 LABORATORY DIAGNOSIS OF BACTERIAL DISEASES

The laboratory diagnosis of bacterial diseases requires that the appropriate specimen is collected, delivered expeditiously to the laboratory in the appropriate transport system, and processed in a manner that will maximize detection of the most likely pathogens. Collection of the proper specimen and its rapid delivery to the clinical laboratory are primarily the responsibility of the patient's physician, whereas the clinical microbiologist selects the appropriate transport systems and detection method (i.e., microscopy, culture, antigen or antibody detection, nucleic acid–based tests). These responsibilities are not mutually exclusive. The microbiologist should be prepared to instruct the physician about what specimens should be collected if a particular diagnosis is suspected, and the physician must provide the microbiologist with information about the clinical diagnosis so that the right tests are selected. This chapter is designed to provide an overview of specimen collection and transport, as well as the methods used in the microbiology laboratory for the detection and identification of bacteria. Because it is beyond the scope of this chapter to cover this subject exhaustively, the student is referred to the citations in the Bibliography and the individual chapters that follow for more detailed information.

• Specimen Collection, Transport, and Processing

Guidelines for proper collection and transport of specimens are summarized in the following text and Table 16-1.

Blood

The culture of blood is one of the most important procedures performed in the clinical microbiology laboratory. The success of this test is directly related to the methods used to collect the blood sample. The most important factor that determines the success of a blood culture is the volume of blood processed. For example, 40% more cultures are positive for organisms if 20 ml rather than 10 ml of blood are cultured, because more than half of all septic patients have less than one organism per milliliter of blood. Approximately 20 ml of blood should be collected from an adult for each blood culture, and proportionally smaller volumes should be collected from children and neonates. Because many hospitalized patients are susceptible to infections with organisms colonizing their skin, careful disinfection of the patient's skin is important.

Bacteremia and **fungemia** are defined as the presence of bacteria and fungi, respectively, in the blood, and these infections are referred to collectively as **septicemia.** Clinical studies have shown that septicemia can be continuous or intermittent. **Continuous septicemia** occurs primarily in patients with intravascular infections (e.g., endocarditis, septic thrombophlebitis, infections associated with intravascular catheter) or with overwhelming sepsis (e.g., septic shock). **Intermittent septicemia** occurs in patients with localized infections (e.g., lungs, urinary tract, soft tissues). The timing of blood collection is not important for patients with continuous septicemia but may be important for patients with intermittent septicemia. In addition, because clinical signs of sepsis (e.g., fever, chills, hypotension) are a response to the release of endotoxins or exotoxins from the organisms, these signs occur as long as 1 hour after the organisms entered the blood. Thus few to no organisms may be in the blood when the patient becomes febrile. For this reason, it is recommended that two to three blood samples should be collected, with the first two simultaneously before antibiotics are administered and the third culture at a random time during a 24-hour period.

Most blood samples are inoculated directly into bottles filled with enriched nutrient broths. To ensure the maximal recovery of important organisms, two bottles of media should be inoculated for each culture (10 ml of blood per bottle). When these inoculated bottles are received in the laboratory, they are incubated at 37° C and inspected at regular intervals for evidence of microbial growth. In most laboratories this is accomplished using automated blood culture instruments. When growth is detected, the broths are subcultured to isolate the organism for identification and antimicrobial susceptibility testing. Most clinically significant isolates are detected within the first 1 to 2 days of incubation; however, all cultures should be incubated for a minimum of 5 to 7 days. More prolonged incubation is generally unnecessary. Because few organisms are typically present in the blood of a septic patient, it is not worthwhile to perform a Gram stain of blood for microscopic analysis.

Cerebrospinal Fluid

Bacterial meningitis is a serious disease associated with high morbidity and mortality if the etiologic diagnosis is delayed. Because some common pathogens are labile (e.g., *Neisseria meningitidis, Streptococcus pneumoniae*), specimens of cerebrospinal fluid should be processed immediately after they are collected. Under no circumstance should the specimen

Table 16-1 Bacteriology Specimen Collection for Bacterial Pathogens

Specimen	Transport System	Specimen Volume	Other Considerations
Blood: routine bacterial culture	Blood culture bottle with nutrient media	Adults: 20 ml/culture Children: 5-10 ml/culture Neonates: 1 ml/culture	Skin should be disinfected with 70% alcohol followed by 0.5%-2% chlorhexidine; 2-3 cultures collected for each septic event; blood is divided equally into two bottles of nutrient media.
Blood: intracellular bacteria (e.g., *Brucella, Francisella, Neisseria* spp.)	Same as that for routine blood cultures; lysis-centrifugation system	Same as that for routine blood cultures	Considerations are same as those for routine blood cultures; release of intracellular bacteria may improve the organism's recovery; *Neisseria* spp. are inhibited by the anticoagulant (sodium polyanetholsulfonate).
Blood: *Leptospira* sp.	Sterile heparinized tube	1-5 ml	The specimen is useful only during the first week of illness; afterward, urine should be cultured.
Cerebrospinal fluid	Sterile screw-capped tube	Bacterial culture: 1-5 ml Mycobacterial culture: as large a volume as possible	The specimen must be collected aseptically and delivered immediately to the laboratory; it should not be exposed to heat or refrigeration.
Other normally sterile fluids (e.g., abdominal, chest, synovial, pericardial)	Small volume: sterile screw-capped tube Large volume: blood culture bottle with nutrient medium	As large a volume as possible	Specimens are collected with a needle and syringe; a swab is not used, because the quantity of collected specimen is inadequate; air should not be injected into culture bottle because it will inhibit growth of anaerobes.
Catheter	Sterile screw-capped tube or specimen cup	N/A	The entry site should be disinfected with alcohol; the catheter should be aseptically removed on receipt of the specimen in the laboratory; the catheter is rolled across a blood agar plate and then discarded.
Respiratory: throat	Swab immersed in transport medium	N/A	The area of inflammation is swabbed; exudate is collected if present; contact with saliva should be avoided because it can inhibit recovery of group A streptococci.
Respiratory: epiglottis	Collection of blood for culture	Same as for blood culture	Swabbing the epiglottis can precipitate complete airway closure; blood cultures should be collected for specific diagnosis.
Respiratory: sinuses	Sterile anaerobic tube or vial	1-5 ml	Specimens must be collected with a needle and syringe; culture of nasopharynx or oropharynx has no value; the specimen should be cultured for aerobic and anaerobic bacteria.
Respiratory: lower airways	Sterile screw-capped bottle; anaerobic tube or vial only for specimens collected by avoiding upper tract flora	1-2 ml	Expectorated sputum: if possible, the patient rinses mouth with water before collection of the specimen; the patient should cough deeply and expectorate lower airway secretions directly into a sterile cup; the collector should avoid contamination with saliva. Bronchoscopy specimen: anesthetics can inhibit growth of bacteria, so specimens should be processed immediately; if a "protected" bronchoscope is used, anaerobic cultures can be performed. Direct lung aspirate: specimens can be processed for aerobic and anaerobic bacteria.
Ear	Capped needleless syringe; sterile screw-capped tube	Whatever volume is collected	The specimen should be aspirated with a needle and syringe; culture of the external ear has no predictive value for otitis media.
Eye	Inoculate plates at bedside (seal and transport to laboratory immediately)	Whatever volume is collected	For infections on surface of eye, specimens are collected with a swab or by corneal scrapings; for deep-seated infections, aspiration of aqueous or vitreous fluid is performed; all specimens should be inoculated onto appropriate media at collection; delays will result in significant loss of organisms.

Table 16-1 Bacteriology Specimen Collection for Bacterial Pathogens—cont'd

Specimen	Transport System	Specimen Volume	Other Considerations
Exudates (transudates, drainage, ulcers)	Swab immersed in transport medium; aspirate in sterile screw-capped tube	Bacteria: 1-5 ml Mycobacteria: 3-5 ml	Contamination with surface material should be avoided; specimens are generally unsuitable for anaerobic culture.
Wounds (abscess, pus)	Aspirate in sterile screw-capped tube or sterile anaerobic tube or vial	1-5 ml of pus	Specimens should be collected with a sterile needle and syringe; a curette is used to collect specimen at base of wound.
Tissues	Sterile screw-capped tube; sterile anaerobic tube or vial	Representative sample from center and border of lesion	The specimen should be aseptically placed into appropriate sterile container; an adequate quantity of specimen must be collected to recover small numbers of organisms.
Urine: midstream	Sterile urine container	Bacteria: 1 ml Mycobacteria: ≥10 ml	Contamination of the specimen with bacteria from the urethra or vagina should be avoided; the first portion of the voided specimen is discarded; organisms can grow rapidly in urine, so specimens must be transported immediately to the laboratory, held in bacteriostatic preservative, or refrigerated.
Urine: catheterized	Sterile urine container	Bacteria: 1 ml Mycobacteria: ≥10 ml	Catheterization is not recommended for routine cultures (risk of inducing infection); the first portion of collected specimen is contaminated with urethral bacteria, so it should be discarded (similar to midstream voided specimen); the specimen must be transported rapidly to the laboratory.
Urine: suprapubic aspirate	Sterile anaerobic tube or vial	Bacteria: 1 ml Mycobacteria: ≥10 ml	This is an invasive specimen, so urethral bacteria are avoided; it is the only valid method available for collecting specimens for anaerobic culture; it is also useful for collection of specimens from children or adults unable to void uncontaminated specimens.
Genitals	Specially designed swabs for *Neisseria gonorrhoeae* and *Chlamydia* probes	N/A	The area of inflammation or exudate should be sampled; the endocervix (not vagina) and urethra should be cultured for optimal detection. The first voided urine specimen can be used for diagnosis of urethritis.
Feces (stool)	Sterile screw-capped container	N/A	Rapid transport to the laboratory is necessary to prevent production of acid (bactericidal for some enteric pathogens) by normal fecal bacteria; it is unsuitable for anaerobic culture; because a large number of different media will be inoculated, a swab should not be used for specimen collection.

N/A, Not applicable.

be refrigerated or placed directly into an incubator. The patient's skin is disinfected before lumbar puncture, and the cerebrospinal fluid is collected into sterile screw-capped tubes. When the specimen is received in the microbiology laboratory, it is concentrated by centrifugation, and the sediment is used to inoculate bacteriologic media and prepare a Gram stain. The laboratory technologist should notify the physician immediately if organisms are observed microscopically or in culture.

Other Normally Sterile Fluids

A variety of other normally sterile fluids may be collected for bacteriologic culture, including abdominal (peritoneal), chest (pleural), synovial, and pericardial fluids. If a large volume of fluid can be collected by aspiration (e.g., abdominal or chest fluids), it should be inoculated into blood culture bottles containing nutrient media. A small portion should also be sent to the laboratory in a sterile tube so that appropriate stains (e.g., Gram, acid-fast) can be prepared. Many organisms are associated with infections at these sites, including polymicrobial mixtures of aerobic and anaerobic organisms. For this reason, biological staining is useful for identifying the organisms responsible for the infection. Because relatively few organisms may be in the sample (because of the dilution of organisms or microbial elimination by the host immune response), it is important to culture as large a volume of fluid as possible. However, if only small quantities of fluid are collected, the specimen can be inoculated directly onto agar media and a tube of enriched broth media. Because anaerobes may also be present in the sample (particularly samples obtained from patients with intraabdominal or pulmonary infections), the specimen should not be exposed to oxygen and should be processed for anaerobes.

Upper Respiratory Tract Specimens

Most bacterial infections of the pharynx are caused by group A *Streptococcus.* Other bacteria that may cause pharyngitis include *Corynebacterium diphtheriae, Bordetella pertussis, Neisseria gonorrhoeae, Chlamydophila pneumoniae,* and *Mycoplasma pneumoniae.* However, special techniques are generally required to recover these organisms. Other potentially pathogenic bacteria, such as *Staphylococcus aureus, Streptococcus pneumoniae, Haemophilus influenzae,* Enterobacteriaceae, and *Pseudomonas aeruginosa,* may be present in the oropharynx but rarely cause pharyngitis.

A Dacron or calcium alginate swab should be used to collect pharyngeal specimens. The tonsillar areas, posterior pharynx, and any exudate or ulcerative area should be sampled. Contamination of the specimen with saliva should be avoided because bacteria in saliva can overgrow or inhibit the growth of group A streptococci. If a pseudomembrane is present (e.g., as with *C. diphtheriae* infections), a portion should be dislodged and submitted for culture. Group A streptococci and *C. diphtheriae* are very resistant to drying, so special precautions are not required for transport of the specimen to the laboratory. In contrast, specimens collected for the recovery of *B. pertussis* and *N. gonorrhoeae* should be inoculated onto culture media immediately after they are collected and before they are sent to the laboratory. Specimens obtained for the isolation of *C. pneumoniae* and *M. pneumoniae* should be transported in a special transport medium.

Group A streptococci can be detected directly in the clinical specimen through the use of immunoassays for the group-specific antigen. Although these tests are very specific and readily available, the older-generation tests were insensitive and could not be used reliably to exclude the diagnosis of group A streptococcal pharyngitis. Newer tests using more sensitive immunoassays and digital reading devices, as well as nucleic acid amplification tests, provide sensitivity equivalent to culture.

Other upper respiratory tract infections can involve the epiglottis and sinuses. Complete airway obstruction can be precipitated by attempts to culture the epiglottis (particularly in children); thus these cultures should never be performed. The specific diagnosis of a sinus infection requires (1) direct aspiration of the sinus, (2) appropriate anaerobic transport of the specimen to the laboratory (using a system that avoids exposing anaerobes to oxygen and drying), and (3) prompt processing. Culture of the nasopharynx or oropharynx is not useful and should not be performed. *S. pneumoniae, H. influenzae, Moraxella catarrhalis, S. aureus,* and anaerobes are the most common pathogens that cause sinusitis.

Lower Respiratory Tract Specimens

A variety of techniques can be used to collect lower respiratory tract specimens; these include expectoration, induction with saline, bronchoscopy, and direct aspiration through the chest wall. Because upper airway bacteria may contaminate expectorated sputa, specimens should be inspected microscopically to assess the magnitude of oral contamination. Specimens containing many squamous epithelial cells and no predominant bacteria in association with neutrophils should not be processed for culture. The presence of squamous epithelial cells indicates that the specimen has been contaminated with saliva. Such contamination can be avoided by obtaining the specimen using specially designed bronchoscopes or direct lung aspiration. If an anaerobic lung infection is suspected, these invasive procedures must be used because contamination of the specimen with upper airway microbes would render the specimen worthless. Most lower respiratory tract pathogens grow rapidly (within 2 to 3 days); however, some slow-growing bacteria, such as mycobacteria or nocardiae, will require extended incubation.

Ear and Eye

Tympanocentesis (i.e., aspiration of fluid from the middle ear) is required to make the specific diagnosis of a middle ear infection. This is unnecessary in most patients because the most common pathogens that cause these infections (*S. pneumoniae, H. influenzae,* and *M. catarrhalis*) can be treated empirically. Outer ear infections are typically caused by *P. aeruginosa* ("swimmer's ear") or *S. aureus*. The proper specimen to be obtained for culture is a scraping of the involved area of the ear.

Collection of specimens for the diagnosis of ocular infections is difficult because the sample obtained is generally very small and relatively few organisms may be present. Samples of the eye surface should be collected by a swab before topical anesthetics are applied, followed by corneal scrapings when necessary. Intraocular specimens are collected by directly aspirating the eye. The culture media should be inoculated when the specimens are collected and before they are sent to the laboratory. Although most common ocular pathogens grow rapidly (e.g., *S. aureus, S. pneumoniae, H. influenzae, P. aeruginosa, Bacillus cereus*), some may require prolonged incubation (e.g., coagulase-negative staphylococci) or use of specialized culture media (*N. gonorrhoeae, Chlamydia trachomatis*).

Wounds, Abscesses, and Tissues

Open, draining wounds can often be contaminated with potentially pathogenic organisms unrelated to the specific infectious process. Therefore it is important to collect samples from deep in the wound after the surface has been cleaned. Whenever possible, a swab should be avoided because it is difficult to obtain a representative sample without contamination with organisms colonizing the surface. Likewise, aspirates from a closed abscess should be collected from both the center and the wall of the abscess. Simply collecting pus from an abscess is generally nonproductive because most organisms actively replicate at the base of the abscess rather than in the center. Drainage from soft-tissue infections can be collected by aspiration. If drainage material is not obtained, a small quantity of saline can be infused into the tissue and then withdrawn for culture. Saline containing a bactericidal preservative should not be used.

Tissues should be obtained from representative portions of the infectious process, with multiple samples collected whenever possible. The tissue specimen should be transported in a sterile screw-capped container, and sterile saline should be added to prevent drying if a small sample (e.g., biopsy specimen) is collected. A sample of tissue should also be submitted for histologic examination. Because collection of tissue specimens requires invasive procedures, every effort should be made to collect the proper specimen and ensure that it is cultured for all clinically significant organisms that may be responsible for the infection. This requires close communication between the physician and microbiologist.

Urine

Urine is one of the most frequently submitted specimens for culture. Because a variety of bacteria colonize the urethra, the first portion of urine collected by voiding or catheterization should be discarded. Urinary tract pathogens can also grow in urine, so there should be no delay in transport of specimens to the laboratory. If the specimen cannot be cultured immediately, it should be refrigerated or placed into a bacteriostatic **urine preservative.** Once the specimen is received in the laboratory, 1 to 10 µl is inoculated onto each culture medium (generally one nonselective agar medium and one selective medium). This is done so that the number of organisms in the urine can be quantitated, which is useful for assessing the significance of an isolate, although small numbers of organisms in a patient with pyuria can be clinically significant. Numerous urine-screening procedures (e.g., biochemical tests, microscopy stains) have been developed and are used widely; however, the current procedures cannot be recommended because they are invariably insensitive in detecting clinically significant, low-grade bacteriuria.

Genital Specimens

Despite the variety of bacteria associated with sexually transmitted diseases, most laboratories concentrate on detecting *N. gonorrhoeae* and *C. trachomatis*. Traditionally this was done by inoculating the specimen into a culture system selective for these organisms; however, this is a slow process, taking 2 or more days for a positive culture to be obtained and even more time for isolates to be identified. Culture was also found to be insensitive because the organisms are extremely labile and die rapidly if transported under less than optimal conditions. For these reasons, a variety of nonculture methods are now used. The most popular methods are nucleic acid amplification procedures (e.g., amplification of species-specific deoxyribonucleic acid [DNA] sequences by the polymerase chain reaction or other methods) for both organisms. Detection of these amplified sequences is both sensitive and specific. Urine can be used for these tests but, in contrast with specimens collected for the diagnosis of cystitis, the first voided portion of urine should be tested for the diagnosis of urethritis.

The other major bacterium that causes sexually transmitted disease is *Treponema pallidum,* the etiologic agent of syphilis. This organism cannot be cultured in the clinical laboratory, so the diagnosis is made using microscopy or serology. Material from lesions must be examined using darkfield microscopy because the organism is too thin to be detected using brightfield microscopy. In addition, the organism dies rapidly when exposed to air and drying conditions, so the microscopic examination must be performed at the time the specimen is collected.

Fecal Specimens

A large variety of bacteria can cause gastrointestinal infections. For these bacteria to be recovered in culture, an adequate stool sample must be collected (generally not a problem in a patient with diarrhea), transported to the laboratory in a manner that ensures viability of the infecting organism, and inoculated onto the appropriate selective media. Rectal swabs should not be submitted because multiple selective media must be inoculated for the various possible pathogens to be recovered. The quantity of feces collected on a swab would be inadequate.

Stool specimens should be collected in a clean pan and then transferred into a tightly sealed waterproof container. The specimens should be transported promptly to the laboratory to prevent acidic changes in the stool (caused by bacterial metabolism), which are toxic for some organisms (e.g., *Shigella*). If a delay is anticipated, the feces should be mixed with a preservative, such as phosphate buffer mixed with glycerol or Cary-Blair transport medium. In general, however, rapid transport of the specimen to the laboratory is always superior to the use of any transport medium.

It is important to notify the laboratory if a particular enteric pathogen is suspected; this will help the laboratory select the appropriate specialized culture medium. For example, although *Vibrio* species can grow on the common media used for the culture of stool specimens, use of media selective for *Vibrio* facilitates rapid isolation and identification of this organism. In addition, some organisms are not isolated routinely by the laboratory procedures (e.g., enterotoxigenic *Escherichia coli* can grow on routine culture media but would not be readily distinguished from nonpathogenic *E. coli*). Likewise, other organisms would not be expected to be in a stool sample because their disease is caused by toxin produced in food, not by growth of the organism in the gastrointestinal tract (e.g., *S. aureus, B. cereus*). The microbiologist should be able to select the appropriate test (e.g., culture, toxin assay, nucleic acid amplification) if the specific pathogen is indicated. *Clostridium difficile* is a significant cause of antibiotic-associated gastrointestinal disease. Although the organism can be cultured from stool specimens if the specimens are delivered promptly to the laboratory, the most specific way to diagnose the infection is by detecting in fecal extracts the *C. difficile* toxins responsible for the disease or the genes that code for these toxins. The most sensitive and specific tests for diagnosing *C. difficile* disease is detection of the toxin genes by nucleic acid amplification tests. These tests are also available as commercial assays for detection of the most common bacterial, viral, and parasitic enteric pathogens.

Because many bacteria, both pathogenic and nonpathogenic, are present in fecal specimens, it often takes at least 3 days for the enteric pathogen to be isolated and identified. For this reason, stool cultures are used to confirm the clinical diagnosis, and therapy, if indicated, should not be delayed pending culture results.

Bacterial Detection and Identification

Detection of bacteria in clinical specimens is accomplished by five general procedures: (1) microscopy, (2) detection of bacterial antigens, (3) detection of specific bacterial nucleic acids, (4) culture, and (5) detection of an antibody response to the bacteria (serology). The specific techniques used for these procedures were presented in the preceding chapters and will not be repeated in this chapter. However, Table 16-2

Table 16-2 Detection Methods for Bacteria

Organism	Detection Methods				
	Microscopy	Antigen Detection	Nucleic Acid–Based Tests	Culture	Antibody Detection
Gram-Positive Cocci					
Staphylococcus aureus	A	B	C	A	D
Streptococcus pyogenes	B	A	A	A	B
Streptococcus agalactiae	B	B	A	A	D
Streptococcus pneumoniae	A	B	C	A	C
Enterococcus spp.	A	D	B	A	D
Gram-Positive Rods					
Bacillus anthracis	B	C	B	A	D
Bacillus cereus	B	D	D	B	D
Listeria monocytogenes	A	D	D	A	D
Erysipelothrix rhusiopathiae	A	D	D	A	D
Corynebacterium diphtheriae	B	D	C	A	D
Corynebacterium, other spp.	A	D	D	A	D
Tropheryma whipplei	B	D	A	D	D
Acid-Fast and Partially Acid-Fast Rods					
Nocardia spp.	A	D	B	A	D
Rhodococcus equi	A	D	D	A	D
Mycobacterium tuberculosis	A	B	A	A	C
Mycobacterium leprae	B	D	D	D	B
Mycobacterium, other spp.	A	D	B	A	D
Gram-Negative Cocci					
Neisseria gonorrhoeae	A	D	A	A	D
Neisseria meningitidis	A	B	D	A	D
Moraxella catarrhalis	A	D	D	A	D
Gram-Negative Rods					
Escherichia coli	A	B	C	A	D
Salmonella spp.	B	D	D	A	B
Shigella spp.	B	D	D	A	D
Yersinia pestis	B	C	B	A	C
Yersinia enterocolitica	B	D	B	A	B
Enterobacteriaceae, other genera	A	D	D	A	D
Vibrio cholerae	B	D	B	A	D
Vibrio, other spp.	B	D	D	A	D
Aeromonas spp.	B	D	B	A	D
Campylobacter spp.	B	A	B	A	D
Helicobacter pylori	B	A	C	B	A
Pseudomonas aeruginosa	A	D	D	A	D
Burkholderia spp.	A	D	D	A	D
Acinetobacter spp.	A	D	D	A	D
Haemophilus influenzae	A	B	C	A	D

Table 16-2 **Detection Methods for Bacteria—cont'd**

Organism	Detection Methods				
	Microscopy	Antigen Detection	Nucleic Acid–Based Tests	Culture	Antibody Detection
Haemophilus ducreyi	B	D	C	A	D
Bordetella pertussis	B	C	A	B	A
Brucella spp.	B	C	D	A	B
Francisella tularensis	B	C	D	A	B
Legionella spp.	B	A	B	A	B
Bartonella spp.	C	D	B	A	A
Anaerobes					
Clostridium perfringens	A	D	D	A	D
Clostridium tetani	B	D	D	A	D
Clostridium botulinum	B	A	D	B	D
Clostridium difficile	C	D	A	B	D
Anaerobic gram-positive cocci	A	D	D	A	D
Anaerobic gram-positive rods	A	D	D	A	D
Anaerobic gram-negative rods	A	D	D	A	D
Spiral-Shaped Bacteria					
Treponema pallidum	B	D	D	D	A
Borrelia burgdorferi	C	A	A	B	A
Borrelia, other spp.	A	D	D	B	D
Leptospira spp.	B	D	B	B	A
Mycoplasma and Obligate Intracellular Bacteria					
Mycoplasma pneumoniae	D	C	A	B	A
Rickettsia spp.	B	D	B	D	A
Orientia spp.	B	C	C	C	A
Ehrlichia spp.	B	C	C	C	A
Anaplasma spp.	B	C	C	C	A
Coxiella burnetii	C	C	B	C	A
Chlamydia trachomatis	B	B	A	B	D
Chlamydophila pneumoniae	D	D	B	C	B
Chlamydophila psittaci	D	D	B	D	A

A, Test generally useful for diagnosis; *B,* test useful under certain circumstances or for the diagnosis of specific forms of disease; *C,* test generally not used in diagnostic laboratories or used only in specialty reference laboratories; *D,* test generally not useful.

summarizes the relative value of each procedure for the detection of organisms discussed in Chapters 18 to 35.

Although many organisms can be specifically identified by a variety of techniques, the most common procedure used in diagnostic laboratories is to identify an organism isolated in culture by biochemical tests. In large teaching hospital laboratories and reference laboratories, many biochemical test procedures have been replaced recently with sequencing bacterial specific genes (e.g., 16S rRNA gene) or using proteomic tools such as mass spectrometry. We believe most students using this textbook are not interested in the details of microbial identification. Those who are interested should refer to textbooks such as *Bailey and Scott's Diagnostic Microbiology,* the *ASM Manual of Clinical Microbiology,* and reviews that specifically cover this topic.

It is important for all students to appreciate that empirical antimicrobial therapy can be refined based on preliminary identification of an organism using microscopic and macroscopic morphology and selected rapid biochemical tests. Refer to Table 16-3 for specific examples.

Antimicrobial Susceptibility Tests

The results of in vitro antimicrobial susceptibility testing are valuable for selecting chemotherapeutic agents active against

Table 16-3 Preliminary Identification of Bacteria Isolated in Culture

Organism	Properties
Staphylococcus aureus	Gram-positive cocci in clusters; large, β-hemolytic colonies; catalase-positive, coagulase-positive
Streptococcus pyogenes	Gram-positive cocci in long chains; small colonies with large zone of β-hemolysis; catalase-negative, PYR-positive (L-pyrrolidonyl arylamidase)
Streptococcus pneumoniae	Gram-positive cocci in pairs and short chains; small, α-hemolytic colonies; catalase-negative, soluble in bile
Enterococcus spp.	Gram-positive cocci in pairs and short chains; large, α- or nonhemolytic colonies; catalase-negative, PYR-positive
Listeria monocytogenes	Small, gram-positive rods; small, weakly β-hemolytic colonies; characteristic (tumbling) motility
Nocardia spp.	Weakly staining (Gram and modified acid-fast), thin, filamentous, branching rods; slow growth; fuzzy colonies (aerial hyphae)
Rhodococcus equi	Weakly staining (Gram and modified acid-fast); initially nonbranching rods, cocci in older cultures; slow growth; pink-red colonies
Mycobacterium tuberculosis	Strongly acid-fast rods; slow growth; nonpigmented colonies; identified using specific molecular probes
Enterobacteriaceae	Gram-negative rods with "bipolar" staining (more intense at ends); typically single cells; large colonies; growth on MacConkey agar (may/may not ferment lactose); oxidase-negative
Pseudomonas aeruginosa	Gram-negative rods with uniform staining; typically in pairs; large spreading, fluorescent green colonies, usually β-hemolytic, fruity smell (grapelike); growth on MacConkey agar (nonfermenter); oxidase-positive
Stenotrophomonas maltophilia	Gram-negative rods with uniform staining; typically in pairs; lavender-green color on blood agar; growth on MacConkey agar (nonfermenter); oxidase-negative
Acinetobacter spp.	Large, gram-negative coccobacilli arranged as single cells or pairs; will retain crystal violet and may resemble fat, gram-positive cocci in pairs; growth on blood agar and MacConkey agar (may oxidize lactose and resemble weakly purple); oxidase-negative
Campylobacter spp.	Thin, curved, gram-negative rods arranged in pairs (S-shaped pairs); growth on highly selective media for *Campylobacter;* no growth on routine media (blood, chocolate, or MacConkey agars)
Haemophilus spp.	Small, gram-negative coccobacilli arranged as single cells; growth on chocolate agar but not blood or MacConkey agars; oxidase-positive
Brucella spp.	Very small, gram-negative coccobacilli arranged as single cells; slow-growing; no growth on MacConkey agar; biohazard
Francisella spp.	Very small, gram-negative coccobacilli arranged as single cells; slow-growing; no growth on blood or MacConkey agars; biohazard
Legionella spp.	Weakly staining, thin, gram-negative rods; slow-growing; growth on specialized agar; no growth on blood, chocolate, or MacConkey agars
Clostridium perfringens	Large, rectangular rods with spores not observed; rapid growth of spreading colonies with "double zone" of hemolysis (large zone of α-hemolysis with inner zone of β-hemolysis); strict anaerobe
Bacteroides fragilis group	Weakly staining, pleomorphic (variable lengths), gram-negative rods; rapid growth stimulated by bile in media; strict anaerobe

the infecting organism. Extensive work has been performed in an effort to standardize testing methods and improve the clinical predictive value of the results. Despite these efforts, in vitro tests are simply a measurement of the effect of the antibiotic against the organism under specific conditions. Selection of an antibiotic and the patient's outcome are influenced by a variety of interrelated factors, including the pharmacokinetic properties of the antibiotic, drug toxicity, the clinical disease, and the patient's general medical status. Thus some organisms that are "susceptible" to an antibiotic will persist in an infection, and some organisms that are "resistant" to an antibiotic will be eliminated. For example, because oxygen is required for aminoglycosides to enter a bacterial cell, these antibiotics are ineffective in an anaerobic abscess. Likewise, very high concentrations of antibiotics can be achieved in urine, so "resistant" bacteria responsible for urinary tract infections can be eliminated by the high urine concentrations of some antibiotics.

Two general forms of antimicrobial susceptibility tests are performed in the clinical laboratory: **broth dilution tests** and **agar diffusion tests.** For broth dilution tests, serial dilutions of an antibiotic are prepared in a nutrient medium and then inoculated with a standardized concentration of the test bacterium. After overnight incubation, the lowest concentration of antibiotic that is able to inhibit the growth of the bacteria is referred to as the **minimum inhibitory concentration (MIC).** For agar diffusion tests, a standardized concentration of bacteria is spread over the surface of an agar medium, and then paper disks or strips impregnated with antibiotics are placed on the agar surface. After overnight incubation, an area of inhibited growth is observed surrounding the paper disks or strips. The size of the area of inhibition corresponds to the activity of the antibiotic—the more susceptible the organism is to the antibiotic, the larger the area of inhibited growth. By standardizing the test conditions for agar diffusion tests, the area of inhibition corresponds to the MIC value. Indeed, one commercial company has developed a test where the MIC value is calculated directly from the zone of inhibited growth around a strip with a gradient of antibiotic concentrations from the top to the bottom of the strip.

Broth dilution tests were originally performed in test tubes and were very labor intensive. Commercially prepared systems are now available where antibiotic dilutions are prepared in microtiter trays and inoculation of the trays and interpretation of MICs are automated. Disadvantages of these systems are that the range of different antibiotics is determined by the manufacturer, and the number of dilutions of an individual antibiotic is limited. Thus results may not be available for newly introduced antibiotics. Diffusion tests are labor intensive and interpretation of the size of the area of inhibition can be subjective; however, the advantage of these tests is that virtually any antibiotic can be tested. The ability of both susceptibility testing methods to predict clinical response to an antibiotic is equivalent, so test selection is determined by practical considerations.

Bibliography

Forbes B, Sahm D, Weissfeld A: *Bailey and Scott's diagnostic microbiology*, ed 12, St Louis, 2007, Mosby.

Mandell G, Bennett J, Dolin R: *Principles and practice of infectious diseases*, ed 7, New York, 2009, Churchill Livingstone.

Versalovic J, Carroll KC, Funke G, et al: *Manual of clinical microbiology*, ed 10, Washington, DC, 2011, American Society for Microbiology Press.

CHAPTER

ANTIBACTERIAL AGENTS

This chapter provides an overview of the mechanisms of action and spectrum of the most commonly used antibacterial antibiotics, as well as a description of the common mechanisms of bacterial resistance. The terminology appropriate for this discussion is summarized in Box 17-1, and the basic mechanisms and sites of antibiotic activity are summarized in Table 17-1 and Figure 17-1, respectively.

The year 1935 was an important one for the chemotherapy of systemic bacterial infections. Although antiseptics had been applied topically to prevent the growth of microorganisms, the existing antiseptics were ineffective against systemic bacterial infections. In 1935, the dye protosil was shown to protect mice against systemic streptococcal infection and to be curative in patients suffering from such infections. It was soon found that protosil was cleaved in the body to release *p*-aminobenzene sulfonamide (sulfanilamide), which was shown to have antibacterial activity. This first "sulfa" drug ushered in a new era in medicine. Compounds produced by microorganisms (antibiotics) were eventually discovered to inhibit the growth of other microorganisms. For example, Alexander Fleming was the first to realize the mold *Penicillium* prevented the multiplication of staphylococci. A concentrate from a culture of this mold was prepared, and the remarkable antibacterial activity and lack of toxicity of the first antibiotic, penicillin, were demonstrated. Streptomycin and the tetracyclines were developed in the 1940s and 1950s, followed rapidly by the development of additional aminoglycosides, semisynthetic penicillins, cephalosporins, quinolones, and other antimicrobials. All these antibacterial agents greatly increased the range of infectious diseases that could be prevented or treated. Although the development of new antibacterial antibiotics has lagged in recent years, some new classes of agents have been introduced, including the ketolides (e.g., **telithromycin**), glycylcyclines **(tigecycline),** lipopeptides **(daptomycin),** streptogramins **(quinupristin-dalfopristin),** and oxazolidinones **(linezolid).**

Unfortunately, with the introduction of new chemotherapeutic agents, bacteria have shown a remarkable ability to develop resistance. Thus antibiotic therapy will not be the magical cure for all infections, as predicted; rather, it is only one weapon, albeit an important one, against infectious diseases. It is also important to recognize that because resistance to antibiotics is often not predictable, physicians must rely on their clinical experience for the initial selection of **empirical therapy** and then refine their treatment by selecting antibiotics demonstrated to be active by in vitro susceptibility tests. Guidelines for the management of infections caused by specific organisms are discussed in the relevant chapters of this text.

Inhibition of Cell Wall Synthesis

The most common mechanism of antibiotic activity is interference with bacterial cell wall synthesis. Most of the cell wall–active antibiotics are classified as β-lactam antibiotics (e.g., penicillins, cephalosporins, cephamycins, carbapenems, monobactams, β-lactamase inhibitors), so named because they share a common β-lactam ring structure. Other antibiotics that interfere with construction of the bacterial cell wall include vancomycin, daptomycin, bacitracin, and the following antimycobacterial agents: isoniazid, ethambutol, cycloserine, and ethionamide.

β-Lactam Antibiotics

The major structural component of most bacterial cell walls is the peptidoglycan layer. The basic structure is a chain of 10 to 65 disaccharide residues consisting of alternating molecules of *N*-acetylglucosamine and *N*-acetylmuramic acid. These chains are then cross-linked with peptide bridges that create a rigid mesh coating for the bacteria. The building of the chains and cross-links is catalyzed by specific enzymes (e.g., transpeptidases, transglycosylases, carboxypeptidases) that are members of a large family of **serine proteases.** These regulatory enzymes are also called **penicillin-binding proteins (PBPs),** because they are the targets of β-lactam antibiotics. When growing bacteria are exposed to these antibiotics, the antibiotic binds to specific PBPs in the bacterial cell wall and inhibits assembly of the peptidoglycan chains. This, in turn, activates autolysins that degrade the cell wall, resulting in bacterial cell death. Thus the β-lactam antibiotics generally act as bactericidal agents.

Bacteria can become resistant to β-lactam antibiotics by three general mechanisms: (1) decreased concentration of the antibiotic at the cell wall target site, (2) decreased binding of the antibiotic to the PBP, and (3) hydrolysis of the antibiotic by bacterial enzymes, **β-lactamases.** The first mechanism of resistance is seen only in gram-negative bacteria. Gram-negative bacteria have an outer membrane that overlies the peptidoglycan layer. Penetration of β-lactam antibiotics into gram-negative rods requires transit through pores in this outer membrane. Changes in the proteins **(porins)** that form the walls of the pores can alter the size of the pore opening or charge of these channels and result in exclusion of the antibiotic. Additionally, active efflux or pumping out

Box 17-1 Terminology

Antibacterial spectrum: Range of activity of an antimicrobial against bacteria. A **broad-spectrum** antibacterial drug can inhibit a variety of gram-positive and gram-negative bacteria, whereas a **narrow-spectrum** drug is active against a limited variety of bacteria.

Bacteriostatic antibiotic: Antibiotic that inhibits the growth of bacteria but does not kill.

Bactericidal antibiotic: Antibiotic that kills bacteria.

Minimum inhibitory concentration (MIC): Determined by exposing a standardized suspension of bacteria to a series of antimicrobial dilutions. The lowest antibiotic concentration that inhibits the growth of the bacteria is the MIC.

Minimum bactericidal concentration (MBC): Determined by exposing a standardized suspension of bacteria to a series of antimicrobial dilutions. The lowest antibiotic concentration that kills 99.9% of the population is referred to as the MBC.

Antibiotic combinations: Combinations of antibiotics that may be used to (1) broaden the antibacterial spectrum for empirical therapy or the treatment of polymicrobial infections, (2) prevent the emergence of resistant organisms during therapy, and (3) achieve a synergistic killing effect.

Antibiotic synergism: Combinations of two antibiotics that have enhanced bactericidal activity when tested together compared with the activity of each antibiotic.

Antibiotic antagonism: Combination of antibiotics in which the activity of one antibiotic interferes with the activity of the other (e.g., the sum of the activity is less than the activity of the most active individual drug).

β-Lactamase: An enzyme that hydrolyzes the β-lactam ring in the β-lactam class of antibiotics, thus inactivating the antibiotic. The enzymes specific for penicillins, cephalosporins, and carbapenems are the **penicillinases, cephalosporinases,** and **carbapenemases,** respectively.

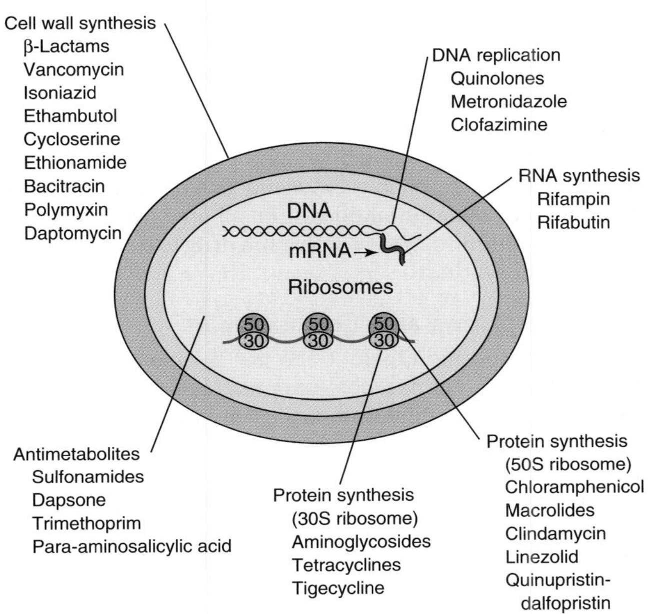

FIGURE 17-1 Basic sites of antibiotic activity.

Table 17-1 Basic Mechanisms of Antibiotic Action

Antibiotic	Action
Disruption of Cell Wall	
Penicillins Cephalosporins Cephamycins Carbapenems Monobactams	Bind PBPs and enzymes responsible for peptidoglycan synthesis
β-Lactam/ β-lactamase inhibitors	Bind β-lactamases and prevent enzymatic inactivation of β-lactam
Vancomycin	Inhibits cross-linkage of peptidoglycan layers
Daptomycin	Causes depolarization of cytoplasmic membrane, resulting in disruption of ionic concentration gradients
Bacitracin	Inhibits bacterial cytoplasmic membrane and movement of peptidoglycan precursors
Polymyxins	Inhibit bacterial membranes
Isoniazid Ethionamide	Inhibit mycolic acid synthesis
Ethambutol	Inhibits arabinogalactan synthesis
Cycloserine	Inhibits cross-linkage of peptidoglycan layers
Inhibition of Protein Synthesis	
Aminoglycosides	Produce premature release of peptide chains from 30S ribosome
Tetracyclines	Prevent polypeptide elongation at 30S ribosome
Glycylcyclines	Bind to 30S ribosome and prevent initiation of protein synthesis
Oxazolidinone	Prevents initiation of protein synthesis at 50S ribosome
Macrolides Ketolides Clindamycin Streptogramins	Prevent polypeptide elongation at 50S ribosome
Inhibition of Nucleic Acid Synthesis	
Quinolones	Bind α subunit of DNA gyrase
Rifampin Rifabutin	Prevent transcription by binding DNA-dependent RNA polymerase
Metronidazole	Disrupts bacteria DNA (is cytotoxic compound)
Antimetabolite	
Sulfonamides	Inhibit dihydropteroate synthase and disrupt folic acid synthesis
Dapsone	Inhibits dihydropteroate synthase
Trimethoprim	Inhibits dihydrofolate reductase and disrupts folic acid synthesis

DNA, Deoxyribonucleic acid; *PBPs,* penicillin-binding proteins; *RNA,* ribonucleic acid.

of the antibiotic can decrease the antibiotic concentration in the cell.

Resistance can also be acquired by modification of the β-lactam antibiotic binding to the PBP. This can be mediated by (1) an overproduction of PBP (a rare occurrence), (2) acquisition of a new PBP (e.g., methicillin resistance in *Staphylococcus aureus*), or (3) modification of an existing PBP through recombination (e.g., penicillin resistance in *Streptococcus pneumoniae*) or a point mutation (penicillin resistance in *Enterococcus faecium*).

Finally, bacteria can produce **β-lactamases** that inactivate the β-lactam antibiotics. Interestingly, the β-lactamases are in the same family of serine proteases as the PBPs. More than 200 different β-lactamases have been described. Some are specific for penicillins (i.e., penicillinases), cephalosporins (i.e., cephalosporinases), or carbapenems (i.e., carbapenemases), whereas others have a broad range of activity, including some that are capable of inactivating most β-lactam antibiotics. An exhaustive discussion of β-lactamases is beyond the scope of this chapter; however, a brief discussion is germane for understanding the limitations of β-lactam antibiotics. By one classification scheme, β-lactamases have been separated into four classes (A to D). The most common class A β-lactamases are SHV-1 and TEM-1, penicillinases found in common gram-negative rods (e.g., *Escherichia, Klebsiella*), with minimal activity against cephalosporins. Unfortunately, simple point mutations in the genes encoding these enzymes have created β-lactamases with activity against all penicillins and cephalosporins. These β-lactamases are referred to as **extended-spectrum β-lactamases (ESBLs)** and are particularly troublesome because most are encoded on plasmids that can be transferred from organism to organism. The class B β-lactamases are zinc-dependent metalloenzymes that have a broad spectrum of activity against all β-lactam antibiotics, including the cephamycins and carbapenems. The **class C β-lactamases** are primarily cephalosporinases that are encoded on the bacterial chromosome. Expression of these enzymes is generally repressed, although this can be altered by exposure to certain "inducing" β-lactam antibiotics or by mutations in the genes controlling expression of the enzymes. Expression of this class of β-lactamases is particularly troublesome because they are active against the most potent expanded-spectrum cephalosporins. The class D β-lactamases are penicillinases found primarily in gram-negative rods.

Penicillins

Penicillin antibiotics (Table 17-2) are highly effective antibiotics with an extremely low toxicity. The basic compound is an organic acid with a β-lactam ring obtained from culture of the mold *Penicillium chrysogenum*. If the mold is grown by a fermentation process, large amounts of 6-aminopenicillanic acid (the β-lactam ring is fused with a thiazolidine ring) are produced. Biochemical modification of this intermediate yields antibiotics that have increased resistance to stomach acids, increased absorption in the gastrointestinal tract, resistance to destruction by penicillinase, or a broader spectrum of activity that includes gram-negative bacteria.

Penicillin G is inactivated by gastric acid; thus it is used mainly as an intravenous drug for the treatment of infections caused by the limited number of susceptible organisms.

Table 17-2 Penicillins

Antibiotics	Spectrum of Activity
Natural penicillins: benzylpenicillin (penicillin G), phenoxymethyl penicillin (penicillin V)	Active against all β-hemolytic streptococci and most other species; limited activity against staphylococci; active against meningococci and most gram-positive anaerobes; poor activity against aerobic and anaerobic gram-negative rods
Penicillinase-resistant penicillins: methicillin, nafcillin, oxacillin, cloxacillin, dicloxacillin	Similar to the natural penicillins, except enhanced activity against staphylococci
Broad-spectrum penicillins: ampicillin, amoxicillin	Activity against gram-positive cocci equivalent to the natural penicillins; active against some gram-negative rods
β-Lactam with β-lactamase inhibitor (ampicillin-sulbactam, amoxicillin-clavulanate, ticarcillin-clavulanate, piperacillin-tazobactam)	Activity similar to natural β-lactams, plus improved activity against β-lactamase–producing staphylococci and selected gram-negative rods; not all β-lactamases are inhibited; piperacillin/tazobactam is the most active

Penicillin V is more resistant to acid and is the preferred oral form for the treatment of susceptible bacteria. **Penicillinase-resistant penicillins** such as methicillin and oxacillin are used to treat infections caused by susceptible staphylococci. Unfortunately, resistance to this group of antibiotics has become commonplace in both hospital-acquired and community-acquired staphylococcal infections. Ampicillin was the first **broad-spectrum penicillin,** although the spectrum of activity against gram-negative rods was limited primarily to *Escherichia, Proteus,* and *Haemophilus* species. Selected penicillins have been combined with **β-lactamase inhibitors.** The β-lactamase inhibitors (e.g., clavulanic acid, sulbactam, tazobactam) are relatively inactive by themselves but when combined with some penicillins (i.e., ampicillin, amoxicillin, ticarcillin, piperacillin) are effective in treating some infections caused by β-lactamase–producing bacteria. The inhibitors irreversibly bind and inactivate susceptible bacterial β-lactamases (although not all are bound by these inhibitors), permitting the companion drug to disrupt bacterial cell wall synthesis.

Cephalosporins and Cephamycins

The cephalosporins (Table 17-3) are β-lactam antibiotics derived from 7-aminocephalosporanic acid (the β-lactam ring is fused with a dihydrothiazine ring) that was originally isolated from the mold *Cephalosporium*. The cephamycins are closely related to the cephalosporins, except that they contain oxygen in place of sulfur in the dihydrothiazine ring, rendering them more stable to β-lactamase hydrolysis. The cephalosporins and cephamycins have the same mechanism of action as the penicillins; however, they have a wider antibacterial spectrum, are resistant to many β-lactamases, and have improved pharmacokinetic properties (e.g., longer half-life).

 Table 17-3 **Selected Examples of Cephalosporins and Cephamycins**

Antibiotics	Spectrum of Activity
Narrow spectrum (cephalexin, cephalothin, cefazolin, cephapirin, cephradine)	Activity equivalent to oxacillin against gram-positive bacteria; some gram-negative activity (e.g., *Escherichia coli, Klebsiella, Proteus mirabilis*)
Expanded-spectrum cephalosporins (cefaclor, cefuroxime)	Activity equivalent to oxacillin against gram-positive bacteria; improved gram-negative activity to include *Enterobacter, Citrobacter,* and additional *Proteus* species
Expanded-spectrum cephamycins (cefotetan, cefoxitin)	Activity similar to expanded-spectrum cephalosporins but less susceptible to β-lactamases
Broad spectrum (cefixime, cefotaxime, ceftriaxone, ceftazidime)	Activity equivalent to oxacillin against gram-positive bacteria; improved gram-negative activity to include *Pseudomonas*
Extended spectrum (cefepime, cefpirome)	Activity equivalent to oxacillin against gram-positive bacteria; marginally improved gram-negative activity

Biochemical modifications in the basic antibiotic molecule resulted in the development of antibiotics with improved activity and pharmacokinetic properties. The cephalosporins have enhanced activity against gram-negative bacteria compared with the penicillins. This activity, in turn, varies among the different "generations" of cephalosporins. The activity of **narrow-spectrum,** first-generation antibiotics is primarily restricted to *Escherichia coli, Klebsiella* species, *Proteus mirabilis,* and oxacillin-susceptible gram-positive cocci. Many of the **expanded-spectrum,** second-generation antibiotics have additional activity against *Haemophilus influenzae, Enterobacter, Citrobacter,* and *Serratia* species, and some anaerobes, such as *Bacteroides fragilis.* The **broad-spectrum,** third-generation antibiotics and **extended-spectrum,** fourth-generation antibiotics are active against most Enterobacteriaceae and *Pseudomonas aeruginosa.* Extended-spectrum antibiotics offer the advantage of increased stability to β-lactamases. Unfortunately, gram-negative bacteria have rapidly developed resistance to most cephalosporins and cephamycins (primarily as the result of β-lactamase production), which has significantly compromised the use of all these agents.

Carbapenems and Monobactams

Other classes of β-lactam antibiotics (Table 17-4) are the **carbapenems** (e.g., imipenem, meropenem, ertapenem, doripenem) and **monobactams** (e.g., aztreonam). The carbapenems are important, widely prescribed broad-spectrum antibiotics that are active against many groups of organisms. In contrast, the monobactams are narrow-spectrum antibiotics that are active only against aerobic, gram-negative bacteria. Anaerobic bacteria and gram-positive bacteria are resistant. The advantage of narrow-spectrum antibiotics is that they can be used to treat susceptible organisms without disruption of the patient's normal, protective bacterial population. Despite this advantage, monobactams are not widely used.

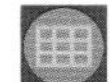 Table 17-4 **Other β-Lactam Antibiotics**

Antibiotics	Spectrum of Activity
Carbapenems (imipenem, meropenem, ertapenem, doripenem)	Broad-spectrum antibiotics active against most aerobic and anaerobic gram-positive and gram-negative bacteria except oxacillin-resistant staphylococci, most *Enterococcus faecium,* and selected gram-negative rods (e.g., some *Burkholderia, Stenotrophomonas,* some *Pseudomonas*)
Monobactam (aztreonam)	Active against selected aerobic gram-negative rods but inactive against anaerobes or gram-positive cocci

In recent years, resistance to carbapenems mediated by production of carbapenemases has become widespread. As mentioned earlier, the β-lactamases are separated into four classes, A to D. The class A carbapenemase has been found in a broad range of bacteria, including *Pseudomonas* and Enterobacteriaceae (the most common one is the *Klebsiella pneumoniae* carbapenemase **[KPC]**), renders organisms producing this carbapenemase resistant to all β-lactams, and is only reliably detected using molecular methods to detect the resistance genes. The class B carbapenemase is a metallo-β-lactamase (requires zinc for activity), is widely distributed in gram-negative bacteria, and also cannot be detected reliably by conventional susceptibility tests. Organisms producing class B carbapenemases (most common is **New Delhi metallo-β-lactamase [NDM],** named for its origin) are resistant to all β-lactam antibiotics, with the possible exception of aztreonam. Finally, the class D carbapenemases are primarily found in *Acinetobacter,* are detected by conventional susceptibility tests, and encode resistance to all β-lactam antibiotics. This group of carbapenemases is important because *Acinetobacter* strains producing this carbapenemase are generally resistant to all antibiotics, with few exceptions.

Glycopeptides

Vancomycin, originally obtained from *Streptomyces orientalis,* is a complex glycopeptide that disrupts cell wall peptidoglycan synthesis in growing gram-positive bacteria. Vancomycin interacts with the D-alanine-D-alanine termini of the pentapeptide side chains, which interferes sterically with formation of the bridges between peptidoglycan chains. Vancomycin is used for the management of infections caused by oxacillin-resistant staphylococci and other gram-positive bacteria resistant to β-lactam antibiotics. Vancomycin is inactive against gram-negative bacteria, because the molecule is too large to pass through the outer membrane pores and reach the peptidoglycan target site. In addition, some organisms are intrinsically resistant to vancomycin (e.g., *Leuconostoc, Lactobacillus, Pediococcus,* and *Erysipelothrix*) because the pentapeptide terminates in D-alanine-D-lactate, which does not bind vancomycin. Intrinsic resistance is also found in some species of enterococci that contain a D-alanine-D-serine terminus (i.e., *Enterococcus gallinarum, Enterococcus casseliflavus*). Finally, some species of enterococci (particularly *E. faecium* and *Enterococcus faecalis*) have acquired resistance to vancomycin. The genes for this resistance (primarily *vanA* and *vanB*), which also mediate changes in the pentapeptide terminus, can be carried on plasmids and have seriously compromised the usefulness of vancomycin for the treatment of enterococcal infections. More importantly, the gene for vancomycin resistance contained within a transposon on a multiresistance conjugative plasmid has been transferred in vivo from *E. faecalis* to a multiresistant *S. aureus.* The transposon then moved from the *E. faecalis* plasmid and recombined and integrated into the *S. aureus* resistance plasmid. This resulted in an *S. aureus* plasmid that encoded resistance to β-lactams, vancomycin, aminoglycosides, and other antibiotics—a plasmid that could be transferred to other staphylococci by conjugation. Interestingly, these resistant strains of *Staphylococcus* have primarily been restricted to Michigan; however, if this resistance becomes widespread, the medical implications are profound.

Lipopeptides

Daptomycin, a naturally occurring cyclic lipopeptide produced by *Streptomyces roseosporus,* binds irreversibly to the cytoplasmic membrane, resulting in membrane depolarization and disruption of the ionic gradients, leading to cell death. It has potent activity against gram-positive bacteria, but gram-negative bacteria are resistant to daptomycin because the drug cannot penetrate through the cell wall to the cytoplasmic membrane. Daptomycin has good activity against multidrug-resistant staphylococci, streptococci, and enterococci (including vancomycin-resistant strains.

Polypeptides

Bacitracin, which was isolated from *Bacillus licheniformis,* is a mixture of polypeptides used in topically applied products (e.g., creams, ointments, sprays) for the treatment of skin infections caused by gram-positive bacteria (particularly those caused by *Staphylococcus* and group A *Streptococcus*). Gram-negative bacteria are resistant to this agent. Bacitracin inhibits cell wall synthesis by interfering with dephosphorylation and recycling of the lipid carrier responsible for moving the peptidoglycan precursors through the cytoplasmic membrane to the cell wall. It may also damage the bacterial cytoplasmic membrane and inhibit ribonucleic acid (RNA) transcription. Resistance to the antibiotic is most likely caused by failure of the antibiotic to penetrate into the bacterial cell.

The **polymyxins** are a group of cyclic polypeptides derived from *Bacillus polymyxa.* These antibiotics insert into bacterial membranes like detergents by interacting with lipopolysaccharides and the phospholipids in the outer membrane, producing increased cell permeability and eventual cell death. **Polymyxins B** and **E (colistin)** are capable of causing serious nephrotoxicity. Thus their use has been limited historically to external treatment of localized infections such as external otitis, eye infections, and skin infections caused by sensitive organisms. However, because some organisms such as *Acinetobacter* and *Pseudomonas* are only susceptible to colistin, this antibiotic is used to treat some systemic infections. These antibiotics are most active against gram-negative rods, because gram-positive bacteria do not have an outer membrane.

Isoniazid, Ethionamide, Ethambutol, and Cycloserine

Isoniazid, ethionamide, ethambutol, and cycloserine are cell wall–active antibiotics used for the treatment of mycobacterial infections. **Isoniazid** (isonicotinic acid hydrazide [INH]) is bactericidal against actively replicating mycobacteria. Although the exact mechanism of action is unknown, the synthesis of mycolic acid is affected (desaturation of the long-chain fatty acids and elongation of fatty acids and hydroxy lipids are disrupted). **Ethionamide,** a derivative of INH, also blocks mycolic acid synthesis. **Ethambutol** interferes with the synthesis of arabinogalactan in the cell wall, and **cycloserine** inhibits two enzymes, D-alanine-D-alanine synthetase and alanine racemase, which catalyze cell wall synthesis. Resistance to these four antibiotics results primarily from reduced drug uptake into the bacterial cell or alteration of the target sites.

Inhibition of Protein Synthesis

The primary action of the agents in the second largest class of antibiotics is inhibition of protein synthesis (see Table 17-1).

Aminoglycosides

The aminoglycoside antibiotics (Table 17-5) consist of amino sugars linked through glycosidic bonds to an aminocyclitol ring. Streptomycin, neomycin, kanamycin, and tobramycin were originally isolated from *Streptomyces* species, and gentamicin and sisomicin were isolated from *Micromonospora* species. Amikacin and netilmicin are synthetic derivatives of kanamycin and sisomicin, respectively. These antibiotics exert their effort by passing through the bacterial outer membrane (in gram-negative bacteria), cell wall, and cytoplasmic membrane to the cytoplasm, where they inhibit bacterial protein synthesis by irreversibly binding to the 30S ribosomal proteins. This attachment to the ribosomes has two effects: production of aberrant proteins as the result of misreading of the messenger RNA (mRNA), and interruption of protein synthesis by causing premature release of the ribosome from mRNA.

The aminoglycosides are bactericidal because of their ability to bind irreversibly to ribosomes and are commonly used to treat serious infections caused by many gram-negative rods (e.g., Enterobacteriaceae, *Pseudomonas, Acinetobacter*) and some gram-positive organisms. Penetration through the cytoplasmic membrane is an aerobic, energy-dependent process, so anaerobes are resistant to aminoglycosides, and susceptible organisms in an anaerobic environment (e.g., abscess) do not respond to treatment. Streptococci and enterococci are resistant to aminoglycosides because the aminoglycosides fail to penetrate through the cell wall of these bacteria. Treatment of these organisms requires coadministration of an aminoglycoside with an inhibitor of cell wall synthesis (e.g., penicillin, ampicillin, vancomycin) that facilitates uptake of the aminoglycoside.

The most commonly used antibiotics in this class are **amikacin, gentamicin,** and **tobramycin.** All three aminoglycosides are used to treat systemic infections caused by susceptible gram-negative bacteria. **Amikacin** has the best activity and is frequently reserved for treatment of infections caused by gram-negative bacteria that are resistant to gentamicin and tobramycin. **Streptomycin** is not readily available but has been used for the treatment of tuberculosis, tularemia, and gentamicin-resistant streptococcal or enterococcal infections (in combination with a penicillin).

Table 17-5 Inhibitors of Protein Synthesis

Antibiotics	Spectrum of Activity
Aminoglycosides (streptomycin, kanamycin, gentamicin, tobramycin, amikacin)	Primarily used to treat infections with gram-negative rods; kanamycin with limited activity; tobramycin slightly more active than gentamicin versus *Pseudomonas;* amikacin most active; streptomycin and gentamicin combined with cell wall–active antibiotic to treat enterococcal infections; streptomycin active versus mycobacteria and selected gram-negative rods
Aminocyclitol (spectinomycin)	Active versus *Neisseria gonorrhoeae*
Tetracyclines (tetracycline, doxycycline, minocycline)	Broad-spectrum antibiotics active against gram-positive and some gram-negative bacteria (*Neisseria,* some Enterobacteriaceae), mycoplasmas, chlamydiae, and rickettsiae
Glycylcyclines (tigecycline)	Spectrum similar to tetracyclines but more active against gram-negative bacteria and rapidly growing mycobacteria
Oxazolidinone (linezolid)	Active against *Staphylococcus* (including methicillin-resistant and vancomycin-intermediate strains), *Enterococcus, Streptococcus,* gram-positive rods, and *Clostridium* and anaerobic cocci; not active against gram-negative bacteria
Macrolides (erythromycin, azithromycin, clarithromycin, roxithromycin)	Broad-spectrum antibiotics active against gram-positive and some gram-negative bacteria, *Neisseria, Legionella, Mycoplasma, Chlamydia, Chlamydophila, Treponema,* and *Rickettsia;* clarithromycin and azithromycin active against some mycobacteria
Ketolides (telithromycin)	Broad-spectrum antibiotic with activity similar to macrolides; active against some macrolide-resistant staphylococci and enterococci
Lincosamide (clindamycin)	Broad-spectrum activity against aerobic gram-positive cocci and anaerobes
Streptogramins (quinupristin-dalfopristin)	Primarily active against gram-positive bacteria; good activity against methicillin-susceptible and -resistant staphylococci, streptococci, vancomycin-susceptible and -resistant *Enterococcus faecium* (no activity against *E. faecalis*), *Haemophilus, Moraxella,* and anaerobes (including *Bacteroides fragilis*); not active against Enterobacteriaceae or other gram-negative rods

Resistance to the antibacterial action of aminoglycosides can develop in one of four ways: (1) mutation of the ribosomal binding site, (2) decreased uptake of the antibiotic into the bacterial cell, (3) increased expulsion of the antibiotic from the cell, or (4) enzymatic modification of the antibiotic. The most common mechanism of resistance is enzymatic modification of aminoglycosides. This is accomplished by the action of phosphotransferases (aminoglycoside phosphotransferases [APHs]), adenyltransferases (adenine nucleotide translocases [ANTs]), and acetyltransferases (acetyl-CoA carboxylases [AACs]) on the amino and hydroxyl groups of the antibiotic. The differences in antibacterial activity among the aminoglycosides are determined by their relative susceptibility to these enzymes. The other mechanisms by which bacteria develop resistance to aminoglycosides are relatively uncommon. Resistance caused by alteration of the bacterial ribosome requires systematic mutation of the multiple copies of the ribosomal genes that exist in the bacterial cell. Resistance caused by inhibited transport of the antibiotic into the bacterial cell is occasionally observed with *Pseudomonas* but is more commonly seen with anaerobic bacteria. This mechanism produces low-level cross-resistance to all aminoglycosides. Active efflux of aminoglycosides occurs only in gram-negative bacteria and is rarely observed.

Tetracyclines

The tetracyclines (see Table 17-5) are broad-spectrum, bacteriostatic antibiotics that inhibit protein synthesis in bacteria by binding reversibly to the 30S ribosomal subunits, thus blocking the binding of aminoacyl-transfer RNA (tRNA) to the 30S ribosome–mRNA complex. Tetracyclines (i.e., **tetracycline, doxycycline, minocycline**) are effective in the treatment of infections caused by *Chlamydia, Mycoplasma,* and *Rickettsia* species and other selected gram-positive and gram-negative bacteria. All tetracyclines have a similar spectrum of activity, with the primary difference among the antibiotics being in their pharmacokinetic properties (doxycycline and minocycline are easily absorbed and have a long half-life). Resistance to the tetracyclines can stem from decreased penetration of the antibiotic into the bacterial cell, active efflux of the antibiotic out of the cell, alteration of the ribosomal target site, or enzymatic modification of the antibiotic. Mutations in the chromosomal gene encoding the outer membrane porin protein, OmpF, can lead to low-level resistance to the tetracyclines, as well as to other antibiotics (e.g., β-lactams, quinolones, chloramphenicol).

Researchers have identified a variety of genes in different bacteria that control active efflux of tetracyclines from the cell. This is the most common cause of resistance. Resistance to the tetracyclines can also result from production of proteins similar to elongation factors that protect the 30S ribosome. When this happens, the antibiotic can still bind to the ribosome, but protein synthesis is not disrupted.

Glycylclines

Tigecycline, the first representative of this new class of antibiotics, is a semisynthetic derivative of minocycline. It inhibits protein synthesis in the same manner as the tetracyclines. Tigecycline has a higher binding affinity for the ribosome and is less affected by efflux or enzymatic modification. It has a broad spectrum of activity against gram-positive, gram-negative, and anaerobic bacteria, although *Proteus, Morganella, Providencia,* and *P. aeruginosa* are generally resistant.

Oxazolidinones

The oxazolidinones are a narrow-spectrum class of antibiotics, with **linezolid** being the agent currently used. Linezolid blocks initiation of protein synthesis by interfering with formation of the initiation complex consisting of tRNA, mRNA, and the ribosome. The drug binds to the 50S ribosomal subunit, which distorts the binding site for tRNA, thus inhibiting formation of the 70S initiation complex. Because of this unique mechanism, cross-resistance with other protein inhibitors does not occur. Linezolid has activity against staphylococci, streptococci, and enterococci (including those strains resistant to penicillins, vancomycin, and the aminoglycosides). Because the multidrug-resistant enterococci are difficult to treat, use of linezolid is generally reserved for these infections.

Chloramphenicol

Chloramphenicol has a broad antibacterial spectrum similar to that of tetracycline but is not commonly used in the United States. The reason for its limited use is that besides interfering with bacterial protein synthesis, it disrupts protein synthesis in human bone marrow cells and can produce blood dyscrasias, such as aplastic anemia. Chloramphenicol exerts its bacteriostatic effect by binding reversibly to the peptidyl transferase component of the 50S ribosomal subunit, thus blocking peptide elongation. Resistance to chloramphenicol is observed in bacteria producing plasmid-encoded chloramphenicol acetyltransferase, which catalyzes the acetylation of the 3-hydroxy group of chloramphenicol. The product is incapable of binding to the 50S subunit. Less commonly, chromosomal mutations alter the outer membrane porin proteins, causing gram-negative rods to be less permeable.

Macrolides

Erythromycin, derived from *Streptomyces erythreus,* is the model macrolide antibiotic (see Table 17-5). The basic structure of this class of antibiotics is a macrocyclic lactone ring bound to two sugars, desosamine and cladinose. Modification of the macrolide structure led to the development of **azithromycin, clarithromycin,** and **roxithromycin.** Macrolides exert their effect by their reversible binding to the 23S ribosomal RNA (rRNA) of the 50S ribosomal subunit, which blocks polypeptide elongation. Resistance to macrolides most commonly stems from methylation of the 23S rRNA, preventing binding by the antibiotic. Other mechanisms of resistance include inactivation of the macrolides by enzymes (e.g., esterases, phosphorylases, glycosidase) or mutations in the 23S rRNA and ribosomal proteins. Macrolides are bacteriostatic antibiotics with a broad spectrum of activity. They have been used to treat pulmonary infections caused by *Mycoplasma, Legionella,* and *Chlamydia* species, as well as to treat infections caused by *Campylobacter* species and gram-positive bacteria in patients allergic to penicillin. Most gram-negative bacteria are resistant to the macrolides. Azithromycin and clarithromycin have also been used to treat infections caused by mycobacteria (e.g., *Mycobacterium avium* complex).

Ketolides

Ketolides are semisynthetic derivatives of erythromycin, modified to increase stability in acid. **Telithromycin** is currently the only ketolide available for use in the United States. As with the macrolides, telithromycin binds to the 50S ribosomal subunit and blocks protein synthesis. Its use is currently restricted to treatment of community-acquired pneumonia. It is active against *S. pneumoniae, Legionella, Mycoplasma,* and *Chlamydia,* but use of the drug is limited by its associated toxicity.

Clindamycin

Clindamycin (in the family of lincosamide antibiotics) is a derivative of lincomycin, which was originally isolated from *Streptomyces lincolnensis.* Like chloramphenicol and the macrolides, clindamycin blocks protein elongation by binding to the 50S ribosome. It inhibits peptidyl transferase by interfering with the binding of the amino acid–acyl-tRNA complex. Clindamycin is active against staphylococci and anaerobic gram-negative rods but is generally inactive against aerobic gram-negative bacteria. Methylation of the 23S rRNA is the source of bacterial resistance. Because both erythromycin and clindamycin can induce this enzymatic resistance (also plasmid mediated), cross-resistance between these two classes of antibiotics is observed.

Streptogramins

The streptogramins are a class of cyclic peptides produced by *Streptomyces* species. These antibiotics are administered as a combination of two components, group A and group B streptogramins, which act synergistically to inhibit protein synthesis. The antibiotic currently available in this class is **quinupristin-dalfopristin.** Dalfopristin binds to the 50S ribosomal subunit and induces a conformational change that facilitates binding of quinupristin. Dalfopristin prevents peptide chain elongation, and quinupristin initiates premature release of peptide chains from the ribosome. This combination drug is active against staphylococci, streptococci, and *E. faecium* (but not *E. faecalis*). Use of the antibiotic has been restricted primarily to treating vancomycin-resistant *E. faecium* infections.

Inhibition of Nucleic Acid Synthesis

Quinolones

The quinolones (Table 17-6) are one of the most widely used classes of antibiotics. These are synthetic chemotherapeutic agents that inhibit bacterial DNA topoisomerase type II (gyrase) or topoisomerase type IV, which are required for DNA replication, recombination, and repair. The DNA gyrase-A subunit is the primary quinolone target in gram-negative bacteria, whereas topoisomerase type IV is the primary target in gram-positive bacteria. The first quinolone used in clinical practice was **nalidixic acid.** This drug was used to treat urinary tract infections caused by a variety of gram-negative bacteria, but resistance to the drug developed rapidly, causing it to fall out of use. This drug has now been replaced by newer, more active quinolones, such as **ciprofloxacin, levofloxacin,** and **moxifloxacin.** Modifying the two-ring quinolone nucleus made these newer quinolones (referred to as *fluoroquinolones*). These antibiotics have

 Table 17-6 Quinolones

Antibiotics	Spectrum of Activity
Narrow spectrum (nalidixic acid)	Active against selected gram-negative rods; no useful gram-positive activity
Broad spectrum (ciprofloxacin, levofloxacin)	Broad-spectrum antibiotics with activity against gram-positive and gram-negative bacteria
Extended spectrum (moxifloxacin)	Broad-spectrum antibiotics with enhanced activity against gram-positive bacteria (particularly streptococci and enterococci) compared with early quinolones; activity against gram-negative rods similar to that of ciprofloxacin and related quinolones

excellent activity against gram-positive and gram-negative bacteria, although resistance can develop rapidly in *Pseudomonas,* oxacillin-resistant staphylococci, and enterococci. In particular, the newer extended-spectrum quinolones have significant activity against gram-positive bacteria.

Resistance to the quinolones is mediated by chromosomal mutations in the structural genes for DNA gyrase and topoisomerase type IV. Other mechanisms include decreased drug uptake caused by mutations in the membrane permeability regulatory genes, and overexpression of efflux pumps that actively eliminate the drug. Each of these mechanisms is primarily chromosomally mediated.

Rifampin and Rifabutin

Rifampin, a semisynthetic derivative of rifamycin B produced by *Streptomyces mediterranei,* binds to DNA-dependent RNA polymerase and inhibits initiation of RNA synthesis. Rifampin is bactericidal for *Mycobacterium tuberculosis* and is very active against aerobic gram-positive cocci, including staphylococci and streptococci.

Because resistance can develop rapidly, rifampin is usually combined with one or more other effective antibiotics. Rifampin resistance in gram-positive bacteria results from a mutation in the chromosomal gene that codes for the beta subunit of RNA polymerase. Gram-negative bacteria are resistant intrinsically to rifampin because of decreased uptake of the hydrophobic antibiotic. **Rifabutin,** a derivative of rifamycin, has a similar mode and spectrum of activity. It is particularly active against *M. avium.*

Metronidazole

Metronidazole was originally introduced as an oral agent for the treatment of *Trichomonas* vaginitis. However, it was also found to be effective in the treatment of amebiasis, giardiasis, and serious anaerobic bacterial infections (including those caused by *B. fragilis*). Metronidazole has no significant activity against aerobic or facultatively anaerobic bacteria. The antimicrobial properties of metronidazole stem from the reduction of its nitro group by bacterial nitroreductase, thereby producing cytotoxic compounds that disrupt the host DNA. Resistance results either from decreased uptake of the antibiotic or from elimination of the cytotoxic compounds before they can interact with host DNA.

Antimetabolites

The **sulfonamides** are antimetabolites that compete with *p*-aminobenzoic acid, thereby preventing synthesis of the folic acid required by certain microorganisms. Because mammalian organisms do not synthesize folic acid (required as a vitamin), sulfonamides do not interfere with mammalian cell metabolism. **Trimethoprim** is another antimetabolite that interferes with folic acid metabolism by inhibiting dihydrofolate reductase, thereby preventing the conversion of dihydrofolate to tetrahydrofolate. This inhibition blocks the formation of thymidine, some purines, methionine, and glycine. Trimethoprim is commonly combined with sulfamethoxazole to produce a synergistic combination active at two steps in the synthesis of folic acid. **Dapsone** and ***p*-aminosalicylic** acid are also antifolates that have proved to be useful for treating mycobacterial infections.

Sulfonamides are effective against a broad range of gram-positive and gram-negative organisms, such as *Nocardia, Chlamydia,* and some protozoa. Short-acting sulfonamides, such as sulfisoxazole, are among the drugs of choice for the treatment of acute urinary tract infections caused by susceptible bacteria, such as *E. coli.* Trimethoprim-sulfamethoxazole is effective against a large variety of gram-positive and gram-negative microorganisms and is the drug of choice for the treatment of acute and chronic urinary tract infections. The combination is also effective in the treatment of infections caused by *Pneumocystis jirovecii,* bacterial infections of the lower respiratory tract, otitis media, and uncomplicated gonorrhea.

Resistance to these antibiotics can stem from a variety of mechanisms. Bacteria such as *Pseudomonas* are resistant as the result of permeability barriers. A decreased affinity of dihydrofolate reductase can be the source of trimethoprim resistance. In addition, bacteria that use exogenous thymidine (e.g., enterococci) are also intrinsically resistant.

Other Antibiotics

Clofazimine is a lipophilic antibiotic that binds to mycobacterial DNA. It is highly active against *M. tuberculosis,* is a first-line drug for the treatment of *Mycobacterium leprae* infections, and has been recommended as a secondary antibiotic for the treatment of infections caused by other mycobacterial species.

Pyrazinamide (PZA) is active against *M. tuberculosis* at a low pH, such as that found in phagolysosomes. The active form of this antibiotic is pyrazinoic acid, produced when PZA is hydrolyzed in the liver. The mechanism by which PZA exerts its effect is unknown.

Bibliography

Bryskier A: *Antimicrobial agents: antibacterials and antifungals,* Washington, DC, 2005, American Society for Microbiology Press.

Kucers A, Bennett NM: *The use of antibiotics: a comprehensive review with clinical emphasis,* ed 4, Philadelphia, 1989, Lippincott.

Mandell GL, Bennett JE, Dolin R: *Principles and practice of infectious diseases,* ed 7, Philadelphia, 2010, Churchill Livingstone.

Versalovic J, Carroll KC, Funke G, et al: *Manual of clinical microbiology,* ed 10, Washington, DC, 2011, American Society for Microbiology Press.

CHAPTER

STAPHYLOCOCCUS AND RELATED GRAM-POSITIVE COCCI

A 26-year-old marine recruit presents to the base medic with large, pus-filled lesions surrounded by erythema on both legs. Infection with *Staphylococcus aureus* is suspected.

1. What structural properties are unique to this species of *Staphylococcus?*
2. How do the cytotoxins produced by this organism produce the clinical manifestations seen in this patient?
3. Three additional distinct toxins are described in strains of *S. aureus*. What diseases are associated with these toxins?
4. Resistance to what major class of antibiotics is now common in community-acquired infections with *S. aureus?*

Answers to these questions are available on StudentConsult.com.

• SUMMARIES CLINICALLY SIGNIFICANT ORGANISMS

Staphylococcus aureus

Trigger Words

Coagulase, cytotoxins, exfoliative toxins, enterotoxins, toxic shock syndrome toxin, MRSA

Biology and Virulence

- Catalase-positive, gram-positive cocci arranged in clusters
- Species characterized by the presence of coagulase, protein A, and species-specific ribitol teichoic acid with *N*-acetylglucosamine residues ("polysaccharide A")
- Virulence factors include structural components that facilitate adherence to host tissues and avoid phagocytosis, and a variety of toxins and hydrolytic enzymes (refer to Table 18-3)
- Hospital- and community-acquired infections with methicillin-resistant *Staphylococcus aureus* (MRSA) are a significant worldwide problem

Epidemiology

- Normal flora on human skin and mucosal surfaces
- Organisms can survive on dry surfaces for long periods (owing to thickened peptidoglycan layer and absence of outer membrane)
- Person-to-person spread through direct contact or exposure to contaminated fomites (e.g., bed linens, clothing)
- Risk factors include presence of a foreign body (e.g., splinter, suture, prosthesis, catheter), previous surgical procedure, and use of antibiotics that suppress the normal microbial flora
- Patients at risk for specific diseases include infants (scalded skin syndrome), young children with poor personal hygiene (impetigo and other cutaneous infections), menstruating women (toxic shock syndrome), patients with intravascular catheters (bacteremia and endocarditis) or shunts (meningitis), and patients with compromised pulmonary function or an antecedent viral respiratory infection (pneumonia)
- MRSA now the most common cause of community-acquired skin and soft-tissue infections

Diseases

- Diseases include toxin-mediated diseases (food poisoning, toxic shock syndrome, scalded skin syndrome), pyogenic diseases (impetigo, folliculitis, furuncles, carbuncles, wound infections), and other systemic diseases

Diagnosis

- Microscopy useful for pyogenic infections but not blood infections or toxin-mediated infections
- Staphylococci grow rapidly when cultured on nonselective media
- Selective media (e.g., mannitol-salt agar) can be used to recover *S. aureus* in contaminated specimens
- Nucleic acid amplification tests are useful for screening patients for carriage of methicillin-sensitive *S. aureus* (MSSA) and MRSA
- *S. aureus* is identified by biochemical tests (e.g., coagulase), molecular probes, or mass spectrometry

Treatment, Prevention, and Control

- Localized infections managed by incision and drainage; antibiotic therapy indicated for systemic infections
- Empirical therapy should include antibiotics active against MRSA strains
- Oral therapy can in include trimethoprim-sulfamethoxazole, doxycycline or minocycline, clindamycin, or linezolid; vancomycin is drug of choice for intravenous therapy, with daptomycin, tigecycline, or linezolid acceptable alternatives
- Treatment is symptomatic for patients with food poisoning (although the source of infection should be identified so that appropriate preventive procedures can be enacted)
- Proper cleansing of wounds and use of disinfectant help prevent infections
- Thorough hand washing and covering of exposed skin helps medical personnel prevent infection or spread to other patients

Coagulase-Negative Staphylococci

Trigger Words

Opportunistic, slime layer, subacute

Biology and Virulence

- Catalase-positive, coagulase-negative, gram-positive cocci arranged in clusters
- Relatively avirulent, although production of a "slime" layer can allow adherence to foreign bodies (e.g., catheters, grafts, prosthetic valves and joints, shunts) and protection from phagocytosis and antibiotics

Epidemiology

- Normal human flora on skin and mucosal surfaces
- Organisms can survive on dry surfaces for long periods
- Person-to-person spread through direct contact or exposure to contaminated fomites, although most infections are with the patient's own organisms
- Patients are at risk when a foreign body is present
- The organisms are ubiquitous, so there are no geographic or seasonal limitations

Diseases

- Infections include subacute endocarditis, infections of foreign bodies, and urinary tract infections

Diagnosis

- As with *S. aureus* infections

Treatment, Prevention, and Control

- The antibiotics of choice are oxacillin (or other penicillinase-resistant penicillin) or vancomycin for oxacillin-resistant strains
- Removal of the foreign body is often required for successful treatment
- Prompt treatment for endocarditis or shunt infections is necessary to prevent further tissue damage or immune complex formation

The gram-positive cocci are a heterogeneous collection of bacteria. Features they have in common are their spherical shape, their Gram-stain reaction, and an absence of endospores. The presence or absence of **catalase,** an enzyme that converts **hydrogen peroxide** into water and oxygen, is used to subdivide the various genera. The most important aerobic catalase-positive genus is *Staphylococcus* (discussed in this chapter), and the most important aerobic catalase-negative genera, *Streptococcus* and *Enterococcus,* are discussed in the next chapter.

Staphylococci are gram-positive cocci that grow in a characteristic pattern resembling a cluster of grapes (Figure 18-1 and Table 18-1), although organisms in clinical specimens may also appear as single cells, pairs, or short chains. Most staphylococci are large, 0.5 to 1.5 µm in diameter, and able to grow and potentially produce disease in a variety of conditions—aerobic and anaerobic atmosphere, in the presence of a high concentration of salt (e.g., 10% sodium chloride), and at temperatures ranging from 18° C to 40° C. The genus currently consists of 49 species and 27 subspecies, many of which are found on the skin and mucous membranes of humans. Some species have very specific niches where they are commonly found. For example, *Staphylococcus aureus* colonizes the anterior nares, *Staphylococcus capitis* is found where sebaceous glands are present (e.g., forehead), and *Staphylococcus haemolyticus* and *Staphylococcus hominis* are found in areas where apocrine glands are present (e.g., axilla). Staphylococci are important pathogens in humans, causing opportunistic infections and a wide spectrum of life-threatening systemic diseases, including infections of the skin, soft tissues, bones, and urinary tract (Table 18-2). The species most commonly associated with human diseases are ***S. aureus*** (the most virulent and best-known member of the genus), ***Staphylococcus epidermidis, S. haemolyticus, Staphylococcus lugdunensis,*** and ***Staphylococcus saprophyticus.*** **Methicillin-resistant *S. aureus* (MRSA)** is notorious for producing serious infections in hospitalized patients and outside the hospital in previously healthy children and adults. *S. aureus* colonies can have a yellow or gold color as the result of the carotenoid pigments that form during their growth, hence the species name. It is also the most common species in humans that produces the enzyme **coagulase,** and therefore this property is a useful diagnostic test. When a colony of *S. aureus* is suspended in plasma, coagulase binds to a serum factor and this complex converts fibrinogen to fibrin, resulting in formation of a clot. Most other staphylococcal species do not produce coagulase and are referred to collectively as **coagulase-negative staphylococci.** This is a useful distinction because the coagulase-negative staphylococci are less virulent and primarily cause opportunistic infections.

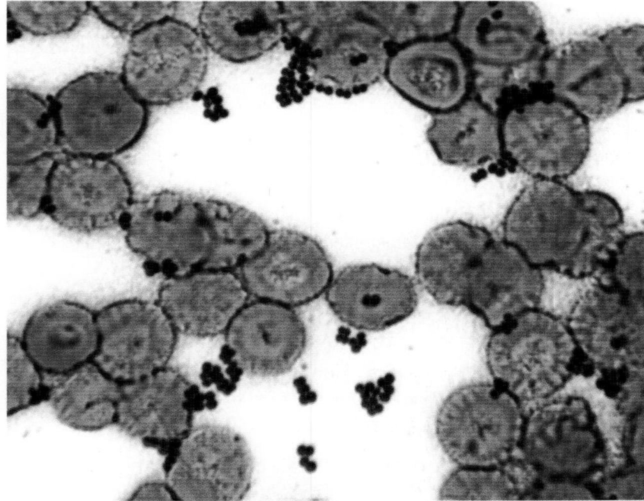

FIGURE 18-1 Gram stain of *Staphylococcus* in a blood culture.

 Table 18-1 **Important Staphylococci**

Organism	Historical Derivation
Staphylococcus	*staphylé,* bunch of grapes; *coccus,* grain or berry (grapelike cocci)
S. aureus	*aureus,* golden (golden or yellow)
S. epidermidis	*epidermidis,* outer skin (of the epidermis or outer skin)
S. lugdunensis	*Lugdunum,* Latin name for Lyon, France, where the organism was first isolated
S. saprophyticus	*sapros,* putrid; *phyton,* plant (saprophytic or growing on dead tissues)

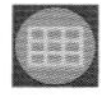 Table 18-2 **Common *Staphylococcus* Species and Their Diseases**

Organism	Diseases
S. aureus	Toxin mediated (food poisoning, scalded skin syndrome, toxic shock syndrome), cutaneous (carbuncles, folliculitis, furuncles, impetigo, wound infections), other (bacteremia, endocarditis, pneumonia, empyema, osteomyelitis, septic arthritis)
S. epidermidis	Bacteremia; endocarditis; surgical wounds; urinary tract infections; opportunistic infections of catheters, shunts, prosthetic devices, and peritoneal dialysates
S. saprophyticus	Urinary tract infections, opportunistic infections
S. lugdunensis	Endocarditis, arthritis, bacteremia, opportunistic infections, urinary tract infections
S. haemolyticus	Bacteremia, endocarditis, bone and joint infections, urinary tract infections, wound infections, opportunistic infections

• Physiology and Structure

Capsule and Slime Layer

The outermost layer of the cell wall of many staphylococci is covered with a **polysaccharide capsule.** Eleven capsular serotypes have been identified in *S. aureus*. Serotypes 1 and 2 are associated with very thick capsules and mucoid-appearing colonies but are rarely associated with human disease. In contrast, serotypes 5 and 8 are associated with the majority of infections in humans. The capsule protects the bacteria by inhibiting phagocytosis of the organisms by polymorphonuclear leukocytes (PMNs). A loose-bound, water-soluble film **(slime layer** or **biofilm)** consisting of monosaccharides, proteins, and small peptides is produced by most staphylococci in varying amounts. This extracellular substance binds the bacteria to tissues and foreign bodies such as catheters, grafts, prosthetic valves and joints, and shunts and is particularly important for the survival of relatively avirulent coagulase-negative staphylococci.

Peptidoglycan and Associated Enzymes

An understanding of the structure of the gram-positive bacterial cell wall is important because this is the target of many important antibiotics. Half of the cell wall by weight is **peptidoglycan,** consisting of layers of glycan chains built with 10 to 12 alternating subunits of *N*-acetylmuramic acid and *N*-acetylglucosamine. Oligopeptide side chains are attached to the *N*-acetylmuramic acid subunits and are then cross-linked with peptide bridges. Unlike gram-negative bacteria, the peptidoglycan layer in gram-positive organisms consists of **many cross-linked layers,** which makes the cell wall more rigid. The **enzymes** that catalyze construction of the peptidoglycan layer are called **penicillin-binding proteins** because these are the targets of penicillins and other β-lactam antibiotics. Bacterial resistance to methicillin and related penicillins and cephalosporins is mediated by acquisition of a gene *(mecA)* that codes for a novel penicillin-binding protein, PBP2a, that has a low affinity for methicillin and related penicillins and cephalosporins (refer to Treatment, Prevention, and Control for additional details). The ***mecA* gene** is located on the staphylococcal cassette chromosome mec (SCC*mec*), and multiple gene sequences of this cassette are described. This information is relevant because **MRSA** strains, previously restricted to hospital-acquired infections, are now present in the community and responsible for the majority of staphylococcal infections. Although the hospital and community strains were initially distinct, movement into and out of the hospital is now common, making control of hospital-acquired infections more difficult.

The peptidoglycan has endotoxin-like activity, stimulating the production of endogenous pyrogens, activation of complement, production of interleukin (IL)-1 from monocytes, and aggregation of PMNs (a process responsible for abscess formation).

Teichoic Acids and Lipoteichoic Acids

Teichoic acids are the other major component of the cell wall. Teichoic acids are **species-specific,** phosphate-containing polymers that are bound covalently to *N*-acetylmuramic acid residues of the peptidoglycan layer or to the lipids in the cytoplasmic membrane **(lipoteichoic acids).** Although the teichoic acids are poor immunogens, a specific antibody response is stimulated when they are bound to peptidoglycan. Although the production of antibodies was used initially as a marker of *S. aureus* infection, this insensitive test has been abandoned in recent years.

Surface Adhesion Proteins

A large collection of surface proteins have been identified in *S. aureus* that are important virulence factors because they adhere to host matrix proteins bound to host tissues (e.g., fibronectin, fibrinogen, elastin, collagen). Most of these surface adhesion proteins are covalently bound to the cell wall peptidoglycan in staphylococci and have been designated **MSCRAMM (*m*icrobial *s*urface *c*omponents *r*ecognizing *a*dhesive *m*atrix *m*olecules) proteins.** The nomenclature for the individual proteins is confusing; for example, staphylococcal protein A *(spa)* binds to the Fc receptor of immunoglobulin (Ig)G1, IgG2, and IgG4; fibronectin-binding protein A binds fibronectin as the name indicates; and *S. aureus* surface protein A has an undetermined function. The best characterized MSCRAMM proteins are staphylococcal protein A, fibronectin-binding proteins A and B, and clumping factor proteins A and B. The clumping factor proteins (also called **coagulase**) bind fibrinogen and convert it to insoluble fibrin, causing the staphylococci to clump or aggregate. Detection of these proteins is the primary **identification test** for *S. aureus.* Two MSCRAMM proteins, *S. aureus* surface proteins G and H, have been associated with invasive disease.

Cytoplasmic Membrane

The **cytoplasmic membrane** is made up of a complex of proteins, lipids, and a small amount of carbohydrates. It serves as an osmotic barrier for the cell and provides an anchorage for the cellular biosynthetic and respiratory enzymes.

Pathogenesis and Immunity

The ability of staphylococci to cause disease depends on the ability of the bacteria to **evade** immune clearance, produce surface proteins that mediate **adherence** of the bacteria to host tissues during colonization, and produce disease through the elaboration of specific toxins and hydrolytic enzymes leading to **tissue destruction** (Table 18-3). These properties—immunologic evasion, adherence, tissue destruction—are common to most pathogenic organisms.

Regulation of Virulence Genes

Expression of virulence factors in staphylococci is under the complex control of the ***agr*** **(accessory gene regulator) operon.** This quorum-sensing (bacterial density) control system allows expression of adhesion proteins and promotes tissue colonization when the density of bacteria is low, and tissue invasion and production of hydrolytic enzymes and toxins when the density is high. The operon encodes autoinducer peptides (AIP1-4) that bind to cell surface receptors and regulate protein expression based on the population density. The innate immune regulation of bacterial virulence is mediated by apolipoprotein B, the major structural protein of very low- and low-density lipoproteins (VLDL, LDL), which binds to AIPs and suppresses *agr* signaling. Thus, under optimal conditions, the bacterial density is maintained at a low concentration, providing the benefits of immune stimulation by colonizing staphylococci without the consequences of tissue invasion and destruction.

Table 18-3 ***Staphylococcus aureus*** **Virulence Factors**

Virulence Factors	Biological Effects
Structural Components	
Capsule	Inhibits chemotaxis and phagocytosis; inhibits proliferation of mononuclear cells
Slime layer	Facilitates adherence to foreign bodies
Peptidoglycan	Provides osmotic stability; stimulates production of endogenous pyrogen (endotoxin-like activity); leukocyte chemoattractant (abscess formation); inhibits phagocytosis
Teichoic acid	Binds to fibronectin
Protein A	Inhibits antibody-mediated clearance by binding IgG1, IgG2, and IgG4 Fc receptors; leukocyte chemoattractant; anticomplementary
Toxins	
Cytotoxins	Toxic for many cells, including erythrocytes, fibroblasts, leukocytes, macrophages, and platelets
Exfoliative toxins (ETA, ETB)	Serine proteases that split the intercellular bridges in the stratum granulosum epidermis
Enterotoxins (A-E, G-I)	Superantigens (stimulate proliferation of T cells and release of cytokines); stimulate release of inflammatory mediators in mast cells, increasing intestinal peristalsis and fluid loss, as well as nausea and vomiting
Toxic shock syndrome toxin-1	Superantigen (stimulates proliferation of T cells and release of cytokines); produces leakage or cellular destruction of endothelial cells
Enzymes	
Coagulase	Converts fibrinogen to fibrin
Hyaluronidase	Hydrolyzes hyaluronic acids in connective tissue, promoting spread of staphylococci in tissue
Fibrinolysin	Dissolves fibrin clots
Lipases	Hydrolyze lipids
Nucleases	Hydrolyze DNA

Defenses Against Innate Immunity

Opsonins (IgG, complement factor C3) in serum bind to encapsulated staphylococci, but the **capsule** protects the bacteria by inhibiting phagocytosis of the organisms by PMNs; however, in the presence of specific antibodies directed against the staphylococci, increased C3 is bound to the bacteria and leads to phagocytosis. The extracellular **slime layer** also interferes with phagocytosis of bacteria. The ability of **protein A** to bind immunoglobulins effectively prevents antibody-mediated immune clearance of the *S. aureus*. Additionally, extracellular protein A can bind antibodies and form immune complexes, with the subsequent consumption of the complement.

Staphylococcal Toxins

S. aureus produces many toxins, including five cytolytic or membrane-damaging toxins (alpha, beta, delta, gamma, and Panton-Valentine [P-V] leukocidin), two exfoliative toxins (A and B), numerous enterotoxins (A to E, G to X, plus multiple variants), and toxic shock syndrome toxin-1 (TSST-1). The cytolytic toxins have been described as hemolysins, but this is a misnomer because the activities of the first four toxins are not restricted solely to red blood cells, and P-V leukocidin is unable to lyse erythrocytes. Cytotoxins can lyse neutrophils, resulting in the release of lysosomal enzymes that subsequently damage surrounding tissues. One cytotoxin, P-V leukocidin, has been linked with severe pulmonary and cutaneous infections.

Exfoliative toxin A, the enterotoxins, and TSST-1 belong to a class of polypeptides known as **superantigens.** These toxins bind to class II major histocompatibility complex (MHC II) molecules on macrophages, which in turn interact with the ***v****ariable regions of the* β subunit of specific ***T****-**c**ell* ***r****eceptors* **(VβTCR).** This results in a massive release of cytokines by both macrophages (IL-1β and tumor necrosis factor [TNF]-α) and T cells (IL-2, interferon [IFN]-γ, and TNF-β).

Release of TNF-α and TNF-β is associated with hypotension and shock, and fever is associated with IL-1β release.

Cytotoxins

Alpha toxin, which can be encoded on both the bacterial chromosome and a plasmid, is a 33,000-Da polypeptide produced by most strains of *S. aureus* that cause human disease. The toxin disrupts the smooth muscle in blood vessels and is toxic to many types of cells, including erythrocytes, leukocytes, hepatocytes, and platelets. Alpha toxin binds to the cell surface, aggregates into a heptamer (7 toxin molecules) forming a 1- to 2-nm pore, and allows the rapid efflux of K^+ and influx of Na^+, Ca^{2+}, and other small molecules, which leads to osmotic swelling and cell lysis. Alpha toxin is believed to be an important mediator of tissue damage in staphylococcal disease.

Beta toxin, also called **sphingomyelinase C,** is a 35,000-Da heat-labile protein produced by most strains of *S. aureus* responsible for disease in humans and animals. This enzyme has a specificity for sphingomyelin and lysophosphatidylcholine and is toxic to a variety of cells, including erythrocytes, fibroblasts, leukocytes, and macrophages. It catalyzes the hydrolysis of membrane phospholipids in susceptible cells, with lysis proportional to the concentration of sphingomyelin exposed on the cell surface. This is believed to be responsible for the differences in species susceptibility to the toxin. The effect on erythrocytes occurs primarily at low temperatures, so this toxin may be less efficient than other hemolysins.

Delta toxin is a 3000-Da polypeptide produced by almost all *S. aureus* strains and other staphylococci (e.g., *S. epidermidis, S. haemolyticus*). The toxin has a wide spectrum of cytolytic activity, affecting erythrocytes, many other mammalian cells, and intracellular membrane structures. This relatively nonspecific membrane toxicity is consistent with the belief that the toxin acts as a surfactant, disrupting cellular membranes by means of a detergent-like action.

Gamma toxin (made by almost all *S. aureus* strains) and **P-V leukocidin** are bicomponent toxins composed of two polypeptide chains: the S (slow-eluting proteins) component and F (fast-eluting proteins) component. Three S proteins (HlgA [hemolysin gamma A], HlgC, LukS-PV) and two F proteins (HlgB, LukF-PV) have been identified. Bacteria capable of producing both toxins can encode all these proteins, with the potential for producing six distinct toxins. All six toxins can lyse neutrophils and macrophages, whereas the greatest hemolytic activity is associated with HlgA/HlgB, HlgC/HlgB, and HlgA/LukF-PV. The PV leukocidin toxin (LukS-PV/LukF-PV) is leukotoxic but has no hemolytic activity. Cell lysis by the gamma and PV leukocidin toxins is mediated by pore formation, with subsequent increased permeability to cations and osmotic instability.

Exfoliative Toxins

Staphylococcal scalded skin syndrome (SSSS), a spectrum of diseases characterized by exfoliative dermatitis, is mediated by exfoliative toxins. The prevalence of toxin production in *S. aureus* strains varies geographically but is generally less than 5%. Two distinct forms of exfoliative toxin (ETA and ETB) have been identified, and either can produce disease. ETA is heat stable and the gene is phage associated, whereas ETB is heat labile and located on a plasmid. The toxins are **serine proteases** that split desmoglein-1, a member of a family of cell adhesion structures (desmosomes) responsible for forming the intercellular bridges in the stratum granulosum epidermis. The toxins are not associated with cytolysis or inflammation, so neither staphylococci nor leukocytes are typically present in the involved layer of the epidermis (this is an important **diagnostic clue**). After exposure of the epidermis to the toxin, protective neutralizing antibodies develop, leading to resolution of the toxic process. SSSS is seen mostly in young children and only rarely in older children and adults.

Enterotoxins

Numerous distinct **staphylococcal enterotoxins** (A to X) have been identified, with enterotoxin A most commonly associated with food poisoning. Enterotoxins C and D are found in contaminated milk products, and enterotoxin B causes staphylococcal pseudomembranous enterocolitis. Less is known about the prevalence or clinical importance of the other enterotoxins. The enterotoxins are designed perfectly for causing foodborne disease—stable to heating at 100° C for 30 minutes and resistant to hydrolysis by gastric and jejunal enzymes. Thus, once a food product has been contaminated with enterotoxin-producing staphylococci and the toxins have been produced, neither mild reheating of the food nor exposure to gastric acids will be protective. These toxins are produced by 30% to 50% of all *S. aureus* strains. The precise mechanism of toxin activity is not understood. These toxins are **superantigens** capable of inducing nonspecific activation of T cells and massive cytokine release. Characteristic histologic changes in the stomach and jejunum include infiltration of neutrophils into the epithelium and underlying lamina propria, with loss of the brush border in the jejunum. Stimulation of release of inflammatory mediators from mast cells is believed to be responsible for the emesis that is characteristic of staphylococcal food poisoning.

Toxic Shock Syndrome Toxin-1

TSST-1 is a 22,000-Da heat- and proteolysis-resistant, chromosomally mediated exotoxin. It is estimated that 90% of *S. aureus* strains responsible for menstruation-associated toxic shock syndrome (TSS) and half of the strains responsible for other forms of TSS produce TSST-1. Enterotoxin B and (rarely) enterotoxin C are responsible for approximately half the cases of nonmenstruation-associated TSS. Expression of TSST-1 in vitro requires an elevated oxygen concentration and neutral pH. This is likely the reason TSS is relatively uncommon compared with the incidence of *S. aureus* wound infections (a setting where the environment of an abscess is relatively anaerobic and acidic). TSST-1 is a **superantigen** that stimulates release of cytokines, producing leakage of endothelial cells at low concentrations and a cytotoxic effect to the cells at high concentrations. The ability of TSST-1 to penetrate mucosal barriers, even though the infection remains localized in the vagina or at the site of a wound, is responsible for the systemic effects of TSS. Death in patients with TSS is caused by hypovolemic shock leading to multiorgan failure.

Staphylococcal Enzymes

S. aureus strains possess two forms of **coagulase:** bound and free. Coagulase bound to the staphylococcal cell wall can directly convert fibrinogen to insoluble fibrin and cause the staphylococci to clump. The cell-free coagulase accomplishes the same result by reacting with a globulin plasma factor **(coagulase-reacting factor)** to form staphylothrombin, a thrombin-like factor. This factor catalyzes the conversion of fibrinogen to insoluble fibrin. The role of coagulase in the pathogenesis of disease is speculative, but coagulase may cause the formation of a fibrin layer around a staphylococcal abscess, thus localizing the infection and protecting the organisms from phagocytosis. Some other species of staphylococci produce coagulase, but these are primarily animal pathogens and uncommonly recovered in human infections.

Staphylococci produce a variety of other enzymes that hydrolyze host tissue components and aid in bacterial spread. **Hyaluronidase** hydrolyzes hyaluronic acids, present in the acellular matrix of connective tissue. **Fibrinolysin,** also called staphylokinase, can dissolve fibrin clots. All strains of *S. aureus* and more than 30% of the strains of coagulase-negative *Staphylococcus* produce several different **lipases** that hydrolyze lipids and ensure survival of staphylococci in the sebaceous areas of the body. *S. aureus* also produces a thermostable **nuclease** that can hydrolyze viscous DNA.

Epidemiology

Staphylococci are **ubiquitous.** All persons have coagulase-negative staphylococci on their skin, and transient colonization of moist skinfolds with *S. aureus* is common. Colonization of the umbilical stump, skin, and perineal area of neonates with *S. aureus* is common. *S. aureus* and coagulase-negative staphylococci are also found in the oropharynx, gastrointestinal tract, and urogenital tract. Short-term or persistent *S. aureus* carriage in older children and adults is more common in the anterior **nasopharynx** than in the oropharynx. Approximately 15% of normal healthy adults are persistent nasopharyngeal carriers of *S. aureus,* with a higher incidence reported for hospitalized patients, medical personnel, persons with eczematous skin diseases, and those who regularly use needles, either illicitly (e.g., drug abusers) or for medical reasons (e.g., patients with insulin-dependent diabetes, patients receiving allergy injections, or those undergoing hemodialysis). Adherence of the organism to the mucosal epithelium is regulated by the staphylococcal cell surface adhesins.

Because staphylococci are found on the skin and in the nasopharynx, shedding of the bacteria is common and is responsible for many hospital-acquired infections. Staphylococci are susceptible to high temperatures and disinfectants and antiseptic solutions; however, the organisms can survive on dry surfaces for long periods. The organisms can be transferred to a susceptible person either through direct contact or through contact with fomites (e.g., contaminated clothing, bed linens). Therefore, medical personnel must use proper hand-washing techniques to prevent transfer of staphylococci from themselves to patients or among patients.

Beginning in the 1980s, strains of MRSA spread rapidly in susceptible hospitalized patients, dramatically changing the therapy available for preventing and treating staphylococcal infections. Although MRSA infections were relatively uncommon among healthy individuals in the community, a dramatic change was observed in 2003 when new strains of MRSA were reported to be responsible for outbreaks of community-acquired cutaneous infections and severe pneumonia. Interestingly, the strains were not related to strains circulating in hospitals, and strains isolated in each country were genetically unique. Unfortunately, the community strains have moved into hospitals in the last decade, complicating control measures previously established. Hospitalized patients are now susceptible to infections caused by strains they were colonized with in the community as well as strains acquired in the hospital.

Clinical Diseases (Box 18-1)

Staphylococcus aureus

S. aureus causes disease through production of toxins or through direct invasion and destruction of tissue. The clinical manifestations of some staphylococcal diseases are almost exclusively the result of toxin activity (e.g., staphylococcal scalded skin syndrome, staphylococcal food poisoning, and toxic shock syndrome), whereas other diseases result from proliferation of the organisms, leading to abscess formation and tissue destruction (e.g., cutaneous infections, endocarditis, pneumonia, empyema, osteomyelitis, septic arthritis) (Figure 18-2). In the presence of a foreign body (e.g., splinter, catheter, shunt, prosthetic valve or joint), significantly fewer staphylococci are necessary to establish disease. Likewise, patients with congenital diseases associated with an impaired chemotactic or phagocytic response (e.g., Job syndrome, Wiskott-Aldrich syndrome, chronic granulomatous disease) are more susceptible to staphylococcal diseases.

Staphylococcal Scalded Skin Syndrome (SSSS)

In 1878, Gottfried Ritter von Rittershain described 297 infants younger than 1 month old who had bullous exfoliative dermatitis. The disease he described, now called **Ritter's disease** or SSSS, is characterized by the abrupt onset of a localized perioral erythema (redness and inflammation around the mouth) that spreads over the entire body within 2 days. Slight pressure displaces the skin (a positive Nikolsky sign), and large bullae or **cutaneous blisters** form soon thereafter, followed by desquamation of the epithelium (Figure 18-3). The blisters contain clear fluid but no organisms or leukocytes, a finding consistent with the fact that the disease is caused by the bacterial toxin. The epithelium becomes intact again within 7 to 10 days, when antibodies against the toxin appear. Scarring does not occur, because only the top layer of epidermis is sloughed. This is a disease primarily of neonates and young children, with the mortality rate less than 5%. When death does occur, it is a result of secondary bacterial infection of the denuded skin areas. Infections in adults usually occur in immunocompromised hosts or patients with renal disease, and mortality is as high as 60%.

Bullous impetigo is a localized form of SSSS. In this syndrome, specific strains of toxin-producing *S. aureus* (e.g., phage type 71) are associated with formation of superficial skin blisters (Figure 18-4). Unlike patients with the disseminated manifestations of SSSS, patients with bullous impetigo have localized blisters that are culture positive. The erythema does not extend beyond the borders of the blister, and the

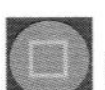

Box 18-1 Staphylococcal Diseases: Clinical Summaries

Staphylococcus aureus

Toxin-Mediated Diseases

Scalded skin syndrome: Disseminated desquamation of epithelium in infants; blisters with no organisms or leukocytes

Food poisoning: After consumption of food contaminated with heat-stable enterotoxin, rapid onset of severe vomiting, diarrhea, and abdominal cramping, with resolution within 24 hours

Toxic shock: multisystem intoxication characterized initially by fever, hypotension, and a diffuse, macular, erythematous rash; high mortality without prompt antibiotic therapy and elimination of the focus of infection

Suppurative Infections

Impetigo: localized cutaneous infection characterized by pus-filled vesicle on an erythematous base

Folliculitis: impetigo involving hair follicles

Furuncles or boils: large, painful, pus-filled cutaneous nodules

Carbuncles: Coalescence of furuncles with extension into subcutaneous tissues and evidence of systemic disease (fever, chills, bacteremia)

Bacteremia and endocarditis: Spread of bacteria into the blood from a focus of infection; endocarditis characterized by damage to the endothelial lining of the heart

Pneumonia and empyema: Consolidation and abscess formation in the lungs; seen in the very young and elderly and in patients with underlying or recent pulmonary disease; a severe form of necrotizing pneumonia with septic shock and high mortality is now recognized

Osteomyelitis: Destruction of bones, particularly the metaphyseal area of long bones

Septic arthritis: Painful erythematous joint with collection of purulent material in the joint space

Coagulase-Negative *Staphylococcus* Species

Wound infections: Characterized by erythema and pus at the site of a traumatic or surgical wound; infections with foreign bodies can be caused by *S. aureus* and coagulase-negative staphylococci

Urinary tract infections: Dysuria and pyuria in young sexually active women (*S. saprophyticus*), in patients with urinary catheters (other coagulase-negative staphylococci), or following seeding of the urinary tract by bacteremia (*S. aureus*)

Catheter and shunt infections: Chronic inflammatory response to bacteria coating a catheter or shunt (most commonly with coagulase-negative staphylococci)

Prosthetic device infections: Chronic infection of device characterized by localized pain and mechanical failure of the device (most commonly with coagulase-negative staphylococci)

Nikolsky sign is not present. The disease occurs primarily in infants and young children and is highly communicable.

Staphylococcal Food Poisoning (Clinical Case 18-1)

Staphylococcal food poisoning, one of the most common foodborne illnesses, is an **intoxication** rather than an infection. Disease is caused by bacterial toxin present in food rather than from a direct effect of the organisms on the patient. The most commonly contaminated foods are **processed meats** such as ham and salted pork, **custard**-filled **pastries, potato salad,** and **ice cream.** Growth of *S. aureus* in salted meats is consistent with the ability of this organ-

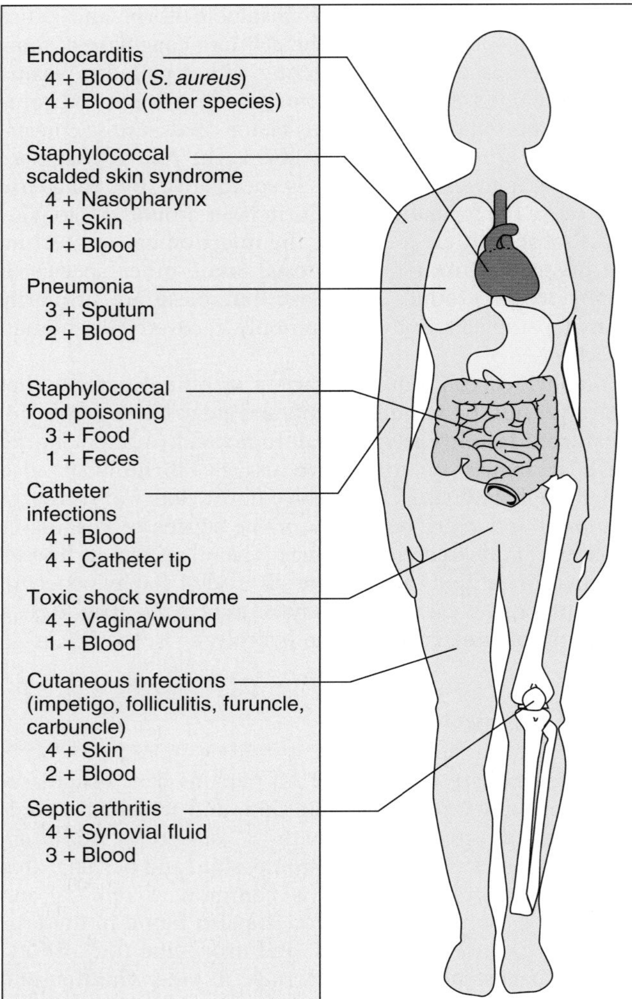

FIGURE 18-2 Staphylococcal diseases. Isolation of staphylococci from sites of infection. *1+*, Less than 10% positive cultures; *2+*, 10% to 50% positive cultures; *3+*, 50% to 90% positive cultures; *4+*, more than 90% positive cultures.

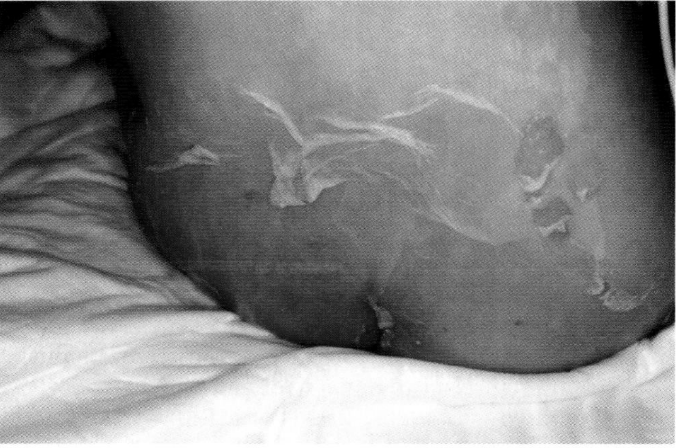

FIGURE 18-3 Staphylococcal scalded skin syndrome. (From Mandell G, Bennett J, Dolin R: *Principles and practice of infectious disease,* ed 6, Philadelphia, 2005, Churchill Livingstone.)

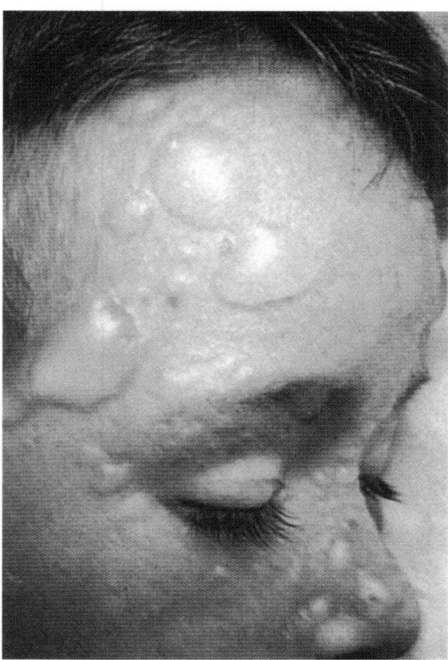

FIGURE 18-4 Bullous impetigo, a localized form of staphylococcal scalded skin syndrome. (From Emond RT, Rowland HAK, Welsby P: *Colour atlas of infectious diseases,* ed 3, London, 1995, Wolfe.)

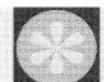

Clinical Case 18-1 Staphylococcal Food Poisoning

A report published in the Centers for Disease Control and Prevention's *Morbidity and Mortality Weekly Report* (*MMWR* 46:1189–1191, 1997) illustrates many important features of staphylococcal food poisoning. A total of 18 persons attending a retirement party became ill approximately 3 to 4 hours after eating. The most common symptoms were nausea (94%), vomiting (89%), and diarrhea (72%). Relatively few individuals had fever or headache (11%). The symptoms lasted a median of 24 hours. The illness was associated with eating ham at the party. A sample of the cooked ham was positive for staphylococcal enterotoxin type A. A food preparer had cooked the ham at home, transported it to her workplace and sliced it while it was still hot, and then refrigerated the ham in a large plastic container covered with foil. The ham was served cold the next day. Cooking the ham would kill any contaminating *S. aureus,* so it is likely the ham was contaminated after it was cooked. The delays involved in refrigerating the ham and the fact it was stored in a single container allowed the organism to proliferate and produce enterotoxin. Type A toxin is the most common toxin associated with human disease. The rapid onset and short duration of nausea, vomiting, and diarrhea is typical of this disease. Care must be used to avoid contamination of salted meats such as ham because reheating the food at a later time will not inactivate the heat-stable toxin.

ism to grow in the presence of high salt concentrations. Unlike many other forms of food poisoning in which an animal reservoir is important, staphylococcal food poisoning results from contamination of the food by a human carrier. Although contamination can be prevented by not allowing individuals with an obvious staphylococcal skin infection to prepare food, approximately half of the infections originate from carriers with asymptomatic nasopharyngeal colonization. After the staphylococci have been introduced into the food (through a sneeze or contaminated hand), the food must remain at room temperature or warmer for the organisms to grow and release the toxin. The contaminated food will not appear or taste tainted. Subsequent heating of the food will kill the bacteria but not inactivate the **heat-stable toxin.**

After ingestion of contaminated food, the onset of disease is abrupt and rapid, with a mean incubation period of 4 hours, which again is consistent with a disease mediated by preformed toxin. Further toxin is not produced by ingested staphylococci, so the disease has a rapid course, with symptoms generally lasting less than 24 hours. Severe vomiting, diarrhea, and abdominal pain or nausea are characteristic of staphylococcal food poisoning. Sweating and headache may occur, but fever is not seen. The diarrhea is watery and nonbloody, and dehydration may result from the considerable fluid loss.

The toxin-producing organisms can be cultured from the contaminated food if the organisms are not killed during food preparation. The enterotoxins are heat-stable, so contaminated food can be tested for toxins at a public health facility; however, these tests are rarely performed.

Treatment is for relief of abdominal cramping and diarrhea and for fluid replacement. Antibiotic therapy is not indicated; as already noted, the disease is mediated by preformed toxin, not by replicating organisms. Neutralizing antibodies to the toxin can be protective, and limited cross-protection occurs among the different enterotoxins. Short-lived immunity means that second episodes of staphylococcal food poisoning can occur, particularly with serologically distinct enterotoxins.

Certain strains of *S. aureus* can also cause **enterocolitis,** which is manifested clinically by watery diarrhea, abdominal cramps, and fever. The majority of strains producing this disease produce both enterotoxin A and the bicomponent leukotoxin LukE/LukD. Enterocolitis occurs primarily in patients who have received broad-spectrum antibiotics that suppress the normal colonic flora and permit the growth of *S. aureus.* The diagnosis of staphylococcal enterocolitis can be confirmed only after more common causes of infection have been excluded (e.g., *Clostridium difficile* colitis). Abundant staphylococci are typically present in the stool of affected patients, and the normal gram-negative bacteria are absent. Fecal leukocytes are observed, and white plaques with ulceration are seen on the colonic mucosa.

Toxic Shock Syndrome (TSS; Clinical Case 18-2)

The first outbreak of this disease occurred in 1928 in Australia, where the disease developed in 21 children, 12 of whom died after an injection with an *S. aureus*–contaminated vaccine. Fifty years later, J.K. Todd observed what he called **toxic shock syndrome** in seven children with systemic disease, and the first reports of TSS in menstruating women were published in the summer of 1980. These reports were followed by a dramatic increase in the incidence of TSS, particularly in women. Subsequently, it was discovered that TSST-1–producing strains of *S. aureus* could multiply rapidly in hyperabsorbent tampons and release toxin. After the recall of these tampons, the incidence of disease—particularly in menstruating women—decreased rapidly. At present, fewer than 100 cases of TSS are reported annually in the United States. Although it was originally reported that

Clinical Case 18-2 Staphylococcal Toxic Shock Syndrome

Todd and associates (*Lancet* 2:1116–1118, 1978) were the first investigators to describe a pediatric disease they called "toxic shock syndrome" (TSS). This patient illustrates the clinical course of the disease. A 15-year-old girl was admitted to the hospital with a 2-day history of pharyngitis and vaginitis associated with vomiting and watery diarrhea. She was febrile and hypotensive on admission, with a diffuse erythematous rash over her entire body. Laboratory tests were consistent with acidosis, oliguria, and disseminated intravascular coagulation with severe thrombocytopenia. Her chest radiograph showed bilateral infiltrates suggestive of "shock lung." She was admitted to the hospital intensive care unit, where she was stabilized and improved gradually over a 17-day period. On the third day, fine desquamation started on her face, trunk, and extremities and progressed to peeling of the palms and soles by the 14th day. All cultures were negative except from the throat and vagina, from which *Staphylococcus aureus* was isolated. This case illustrates the initial presentation of TSS, the multiorgan toxicity, and the protracted period of recovery.

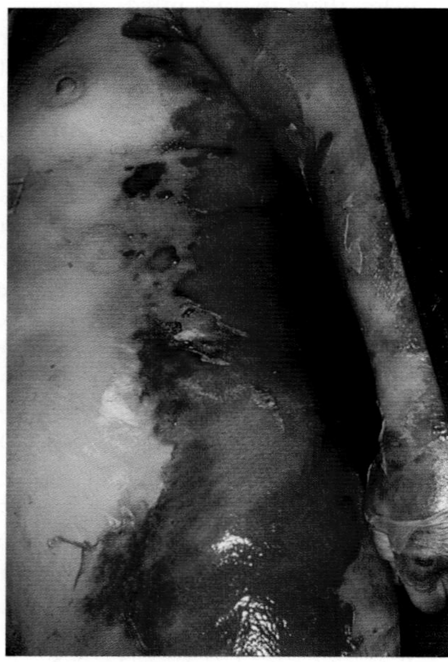

FIGURE 18-5 Toxic shock syndrome. A case of fatal infection with cutaneous and soft-tissue involvement is shown.

coagulase-negative staphylococci could cause TSS, it is now believed that this disease is restricted to *S. aureus.*

The disease is initiated with the localized growth of toxin-producing strains of *S. aureus* in the vagina or a wound, followed by release of the toxin into blood. Toxin production requires an aerobic atmosphere and neutral pH. Clinical manifestations start abruptly and include fever, hypotension, and a diffuse, macular, erythematous rash. Multiple organ systems (e.g., central nervous, gastrointestinal, hematologic, hepatic, musculature, renal) are also involved, and the entire skin, including the palms and soles, desquamates (Figure 18-5). A particularly virulent form of toxic shock syndrome is **purpura fulminans.** This disease is characterized by large purpuric skin lesion, fever, hypotension, and disseminated intravascular coagulation. Previously, purpura fulminans was primarily associated with overwhelming *Neisseria meningitidis* infections.

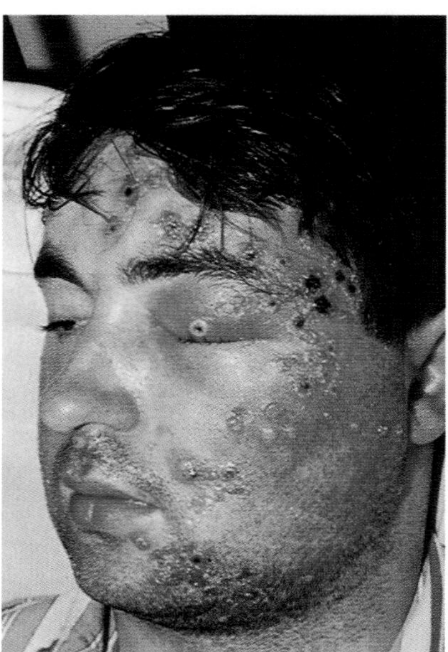

FIGURE 18-6 Pustular impetigo. Note the vesicles at different stages of development, including pus-filled vesicles on an erythematous base and dry, crusted lesions. (From Emond RT, Rowland HAK, Welsby P: *Colour atlas of infectious diseases,* ed 3, London, 1995, Wolfe.)

As the etiology and epidemiology of this disease have become better understood, the initially high-fatality rate has been decreased to approximately 5%. Unless the patient is specifically treated with an effective antibiotic, however, the risk of recurrent disease is as high as 65%. Serologic studies have demonstrated that more than 90% of adults have antibodies to TSST-1; however, more than 50% of patients with TSS fail to develop protective antibodies after their disease resolves. These unprotected patients are at significant risk for **recurrent disease.**

Cutaneous Infections

Localized **pyogenic staphylococcal infections** include impetigo, folliculitis, furuncles, and carbuncles. **Impetigo,** a superficial infection that mostly affects young children, occurs primarily on the face and limbs. Initially, a small macule (flattened red spot) is seen, and then a pus-filled vesicle (pustule) on an erythematous base develops. Crusting occurs after the pustule ruptures. Multiple vesicles at different stages of development are common, owing to the secondary spread of the infection to adjacent skin sites (Figure 18-6). Impetigo is usually caused by *S. aureus,* although group A streptococci, either alone or with *S. aureus,* are responsible for 20% of cases.

Folliculitis is a pyogenic infection in the hair follicles. The base of the follicle is raised and reddened, and there is a small collection of pus beneath the epidermal surface. If this occurs at the base of the eyelid, it is called a **stye. Furuncles** (boils), an extension of folliculitis, are large, painful, raised nodules that have an underlying collection of dead and necrotic tissue. These can drain spontaneously or after surgical incision.

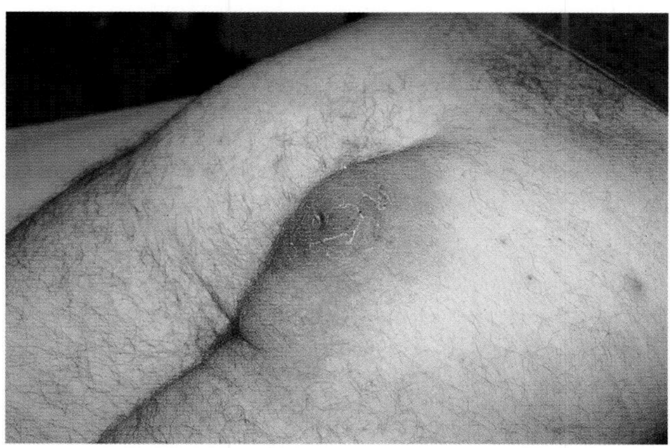

FIGURE 18-7 *Staphylococcus aureus* carbuncle. This carbuncle developed on the buttock over a 7- to 10-day period and required surgical drainage plus antibiotic therapy. (From Cohen J, Powderly WG, Opal SM: *Infectious diseases,* ed 3, Philadelphia, 2010, Mosby.)

Carbuncles occur when furuncles coalesce and extend to the deeper subcutaneous tissue (Figure 18-7). Multiple sinus tracts are usually present. Unlike patients with folliculitis and furuncles, patients with carbuncles have chills and fevers, indicating the systemic spread of staphylococci via bacteremia to other tissues.

Staphylococcal **wound infections** can also occur in patients after a surgical procedure or after trauma, with organisms colonizing the skin introduced into the wound. The staphylococci are generally not able to establish an infection in an immunocompetent person unless a foreign body (e.g., stitches, a splinter, dirt) is present in the wound. Infections are characterized by edema, erythema, pain, and an accumulation of purulent material. The infection can be easily managed if the wound is reopened, the foreign matter removed, and the purulence drained. If signs such as fever and malaise are observed or if the wound does not clear in response to localized management, antibiotic therapy directed against *S. aureus* is indicated.

With the spread of **MRSA strains in the community,** these organisms are now the most common cause of skin and soft-tissue infections in patients presenting to U.S. hospital emergency departments. This problem is complicated by the fact that the majority of these patients are initially treated with a penicillin, cephalosporin, or other equally ineffective antibiotic.

Bacteremia and Endocarditis (Clinical Case 18-3)

S. aureus is a common cause of **bacteremia.** Although bacteremias caused by most other organisms originate from an identifiable focus of infection (e.g., infection of the lungs, urinary tract, gastrointestinal tract), the initial foci of infection in approximately a third of patients with *S. aureus* bacteremias are not known. Most likely, the infection spreads to the blood from an innocuous-appearing skin infection. More than 50% of the cases of *S. aureus* bacteremia are acquired in the hospital after a surgical procedure or result from continued use of a contaminated intravascular catheter. *S. aureus* bacteremias, particularly prolonged episodes, are associated with dissemination to other body sites, including the heart.

Acute **endocarditis** caused by *S. aureus* is a serious disease, with a mortality rate approaching 50%. Although patients with *S. aureus* endocarditis may initially have nonspecific influenza-like symptoms, their condition can deteriorate rapidly and include disruption of cardiac output and peripheral evidence of septic embolization. Unless appropriate medical and surgical intervention is instituted immediately, the patient's prognosis is poor. An exception to this is *S. aureus* endocarditis in parenteral drug abusers, whose disease normally involves the right side of the heart (tricuspid valve) rather than the left. The initial symptoms may be mild, but fever, chills, and pleuritic chest pain caused by pulmonary emboli are generally present. Clinical cure of the endocarditis is the rule, although it is common for complications to occur as the result of secondary spread of the infection to other organs.

Pneumonia and Empyema

S. aureus respiratory disease can develop after the aspiration of oral secretions or from the hematogenous spread of the organism from a distant site. **Aspiration pneumonia** is seen primarily in the very young, the elderly, and patients with cystic fibrosis, influenza, chronic obstructive pulmonary disease, and bronchiectasis. The clinical and radiographic presentations of the pneumonia are not unique. Radiographic examination reveals the presence of patchy infiltrates with consolidation or abscesses, the latter consistent with the organism's ability to secrete cytotoxic toxins and enzymes and to form localized abscesses. **Hematogenous pneumonia** is common for patients with bacteremia or endocarditis. Community-acquired MRSA is responsible for a severe form of **necrotizing pneumonia** with massive hemoptysis, septic shock, and a high mortality rate. Although this disease is reported most commonly in children and young adults, it is not restricted to these age groups.

Empyema occurs in 10% of patients with pneumonia, and *S. aureus* is responsible for a third of all cases. Because the organism can become consolidated in loculated areas, drainage of the purulent material is sometimes difficult.

Osteomyelitis and Septic Arthritis

S. aureus **osteomyelitis** can result from hematogenous dissemination to bone, or it can be a secondary infection resulting from trauma or the extension of disease from an adjacent area. Hematogenous spread in children generally results from a cutaneous staphylococcal infection and usually involves the metaphyseal area of long bones, a highly vascularized area of bony growth. This infection is characterized by the sudden onset of localized pain over the involved bone and by high fever. Blood cultures are positive in approximately 50% of cases.

The hematogenous osteomyelitis seen in adults commonly occurs in the form of vertebral osteomyelitis and rarely in the form of an infection of the long bones. Intense back pain with fever is the initial symptom. Radiographic evidence of osteomyelitis in children and adults is not seen until 2 to 3 weeks after the initial symptoms appear. A **Brodie abscess** is a sequestered focus of staphylococcal osteomyelitis that arises in the metaphyseal area of a long bone and occurs only in adults. The staphylococcal osteomyelitis that

Clinical Case 18-3 *Staphylococcus aureus* Endocarditis

Chen and Li (*N Engl J Med* 355:e27, 2006) described a 21-year-old woman with a history of intravenous drug abuse, HIV, and a CD4 count of 400 cells/mm^3 who developed endocarditis caused by *S. aureus*. The patient had a 1-week history of fever, chest pain, and hemoptysis. Physical exam revealed a 3/6 pansystolic murmur and rhonchi in both lung fields. Multiple bilateral cavitary lesions were observed by chest radiography, and cultures of blood and sputum were positive for methicillin-susceptible *S. aureus*. The patient was treated with oxacillin for 6 weeks, with resolution of the endocarditis and pulmonary abscesses. This case illustrated the acute onset of *S. aureus* endocarditis, risk factors of intravenous drug abuse, and the frequency of complications caused by septic emboli.

occurs after trauma or a surgical procedure is generally accompanied by inflammation and purulent drainage from the wound or the sinus tract overlying the infected bone. Because the staphylococcal infection may be restricted to the wound, isolation of the organism from this site is not conclusive evidence of bony involvement. With appropriate antibiotic therapy and surgery, the cure rate for staphylococcal osteomyelitis is excellent.

S. aureus is the primary cause of **septic arthritis** in young children and in adults who are receiving intraarticular injections or who have mechanically abnormal joints. Secondary involvement of multiple joints is indicative of hematogenous spread from a localized focus. *S. aureus* is replaced by *Neisseria gonorrhoeae* as the most common cause of septic arthritis in sexually active persons. Staphylococcal arthritis is characterized by a painful erythematous joint, with purulent material obtained on aspiration. Infection is usually demonstrated in the large joints (e.g., shoulder, knee, hip, elbow). The prognosis in children is excellent, but in adults it depends on the nature of the underlying disease and the occurrence of any secondary infectious complications.

Staphylococcus epidermidis and Other Coagulase-Negative Staphylococci

Endocarditis (Clinical Case 18-4)

S. epidermidis, S. lugdunensis, and related coagulase-negative staphylococci can infect prosthetic and, less commonly, native heart valves. Infections of native valves are believed to result from the inoculation of organisms onto a damaged heart valve (e.g., a congenital malformation, damage resulting from rheumatic heart disease). ***S. lugdunensis*** is the staphylococcal species most commonly associated with native valve endocarditis, although this disease is more commonly caused by streptococci. In contrast, staphylococci are a major cause of **endocarditis of artificial valves.** The organisms are introduced at the time of valve replacement, and the infection characteristically has an indolent course, with clinical signs and symptoms not developing for as long as 1 year after the procedure. Although the heart valve can be infected, more commonly the infection occurs at the site where the valve is sewn to the heart tissue. Thus infection with abscess formation can lead to separation of the valve at the suture line and to mechanical heart failure. The prognosis is guarded for patients who have this infection, and prompt medical and surgical management is critical.

Clinical Case 18-4 *Staphylococcus lugdunensis* Endocarditis

Seenivasan and Yu (*Eur J Clin Microbiol Infect Dis* 22:489–491, 2003) described a typical report of native valve endocarditis caused by *S. lugdunensis*, a coagulase-negative *Staphylococcus* with a predilection for causing endocarditis. The 36-year-old woman was an active cocaine user who presented with an acute onset of weakness in the right extremities. She reported fever with chills, malaise, and shortness of breath over the preceding 10 weeks. Upon admission to the hospital, she had tachycardia, hypotension, a temperature of 39° C, a pansystolic murmur, and right-sided hemiparesis. A computed tomography scan of the brain revealed a large infarct in the left basal ganglia. Four sets of blood cultures were positive with *S. lugdunensis*. The isolate was penicillin resistant and susceptible to all other tested antibiotics. Because the patient had a penicillin allergy, treatment was initiated with vancomycin and gentamicin. The patient became afebrile at 3 days, and subsequent blood cultures were negative. Gentamicin was discontinued after 1 week, and the patient received a total of 6 weeks of therapy with vancomycin. Over the next 7 months, the patient developed progressive mitral regurgitation that necessitated mitral valve replacement. *S. lugdunensis* is more virulent compared with other coagulase-negative staphylococci, causing disease most commonly in native heart valves and with secondary complications (e.g., a brain infarct caused by septic emboli) more frequently reported. Persistent bacteremia is characteristic of intravascular infections such as endocarditis.

Catheter and Shunt Infections

More than 50% of all infections of catheters and shunts are caused by coagulase-negative staphylococci. These infections have become a major medical problem because long-dwelling catheters and shunts are used commonly for the medical management of critically ill patients. The coagulase-negative staphylococci are particularly well adapted for causing these infections, because they can produce a polysaccharide slime that bonds them to catheters and shunts and protects them from antibiotics and inflammatory cells. A persistent bacteremia is generally observed in patients with infections of shunts and catheters, because the organisms have continual access to the blood. Immune complex–mediated glomerulonephritis occurs in patients with long-standing disease.

Prosthetic Joint Infections

Infections of artificial joints, particularly the hip, can be caused by coagulase-negative staphylococci. The patient usually experiences only localized pain and mechanical failure of the joint. Systemic signs such as fever and leukocytosis are not prominent, and blood cultures are usually negative. Treatment consists of joint replacement and antimicrobial therapy. The risk of reinfection of the new joint is considerably increased in such patients.

Urinary Tract Infections

S. saprophyticus has a predilection for causing urinary tract infections in young, sexually active women and is rarely responsible for infections in other patients. It is also infrequently found as an asymptomatic colonizer of the urinary tract. Infected women usually have dysuria (pain on urination), pyuria (pus in urine), and numerous organisms in the urine. Typically, patients respond rapidly to antibiotics, and reinfection is uncommon.

Laboratory Diagnosis

Microscopy

Staphylococci are **gram-positive cocci** that form **clusters** when grown on agar media but commonly appear as single cells or small groups of organisms in clinical specimens. Successful detection of organisms in a clinical specimen depends on the type of infection (e.g., abscess, bacteremia, impetigo) and the quality of the material submitted for analysis. If the clinician scrapes the base of the abscess with a swab or curette, then an abundance of organisms should be observed in the Gram-stained specimen. Aspirated pus or superficial specimens collected with swabs consist primarily of necrotic material with relatively few organisms, so these specimens are not as useful. Relatively few organisms are generally present in the blood of bacteremic patients (an average of <1 organism per milliliter of blood), so blood specimens should be cultured, but blood examined by Gram stain is not useful. Staphylococci are seen in the nasopharynx of patients with SSSS and in the vagina of patients with TSS, but these staphylococci cannot be distinguished from the organisms that normally colonize these sites. Diagnosis of these diseases is made by the clinical presentation of the patient, with isolation of *S. aureus* in culture confirmatory. Staphylococci are implicated in food poisoning by the clinical presentation of the patient (e.g., rapid onset of vomiting and abdominal cramps) and a history of specific food ingestion (e.g., salted ham). Gram stains of the food or patient stool specimens are generally not useful.

Nucleic Acid–Based Tests

Commercial nucleic acid amplification tests are available for the direct detection and identification of *S. aureus* in clinical specimens. Whereas the earlier versions of these tests required manual extraction of bacterial DNA and testing multiple specimens in large batches, integrated processing of specimens (extraction, gene amplification, target detection) is now performed on highly automated platforms with disposable reagent strips or cartridges. These tests are useful for the detection of methicillin-sensitive *S. aureus* (MSSA) and MRSA in wound specimens and screening nasal specimens for carriage of these bacteria.

Culture

Clinical specimens should be inoculated onto nutritionally enriched agar media supplemented with sheep blood. Staphylococci grow rapidly on nonselective media incubated aerobically or anaerobically, with large, smooth colonies seen within 24 hours (Figure 18-8). As noted earlier, *S. aureus* colonies will gradually turn **yellow,** particularly when the cultures are incubated at room temperature. Almost all isolates of *S. aureus* and some strains of coagulase-negative staphylococci produce hemolysis on sheep blood agar. The hemolysis is caused by cytotoxins, particularly alpha toxin. If there is a mixture of organisms in the specimen (e.g., wound or respiratory specimen), *S. aureus* can be isolated selectively on a variety of special media including **chromogenic agar** (where *S. aureus* colonies are a characteristic color) or **mannitol-salt agar,** which is supplemented with mannitol (fermented by *S. aureus* but not by most other staphylococci) and 7.5% sodium chloride (inhibits the growth of most other organisms).

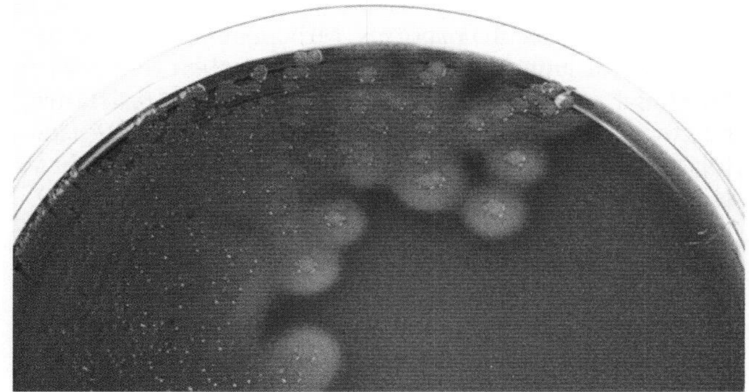

FIGURE 18-8 *Staphylococcus aureus* grown on a sheep blood agar plate. Note the colonies are large and β-hemolytic.

Identification

Relatively simple biochemical tests (e.g., positive reactions for **coagulase,** protein A, heat-stable nuclease, and mannitol fermentation) can be used to identify *S. aureus.* Colonies resembling *S. aureus* are identified in most laboratories by mixing a suspension of organisms with a drop of plasma and observing clumping of the organisms (positive coagulase test). Alternatively, plasma placed in a test tube can be inoculated with the organism and examined at 4 and 24 hours for formation of a clot (positive tube coagulase test). Identification of the coagulase-negative staphylococci is more complex, traditionally requiring the use of commercial identification systems or detection of species-specific genes by nucleic acid sequencing techniques. More recently mass spectrometry has been used to identify these bacteria, as well as many other species of organisms, with a high level of accuracy and rapid time to results (generally identified in minutes). Historically, the analysis of genomic DNA by pulsed-field gel electrophoresis or similar technique was the most commonly used method for characterizing isolates at the subspecies levels; however, whole genome sequencing is rapidly becoming the preferred tool for subtyping organisms for epidemiologic studies.

Antibody Detection

Antibodies to cell wall teichoic acids are present in many patients with long-standing *S. aureus* infections. However, this test has been discontinued in most hospitals because it is less sensitive than culture and nucleic acid–based tests.

Treatment, Prevention, and Control

Staphylococci quickly developed drug resistance after penicillin was introduced, and today less than 10% of the strains are susceptible to this antibiotic. This resistance is mediated by **penicillinase** (β-lactamase specific for penicillins), which hydrolyzes the β-lactam ring of penicillin. Because of the problems with penicillin-resistant staphylococci, **semisynthetic penicillins** resistant to β-lactamase hydrolysis (e.g., methicillin, nafcillin, oxacillin, dicloxacillin) were developed. Unfortunately, staphylococci developed resistance to these antibiotics as well. Currently, the majority of *S. aureus* responsible for hospital- and community-acquired infections are resistant to these semisynthetic penicillins, and these MRSA strains are resistant to all β-lactam antibiotics (i.e., penicillins, cephalosporins, carbapenems). Not all bacteria in a resistant population may express their resistance in traditional susceptibility tests **(heterogeneous resistance);** therefore the definitive method for identifying a resistant isolate is detection of the *mecA* or *mecC* genes that code for the penicillin-binding proteins that confer resistance.

Patients with localized skin and soft-tissue infections can generally be managed by incision and drainage of the abscesses. If the infection involves a larger area or systemic signs are present, then antibiotic therapy is indicated. Because MRSA strains are responsible for a significant proportion of hospital- and community-acquired infections, empirical therapy should include antibiotics active against MRSA strains. Oral therapy can include trimethoprim-sulfamethoxazole, a long-acting tetracycline such as doxycycline or minocycline, clindamycin, or linezolid. Resistance to clindamycin is common in some communities, and use of linezolid is limited by its cost and toxicity. Vancomycin is the drug of choice for intravenous therapy, with daptomycin, tigecycline, or linezolid acceptable alternatives.

Staphylococci have demonstrated the remarkable ability to develop resistance to most antibiotics. Until recently, the one antibiotic that remained uniformly active against staphylococci was vancomycin, the current antibiotic of choice for treating serious infections caused by staphylococci resistant to methicillin. Unfortunately, isolates of *S. aureus* have now been found with two forms of **resistance to vancomycin.** Low-level resistance is observed in *S. aureus* strains with a thicker, more disorganized cell wall. It is postulated that vancomycin is trapped in the cell wall matrix and is unable to reach the cytoplasmic membrane, where it can disrupt cell wall synthesis. High-level resistance is mediated by the *vanA* gene operon that was acquired from vancomycin-resistant enterococci. These bacteria have a modified peptidoglycan layer that does not bind vancomycin. Presently, this resistance is uncommon; however, if these resistant staphylococci become widespread, then antibiotic treatment of these highly virulent bacteria could be difficult.

Staphylococci are ubiquitous organisms present on the skin and mucous membranes, and their introduction through breaks in the skin occurs often. However, the number of organisms required to establish an infection **(infectious dose)** is generally large unless a foreign body (e.g., dirt, a splinter, stitches) is present in the wound. Proper cleansing of the wound and application of an appropriate disinfectant (e.g., germicidal soap, iodine solution, hexachlorophene) will prevent most infections in healthy individuals.

The spread of staphylococci from person to person is more difficult to prevent. An example of this is surgical wound infections, which can be caused by relatively few organisms, because foreign bodies and devitalized tissue may be present. Although it is unrealistic to sterilize operating room personnel and the environment, the risk of contamination during an operative procedure can be minimized through proper hand washing and the covering of exposed skin surfaces. The spread of methicillin-resistant organisms can also be difficult to control because asymptomatic nasopharyngeal carriage is the most common source of these organisms.

Bibliography

Bukowski M, Wladyka B, Dubin G: Exfoliative toxins of *Staphylococcus aureus*, *Toxins* 2:1148–1165, 2010.

Fournier B, Philpott D: Recognition of *Staphylococcus aureus* by the innate immune system, *Clin Microbiol Rev* 18:521–540, 2005.

Frank K, del Pozo J, Patel R: From clinical microbiology to infection pathogenesis: how daring to be different works for *Staphylococcus lugdunensis*, *Clin Microbiol Rev* 21:111–133, 2008.

Gravet A, Rondeau M, Harf-Monteil C, et al: Predominant *Staphylococcus aureus* isolated from antibiotic-associated diarrhea is clinically relevant and produces enterotoxin A and the bicomponent toxin LukE-LukD, *J Clin Microbiol* 37:4012–4019, 1999.

Hall PR, Elmore BO, Spang CH, et al: Nox2 modification of LDL is essential for optimal apolipoprotein B-mediated control of *agr* Type III *Staphylococcus aureus* quorum-sensing, *PLoS Pathog* 9:e1003166, 2013.

Ippolito G, Leone S, Lauria FN, et al: Methicillin-resistant *Staphylococcus aureus*: the superbug, *Int J Infect Dis* 14(Suppl 4):S7–S11, 2010.

James E, Edwards A, Wigneshweraraj S: Transcriptional downregulation of *agr* expression in *Staphylococcus aureus* during growth in human serum can be overcome by constitutively active mutant forms of the sensor kinase AgrC, *FEMS Microbiol Lett* 349:153–162, 2013.

Krakauer T, Stiles B: The staphylococcal enterotoxin (SE) family, *Virulence* 4:759–773, 2013.

Kurlenda J, Grinholc M: Current diagnostic tools for methicillin-resistant *Staphylococcus aureus* infections, *Mol Diagn Ther* 14:73–80, 2010.

Limbago BM, Kallen AJ, Zhu W, et al: Report of the 13th vancomycin-resistant *Staphylococcus aureus* isolate from the United States, *J Clin Microbiol* 52:998–1002, 2014.

Los FC, Randis TM, Aroian RV, et al: Role of pore-forming toxins in bacterial infectious diseases, *Microbiol Mol Biol Rev* 2:173–207, 2013.

Moran GJ, Krishnadasan A, Gorwitz RJ, et al: Methicillin-resistant *S. aureus* infections among patients in the emergency department, *N Engl J Med* 355:666–674, 2006.

Novick RP, Geisinger E: Quorum sensing in staphylococci, *Annu Rev Genet* 42:541–564, 2008.

Otto M: Basis of virulence in community-associated methicillin-resistant *Staphylococcus aureus*, *Annu Rev Microbiol* 64:143–162, 2010.

Pannaraj PS, Hulten KG, Gonzalez BE, et al: Infective pyomyositis and myositis in children in the era of community-acquired, methicillin-resistant *Staphylococcus aureus* infection, *Clin Infect Dis* 43:953–960, 2006.

Seybold U, Kourbatova EV, Johnson JG, et al: Emergence of community-associated methicillin-resistant *Staphylococcus aureus* USA300 genotype as a major cause of health care associated blood stream infections, *Clin Infect Dis* 42:647–656, 2006.

Silversides J, Lappin E, Ferguson A: Staphylococcal toxic shock syndrome: mechanisms and management, *Curr Infect Dis Rep* 12:392–400, 2010.

Singer A, Talan D: Management of skin abscesses in the era of methicillin-resistant *Staphylococcus aureus*, *N Engl J Med* 370:1039–1047, 2014.

Srinivasan A, Dick JD, Perl TM: Vancomycin resistance in staphylococci, *Clin Microbiol Rev* 15:430–438, 2002.

Stanley J, Amagai M: Pemphigus, bullous impetigo, and the staphylococcal scalded-skin syndrome, *N Engl J Med* 355:1800–1810, 2006.

Tang Y, Stratton C: *Staphylococcus aureus*: an old pathogen with new weapons, *Clin Lab Med* 30:179–208, 2010.

Uhlemann AC, Otto M, Lowy FD, et al: Evolution of community- and healthcare-associated methicillin-resistant *Staphylococcus aureus*, *Infect Genet Evol* 21:563–574, 2014.

Vandenesch F, Lina G, Henry T: *Staphylococcus aureus* hemolysins, bi-component leukocidins, and cytolytic peptides: a redundant arsenal of membrane-damaging virulence factors? *Front Cell Infect Microbiol* 2:12, 2012.

Zhu W, Murray PR, Huskins WC, et al: Dissemination of an *Enterococcus* Inc18-Like vanA plasmid associated with vancomycin-resistant *Staphylococcus aureus*, *Antimicrob Agents Chemother* 54:4314–4320, 2010.

CHAPTER

19 STREPTOCOCCUS AND ENTEROCOCCUS

An 8-year-old boy presented to his pediatrician with a low-grade fever and a diffuse erythematous rash over his chest, which developed 2 days after he complained of a painful sore throat. An exudate was present over the tonsillar area of the throat and covered his tongue. The clinical diagnosis of scarlet fever was confirmed by positive antigen test for group A *Streptococcus* from a throat specimen. The genera *Streptococcus* and *Enterococcus* include a large number of species capable of causing a wide spectrum of diseases.

1. What sites of the human body are normally colonized with *Streptococcus pyogenes, Streptococcus agalactiae,* and *Streptococcus pneumoniae*? How does this relate to infections caused by these bacteria?
2. The viridans streptococci (i.e., α-hemolytic and nonhemolytic streptococci) are subdivided into five groups. What are the groups and the specific diseases associated with each group?
3. Enterococci, like many other bacteria, can cause urinary tract infections but primarily in hospitalized patients. What characteristics of this bacterium are responsible for the predilection for disease in this population?
4. What biochemical properties are used to separate enterococci from the staphylococci and streptococci?

Answers to these questions are available on StudentConsult.com.

• SUMMARIES CLINICALLY SIGNIFICANT ORGANISMS

Streptococcus pyogenes (Group A)

Trigger Words

Group A, pharyngitis, pyoderma, rheumatic fever, glomerulonephritis

Biology and Virulence

- Rapidly growing gram-positive cocci arranged in chains; group-specific carbohydrate (A antigen) and type-specific proteins (M protein) in cell wall
- Virulence determined by ability to avoid phagocytosis (mediated primarily by capsule, M and M-like proteins, C5a peptidase), adhere to and invade host cells (M protein, lipoteichoic acid, F protein), and produce toxins (streptococcal pyrogenic exotoxins, streptolysin S, streptolysin O, streptokinase, DNases)

Epidemiology

- Transient colonization in upper respiratory tract and skin surface, with disease caused by recently acquired strains (before protective antibodies are produced)
- Pharyngitis and soft-tissue infections typically caused by strains with different M proteins
- Person-to-person spread by respiratory droplets (pharyngitis) or through breaks in skin after direct contact with infected person, fomite, or arthropod vector
- Individuals at higher risk for disease include children 5 to 15 years old (pharyngitis); children 2 to 5 years old with poor personal hygiene (pyoderma); patients with soft-tissue infection (streptococcal toxic shock syndrome); patients with prior streptococcal pharyngitis (rheumatic fever, glomerulonephritis) or soft-tissue infection (glomerulonephritis)

Diseases

- Responsible for suppurative diseases (pharyngitis, soft-tissue infections, streptococcal toxic shock) and nonsuppurative diseases (rheumatic fever, glomerulonephritis)

Diagnosis

- Microscopy is useful in soft-tissue infections but not pharyngitis or nonsuppurative complications
- Direct tests for the group A antigen are useful for the diagnosis of streptococcal pharyngitis
- Isolates identified by catalase (negative), positive PYR (L-pyrrolidonyl arylamidase) reaction, susceptibility to bacitracin, and presence of group-specific antigen (group A antigen)
- Antistreptolysin O test is useful for confirming rheumatic fever or glomerulonephritis associated with streptococcal pharyngitis; anti-DNase B test should be performed for glomerulonephritis associated with pharyngitis or soft-tissue infections

Treatment, Prevention, and Control

- Penicillin V or amoxicillin used to treat pharyngitis; oral cephalosporin or macrolide for penicillin-allergic patients; intravenous penicillin plus clindamycin used for systemic infections

- Oropharyngeal carriage occurring after treatment can be re-treated; treatment is not indicated for prolonged asymptomatic carriage, because antibiotics disrupt normal protective flora
- Starting antibiotic therapy within 10 days in patients with pharyngitis prevents rheumatic fever
- For glomerulonephritis, no specific antibiotic treatment or prophylaxis is indicated
- For patients with a history of rheumatic fever, antibiotic prophylaxis is required before procedures (e.g., dental) that can induce bacteremias leading to endocarditis

Streptococcus agalactiae (Group B)

Trigger Words

Group B, neonatal disease, screening pregnant women

Biology and Virulence

- Rapidly growing gram-positive cocci arranged in chains; group-specific carbohydrate (B antigen) and type-specific capsular carbohydrates (Ia, Ib, II-VIII)
- Virulence determined primarily by ability to avoid phagocytosis (mediated by capsule)

Epidemiology

- Asymptomatic colonization of the upper respiratory tract and genitourinary tract
- Early-onset disease acquired by neonates from mother during pregnancy or at time of birth
- Neonates are at higher risk for infection if (1) there is premature rupture of membranes, prolonged labor, preterm birth, or disseminated maternal group B streptococcal disease, and (2) mother is without type-specific antibodies and has low complement levels
- Women with genital colonization are at risk for postpartum disease
- Men and nonpregnant women with diabetes mellitus, cancer, or alcoholism are at increased risk for disease
- No seasonal incidence

Diseases

- Responsible for neonatal disease (early-onset and late-onset disease with meningitis, pneumonia, bacteremia), infections in pregnant women (endometritis, wound infections, urinary tract infections), and other adults (bacteremia, pneumonia, bone and joint infections, skin and soft-tissue infections)

Diagnosis

- Microscopy useful for meningitis (cerebrospinal fluid), pneumonia (lower respiratory secretions), and wound infections (exudates)
- Antigen tests are less sensitive than microscopy and should not be used
- Culture most sensitive test; a selective broth (i.e., LIM) is needed for optimal detection of vaginal carriage
- Polymerase chain reaction–based assays to detect vaginal carriage in pregnant women are commercially available; currently require use of enrichment broth for optimum sensitivity
- Isolates identified by demonstration of group-specific cell wall carbohydrate or positive nucleic acid amplification test

Treatment, Prevention, and Control

- Penicillin G is the drug of choice; empirical therapy with broad-spectrum antibiotics (broad-spectrum cephalosporin plus aminoglycoside) used until specific pathogen identified; combination of penicillin and aminoglycoside is used in patients with serious infections; a cephalosporin or vancomycin is used for patients allergic to penicillin
- For high-risk babies, penicillin is given at least 4 hours before delivery
- No vaccine is currently available

Streptococcus pneumoniae

Trigger Words

Diplococci, capsule, pneumonia, meningitis, vaccine

Biology and Virulence

- Elongated gram-positive cocci arranged in pairs (diplococci) and short chains; cell wall includes teichoic acid rich in phosphorylcholine (C polysaccharide), which is required for the activity of an autolytic enzyme, amidase
- Virulence determined by ability to colonize oropharynx (surface protein adhesions), spread into normally sterile tissues (pneumolysin, immunoglobulin [Ig]A protease), stimulate local inflammatory response (teichoic acid, peptidoglycan fragments, pneumolysin), and evade phagocytic killing (polysaccharide capsule)
- Responsible for pneumonia, sinusitis and otitis media, meningitis, and bacteremia

Epidemiology

- Most infections are caused by endogenous spread from the colonized nasopharynx or oropharynx to distal site (e.g., lungs, sinuses, ears, blood, meninges); person-to-person spread through infectious droplets is rare
- Colonization is highest in young children and their contacts
- Individuals with antecedent viral respiratory tract disease or other conditions that interfere with bacterial clearance from respiratory tract are at increased risk for pulmonary disease
- Children and the elderly are at greatest risk for meningitis
- People with hematologic disorder (e.g., malignancy, sickle cell disease) or functional asplenia are at risk for fulminant sepsis
- Although the organism is ubiquitous, disease is more common in cool months

Diagnosis

- Microscopy is highly sensitive, as is culture, unless the patient has been treated with antibiotics
- Antigen tests for pneumococcal C polysaccharide are sensitive with cerebrospinal fluid (meningitis) but not with urine (meningitis, pneumonia, other infections)
- Nucleic acid–based tests are not commonly used for diagnosis
- Culture requires use of enriched-nutrient media (e.g., sheep blood agar); organism highly susceptible to many antibiotics, so culture can be negative in partially treated patients
- Isolates identified by catalase (negative), susceptibility to optochin, and solubility in bile

Treatment, Prevention, and Control

- Penicillin is the drug of choice for susceptible strains, although resistance is increasingly common
- Vancomycin combined with ceftriaxone is used for empirical therapy; monotherapy with a cephalosporin, fluoroquinolone, or vancomycin can be used in patients with susceptible isolates
- Immunization with 13-valent conjugated vaccine is recommended for all children younger than 2 years; a 23-valent polysaccharide vaccine is recommended for adults at risk for disease

Enterococcus

Trigger Words

Diplococci, gastrointestinal carriage, drug-resistant, urinary tract infections, peritonitis

Biology and Virulence

- Gram-positive cocci arranged in pairs and short chains (morphologically similar to *Streptococcus pneumoniae*)
- Cell wall with group-specific antigen (group D glycerol teichoic acid)
- Virulence mediated by ability to adhere to host surfaces and form biofilms and by antibiotic resistance

Epidemiology

- Colonizes the gastrointestinal tracts of humans and animals; spreads to other mucosal surfaces if broad-spectrum antibiotics eliminate the normal bacterial population
- Cell wall structure typical of gram-positive bacteria, which allows survival on environmental surfaces for prolonged periods
- Most infections endogenous (from patient's bacterial flora); some caused by patient-to-patient spread
- Patients at increased risk include those hospitalized for prolonged periods and treated with broad-spectrum antibiotics (particularly cephalosporins, to which enterococci are naturally resistant)

Diseases

- Diseases include urinary tract infections, peritonitis (usually polymicrobic), wound infections, and bacteremia with or without endocarditis

Diagnosis

- Grows readily on common nonselective media; differentiated from related organisms by simple tests (catalase negative, L-pyrrolidonyl arylamidase–positive, resistant to bile and optochin)

Treatment, Prevention, and Control

- Therapy for serious infections requires combination of an aminoglycoside with a cell wall–active antibiotic (penicillin, ampicillin, or vancomycin); newer agents used for antibiotic-resistant bacteria include linezolid, daptomycin, tigecycline, and quinupristin/dalfopristin
- Antibiotic resistance to each of these drugs is becoming increasingly common, and infections with many isolates (particularly *Enterococcus faecium*) are not treatable with any antibiotics
- Prevention and control of infections require careful restriction of antibiotic use and implementation of appropriate infection-control practices

The genera *Streptococcus* and *Enterococcus* are a diverse collection of **gram-positive cocci** typically arranged in **pairs or chains** (in contrast to the clusters formed by *Staphylococcus*) (Table 19-1). Most species are facultative anaerobes, and some grow only in an atmosphere enhanced with carbon dioxide **(capnophilic growth).** Their nutritional requirements are complex, necessitating the use of blood- or serum-enriched media for isolation. Carbohydrates are fermented, resulting in the production of lactic acid, and unlike *Staphylococcus* species, streptococci and enterococci are **catalase negative.** The number of genera of catalase-negative, gram-positive cocci that are recognized as human pathogens continues to increase; however, *Streptococcus* and *Enterococcus* are the genera most frequently isolated and most commonly responsible for human disease. The other genera are relatively uncommon and are listed in Table 19-2 but are not discussed further.

The classification of more than 100 species within the genus *Streptococcus* is complicated because three different overlapping schemes are used: (1) serologic properties: **Lancefield groupings** (originally A to W); (2) **hemolytic patterns:** complete (beta [β]) hemolysis, incomplete (alpha [α]) hemolysis, and no (gamma [γ]) hemolysis; and (3) **biochemical (physiologic) properties.** Although this is an oversimplification, it is practical to think that the streptococci are divided into two groups: (1) the β-hemolytic streptococci, which are classified by Lancefield grouping, and (2) the α-hemolytic and γ-hemolytic streptococci, which are classified by biochemical testing. The latter group is referred to collectively as **viridans streptococci,** a name derived from *viridis* (Latin for "green"), referring to the green pigment formed by the partial hemolysis of blood agar.

Rebecca Lancefield developed the serologic classification scheme in 1933. β-Hemolytic strains possess group-specific cell wall antigens, most of which are carbohydrates. These antigens can be readily detected by immunologic assays and have been useful for the rapid identification of some important streptococcal pathogens. For example, one disease caused by *Streptococcus pyogenes* (classified as group A *Streptococcus* in the Lancefield typing scheme) is streptococcal pharyngitis ("strep throat"). The group antigen for this organism can be detected directly from throat swab specimens by a variety of rapid immunoassays and is a commonly used diagnostic test in hospital and physician office laboratories. The Lancefield typing scheme is primarily used today for only a few species of streptococci (e.g., those classified in groups A, B, C, F, and G; Table 19-3).

The enterococci ("enteric cocci") were previously classified as **group D streptococci** because they share the **group D cell wall antigen,** a glycerol teichoic acid, with other streptococci. In 1984, the enterococci were reclassified into the new genus *Enterococcus,* and there are currently 54 species in this genus; however, relatively few species are important human pathogens. The most commonly isolated and

Table 19-1 Important Streptococci and Enterococci

Organism	Historical Derivation
Streptococcus	*streptus,* pliant; *coccus,* grain or berry (a pliant berry or coccus; refers to the appearance of long, flexible chains of cocci)
S. agalactiae	*agalactia,* want of milk (original isolate [called *S. mastitidis*] was responsible for bovine mastitis)
S. anginosus	*anginosus,* pertaining to angina
S. constellatus	*constellatus,* studded with stars (original isolate embedded in agar with smaller colonies surrounding the large colony; satellite formation does not occur around colonies on the surface of an agar plate)
S. dysgalactiae	*dys,* ill, hard; *galactia,* pertaining to milk (loss of milk secretion; isolates associated with bovine mastitis)
S. gallolyticus	*gallatum,* gallate; *lyticus,* to loosen (able to digest or hydrolyze methyl gallate)
S. intermedius	*intermedius,* intermediate (initial confusion about whether this was an aerobic or an anaerobic bacterium)
S. mitis	*mitis,* mild (incorrectly thought to cause mild infections)
S. mutans	*mutans,* changing (cocci that may appear rodlike, particularly when initially isolated in culture)
S. pneumoniae	*pneumon,* the lungs (causes pneumonia)
S. pyogenes	*pyus,* pus; *gennaio,* beget or producing (pus producing; typically associated with formation of pus in wounds)
S. salivarius	*salivarius,* salivary (found in the mouth in saliva)
Enterococcus	*enteron,* intestine; *coccus,* berry (intestinal coccus)
E. faecalis	*faecalis,* relating to feces
E. faecium	*faecium,* of feces
E. gallinarum	*gallinarum,* of hens (original source was intestines of domestic fowl)
E. casseliflavus	*casseli,* Kassel's; *flavus,* yellow (Kassel's yellow)

clinically important species are ***Enterococcus faecalis*** and ***Enterococcus faecium. Enterococcus gallinarum*** and ***Enterococcus casseliflavus*** are also common colonizers of the human intestinal tract and are important because these species are inherently vancomycin resistant.

The viridans streptococci are subdivided into five clinically distinct groups (Table 19-4). Some species of the viridans streptococci can be β-hemolytic as well as α-hemolytic and nonhemolytic, which unfortunately has resulted in classifying these bacteria by both their Lancefield grouping and as viridans streptococci. Although the classification of the streptococci is somewhat confusing, clinical disease is well defined for individual species, which will be the emphasis for the remainder of this chapter.

Streptococcus pyogenes

S. pyogenes causes a variety of suppurative and nonsuppurative diseases (Box 19-1). Although this organism is the most common cause of bacterial pharyngitis, the notoriety of *S. pyogenes,* popularly called "flesh-eating" bacteria, results from life-threatening myonecrosis caused by this organism.

Table 19-2 Catalase-Negative, Gram-Positive Cocci and Their Diseases

Organism	Diseases
Abiotrophia	Bacteremia, endocarditis (native and prosthetic valves), nosocomial brain abscesses and meningitis, eye infections
Aerococcus	Bacteremia, endocarditis, urinary tract infections
Enterococcus	Bacteremia, endocarditis, urinary tract infections, peritonitis, wound infections
Granulicatella	Bacteremia, endocarditis (native and prosthetic valves), eye infections
Lactococcus	Bacteremia in immunocompromised patients, endocarditis (native and prosthetic valves), urinary tract infections, osteomyelitis
Leuconostoc	Opportunistic infections, including bacteremia, wound infections, central nervous system infections, and peritonitis
Pediococcus	Opportunistic infections, including bacteremia in severely immunocompromised patients
Streptococcus	Refer to Tables 19-3 and 19-4

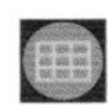

Table 19-3 Classification of Common β-Hemolytic Streptococci

Group	Representative Species	Diseases
A	*S. pyogenes*	Pharyngitis, skin and soft-tissue infections, bacteremia, rheumatic fever, acute glomerulonephritis
	S. anginosus group	Abscesses
B	*S. agalactiae*	Neonatal disease, endometritis, wound infections, urinary tract infections, bacteremia, pneumonia, skin and soft-tissue infections
C	*S. dysgalactiae*	Pharyngitis, acute glomerulonephritis
F, G	*S. anginosus* group	Abscesses
	S. dysgalactiae	Pharyngitis, acute glomerulonephritis

Physiology and Structure

Isolates of *S. pyogenes* are spherical cocci, 1 to 2 μm in diameter, arranged in short chains in clinical specimens and longer chains when grown in liquid media (Figure 19-1). Growth is optimal on enriched-blood agar media but is inhibited if the medium contains a high concentration of glucose. After 24 hours of incubation, 1- to 2-mm white colonies with large zones of β-hemolysis are observed (Figure 19-2).

The antigenic structure of *S. pyogenes* has been extensively studied. The basic structural framework of the cell wall

 **Table 19-4 Classification of Viridans Group of *Streptococcus***

Group	Representative Species	Diseases
Anginosus	*S. anginosus, S. constellatus, S. intermedius*	Abscesses in brain, oropharynx, or peritoneal cavity
Mitis	*S. mitis, S. pneumoniae, S. oralis*	Subacute endocarditis; sepsis in neutropenic patients; pneumonia; meningitis
Mutans	*S. mutans, S. sobrinus*	Dental caries; bacteremia
Salivarius	*S. salivarius*	Bacteremia; endocarditis
Bovis	*S. gallolyticus* subsp. *gallolyticus,* subsp. *pasteurianus*	Bacteremia associated with gastrointestinal cancer (subsp. *gallolyticus*); meningitis (subsp. *pasteurianus*)
Ungrouped	*S. suis*	Meningitis; bacteremia; streptococcal toxic shock syndrome

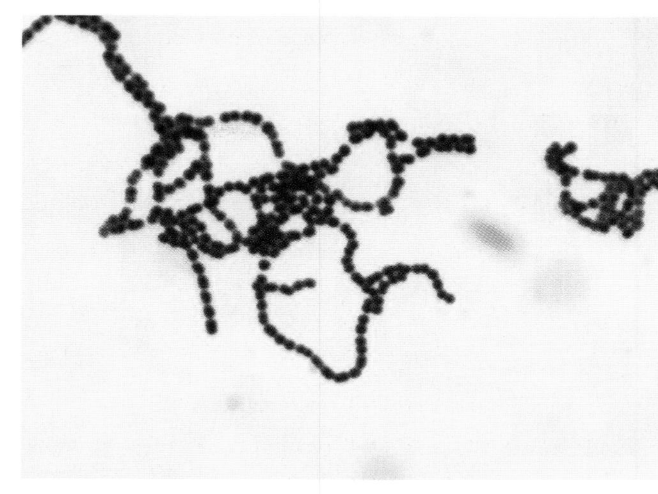

FIGURE 19-1 Gram stain of *Streptococcus pyogenes.*

 **Box 19-1 Streptococcal and Enterococcal Diseases: Clinical Summaries**

***Streptococcus pyogenes* (Group A)**

Suppurative Infections

Pharyngitis: reddened pharynx with exudates generally present; cervical lymphadenopathy can be prominent

Scarlet fever: diffuse erythematous rash beginning on the chest and spreading to the extremities; complication of streptococcal pharyngitis

Pyoderma: localized skin infection with vesicles progressing to pustules; no evidence of systemic disease

Erysipelas: localized skin infection with pain, inflammation, lymph node enlargement, and systemic symptoms

Cellulitis: infection of the skin that involves the subcutaneous tissues

Necrotizing fasciitis: deep infection of skin that involves destruction of muscle and fat layers

Streptococcal toxic shock syndrome: multiorgan systemic infection resembling staphylococcal toxic shock syndrome; however, most patients are bacteremic and with evidence of fasciitis

Other suppurative diseases: variety of other infections recognized including puerperal sepsis, lymphangitis, and pneumonia

Nonsuppurative Infections

Rheumatic fever: characterized by inflammatory changes of the heart (pancarditis), joints (arthralgias to arthritis), blood vessels, and subcutaneous tissues

Acute glomerulonephritis: acute inflammation of the renal glomeruli with edema, hypertension, hematuria, and proteinuria

***Streptococcus agalactiae* (Group B)**

Early-onset neonatal disease: within 7 days of birth, infected newborns develop signs and symptoms of pneumonia, meningitis, and sepsis

Late-onset neonatal disease: more than 1 week after birth, neonates develop signs and symptoms of bacteremia with meningitis

Infections in pregnant women: most often present as postpartum endometritis, wound infections, and urinary tract infections; bacteremia and disseminated complications may occur

Infections in other adult patients: most common diseases include bacteremia, pneumonia, bone and joint infections, and skin and soft-tissue infections

Other β-Hemolytic Streptococci

Abscess formation in deep tissues: associated with *S. anginosus* group

Pharyngitis: associated with *S. dysgalactiae;* disease resembles that caused by *S. pyogenes;* can be complicated with acute glomerulonephritis

Viridans Streptococci

Abscess formation in deep tissues: associated with *S. anginosus* group

Septicemia in neutropenic patients: associated with *S. mitis* group

Subacute endocarditis: associated with *S. mitis* and *S. salivarius* groups

Dental caries: associated with *S. mutans* group

Malignancies of gastrointestinal tract: associated with *S. bovis* group (*S. gallolyticus* subsp. *gallolyticus*)

Meningitis: associated with *S. gallolyticus* subsp. *pasteurianus, S. suis,* and *S. mitis* group

Streptococcus pneumoniae

Pneumonia: acute onset with severe chills and sustained fever; productive cough with blood-tinged sputum; lobar consolidation

Meningitis: severe infection involving the meninges, with headache, fever, and sepsis; high mortality and severe neurologic deficits in survivors

Bacteremia: more common in patients with meningitis than with pneumonia, otitis, media, or sinusitis; overwhelming sepsis in asplenic patients

Enterococcus faecalis* and *Enterococcus faecium

Urinary tract infection: dysuria and pyuria, most commonly in hospitalized patients with an indwelling urinary catheter and receiving broad-spectrum cephalosporin antibiotics

Peritonitis: abdominal swelling and tenderness after abdominal trauma or surgery; patients typically are acutely ill and febrile and have positive blood cultures; typically a polymicrobic infection

Bacteremia: associated with either a localized infection or endocarditis

Endocarditis: infection of the heart endothelium or valves; associated with persistent bacteremia; can present acutely or chronically

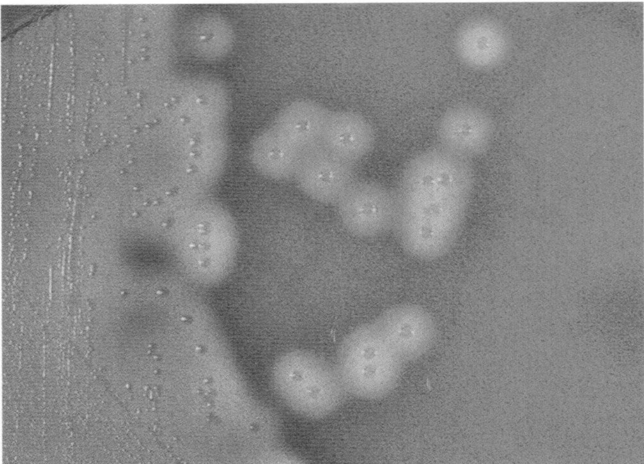

FIGURE 19-2 *Streptococcus pyogenes* (group A) typically appears as small colonies with a large zone of hemolysis.

is the peptidoglycan layer, which is similar in composition to that found in other gram-positive bacteria. Within the cell wall are group-specific and type-specific antigens. The **group-specific carbohydrate** that constitutes approximately 10% of the dry weight of the cell **(Lancefield group A antigen)** is a dimer of *N*-acetylglucosamine and rhamnose. This antigen is used to classify group A streptococci and distinguish them from other streptococcal groups. **M protein** is the major type-specific protein associated with virulent strains. It consists of two polypeptide chains complexed in an alpha helix. The protein is anchored in the cytoplasmic membrane, extends through the cell wall, and protrudes above the cell surface. The carboxyl terminus, which is anchored in the cytoplasmic membrane, and the portion of the molecule in the cell wall are highly conserved (by amino acid sequence) among all group A streptococci. The amino terminus, which extends above the cell surface, is responsible for the antigenic differences observed among the unique serotypes of M proteins. M proteins are subdivided into class I and class II molecules. The class I M proteins share exposed antigens, whereas the class II M proteins do not have exposed shared antigens. Although strains with both classes of antigens can cause suppurative infections and glomerulonephritis, only bacteria with class I (exposed shared antigen) M proteins cause rheumatic fever. The epidemiologic classification of *S. pyogenes* is based on sequence analysis of the *emm* gene that encodes the M proteins.

Other important components in the cell wall of *S. pyogenes* include **M-like surface proteins, lipoteichoic acid,** and **F protein.** A complex of more than 20 genes that comprise the *emm* gene superfamily encode the M-like proteins as well as the M proteins and immunoglobulin-binding proteins. Lipoteichoic acid and F protein facilitate binding of host cells by complexing with fibronectin, which is present on the host cell surface.

Some strains of *S. pyogenes* have an outer hyaluronic acid **capsule** that is antigenically indistinguishable from hyaluronic acid in mammalian connective tissues. Because the capsule can protect the bacteria from phagocytic clearance, encapsulated strains are more likely to be responsible for severe systemic infections.

Pathogenesis and Immunity

The virulence of group A streptococci is determined by the ability of the bacteria to avoid opsonization and phagocytosis, adhere to and invade host cells, and produce a variety of toxins and enzymes.

Initial Host-Parasite Interactions

S. pyogenes has multiple mechanisms for **avoiding opsonization and phagocytosis.** The **hyaluronic acid capsule** is a poor immunogen and interferes with phagocytosis. The **M proteins** also interfere with phagocytosis by blocking the binding of the complement component C3b, an important mediator of phagocytosis. C3b may also be degraded by factor H, which binds to the cell surface of the M protein. M-like proteins resemble M proteins in structure and are under the same regulatory control. These proteins interfere with phagocytosis by binding either the Fc fragment of antibodies or fibronectin, which blocks activation of complement by the alternate pathway and reduces the amount of bound C3b. Finally, *S. pyogenes* has **C5a peptidase** on the surface. This serine protease inactivates C5a, a chemoattractant of neutrophils and mononuclear phagocytes, and protects the bacteria from early clearance from infected tissues.

Many different bacterial antigens have been demonstrated to mediate **adherence to host cells,** with lipoteichoic acid, M proteins, and F protein the most important. The initial adherence is a weak interaction between **lipoteichoic acid** and fatty acid binding sites on fibronectin and epithelial cells. Subsequent adherence involves **M protein, F protein,** and other adhesins that interact with specific host cell receptors.

S. pyogenes can **invade into epithelial cells,** a process that is mediated by **M protein** and **F protein** and other bacterial antigens. This internalization is believed to be important for maintenance of persistent infections (e.g., recurrent streptococcal pharyngitis) and invasion into deep tissues.

Toxins and Enzymes

The **streptococcal pyrogenic exotoxins (Spe),** originally called *erythrogenic toxins,* are produced by lysogenic strains of streptococci and are similar to the toxin produced in *Corynebacterium diphtheriae.* Four immunologically distinct heat-labile toxins (SpeA, SpeB, SpeC, and SpeF) have been described in *S. pyogenes* and in rare strains of groups C and G streptococci. The toxins act as superantigens, interacting with both macrophages and helper T cells, with the enhanced release of proinflammatory cytokines. This family of exotoxins is believed responsible for many of the clinical manifestations of severe streptococcal diseases, including necrotizing fasciitis and streptococcal toxic shock syndrome, as well as the rash observed in patients with scarlet fever. It is unclear whether the rash results from the direct effect of the toxin on the capillary bed or, more likely, is secondary to a hypersensitivity reaction.

Streptolysin S is an oxygen-stable, nonimmunogenic, cell-bound hemolysin that can lyse erythrocytes, leukocytes, and platelets. It can also stimulate the release of lysosomal contents after engulfment, with subsequent death of the phagocytic cell. Streptolysin S is produced in the presence of serum (the S indicates serum stable) and is responsible for the characteristic β-hemolysis seen on blood agar media.

Streptolysin O is an oxygen-labile hemolysin capable of lysing erythrocytes, leukocytes, platelets, and cultured cells. This hemolysin is antigenically related to oxygen-labile toxins produced by *Streptococcus pneumoniae, Clostridium tetani, Clostridium perfringens, Bacillus cereus,* and *Listeria monocytogenes.* Antibodies are readily formed against streptolysin O **(antistreptolysin O [ASO] antibodies),** a feature differentiating it from streptolysin S, and are useful for documenting recent group A streptococcal infection (ASO test). Streptolysin O is irreversibly **inhibited by cholesterol** in skin lipids, so patients with cutaneous infections do not develop ASO antibodies.

At least two forms of **streptokinase (A and B)** have been described. These enzymes mediate the cleavage of plasminogen, releasing the protease plasmin that, in turn, cleaves fibrin and fibrinogen. Thus these enzymes can lyse blood clots and fibrin deposits and facilitate the rapid spread of *S. pyogenes* in infected tissues. Antibodies directed against these enzymes **(anti-streptokinase antibodies)** are a useful marker for infection.

Four immunologically distinct deoxyribonucleases **(DNases A to D)** have been identified. These enzymes are not cytolytic but can depolymerize free deoxyribonucleic acid (DNA) present in pus. This process reduces the viscosity of the abscess material and facilitates spread of the organisms. Antibodies developed against DNase B are an important marker of *S. pyogenes* infections **(anti-DNase B test),** particularly for patients with cutaneous infections, because they fail to make antibodies against streptolysin O (see preceding text).

Epidemiology

The Centers for Disease Control and Prevention (CDC) has estimated that at least 10 million cases of noninvasive disease occur annually, with pharyngitis and pyoderma the most common infections. Group A streptococci can colonize the oropharynx of healthy children and young adults in the absence of clinical disease. However, isolation of *S. pyogenes* in a patient with pharyngitis is generally considered significant. Asymptomatic colonization with *S. pyogenes* is transient, regulated by the person's ability to mount specific immunity to the M protein of the colonizing strain and the presence of competitive organisms in the oropharynx. Untreated patients produce antibodies against the specific bacterial M protein that can result in long-lived immunity; however, this antibody response is diminished in treated patients.

In general, *S. pyogenes* disease is caused by recently acquired strains that can establish an infection of the pharynx or skin before specific antibodies are produced or competitive organisms are able to proliferate. Pharyngitis caused by *S. pyogenes* is primarily a disease of children between the ages of 5 and 15 years, but infants and adults are also susceptible. The pathogen is spread from person to person through respiratory droplets. Crowding, such as in classrooms and day-care facilities, increases the opportunity for the organism to spread, particularly during the winter months. Soft-tissue infections (i.e., pyoderma, erysipelas, cellulitis, fasciitis) are typically preceded by initial skin colonization with group A streptococci, after which the organisms are introduced into the superficial or deep tissues through a break in the skin.

Clinical Diseases

Suppurative Streptococcal Disease

Pharyngitis

Pharyngitis generally develops 2 to 4 days after exposure to the pathogen, with an abrupt onset of sore throat, fever, malaise, and headache. The posterior pharynx can appear erythematous with an exudate, and cervical lymphadenopathy can be prominent. Despite these clinical signs and symptoms, differentiating streptococcal pharyngitis from viral pharyngitis is difficult. An accurate diagnosis can be made only with specific laboratory tests.

Scarlet fever is a complication of streptococcal pharyngitis that occurs when the infecting strain is lysogenized by a bacteriophage that mediates production of a pyrogenic exotoxin. Within 1 to 2 days after the initial clinical symptoms of pharyngitis develop, a diffuse erythematous rash initially appears on the upper chest and then spreads to the extremities. The area around the mouth is generally spared **(circumoral pallor),** as are the palms and soles. A yellowish-white coating initially covers the tongue and is later shed, revealing a red, raw surface beneath **("strawberry tongue").** The rash, which blanches when pressed, is best seen on the abdomen and in skinfolds **(Pastia lines).** The rash disappears over the next 5 to 7 days and is followed by desquamation of the superficial skin layer. Suppurative complications of streptococcal pharyngitis (e.g., peritonsillar and retropharyngeal abscesses) are rare since the advent of antimicrobial therapy.

Pyoderma

Pyoderma (impetigo) is a confined, purulent *("pyo")* infection of the skin *("derma")* that primarily affects exposed areas (i.e., face, arms, legs). Infection begins when the skin is colonized with *S. pyogenes* after direct contact with an infected person or fomites. The organism is introduced into the subcutaneous tissues through a break in the skin (e.g., scratch, insect bite). Vesicles develop, progressing to pustules (pus-filled vesicles), and then rupture and crust over. The regional lymph nodes can become enlarged, but systemic signs of infection (e.g., fever, sepsis, involvement of other organs) are uncommon. Secondary dermal spread of the infection caused by scratching is typical.

Pyoderma is seen primarily during the warm, moist months in young children with poor personal hygiene. Although *S. pyogenes* is responsible for most streptococcal skin infections, groups C and G streptococci have also been implicated. *Staphylococcus aureus* is also commonly present in the lesions. The strains of streptococci that cause skin infections differ from those that cause pharyngitis, although pyoderma serotypes can colonize the pharynx and establish a persistent carriage state.

Erysipelas

Erysipelas (*erythros,* "red"; *pella,* "skin") is an acute infection of the skin. Patients experience localized pain, inflammation (erythema, warmth), lymph node enlargement, and systemic signs (chills, fever, leukocytosis). The involved skin area is typically raised and distinctly differentiated from the uninvolved skin (Figure 19-3). Erysipelas occurs most commonly in young children or older adults, historically on the face but now more commonly on the legs, and usually is preceded by infections of the respiratory tract or skin with *S. pyogenes* (less commonly with group C or G streptococci).

Cellulitis

Unlike erysipelas, **cellulitis** typically involves both the skin and deeper subcutaneous tissues, and the distinction between infected and noninfected skin is not as clear. As in erysipelas, local inflammation and systemic signs are observed. Precise identification of the offending organism is necessary because many different organisms can cause cellulitis.

Necrotizing Fasciitis

Necrotizing fasciitis (also called *streptococcal gangrene*) is an infection that occurs deep in the subcutaneous tissue, spreads along the fascial planes, and is characterized by an extensive destruction of muscle and fat (Figure 19-4). The organism (referred to by the news media as "flesh-eating bacteria") is introduced into the tissue through a break in the skin (e.g., minor cut or trauma, vesicular viral infection, burn, surgery). Initially, there is evidence of cellulitis, after which bullae form and gangrene (tissue necrosis associated with obstructed blood flow) and systemic symptoms develop. Toxicity, multiorgan failure, and death are the hallmarks of this disease; thus prompt medical intervention is necessary to save the patient. Unlike cellulitis, which can be treated with antibiotic therapy, fasciitis must also be treated aggressively with surgical debridement of infected tissue.

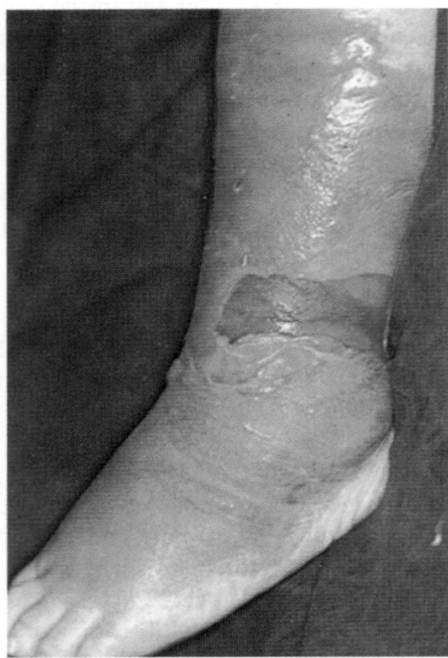

FIGURE 19-3 Acute stage of erysipelas of the leg. Note the erythema in the involved area and bullae formation. (From Emond RT, Rowland HAK, Welsby P: *Colour atlas of infectious diseases,* ed 3, London, 1995, Wolfe.)

Streptococcal Toxic Shock Syndrome (Clinical Case 19-1)

Although the incidence of severe *S. pyogenes* disease declined steadily after the advent of antibiotics, this trend changed dramatically in the late 1980s, when infections characterized by multisystem toxicity were reported. Patients with this syndrome initially experience soft-tissue inflammation at the site of the infection, pain, and nonspecific symptoms such as fever, chills, malaise, nausea, vomiting, and diarrhea. The pain intensifies as the disease progresses to shock and organ failure (e.g., kidney, lungs, liver, heart)—features similar to those of staphylococcal toxic shock syndrome. However, in contrast with staphylococcal disease, most patients with streptococcal disease are bacteremic, and many have necrotizing fasciitis.

Although people of all age groups are susceptible to **streptococcal toxic shock syndrome,** increased risk for disease is observed for patients with human immunodeficiency virus (HIV) infection, cancer, diabetes mellitus, heart or pulmonary disease, and varicella-zoster virus infection, as well as intravenous drug abusers and those who abuse alcohol. The strains of *S. pyogenes* responsible for this syndrome differ from the strains causing pharyngitis in that most of the former are M serotypes 1 or 3 and many have prominent mucopolysaccharide hyaluronic acid capsules (mucoid strains). The production of pyrogenic exotoxins, particularly SpeA and SpeC, is also a prominent feature of these organisms.

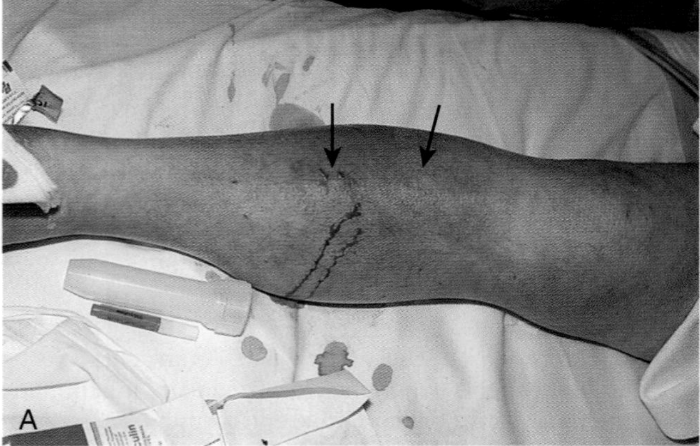

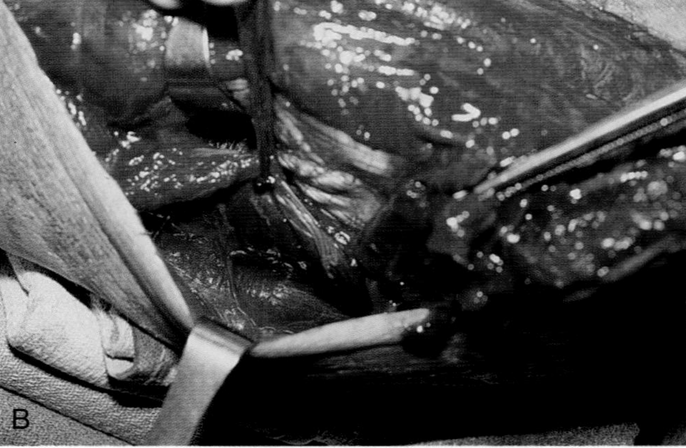

FIGURE 19-4 Necrotizing fasciitis caused by *Streptococcus pyogenes.* The patient presented with a 3-day history of malaise, diffuse myalgia, and low-grade fever. Over 3 hours, the pain became excruciating and was localized to the calf. **A,** Note the two small, purple bullae over the calf *(arrows).* **B,** Extensive necrotizing fasciitis was present on surgical exploration. The patient died despite aggressive surgical and medical management. (From Cohen J, Powderly WG, Opal SM: *Infectious diseases,* ed 3, Philadelphia, 2010, Mosby.)

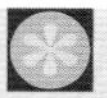

Clinical Case 19-1 Streptococcal Toxic Shock Syndrome

Streptococcal toxic shock syndrome is a frightening, deadly infection. This is illustrated by a patient reported by Cone and associates in 1987 (*N Engl J Med* 317:146–149, 1987). The patient was a 46-year-old man who was scratched on his forearm by his German shepherd dog and then reopened the wound while at work the next day. The following evening, he developed a low-grade fever, chills, backache, and myalgia. When he presented to the local emergency department, minimal erythema and a thin serous discharge were noted at the wound site. Cultures of the wound and blood were collected, and intravenous antibiotics were started. Within 10 hours, the patient became confused and hypotensive. He was transferred to the intensive care unit. Because the erythema over the wound had spread and multiple bullae formed on the wound surface, the patient was taken to surgery, where yellowish fluid in the muscle tissues was drained. Cultures from the surgical site, as well as the original wound cultures, grew *Streptococcus pyogenes*. Following surgical debridement, the patient continued to decline, with the development of abnormal liver function, renal failure, pulmonary distress, and cardiac abnormalities. The patient developed persistent hypotension and died 3 days after admission to the hospital. The fulminant progression of this disease and multiorgan failure underlines the need for aggressive medical intervention.

Other Suppurative Diseases

S. pyogenes has been associated with a variety of other suppurative infections, including puerperal sepsis, lymphangitis, and pneumonia. Although these infections are still seen, they became less common after the introduction of antibiotic therapy.

Bacteremia

S. pyogenes is one of the most common β-hemolytic streptococci isolated in blood cultures. Patients with localized infections (e.g., pharyngitis, pyoderma, erysipelas) rarely are bacteremic, but blood cultures are positive in most patients with necrotizing fasciitis or toxic shock syndrome. The mortality in this population of patients approaches 40% in countries with a sophisticated medical infrastructure and is much higher in resource-limited countries.

Nonsuppurative Streptococcal Disease

Rheumatic Fever

Rheumatic fever is a nonsuppurative complication of *S. pyogenes* pharyngitis. It is characterized by inflammatory changes involving the heart, joints, blood vessels, and subcutaneous tissues. Involvement of the heart manifests as a pancarditis (endocarditis, pericarditis, myocarditis) and is often associated with subcutaneous nodules. Chronic progressive damage to the heart valves may occur. Joint manifestations can range from arthralgias to frank arthritis, with multiple joints involved in a migratory pattern (i.e., involvement shifts from one joint to another).

The incidence of rheumatic fever in the United States has decreased from a peak of more than 10,000 cases per year reported in 1961 to 112 cases reported in 1994 (the last year of mandatory reporting). In contrast, disease in developing countries is much more common, with an estimated 100 cases per 100,000 children per year. Specific class I M protein types (e.g., types 1, 3, 5, 6, and 18) with an exposed shared antigenic site are responsible for rheumatic fever. In addition, rheumatic fever is associated with streptococcal pharyngitis but not cutaneous streptococcal infections. As would be expected, the epidemiologic characteristics of the disease mimic those of streptococcal pharyngitis. It is most common in young school-age children, with no male or female predilection, and occurs primarily during the cooler months of the fall or winter. The disease occurs most commonly in patients with severe streptococcal pharyngitis; however, as many as one third of patients have asymptomatic or mild infection. Rheumatogenic strains induce a vigorous antibody response in all patients with pharyngitis. Rheumatic fever can recur with a subsequent streptococcal infection if antibiotic prophylaxis is not used. The risk for recurrence decreases with time.

Because no specific diagnostic test can identify patients with rheumatic fever, the diagnosis is made on the basis of clinical findings and documented evidence of a recent *S. pyogenes* infection, such as (1) positive throat culture or specific nucleic acid–based test, (2) detection of the group A antigen in a throat swab, or (3) an elevation of ASO, anti-DNase B, or anti-hyaluronidase antibodies. The absence of an elevated or rising antibody titer would be strong evidence against rheumatic fever.

Acute Glomerulonephritis

The second nonsuppurative complication of streptococcal disease is **glomerulonephritis,** which is characterized by acute inflammation of the renal glomeruli with edema, hypertension, hematuria, and proteinuria. Specific nephritogenic strains of group A streptococci are associated with this disease. In contrast with rheumatic fever, acute glomerulonephritis is a sequela of both pharyngeal and pyodermal streptococcal infections; however, the nephrogenic M serotypes differ for the two primary diseases. The epidemiologic characteristics of the disease are similar to those of the initial streptococcal infection. Diagnosis is determined on the basis of the clinical presentation and the finding of evidence of a recent *S. pyogenes* infection. Young patients generally have an uneventful recovery, but the long-term prognosis for adults is unclear. Progressive irreversible loss of renal function has been observed in adults.

Laboratory Diagnosis

Microscopy

Gram stains of affected tissue can be used to make a rapid preliminary diagnosis of *S. pyogenes* soft-tissue infections or pyoderma. Because streptococci are not observed in Gram stains of uninfected skin, the finding of gram-positive cocci in pairs and chains in association with leukocytes is important. In contrast, many species of streptococci are part of the normal oropharyngeal flora, so observation of streptococci in a respiratory specimen from a patient with pharyngitis has no diagnostic significance.

Antigen Detection

A variety of immunologic tests using antibodies that react with the group-specific carbohydrate in the bacterial cell wall can be used to detect group A streptococci directly in throat swabs. These tests are rapid, inexpensive, and specific. Antigen tests are not used for cutaneous or nonsuppurative diseases.

Nucleic Acid–Based Tests

Commercial nucleic acid probe assay and nucleic acid amplification assays are available for the detection of *S. pyogenes* in pharyngeal specimens. Probe assays are less sensitive than culture, but amplification assays are as sensitive as culture and are the test of choice where available.

Culture

Despite the difficulty of collecting throat swab specimens from children, specimens must be obtained from the posterior oropharynx (e.g., tonsils). Fewer bacteria are present in the anterior areas of the mouth, and because the mouth (particularly saliva) is colonized with bacteria that inhibit the growth of *S. pyogenes,* contamination of even a properly collected specimen may obscure or suppress the growth of *S. pyogenes.* The recovery of *S. pyogenes* from patients with impetigo is not a problem. The crusted top of the lesion is raised, and the purulent material and base of the lesion are cultured. Culture specimens should not be obtained from open draining skin pustules, because they might be superinfected with staphylococci. Organisms are readily recovered in the tissues and blood cultures obtained from patients with necrotizing fasciitis; however, relatively few organisms may be present in the skin of patients with erysipelas or cellulitis. As mentioned previously, streptococci have fastidious growth requirements and growth on the plates may be delayed, so prolonged incubation (2 to 3 days) should be used before a culture is considered negative.

Identification

Group A streptococci are identified definitively through the demonstration of the **group-specific carbohydrate,** a technique that was not practical until the introduction of direct antigen detection tests. Differentiation of *S. pyogenes* from other species of streptococci with the group-specific A antigen can be determined by their susceptibility to **bacitracin** or the presence of the enzyme **L-pyrrolidonyl arylamidase (PYR).** Susceptibility to bacitracin is determined by placing a disk saturated with bacitracin onto a plate inoculated with group A streptococci; after overnight incubation, strains inhibited by bacitracin are considered group A streptococci. The PYR test measures hydrolysis L-pyrrolindonyl-β-naphthylamide, releasing β-naphthylamine, which, in the presence of *p*-dimethylaminocinnamaldehyde, forms a red compound. The advantage of this specific test is that it takes less than 1 minute to determine whether the reaction is positive *(S. pyogenes)* or negative (all other streptococci). Enterococci are PYR positive but do not react with group A antisera.

Antibody Detection

Patients with *S. pyogenes* disease produce antibodies to specific streptococcal enzymes. Although antibodies against the M protein are produced and are important for maintaining immunity, these type-specific antibodies appear late in the clinical course of the disease and are not useful for diagnosis. In contrast, the measurement of antibodies against streptolysin O **(ASO test)** is useful for confirming rheumatic fever or acute glomerulonephritis resulting from a recent streptococcal pharyngeal infection. These antibodies appear 3 to 4 weeks after the initial exposure to the organism and then persist. An elevated ASO titer is not observed in patients with streptococcal pyoderma (see previous discussion). The production of antibodies against other streptococcal enzymes, particularly DNase B, has been documented in patients with either streptococcal pyoderma or pharyngitis. The **anti-DNase B test** should be performed if streptococcal glomerulonephritis is suspected.

Treatment, Prevention, and Control

S. pyogenes is very sensitive to penicillin, so oral penicillin V or amoxicillin can be used to treat streptococcal pharyngitis. For penicillin-allergic patients, an oral cephalosporin or macrolide may be used. The combined use of intravenous penicillin with a protein synthesis–inhibiting antibiotic (e.g., clindamycin) is recommended for severe systemic infections. Resistance or poor clinical response has limited the usefulness of the tetracyclines and sulfonamides, and resistance to erythromycin and the newer macrolides (e.g., azithromycin, clarithromycin) is increasing in frequency. Drainage and aggressive surgical debridement must be promptly initiated in patients with serious soft-tissue infections.

Persistent oropharyngeal carriage of *S. pyogenes* can occur after a complete course of therapy. This state may stem from poor compliance with the prescribed course of therapy, reinfection with a new strain, or persistent carriage in a sequestered focus. Because penicillin resistance has not been observed in patients with oropharyngeal carriage, penicillin can be given for an additional course of treatment. If carriage persists, re-treatment is not indicated, because prolonged antibiotic therapy can disrupt the normal bacterial flora. Antibiotic therapy in patients with pharyngitis speeds the relief of symptoms and, if initiated within 10 days of the initial clinical disease, prevents rheumatic fever. Antibiotic therapy does not appear to influence the progression to acute glomerulonephritis.

Patients with a history of rheumatic fever require long-term **antibiotic prophylaxis** to prevent recurrence of the disease. Because damage to the heart valve predisposes these patients to endocarditis, they also require antibiotic prophylaxis before they undergo procedures that can induce transient bacteremias (e.g., dental procedures). Specific antibiotic therapy does not alter the course of acute glomerulonephritis, and prophylactic therapy is not indicated because recurrent disease is not observed in these patients.

Streptococcus agalactiae

S. agalactiae is the only species that has the group B antigen. This organism was first recognized as a cause of puerperal sepsis. Although this disease is now relatively uncommon, *S. agalactiae* has become better known as an important cause of septicemia, pneumonia, and meningitis in newborn children, as well as a cause of serious disease in adults (see Box 19-1).

Physiology and Structure

Group B streptococci are gram-positive cocci (0.6 to 1.2 μm) that form short chains in clinical specimens and longer chains in culture, features that make them indistinguishable on Gram stain from *S. pyogenes.* They grow well on nutritionally enriched media and, in contrast with the colonies of

S. pyogenes, the colonies of *S. agalactiae* are large with a narrow zone of β-hemolysis. Some strains (1% to 2%) are nonhemolytic, although their prevalence may be underestimated because nonhemolytic strains are not commonly screened for the group B antigen.

Strains of *S. agalactiae* can be characterized on the basis of three serologic markers: (1) the **group-specific cell wall polysaccharide B antigen** (Lancefield grouping antigen); (2) nine **type-specific capsular polysaccharides** (Ia, Ib, and II to VIII); and (3) **surface proteins** (the most common is the **c antigen**). The type-specific polysaccharides are important epidemiologic markers, with serotypes Ia, Ib, II, III, and V most commonly associated with colonization and disease. Knowledge of the specific serotypes associated with disease and of shifting patterns of serotype prevalence is important for vaccine development.

Pathogenesis and Immunity

The most important virulence factor of *S. agalactiae* is the **polysaccharide capsule** that interferes with phagocytosis until the patient develops type-specific antibodies. Antibodies against the type-specific capsular antigens are protective, a factor that partly explains the predilection of this organism for neonates. In the absence of maternal antibodies, the neonate is at risk for disease. In addition, genital colonization with group B streptococci has been associated with increased risk of premature delivery, and premature infants are at greater risk of disease. Functional classical and alternative complement pathways are required for killing group B streptococci, particularly types Ia, III, and V. As a result, there is a greater likelihood of systemic spread of the organism in colonized premature infants with physiologically **low complement levels** or for infants in whom the receptors for complement, or for the Fc fragment of immunoglobulin (Ig)G antibodies, are not exposed on neutrophils. It has also been found that the type-specific capsular polysaccharides of types Ia, Ib, and II streptococci have a terminal residue of sialic acid. **Sialic acid** can inhibit activation of the alternative complement pathway, thus interfering with the phagocytosis of these strains of group B streptococci.

Epidemiology

Group B streptococci colonize the lower gastrointestinal tract and the genitourinary tract. Transient vaginal carriage has been observed in 10% to 30% of pregnant women, although the observed incidence depends on the time during the gestation period when the sampling is done and the culture techniques used.

Approximately 60% of infants born to colonized mothers become colonized with their mothers' organisms. The likelihood of colonization at birth is higher when the mother is colonized with large numbers of bacteria. Other associations for neonatal colonization are premature delivery, prolonged membrane rupture, and intrapartum fever. Disease in infants younger than 7 days of age is called **early-onset disease;** disease appearing between 1 week and 3 months of life is considered **late-onset disease.** The serotypes most commonly associated with early-onset disease are Ia (35% to 40%), III (30%), and V (15%). Serotype III is responsible for most late-onset disease. Serotypes Ia and V are the most common in adult disease.

Colonization with subsequent development of disease in the neonate can occur in utero, at birth, or during the first few months of life. *S. agalactiae* is the most common cause of bacterial septicemia and meningitis in newborns. The use of intrapartum antibiotic prophylaxis is responsible for a dramatic decline in neonatal disease—from approximately 8000 infections in 1993 to 1800 infections in 2002.

The risk of invasive disease in adults is greater in pregnant women than in men and nonpregnant women. Urinary tract infections, amnionitis, endometritis, and wound infections are the most common manifestations in pregnant women. Infections in men and nonpregnant women are primarily skin and soft-tissue infections, bacteremia, urosepsis (urinary tract infection with bacteremia), and pneumonia. Conditions that predispose to the development of disease in nonpregnant adults include diabetes mellitus, chronic liver or renal disease, cancer, and HIV infection.

Clinical Diseases

Early-Onset Neonatal Disease

Clinical symptoms of group B streptococcal disease acquired in utero or at birth develop during the first week of life. Early-onset disease, characterized by **bacteremia, pneumonia,** or **meningitis,** is indistinguishable from sepsis caused by other organisms. Because pulmonary involvement is observed in most infants and meningeal involvement may be initially inapparent, examination of cerebrospinal fluid (CSF) is required for all infected children. The mortality rate has decreased to less than 5% because of rapid diagnosis and better supportive care; however, 15% to 30% of infants who survive meningitis have severe neurologic sequelae, including blindness, deafness, and mental retardation.

Late-Onset Neonatal Disease (Clinical Case 19-2)

Late-onset disease is acquired from an exogenous source (e.g., mother, another infant) and develops between 1 week and 3 months of age. The predominant manifestation is **bacteremia with meningitis,** which resembles disease caused by other bacteria. Although the mortality rate is low (e.g., 3%), neurologic complications are common in children with meningitis (e.g., 25% to 50%).

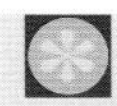

Clinical Case 19-2 Group B Streptococcal Disease in a Neonate

The following is a description of late-onset group B streptococcal disease in a neonate (Hammersen et al: *Eur J Pediatr* 126:189–197, 1977). An infant male weighing 3400 grams was delivered spontaneously at term. Physical examinations of the infant were normal during the first week of life; however, the child started feeding irregularly during the second week. On day 13, the baby was admitted to the hospital with generalized seizures. A small amount of cloudy cerebrospinal fluid was collected by lumbar puncture, and *Streptococcus agalactiae* serotype III was isolated from culture. Despite prompt initiation of therapy, the baby developed hydrocephalus, necessitating implantation of an atrioventricular shunt. The infant was discharged at age 3.5 months with retardation of psychomotor development. This patient illustrates neonatal meningitis caused by the most commonly implicated serotype of group B streptococci in late-onset disease and the complications associated with this infection.

Infections in Pregnant Women

Postpartum endometritis, wound infection, and **urinary tract infections** occur in women during and immediately after pregnancy. Because childbearing women are generally in good health, the prognosis is excellent for those who receive appropriate therapy. Secondary complications of bacteremia such as endocarditis, meningitis, and osteomyelitis are rare.

Infections in Men and Nonpregnant Women

Compared with pregnant women who acquire group B streptococcal infection, men and nonpregnant women with group B streptococcal infections are generally older and have debilitating underlying conditions. The most common presentations are **bacteremia, pneumonia, bone and joint infections,** and **skin and soft-tissue infections.** Because these patients often have compromised immunity, mortality is higher in this population.

Laboratory Diagnosis

Antigen Detection

Tests for the direct detection of group B streptococci in urogenital specimens are available but are too insensitive to be used to screen mothers and predict which newborns are at increased risk for acquiring neonatal disease. Likewise, the antigen tests are too insensitive (<30%) to be used with CSF. A Gram stain of CSF has much better sensitivity and should be used.

Nucleic Acid–Based Tests

Polymerase chain reaction (PCR)–based nucleic acid amplification assays are approved by the U.S. Food and Drug Administration (FDA) for rectal/vaginal swabs from pregnant women. The tests are relatively insensitive, so testing must be performed using a selective enrichment broth (e.g., Lim broth) rather than directly with the clinical specimen.

Culture

Group B streptococci readily grow on a nutritionally enriched medium, producing large colonies after 24 hours of incubation; however, β-hemolysis may be difficult to detect or absent, posing a problem in the detection of the organism when other organisms are present in the culture (e.g., vaginal culture). Thus use of a selective enrichment broth medium with antibiotics added to suppress the growth of other organisms (e.g., LIM broth with colistin and nalidixic acid) followed by subculture to nonselective media such as a blood agar plate is currently recommended by the CDC for the detection of group B streptococci in women between weeks 35 and 37 of pregnancy.

Identification

Isolates of *S. agalactiae* are identified definitively by the demonstration of the group-specific cell wall carbohydrate.

Treatment, Prevention, and Control

Group B streptococci are susceptible to **penicillin,** which is the drug of choice. Because other bacteria can be responsible for neonatal disease (e.g., *S. pneumoniae, Listeria,* gram-negative rods), broad-spectrum therapy should be selected for empirical therapy. A cephalosporin or vancomycin can be used in penicillin-allergic patients. Resistance to macrolides, clindamycin, and tetracyclines is common, so these drugs should not be selected unless demonstrated to be active in vitro.

In an effort to prevent neonatal disease, it is recommended that all pregnant women should be **screened for colonization** with group B streptococci at 35 to 37 weeks' gestation (refer to the following CDC document for additional information: www.cdc.gov/groupbstrep/guidelines/index.html). **Chemoprophylaxis** should be used for all women who are either colonized or at high risk. A pregnant woman is considered to be at high risk to give birth to a baby with invasive group B disease if she has previously given birth to an infant with the disease or risk factors for the disease are present at birth. These risk factors are (1) intrapartum temperature of at least 38° C, (2) membrane rupture at least 18 hours before delivery, and (3) vaginal or rectal culture positive for organisms at 35 to 37 weeks' gestation. Intravenous penicillin G or ampicillin administered at least 4 hours before delivery is recommended; cefazolin is used for penicillin-allergic women or clindamycin (if susceptible) or vancomycin for mothers at high risk for anaphylaxis. This approach ensures high protective antibiotic levels in the infant's circulatory system at the time of birth.

Because newborn disease is associated with decreased circulating antibodies in the mother, efforts have been directed at developing a polyvalent vaccine against serotypes Ia, Ib, II, III, and V. The capsular polysaccharides are poor immunogens; however, complexing them with tetanus toxoid has improved the immunogenicity of the vaccine. Trials with this polyvalent vaccine demonstrated that protective levels of antibodies are induced in animal models; however, no licensed vaccine is currently available.

Other β-Hemolytic Streptococci

Among the other β-hemolytic streptococci, groups C, F, and G are most commonly associated with human disease. Organisms of particular importance are the *Streptococcus anginosus* group (includes *S. anginosus, Streptococcus constellatus,* and *Streptococcus intermedius*) and *Streptococcus dysgalactiae*. β-Hemolytic members of the *S. anginosus* group can possess the group A, C, F, or G polysaccharide antigen (or not have any group-specific antigen), and *S. dysgalactiae* can have either the group C or G antigen. It should be noted that an individual isolate possesses only one group antigen. Isolates of the *S. anginosus* group grow as small colonies (requiring 2 days of incubation) with a narrow zone of β-hemolysis (Figure 19-5A). These species are primarily associated with abscess formation and not pharyngitis, in contrast with the other group A *Streptococcus, S. pyogenes*. *S. dysgalactiae* produces large colonies with a large zone of β-hemolysis on blood agar media (see Figure 19-5B), resembling *S. pyogenes*. Additionally, *S. dysgalactiae* causes pharyngitis, which is sometimes complicated by acute glomerulonephritis but never rheumatic fever.

Viridans Streptococci

The viridans group of streptococci is a heterogeneous collection of α-hemolytic and nonhemolytic streptococci

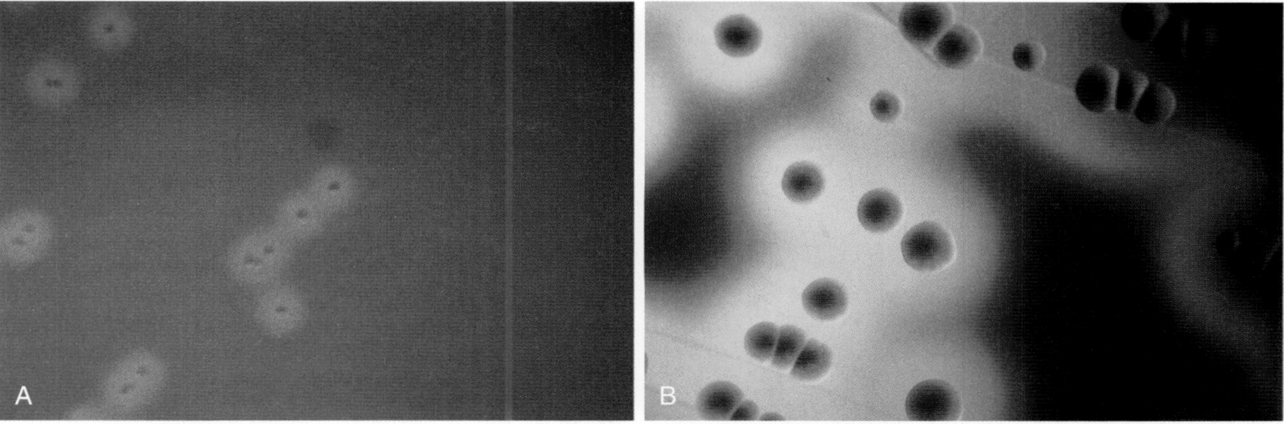

FIGURE 19-5 Group C *Streptococcus.* **A,** *S. anginosus,* small-colony species. **B,** *S. dysgalactiae,* large-colony species.

(Figure 19-6). Many species and subspecies have been identified, and most are classified into five subgroups. This classification scheme is clinically important because many of the species in the five subgroups are responsible for specific diseases (see Table 19-4). Some members of the viridans streptococci (e.g., *S. anginosus* group) can have β-hemolytic strains with the group-specific cell wall polysaccharides (thus contributing to the confusing taxonomy of this genus). In addition, *S. pneumoniae* is a member of the *Streptococcus mitis* subgroup, although most physicians and microbiologists do not think of *S. pneumoniae* as viridans streptococci; it will be discussed separately in this chapter.

The viridans streptococci colonize the oropharynx, gastrointestinal tract, and genitourinary tract. Similar to most other streptococci, viridans species are nutritionally fastidious, requiring complex media supplemented with blood products and, frequently, an incubation atmosphere with 5% to 10% carbon dioxide.

Although most viridans streptococci are highly susceptible to penicillin, with minimum inhibitory concentrations (MICs) of less than 0.1 μg/ml, moderately resistant (penicillin MIC of 0.2 to 2 μg/ml) and highly resistant (MIC >2 μg/ml) streptococci have become common in the *S. mitis* group. Infections with isolates that are moderately resistant can generally be treated with a combination of penicillin and an aminoglycoside; however, alternative antibiotics such as a broad-spectrum cephalosporin or vancomycin must be used to treat serious infections.

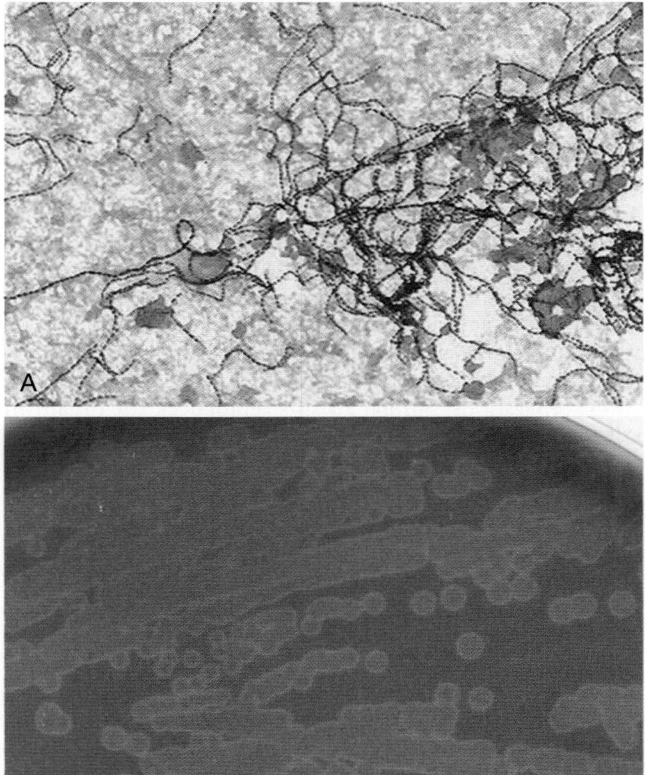

FIGURE 19-6 *Streptococcus mitis.* **A,** Gram stain from blood culture. **B,** α-Hemolytic colonies.

Streptococcus pneumoniae

S. pneumoniae was isolated independently by Pasteur and Steinberg more than 100 years ago. Since that time, research with this organism has led to a greater understanding of molecular genetics, antibiotic resistance, and vaccine-related immunoprophylaxis. Unfortunately, pneumococcal disease is still a leading cause of morbidity and mortality.

Physiology and Structure

The pneumococcus is an **encapsulated** gram-positive coccus. The cells are 0.5 to 1.2 μm in diameter, oval, and arranged in pairs (commonly referred to as **diplococci**) or short chains (Figure 19-7). Older cells decolorize readily and can stain gram-negative. Colonial morphology varies, with colonies of encapsulated strains generally large (1 to 3 mm in diameter on blood agar; smaller on chocolatized or heated blood agar), round, and mucoid, and colonies of nonencapsulated strains smaller and flat. All colonies undergo autolysis with aging—that is, the central portion of the colony dissolves, leaving a dimpled appearance. Colonies appear α-hemolytic on blood agar if incubated aerobically and may be β-hemolytic

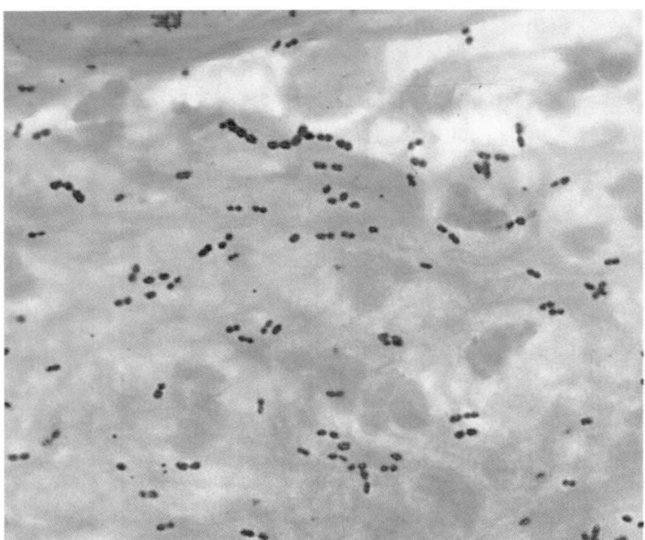

FIGURE 19-7 Gram stain of *Streptococcus pneumoniae.*

if grown anaerobically. The α-hemolytic appearance results from production of **pneumolysin,** an enzyme that degrades hemoglobin, producing a green product.

The organism has fastidious nutritional requirements and can grow only on enriched media supplemented with blood products. *S. pneumoniae* can ferment carbohydrates, producing lactic acid as the primary metabolic byproduct. *S. pneumoniae* grows poorly in media with high glucose concentrations because lactic acid rapidly reaches toxic levels in such preparations. Similar to all streptococci, the organism lacks catalase. Unless an exogenous source of catalase is provided (e.g., from blood), the accumulation of hydrogen peroxide inhibits the growth of *S. pneumoniae,* as observed on chocolatized blood agar.

Virulent strains of *S. pneumoniae* are covered with a complex **polysaccharide capsule.** The capsular polysaccharides have been used for the serologic classification of strains; currently, 94 serotypes are recognized. Purified capsular polysaccharides from the most commonly isolated serotypes are used in a **polyvalent vaccine.** Individual strains of *S. pneumoniae* can switch capsular serotypes through genomic recombination and point mutations in the capsular genes. Recombination is also associated with acquisition of genes encoding penicillin resistance, so use of vaccines or antibiotic therapy can facilitate the selection and dissemination of new capsular serotypes.

The peptidoglycan layer of the cell wall of the pneumococcus is typical of gram-positive cocci. Attached to alternating subunits of *N*-acetylglucosamine and *N*-acetylmuramic acid are oligopeptide chains, which, in turn, are cross-linked by pentaglycine bridges. The other major component of the cell wall is teichoic acid. Two forms of teichoic acid exist in the pneumococcal cell wall, one exposed on the cell surface and a similar structure covalently bound to the plasma membrane lipids. The exposed teichoic acid is linked to the peptidoglycan layer and extends through the overlying capsule. This species-specific structure, called the **C polysaccharide,** is unrelated to the group-specific carbohydrate observed by Lancefield in β-hemolytic streptococci. The C polysaccharide precipitates a serum globulin fraction (**C-reactive protein [CRP]**) in the presence of calcium. CRP is present in low concentrations in healthy people but in elevated concentrations in patients with acute inflammatory diseases (hence, monitoring levels of CRP is used to predict inflammation). The teichoic acid bound to lipids in the bacterial cytoplasmic membrane is called the **F antigen** because it can cross-react with the Forssman surface antigens on mammalian cells. Both forms of teichoic acid are associated with phosphorylcholine residues. **Phosphorylcholine** is unique to the cell wall of *S. pneumoniae* and plays an important regulatory role in cell wall hydrolysis. Phosphorylcholine must be present for activity of the pneumococcal autolysin, **amidase,** during cell division.

Pathogenesis and Immunity

Although *S. pneumoniae* has been extensively studied, much remains to be learned about the pathogenesis of pneumococcal disease. The disease manifestations are caused primarily by the host response to infection rather than the production of organism-specific toxic factors. However, an understanding of how *S. pneumoniae* colonizes the oropharynx, spreads into normally sterile tissues, stimulates a localized inflammatory response, and evades being killed by phagocytic cells is crucial.

Colonization and Migration

S. pneumoniae is a human pathogen that colonizes the oropharynx and then, in specific situations, is able to spread to the lungs, paranasal sinuses, or middle ear. It can also be transported in the blood to distal sites such as the brain. The initial colonization of the oropharynx is mediated by the binding of the bacteria to epithelial cells by means of **surface protein adhesins.** Subsequent migration of the organism to the lower respiratory tract can be prevented if the bacteria are enveloped in mucus and removed from the airways by the action of ciliated epithelial cells. The bacteria counteract this envelopment by producing **secretory IgA protease** and **pneumolysin.** Secretory IgA traps bacteria in mucus by binding the bacteria to mucin with the Fc region of the antibody. The bacterial IgA protease prevents this interaction. **Pneumolysin,** a cytotoxin similar to the streptolysin O in *S. pyogenes,* binds cholesterol in the host cell membrane and creates pores. This activity can destroy the ciliated epithelial cells and phagocytic cells.

Tissue Destruction

A characteristic of pneumococcal infections is the mobilization of inflammatory cells to the focus of infection. Pneumococcal teichoic acid, peptidoglycan fragments, and pneumolysin mediate the process. **Teichoic acid** and the **peptidoglycan fragments** activate the alternative complement pathway, producing C5a, which mediates the inflammatory process. This activity is augmented by the bacterial enzyme **amidase,** which enhances release of the cell wall components. **Pneumolysin** activates the classic complement pathway, resulting in the production of C3a and C5a. In turn, cytokines such as interleukin (IL)-1 and tumor necrosis factor (TNF)-α are produced by the activated leukocytes, leading to the further migration of inflammatory cells to the site of infection, fever, tissue damage, and other signs characteristic of pneumococcal infection. The production of

hydrogen peroxide by *S. pneumoniae* can also lead to tissue damage caused by reactive oxygen intermediates.

Finally, **phosphorylcholine** present in the bacterial cell wall can bind to receptors for platelet-activating factor that are expressed on the surface of endothelial cells, leukocytes, platelets, and tissue cells, such as those in the lungs and meninges. By binding these receptors, the bacteria can enter the cells, where they are protected from opsonization and phagocytosis, and pass into sequestered areas, such as blood and the central nervous system. This activity facilitates the spread of disease.

Phagocytic Survival

S. pneumoniae survives phagocytosis because of the antiphagocytic protection afforded by its **capsule** and the pneumolysin-mediated suppression of the phagocytic cell oxidative burst, which is required for intracellular killing. The virulence of *S. pneumoniae* is a direct result of this capsule. Encapsulated (smooth) strains can cause disease in humans and experimental animals, whereas nonencapsulated (rough) strains are avirulent. Antibodies directed against the type-specific capsular polysaccharides protect against disease caused by immunologically related strains, so capsular switching allows a strain to avoid immune clearance. The capsular polysaccharides are soluble and have been called **specific soluble substances.** Free polysaccharides can protect viable organisms from phagocytosis by binding with opsonic antibodies.

Epidemiology

S. pneumoniae is a common inhabitant of the throat and nasopharynx in healthy people, with colonization more common in children than in adults and more common in adults living in a household with children. Colonization initially occurs at approximately 6 months of age. Subsequently, the child is transiently colonized with other serotypes of the organism. The duration of carriage decreases with each successive serotype carried, in part because of the development of serotype-specific immunity. Although new serotypes are acquired throughout the year, the incidence of carriage and associated disease is highest during the cool months. The strains of pneumococci that cause disease are the same as those associated with carriage.

Pneumococcal disease occurs when organisms colonizing the nasopharynx and oropharynx spread to the lungs (pneumonia), paranasal sinuses (sinusitis), ears (otitis media), or meninges (meningitis). Spread of *S. pneumoniae* in blood to other body sites can occur with all of these diseases. It is recognized that some serotypes have a higher predilection for invasive pneumococcal disease.

Although the introduction of vaccines for pediatric and adult populations has reduced the incidence of disease caused by *S. pneumoniae,* the organism is still a common cause of bacterial pneumonia acquired outside the hospital, meningitis, otitis media and sinusitis, and bacteremia. Disease is most common in children and the elderly with low levels of protective antibodies directed against the pneumococcal capsular polysaccharides. The World Health Organization (WHO) estimates that more than 200,000 children younger than age 5 years die each year of pneumococcal pneumonia.

Pneumonia occurs when the endogenous oral organisms are aspirated into the lower airways. Although strains can spread on airborne droplets from one person to another in a closed population, epidemics are rare. Disease occurs when the natural defense mechanisms (e.g., epiglottal reflex, trapping of bacteria by the mucus-producing cells lining the bronchus, removal of organisms by the ciliated respiratory epithelium, and cough reflex) are circumvented, permitting organisms colonizing the oropharynx to gain access to the lungs. Pneumococcal disease is most commonly associated with an antecedent viral respiratory disease, such as influenza, or with other conditions that interfere with bacterial clearance, such as chronic pulmonary disease, alcoholism, congestive heart failure, diabetes mellitus, chronic renal disease, and splenic dysfunction or splenectomy.

Clinical Diseases

Pneumonia (Clinical Case 19-3)

Pneumococcal **pneumonia** develops when the bacteria multiply in the alveolar spaces. After aspiration, the bacteria grow rapidly in the nutrient-rich edema fluid. Erythrocytes leaking from congested capillaries accumulate in the alveoli, followed by the neutrophils, and then the alveolar macrophages. Resolution occurs when specific anticapsular antibodies develop, facilitating phagocytosis of the organism and microbial killing.

The onset of the clinical manifestations of pneumococcal pneumonia is abrupt, consisting of a severe shaking chill and sustained fever of 39° C to 41° C. The patient often has symptoms of a viral respiratory tract infection 1 to 3 days before the onset. Most patients have a productive cough with blood-tinged sputum, and they commonly have chest pain **(pleurisy)**. Because the disease is associated with aspiration, it is generally localized in the lower lobes of the lungs (hence the name **lobar pneumonia;** Figure 19-8). However, children and the elderly can have a more generalized bronchopneumonia. Patients usually recover rapidly after the initiation of appropriate antimicrobial therapy, with complete radiologic resolution in 2 to 3 weeks.

The overall mortality rate is 5%, although the likelihood of death is influenced by the serotype of the organism and the age and underlying disease of the patient. The mortality rate is considerably higher in patients with disease caused by

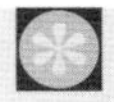

Clinical Case 19-3 *Streptococcus pneumoniae* Pneumonia

Costa and associates (*Am J Hematol* 77:277–281, 2004) described a 68-year-old woman who was in good health until 3 days before hospitalization. She developed fever, chills, increased weakness, and a productive cough with pleuritic chest pain. On admission, she was febrile, had an elevated pulse and respiration rate, and was in moderate respiratory distress. Initial laboratory values showed leucopenia, anemia, and acute renal failure. Chest radiograph demonstrated infiltrates in the right and left lower lobes, with pleural effusions. Therapy with a fluoroquinolone was initiated, and blood and respiratory cultures were positive for *S. pneumoniae.* Additional tests (serum and urine protein electrophoresis) revealed the patient had multiple myeloma. The patient's infection resolved with a 14-day course of antibiotics. This patient illustrates the typical picture of pneumococcal lobar pneumonia and the increased susceptibility to infection in patients with defects in their ability to clear encapsulated organisms.

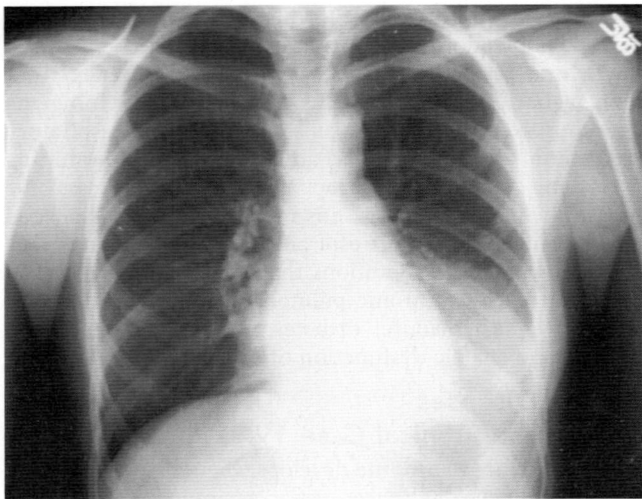

FIGURE 19-8 Dense consolidation of left lower lobe in patient with pneumonia caused by *Streptococcus pneumoniae.* (From Mandell G, Bennett J, Dolin R: *Principles and practice of infectious diseases,* ed 8, Philadelphia, 2015, Elsevier.)

S. pneumoniae type 3, as well as in elderly patients and patients with documented bacteremia. Patients with splenic dysfunction or splenectomy can also have severe pneumococcal disease because of decreased bacterial clearance from the blood and the defective production of early antibodies. In these patients, disease can be associated with a fulminant course and high mortality rate.

Abscesses do not commonly form in patients with pneumococcal pneumonia, except in those infected with specific serotypes (e.g., serotype 3). Pleural effusions are seen in approximately 25% of patients with pneumococcal pneumonia, and empyema (purulent effusion) is a rare complication.

Sinusitis and Otitis Media

S. pneumoniae is a common cause of acute infections of the paranasal sinuses and ear. The disease is usually preceded by a viral infection of the upper respiratory tract, after which polymorphonuclear neutrophils (leukocytes) (PMNs) infiltrate and obstruct the sinuses and ear canal. Middle ear infection **(otitis media)** is primarily seen in young children, but bacterial **sinusitis** can occur in patients of all ages.

Meningitis

S. pneumoniae can spread into the central nervous system after bacteremia, infections of the ear or sinuses, or head trauma that causes a communication between the subarachnoid space and the nasopharynx. Although **pneumococcal meningitis** is relatively uncommon in neonates, *S. pneumoniae* is now a leading cause of disease in children and adults. Mortality and severe neurologic deficits are 4 to 20 times more common in patients with meningitis caused by *S. pneumoniae* than in those with meningitis resulting from other organisms.

Bacteremia

Bacteremia occurs in 25% to 30% of patients with pneumococcal pneumonia and in more than 80% of patients with meningitis. In contrast, bacteria are generally not present in the blood of patients with sinusitis or otitis media. Endocarditis can occur in patients with normal or previously damaged heart valves. Destruction of valve tissue is common.

Laboratory Diagnosis

Microscopy

Gram stain of sputum specimens is a rapid way to diagnose pneumococcal pneumonia and meningitis. The organisms characteristically appear as elongated pairs of gram-positive cocci surrounded by an unstained capsule; however, they may also appear to be gram negative because they tend not to stain well (particularly in older cultures). In addition, their morphology may be distorted in a patient receiving antibiotic therapy. A Gram stain consistent with *S. pneumoniae* can be confirmed with the **quellung** (German for "swelling") reaction. In this test, polyvalent anticapsular antibodies are mixed with the bacteria, and then the mixture is examined microscopically. A greater refractiveness around the bacteria is a positive reaction for *S. pneumoniae*. An alternative test is to mix a drop of bile with a suspension of bacteria. Bile will dissolve *S. pneumoniae* and no organisms will be seen in the Gram stain.

Antigen Detection

Pneumococcal C polysaccharide is excreted in urine and can be detected using a commercially prepared immunoassay. Maximum sensitivity requires that the urine be concentrated by ultrafiltration before it is assayed. Sensitivity has been reported to be 70% in patients with bacteremic pneumococcal pneumonia; however, specificity can be low, particularly in pediatric patients. For this reason, the test is not recommended for children with suspected infections. The test has a sensitivity approaching 100% for patients with pneumococcal meningitis if CSF is tested; however, the test has poor sensitivity and specificity if urine is tested in these patients.

Nucleic Acid–Based Tests

PCR assays have been developed for identification of *S. pneumoniae* isolates in clinical specimens such as CSF but are not widely used.

Culture

Sputum specimens should be inoculated onto an enriched nutrient medium supplemented with blood. *S. pneumoniae* is recovered in the sputum cultures from only half of the patients who have pneumonia, because the organism has fastidious nutritional requirements and is rapidly overgrown by contaminating oral bacteria. Selective media have been used with some success to isolate the organism from sputum specimens, but it takes some technical skill to distinguish *S. pneumoniae* from the other α-hemolytic streptococci that are often present in the specimen. An aspirate must be obtained from the sinus or middle ear for the organism responsible for sinusitis or otitis to be diagnosed definitively. Specimens taken from the nasopharynx or outer ear should not be cultured. It is not difficult to isolate *S. pneumoniae* from specimens of CSF if antibiotic therapy has not been initiated before the specimen is collected; however, as many as half of infected patients who have received even a single dose of antibiotics will have negative cultures.

Identification

Isolates of *S. pneumoniae* are lysed rapidly when the autolysins are activated after exposure to bile **(bile solubility test).** Thus the organism can be identified by placing a drop of bile on an isolated colony. Most colonies of *S. pneumoniae* are dissolved within a few minutes, whereas other α-hemolytic streptococci remain unchanged. *S. pneumoniae* can also be identified by its susceptibility to **optochin** (ethylhydrocupreine dihydrochloride). The isolate is streaked onto a blood agar plate and a disk saturated with optochin is placed in the middle of the inoculum. A zone of inhibited bacterial growth is seen around the disk after overnight incubation. Additional biochemical, serologic, or molecular diagnostic tests can be performed for a definitive identification.

Treatment, Prevention, and Control

Historically **penicillin** was the treatment of choice for pneumococcal disease; however, in 1977, researchers in South Africa reported isolates of *S. pneumoniae* that were resistant to multiple antibiotics, including penicillin. Although high-level resistance to penicillin (MIC of at least 2 μg/ml) was relatively uncommon, this situation changed dramatically beginning in 1990. Now resistance to penicillin is observed for as many as half of the strains isolated in the United States and in other countries. Resistance to penicillins is associated with a decreased affinity of the antibiotic for the penicillin-binding proteins present in the bacterial cell wall, and patients infected with resistant bacteria have an increased risk of an adverse outcome. Resistance to macrolides (e.g., erythromycin), tetracyclines, and to a lesser extent cephalosporins (e.g., ceftriaxone) has also become commonplace. Thus, for serious pneumococcal infections, treatment with a combination of antibiotics is recommended until in vitro susceptibility results are available. **Vancomycin** combined with **ceftriaxone** is used commonly for empirical treatment, followed by monotherapy with an effective cephalosporin, fluoroquinolone, or vancomycin.

Efforts to prevent or control the disease have focused on the development of effective anticapsular vaccines. A **23-valent pneumococcal polysaccharide vaccine** (with 23 different capsular polysaccharides) is recommended for children older than 2 years and adults. Polysaccharides are T-independent antigens, stimulating mature B lymphocytes but not T lymphocytes. Very young children respond poorly to T-independent antigens, so these polysaccharide vaccines are ineffective for this population. In contrast, conjugation of polysaccharides to proteins stimulates a T-helper cell response, resulting in a strong primary response among infants and effective booster response when reimmunized. This approach of using conjugated vaccines for pediatric immunizations has also been used for other neonatal pathogens, such as *Haemophilus influenzae.* Immunization with the **13-valent conjugated pneumococcal vaccine** is currently recommended for infants younger than 2 years. Whereas a single dose of the 23-valent vaccine is generally effective, a series of four doses (at 2, 4, 6, and 12 to 15 months) is recommended for the 13-valent conjugated vaccine. The effectiveness of these vaccines is determined by the prevalent serotypes of *S. pneumoniae* responsible for invasive disease in the population. Whereas these vaccines are generally effective in the United States and European populations, they are less effective in developing countries because the prevalent serotypes are not represented in the vaccines. Additionally, although the 23-valent vaccine is immunogenic in normal adults and immunity is long lived, the vaccine is less effective in some patients at high risk for pneumococcal disease, including: (1) patients with asplenia, sickle cell disease, hematologic malignancy, and HIV infection; (2) patients who have undergone renal transplant; and (3) the elderly.

• *Enterococcus*

Physiology and Structure

The enterococci are gram-positive cocci, typically arranged in **pairs and short chains** (Figure 19-9). The microscopic morphology of these isolates cannot be differentiated reliably from that of *S. pneumoniae.* The cocci grow both aerobically and anaerobically in a broad temperature range (10° C to 45° C), in a wide pH range (4.6 to 9.9), and in the presence of high concentrations of sodium chloride **(NaCl)** and **bile salts.** Thus there are very few clinical conditions that inhibit the growth of enterococci. Glucose is fermented with L-lactic acid as the predominant end product (enterococci are commonly referred to as *lactic acid bacteria*). After 24 hours of incubation, colonies on enriched sheep blood agar are large and can appear nonhemolytic, α-hemolytic, or, rarely, β-hemolytic.

Pathogenesis and Immunity

Although enterococci do not possess the broad range of virulence factors found in staphylococci or streptococci, life-threatening disease with antibiotic-resistant strains has become a serious problem in hospitalized patients. Virulence is mediated by two general properties: (1) ability to adhere to tissues and form biofilms and (2) antibiotic resistance. A number of factors have been described that mediate adherence and biofilm formation, including surface proteins, membrane glycolipids, gelatinase, and pili. In addition, the enterococci either are **inherently resistant to many commonly used antibiotics** (e.g., oxacillin, cephalosporins) or

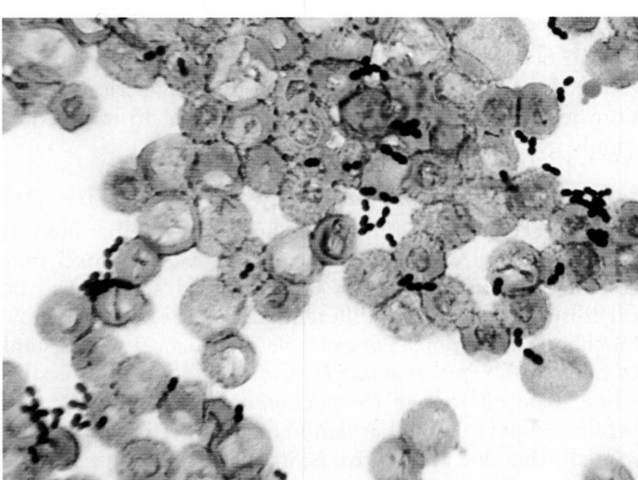

FIGURE 19-9 Gram stain of blood culture with *Enterococcus faecalis.*

have acquired resistance genes (e.g., to aminoglycosides, vancomycin). Clearance of enterococci from blood and tissues is mediated by the rapid influx of neutrophils and opsonization of the bacteria, so patients who are immunocompromised are particularly susceptible to enterococcal infections.

Epidemiology

As their name implies, enterococci are enteric bacteria that are commonly recovered in feces collected from humans and from a variety of animals. *E. faecalis* is found in the large intestine in high concentrations (e.g., 10^5 to 10^7 organisms per gram of feces) and in the genitourinary tract. The distribution of *E. faecium* is similar to that of *E. faecalis* but is found in lower concentrations. Significant risk factors for enterococcal infections include use of urinary or intravascular catheters, prolonged hospitalization, and use of **broad-spectrum antibiotics,** particularly antibiotics that are inherently inactive against enterococci.

The prevalence of the many other enterococcal species is unknown, although they are believed to colonize the intestines in small numbers. Two species that are commonly recovered in the human intestines are *E. gallinarum* and *E. casseliflavus.* These relatively avirulent species are important because, although they are rarely associated with human disease, they are inherently resistant to vancomycin and can be confused with the more important species, *E. faecalis* and *E. faecium.*

Clinical Diseases (See Box 19-1)

Enterococci are important pathogens, particularly in hospitalized patients; indeed, enterococci are one of the most common causes of infections acquired in the hospital **(nosocomial infection).** The urinary tract is the most common site of enterococcal infections, and infections are frequently associated with urinary catheterization or instrumentation. These infections may be asymptomatic, uncomplicated cystitis, or cystitis associated with pyelonephritis. Peritoneal infections are typically polymicrobic (i.e., associated with other aerobic and anaerobic bacteria) and associated with leakage of intestinal bacteria either from trauma or due to disease that compromises the intestinal lining. Enterococci recovered in the blood may either be dissemination from a localized infection of the urinary tract, the peritoneum, or a wound or represent primary infection of the endocardium (endocarditis). Endocarditis is a particularly serious infection because many enterococci are resistant to most commonly used antibiotics (Clinical Case 19-4).

Laboratory Diagnosis

Enterococci grow readily on nonselective media such as blood agar and chocolate agar. Although enterococci may resemble *S. pneumoniae* on Gram-stained specimens, the organisms can be readily differentiated on the basis of simple biochemical reactions. For example, enterococci are resistant to optochin (*S. pneumoniae* is susceptible), do not dissolve when exposed to bile (*S. pneumoniae* is dissolved), and produce L-pyrrolidonyl arylamidase (PYR) (the only *Streptococcus* that is PYR positive is *Streptococcus pyogenes*). The **PYR test** is a commonly performed "5-minute spot" test. Catalase-negative, PYR-positive cocci arranged in pairs and short chains can be presumptively identified as enterococci.

Clinical Case 19-4 Enterococcal Endocarditis

Zimmer and associates (*Clin Infect Dis* 37:e29–e30, 2003) described the epidemiology of enterococcal infections and the difficulties in treating a patient with endocarditis. The patient was a 40-year-old man with hepatitis C, hypertension, and end-stage renal disease who developed fevers and chills during hemodialysis. In the 2 months before this episode, he was treated with ampicillin, levofloxacin, and gentamicin for group B streptococcal endocarditis. Cultures performed during the hemodialysis grew *Enterococcus faecalis* resistant to levofloxacin and gentamicin. Because the patient had an allergic reaction to ampicillin, he was treated with linezolid. Echocardiography showed vegetation on the mitral and tricuspid valves. Over a 3-week period, the patient's cardiac output deteriorated, so the patient was desensitized to ampicillin and therapy was switched to ampicillin and streptomycin. After 25 days of hospitalization, the patient's damaged heart valves were replaced, and therapy was extended for an additional 6 weeks. Thus use of broad-spectrum antibiotics predisposed this patient with previously damaged heart valves to endocarditis caused by *Enterococcus,* and treatment was complicated by resistance of the isolate to many commonly used antibiotics.

Phenotypic properties (e.g., pigment production, motility), biochemical tests, and nucleic acid sequencing are necessary to differentiate among *E. faecalis, E. faecium,* and the other *Enterococcus* species, but this topic is beyond the scope of this text.

Treatment, Prevention, and Control

Antimicrobial therapy for enterococcal infections is complicated because most antibiotics are not bactericidal at clinically relevant concentrations. Therapy for serious infections has traditionally consisted of the synergistic **combination of an aminoglycoside and a cell wall–active antibiotic** (e.g., ampicillin, vancomycin). However, some cell wall antibiotics have no activity against enterococci (e.g., nafcillin, oxacillin, cephalosporins), ampicillin and penicillin are generally ineffective against *E. faecium*, and vancomycin resistance (particularly in *E. faecium*) is commonplace. In addition, more than 25% of enterococci are resistant to the aminoglycosides, and resistance to aminoglycosides and vancomycin is particularly troublesome because it is mediated by plasmids and can be transferred to other bacteria.

Newer antibiotics have been developed that can treat enterococci resistant to ampicillin, vancomycin, or the aminoglycosides. They include linezolid, daptomycin, tigecycline, and quinupristin/dalfopristin. Unfortunately, resistance to linezolid is steadily increasing, and quinupristin/dalfopristin is not active against *E. faecalis* (the most commonly isolated enterococcal species). Enterococci susceptible to ampicillin and resistant to aminoglycosides can be treated with ampicillin plus daptomycin, imipenem, or linezolid. Enterococci resistant to ampicillin and susceptible to aminoglycosides can be treated with an aminoglycoside combined with vancomycin (if active), linezolid, or daptomycin. If the isolate is resistant to both ampicillin and aminoglycosides, then treatment can include daptomycin, linezolid, or vancomycin combined with another active agent.

It is difficult to prevent and control enterococcal infections. Careful restriction of antibiotic usage and the implementation of appropriate infection-control practices (e.g., isolation of infected patients, use of gowns and gloves by anyone in contact with patients) can reduce the risk of colonization with these bacteria, but the complete elimination of infections is unlikely. Additionally, it is extremely difficult to eradicate a vancomycin-resistant strain of *E. faecium* or *E. faecalis* once a patient is colonized.

Bibliography

Arias C, Contreras G, Murray B: Management of multidrug-resistant enterococcal infections, *Clin Microbiol Infect* 16:555–562, 2010.

Centers for Disease Control and Prevention: Prevention of perinatal group B streptococcal disease, *MMWR Morb Mortal Wkly Rep* 59(RR–10):1–32, 2010.

Fisher K, Phillips C: The ecology, epidemiology and virulence of *Enterococcus*, *Microbiol* 155:1749–1757, 2009.

Harboe ZB, Thomsen RW, Riis A, et al: Pneumococcal serotypes and mortality following invasive pneumococcal disease: a population-based cohort study, *PLoS Med* 6:e1000081, 2009.

Hegstad K, Mikalsen T, Coque TM, et al: Mobile genetic elements and their contribution to the emergence of antimicrobial resistant *Enterococcus faecalis* and *Enterococcus faecium*, *Clin Microbiol Infect* 16:541–554, 2010.

Johansson L, Thulin P, Low DE, et al: Getting under the skin: the immunopathogenesis of *Streptococcus pyogenes* deep tissue infections, *Clin Infect Dis* 51:58–65, 2010.

Johnson DR, Kurlan R, Leckman J, et al: The human immune response to streptococcal extracellular antigens: clinical, diagnostic, and potential pathogenetic implications, *Clin Infect Dis* 50:481–490, 2010.

Kanjanabuch T, Kittikowit W, Eiam-Ong S: An update on acute postinfectious glomerulonephritis worldwide, *Nat Rev Nephrol* 5:259–269, 2009.

Krzysciak W, Pluskwa KK, Jurczak A, et al: The pathogenicity of the *Streptococcus* genus, *Eur J Clin Microbiol Infect Dis* 32:1361–1376, 2013.

Le Doare K, Heath PT: An overview of global GBS epidemiology, *Vaccine* 31(Suppl 4):D7–D12, 2013.

Mitchell A, Mitchell T: *Streptococcus pneumoniae*: virulence factors and variation, *Clin Microbiol Infect* 16:411–418, 2010.

Sava IG, Heikens E, Huebner J: Pathogenesis and immunity in enterococcal infections, *Clin Microbiol Infect* 16:533–540, 2010.

Walker MJ, Barnett TC, McArthur JD, et al: Disease manifestations and pathogenic mechanisms of group A *Streptococcus*, *Clin Microbiol Rev* 27:264–301, 2014.

Wessels M: Streptococcal pharyngitis, *N Engl J Med* 364:648–655, 2011.

Wyres KL, Lambertsen LM, Croucher NJ, et al: Pneumococcal capsular switching: a historical perspective, *J Infect Dis* 207:439–449, 2013.

CHAPTER

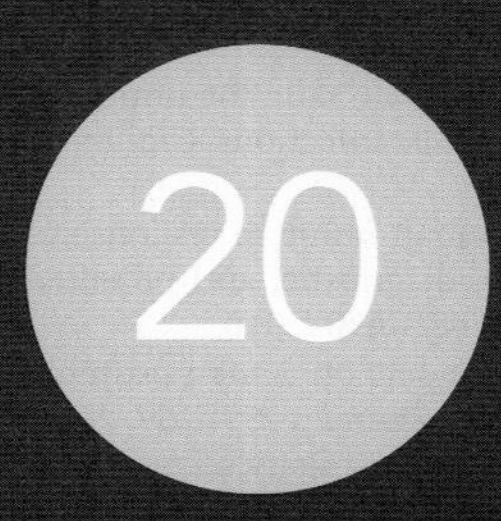

BACILLUS

Two hours after a dinner, **a family of four developed acute abdominal cramps with nausea and vomiting. The illness lasted for less than a day.**

1. *Bacillus cereus* is associated with two forms of food poisoning. Discuss the epidemiology and clinical presentation of each.
2. *B. cereus* is also associated with eye infections. Discuss the epidemiology and clinical presentation. What virulence factor is important in these infections?

Answers to these questions are available on StudentConsult.com.

• SUMMARIES CLINICALLY SIGNIFICANT ORGANISMS

Bacillus anthracis

Trigger Words

Spore-former, capsule, edema toxin, lethal toxin, anthrax, bioterrorism

Biology and Virulence

- Spore-forming, nonmotile, nonhemolytic gram-positive rods
- Polypeptide capsule consisting of poly-D-glutamic acid observed in clinical specimens
- Virulent strains produce three exotoxins that combine to form edema toxin (combination of protective antigen and edema factor) and lethal toxin (protective antigen with lethal factor)
- The polypeptide capsule inhibits phagocytosis of bacteria

Epidemiology

- *B. anthracis* primarily infects herbivores, with humans as accidental hosts
- Rarely isolated in developed countries but is prevalent in impoverished areas where vaccination of animals is not practiced
- The greatest danger of anthrax in industrial countries is the use of *B. anthracis* as an agent of bioterrorism

Diseases

- Three forms of anthrax are recognized: cutaneous (most common in humans), gastrointestinal (most common in herbivores), and inhalation (bioterrorism)

Diagnosis

- Organism is present in high concentrations in clinical specimens (microscopy typically positive) and grows readily in culture
- Preliminary identification is based on microscopic (gram-positive, nonmotile rods) and colonial (nonhemolytic, adherent colonies) morphology; confirmed by demonstrating capsule and either lysis with gamma phage, a positive direct fluorescent antibody test for the specific cell wall polysaccharide, or positive nucleic acid amplification assay

Treatment, Prevention, and Control

- Inhalation or gastrointestinal anthrax or bioterrorism-associated anthrax should be treated with ciprofloxacin or doxycycline, combined with one or two additional antibiotics (e.g., rifampin, vancomycin, penicillin, imipenem, clindamycin, clarithromycin)
- Naturally acquired cutaneous anthrax can be treated with amoxicillin
- Vaccination of animal herds and people in endemic areas can control disease, but spores are difficult to eliminate from contaminated soils
- Vaccination of animal herds and at-risk humans is effective, although the development of a less toxic vaccine is desired
- Alternative treatments interfering with the activity of anthrax toxins are under investigation

Bacillus cereus

Trigger Words

Spore-former, enterotoxin, gastroenteritis, eye infections

Biology and Virulence

- Spore-forming, motile, gram-positive rods
- Heat-stable and heat-labile enterotoxin
- Tissue destruction is mediated by cytotoxic enzymes, including cereolysin and phospholipase C

Epidemiology

- Ubiquitous in soils throughout the world
- People at risk include those who consume food contaminated with the bacterium (e.g., rice, meat, vegetables, sauces), those with penetrating injuries (e.g., to eye), those who receive intravenous injections, and immunocompromised patients exposed to *B. cereus*

Diseases

- Capable of causing gastrointestinal diseases (emetic and diarrheal forms), ocular infections, and an anthrax-like disease in immunocompetent patients

Diagnosis

- Isolation of the organism in implicated food product or nonfecal specimens (e.g., eye, wound)

Treatment, Prevention, and Control

- Gastrointestinal infections are treated symptomatically
- Ocular infectious or other invasive diseases require removal of foreign bodies and treatment with vancomycin, clindamycin, ciprofloxacin, or gentamicin
- Gastrointestinal disease is prevented by proper preparation of food (e.g., foods should be consumed immediately after preparation or refrigerated)

The family Bacillaceae consists of a diverse collection of more than 50 genera that share one common feature: the ability to form endospores (Figure 20-1). For practical purposes, the students need to know only one clinically important genus—*Bacillus*—and although there are almost 300 species in this genus, only two will be the focus of this chapter: *Bacillus anthracis* and *Bacillus cereus* (Table 20-1). *Bacillus anthracis,* the organism responsible for anthrax, is considered one of the most feared agents of biological warfare, and since the release of *B. anthracis* spores in the U.S. Postal Service in 2001, the potential danger associated with this organism is well known. *Bacillus cereus,* the other clinically important species in this genus, is an organism responsible for gastroenteritis, traumatic eye infections, catheter-associated sepsis, and, rarely, severe pneumonia.

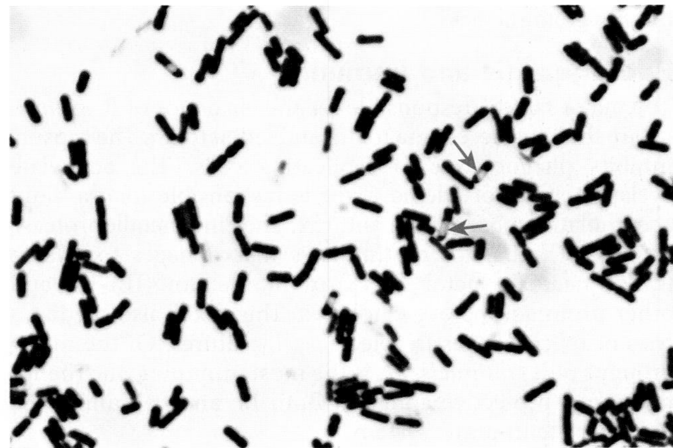

FIGURE 20-1 *Bacillus cereus.* The clear areas in the gram-positive rods are unstained spores *(arrows).*

Bacillus anthracis

Physiology and Structure

B. anthracis is a large (1×3 to 8 μm) organism arranged as single or paired rods (Figure 20-2) or as long, serpentine chains. Although spores are readily observed in 2- to 3-day-old cultures, they are not seen in clinical specimens.

Because of the unique medical importance of *B. anthracis,* it is important to understand the functional details of this organism's toxins. Virulent *B. anthracis* carries genes for three toxin protein components on a large plasmid, pXO1. The individual proteins, **protective antigen (PA), edema factor (EF),** and **lethal factor (LF),** are nontoxic individually but form important toxins when combined: PA plus EF forms **edema toxin,** and PA plus LF forms **lethal toxin.** PA is an 83-kDa protein that binds to one of two receptors on host cell surfaces that are present on many cells and tissues (e.g., brain, heart, intestine, lung, skeletal muscle, pancreas, macrophages). After PA binds to its receptor, host proteases cleave PA, releasing a small fragment and retaining the 63-kDa fragment (PA_{63}) on the cell surface. The PA_{63} fragments self-associate on the cell surface, forming a ring-shaped complex of seven fragments (pore precursor or "prepore"). This heptameric complex can then bind up to three molecules of LF and/or EF. Both factors recognize the same binding site of PA_{63}, so the binding is competitive. Formation of the complex stimulates endocytosis and movement to an acidic compartment. In this environment, the heptameric complex forms a transmembrane pore and releases LF and EF into the cell interior. **LF is a zinc-dependent protease** that is capable of cleaving mitogen-activated protein (MAP) kinase, leading to cell death. **EF is**

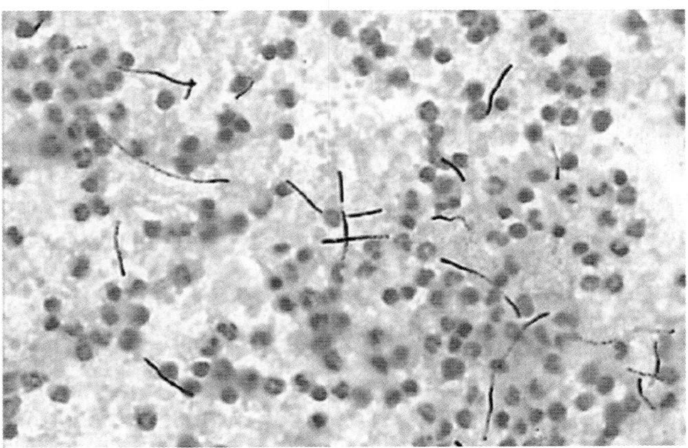

FIGURE 20-2 *Bacillus anthracis* in the blood of a patient with inhalation anthrax.

Table 20-1 Important *Bacillus* Species

Organism	Historical Derivation
Bacillus	*bacillum,* a small rod
B. anthracis	*anthrax,* charcoal, a carbuncle (refers to the black necrotic wound associated with cutaneous anthrax)
B. cereus	*cereus,* waxen, wax-colored (refers to colonies with a typical dull or frosted-glass surface)

a **calmodulin-dependent adenylate cyclase** that increases the intracellular cyclic adenosine monophosphate (cAMP) levels and results in edema. EF is related to the adenylate cyclases produced by *Bordetella pertussis* and *Pseudomonas aeruginosa.*

The other important virulence factor carried by *B. anthracis* is a prominent polypeptide **capsule** (consisting of poly-D-glutamic acid). The capsule is observed in clinical specimens but is not produced in vitro unless special growth conditions are used. Three genes (*capA, capB,* and *capC*) are responsible for synthesis of this capsule and are carried on a second plasmid (pXO2). Only one serotype of capsule has been identified, presumably because the capsule is composed of only glutamic acid.

Pathogenesis and Immunity

The major factors responsible for the virulence of *B. anthracis* are the capsule, edema toxin, and lethal toxin. The capsule inhibits phagocytosis of replicating cells. The adenylate cyclase activity of edema toxin is responsible for the fluid accumulation observed in anthrax. The zinc metalloprotease activity of lethal toxin stimulates macrophages to release tumor necrosis factor (TNF)-α, interleukin (IL)-1β, and other proinflammatory cytokines. This toxin also mediates lysis of macrophages in selected cell cultures. Of the major proteins of *B. anthracis,* PA is the most immunogenic (hence the name, protective antigen). Both LF and EF inhibit the host's innate immune system.

Epidemiology

Anthrax is primarily a disease of herbivores; humans are infected through exposure to contaminated animals or animal products. The disease is a serious problem in countries where animal vaccination is not practiced or is impractical (e.g., disease is established in African wildlife). In contrast, natural infections with *B. anthracis* are rarely seen in the United States, with only five cases reported between 1981 and 1999. This statistic may now be meaningless, with the deliberate contamination of the U.S. Postal Service with *B. anthracis* spores in 2001. The risk of exposing a large population to the dangerous pathogen has increased dramatically in this era of bioterrorism. A number of nations and independent terrorist groups have biological warfare programs and have experimented with using *B. anthracis* as a weapon. Indeed, much of what we know about anthrax acquired via the inhalation route was learned from the accidental release in 1979 of spores in Sverdlovsk in the former Soviet Union (at least 79 cases of anthrax, with 68 deaths) and the terrorist contamination of employees of the U.S. Postal Service with letters containing *B. anthracis* (11 patients with inhalation anthrax and 11 patients with cutaneous anthrax).

Human *B. anthracis* disease (Box 20-1) is acquired by one of three routes: **inoculation, ingestion,** and **inhalation.** Approximately 95% of naturally acquired anthrax infections in humans result from inoculation of *Bacillus* spores through exposed skin from either contaminated soil or infected animal products, such as hides, goat hair, and wool.

Ingestion anthrax is very rare in humans, but ingestion is a common route of infection in herbivores. Because the organism can form resilient spores, contaminated soil or animal products can remain infectious for many years.

Box 20-1 *Bacillus* Diseases: Clinical Summaries

Bacillus anthracis

Cutaneous anthrax: painless papule progresses to ulceration with surrounding vesicles and then to eschar formation; painful lymphadenopathy, edema, and systemic signs may develop

Gastrointestinal anthrax: ulcers form at site of invasion (e.g., mouth, esophagus, intestine), leading to regional lymphadenopathy, edema, and sepsis

Inhalation anthrax: initial nonspecific signs followed by rapid onset of sepsis with fever, edema, and lymphadenopathy (mediastinal lymph nodes); meningeal symptoms in half the patients, and most patients with inhalation anthrax will die unless treatment is initiated immediately

Bacillus cereus

Gastroenteritis: emetic form characterized by rapid onset of vomiting and abdominal pain and a short duration; diarrheal form characterized by a longer onset and duration of diarrhea and abdominal cramps

Ocular infections: rapid, progressive destruction of the eye after traumatic introduction of the bacteria into the eye

Severe pulmonary disease: severe anthrax-like pulmonary disease in immunocompetent patients

Inhalation anthrax was historically called **wool-sorters' disease** because most human infections resulted from inhalation of *B. anthracis* spores during the processing of goat hair. This is currently an uncommon source for human infections; however, inhalation is the most likely route of infection with biological weapons, and the infectious dose of the organism is believed to be low. Person-to-person transmission does not occur because bacterial replication occurs in the mediastinal lymph nodes rather than the bronchopulmonary tree.

Clinical Diseases (Clinical Case 20-1)

Typically, **cutaneous anthrax** starts with the development of a painless papule at the site of inoculation that rapidly progresses to an ulcer surrounded by vesicles and then to a necrotic eschar (Figure 20-3). Systemic signs, painful lymphadenopathy, and massive edema may develop. The mortality rate in patients with untreated cutaneous anthrax is 20%.

Clinical symptoms of **gastrointestinal anthrax** are determined by the site of the infection. If organisms invade the upper intestinal tract, ulcers form in the mouth or esophagus, leading to regional lymphadenopathy, edema, and sepsis. If the organism invades the cecum or terminal ileum, the patient presents with nausea, vomiting, and malaise, which rapidly progress to systemic disease. The mortality associated with gastrointestinal anthrax is believed to approach 100%.

Unlike the other two forms of anthrax, **inhalation anthrax** can be associated with a prolonged latent period (2 months or more), during which the infected patient remains asymptomatic. Spores can remain latent in the nasal passages or reach the lower airways, where alveolar macrophages ingest the inhaled spores and transport them to the mediastinal lymph nodes. The initial clinical symptoms of disease are nonspecific—fever, myalgias, nonproductive cough, and malaise. The second stage of disease is more dramatic, with

Clinical Case 20-1 Inhalation Anthrax

Bush and associates (*N Engl J Med* 345:1607–1610, 2001) reported the first case of inhalation anthrax in the 2001 bioterrorism attack in the United States. The patient was a 63-year-old man living in Florida who had a 4-day history of fever, myalgias, and malaise without localizing symptoms. His wife brought him to the regional hospital because he awoke from sleep with fever, emesis, and confusion. On physical examination, he had a temperature of 39° C, blood pressure of 150/80 mm Hg, pulse of 110 beats/min, and respiration of 18 breaths/min. No respiratory distress was noted. Treatment was initiated for presumed bacterial meningitis. Basilar infiltrates and a widened mediastinum were noted on the initial chest radiograph. Gram stain of cerebrospinal fluid (CSF) revealed many neutrophils and large gram-positive rods. Anthrax was suspected, and penicillin treatment was initiated. Within 24 hours of admission, CSF and blood cultures were positive for *Bacillus anthracis.* During the first day of hospitalization, the patient had a grand mal seizure and was intubated. On the second hospital day, hypotension and azotemia developed, with subsequent renal failure. On the third hospital day, refractory hypotension developed and the patient had a fatal cardiac arrest. This patient illustrates the rapidity with which patients with inhalation anthrax can deteriorate despite a rapid diagnosis and appropriate antimicrobial therapy. Although the route of exposure is via the respiratory tract, patients do not develop pneumonia; rather, the abnormal chest radiograph is caused by hemorrhagic mediastinitis.

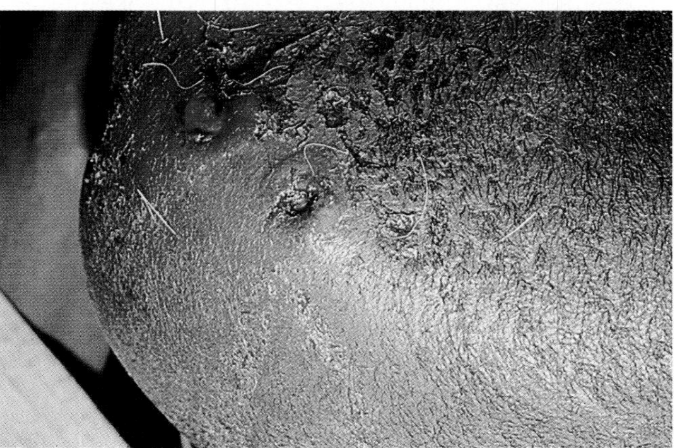

FIGURE 20-3 Cutaneous anthrax demonstrating marked erythema, edema, and vesicle rupture. (From Cohen J, Powderly WG: *Infectious diseases,* ed 2, St Louis, 2004, Mosby.)

a rapidly worsening course of fever, edema, massive enlargement of the mediastinal lymph nodes (this is responsible for the widened mediastinum observed on chest radiography [Figure 20-4]), respiratory failure, and sepsis. Although the route of infection is by inhalation, pneumonia rarely develops. Meningeal symptoms are seen in half of patients with inhalation anthrax. Almost all cases progress to shock and death within 3 days of initial symptoms unless anthrax is suspected and treatment is initiated immediately. Serologic evidence indicates that a subclinical or asymptomatic form of inhalation anthrax does not exist. Virtually all patients who develop disease progress to a fatal outcome unless there is immediate medical intervention.

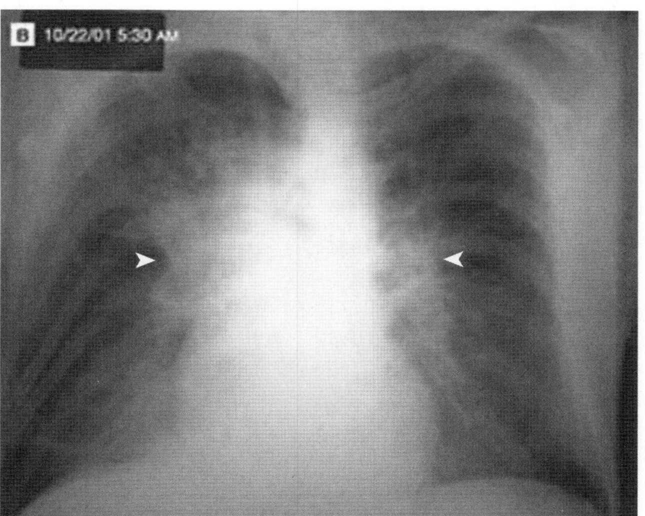

FIGURE 20-4 Inhalation anthrax demonstrating enlarged mediastinal lymph nodes *(arrowheads).*

Laboratory Diagnosis

Infections with *B. anthracis* are characterized by overwhelming numbers of organisms present in wounds, involved lymph nodes, and blood. Anthrax is one of the few bacterial diseases where organisms can be seen when peripheral blood is Gram stained (see Figure 20-2). Therefore the detection of organisms by microscopy and culture is not a problem. The diagnostic difficulty is distinguishing *B. anthracis* from other members of the taxonomically related *B. cereus* group. A preliminary identification of *B. anthracis* is based on microscopic and colonial morphology. The organisms appear as long, thin, gram-positive rods arranged singly or in long chains. Spores are not observed in clinical specimens but only in cultures incubated in a low carbon dioxide (CO_2) atmosphere and can be best seen with the use of a special spore stain (e.g., malachite green stain; Figure 20-5). The **capsule** of *B. anthracis* is produced in vivo but is not typically observed in culture. The capsule can be observed with a contrasting stain, such as India ink (the ink particles are excluded by the capsule so that the background, but not the area around bacteria, appears black), M'Fadyean methylene blue stain, or a direct fluorescent antibody (DFA) test developed against the capsular polypeptide. Colonies cultured on sheep blood agar are characteristically large and nonpigmented and have a dry "ground-glass" surface and irregular edges. The colonies are quite sticky and adherent to the agar, and if the edge is lifted with a bacteriologic loop, it will remain standing like beaten egg whites. Colonies are **not hemolytic,** in contrast with *B. cereus. B. anthracis* will appear **nonmotile** in motility tests such as the microscopic observation of individual rods in a suspended drop of culture medium. The definitive identification of nonmotile, nonhemolytic organisms resembling *B. anthracis* is made in a public health reference laboratory. This is accomplished by demonstrating capsule production (by microscopy or DFA) and either lysis of the bacteria with gamma phage or a positive DFA test for a specific *B. anthracis* cell wall polysaccharide. In addition, nucleic acid amplification tests (e.g., polymerase chain reaction [PCR]) have been developed and

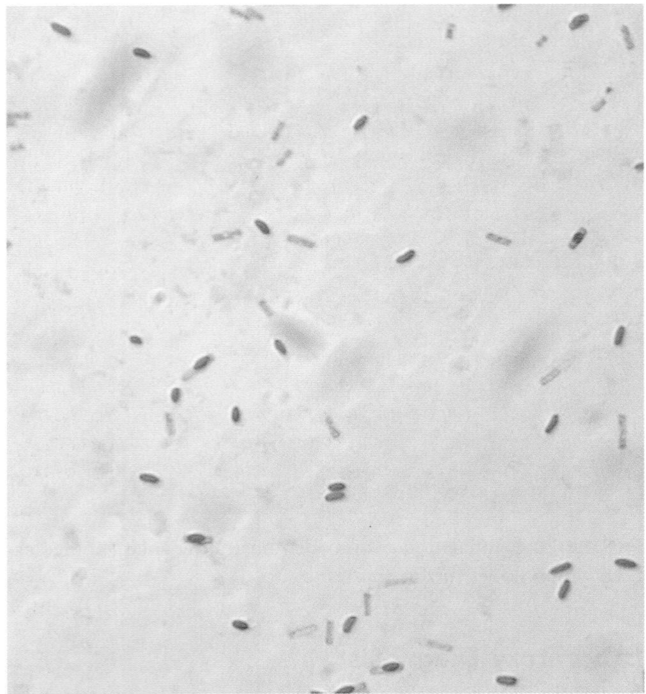

FIGURE 20-5 *Bacillus cereus.* Spores retain the malachite green dye in this special spore stain, and the vegetative cells are gray or colorless.

are performed in reference laboratories. The PCR tests are also commercially available.

Treatment, Prevention, and Control

Although penicillin was the drug of choice for *B. anthracis,* resistance in naturally occurring strains has been observed, as well as resistance to sulfonamides and extended-spectrum cephalosporins. In addition, resistance to other antibiotics can be selected in laboratory-derived strains, so this must be considered for treatment of bioterrorism-associated anthrax. The current empirical treatment recommendation is use of **ciprofloxacin** or **doxycycline** combined with one or two additional antibiotics (e.g., rifampin, vancomycin, penicillin, imipenem, clindamycin, clarithromycin). Although penicillin resistance is observed for naturally acquired anthrax, oral penicillin **(amoxicillin)** is still recommended for naturally acquired cutaneous anthrax.

Control of naturally acquired human disease requires control of animal disease, which involves **vaccination of animal herds** in endemic regions and burning or burial of animals that die of anthrax. Complete eradication of anthrax is unlikely because the spores of the organism can exist for many years in soil. Furthermore, complete eradication of anthrax infections is unlikely with the threat of bioterrorist-related infections a current reality.

Vaccination has also been used to protect (1) people who live in areas where the disease is endemic, (2) people who work with animal products imported from countries with endemic anthrax, and (3) military personnel. Although the current vaccine appears to be effective, research to develop a less toxic vaccine is under way. Alternative approaches to inactivating anthrax toxins have focused on PA and its receptor target. Passive infusion of human monoclonal antibodies against *B. anthracis* PA prevented death in an animal model of inhalation anthrax and was well tolerated in human volunteers. Synthetic peptide complexes that target the cell surface receptors for PA have also been used to neutralize anthrax toxin in animal models. How these alternative approaches can be used to treat human disease remains to be demonstrated.

 Table 20-2 ***Bacillus cereus* Food Poisoning**

Disease Features	Emetic Form	Diarrheal Form
Implicated food	Rice	Meat, vegetables
Incubation period (hours)	<6 (mean, 2)	>6 (mean, 9)
Symptoms	Vomiting, nausea, abdominal cramps	Diarrhea, nausea, abdominal cramps
Duration (hours)	8-10 (mean, 9)	20-36 (mean, 24)
Enterotoxin	Heat stable	Heat labile

Bacillus cereus

Bacillus species other than *B. anthracis* are primarily opportunistic pathogens that have relatively low capacities for virulence. Although most of these species have been found to cause disease, *B. cereus* is clearly the most important pathogen, with gastroenteritis, ocular infections, and intravenous catheter-related sepsis being the diseases most commonly observed, as well as rare cases of severe pneumonia.

Pathogenesis and Immunity

Gastroenteritis caused by *B. cereus* is mediated by one of **two enterotoxins** (Table 20-2). The **heat-stable,** proteolysis-resistant enterotoxin causes the **emetic form** of the disease, and the **heat-labile** enterotoxin causes the **diarrheal form** of the disease. The heat-labile enterotoxin is similar to the enterotoxins produced by *Escherichia coli* and *Vibrio cholerae;* each stimulates the adenylate cyclase–cyclic adenosine monophosphate system in intestinal epithelial cells, leading to profuse watery diarrhea. The mechanism of action of the heat-stable enterotoxin is unknown.

The pathogenesis of *B. cereus* ocular infections is also incompletely defined. At least three toxins have been implicated: **necrotic toxin** (a heat-labile enterotoxin), **cereolysin** (a potent hemolysin named after the species), and **phospholipase C** (a potent lecithinase). It is likely that the rapid destruction of the eye that is characteristic of *B. cereus* infections results from the interaction of these toxins and other unidentified factors.

Bacillus species can colonize skin transiently and can be recovered as insignificant contaminants in blood cultures. In the presence of an intravascular foreign body, however, these organisms can be responsible for persistent bacteremia and signs of sepsis (i.e., fever, chills, hypotension, shock).

Epidemiology

B. cereus and other *Bacillus* species are ubiquitous organisms, present in virtually all environments. Nearly all infections originate from an environmental source (e.g., contaminated soil). Isolation of bacteria from clinical specimens in the absence of characteristic disease usually represents insignificant contamination.

Clinical Diseases

As mentioned previously, *B. cereus* is responsible for two forms of food poisoning: **vomiting disease (emetic form)** and **diarrheal disease (diarrheal form).** In most patients, the emetic form of disease results from consumption of **contaminated rice.** Most bacteria are killed during the initial cooking of the rice, but the heat-resistant spores survive. If the cooked rice is not refrigerated, the spores germinate and the bacteria can multiply rapidly. The heat-stable enterotoxin that is released is not destroyed when the rice is reheated. The emetic form of disease is an intoxication caused by ingestion of the enterotoxin, not the bacteria. Thus the incubation period after eating the contaminated rice is short (1 to 6 hours), and the duration of illness is also short (<24 hours). Symptoms consist of vomiting, nausea, and abdominal cramps. Fever and diarrhea are generally absent. Fulminant liver failure has also been associated with consumption of food contaminated with large amounts of emetic toxin, which impairs mitochondrial fatty acid metabolism. Fortunately, this is a rare complication.

The diarrheal form of *B. cereus* food poisoning is a true infection resulting from ingestion of the bacteria in contaminated meat, vegetables, or sauces. There is a longer incubation period during which the organism multiplies in the patient's intestinal tract, and the release of the heat-labile enterotoxin follows. This enterotoxin is responsible for the diarrhea, nausea, and abdominal cramps that develop. This form of disease generally lasts 1 day or longer.

B. cereus **ocular infections** usually occur after traumatic, penetrating injuries of the eye with a soil-contaminated object (Clinical Case 20-2). *Bacillus* panophthalmitis is a rapidly progressive disease that almost universally results in complete eye loss within 48 hours of the injury. Disseminated infections with ocular manifestations can also develop in intravenous drug abusers.

Other common infections with *B. cereus* and other *Bacillus* species are intravenous catheter and central nervous system shunt infections and endocarditis (most common in drug abusers), as well as pneumonitis, bacteremia, and meningitis in severely immunosuppressed patients. It has also been reported that ingestion of **tea** by immunocompromised patients is associated with an increased risk for invasive *B. cereus* disease.

One rare disease of *B. cereus* deserves special attention—**severe pneumonia mimicking anthrax in immunocompetent patients.** Four patients with this disease, all metal workers residing in Texas or Louisiana, have been described in the literature. Most interesting is that the strains contained the ***B. anthracis*** **pXO1 toxin genes** and all were **encapsulated,** although this was not the typical *B. anthracis* poly-γ-D-glutamic acid capsule. These strains demonstrate the potential danger and presumed ease of transferring *B. anthracis* virulence genes into the ubiquitous *B. cereus*.

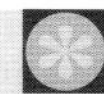

Clinical Case 20-2 *Bacillus cereus* Traumatic Endophthalmitis

Endophthalmitis caused by the traumatic introduction of *Bacillus cereus* into the eye is unfortunately not uncommon. This is a typical presentation. A 44-year-old man suffered a traumatic eye injury while working in a vegetable garden, when a piece of metal was deflected into his left eye, damaging the cornea and anterior and posterior lens capsule. Over the next 12 hours, he developed increasing pain and purulence in his eye. He underwent surgery to relieve the ocular pressure, drain the purulence, and introduce intravitreal antibiotics (vancomycin, ceftazidime) and dexamethasone. Culture of the aspirated fluid was positive for *B. cereus*. Ciprofloxacin was added to his therapeutic regimen postoperatively. Despite the prompt surgical and medical intervention and subsequent intravitreal antibiotic injections, the intraocular inflammation persisted and evisceration was required. This patient illustrates the risks involved with penetrating eye injuries and the need to intervene aggressively if the eye is to be saved.

Laboratory Diagnosis

Similar to *B. anthracis, B. cereus* and other species can be readily cultured from clinical specimens collected from patients with the emetic form of food poisoning. Because individuals can be transiently colonized with *B. cereus,* the implicated food (e.g., rice, meat, vegetables) must be cultured for confirmation of the existence of foodborne disease. In practice, neither cultures nor tests to detect the heat-stable or heat-labile enterotoxins are commonly performed, so most cases of *B. cereus* gastroenteritis are diagnosed by epidemiologic criteria. *Bacillus* organisms grow rapidly and are readily detected with the Gram stain and culture of specimens collected from infected eyes, intravenous culture sites, and other locations.

Treatment, Prevention, and Control

Because the course of *B. cereus* gastroenteritis is short and uncomplicated, symptomatic treatment is adequate. The treatment of other *Bacillus* infections is complicated because they have a rapid and progressive course and a high incidence of multiple-drug resistance (e.g., *B. cereus* carries genes for resistance to penicillins and cephalosporins). **Vancomycin, clindamycin, ciprofloxacin,** and **gentamicin** can be used to treat infections. Penicillins and cephalosporins are ineffective. Eye infections must be treated rapidly. Rapid consumption of foods after cooking and proper refrigeration of uneaten foods can prevent food poisoning.

Bibliography

Avashia SB, Riggins WS, Lindley C, et al: Fatal pneumonia among metalworkers due to inhalation exposure to *Bacillus cereus* containing *Bacillus anthracis* toxin genes, *Clin Infect Dis* 44:414–416, 2007.

Baggett HC, Rhodes JC, Fridkin SK, et al: No evidence of a mild form of inhalational *Bacillus anthracis* infection during a bioterrorism-related inhalational anthrax outbreak in Washington, D.C., in 2001, *Clin Infect Dis* 41:991–997, 2005.

Basha S, Rai P, Poon V, et al: Polyvalent inhibitors of anthrax toxin that target host receptors, *Proc Natl Acad Sci U S A* 103:13509–13513, 2006.

Bottone E: *Bacillus cereus,* a volatile human pathogen, *Clin Microbiol Rev* 23:382–398, 2010.

Collier RJ, Young JAT: Anthrax toxin, *Annu Rev Cell Dev Biol* 19:45–70, 2003.

Doganay M, Metan G, Alp E: A review of cutaneous anthrax and its outcome, *J Infect Public Health* 3:98–105, 2010.

El Saleeby CM, Howard SC, Hayden RT, et al: Association between tea ingestion and invasive *Bacillus cereus* infection among children with cancer, *Clin Infect Dis* 39:1536–1539, 2004.

Hoffmaster AR, Hill KK, Gee JE, et al: Characterization of *Bacillus cereus* isolates associated with fatal pneumonias: strains are closely related to *Bacillus anthracis* and harbor *B. anthracis* virulence genes, *J Clin Microbiol* 44:3352–3360, 2006.

Krantz BA, Melnyk RA, Zhang S, et al: A phenylalanine clamp catalyzes protein translocation through the anthrax toxin pore, *Science* 309:777–781, 2005.

Mahtab M, Leppla SH: The roles of anthrax toxin in pathogenesis, *Curr Opin Microbiol* 7:19–24, 2004.

Melnyk RA, Hewitt KM, Lacy DB, et al: Structural determinants for the binding of anthrax lethal factor to oligomeric protective antigen, *J Biol Chem* 281:1630–1635, 2006.

Pickering AK, Merkel TJ: Macrophages release tumor necrosis factor alpha and interleukin-12 in response to intracellular *Bacillus anthracis* spores, *Infect Immun* 72:3069–3072, 2004.

Turnbull PC: Introduction: anthrax history, disease and ecology, *Curr Top Microbiol Immunol* 271:1–19, 2002.

CHAPTER

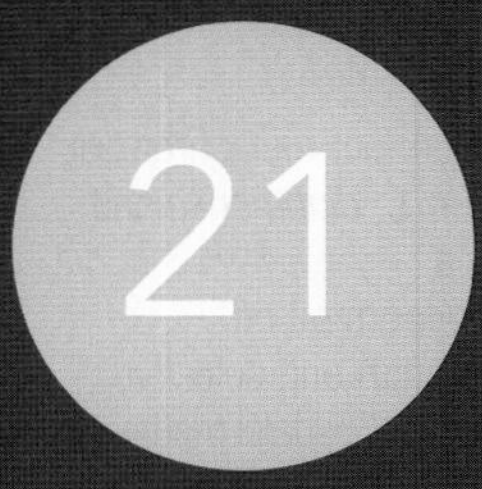

LISTERIA AND RELATED GRAM-POSITIVE BACTERIA

Listeria monocytogenes, Erysipelothrix rhusiopathiae, and Corynebacterium diphtheriae are three medically important gram-positive rods that produce very dissimilar diseases.

1. What patient populations are most susceptible to infections caused by *Listeria* and *Erysipelothrix,* and how are these infections acquired?
2. Treatment of *Listeria* infections is most similar to what other gram-positive pathogen?
3. Why is the laboratory diagnosis of *Erysipelothrix* infections difficult to make?
4. Why is diphtheria not seen in the United States but still found in other countries?
5. Why is a Gram stain of a throat exudate or blood culture not useful for the diagnosis of diphtheria? How would the diagnosis be made if diphtheria is suspected?
6. What virulence factor is responsible for the clinical manifestations of diphtheria?

Answers to these questions are available on StudentConsult.com.

• SUMMARIES CLINICALLY SIGNIFICANT ORGANISMS

Listeria monocytogenes

Trigger Words

Coccobacilli, beta-hemolytic, meningitis, opportunistic

Biology and Virulence

- Gram-positive coccobacilli, often arranged in pairs resembling *Streptococcus pneumoniae*
- Facultative intracellular pathogen that can avoid antibody-mediated clearance
- Ability to grow at 4° C, in a wide pH range, and in the presence of salt can lead to high concentrations of the bacteria in contaminated foods
- Virulent strains produce cell attachment factors (internalins), hemolysins (listeriolysin O, two phospholipase C enzymes), and a protein that mediates actin-directed intracellular motility (ActA)

Epidemiology

- Isolated in soil, water, and vegetation and from a variety of animals, including humans (low-level gastrointestinal carriage)
- Disease associated with consumption of contaminated food products (e.g., contaminated milk and cheese, processed meats, raw vegetables [especially cabbage]) or transplacental spread from mother to neonate; sporadic cases and epidemics occur throughout the year
- Neonates, elderly, pregnant women, and patients with defects in cellular immunity are at increased risk for disease

Diseases

- Neonatal disease can result in in utero death or multiorgan abscesses, meningitis, and septicemia
- Other diseases include influenza-like symptoms, self-limited gastroenteritis, and meningitis in patients with defects in cell-mediated immunity

Diagnosis

- Microscopy is insensitive; culture may require incubation for 2 to 3 days or enrichment at 4° C
- Characteristic properties include motility at room temperature, weak β-hemolysis, and growth at 4° C and at high-salt concentrations

Treatment, Prevention, and Control

- The treatment of choice for severe disease is penicillin or ampicillin, alone or in combination with gentamicin
- People at high risk should avoid eating raw or partially cooked foods of animal origin, soft cheese, and unwashed raw vegetables

Erysipelothrix rhusiopathiae

Trigger Words

Pleomorphic rod, zoonotic, cutaneous infection, endocarditis

Biology and Virulence

- Slender, pleomorphic, gram-positive rods that form long (e.g., 60 μm) filaments
- Production of neuraminidase believed to be important for attachment and penetration into epithelial cells, and polysaccharide-like capsule protects the bacteria from phagocytosis

Epidemiology

- Colonizes a variety of organisms, particularly swine and turkey
- Found in soil rich in organic matter or groundwater contaminated with wastes from colonized animals
- Uncommon pathogen in the United States
- Occupational disease of butchers, meat processors, farmers, poultry workers, fish handlers, and veterinarians

Diseases

- Disease in humans most commonly (1) localized cutaneous infection, (2) generalized cutaneous disease, or (3) septicemia associated with subacute endocarditis involving previously undamaged heart valves

Diagnosis

- Long, filamentous, gram-positive rods seen on Gram stain of a biopsy collected at the advancing edge of the lesion
- Grows slowly on blood and chocolate agars incubated in 5% to 10% carbon dioxide

Treatment, Prevention, and Control

- Penicillin is drug of choice for both localized and systemic diseases; ciprofloxacin or clindamycin can be used for localized cutaneous infections for patients allergic to penicillin, and ceftriaxone or imipenem can be considered for disseminated infections
- Workers should cover exposed skin when handling animals and animal products
- Swineherds should be vaccinated

Corynebacterium diphtheriae

Trigger Words

Diphtheria toxin, pharyngitis, selective culture, vaccine

Biology and Virulence

- Gram-positive pleomorphic rods
- The major virulence factor is the diphtheria toxin, an A-B exotoxin; inhibits protein synthesis

Epidemiology

- Worldwide distribution maintained in asymptomatic carriers and infected patients
- Humans are the only known reservoir, with carriage in oropharynx or on skin surface
- Spread person to person by exposure to respiratory droplets or skin contact
- Disease observed in unvaccinated or partially immune children or adults traveling to countries with endemic disease
- Diphtheria is very uncommon in the United States and other countries with active vaccination programs

Diseases

- Etiologic agent of diphtheria: respiratory and cutaneous forms

Diagnosis

- Microscopy is nonspecific; metachromatic granules observed in *C. diphtheriae* and other corynebacteria
- Culture should be performed on nonselective (blood agar) and selective (cysteine-tellurite agar, Tinsdale medium, colistin-nalidixic agar) media
- Presumptive identification of *C. diphtheriae* can be based on the presence of cystinase and absence of pyrazinamidase; definitive identification by biochemical tests or species-specific gene sequencing
- Demonstration of exotoxin is performed by Elek test or polymerase chain reaction assay

Treatment, Prevention, and Control

- Infections treated with diphtheria antitoxin to neutralize exotoxin, penicillin or erythromycin to eliminate *C. diphtheriae* and terminate toxin production, and immunization of convalescing patients with diphtheria toxoid to stimulate protective antibodies
- Administration of diphtheria vaccine and booster shots to susceptible population

The aerobic, non–spore-forming, gram-positive rods are a heterogeneous group of bacteria. Some are well-recognized human pathogens (e.g., *Listeria monocytogenes, Corynebacterium diphtheriae*); others are primarily animal pathogens that can cause human disease (e.g., *Erysipelothrix rhusiopathiae*); and some are opportunistic pathogens that typically infect hospitalized or immunocompromised patients (e.g., *Corynebacterium jeikeium* [Figure 21-1]). Although the clinical presentation of the diseases can be characteristic, detection and identification of the organisms in the laboratory can be problematic. One technique that is useful for the preliminary identification of these bacteria involves their **microscopic morphology.** Gram-positive rods that are uniform in shape include ***Listeria*** and ***Erysipelothrix;*** irregularly shaped gram-positive rods typically are members of the genus *Corynebacterium* or closely related genera (Table 21-1). This chapter will focus on three species of gram-positive rods: *Listeria monocytogenes, Erysipelothrix rhusiopathiae,* and *Corynebacterium diphtheriae*. The diseases caused by these and related bacteria are summarized in Table 21-2.

Listeria monocytogenes

The genus *Listeria* consists of 19 species, with ***L. monocytogenes*** the most significant human pathogen. *L. monocytogenes* is a short (0.4 to 0.5 × 0.5 to 2 μm), nonbranching, gram-positive, facultatively anaerobic rod capable of growth at a broad temperature range (1° C to 45° C) and in a high concentration of salt. The **short rods** appear singly, in pairs, or in short chains (Figure 21-2) and can be mistaken for *Streptococcus pneumoniae*. This is important because both *S. pneumoniae* and *L. monocytogenes* can cause meningitis. The organisms are **motile** at room temperature but less so at 37° C, and they exhibit a characteristic end-over-end tumbling motion when a drop of broth is examined microscopically. *L. monocytogenes* exhibits **weak β-hemolysis** when grown on sheep blood agar plates. These differential characteristics (i.e., Gram-stain morphology, motility, β-hemolysis) are useful for the preliminary identification of *Listeria*. Although the bacteria are widely distributed in nature, human disease is uncommon and is restricted primarily to several well-defined populations: neonates, the elderly, pregnant women, and patients with defective cellular immunity.

Pathogenesis and Immunity

L. monocytogenes is a **facultative intracellular pathogen.** Following ingestion of contaminated food, *L. monocytogenes* is able to survive exposure to proteolytic enzymes, stomach acid, and bile salts through the protective action of stress-response genes. The bacteria are then able to **adhere to host cells** via the interaction of proteins on the surface of the bacteria (i.e., internalin A [InlA]) with glycoprotein receptors on the host cell surface (e.g., epithelial cadherin [calcium-dependent adhesin]). Other internalins (e.g., InlB) can recognize receptors on a wider range of host cells. Studies with animal models have shown that infection is initiated in the enterocytes or M cells in Peyer patches. After penetration into the cells, the acid pH of the phagolysosome that surrounds the bacteria activates a bacterial pore-forming cytolysin **(listeriolysin O)** and two different **phospholipase C** enzymes, leading to release of the bacteria into the cell cytosol. The bacteria proceed to replicate and then move to the cell membrane. This movement is mediated by a bacterial protein, **ActA** (localized on the cell surface at one end of a bacterium), that coordinates **assembly of actin.** The distal ends of the actin tail remain fixed while assembly occurs adjacent to the end of the bacterium. Thus the bacterium is pushed to the cell membrane and a protrusion (filopod) is formed, pushing the bacterium into the adjacent cell. After the adjacent cell ingests the bacterium, the process of **phagolysosome lysis, bacterial replication,** and **directional movement** repeats. Entry into macrophages after passage through the intestinal lining carries the bacteria to the liver and spleen, leading to disseminated disease. The genes responsible for membrane lysis, intracellular replication, and directional movement are clustered together and regulated by a single gene, ***prfA*** or the **"positive regulatory factor" gene.**

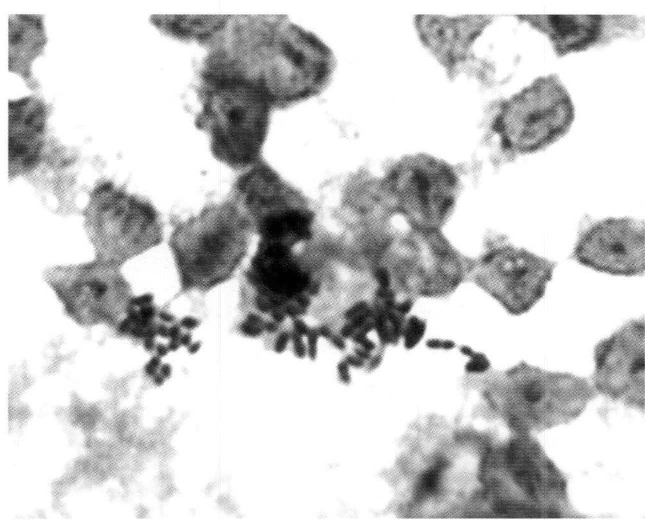

FIGURE 21-1 Gram stain of *Corynebacterium jeikeium* from a blood culture; small, nondescript coccobacilli.

Humoral immunity is relatively unimportant for management of infections with *L. monocytogenes*. These bacteria can replicate in macrophages and move within cells, thus avoiding antibody-mediated clearance. For this reason, patients with defects in **cellular immunity,** but not in humoral immunity, are particularly susceptible to severe infections.

Epidemiology

L. monocytogenes is isolated from a variety of environmental sources and from the feces of mammals, birds, fish, and other animals. The primary source of infection with this organism is consumption of contaminated food; however, human-to-human transmission can occur primarily from mother to child in utero or at birth. Fecal carriage is estimated to occur in 1% to 5% of healthy people. Because the organism is ubiquitous, exposure and transient colonization are likely to occur in most individuals. Approximately 850 infections are reported annually in the United States; however, many mild infections are not reported. Large outbreaks associated with **contaminated food products** are well documented. For example, 30 million pounds of contaminated meat were recalled in one outbreak in 1999, and 16 million pounds of processed turkey and chicken meat were recalled in a second multistate outbreak in 2000. Many people were exposed to the bacteria before the recall could be accomplished. The incidence of disease is also disproportionate in **high-risk populations,** such as neonates, the elderly, pregnant women, and patients with severe defects in cell-mediated immunity (e.g., transplants, lymphomas, acquired immunodeficiency syndrome [AIDS]).

Table 21-1 *Listeria* and Related Bacteria

Organism	Historical Derivation
Listeria	*Listeria,* named after the English surgeon Lord Joseph Lister
L. monocytogenes	*monocytum,* a blood cell or monocyte; *gennaio,* produce (monocyte producing; membrane extracts stimulate monocyte production in rabbits, but this is not seen in human disease)
Erysipelothrix	*erythros,* red; *pella,* skin; *thrix,* hair (thin, hairlike organism that produces a red or inflammatory skin lesion)
E. rhusiopathiae	*rhusios,* red; *pathos,* disease (red disease)
Corynebacterium	*coryne,* a club; *bakterion,* a small rod (a small, club-shaped rod)
C. diphtheriae	*diphthera,* leather or skin (reference to the leathery membrane that forms initially on the pharynx)
C. jeikeium	*jeikeium* (species originally classified as group JK)
C. urealyticum	*urea,* urea; *lyticum,* lyse (capable of lysing urea; species rapidly hydrolyzes urea)
C. amycolatum	*a,* without; *mycolatum,* pertaining to mycolic acids (species does not have mycolic acids in the cell wall)
C. pseudotuberculosis	*pseudo,* like; *tuberculosis* (produces chronic purulent infections [e.g., tuberculosis] in sheep and other warm-blooded animals)
C. ulcerans	*ulcerans* (can produce pharyngeal ulcers like *C. diphtheriae*)
Arcanobacterium	*arcanus,* secretive; *bacterium,* rod (secretive bacterium; a slow-growing organism that can prove difficult to isolate)
Rothia mucilaginosa	Named after Roth, the bacteriologist who originally studied this group of organisms; *mucilaginosa,* slimy (slimy or mucoid organisms)
Tropheryma whipplei	*trophe,* nourishment; *eryma,* barrier; *whipple,* named after George Whipple who described in 1907 a malabsorption disease; also called Whipple disease

Table 21-2 **Human Disease Associated with *Listeria* and Related Bacteria**

Organism	Diseases
Listeria monocytogenes	Neonatal disease (spontaneous abortion, disseminated abscesses and granulomas, meningitis, septicemia); influenza-like illness in healthy adults; bacteremia or disseminated disease with meningitis in pregnant women and patients with cell-mediated immune defects
Erysipelothrix rhusiopathiae	Erysipeloid (painful, pruritic inflammatory skin lesion); generalized cutaneous disease: a diffuse cutaneous infection with fever and arthralgias; septicemia typically associated with endocarditis
Corynebacterium diphtheriae	Diphtheria (respiratory, cutaneous); pharyngitis and endocarditis (nontoxigenic strains)
C. jeikeium (group JK)	Septicemia, endocarditis, wound infections, foreign body (catheter, shunt, prosthesis) infections
C. urealyticum	Urinary tract infections (including pyelonephritis and alkaline-encrusted cystitis), septicemia, endocarditis, wound infections
C. amycolatum	Wound infections, foreign body infections, septicemia, urinary tract infections, respiratory tract infections
C. pseudotuberculosis	Lymphadenitis, ulcerative lymphangitis, abscess formation, respiratory diphtheria
C. ulcerans	Respiratory diphtheria
Arcanobacterium	Pharyngitis, cellulitis, wound infections, abscess formation, septicemia, endocarditis
Rothia	Endocarditis, foreign-body infections
Tropheryma	Whipple disease

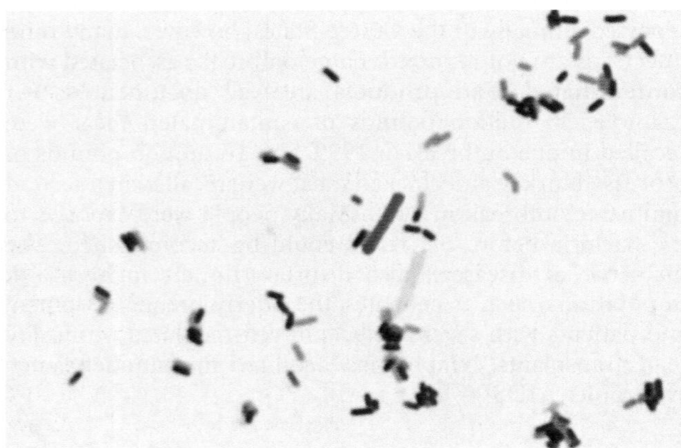

FIGURE 21-2 Gram stain of *Listeria monocytogenes* in culture. *Listeria* appear as small gram-positive rods; some readily decolorize and appear gram-negative. The much larger gram-negative rod in the center of the photograph is *Escherichia coli.*

Human listeriosis is a sporadic disease seen throughout the year, with focal epidemics and sporadic cases of listeriosis associated with consumption of undercooked processed meat (e.g., turkey franks, cold cuts), unpasteurized or contaminated milk or cheese, and unwashed raw vegetables, including cabbage. Although fresh produce is an uncommon cause of outbreaks, disease associated with consumption of contaminated cantaloupe was reported in 147 individuals in 2011 (86% were 60 years of age or older; 22% fatality rate). Because *Listeria* can grow in a wide pH range and at cold temperatures, foods with small numbers of organisms can become heavily contaminated during prolonged refrigeration. Disease can occur if the food is uncooked or inadequately cooked (e.g., microwaved beef and turkey franks) before consumption. Although *Listeria* infections are relatively uncommon, it is the leading cause of deaths attributed to foodborne illnesses in the United States.

Clinical Diseases (see Table 21-2)

Neonatal Disease

Two forms of neonatal disease have been described: (1) **early-onset disease,** acquired transplacentally in utero, and (2) **late-onset disease,** acquired at or soon after birth. Early-onset disease can result in abortion, stillbirth, or premature birth. **Granulomatosis infantiseptica** is a severe form of early-onset listeriosis characterized by the formation of abscesses and granulomas in multiple organs and a high mortality rate unless treated promptly.

Late-onset disease occurs 2 to 3 weeks after birth in the form of meningitis or meningoencephalitis with septicemia. The clinical signs and symptoms are not unique; thus other causes of neonatal central nervous system disease, such as group B streptococcal disease, must be excluded.

Infections in Pregnant Women

Most infections in pregnant women occur during the third trimester when cellular immunity is most impaired. Infected women typically develop nonspecific influenza-like symptoms that may resolve without treatment. Unless blood cultures are collected in pregnant febrile women without another source of infection (e.g., urinary tract infection), *Listeria* bacteremia and the associated neonatal risk may be unappreciated.

Disease in Healthy Adults

Most *Listeria* infections in healthy adults are asymptomatic or occur in the form of a mild influenza-like illness. An acute self-limited gastroenteritis develops in some patients, characterized by a 1-day incubation period followed by 2 days of symptoms, including watery diarrhea, fever, nausea, headache, myalgias, and arthralgias. In contrast to these self-limited illnesses, listeriosis in elderly patients and those with compromised cellular immunity is more severe.

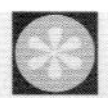

Clinical Case 21-1 *Listeria* Meningitis in Immunocompromised Man

The following patient described by Bowie and associates (*Ann Pharmacother* 38:58–61, 2004) illustrates the clinical presentation of *Listeria* meningitis. A 73-year-old man with refractory rheumatoid arthritis was brought by his family to the local hospital because he had a decreased level of consciousness and a 3-day history of headache, nausea, and vomiting. His current medications were infliximab, methotrexate, and prednisone for his rheumatoid arthritis. On physical examination, the patient had a stiff neck and was febrile, had a pulse of 92 beats/min, and had a blood pressure of 179/72 mm Hg. Because meningitis was suspected, blood and cerebrospinal fluid (CSF) were collected for culture. The Gram stain of the CSF was negative, but *Listeria* grew from both blood and CSF cultures. The patient was treated with vancomycin, the infliximab was discontinued, and he made an uneventful recovery despite using less-than-optimal antimicrobial therapy. Infliximab has been associated with a dose-dependent monocytopenia. Because monocytes are key effectors for clearance of *Listeria,* this immunocompromised patient was specifically at risk for infection with this organism. Failure to detect *Listeria* in CSF by Gram stain is typical of this disease because the bacteria fail to multiply to detectable levels.

Meningitis in Adults (Clinical Case 21-1)

Meningitis is the most common form of disseminated *Listeria* infection in adults. Although the clinical signs and symptoms of meningitis caused by this organism are not specific, *Listeria* should always be suspected in patients with organ transplants or cancer and in pregnant women in whom meningitis develops. Disease is associated with high mortality (20% to 50%) and significant neurologic sequelae among the survivors.

Primary Bacteremia

Patients with bacteremia may have an unremarkable history of chills and fever (commonly observed in pregnant women) or a more acute presentation with high-grade fever and hypotension. Only severely immunocompromised patients and the infants of pregnant women with sepsis appear to be at risk of death.

Laboratory Diagnosis

Microscopy

Gram-stain preparations of cerebrospinal fluid (CSF) typically show no organisms because the bacteria are generally present in concentrations below the limit of detection (e.g., 10^4 bacteria per milliliter CSF or less). This is in contrast with most other bacterial pathogens of the central nervous system, which are present in concentrations of 100-fold to 1000-fold higher. If the Gram stain shows organisms, they are intracellular and extracellular gram-positive coccobacilli. Care must be used to distinguish them from other bacteria such as *S. pneumoniae, Enterococcus,* and *Corynebacterium.*

Culture

Listeria grows on most conventional laboratory media, with small, round colonies observed on agar media after incubation for 1 to 2 days. It may be necessary to use selective media and **cold enrichment** (storage of the specimen in the refrigerator for a prolonged period) to detect listeriae in specimens contaminated with rapidly growing bacteria. β-Hemolysis on sheep blood agar media can serve to distinguish *Listeria* from morphologically similar bacteria; however, hemolysis is generally weak and may not be observed initially. Hemolysis is enhanced when the organisms are grown next to β-hemolytic *Staphylococcus aureus.* This enhanced hemolysis is referred to as a positive CAMP (Christie, Atkins, Munch-Petersen) test. The characteristic motility of the organism in a liquid medium or semisolid agar is also helpful for the preliminary identification of listeriae. All gram-positive rods isolated from blood and CSF should be identified to distinguish between *Corynebacterium* (presumably a contaminant) and *Listeria.*

Identification

Selected biochemical tests are used to identify the pathogen definitively, which is important because *L. monocytogenes,* the only species responsible for human disease, must be differentiated from other *Listeria* species that may contaminate food products. Serologic and molecular typing methods are used for epidemiologic investigations. A total of 13 serotypes have been described; however, serotypes 1/2a, 1/2b, and 4b are responsible for most infections in neonates and adults, so serotyping is generally not useful in epidemiologic investigations. Pulsed-field gel electrophoresis (PFGE) and more recently whole genome sequence analysis are the most commonly used molecular methods for epidemiologic investigations of suspected outbreaks.

Treatment, Prevention, and Control

Because most antibiotics are only bacteriostatic with *L. monocytogenes,* the combination of **gentamicin with either penicillin or ampicillin** is the treatment of choice for serious infections. Listeriae are naturally resistant to cephalosporins, and resistance to macrolides, fluoroquinolones, and tetracyclines has been observed, which can limit the utility of these drugs. Trimethoprim-sulfamethoxazole is bactericidal to *L. monocytogenes* and has been used successfully. Other antibiotics, such as linezolid, daptomycin, and tigecycline, have good in vitro activity but have not been used extensively to treat patients.

Because listeriae are ubiquitous and most infections are sporadic, prevention and control are difficult. People at high risk of infection should avoid eating raw or partially cooked foods of animal origin, soft cheeses, and unwashed raw vegetables. A vaccine is not available, and prophylactic antibiotic therapy for high-risk patients has not been evaluated.

Erysipelothrix rhusiopathiae

Physiology and Structure

E. rhusiopathiae is a gram-positive, non–spore-forming rod that is distributed worldwide in wild and domestic animals. The rods are slender (0.2 to 0.5 × 0.8 to 2.5 μm) and sometimes pleomorphic, with a tendency to form "hairlike" filaments as long as 60 μm. They decolorize readily and may appear gram-negative (Figure 21-3). The organisms are microaerophilic, with growth best in an atmosphere of reduced oxygen and supplemented carbon dioxide (5% to 10% CO_2). A mixture of tiny, smooth colonies and larger, rough colonies are observed after 2 to 3 days of incubation.

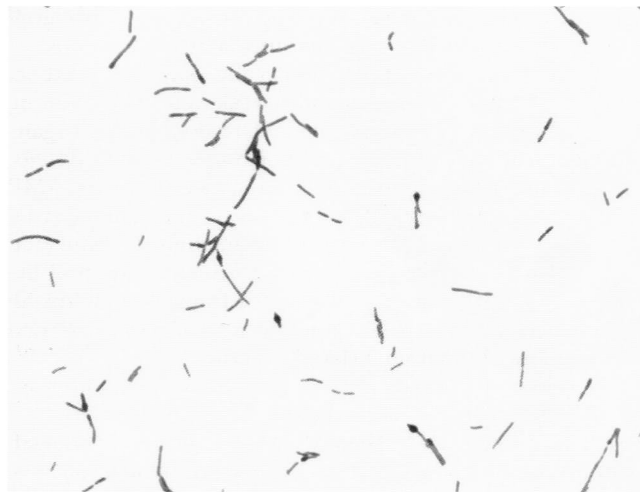

FIGURE 21-3 Gram stain of *Erysipelothrix rhusiopathiae* in culture. Note the variable lengths of the rods and the "gram-negative" appearance.

Clinical Case 21-2 *Erysipelothrix* Endocarditis

Endocarditis caused by *Erysipelothrix rhusiopathiae* is an uncommon but well-recognized disease. The following case history reported by Artz and associates (*Eur J Clin Microbiol Infect Dis* 20:587–588, 2001) is typical of this disease. A 46-year-old man who worked as a butcher and had a history of alcoholism was admitted to the hospital with an erythematous rash over his upper body and a complaint of arthralgias of both shoulders. Medical history revealed a 4-week history of night sweats and daily recurring chills, which the patient attributed to his drinking. Physical examination revealed hepatosplenomegaly, a systolic murmur detected on auscultation, and a calcified aortic valve with mild regurgitation but no vegetations on echocardiography. Five blood cultures were collected, and all were positive for *E. rhusiopathiae* after 2 days. The patient was transferred to surgery for valve replacement, and paravalvular abscesses were detected intraoperatively. After surgical repair, the patient was treated with clindamycin and penicillin and made a complete recovery. This case illustrates risk factors (i.e., butcher, alcoholism), a chronic course, and the value of surgery combined with treatment with effective antibiotics (i.e., penicillin, clindamycin).

If the rough colonies are absent, the small smooth colonies may be overlooked unless the culture plates are examined carefully.

Pathogenesis

Little is known about specific virulence factors in *Erysipelothrix*. Production of neuraminidase is believed to be important for attachment and penetration into epithelial cells, and a polysaccharide-like capsule protects the bacteria from phagocytosis.

Epidemiology

Erysipelothrix is a ubiquitous organism that is distributed worldwide. It can be recovered on the tonsils or in the digestive tracts of many wild and domestic animals, including mammals, birds, and fish. Colonization is particularly high in **swine** and **turkeys.** Soil rich in organic matter or groundwater contaminated with animal wastes can facilitate spread in an animal population. The bacteria are resistant to drying and can survive in soil for months to years. In addition, *E. rhusiopathiae* is resistant to high concentrations of salt, pickling, and smoking. *Erysipelothrix* disease in humans is **zoonotic** (spread from animals to humans) and primarily occupational. Butchers, meat processors, farmers, poultry workers, fish handlers, and veterinarians are at greatest risk. Cutaneous infections typically develop after the organism is inoculated subcutaneously through an abrasion or puncture wound during the handling of contaminated animal products or soil. The incidence of human disease is unknown because *Erysipelothrix* infection is not a reportable disease.

Clinical Diseases (see Table 21-2; Clinical Case 21-2)

Animal disease, particularly in swine, is widely recognized, but human disease is less common. Three primary forms of human infection with *E. rhusiopathiae* have been described: (1) a localized skin infection, **erysipeloid** (not to be confused with streptococcal erysipelas), (2) generalized cutaneous disease, and (3) **septicemia.** Erysipeloid is an inflammatory skin lesion that develops at the site of trauma after 2 to 7 days of incubation. The lesion most commonly presents on the fingers or hands and appears violaceous with a raised edge. It slowly spreads peripherally as the discoloration in the central area fades. The painful lesion is pruritic, and the patient experiences a burning or throbbing sensation. Suppuration is uncommon, a feature distinguishing erysipeloid from streptococcal erysipelas. The resolution can be spontaneous but can be hastened with appropriate antibiotic therapy. The diffuse cutaneous infection is characterized by development of lesions either in the general area of the initial lesion or at other skin locations. The systemic signs of fever and arthralgias are common, but blood cultures are typically negative.

The septicemic form of *Erysipelothrix* infections is uncommon, but when present, it is frequently associated with endocarditis. *Erysipelothrix* endocarditis may have an acute onset but is usually subacute. Involvement of previously undamaged heart valves (particularly the aortic valve) is common. Other systemic complications (e.g., abscess formation, meningitis, osteomyelitis) are relatively uncommon.

Laboratory Diagnosis

The rods are located only in the deep tissue of the lesion. Thus full-thickness biopsy specimens or deep aspirates must be collected from the margin of the lesion. A Gram stain of the specimen is typically negative, although the presence of **thin, gram-positive rods** associated with a characteristic lesion and clinical history can be diagnostic. *E. rhusiopathiae* is not fastidious and grows on most conventional laboratory media incubated in the presence of 5% to 10% CO_2; however, growth is slow, and cultures must be incubated for 3 days or longer before considered negative. The absence of both motility and catalase production distinguishes this organism from *Listeria*. The organism is weakly fermentative and produces hydrogen sulfide on triple-sugar iron agar. Serology is not useful for diagnosis because an antibody response is weak in human infections.

Treatment, Prevention, and Control

Erysipelothrix is susceptible to **penicillin,** which is the antibiotic of choice for both localized and systemic diseases. Cephalosporins, carbapenems, fluoroquinolones, and clindamycin are also active in vitro, but the organism has variable susceptibility to macrolides, sulfonamides, and aminoglycosides and is resistant to vancomycin. For patients allergic to penicillin, ciprofloxacin or clindamycin can be used for localized cutaneous infections, and ceftriaxone or imipenem can be considered for disseminated infections. Infections in people at a higher occupational risk are prevented by the use of gloves and other appropriate coverings on exposed skin. Vaccination is used to control disease in swine.

• *Corynebacterium diphtheriae*

The genus *Corynebacterium* is a large, heterogeneous collection of more than 100 species and subspecies that have a cell wall with arabinose, galactose, *meso*-diaminopimelic acid (*meso*-DAP), and (in most species) **short-chain mycolic acids** (22 to 36 carbon atoms). Although organisms with medium- and long-chain mycolic acids stain with acid-fast stains (see Chapter 22), *Corynebacterium* organisms are not acid-fast. Gram stains of these bacteria reveal clumps and short chains of irregularly shaped (club-shaped) rods (Figure 21-4). Corynebacteria are aerobic or facultatively anaerobic, nonmotile, and catalase positive. Most (but not all) species ferment carbohydrates, producing lactic acid as a byproduct. Many species grow well on common laboratory media; however, some species form small colonies because they require lipid supplemented media for good growth (**lipophilic** strains).

Corynebacteria are ubiquitous in plants and animals, and they normally colonize the skin, upper respiratory tract, gastrointestinal tract, and urogenital tract in humans. Although all species of corynebacteria can function as opportunistic pathogens, relatively few are associated with human disease (see Table 21-2). The most famous of these is *C. diphtheriae*, the etiologic agent of **diphtheria.** A number of other genera of coryneform bacteria have been characterized. Three genera associated with human disease (*Arcanobacterium, Rothia, Tropheryma*) are listed in Table 21-2 but will not be discussed further.

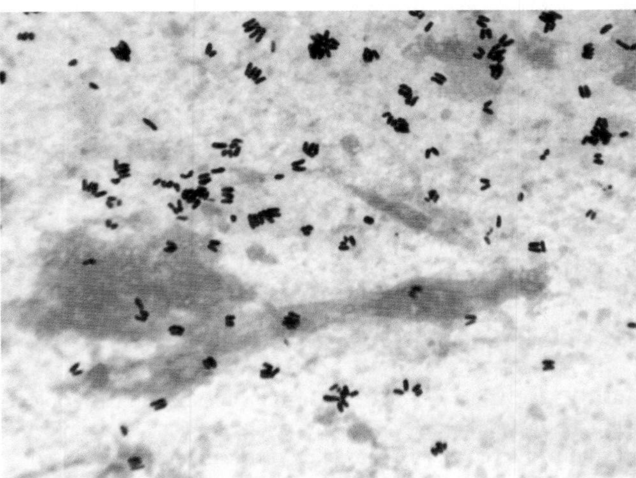

FIGURE 21-4 Gram stain of *Corynebacterium* species in sputum specimen.

Physiology and Structure

C. diphtheriae is an irregularly staining, pleomorphic rod (0.3 to 0.8 × 1.0 to 8.0 μm). After overnight incubation, large 1- to 3-mm colonies are observed on blood agar medium. More selective, differential media can be used to recover this pathogen from specimens with other organisms present, such as pharyngeal specimens. This species is subdivided into four biotypes based on their colonial morphology and biochemical properties: *belfanti, gravis, intermedius,* and *mitis,* with most disease caused by **biotype *mitis*.**

Pathogenesis and Immunity

Diphtheria toxin is the major virulence factor of *C. diphtheriae*. The *tox* gene that codes for the exotoxin is introduced into strains of *C. diphtheriae* by a lysogenic bacteriophage, **β-phage.** Two processing steps are necessary for the active gene product to be secreted: (1) proteolytic cleavage of the leader sequence from the Tox protein during secretion from the bacterial cell and (2) cleavage of the toxin molecule into two polypeptides (A and B) that remain attached by a disulfide bond. This 58,300-Da protein is an example of the classic **A-B exotoxin.**

Three functional regions exist on the toxin molecule: a **catalytic region** on the A subunit and a **receptor-binding region** and a **translocation region** on the B subunit. The receptor for the toxin is **heparin-binding epidermal growth factor,** which is present on the surface of many eukaryotic cells, particularly heart and nerve cells; its presence explains the cardiac and neurologic symptoms observed in patients with severe diphtheria. After the toxin becomes attached to the host cell, the translocation region is inserted into the endosomal membrane, facilitating the movement of the catalytic region into the cell cytosol. The A subunit then terminates host cell protein synthesis by inactivating **elongation factor-2 (EF-2),** a factor required for the movement of nascent peptide chains on ribosomes. Because the turnover of EF-2 is very slow and approximately only one molecule per ribosome is present in a cell, it has been estimated that one exotoxin molecule can inactivate the entire EF-2 content in a cell, completely terminating host cell protein synthesis. Toxin synthesis is regulated by a chromosomally encoded element, **diphtheria toxin repressor (DTxR).** This protein, activated in the presence of high iron concentrations, can bind to the toxin gene operator and prevent toxin production.

Epidemiology

Diphtheria is a disease found worldwide, particularly in poor urban areas where there is crowding and the protective level of vaccine-induced immunity is low. The largest outbreak in the latter part of the 20th century occurred in the former Soviet Union, where in 1994 almost 48,000 cases were documented, with 1746 deaths. *C. diphtheriae* is maintained in the population by **asymptomatic carriage** in the oropharynx or on the skin of immune people. Respiratory droplets or skin contact transmits it from person to person. **Humans** are the **only known reservoir** for this organism.

Diphtheria has become uncommon in the United States because of an active immunization program, as shown by the fact that more than 200,000 cases were reported in 1921 but no cases have been reported since 2003. An analysis of *C. diphtheriae* infections in the United Kingdom between 1986 and 2008 identified that the major risk factor for infection was travel of nonimmune individuals to countries with endemic disease (e.g., Indian subcontinent, Africa, Southeast Asia). Diphtheria is primarily a pediatric disease, but the highest incidence has shifted toward older age groups in areas where there are active immunization programs for children. Skin infection with toxigenic *C. diphtheriae* (cutaneous diphtheria) also occurs, but it is not a reportable disease in the United States, so its incidence is unknown.

Clinical Diseases

The clinical presentation of diphtheria is determined by the (1) site of infection, (2) immune status of the patient, and (3) virulence of the organism. Exposure to *C. diphtheriae* may result in asymptomatic colonization in fully immune people, mild respiratory disease in partially immune patients, or a fulminant, sometimes fatal, disease in nonimmune patients. Diphtheria toxin is produced at the site of the infection and then disseminates through the blood to produce the systemic signs of diphtheria. The organism does not need to enter the blood to produce disease.

Respiratory Diphtheria (Clinical Case 21-3)

The symptoms of diphtheria involving the respiratory tract develop after a 2- to 4-day incubation period. Organisms multiply locally on epithelial cells in the pharynx or adjacent surfaces and initially cause localized damage as a result of exotoxin activity. The onset is sudden, with malaise, sore throat, **exudative pharyngitis,** and a low-grade fever. The exudate evolves into a thick **pseudomembrane** composed of bacteria, lymphocytes, plasma cells, fibrin, and dead cells that can cover the tonsils, uvula, and palate and can extend up into the nasopharynx or down into the larynx (Figure 21-5). The pseudomembrane firmly adheres to the underlying tissue and is difficult to dislodge without making the tissue bleed (unique to diphtheria). As the patient recovers after the approximately 1-week course of the disease, the membrane dislodges and is expectorated. Systemic complications in patients with severe disease primarily involve the heart and nervous system. Evidence of **myocarditis** can be detected in the majority of patients with diphtheria, typically developing 1 to 2 weeks into the illness and at a time when the pharyngeal symptoms are improving. Symptoms can present acutely or gradually, progressing in severe disease to congestive heart failure, cardiac arrhythmias, and death. **Neurotoxicity** is proportional to the severity of the primary disease, which is influenced by the patient's immunity. The majority of patients with severe primary disease develop neuropathy, initially localized to the soft palate and pharynx, later involving oculomotor and ciliary paralysis, with progression to peripheral neuritis.

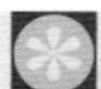

Clinical Case 21-3 Respiratory Diphtheria

Lurie and associates (*JAMA* 291:937–938, 2004) reported the last patient with respiratory diphtheria seen in the United States. An unvaccinated 63-year-old man developed a sore throat while on a week-long trip in rural Haiti. Two days after he returned home to Pennsylvania, he visited a local hospital with complaints of a sore throat and difficulties in swallowing. He was treated with oral antibiotics but returned 2 days later with chills, sweating, difficulty swallowing and breathing, nausea, and vomiting. He had diminished breath sounds in the left lung, and radiographs confirmed pulmonary infiltrates as well as enlargement of the epiglottis. Laryngoscopy revealed yellow exudates on the tonsils, posterior pharynx, and soft palate. He was admitted to the intensive care unit and treated with azithromycin, ceftriaxone, nafcillin, and steroids, but over the next 4 days he became hypotensive with a low-grade fever. Cultures were negative for *Corynebacterium diphtheriae*. By the eighth day of illness, a chest radiograph showed infiltrates in the right and left lung bases, and a white exudate consistent with *C. diphtheriae* pseudomembrane was observed over the supraglottic structures. Cultures at this time remained negative for *C. diphtheriae,* but polymerase chain reaction testing for the exotoxin gene was positive. Despite aggressive therapy the patient continued to deteriorate, and on the seventeenth day of hospitalization he developed cardiac complications and died. This patient illustrates (1) the risk factor of an unimmunized patient traveling to an endemic area, (2) the classic presentation of severe respiratory diphtheria, (3) delays associated with diagnosis of an uncommon disease, and (4) the difficulties most laboratories would now have isolating the organism in culture.

Cutaneous Diphtheria

Cutaneous diphtheria is acquired through skin contact with other infected persons. The organism colonizes the skin and gains entry into the subcutaneous tissue through breaks in the skin. A papule develops first and then evolves into a **chronic, nonhealing ulcer,** sometimes covered with a grayish membrane. *Staphylococcus aureus* or *Streptococcus pyogenes* is also frequently present in the wound.

Laboratory Diagnosis

The initial treatment of a patient with diphtheria is instituted on the basis of the clinical diagnosis, not laboratory results, because definitive results are not available for at least a week.

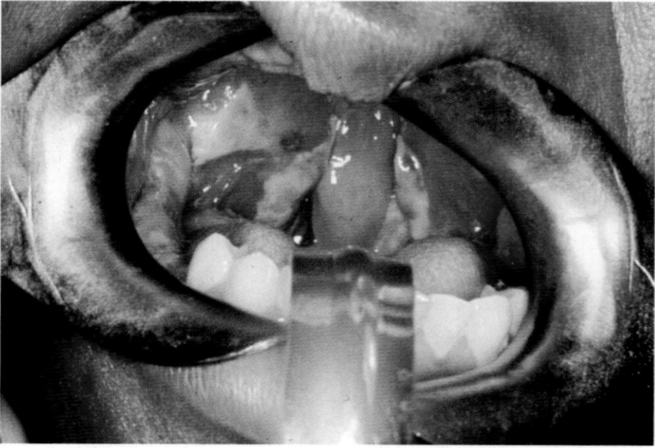

FIGURE 21-5 Pharynx of a 39-year-old woman with bacteriologically confirmed diphtheria. The photograph was taken 4 days after the onset of fever, malaise, and sore throat. Hemorrhage caused by removal of the membrane by swabbing appears as a dark area on the left. (From Mandell G, Bennett J, Dolin R: *Principles and practice of infectious diseases,* ed 8, Philadelphia, 2015, Elsevier.)

Microscopy

The results of microscopic examination of clinical material are unreliable. Metachromatic granules in bacteria stained with methylene blue have been described, but this appearance is not specific to *C. diphtheriae*.

Culture

Specimens for the recovery of *C. diphtheriae* should be collected from both the nasopharynx and throat and should be inoculated onto a nonselective, enriched blood agar plate and a selective medium (e.g., cysteine-tellurite blood agar [CTBA], Tinsdale medium, colistin-nalidixic agar [CNA]). Tellurite inhibits the growth of most upper respiratory tract bacteria and gram-negative rods and is reduced by *C. diphtheriae,* producing a characteristic gray to black color on agar. Degradation of cysteine by *C. diphtheriae* cysteinase activity produces a brown halo around the colonies. CTBA has a long shelf life (practical for cultures that are infrequently performed) but inhibits some strains of *C. diphtheriae*. Tinsdale medium is the best medium for recovering *C. diphtheriae* in clinical specimens, but it has a short shelf life and requires addition of horse serum. Because infections caused by *C. diphtheriae* are rarely seen or suspected in nonendemic areas, CTBA and Tinsdale medium are not commonly available in most laboratories. CNA is commonly used for the selective recovery of gram-positive bacteria; therefore this is a practical alternative medium. Regardless of the media used, all isolates resembling *C. diphtheriae* must be identified by biochemical testing and the presence of the diphtheria exotoxin confirmed because nontoxigenic strains occur.

Identification

The presumptive identification of *C. diphtheriae* can be based on the presence of cystinase and absence of pyrazinamidase (two enzyme reactions that can be rapidly determined). More extensive biochemical tests or nucleic acid sequencing of species-specific genes is required for identification at the species level.

Toxigenicity Testing

All isolates of *C. diphtheriae* should be tested for the production of exotoxin. The gold standard for detection of diphtheria toxin is an in vitro immunodiffusion assay **(Elek test).** An alternative method is detection of the exotoxin gene using a **polymerase chain reaction (PCR)–based nucleic acid amplification method.** This test can detect the *tox* gene in clinical isolates and directly in clinical specimens (e.g., swabs from the diphtheritic membrane or biopsy material). Although this test is rapid and specific, strains in which the *tox* gene is not expressed (presumably because the **diphtheria toxin repressor** is expressed) can give a positive signal. Nontoxigenic strains of *C. diphtheriae* do not produce classic diphtheria; however, they should not be ignored, because these strains have been associated with other significant diseases, including septicemia, endocarditis, septic arthritis, osteomyelitis, and abscess formation.

Treatment, Prevention, and Control

The most important aspect of the treatment for diphtheria is early administration of **diphtheria antitoxin** to specifically neutralize the exotoxin before it is bound by the host cell. Once the cell internalizes the toxin, cell death is inevitable. Unfortunately, because diphtheria may not be suspected initially, significant progression of disease can occur before the antitoxin is administered. Antibiotic therapy with **penicillin or erythromycin** is also used to eliminate *C. diphtheriae* and terminate toxin production. Bed rest, isolation to prevent secondary spread, and maintenance of an open airway in patients with respiratory diphtheria are all important. After the patient has recovered, **immunization with toxoid** is required because most patients fail to develop protective antibodies after a natural infection.

Symptomatic diphtheria can be prevented by actively immunizing people with diphtheria toxoid. The nontoxic, immunogenic toxoid is prepared by formalin treatment of the toxin. Initially, children are given five injections of this preparation with pertussis and tetanus antigens **(DPT vaccine)** at ages 2, 4, 6, 15 to 18 months, and 4 to 6 years. After that time, it is recommended that booster vaccinations with diphtheria toxoid combined with tetanus toxoid be given every 10 years. The effectiveness of immunization is well documented, with disease restricted to nonimmune or incompletely immunized individuals.

People in close contact with patients who have documented diphtheria are at risk for acquiring the disease. Nasopharyngeal specimens for culture should be collected from all close contacts and antimicrobial prophylaxis with erythromycin or penicillin started immediately. Any contact who has not completed the series of diphtheria immunizations or who has not received a booster dose within the previous 5 years should receive a booster dose of toxoid. People exposed to cutaneous diphtheria should be managed in the same manner because it is reported that they are more contagious than patients with respiratory diphtheria. If the respiratory or cutaneous infection is caused by a nontoxigenic strain, it is unnecessary to institute prophylaxis in contacts.

Bibliography

Allerberger F, Wagner M: Listeriosis: a resurgent foodborne infection, *Clin Microbiol Infect* 16:16–23, 2010.

Fenollar F, Puechal X, Raoult D: Whipple's disease, *N Engl J Med* 356:55–66, 2007.

Freitag N, Port G, Miner M: *Listeria monocytogenes*—from saprophyte to intracellular pathogen, *Nat Rev Microbiol* 7:623–628, 2009.

Funke G, von Graevenitz A, Clarridge JE 3rd, et al: Clinical microbiology of coryneform bacteria, *Clin Microbiol Rev* 10:125–159, 1997.

Gorby GL, Peacock JE Jr: *Erysipelothrix rhusiopathiae* endocarditis: microbiologic, epidemiologic, and clinical features of an occupational disease, *Rev Infect Dis* 10:317–325, 1988.

Gray MJ, Freitag NE, Boor KJ: How the bacterial pathogen *Listeria monocytogenes* mediates the switch from environmental Dr. Jekyll to pathogenic Mr. Hyde, *Infect Immun* 74:2505–2512, 2006.

McCollum JT, Cronquist AB, Silk BJ, et al: Multistate outbreak of listeriosis associated with cantaloupe, *N Engl J Med* 369:944–953, 2013.

Pamer EG: Immune responses to *Listeria monocytogenes*, *Nat Rev Immunol* 4:812–823, 2004.

Popovic T, Kombarova SY, Reeves MW, et al: Molecular epidemiology of diphtheria in Russia, 1985-1994, *J Infect Dis* 174:1064–1072, 1996.

Wagner KS, White JM, Crowcroft NS, et al: Diphtheria in the United Kingdom, 1986-2008: the increasing role of *Corynebacterium ulcerans*, *Epidemiol Infect* 138:1519–1530, 2010.

Wang Q, Chang BJ, Riley TV: *Erysipelothrix rhusiopathiae*, *Vet Microbiol* 140:405–417, 2010.

Wing E, Gregory S: *Listeria monocytogenes:* clinical and experimental update, *J Infect Dis* 185(Suppl 1):S18–S24, 2002.

CHAPTER

22 MYCOBACTERIUM AND RELATED ACID-FAST BACTERIA

A 47-year-old renal transplant recipient who had been receiving prednisone and azathioprine for 2 years was admitted to the university medical center. Two weeks earlier, the patient had noticed the development of a dry, persistent cough. Five days before admission, the cough became productive and pleuritic chest pain developed. On the day of admission, the patient was in mild respiratory distress, and chest radiographs revealed a patchy right upper lobe infiltrate. Sputum specimens were initially sent for bacterial culture, and the modified acid-fast stain was positive.

1. What genera of bacteria will stain with the modified acid-fast stain?
2. If this patient has no travel history outside the United States, what would be the most likely cause of the respiratory illness?
3. What are the most common diseases caused by the genera of acid-fast bacteria?
4. What characteristic morphologic properties and growth properties will help differentiate the most common acid-fast bacteria?

Answers to these questions are available on StudentConsult.com.

• SUMMARIES CLINICALLY SIGNIFICANT ORGANISMS

Mycobacterium tuberculosis

Trigger Words

Acid-fast, lipid-rich cell wall, intracellular, PPD, drug-resistant

Biology and Virulence

- Weakly gram-positive, strongly acid-fast, aerobic rods
- Lipid-rich cell wall, making the organism resistant to traditional stains, disinfectants, detergents, common antibacterial antibiotics, and host immune response
- Capable of intracellular growth in alveolar macrophages
- Disease primarily from host response to infection

Epidemiology

- Worldwide; one third of the world's population is infected with this organism
- A total of 8.6 million new cases each year and 1.3 million deaths
- Disease most common in China, India, Eastern Europe, Pakistan, sub-Saharan Africa, and South Africa
- 9945 new cases in United States in 2012
- Populations at greatest risk for disease are immunocompromised patients (particularly those with HIV infection), drug or alcohol abusers, homeless persons, and individuals exposed to diseased patients
- Humans are the only natural reservoir
- Person-to-person spread by infectious aerosols

Diseases

- Primary infection is pulmonary
- Dissemination to any body site occurs most commonly in immunocompromised patients

Diagnosis

- Tuberculin skin test and interferon (IFN)-γ release tests are sensitive markers for exposure to organism
- Microscopy and culture are sensitive and specific
- Direct detection by molecular probes is relatively insensitive except for acid-fast smear-positive specimens
- Nucleic acid amplification tests important where culture is not available and microscopy is inaccurate
- Identification most commonly made using species-specific molecular probes, sequencing, or mass spectrometry

Treatment, Prevention, and Control

- Prolonged treatment with multiple drugs is required to prevent development of drug-resistant strains
- Isoniazid (INH), ethambutol, pyrazinamide, and rifampin for 2 months followed by 4 to 6 months of INH and rifampin or alternative combination drugs
- Prophylaxis for exposure to tuberculosis can include INH for 6 to 9 months or daily rifampin for 4 months; pyrazinamide and ethambutol or levofloxacin are used for 6 to 12 months after exposure to drug-resistant *M. tuberculosis*
- Immunoprophylaxis with bacille Calmette-Guérin (BCG) in endemic countries
- Control of disease through active surveillance, prophylactic and therapeutic intervention, and careful case monitoring

Mycobacterium leprae

Trigger Words

Acid-fast, leprosy, nonculturable, skin test, IFN-γ release assays

Biology and Virulence

- Weakly gram-positive, strongly acid-fast rods
- Lipid-rich cell wall
- Unable to be cultured on artificial media
- Disease primarily from host response to infection

Epidemiology

- Fewer than 300,000 new cases were reported in 2005, with most cases in India, Nepal, and Brazil
- 64 new cases reported in United States in 2013
- Lepromatous form of disease, but not the tuberculoid form, is highly infectious
- Person-to-person spread by direct contact or inhalation of infectious aerosols

Diseases

- Tuberculoid (paucibacillary) and lepromatous (multibacillary) forms of leprosy

Diagnosis

- Microscopy is sensitive for the lepromatous form but not the tuberculoid form
- Skin testing is required to confirm tuberculoid leprosy
- Culture is not useful

Treatment, Prevention, and Control

- Tuberculoid form is treated with rifampicin and dapsone for 6 months; clofazimine is added to this regimen for treatment of the lepromatous form, and therapy is extended to a minimum of 12 months
- Disease is controlled through prompt recognition and treatment of infected people

Mycobacterium avium Complex

Trigger Words

Acid-fast, pulmonary infections, AIDS, prophylaxis

Biology and Virulence

- Weakly gram-positive, strongly acid-fast aerobic rods
- Lipid-rich cell wall
- Disease primarily from host response to infection

Epidemiology

- Worldwide distribution, but disease is seen most commonly in countries where tuberculosis is less common
- Acquired primarily through ingestion of contaminated water or food; inhalation of infectious aerosols is believed to play a minor role in transmission
- Patients at greatest risk for disease are those who are immunocompromised (particularly patients with AIDS) and those with long-standing pulmonary disease

Diseases

- Disease includes asymptomatic colonization, chronic localized pulmonary disease, solitary nodule, or disseminated disease, particularly in patients with acquired immunodeficiency syndrome (AIDS)

Diagnosis

- Microscopy and culture are sensitive and specific

Treatment, Prevention, and Control

- Infections treated for prolonged period with clarithromycin or azithromycin combined with ethambutol and rifabutin
- Prophylaxis in AIDS patients who have a low CD4 cell count consists of clarithromycin or azithromycin or rifabutin, and such treatment has greatly reduced the incidence of disease

Nocardia

Trigger Words

Modified acid-fast, filamentous, bronchopulmonary or cutaneous disease, opportunistic

Biology and Virulence

- Gram-positive, partially acid-fast, filamentous rods; cell wall with mycolic acid
- Strict aerobe capable of growth on most nonselective bacteria, fungal, and mycobacterial media; however, prolonged incubation (2 days or more) may be required
- Virulence associated with ability to avoid intracellular killing
- Catalase and superoxide dismutase inactivate toxic oxygen metabolites (e.g., hydrogen peroxide, superoxide)
- Cord factor prevents intracellular killing in phagocytes by interfering with fusion of phagosomes with lysosomes

Epidemiology

- Worldwide distribution in soil rich with organic matter
- Exogenous infections acquired by inhalation (pulmonary) or traumatic introduction (cutaneous)
- Opportunistic pathogen causing disease most commonly in immunocompromised patients with T-cell deficiencies (transplant recipients, patients with malignancies, patients infected with the human immunodeficiency virus, patients receiving corticosteroids)

Diseases

- Primary disease most commonly bronchopulmonary (e.g., cavitary disease) or primary cutaneous infections (e.g., mycetoma, lymphocutaneous infection, cellulitis, subcutaneous abscesses)
- Dissemination most commonly to central nervous system (e.g., brain abscesses) or skin

Diagnosis

- Microscopy is sensitive and relatively specific when branching, partially acid-fast organisms are seen
- Culture is slow, requiring incubation for up to 1 week; selective media (e.g., buffered charcoal yeast extract agar) may be required for isolating *Nocardia* in mixed cultures
- Identification at the genus level can be made by the microscopic and macroscopic appearances (branching, weakly acid-fast rods forming colonies with aerial hyphae)
- Identification at the species level requires genomic analysis for most isolates

Treatment, Prevention, and Control

- Infections are treated with antibiotics and proper wound care
- Trimethoprim-sulfamethoxazole (TMP-SMX) used as initial empirical therapy for cutaneous infections in immunocompetent patients; therapy for severe infections and cutaneous infections in immunocompromised patients should include TMP-SMX plus amikacin for pulmonary or cutaneous infections and TMP-SMX plus imipenem or a cephalosporin for central nervous system infections; prolonged treatment (up to 12 months) is recommended
- Exposure cannot be avoided because nocardiae are ubiquitous

The genera discussed in this chapter are nonmotile, non–spore-forming, aerobic gram-positive rods that stain **acid-fast** (i.e., resist decolorization with weak to strong acid solutions) due to the presence of medium to long chains of mycolic acids in their cell wall. This staining property is important because only five genera of acid-fast bacteria are medically important (Table 22-1). All acid-fast organisms are relatively slow-growing bacteria, requiring incubation for 2 to 7 days *(Nocardia, Rhodococcus, Gordonia, Tsukamurella)* to as long as 1 month or more *(Mycobacteria)*. Currently, more than 350 species of acid-fast bacteria have been described; however, the number associated commonly with human disease is relatively limited (Table 22-2). The spectrum of the infections associated with the acid-fast genera is extensive and includes insignificant colonization, cutaneous infections, pulmonary disease, systemic infections, and opportunistic infections. *Mycobacteria* and *Nocardia* will be the emphasis of this chapter because these are the most common acid-fast bacteria responsible for human disease.

• Physiology and Structure of Mycobacteria

Bacteria are classified in the genus *Mycobacterium* on the basis of (1) their acid-fastness, (2) the presence of cell wall

Table 22-1 Important Acid-Fast Bacteria

Organism	Historical Derivation
Mycobacterium	*myces,* a fungus; *bakterion,* a small rod (fungus-like rod)
M. abscessus	*abscessus,* of abscesses (causes abscess formation)
M. avium	*avis,* of birds (causes tuberculosis-like illness in birds)
M. chelonae	*chelone,* a tortoise (initial source)
M. fortuitum	*fortuitum,* casual, accidental (refers to fact this is an opportunistic pathogen)
M. haemophilum	*haema,* blood; *philos,* loving (blood loving; refers to requirement for blood or hemin for in vitro growth)
M. intracellulare	*intra,* within; *cella,* small room (within cells; refers to the intracellular location of this and all mycobacteria)
M. kansasii	*kansasii,* of Kansas (where the organism was originally isolated)
M. leprae	*lepra,* of leprosy (the cause of leprosy)
M. marinum	*marinum,* of the sea (bacterium associated with contaminated freshwater and saltwater)
M. tuberculosis	*tuberculum,* a small swelling or tubercle; *osis* (characterized by tubercles; refers to the formation of tubercles in the lungs of infected patients)
Nocardia	Named after the French veterinarian Edmond Nocard
Rhodococcus	*rhodo,* rose or red colored; *coccus,* berry (red-colored coccus)
Gordonia	Named after the American microbiologist Ruth Gordon
Tsukamurella	Honoring the Japanese microbiologist Michio Tsukamura, who first described the original isolate of this genus

Table 22-2 Classification of Selected Acid-Fast Bacteria Pathogenic for Humans

Organism	Pathogenicity	Frequency in United States
***Mycobacterium tuberculosis* Complex**		
M. tuberculosis	Strictly pathogenic	Common
M. leprae	Strictly pathogenic	Uncommon
M. africanum	Strictly pathogenic	Rare
M. bovis	Strictly pathogenic	Rare
M. bovis BCG (bacille Calmette-Guérin strain)	Sometimes pathogenic	Rare
Slow-Growing Nontuberculous Mycobacteria		
M. avium complex	Usually pathogenic	Common
M. kansasii	Usually pathogenic	Common
M. marinum	Usually pathogenic	Uncommon
M. simiae	Usually pathogenic	Uncommon
M. szulgai	Usually pathogenic	Uncommon
M. genavense	Usually pathogenic	Uncommon
M. haemophilum	Usually pathogenic	Uncommon
M. malmoense	Usually pathogenic	Uncommon
M. ulcerans	Usually pathogenic	Uncommon
M. scrofulaceum	Sometimes pathogenic	Uncommon
M. xenopi	Sometimes pathogenic	Uncommon
Rapidly Growing Nontuberculous Mycobacteria		
M. abscessus	Sometimes pathogenic	Common
M. chelonae	Sometimes pathogenic	Common
M. fortuitum	Sometimes pathogenic	Common
M. mucogenicum	Sometimes pathogenic	Common
Nocardia		
N. cyriacigeorgica	Usually pathogenic	Common
N. farcinica	Usually pathogenic	Common
N. abscessus	Usually pathogenic	Uncommon
N. beijingensis	Usually pathogenic	Uncommon
N. brasiliensis	Usually pathogenic	Uncommon
N. nova	Usually pathogenic	Uncommon
N. otitidiscaviarum	Usually pathogenic	Uncommon
Nocardia spp.	Sometimes pathogenic	Rare
Rhodococcus equi	Usually pathogenic	Common
Gordonia bronchialis	Sometimes pathogenic	Rare
G. otitidis	Sometimes pathogenic	Rare
G. sputi	Sometimes pathogenic	Rare
Gordonia spp.	Sometimes pathogenic	Rare
Tsukamurella pulmonis	Sometimes pathogenic	Rare
T. tyrosinosolvens	Sometimes pathogenic	Rare
Tsukamurella spp.	Sometimes pathogenic	Rare

mycolic acids containing 70 to 90 carbons, and (3) a high (61% to 71% mol) guanine plus cytosine (G+C) content in their deoxyribonucleic acid (DNA). Mycobacteria possess a complex, **lipid-rich cell wall** that is responsible for many of the characteristic properties of the bacteria (e.g., acid-fastness; slow growth; resistance to detergents, common antibacterial antibiotics, and the host immune response; antigenicity). The proteins associated with the cell wall are biologically important antigens, stimulating the patient's cellular immune response. Extracted and partially purified preparations of these proteins **(purified protein derivatives [PPDs])** are used as specific diagnostic skin test reagents to measure exposure to *M. tuberculosis.*

Growth properties and colonial morphology are used for the preliminary classification of mycobacteria. As noted earlier, *M. tuberculosis* and closely related species in the *M. tuberculosis* complex are slow-growing bacteria. The colonies of these mycobacteria are either nonpigmented or a light tan color (Figure 22-1). The other mycobacteria, referred to as "nontuberculous mycobacteria" (NTM), were classified originally by Runyon by their rate of growth (see Table 22-2) and pigmentation. The pigmented mycobacteria produce intensely **yellow carotenoids,** which may be stimulated by exposure to light (photochromogenic organisms, Figure 22-2) or are produced in the absence of light (scotochromogenic organisms). The **Runyon classification** scheme of NTM consists of four groups: slow-growing photochromogens (e.g., *M. kansasii, M. marinum*), slow-growing scotochromogens (e.g., *M. gordonae*—a commonly isolated nonpathogen), slow-growing nonpigmented mycobacteria (e.g., *M. avium, M. intracellulare*), and rapidly growing mycobacteria (e.g., *M. fortuitum, M. chelonae, M. abscessus, M. mucogenicum*). Currently used methods for rapid detection and identification of mycobacteria have made this scheme less important. Nonetheless, a pigmented or rapidly growing *Mycobacterium* should never be mistaken for *M. tuberculosis.*

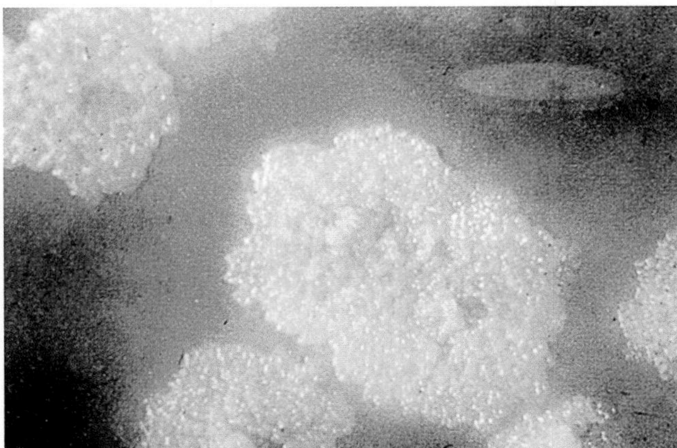

FIGURE 22-1 *Mycobacterium tuberculosis* colonies on Löwenstein-Jensen agar after 8 weeks of incubation. (From Baron EJ, Peterson LR, Finegold SM: *Bailey and Scott's diagnostic microbiology,* ed 9, St Louis, 1994, Mosby.)

Mycobacterium tuberculosis

Pathogenesis and Immunity

M. tuberculosis is an intracellular pathogen that is able to establish lifelong infection. Maintenance of persistent infection without progression to disease involves a delicate balance between growth of the bacteria and immunologic regulation. At the time of exposure, *M. tuberculosis* enters the respiratory airways, and infectious particles penetrate to the alveoli where they are phagocytized by alveolar macrophages. In contrast with most phagocytized bacteria, *M. tuberculosis* **prevents fusion of the phagosome with lysosomes** (by blocking the specific bridging molecule, early endosomal autoantigen 1 [EEA1]). At the same time, the phagosome is able to fuse with other intracellular vesicles, permitting access to nutrients and facilitating intravacuole replication. Phagocytized bacteria are also able to evade macrophage killing mediated by reactive nitrogen intermediates formed between nitric oxide and superoxide anions by catalytically catabolizing the oxidants that are formed. So in this state, the bacteria are able to evade the immune system and replicate. However, in response to infection with *M. tuberculosis,* macrophages secrete **interleukin (IL)-12** and **tumor necrosis factor (TNF)-α.** These cytokines increase localized inflammation with the recruitment of T cells and natural killer (NK) cells into the area of the infected macrophages, inducing T-cell differentiation into **TH1 cells (T-helper cells),** with subsequent secretion of **interferon (IFN)-γ.** In the presence of IFN-γ, the infected macrophages are activated, leading to increased phagosome-lysosome fusion and intracellular killing. In addition, TNF-α stimulates production of nitric oxide and related reactive nitrogen intermediates, leading to enhanced intracellular killing. Patients with decreased production of IFN-γ or TNF-α, or who have defects in the receptors for these cytokines, are at increased risk for severe progressive mycobacterial infections.

The effectiveness of bacterial elimination is in part related to the size of the focus of infection. Alveolar macrophages, epithelioid cells, and **Langhans giant cells** (fused epithelioid cells) with intracellular mycobacteria form the central core

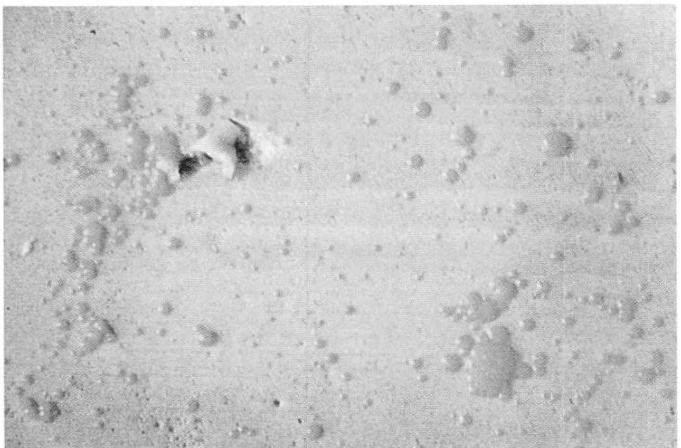

FIGURE 22-2 *Mycobacterium kansasii* colonies on Middlebrook agar; yellow pigment develops after brief exposure to light.

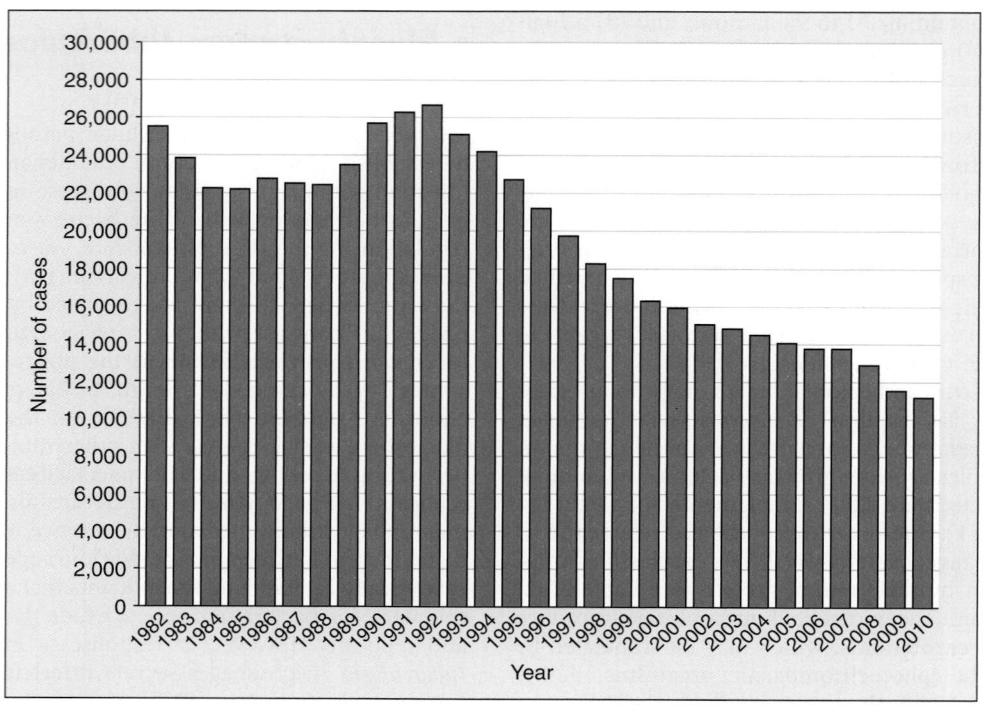

FIGURE 22-3 Incidence of *Mycobacterium tuberculosis* infections in the United States, 1982-2010.

of a necrotic mass that is surrounded by a dense wall of macrophages and CD4, CD8, and NK T cells. This structure, a **granuloma,** prevents further spread of the bacteria. If a small antigenic burden is present at the time the macrophages are stimulated, the granuloma is small and the bacteria are destroyed with minimal tissue damage. However, if many bacteria are present, the large necrotic or caseous granulomas become encapsulated with fibrin that effectively protects the bacteria from macrophage killing. The bacteria can remain dormant in this stage or can be reactivated years later when the patient's immunologic responsiveness wanes as the result of old age or immunosuppressive disease or therapy. This process is the reason that disease may not develop until late in life in patients exposed to *M. tuberculosis.*

Clinical Case 22-1 Drug-Resistant *Mycobacterium tuberculosis*

The risk of active tuberculosis is significantly increased in HIV-infected individuals. Unfortunately, this problem is complicated by the development of drug-resistant *M. tuberculosis* strains in this population. This was illustrated by the report by Gandhi and associates (*Lancet* 368:1575–1580, 2006), who studied the prevalence of tuberculosis in South Africa from January 2005 to March 2006. They identified 475 patients with culture-confirmed tuberculosis, of whom 39% had multidrug-resistant strains (MDR TB) and 6% had extensively drug-resistant strains (XDR TB). All patients with XDR TB were co-infected with HIV, and 98% of these patients died. The high prevalence of MDR TB and the evolution of XDR TB pose a serious challenge for tuberculosis treatment programs and emphasize the need for rapid diagnostic tests.

Epidemiology

Although tuberculosis can be established in primates and laboratory animals, such as guinea pigs, **humans are the only natural reservoir.** The disease is spread by close person-to-person contact through the inhalation of infectious aerosols. Large particles are trapped on mucosal surfaces and removed by the ciliary action of the respiratory tree. However, small particles containing one to three tubercle bacilli can reach the alveolar spaces and establish infection.

The World Health Organization (WHO) estimates that one third of the world's population is infected with *M. tuberculosis.* In 2012, there were 8.6 million new cases of tuberculosis and 1.3 million deaths. Despite these grim statistics, the number of new cases worldwide is declining and the death rate decreased by 45% between 1990 and 2012. Regions with the highest incidence of disease are China, India, Eastern Europe, Pakistan, sub-Saharan Africa, and South Africa. In the United States, the incidence of tuberculosis has decreased steadily since 1992 (Figure 22-3). A total of 9945 cases were reported in 2012 (3.2 cases per 100,000 individuals), with almost 60% of the infections in foreign-born persons. Other populations at increased risk for *M. tuberculosis* disease are homeless persons, drug and alcohol abusers, prisoners, and people infected with the human immunodeficiency virus (HIV). Because it is difficult to eradicate disease in these patients, spread of the infection to other populations, including health care workers, poses a significant public health problem. This is particularly true for drug-resistant *M. tuberculosis,* because patients who receive inadequate treatment may remain infectious for a long time.

Clinical Diseases (Clinical Case 22-1)

Although tuberculosis can involve any organ, most infections in immunocompetent patients are restricted to the lungs. The initial pulmonary focus is the middle or lower lung fields, where the tubercle bacilli can multiply freely. The patient's cellular immunity is activated and mycobacterial replication ceases in most patients within 3 to 6 weeks after exposure to the organism. Approximately 5% of patients exposed to *M. tuberculosis* progress to having active disease within 2 years, and another 5% experience disease sometime later in life.

The likelihood that infection will progress to active disease is a function of both the infectious dose and the patient's immune competence. For example, active disease develops within 1 year of exposure in approximately 10% of patients who are infected with HIV and have a low CD4 T-cell count, usually appears before the onset of other opportunistic infections, is twice as likely to spread to extrapulmonary sites, and can progress rapidly to death. Indeed, tuberculosis is the leading cause of death in HIV-infected patients. Because these patients have compromised immunity, they commonly present with asymptomatic, subclinical disease and negative chest radiography despite widespread dissemination of the bacteria.

The clinical signs and symptoms of tuberculosis reflect the site of infection, with primary disease usually restricted to the lower respiratory tract. The disease is insidious at onset. Patients typically have nonspecific complaints of malaise, weight loss, cough, and night sweats. Sputum may be scant or bloody and purulent. Blood-streaked sputum production (hemoptysis) is associated with tissue destruction (e.g., **cavitary disease**). The clinical diagnosis is supported by (1) radiographic evidence of pulmonary disease (Figure 22-4), (2) positive skin test reactivity, and (3) the laboratory detection of mycobacteria, either with microscopy or in cultures. One or both upper lobes of the lungs are usually involved in patients with active disease that includes either pneumonitis or abscess formation and cavitation.

Extrapulmonary tuberculosis can occur as the result of the hematogenous spread of the bacilli during the initial phase of multiplication. There may be no evidence of pulmonary disease in patients with **disseminated tuberculosis.**

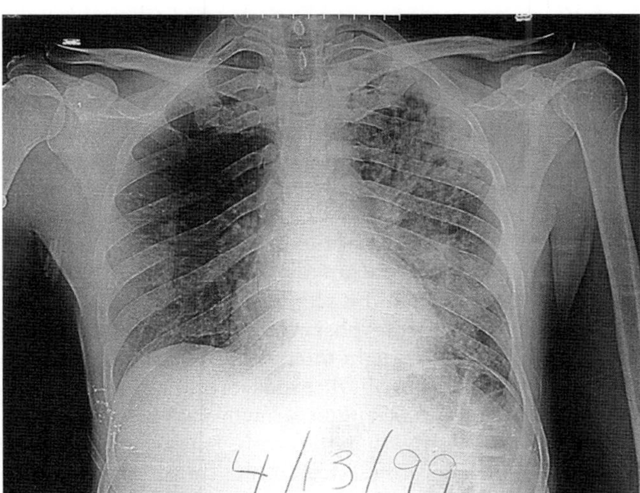

FIGURE 22-4 Pulmonary tuberculosis.

Laboratory Diagnosis (Box 22-1)

Immunodiagnosis

The traditional test to assess the patient's response to exposure to *M. tuberculosis* is the **tuberculin skin test.** Reactivity to an intradermal injection of mycobacterial antigens (purified protein derivative [PPD]) can differentiate between infected and noninfected people, with a positive reaction usually developing 3 to 4 weeks after exposure to *M. tuberculosis.* The only evidence of infection with mycobacteria in most patients is a lifelong positive skin test reaction and radiographic evidence of calcification of granulomas in the lungs or other organs. In this test, a specific amount of the antigen (5 tuberculin units of PPD) is inoculated into the intradermal layer of the patient's skin. Skin test reactivity (defined by the diameter of the area of induration) is measured 48 hours later. Patients infected with *M. tuberculosis* may not show a response to the tuberculin skin test if they are anergic (nonreactive to antigens; particularly true of HIV-infected patients); thus, control antigens should always be used with tuberculin tests. Additionally, individuals from countries where vaccination with attenuated *M. bovis* **(bacille Calmette-Guérin [BCG])** is widespread will have a positive skin test reaction, so this test is not helpful.

In vitro IFN-γ release assays have been introduced as an alternative to the PPD skin test. The tests use immunoassays to measure IFN-γ produced by sensitized T cells stimulated by *M. tuberculosis* antigens. If an individual was previously infected with *M. tuberculosis,* exposure of sensitized T cells present in whole blood to *M. tuberculosis*–specific antigens results in IFN-γ production. The initial assays that used PPD as the stimulating antigen have been replaced with second-generation assays that use more specific antigens (i.e., **early secreted antigenic target-6 [ESAT-6], culture filtrate protein-10 [CFP-10]**) and can be used to discriminate between infections with *M. tuberculosis* and BCG

Box 22-1 Laboratory Diagnosis of Mycobacterial Disease

Immunodiagnosis
Tuberculin skin test
Interferon-γ release assays

Microscopy
Ziehl-Neelsen (hot acid-fast) stain
Kinyoun (cold acid-fast) stain
Truant fluorochrome acid-fast stain

Nucleic Acid–Based Tests
Nucleic acid amplification tests

Culture
Agar- or egg-based media
Broth-based media

Identification
Morphologic properties
Biochemical reactions
Analysis of cell wall lipids
Nucleic acid probes
Nucleic acid sequencing

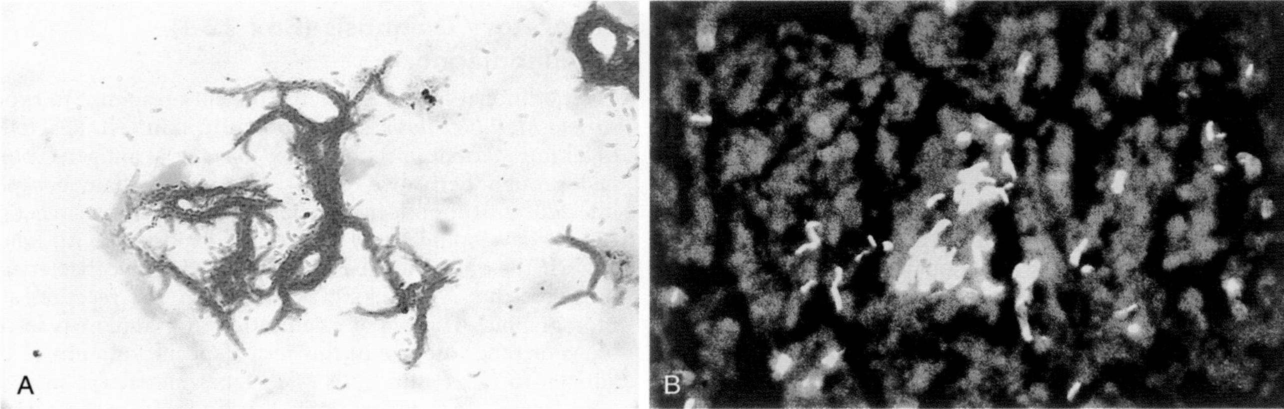

FIGURE 22-5 Acid-fast stains of *Mycobacterium tuberculosis.* **A,** Stained with carbolfuchsin using the Kinyoun method. **B,** Stained with the fluorescent dyes auramine and rhodamine using the Truant fluorochrome method.

vaccination. Although the tests are sensitive and highly specific, the technical complexity of the assays currently limits their use.

Microscopy

Microscopic detection of acid-fast bacteria in clinical specimens is the most rapid way to confirm mycobacterial disease. The clinical specimen is stained with carbolfuchsin (**Ziehl-Neelsen** or **Kinyoun** methods) or fluorescent auramine-rhodamine dyes (**Truant fluorochrome** method), decolorized with an acid-alcohol solution, and then counterstained. The specimens are examined with a light microscope or, if fluorescent dyes are used, a fluorescent microscope (Figure 22-5). The **fluorochrome method is the most sensitive method** because the specimen can be scanned rapidly under low magnification for fluorescent areas, and then the presence of acid-fast bacteria can be confirmed with higher magnification.

In approximately half of all culture-positive specimens, acid-fast bacteria are detected by microscopy. The sensitivity of this test is high for (1) respiratory specimens (particularly from patients with radiographic evidence of cavitation) and (2) specimens for which many mycobacteria are isolated in culture. Thus a positive acid-fast stain reaction corresponds to higher infectivity. The specificity of the test is greater than 95% when it is performed carefully.

Nucleic Acid–Based Tests

Although microscopy provides useful information regarding the presence of mycobacterial disease, it cannot identify the particular mycobacterial species involved. For this reason, techniques have been developed to detect specific mycobacterial nucleic acid sequences present in clinical specimens. Because only a few bacteria may be present, commercial companies have developed a variety of nucleic acid amplification techniques (e.g., polymerase chain reaction [PCR]). The commercial assays currently used are specific for *M. tuberculosis* and one currently available assay can detect *M. tuberculosis* in clinical specimens as well as determine susceptibility to rifampin, a surrogate marker for multidrug-resistant strains. Although this test is expensive and use in resource-limited countries is subsidized by global funding programs, the test allows rapid, routine testing in countries with a high incidence of disease and where microscopy is inaccurate and culture is impractical.

Culture

Mycobacteria that cause pulmonary disease, particularly in patients with evidence of cavitation, are abundant in the respiratory secretions (e.g., 10^8 bacilli per milliliter or more). Recovery of the organisms is virtually assured in patients from whom early morning respiratory specimens are collected for 3 consecutive days; however, it is more difficult to isolate *M. tuberculosis* from other sites in patients with disseminated disease (e.g., genitourinary tract, tissues, cerebrospinal fluid). In such cases, additional specimens must be collected for cultures, and a large volume of fluid or tissue must be processed.

The in vitro growth of mycobacteria is complicated by the fact that most isolates grow slowly and can be obscured by the rapidly growing bacteria that normally colonize people. Thus specimens such as sputum are initially treated with a **decontaminating reagent** (e.g., 2% sodium hydroxide) to eliminate organisms that could confound results. Mycobacteria can tolerate brief alkali treatment that kills the rapidly growing bacteria and permits selective isolation of mycobacteria. Extended decontamination of the specimen kills mycobacteria, so the procedure is not performed when normally sterile specimens are being tested or when few mycobacteria are expected.

Specimens inoculated onto egg-based (e.g., **Löwenstein-Jensen**) and agar-based (e.g., **Middlebrook**) media generally take 4 or more weeks for *M. tuberculosis* to be detected. However, this time has been shortened approximately 2 weeks through the use of specially formulated **broth cultures** that support the rapid growth of most mycobacteria. The ability of *M. tuberculosis* to grow rapidly in broth cultures has been used for performing rapid susceptibility tests. The technique, **MODS** or ***m**icroscopic **o**bservation **d**rug **s**usceptibility* **assay,** uses an inverted light microscope to examine 24-well plates inoculated with Middlebrook broth and decontaminated sputum. *M. tuberculosis* growth can be detected as tangles or cords of growth in the broth, generally after 1 week of incubation. Incorporation of antimycobacterial drugs in the broth enables rapid, direct susceptibility testing with clinical specimens. This technique is widely available in laboratories servicing resource-limited countries where drug-resistant strains of *M. tuberculosis* are widespread.

Identification

Growth properties and colonial morphology can be used for the preliminary identification of the most common species of mycobacteria. The definitive identification of mycobacteria can be made using a variety of techniques. Biochemical tests were the standard method for identifying mycobacteria; however, the results are not available for at least 3 weeks or more, and many species cannot be differentiated by this approach. Species-specific molecular probes, amplification of species-specific target genes (e.g., *16S rRNA* gene, *SecA* gene), and most recently mass spectrometry are used now for mycobacterial identification. It is likely that mass spectrometry will become the identification test of choice because of the rapid time to results (<1 hour), low cost, and ability to identify virtually all species of acid-fast organisms.

Treatment, Prevention, and Control

Treatment

Treatment of *M. tuberculosis* infections, unlike those for most other bacterial infections, is complex. Slow-growing mycobacteria are resistant to most antibiotics used to treat other bacterial infections, and in general, patients must take multiple antibiotics for an extended period (e.g., minimum of 6 to 9 months) or else antibiotic-resistant strains will develop. In 1990, the first outbreaks of **multidrug-resistant *M. tuberculosis* (MDR TB;** resistant to at least isoniazid and rifampin) were observed in patients with acquired immunodeficiency syndrome (AIDS) and in homeless persons in New York City and Miami. Although there has been a reduction in the United States of infections with these resistant strains, they are increasing dramatically in prevalence in resource-limited countries. In addition, strains of highly resistant *M. tuberculosis* called **extensively drug-resistant (XDR) TB** have emerged in most regions of the world. These strains, defined as MDR TB that are resistant to fluoroquinolones and at least one of the second-line drugs (e.g., kanamycin, amikacin, capreomycin), are potentially untreatable.

The various treatment regimens that have been developed for drug-susceptible and drug-resistant tuberculosis are too complex to review here comprehensively (refer to the reference citations and the Centers for Disease Control and Prevention [CDC] website: www.cdc.gov/tb/). Most treatment regimens begin with 2 months of isoniazid (isonicotinylhydrazine [INH]), ethambutol, pyrazinamide, and rifampin, followed by 4 to 6 months of INH and rifampin or alternative combination drugs. Modifications to this treatment scheme are dictated by the drug susceptibility of the isolate and the patient population.

Chemoprophylaxis

The American Thoracic Society and the CDC have examined a number of prophylactic regimens for use in patients (HIV positive and HIV negative) exposed to *M. tuberculosis.* The regimens that have been recommended include daily or twice weekly INH for 6 to 9 months, or daily rifampin for 4 months. Patients who have been exposed to drug-resistant *M. tuberculosis* should receive prophylaxis with pyrazinamide and either ethambutol or levofloxacin for 6 to 12 months.

Immunoprophylaxis

Vaccination with attenuated *M. bovis* **(BCG)** is commonly used in countries where tuberculosis is endemic and is responsible for significant morbidity and mortality. This practice can lead to a significant reduction in the incidence of tuberculosis if BCG is administered to people when they are young (it is less effective in adults). Unfortunately, BCG immunization cannot be used in immunocompromised patients (e.g., those with HIV infection). Thus it is unlikely to be useful in countries with a high prevalence of HIV infections (e.g., Africa) or to control the spread of drug-resistant tuberculosis. An additional problem with BCG immunization is that positive skin test reactivity develops in all patients and may persist for a prolonged time. However, skin test reactivity is generally low, so a strongly reactive skin test (e.g., >20 mm of induration) is generally significant for recent exposure to *M. tuberculosis.* The second-generation IFN-γ release assays are not affected by BCG immunization, so they can be used for screening this population. BCG immunization is not widely used in the United States or in other countries where the incidence of tuberculosis is low.

Control

Because one third of the world's population is infected with *M. tuberculosis,* elimination of this disease is highly unlikely. Disease can be controlled, however, with a combination of active surveillance, prophylactic and therapeutic intervention, and careful case monitoring.

Other Slow-Growing Mycobacteria

Leprosy (also called **Hansen disease**) is caused by ***Mycobacterium leprae.*** Leprosy was first described in 600 BC and was recognized in the ancient civilizations of China, Egypt, and India. The global **prevalence of leprosy has fallen dramatically** with widespread use of effective therapy. More than 5 million cases were documented in 1985 and fewer than 300,000 cases 20 years later. Currently, 90% of the cases are in Brazil, Madagascar, Mozambique, Tanzania, and Nepal. In the United States, leprosy is uncommon, with only 64 cases reported in 2013. Most cases occur in California and Hawaii and primarily in immigrants from Mexico, Asia, Africa, and the Pacific Islands. Interestingly, leprosy is endemic in **armadillos** found in Texas and Louisiana, producing a disease similar to the highly infectious lepromatous form of leprosy in humans. Thus these armadillos represent a potential endemic focus in this country.

Leprosy is spread by person-to-person contact. Although the most important route of infection is unknown, it is believed that *M. leprae* is spread either through the inhalation of infectious aerosols or through skin contact with respiratory secretions and wound exudates. Because the bacteria multiply very slowly, the incubation period is prolonged, with symptoms developing as long as 20 years after infection. The clinical presentation of leprosy ranges from the tuberculoid form to the lepromatous form (Table 22-3). Patients with **tuberculoid leprosy** (also called **paucibacillary Hansen disease**) have a strong cellular immune reaction to the bacteria, with the induction of cytokine production that mediates macrophage activation, phagocytosis, and bacillary clearance. The tuberculoid form (Figure 22-6) is

Table 22-3 Clinical and Immunologic Manifestations of Leprosy

Features	Tuberculoid Leprosy	Lepromatous Leprosy
Skin lesions	Few erythematous or hypopigmented plaques with flat centers and raised, demarcated borders; peripheral nerve damage with complete sensory loss; visible enlargement of nerves	Many erythematous macules, papules, or nodules; extensive tissue destruction (e.g., nasal cartilage, bones, ears); diffuse nerve involvement with patchy sensory loss; lack of nerve enlargement
Histopathology	Infiltration of lymphocytes around center of epithelial cells; presence of Langhans cells; few or no acid-fast rods observed	Predominantly "foamy" macrophages with few lymphocytes; lack of Langhans cells; numerous acid-fast rods in skin lesions and internal organs
Infectivity	Low	High
Immune response	Delayed hypersensitivity reactivity to lepromin	Nonreactivity to lepromin
Immunoglobulin levels	Normal	Hypergammaglobulinemia
Erythema nodosum	Absent	Usually present

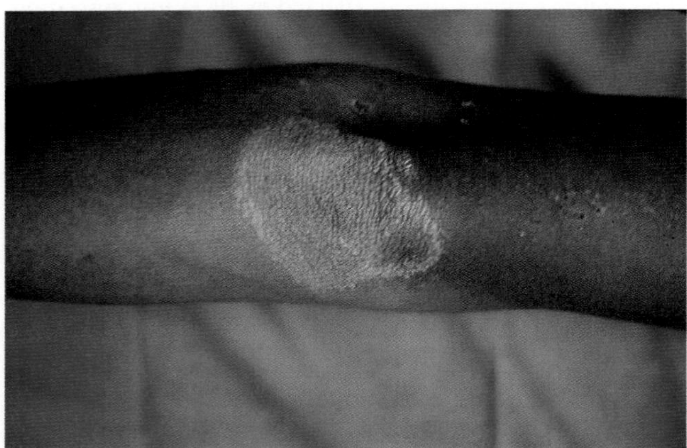

FIGURE 22-6 Tuberculoid leprosy. Early tuberculoid lesions are characterized by anesthetic macules with hypopigmentation. (From Cohen J, Powderly WG, Opal SM: *Infectious diseases,* ed 3, Philadelphia, 2010, Mosby.)

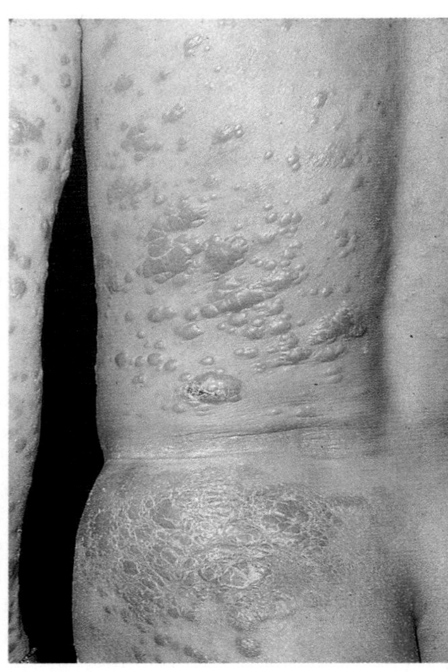

FIGURE 22-7 Lepromatous leprosy. Diffuse infiltration of the skin by multiple nodules of varying size, each with many bacteria. (From Cohen J, Powderly WG, Opal SM: *Infectious diseases,* ed 3, Philadelphia, 2010, Mosby.)

characterized by hypopigmented skin macules and diagnosed by reactive in skins tests to mycobacterial antigen (lepromin); acid-fast stains are generally negative. *M. leprae* cannot grow in cell-free cultures. Patients with **lepromatous leprosy (multibacillary Hansen disease)** have a strong antibody response but a specific defect in the cellular response to *M. leprae* antigens; thus an abundance of bacteria are typically observed in dermal macrophages and the Schwann cells of the peripheral nerves. As would be expected, this is the most infectious form of leprosy. The lepromatous form (Figure 22-7) is associated with disfiguring skin lesions, nodules, plaques, thickened dermis, and involvement of the nasal mucosa.

In the last decade, treatment of leprosy has successfully reduced the overall incidence of disease. The treatment regimens advanced by the WHO (http://WHO.int/lep) have distinguished between patients with the tuberculoid (paucibacillary) form and the lepromatous (multibacillary) form. The paucibacillary form should be treated with rifampicin and dapsone for a minimum of 6 months, whereas the multibacillary form should have clofazimine added to the regimen, and treatment should be extended to 12 months. It should be noted that many investigators believe much longer therapy is required for optimum management of patients. Single-drug treatment should not be used for either form.

Members of the ***Mycobacterium avium*** complex are among the most common pathogenic acid-fast species, particularly in immunocompromised patients, so a brief discussion of the taxonomy of this complex is important. Two species, *M. avium* and *M. intracellulare,* and four subspecies are recognized currently (Table 22-4). Most reports in the literature refer to *M. avium* or *M. avium* complex as a cause of human disease; however, it appears that the strains responsible for avian disease (*M. avium* subsp. *avium*) are distinct from the strains responsible for most human disease (*M. avium* subsp. *hominissuis*). *M. avium* subsp. *silvaticum* has not been implicated in human disease, and a large body of literature has debated the role of *M. avium* subsp. *paratuberculosis,* the etiologic agent of chronic granulomatous

Table 22-4 *Mycobacterium avium* Complex Diseases

Species	Disease
M. avium subsp. *avium*	Avian tuberculosis
M. avium subsp. *hominissuis*	Disease in humans and pigs; disseminated disease in HIV-infected patients; cervical lymphadenitis in children; chronic pulmonary disease in adolescents with cystic fibrosis and older adults with underlying pulmonary disease
M. avium subsp. *silvaticum*	Disease in wood pigeons
M. avium subsp. *paratuberculosis*	Chronic granulomatous enteric disease in ruminants (Johne disease) and possibly in humans (Crohn disease)
M. intracellulare	Pulmonary disease in immunocompetent patients

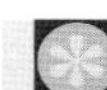

Clinical Case 22-2 *Mycobacterium avium* Infections

Woods and Goldsmith (*Chest* 95:1355–1357, 1989) described a patient with advanced AIDS who died of disseminated *M. avium* infection. The patient was a 27-year-old man who initially presented in October 1985 with a 2-week history of progressive dyspnea and a nonproductive cough. *Pneumocystis* was detected in a bronchoalveolar lavage, and serology confirmed the patient had an HIV infection. The patient was successfully treated with trimethoprim-sulfamethoxazole and discharged. The patient remained stable until May 1987, when he presented with persistent fever and dyspnea. Over the next week, he developed severe substernal chest pain and a pericardial friction rub. Echocardiogram revealed a small effusion. The patient left the hospital against medical advice but returned 1 week later with a persistent cough, fever, and pain in the chest and left arm. A diagnostic pericardiocentesis was performed, and 220 ml of fluid was aspirated. Tuberculous pericarditis was suspected, and appropriate antimycobacterial therapy was initiated. However, over the next 3 weeks, the patient developed progressive cardiac failure and died. *M. avium* was recovered from the pericardial fluid, as well as autopsy cultures of the pericardium, spleen, liver, adrenal glands, kidneys, small intestine, lymph nodes, and pituitary gland. Although *M. avium* pericarditis was unusual, the extensive dissemination of the mycobacteria in patients with advanced AIDS was common before azithromycin prophylaxis became widely used.

enteritis (Johne disease) in ruminants, as a cause of chronic granulomatous enteritis in humans (Crohn disease). These taxonomic differences are important for understanding the epidemiology and pathogenesis of the *M. avium* complex strains responsible for human disease. However, for the purpose of this text, I will only use the terms *M. avium* (*M. avium* subsp. *hominissuis*) and *M. avium* complex (*M. avium* and *M. intracellulare*).

Both species in the *M. avium* complex (MAC, a term commonly used today) produce disease in immunocompetent patients, whereas disease in HIV-infected patients is primarily caused by *M. avium*. Before the HIV epidemic, recovery of the organisms in clinical specimens typically represented transient colonization or, less commonly, chronic pulmonary disease. Pulmonary disease in immunocompetent patients presents in one of three forms. Most commonly, disease is seen in middle-age or older men with a history of smoking and **underlying pulmonary disease.** These patients typically have a slowly evolving cavitary disease that resembles tuberculosis on chest radiography. The second form of MAC infection is observed in elderly female nonsmokers. These patients have lingular or middle lobe infiltrates with a patchy, nodular appearance on radiography and associated bronchiectasis (chronically dilated bronchi). This form of disease is indolent and has been associated with significant morbidity and mortality. It has been postulated that this disease is seen primarily in fastidious elderly women who chronically suppress their cough reflex, leading to nonspecific inflammatory changes in the lungs and predisposing them to superinfection with MAC. This specific disease has been called **Lady Windermere syndrome,** the name of the principle character in an Oscar Wilde play. The third form of MAC disease is formation of a **solitary pulmonary nodule.** *M. avium* complex is the most common mycobacterial species that causes solitary the pulmonary nodules.

A different spectrum of disease develops in **patients with AIDS.** In contrast to disease in other groups of patients, MAC infection in patients with AIDS is typically disseminated, with virtually no organ spared (Clinical Case 22-2). The magnitude of these infections is remarkable; the tissues of some patients are literally filled with the mycobacteria (Figure 22-8), and there are hundreds to thousands of bacteria per milliliter of blood. Overwhelming disseminated infections with *M. avium* are particularly common in patients who are in the terminal stages of their immune disorder, when their CD4 T-lymphocyte counts fall to less than 10 cells/mm^3. Fortunately, with more effective antiretroviral therapy and the routine use of prophylactic antibiotics, *M. avium* disease infection in HIV-infected patients has become much less common. Although some patients with AIDS develop *M. avium* disease after pulmonary exposure (e.g., infectious aerosols of contaminated water), most infections are believed to develop after ingestion of the bacteria. Person-to-person transmission has not been demonstrated. After exposure to the mycobacteria, replication is initiated in localized lymph nodes followed by systemic spread. The clinical manifestations of disease are not observed until the mass of replicating bacteria impairs normal organ function.

M. avium complex and many other slow-growing mycobacteria are resistant to common antimycobacterial agents. One regimen recommended currently for MAC infections is clarithromycin or azithromycin, combined with ethambutol and rifampin. The duration of treatment and final selection of drugs for these species and other slow-growing mycobacteria are determined by (1) the response to therapy and (2) interactions among these drugs and other drugs the patient is receiving (e.g., toxic and pharmacokinetic interactions of these drugs with protease inhibitors used to treat HIV infection). Refer to the publication by Griffith and associates cited in the Bibliography for additional information about treating *M. avium* complex and other NTM infections. Because *M. avium* complex intracellular infections are common in patients with AIDS, chemoprophylaxis is recommended for patients whose CD4 T-cell counts fall to less than 50 cells/µl. Prophylaxis with clarithromycin or azithromycin is recommended. Combinations of these drugs with rifabutin have

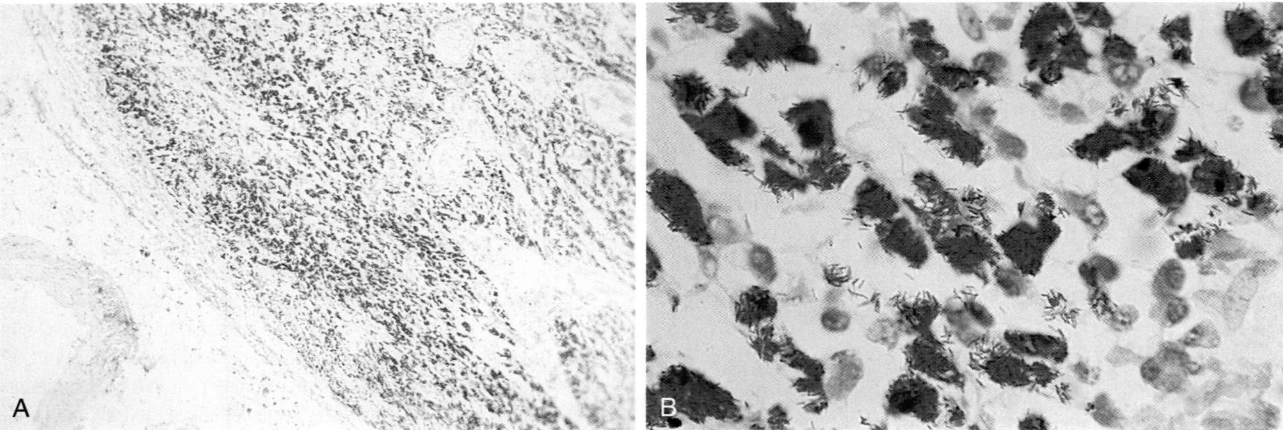

FIGURE 22-8 Tissue from a patient with acquired immunodeficiency syndrome who is infected with *Mycobacterium avium* complex, photographed under low **(A)** and high **(B)** magnification.

been used, but they are generally more toxic and no more effective than the single agent.

Many **other slow-growing mycobacteria** can cause human disease and new species continue to be reported as better diagnostic test methods are developed. The spectrum of diseases produced by these mycobacteria also continues to expand, in large part because diseases such as AIDS, malignancies, and organ transplantation with concomitant use of immunosuppressive drugs have created a population of patients who are highly susceptible to organisms with relatively low virulence potential. Some mycobacteria produce disease identical to pulmonary tuberculosis (e.g., *Mycobacterium bovis, M. kansasii*), other species commonly cause infections localized to lymphatic tissue *(Mycobacterium scrofulaceum)*, and others that grow optimally at cool temperatures primarily produce cutaneous infections *(Mycobacterium ulcerans, M. marinum, Mycobacterium haemophilum)*. However, disseminated disease can be observed in patients with AIDS who are infected with these same species, as well as with relatively uncommon mycobacteria (e.g., *Mycobacterium genavense, Mycobacterium simiae*). With the exception of *M. bovis* and other mycobacteria closely related to *M. tuberculosis*, person-to-person spread of these mycobacteria does not occur.

Clinical Case 22-3 Mycobacterial Infections Associated with Nail Salons

In September 2000 (Winthrop KL et al: *N Engl J Med* 346:1366–1371, 2002) a physician reported to the California Department of Health four female patients who developed lower extremity furunculosis. Each patient presented with small erythematous papules that became large, tender, fluctuant, violaceous boils over several weeks. Bacterial cultures of the lesions were negative, and the patients failed empirical antibacterial therapy. All of the patients had visited the same nail salon before the furuncles developed. As a result of the investigation of the nail salon, a total of 110 patients with furunculosis were identified. *Mycobacterium fortuitum* was cultured from the lesions from 32 patients, as well as from the footbaths used by the patients before their pedicures. Shaving the legs was identified as a risk factor for disease. Similar outbreaks have been reported in the literature, which illustrates the risks associated with contamination of waters with rapidly growing mycobacteria; the difficulties of confirming these infections by routine bacterial cultures, which are typically incubated for only 1 to 2 days; and the need for effective antibiotic therapy.

• Rapidly Growing Mycobacteria

As discussed previously, NTM can be subdivided into slow-growing species and rapidly growing species (growth in <7 days). This distinction is important because the rapidly growing species have a relatively low virulence potential, stain irregularly with traditional mycobacterial stains, and are more susceptible to "conventional" antibacterial antibiotics than to drugs used to treat other mycobacterial infections. The most common species associated with disease are *M. fortuitum, M. chelonae, M. abscessus,* and *M. mucogenicum*.

The rapidly growing mycobacteria rarely cause disseminated infections. Rather, they are most commonly associated with disease occurring after bacteria are introduced into the deep subcutaneous tissues by **trauma or iatrogenic infections** (e.g., infections associated with an intravenous catheter, contaminated wound dressing, prosthetic device such as a heart valve, peritoneal dialysis, or bronchoscopy). Unfortunately, the incidence of infections with these organisms is increasing as more invasive procedures are performed in hospitalized patients and advanced medical care lengthens the life expectancy of immunocompromised patients. Opportunistic infections in immunocompetent patients are becoming commonplace (Clinical Case 22-3).

Unlike the slow-growing mycobacteria, the rapidly growing species are resistant to most commonly used antimycobacterial agents but are susceptible to antibiotics such as clarithromycin, imipenem, amikacin, cefoxitin, and the sulfonamides. The specific activity of these agents must be determined with in vitro tests. Because infections with these mycobacteria are generally confined to the skin or are associated with prosthetic devices, surgical debridement or removal of the prosthesis is also necessary.

Nocardia

Physiology and Structure

Nocardiae are strict aerobic rods that form branched filaments in tissues and culture. These filaments resemble the hyphae formed by molds, and at one time *Nocardia* was thought to be a fungus; however, the organisms have a gram-positive cell wall and other cellular structures that are characteristic of bacteria. Most isolates stain poorly with the Gram stain and appear to be gram-negative, with intracellular gram-positive beads (Figure 22-9). The reason for this staining property is that nocardiae have a cell wall structure with branched-chain fatty acids (e.g., **tuberculostearic acid,** *meso*-diaminopimelic acid [*meso*-DAP], mycolic acids). The length of the mycolic acids in nocardiae (50 to 62 carbon atoms) is shorter than in mycobacteria (70 to 90 carbon atoms). This difference may explain why even though both genera stain acid-fast, *Nocardia* is described as **"weakly acid-fast"**; that is, a weak decolorizing solution of hydrochloric acid must be used to demonstrate the acid-fast property of nocardiae (Figure 22-10). This acid-fastness is also a helpful characteristic for distinguishing *Nocardia* organisms from morphologically similar organisms such as *Actinomyces.*

Nocardia species are catalase-positive, use carbohydrates oxidatively, and can grow on most nonselective laboratory media used for the isolation of bacteria, mycobacteria, and fungi. However, their growth is slow, requiring 3 to 5 days of incubation before colonies may be observed on the culture plates, so the laboratory should be notified that the cultures should be incubated beyond the normal 1 to 2 days. The colonies initially appear white but can be quite variable (e.g., dry to waxy, white to orange; Figure 22-11). Aerial hyphae (hyphae that protrude upward from the surface of a colony) are usually observed when the colonies are viewed with a dissecting microscope (Figure 22-12). The combination of both **presence of aerial hyphae and acid-fastness is unique** to the genus *Nocardia* and can be used as a rapid test for identification of the genus.

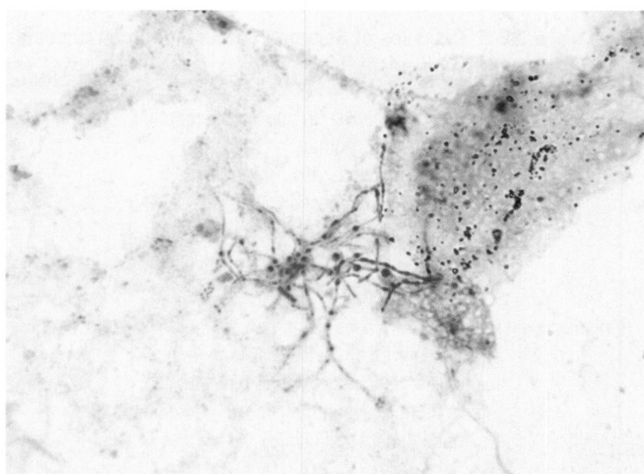

FIGURE 22-10 Acid-fast stain of *Nocardia* species in expectorated sputum. In contrast with the mycobacteria, members of the genus *Nocardia* do not uniformly retain the stain ("partially acid-fast").

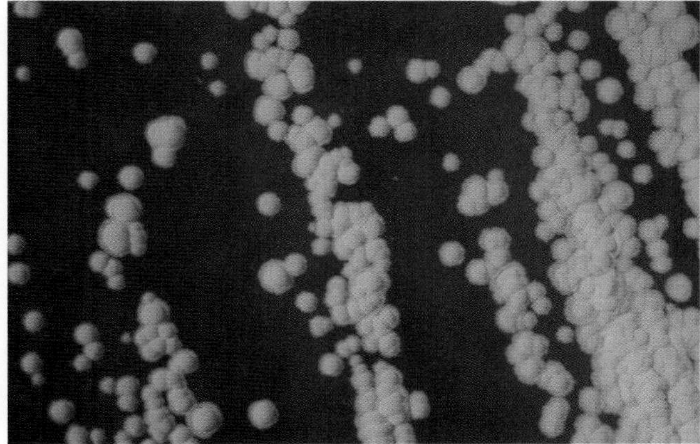

FIGURE 22-11 Colonies of *Nocardia.*

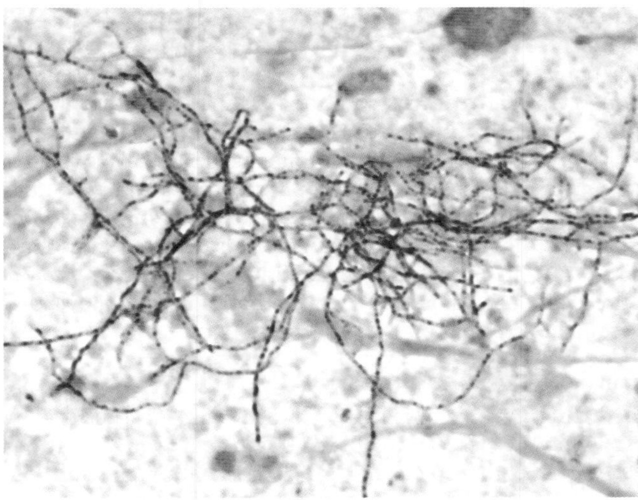

FIGURE 22-9 Gram stain of *Nocardia* in expectorated sputum. Note the delicate beaded filaments.

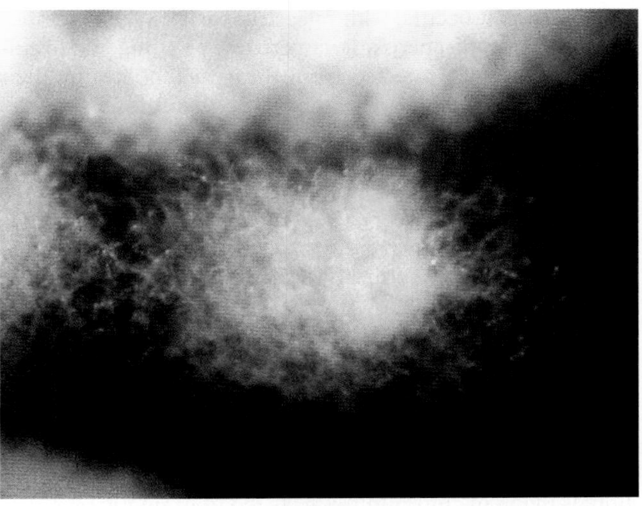

FIGURE 22-12 Aerial hyphae of *Nocardia.*

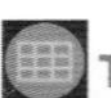 Table 22-5 Diseases of Selected Pathogenic Actinomycetes

Organism	Diseases	Frequency
Nocardia	Pulmonary diseases (bronchitis, pneumonia, lung abscesses); primary or secondary cutaneous infections (e.g., mycetoma, lymphocutaneous infections, cellulitis, subcutaneous abscesses); secondary central nervous system infections (e.g., meningitis, brain abscesses)	Common
Rhodococcus	Pulmonary diseases (pneumonia, lung abscesses); disseminated diseases (e.g., meningitis, pericarditis); opportunistic infections (e.g., wound infections, peritonitis, traumatic endophthalmitis)	Uncommon
Gordonia	Opportunistic infections	Rare
Tsukamurella	Opportunistic infections	Rare

 Box 22-2 Nocardiosis: Clinical Summaries

Bronchopulmonary disease: indolent pulmonary disease with necrosis and abscess formation; dissemination to central nervous system or skin is common

Mycetoma: chronic destructive progressive disease, generally of extremities, characterized by suppurative granulomas, progressive fibrosis and necrosis, and sinus tract formation

Lymphocutaneous disease: primary infection or secondary spread to cutaneous site, characterized by chronic granuloma formation and erythematous subcutaneous nodules, with eventual ulcer formation

Cellulitis and subcutaneous abscesses: granulomatous ulcer formation with surrounding erythema but minimal or no involvement of the draining lymph nodes

Brain abscess: chronic infection with fever, headache, and focal deficits related to the location of the slowly developing abscess(es)

The taxonomic classification of this genus is—simply stated—a mess, with most of the organisms described in the literature now recognized as incorrectly identified. Historically, these organisms were classified by their ability to utilize carbohydrates and decompose a variety of substrates, as well as their antimicrobial susceptibility patterns. The true taxonomic relationships among the members of the genus were appreciated only recently through the use of gene sequencing. Currently, more than 150 species have been identified, far more than what is identified by biochemical testing. Fortunately, most infections are caused by a relatively few species, and identification of this group of organisms at the genus level combined with in vitro susceptibility testing is sufficient for the management of most patients (Table 22-5).

Pathogenesis and Immunity

Although toxins and hemolysins have been described for nocardiae, the role these factors play in disease has not been defined. It would appear that the primary factor associated with virulence is the ability of pathogenic strains to **avoid phagocytic killing.** When phagocytes contact microbes, an oxidative burst occurs, with release of toxic oxygen metabolites (i.e., hydrogen peroxide, superoxide). Pathogenic strains of nocardiae are protected from these metabolites by their secretion of **catalase** and **superoxide dismutase.** Surface-associated superoxide dismutase also protects the bacteria. Nocardiae are also able to survive and **replicate in macrophages** by (1) preventing fusion of the phagosome-lysosome (mediated by **cord factor**), (2) preventing acidification of the phagosome, and (3) avoiding acid phosphatase–mediated killing by metabolic utilization of the enzyme as a carbon source.

Epidemiology

Nocardia infections are **exogenous** (i.e., caused by organisms not normally part of the normal human flora). The ubiquitous presence of the organism in soil rich with organic matter and the increasing numbers of immunocompromised individuals living in communities have led to dramatic increases in disease caused by this organism. The increase is particularly noticeable in high-risk populations, such as ambulatory patients who are infected with HIV or have other T-cell deficiencies, patients receiving immunosuppressive therapy for bone marrow or solid organ transplants, and immunocompetent patients with pulmonary function compromised by bronchitis, emphysema, asthma, bronchiectasis, and alveolar proteinosis. Bronchopulmonary disease develops after the initial colonization of the upper respiratory tract by inhalation and then aspiration of oral secretions into the lower airways. Primary cutaneous nocardiosis develops after traumatic introduction of organisms into subcutaneous tissues, and secondary cutaneous involvement typically follows dissemination from a pulmonary site.

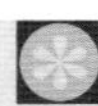 Clinical Case 22-4 Disseminated Nocardiosis

Shin and associates (*Transplant Infect Dis* 8:222–225, 2006) described a 63-year-old man who received a liver transplant for liver cirrhosis caused by hepatitis C. The patient was treated with immunosuppressive drugs, including tacrolimus and prednisone for 4 months, at which time he returned to the hospital with fever and lower leg pain. Although the chest radiograph was normal, ultrasound revealed an abscess in the soleus muscle. Poorly staining gram-positive rods were observed in the Gram stain of the pus aspirated from the abscess, and *Nocardia* grew after 3 days of incubation. Treatment with imipenem was started; however, the patient developed convulsions 10 days later and partial left-sided paralysis. Brain imaging studies revealed three lesions. Treatment was switched to ceftriaxone and amikacin. The subcutaneous abscess and brain lesions gradually improved, and the patient was discharged after 55 days of hospitalization. This patient illustrates the propensity of *Nocardia* to infect immunocompromised patients and disseminate to the brain, the slow rate of growth of the organism in culture, and the related need for prolonged treatment.

Clinical Diseases (Box 22-2)

Bronchopulmonary disease (Clinical Case 22-4) caused by *Nocardia* species cannot be distinguished from infections caused by other pyogenic organisms, although *Nocardia* infections tend to develop more slowly, and primary pulmonary disease caused by *Nocardia* occurs almost always in immunocompromised patients. Signs such as cough, dyspnea, and fever are usually present but are not diagnostic. Cavitation and spread into the pleura are common. Although the clinical picture is not specific for *Nocardia,* these organisms should be considered when immunocompromised patients experience pneumonia with cavitation, particularly if there is evidence of dissemination to the central nervous system (CNS) or subcutaneous tissues. If a pulmonary or disseminated *Nocardia* infection is diagnosed in an individual with no underlying disease, then a comprehensive immunologic workup is indicated.

Cutaneous infections may be primary infections (e.g., mycetoma, lymphocutaneous infections, cellulitis, subcutaneous abscesses) or from the result of the secondary spread of organisms from a primary pulmonary infection. **Mycetoma** is a painless, chronic infection primarily of the feet, characterized by localized subcutaneous swelling with involvement of the underlying tissues, muscle, and bone; suppuration; and the formation of multiple sinus tracts (narrow path from the focus of infection to the skin surface). A variety of organisms can cause mycetoma, although *Nocardia brasiliensis* is the most common cause in North America, Central America, and South America. **Lymphocutaneous infections** can manifest as cutaneous nodules and ulcerations along the lymphatics and regional lymph node involvement. These infections resemble cutaneous infections caused by some species of mycobacteria and by the fungus *Sporothrix schenckii. Nocardia* can also cause **chronic ulcerative lesions, subcutaneous abscesses,** and **cellulitis** (Figure 22-13).

As many as one third of all patients with *Nocardia* infections have dissemination to the brain, most commonly involving the formation of single or multiple **brain abscesses.** The disease can present initially as chronic meningitis.

Laboratory Diagnosis

Multiple sputum specimens should be collected from patients with pulmonary disease. Because nocardiae are usually distributed throughout the tissue and abscess material, it is relatively easy to detect them by microscopy and to recover them in culture of specimens from patients with pulmonary, cutaneous, or CNS disease. The delicate hyphae of *Nocardia* in tissues cause them to resemble *Actinomyces* organisms; however, in contrast with *Actinomyces*, nocardiae are typically weakly acid-fast (see Figure 22-10).

The organisms grow on most laboratory media incubated in an atmosphere of 5% to 10% carbon dioxide, but the presence of these slow-growing organisms may be obscured by more rapidly growing commensal bacteria. If a specimen is potentially contaminated with other bacteria (e.g., oral bacteria in sputum), selective media should be inoculated. Success has been achieved with the medium used for the isolation of *Legionella* species **(buffered charcoal yeast extract [BCYE] agar).** Indeed, this medium can be used to recover both *Nocardia* and *Legionella* from pulmonary specimens. *Nocardia* occasionally grows on media used for the isolation of mycobacteria and fungi; however, this method is less reliable than the use of special bacterial media. It is important to notify the laboratory that nocardiosis is suspected so the culture plates are held for additional days.

The preliminary identification of *Nocardia* is uncomplicated. Members of the genus can be classified initially on the basis of the presence of **filamentous, weakly acid-fast bacilli** and **aerial hyphae** on the colony surface. Definitive identification at the species level is more difficult because most species cannot be identified accurately by biochemical tests, although many laboratories continue to use these tests. Accurate identification of *Nocardia* requires molecular analysis of ribosomal ribonucleic acid (RNA) genes and "housekeeping" genes (e.g., heat shock protein gene) or use of mass spectrometry. Although mass spectrometry has only recently been introduced into diagnostic microbiology laboratories, this is rapidly becoming the method of choice for identification of these organisms.

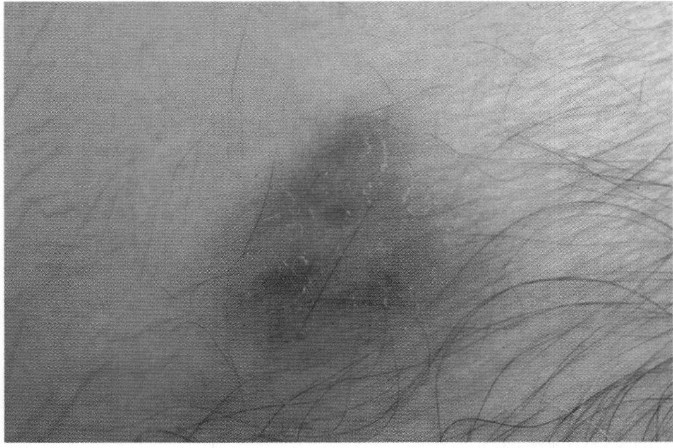

FIGURE 22-13 Cutaneous lesion caused by *Nocardia.* (From Cohen J, Powderly WG, Opal SM: *Infectious diseases,* ed 3, Philadelphia, 2010, Mosby.)

Treatment, Prevention, and Control

Antibiotics with activity against *Nocardia* include trimethoprim-sulfamethoxazole (TMP-SMX), amikacin, imipenem, and broad-spectrum cephalosporins (e.g., ceftriaxone, cefotaxime). Because antibiotic susceptibility can vary among individual isolates, antimicrobial susceptibility tests should be performed to guide specific therapy. TMP-SMX can be used as initial empirical therapy for cutaneous infections in immunocompetent patients. Antibiotic therapy for severe infections and cutaneous infections in immunocompromised patients should include two or three antibiotics, such as TMP-SMX plus amikacin for pulmonary or cutaneous infections and TMP-SMX plus imipenem or a cephalosporin for CNS infections. Because *Nocardia* grows slowly and is associated with therapeutic relapses, prolonged treatment (up to 12 months) is recommended. Whereas the clinical response is favorable in patients with localized infections, the prognosis is poor for immunocompromised patients with disseminated disease.

Nocardiae are ubiquitous, so it is impossible to avoid exposure to them. However, bronchopulmonary disease caused by nocardiae is uncommon in immunocompetent persons, and primary cutaneous infections can be prevented with proper wound care. The complications associated with disseminated disease can be minimized if nocardiosis is considered in the differential diagnosis for immunocompromised patients with cavitary pulmonary disease and promptly treated.

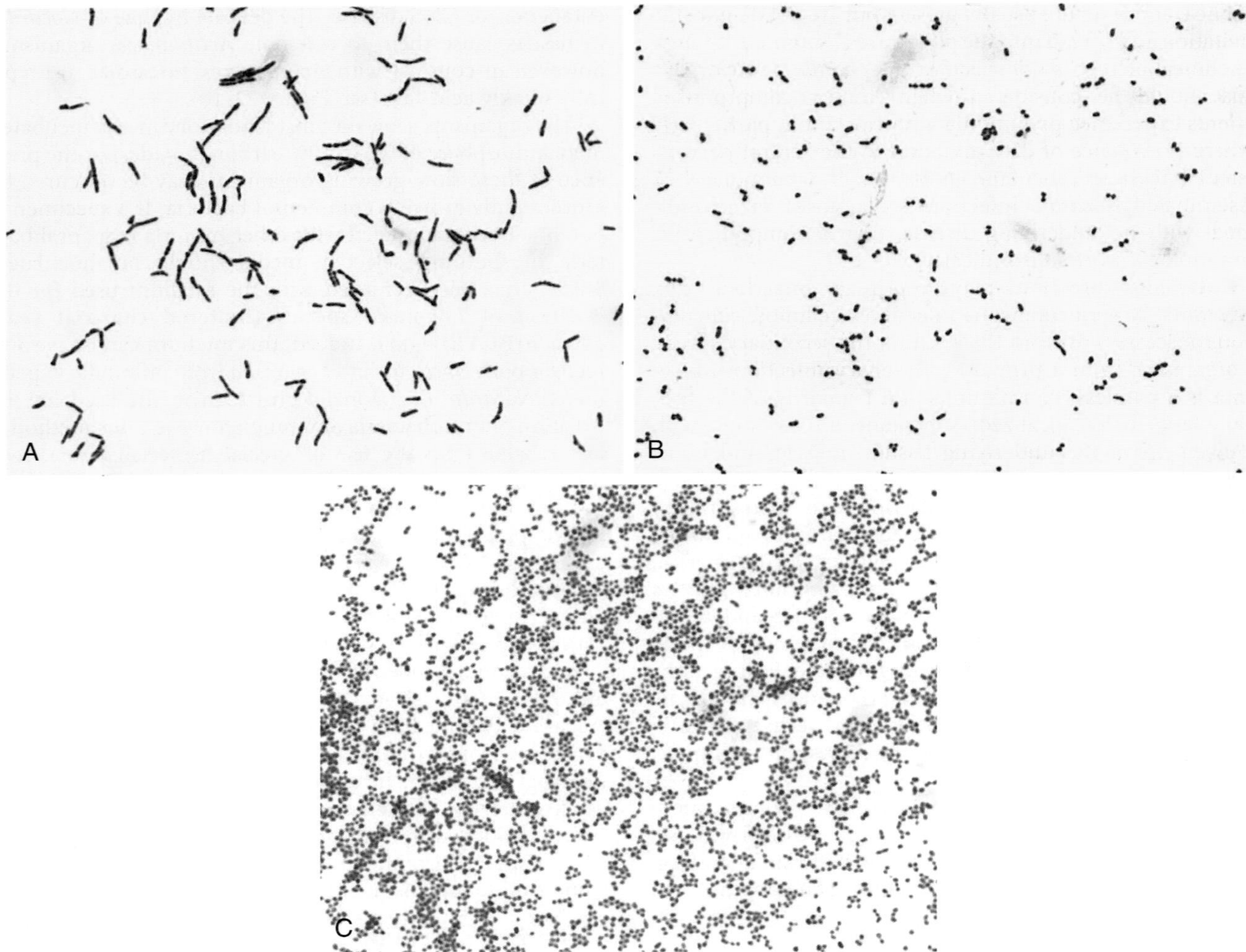

FIGURE 22-14 *Rhodococcus.* **A,** Gram stain after growth in nutrient broth for 4 hours. **B,** Gram stain after growth in nutrient broth for 18 hours. **C,** Acid-fast stain of organisms grown on mycobacterial Middlebrook agar for 2 days (note the paucity of red "acid-fast" cells).

• Other Weakly Acid-Fast Bacteria

The genus *Rhodococcus* consists of gram-positive acid-fast bacteria that initially appear rodlike and then revert to coccoid forms (Figure 22-14). Rudimentary branching may be present, but the delicate, branching, filamentous forms commonly seen with nocardiae are not observed with rhodococci. Of the species currently recognized, ***Rhodococcus equi*** is the most important human pathogen. Originally, *R. equi* (formerly *Corynebacterium equi*) was considered a veterinary pathogen, particularly in herbivores, that occasionally caused occupational disease in farmers and veterinarians. However, this organism has become an increasingly more common **pathogen of immunocompromised patients** (e.g., patients infected with HIV, transplant recipients). Interestingly, most infected patients do not have a history of contact with grazing animals or of exposure to soil contaminated with herbivore manure. The rise in the incidence of human infection is most likely related to the increase in the number of patients with immunosuppressive diseases, particularly AIDS, and to the enhanced awareness of the organism. It is likely that many isolates were ignored previously or were misidentified as insignificant coryneform bacteria.

Similar to *Nocardia, R. equi* is a facultative, intracellular organism that survives in macrophages and causes granulomatous inflammation that leads to **abscess formation.** Although numerous putative virulence factors have been identified, the precise pathophysiology of the infection is incompletely understood. Individuals with depressed production of IFN-γ appear to be unable to clear bacteria from lung infections.

Immunocompromised patients most typically present with **invasive pulmonary disease** (e.g., pulmonary nodules, consolidation, lung abscesses), and evidence of dissemination in the blood to distal sites (lymph nodes, meninges, pericardium, and skin) is commonly observed. Rhodococci usually cause **opportunistic infections in immunocompetent patients** (e.g., posttraumatic cutaneous infections, peritonitis in patients undergoing long-term dialysis, traumatic endophthalmitis).

Rhodococci grow on nonselective media incubated aerobically, but the characteristic salmon-pink pigment may not be obvious for at least 4 days. Colonies are typically **mucoid,** although dry forms may also be seen. The organisms can be identified initially by their slow growth, macroscopic and microscopic morphology, and ability to weakly retain the **acid-fast** stain (acid-fastness observed primarily when organisms are grown on media for mycobacteria). Definitive identification at the species level is problematic; organisms are relatively inert, so biochemical tests are not useful. Similar to *Nocardia,* accurate identification at the species level requires either gene sequencing or protein profiling by mass spectrometry.

Rhodococcus infections are difficult to treat. Although in vitro tests and tests in animal models have identified specific combinations of effective drugs, only limited success has been realized in the treatment of human infections, particularly in immunocompromised patients with low CD4 cell counts (50% mortality) compared with immunocompetent patients (20% mortality). The current recommendation for treating localized infections in immunocompetent patients is to use either an extended-spectrum macrolide (e.g., azithromycin, clarithromycin) or fluoroquinolone (e.g., levofloxacin). Disseminated infections and infections in immunocompromised patients should be managed with combinations of two or more antibiotics, with at least one with excellent penetration into macrophages (e.g., vancomycin, imipenem, aminoglycosides, levofloxacin, rifampin, ciprofloxacin). Penicillins and cephalosporins should not be used, because resistance to these agents is common in rhodococci, and the effectiveness of any antibiotic must be confirmed by in vitro testing.

Gordonia and ***Tsukamurella*** were previously classified with *Rhodococcus* because they are morphologically similar, contain mycolic acids, and are **partially acid-fast.** The organisms are present in soil and are rare opportunistic pathogens in humans. *Gordonia* has been associated with pulmonary and cutaneous infections, as well as nosocomial infections, such as those resulting from contaminated intravascular catheters. *Tsukamurella* has been associated with catheter infections. The significance of isolating either organism in clinical specimens must be evaluated carefully.

Bibliography

Ambrosioni J, Lew D, Garbino J: Nocardiosis: updated clinical review and experience at a tertiary center, *Infection* 38:89–97, 2010.

Appelberg R: Pathogenesis of *Mycobacterium avium* infection, *Immunol Res* 35:179–190, 2006.

Bouza E, Perez-Parra A, Rosal M, et al: *Tsukamurella*: a cause of catheter-related blood stream infections, *Eur J Clin Microbiol Infect Dis* 28:203–210, 2009.

Conville PS, Witebsky FG: *Nocardia, Rhodococcus, Gordonia, Actinomadura, Streptomyces,* and other aerobic actinomycetes. In Murray PR, et al, editors: *ASM manual of clinical microbiology*, ed 9, Washington, DC, 2007, American Society for Microbiology Press.

De Groote M, Huitt G: Infections due to rapidly growing mycobacteria, *Clin Infect Dis* 42:1756–1763, 2006.

Dodiuk-Gad R, Cohen E, Ziv M, et al: Cutaneous nocardiosis: report of two cases and review of the literature, *Internatl J Derm* 49:1380–1385, 2010.

Griffith DE, Aksamit T, Brown-Elliott BA, et al: An official ATS/IDSA statement: diagnosis, treatment, and prevention of nontuberculous mycobacterial diseases, *Am J Respir Crit Care Med* 175:367–416, 2007.

Ioerger TR, O'Malley T, Liao R, et al: Identification of new drug targets and resistance mechanisms in *Mycobacterium tuberculosis*, *PLoS ONE* 8:e75245, 2013.

Martinez R, Reyes S, Menendez R: Pulmonary nocardiosis: risk factors, clinical features, diagnosis and prognosis, *Curr Opin Pulm Med* 14:219–227, 2008.

Mazurek GH, Jereb J, Vernon A, et al: Updated guidelines for using interferon gamma release assays to detect *Mycobacterium tuberculosis* infection—United States, 2010, *MMWR Recomm Rep* 59(RR–5):1–25, 2010.

Perez-Velez C, Marais B: Tuberculosis in children, *N Engl J Med* 367:348–361, 2012.

Ramanan P, Deziel P, Wengenack N: *Gordonia* bacteremia, *J Clin Microbiol* 51:3443–3447, 2013.

See I, Nguyen DB, Chatterjee S, et al: Outbreak of *Tsukamurella* species bloodstream infection among patients at an oncology clinic, West Virginia, 2011-2012, *Infect Control Hosp Epidemiol* 35:300–306, 2014.

Turenne CY, Wallace R Jr, Behr MA: *Mycobacterium avium* in the postgenomic era, *Clin Microbiol Rev* 20:205–229, 2007.

Ulrichs T, Kaufmann S: New insights into the function of granulomas in human tuberculosis, *J Pathol* 208:261–269, 2006.

Wells CD, Cegielski JP, Nelson LJ, et al: HIV infection and multidrug-resistant tuberculosis—the perfect storm, *J Infect Dis* 196:S86–S107, 2007.

Yew W, Leung C: Update in tuberculosis 2006, *Am J Respir Crit Care Med* 175:541–546, 2007.

Zumla A, Raviglione M, Hafner R, et al: Tuberculosis, *N Engl J Med* 368:745–755, 2013.

CHAPTER 23 NEISSERIA AND RELATED GENERA

A 22-year-old woman was admitted to the hospital with a 1-day history of high fever, chills, and an erythematous maculopapular rash over her chest, arms, and legs. She had an elevated leukocyte count and sedimentation rate. Blood cultures drawn at the time of admission were positive 10 hours later with gram-negative diplococci. This patient most likely has an infection with either *Neisseria gonorrhoeae* or *Neisseria meningitidis,* because no other gram-negative bacteria will look like this. Additional tests will be required to determine which bacterium is responsible for this infection.

1. *N. gonorrhoeae* and *N. meningitidis* are the most important members of the genus *Neisseria.* How is this genus differentiated from other bacteria, and what growth properties distinguish these two species from other members of the genus?
2. What are the major virulence factors for each organism?
3. Why does a vaccine exist for *N. meningitidis* but not *N. gonorrhoeae?* What serogroup is not covered by the *N. meningitidis* vaccine, and why is this important?

Answers to these questions are available on StudentConsult.com.

• SUMMARIES CLINICALLY SIGNIFICANT ORGANISMS

Neisseria gonorrhoeae

Trigger Words

Diplococci, person-to-person, gonorrhea, arthritis, ophthalmia, drug resistance

Biology and Virulence

- Gram-negative diplococci with fastidious growth requirements
- Growth best at 35° C to 37° C in a humid atmosphere supplemented with CO_2
- Oxidase and catalase positive; acid produced from glucose oxidatively
- Outer surface with multiple antigens: pili protein; Por proteins; Opa proteins; Rmp protein; protein receptors for transferrin, lactoferrin, and hemoglobin; lipooligosaccharide; immunoglobulin protease; β-lactamase
- Refer to Table 23-2 for summary of virulence factors

Epidemiology

- Humans are the only natural hosts
- Carriage can be asymptomatic, particularly in women
- Transmission is primarily by sexual contact
- Almost 335,000 cases reported in United States in 2012 (true incidence of disease believed to be at least twice that); estimated 100 million new cases worldwide
- Disease most common in blacks, people aged 15 to 24 years, residents of southeastern United States, people who have multiple sexual encounters
- Higher risk of disseminated disease in patients with deficiencies in late components of complement

Diseases

- Refer to Box 23-1 for summary of clinical diseases

Diagnosis

- Gram stain of urethral specimens is accurate for symptomatic males only
- Culture is sensitive and specific but has been replaced with nucleic acid amplification assays in most laboratories

Treatment, Prevention, and Control

- Ceftriaxone with either azithromycin or doxycycline is currently the treatment of choice, although high-level resistance to cephalosporins has been observed
- For neonates, prophylaxis with 1% silver nitrate; ophthalmia neonatorum is treated with ceftriaxone
- Prevention consists of patient education, use of condoms or spermicides with nonoxynol-9 (only partially effective), and aggressive follow-up of sexual partners of infected patients
- Effective vaccines are not available

Neisseria meningitidis

Trigger Words

Diplococci, person-to-person, meningitis, meningococcemia, pneumonia, vaccine

Biology and Virulence

- Gram-negative diplococci with fastidious growth requirements
- Grows best at 35° C to 37° C in a humid atmosphere

- Oxidase and catalase positive; acid produced from carbohydrates oxidatively
- Outer surface antigens include polysaccharide capsule, pili, and lipooligosaccharides
- Capsule protects bacteria from antibody-mediated phagocytosis
- Specific receptors for meningococcal pili allow colonization of nasopharynx and replication; posttranslational modification of the pili enhances host cell penetration and person-to-person spread
- Bacteria can survive intracellular killing in the absence of humoral immunity
- Endotoxin mediates most clinical manifestations

Epidemiology

- Humans are the only natural hosts
- Person-to-person spread occurs via aerosolization of respiratory tract secretions
- Highest incidence of disease is in children younger than 5 years (particularly infants < 6 months of age), institutionalized people, and patients with late complement deficiencies
- Endemic and epidemic disease most commonly caused by serogroups A, B, C, W135, X, and Y; pneumonia most commonly caused by serogroups Y and W135; serogroups A and W135 associated with disease in underdeveloped countries
- Disease occurs worldwide, most commonly in the dry, cold months of the year

Diseases

- Refer to Box 23-1 for summary of clinical diseases

Diagnosis

- Gram stain of cerebrospinal fluid is sensitive and specific but is of limited value for blood specimens (too few organisms are generally present, except in overwhelming sepsis)
- Culture is definitive, but organism is fastidious and dies rapidly when exposed to cold or dry conditions
- Tests to detect meningococcal antigens are insensitive and nonspecific

Treatment, Prevention, and Control

- Breast-feeding infants have passive immunity (first 6 months)
- Empirical treatment of patients with suspected meningitis or bacteremia should be initiated with ceftriaxone; if the isolate is penicillin susceptible, treatment can be changed to penicillin G
- Chemoprophylaxis for contact with persons with the disease is with rifampin, ciprofloxacin, or ceftriaxone
- For immunoprophylaxis, vaccination is an adjunct to chemoprophylaxis; it is used only for serogroups A, C, Y, and W135; no effective vaccine is available for serogroup B; vaccination for serogroup A has been introduced in Africa

Three genera of medically important bacteria are in the family Neisseriaceae: ***Neisseria, Eikenella,*** and ***Kingella*** (Table 23-1). Other genera in the family are rarely associated with human disease and will not be discussed in this chapter. The genus *Neisseria* consists of 29 species with two species, ***Neisseria gonorrhoeae*** and ***Neisseria meningitidis,*** strictly human pathogens. Additional species are commonly present on mucosal surfaces of the oropharynx and nasopharynx and occasionally colonize the anogenital mucosal membranes. Diseases caused by *N. gonorrhoeae* and *N. meningitidis* are well known; the other *Neisseria* species have limited virulence and generally produce opportunistic infections (Box 23-1). ***Eikenella corrodens*** and ***Kingella kingae*** colonize the human oropharynx and are also opportunistic pathogens.

Neisseria gonorrhoeae and *Neisseria meningitidis*

Infections caused by *N. gonorrhoeae,* particularly the sexually transmitted disease gonorrhea, have been recognized for centuries. Despite effective antibiotic therapy, gonorrhea is still one of the most common sexually transmitted diseases in the United States. The presence of *N. gonorrhoeae* in a clinical specimen is always considered significant. In contrast, strains of *N. meningitidis* can colonize the nasopharynx of healthy people without producing disease or can cause community-acquired meningitis, overwhelming and rapidly fatal sepsis, or bronchopneumonia. The swift progression from good health to life-threatening disease produces fear and panic in communities, unlike the reaction to almost any other pathogen.

Physiology and Structure

Neisseria species are aerobic **gram-negative** bacteria, typically coccoid shaped (0.6 to 1.0 µm in diameter) and arranged in pairs **(diplococci)** with adjacent sides flattened together (resembling coffee beans [Figure 23-1]). All species are oxidase positive and most produce catalase, properties that combined with the Gram stain morphology allow a rapid, presumptive identification of a clinical isolate. Acid is produced by oxidation of carbohydrates (not by fermentation), a property that was historically used to differentiate *Neisseria* species. More rapid methods such as mass spectrometry are now used to identify these bacteria.

Pathogenic and nonpathogenic species of *Neisseria* can also be differentiated by their growth on blood agar and nutrient agar. Nonpathogenic strains grow on both media, *N. meningitidis* grows on blood agar and has variable growth on nutrient agar, and *N. gonorrhoeae* cannot grow on either media. All strains of *N. gonorrhoeae* require cystine and an energy source (e.g., glucose, pyruvate, lactate) for growth, and many strains require supplementation of media with amino acids, purines, pyrimidines, and vitamins. Soluble starch is added to the media to neutralize the toxic effect of the fatty acids. Thus *N. gonorrhoeae* only grows on enriched **chocolate agar** and other supplemented media. The optimum growth temperature is **35° C to 37° C**, with poor survival of the organism at cooler temperatures. A humid atmosphere supplemented with **5% carbon dioxide** is either required or enhances growth of *N. gonorrhoeae.* These growth properties have practical importance: unless the specimen is processed on appropriate enriched media, *N. gonorrhoeae* will not be recovered. Although the fastidious nature of this organism makes recovery from clinical specimens difficult, it is nevertheless easy for the organism to be transmitted sexually from person to person.

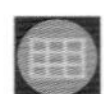

Table 23-1 Important Neisseriaceae

Organism	Historical Derivation
Neisseria	Named after the German physician Albert Neisser, who originally described the organism responsible for gonorrhea
N. gonorrhoeae	*gone,* seed; *rhoia,* a flow (a flow of seeds; reference to the disease gonorrhea)
N. meningitidis	*meningis,* the covering of the brain; *itis,* inflammation (inflammation of the meninges as in meningitis)
Eikenella	Named after M. Eiken, who first named the type species in this genus
E. corrodens	*corrodens,* gnawing or eating (reference to the observation that colonies of this species eat into the agar)
Kingella	Named after the American bacteriologist Elizabeth King

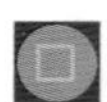

Box 23-1 Neisseriaceae: Clinical Summaries

Neisseria gonorrhoeae

Gonorrhea: characterized by purulent discharge for involved site (e.g., urethra, cervix, epididymis, prostate, rectum) after 2- to 5-day incubation period

Disseminated infections: spread of infection from genitourinary tract through blood to skin or joints; characterized by pustular rash with erythematous base and suppurative arthritis in involved joints

Ophthalmia neonatorum: purulent ocular infection acquired by neonate at birth

Neisseria meningitidis

Meningitis: purulent inflammation of meninges associated with headache, meningeal signs, and fever; high mortality rate unless promptly treated with effective antibiotics

Meningococcemia: disseminated infection characterized by thrombosis of small blood vessels and multiorgan involvement; small petechial skin lesions coalesce into larger hemorrhagic lesions

Pneumonia: milder form of meningococcal disease characterized by bronchopneumonia in patients with underlying pulmonary disease

Eikenella corrodens

Human bite wounds: infection associated with traumatic (e.g., bite, fistfight injury) introduction of oral organisms into deep tissue

Subacute endocarditis: infection of endocardium characterized by gradual onset of low-grade fevers, night sweats, and chills

Kingella kingae

Subacute endocarditis: as with *E. corrodens*

The cell wall structure of *N. gonorrhoeae* and *N. meningitidis* is typical of gram-negative bacteria, with the thin peptidoglycan layer sandwiched between the inner cytoplasmic membrane and the outer membrane. The major virulence factor for *N. meningitidis* is the polysaccharide capsule. Although the outer surface of *N. gonorrhoeae* is not covered with a true carbohydrate capsule, the cell surface of *N. gonorrhoeae* has a capsule-like negative charge. Antigenic differences in the **polysaccharide capsule** of *N. meningitidis* are the basis for serogrouping these bacteria in vitro and play a

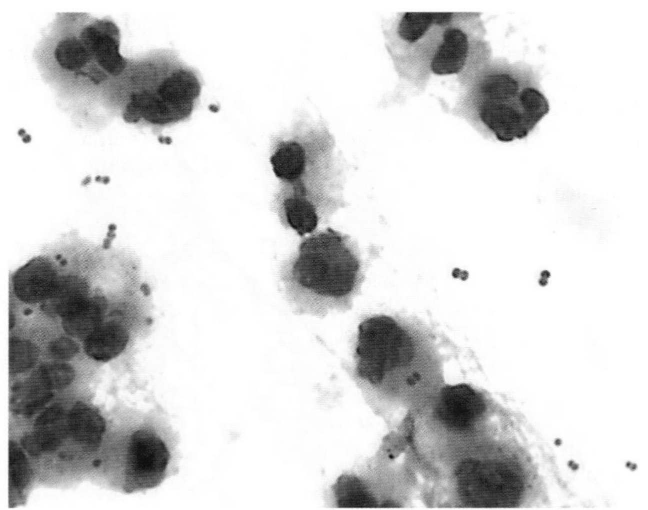

FIGURE 23-1 *Neisseria meningitidis* in cerebrospinal fluid. Note the spatial arrangement of the pairs of cocci with sides pressed together, which is characteristic of this genus.

prominent role in determining if an individual strain will cause disease. Thirteen serogroups are currently recognized, with 6 serogroups (A, B, C, W135, X, and Y) associated with endemic and epidemic disease.

Pathogenic and nonpathogenic strains of *Neisseria* have **pili** that extend from the cytoplasmic membrane through the outer membrane. Pili mediate a number of functions, including attachment to host cells, transfer of genetic material, and motility, and the presence of pili in *N. gonorrhoeae* and *N. meningitidis* appears to be important for pathogenesis, in part because the pili mediate attachment to nonciliated epithelial cells and provide resistance to killing by neutrophils. The pili are composed of repeating protein subunits **(pilins)** that have a conserved region at one end and a highly variable region at the exposed carboxyl terminus. The lack of immunity to reinfection with *N. gonorrhoeae* results partially from the antigenic variation among the pilin proteins and partially from the phase variation in pilin expression, factors that complicate attempts to develop effective vaccines for gonorrhea.

Other prominent families of proteins are present in the outer membrane. The **porin proteins** are integral outer membrane proteins that form pores or channels for nutrients to pass into the cell and waste products to exit. *N. gonorrhoeae* and *N. meningitidis* have two porin genes, *porA* and *porB.* The gene products, **PorA and PorB proteins,** are both expressed in *N. meningitidis,* but the *porA* gene is silent in *N. gonorrhoeae.* Thus not only is PorB the major outer membrane protein in *N. gonorrhoeae* (an estimated 60% of the gonococcal outer membrane proteins), but it must also be functionally active for *N. gonorrhoeae* to survive. This would seem to be a logical target for a vaccine; however, PorB is expressed as two distinct classes of antigens, PorB1A and PorB1B, with many distinct serologic variants. Thus, although the PorB protein is expressed in all gonococci, the large number of antigens and antigenic variation of this protein make it a poor target for vaccine development.

PorB is important for the virulence of *N. gonorrhoeae* because these proteins can interfere with degranulation of neutrophils (i.e., phagolysosome fusion that would lead to killing of intracellular bacteria) and presumably protect the bacteria from the host's inflammatory response. Additionally, PorB with other adhesins facilitates the bacterial invasion into epithelial cells. Finally, expression of some PorB antigens makes the bacteria resistant to complement-mediated serum killing.

Opa proteins (opacity proteins) are a family of membrane proteins that mediate intimate binding to epithelial and phagocytic cells and are important for cell-to-cell signaling. Multiple alleles of these proteins can be expressed by individual isolates. *N. gonorrhoeae* expressing the Opa proteins appear opaque when grown in culture (thus the source of the name). Opaque colonies are recovered most commonly in patients with localized disease (i.e., endocervicitis, urethritis, pharyngitis, proctitis), whereas transparent colonies are more commonly associated with pelvic inflammatory disease and disseminated infections.

The third group of proteins in the outer membrane is the highly conserved **Rmp proteins** (reduction-modifiable proteins). These proteins stimulate antibodies that interfere with the serum bactericidal activity against pathogenic neisseriae.

Iron is essential for the growth and metabolism of *N. gonorrhoeae* and *N. meningitidis.* These pathogenic neisseriae are able to compete with their human hosts for iron by **binding host cell transferrin** to specific bacterial surface receptors. The specificity of this binding for human transferrin is likely the reason these bacteria are strict human pathogens. The presence of this receptor is fundamentally different from most bacteria that synthesize siderophores to scavenge iron. The gonococci also have a variety of additional surface receptors for other host iron complexes, such as lactoferrin and hemoglobin.

Another major antigen in the cell wall is **lipooligosaccharide (LOS).** This antigen is composed of lipid A and a core oligosaccharide but lacks the O-antigen polysaccharide found in lipopolysaccharide (LPS) in most gram-negative rods. The lipid A moiety possesses endotoxin activity. Both *N. gonorrhoeae* and *N. meningitidis* spontaneously release **outer membrane blebs** during rapid cell growth. These blebs contain LOS and surface proteins and may act to both enhance endotoxin-mediated toxicity and protect replicating bacteria by binding protein-directed antibodies.

N. gonorrhoeae and *N. meningitidis* produce **immunoglobulin (Ig)A1 protease,** which cleaves the hinge region in IgA1. This action creates immunologically inactive Fc and Fab fragments. Some strains of *N. gonorrhoeae* also produce **β-lactamases** that can degrade penicillin.

Pathogenesis and Immunity (Table 23-2)

Gonococci attach to mucosal cells, penetrate into the cells and multiply, and then pass through the cells into the subepithelial space where infection is established. Pili, PorB, and Opa proteins mediate attachment and penetration into host cells. The gonococcal LOS stimulates release of the proinflammatory cytokine **tumor necrosis factor (TNF)-α,** which causes most of the symptoms associated with gonococcal disease.

IgG3 is the predominant IgG antibody formed in response to gonococcal infection. Although the antibody response to PorB is minimal, serum antibodies to pilin, Opa protein, and LOS are readily detected. Antibodies to LOS can activate complement, releasing complement component C5a, which has a chemotactic effect on neutrophils; however, IgG and secretory IgA1 antibodies directed against Rmp protein can block this bactericidal antibody response.

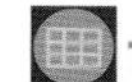
Table 23-2 Virulence Factors in *Neisseria gonorrhoeae*

Virulence Factor	Biological Effect
Pilin	Protein that mediates initial attachment to nonciliated human cells (e.g., epithelium of vagina, fallopian tube, and buccal cavity); interferes with neutrophil killing
Por protein	Porin protein: promotes intracellular survival by preventing phagolysosome fusion in neutrophils
Opa protein	Opacity protein: mediates firm attachment to eukaryotic cells
Rmp protein	Reduction-modifiable protein: protects other surface antigens (Por protein, lipooligosaccharide) from bactericidal antibodies
Transferrin-, lactoferrin-, and hemoglobin-binding proteins	Mediate acquisition of iron for bacterial metabolism
LOS	Lipooligosaccharide: has endotoxin activity
IgA1 protease	Destroys immunoglobulin A1 (role in virulence is unknown)
β-Lactamase	Hydrolyzes the β-lactam ring in penicillin

Experiments with nasopharyngeal tissue organ cultures have shown that meningococci attach selectively to specific receptors on nonciliated columnar cells of the nasopharynx. Presence of the capsule interferes with epithelial cell attachment, so synthesis is down-regulated before attachment. Following attachment, meningococci are able to multiply, forming large aggregates of bacteria anchored to the host cells. Within a few hours of attachment, the pili undergo posttranslational modification, leading to destabilization of the aggregates. This results in the enhanced ability of the bacteria to both penetrate into the host cells and release into the airways, and thus person-to-person spread is potentially increased.

Meningococcal disease occurs in patients who lack specific antibodies directed against the polysaccharide capsule and other expressed bacterial antigens. Infants are initially afforded protection by the passive transfer of maternal antibodies. When the infant has reached age 6 months, however, this protective immunity has waned, a finding consistent with the observation that the incidence of disease is greatest in children younger than 2 years. Immunity can be stimulated by colonization with *N. meningitidis* or other bacteria with cross-reactive antigens (e.g., colonization with nonencapsulated *Neisseria* species; exposure to *Escherichia coli* K1 antigen that cross-reacts with the group B capsular polysaccharide). Bactericidal activity also requires the existence of complement. Patients with **deficiencies in C5, C6, C7, or C8** of the complement system are estimated to be at a 6000-fold greater risk for meningococcal disease. Although immunity is mediated primarily by the humoral immune response, lymphocyte responsiveness to meningococcal antigens is markedly depressed in patients with acute disease.

Similar to *N. gonorrhoeae,* meningococci are internalized into phagocytic vacuoles and are able to avoid intracellular death, replicate, and then migrate to the subepithelial spaces. The polysaccharide capsule protects *N. meningitidis* from phagocytic destruction. The diffuse vascular damage associated with meningococcal infections (e.g., endothelial damage, inflammation of vessel walls, thrombosis, disseminated intravascular coagulation [DIC]) is largely attributed to the action of the **LOS endotoxin** present in the outer membrane.

Epidemiology

Gonorrhea occurs naturally only in humans; it has no other known reservoir. It is second only to chlamydia as the most commonly reported sexually transmitted disease in the United States. Infection rates are the same in males and females, are disproportionately higher in blacks than in Hispanic Americans and whites, and are highest in the southeastern United States. The peak incidence of the disease is in the age group 15 to 24 years. The incidence of disease generally declined after 1978, but the decrease slowed around 1996, and gonococcal infections have increased since 2010. In 2012, almost 335,000 new infections were reported in the United States. However, even this large number is an underestimation of the true incidence of disease, because diagnosis and reporting of infections are incomplete. Public health officials believe that at least half of new infections are not reported. The U.S. experience also pales in comparison with an estimate of greater than 100 million new cases of gonorrhea worldwide.

N. gonorrhoeae is transmitted primarily by sexual contact. Women have a 50% risk of acquiring the infection as the result of a single exposure to an infected man, whereas men have a risk of approximately 20% as the result of a single exposure to an infected woman. The risk of infection rises as the person has more sexual encounters with infected partners.

The major reservoir for gonococci is the asymptomatically infected person. Asymptomatic carriage is more common in women than in men. As many as half of all infected women have mild or asymptomatic infections, whereas most men are initially symptomatic. The symptoms generally clear within a few weeks in individuals with untreated disease, and asymptomatic carriage may then become established. The site of infection also determines whether carriage occurs, with rectal and pharyngeal infections more commonly asymptomatic than genital infections.

Endemic meningococcal disease occurs worldwide, and epidemics are common in developing countries. Epidemic spread of disease results from the introduction of a new virulent strain into an immunologically naïve population. Endemic disease and pandemics have been uncommon in developed countries since World War II. For example, in 2011 fewer than 800 cases of invasive meningococcal disease were reported in the United States; in contrast, almost 90,000 cases of meningitis were reported in 14 African countries in 2009. Of the 13 serogroups, almost all infections are caused by serogroups A, B, C, W135, X, and Y. In Europe and the Americas, serogroups B, C, and Y predominate in meningitis or meningococcemia; serogroup A is responsible for 80% to 85% of disease in the 26 countries comprising the sub-Saharan African meningitis belt (stretching from Senegal to Ethiopia); and W135 is responsible for an ongoing outbreak of meningitis in Chile. Serogroups Y and W135 are most commonly associated with meningococcal pneumonia.

N. meningitidis is transmitted by respiratory droplets among people in prolonged close contact, such as family members living in the same household and soldiers living together in military barracks. Classmates in schools and hospital employees are not considered close contacts and are not at significantly higher risk of acquiring the disease unless they are in direct contact with the respiratory secretions of an infected person.

Humans are the only natural carriers for *N. meningitidis.* Studies of asymptomatic carriage of *N. meningitidis* have shown tremendous variation in its prevalence, from less than 1% to almost 40%. The oral and nasopharyngeal carriage rates are highest for school-age children and young adults, are higher in lower socioeconomic populations (caused by person-to-person spread in crowded areas), and do not vary with the seasons, even though disease is most common during the dry, cold months of the year. Carriage is typically transient, with clearance occurring after specific antibodies develop. Disease is most common in children younger than age 5 (particularly infants less than age 6 months) and teenagers and young adults. People who are immunocompromised, the elderly, or those who live in closed populations (e.g., military barracks, prisons) are prone to infection during epidemics.

Clinical Diseases (see Box 23-1)

Neisseria gonorrhoeae

Gonorrhea

Genital infection in men is primarily restricted to the **urethra.** A purulent urethral discharge (Figure 23-2) and dysuria develop after a 2- to 5-day incubation period. Virtually all infected men have acute symptoms. Although complications are rare, epididymitis, prostatitis, and periurethral

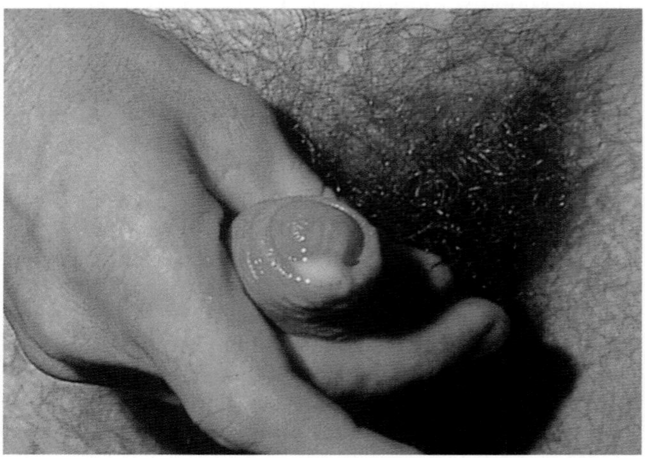

FIGURE 23-2 Purulent urethral discharge in man with urethritis. (From Morse SA, Ballard RC, Holmes KK, et al: *Atlas of sexually transmitted diseases and AIDS,* ed 4, London, 2010, Saunders.)

Clinical Case 23-1 Gonococcal Arthritis

Gonococcal arthritis is a common presentation of disseminated *Neisseria gonorrhoeae* infection. Fam and associates (*Can Med Assoc J* 108:319–325, 1973) described six patients with this disease, including the following patient, who has a typical presentation. A 17-year-old girl was admitted to the hospital with a 4-day history of fever, chills, malaise, sore throat, skin rash, and polyarthralgia. She reported being sexually active and having a 5-week history of a profuse yellowish vaginal discharge that was untreated. Upon presentation, she had erythematous maculopapular skin lesions over her forearm, thigh, and ankle, and her metacarpophalangeal joint, wrist, knee, ankle, and midtarsal joints were acutely inflamed. She had an elevated leukocyte count and sedimentation rate. Cultures of her cervix were positive for *N. gonorrhoeae,* but blood specimens, exudates for the skin lesions, and synovial fluid were all sterile. The diagnosis of disseminated gonorrhea with polyarthritis was made, and she was successfully treated with penicillin G for 2 weeks. This case illustrates the limitations of culture in disseminated infections and the value of a careful history.

abscesses may occur. The primary site of infection in women is the cervix because the bacteria infect the endocervical columnar epithelial cells. The organism cannot infect the squamous epithelial cells that line the vagina of postpubescent women. Symptomatic patients commonly experience vaginal discharge, dysuria, and abdominal pain. Ascending genital infections, including salpingitis, tuboovarian abscesses, and pelvic inflammatory disease, are observed in 10% to 20% of women.

Gonococcemia (Clinical Case 23-1)

Disseminated infections with **septicemia** and **infection of skin and joints** occur in 1% to 3% of infected women and in a much lower percentage of infected men. The greater proportion of disseminated infections in women is caused by the numerous untreated asymptomatic infections in this population. The clinical manifestations of disseminated disease include fever; migratory arthralgias; suppurative arthritis in the wrists, knees, and ankles; and a pustular rash on an erythematous base (Figure 23-3) over the extremities but not on the head and trunk. *N. gonorrhoeae* is a leading cause of **purulent arthritis** in adults.

Other Neisseria gonorrhoeae *Syndromes*

Other diseases associated with *N. gonorrhoeae* are perihepatitis **(Fitz-Hugh–Curtis syndrome);** purulent conjunctivitis (Figure 23-4), particularly in newborns infected during vaginal delivery (ophthalmia neonatorum); anorectal gonorrhea in homosexual men; and pharyngitis.

Neisseria meningitidis

Meningitis

The disease usually begins abruptly with headache, meningeal signs, and fever; however, very young children may have only nonspecific signs such as fever and vomiting. Mortality approaches 100% in untreated patients but is less than 10% in patients in whom appropriate antibiotic therapy is instituted promptly. The incidence of neurologic sequelae is low, with hearing deficits, learning disabilities, and arthritis most common.

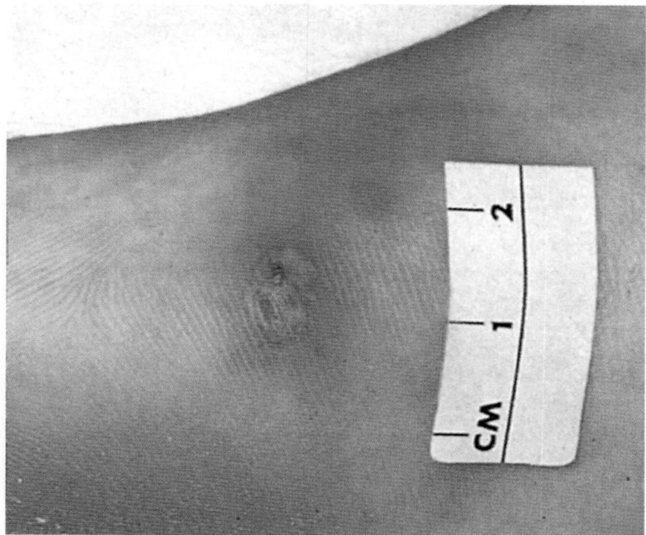

FIGURE 23-3 Skin lesions of disseminated gonococcal infection. Classic large lesions with a necrotic, grayish central lesion on an erythematous base. (From Morse SA, Ballard RC, Holmes KK, et al: *Atlas of sexually transmitted diseases and AIDS,* ed 4, London, 2010, Saunders.)

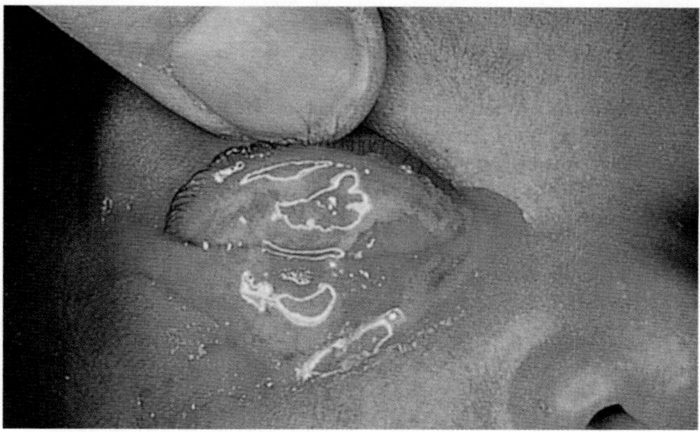

FIGURE 23-4 Gonococcal ophthalmia neonatorum. Lid edema, erythema, and marked purulent discharge are seen. A Gram-stained smear would reveal abundant organisms and inflammatory cells. (From Morse SA, Ballard RC, Holmes KK, et al: *Atlas of sexually transmitted diseases and AIDS,* ed 4, London, 2010, Saunders.)

Meningococcemia (Clinical Case 23-2)

Septicemia (meningococcemia) with or without meningitis is a life-threatening disease. Thrombosis of small blood vessels and multiorgan involvement are the characteristic clinical features. Small, petechial skin lesions on the trunk and lower extremities are common and may coalesce to form larger hemorrhagic lesions (Figure 23-5). Overwhelming DIC with shock, together with bilateral destruction of the adrenal glands **(Waterhouse-Friderichsen syndrome),** may ensue. A milder, chronic septicemia has also been observed. Bacteremia can persist for days or weeks, and the only signs of infection are a low-grade fever, arthritis, and petechial skin lesions. The response to antibiotic therapy in patients with this form of the disease is generally excellent.

 **Clinical Case 23-2 Meningococcal Disease**

Gardner (*N Engl J Med* 355:1466–1473, 2006) described a previously healthy 18-year-old man who presented to a local emergency department with the acute onset of fever and headache. His temperature was elevated (40° C), and he was tachycardic (pulse of 140 beats/min) and hypotensive (blood pressure 70/40 mm Hg). Petechiae were noted over his chest. Although the result of a cerebrospinal fluid culture was not reported, *Neisseria meningitidis* was recovered in the patient's blood cultures. Despite prompt administration of antibiotics and other support measures, the patient's condition rapidly deteriorated, and he died 12 hours after arrival in the hospital. This patient illustrates the rapid progression of meningococcal disease, even in healthy young adults.

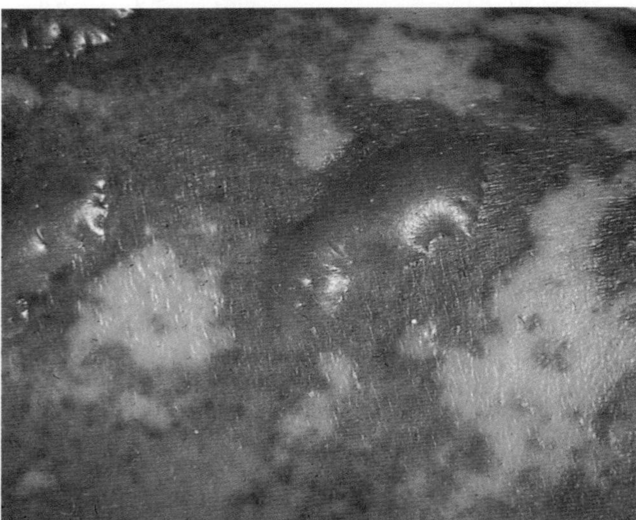

FIGURE 23-5 Skin lesions in a patient with meningococcemia. Note that the petechial lesions have coalesced and formed hemorrhagic bullae.

Other Neisseria meningitidis *Syndromes*

Additional infections caused by *N. meningitidis* are pneumonia, arthritis, and urethritis. Meningococcal pneumonia is usually preceded by a respiratory tract infection. Symptoms include cough, chest pain, rales, fever, and chills. Evidence of pharyngitis is observed in most affected patients. The prognosis in patients with meningococcal pneumonia is good.

Laboratory Diagnosis

Microscopy

Gram stain is very sensitive (>90%) and specific (98%) in detecting gonococcal infection in men with purulent urethritis. However, its sensitivity in detecting infection in asymptomatic men is 60% or less. The test is also relatively insensitive in detecting gonococcal cervicitis in both symptomatic and asymptomatic women, although a positive result is considered reliable when an experienced microscopist sees gram-negative diplococci within polymorphonuclear leukocytes. Thus all negative Gram stain results in women and asymptomatic men must be confirmed.

The Gram stain is also useful for early diagnosis of purulent arthritis but is insensitive and nonspecific for detection of *N. gonorrhoeae* in patients with skin lesions, anorectal infections, or pharyngitis. Commensal *Neisseria* species in the oropharynx and morphologically similar bacteria in the gastrointestinal tract can be confused with *N. gonorrhoeae.*

N. meningitidis can be readily seen in the cerebrospinal fluid (CSF) of patients with meningitis (see Figure 23-1) unless the patient has received antimicrobial therapy before the clinical specimen is collected. Most patients with bacteremia caused by other organisms have so few organisms present in their blood that the Gram stain has no value; however, patients with overwhelming meningococcal disease commonly have large numbers of organisms in their blood, which can be seen when the peripheral blood leukocytes are Gram stained.

Antigen Detection

Antigen testing for the detection of *N. gonorrhoeae* is less sensitive than culture or nucleic acid amplification tests and is not recommended unless confirmatory tests are performed on negative specimens. Commercial tests to detect *N. meningitidis* capsular antigens in CSF, blood, and urine (where the antigens are excreted) were widely used in the past but have fallen into disfavor in recent years because the tests are less sensitive than the Gram stain and false-positive reactions, particularly with urine specimens, can occur.

Nucleic Acid–Based Tests

Nucleic acid amplification (NAA) assays specific for *N. gonorrhoeae* have been developed for the direct detection of bacteria in clinical specimens. Tests using these assays are rapid (results are available in 1 to 2 hours), sensitive, and generally specific, although confirmatory tests are recommended for positive results with nongenital specimens (e.g., throat, rectum). Combination NAA assays for both *N. gonorrhoeae* and *Chlamydia* organisms are available and have replaced culture or other diagnostic tests in most laboratories. The primary problem with this approach is that it cannot be used to monitor antibiotic resistance of the identified pathogens.

Culture

N. gonorrhoeae can be readily isolated from genital specimens if care is taken in collecting and processing the specimens (Figure 23-6). Because other commensal organisms normally colonize mucosal surfaces, all genital, rectal, and pharyngeal specimens must be inoculated onto both **nonselective media** (e.g., chocolate blood agar) and **selective media** that suppress the growth of contaminating organisms (e.g., modified Thayer-Martin medium). A nonselective medium should be used because some gonococcal strains are inhibited by the vancomycin present in most selective media. The organisms are also inhibited by the fatty acids and trace metals present in the peptone hydrolysates and agar in other common laboratory media (e.g., blood agar, nutrient agar). Gonococci die rapidly if specimens are allowed to dry, so drying and cold temperatures should be avoided by directly inoculating the specimen onto prewarmed media at the time of collection.

The endocervix must be properly exposed to ensure that an adequate specimen is collected. Although bacteria can be recovered in endocervical exudate present in the vagina, a vaginal specimen is inadequate from asymptomatic women.

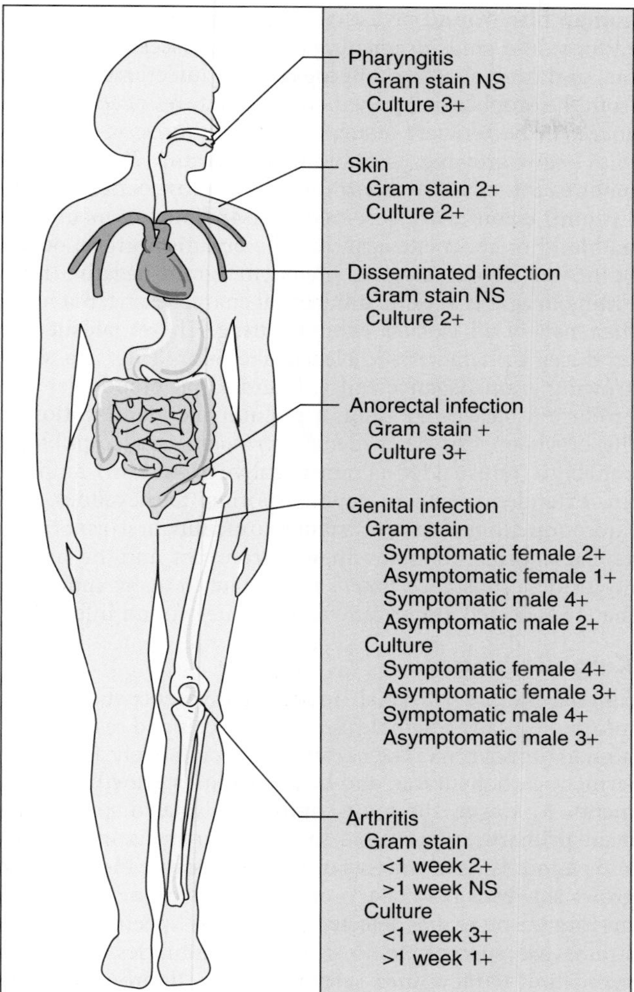

FIGURE 23-6 Laboratory detection of *Neisseria gonorrhoeae. NS,* Not specific or sensitive.

Although the endocervix is the most common site of infection in women, rectal cultures may be the only positive specimens in women who have asymptomatic infections, as well as in homosexual and bisexual men. Blood culture results are generally positive for gonococci only during the first week of the infection in patients with disseminated disease. In addition, special handling of blood specimens is required to ensure adequate recovery of gonococci, because supplements present in the blood culture media can be toxic to *Neisseria.* Cultures of specimens from infected joints are positive for the organism if the specimens are collected at the time the arthritis develops, but cultures of skin specimens are usually negative.

N. meningitidis is generally present in large numbers in CSF, blood, and sputum. Although the organism is inhibited by toxic factors in media and by the anticoagulant in blood cultures, this appears to be less of a problem than with *N. gonorrhoeae.* Care should be used in processing CSF and blood specimens because bacterial strains responsible for disseminated disease are more virulent and pose a safety risk for laboratory technologists.

Identification

Pathogenic *Neisseria* species are identified preliminarily on the basis of the isolation of oxidase-positive, gram-negative diplococci that grow on chocolate blood agar or on media that are selective for pathogenic *Neisseria* species. Definitive identification is guided by the pattern of oxidation of carbohydrates or other tests such as MALDI mass spectrometry.

Treatment, Prevention, and Control

Penicillin was historically the antibiotic of choice for treatment of gonorrhea; however, penicillin is not used today because the concentration of drug required to kill "susceptible" strains has steadily increased and frank resistance has become common. Resistance to tetracycline and ciprofloxacin has also become prevalent. In 2010 it was observed that 27% of isolates in the United States were resistant to penicillin, tetracycline, or ciprofloxacin, and 7% of the isolates were resistant to all three antibiotics. Currently the Centers for Disease Control and Prevention (CDC) recommends dual therapy with **ceftriaxone** and either azithromycin or doxycycline. Unfortunately, it is unclear how long this therapeutic approach will be effective. Strains of *N. gonorrhoeae* with decreased susceptibility to cephalosporins are reported with increased frequency in countries in Asia and the Pacific, as well as Europe, Canada, and the United States, and recently strains with high-level cephalosporin resistance have been identified in Asia, Africa, Europe, and North America.

Major efforts to stem the epidemic of gonorrhea encompass education, aggressive detection, and follow-up screening of sexual contacts. It is important to realize that gonorrhea is a significant disease. Chronic infections can lead to sterility, and asymptomatic infections perpetuate the reservoir of disease and lead to a higher incidence of disseminated infections. Chemoprophylaxis with 1% silver nitrate, 1% tetracycline, or 0.5% erythromycin eye ointment is routinely used to protect newborns against gonococcal eye infections (ophthalmia neonatorum); however, prophylactic use of antibiotics to prevent genital disease is ineffective and not recommended. Although there is interest in developing a vaccine against ***N. gonorrhoeae,*** an **effective vaccine is not yet available.** Immunity to infection with *N. gonorrhoeae* is poorly understood. Antibodies to pili antigens, Por proteins, and LOS can be detected; however, multiple infections are common in sexually promiscuous people. This lack of protective immunity is explained in part by the antigenic diversity of gonococcal strains. The variable region at the carboxyl terminus of the pilin proteins is the immunodominant portion of the molecule. Antibodies developed against this region protect against reinfection with a homologous strain, but cross-protection against heterologous strains is incomplete. This antigenic diversity also explains the ineffectiveness of vaccines developed against pilin proteins.

Cefotaxime or ceftriaxone should be used initially to treat *N. meningitidis* infections. If the organism is demonstrated to be penicillin susceptible, treatment can be changed to penicillin G. Chemoprophylaxis is recommended for contacts with significant exposure to patients with meningococcal disease (defined as individuals with direct exposure to respiratory secretions or >8 hours of close contact with the patient). Currently, rifampin, ciprofloxacin, or ceftriaxone is recommended for prophylaxis.

Antibiotic eradication of *N. meningitidis* in healthy carriers is ineffective, so prevention of disease has focused on enhancement of immunity through the use of vaccines directed against the serogroups most commonly associated with disease. Two tetravalent vaccines effective against serogroups A, C, Y, and W135 are currently licensed in the United States—a polysaccharide vaccine and a polysaccharide-protein conjugate vaccine. The conjugate vaccine is recommended for all adolescents aged 11 or 12 years, with a booster dose given at age 16. Other adults at increased risk for meningococcal disease should be vaccinated with either tetravalent vaccine. Unfortunately, the group B polysaccharide is a weak immunogen and is antigenically related to a polysaccharide in human neurologic tissues. Efforts to develop group B protein vaccines are ongoing. In December 2010 a new meningococcal A conjugate vaccine was introduced successfully in Africa, and a decreased incidence of meningitis was observed in the regions where the vaccine was used. It is planned that by 2016 all 26 countries in the African meningitis belt will have introduced this vaccine.

Other *Neisseria* Species

Neisseria species such as *Neisseria sicca* and *Neisseria mucosa* are commensal organisms in the oropharynx. These organisms have been implicated in isolated cases of meningitis, osteomyelitis, endocarditis, bronchopulmonary infections, acute otitis media, and acute sinusitis. The true incidence of respiratory tract infections caused by these organisms is not known because most specimens are contaminated with oral secretions. However, the observation of many gram-negative diplococci associated with inflammatory cells in a well-collected respiratory specimen would support the etiologic role of these organisms. Most isolates of *N. sicca* and *N. mucosa* are susceptible to penicillin, although low-level resistance caused by altered penicillin-binding protein (i.e., PBP2) has been observed.

Eikenella corrodens

In the early 1960s, a collection of small, fastidious, gram-negative rods were classified by workers at the CDC as members of the HB group (named after the patient infected with the original isolate). The organisms were subsequently subdivided into subgroup HB-1 (now known as *E. corrodens*), subgroup HB-2 (*Aggregatibacter [Haemophilus] aphrophilus;* see Chapter 24), and subgroups HB-3 and HB-4 (*Aggregatibacter [Actinobacillus] actinomycetemcomitans;* see Chapter 24). In addition to being morphologically similar, these organisms colonize the human oropharynx and, in the setting of preexisting heart disease, can cause subacute bacterial endocarditis.

E. corrodens is a moderate-sized (0.2×2.0 µm), nonmotile, non–spore-forming, facultatively anaerobic, gram-negative rod. The organism is named after Eiken, who characterized the bacterium and observed the ability of the organism to pit or "corrode" agar. *E. corrodens* is a normal inhabitant of the human upper respiratory tract, but because of its fastidious growth requirements it is difficult to detect unless specific selective culture media are used. It is an opportunistic pathogen that causes infections in patients who are immunocompromised or have diseases or trauma of the oral cavity. *E. corrodens* is most commonly isolated in the settings of a **human bite wound** or fistfight injury. Other infections are endocarditis, sinusitis, meningitis, brain abscesses, pneumonia, and lung abscesses. Because most infections originate from the oropharynx, polymicrobial mixtures of aerobic and anaerobic bacteria are often present in cultures.

A slow-growing, fastidious organism, *E. corrodens* requires 5% to 10% carbon dioxide to grow. Small (0.5- to 1.0-mm) colonies are observed after 48 hours of incubation on blood or chocolate agar, but the organism grows poorly or not at all on selective media for gram-negative rods. Pitting in agar is a useful differential characteristic, but fewer than half of all isolates exhibit pitting. The organism also produces a characteristic bleach-like odor. Thus if a slow-growing gram-negative rod is found to pit blood agar and produce a bleach-like odor, a preliminary identification of the organism can be made. *E. corrodens* is susceptible to penicillin (unusual for a gram-negative bacterium), ampicillin, extended-spectrum cephalosporins, tetracyclines, and fluoroquinolones but is resistant to oxacillin, first-generation cephalosporins, clindamycin, erythromycin, and the aminoglycosides. Thus *E. corrodens* is resistant to many antibiotics that are selected empirically to treat bite-wound infections.

Kingella kingae

Kingella species are small gram-negative coccobacilli that morphologically resemble *Neisseria* species and reside in the human oropharynx. The bacteria are facultatively anaerobic, ferment carbohydrates, and have fastidious growth requirements. *K. kingae,* the most commonly isolated species, has been primarily responsible for septic arthritis in children and endocarditis in patients of all ages. Because the organism grows slowly, it may take 3 or more days of incubation for the organism to be detected in clinical specimens. Most strains are susceptible to β-lactam antibiotics, including penicillin, tetracyclines, erythromycin, fluoroquinolones, and aminoglycosides.

Bibliography

Cohn AC, MacNeil JR, Harrison LH, et al: Changes in *Neisseria meningitidis* disease epidemiology in the United States, 1998-2007: implications for prevention of meningococcal disease, *Clin Infect Dis* 50:184–191, 2010.

Gardner P: Clinical practice: prevention of meningococcal disease, *N Engl J Med* 355:1466–1473, 2006.

Harrison L: Epidemiological profile of meningococcal disease in the United States, *Clin Infect Dis* 50:S37–S44, 2010.

Kirkcaldy RD, Kidd S, Weinstock HS, et al: Trends in antimicrobial resistance in *Neisseria gonorrhoeae* in the USA: the Gonococcal Isolate Surveillance Project (GISP), January 2006–June 2012, *Sex Transmit Infect* 89(Suppl 4):5–10, 2013.

Milonovich L: Meningococcemia: epidemiology, pathophysiology, and management, *J Pediatr Health Care* 21:75–80, 2007.

Ohnishi M, Golparian D, Shimuta K, et al: Is *Neisseria gonorrhoeae* Initiating a future era of untreatable gonorrhea: detailed characterization of the first strain with high level resistance to ceftriaxone, *Antimicrob Agents Chemother* 55:3538–3545, 2011.

Quagliarella V: Dissemination of *Neisseria meningitidis*, *N Engl J Med* 364:1573–1575, 2011.

Schielke S, Frosch M, Kurzai O: Virulence determinants involved in differential host niche adaptation of *Neisseria meningitidis* and *Neisseria gonorrhoeae*, *Med Microbiol Immunol* 199:185–196, 2010.

Stephens D: Conquering the meningococcus, *FEMS Microbiol Rev* 31:3–14, 2007.

Tan L, Carlone G, Borrow R: Advances in the development of vaccines against *Neisseria meningitidis*, *N Engl J Med* 362:1511–1520, 2010.

Winstead JM, McKinsey DS, Tasker S, et al: Meningococcal pneumonia: characterization and review of cases seen over the past 25 years, *Clin Infect Dis* 30:87–94, 2000.

CHAPTER 24

HAEMOPHILUS AND RELATED BACTERIA

A 10-year-old boy was catching and throwing a baseball with a friend. When he missed catching the ball, he ran into a neighbor's yard to retrieve the ball. His motion surprised a sleeping dog who then barked and bit the boy in the leg. The bite broke the skin but otherwise did not hurt the boy. He ran back to his friend and continued tossing the ball, not terribly concerned by the bite. Two days later the bite wound became erythematous and painful, and a serous discharge was present. His mother took the boy to the local emergency clinic, where cultures were performed and antibiotics started. The next day the laboratory reported that it had isolated a gram-negative rod that was subsequently identified as *Pasteurella multocida*. This organism is a member of the family Pasteurellaceae, a heterogeneous collection of small gram-negative rods.

1. What are the most common infections associated with *Haemophilus influenzae* type b, *Actinobacillus, Aggregatibacter,* and *Pasteurella?*
2. Why is disease with *H. influenzae* type b uncommon in the United States?
3. Why is detection of the capsular polysaccharide (i.e., polyribitol phosphate [PRP]) in *H. influenzae* of limited value?
4. What is the treatment of choice for *Pasteurella* infections?

Answers to these questions are available on StudentConsult.com.

• SUMMARIES CLINICALLY SIGNIFICANT ORGANISMS

Haemophilus

Trigger Words

Small coccobacilli, type b, PRP, meningitis, chancroid, vaccine

Biology and Virulence

- Small, pleomorphic, gram-negative rods or coccobacilli
- Facultative anaerobes, fermentative
- Most species require X and/or V factor for growth
- *H. influenzae* subdivided serologically (types a to f) and biochemically (biotypes I to VIII)
- *H. influenzae* type b is clinically most virulent (with polyribitol phosphate [PRP] in capsule)
- *Haemophilus* adhere to host cells via pili and nonpilus structures

Epidemiology

- *Haemophilus* species commonly colonized in humans, although encapsulated *Haemophilus* species, particularly *H. influenzae* type b, are uncommon members of normal flora
- Disease caused by *H. influenzae* type b was primarily a pediatric problem; eliminated in immunized populations
- *H. ducreyi* disease is uncommon in the United States
- With the exception of *H. ducreyi,* which is spread by sexual contact, most *Haemophilus* infections are caused by the patient's oropharyngeal flora (endogenous infections)
- Patients at greatest risk for disease are those with inadequate levels of protective antibodies, those with depleted complement, and those who have undergone splenectomy

Diseases

- Refer to Table 24-2 for a summary of diseases

Diagnosis

- Microscopy is a sensitive test for detecting *H. influenzae* in cerebrospinal fluid, synovial fluid, and lower respiratory specimens but not from other sites
- Culture is performed using chocolate agar
- Antigen tests are specific for *H. influenzae* type b; therefore these tests are nonreactive for infections caused by other organisms

Treatment, Prevention, and Control

- *Haemophilus* infections are treated with broad-spectrum cephalosporins, amoxicillin, azithromycin, doxycycline, or fluoroquinolones; susceptibility to amoxicillin should be documented
- Active immunization with conjugated PRP vaccines prevents most *H. influenzae* type b infections

The four most important genera in the family Pasteurellaceae are ***Haemophilus, Actinobacillus, Aggregatibacter,*** and ***Pasteurella*** (Table 24-1), and they are responsible for a broad spectrum of diseases (Box 24-1). The members of this family are small (0.2 to 0.3 × 1.0 to 2.0 µm), facultative anaerobic, gram-negative rods. Most have fastidious properties, requiring enriched media for isolation. Members of the genus *Haemophilus,* particularly *H. influenzae,* are the most common pathogens in this family and will be the main focus of this chapter (Table 24-2).

Haemophilus

Haemophilae are small, sometimes pleomorphic, gram-negative rods present on the mucous membranes of humans (Figure 24-1). ***Haemophilus influenzae*** is the species most commonly associated with disease, although introduction of the *H. influenzae* type b vaccine has dramatically reduced the incidence of disease, particularly in the pediatric population. ***Haemophilus aegyptius*** is an important cause of acute purulent conjunctivitis. ***Haemophilus ducreyi*** is well recognized as the etiologic agent of the sexually transmitted disease **soft chancre** or **chancroid.** The other members of the genus are commonly isolated in clinical specimens (e.g., *Haemophilus parainfluenzae* is the most common species in the mouth) but are rarely pathogenic, being responsible primarily for opportunistic infections.

Physiology and Structure

The growth of most species of *Haemophilus* requires supplementation of media with one or both of the following growth-stimulating factors: (1) **hemin** (also called **X factor** for "unknown factor") and (2) **nicotinamide adenine dinucleotide** (**NAD;** also called **V factor** for "vitamin"). Although both factors are present in blood-enriched media, sheep blood agar must be gently heated to destroy the inhibitors of V factor. For this reason, heated blood ("chocolate") agar is used for the isolation of *Haemophilus* in culture.

The cell wall structure of *Haemophilus* is typical of other gram-negative rods. Lipopolysaccharide with endotoxin activity is present in the cell wall, and strain-specific and species-specific proteins are found in the outer membrane. Analysis of these strain-specific proteins is valuable in epidemiologic investigations. The surface of many, but not all, strains of *H. influenzae* is covered with a **polysaccharide capsule,** and six antigenic **serotypes** (**a** through **f**) have been identified. Before the introduction of the *H. influenzae* type b vaccine, *H. influenzae* serotype b was responsible for more than 95% of all invasive *Haemophilus* infections. After introduction of the vaccine, most disease caused by this serotype disappeared in vaccinated populations, and more than half of all invasive disease is now caused by nonencapsulated (nontypeable) strains. A 2014 study reported that serogroup A was responsible for an increase in *H. influenzae* invasive disease, so a reemergence of this pathogen may be observed in the future.

Table 24-1 Important Pasteurellaceae

Organism	Historical Derivation
Haemophilus	*haemo,* blood; *hilos,* lover ("blood lover"; requires blood for growth on agar media)
H. influenzae	Originally thought to be the cause of influenza
H. aegyptius	*aegyptius,* Egyptian (observed by Robert Koch in 1883 in exudates from Egyptians with conjunctivitis)
H. ducreyi	Named after the bacteriologist Ducrey, who first isolated this organism
Actinobacillus	*actinis,* ray; *bacillus,* small staff or rod ("ray bacillus"; refers to the growth of filamentous forms [rays])
Aggregatibacter	*aggregare,* to come together; *bacter,* bacterial rod; rod-shaped bacteria that aggregate or clump together
A. actinomycetemcomitans	*comitans,* accompanying ("accompanying an actinomycete"; isolates are frequently associated with *Actinomyces*)
A. aphrophilus	*aphros,* foam; *philos,* loving ("foam loving")
Pasteurella	Named after Louis Pasteur
P. multocida	*multus,* many; *cidus,* to kill ("many-killing"; pathogenic for many species of animals)
P. canis	*canis,* dogs (isolated from the mouths of dogs)

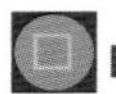

Box 24-1 Pasteurellaceae: Clinical Summaries

Haemophilus influenzae

Meningitis: a disease primarily of unimmunized children characterized by fever, severe headache, and systemic signs

Epiglottitis: a disease primarily of unimmunized children characterized by initial pharyngitis, fever, and difficulty breathing, and progressing to cellulitis and swelling of the supraglottic tissues, with obstruction of the airways possible

Pneumonia: inflammation and consolidation of the lungs observed primarily in the elderly with underlying chronic pulmonary disease; typically caused by nontypeable strains

Haemophilus aegyptius

Conjunctivitis: an acute purulent conjunctivitis ("pink eye")

Haemophilus ducreyi

Chancroid: sexually transmitted disease characterized by a tender papule with an erythematous base that progresses to painful ulceration with associated lymphadenopathy

Aggregatibacter actinomycetemcomitans

Endocarditis: responsible for subacute form of endocarditis in patients with underlying damage to the heart valve

Aggregatibacter aphrophilus

Endocarditis: as with *A. actinomycetemcomitans*

Pasteurella multocida

Bite wound: most common manifestation is infected cat or dog bite wound; particularly common with cat bites because the wounds are deep and difficult to disinfect

Table 24-2 ***Haemophilus* Species Associated with Human Disease**

Species	Primary Diseases	Frequency
H. influenzae	Pneumonia, sinusitis, otitis, meningitis, epiglottitis, cellulitis, bacteremia	Common worldwide; uncommon in United States
H. aegyptius	Conjunctivitis	Uncommon
H. ducreyi	Chancroid	Uncommon in United States
H. parainfluenzae	Bacteremia, endocarditis, opportunistic infections	Rare
H. haemolyticus	Opportunistic infections	Rare
H. parahaemolyticus	Opportunistic infections	Rare

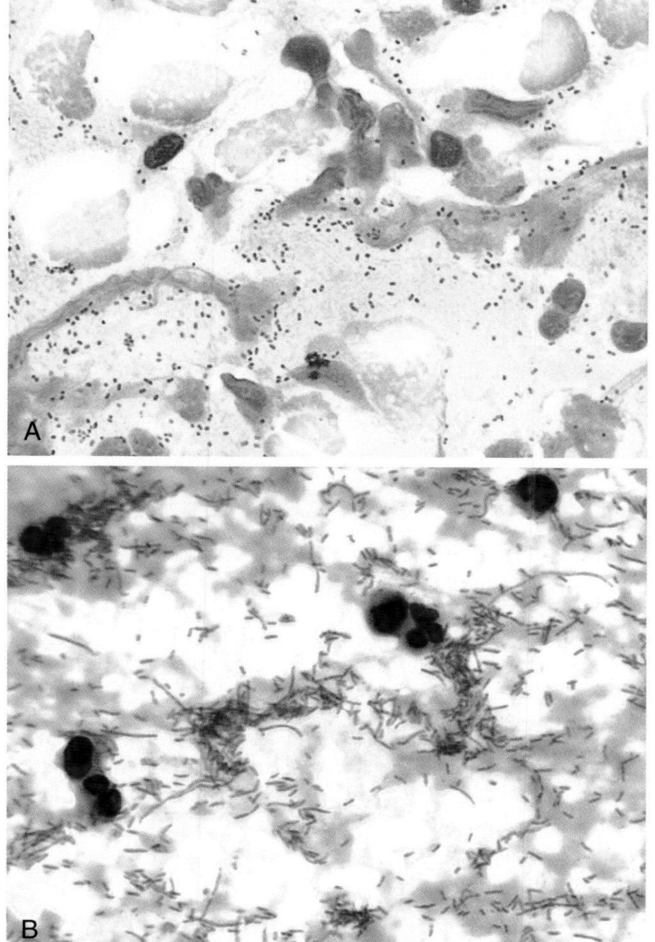

FIGURE 24-1 Gram stains of *Haemophilus influenzae.* **A,** Small coccobacilli forms seen in sputum from patient with pneumonia. **B,** Thin pleomorphic forms seen in a 1-year-old unvaccinated child in Africa with overwhelming meningitis.

In addition to the serologic differentiation of *H. influenzae,* the species is subdivided into eight **biotypes** (I through VIII) as determined by three biochemical reactions: indole production, urease activity, and ornithine decarboxylase activity. The separation of these biotypes is useful for epidemiologic purposes.

Pathogenesis and Immunity

Haemophilus species, particularly *H. parainfluenzae* and nonencapsulated *H. influenzae,* colonize the upper respiratory tract in virtually all people within the first few months of life. These organisms can spread locally and cause disease in the ears (otitis media), sinuses (sinusitis), and lower respiratory tract (bronchitis, pneumonia). Disseminated disease, however, is relatively uncommon. In contrast, encapsulated *H. influenzae* (particularly serotype b [biotype I]) is uncommon in the upper respiratory tract or is present in only very small numbers but is a common cause of **disease in unvaccinated children** (i.e., meningitis, epiglottitis [obstructive laryngitis], cellulitis). Pili and nonpilus adhesins mediate colonization of the oropharynx with *H. influenzae.* Cell wall components of the bacteria (e.g., lipopolysaccharide and a low-molecular-weight glycopeptide) impair ciliary function, leading to damage of the respiratory epithelium. The bacteria can then be translocated across both epithelial and endothelial cells and can enter the blood. In the absence of specific opsonic antibodies directed against the polysaccharide capsule, high-grade bacteremia can develop, with dissemination to the meninges or other distal foci.

The major virulence factor in *H. influenzae* type b is the antiphagocytic polysaccharide capsule, which contains ribose, ribitol, and phosphate (commonly referred to as **polyribitol phosphate [PRP]**). Antibodies directed against the capsule greatly stimulate bacterial phagocytosis and complement-mediated bactericidal activity. These antibodies develop because of natural infection, vaccination with purified PRP, or the passive transfer of maternal antibodies. The severity of systemic disease is inversely related to the rate of clearance of bacteria from the blood. The risk of meningitis and epiglottitis is significantly greater in patients with no anti-PRP antibodies, those with depletion of complement, and those who have undergone splenectomy. The lipopolysaccharide **lipid A** component induces meningeal inflammation in an animal model and may be responsible for initiating this response in humans. Immunoglobulin **IgA1 proteases** are produced by *H. influenzae* (both encapsulated and nonencapsulated strains) and may facilitate colonization of the organisms on mucosal surfaces by interfering with humoral immunity.

Epidemiology

Haemophilus species are present in almost all individuals, primarily colonizing the mucosal membranes of the respiratory tract. *H. parainfluenzae* is the predominant *Haemophilus* species in the mouth. Nonencapsulated strains of

H. influenzae are also commonly found in the upper respiratory tract; however, encapsulated strains are detectable only in small numbers and only when highly selective culture methods are used. Before the introduction of the *H. influenzae* vaccine, even though *H. influenzae* type b was the most common serotype that caused systemic disease, it was rarely isolated in healthy children (a fact that emphasizes the virulence of this bacterium).

The epidemiology of *Haemophilus* disease has changed dramatically. Before the introduction of **conjugated *H. influenzae* type b vaccines,** an estimated 20,000 cases of invasive *H. influenzae* type b disease occurred annually in children younger than age 5 years in the United States. The first polysaccharide vaccines for *H. influenzae* type b were not protective for children younger than 18 months (the population at greatest risk for disease) because there is a natural delay in the maturation of the immune response to polysaccharide antigens. When vaccines containing purified PRP antigens conjugated to protein carriers (i.e., diphtheria toxoid, tetanus toxoid, meningococcal outer membrane protein) were introduced in December 1987, a protective antibody response in infants aged 2 months and older was produced, and systemic disease in children younger than age 5 was virtually eliminated in the United States, with only 14 cases reported in 2011. Most of the *H. influenzae* type b infections now occur in children who are not immune (because of incomplete vaccination or a poor response to the vaccine) and in elderly adults with waning immunity. In addition, invasive *H. influenzae* disease caused by other serotypes of encapsulated bacteria and by nonencapsulated strains has now become proportionally more common than that resulting from serotype b. It should be noted that successful elimination of *H. influenzae* type b disease in the United States has not been seen in many developing countries where vaccination programs have been difficult to implement. Thus *H. influenzae* type b remains the most significant pediatric pathogen in many countries of the world. It is estimated that 3 million cases of serious disease and up to 700,000 fatalities occur in children each year worldwide, a tragedy considering that vaccination could eliminate virtually all disease. The epidemiology of disease caused by nonencapsulated *H. influenzae* and other *Haemophilus* species is distinct. Ear and sinus infections caused by these organisms are primarily pediatric diseases but can occur in adults. Pulmonary disease most commonly affects elderly people, particularly those with a history of underlying chronic obstructive pulmonary disease (COPD) or conditions predisposing to aspiration (e.g., alcoholism, altered mental state).

H. ducreyi is an important cause of genital ulcers (chancroid) in Africa and Asia but is less common in Europe and North America. The incidence of disease in the United States is cyclic. A peak incidence of more than 5000 cases was reported in 1988, which decreased to 8 cases in 2011. Despite this favorable trend, the Centers for Disease Control and Prevention has documented that the disease is significantly unrecognized and underreported, making the true incidence unknown.

Clinical Diseases (see Table 24-2)

The clinical syndromes seen in patients with *H. influenzae* infections are represented in Figure 24-2. The diseases caused by all *Haemophilus* species are described in the following sections.

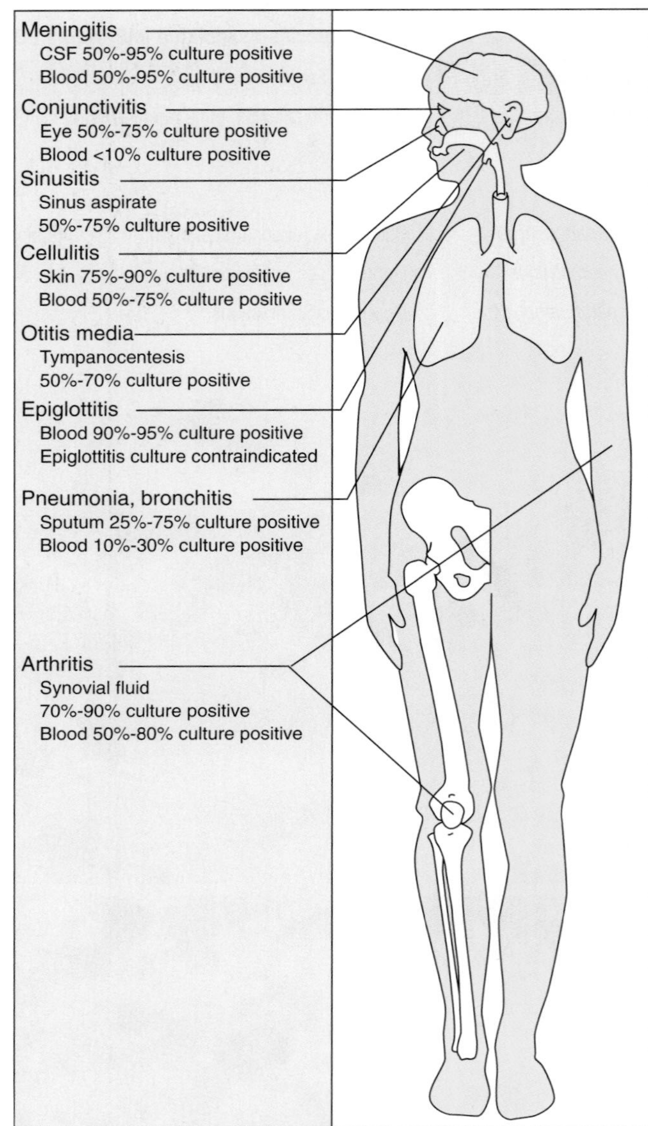

FIGURE 24-2 Infections caused by *Haemophilus influenzae.* With the advent of the conjugated vaccine, most infections in adults involve areas contiguous with the oropharynx (i.e., lower respiratory tract, sinuses, ears). Serious systemic infections (e.g., meningitis, epiglottitis) can occur in nonimmune patients. *CSF,* Cerebrospinal fluid.

Meningitis

H. influenzae type b was the most common cause of pediatric meningitis, but this situation changed rapidly when the conjugated vaccines became widely used. Disease in nonimmune patients results from bacteremic spread of the organisms from the nasopharynx and cannot be differentiated clinically from other causes of bacterial meningitis. The initial presentation is a 1- to 3-day history of mild upper respiratory disease, after which the typical signs and symptoms of meningitis appear. Mortality is less than 10% in patients who receive prompt therapy, and carefully designed studies have documented a low incidence of serious neurologic sequelae (in contrast with the 50% incidence of severe residual damage reported in nonimmune children seen in early studies). Person-to-person spread in a nonimmune population is well documented, so appropriate epidemiologic precautions must be used.

Epiglottitis

Epiglottitis, characterized by cellulitis and the swelling of the supraglottic tissues, represents a life-threatening emergency. Although epiglottitis is a pediatric disease, the peak incidence of this disease during the prevaccine era occurred in children 2 to 4 years of age; in contrast, the peak incidence of meningitis was seen in children 3 to 18 months of age. Children with epiglottitis have pharyngitis, fever, and difficulty breathing, which can progress rapidly to obstruction of the airway and death. Since the introduction of the vaccine, the incidence of this disease has also decreased dramatically in children and remains relatively rare in adults.

Cellulitis

Like meningitis and epiglottitis, cellulitis is a pediatric *H. influenzae* disease that has largely been eliminated by vaccination. When it is observed, patients have fever and cellulitis characterized by the development of reddish-blue patches on the cheeks or periorbital areas. The diagnosis is strongly suggested by the typical clinical presentation, cellulitis proximal to the oral mucosa, and lack of documented vaccination in the child.

Arthritis

Before the advent of conjugated vaccines, the most common form of arthritis in children younger than 2 years was an infection of a single, large joint secondary to bacteremic spread of *H. influenzae* type b. Disease does occur in older children and adults, but it is very uncommon and generally affects immunocompromised patients and patients with previously damaged joints.

Otitis, Sinusitis, and Lower Respiratory Tract Disease (Clinical Case 24-1)

Nonencapsulated strains of *H. influenzae* are opportunistic pathogens that can cause infections of the upper and lower airways. Most studies have shown that *H. influenzae* and *Streptococcus pneumoniae* are the two most common causes of acute and chronic otitis and sinusitis. Primary pneumonia is uncommon in children and adults who have normal pulmonary function. These organisms commonly colonize patients who have chronic pulmonary disease (including cystic fibrosis), and frequently are associated with exacerbation of bronchitis and frank pneumonia.

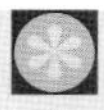

Clinical Case 24-1 Pneumonia Caused by *Haemophilus influenzae*

Holmes and Kozinn (*J Clin Microbiol* 18:730–732, 1983) described a 61-year-old woman with pneumonia caused by *Haemophilus influenzae* serotype d. The patient had a long history of smoking, chronic obstructive lung disease, diabetes mellitus, and congestive heart failure. She presented with left upper lobe pneumonia, producing purulent sputum with many gram-negative coccobacilli. Both sputum and blood cultures were positive for *H. influenzae* serotype d. The organism was susceptible to ampicillin, to which the patient responded. This case illustrates the susceptibility of patients with chronic underlying pulmonary disease to infections with non–serotype b strains of *H. influenzae*.

Conjunctivitis

H. aegyptius, also called the **Koch-Weeks bacillus,** causes an acute purulent conjunctivitis. This contagious organism is associated with epidemics, particularly during the warm months of the year.

Chancroid

Chancroid is a sexually transmitted disease that is most commonly diagnosed in men, presumably because women can have asymptomatic or inapparent disease. Approximately 5 to 7 days after exposure, a tender papule with an erythematous base develops on the genitalia or perianal area. Within 2 days the lesion ulcerates and becomes **painful,** and inguinal **lymphadenopathy** is commonly present. Other causes of genital ulcers, such as syphilis and herpes simplex disease, must be excluded to confirm the diagnosis of chancroid.

Other Infections

Other species of *Haemophilus* can cause opportunistic infections such as otitis media, conjunctivitis, sinusitis, endocarditis, meningitis, and dental abscesses.

Laboratory Diagnosis

Specimen Collection and Transport

Because most *Haemophilus* infections in vaccinated individuals originate from the oropharynx and are restricted to the upper and lower respiratory tract, contamination of the specimen with oral secretions should be avoided. Direct needle aspiration should be used for the microbiological diagnosis of sinusitis or otitis, and sputum produced from the lower airways is used for the diagnosis of pneumonia. Culture of blood for patients with pneumonia may be useful but would be predictably negative in patients with upper respiratory infections. Both blood and cerebrospinal fluid (CSF) should be collected from patients with the diagnosis of meningitis. Because there are approximately 10^7 bacteria per ml of CSF in patients with untreated meningitis, 1 to 2 ml of fluid is generally adequate for microscopy, culture, and antigen-detection tests. Microscopy and culture are less sensitive if the patient has been exposed to antibiotics before the CSF is collected. Blood cultures should also be collected for the diagnosis of epiglottitis, cellulitis, and arthritis. Specimens should not be collected from the posterior pharynx in patients with suspected epiglottitis because the procedure may stimulate coughing and obstruct the airway. Specimens for the detection of *H. ducreyi* should be collected with a moistened swab from the base or margin of the ulcer. Culture of pus collected by aspiration from an enlarged lymph node can be performed but is generally less sensitive than culture of the ulcer. The laboratory should be notified that *H. ducreyi* is suspected, because special culture techniques must be used for recovery of the organism.

Microscopy

If microscopy is performed carefully, the detection of *Haemophilus* species in clinical specimens is both sensitive and specific. Gram-negative rods ranging in shape from coccobacilli to long, pleomorphic filaments can be detected in more than 80% of CSF specimens from patients with untreated *Haemophilus* meningitis (see Figure 24-1). Microscopic examination of Gram-stained specimens is also useful for the rapid diagnosis of the organism in arthritis and lower respiratory tract disease.

Antigen Detection

The immunologic detection of *H. influenzae* antigen, specifically the PRP capsular antigen, is a rapid and sensitive way to diagnose *H. influenzae* type b disease. PRP can be detected with the particle agglutination test, which can detect less than 1 ng/ml of PRP in a clinical specimen. In this test, antibody-coated latex particles are mixed with the clinical specimen; agglutination occurs if PRP is present. Antigen can be detected in CSF and urine (in which the antigen is eliminated intact). However, this test has limited use because it can detect only *H. influenzae* type b, which is now uncommon in the United States and other countries with an established vaccine program. Other capsular serotypes and nonencapsulated strains do not give a positive reaction.

Culture

It is relatively easy to isolate *H. influenzae* from clinical specimens inoculated onto media supplemented with the appropriate growth factors. Chocolate agar is used in most laboratories. However, if chocolate agar is overheated during preparation, V factor is destroyed, and *Haemophilus* species requiring this growth factor (e.g., *H. influenzae, H. aegyptius, H. parainfluenzae*) will not grow. The bacteria appear as 1- to 2-mm, smooth, opaque colonies after 24 hours of incubation. They can also be detected growing around colonies of *Staphylococcus aureus* on unheated blood agar (**satellite phenomenon** [Figure 24-3]). The staphylococci provide the requisite growth factors by lysing the erythrocytes in the medium and releasing intracellular heme (X factor) and excreting NAD (V factor). The colonies of *H. influenzae* in these cultures are much smaller than they are on chocolate agar because the V factor inhibitors present in blood are not inactivated.

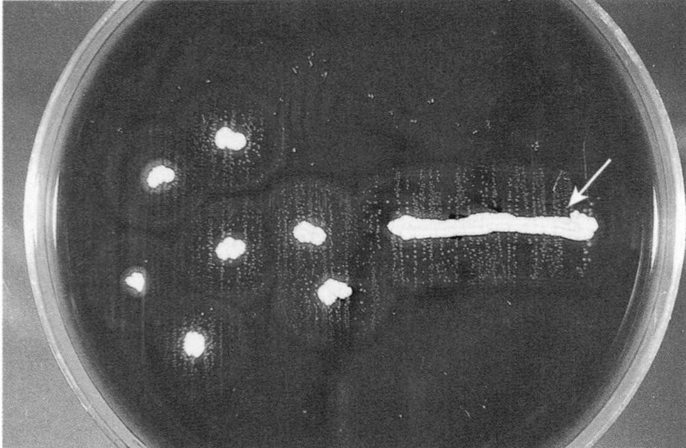

FIGURE 24-3 Satellite phenomenon. *Staphylococcus aureus* excretes nicotinamide adenine dinucleotide (NAD, or V factor) into the medium, providing a growth factor required for *Haemophilus influenzae* (small colonies surrounding *S. aureus* colonies *[arrow]*).

The growth of *Haemophilus* in blood cultures is generally delayed because most commercially prepared blood culture broths are not supplemented with optimum concentrations of X and V factors and inhibitors of V factor. Furthermore, the growth factors are released only when the blood cells lyse. Isolates of *H. influenzae* often grow better in anaerobically incubated blood cultures because, under these conditions, the organisms do not require X factor for growth.

H. aegyptius and *H. ducreyi* are fastidious and require specialized growth conditions. *H. aegyptius* grows best on chocolate agar supplemented with 1% IsoVitaleX (mixture of chemically defined supplements), with growth detected after incubation in a carbon dioxide atmosphere for 2 to 4 days. Culture for *H. ducreyi* is relatively insensitive (<85% of cultures yield organisms under optimal conditions) but reportedly is best on gonococcal (GC) agar supplemented with 1% to 2% hemoglobin, 5% fetal bovine serum, IsoVitaleX enrichment, and vancomycin (3 μg/ml). Cultures should be incubated at 33° C in 5% to 10% carbon dioxide for 7 days or more. Because the media and incubation conditions are not used for other bacterial cultures, success in recovering *H. ducreyi* requires that the microbiologist look specifically for this organism.

Identification

A presumptive identification of *H. influenzae* can be made by the Gram stain morphology and demonstration of a requirement for both X and V factors. Further subgrouping of *H. influenzae* can be done with biotyping, electrophoretic characterization of the membrane protein antigens, and analysis of the strain-specific nucleic acid sequences. Biochemical tests, nucleic acid analysis, or mass spectrometry is used to identify other species in this genus.

Treatment, Prevention, and Control

Patients with systemic *H. influenzae* infections require prompt antimicrobial therapy because the mortality rate in patients with untreated meningitis or epiglottitis approaches 100%. Serious infections are treated with **broad-spectrum cephalosporins.** Less severe infections, such as sinusitis and otitis, can be treated with amoxicillin (if susceptible; approximately 30% of strains are resistant), an active cephalosporin, azithromycin, doxycycline, or a fluoroquinolone. Most isolates of *H. ducreyi* are susceptible to **erythromycin,** the drug recommended for treatment.

The primary approach to preventing *H. influenzae* type b disease is through active immunization with purified capsular PRP. As discussed previously, the use of conjugated vaccines has been remarkably successful in reducing the incidences of *H. influenzae* type b disease and colonization. Currently, it is recommended that children receive two or three doses of vaccine against *H. influenzae* type b disease before the age of 6 months, followed by a booster dose at age 12 to 15 months.

Antibiotic chemoprophylaxis is used to eliminate the carriage of *H. influenzae* type b in children at high risk for disease (e.g., children <2 years in a family or day-care center where systemic disease is documented). Rifampin prophylaxis has been used in these settings.

Actinobacillus

Actinobacillus species are small, facultatively anaerobic, gram-negative rods that grow slowly (generally requiring 2 to 3 days of incubation). *Actinobacillus actinomycetemcomitans* was the most important human pathogen in this genus; however, in 2006 this species and *Haemophilus aphrophilus* were transferred into a new genus, *Aggregatibacter*. The remaining members of the genus *Actinobacillus* colonize the oropharynx of humans and animals and are causes of periodontitis and rarely endocarditis, bite wound infections, and opportunistic infections (Table 24-3).

Aggregatibacter (Clinical Case 24-2)

Two members of this genus are important human pathogens: ***A. actinomycetemcomitans*** and ***A. aphrophilus*** (Table 24-4). Both species colonize the human mouth and can spread from the mouth into the blood and then stick to a previously damaged heart valve or artificial valve, leading to the development of endocarditis. **Endocarditis** caused by these bacteria is particularly difficult to diagnose because clinical signs and symptoms develop slowly **(subacute endocarditis)** and the bacteria grow slowly in blood cultures. Both species form adherent colonies that can be observed on the glass surface of blood culture bottles and on agar media. The treatment of choice for endocarditis caused by these organisms is a cephalosporin such as ceftriaxone.

Pasteurella (Clinical Case 24-3)

Pasteurella are small, facultatively anaerobic, fermentative coccobacilli (Figure 24-4) commonly found as commensals in the oropharynx of healthy animals. Most human infections result from animal contact (e.g., animal bites, scratches, shared food). ***Pasteurella multocida*** (the most common isolate) and ***Pasteurella canis*** are human pathogens; the other *Pasteurella* species are rarely associated with human infections (Table 24-5). The following three general forms of disease are reported: (1) localized **cellulitis** and **lymphadenitis** that occur after an animal bite or scratch (*P. multocida* from contact with cats or dogs; *P. canis* from dogs), (2) an exacerbation of chronic **respiratory disease** in patients with underlying pulmonary dysfunction (presumably related to colonization of the patient's oropharynx followed by the aspiration of oral secretions), and (3) a **systemic infection in immunocompromised patients,** particularly those with underlying hepatic disease. Production of a polysaccharide

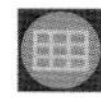

Table 24-3 *Actinobacillus* Species Associated with Human Disease

Species	Primary Diseases	Frequency
A. equuli	Bite wound infections	Rare
A. hominis	Opportunistic infections (bacteremia, pneumonia)	Rare
A. lignieresii	Bite wound infections	Rare
A. ureae	Opportunistic infections (bacteremia, meningitis, pneumonia)	Rare

Table 24-4 *Aggregatibacter* Species Associated with Human Disease

Species	Primary Diseases	Frequency
A. actinomycetemcomitans	Periodontitis, endocarditis, bite wound infections	Common
A. aphrophilus	Endocarditis, opportunistic infections	Uncommon

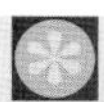

Clinical Case 24-2 Endocarditis Caused by *Aggregatibacter actinomycetemcomitans*

Steitz and associates (*Clin Infect Dis* 27:224–225, 1998) described a 54-year-old woman who was admitted to their hospital with a history of fever, night sweats, and fatigue. Physical examination revealed a tricuspid systolic murmur and splenomegaly, and echocardiography revealed vegetation on the tricuspid valve. Cultures of blood collected on admission were positive after 5 days of incubation for *Aggregatibacter (Actinobacillus) actinomycetemcomitans*. Her clinical history was incomplete because it was not known how chronic her course was; however, this case illustrates the slow growth of the organism in routine culture.

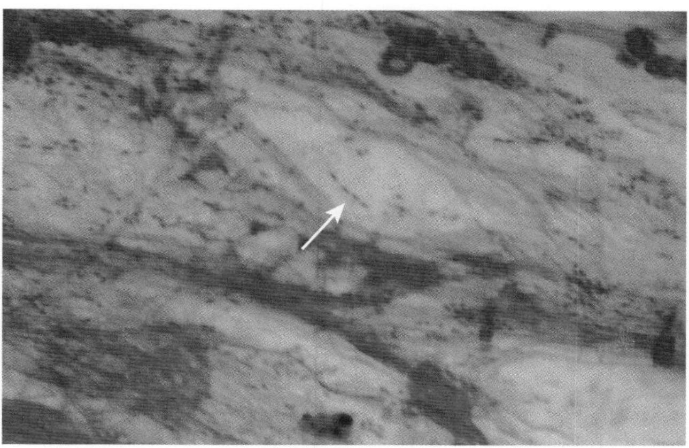

FIGURE 24-4 *Pasteurella multocida* in respiratory specimen from patient with pneumonia *(arrow)*.

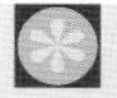

Clinical Case 24-3 Fatal *Pasteurella multocida* Infection

Chang and associates (*Scan J Infect Dis* 39:167–192, 2007) described a fatal case of *Pasteurella multocida* bacteremia and necrotizing fasciitis. The 58-year-old man had a history of chronic renal insufficiency, gouty arthritis, and Cushing syndrome treated with steroids. Upon admission to the hospital, his left hand was erythematous, warm, and tender with reddish to purplish macules over the surface. Over a 2-day period, bullae developed and extended rapidly to the left arm, left calf, and right foot, and the patient had systemic signs of shock and gastrointestinal bleeding. Blood cultures collected at the time of admission were positive for *P. multocida*. Despite aggressive antibiotic and surgical treatment, the lesions progressed rapidly and the patient eventually expired. A careful history at the time of admission revealed that the patient allowed his pet dog to lick his open wounds. This was the likely source of the bacteria, and the steroid treatments allowed the organism to invade the wound and rapidly spread in the tissues.

Table 24-5 *Pasteurella* Species Associated with Human Disease

Species	Primary Disease	Frequency
P. multocida	Bite wound infections, chronic pulmonary disease, bacteremia, meningitis	Common
P. canis	Bite wound infections	Uncommon
P. bettyae	Opportunistic infections (abscesses, bite wound infections, urogenital infections, bacteremia)	Rare
P. dagmatis	Bite wound infections	Rare
P. stomatis	Bite wound infections	Rare

capsule composed of hyaluronic acid is an important virulence factor in *Pasteurella* strains responsible for animal diseases and likely to be important in human infections.

P. multocida grows well on blood and chocolate agars but poorly on MacConkey agar and other media typically selective for gram-negative rods. After overnight incubation on blood agar, large buttery colonies (resulting from the polysaccharide capsule) with a characteristic musty odor caused by the production of indole are present. *P. multocida* is susceptible to a variety of antibiotics. **Penicillin** is the antibiotic of choice, and expanded-spectrum cephalosporins, macrolides, tetracyclines, or fluoroquinolones are acceptable alternatives. Semisynthetic penicillins (e.g., oxacillin), first-generation cephalosporins, and aminoglycosides have poor activity.

Bibliography

Briere EC, Rubin L, Moro PL, et al: Prevention and control of *Haemophilus influenzae* type b disease: recommendations of the Advisory Committee on Immunization Practices, *MMWR Recomm Rep* 63:1–14, 2014.

Bruce MG, Zulz T, DeByle C, et al: *Haemophilus influenza* serotype A invasive disease, Alaska, USA, 1983–2011, *Emerg Infect Dis* 19:932–937, 2013.

Davis S, Feikin D, Johnson H: The effect of *Haemophilus influenzae* type B and pneumococcal conjugate vaccines on childhood meningitis mortality: a systematic review, *BMC Public Health* 13:3–21, 2013.

Dworkin M, Park L, Borchardt S: The changing epidemiology of invasive *Haemophilus influenzae* disease, especially in persons >65 years old, *Clin Infect Dis* 44:810–816, 2007.

Hallstrom T, Riesbeck K: *Haemophilus influenzae* and the complement system, *Trends Microbiol* 18:258–265, 2010.

Norskov-Lauritsen N, Kilian M: Reclassification of *Actinobacillus actinomycetemcomitans, Haemophilus aphrophilus, Haemophilus paraphrophilus,* and *Haemophilus segnis* as *Aggregatibacter actinomycetemcomitans, Aggregatibacter aphrophilus,* and *Aggregatibacter segnis,* respectively, and emended description of *Aggregatibacter aphrophilus* to include V factor–dependent and V factor–independent isolates, *Int J System Evol Microbiol* 56:2135–2146, 2006.

O'Loughlin RE, Edmond K, Mangtani P, et al: Methodology and measurement of the effectiveness of *Haemophilus influenzae* type b vaccine: systematic review, *Vaccine* 28:6128–6136, 2010.

Peltola H: Worldwide *Haemophilus influenzae* type b disease at the beginning of the 21st century: global analysis of the disease burden 25 years after the use of the polysaccharide vaccine and a decade after the advent of conjugates, *Clin Microbiol Rev* 13:302–317, 2000.

Trees D, Morse S: Chancroid and *Haemophilus ducreyi:* an update, *Clin Microbiol Rev* 8:357–375, 1995.

Tristram S, Jacobs M, Appelbaum P: Antimicrobial resistance in *Haemophilus influenzae, Clin Microbiol Rev* 20:368–389, 2007.

Wang CY, Wang HC, Li JM, et al: Invasive infections of *Aggregatibacter actinomycetemcomitans, J Microbiol Immunol Infect* 43:491–497, 2010.

CHAPTER

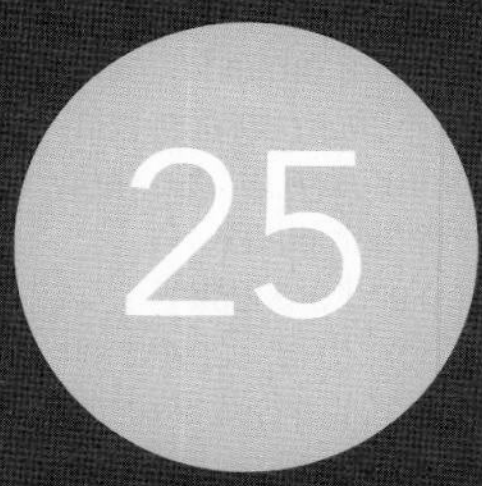

25 ENTEROBACTERIACEAE

This chapter covers **the largest family of clinically important bacteria. This is a heterogeneous collection of organisms responsible for virtually all types of infections that would be seen in a clinical practice.**

1. Many of the members of the Enterobacteriaceae are part of the normal population of bacteria that colonize the human body. Give three examples of organisms that are normal flora in healthy individuals and an example of disease caused by each organism. What condition leads to disease with each?
2. Some Enterobacteriaceae are normally found in animals but cause disease when humans are exposed. Give three examples and the diseases they cause.
3. Some Enterobacteriaceae are strict human pathogens. Give two examples and the diseases they cause.

Answers to these questions are available on StudentConsult.com.

• SUMMARIES CLINICALLY SIGNIFICANT ORGANISMS

Escherichia coli

Trigger Words

Gastroenteritis (EAEC, EIEC, EPEC, ETEC, STEC), neonatal meningitis, urinary tract infection

Biology and Virulence

- Gram-negative, facultative anaerobic rods
- Fermenter; oxidase negative
- Lipopolysaccharide consists of outer somatic O polysaccharide, core polysaccharide (common antigen), and lipid A (endotoxin)
- Virulence—refer to Box 25-2 and Table 25-2

Epidemiology

- Most common aerobic gram-negative rods in the gastrointestinal tract
- Most infections are endogenous (patient's microbial flora), although strains causing gastroenteritis are generally acquired exogenously

Diseases

- At least five different pathogenic groups cause gastroenteritis: EAEC, enteroaggregative *E. coli;* EIEC, enteroinvasive *E. coli;* EPEC, enteropathogenic *E. coli;* ETEC, enterotoxigenic *E. coli;* STEC, Shiga toxin–producing *E. coli.*
- Most cause diseases in developing countries, although STEC is an important cause of hemorrhagic colitis and hemolytic uremic syndrome in the United States
- Extraintestinal disease includes bacteremia, neonatal meningitis, urinary tract infections, and intraabdominal infections

Diagnosis

- Organisms grow rapidly on most culture media
- Enteric pathogens, with the exception of STEC, are detected only in reference or research laboratories

Treatment, Prevention, and Control

- Enteric pathogens are treated symptomatically unless disseminated disease occurs
- Antibiotic therapy is guided by in vitro susceptibility tests; increased resistance to penicillins and cephalosporins mediated by extended-spectrum β-lactamases (ESBLs)
- Appropriate infection-control practices are used to reduce the risk of nosocomial infections (e.g., restricting use of antibiotics, avoiding unnecessary use of urinary tract catheters)
- Maintenance of high hygienic standards to reduce the risk of exposure to gastroenteritis strains
- Proper cooking of beef products to reduce risk of STEC infections

Salmonella

Trigger Words

Gastroenteritis, enteric fever, poultry, antibiotic treatment

Biology and Virulence

- Gram-negative, facultative anaerobic rods
- Fermenter; oxidase negative
- Lipopolysaccharide consists of outer somatic O polysaccharide, core polysaccharide (common antigen), and lipid A (endotoxin)
- More than 2500 O serotypes
- Virulence—refer to Box 25-2; tolerant of acids in phagocytic vesicles
- Can survive in macrophages and spread from the intestine to other body sites

Epidemiology

- Most infections are acquired by eating contaminated food products (poultry, eggs, and dairy products are the most common sources of infection)
- Direct fecal-oral spread in children
- *Salmonella* Typhi and *Salmonella* Paratyphi are strict human pathogens (no other reservoirs); these infections are passed person to person; asymptomatic long-term colonization occurs commonly

- Individuals at risk for infection include those who eat improperly cooked poultry or eggs, patients with reduced gastric acid levels, and immunocompromised patients
- Infections occur worldwide, particularly in the warm months of the year

Diseases

- Diseases: enteritis (fever, nausea, vomiting, bloody or nonbloody diarrhea, abdominal cramps); enteric fever (typhoid fever, paratyphoid fever); bacteremia (most commonly seen with *Salmonella* serotype Typhi, *Salmonella* serotype Paratyphi, *Salmonella* serotype Choleraesuis); asymptomatic colonization (primarily with *Salmonella* Typhi and *Salmonella* Paratyphi)

Diagnosis

- Isolation from stool specimens requires use of selective media

Treatment, Prevention, and Control

- Antibiotic treatment not recommended for enteritis because this may prolong the duration of disease
- Infections with *Salmonella* Typhi and *Salmonella* Paratyphi or disseminated infections with other organisms should be treated with an effective antibiotic (selected by in vitro susceptibility tests); fluoroquinolones (e.g., ciprofloxacin), chloramphenicol, trimethoprim-sulfamethoxazole, or a broad-spectrum cephalosporin may be used
- Most infections can be controlled by proper preparation of poultry and eggs (completely cooked) and avoidance of contamination of other foods with uncooked poultry products
- Carriers of *Salmonella* Typhi and *Salmonella* Paratyphi should be identified and treated
- Vaccination against *Salmonella* Typhi can reduce the risk of disease for travelers into endemic areas

Shigella

Trigger Words

Gastroenteritis, dysentery, person-to-person, Shiga toxin, antibiotic treatment

Biology and Virulence

- Gram-negative, facultatively anaerobic rods
- Fermenter; oxidase negative
- Lipopolysaccharide consists of somatic O polysaccharide, core polysaccharide (common antigen), and lipid A (endotoxin)
- Four species recognized: *S. sonnei* responsible for most infections in developed countries, *S. flexneri* for infections in developing countries, *S. dysenteriae* for the most severe infections, and *S. boydii* not commonly isolated
- Virulence—refer to Box 25-2; exotoxin (Shiga toxin) produced by *S. dysenteriae* disrupts protein synthesis and produces endothelial damage

Epidemiology

- Humans are the only reservoir for these bacteria
- Disease spread person to person by fecal-oral route
- Patients at highest risk for disease are young children in day-care centers, nurseries, and custodial institutions; siblings and parents of these children; male homosexuals
- Relatively few organisms can produce disease (highly infectious)
- Disease occurs worldwide with no seasonal incidence (consistent with person-to-person spread involving a low inoculum)

Diseases

- Disease—most common form of disease is gastroenteritis (shigellosis), an initial watery diarrhea progressing within 1 to 2 days to abdominal cramps and tenesmus (with or without bloody stools); severe form of disease is caused by *S. dysenteriae* (bacterial dysentery); asymptomatic carriage develops in a small number of patients (reservoir for future infections)

Diagnosis

- Isolation from stool specimens requires use of selective media

Treatment, Prevention, and Control

- Antibiotic therapy shortens the course of symptomatic disease and fecal shedding
- Treatment should be guided by in vitro susceptibility tests
- Empirical therapy can be initiated with a fluoroquinolone or trimethoprim-sulfamethoxazole
- Appropriate infection control measures should be instituted to prevent spread of the organism, including hand washing and proper disposal of soiled linens

Yersinia

Trigger Words

Bubonic plague, pneumonic plague, gastroenteritis, transfusion sepsis, zoonotic

Biology and Virulence

- Gram-negative, facultatively anaerobic rods
- Fermenter; oxidase negative
- Lipopolysaccharide consists of somatic O polysaccharide, core polysaccharide (common antigen), and lipid A (endotoxin)
- *Y. pestis* is covered with a protein capsule
- Some species (e.g., *Y. enterocolitica*) can grow at cold temperatures (e.g., can grow to high numbers in contaminated refrigerated food or blood products)
- Virulence—refer to Box 25-2; capsule on *Y. pestis* is antiphagocytic; *Y. pestis* is resistant to serum killing; *Yersinia* with genes for adherence, cytotoxic activity, inhibition of phagocytic migration and engulfment, and inhibition of platelet aggregation

Epidemiology

- *Y. pestis* is a zoonotic infection, with humans the accidental host; natural reservoirs include rats, squirrels, rabbits, and domestic animals
- Disease is spread by flea bites or direct contact with infected tissues or person to person by inhalation of infectious aerosols from a patient with pulmonary disease
- Other *Yersinia* infections are spread through exposure to contaminated food products or blood products *(Y. enterocolitica)*
- Colonization with other *Yersinia* species can occur

Diseases

- *Y. pestis* causes bubonic plague (most common) and pulmonary plague, both having a high mortality rate; other *Yersinia* species cause gastroenteritis (acute watery diarrhea or chronic diarrhea) and transfusion-related sepsis; enteric disease in children may manifest as enlarged mesenteric lymph nodes and mimic acute appendicitis

Diagnosis

- Organisms grow on most culture media; prolonged storage at 4° C can selectively enhance isolation

Treatment, Prevention, and Control

- *Y. pestis* infections are treated with streptomycin; tetracyclines, chloramphenicol, or trimethoprim-sulfamethoxazole can be administered as alternative therapy
- Enteric infections with other *Yersinia* species are usually self-limited; if antibiotic therapy is indicated, most organisms are susceptible to broad-spectrum cephalosporins, aminoglycosides, chloramphenicol, tetracyclines, and trimethoprim-sulfamethoxazole
- Plague is controlled by reduction of the rodent population and vaccination of individuals at risk
- Other *Yersinia* infections are controlled by proper preparation of food products

The family Enterobacteriaceae is the largest, most heterogeneous collection of medically important **gram-negative rods**. More than 50 genera and hundreds of species and subspecies have been described (Table 25-1). These genera have been classified based on biochemical properties, antigenic structure, and molecular analysis of their genomes by gene sequencing and protein composition by mass spectrometry. Despite the complexity of this family, most human infections are caused by relatively few genera and species (Box 25-1).

Table 25-1 Important Enterobacteriaceae

Organism	Historical Derivation
Escherichia coli	*escherichia*, named after Escherich; *coli*, of the colon
Salmonella enterica	*salmonella*, named after Salmon; *enteron*, gut; pertaining to the gut
Salmonella Typhi	*typhi*, of typhoid; disease is typhoid fever
Salmonella Paratyphi	*paratyphi*, of a typhoid-like infection
Salmonella Choleraesuis	*cholera*, cholera; *sus*, hog; cholera of a hog
Salmonella Typhimurium	*typhi*, of typhoid; *murium*, of mice; *typhimurium*, typhoid of mice
Salmonella Enteritidis	*enteris*, gut; *idis*, inflammation
Shigella dysenteriae	*shigella*, named after Shiga; *dysenteriae*, dysentery
Shigella flexneri	*flexneri*, named after Flexner
Shigella boydii	*boydii*, named after Boyd
Shigella sonnei	*sonnei*, named after Sonne
Yersinia pestis	*yersinia*, named after Yersin; *pestis*, plague
Yersinia enterocolitica	*enterocolitica*, pertaining to the intestine and colon
Yersinia pseudotuberculosis	*tuberculum*, a small swelling; *pseudotuberculosis*, false swelling
Klebsiella pneumoniae	*klebsiella*, named after Klebs; *pneumoniae*, inflammation of the lungs
Klebsiella oxytoca	*oxus*, acid; *tokos*, producing; acid-producing (refers to biochemical properties)
Proteus mirabilis	*proteus*, a god able to change himself into different shapes; *mirabilis*, surprising; refers to pleomorphic colony forms
Citrobacter freundii	*citrus*, lemon; *bacter*, a rod; citrate-utilizing rod; *freundii*, named after Freund
Citrobacter koseri	*koseri*, named after Koser
Enterobacter aerogenes	*enteron*, intestine; *bacter*, a small rod; *aeros*, air; *genes*, producing; small gas-producing intestinal rod
Enterobacter cloacae	*cloacae*, of a sewer; originally isolated in sewage
Serratia marcescens	*serratia*, named after Serrati; *marcescens*, becoming weak, fading away; originally believed not virulent

Enterobacteriaceae are **ubiquitous** organisms found worldwide in soil, water, and vegetation and are part of the normal intestinal flora of most animals, including humans. These bacteria cause a variety of human diseases, including one quarter to one third of all bacteremias, more than 70% of urinary tract infections (UTIs), and many intestinal infections. Some organisms (e.g., *Salmonella* serotype Typhi, *Shigella* species, *Yersinia pestis*) are **always associated with human disease** when present in clinical specimens, whereas others (e.g., *Escherichia coli, Klebsiella pneumoniae, Proteus mirabilis*) are members of the normal commensal flora that can cause **opportunistic infections.** A third group of Enterobacteriaceae exists—those normally commensal organisms that become pathogenic when they acquire virulence genes present on plasmids, bacteriophages, or pathogenicity islands (e.g., *E. coli*). Infections with the Enterobacteriaceae can originate from an animal reservoir (e.g., most *Salmonella* species, *Yersinia* species), from a human carrier (e.g., *Shigella* species, *Salmonella* Typhi), or through the endogenous spread of organisms (e.g., spread of *E. coli* from the intestine to the peritoneal cavity following perforation of the intestine).

General Properties

Physiology and Structure

Members of the family Enterobacteriaceae are moderate-sized (0.3 to 1.0 × 1.0 to 6.0 μm), non–spore-forming, gram-negative rods (Figure 25-1) that share a common antigen **(enterobacterial common antigen).** All members can grow rapidly, aerobically and anaerobically **(facultative anaerobes),** on a variety of nonselective (e.g., blood agar) and selective (e.g., MacConkey agar) media. The Enterobacteriaceae have simple nutritional requirements, ferment glucose, reduce nitrate, and are catalase positive and oxidase negative. The absence of cytochrome oxidase activity is an important characteristic because it can be measured rapidly with a simple test and is used to distinguish the Enterobacteriaceae from many other fermentative and nonfermentative gram-negative rods (e.g., *Vibrio*, *Pseudomonas*).

The appearance of the bacteria on culture media has been used to differentiate common members of the Enterobacteriaceae. For example, **fermentation of lactose** (detected by

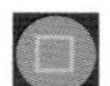

Box 25-1 Common Medically Important Enterobacteriaceae

Citrobacter freundii, Citrobacter koseri
Enterobacter aerogenes, Enterobacter cloacae
Escherichia coli
Klebsiella pneumoniae, Klebsiella oxytoca
Morganella morganii
Proteus mirabilis
Salmonella serotype Typhi, *Salmonella* nontyphoidal serotypes
Serratia marcescens
Shigella sonnei, Shigella flexneri
Yersinia pestis, Yersinia enterocolitica, Yersinia pseudotuberculosis

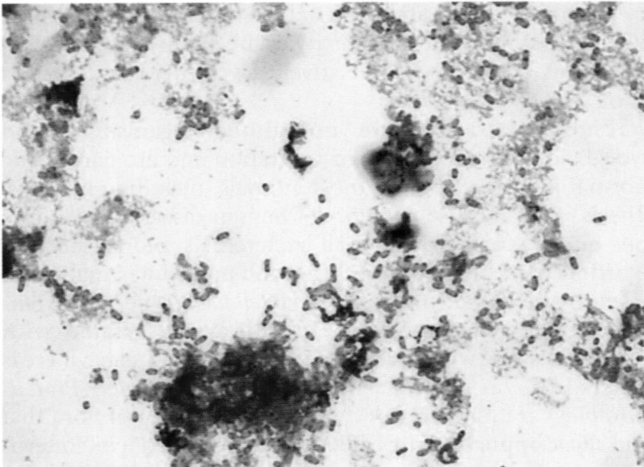

FIGURE 25-1 Gram stain of *Salmonella* Typhi from a positive blood culture. Note the intense staining at the ends of the bacteria. This "bipolar staining" is characteristic of the Enterobacteriaceae.

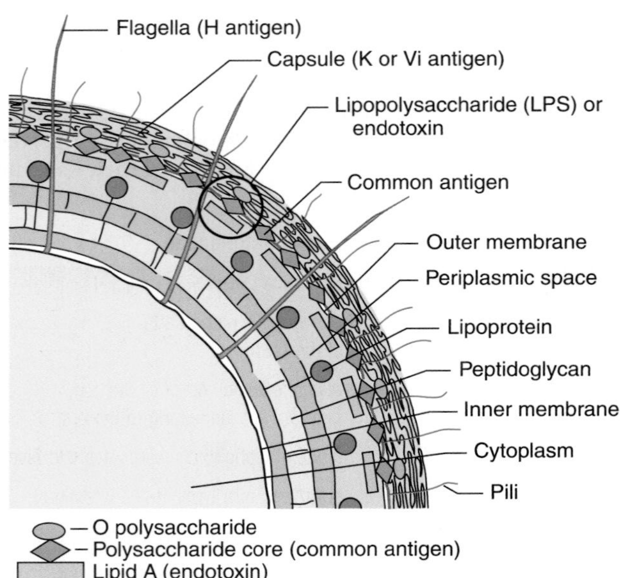

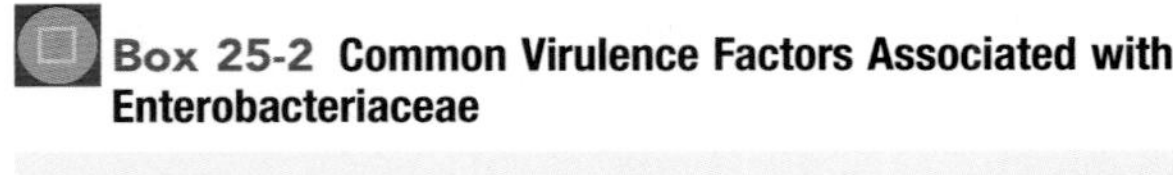

FIGURE 25-2 Antigenic structure of Enterobacteriaceae cell wall.

color changes in lactose-containing media such as the commonly used MacConkey agar) has been used to differentiate some enteric pathogens that do not ferment lactose or do so slowly (e.g., *Salmonella, Shigella,* and *Yersinia* spp.—colorless colonies on MacConkey agar) from lactose-fermenting species (e.g., *Escherichia, Klebsiella, Enterobacter, Citrobacter,* and *Serratia*—pink-purple colonies on MacConkey agar). **Resistance to bile salts** in some selective media has also been used to separate enteric pathogens (e.g., *Shigella, Salmonella*) from commensal organisms that are inhibited by bile salts (e.g., gram-positive and some gram-negative bacteria present in the gastrointestinal [GI] tract). In this way, use of culture media that assess lactose fermentation and resistance to bile salts is a rapid screening test for enteric pathogens that would be otherwise difficult to detect in diarrheal stool specimens, where many different organisms may be present. Some Enterobacteriaceae such as *Klebsiella* are also characteristically mucoid (wet, heaped, viscous colonies with prominent **capsules,** whereas a loose-fitting, diffusible slime layer surrounds other strains.

The heat-stable **lipopolysaccharide (LPS)** is the major cell wall antigen and consists of three components: the outermost somatic **O polysaccharide,** a **core polysaccharide** common to all Enterobacteriaceae (enterobacterial common antigen mentioned earlier), and **lipid A** (Figure 25-2). The core polysaccharide is important for classifying an organism as a member of the Enterobacteriaceae, the O polysaccharide is important for the epidemiologic classification of strains within a species, and the lipid A component of LPS is responsible for endotoxin activity, an important virulence factor.

The epidemiologic (serologic) classification of the Enterobacteriaceae is based on three major groups of antigens: **somatic O polysaccharides, K antigens** in the capsule (type-specific polysaccharides), and **H proteins** in the bacterial flagella. Strain-specific O antigens are present in each genus and species, although cross-reactions between closely related genera are common (e.g., *Salmonella* with *Citrobacter, Escherichia* with *Shigella*). The K antigens are not commonly used for strain typing but are important because they may interfere with detection of the O antigens. The H antigens are heat-labile flagellin proteins. Detection of these various antigens has important clinical significance beyond epidemiologic investigations—some pathogenic species of bacteria are associated with specific O and H serotypes (e.g., *E. coli* O157:H7 is associated with hemorrhagic colitis).

Most Enterobacteriaceae are motile, with the exception of some common genera (e.g., *Klebsiella, Shigella, Yersinia*). The motile strains are coated with **flagella** (peritrichous). Many Enterobacteriaceae also possess fimbriae (also referred to as pili), which have been subdivided into two general classes: chromosomally mediated common fimbriae and plasmid-encoded sex pili. The **common fimbriae** are important for the ability of bacteria to adhere to specific host cell receptors, whereas the **sex** or **conjugative pili** facilitate genetic transfer between bacteria.

Box 25-2 Common Virulence Factors Associated with Enterobacteriaceae

Endotoxin
Capsule
Antigenic phase variation
Type III secretion systems
Sequestration of growth factors
Resistance to serum killing
Antimicrobial resistance

Pathogenesis and Immunity

Numerous virulence factors have been identified in the members of the family Enterobacteriaceae. Some are common to all genera (Box 25-2), and others are unique to specific virulent strains.

Endotoxin

Endotoxin is a virulence factor shared among aerobic and some anaerobic gram-negative bacteria. The activity of this toxin depends on the **lipid A** component of LPS, which is released at cell lysis. Many of the systemic manifestations of gram-negative bacterial infections are initiated by endotoxin: activation of complement, release of cytokines, leukocytosis, thrombocytopenia, disseminated intravascular coagulation, fever, decreased peripheral circulation, shock, and death.

Capsule

Encapsulated Enterobacteriaceae are protected from phagocytosis by the hydrophilic capsular antigens, which repel the hydrophobic phagocytic cell surface. These antigens interfere with the binding of antibodies to the bacteria and are poor immunogens or activators of complement. The protective role of the capsule is diminished, however, if the patient develops specific anticapsular antibodies.

Antigenic Phase Variation

The expression of the somatic O antigens, capsular K antigens, and flagellar H antigens is under the genetic control of the organism. Each of these antigens can be alternately expressed or not expressed (phase variation), a feature that protects the bacteria from antibody-mediated cell death.

Type III Secretion Systems

A variety of bacteria (e.g., *Yersinia, Salmonella, Shigella,* enteropathogenic *Escherichia, Pseudomonas, Chlamydia*) have a common effector system for delivering their virulence factors into targeted eukaryotic cells. Think of the **type III secretion system** as a molecular syringe consisting of approximately 20 proteins that facilitate transfer of bacterial virulence factors into the targeted host cells. Although the virulence factors and their effects differ among the various gram-negative rods, the general mechanism by which the virulence factors are introduced is the same. In the absence of the type III secretion system, the bacteria have diminished virulence.

Sequestration of Growth Factors

Nutrients are provided to the organisms in enriched culture media, but the bacteria must become nutritional scavengers when growing in vivo. Iron is an important growth factor required by bacteria, but it is bound in **heme proteins** (e.g., hemoglobin, myoglobin) or in **iron-chelating proteins** (e.g., transferrin, lactoferrin). The bacteria counteract the binding by producing their own competitive **siderophores** or iron-chelating compounds (e.g., **enterobactin, aerobactin**). Iron can also be released from host cells by hemolysins produced by the bacteria.

Resistance to Serum Killing

Whereas many bacteria can be rapidly cleared from blood, virulent organisms capable of producing systemic infections are often resistant to serum killing. The bacterial capsule can protect the organism from serum killing as well as other factors that prevent the binding of complement components to the bacteria and subsequent complement-mediated clearance.

Antimicrobial Resistance

As rapidly as new antibiotics are introduced, organisms can develop resistance to them. This resistance can be encoded on transferable plasmids and exchanged among species, genera, and even families of bacteria.

• *Escherichia coli*

E. coli is the most common and important member of the genus *Escherichia.* This organism is associated with a variety of diseases, including gastroenteritis and extraintestinal infections such as UTIs, meningitis, and sepsis. A multitude of strains are capable of causing disease, with some serotypes associated with greater virulence (e.g., *E. coli* O157 is the most common cause of hemorrhagic colitis and hemolytic uremic syndrome).

Pathogenesis and Immunity

E. coli possesses a broad range of virulence factors (Table 25-2). In addition to the general factors possessed by all members of the family Enterobacteriaceae, *Escherichia* strains possess specialized virulence factors that can be placed into two general categories: adhesins and exotoxins. The function of these factors will be discussed in greater detail in the following sections.

Epidemiology

Large numbers of *E. coli* are present in the GI tract. Although these organisms can be opportunistic pathogens when the intestines are perforated and the bacteria enter the peritoneal cavity, most *E. coli* that cause GI and extraintestinal disease do so because they have acquired specific virulence factors encoded on plasmids or in bacteriophage DNA. The effectiveness of *E. coli* as a pathogen is illustrated by the fact that the bacteria are (1) the most common gram-negative rods isolated from patients with sepsis (Figure 25-3), (2) responsible for causing more than 80% of all community-acquired UTIs as well as many hospital-acquired infections, and (3) a prominent cause of gastroenteritis. Most infections (with the exception of neonatal meningitis and gastroenteritis) are endogenous; that is, the *E. coli* that are part of the patient's normal microbial flora are able to establish infection when

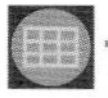

Table 25-2 Specialized Virulence Factors Associated with *Escherichia coli*

Bacteria	Adhesins	Exotoxins
ETEC	Colonization factor antigens (CFA/I, CFA/II, CFA/III)	Heat-labile toxin (LT-1); heat-stable toxin (STa)
EPEC	BFP; intimin	
EAEC	Aggregative adherence fimbriae (AAF/I, AAF/II, AAF/III)	Enteroaggregative heat-stable toxin; plasmid-encoded toxin
STEC	BFP; intimin	Shiga toxins (Stx1, Stx2)
EIEC	Invasive plasmid antigen	Hemolysin (HlyA)
Uropathogens	P pili; Dr fimbriae	

BFP, Bundle-forming pili; *EAEC,* enteroaggregative *E. coli; EIEC,* enteroinvasive *E. coli; EPEC,* enteropathogenic *E. coli; ETEC,* enterotoxigenic *E. coli; STEC,* Shiga toxin–producing *E. coli.*

the patient's defenses are compromised (e.g., through trauma or immune suppression).

Clinical Diseases

Gastroenteritis

The strains of *E. coli* that cause gastroenteritis are subdivided into a number of groups. Five of these groups will be the focus of this chapter: enterotoxigenic, enteropathogenic, enteroaggregative, Shiga toxin–producing, and enteroinvasive *E. coli* (Table 25-3). The first three groups primarily cause a secretory diarrhea involving the small intestine, and the last two groups primarily involve the large intestine.

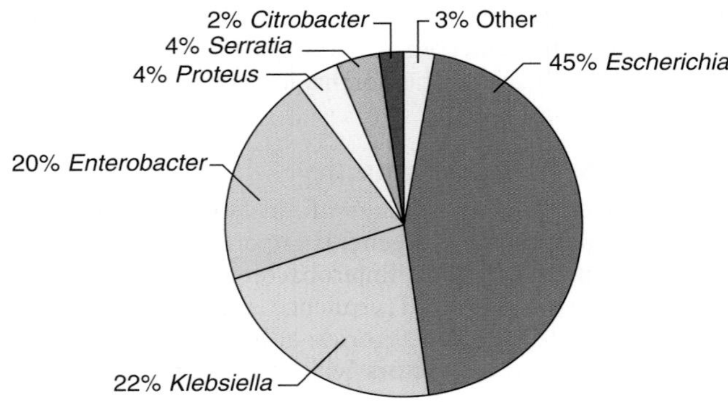

FIGURE 25-3 Incidence of Enterobacteriaceae associated with bacteremia. (Data courtesy Barnes-Jewish Hospital, St Louis, Mo.)

Enterotoxigenic E. coli

Enterotoxigenic *E. coli* (ETEC) is one of the most common causes of bacterial diarrheal disease in developing countries (estimated 840 million cases annually) and in an estimated 30% of travelers to these countries with diarrheal disease. Because the inoculum for disease is high, infections are primarily **acquired through consumption of fecally contaminated food or water.** Person-to-person spread does not occur. **Secretory diarrhea** caused by ETEC develops after a 1- to 2-day incubation period and persists for an average of 3 to 5 days. The symptoms (watery, nonbloody diarrhea and abdominal cramps; less commonly nausea and vomiting) are similar to those of cholera but are usually milder, although mortality is high in malnourished individuals and in those with underlying diseases, particularly children and the elderly.

Disease requires bacterial attachment to the small bowel epithelium by bacterial surface proteins (colonization factors

Table 25-3 Gastroenteritis Caused by *Escherichia coli*

Organism	Site of Action	Disease	Pathogenesis	Diagnosis
Enterotoxigenic *E. coli* (ETEC)	Small intestine	Traveler's diarrhea; infant diarrhea in developing countries; watery diarrhea, vomiting, cramps, nausea, low-grade fever	Plasmid-mediated, heat-stable (ST) and heat-labile (LT) enterotoxins that stimulate hypersecretion of fluids and electrolytes	Most U.S. outbreaks caused by ST-producing strains; commercial immunoassays available for detecting ST in clinical specimens and cultures; PCR assays used with clinical specimens
Enteropathogenic *E. coli* (EPEC)	Small intestine	Infant diarrhea in developing countries; watery diarrhea and vomiting, nonbloody stools; believed to be rare in United States	Plasmid-mediated A/E histopathology, with disruption of normal microvillus structure resulting in malabsorption and diarrhea	Characteristic adherence to HEp-2 or HeLa cells; probes and amplification assays developed for the plasmid-encoded bundle-forming pili and gene targets on the "locus of enterocyte effacement" pathogenicity island
Enteroaggregative *E. coli* (EAEC)	Small intestine	Infant diarrhea in developing and probably developed countries; traveler's diarrhea; persistent watery diarrhea with vomiting, dehydration, and low-grade fever	Plasmid-mediated aggregative adherence of rods ("stacked bricks") with shortening of microvilli, mononuclear infiltration, and hemorrhage; decreased fluid absorption	Characteristic adherence to HEp-2 cells; DNA probe and amplification assays developed for conserved plasmid
Shiga toxin–producing *E. coli* (STEC)	Large intestine	Initial watery diarrhea followed by grossly bloody diarrhea (hemorrhagic colitis) with abdominal cramps; little or no fever; may progress to hemolytic uremic syndrome	STEC evolved from EPEC; A/E lesions with destruction of intestinal microvilli, resulting in decreased absorption; pathology mediated by cytotoxic Shiga toxins (Stx1, Stx2), which disrupt protein synthesis	Screen for O157:H7 with sorbitol-MacConkey agar; confirm by serotyping; immunoassays (ELISA, latex agglutination) for detection of the Stx toxins in stool specimens and cultured bacteria; DNA amplification assays developed for Stx genes
Enteroinvasive *E. coli* (EIEC)	Large intestine	Rare in developing and developed countries; fever, cramping, watery diarrhea; may progress to dysentery with scant bloody stools	Plasmid-mediated invasion and destruction of epithelial cells lining colon	Sereny (guinea pig keratoconjunctivitis) test; plaque assay in HeLa cells; probes and amplification assays for genes regulating invasion (cannot discriminate between EIEC and *Shigella*)

A/E, Attachment/effacement; *DNA*, deoxyribonucleic acid; *ELISA*, enzyme-linked immunosorbent assay; *LT*, labile toxin; *PCR*, polymerase chain reaction; *ST*, stable toxin.

[CF]) and elaboration of heat-stable and heat-labile enterotoxins. The genes for the colonization factors and enterotoxins are encoded on a transmissible plasmid. The colonization factors are subdivided into families (CFA/I, CFA/II, CFA/IV are the most common) and further subdivided by their antigenic properties (coli surface antigens [CS]). More than 20 CS colonization factors have been described, and host specificity is defined by their affinity for receptors on host cells.

ETEC produce two classes of enterotoxins: **heat-stable toxins (STa and STb)** and **heat-labile toxins (LT-I, LT-II).** Heat-stable toxin STa but not STb is associated with human disease, is found in 75% to 80% of ETEC either alone or associated with LT, and is responsible more commonly for severe disease than LT-only ETEC strains. STa is a small monomeric peptide that binds to the transmembrane guanylate cyclase C receptor on the intestinal epithelium, leading to an **increase in cyclic guanosine monophosphate (cGMP)** and subsequent hypersecretion of fluids well as inhibition of fluid absorption. Of the heat-labile toxins, LT-I is more commonly associated with human disease. LT-I is functionally and structurally similar to cholera toxin (80% homology) and consists of one A subunit and five identical B subunits. The B subunits bind to the same receptor as cholera toxin (GM_1 gangliosides), as well as other surface glycoproteins on epithelial cells in the small intestine. After endocytosis, the A subunit moves across the membrane of the vacuole and interacts with a membrane protein (Gs) that regulates adenylate cyclase. The net effect of this interaction is an **increase in cyclic adenosine monophosphate (cAMP)** levels, resulting in enhanced secretion of chloride and decreased absorption of sodium and chloride. These changes are manifested in a watery diarrhea. Exposure to the toxin also stimulates prostaglandin secretion and production of inflammatory cytokines, resulting in further fluid loss.

Enteropathogenic E. coli

Two groups of *E. coli* responsible for enteric disease (Enteropathogenic *E. coli* [EPEC] and some Shiga toxin–producing *E. coli* [STEC]) possess a cluster of virulence genes located on a chromosomal pathogenicity island called the **locus of enterocyte effacement (LEE).** Bacteria in the heterogeneous EPEC group were the first *E. coli* strains associated with outbreaks of diarrheal disease reported in the 1940s and 1950s. They were originally characterized by the specific serotypes responsible for each outbreak but are now defined by (1) presence of LEE and (2) absence of Shiga toxin. EPEC are further subdivided into typical and atypical strains based on the presence or absence of the ***E. coli* adherence factor (EAF) plasmid**. Sporadic disease and outbreaks are relatively uncommon in developed countries and are now reported only sporadically in impoverished countries, with disease primarily in infants and most commonly associated with the atypical strains. Disease is transmitted by fecal-oral exposure to contaminated surfaces or food products. Humans are the only source of typical strains, whereas both humans and a variety of animal hosts are reservoirs of atypical strains.

Infection is initiated by bacterial attachment to epithelial cells of the small intestine, with subsequent effacement (destruction) of the microvillus **(attachment/effacement [A/E] histopathology).** The initial aggregation of typical EPEC leading to the formation of microcolonies on the epithelial cell surface is mediated by plasmid-encoded **bundle-forming pili (BFP);** however, this plasmid is not present in atypical EPEC. The subsequent stages of attachment are regulated by genes encoded on the **LEE pathogenicity island.** This island of more than 40 genes is responsible for attachment and destruction of the host cell surface. Following the loose attachment, active secretion of bacterial proteins into the host epithelial cell occurs by the bacterial type III secretion system. One protein, **translocated intimin receptor (Tir),** is inserted into the epithelial cell membrane and functions as a receptor for an outer membrane bacterial adhesin, **intimin.** Binding of intimin to Tir results in polymerization of actin, accumulation of cytoskeletal elements beneath the attached bacteria, loss of cell surface integrity, and eventual cell death.

Disease occurs primarily in children younger than 2 years and is characterized by **watery diarrhea** that may be severe and protracted and is often accompanied by fever and vomiting. The onset of disease may be as rapid as a few hours after ingestion of EPEC, and although most infections resolve after a few days, persistent diarrhea requiring hospitalization can occur.

Enteroaggregative E. coli

Enteroaggregative *E. coli* (EAEC) are a heterogeneous collection of strains characterized by their autoagglutination in a "stacked-brick" arrangement over the epithelium of the small intestine and, in some cases, the colon. The prevalence of disease caused by EAEC is unclear because a single molecular marker for these bacteria has not been discovered. Genes encoding adhesins, toxins including Shiga toxin, and other virulence proteins are highly variable among EAEC. However, comprehensive analyses of outbreaks in both developed and developing countries have demonstrated these bacteria are common. Outbreaks of gastroenteritis caused by EAEC have also been reported in the United States, Europe, and Japan and are likely an important cause of childhood diarrhea in developed countries. These are one of the few bacteria associated with **chronic diarrhea and growth retardation** in children. Characteristically, following adherence to the epithelium, cytokine release is stimulated, which results in neutrophil recruitment and progression to an inflammatory diarrhea. Disease is characterized by a watery secretory diarrhea, often with inflammatory cells and accompanied by fever, nausea, vomiting, and abdominal pain. This process can be either acute or progress to a persistent diarrhea, particularly in children and HIV-infected patients.

Shiga Toxin–Producing E. coli (Clinical Case 25-1)

Nomenclature for this group of *E. coli* is confusing, referring to them as **Shiga toxin–producing *E. coli* (STEC)**, verocytotoxin-producing *E. coli* (VTEC), and enterohemorrhagic *E. coli* (EHEC). To provide some clarity, consider VTEC an outdated name and EHEC a subset of STEC. All members of this group are defined by the presence of Shiga toxin 1 (Stx1) or 2 (Stx2). Some but not all EHEC strains are LEE positive and form A/E cytopathology, resembling EPEC strains. Classification of STEC is further complicated because the most common serotype associated with human disease is O157:H7, and initial efforts to diagnose disease were to determine if the suspected pathogen was this serotype. It is

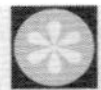 **Clinical Case 25-1 Multistate Outbreak of Shiga Toxin–Producing *Escherichia coli* (STEC) Infections**

In 2006, *E. coli* O157 was responsible for a large multistate outbreak of gastroenteritis. The outbreak was linked to contamination of spinach, with a total of 173 cases reported in 25 states, primarily over an 18-day period. The outbreak resulted in hospitalization of more than 50% of the patients with documented disease, a 16% rate of hemolytic uremic syndrome, and one death. Despite the wide distribution of the contaminated spinach, publication of the outbreak and the rapid determination that spinach was responsible resulted in prompt removal of spinach from grocery stores and termination of the outbreak. This outbreak illustrates how contamination of a food product, even with small numbers of organisms, can lead to a widespread outbreak with a particularly virulent organism, such as strains of STEC.

now appreciated that although O157:H7 is the most common serotype associated with severe human disease, it represents less than 50% of the responsible serotypes. Additionally, the prevalent serotypes will vary geographically. Thus diagnosis of STEC disease is now based on detection of the Shiga toxins rather than serotyping suspected isolates.

Various national programs have been established in the United States, Canada, Europe, and Australia to monitor foodborne diseases and have documented widespread prevalence of STEC disease in these countries, as well as in other countries where outbreaks have been documented. It is estimated that these bacteria cause 73,000 infections and 60 deaths each year in the United States, although awareness of these pathogens are now associated with an overall decrease in prevalence. STEC disease is most common in the warm months, and the highest incidence is in children younger than 5 years. Most infections are attributed to the consumption of undercooked ground beef or other meat products, water, unpasteurized milk or fruit juices (e.g., cider made from apples contaminated with feces from cattle), uncooked vegetables such as spinach, and fruits. **Ingestion of fewer than 100 bacteria can produce disease,** and person-to-person spread occurs.

Disease caused by STEC ranges from mild uncomplicated diarrhea to **hemorrhagic colitis** with severe abdominal pain and bloody diarrhea. Severe disease is more commonly associated with STEC O157:H7. Initially, diarrhea with abdominal pain develops in patients after 3 to 4 days of incubation. Vomiting is observed in approximately half the patients, but a high fever is generally absent. Within 2 days of onset, disease in 30% to 65% of patients progresses to a bloody diarrhea with severe abdominal pain. Complete resolution of symptoms typically occurs after 4 to 10 days in most untreated patients. **Hemolytic uremic syndrome (HUS),** a disorder characterized by acute renal failure, thrombocytopenia, and microangiopathic hemolytic anemia, is a complication in 5% to 10% of infected children younger than 10 years. Resolution of symptoms occurs in uncomplicated disease after 4 to 10 days in most untreated patients; however, death can occur in 3% to 5% of patients with HUS, and severe sequelae (e.g., renal impairment, hypertension, central nervous system [CNS] manifestations) can occur in as many as 30% of HUS patients.

Stx1 is essentially identical to the Shiga toxin produced by *Shigella dysenteriae* (thus the source of the name); Stx2 has 60% homology. Both toxins are acquired by lysogenic bacteriophages. Both have one A subunit and five B subunits, with the B subunits binding to a specific glycolipid on the host cell (globotriaosylceramide [Gb3]). A high concentration of Gb3 receptors is found in the intestinal villi and renal endothelial cells. After the A subunit is internalized, it is cleaved into two molecules, and the A_1 fragment binds to 28S rRNA and causes a cessation of protein synthesis. STEC strains with both Shiga toxins and attaching and effacing activity are more pathogenic than strains producing only one Shiga toxin.

HUS has been preferentially associated with the production of Stx2, which has been shown to destroy glomerular endothelial cells. Damage to the endothelial cells leads to platelet activation and thrombin deposition which results in decreased glomerular filtration and acute renal failure. The Shiga toxins also stimulate expression of inflammatory cytokines (e.g., tumor necrosis factor [TNF]-γ, interleukin [IL]-6), enhancing expression of the B subunit receptor Gb3.

Enteroinvasive E. coli

Enteroinvasive *E. coli* (EIEC) strains are rare in both developed and developing countries. Pathogenic strains are primarily associated with a few restricted O serotypes: O124, O143, and O164. The strains are closely related by phenotypic and pathogenic properties to *Shigella.* The bacteria are able to invade and destroy the colonic epithelium, producing a disease characterized initially by **watery diarrhea.** A minority of patients progress to the dysenteric form of disease, consisting of fever, abdominal cramps, and blood and leukocytes in stool specimens.

A series of genes on a plasmid mediate bacterial invasion **(*pInv* genes)** into the colonic epithelium. The bacteria then lyse the phagocytic vacuole and replicate in the cell cytoplasm. Movement within the cytoplasm and into adjacent epithelial cells is regulated by formation of actin tails (similar to that observed with *Listeria*). This process of epithelial cell destruction with inflammatory infiltration can progress to colonic ulceration.

Extraintestinal Infections

Urinary Tract Infection

Most gram-negative rods that produce UTIs originate in the colon, contaminate the urethra, ascend into the bladder, and may migrate to the kidney or prostate. Although most strains of *E. coli* can produce UTIs, disease is more common with certain specific serogroups. These bacteria are particularly virulent because of their ability to produce **adhesins** (primarily P pili, AAF/I, AAF/III, and Dr) that bind to cells lining the bladder and upper urinary tract (preventing elimination of the bacteria in voided urine) and **hemolysin HlyA** that lyses erythrocytes and other cell types (leading to cytokine release and stimulation of an inflammatory response).

Neonatal Meningitis

E. coli and group B streptococci cause the majority of CNS infections in infants younger than 1 month. Approximately 75% of the *E. coli* strains possess the **K1 capsular antigen.** This serogroup is also commonly present in the GI tracts of pregnant women and newborn infants. However, the reason this serogroup has a predilection for crossing the blood-brain barrier and causing meningitis in newborns is not understood.

Septicemia

Typically, septicemia caused by gram-negative rods, such as *E. coli,* most commonly originates from infections in the urinary or GI tract (e.g., intestinal leakage leading to an intraabdominal infection). The mortality associated with *E. coli* septicemia is high for patients in whom immunity is compromised or the primary infection is in the abdomen or CNS.

Salmonella

The taxonomic classification of the genus *Salmonella* is problematic. DNA homology studies have revealed that most clinically significant isolates belong to the species *Salmonella enterica.* More than 2500 unique serotypes have been described for this single species; however, these serotypes are commonly listed as individual species (e.g., *Salmonella typhi, Salmonella choleraesuis, Salmonella typhimurium, Salmonella enteritidis*). These designations are incorrect—for example, the correct nomenclature is *Salmonella enterica,* serovar. Typhi. In an effort to prevent confusion and still retain the historical terms, individual serotypes are now commonly written with the serotype name capitalized and not in italics. For example, *Salmonella enterica*, serovar. Typhi is commonly designated as *Salmonella* Typhi. For the sake of consistency, this nomenclature will be used in this chapter.

Pathogenesis and Immunity

After ingestion and passage through the stomach, salmonellae attach to the mucosa of the **small intestine** and invade into the **M (microfold) cells** located in Peyer patches, as well as into enterocytes. The bacteria remain in endocytic vacuoles, where they replicate. The bacteria can also be transported across the cytoplasm and released into the blood or lymphatic circulation. Regulation of attachment, engulfment, and replication is controlled primarily by two large clusters of genes **(pathogenicity island I and II)** on the bacterial chromosome. Pathogenicity island I encodes **salmonella-secreted invasion proteins (Ssps)** and a **type III secretion system** that injects the proteins into the host cell. Pathogenicity island II contains genes that allow the bacteria to evade the host's immune response and encodes a second type III secretion system for this function. The inflammatory response confines the infection to the GI tract, mediates the release of prostaglandins, and stimulates cAMP and active fluid secretion.

Epidemiology

Salmonella can colonize virtually all animals, including poultry, reptiles, livestock, rodents, domestic animals, birds, and humans. Animal-to-animal spread and the use of *Salmonella*-contaminated animal feeds maintain an **animal reservoir.** Serotypes such as *Salmonella* Typhi and *Salmonella* Paratyphi are highly **adapted to humans** and do not cause disease in nonhuman hosts. Other *Salmonella* serotypes (e.g., *Salmonella* Choleraesuis) are adapted to animals and, when they infect humans, can cause severe disease. In addition, in contrast with other *Salmonella* serotypes, strains that are highly adapted to humans (i.e., *Salmonella* Typhi, *Salmonella* Paratyphi) can survive in the gallbladder and establish chronic carriage. Finally, many *Salmonella* strains have no host specificity and cause disease in both human and nonhuman hosts.

Most infections result from **ingestion** of contaminated food products and, in children, from direct fecal-oral spread. The incidence of disease is greatest in children younger than 5 years and adults older than 60 years, who are infected during the summer and autumn months when contaminated foods are consumed at outdoor social gatherings. The most common sources of human infections are **poultry, eggs, dairy products,** and foods prepared on contaminated work surfaces (e.g., cutting boards where uncooked poultry was prepared). Approximately 50,000 cases of nontyphoidal *Salmonella* infections are reported annually in the United States, although it has been estimated that 1.2 million infections and 400 deaths occur each year. *Salmonella* Typhi infections occur when food or water contaminated by infected food handlers is ingested. There is no animal reservoir. An average of 400 to 500 *Salmonella* Typhi infections are reported annually in the United States, most of which are acquired during foreign travel. In contrast, it is estimated that 27 million *Salmonella* Typhi and *Salmonella* Paratyphi infections and more than 200,000 deaths occur each year worldwide. The risk of disease is highest in children living in poverty in a developing country.

The infectious dose for *Salmonella* Typhi infections is low, so person-to-person spread is common. In contrast, a large inoculum (e.g., 10^6 to 10^8 bacteria) is required for symptomatic disease to develop with most other *Salmonella* serotypes. The organisms can multiply to this high density if contaminated food products are improperly stored (e.g., left at room temperature). The infectious dose is lower for people at high risk for disease because of age, immunosuppression or underlying disease (leukemia, lymphoma, sickle cell disease), or reduced gastric acidity.

Clinical Diseases

The following four forms of *Salmonella* infection exist: gastroenteritis, septicemia, enteric fever, and asymptomatic colonization.

Gastroenteritis

Gastroenteritis is the **most common form of salmonellosis** in the United States. Symptoms generally appear 6 to 48 hours after the consumption of contaminated food or water, with the initial presentation consisting of **nausea, vomiting, and nonbloody diarrhea.** Fever, abdominal cramps, myalgias, and headache are also common. Colonic involvement can be demonstrated in the acute form of the disease. Symptoms can persist for 2 to 7 days before spontaneous resolution.

Septicemia

All *Salmonella* species can cause bacteremia, although infections with *Salmonella* Typhi, *Salmonella* Paratyphi, and *Salmonella* Choleraesuis more commonly lead to a bacteremic phase. The risk for *Salmonella* bacteremia is higher in pediatric and geriatric patients and in immunocompromised

Clinical Case 25-2 *Salmonella* Typhi Infection

Scully and associates (*N Engl J Med* 345:201–205, 2007) described a 25-year-old woman who was admitted to a Boston hospital with a history of persistent fever that did not respond to amoxicillin or acetaminophen or ibuprofen. She was a resident of the Philippines who had been traveling in the United States for the previous 11 days. On physical examination, she was febrile and had an enlarged liver, abdominal pain, and an abnormal urinalysis. Blood cultures were collected upon admission to the hospital and were positive the next day with *Salmonella* Typhi. Because the organism was susceptible to fluoroquinolones, this therapy was selected. Within 4 days, she had defervesced and was discharged to return home to the Philippines. Although typhoid fever can be a very serious life-threatening illness, it can initially present with nonspecific symptoms, as was seen in this woman.

patients (HIV infections, sickle cell disease, congenital immunodeficiencies). The clinical presentation of *Salmonella* bacteremia is like that of other gram-negative bacteremias; however, localized suppurative infections (e.g., osteomyelitis, endocarditis, arthritis) can occur in as many as 10% of patients.

Enteric Fever (Clinical Case 25-2)

Salmonella Typhi produces a febrile illness called **typhoid fever.** A milder form of this disease, referred to as **paratyphoid fever,** is produced by *Salmonella* Paratyphi A, *Salmonella* Schottmuelleri (formerly *Salmonella* Paratyphi B), and *Salmonella* Hirschfeldii (formerly *Salmonella* Paratyphi C). Other *Salmonella* serotypes can rarely produce a similar syndrome. The bacteria responsible for enteric fever pass through the cells lining the intestines and are engulfed by macrophages. They replicate after being transported to the liver, spleen, and bone marrow. Ten to 14 days after ingestion of the bacteria, patients experience gradually increasing fever, with nonspecific complaints of headache, myalgias, malaise, and anorexia. These symptoms persist for 1 week or longer and are followed by GI symptoms. This cycle corresponds to an initial bacteremic phase that is followed by colonization of the gallbladder and then reinfection of the intestines. Enteric fever is a serious clinical disease and must be suspected in febrile patients who have recently traveled to developing countries where disease is endemic.

Asymptomatic Colonization

The strains of *Salmonella* responsible for causing typhoid and paratyphoid fevers are maintained by human colonization. **Chronic colonization** for more than 1 year after symptomatic disease develops in 1% to 5% of patients, with the gallbladder being the reservoir in most patients. Chronic colonization with other species of *Salmonella* occurs in less than 1% of patients and does not represent an important source of human infection.

Shigella

The commonly used taxonomic classification of *Shigella* is simple, although technically incorrect. Four species consisting of almost 50 O-antigen–based serogroups have been described: *S. dysenteriae, Shigella flexneri, Shigella boydii,* and *Shigella sonnei.* However, analysis of DNA has determined that these four species are actually biogroups within the species *E. coli.* Because it would be confusing to refer to these bacteria as *E. coli,* their historical names have been retained.

Pathogenesis and Immunity

Shigellae cause disease by invading and replicating in cells lining the **colon.** Structural gene proteins mediate the adherence of the organisms to the cells, as well as their invasion, intracellular replication, and cell-to-cell spread. These genes are carried on a large virulence plasmid but are regulated by chromosomal genes. Thus the presence of the plasmid does not ensure functional gene activity.

Shigella species appear unable to attach to differentiated mucosal cells; rather, they first attach to and invade the M cells located in Peyer patches. The **type III secretion system** mediates secretion of four proteins **(IpaA, IpaB, IpaC, IpaD)** into epithelial cells and macrophages. These proteins induce membrane ruffling on the target cell, leading to engulfment of the bacteria. Shigellae lyse the phagocytic vacuole and replicate in the host cell cytoplasm (unlike *Salmonella,* which replicate in the vacuole). With the rearrangement of actin filaments in the host cells, the bacteria are propelled through the cytoplasm to adjacent cells, where **cell-to-cell passage** occurs. In this way, *Shigella* organisms are protected from immune-mediated clearance. Shigellae survive phagocytosis by inducing programmed cell death **(apoptosis).** This process also leads to the release of IL-1β, resulting in the attraction of polymorphonuclear leukocytes into the infected tissues. This, in turn, destabilizes the integrity of the intestinal wall and allows the bacteria to reach the deeper epithelial cells.

S. dysenteriae strains produce an exotoxin, **Shiga toxin.** Similar to Shiga toxin produced by STEC, this toxin has one A subunit and five B subunits. The B subunits bind to a host cell glycolipid (Gb3) and facilitate transfer of the A subunit into the cell. The A subunit cleaves the 28S rRNA in the 60S ribosomal subunit, thereby preventing the binding of aminoacyl-transfer RNA and disrupting protein synthesis. The primary manifestation of toxin activity is damage to the intestinal epithelium; however, in a small subset of patients, the Shiga toxin can mediate damage to the glomerular endothelial cells, resulting in renal failure (HUS).

Epidemiology

Humans are the only reservoir for *Shigella.* It is estimated that almost 500,000 cases of *Shigella* infections occur each year in the United States. This figure pales in comparison with the estimated 90 million cases that occur annually worldwide. ***S. sonnei*** is responsible for almost 85% of U.S. infections, whereas ***S. flexneri*** predominates in developing countries. Epidemics of ***S. dysenteriae*** infections occur periodically, most recently in West Africa and Central America, and are associated with case fatality rates of 5% to 15%.

Shigellosis is primarily a pediatric disease, with 60% of all infections in children younger than 10 years. Endemic disease in adults is common in male homosexuals and in household contacts of infected children. Epidemic outbreaks of disease occur in day-care centers, nurseries, and custodial institutions. Shigellosis is **transmitted person to person** by

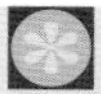

Clinical Case 25-3 *Shigella* Infections in Day-Care Centers

In 2005, three states reported outbreaks of multidrug-resistant *Shigella* infections in day-care centers. A total of 532 infections were reported in the Kansas City area, with the median age of patients 6 years old (Centers for Disease Control and Prevention: *MMWR Morb Mortal Wkly Rep* 55:1068–1071, 2006). The predominant pathogen was a multidrug-resistant strain of *Shigella sonnei,* with 89% of the isolates resistant to ampicillin and trimethoprim-sulfamethoxazole. Shigellosis spreads easily in day-care centers because of the increased risk of fecal contamination and the low infectious dose responsible for disease. Parents and teachers, as well as classmates, are at significant risk for disease.

the fecal-oral route, primarily by people with contaminated hands and less commonly in water or food. Because as few as 100 to 200 bacteria can establish disease, shigellosis spreads rapidly in communities where sanitary standards and the level of personal hygiene are low.

Clinical Diseases (Clinical Case 25-3)

Shigellosis is characterized by **abdominal cramps, diarrhea, fever,** and **bloody stools.** The clinical signs and symptoms of the disease appear 1 to 3 days after the bacteria are ingested. Shigellae initially colonize the small intestine and begin to multiply within the first 12 hours. The first sign of infection (profuse watery diarrhea without histologic evidence of mucosal invasion) is mediated by an enterotoxin. However, the cardinal feature of shigellosis is lower abdominal cramps and tenesmus (straining to defecate), with abundant pus and blood in the stool. It results from invasion of the colonic mucosa by the bacteria. Abundant neutrophils, erythrocytes, and mucus are found in the stool. Infection is generally self-limited, although antibiotic treatment is recommended to reduce the risk of secondary spread to family members and other contacts. Asymptomatic colonization of the organism in the colon develops in a small number of patients and represents a persistent reservoir for infection.

Yersinia

The best known human pathogens within the genus *Yersinia* are ***Y. pestis, Yersinia enterocolitica,*** and ***Yersinia pseudotuberculosis.*** *Y. pestis* is a highly virulent pathogen that causes the highly fatal systemic disease known as **plague;** *Y. enterocolitica* and *Y. pseudotuberculosis* are primarily enteric pathogens that are relatively uncommon and rarely cultured from blood.

Pathogenesis and Immunity

A common characteristic of the pathogenic *Yersinia* species is their ability to **resist phagocytic killing.** The type III secretion system mediates this property. On contact with phagocytic cells, the bacteria secrete proteins into the phagocyte that dephosphorylate several proteins required for phagocytosis (YopH gene product), induce cytotoxicity by disrupting actin filaments (YopE gene product), and initiate apoptosis in macrophages (YopJ/P gene product). The type III secretion system also suppresses cytokine production, in turn diminishing the inflammatory immune response to infection.

Y. pestis has two plasmids that encode virulence genes: (1) fraction 1 *(f1)* gene, which codes for an antiphagocytic **protein capsule,** and (2) **plasminogen activator *(pla)* protease** gene, which degrades complement components C3b and C5a, preventing opsonization and phagocytic migration, respectively. The *pla* gene also degrades fibrin clots, permitting *Y. pestis* to spread rapidly. Other virulence factors specifically associated with *Y. pestis* are serum resistance and the ability of the organism to absorb organic iron as a result of a siderophore-independent mechanism.

Epidemiology

All *Yersinia* infections are **zoonotic,** with humans the accidental hosts. There are two forms of *Y. pestis* infection: **urban plague,** for which rats are the natural reservoirs, and **sylvatic plague,** which causes infections in squirrels, rabbits, field rats, and domestic cats. Pigs, rodents, livestock, and rabbits are the natural reservoirs for *Y. enterocolitica,* whereas rodents, wild animals, and game birds are the natural reservoirs for *Y. pseudotuberculosis.*

Plague, caused by *Y. pestis,* was one of the most devastating diseases in history. Epidemics of the plague were recorded in the Old Testament. The first of three major pandemics (urban plague) started in Egypt in 541 AD and spread throughout North Africa, Europe, central and southern Asia, and Arabia. By the time this pandemic ended in the mid-700s, a major proportion of the population in these countries had died from the plague. The second pandemic, which started in the 1320s, resulted (over a 5-year period) in more than 25 million deaths in Europe alone (30% to 40% of the population). The third pandemic began in China in the 1860s and spread to Africa, Europe, and the Americas. Epidemic and sporadic cases of the disease continue to this day. In recent years, fewer than 10 cases are reported annually in the United States, with disease primarily sylvatic plague and present in western states.

Urban plague is maintained in rat populations and is spread among **rats** or between rats and humans by infected **fleas.** Fleas become infected during a blood meal from a bacteremic rat. After the bacteria replicate in the flea gut, the organisms can be transferred to another rodent or to humans. Urban plague has been eliminated from most communities by the effective control of rats and better hygiene. In contrast, **sylvatic plague** is difficult or impossible to eliminate because the **mammalian reservoirs** and **flea vectors** are widespread. *Y. pestis* produces a fatal infection in the animal reservoir, so cyclic patterns of human disease occur as the number of infected reservoir hosts increases or decreases. Infections can also be acquired through ingestion of contaminated animals or handling of contaminated animal tissues. Although the organism is highly infectious, human-to-human spread is uncommon unless the patient has pulmonary involvement.

Y. enterocolitica is a common cause of enterocolitis in Scandinavian and other northern European countries and in the colder areas of North America. In the United States, approximately one culture-confirmed infection occurs per 100,000 persons each year, with 90% of the infections being associated with consumption of contaminated meat, milk, or water. Most studies show that infections are more common

Clinical Case 25-4 Human Plague in the United States

In 2006, a total of 13 human plague cases were reported in the United States—7 in New Mexico, 3 in Colorado, 2 in California, and 1 in Texas (Centers for Disease Control and Prevention: *MMWR Morb Mortal Wkly Rep* 55:940–943, 2006). The following is a description of a 30-year-old man with a classic presentation of bubonic plague. On July 9, the man presented to his local hospital with a 3-day history of fever, nausea, vomiting, and right inguinal lymphadenopathy. He was discharged without treatment. Three days later, he returned to the hospital and was admitted with sepsis and bilateral pulmonary infiltrates. He was placed on respiratory isolation and treated with gentamicin, to which he responded. Cultures of his blood and enlarged lymph node were positive for *Yersinia pestis*. The bacteria were also recovered in fleas collected near the patient's home. Typically the reservoirs for sylvatic plague are small mammals, and the vectors are fleas. When the mammals die off, the fleas will seek human hosts.

during the cold months. Virulence with this organism is associated with specific serogroups. The most common serogroups found in Europe, Africa, Japan, and Canada are O3 and O9. Serogroup O8 has been identified in the United States. *Y. pseudotuberculosis* is a relatively uncommon cause of human disease.

Clinical Diseases (Clinical Case 25-4)

The two clinical manifestations of *Y. pestis* infection are bubonic plague and pneumonic plague. **Bubonic plague** is characterized by an incubation period of no more than 7 days after a person has been bitten by an infected flea. Patients have a high fever and a painful **bubo** (inflammatory swelling of the lymph nodes) in the groin or axilla. Bacteremia develops rapidly if patients are not treated, and as many as 75% die. The incubation period (2 to 3 days) is shorter in patients with **pneumonic plague.** Initially these patients experience fever and malaise, and pulmonary signs develop within 1 day. The patients are highly infectious; person-to-person spread occurs by aerosols. The mortality rate in untreated patients with pneumonic plague exceeds 90%.

Approximately two thirds of all *Y. enterocolitica* infections are **enterocolitis,** as the name implies. The gastroenteritis is typically associated with ingestion of contaminated food products or water. After an incubation period of 1 to 10 days (average, 4 to 6 days), the patient experiences disease characterized by diarrhea, fever, and abdominal pain that last as long as 1 to 2 weeks. A chronic form of the disease can also develop and persist for months. Disease involves the terminal ileum and, if the mesenteric lymph nodes become enlarged, can mimic acute appendicitis. *Y. enterocolitica* infection is most common in children, with **pseudoappendicitis** posing a particular problem in this age group. *Y. pseudotuberculosis* can also produce an enteric disease with the same clinical features. Other manifestations seen in adults are septicemia, arthritis, intraabdominal abscess, hepatitis, and osteomyelitis.

In 1987, *Y. enterocolitica* was first reported to cause **blood transfusion–related bacteremia** and endotoxic shock. Because *Yersinia* organisms **can grow at 4° C,** this organism can multiply to high concentrations in nutritionally rich blood products that are stored in a refrigerator.

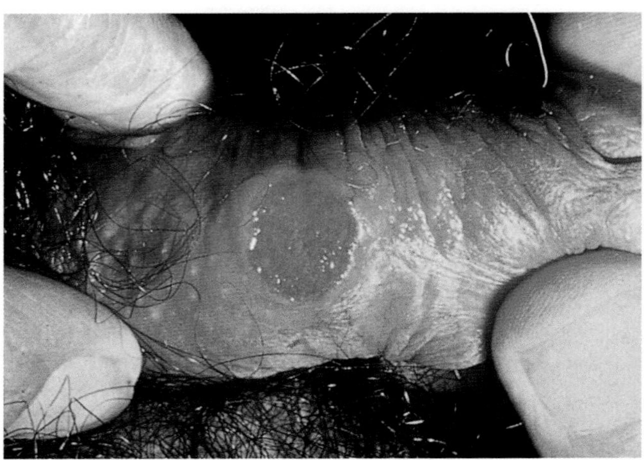

FIGURE 25-4 Penile ulcer caused by *Klebsiella granulomatis.* This can mimic the chancre of syphilis. (From Morse SA, Ballard RC, Holmes KK, et al: *Atlas of sexually transmitted diseases and AIDS,* ed 4, London, 2010, Saunders.)

Other Enterobacteriaceae

Klebsiella

Members of the genus *Klebsiella* have a prominent capsule that is responsible for the mucoid appearance of isolated colonies and the enhanced virulence of the organisms in vivo. The most commonly isolated members of this genus are ***K. pneumoniae*** and ***Klebsiella oxytoca,*** which can cause community- or hospital-acquired primary **lobar pneumonia.** Pneumonia caused by *Klebsiella* species frequently involves necrotic destruction of alveolar spaces, formation of cavities, and production of blood-tinged sputum. These bacteria also cause wound and soft-tissue infections and UTIs.

The organism formerly called *Donovania granulomatis* and then *Calymmatobacterium granulomatis* has been reclassified as ***Klebsiella granulomatis.*** *K. granulomatis* is the etiologic agent of **granuloma inguinale,** a granulomatous disease affecting the genitalia and inguinal area (Figures 25-4 and 25-5). Unfortunately, this disease is commonly called **donovanosis** in reference to the historical origin of the genus name. Granuloma inguinale is a rare disease in the United States but is endemic in parts of Papua New Guinea, the Caribbean, South America, India, southern Africa, Vietnam, and Australia. It can be transmitted after repeated exposure through sexual intercourse or nonsexual trauma to the genitalia. After a prolonged incubation of weeks to months, subcutaneous nodules appear on the genitalia or in the inguinal area. The nodules subsequently break down, revealing one or more painless granulomatous lesions that can extend and coalesce into ulcers resembling syphilitic lesions.

Two other *Klebsiella* species of clinical importance are ***Klebsiella rhinoscleromatis,*** cause of a granulomatous disease of the nose, and ***Klebsiella ozaenae,*** cause of chronic atrophic rhinitis. Both diseases are relatively uncommon in the United States.

Proteus

P. mirabilis, the most common member of this genus, primarily produces infections of the urinary tract (e.g., bladder

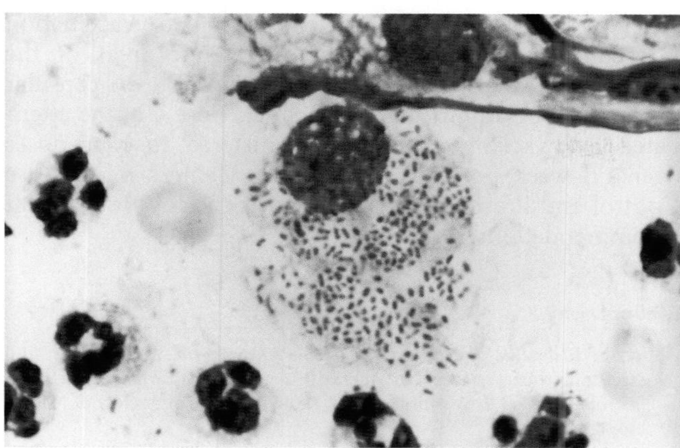

FIGURE 25-5 Light microscopy of impression smear of granulation tissue from genital lesion of patient infected with *Klebsiella granulomatis.* Note the numerous bacteria in the cytoplasmic vacuole of the mononuclear cell (modified Giemsa stain). (From Morse SA, Ballard RC, Holmes KK, et al: *Atlas of sexually transmitted diseases and AIDS,* ed 4, London, 2010, Saunders.)

infection or cystitis; kidney infection or pyelonephritis). *P. mirabilis* produces large quantities of urease, which splits urea into carbon dioxide and ammonia. This process raises the urine pH, precipitating magnesium and calcium in the form of struvite and apatite crystals, respectively, and results in the formation of **renal (kidney) stones.** The increased alkalinity of the urine is also toxic to the uroepithelium.

Enterobacter, Citrobacter, Morganella, and *Serratia*

Primary infections caused by *Enterobacter, Citrobacter, Morganella,* and *Serratia* are rare in immunocompetent patients. They are more common causes of hospital-acquired infections in neonates and immunocompromised patients. For example, ***Citrobacter koseri*** has been recognized to have a predilection for causing meningitis and brain abscesses in neonates.

• Other General Properties

Laboratory Diagnosis

Culture

Members of the family Enterobacteriaceae grow readily on culture media. Specimens of normally sterile material, such as spinal fluid and tissue collected at surgery, can be inoculated onto nonselective blood agar media. Selective media (e.g., MacConkey agar, eosin-methylene blue [EMB] agar) are used for the culture of specimens normally contaminated with other organisms (e.g., sputum, feces). Use of these selective differential agars enables the separation of lactose-fermenting Enterobacteriaceae from nonfermenting strains, thereby providing information that can be used to guide empirical antimicrobial therapy.

Diagnosis of *E. coli* strains responsible for gastroenteritis is most commonly performed by reference laboratories. The exception is detection of STEC. Two approaches have been used: culture and toxin detection. In contrast with most *E. coli,* many strains of STEC, particularly O157:H7, do not ferment sorbitol. Thus **sorbitol-containing MacConkey agar** (S-MAC) has been used to screen stool specimens for sorbitol-negative (colorless), gram-negative bacteria that are then confirmed by serogrouping and biochemical tests to be *E. coli* O157. The limitation to this approach is that some strains of O157 and many other STEC serotypes ferment sorbitol and would be missed by this screening approach. The preferred method to detect STEC is to test stool specimens directly for the presence of Shiga toxin by use of commercial immunoassays or molecular tests for the Shiga toxin (Stx1 and Stx2) genes. These tests are rapid and sensitive.

Highly selective or organism-specific media are useful for the recovery of organisms such as *Salmonella* and *Shigella* in stool specimens, where an abundance of normal flora can obscure the presence of these important pathogens.

It is difficult to recover *Y. enterocolitica* because this organism grows slowly at traditional incubation temperatures and prefers cooler temperatures, at which it is more active metabolically. Clinical laboratories have exploited this property, however, by mixing the fecal specimen with saline and then storing the specimen at 4° C for 2 weeks or more before subculturing it to agar media. This **cold enrichment** permits the growth of *Yersinia* but inhibits or kills other organisms in the specimen. Although use of the cold enrichment method does not aid in the initial management of a patient with *Yersinia* gastroenteritis, it has helped elucidate the role of this organism in chronic intestinal disease.

Biochemical Identification

There are many diverse species in the family Enterobacteriaceae. The citations listed in the Bibliography at the end of this chapter provide additional information about their biochemical identification. Biochemical test systems have become increasingly sophisticated, and the most common members of the family can be identified accurately in less than 24 hours with one of the many commercially available identification systems. Sequencing of species-specific genes (e.g., 16S rRNA gene) or detection of characteristic protein profiles by mass spectrometry is used to identify the less common species.

Serologic Classification

Serologic testing is very useful for determining the clinical significance of an isolate (e.g., serotyping specific pathogenic strains such as *E. coli* O157 or *Y. enterocolitica* O8) and for classifying isolates for epidemiologic purposes. The usefulness of this procedure is limited, however, by cross-reactions with antigenically related Enterobacteriaceae and with organisms from other bacterial families.

Treatment, Prevention, and Control

Antibiotic therapy for infections with Enterobacteriaceae must be guided by in vitro susceptibility test results and clinical experience. Some organisms, such as *E. coli* and *P. mirabilis,* are susceptible to many antibiotics, but others can be highly resistant. Production of enzymes that inactivate all the penicillins and cephalosporins (e.g., extended-spectrum β-lactamases [ESBLs]) is now widespread in *E. coli, Klebsiella,* and *Proteus.* Additionally, use of carbapenems (e.g., imipenem, meropenem, ertapenem) was once a mainstay of treatment; however, the recent recovery of carbapenemase-producing bacteria has limited the empirical use of carbapenems and all other β-lactam antibiotics for many regions of the world. In general, **antibiotic resistance** is more common in hospital-acquired infections than in community-acquired infections. Antibiotic therapy is not recommended for some infections. For example, symptomatic relief but not antibiotic treatment is usually recommended for patients with Shiga toxin–producing *E. coli* and *Salmonella* gastroenteritis, because antibiotics can prolong the fecal carriage of these organisms or increase the risk of secondary complications (e.g., HUS with STEC infections in children). Treatment of *Salmonella* Typhi infections or other systemic *Salmonella* infections is indicated; however, increasing resistance to antibiotics, such as the fluoroquinolones, has complicated therapy.

It is difficult to prevent infections with Enterobacteriaceae because these organisms are a major part of the endogenous microbial population. However, some risk factors for the infections should be avoided. These include the unrestricted use of antibiotics that can select for resistant bacteria, performance of procedures that traumatize mucosal barriers without prophylactic antibiotic coverage, and use of urinary catheters. Unfortunately, many of these factors are present in patients at greatest risk for infection (e.g., immunocompromised patients confined to the hospital for extended periods).

Exogenous infection with Enterobacteriaceae is theoretically easier to control. For example, the source of infections with organisms such as *Salmonella* is well defined. However, these bacteria are ubiquitous in poultry and eggs. Unless care is taken in the preparation and refrigeration of such foods, little can be done to control these infections. *Shigella* organisms are predominantly transmitted in young children, but it is difficult to interrupt the fecal-hand-mouth transmission responsible for spreading the infection in this population. Outbreaks of these infections can be effectively prevented and controlled only through education and the introduction of appropriate infection-control procedures (e.g., hand washing, proper disposal of soiled diapers and linens) in the settings where these infections typically occur.

A vaccine for *Y. pestis* is no longer available, although this is likely to change in light of the concern that this organism can be used by bioterrorists. Two vaccines for *Salmonella* Typhi are available—an oral, live, attenuated vaccine and a Vi capsular polysaccharide vaccine. Both vaccines protect 40% to 70% of the recipients. Vaccination is recommended for travelers to endemic areas of the world (e.g., Africa, Asia, Latin America). The Vi capsular vaccine can be administered in a single dose, but the attenuated live vaccine must be administered in four doses over a 1-week period. Refer to the Centers for Disease Control and Prevention website (www.cdc.gov) for current recommendations.

Bibliography

Abbott S: *Klebsiella, Enterobacter, Citrobacter, Serratia, Plesiomonas*, and other Enterobacteriaceae. In Murray PR, et al, editors: *Manual of clinical microbiology*, ed 9, Washington, DC, 2007, American Society of Microbiology Press.

Ackers ML, Puhr ND, Tauxe RV, et al: Laboratory-based surveillance of *Salmonella* serotype Typhi infections in the United States: antimicrobial resistance on the rise, *JAMA* 283:2668–2673, 2000.

Croxen MA, Law RJ, Scholz R, et al: Recent advances in understanding enteric pathogenic *Escherichia coli*, *Clin Microbiol Rev* 26:822–880, 2013.

Darwin KH, Miller VL: Molecular basis of the interaction of *Salmonella* with the intestinal mucosa, *Clin Microbiol Rev* 12:405–428, 1999.

Farmer JJ, et al: Enterobacteriaceae: introduction and identification. In Murray PR, et al, editors: *Manual of clinical microbiology*, ed 9, Washington, DC, 2007, American Society of Microbiology Press.

Jackson BR, Iqbal S, Mahon B: Updated recommendations for the use of typhoid vaccine—Advisory Committee on Immunization Practices, United States, *MMWR Morb Mortal Wkly Rep* 64(11):305–308, 2015.

Kotloff KL, Nataro JP, Blackwelder WC, et al: Burden and etiology of diarrhoeal disease in infants and young children in developing countries (the Global Enteric Multicenter Study, GEMS): a prospective, case-control study, *Lancet* 382:209–222, 2013.

Lamberti LM, Bourgeois AL, Fischer Walker CL, et al: Estimating diarrheal illness and deaths attributable to *Shigella* and enterotoxigenic *Escherichia coli* among older children, adolescents, and adults in South Asia and Africa, *PLoS Negl Trop Dis* 8:e2705, 2014.

Nataro J, et al: *Escherichia, Shigella,* and *Salmonella*. In Murray PR, et al, editors: *Manual of clinical microbiology*, ed 9, Washington, DC, 2007, American Society of Microbiology Press.

Ross AG, Olds GR, Cripps AW, et al: Enteropathogens and chronic illness in returning travelers, *N Engl J Med* 368:1817–1825, 2013.

Wanger A: *Yersinia*. In Murray PR, et al, editors: *Manual of clinical microbiology*, ed 9, Washington, DC, 2007, American Society of Microbiology Press.

Wong CS, Jelacic S, Habeeb RL, et al: The risk of the hemolytic-uremic syndrome after antibiotic treatment of *Escherichia coli* O157:H7 infections, *N Engl J Med* 342:1930–1936, 2000.

Zaharik ML, Gruenheid S, Perrin AJ, et al: Delivery of dangerous goods: type III secretion in enteric pathogens, *Int J Med Microbiol* 291:593–603, 2002.

CHAPTER

26 VIBRIO AND RELATED BACTERIA

A 67-year-old woman living in Louisiana developed massive watery diarrhea 2 days after she ate crabs. She was admitted to the local hospital's intensive care unit with hypotension and bradycardia. She was resuscitated after a large volume of fluid (≈22 liters of fluids over 24 hours) was administered. Stool cultures grew *Vibrio cholerae* 01 biotype El Tor, serotype Inaba, and treatment with intravenous doxycycline was initiated. Over the next week her diarrhea resolved, and her recovery was uneventful.

1. *Vibrio* and *Aeromonas* are important gram-negative rods that cause significant enteric disease and wound infections. What properties do these genera share with the Enterobacteriaceae, and how would they be differentiated from this family?
2. How do certain strains of *Vibrio cholerae* produce cholera, and what other organism has a similar virulence factor?
3. What disease does *Vibrio vulnificus* produce, and who is at greatest risk for serious disease?
4. What diseases are associated with *Aeromonas*?

Answers to these questions are available on StudentConsult.com.

• SUMMARIES CLINICALLY SIGNIFICANT ORGANISMS

Vibrio cholerae

Trigger Words

Serogroup 01, cholera, cholera toxin, shellfish, fluid replacement

Biology and Virulence

- Curved gram-negative rods
- Fermentative, facultative anaerobic; require salt for growth
- Strains subdivided into more than 200 serogroups (O–cell wall antigens)
- *V. cholerae* serogroup 01 is further subdivided into serotypes (Inaba, Ogawa, Hikojima) and biotypes (Classical, El Tor)
- Disease mediated by cholera toxin (complex A-B toxin) and toxin co-regulated pilus

Epidemiology

- Serotype 01 is responsible for major pandemics (worldwide epidemics), with significant mortality in developing countries; 0139 can cause similar diseases
- Organism found in estuarine and marine environments worldwide (including along the coast of the United States); associated with chitinous shellfish
- Organism can multiply freely in water
- Bacterial levels in contaminated waters increase during the warm months
- Most commonly spread by consumption of freshly contaminated water
- Direct person-to-person spread is rare because the infectious dose is high; the infectious dose is high because most organisms are killed by stomach acids

Diseases

- Infection can range from asymptomatic colonization or mild diarrhea to severe, rapidly fatal diarrhea

Diagnosis

- Microscopic examination of stool can be useful in acute infections in the setting of an epidemic but rapidly becomes negative as the disease progresses
- Immunoassays for cholera toxin or 01 and 0139 lipopolysaccharides can be useful, although the analytical performance of the assays is quite variable
- Culture should be performed early in course of disease with fresh stool specimens maintained in a neutral to alkaline pH

Treatment, Prevention, and Control

- Fluid and electrolyte replacement are crucial
- Antibiotics (e.g., azithromycin) reduce the bacterial burden and exotoxin production, as well as duration of diarrhea
- Improved hygiene is critical for control
- Combination inactivated whole cell and cholera toxin B subunit vaccines provide limited protection and herd immunity

Vibrio parahaemolyticus

Trigger Words

Kanagawa hemolysin, shellfish, gastroenteritis

Biology and Virulence

- Curved gram-negative rods
- Fermentative, facultative anaerobic; require salt for growth
- Production of thermostable direct hemolysin (Kanagawa hemolysin) associated with pathogenic strains

Epidemiology

- Organism found in estuarine and marine environments worldwide

- Associated with consumption of contaminated raw shellfish
- Most common cause of bacterial gastroenteritis in Japan and Southeast Asia
- Most common cause of seafood-associated gastroenteritis in United States

Diseases

- Most symptomatic infections are self-limited diarrhea

Diagnosis

- Culture should be performed as with *V. cholerae*

Treatment, Prevention, and Control

- Self-limited disease, although antibiotics can shorten length of symptoms and fluid loss
- Disease prevented by proper cooking of shellfish
- No vaccine is available

Vibrio vulnificus

Trigger Words

Septicemia, wound infections, hepatic disease, life-threatening

Biology and Virulence

- Curved gram-negative rods
- Fermentative, facultative anaerobic; require salt for growth
- Virulence associated with presence of polysaccharide capsule and hydrolytic enzymes

Epidemiology

- Infection associated with exposure of a wound to contaminated salt water or ingestion of improperly prepared shellfish

Diseases

- High mortality associated with primary septicemia and wound infections, particularly in patients with underlying hepatic disease

Diagnosis

- Culture wounds and blood

Treatment, Prevention, and Control

- Life-threatening illnesses that must be promptly treated with antibiotics
- Minocycline or doxycycline combined with a ceftriaxone or cefotaxime is the treatment of choice
- No vaccine is available

The second major group of **gram-negative, facultatively anaerobic, fermentative rods** are the genera *Vibrio* and *Aeromonas.* These organisms were at one time classified together in the family Vibrionaceae and were separated from the Enterobacteriaceae on the basis of a **positive oxidase reaction** and the presence of **polar flagella.** These organisms were also classified together because they are primarily found in water and are able to cause gastrointestinal disease. However, DNA sequencing has established that these genera are only distantly related and belong in separate families: *Vibrio* and *Aeromonas* are now classified in the families Vibrionaceae and Aeromonadaceae, respectively (Table 26-1). Despite this taxonomic reorganization, it is appropriate to consider these bacteria together because their epidemiology and range of diseases are similar.

Vibrio

The genus *Vibrio* has undergone numerous changes in recent years, with a number of less common species described or reclassified. Currently the genus is composed of 119 species of **curved rods.** Three species are particularly important human pathogens (Table 26-2): ***Vibrio cholerae, Vibrio parahaemolyticus,*** and ***Vibrio vulnificus.***

Physiology and Structure

Vibrio species can grow on a variety of simple media within a broad temperature range (from 14° C to 40° C). All species of *Vibrio* **require sodium chloride (NaCl)** for growth. *V. cholerae* can grow on most media without additional salt, but most other halophilic ("salt-loving") species require supplementation with NaCl. Vibrios tolerate a wide range of pH (e.g., pH of 6.5 to 9.0) but are **susceptible to stomach acids.** Generally, exposure to a large inoculum of organisms is required for disease, but if gastric acid production is reduced or neutralized, patients are more susceptible to *Vibrio* infections.

Most vibrios have **polar flagella** (important for motility) as well as various pili that are important for virulence (e.g., **toxin co-regulated pilus** in epidemic strains of *V. cholera*). The cell wall structure of vibrios is also important. All strains possess **lipopolysaccharides** consisting of lipid A (endotoxin), core polysaccharide, and an O polysaccharide side chain. The O polysaccharide is used to subdivide *Vibrio* species into **serogroups:** There are more than 200 serogroups of *V. cholerae* plus multiple serogroups of *V. vulnificus* and *V. parahaemolyticus.* The interest in this classification scheme is more than academic—***V. cholerae*** **O1 and O139** produce **cholera toxin** and are associated with epidemics of cholera. Other strains of *V. cholerae* generally do not produce cholera toxin and do not cause epidemic disease. *V. cholerae* serogroup O1 is further subdivided into serotypes **(Inaba, Ogawa,** and **Hikojima)** and biotypes **(Classical** and **El Tor).** Strains can shift between serotype Inaba and serotype Ogawa, with Hikojima a transitional state in which both Inaba and Ogawa antigens are expressed. Seven worldwide pandemics of *V. cholerae* infections have been documented since 1817. *V. cholerae* strains responsible for the sixth worldwide pandemic of cholera were of the Classical biotype, whereas strains responsible for the current seventh pandemic are of the El Tor biotype.

V. vulnificus and non-O1 *V. cholerae* produce acidic **polysaccharide capsules** that are important for disseminated infections. *V. cholerae* O1 does not produce a capsule, so infections with this organism do not spread beyond the confines of the intestine.

V. cholerae and *V. parahaemolyticus* possess two circular chromosomes, each of which carries essential genes for these bacteria. Plasmids, including those encoding antimicrobial resistance, are also commonly found in *Vibrio* species.

Pathogenesis and Immunity (Table 26-3)

Virulence of *V. cholerae* involved acquisition of first a sequence of genes including the **toxin co-regulated pilus**

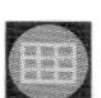

Table 26-1 Important *Vibrio* and *Aeromonas* Species

Organism	Historical Derivation
Vibrio	*vibrio,* move rapidly or vibrate (rapid movement caused by polar flagella)
V. cholerae	*cholera,* cholera or an intestinal disease
V. parahaemolyticus	*para,* by the side of; *haema,* blood; *lyticus,* dissolving (dissolving blood; Kanagawa toxin–positive strains are hemolytic)
V. vulnificus	*vulnificus,* inflicting wounds (associated with prominent wound infections)
Aeromonas	*aero,* gas or air; *monas,* unit or monad (gas-producing bacteria)
A. caviae	*cavia,* guinea pig (first isolated in guinea pigs)
A. hydrophila	*hydro,* water; *phila,* loving (water loving)
A. veronii	*veron,* named after the bacteriologist Veron

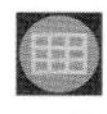

Table 26-2 *Vibrio* Species Most Commonly Associated with Human Disease

Species	Source of Infection	Clinical Disease
V. cholerae	Water, food	Gastroenteritis, bacteremia
V. parahaemolyticus	Shellfish, seawater	Gastroenteritis, wound infection, bacteremia
V. vulnificus	Shellfish, seawater	Bacteremia, wound infection

Table 26-3 Virulence Factors of *Vibrio* Species

Species	Virulence Factor	Biological Effect
V. cholerae	Cholera toxin	Hypersecretion of electrolytes and water
	Toxin co-regulated pilus	Surface binding site receptor for bacteriophage CTXΦ; mediates bacterial adherence to intestinal mucosal cells
	Chemotaxis protein	Adhesin factor
	Accessory cholera enterotoxin	Increases intestinal fluid secretion
	Zonula occludens toxin	Increases intestinal permeability
	Neuraminidase	Modifies cell surface to increase GM_1 binding sites for cholera toxin
V. parahaemolyticus	Kanagawa hemolysin	Enterotoxin that induces chloride ion secretion (watery diarrhea)
V. vulnificus	Polysaccharide capsule	Antiphagocytic
	Cytolysins, proteases, collagenase	Mediates tissue destruction

(TCP) on what is termed the **vibrio pathogenicity island (VPI-1),** followed by infection with the **bacteriophage CTXΦ** that encodes the genes for the two subunits of **cholera toxin** (*ctxA* and *ctxB*). TCP serves as the cell surface receptor for the bacteriophage, permitting it to move into the bacterial cell, where it becomes integrated into the *V. cholerae* genome. The lysogenic bacteriophage chromosomal locus also contains other virulence factors, including the *ace* gene for **accessory cholera enterotoxin,** *zot* gene for **zonula occludens toxin,** and *cep* gene for **chemotaxis proteins.** Multiple copies of these genes are found in *V. cholerae* O1 and O139, and their expression is coordinated by regulatory genes.

The cholera toxin is a **complex A-B toxin** that is structurally and functionally similar to the heat-labile enterotoxin of *Escherichia coli.* A ring of five identical B subunits of cholera toxin binds to the ganglioside GM_1 receptors on the intestinal epithelial cells. The active portion of the A subunit is internalized and interacts with G proteins that control adenylate cyclase, leading to the catabolic conversion of adenosine triphosphate (ATP) to cyclic adenosine monophosphate (cAMP). This results in a hypersecretion of water and electrolytes. Severely infected patients can lose as much as 1 liter of fluid per hour during the height of the disease. Such a tremendous loss of fluid would normally flush the organisms out of the gastrointestinal tract; however, *V. cholerae* are able to **adhere to the mucosal cell layer** by means of (1) the **TCP** encoded by the *tcp* gene complex and (2) the *cep*-encoded **chemotaxis proteins.** Nonadherent strains are unable to establish infection.

In the absence of cholera toxin, *V. cholerae* O1 can still produce significant diarrhea through the action of the **accessory cholera enterotoxin** and **zonula occludens toxin.** The enterotoxin produces increased fluid secretion, and the zonula occludens toxin loosens the tight junctions (zonula occludens) of the small intestine mucosa, leading to increased intestinal permeability.

Unlike other non-O1 serotypes, *V. cholerae* O139 possesses the same virulence complex as the O1 strains. Thus the ability of the O139 strains to adhere to the intestinal mucosa and produce cholera toxin is the reason these strains can produce a watery diarrhea similar to cholera.

The means by which other *Vibrio* species cause disease is less clearly understood, although a variety of potential virulence factors have been identified. Most virulent strains of *V. parahaemolyticus* produce adhesins, a thermostable direct hemolysin (TDH, also called **Kanagawa hemolysin**), and type III secretion systems that mediate bacterial survival and expression of virulence factors. TDH is an enterotoxin that induces chloride ion secretion in epithelial cells by increasing intracellular calcium. An important method for classifying virulent strains of *V. parahaemolyticus* is detection of this hemolysin, which produces β-hemolytic colonies on agar media with human blood but not sheep blood. These virulent strains are referred to as **Kanagawa positive.** In the presence of gastric acids, *V. vulnificus* rapidly degrades lysine, producing alkaline byproducts. In addition, the bacteria are able to evade the host immune response by inducing macrophage apoptosis and to avoid phagocytosis by expression of a polysaccharide capsule. *V. vulnificus* also possesses surface proteins that mediate attachment to host cells and secretes cytolytic toxins leading to tissue necrosis.

Epidemiology

Vibrio species, including *V. cholerae,* grow naturally in **estuarine and marine environments** worldwide. All *Vibrio* species are able to survive and replicate in contaminated waters with increased salinity. Pathogenic vibrios can also flourish in waters with chitinous **shellfish** (e.g., oysters, clams, mussels)—hence the association between *Vibrio* infections and the consumption of shellfish. Asymptomatically infected humans can also be an important reservoir for this organism in areas where *V. cholerae* disease is endemic.

Seven major pandemics of cholera have occurred since 1817, resulting in thousands of deaths and major socioeconomic changes. Sporadic disease and epidemics occurred before this time, but worldwide spread of the disease became possible with intercontinental travel resulting from increased commerce and wars.

The seventh pandemic, which was caused by ***V. cholerae* O1 biotype El Tor,** began in Asia in 1961 and spread to Africa, Europe, and Oceania in the 1970s and 1980s. In 1991, the pandemic strain spread to Peru and subsequently has caused disease in most countries in South and Central America, as well as in the United States and Canada. A second epidemic strain emerged in 1992 in India and rapidly spread across Asia but now remains primarily restricted to this area. This strain, ***V. cholerae* O139 Bengal,** produces the cholera toxin and shares other traits with *V. cholerae* O1. This is the first non-O1 strain capable of causing epidemic disease, and it is capable of producing disease in adults who were previously infected with the O1 strain (showing that no protective immunity is conferred).

It is estimated that 3 to 5 million cases of cholera and 120,000 deaths occur worldwide each year. The most recent epidemics occurred in 2004 in Bangladesh following flooding, in 2008 to 2009 in Zimbabwe, and in 2010 in Haiti following the devastating earthquake. Cholera is spread by **contaminated water and food** rather than direct person-to-person spread, because a high inoculum (e.g., $>10^8$ organisms) is required to establish infection in a person with normal gastric acidity. In a person with achlorhydria or hypochlorhydria, the infectious dose can be as low as 10^3 to 10^5 organisms. Strains shed from patients are 10- to 100-fold more infectious than environmental strains, although this hyperinfectivity is lost within 24 hours of shedding. Thus cholera is usually seen in communities with **poor sanitation.** Indeed, one outcome from the cholera pandemics was recognition of the role of contaminated water in the spread of disease and the need to improve community sanitation systems so that the disease could be controlled. Thus it is not surprising to observe cholera outbreaks when natural disasters, such as the earthquake in Haiti, compromise the control of sanitary wastes. DNA sequencing of the genomes of epidemic strains has helped us to understand how epidemics develop and are maintained. *V. cholerae* stains in contaminated waters are typically polyclonal. In contrast, epidemic strains are monoclonal, able to initiate disease by specific virulence properties. Thus exposure to *V. cholerae* whose concentration in water may fluctuate during the seasons or following a natural disaster is not sufficient to maintain an epidemic. Exposure must be with the specific clone responsible for disease.

Infections caused by *V. parahaemolyticus, V. vulnificus,* and other pathogenic vibrios result from consumption of improperly cooked seafood, particularly oysters, or exposure to contaminated seawater. ***V. parahaemolyticus*** is the most common cause of bacterial gastroenteritis in Japan and Southeast Asia and is the most common *Vibrio* species responsible for gastroenteritis in the United States. ***V. vulnificus*** is not frequently isolated but is responsible for severe wound infections and a high incidence of fatal outcomes. *V. vulnificus* is the most common cause of *Vibrio* septicemia. Gastroenteritis caused by vibrios occurs throughout the year because oysters are typically contaminated with abundant organisms year-round. In contrast, septicemia and wound infections with *Vibrio* occur during the warm months, when the organisms in seawater can multiply to high numbers.

Clinical Diseases (Box 26-1)

Vibrio cholerae (Clinical Case 26-1)

The majority of individuals exposed to toxigenic ***V. cholerae* O1** have asymptomatic infections or self-limited diarrhea; however, some individuals develop severe, rapidly fatal diarrhea. The clinical manifestations of cholera begin an average of 2 to 3 days after ingestion of the bacteria (can be <12 hours), with the abrupt onset of watery diarrhea and vomiting. Fever is rare and may be indicative of a secondary infection. As more fluid is lost, the feces-streaked stool specimens become colorless and odorless, free of protein, and speckled with mucus **("rice-water" stools).** The resulting severe fluid and electrolyte loss can lead to dehydration, painful muscle cramps, metabolic acidosis (bicarbonate loss), and hypokalemia and hypovolemic shock (potassium loss), with cardiac arrhythmia and renal failure. The mortality rate is as high as 70% in untreated patients but less than 1% in patients who are promptly treated with replacement of lost fluids and electrolytes. Disease caused by ***V. cholerae* O139** can be as severe as disease caused by *V. cholerae* O1. Other serotypes of *V. cholerae* (commonly called ***V. cholerae* non-O1**) do not produce cholera toxin and are usually responsible for mild watery diarrhea. These strains can also cause extraintestinal infections such as septicemia, particularly in patients with liver disease or hematologic malignancies.

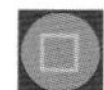

Box 26-1 *Vibrio* Clinical Summaries

Vibrio cholerae

Cholera: begins with an abrupt onset of watery diarrhea and vomiting and can progress to severe dehydration, metabolic acidosis and hypokalemia, and hypovolemic shock

Gastroenteritis: milder forms of diarrheal disease can occur in toxin-negative strains of *V. cholerae* O1 and in non-O1 serotypes

Vibrio parahaemolyticus

Gastroenteritis: generally self-limited, with an explosive onset of watery diarrhea and nausea, vomiting, abdominal cramps, headache, and low-grade fever

Wound infection: associated with exposure to contaminated water

Vibrio vulnificus

Wound infection: severe, potentially fatal infections characterized by erythema, pain, bullae formation, tissue necrosis, and septicemia

 **Clinical Case 26-1 Cholera Caused by *Vibrio cholerae***

Although cholera is widespread in Africa, Asia, and Latin America, toxigenic *V. cholerae* 01 is also endemic along the U.S. Gulf Coast. Most disease reported in the United States occurs in travelers to countries with an active cholera outbreak in the community; however, after Hurricane Katrina and Hurricane Rita, unsanitary conditions in coastal communities along the Gulf increased the risk of cholera, as illustrated by the following report (Centers for Disease Control and Prevention, *MMWR Morb Mortal Wkly Rep* 55:31–32, 2006). Three weeks after extensive damage to their southeastern Louisiana community by Hurricane Rita, a 43-year-old man and his 46-year-old wife developed diarrhea. Whereas the woman had only mild diarrhea, the man was hospitalized the next day with low-grade fever, muscle pains, nausea, vomiting, abdominal cramps, and severe diarrhea and dehydration. He rapidly progressed to complete loss of renal function and respiratory and cardiac failure. With antibiotic therapy and aggressive rehydration therapy, he eventually recovered to his previous state of health. Toxigenic *V. cholerae* 01, serotype Inaba, biotype El Tor, was isolated at the hospital from stool specimens of the two patients. The isolates were indistinguishable from each other and from other isolates previously associated with the Gulf Coast by use of pulsed-field gel electrophoresis. This case illustrates the rapid progression of cholera resulting from severe diarrhea and dehydration, the need for aggressive rehydration therapy, and the association with deterioration of the public health infrastructure following a natural disaster.

Vibrio parahaemolyticus (Clinical Case 26-2)

The severity of gastroenteritis caused by *V. parahaemolyticus* can range from a self-limited diarrhea to a mild, cholera-like illness. In general, the disease develops after a 5- to 72-hour incubation period (mean, 24 hours), with explosive **watery diarrhea.** No grossly evident blood or mucus is found in stool specimens except in severe cases. Headache, abdominal cramps, nausea, vomiting, and low-grade fever may persist for 72 hours or more. The patient usually experiences an uneventful recovery. Wound infections with this organism can occur in people exposed to contaminated seawater.

Vibrio vulnificus (Clinical Case 26-3)

V. vulnificus is a particularly virulent species of *Vibrio* responsible for more than 90% of the *Vibrio*-related deaths in the United States. The most common presentations are **primary septicemia** after consumption of contaminated raw oysters or rapidly progressive **wound infection** after exposure to contaminated seawater. Patients with primary septicemia present with a sudden onset of fever and chills, vomiting, diarrhea, and abdominal pain. Secondary skin lesions with tissue necrosis are often present. The mortality in patients with *V. vulnificus* septicemia can be as high as 50%. The wound infections are characterized by initial swelling, erythema, and pain at the wound site, followed by the development of vesicles or bullae and eventual tissue necrosis together with systemic signs of fever and chills. Mortality associated with wound infections ranges from 20% to 30%. *V. vulnificus* infections are most severe in patients with hepatic disease, hematopoietic disease, or chronic renal failure and in those receiving immunosuppressive drugs.

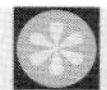 **Clinical Case 26-2 *Vibrio parahaemolyticus* Disease**

One of the largest known outbreaks of *V. parahaemolyticus* in the United States was reported in 2005 (McLaughlin et al, *N Engl J Med* 353:1463–1470, 2005). On July 19, the Nevada Office of Epidemiology reported isolation of *V. parahaemolyticus* from a person who developed gastroenteritis 1 day after eating raw oysters served on an Alaskan cruise ship. Epidemiologic investigations determined that 62 individuals (29% attack rate) developed gastroenteritis following consumption of as few as one raw oyster. In addition to watery diarrhea, the ill individuals reported abdominal cramping (82%), chills (44%), myalgias (36%), headache (32%), and vomiting (29%), with symptoms lasting a median of 5 days. None of the persons required hospitalization. All of the oysters were harvested from a single farm where the water temperatures in July and August were recorded at 16.6° C and 17.4° C. Water temperatures above 15° C are considered favorable for growth of *V. parahaemolyticus.* Since 1997, the mean water temperatures at the oyster farm have increased 0.21° C per year, and they now remain consistently above 15° C. Thus this seasonal warming has extended the range of *V. parahaemolyticus* and the associated gastrointestinal disease. This outbreak illustrates the role of contaminated shellfish in *V. parahaemolyticus* disease and the clinical symptoms typically observed.

 **Clinical Case 26-3 *Vibrio vulnificus* Septicemia**

Septicemia and wound infections are well-known complications following exposure to *V. vulnificus.* The following clinical case published in *Morbidity and Mortality Weekly Report* (*MMWR* 45:621–624, 1996) illustrates typical features of these diseases. A 38-year-old man with a history of alcoholism and insulin-dependent diabetes developed fever, chills, nausea, and myalgia 3 days after eating raw oysters. He was admitted to the local hospital the next day with high fevers and two necrotic lesions on his left leg. The clinical diagnosis of sepsis was made, and the patient was transferred to the intensive care unit. Antibiotic therapy was initiated, and on the second hospital day *V. vulnificus* was isolated from blood specimens collected at the time of admission. Despite aggressive medical management, the patient continued to deteriorate and died on the third day of hospitalization. This case illustrates the rapid, often fatal progression of *V. vulnificus* disease and the risk factor of eating raw shellfish, particularly for individuals with liver disease. A similar progression of disease could have been observed if this individual had been exposed to *V. vulnificus* through a contaminated superficial wound.

Laboratory Diagnosis

Microscopy

Vibrio species are small (0.5 to 1.5 to 3 μm), curved, gram-negative rods. Large numbers of organisms are typically present in the stools of patients at the onset of cholera, so the direct microscopic examination of stool specimens can provide a rapid, presumptive diagnosis in cholera outbreaks; however, as disease progresses the organisms are diluted with massive fluid loss, and microscopy is less useful. Examination of Gram-stained wound specimens may also be useful in a setting suggestive of *V. vulnificus* infection (e.g., exposure of susceptible individual to seafood or seawater).

Immunoassays

Immunoassays for the detection of cholera toxin or the O1 and O139 lipopolysaccharides are used for the diagnosis of cholera in endemic areas. These tests have variable sensitivity (as high as 97%) and specificity and have decreasing value as the disease progresses, because fewer organisms are present in the clinical specimens.

Culture

Vibrio organisms survive poorly in an acidic or dry environment. Specimens must be collected early in the disease and inoculated promptly onto culture media. If culture will be delayed, the specimen should be mixed in a Cary-Blair transport medium and refrigerated. Vibrios have low survival rates in buffered glycerol-saline, the transport medium used for most enteric pathogens.

Vibrios grow on most media used in clinical laboratories for stool and wound cultures, including blood agar and MacConkey agar. Special selective agar for vibrios (e.g., thiosulfate citrate bile salts sucrose **[TCBS]** agar), as well as an enrichment broth (e.g., **alkaline peptone broth,** pH 8.6), can also be used to recover vibrios in specimens with a mixture of organisms (e.g., stools). Isolates are identified with selective biochemical tests and serotyped using polyvalent antisera. In tests performed to identify halophilic vibrios, the media for biochemical testing must be supplemented with 1% NaCl.

Treatment, Prevention, and Control

Patients with cholera must be promptly treated with **fluid and electrolyte replacement** before the resultant massive fluid loss leads to hypovolemic shock. Antibiotic therapy, although of secondary value, can reduce toxin production and clinical symptoms as well as decrease transmission by the more rapid elimination of the organism. A single dose of **azithromycin** is currently the drug of choice for children and adults because macrolide resistance is relatively uncommon. A single dose of doxycycline or ciprofloxacin in nonpregnant adults can be used as alternative therapy if demonstrated to be active in vitro; however, resistance to the tetracycline and fluoroquinolones is relatively common.

V. parahaemolyticus gastroenteritis is usually a self-limited disease, although antibiotic therapy can be used in addition to fluid and electrolyte therapy in patients with severe infections. *V. vulnificus* wound infections and septicemia must be promptly treated with antibiotic therapy. The combination of minocycline or doxycycline with ceftriaxone or cefotaxime appears to be the most effective treatment.

People infected with *V. cholerae* can shed bacteria for the first few days of acute illness and represent important sources of new infections. Although long-term carriage of *V. cholerae* does not occur, vibrios are free living in estuarine and marine reservoirs. Only improvements in sanitation can lead to effective control of the disease. This involves adequate sewage management, use of purification systems to eliminate contamination of the water supply, and implementation of appropriate steps to prevent contamination of food.

Although no oral cholera vaccine is available in the United States, a variety of killed oral **vaccines** are available outside the United States; however, none of the vaccines provide long-term protection. A killed vaccine consisting of whole cells of *V. cholerae* O1 plus recombinant cholera toxin B subunit or a bivalent killed vaccine of whole cells of *V. cholerae* O1 and O139 is recommended for short-term protection of travelers in high-risk settings (e.g., exposure to untreated water or care of ill patients) and endemic regions of the world. Antibiotic prophylaxis of contacts to household patients with cholera can limit the spread but is generally ineffective in communities where disease occurs.

Aeromonas

Aeromonas is a **gram-negative, facultative anaerobic, fermentative rod** that morphologically resembles members of the family Enterobacteriaceae. As with *Vibrio,* extensive reorganization of the taxonomy of these bacteria has occurred. More than 30 species of *Aeromonas* have been described, many of which are associated with human disease. The most important pathogens are ***Aeromonas hydrophila, Aeromonas caviae,*** and ***Aeromonas veronii*** biovar. sobria. The organisms are ubiquitous in fresh and brackish water.

Aeromonas species cause three forms of disease: (1) **diarrheal disease** in otherwise healthy people, (2) **wound infections,** and (3) **opportunistic systemic disease** in immunocompromised patients (particularly those with hepatobiliary disease or an underlying malignancy). Intestinal disease can present as acute watery diarrhea, dysenteric diarrhea characterized by severe abdominal pain and blood and leukocytes in the stools, or a chronic illness with intermittent diarrhea. Gastrointestinal carriage has been observed in individuals, with the highest carriage in the warm months. Thus the significance of isolating *Aeromonas* in enteric specimens must be determined by the clinical presentation of the patient. Gastroenteritis typically occurs after the ingestion of contaminated water or food (e.g., fresh produce, meats, dairy products), whereas wound infections most commonly result from a traumatic injury associated with exposure to contaminated water. One unusual form of *Aeromonas* wound infections is associated with the use of medicinal leeches whose gut is colonized with *A. veronii* biovar. sobria (Clinical Case 26-4).

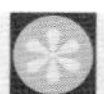

Clinical Case 26-4 *Aeromonas* Wound Infections

Medicinal leeches *(Hiruda medicinalis)* are sometimes used in plastic surgery to stimulate blood flow in surgical skin grafts. Leeches remove stagnant blood and stimulate oozing of blood into the skin graft for up to 48 hours after removal of the leech. This bleeding is mediated by an inhibitor of thrombin, hirudin (source of the genus name), that is present in the saliva of leeches. *Aeromonas* is present in the leech gut and produces proteolytic enzymes used by the leech to digest blood. One complication of using leeches is wound infections with *Aeromonas,* as illustrated by the patient described by Snower and associates (*J Clin Microbiol* 27:1421–1422, 1989). A 62-year-old woman had basal cell epitheliomas removed from her forehead, with the surgical site covered with skin grafts. Medicinal leeches were used to relieve swelling at the graft site. The leeches were removed from a leech tank and applied to the wound for 1 hour on four separate occasions. Eleven days after the initial surgery, the graft appeared infected and was removed. Cultures of this graft, as well as leeches and water from the leech tank, were positive for *Aeromonas.* The patient was treated with parenteral antibiotics, and regrafting without the use of leeches was successful.

Although numerous potential virulence factors (e.g., endotoxin, hemolysins, heat-labile and heat-stable enterotoxins) have been identified for *Aeromonas,* their precise role in disease is unknown.

Acute diarrheal disease is self-limited, and only supportive care is indicated in affected patients. Antimicrobial therapy is necessary in patients with chronic diarrheal disease, wound infections, or systemic disease. *Aeromonas* species are resistant to penicillins, most cephalosporins, and erythromycin. Fluoroquinolones (e.g., levofloxacin, ciprofloxacin) are almost uniformly active against *Aeromonas* strains isolated in the United States and Europe; however, resistance has been reported in strains recovered in Asia. Thus the long-term effectiveness of fluoroquinolones remains to be seen. A fluoroquinolone can be used initially for empirical therapy, but activity should be confirmed with in vitro susceptibility tests.

Bibliography

Albert MJ, Nair GB: *Vibrio cholerae* O139-10 years on, *Rev Med Microbiol* 16:135–143, 2005.

Dick MH, Guillerm M, Moussy F, et al: Review of two decades of cholera diagnostics—how far have we really come?, *PLoS Negl Trop Dis* 6:e1845, 2012.

Harris JB, LaRocque RC, Qadri F, et al: Cholera, *Lancet* 379:2466–2476, 2012.

Janda JM, Abbott S: The genus *Aeromonas*: taxonomy, pathogenicity, and infection, *Clin Microbiol Rev* 23:35–73, 2010.

Jones M, Oliver J: *Vibrio vulnificus*: disease and pathogenesis, *Infect Immun* 77:1723–1733, 2009.

Kitaoka M, Miyata ST, Unterweger D, et al: Antibiotic resistance mechanisms of *Vibrio cholerae, J Med Microbiol* 60:397–407, 2011.

Miyata ST, Bachmann V, Pukatzki S: Type VI secretion system regulation as a consequence of evolutionary pressure, *J Med Microbiol* 62:663–676, 2013.

Moore S, Thomson N, Mutreja A, et al: Widespread epidemic cholera due to a restricted subset of *Vibrio cholerae* clones, *Clin Microbiol Infect* 20:373–379, 2014.

Parker J, Shaw J: *Aeromonas* spp. clinical microbiology and disease, *J Infect* 62:109–118, 2011.

Pastor M, Pedraz J, Esquisabela A: The state-of-the-art of approved and under-development cholera vaccines, *Vaccine* 31:4069–4078, 2013.

Snower DP, Ruef C, Kuritza AP, et al: *Aeromonas hydrophila* infection associated with the use of medicinal leeches, *J Clin Microbiol* 27:1421–1422, 1989.

Zhang L, Orth K: Virulence determinants for *Vibrio parahaemolyticus* infection, *Curr Opin Microbiol* 16:70–77, 2013.

CHAPTER

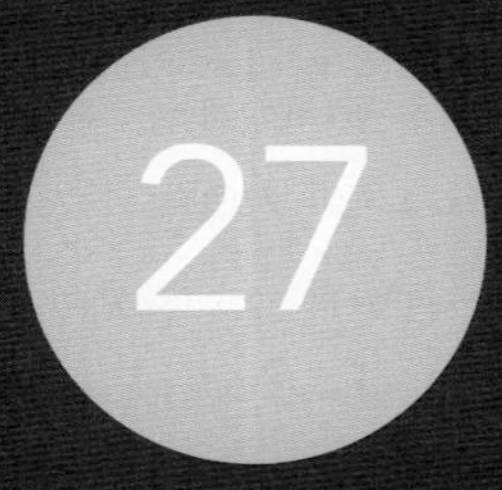

PSEUDOMONAS AND RELATED BACTERIA

A 70-year-old man who had been admitted 7 days previously to the intensive care unit for acute shortness of breath and a temperature of 39° C developed a new productive cough and associated pleuritic chest pain. Examination of his chest revealed crackles at the bases of both lungs, with rhonchi present in both upper lobes; the chest radiograph indicated bilateral opacities consistent with bronchopneumonia. Sputum and blood cultures were performed, and 24 hours later the laboratory reported isolation of *Pseudomonas aeruginosa. Pseudomonas* and the other nonfermentative rods discussed in this chapter are primarily opportunistic pathogens responsible for infections in hospitalized patients, in patients with innate immunity defects (e.g., compromised pulmonary function), or after trauma (e.g., contamination of a wound).

1. *Pseudomonas, Burkholderia,* and *Stenotrophomonas* share what epidemiologic factors?
2. What is the most important virulence factor in *Pseudomonas aeruginosa,* and how does it function?
3. What patient population is at risk for infections with *Burkholderia cepacia?* What is the infection in these patients?
4. Which antibiotics are generally effective against *Pseudomonas* but not *Stenotrophomonas,* and against *Stenotrophomonas maltophilia* but not *P. aeruginosa?*

Answers to these questions are available on StudentConsult.com.

• SUMMARIES CLINICALLY SIGNIFICANT ORGANISMS

Pseudomonas aeruginosa

Trigger Words

Capsule, exotoxin A, environmental, opportunistic, nosocomial infections

Biology and Virulence

- Small gram-negative rods typically arranged in pairs
- Obligate aerobe; glucose oxidizer; simple nutritional needs
- Mucoid polysaccharide capsule
- Multiple virulence factors, including adhesins (e.g., flagella, pili, lipopolysaccharide, alginate capsule), secreted toxins and enzymes (e.g., exotoxin A, pyocyanin, pyoverdin, elastases, proteases, phospholipase C, exoenzymes S and T), and antimicrobial resistance (intrinsic, acquired, and adaptive)

Epidemiology

- Ubiquitous in nature and moist environmental hospital sites (e.g., flowers, sinks, toilets, mechanical ventilation, and dialysis equipment)
- No seasonal incidence of disease
- Can transiently colonize the respiratory and gastrointestinal tracts of hospitalized patients, particularly those treated with broad-spectrum antibiotics, exposed to respiratory therapy equipment, or hospitalized for extended periods
- Patients at high risk for developing infections include neutropenic or immunocompromised patients, cystic fibrosis patients, and burn patients

Diseases

- Diseases include infections of the respiratory tract, urinary tract, skin and soft tissues, ears, and eyes, as well as bacteremia and endocarditis

Diagnosis

- Grows rapidly on common laboratory media
- Identified by colonial characteristics (e.g., β-hemolysis, green pigment, grapelike odor) and simple biochemical tests (e.g., positive oxidase reaction, oxidative utilization of carbohydrates)

Treatment, Prevention, and Control

- Combined use of effective antibiotics (e.g., aminoglycoside and β-lactam antibiotics) frequently required; monotherapy is generally ineffective and can select for resistant strains
- Hospital infection-control efforts should concentrate on preventing contamination of sterile medical equipment and nosocomial transmission; unnecessary use of broad-spectrum antibiotics can select for resistant organisms

Pseudomonas and related nonfermentative rods are opportunistic pathogens of plants, animals, and humans. To complicate our understanding of these organisms, their taxonomic classification has undergone numerous changes in recent years. Despite the many genera, most clinically significant isolates are members of five genera: *Pseudomonas, Burkholderia, Stenotrophomonas, Acinetobacter,* and *Moraxella* (Table 27-1). These organisms will be the focus of this chapter.

Pseudomonas

The genus *Pseudomonas* originally consisted of a large heterogeneous collection of nonfermentative bacteria that were grouped together because of their morphologic similarity. They were referred to as pseudomonads because they are commonly arranged in pairs of cells that resemble a single cell (Figure 27-1). In 1992, this genus was subdivided into a number of new genera (including *Burkholderia* and *Stenotrophomonas*); however, there are still more than 200 species in *Pseudomonas*. ***Pseudomonas aeruginosa*** is the most important species and the one discussed here.

Members of the genus are found in soil, decaying organic matter, vegetation, and water. Unfortunately, they are also found throughout the hospital environment in moist reservoirs such as food, cut flowers, sinks, toilets, floor mops, respiratory therapy and dialysis equipment, and even disinfectant solutions. It is uncommon for carriage to persist in humans as part of the normal microbial flora, except in hospitalized patients and ambulatory, immunocompromised hosts.

The broad environmental distribution of *Pseudomonas* is made possible by their simple growth requirements and nutritional versatility. They are capable of using many organic compounds as sources of carbon and nitrogen, and some strains can even grow in distilled water by using trace nutrients. These organisms also possess many structural factors, enzymes, and toxins that enhance their virulence and render them resistant to most commonly used antibiotics. Indeed, it is surprising that they are not more common pathogens, considering their ubiquitous presence, ability to grow in virtually any environment, virulence properties, and resistance to many antibiotics. Fortunately, *Pseudomonas* infections are **primarily opportunistic** (i.e., restricted to patients receiving broad-spectrum antibiotics that suppress the normal intestinal bacterial population or patients with compromised host defenses). Additionally, expression of virulence traits is regulated by complex cell-density signaling (quorum sensing) systems that in turn are influenced by host factors such as the presence of serum and cytokines.

Physiology and Structure

Pseudomonas species are usually motile, straight or slightly curved, gram-negative rods (0.5 to 1.0 × 1.5 to 5.0 μm) typically **arranged in pairs** (see Figure 27-1). The organisms utilize carbohydrates through **aerobic respiration,** with oxygen the terminal electron acceptor. Although described as obligate aerobes, they can grow anaerobically using nitrate or arginine as an alternate electron acceptor. The presence of **cytochrome oxidase** (detected in a rapid 5-minute test) in *Pseudomonas* species is used to differentiate them from the Enterobacteriaceae and *Stenotrophomonas*. Some strains appear **mucoid** because of the abundance of a polysaccharide capsule (Figure 27-2); these strains are particularly common in patients with cystic fibrosis (CF). Some species produce **diffusible pigments** (e.g., pyocyanin [blue], pyoverdin [yellow-green], pyorubin [reddish-brown]) that give them a characteristic appearance in culture and simplify the preliminary identification.

Pathogenesis and Immunity

P. aeruginosa has many virulence factors, including adhesins, toxins, and enzymes. In addition, the delivery system used by *Pseudomonas*, the type III secretion system, is particularly effective in injecting toxins into the host cell. Despite the diversity of virulence factors, most experts believe that multiple factors must work together for *P. aeruginosa* to cause disease.

Adhesins

As with many bacteria, adherence to host cells is critical for establishing infection. At least four surface components of *P. aeruginosa* facilitate this adherence: (1) flagella, (2) pili, (3) lipopolysaccharide (LPS), and (4) alginate. Flagella and pili also mediate motility in *P. aeruginosa,* and the lipid A component of LPS is responsible for endotoxin activity. Alginate is a mucoid exopolysaccharide that forms a prominent **capsule** on the bacterial surface and protects the organism from phagocytosis and antibiotic killing. Production of this mucoid polysaccharide is under complex regulation. The genes controlling production of the alginate polysaccharide can be activated in patients such as those with CF or other chronic respiratory diseases, who are predisposed to long-term colonization with these mucoid strains of *P. aeruginosa.*

Secreted Toxins and Enzymes

Exotoxin A (ETA) is believed to be one of the most important virulence factors produced by pathogenic strains of *P. aeruginosa.* This toxin **disrupts protein synthesis** by blocking peptide chain elongation in eukaryotic cells, much like the diphtheria toxin produced by *Corynebacterium diphtheriae.* However, the toxins produced by these two organisms are structurally and immunologically different, and ETA is less potent than diphtheria toxin. ETA most likely contributes to the dermatonecrosis that occurs in burn wounds, corneal damage in ocular infections, and tissue damage in chronic pulmonary infections.

A blue pigment, **pyocyanin,** produced by *P. aeruginosa* catalyzes the production of superoxide and hydrogen peroxide, toxic forms of oxygen. This pigment also stimulates interleukin (IL)-8 release, leading to enhanced attraction of neutrophils. A yellow-green pigment, **pyoverdin,** is a siderophore that binds iron for use in metabolism. This pigment also regulates secretion of other virulence factors including ETA.

Two elastases, LasA **(serine protease)** and LasB **(zinc metalloprotease),** act synergistically to degrade elastin, resulting in damage to elastin-containing tissues and producing the lung parenchymal damage and hemorrhagic lesions **(ecthyma gangrenosum)** associated with disseminated *P. aeruginosa* infections. These enzymes can also degrade complement components and inhibit neutrophil

Table 27-1 Important Nonfermentative Gram-Negative Rods

Organism	Historical Derivation
Acinetobacter	*akinetos,* unable to move; *bactrum,* rod (nonmotile rods)
A. baumannii	*baumannii,* named after the microbiologist Baumann
A. lwoffii	*lwoffii,* named after the microbiologist Lwoff
Burkholderia	*Burkholderia,* named after the microbiologist Burkholder
B. cepacia	*cepacia,* like an onion (original strains isolated from rotten onions)
B. mallei	*mallei,* the disease glanders
B. pseudomallei	*pseudes,* false; *mallei* (refers to the fact this species closely resembles *B. mallei*)
Moraxella	*Moraxella,* named after the Swiss ophthalmologist Morax, who first recognized the species
M. catarrhalis	*catarrhus,* downflowing or catarrh (refers to inflammation of the respiratory tract mucus membranes)
Pseudomonas	*pseudes,* false; *monas,* a unit (refers to Gram-stain appearance of pairs of organisms that resemble a single cell)
P. aeruginosa	*aeruginosa,* full of copper rust or green (refers to blue and yellow pigments produced by this species that appear green)
Stenotrophomonas	*stenos,* narrow; *trophos,* one who feeds; *monas,* unit (refers to observation that these are narrow bacteria that require few substrates for growth)
S. maltophilia	*malt,* malt; *philia,* friend (friend of malt)

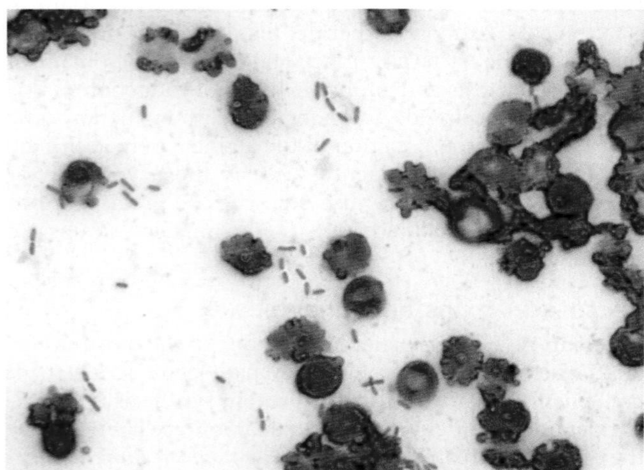

FIGURE 27-1 Gram stain of *Pseudomonas aeruginosa* with cells arranged singly and in pairs.

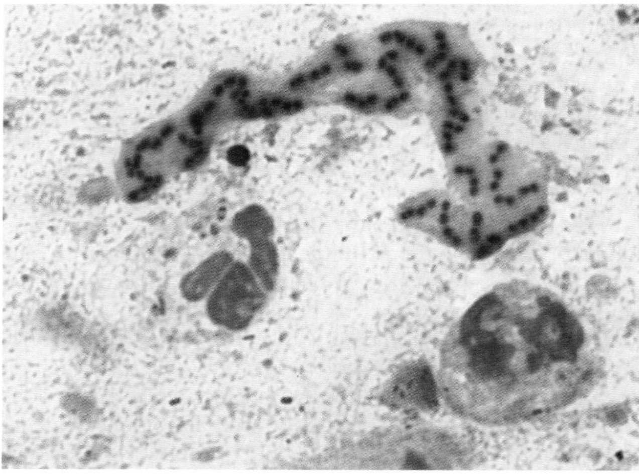

FIGURE 27-2 Gram stain of *Pseudomonas aeruginosa* surrounded by mucoid capsular material in cystic fibrosis patient.

chemotaxis and function, leading to further spread and tissue damage in acute infections. Chronic *Pseudomonas* infections are characterized by the formation of antibodies to LasA and LasB, with the deposition of immune complexes in the infected tissues. Similar to the elastases, **alkaline protease** contributes to tissue destruction and spread of *P. aeruginosa.* It also interferes with the host immune response.

Phospholipase C is a heat-labile hemolysin that breaks down lipids and lecithin, facilitating tissue destruction. The exact role of this enzyme in respiratory and urinary tract infections (UTIs) is unclear, although an important association between hemolysin production and disease has been recognized.

Exoenzymes S and **T** are extracellular toxins produced by *P. aeruginosa.* When the type III secretion system introduces the proteins into their target eukaryotic cells, epithelial cell damage occurs, facilitating bacterial spread, tissue invasion, and necrosis. This cytotoxicity is mediated by actin rearrangement.

Antibiotic Resistance

P. aeruginosa is intrinsically **resistant to many antibiotics** and can acquire resistance to additional antibiotics through horizontal transfer of resistance genes and mutations. The main mechanisms responsible for **intrinsic resistance** are the low rate of movement of antibiotics through the outer membrane pores into the bacterial cell, combined with the rapid efflux of antibiotics due to intrinsic regulation of efflux pumps. Resistance to additional antibiotics such as aminoglycosides and β-lactams can be acquired **(acquired resistance)** through horizontal transfer of resistance genes on plasmids and other genetic elements or mutations of genes that increase expression of resistance. A third form of resistance, **adaptive resistance,** is induced when *Pseudomonas* is exposed to environmental stimuli or specific antibiotics. For example, biofilm formation, such as in the lungs of a CF patient or on the surface of catheters, can trigger bacterial regulatory genes that permit expression of resistance. In the same way, exposure to some β-lactam antibiotics (e.g., ceftazidime) triggers the expression of the ampC gene in *Pseudomonas* that results in inactivation of many β-lactam antibiotics. It is important to recognize that in vitro susceptibility tests can identify resistance due to intrinsic and acquired mechanisms but would likely not be able to predict adaptive resistance, underlying the limitations of these lab tests.

Epidemiology

Pseudomonas is an opportunistic pathogen present in a variety of environments. The ability to isolate this organism from moist surfaces may be limited only by the efforts to look for the organism. *Pseudomonas* has minimal nutritional requirements, tolerates a wide range of temperatures (4° C to 42° C), and is resistant to many antibiotics and disinfectants. Indeed, the recovery of *Pseudomonas* from an environmental source (e.g., hospital sink or floor) means very little unless there is epidemiologic evidence that the contaminated site is a reservoir for infection.

Furthermore, isolation of *Pseudomonas* from a hospitalized patient is worrisome but does not normally justify therapeutic intervention unless there is evidence of disease. The recovery of *Pseudomonas,* particularly species other than *P. aeruginosa,* from a clinical specimen may represent transient colonization of the patient or environmental contamination of the specimen during collection or laboratory processing. Patients at high risk for developing infections with *P. aeruginosa* include neutropenic or immunocompromised patients, CF patients, burn patients, and individuals receiving broad-spectrum antibiotics.

Clinical Diseases (Box 27-1)

Pulmonary Infections

P. aeruginosa infections of the lower respiratory tract can range in severity from **asymptomatic colonization** or benign inflammation of the bronchials **(tracheobronchitis)** to severe **necrotizing bronchopneumonia.** Colonization is seen in patients with CF, other chronic lung diseases, or neutropenia. Infections in patients with CF have been associated with exacerbation of the underlying disease and invasive pulmonary disease. Mucoid strains are commonly isolated from these patients and are difficult to eradicate because chronic infections with these bacteria are associated with progressive increase in acquired antibiotic resistance and expression of adaptive resistance (see earlier discussion).

Conditions that predispose immunocompromised patients to infections with *Pseudomonas* include (1) previous therapy with broad-spectrum antibiotics that eliminate the normal, protective bacterial population and (2) use of mechanical ventilation equipment, which may introduce the organism to the lower airways. Invasive disease in this population is characterized by a diffuse, typically bilateral bronchopneumonia with microabscess formation and tissue necrosis. The mortality rate is as high as 70%.

Box 27-1 Clinical Summaries for Nonfermentative Gram-Negative Rods

Pseudomonas aeruginosa

Pulmonary infections: range from mild irritation of the bronchi (tracheobronchitis) to necrosis of the lung parenchyma (necrotizing bronchopneumonia)

Primary skin infections: opportunistic infections of existing wounds (e.g., burns) to localized infections of hair follicles (e.g., associated with immersion in contaminated waters such as hot tubs)

Urinary tract infections: opportunistic infections in patients with indwelling urinary catheters and following exposure to broad-spectrum antibiotics (selects for these antibiotic-resistant bacteria)

Ear infections: can range from mild irritation of external ear ("swimmer's ear") to invasive destruction of cranial bones adjacent to the infected ear

Eye infections: opportunistic infections of mildly damaged corneas

Bacteremia: dissemination of bacteria from primary infection (e.g., pulmonary) to other organs and tissues; can be characterized by necrotic skin lesions (ecthyma gangrenosum)

***Burkholderia cepacia* Complex**

Pulmonary infections: most worrisome infections are in patients with chronic granulomatous disease or cystic fibrosis, in whom infections can progress to significant destruction of pulmonary tissue

Opportunistic infections: urinary tract infections in catheterized patients; bacteremia in immunocompromised patients with contaminated intravascular catheters

Burkholderia pseudomallei

Pulmonary infections: can range from asymptomatic colonization to abscess formation

Stenotrophomonas maltophilia

Opportunistic infections: a variety of infections (most commonly bacteremia and pneumonia) in immunocompromised patients previously exposed to broad-spectrum antimicrobial therapy

***Acinetobacter* Species**

Pulmonary infections: opportunistic pathogen in patients receiving respiratory therapy

Wound infections: traumatic (e.g., resulting from military conflicts) and nosocomial wounds

Moraxella catarrhalis

Pulmonary infections: tracheobronchitis or bronchopneumonia in patients with chronic pulmonary diseases

Primary Skin and Soft-Tissue Infections

P. aeruginosa can cause a variety of primary skin infections. The most recognized are infections of **burn wounds** (Figure 27-3). Colonization of a burn wound, followed by localized vascular damage, tissue necrosis, and ultimately bacteremia, is common in patients with severe burns. The moist surface of the burn and inability of neutrophils to penetrate into the wounds predispose patients to such infections. Wound management with topical antibiotic creams has had only limited success in controlling these infections.

Folliculitis (Figure 27-4; Clinical Case 27-1) is another common infection caused by *Pseudomonas,* resulting from immersion in contaminated water (e.g., hot tubs, whirlpools, swimming pools). Secondary infections with *Pseudomonas* also occur in people who have acne or who depilate their

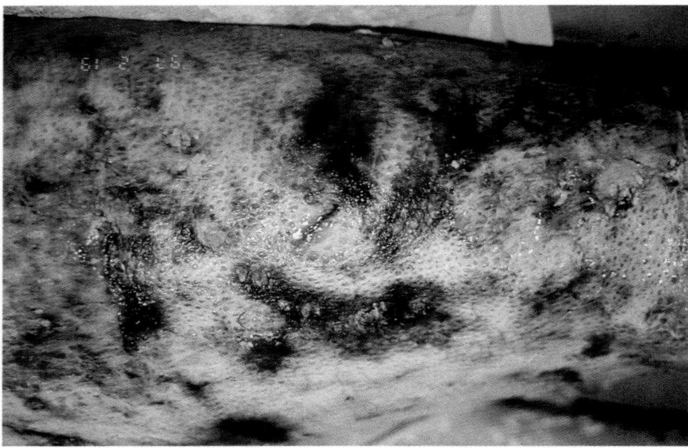

FIGURE 27-3 *Pseudomonas* infection of burn wound. (From Cohen J, Powderly WB: *Infectious diseases,* ed 2, St Louis, 2004, Mosby.)

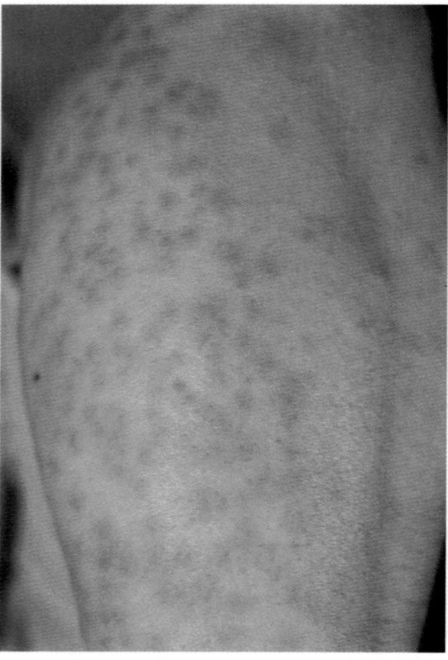

FIGURE 27-4 *Pseudomonas* folliculitis. (From Cohen J, Powderly WB: *Infectious diseases,* ed 2, St Louis, 2004, Mosby.)

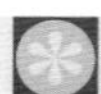

Clinical Case 27-1 *Pseudomonas* Folliculitis

Ratnam and associates (*J Clin Microbiol* 23:655–659, 1986) described an outbreak of folliculitis caused by *P. aeruginosa* in guests of a Canadian hotel. A number of guests complained of a skin rash that began as pruritic erythematous papules and progressed to erythematous pustules distributed in the axilla and over the abdomen and buttocks. For most patients, the rash resolved spontaneously over a 5-day period. The local health department investigated the outbreak and determined the source was a whirlpool contaminated with a high concentration of *P. aeruginosa.* The outbreak was terminated when the whirlpool was drained, cleaned, and superchlorinated. Skin infections such as this are common in individuals with extensive exposure to contaminated water.

legs. Finally, *P. aeruginosa* can cause fingernail infections in people whose hands are frequently exposed to water or who frequent "nail salons."

P. aeruginosa is also the most common cause of **osteochondritis** (inflammation of bone and cartilage) of the foot after a penetrating injury (e.g., associated with stepping on a nail).

Urinary Tract Infections

Infection of the urinary tract is seen primarily in patients with long-term **indwelling urinary catheters.** Typically, such patients are treated with multiple courses of antibiotics, which tend to select for the more resistant strains of bacteria, such as *Pseudomonas.*

Ear Infections

External otitis is frequently caused by *P. aeruginosa,* with swimming an important risk factor **("swimmer's ear").** This localized infection can be managed with topical antibiotics and drying agents. **Malignant external otitis** is a virulent form of disease seen primarily in persons with diabetes and elderly patients. It can invade the underlying tissues, damage the cranial nerves and bones, and be life threatening. Aggressive antimicrobial and surgical intervention is required for patients with the latter disease. *P. aeruginosa* is also associated with **chronic otitis media.**

Eye Infections

Infections of the eye occur after initial trauma to the cornea (e.g., abrasion from contact lens, scratch on the eye surface) and then exposure to *P. aeruginosa* in contaminated water. **Corneal ulcers** develop and can progress to rapidly progressive, eye-threatening disease unless prompt treatment is instituted.

Bacteremia and Endocarditis

Bacteremia caused by *P. aeruginosa* is clinically indistinguishable from that caused by other gram-negative bacteria. However, the mortality rate in affected patients is higher with *P. aeruginosa* bacteremia because of (1) the predilection of the organism for immunocompromised patients, (2) difficulty in treating antibiotic-resistant strains, and (3) the inherent virulence of *Pseudomonas.* Bacteremia occurs most often in patients with neutropenia, diabetes mellitus, extensive burns, and hematologic malignancies. Most bacteremias originate from infections of the lower respiratory tract, urinary tract, and skin and soft tissue (particularly burn wound infections). Although seen in a minority of bacteremic patients, characteristic skin lesions **(ecthyma gangrenosum)** may develop. The lesions manifest as erythematous vesicles that become hemorrhagic, necrotic, and ulcerated. Microscopic examination of the lesion shows abundant organisms, vascular destruction (which explains the hemorrhagic nature of the lesions), and an absence of neutrophils, as would be expected in neutropenic patients.

Pseudomonas **endocarditis** is uncommon and is primarily seen in intravenous drug abusers. These patients acquire the infection from the use of drug paraphernalia contaminated with the waterborne organisms. The tricuspid valve is often involved, and the infection is associated with a chronic course but with a more favorable prognosis than that in patients who have infections of the aortic or mitral valve.

Other Infections

P. aeruginosa is also the cause of a variety of other infections, including those localized in the gastrointestinal tract, central nervous system, and musculoskeletal system. The underlying conditions required for most infections are (1) the presence of the organism in a moist reservoir and (2) compromised host defenses (e.g., cutaneous trauma, elimination of normal microbial flora as a result of antibiotic usage, neutropenia).

Laboratory Diagnosis

Microscopy

Observation of thin gram-negative rods arranged singly and in pairs is suggestive of *Pseudomonas* but not definitive—*Burkholderia, Stenotrophomonas,* and other pseudomonads have a similar morphology.

Culture

Because *Pseudomonas* has simple nutritional requirements, the bacteria are readily recovered on common isolation media such as blood agar and MacConkey agar. They do require aerobic incubation (unless nitrate is available), so their growth in broth is generally confined to the broth-air interface, where the oxygen concentration is the highest.

Identification

The colonial morphology (Figure 27-5), odor, and results of selected rapid biochemical tests (e.g., positive **oxidase** reaction) are sufficient for the preliminary identification of these isolates. For example, *P. aeruginosa* grows rapidly and has flat colonies with a spreading border, **β-hemolysis,** a **green pigmentation** caused by the production of the blue (pyocyanin) and yellow-green (pyoverdin) pigments, and a characteristic sweet, **grapelike odor.** Although definitive identification of *P. aeruginosa* is relatively easy, an extensive battery of physiologic tests may be required to identify other species.

Treatment, Prevention, and Control

The antimicrobial therapy for *Pseudomonas* infections is frustrating because (1) the bacteria are typically resistant to most antibiotics and (2) the infected patient with compromised host defenses cannot augment the antibiotic activity. A **combination of active antibiotics** is generally required for therapy to be successful in patients with serious infections.

Attempts to eliminate *Pseudomonas* from the hospital environment are practically useless given the ubiquitous presence of the organism in water supplies. Effective infection-control practices should concentrate on **preventing the contamination of sterile equipment,** such as mechanical ventilation equipment and dialysis machines, and the cross-contamination of patients by medical personnel. Inappropriate use of broad-spectrum antibiotics should also be avoided because such use can suppress the normal microbial flora and permit overgrowth of resistant strains of *Pseudomonas*.

Burkholderia

In 1992, seven species formerly classified as *Pseudomonas* were reclassified as members of the new genus *Burkholderia.* It was subsequently appreciated that the most common species, *B. cepacia,* was actually a complex of 17 species. Because most laboratories cannot identify the individual species, the collection is commonly referred to as *B. cepacia* complex. ***B. cepacia* complex, *Burkholderia gladioli,*** and ***Burkholderia pseudomallei*** are important human pathogens in this genus (see Box 27-1); other species (e.g., *Burkholderia mallei*) are less commonly associated with human disease.

Like *P. aeruginosa, Burkholderia* species can colonize a variety of moist environmental surfaces and are **opportunistic pathogens** (Clinical Case 27-2). Patients particularly susceptible to pulmonary infections with *B. cepacia* complex and *B. gladioli* are those with CF or chronic granulomatous disease (CGD, a primary immunodeficiency in which white blood cells have defective intracellular microbicidal activity). Colonization of the respiratory tract of CF patients with *B. cepacia* complex has such a poor prognosis that this is a contraindication for lung transplantation. *B. cepacia* complex

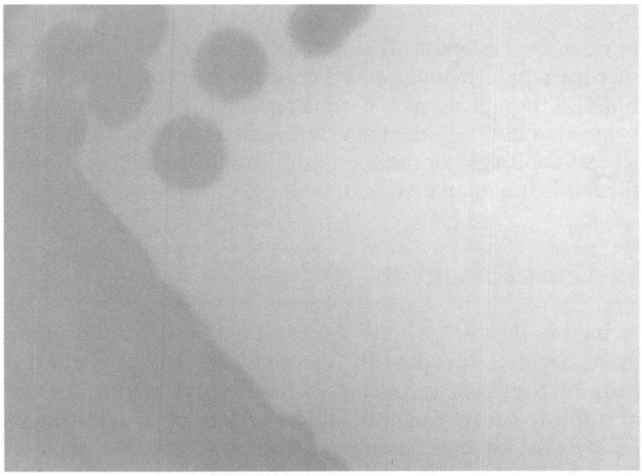

FIGURE 27-5 Colonial morphology of *Pseudomonas aeruginosa;* note the green pigmentation that results from the production of two water-soluble dyes: blue pyocyanin and yellow fluorescein.

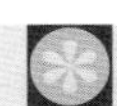

Clinical Case 27-2 *Burkholderia* Granulomatous Disease

Mclean-Tooke and associates (*BMC Clin Pathol* 7:1–5, 2007) described a 21-year-old man with granulomatous lymphadenitis. The man presented with a history of weight loss, fevers, hepatosplenomegaly, and cervical lymphadenopathy. During the preceding 3 years he had presented on two occasions with enlarged lymph nodes that were biopsied, and histologic examination revealed granulomatous lymphadenitis. A clinical diagnosis of sarcoidosis was made, and the man was discharged on 20 mg prednisolone. Over the next 24 months, the patient remained clinically well; however, he developed pancytopenia, and granulomas were observed on a bone marrow biopsy. During the current hospitalization, the patient developed a cough. Chest radiograph revealed consolidation in the base of the lungs. A lung biopsy and bronchoalveolar lavage was submitted for culture, and *B. cepacia* was isolated from both specimens. A subsequent immunologic evaluation of the patient confirmed that he had a genetic disease, chronic granulomatous disease (CGD). This case illustrates the susceptibility of CGD patients to infections with *Burkholderia*.

is also responsible for UTIs in catheterized patients, septicemia (particularly in patients with contaminated intravascular catheters), and other opportunistic infections. With the exception of pulmonary infections, *B. cepacia* complex has a relatively low level of virulence, and infections with the organism do not commonly result in death.

B. pseudomallei is a saprophyte found in soil, water, and vegetation. It is endemic in Southeast Asia, India, Africa, and Australia. Infections are acquired by either inhalation or less commonly by percutaneous inoculation. Most persons exposed to *B. pseudomallei* remain asymptomatic; however, alcoholics, diabetics, and individuals with chronic renal or lung disease are susceptible to opportunistic infections caused by this organism. Infections are called **melioidosis** (*melis*, distemper; *eidos,* resemblance; *osis,* condition: disease resembling equine distemper or glanders caused by *B. mallei*). Exposure by the percutaneous route presents as a localized, suppurative **cutaneous infection** accompanied by regional lymphadenitis, fever, and malaise. This form of disease can resolve without incident or can progress rapidly to overwhelming sepsis. **Pulmonary disease** that develops after respiratory exposure may range in severity from a mild bronchitis to necrotizing pneumonia. Cavitation progressing to overwhelming sepsis and death can develop if appropriate antimicrobial therapy is not instituted. *B. pseudomallei* has been used in biological weapons programs, so work with this organism is restricted to appropriately licensed laboratories, and its recovery from a patient justifies intervention by the public health department. Isolation of *B. pseudomallei* for diagnostic purposes should be approached carefully because the organism is highly infectious, similar to respiratory pathogens such as *Mycobacterium tuberculosis.*

Burkholderia species are susceptible to **trimethoprim-sulfamethoxazole (TMP-SMX),** which distinguishes them from *P. aeruginosa,* which is uniformly resistant. Although the organisms appear to be susceptible in vitro to piperacillin, broad-spectrum cephalosporins, and ciprofloxacin, the clinical response is generally poor.

Stenotrophomonas maltophilia

S. maltophilia was originally classified in the genus *Pseudomonas,* moved to the genus *Xanthomonas,* and then transferred to the genus *Stenotrophomonas.* Despite the confusion created by these taxonomic changes, the clinical importance of this opportunistic pathogen is well known. It is responsible for infections in debilitated patients with impaired host defense mechanisms. Also, because *S. maltophilia* is resistant to most commonly used β-lactam and aminoglycoside antibiotics, patients receiving long-term antibiotic therapy with these drugs are particularly at risk for acquiring infections.

The most common nosocomial infections caused by *S. maltophilia* are bacteremia and pneumonia, with both associated with a high incidence of complications and death (Clinical Case 27-3). Hospital infections with this organism have been traced to contaminated intravenous catheters, disinfectant solutions, mechanical ventilation equipment, and ice machines.

Antimicrobial therapy is complicated because the organism is resistant to many commonly used drugs. In contrast with most gram-negative rods, *Stenotrophomonas* is uniformly **resistant to carbapenems** (e.g., imipenem, meropenem, ertapenem) and typically susceptible to **TMP-SMX,** although increased resistance has been reported in some studies. Treatment is usually effective with TMP-SMX (if susceptible) or with ciprofloxacin combined with ticarcillin-clavulanate or ceftazidime.

Clinical Case 27-3 Disseminated *Stenotrophomonas* Infection in a Neutropenic Patient

Wan-Yee and associates (*Ann Acad Med Singapore* 35:897–900, 2006) described an 8-year-old Chinese girl with acute myeloid leukemia and a complex history of recurrent fungal and bacterial infections during treatment of her leukemia. Infections included pulmonary aspergillosis and septicemia with *Klebsiella, Enterobacter, Staphylococcus, Streptococcus,* and *Bacillus.* While receiving treatment with meropenem (a carbapenem antibiotic) and amikacin (an aminoglycoside), and during a period of severe neutropenia, she became bacteremic with *Stenotrophomonas maltophilia* that was sensitive to trimethoprim-sulfamethoxazole (TMP-SMX). Over the next few days, she developed painful, erythematous, nodular skin lesions. *S. maltophilia* was isolated from a biopsy of one of the lesions. Treatment with intravenous TMP-SMX led to gradual resolution of the skin lesions. This case illustrates the predilection for *Stenotrophomonas* to cause disease in immunocompromised patients receiving a carbapenem antibiotic. Characteristically, *Stenotrophomonas* is one of the few gram-negative bacteria that is inherently resistant to carbapenems and aminoglycoside and susceptible to TMP-SMX.

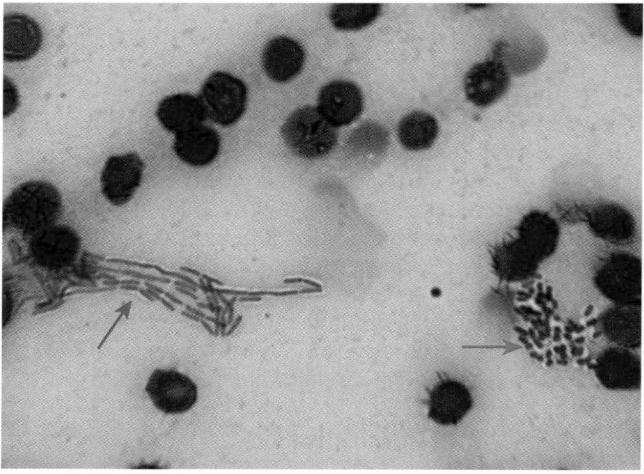

FIGURE 27-6 Gram stain of *Acinetobacter baumannii (blue arrow)* and *Pseudomonas aeruginosa (red arrow).*

Acinetobacter

Acinetobacters are strictly aerobic, oxidase-negative, plump gram-negative coccobacilli (Figure 27-6). They are **ubiquitous** saprophytes, recovered in nature and in the hospital and able to survive on both moist surfaces, such as mechanical ventilation equipment, and on dry surfaces, such as human skin (the latter feature is unusual for gram-negative rods). These bacteria are also part of the normal oropharyngeal flora of a small number of healthy people and can proliferate to large numbers during hospitalization. The genus

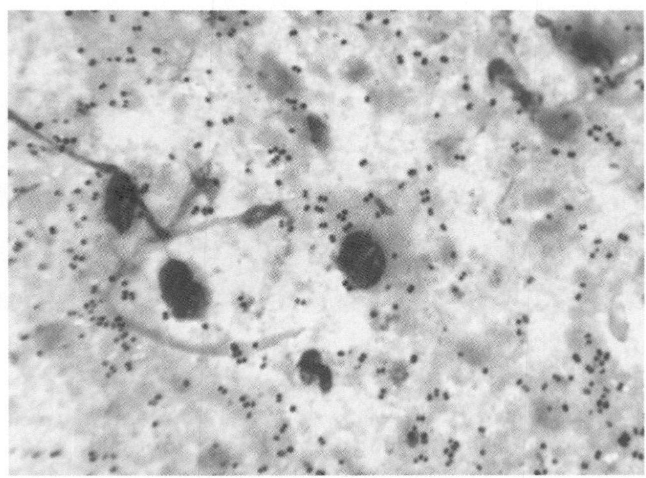

FIGURE 27-7 Gram stain of *Moraxella catarrhalis.*

Acinetobacter is subdivided into two groups: glucose-oxidizing species (***A. baumannii*** is the most common) and glucose nonoxidizing species (***A. lwoffii*** and ***A. haemolyticus*** are the most common). Most human infections are caused by *A. baumannii.*

Acinetobacters are **opportunistic pathogens** (see Box 27-1) that cause infections in the respiratory tract, urinary tract, and wounds; they also cause septicemia. Patients at risk for *Acinetobacter* infections are those receiving broad-spectrum antibiotics, recovering from surgery, or on respiratory ventilation. Nosocomial wound and pulmonary infections in hospitalized patients have become a significant problem because many of the infections are caused by strains resistant to most antibiotics, including the carbapenems. Specific therapy must be guided by in vitro susceptibility tests. Care must be taken when carbapenems or colistin are selected, because in vitro tests may not reliably detect heteroresistant strains (i.e., a highly resistant subpopulation of organisms).

Moraxella

Like other genera discussed in this chapter, the genus *Moraxella* was reorganized on the basis of nucleic acid analysis. Although the species classified in this genus continue to change, *M. catarrhalis* is the most important pathogen. ***M. catarrhalis*** is a strictly aerobic, oxidase-positive, gram-negative diplococci (Figure 27-7). This organism is a common cause of bronchitis and bronchopneumonia (in elderly patients with chronic pulmonary disease), sinusitis, and otitis (see Box 27-1). The latter two infections occur most commonly in previously healthy people. Most isolates produce β-lactamases and are **resistant to penicillins;** however, these bacteria are uniformly susceptible to most other antibiotics, including cephalosporins, erythromycin, tetracycline, TMP-SMX, and the combination of penicillins with a β-lactamase inhibitor (e.g., clavulanic acid).

Bibliography

Breidenstein E, de la Fuente-Nunez C, Hancock R: *Pseudomonas aeruginosa*: all roads lead to resistance, *Trends Microbiol* 19:419–426, 2011.

Broides A, Dagan R, Greenberg D, et al: Acute otitis media caused by *Moraxella catarrhalis:* epidemiology and clinical characteristics, *Clin Infect Dis* 49:1641–1647, 2009.

Brooke J: *Stenotrophomonas maltophilia:* an emerging global opportunistic pathogen, *Clin Microbiol Rev* 25:2–41, 2012.

Dijkshoorn L, Nemec A, Seifert H: An increasing threat in hospitals: multidrug-resistant *Acinetobacter baumannii, Nat Rev Microbiol* 5:939–951, 2007.

Hauser A: The type III secretion system of *Pseudomonas aeruginosa*: infection by injection, *Nat Rev Microbiol* 7:654–665, 2009.

Ikonomidis A, Neou E, Gogou V, et al: Heteroresistance to meropenem in carbapenem-susceptible *Acinetobacter baumannii, J Clin Microbiol* 47:4055–4059, 2009.

Jimenez PN, Koch G, Thompson JA, et al: The multiple signaling systems regulating virulence in *Pseudomonas aeruginosa, Microbiol Mol Biol Rev* 76:46–65, 2012.

Karthikeyan RS, Priya JL, Leal SM Jr, et al: Host response and bacterial virulence factor expression in *Pseudomonas aeruginosa* and *Streptococcus pneumoniae* corneal ulcers, *PLoS ONE* 8:e64867, 2013.

Kipnis E, Sawa T, Wiener-Kronish J: Targeting mechanisms of *Pseudomonas aeruginosa* pathogenesis, *Med Mal Infect* 36:78–91, 2006.

Kruczek C, Qaisar U, Comer-Hamood JA, et al: Serum influences the expression of *Pseudomonas aeruginosa* quorum-sensing genes and QS-controlled virulence genes during early and late stages of growth, *Microbiologyopen* 3:64–79, 2014.

Ledizet M, Murray TS, Puttagunta S, et al: The ability of virulence factor expression by *Pseudomonas aeruginosa* to predict clinical disease in hospitalized patients, *PLoS ONE* 7:e49578, 2012.

Looney WJ, Narita M, Muhlemann K: *Stenotrophomonas maltophilia*: an emerging opportunist human pathogen, *Lancet Infect Dis* 9:312–323, 2009.

McGregor K, Chang BJ, Mee BJ, et al: *Moraxella catarrhalis:* clinical significance, antimicrobial susceptibility and BRO beta-lactamases, *Eur J Clin Microbiol Infect Dis* 17:219–234, 1998.

Peleg A, Seifert H, Paterson D: *Acinetobacter baumannii*: emergence of a successful pathogen, *Clin Microbiol Rev* 21:538–582, 2008.

Voor AF, Severin JA, Lesaffre EM, et al: A systematic review and meta-analyses show that carbapenems use and medical devices are the leading risk factors for carbapenem-resistant *Pseudomonas aeruginosa, Antimicrob Agents Chemother* 58:2626–2637, 2014.

Yates SP, Jorgensen R, Andersen GR, et al: Stealth and mimicry by deadly bacterial toxins, *Trends Biochem Sci* 31:123–133, 2006.

CHAPTER

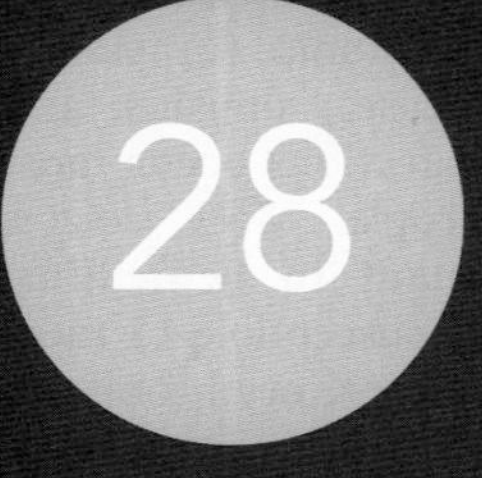

CAMPYLOBACTER AND HELICOBACTER

A 26-year-old woman was admitted to the hospital with a 48-hour history of colicky lower abdominal pain associated with about 20 watery stools per day, which contained mucus and blood. She was afebrile and had diffuse abdominal tenderness. No pathogens were isolated on routine stool culture, but specimens were also inoculated on a *Campylobacter*-selective medium and incubated microaerophilically at 40° C. Examination of the plates after 42 hours revealed the presence of flat, nonhemolytic, mucoid colonies that were subsequently identified as *Campylobacter jejuni. Campylobacter* and *Helicobacter* are now widely recognized as significant human pathogens; however, they were only discovered in the last 20 to 30 years.

1. What properties of *Campylobacter* and *Helicobacter* led to their delayed discovery?
2. *Campylobacter* is associated with what two immune disorders?
3. How does *Helicobacter pylori* survive in the stomach?

Answers to these questions are available on StudentConsult.com.

• SUMMARIES CLINICALLY SIGNIFICANT ORGANISMS

Campylobacter

Trigger Words

Curved rods, gastroenteritis, Guillain-Barré syndrome, poultry

Biology and Virulence

- Thin, curved, gram-negative rods
- Factors that regulate adhesion, motility, and invasion into intestinal mucosa are poorly defined

Epidemiology

- Zoonotic infection; improperly prepared poultry is a common source of human infections
- Infections acquired by ingestion of contaminated food, unpasteurized milk, or contaminated water
- Person-to-person spread is unusual
- Dose required to establish disease is high unless the gastric acids are neutralized or absent
- Worldwide distribution with enteric infections seen throughout the year

Diseases

- Most common disease is acute enteritis with diarrhea, malaise, fever, and abdominal pain
- Guillain-Barré syndrome is believed to be an autoimmune disease caused by antigenic cross-reactivity between oligosaccharides in the bacterial capsule and glycosphingolipids on the surface of neural tissues
- Most infections are self-limited but can persist for a week or more
- *C. fetus* is associated with septicemia and is disseminated to multiple organs

Diagnosis

- Microscopic detection of thin, S-shaped, gram-negative rods in stool specimens is specific but insensitive
- Commercial multiplex nucleic acid amplification assays are highly sensitive and specific for enteric pathogens and particularly useful for detection of *C. jejuni* and *C. coli* infections
- Culture requires use of specialized media incubated with reduced oxygen, increased carbon dioxide, and (for thermophilic species) elevated temperatures; requires incubation for 2 or more days and is relatively insensitive unless fresh media are used
- Detection of *Campylobacter* antigens in stool specimens is moderately sensitive and very specific compared with culture

Treatment, Prevention, and Control

- For gastroenteritis, infection is self-limited and is managed by fluid and electrolyte replacement
- Severe gastroenteritis and septicemia are treated with erythromycin or azithromycin
- Gastroenteritis is prevented by proper preparation of food and consumption of pasteurized milk; preventing contamination of water supplies also controls infection
- Experimental vaccines targeting the outer capsular polysaccharides are promising for control of infections in animal reservoirs

Helicobacter pylori

Trigger Words

Gastritis, peptic ulcers, gastric cancer, urease, person-to-person

Biology and Virulence

- Curved gram-negative rods
- Urease production at very high levels is typical of gastric helicobacters (e.g., *H. pylori;* important diagnostic test for *H. pylori*) and uncommon in intestinal helicobacters
- Multiple factors contribute to gastric colonization, inflammation, alteration of gastric acid production, and tissue destruction

Epidemiology

- Infections are common, particularly in people in a low socioeconomic class or in developing nations
- Humans are the primary reservoir
- Person-to-person spread is important (typically fecal-oral)
- Ubiquitous and worldwide, with no seasonal incidence of disease

Diseases

- *H. pylori* is an important cause of acute and chronic gastritis, peptic ulcers, gastric adenocarcinoma, and mucosa-associated lymphoid tissue lymphoma

Diagnosis

- Microscopy: histologic examination of biopsy specimens is sensitive and specific
- Urease test relatively sensitive and highly specific; urea breath test is a noninvasive test
- *H. pylori* antigen test is sensitive and specific; performed with stool specimens
- Culture requires incubation in microaerophilic conditions; growth is slow; relatively insensitive unless multiple biopsies are cultured
- Serology useful for demonstrating exposure to *H. pylori*

Treatment, Prevention, and Control

- Multiple regimens have been evaluated for treatment of *H. pylori* infections. Combined therapy with a proton pump inhibitor (e.g., omeprazole), a macrolide (e.g., clarithromycin), and a β-lactam (e.g., amoxicillin) for 2 weeks has had a high success rate
- Prophylactic treatment of colonized individuals has not been useful and potentially has adverse effects, such as predisposing patients to adenocarcinomas of the lower esophagus
- Human vaccines are not currently available

There are two families of related spiral-shaped gram-negative bacteria of clinical importance: **Campylobacteraceae,** which includes the genera *Campylobacter, Arcobacter,* and *Sulfurospirillum,* and **Helicobacteraceae,** which includes *Helicobacter* and *Wolinella*.

Members of these families share two important properties that contribute to problems with recovering the organisms in culture and identification by traditional biochemical testing: (1) microaerophilic growth requirements (i.e., growth only in the presence of reduced oxygen and increased carbon dioxide) and (2) inability to ferment or oxidize carbohydrates. Because of this, the clinical significance of two important human pathogens, *Campylobacter* and *Helicobacter* (Table 28-1), was only recently appreciated.

Campylobacter

The genus *Campylobacter* consists of small (0.2 to 0.5 μm wide and 0.5 to 5.0 μm long), motile, **comma-shaped, gram-negative rods** (Figure 28-1). Bacteria in older colonies may appear coccoid rather than rodlike. A total of 33 species and 14 subspecies are now recognized, many of which are associated with human disease, but only four species are common human pathogens (Table 28-2).

The primary diseases caused by campylobacters are gastroenteritis and septicemia. *Campylobacter* is the most common cause of bacterial gastroenteritis in both developed and developing countries, with ***Campylobacter jejuni*** responsible for most infections and ***Campylobacter coli*** associated with a minority of cases of *Campylobacter* gastroenteritis in the United States (more commonly observed in developing countries). The incidence of gastroenteritis caused by ***Campylobacter upsaliensis*** is unknown because the organism is inhibited by the antibiotics used in isolation media for other campylobacters; however, some have estimated that 10% of *Campylobacter* gastroenteritis is caused by this bacterium. A variety of other species are rare causes of gastroenteritis or systemic infections, with one exception. Unlike other *Campylobacter* species, ***Campylobacter fetus*** is primarily responsible for causing systemic infections such as bacteremia, septic thrombophlebitis, arthritis, septic abortion, and meningitis.

Physiology and Structure

Recognition of the role of campylobacters in gastrointestinal (GI) disease was delayed because the organisms grow best in an atmosphere of reduced oxygen (5% to 7%) and increased carbon dioxide (5% to 10%). In addition, ***C. jejuni* grows better at 42° C** than at 37° C. These properties have been exploited for the selective isolation of pathogenic campylobacters in stool specimens. The **small size** of the organisms (0.2 to 0.5 μm in diameter) has also been used to recover the bacteria by filtration of stool specimens. Campylobacters pass through 0.45-μm filters, whereas other bacteria are retained. Although this property led to the initial discovery of campylobacters (stools were filtered looking for viruses), filtration of stool specimens is a cumbersome procedure and is not used in clinical laboratories. Campylobacters have a gram-negative cell wall structure with an outer polysaccharide capsule; however, instead of cell wall lipopolysaccharides (LPS) with endotoxin activity found in other gram-negative bacteria, they express lipooligosaccharides. The capsular polysaccharides (CPS) contribute to the virulence of the bacteria and are the targets of vaccine development.

Pathogenesis and Immunity

Although adhesins, cytotoxic enzymes, and enterotoxins have been detected in *C. jejuni,* their specific role in disease remains poorly defined. It is clear that the risk of disease is influenced by the infectious dose. The organisms are killed when exposed to gastric acids, so conditions that decrease or neutralize gastric acid secretion favor disease. The patient's immune status also affects the severity of disease. People living in a population of high endemic disease develop measurable levels of specific serum and secretory antibodies and have less severe disease. As would be expected, patients with hypogammaglobulinemia have prolonged severe disease with *C. jejuni*.

C. jejuni GI disease characteristically produces **histologic damage to the mucosal surfaces of the jejunum** (as implied by the name of the species), ileum, and colon. The mucosal surface appears ulcerated, edematous, and bloody, with crypt abscesses in the epithelial glands and infiltration of the lamina propria with neutrophils, mononuclear cells, and eosinophils. This inflammatory process is consistent with

Table 28-1 Important *Campylobacter* and *Helicobacter* Species

Organism	Historical Derivation
Campylobacter	*kampylos*, curved; *bacter*, rod (a curved rod)
C. jejuni	*jejuni*, of the jejunum
C. coli	*coli*, of the colon
C. fetus	*fetus*, refers to the initial observation that these bacteria caused fetal infections
C. upsaliensis	*upsaliensis*, original isolates recovered from the feces of dogs at an animal clinic in Uppsala, Sweden
Helicobacter	*helix*, spiral; *bacter*, rod (a spiral rod)
H. pylori	*pylorus*, lower part of the stomach
H. cinaedi	*cinaedi*, of a homosexual (the organism was first isolated from homosexuals with gastroenteritis)
H. fennelliae	*fennelliae*, named after C. Fennell, who first isolated the organism

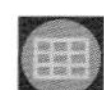

Table 28-2 Common *Campylobacter* Species Associated with Human Disease

Species	Common Reservoir Hosts	Human Disease
C. jejuni	**Poultry,** cattle, sheep	**Gastroenteritis,** extraintestinal infections, **Guillain-Barré syndrome, reactive arthritis**
C. coli	**Pigs,** poultry, sheep, birds	**Gastroenteritis,** extraintestinal infections
C. fetus	**Cattle, sheep**	**Vascular infections** (e.g., septicemia, septic thrombophlebitis, endocarditis), meningoencephalitis, gastroenteritis
C. upsaliensis	**Dogs,** cats	**Gastroenteritis,** extraintestinal infections, Guillain-Barré syndrome

Bold type signifies the most common hosts and diseases.

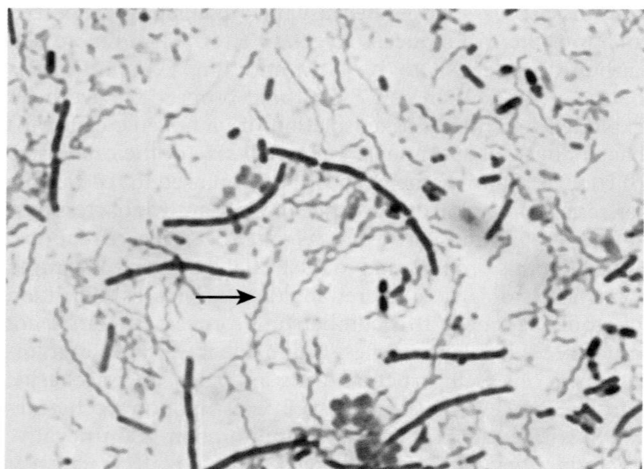

FIGURE 28-1 Mixed culture of bacteria from a fecal specimen. *Campylobacter jejuni* is the thin, curved, gram-negative bacteria (arrow).

invasion of the organisms into the intestinal tissue. However, the precise roles of cytopathic toxins, enterotoxins, and endotoxic activity that have been detected in *C. jejuni* isolates have not been defined. For example, strains lacking enterotoxin activity are still fully virulent.

C. jejuni and *C. upsaliensis* have been associated with **Guillain-Barré syndrome,** an autoimmune disorder of the peripheral nervous system characterized by development of symmetric weakness over several days and recovery requiring months or longer. Although this is an uncommon complication of *Campylobacter* disease (≈1 in 1000 diagnosed infections), the syndrome has been associated with specific serotypes (primarily *C. jejuni* serotype O:19). It is believed that the pathogenesis of this disease is related to **antigenic cross-reactivity** between the surface lipooligosaccharides of some strains of *Campylobacter* and peripheral nerve gangliosides. Thus antibodies directed against specific strains of *Campylobacter* can damage neural tissue in the peripheral nervous system. Another immune-related late complication of *Campylobacter* infections is **reactive arthritis,** a condition characterized by joint pain and swelling involving the hands, ankles, and knees and persisting from 1 week to several months. Reactive arthritis is unrelated to the severity of the diarrheal disease but is more common in patients who have the HLA-B27 phenotype.

C. jejuni and *C. coli* rarely cause bacteremia (1.5 cases per 1000 intestinal infections); however, *C. fetus* has a propensity to spread from the GI tract to the blood and distal foci. In vitro studies provide an explanation for this observation: *C. fetus* is resistant to complement- and antibody-mediated serum killing, and *C. jejuni* and most other *Campylobacter* species are killed rapidly. *C. fetus* is covered with a heat-stable, capsule-like protein **(S protein)** that prevents C3b binding to the bacteria and subsequent complement-mediated killing in serum. *C. fetus* loses its virulence if this protein layer is removed. Bacteremia is particularly common in debilitated and immunocompromised patients, such as those with liver disease, diabetes mellitus, chronic alcoholism, or malignancies.

Epidemiology

Campylobacter infections are **zoonotic,** with a variety of animals serving as reservoirs (see Table 28-2). Humans acquire the infections with *C. jejuni* and *C. coli* after consumption of contaminated food, milk, or water; **contaminated poultry** are responsible for more than half of the *Campylobacter* infections in developed countries. In contrast, *C. upsaliensis* infections are acquired primarily after contact with domestic dogs (either healthy carriers or pets with diarrheal disease). Food products that neutralize gastric acids (e.g., milk) effectively reduce the infectious dose. Fecal-oral transmission from person-to-person contact may also occur, but it is **uncommon for the disease to be transmitted by food handlers.**

The actual incidence of *Campylobacter* infections is unknown because disease is not reported to public health officials. Epidemiologic surveys indicate that the incidence of disease has decreased in the last decade, most likely owing to improved food handling techniques. However, it is estimated that between 1.4 and 2 million infections occur annually in the United States, and these infections are more common than *Salmonella* and *Shigella* infections combined. The number of *Campylobacter* infections may be even higher because *C. upsaliensis* is not isolated by commonly used techniques. Disease occurs sporadically through the year, with a peak incidence during the summer months. Disease is most commonly observed in **infants and young children,** with a second peak of disease in 20- to 40-year-old adults. The incidence of disease is higher in developing countries, with symptomatic disease in infants and young children and asymptomatic carriage frequently observed in adults.

C. fetus infections are relatively uncommon, with fewer than 250 cases reported in the United States annually. Unlike *C. jejuni, C. fetus* primarily infects immunocompromised or elderly people.

Clinical Diseases (Clinical Case 28-1)

GI infections with *C. jejuni, C. coli,* and *C. upsaliensis* present most commonly as **acute enteritis** with diarrhea, fever, and severe abdominal pain. Affected patients can have 10 or more bowel movements per day during the peak of disease, and stools may be bloody on gross examination. The disease is generally self-limited, although symptoms may last for a week or longer. The range of clinical manifestations includes acute colitis, **abdominal pain mimicking acute appendicitis,** and chronic enteric infections that develop most commonly in immunocompromised patients (e.g., patients with acquired immunodeficiency syndrome [AIDS]). Various extraintestinal infections are reported but are relatively uncommon. **Guillain-Barré syndrome** and **reactive arthritis** are well-recognized complications of *Campylobacter* infections. *C. fetus* differs from other *Campylobacter* species in that this species is primarily responsible for **intravascular** (e.g., septicemia, endocarditis, septic thrombophlebitis) and **extraintestinal** (e.g., meningoencephalitis, abscesses) **infections.**

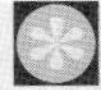

Clinical Case 28-1 *Campylobacter jejuni* Enteritis and Guillain-Barré Syndrome

Scully and associates (*N Engl J Med* 341:1996–2003, 1999) described the clinical history of a 74-year-old woman who developed Guillain-Barré syndrome following an episode of *C. jejuni* enteritis. After 1 week of fever, watery diarrhea, nausea, abdominal pain, weakness, and fatigue, the patient's speech was noted to be severely slurred. She was taken to the hospital, where it was noted she was unable to speak, although she was oriented and able to write coherently. She had perioral numbness, bilateral ptosis and facial weakness were noted, and her pupils were nonreactive. Neurologic examination revealed bilateral muscle weakness in her arms and chest. On the second hospital day, the muscle weakness extended to her upper legs. On the third hospital day, the patient's mental status remained normal, but she could only move her thumb minimally and could not lift her legs. Sensation to light touch was normal, but deep-tendon reflexes were absent. *C. jejuni* was recovered from this patient's stool culture, collected at the time of admission, and the clinical diagnosis of Guillain-Barré syndrome was made. Despite aggressive medical treatment, the patient had significant neurologic deficits 3 months after discharge to a rehabilitation facility. This woman illustrates one of the significant complications of *Campylobacter* enteritis.

Laboratory Diagnosis

Microscopy

Campylobacters are thin and not easily seen when specimens are Gram stained. Despite the low sensitivity of a Gram stain, observation of the characteristic **thin, S-shaped organisms** in a stool specimen (see Figure 28-1) is useful for a presumptive confirmation of *Campylobacter* infection.

Antigen Detection

A commercial immunoassay for detection of *C. jejuni* and *C. coli* is available. When compared with culture, the test has a sensitivity of 80% to 90% and a specificity of greater than 95%. Some strains of *C. upsaliensis* are also reactive in this test.

Nucleic Acid–Based Tests

Commercial multiplex nucleic acid amplification tests for enteric pathogens are rapidly gaining acceptance because they can rapidly detect a comprehensive spectrum of bacterial, viral, and parasitic pathogens with a sensitivity superior to culture. This is particularly true for *Campylobacter* infections, although these molecular assays are generally restricted to detection of *C. jejuni* and *C. coli* and not the other *Campylobacter* species.

Culture

C. jejuni, C. coli, and *C. upsaliensis* went unrecognized for many years because their isolation requires growth in a **microaerophilic atmosphere** (i.e., 5% to 7% oxygen, 5% to 10% carbon dioxide), at an **elevated incubation temperature** (i.e., 42° C), and on selective agar media to suppress nonpathogenic enteric bacteria. The appropriate atmosphere for growing campylobacters can be produced by disposable commercial gas generator systems that are added to an incubation jar with the inoculated culture media. The selective media must contain blood or charcoal to remove toxic oxygen radicals, and antibiotics are added to inhibit the growth of contaminating organisms. Unfortunately, the antibiotics used in most *Campylobacter* media may inhibit some species (e.g., *C. upsaliensis*). Campylobacters are **slow-growing** organisms, usually requiring incubation for 48 hours or longer. *C. fetus* is not thermophilic and cannot grow at 42° C; however, its isolation requires a microaerophilic atmosphere.

Identification

A presumptive identification of isolates is based on growth under selective conditions, typical microscopic morphology, and positive oxidase and catalase tests.

Antibody Detection

Serologic testing for immunoglobulin (Ig)M and IgG is useful for epidemiologic surveys but is not used for diagnosis in an individual patient.

Treatment, Prevention, and Control

Campylobacter gastroenteritis is typically a self-limited infection managed by the replacement of lost fluids and electrolytes. Antibiotic therapy may be used in patients with severe infections or septicemia. Campylobacters are susceptible to a variety of antibiotics, including macrolides (i.e., erythromycin, azithromycin, clarithromycin), tetracyclines, aminoglycosides, chloramphenicol, fluoroquinolones, clindamycin, amoxicillin/clavulanic acid, and imipenem. Most isolates are resistant to penicillins, cephalosporins, and sulfonamide antibiotics. **Erythromycin** or **azithromycin** are the antibiotics of choice for the treatment of enteritis, with tetracycline or fluoroquinolones used as secondary antibiotics. Resistance to fluoroquinolones has increased, so these drugs may be less effective. Amoxicillin/clavulanic acid can be used in place of tetracycline, which is contraindicated in young children. Systemic infections are treated with an aminoglycoside, chloramphenicol, or imipenem.

Exposure to enteric campylobacters is prevented by proper food preparation (particularly poultry), avoidance of unpasteurized dairy products, and implementation of safeguards to prevent contamination of water supplies. Almost 50 capsular serotypes of *C. jejuni* are recognized, although the majority of strains associated with disease are restricted to a limited number of serotypes. Preliminary studies demonstrate these are attractive targets for vaccines and potentially could reduce the colonization rate in food animals such as chickens and turkeys.

Helicobacter

In 1983, **spiral gram-negative rods** resembling campylobacters were found in patients with type B gastritis (chronic inflammation of the stomach antrum [pyloric end]). The organisms were originally classified as *Campylobacter* but were subsequently reclassified as a new genus, *Helicobacter.* Helicobacters were subsequently subdivided into species that primarily colonize the stomach **(gastric helicobacters)** and those that colonize the intestines **(enterohepatic helicobacters).** The most important species is ***Helicobacter pylori,*** a gastric helicobacter associated with **gastritis, peptic ulcers, gastric adenocarcinoma,** and **gastric mucosa–associated lymphoid tissue (MALT) B-cell lymphomas** (Table 28-3). The most important enterohepatic helicobacters associated with **gastroenteritis** and **bacteremia** are ***Helicobacter cinaedi*** and ***Helicobacter fennelliae,*** which have been isolated most commonly in immunocompromised patients (e.g., homosexual men with human immunodeficiency virus [HIV] infections). Another species of uncertain taxonomy, currently termed "*Helicobacter* species flexispira" causes bacteremia with cellulitis and wound infections in immunocompromised patients (e.g., patients with Bruton X-linked agammaglobulinemia). The discussion in this chapter will be restricted to the gastric helicobacter, *H. pylori.*

Table 28-3 *Helicobacter* Species Associated with Human Disease

Species	Common Reservoir Hosts	Human Disease
H. pylori	**Humans,** primates, pigs	**Gastritis, peptic ulcers, gastric adenocarcinoma,** mucosa-associated lymphoid tissue B-cell lymphomas
H. cinaedi	**Humans,** hamster	**Gastroenteritis,** septicemia, proctocolitis
H. fennelliae	**Humans**	**Gastroenteritis,** septicemia, proctocolitis

Bold type signifies the most common hosts and diseases.

Physiology and Structure

Helicobacter species are characterized according to sequence analysis of their 16S rRNA genes, their cellular fatty acids, and the presence of polar flagella. Currently, 35 species have been characterized, but this taxonomy is changing rapidly. Helicobacters have a bacillary or **spiral shape** in young cultures (0.5 to 1.0 µm wide × 2 to 4 µm long) and, like campylobacters, can assume coccoid forms in older cultures (Figure 28-2).

All gastric helicobacters, including *H. pylori,* are highly **motile** (corkscrew motility) and produce an abundance of **urease.** These properties are believed to be important for survival in gastric acids and rapid movement through the viscous mucus layer toward a neutral pH environment. Most helicobacters are catalase- and oxidase-positive and do not ferment or oxidize carbohydrates, although they can metabolize amino acids by fermentative pathways. Lipopolysaccharide (LPS), consisting of lipid A, core oligosaccharide, and an O side chain, is present in the outer membrane. *H. pylori* lipid A has low endotoxin activity compared with other gram-negative bacteria, and the O side chain is antigenically similar to the Lewis blood group antigens, which may protect the bacteria from immune clearance.

Growth of *H. pylori* and other helicobacters requires a complex medium supplemented with blood, serum, charcoal, starch, or egg yolk in microaerophilic conditions (decreased oxygen and increased carbon dioxide) and in a temperature range between 30° C and 37° C. Because helicobacters are relatively difficult to isolate in culture and identify by biochemical testing, most diseases caused by *H. pylori* are confirmed by nonculture techniques (see later).

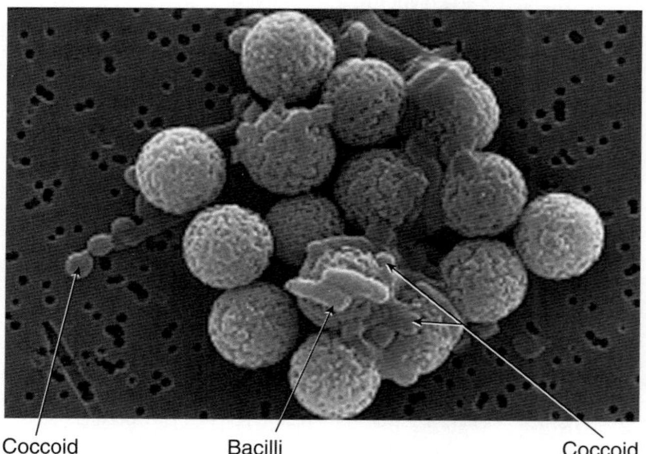

FIGURE 28-2 Scanning electron micrograph of *Helicobacter pylori* in a 7-day culture. Bacillary and coccoid forms are bound to paramagnetic beads used in immunomagnetic separation. (Courtesy Dr. L. Engstrand, Uppsala, Sweden.)

Pathogenesis and Immunity

H. pylori is a remarkable bacterium in its ability to establish lifelong colonization in the stomach of untreated humans. Most research into the virulence factors in helicobacters has focused on *H. pylori.* Multiple factors contribute to the gastric colonization, inflammation, alteration of gastric acid production, and tissue destruction that are characteristic of *H. pylori* disease. Initial colonization is facilitated by (1) blockage of acid production by a bacterial acid–inhibitory protein and (2) neutralization of gastric acids with the ammonia produced by bacterial urease activity. The actively motile helicobacters can then pass through the gastric mucus and adhere to the gastric epithelial cells by multiple surface adhesion proteins. Surface proteins can also bind host proteins and help the bacteria evade the immune system. Localized tissue damage is mediated by urease byproducts, **mucinase, phospholipases,** and the activity of **vacuolating cytotoxin A (VacA),** a protein that after penetration into epithelial cells damages the cells by producing vacuoles. Another important virulence factor of *H. pylori* is the **cytotoxin-associated gene *(cagA)*** that resides on a pathogenicity island containing approximately 30 genes. These genes encode a structure (type VI secretion system) that acts like a syringe to inject the CagA protein into the host epithelial cells, which interferes with the normal cytoskeletal structure of the epithelial cells. The *cag* *p*hosphoribosyl*a*nthranilate *i*somerase (PAI) genes also induce **interleukin (IL)-8 production,** which attracts neutrophils. Release of proteases and reactive oxygen molecules by these neutrophils is believed to contribute to gastritis and gastric ulcers.

Epidemiology

An enormous amount of information about the prevalence of *H. pylori* has been collected since 1984 when the organism was first isolated in culture. The highest incidence of carriage is found in developing countries, where 70% to 90% of the population is colonized, most before the age of 10 years. The prevalence of *H. pylori* in industrial countries such as the United States is less than 40% and is decreasing because of improved hygiene and active treatment of colonized individuals. These studies have also demonstrated that 70% to 100% of patients with gastritis, gastric ulcers, or duodenal ulcers are infected with *H. pylori.* **Humans are the primary reservoir for *H. pylori,*** and colonization is believed to persist for life unless the host is specifically treated. Transmission is most likely via the **fecal-oral route.**

An interesting observation about *H. pylori* colonization has been made. This organism is clearly associated with diseases such as gastritis, gastric ulcers, gastric adenocarcinoma, and gastric MALT lymphomas. It is anticipated that treatment of colonized or infected individuals will lead to a reduction of these diseases. However, colonization with *H. pylori* appears to offer protection from gastroesophageal reflux disease and adenocarcinomas of the lower esophagus and gastric cardia. Thus it may be unwise to eliminate *H. pylori* in patients without symptomatic disease. Certainly, the complex relationship between *H. pylori* and its host remains to be defined.

Clinical Diseases (Clinical Case 28-2)

Disease caused by helicobacters is directly related to their site of colonization. For example, *H. pylori* is associated with gastritis, whereas the enterohepatic species cause gastroenteritis. Colonization with *H. pylori* invariably leads to histologic evidence of **gastritis** (i.e., infiltration of neutrophils and mononuclear cells into the gastric mucosa). The acute phase of gastritis is characterized by a feeling of fullness, nausea, vomiting, and hypochlorhydria (decreased acid production in the stomach). This can evolve into chronic gastritis, with disease confined to the gastric antrum (where few acid-secreting parietal cells are present) in individuals with normal acid secretion, or involve the entire stomach (pangastritis) if acid secretion is suppressed. Approximately 10% to 15% of patients with chronic gastritis will progress to develop peptic ulcers. The ulcers develop at the sites of intense inflammation, commonly involving the junction between the corpus and antrum **(gastric ulcer)** or the proximal duodenum **(duodenal ulcer).** *H. pylori* is responsible for 85% of the gastric ulcers and 95% of the duodenal ulcers. Recognition of the role of *H. pylori* has dramatically changed the treatment and prognosis of peptic ulcer disease.

Chronic gastritis eventually leads to replacement of the normal gastric mucosa with fibrosis and proliferation of intestinal-type epithelium. This process increases the patient's risk for **gastric cancer** by almost 100-fold. This risk is influenced by the strain of *H. pylori* and the host's response (*cagA*-positive strains and high levels of IL-1 production are associated with a higher risk for cancer). Infection with *H. pylori* is also associated with infiltration of lymphoid tissue into the gastric mucosa. In a small number of patients, a monoclonal population of B cells may develop and evolve into a **MALT lymphoma.**

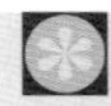

Clinical Case 28-2 The Discovery of *Helicobacter pylori*

In 1984, Australian physicians Marshall and Warren reported a discovery that completely changed the approach to treatment of gastritis and peptic ulcer disease, as well as set the foundation for understanding the cause of gastric adenocarcinomas and mucosa-associated lymphoid tissue lymphomas (*Lancet* i:1311–1315, 1984). In an analysis of gastric biopsy specimens from 100 consecutive patients presenting for gastroscopy, they demonstrated curved gram-negative rods resembling *Campylobacter* in 58 patients. The bacteria were observed in most patients with active gastritis, gastric ulcers, and duodenal ulcers. Although similar organisms were observed associated with gastric tissues 45 years earlier, this report stimulated resurgence in investigations of the role of this "new" organism in gastric diseases. Despite the skepticism that greeted their initial report, the significance of their work with *Campylobacter* was recognized in 2005 when Marshall and Warren received the Nobel Prize in Medicine.

Laboratory Diagnosis

Microscopy

H. pylori is detected by histologic examination of gastric biopsy specimens. Although the organism can be seen in specimens stained with hematoxylin-eosin or Gram stain, the Warthin-Starry silver stain is the most sensitive. When an adequate specimen is collected and examined by an experienced microscopist, the test sensitivity and specificity approaches 100% and is considered diagnostic. Because this is an invasive test, alternative test procedures are preferred for routine diagnosis. The microscopic examination of stool specimens for helicobacters is not reliable, because the organisms are difficult to see and nonpathogenic helicobacters may be present.

Antigen Detection

Biopsy specimens can also be tested for the presence of bacterial urease activity. The abundance of urease produced by *H. pylori* permits detection of the alkaline byproduct in less than 2 hours. The sensitivity of the direct test with biopsy specimens varies from 75% to 95%; however, the specificity approaches 100%. Thus a positive reaction is compelling evidence of an active infection. As with microscopy, the limitation of this method is the requirement for a biopsy specimen. Noninvasive urease testing of human breath (urea breath test) following consumption of an isotopically labeled urea solution has excellent sensitivity and specificity. Unfortunately, this assay is relatively expensive because of the cost of the detection instruments.

A number of polyclonal and monoclonal immunoassays for *H. pylori* antigens excreted in stool have been developed and demonstrated to have sensitivities and specificities exceeding 95%. These tests are easy to perform, inexpensive, and able to be used on stool specimens rather than biopsies. These assays are now widely recommended for both detection of *H. pylori* infections and confirmation of cure after antibiotic treatment.

Nucleic Acid–Based Tests

Currently, nucleic acid–based amplification tests for *H. pylori* and enterohepatic helicobacters are restricted to research laboratories and not used in clinical laboratories.

Culture

H. pylori adheres to gastric mucosa and is not recovered in stool or blood specimens. The bacteria can be isolated in culture if the specimen is inoculated onto an enriched medium supplemented with blood, hemin, or charcoal and incubated in a microaerophilic atmosphere for up to 2 weeks. However, diagnosis of *H. pylori* infections is most commonly by noninvasive methods (e.g., immunoassay), with culture reserved for antibiotic susceptibility tests.

Identification

Presumptive identification of isolates is based on their growth characteristics under selective conditions, typical microscopic morphologic findings, and detection of oxidase, catalase, and urease activity.

Antibody Detection

Serology is an important screening test for the diagnosis of *H. pylori,* with a variety of commercial tests available. Although IgM antibodies disappear rapidly, IgA and IgG antibodies can persist for months to years. Because the **antibody titers persist** for many years, the test cannot be used to discriminate between past and current infection. Furthermore, the titer of antibodies measured does not correlate with the severity of disease or the response to therapy. However, the tests are useful for documenting exposure to the bacteria, either for epidemiologic studies or for the initial evaluation of a symptomatic patient.

Treatment, Prevention, and Control

Numerous antibiotic regimens have been evaluated for treating *H. pylori* infections. Use of a single antibiotic or an antibiotic combined with bismuth is ineffective. The greatest success in curing gastritis or peptic ulcer disease has been accomplished with the combination of a **proton pump inhibitor** (e.g., omeprazole), a **macrolide** (e.g., clarithromycin), and a **β-lactam** (e.g., amoxicillin), with administration for 7 to 10 days initially. Treatment failure is most commonly associated with clarithromycin resistance. Susceptibility testing should be performed if the patient does not respond to therapy. Metronidazole can also be used in combination therapy, but resistance is commonplace.

Infection with *H. pylori* stimulates a strong TH1 cell–mediated inflammatory response. Use of *H. pylori* antigens in experimental vaccines that stimulate TH1 cells leads to enhanced inflammation. In contrast, use of antigens in combination with mucosal adjuvants that induce a TH2 cell response is protective in an animal model and can eradicate existing infections. The effectiveness of these vaccines in humans remains to be demonstrated.

Bibliography

Algood H, Cover T: *Helicobacter pylori* persistence: an overview of interactions between *H. pylori* and host immune defenses, *Clin Microbiol Rev* 19:597–613, 2006.

Farinha P, Gascoyne R: *Helicobacter pylori* and MALT lymphoma, *Gastroenterology* 128:1579–1605, 2005.

Garza-Gonzalez E, Perez-Perez GI, Maldonado-Garza HJ, et al: A review of *Helicobacter pylori* diagnosis, treatment, and methods to detect eradication, *World J Gastroenterol* 20:1438–1449, 2014.

Iovine N: Resistance mechanisms in *Campylobacter jejuni*, *Virulence* 4:230–240, 2013.

Kabir S: The current status of *Helicobacter pylori* vaccines: a review, *Helicobacter* 12:89–102, 2007.

Kusters JG, van Vliet A, Kuipers EJ: Pathogenesis of *Helicobacter pylori* infection, *Clin Microbiol Rev* 19:449–490, 2006.

Nachamkin I, Allos BM, Ho T: *Campylobacter* species and Guillain-Barré syndrome, *Clin Microbiol Rev* 11:555–567, 1998.

Passaro D, Chosy EJ, Parsonnet J: *Helicobacter pylori:* consensus and controversy, *Clin Infect Dis* 35:298–304, 2002.

Pike B, Guerry P, Poly F: Global distribution of *Campylobacter jejuni* Penner serotypes: a systematic review, *PLoS ONE* 8:1–8, 2013.

Plummer P: LuxS and quorum-sensing in *Campylobacter*, *Front Cell Infect Microbiol* 2:1–9, 2012.

Solnick J: Clinical significance of *Helicobacter* species other than *Helicobacter pylori*, *Clin Infect Dis* 36:348–354, 2003.

CHAPTER

MISCELLANEOUS GRAM-NEGATIVE RODS

The gram-negative rods discussed in this chapter are a miscellaneous collection of clinically important bacteria.

1. Which *Bartonella* species are associated with disease in immunocompromised patients, and how do these infections present?
2. What is the epidemiologic source of *Bordetella pertussis* infections?
3. Why is culture not a good diagnostic test for *B. pertussis?*
4. What is the most common source of human infections with *Francisella* and *Brucella?*
5. What disease is produced by *Cardiobacterium* species?
6. Why had *Legionella* not been recognized before the 1976 outbreak in Philadelphia at the American Legion convention?

Answers to these questions are available on StudentConsult.com.

• SUMMARIES CLINICALLY SIGNIFICANT ORGANISMS

Bordetella pertussis

Trigger Words

Slow-growing, whooping cough, pertussis toxin, person-to-person, vaccination

Biology and Virulence

- Very small gram-negative coccobacilli
- Nonfermentative but can oxidize amino acids as an energy source
- Strict aerobe
- Growth in vitro requires prolonged incubation in media supplemented with charcoal, starch, blood, or albumin
- Adherence to eukaryotic cells mediated by pertactin, filamentous hemagglutinin, and fimbria; localized tissue destruction mediated by dermonecrotic toxin and tracheal cytotoxin; systemic toxicity produced by pertussis toxin

Epidemiology

- Pertussis is a human disease with no known animal or environmental reservoir
- Worldwide distribution with a high prevalence in unvaccinated populations
- Children younger than 1 year are at greatest risk for infection and mortality
- In vaccinated populations, disease is observed in older children and young adults
- Unvaccinated individuals are at greatest risk for disease
- Disease spread person to person by infectious aerosols

Diseases

- Pertussis characterized by three stages: catarrhal, paroxysmal, and convalescent
- Most severe disease is in unvaccinated individuals, particularly children

Diagnosis

- Microscopy is insensitive and nonspecific
- Culture is specific but insensitive
- Nucleic acid amplification tests are the most sensitive and specific tests
- Detection of immunoglobulin (Ig)G or IgA can be used as a confirmatory test

Treatment, Prevention, and Control

- Treatment with macrolide (i.e., azithromycin, clarithromycin) is effective in eradicating organisms and reducing length of infectious stage
- Azithromycin is used for prophylaxis
- Vaccines containing inactivated pertussis toxin, filamentous hemagglutinin, and pertactin are effective
- Pediatric vaccine administered in 5 doses (at ages 2, 4, 6, and 15 to 18 months, and between ages 4 and 6 years); adult vaccine administered at ages 11 to 12 years and between 19 to 65 years

Brucella

Trigger Words

Small coccobacilli, slow-growing, zoonotic, undulant fever

Biology and Virulence

- Very small gram-negative coccobacilli (0.5 × 0.6 to 1.5 μm)
- Strict aerobe; does not ferment carbohydrates
- Requires complex media and prolonged incubation for in vitro growth
- Intracellular pathogen that is resistant to killing in serum and by phagocytes
- Smooth colonies associated with virulence

Epidemiology

- Animal reservoirs are goats and sheep *(Brucella melitensis);* cattle and American bison *(Brucella abortus);* swine, reindeer, and caribou *(Brucella suis);* and dogs, foxes, and coyotes *(Brucella canis)*
- Infects animal tissues rich in erythritol (e.g., breast, uterus, placenta, epididymis)
- Worldwide distribution, particularly in Latin America, Africa, the Mediterranean basin, the Middle East, and Western Asia
- Vaccination of herds has controlled disease in the United States
- Most disease in the United States is reported in California and Texas in travelers from Mexico
- Individuals at greatest risk for disease are people who consume unpasteurized dairy products, people in direct contact with infected animals, and laboratory workers

Diseases

- Refer to Box 29-1 for diseases

Diagnosis

- Microscopy is insensitive
- Culture (blood, bone marrow, infected tissue if localized infection) is sensitive and specific if prolonged incubation is used (minimum of 3 days to 2 weeks)
- Serology can be used to confirm the clinical diagnosis; fourfold increase in titer or single titer ≥ 1 : 160; high titers can persist for months to years

Treatment, Prevention, and Control

- Recommended treatment is doxycycline combined with rifampin for a minimum of 6 weeks for nonpregnant adults; trimethoprim-sulfamethoxazole for pregnant women and for children younger than 8 years
- Human disease is controlled by eradication of the disease in the animal reservoir through vaccination and serologic monitoring of the animals for evidence of disease, pasteurization of dairy products, and use of proper safety techniques in clinical laboratories working with this organism

Francisella tularensis

Trigger Words

Small coccobacilli, slow-growing, cysteine-supplemented media, zoonotic, ulceroglandular, oculoglandular, pneumonic

Biology and Virulence

- Very small gram-negative coccobacilli (0.2 × 0.2 to 0.7 μm)
- Strict aerobe; do not ferment carbohydrates
- Antiphagocytic capsule
- Intracellular pathogen resistant to killing in serum and by phagocytes

Epidemiology

- Wild mammals, domestic animals, birds, fish, and blood-sucking arthropods are reservoirs; rabbits, cats, hard ticks, and biting flies are most commonly associated with human disease; humans are accidental hosts
- Worldwide distribution; most common in United States in Oklahoma, Missouri, and Arkansas
- Approximately 1050 cases seen in United States, although the actual number may be much higher
- Infectious dose is small when exposure is by arthropod, through skin, or by inhalation; large numbers of organisms must be ingested for infection by this route

Diseases

- Clinical symptoms and prognosis determined by route of infection: ulceroglandular, oculoglandular, glandular, typhoidal, oropharyngeal, gastrointestinal, pneumonic (see Box 29-1)

Diagnosis

- Microscopy is insensitive
- Culture on cysteine-supplemented media (e.g., chocolate agar, buffered charcoal yeast extract agar) is sensitive if prolonged incubation is used
- Serology can be used to confirm clinical diagnosis; fourfold increase in titer or single titer ≥ 1 : 160; high titers can persist for months to years

Treatment, Prevention, and Control

- Gentamicin is the antibiotic of choice; fluoroquinolones (e.g., ciprofloxacin) and doxycycline have good activity; penicillins and some cephalosporins are ineffective
- Disease prevented by avoiding reservoirs and vectors of infection; clothing and gloves are protective
- Live attenuated vaccine available but rarely used for human disease

Legionella pneumophila

Trigger Words

Poor-staining slender rods, legionnaires disease, Pontiac fever, contaminated water, BCYE agar

Biology and Virulence

- Slender, pleomorphic, nonfermentative, gram-negative rods
- Stains poorly with common reagents
- Nutritionally fastidious, with requirement for L-cysteine and enhanced growth with iron salts
- Capable of replication in alveolar macrophages (and in amebae in nature)
- Prevents phagolysosome fusion

Epidemiology

- Capable of sporadic, epidemic, and nosocomial infections
- Commonly found in natural bodies of water, cooling towers, condensers, and water systems (including hospital systems)
- Estimated to be between 10,000 and 20,000 cases of infection in United States annually
- Patients at high risk for symptomatic disease include patients with compromised pulmonary function and patients with decreased cellular immunity (particularly transplant patients)

Diseases

- Responsible for legionnaires disease and Pontiac fever

Diagnosis

- Microscopy is insensitive
- Antigen tests are sensitive for *L. pneumophila* serogroup 1 but have poor sensitivity for other serogroups and species
- Culture on buffered charcoal yeast extract agar is the diagnostic test of choice
- Seroconversion must be demonstrated; this can take as long as 6 months to develop; positive serology may persist for months
- Nucleic acid amplification assays are as sensitive and specific as culture

Treatment, Control, and Prevention

- Macrolides (e.g., azithromycin, clarithromycin) or fluoroquinolones (e.g., ciprofloxacin, levofloxacin) are the treatment of choice
- Decrease environmental exposure to reduce risk of disease
- For environmental sources associated with disease, treat with hyperchlorination, superheating, or copper-silver ionization

A few medically important gram-negative rods have not been discussed in the preceding chapters and are the subject of this chapter (Table 29-1).

• *Bartonella*

As with many groups of bacteria studied in recent years, analysis of the 16S ribosomal ribonucleic acid (rRNA) gene has led to reorganization of the genus *Bartonella.* Currently, 29 species are included in the genus, with 3 species most commonly associated with human disease: ***B. bacilliformis, B. henselae,*** and ***B. quintana*** (Box 29-1). Members of the genus are short (0.2 to 0.6 × 0.5 to 1.0 μm), gram-negative, coccobacillary or bacillary rods with fastidious growth requirements, requiring prolonged incubation (2 to 6 weeks) for their initial recovery in culture.

Members of the genus *Bartonella* are found in a variety of animal reservoirs and are typically present without evidence of disease. Spread of most *Bartonella* species from colonized animals to humans is either by direct contact or **insect vectors** (e.g., *B. bacilliformis*—**sandflies;** *B. quintana*—**lice;** *B. henselae*—**fleas**). Most infections with *Bartonella* are characterized by **recurrent fevers** and/or **angioproliferative lesions** (blood-filled cysts).

B. bacilliformis, the original member of the genus, is responsible for **Carrión disease,** an acute hemolytic bacteremia consisting of fevers and severe anemia **(Oroya fever)** followed by the development of chronic vasoproliferative nodules (**verruga peruana,** "Peruvian wart"). The disease is restricted to the Andes mountain regions of Peru, Ecuador, and Colombia, the endemic area of the sandfly vector *Phlebotomus.* After the bite of an infected sandfly, the bacteria enter the blood, multiply, and penetrate into erythrocytes and endothelial cells. This process increases the fragility of the infected cells and facilitates their clearance by the reticuloendothelial system, leading to acute anemia. Myalgia, arthralgia, and headache are also common. This stage of illness ends with the development of humoral immunity. In the chronic stage of Carrión disease, 1- to 2-cm cutaneous nodules, often engorged with blood ("angioproliferative"), appear over the course of 1 to 2 months and may persist for months to years. The link between verruga peruana skin lesions and Oroya fever was demonstrated by a medical student, Carrión, who infected himself with aspirates from the skin lesions and died of Oroya fever. This act of scientific recklessness immortalized him and illustrates the high mortality associated with this disease if untreated, so it is recommended that *B. bacilliformis* infections should be treated with chloramphenicol or ciprofloxacin.

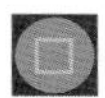
Box 29-1 Clinical Summaries

Bartonella bacilliformis

Carrión disease: febrile disease characterized by acute hemolytic bacteremia (Oroya fever) followed by the development of chronic cutaneous blood-filled nodules (verruga peruana)

Bartonella quintana

Trench fever: disease characterized by severe headache, fever, weakness, and pain in the long bones; the fever recurs at 5-day intervals

Chronic bacteremia: malaise, myalgias, fatigue, weight loss, headaches, and recurrent fevers in immunocompromised patients

Subacute endocarditis: mild but progressive infection of the endocardium

Bacillary angiomatosis: vascular proliferative disease in immunocompromised patients with blood-filled nodules involving the skin, subcutaneous tissues, and bones

Bartonella henselae

Bacillary angiomatosis: same as above, except primarily involving the skin, lymph nodes, or liver and spleen

Subacute endocarditis: same as above

Cat-scratch disease: chronic regional lymphadenopathy associated with cat scratch

Bordetella pertussis

Pertussis: after a 7- to 10-day incubation period, disease is characterized by the catarrhal stage (resembles the common cold), progressing to the paroxysmal stage (repetitive coughs followed by inspiratory whoops), then the convalescence stage (diminishing paroxysms and secondary complication)

Bordetella parapertussis: produces a milder form of pertussis

Bordetella bronchiseptica: primarily a respiratory disease of animals but can cause bronchopneumonia in humans

Bordetella holmesii: uncommon cause of sepsis

Brucella

Brucellosis: initial nonspecific symptoms of malaise, chills, sweats, fatigue, myalgias, weight loss, arthralgias, and fever; can be intermittent (undulant fever); can progress to systemic involvement (gastrointestinal tract, bones or joints, respiratory tract, other organs)

Brucella melitensis: severe, acute systemic disease, with complications common

Brucella abortus: mild disease with suppurative complications

Brucella suis: chronic, suppurative, destructive disease

Brucella canis: mild disease with suppurative complications

Cardiobacterium hominis

Subacute endocarditis: same as above

Francisella tularensis

Ulceroglandular tularemia: painful papule develops at the site of inoculation that progresses to ulceration; localized lymphadenopathy

Oculoglandular tularemia: after inoculation into the eye (e.g., rubbing eye with a contaminated finger), painful conjunctivitis develops, with regional lymphadenopathy

Pneumonic tularemia: pneumonitis with signs of sepsis develops rapidly after exposure to contaminated aerosols; high mortality unless promptly diagnosed and treated

Legionella pneumophila

Pontiac fever: self-limited febrile disease with chills, myalgias, malaise, and headache but no evidence of pneumonia

Legionnaires disease: severe pneumonia with acute onset of fever, chills, nonproductive cough, and headache progressing to multilobar consolidation of the lungs and multiorgan failure

Streptobacillus moniliformis

Rat-bite fever: irregular fever, headache, chills, myalgia, and arthralgia associated with rodent bite; pharyngitis and vomiting associated with exposure to bacteria in food or water

 Table 29-1 **Important Miscellaneous Gram-Negative Rods**

Organism	Historical Derivation
Bartonella	Named after Barton, who originally described *B. bacilliformis*
B. bacilliformis	*bacillus,* rod; *forma,* shape (rod shaped)
B. henselae	*hensel,* named after D.M. Hensel, who worked with this organism
B. quintana	*quintana,* fifth (refers to 5-day fever)
Bordetella	Named after Jules Bordet, who first isolated the organism responsible for pertussis
B. pertussis	*per,* very or severe; *tussis,* cough (a severe cough)
B. parapertussis	*para,* resembling (resembling pertussis)
B. bronchiseptica	*bronchus,* the trachea; *septicus,* septic (an infected bronchus)
B. holmesii	Named after the microbiologist Barry Holmes
Brucella	Named after Sir David Bruce, who first recognized the organism as a cause of "undulant fever"
B. abortus	*abortus,* abortion or miscarriage (this organism is responsible for abortion in infected animals)
B. melitensis	*melitensis,* pertaining to the Island of Malta (Melita), where the first outbreak was recognized by Bruce
B. suis	*suis,* of the pig (a swine pathogen)
B. canis	*canis,* of the dog (a dog pathogen)
Cardiobacterium hominis	*cardia,* heart; *bakterion,* small rod; *hominis,* of man (small rod of the hearts of men; refers to the predilection of this bacterium to cause endocarditis in humans)
Francisella	Named after the American microbiologist Edward Francis, who first described tularemia
F. tularensis subsp. *tularensis* (type A)	*tularensis,* pertaining to Tulare County, California, where the disease was first described
F. tularensis subsp. *holarctica* (type B)	*holos,* whole; *arctos,* northern regions (reference to distribution in the arctic or northern regions)
F. tularensis subsp. *mediaasiatica*	*media,* middle; *asiatica,* Asian (pertaining to middle Asia)
F. tularensis subsp. *novicida*	*novus,* new; *cida,* to cut (a "new killer")
F. philomiragia	*philos,* loving; *miragia,* mirage ("loving of mirages," reference to presence in water)
Legionella pneumophila	*Legionella,* first recognized outbreak was at an American Legion convention; *pneumôn,* lung; *phila,* loving; *pneumophila,* lung-loving.
Streptobacillus moniliformis	*streptos,* twisted or curved; *bacillus,* rod; *monile,* necklace; *forma,* shape (twisted, necklace-shaped bacillus; refers to the pleomorphic morphology of the bacteria)

Bartonella quintana was originally described as the causative organism of **trench fever** (also called **"5-day" fever**), a disease prevalent during World War I. Infection can vary from asymptomatic to a severe, debilitating illness. Typically, patients have severe headache, fever, weakness, and pain in the long bones (particularly the tibia). The fever can recur at 5-day intervals, hence the name of the disease. Although trench fever does not cause death, the illness can be very severe. No animal reservoir for this disease has been identified; rather, exposure to contaminated feces of the **human body louse** spreads disease from person to person. *B. quintana* is also associated with disease in immunocompromised patients, particularly patients infected with the human immunodeficiency virus (HIV): **recurrent fevers with bacteremia** (Clinical Case 29-1) and **bacillary angiomatosis.** Bacteremia is characterized by an insidious onset of malaise, body aches, fatigue, weight loss, headaches, and recurrent fevers. This can lead to endocarditis or more commonly vascular proliferative diseases of the skin (bacillary angiomatosis; Figure 29-1), subcutaneous tissues, or bone. The vascular

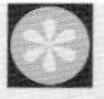 Clinical Case 29-1 **Fever and Bacteremia Caused by *Bartonella***

Slater and associates (*N Engl J Med* 3323:1587–1593, 1990) described the first *Bartonella henselae* infection in an HIV-infected patient. A 31-year-old man with advanced HIV infection presented with high fevers, chills, sweats, and weight loss. Blood cultures were negative after 2 days of incubation, and despite an initial response to oral antibiotic therapy, the fevers returned after 2 weeks. The patient was pancytopenic and had elevated liver enzyme levels. Hepatomegaly was the only abnormality detected by computed tomography. All diagnostic tests were negative until after more than 2 weeks of incubation; gram-negative rods were recovered from the blood cultures. Subsequent studies characterized this as a newly discovered organism and named it *B. henselae.* The patient was treated with parenteral erythromycin and, despite recurrent fevers, subsequently became culture negative. This patient illustrates the susceptibility of HIV patients to this organism and the insidious onset and prolonged course of the disease.

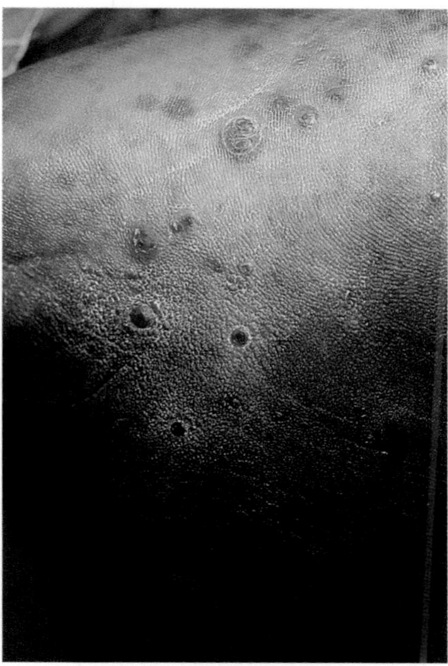

FIGURE 29-1 Skin lesions of bacillary angiomatosis caused by *Bartonella henselae.* (From Cohen J, Powderly WG: *Infectious diseases,* ed 2, St Louis, 2004, Mosby.)

lesions appear as multiple blood-filled nodules (resembling verruga peruana). As with trench fever, the vector of these diseases appears to be the human body louse, and disease is primarily restricted to the homeless population, in whom personal hygiene is substandard. Oral erythromycin, doxycycline, or azithromycin is most commonly used for treatment of *B. quintana* infections.

B. henselae is also responsible for bacillary angiomatosis; however, it primarily involves the skin, lymph nodes, liver **(peliosis hepatis),** or spleen **(splenic peliosis).** The reasons for this differential tissue affinity are not known. Also like *B. quintana, B. henselae* can cause subacute endocarditis. The reservoirs for *B. henselae* are cats and their fleas. The bacteria are carried asymptomatically in the feline oropharynx and can cause transient bacteremia, particularly in young or feral cats. *B. henselae* is responsible for another disease acquired after exposure to cats (e.g., scratches, bites, contact with the contaminated feces of cat fleas): **cat-scratch disease.** Typically, cat-scratch disease is a benign infection in children, characterized by **chronic regional adenopathy** of the lymph nodes draining the site of contact. Although most infections are self-limited, dissemination can occur to the liver, spleen, eye, or central nervous system. Bacteria may be seen in the lymph node tissues; however, culture is virtually always negative. A definitive diagnosis is based on the characteristic presentation and serologic evidence of a recent infection. Cultures are not useful because relatively few organisms are present in the tissues as a result of the vigorous cellular immune reaction in immunocompetent patients. In contrast, *B. henselae* can be isolated from blood collected from immunocompromised patients with chronic bacteremia if the cultures are incubated for 4 weeks or more (Figure 29-2).

The effectiveness of treating cat-scratch disease with antibiotics has not been demonstrated, although azithromycin is recommended if treatment is used. Oral erythromycin, doxycycline, or azithromycin is used for treatment of other *B. henselae* infections. Penicillinase-resistant penicillins, first-generation cephalosporins, and clindamycin do not appear active in vitro against *Bartonella.* The incidence of *Bartonella* infections in HIV-infected patients has declined in recent years because these patients are treated routinely with azithromycin or clarithromycin for prevention of *Mycobacterium avium* infections.

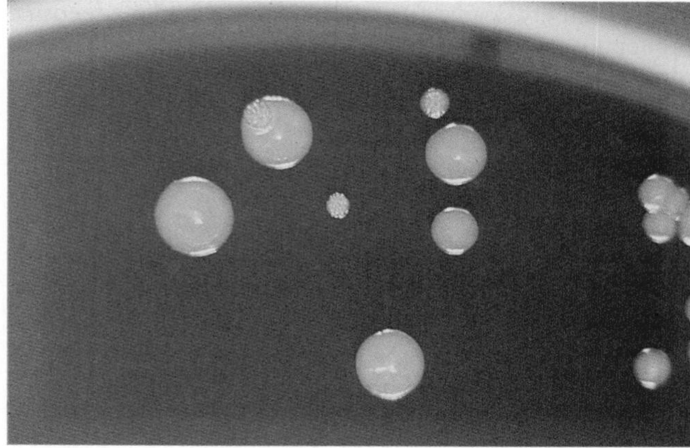

FIGURE 29-2 *Bartonella henselae* growing on blood agar plates; note the two typical colonial morphologies. (From Cohen J, Powderly WG: *Infectious diseases,* ed 2, St Louis, 2004, Mosby.)

Bordetella

Bordetella is an extremely **small** (0.2 to 0.5 × 1 μm), **strictly aerobic, gram-negative coccobacillus.** Eight species are currently recognized, with four species responsible for human disease (see Box 29-1): ***Bordetella pertussis,*** the agent responsible for pertussis or whooping cough; ***Bordetella parapertussis,*** responsible for a milder form of pertussis; ***Bordetella bronchiseptica,*** responsible for respiratory disease in dogs, swine, laboratory animals, and occasionally humans; and ***Bordetella holmesii,*** an uncommon cause of sepsis. *Bordetella* species are differentiated on the basis of their growth characteristics, biochemical reactivity, and antigenic properties. Despite phenotypic differences, genetic studies have shown that the four species pathogenic for humans are closely related or identical species, differing only in the expression of virulence genes.

Infection with *B. pertussis* and the development of whooping cough require exposure to the organism, bacterial attachment to the ciliated epithelial cells of the respiratory tract, proliferation of the bacteria, and production of localized tissue damage and systemic toxicity. Attachment of the organisms to ciliated epithelial cells is mediated by protein adhesins: **pertactin, filamentous hemagglutinin,** and **fimbria.** Similar proteins are also found in *B. parapertussis* and *B. bronchiseptica.* Localized tissue damage is mediated by **dermonecrotic toxin** (produces localized ischemia in mouse model) and **tracheal cytotoxin** (inhibits cilia movement, disrupting normal clearance mechanisms in the respiratory tree leading to the characteristic pertussis cough). Systemic toxicity is produced primarily by **pertussis toxin.** This toxin inactivates the protein that controls adenylate cyclase activity, leading to an increase in cyclic adenosine monophosphate (cAMP) levels and a subsequent increase in respiratory secretions and mucus production, characteristic of the paroxysmal stage of pertussis.

Pertussis is a **human disease** with no other recognized animal or environmental reservoir. Although the incidence of pertussis, with its associated morbidity and mortality, was reduced considerably after the introduction of vaccines in 1949, the disease is still endemic worldwide, with an estimated 16 million infections and 200,000 deaths each year, primarily in unvaccinated children. The incidence of reported disease in the United States has steadily increased over the last 25 years, with more than 48,000 cases reported in 2012; however, this is an underestimation of the true incidence of disease. Historically, pertussis was considered a pediatric disease, but now a significant proportion of infections are found in **adolescents and adults** (Clinical Case 29-2). The recognition of milder forms of disease in older children and adults and improved diagnostic tests have contributed to the increase in reported disease.

Infection is initiated when infectious aerosols are inhaled and the bacteria become attached to and proliferate on ciliated epithelial cells. After a 7- to 10-day incubation period, the classical presentation of pertussis proceeds through three stages (Figure 29-3). The first stage, the **catarrhal stage,** resembles a common cold, with serous rhinorrhea, sneezing, malaise, anorexia, and low-grade fever. Because the peak number of bacteria is produced during this stage and the cause of the disease is not yet recognized, patients in the catarrhal stage pose the highest risk to their contacts. After 1 to 2 weeks, the **paroxysmal stage** begins. During this time, ciliated epithelial cells are extruded from the respiratory tract, and the clearance of mucus is impaired. This stage is characterized by the **classic whooping cough paroxysms** (i.e., a series of repetitive coughs followed by an inspiratory whoop). Mucus production in the respiratory tract is common and is partially responsible for causing airway restriction. The paroxysms are frequently terminated with vomiting and exhaustion. A marked lymphocytosis is also prominent during this stage. Affected patients may experience as many as 40 to 50 paroxysms daily during the height of the illness. After 2 to 4 weeks, the disease enters the **convalescent stage;** at this time, the paroxysms diminish in number and severity, but secondary complications can occur. It is now appreciated that this classic presentation of pertussis may not be seen in patients with partial immunity or in adults. Such patients may have a history of a chronic persistent cough without whooping or vomiting. Because this presentation is not distinctive, appropriate diagnostic tests should be performed for *Bordetella* as well as other bacterial (e.g., *Mycoplasma pneumoniae, Chlamydophila pneumoniae, Legionella pneumophila*) and viral respiratory pathogens.

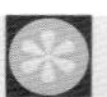

Clinical Case 29-2 Pertussis Outbreak in Health Care Workers

Pascual and associates (*Infect Control Hosp Epidemiol* 27:546–552, 2006) reported an outbreak of pertussis among hospital workers. The index case, a nurse anesthetist, presented acutely with coughing paroxysms followed by vomiting and apneic episodes that led to loss of consciousness. Surgical service personnel and exposed patients and family members were surveyed, with cultures, polymerase chain reaction testing, and serology obtained from patients with respiratory symptoms. Twelve (23%) health care workers and 0 of 146 patients had clinical pertussis. The lack of disease in patients was attributed to mask use, cough etiquette, and limited face-to-face contact. This outbreak emphasizes the susceptibility of adults to infection and the highly infectious nature of *Bordetella pertussis.*

	Incubation	Catarrhal	Paroxysmal	Convalescent
Duration	7-10 days	1-2 weeks	2-4 weeks	3-4 weeks (or longer)
Symptoms	None	Rhinorrhea, malaise, fever, sneezing, anorexia	Repetitive cough with whoops, vomiting, leukocytosis	Diminished paroxysmal cough, development of secondary complications (pneumonia, seizures, encephalopathy)
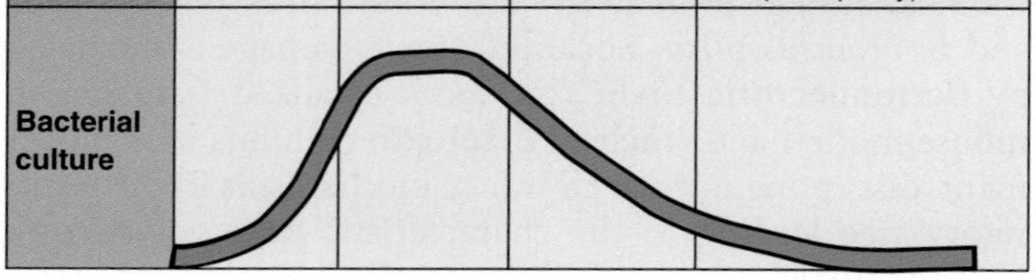 Bacterial culture				

FIGURE 29-3 Clinical presentation of *Bordetella pertussis* disease.

The laboratory diagnosis of *B. pertussis* infections has changed in recent years. The bacteria are extremely sensitive to drying and do not survive unless care is taken during collection and transport of the specimen to the laboratory. Although *Bordetella* species have simple nutritional requirements, some species are highly **susceptible to toxic substances and metabolites** present in common laboratory media. These species (particularly *B. pertussis*) require media supplemented with charcoal, starch, blood, or albumin to absorb these toxic substances. The more fastidious species also grow slowly in culture, and all require freshly prepared media. Even under ideal conditions, recovery of *B. pertussis* in culture is difficult. For these reasons, a number of nucleic acid amplification assays targeting a variety of genes have been developed. The performance characteristics of these assays (e.g., sensitivity, specificity) are superior to microscopy and culture. It is difficult to interpret the results of serologic tests because microscopy and culture techniques are relatively insensitive standards by which these tests have been evaluated. Enzyme-linked immunosorbent assay (ELISA) tests have been developed to detect antibodies against pertussis toxin, filamentous hemagglutinin, pertactin, and fimbriae.

Treatment for pertussis is primarily supportive, with nursing supervision during the paroxysmal and convalescent stages of the illness. Antibiotics can ameliorate the clinical course and reduce infectivity, particularly during the early stages of disease, but convalescence depends primarily on the rapidity and degree to which the layer of ciliated epithelial cells regenerates. **Macrolides** (i.e., erythromycin, azithromycin, clarithromycin) are effective in eradicating the organisms; however, this effect has limited value because the illness is usually unrecognized during the peak of contagiousness. Azithromycin and clarithromycin are generally better tolerated and the preferred macrolides.

Trimethoprim-sulfamethoxazole or fluoroquinolones can be used in patients unable to tolerate macrolides.

Two **acellular vaccines** (one for children, one for adults) administered in combination with vaccines for tetanus and diphtheria are currently approved in the United States. Both vaccines contain inactivated pertussis toxin, filamentous hemagglutinin, and pertactin. The pediatric vaccine is administered to children at the ages of 2, 4, 6, and 15 to 18 months, with the fifth dose between the ages of 4 and 6 years. The current recommendation for the adult vaccine is to administer it at 11 or 12 years of age, and then again between the ages of 19 and 65. Because pertussis is highly contagious in a susceptible population, and unrecognized infections in family members of a symptomatic patient can maintain disease in a community, azithromycin has been used for prophylaxis in select instances.

Other *Bordetella* Species

B. parapertussis is responsible for causing 10% to 20% of the cases of mild pertussis occurring annually in the United States. *B. bronchiseptica* causes respiratory disease primarily in animals but has been associated with human respiratory tract colonization and bronchopulmonary disease. Investigators at the Centers for Disease Control and Prevention (CDC) in Atlanta reported that *B. holmesii* is primarily associated with septicemia.

Brucella

Molecular studies of the genus *Brucella* demonstrate a close relationship among the strains and are consistent with a single species; however, the genus is subdivided into 10 species, with 4 species most commonly associated with human disease: ***Brucella abortus, Brucella melitensis, Brucella suis,*** and ***Brucella canis*** (see Box 29-1). The diseases caused by members of this genus are characterized by a number of names based on the original microbiologists who isolated and described the organisms (e.g., Sir David Bruce [**brucellosis**], Bernhard Bang [**Bang disease**]), their clinical presentation **(undulant fever)**, and the sites of recognized outbreaks (e.g., Malta fever, Mediterranean remittent fever, rock fever of Gibraltar, county fever of Constantinople, fever of Crete). The most commonly used term is *brucellosis.*

Brucellae are small (0.5 × 0.6 to 1.5 μm), nonmotile, nonencapsulated, gram-negative coccobacilli. The organism grows slowly in culture (taking a week or more) and generally requires complex growth media; is strictly aerobic, with some strains requiring supplemental carbon dioxide for growth; and does not ferment carbohydrates.

Colonies can assume both smooth (translucent, homogeneous) and rough (opaque, granular, or sticky) forms, as determined by the O antigen of the cell wall lipopolysaccharide (LPS). Antisera to one form (e.g., smooth) do not cross-react with the other form (e.g., rough).

Brucella does not produce a detectable exotoxin, and the endotoxin is less toxic than that produced by other gram-negative rods. Reversion of smooth strains to the rough morphology is associated with greatly reduced virulence, so the O chain of the smooth LPS is an important marker for virulence. *Brucella* is also an **intracellular parasite** of the **reticuloendothelial system.** After the initial exposure, the organisms are phagocytosed by macrophages and monocytes, where the bacteria survive and replicate. Phagocytosed bacteria are carried to the spleen, liver, bone marrow, lymph nodes, and kidneys. The bacteria secrete proteins that induce granuloma formation in these organs, and destructive changes in these and other tissues occur in patients with advanced disease.

Brucella infections have a **worldwide distribution,** with endemic disease most common in countries that do not have domestic animal vaccination programs, such as Latin America, Africa, the Mediterranean basin, the Middle East, and Western Asia. More than 500,000 documented cases are reported annually worldwide. In contrast, the incidence of disease in the United States is much lower (79 reported infections in 2011). The highest numbers of U.S. cases are reported in **California** and **Texas,** and most of these infections occur in residents from Mexico or visitors to that country. Laboratory personnel are also at significant risk for infection through direct contact or inhalation of the organism. Disease in cattle, swine, sheep, and goats in the United States has been eliminated effectively through the destruction of infected animals and the vaccination of disease-free animals.

Brucellosis in humans can be acquired by direct contact with the organism (e.g., a laboratory exposure), ingestion (e.g., consumption of contaminated food products), or inhalation. Of particular concern is the potential use of *Brucella* as a biological weapon, in which exposure would most likely be by inhalation.

Brucella causes mild or asymptomatic disease in the natural host: *B. abortus* infects cattle and American bison; *B. melitensis,* goats and sheep; *B. suis,* swine, reindeer, and caribou; and *B. canis,* dogs, foxes, and coyotes. The organism has a predilection for infecting organs rich in **erythritol,** a sugar metabolized by many *Brucella* strains in preference to glucose. Animal (but not human) tissues, including breast, uterus, placenta, and epididymis, are rich in erythritol. The organisms thus localize in these tissues in nonhuman reservoirs and can cause sterility, abortions, or asymptomatic lifelong carriage. Brucellae are shed in high numbers in milk, urine, and birth products. Human disease in the United States is most commonly caused by ***B. melitensis*** and results primarily from consumption of contaminated, unpasteurized milk and other **dairy products.**

Clinical Diseases

The disease spectrum of **brucellosis** (Clinical Case 29-3; see Box 29-1) depends on the infecting organism. *B. abortus* and

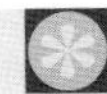

Clinical Case 29-3 Brucellosis

Lee and Fung (*Hong Kong Med J* 11:403–406, 2005) described a 34-year-old woman who developed brucellosis caused by *Brucella melitensis.* The woman presented with recurrent headaches, fever, and malaise that developed after she had handled goat placenta in China. Blood cultures were positive for *B. melitensis* after extended incubation. She was treated for 6 weeks with doxycycline and rifampicin and had a successful response. The case was a classical description of exposure to contaminated tissues high in erythritol, a presentation of recurrent fevers and headaches, and response to the combination of doxycycline and rifampicin.

B. canis tend to produce mild disease with rare suppurative complications. In contrast, *B. suis* causes the formation of destructive lesions and has a prolonged course. *B. melitensis* also causes severe disease with a high incidence of serious complications because the organisms can multiply to high concentrations in phagocytic cells.

Acute disease develops in approximately half of the patients infected with *Brucella,* with symptoms first appearing typically 1 to 3 weeks after exposure. Initial symptoms are nonspecific and consist of malaise, chills, sweats, fatigue, weakness, myalgias, weight loss, arthralgias, and nonproductive cough. Almost all patients have fever, and this can be intermittent in untreated patients, hence the name **undulant fever.** Patients with advanced disease can have gastrointestinal tract symptoms, osteolytic lesions or joint effusions, respiratory tract symptoms, and less commonly, cutaneous, neurologic, or cardiovascular manifestations. Chronic infections can also develop in inadequately treated patients, with symptoms developing within 3 to 6 months after discontinuing antibiotic therapy. Relapses are associated with a persistent focus on infections (e.g., in bone, spleen, liver) and not with the development of antibiotic resistance.

For the laboratory diagnosis of brucellosis, several blood samples should be collected for culture and serologic testing. Bone marrow cultures and cultures of infected tissues may also be useful. To ensure safe handling of the specimen, the laboratory should be notified if brucellosis is suspected. *Brucella* organisms are readily stained using conventional techniques, but their intracellular location and small size make them difficult to detect in clinical specimens. The organisms grow slowly in culture, requiring enriched blood agars and extended incubation (3 days or more). **Blood cultures should be incubated for 2 weeks** before they are considered negative. Preliminary identification of *Brucella* is based on the isolate's microscopic and colonial morphology, positive oxidase and urease reactions, and reactivity with specific antibodies. Identification at the genus level can also be accomplished by sequencing the 16S ribosomal ribonucleic acid (rRNA) gene. Subclinical brucellosis and many cases of acute and chronic diseases are identified by a specific antibody response in the infected patient. Antibodies are detected in virtually all patients and can persist for many months or years; thus a significant increase in the antibody titer is required to provide definitive serologic evidence of current disease. A **presumptive diagnosis** can be made if there is a fourfold increase in the titer or a single titer is 1:160 or greater.

Tetracyclines, with **doxycycline** the preferred agent, are generally active against most strains of *Brucella;* however, because this is a bacteriostatic drug, relapse is common after an initially successful response. The World Health Organization currently recommends the combination of **doxycycline with rifampin.** Because the tetracyclines are toxic to young children and fetuses, doxycycline should be replaced with trimethoprim-sulfamethoxazole for pregnant women and for children younger than 8 years. Treatment must be continued for 6 weeks or longer for it to be successful. Fluoroquinolones, macrolides, penicillins, and cephalosporins are either ineffective or have unpredictable activity. Relapse of disease is caused by inadequate therapy and not the development of antibiotic resistance.

Control of human brucellosis is accomplished through control of the disease in livestock, as demonstrated in the United States. This requires systematic identification (by serologic testing) and elimination of infected herds and **animal vaccination** (currently with the rough strain of *B. abortus* strain RB51). The avoidance of unpasteurized dairy products, the observance of appropriate safety procedures in the clinical laboratory, and the wearing of protective clothing by abattoir workers are further ways to prevent brucellosis. The live attenuated *B. abortus* and *B. melitensis* vaccines have been used successfully to prevent infection in animal herds. Vaccines have not been developed against *B. suis* or *B. canis,* and the existing vaccines cannot be used in humans because they produce symptomatic disease. Lack of an effective human vaccine is of concern because *Brucella* could be used as an agent of bioterrorism.

Cardiobacterium

Cardiobacterium hominis is named for the predilection of this bacterium to cause endocarditis in humans (see Box 29-1). These bacteria are nonmotile, facultatively anaerobic, and characteristically small (1 × 1 to 2 μm) pleomorphic gram-negative or gram-variable rods. The bacteria are fermentative, oxidase positive, and catalase negative. *C. hominis* is present in the upper respiratory tract of most healthy people.

Endocarditis is the primary human disease caused by *C. hominis* and the related species *Cardiobacterium valvarum* (Clinical Case 29-4). Many infections are likely to be unreported or undiagnosed because of the low virulence of this organism and its slow growth in vitro. Most patients with *Cardiobacterium* endocarditis have **preexisting heart disease** and either a history of oral disease or have undergone a dental procedure before the clinical symptoms developed. The organisms are able to enter the blood from the oropharynx, adhere to the damaged heart tissue, and then slowly multiply. The course of disease is insidious and subacute; patients typically have symptoms (e.g., fatigue, malaise, and low-grade fever) for months before seeking medical care.

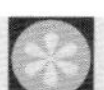

Clinical Case 29-4 *Cardiobacterium* Endocarditis

Hoover and associates (*Ann Intern Med* 142:229–230, 2005) described the first patient infected with *Cardiobacterium valvarum* (a newly described species in the genus *Cardiobacterium*). The patient was a 46-year-old man who, over the course of 1 month, developed anorexia and fatigue. The symptoms developed 2 weeks after a dental extraction. His physical examination was notable for fatigue, lower extremity edema, and a new heart murmur. Bilateral pleural effusions were revealed on chest radiography. All blood cultures collected over a 24-hour period were positive for a pleomorphic gram-negative rod that was subsequently identified as *C. valvarum.* Management of the patient involved replacement of the aortic valve with a prosthetic valve and 4 weeks of treatment with ceftriaxone. Follow-up visits with the patient documented complete recovery. This case illustrates the subacute presentation and generally successful outcome for patients with *Cardiobacterium* endocarditis. What is unique is that the patient did not have a history of previous heart disease, although it is likely to have been present.

Complications are rare, and complete recovery after appropriate antibiotic therapy is common.

The isolation of *C. hominis* from blood cultures confirms the diagnosis of endocarditis. The organism grows slowly in culture, requiring 1 week or more for growth to be detected. The organism requires enhanced carbon dioxide and humidity levels to grow on agar media, with 1-mm pinpoint colonies seen on blood or chocolate agar plates after 2 days of incubation. The organism does not grow on MacConkey agar or other selective media commonly used for gram-negative rods. *C. hominis* can be readily identified from its growth properties, microscopic morphology, and reactivity in biochemical tests.

C. hominis is susceptible to many antibiotics, and most infections are treated successfully with **penicillin or ampicillin** for 2 to 6 weeks, although penicillin-resistant strains have been reported. *C. hominis* endocarditis in people with preexisting heart disease is prevented by maintenance of good oral hygiene and use of antibiotic prophylaxis at the time of dental procedures. Long-acting penicillin is effective prophylaxis. Erythromycin should not be used, because *C. hominis* is commonly resistant to it.

Francisella

Francisella is an important **zoonotic pathogen** that can cause significant human disease. Three species of the genus *Francisella* are associated with human disease: *Francisella tularensis, Francisella novicida,* and *Francisella philomiragia.* *F. tularensis* (see Box 29-1) is the causative agent of **tularemia** (also called **glandular fever, rabbit fever, tick fever,** and **deerfly fever**) in animals and humans. *F. tularensis* is subdivided into three subspecies based on their biochemical properties. **Subspecies *tularensis* (type A)** and **subspecies *holarctica* (type B)** are the most important, whereas *F. tularensis* subsp. *mediaasiatica* is rarely associated with human disease. *F. novicida* and *F. philomiragia* are uncommon, opportunistic pathogens that have a predilection for patients with immunologic deficiencies (i.e., chronic granulomatous disease, myeloproliferative diseases).

F. tularensis is a **very small** (0.2 × 0.2 to 0.7 μm), faintly staining, gram-negative coccobacillus (Figure 29-4). The organism is nonmotile, has a thin lipid capsule, and has fastidious growth requirements (i.e., most strains **require cysteine** for growth). It is **strictly aerobic** and requires 3 or more days before growth is detected in culture.

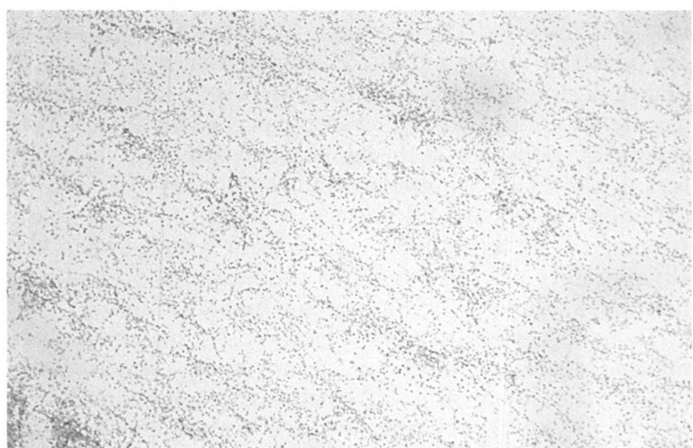

FIGURE 29-4 Gram stain of *Francisella tularensis* isolated in culture; note the extremely small, dotlike coccobacilli.

F. tularensis is an **intracellular pathogen** that can replicate in macrophages, neutrophils, epithelial cells, and endothelial cells. The organism inhibits phagosome-lysosome fusion through secretion of proteins that facilitate bacterial escape from the phagosome and subsequent replication in the cytosol. Pathogenic strains possess an antiphagocytic, **polysaccharide-rich capsule,** and loss of the capsule is associated with decreased virulence. The capsule protects the bacteria from complement-mediated killing during the bacteremia phase of disease. This organism has an endotoxin, but it is considerably less active than the endotoxin found in other gram-negative rods.

A strong, innate immune response with production of interferon (IFN)-γ and tumor necrosis factor is important for controlling bacterial replication in macrophages in the early phase of infection. Specific T-cell immunity is required for activation of macrophages for intracellular killing in the late stages of disease. B cell–mediated immunity is less important for elimination of this facultative intracellular pathogen.

F. tularensis subsp. *tularensis* (type A) is restricted to North America, whereas subsp. *holarctica* (type B) is endemic throughout the Northern Hemisphere. Type A strains are further subdivided into **type A–west,** which predominates in the arid region from the Rocky Mountains to the Sierra Nevada Mountains, and **type A–east,** which occurs in the central southeast states of Arkansas, Missouri, and Oklahoma and along the Atlantic Coast. **Type B** strains cluster along major waterways, such as the upper Mississippi River, and in areas with high rainfall, such as the Pacific Northwest. The distribution of these strains is important because the epidemiologic features of the individual diseases are distinct and the course of clinical disease is significantly different. The geographic distribution of type A–west, type A–east, and type B strains is defined by the distribution of the natural reservoirs and vectors of *F. tularensis.* More than 200 species of mammals, as well as birds and blood-sucking arthropods, are infected naturally with *F. tularensis.* Type A infections are most commonly associated with exposure to **lagomorphs** (rabbits, hares) and **cats;** type B infections are associated with **rodents** and cats, but not lagomorphs. Infections caused by **biting arthropods** (e.g., hard ticks [*Ixodes, Dermacentor, Amblyomma* spp.], deerflies) are more common with type A than with type B strains. The spread to type A–east strains from the central southeast states to the Atlantic Coast states occurred when infected rabbits were imported from the central states to East Coast hunting clubs in the 1920s and 1930s. Type A–east infections are more commonly associated with disseminated disease and a high mortality rate when compared with disease caused by type A–west strains; the course of disease caused by type B stains is intermediate.

The reported incidence of disease is low. In 2012, 149 cases were reported in the United States; however, the actual number of infections is likely to be much higher because tularemia is frequently unsuspected and is difficult to confirm by laboratory tests. Most of the infections occur during the summer (when exposure to infected ticks is greatest). The incidence of disease increases dramatically when a relatively

Clinical Case 29-5 Cat-Associated Tularemia

Capellan and Fong (*Clin Infect Dis* 16:472–475, 1993) described a 63-year-old man who developed ulceroglandular tularemia complicated by pneumonia after a cat bite. He initially presented with pain and localized swelling of his thumb 5 days after the bite. Oral penicillins were prescribed, but the patient's condition worsened, with increased local pain, swelling and erythema at the wound site, and systemic signs (fever, malaise, vomiting). Incision of the wound was performed, but no abscess was found; culture of the wound was positive for a light growth of coagulase-negative staphylococci. Intravenous penicillins were prescribed, but the patient continued to deteriorate, with the development of tender axillary lymphadenopathy and pulmonary symptoms. A chest radiograph revealed pneumonic infiltrates in the right middle and lower lobes of the lung. The patient's therapy was changed to clindamycin and gentamicin, which was followed by defervescence and improvement of his clinical status. After 3 days of incubation, tiny colonies of faintly staining gram-negative coccobacilli were observed on the original wound culture. The organism was referred to a national reference laboratory, where it was identified as *Francisella tularensis*. A more complete history revealed the patient's cat lived outdoors and fed on wild rodents. This case illustrates the difficulty in making the diagnosis of tularemia and the lack of responsiveness to penicillins.

warm winter is followed by a wet summer, causing the tick population to proliferate. People at greatest risk for infection are hunters, laboratory personnel, and those exposed to ticks and other biting arthropods. In areas where the organism is endemic, it is said that if a rabbit is moving so slowly that it can be shot by a hunter or caught by a pet, the rabbit could be infected (Clinical Case 29-5).

Disease caused by *F. tularensis* is subdivided into several forms based on the clinical presentation: **ulceroglandular** (cutaneous ulcer and swollen lymph node), **oculoglandular** (eye involvement and swollen cervical lymph nodes), **glandular** (primarily swollen lymph nodes with no other localized symptoms), **typhoidal** (systemic signs of sepsis), **pneumonic** (pulmonary symptoms), and **oropharyngeal** and **gastrointestinal** disease after ingestion of *F. tularensis*. Variations of these presentations are also common (e.g., pneumonic tularemia typically has systemic signs of sepsis).

Ulceroglandular tularemia is the most common manifestation. The skin lesion, which starts as a painful papule, develops at the site of the tick bite or direct inoculation of the organism into the skin (e.g., a laboratory accident). The papule then ulcerates and has a necrotic center and raised border. Localized lymphadenopathy and bacteremia are also typically present (although bacteremia may be difficult to document).

Oculoglandular tularemia (Figure 29-5) is a specialized form of the disease and results from direct contamination of the eye. The organism can be introduced into the eyes, for example, by contaminated fingers or through exposure to water or aerosols. Affected patients have a painful conjunctivitis and regional lymphadenopathy.

Pneumonic tularemia (Figure 29-6) results from inhalation of infectious aerosols and is associated with high morbidity and mortality unless the organism is recovered rapidly in blood cultures (it is generally difficult to detect in respiratory cultures). There is also concern that *F. tularensis* could be used as a biological weapon. As such, creation of an infectious aerosol would be the most likely method of dispersal.

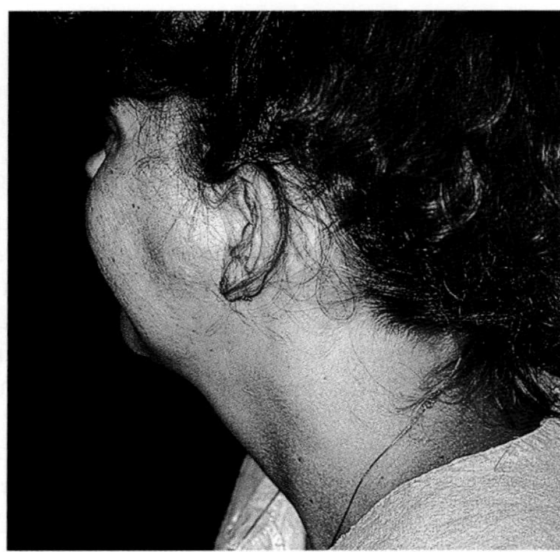

FIGURE 29-5 Patient with oculoglandular tularemia (note swelling beside the ear).

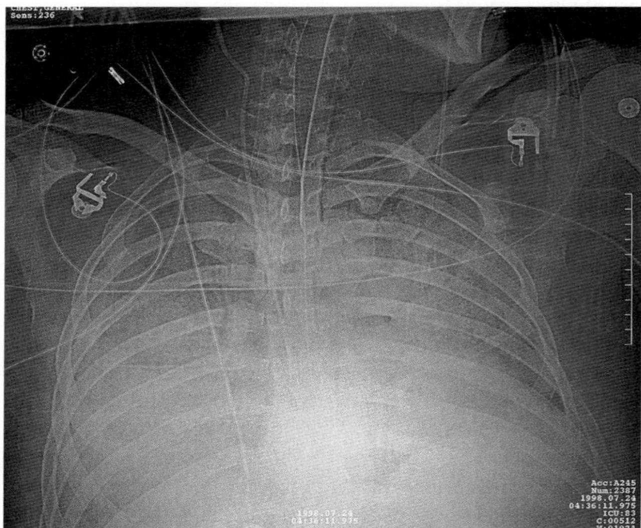

FIGURE 29-6 Chest radiograph of patient with pulmonary tularemia.

Collection and processing of specimens for the isolation of *F. tularensis* are hazardous for both the physician and the laboratory worker. The organism, by virtue of its small size, can penetrate through unbroken skin and the mucous membranes during collection of the sample, or it can be inhaled if aerosols are produced (a particular concern during processing of specimens in the laboratory). Although tularemia is rare, laboratory-acquired infections are disproportionately common. Gloves should be worn during collection of the specimen (e.g., aspiration of an ulcer or lymph node), and all laboratory work (both initial processing and identification tests) should be performed in a biohazard hood.

Detection of *F. tularensis* in Gram-stained aspirates from infected nodes or ulcers is almost always **unsuccessful** because the organism is extremely small and stains faintly (see Figure 29-4). Polymerase chain reaction (PCR)-based assays are not widely available at this time, although this may change with the increased interest in the development of diagnostic tests for this organism in the event of a bioterrorist attack. It has been stated that *F. tularensis* cannot be reliably recovered on common laboratory media because the organism requires sulfhydryl-containing substances (e.g., **cysteine**) for growth. However, *F. tularensis* can grow on **chocolate agar** or **buffered charcoal yeast extract (BCYE)** agar, media supplemented with cysteine that are used in most laboratories. If infection with *F. tularensis* is suspected, the laboratory should be notified because *F. tularensis* grows slowly and may be overlooked if the cultures are not incubated for a prolonged period. In addition, because this organism is highly infectious, special care is required for microbiological testing. Blood cultures are generally negative for the organism unless the cultures are incubated for a week or longer. Cultures of respiratory specimens will be positive if appropriate selective media are used to suppress the more rapidly growing bacteria from the upper respiratory tract. *F. tularensis* also grows on the selective media used for *Legionella* (e.g., BCYE agar). Aspirates of lymph nodes or draining sinuses are usually positive if the cultures are incubated for 3 days or longer.

Preliminary identification of *F. tularensis* is based on the slow growth of very small gram-negative coccobacilli on chocolate agar but not blood agar (blood agar is not supplemented with cysteine). The identification is confirmed by demonstrating the reactivity of the bacteria with specific antiserum (i.e., agglutination of the organism with antibodies against *Francisella*).

Tularemia is diagnosed in most patients by the finding of a fourfold or greater increase in the titer of antibodies during the illness or a single titer of 1:160 or greater. However, antibodies (including immunoglobulin [Ig]G, IgM, and IgA) can persist for many years, making it difficult to differentiate between past and current disease.

Gentamicin is considered the antibiotic of choice. Doxycycline and ciprofloxacin can be used to treat mild infections. *F. tularensis* strains produce β-lactamase, which renders penicillins and cephalosporins ineffective. The mortality rate is less than 1% if patients are treated promptly but is much higher in untreated patients, particularly those infected with type A–east strains.

To prevent infection, people should avoid the reservoirs and vectors of infection (e.g., rabbits, ticks, biting insects), but this is often difficult. At a minimum, people should not handle ill-appearing rabbits and should wear gloves when skinning and eviscerating animals. Because the organism is present in the arthropod's feces and not saliva, the tick must feed for a prolonged time before the infection is transmitted. Prompt removal of the tick can therefore prevent infection. Wearing protective clothing and using insect repellents reduce the risk of exposure. Persons who have a high-risk exposure (e.g., exposure to an infectious aerosol) should be treated with prophylactic antibiotics. Interest in developing a live attenuated vaccine is motivated by fear of exposure to the bacteria as a bioterrorism agent; however, an effective vaccine is not currently available. Inactivated vaccines do not elicit protective cellular immunity.

Legionella

In the summer of 1976, public attention was focused on an outbreak of severe pneumonia that caused many deaths among American Legion members attending a convention in Philadelphia. After months of intensive investigations, a previously unknown gram-negative rod was isolated. Subsequent studies found this organism, named ***Legionella pneumophila,*** to be the cause of multiple epidemics and sporadic infections. The organism was not previously recognized because it stains poorly with conventional dyes and does not grow on common laboratory media. Despite initial problems with the isolation of *Legionella* organisms, it is now known to be a ubiquitous aquatic saprophyte.

The family Legionellaceae consists of four genera: *Legionella, Fluoribacter, Tatlockia,* and *Sarcobium. Legionella* is the most important genus, with 58 species and 3 subspecies. Approximately half of these species have been implicated in human disease, with the others found in environmental sources. *L. pneumophila* is the cause of 90% of all infections; serotypes 1 and 6 are most commonly isolated. *Fluoribacter* consists of 3 species, *Tatlockia* contains 2 species and *Sarcobium* has 1 species. *Fluoribacter bozemanae* and *Tatlockia micdadei*, formerly members of the genus *Legionella,* cause disease similar to *L. pneumophila* and are commonly referred to in the literature by their historical names.

Members of the genus *Legionella* are **slender, pleomorphic, gram-negative rods** measuring 0.3 to 0.9 × 2 μm in size. The organisms characteristically appear as short coccobacilli when observed in tissue but are very pleomorphic (up to 20 μm long) on artificial media (Figure 29-7). Legionellae in clinical specimens do not stain with common reagents but can be seen in tissues stained with Dieterle silver stain. One species, *T. micdadei,* can also be stained with acid-fast stains, but the organism loses this property when grown in vitro.

Legionellae are obligatively aerobic and nutritionally fastidious. They require media supplemented with L-cysteine, and growth is enhanced by iron. Growth of these bacteria on supplemented media but not on conventional blood agar media has been used as the basis for the preliminary identification of clinical isolates. The bacteria have developed multiple methods to acquire iron from their host cells or in vitro media, and loss of this ability is associated with loss of virulence. The organisms derive energy from the metabolism of amino acids but not carbohydrates.

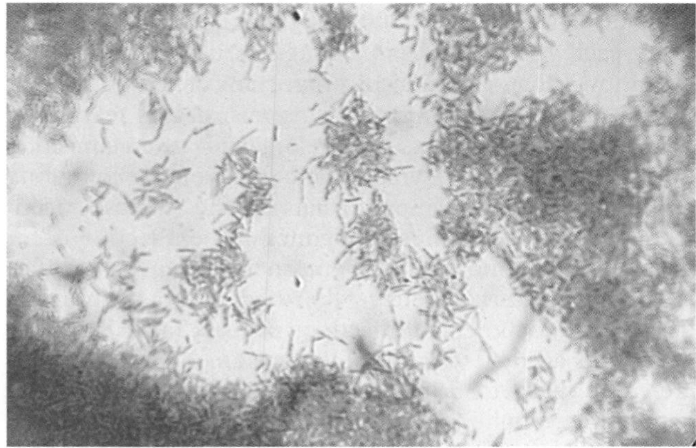

FIGURE 29-7 Gram stain of *Legionella pneumophila* grown on buffered charcoal yeast extract agar. Note the pleomorphic forms characteristic of *Legionella.* (Courtesy Dr. Janet Stout, Pittsburgh, Penn.)

Respiratory tract disease caused by *Legionella* species develops in susceptible people who inhale infectious aerosols. Legionellae are facultative **intracellular bacteria** that multiply in free-living amebae in nature, and in alveolar macrophages, monocytes, and alveolar epithelial cells in infected hosts. This ability to infect and replicate in macrophages is mediated by first binding complement component C3b to an outer membrane porin protein on the bacterial surface and then binding to the CR3 complement receptor on the mononuclear phagocyte surface. The organisms then penetrate the cell through endocytosis and initiate replication. The bacteria are not killed in the cells by exposure to toxic superoxide, hydrogen peroxide, and hydroxyl radicals, because phagolysosome fusion is inhibited. Chemokines and cytokines released by the infected macrophages stimulate a robust inflammatory response that is characteristic of infections with *Legionella*. The organisms proliferate in their intracellular vacuole and produce proteolytic enzymes (phosphatase, lipase, and nuclease) that eventually kill the host cell when the vacuole is lysed. Immunity to disease is primarily cell mediated, with humoral immunity playing a minor role. The bacteria are not killed until sensitized helper T cells (TH1 cells) activate the parasitized macrophages. Production of IFN-γ is critical for elimination of *Legionella* organisms.

Legionellae have a **worldwide distribution,** commonly present in natural bodies of water such as lakes and streams, as well as in air conditioning cooling towers and condensers and in water systems (e.g., showers, hot tubs). Human infections are most commonly associated with **exposure to contaminated aerosols** (e.g., air conditioning cooling towers, whirlpool spas, showerheads, water misters). The organisms can survive in moist environments for a long time, at relatively high temperatures, and in the presence of disinfectants such as chlorine. One reason for their survival is that the bacteria parasitize amebae in the water and replicate in this protected environment (similar to their replication in human macrophages). The bacteria also survive in biofilms that develop in the pipes of water systems.

The incidence of infections caused by *Legionella* species is unknown because disease is difficult to document. The number of reported cases has steadily risen since 2000, with more than 4200 cases reported in 2011. However, the CDC estimates that up to 18,000 cases of legionnaires disease occur each year in the United States. Serologic studies have also shown that a significant proportion of the population has acquired immunity to these organisms. It is reasonable to conclude that contact with the organism and acquisition of immunity after an asymptomatic infection are common.

Although sporadic outbreaks of the disease occur throughout the year, most epidemics of the infection occur in late summer and autumn because the organism proliferates in water reservoirs during the warm months. More than 90% of the documented infections in the United States are in persons aged 40 years or older, presumably because they are more likely to have decreased cellular immunity and compromised pulmonary function. A significant proportion of reported cases are acquired in hospitals because of the predominance of high-risk patients. Person-to-person spread or an animal reservoir has not been demonstrated.

Asymptomatic *Legionella* infections are believed to be relatively common. Symptomatic infections primarily affect the lungs and present in one of two forms (see Box 29-1): (1) an influenza-like illness (referred to as **Pontiac fever**) and (2) a severe form of pneumonia (i.e., **legionnaires disease**).

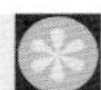

Clinical Case 29-6 Outbreak of Legionnaires Disease

Kirrage and associates (*Respir Med* 101:1639–1644, 2007) described an outbreak of legionnaires disease (LD) that occurred in Hereford, England. On October 24, 2003, the public health agency was notified that an elderly man had died of LD. Three days later, the agency was notified that an elderly woman had also died of LD. As part of an active surveillance investigation, two additional patients with positive *Legionella* urine antigen tests were identified in a local hospital. Further investigations revealed 28 epidemiologically linked patients with the onset of disease from October 8 to November 20. All patients had positive urine antigen tests, four had high antibody titers, and two were culture positive. The implicated source of the outbreak was a cooling tower that had recently been restarted after a period of inactivity. After the tower was closed and recleaned, the epidemic was terminated. This outbreak illustrates the difficulty of recognizing the problem when the individuals infected may present to different hospitals. This is particularly a problem when the source is located in a hotel or vacation place.

L. pneumophila was responsible for causing a self-limited, febrile illness in people working at the Pontiac, Michigan, Public Health Department in 1968. Fever, chills, myalgia, malaise, and headache, but no clinical evidence of pneumonia, are characteristic of the disease. The symptoms developed over 12 hours, persisted for 2 to 5 days, and then resolved spontaneously without antibiotic treatment and with minimal morbidity and no deaths. Other outbreaks of Pontiac fever, with and without *Legionella* pneumonia, have been reported. The precise pathogenesis of this syndrome is unknown, although it is believed that this disease is caused by a hypersensitivity reaction to bacterial toxin (e.g., endotoxin).

Legionnaires disease (legionellosis; Clinical Case 29-6) is characteristically more severe and, if untreated, promptly causes considerable morbidity, often leading to death in 15% of previously healthy individuals and up to 75% of immunocompromised patients. After an incubation period of 2 to 10 days, systemic signs of an acute illness appear abruptly (e.g., fever and chills, a dry, nonproductive cough, headache). Multiorgan disease involving the gastrointestinal tract, central nervous system, liver, and kidneys is common. The primary manifestation is pneumonia, with multilobar consolidation and inflammation and microabscesses in lung tissue observed on histopathologic studies. Pulmonary function steadily deteriorates in susceptible patients with untreated disease. The clinical presentation of pneumonia caused by *Legionella* is not unique, so laboratory tests are required to confirm the diagnosis.

Since *Legionella* was first isolated, the laboratory diagnosis of infections caused by this organism has undergone a significant transition. Initial testing depended on microscopy, culture, and serology. Although culture remains the gold standard for diagnosis, microscopy and serology have been replaced by immunoassays for the detection of *Legionella*-specific antigens in urine, and nucleic acid amplification assays have replaced microscopy and serology. The bacteria stain poorly with Gram stain and are rarely observed in clinical specimens; serology is insensitive and nonspecific.

Immunoassays are used to detect soluble ***Legionella*** **serogroup 1–specific lipopolysaccharide antigens** excreted in the urine of infected patients. The sensitivity of these assays for *L. pneumophila* serogroup 1 is relatively high (up to 90%), particularly with concentrated urines, but the assays do not reliably detect other serogroups or *Legionella* species. This is an important distinction because *L. pneumophila* serogroup 1 is responsible for 80% to 90% of community-acquired infections but is responsible for less than 50% of hospital-acquired infections. Antigens persist in the urine of treated patients, with almost 50% of patients remaining positive at 1 month and 25% at 2 months. Persistence is particularly common with immunosuppressed patients, in which antigens can persist for up to 1 year.

Nucleic acid amplification assays are highly specific and have a sensitivity equivalent to culture for detection of *Legionella* species in respiratory secretions (i.e., bronchial alveolar lavage fluid). The presence of inhibitors in respiratory secretions may cause false-negative reactions, so all specimens should still be cultured.

Although legionellae were difficult to grow initially, commercially available media now make culture easy (test sensitivity, 80% to > 90%). As mentioned, legionellae require L-cysteine, and recovery is enhanced in the presence of iron salts (supplied in hemoglobin or ferric pyrophosphate). The medium most commonly used for the isolation of legionellae is **buffered charcoal yeast extract (BCYE) agar,** although other supplemented media have been used. Antibiotics can be added to suppress the growth of rapidly growing, contaminating bacteria. Legionellae grow in air or 3% to 5% carbon dioxide at 35° C after 3 to 5 days. The small (1 to 3 mm) colonies have a characteristic ground-glass appearance.

It is easy to identify an isolate as *Legionella* from the findings of typical morphology and specific growth requirements. Legionellae appear as weakly staining, pleomorphic, thin, gram-negative rods. Their growth on BCYE agar, but not on media without L-cysteine, is presumptive evidence that the organism is *Legionella.* In contrast to identification of the genus, species classification is problematic and generally relegated to reference laboratories. Although biochemical tests are useful for differentiating species, the species can be identified definitively only through sequencing species-specific gene targets or assessment of protein profiles using mass spectrometry.

In vitro susceptibility tests are not performed with legionellae because the organisms grow poorly on the media commonly used for these tests. In addition, some antibiotics that appear active in vitro are ineffective in treating infections. One explanation is that these antibiotics cannot penetrate the macrophages where the legionellae survive and multiply. Accumulated clinical experience indicates that **macrolides** (e.g., azithromycin, clarithromycin) or **fluoroquinolones** (e.g., ciprofloxacin, levofloxacin) should be used to treat *Legionella* infections. β-Lactam antibiotics are ineffective because most isolates produce β-lactamases, and these antibiotics do not penetrate macrophages. Specific therapy for Pontiac fever is generally unnecessary because it is a self-limited hypersensitivity disease.

Prevention of legionellosis requires identification of the environmental source of the organism and reduction of the microbial burden. Hyperchlorination of the water supply and maintenance of elevated water temperatures have proved moderately successful. However, elimination of *Legionella* organisms from a water supply is often difficult or impossible to achieve. Because the organism has a low potential for causing disease, reducing the number of organisms in the water supply is often an adequate control measure. Hospitals with patients at high risk for disease should monitor their water supply on a regular basis for the presence of *Legionella* and their hospital population for disease. If hyperchlorination or superheating of the water does not eliminate disease (complete elimination of the organisms in the water supply is probably not possible), continuous copper-silver ionization of the water supply may be necessary.

Streptobacillus

Streptobacillus moniliformis, the causative agent of **rat-bite fever,** is a long, thin (0.1 to 0.5 × 1 to 5 μm), gram-negative rod that tends to stain poorly and to be more pleomorphic in older cultures. Granules, bulbous swellings resembling a string of beads, and extremely long filaments may be seen (Figure 29-8).

Streptobacillus is found in the nasopharynx of rats and other small rodents, as well as transiently in animals that feed on rodents (e.g., dogs, cats). Human infections result from rodent bites (**rat-bite fever;** Clinical Case 29-7) or much less commonly from consumption of contaminated food or water (**Haverhill fever**) (see Box 29-1). Most cases of rat-bite fever in the United States are in children with pet rats, laboratory workers, and pet shop employees. After a 2- to 10-day incubation period, the onset of rat-bite fever is abrupt, characterized by irregular fever, headache, chills, muscle pain, and migratory pain in multiple joints (polyarthralgias). A maculopapular or petechial rash develops a few days later, with involvement extending to the hands and feet. This hemorrhagic rash in a patient with a recent history of a rat bite and migratory polyarthralgias is diagnostic. In the absence of effective antibiotics, rat-bite fever is associated with a 10% mortality rate. Despite effective treatment, some patients have persistent polyarthralgias, fatigue, and a slowly resolving rash.

Laboratory confirmation of *Streptobacillus* infections is difficult. Blood and joint fluid should be collected, and the

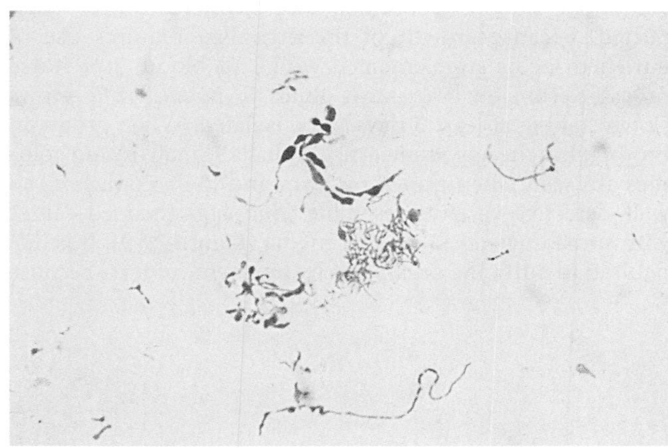

FIGURE 29-8 Gram stain of *Streptobacillus moniliformis;* note the pleomorphic forms and bulbous swellings.

Clinical Case 29-7 Rat-Bite Fever

Irvine (*Clin Microbiol Newslett* 28:15–17, 2006) described a 60-year-old man who developed rat-bite fever. The patient was admitted to the hospital complaining of fever, confusion, headaches, and pustular lesions on both hands. The diagnosis of sepsis was made, and blood cultures, cerebrospinal fluid (CSF), and the purulent material from the lesions were collected. Lymphocytes were the predominant cells in the CSF, and no bacteria were seen on Gram stain, consistent with aseptic meningitis. A Gram stain of purulent material revealed pleomorphic gram-negative rods. After 3 days of incubation, the bacteria grew from both the blood and wound cultures. Growth in the blood culture broths appeared as clumps of organisms resembling "bread crumbs." The organism was subsequently identified as *Streptobacillus moniliformis*. The patient was treated with penicillin, and within 24 hours, his fever resolved and sensorium cleared. A more complete social history revealed that the patient had a pet snake and maintained mice to feed the snake. Although he did not remember recent bites from the mice, exposure of open cuts on his hands to the rodents would have been sufficient for an infection to develop.

FIGURE 29-9 Methylene blue stain of *Streptobacillus moniliformis* from a positive blood culture of a 2-year-old Kuwaiti girl following exposure to rodents. (Courtesy Dr. R.M. Joshi, Safat, Kuwait.)

laboratory should be notified that *S. moniliformis* is suspected, because growth of the organism requires use of enriched media supplemented with 15% blood, 20% horse or calf serum, or 5% ascitic fluid. *S. moniliformis* grows slowly, taking at least 3 days to be isolated. When grown in broth, it has the appearance of "puffballs." Small, round colonies are seen when grown on agar, and the colonies of cell wall–defective variants resemble fried eggs (heaped center with spreading edges) on agar media (Figure 29-9). It is difficult to identify the organisms by biochemical tests because they are relatively inactive metabolically. The most reliable method for identifying isolates is to sequence the 16S rRNA gene. *S. moniliformis* is susceptible to many antibiotics, including **penicillin** (not active against cell wall–defective variants) and **tetracycline.**

Bibliography

Barker JR, Chong A, Wehrly TD, et al: The *Francisella tularensis* pathogenicity island encodes a secretion system that is required for phagosome escape and virulence, *Mol Microbiol* 74:1459–1470, 2009.

Carbonetti N: Pertussis toxin and adenylate cyclase toxin: key virulence factors of *Bordetella pertussis* and cell biology tools, *Future Microbiol* 5:455–469, 2010.

de Gouw D, Diavatopoulos DA, Bootsma HJ, et al: Pertussis: a matter of immune modulation, *FEMS Microbiol Rev* 35:441–474, 2011.

Elliott S: Rat bite fever and *Streptobacillus moniliformis*, *Clin Microbiol Rev* 20:13–22, 2007.

Fields BS, Benson RF, Besser RE: *Legionella* and Legionnaires' disease: 25 years of investigation, *Clin Microbiol Rev* 15:506–526, 2002.

Guiso N: *Bordetella pertussis* and pertussis vaccines, *Clin Infect Dis* 49:1565–1569, 2009.

Hayden RT, Uhl JR, Qian X, et al: Direct detection of *Legionella* species from bronchoalveolar lavage and open lung biopsy specimens: comparison of LightCycler PCR, in situ hybridization, direct fluorescence antigen detection, and culture, *J Clin Microbiol* 39:2618–2626, 2001.

Helbig JH, Uldum SA, Bernander S, et al: Clinical utility of urinary antigen detection for diagnosis of community-acquired, travel-associated, and nosocomial legionnaires' disease, *J Clin Microbiol* 41:838–840, 2003.

Jones BD, Faron M, Rasmussen JA, et al: Uncovering the components of the *Francisella tularensis* virulence stealth strategy, *Front Cell Infect Microbiol* 4:32, 2014.

Koehler JE, Sanchez MA, Tye S, et al: Prevalence of *Bartonella* infection among human immunodeficiency virus–infected patients with fever, *Clin Infect Dis* 37:559–566, 2003.

Malani AN, Aronoff DM, Bradley SF, et al: *Cardiobacterium hominis* endocarditis: two cases and a review of the literature, *Eur J Clin Microbiol Infect Dis* 25:587–595, 2006.

Mattoo S, Cherry J: Molecular pathogenesis, epidemiology, and clinical manifestations of respiratory infections due to *Bordetella pertussis* and other *Bordetella* subspecies, *Clin Microbiol Rev* 18:326–382, 2005.

Melvin JA, Scheller EV, Miller JF, et al: *Bordetella pertussis* pathogenesis: current and future challenges, *Nat Rev Microbiol* 12:274–284, 2014.

Metzkor-Cotter E, Kletter Y, Avidor B, et al: Long-term serological analysis and clinical follow-up of patients with cat scratch disease, *Clin Infect Dis* 37:1149–1154, 2003.

Modol J, Sabria M, Reynaga E, et al: Hospital-acquired legionnaires disease in a university hospital: impact of the copper-silver ionization system, *Clin Infect Dis* 44:263–265, 2007.

Newton HJ, Ang DK, van Driel IR, et al: Molecular pathogenesis of infections caused by *Legionella pneumophila*, *Clin Microbiol Rev* 23:274–298, 2010.

Pappas G, Akritidis N, Bosilkovski M, et al: Brucellosis, *N Engl J Med* 352:2325–2336, 2005.

Prutsky G, Domecq JP, Mori L, et al: Treatment outcomes of human bartonellosis: a systematic review and meta-analysis, *Int J Infect Dis* 17:e811–e819, 2013.

Resto-Ruiz S, Burgess A, Anderson B: The role of the host immune response in pathogenesis of *Bartonella henselae*, *DNA Cell Biol* 22:431–440, 2003.

Staples JE, Kubota KA, Chalcraft LG, et al: Epidemiologic and molecular analysis of human tularemia, United States, 1964–2004, *Emerg Infect Dis* 12:1113–1118, 2006.

Starr T, Ng TW, Wehrly TD, et al: *Brucella* intracellular replication requires trafficking through the late endosomal/lysosomal compartment, *Traffic* 9:678–694, 2008.

CHAPTER

CLOSTRIDIUM

The genus *Clostridium* consists of a large heterogeneous collection of spore-forming anaerobic rods. Pathogens such as *Clostridium tetani* and *Clostridium botulinum,* the agents responsible for tetanus and botulism, respectively, are well recognized and have historical significance, and disease caused by *Clostridium difficile* has evolved in recent years as an infectious complication of antibiotic usage, in both the hospital and the community. Other species of clostridia are also well-recognized pathogens.

1. *Clostridium perfringens* is an important cause of myonecrosis. What virulence factors are responsible for this disease?
2. Food poisoning caused by *C. perfringens* and *C. botulinum* is caused by ingestion of toxins (intoxication). Compare the clinical manifestations of these two diseases.
3. What disease is caused by *Clostridium septicum,* and what patient population is most susceptible?

Answers to these questions are available on StudentConsult.com.

SUMMARIES CLINICALLY SIGNIFICANT ORGANISMS

Clostridium difficile

Trigger Words

Spore-former, fecal carriage, antibiotic-associated diarrhea, toxins A and B

Biology and Virulence

- Large anaerobic rod characterized by abundant spore formation, rapid growth, and production of volatile fatty acids
- Most strains produce two toxins: an enterotoxin that attracts neutrophils and stimulates their release of cytokines, and a cytotoxin that increases permeability of the intestinal wall and subsequent diarrhea
- Spore formation allows the organism to persist in the hospital environment and resist decontamination efforts
- Resistance to antibiotics such as clindamycin, cephalosporins, and fluoroquinolones allows *C. difficile* to overgrow the normal intestinal bacteria in patients exposed to these antibiotics and produce disease

Epidemiology

- Colonizes the intestines of a small proportion of healthy individuals (<5%)
- Exposure to antibiotics is associated with overgrowth of *C. difficile* and subsequent disease (endogenous infection)
- Spores can be detected in hospital rooms of infected patients (particularly around beds and in bathrooms); these can be an exogenous source of infection
- A highly virulent strain of *C. difficile* currently causes disease in communities and hospitals in Canada, the United States, and Europe

Diseases

- Antibiotic-associated diarrhea: acute diarrhea generally developing 5 to 10 days after initiation of antibiotic treatment; may be brief and self-limited or more protracted
- Pseudomembranous colitis: most severe form of *C. difficile* disease, with profuse diarrhea, abdominal cramping, and fever; whitish plaques (pseudomembranes) form over intact colonic tissue

Diagnosis

- *C. difficile* disease is confirmed by detecting cytotoxin or enterotoxin or the toxin genes in the patient's feces

Treatment, Prevention, and Control

- The implicated antibiotic should be discontinued
- Treatment with metronidazole or vancomycin should be used in severe disease; fecal transplants have been used to treat recurrent disease
- Relapse is common because antibiotics do not kill spores; a second course of therapy with the same antibiotic is usually successful, although multiple courses may be necessary
- The hospital room should be carefully cleaned after the infected patient is discharged

Clostridium perfringens

Trigger Words

Weak spore-former, environmental, myonecrosis, sepsis, food poisoning, surgical debridement

Biology and Virulence

- Large gram-positive rods with spores rarely observed
- Distinct colony morphology and rapid growth
- Produces many toxins and enzymes that lyse blood cells and destroy tissues, leading to diseases such as overwhelming sepsis, massive hemolysis, and myonecrosis
- Produces a heat-sensitive enterotoxin that binds to receptors on the epithelium of the small intestine, leading to loss of fluids and ions (watery diarrhea)

Epidemiology

- Ubiquitous; present in soil, water, and intestinal tract of humans and animals
- Type A strains are responsible for most human infections

Diseases

- Food poisoning associated with contaminated meat products (beef, poultry, gravy) held at temperatures between 5° C and 60° C, which allows the organisms to grow to large numbers
- Soft-tissue infections typically associated with bacterial contamination of wounds or localized trauma

Diagnosis

- Reliably seen in Gram-stained tissue specimens (large, gram-positive rods)
- Grows rapidly in culture

Treatment, Prevention, and Control

- Rapid treatment is essential for serious infections
- Severe infections require surgical debridement and high-dose penicillin therapy
- Symptomatic treatment for food poisoning
- Proper wound care and judicious use of prophylactic antibiotics will prevent most infections

Clostridium tetani

Trigger Words

Spore-former, environmental, neurotoxin blocks GABA and glycine, contaminated wounds, tetanus, vaccine

Biology and Virulence

- Organism extremely oxygen sensitive, which makes detection by culture difficult
- The primary virulence factor is tetanospasmin, a heat-labile neurotoxin that blocks release of neurotransmitters (i.e., gamma-aminobutyric acid, glycine) for inhibitory synapses

Epidemiology

- Ubiquitous; spores are found in most soils and can colonize gastrointestinal tract of humans and animals
- Exposure to spores is common, but disease is uncommon, except in developing countries where there is poor access to vaccine and medical care
- Risk is greatest for people with inadequate vaccine-induced immunity
- Disease does not induce immunity

Diseases

- Disease is characterized by muscle spasms and involvement of the autonomic nervous system

Diagnosis

- Diagnosis is based on clinical presentation and not laboratory tests
- Microscopy and culture are insensitive, and neither tetanus toxin nor antibodies are typically detected

Treatment, Prevention, and Control

- Treatment requires debridement, antibiotic therapy (penicillin, metronidazole), passive immunization with antitoxin globulin, and vaccination with tetanus toxoid
- Prevention through use of vaccination, consisting of three doses of tetanus toxoid followed by booster doses every 10 years

Clostridium botulinum

Trigger Words

Spore-former, environmental, neurotoxin blocks acetylcholine, contaminated foods, foodborne and infant botulism, no vaccine

Biology and Virulence

- Seven distinct botulinum toxins (A to G) are produced, with human disease caused most commonly by types A and B; types E and F are also associated with human disease
- Botulinum toxin prevents release of the neurotransmitter acetylcholine, thus blocking neurotransmission at peripheral cholinergic synapses, leading to a flaccid paralysis

Epidemiology

- *C. botulinum* spores are found in soil worldwide
- Relatively few cases of botulism in the United States but prevalent in developing countries
- Infant botulism more common than other forms in the United States

Diseases

- Foodborne botulism is characterized by blurred vision, dry mouth, constipation, and abdominal pain, with progressive weakness of the peripheral muscles and flaccid paralysis
- Infant botulism begins with nonspecific symptoms but progresses to flaccid paralysis
- Other forms of botulism include wound botulism and inhalation botulism

Diagnosis

- Diagnosis of foodborne botulism is confirmed if toxin activity is demonstrated in the implicated food or in the patient's serum, feces, or gastric fluid
- Infant botulism is confirmed if toxin is detected in the infant's feces or serum, or the organism cultured from feces
- Wound botulism is confirmed if toxin is detected in the patient's serum or wound, or the organism cultured from the wound

Treatment, Prevention, and Control

- Treatment involves administration of metronidazole or penicillin, trivalent botulinum antitoxin, and ventilatory support
- Spore germination in foods prevented by maintaining food at an acid pH, by high sugar content (e.g., fruit preserves), or by storing the foods at 4° C or colder
- Toxin is heat labile and therefore can be destroyed by heating of food for 10 minutes at 60° C to 100° C
- Infant botulism associated with ingestion of contaminated soil or consumption of contaminated foods (particularly honey)

Historically, the collection of all anaerobic gram-positive rods capable of forming **endospores** was placed in the genus *Clostridium;* however, clinically significant members of the genus can be misclassified. Spores are only rarely demonstrated in some species *(Clostridium perfringens, Clostridium ramosum),* some species are aerotolerant and can grow on agar media exposed to air (e.g., *Clostridium tertium, Clostridium histolyticum*), and some clostridia consistently stain gram-negative (e.g., *C. ramosum, Clostridium clostridioforme*). It should not be surprising that the use of gene-sequencing techniques has led to reorganization of this heterogeneous collection of organisms into many new genera; however, most clinically significant species cluster in homology group I and remain in the genus

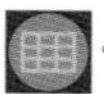

Table 30-1 Important Clostridia

Organism	Historical Derivation
Clostridium	*closter,* a spindle
C. botulinum	*botulus,* sausage (the first major outbreak was associated with insufficiently smoked sausage)
C. difficile	*difficile,* difficult (difficult to isolate and grow; refers to the extreme oxygen sensitivity of this organism)
C. perfringens	*perfringens,* breaking through (associated with highly invasive tissue necrosis)
C. septicum	*septicum,* putrefactive (associated with sepsis and a high mortality)
C. sordellii	*sordellii,* named after the bacteriologist Sordelli, who first described the organism
C. tertium	*tertium,* third (historically, the third most commonly isolated anaerobe from war wounds)
C. tetani	*tetani,* related to tension (disease caused by this organism characterized by muscle spasms)

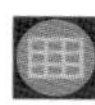

Table 30-2 Pathogenic Clostridia and Their Associated Human Diseases*

Species	Human Disease	Frequency
C. difficile	Antibiotic-associated diarrhea, pseudomembranous colitis	Common
C. perfringens	Soft-tissue infections (e.g., cellulitis, suppurative myositis, myonecrosis, gas gangrene), food poisoning, enteritis necroticans, septicemia	Common
C. septicum	Gas gangrene, septicemia	Uncommon
C. botulinum	Botulism	Uncommon
C. tetani	Tetanus	Uncommon
C. tertium	Opportunistic infections	Uncommon
C. baratii	Botulism	Rare
C. butyricum	Botulism	Rare
C. clostridioforme	Opportunistic infections	Rare
C. histolyticum	Gas gangrene	Rare
C. innocuum	Opportunistic infections	Rare
C. novyi	Gas gangrene	Rare
C. ramosum	Opportunistic infections	Rare
C. sordellii	Gas gangrene, septic shock syndrome	Rare
C. sporogenes	Opportunistic infections	Rare

*Other clostridial species have been associated with human disease but primarily as opportunistic pathogens. In addition, some species (e.g., *C. clostridioforme, C. innocuum, C. ramosum*) are commonly isolated but rarely associated with disease.

Clostridium. These bacteria are the focus of this chapter (Table 30-1).

The clostridia are **ubiquitous** in soil, water, and sewage and are part of the normal microbial population in the gastrointestinal (GI) tracts of animals and humans. Most clostridia are harmless saprophytes, but some are well-recognized human pathogens with a clearly documented history of causing diseases such as **food poisoning** *(C. perfringens),* **diarrhea** and **colitis** *(Clostridium difficile),* **tetanus** *(Clostridium tetani),* **botulism** *(Clostridium botulinum, Clostridium baratii, Clostridium butyricum),* and **myonecrosis (gas gangrene)** *(C. perfringens, Clostridium novyi, Clostridium septicum, C. histolyticus)* (Table 30-2; Box 30-1). The remarkable ability of clostridia to cause diseases is attributed to their (1) ability to survive adverse environmental conditions through spore formation, (2) rapid growth in a nutritionally enriched, oxygen-deprived environment, and (3) production of numerous histolytic toxins, enterotoxins, and neurotoxins.

Box 30-1 Clostridial Diseases: Clinical Summaries

Clostridium difficile

Antibiotic-associated diarrhea: acute diarrhea generally developing 5 to 10 days after initiation of antibiotic treatment (particularly clindamycin, penicillins, cephalosporins, fluoroquinolones); may be brief and self-limited or more protracted

Pseudomembranous colitis: most severe form of *C. difficile* disease, with profuse diarrhea, abdominal cramping, and fever; whitish plaques (pseudomembranes) over intact colonic tissue seen on colonoscopy

Clostridium perfringens

Soft-Tissue Infections

Cellulitis: localized edema and erythema with gas formation in the soft tissue; generally nonpainful

Suppurative myositis: accumulation of pus (suppuration) in the muscle planes, without muscle necrosis or systemic symptoms

Myonecrosis: painful, rapid destruction of muscle tissue; systemic spread with high mortality

Gastroenteritis

Food poisoning: rapid onset of abdominal cramps and watery diarrhea with no fever, nausea, or vomiting; short duration and self-limited

Necrotizing enteritis: acute, necrotizing destruction of jejunum, with abdominal pain, vomiting, bloody diarrhea, and peritonitis

Clostridium tetani

Generalized tetanus: generalized musculature spasms and involvement of the autonomic nervous system in severe disease (e.g., cardiac arrhythmias, fluctuations in blood pressure, profound sweating, dehydration)

Localized tetanus: musculature spasms restricted to localized area of primary infection

Neonatal tetanus: neonatal infection primarily involving the umbilical stump; very high mortality

Clostridium botulinum

Foodborne botulism: initial presentation of blurred vision, dry mouth, constipation, and abdominal pain; progresses to bilateral descending weakness of the peripheral muscles, with flaccid paralysis

Infant botulism: initially nonspecific symptoms (e.g., constipation, weak cry, failure to thrive) that progress to flaccid paralysis and respiratory arrest

Wound botulism: clinical presentation same as with foodborne disease, although the incubation period is longer and fewer gastrointestinal symptoms are reported

Inhalation botulism: rapid onset of symptoms (flaccid paralysis, pulmonary failure) and high mortality from inhalation exposure to botulinum toxin

Clostridium difficile (Clinical Case 30-1)

Physiology and Structure

C. difficile is a large (0.5 to 1.9 by 3.0 to 17 µm) anaerobic rod that freely forms spores in vivo and in culture. The organism grows rapidly in culture, although the vegetative cells die rapidly when exposed to oxygen. *C. difficile* produces a variety of volatile fatty acids that produce a characteristic "barnyard" smell in culture.

Pathogenesis and Immunity

C. difficile produces two toxins: an **enterotoxin (toxin A)** and a **cytotoxin (toxin B).** The enterotoxin is chemotactic for neutrophils, stimulating the infiltration of polymorphonuclear neutrophils into the ileum with release of cytokines. Toxin A also produces a cytopathic effect, resulting in disruption of the tight cell-to-cell junction, increased permeability of the intestinal wall, and subsequent diarrhea. The cytotoxin causes actin to depolymerize, with resultant destruction of the cellular cytoskeleton both in vivo and in vitro. Although both toxins appear to interact synergistically in the pathogenesis of disease, enterotoxin A–negative isolates can still produce disease. In addition, production of one or both toxins alone does not appear to be sufficient for disease (e.g., carriage of *C. difficile* and high levels of toxins are common in young children, although disease is rare). Bacterial "surface layer proteins" are important for the binding of *C. difficile* to the intestinal epithelium, leading to localized production of toxins and subsequent tissue damage.

Epidemiology

C. difficile is part of the normal intestinal flora in a small number of healthy people and hospitalized patients. In contrast with the original belief that *C. difficile* disease is restricted to hospitalized patients, it is now recognized that a significant proportion of individuals with *C. difficile* disease develops symptomatic disease outside the hospital. For most of these patients, they have a recent history of exposure to a health care facility, where they were presumably exposed to *C. difficile*, and antibiotic use. The disease develops in people taking antibiotics, because the drugs alter the normal enteric flora, either permitting overgrowth of these relatively resistant organisms or making the patient more susceptible to exogenous acquisition of *C. difficile*. The disease occurs if the organisms proliferate in the colon and produce their toxins.

Clinical Diseases (see Box 30-1)

Until the mid-1970s, the clinical importance of *C. difficile* was not appreciated. This organism was infrequently isolated in fecal cultures, and its role in human disease was unknown. Systematic studies now clearly show, however, that toxin-producing *C. difficile* is responsible for antibiotic-associated GI diseases ranging from a relatively benign, self-limited diarrhea to severe, life-threatening pseudomembranous colitis (Figures 30-1 and 30-2).

In 2003, disease caused by a highly virulent strain of *C. difficile* was reported in communities and hospitals in Canada, the United States, and Europe. This strain is responsible for more severe disease, a high mortality rate, increased risk of relapse, and more complications. The increased virulence of this strain is the result of a mutation in the gene that regulates production of the enterotoxin and cytotoxin. Because the regulatory gene is nonfunctional, there is a significant **increase in toxin production.** This new strain of *C. difficile* also produces another toxin, binary toxin, that is a useful marker for this strain and has been shown to facilitate adherence of the bacteria to the surface of epithelial cells. Unlike most isolates of *C. difficile,* this strain is resistant to fluoroquinolone antibiotics. Because fluoroquinolones are widely used in the community and hospitals, it is believed that this practice has selected for this virulent strain.

Clinical Case 30-1 *Clostridium difficile* Colitis

Limaye and colleagues (*J Clin Microbiol* 38:1696, 2000) presented a classic presentation of *C. difficile* disease in a 60-year-old man who received a transplanted liver 5 years previous to his hospital admission for evaluation of crampy abdominal pain and severe diarrhea. Three weeks prior to admission he received a 10-day course of oral trimethoprim-sulfamethoxazole for sinusitis. On physical examination, the patient was febrile and had moderate abdominal tenderness. Abdominal computed tomography scan revealed right colon thickening but no abscess. Colonoscopy showed numerous whitish plaques and friable erythematous mucosa consistent with pseudomembranous colitis. Empirical therapy with oral metronidazole and intravenous levofloxacin was initiated. A stool immunoassay for *C. difficile* toxin A was negative, but *C. difficile* toxin was detected by both culture and cytotoxicity assay (demonstration stool filtrate causes cytotoxicity to cell cultures that is neutralized by specific antisera against *C. difficile* toxins). Therapy was changed to oral vancomycin, and the patient responded with resolution of diarrhea and abdominal pain. This is an example of severe *C. difficile* disease following antibiotic exposure in an immunocompromised patient, with a characteristic presentation of pseudomembranous colitis. The diagnostic problems with immunoassays are well known and have now been replaced by polymerase chain reaction assays that target the toxin genes. Treatment with metronidazole is currently preferred, although vancomycin is an acceptable alternative.

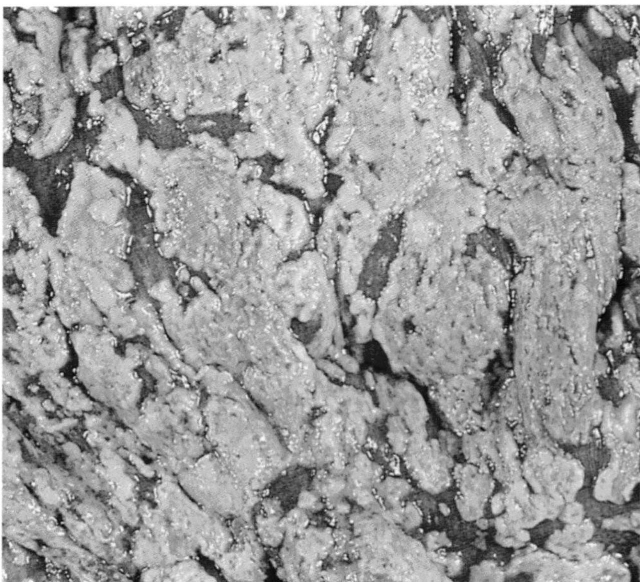

FIGURE 30-1 Antibiotic-associated colitis: gross section of the lumen of the colon. Note the white plaques of fibrin, mucus, and inflammatory cells overlying the normal red intestinal mucosa.

Laboratory Diagnosis

Isolation of the *C. difficile* in stool culture documents colonization but not disease, so the diagnosis of disease is confirmed by demonstration of the enterotoxin or cytotoxin in a stool specimen from a patient with compatible clinical symptoms or detection of the *C. difficile* toxin genes directly in clinical specimens by nucleic acid amplification techniques. Commercial assays with high sensitivity and specificity are now available that provide results within a few hours of sample collection.

Treatment, Prevention, and Control

Discontinuation of the implicated antibiotic (e.g., ampicillin, clindamycin, fluoroquinolones) is generally sufficient to alleviate mild disease. However, specific therapy with **metronidazole** or **vancomycin** is necessary for the management of severe diarrhea or colitis. Relapses may occur in as many as 20% to 30% of patients after completion of therapy, because only the vegetative forms of *C. difficile* are killed by the antibiotics; the spores are resistant. A second course of treatment with the same antibiotic is frequently successful, although multiple relapses are well documented in some patients. One novel approach to treat recurrent disease is to infuse fecal contents from a healthy donor ("rePOOPulate") into the intestines of the ill patient. Remarkable success with these "fecal transplants" has been demonstrated, illustrating the fact that *C. difficile* does not become established when a healthy enteric population of bacteria is present. It is difficult to prevent the disease, because the organism commonly exists in hospitals, particularly in areas adjacent to infected patients (e.g., beds, bathrooms). The spores of *C. difficile* are difficult to eliminate unless thorough housekeeping measures are used. Thus the organism can contaminate an environment for many months and can be a major source of nosocomial outbreaks of *C. difficile* disease.

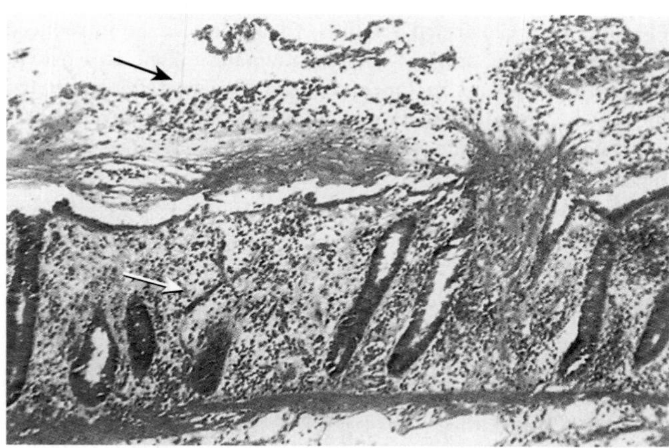

FIGURE 30-2 Antibiotic-associated colitis caused by *Clostridium difficile.* A histologic section of colon shows an intense inflammatory response, with the characteristic "plaque" *(black arrow)* overlying the intact intestinal mucosa *(white arrow)* (hematoxylin and eosin stain). (From Lambert HP, Farrar WE, editors: *Infectious diseases illustrated,* London, 1982, Gower.)

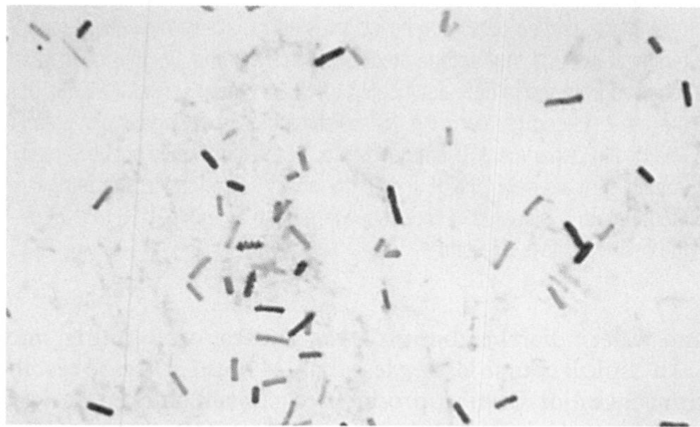

FIGURE 30-3 Gram stain of *Clostridium perfringens* in a wound specimen. Note the rectangular shape of the rods, the presence of many decolorized rods appearing gram-negative, and the absence of spore and blood cells.

• *Clostridium perfringens*

Physiology and Structure

C. perfringens is a large (0.6 to 2.4 × 1.3 to 19.0 μm), rectangular, gram-positive rod (Figure 30-3), with **spores rarely observed** either in vivo or after in vitro cultivation, an important characteristic that differentiates this species from most other clostridia. Colonies of *C. perfringens* are also distinctive, with their rapid, spreading growth on laboratory media and β-hemolysis on blood-containing media (Figure 30-4). The production of one or more "major lethal" toxins by *C. perfringens* (alpha, beta, epsilon, and iota toxins) is used to subdivide isolates into five types (A through E).

Pathogenesis and Immunity

Alpha toxin, produced by all five types of *C. perfringens,* is a lecithinase (phospholipase C) that lyses erythrocytes, platelets, leukocytes, and endothelial cells. This toxin mediates

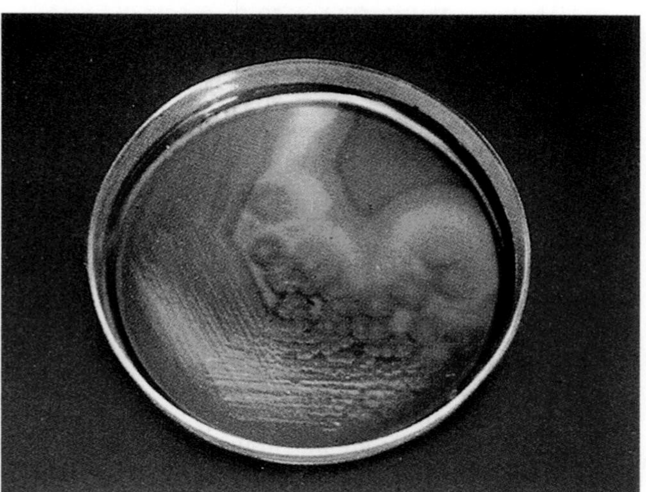

FIGURE 30-4 Growth of *Clostridium perfringens* on sheep blood agar. Note the flat, spreading colonies and the hemolytic activity of the organism. A presumptive identification of *C. perfringens* can be made by detection of a zone of complete hemolysis (caused by the theta toxin) and a wider zone of partial hemolysis (caused by the alpha toxin), combined with the characteristic microscopic morphology.

massive hemolysis, increased vascular permeability and bleeding (augmented by destruction of platelets), tissue destruction, hepatic toxicity, and myocardial dysfunction (bradycardia, hypotension). **Beta toxin** is responsible for intestinal stasis, loss of mucosa with formation of necrotic lesions, and progression to necrotizing enteritis. **Epsilon toxin,** a protoxin, is activated by trypsin and increases the vascular permeability of the gastrointestinal wall. **Iota toxin,** produced by type E *C. perfringens,* has necrotic activity and increases vascular permeability.

C. perfringens produces **enterotoxin,** primarily by type A strains, whose activity is enhanced by exposure to trypsin. The enterotoxin is produced during the phase transition from vegetative cells to spores and is released in the alkaline environment of the small intestine when the cells undergo the terminal stages of spore formation **(sporulation).** The released enterotoxin binds to receptors on the brush border membrane of the small intestine epithelium in the ileum (primarily) and jejunum but not duodenum. Insertion of the toxin into the cell membrane leads to altered membrane permeability and loss of fluids and ions. The enterotoxin also acts as a superantigen, stimulating T-lymphocyte activity.

Epidemiology

Type A *C. perfringens* commonly inhabits the intestinal tract of humans and animals and is widely distributed in nature, particularly in soil and water contaminated with feces. Spores are formed under adverse environmental conditions and can survive for prolonged periods. Strains of types B through E do not survive in soil but colonize the intestinal tracts of animals and occasionally humans. *C. perfringens,* particularly type A, is responsible for a variety of diseases including soft-tissue infections, food poisoning, necrotizing enteritis, and septicemia.

Clinical Diseases (see Box 30-1)

C. perfringens is responsible for a range of soft-tissue infections including **cellulitis** (Figure 30-5), fasciitis or suppurative **myositis,** and **myonecrosis** with gas formation in the soft tissue (gas gangrene). Clostridial myonecrosis is most commonly caused by *C. perfringens,* although other species (e.g., *C. septicum, C. histolyticum, C. novyi*) can also produce this disease. This is a life-threatening disease that illustrates the full virulence potential of histotoxic clostridia. The onset of disease, characterized by intense pain, generally develops within a week after clostridia are introduced into tissue by trauma or surgery. The onset is followed rapidly by extensive muscle necrosis, shock, renal failure, and death, often within 2 days of initial onset. Macroscopic examination of muscle reveals devitalized necrotic tissue. Gas found in the tissue is caused by the metabolic activity of the rapidly dividing bacteria (hence the name **gas gangrene**). Gram stain of tissue or exudate collected from the wound of a patient with *C. perfringens* myonecrosis will reveal abundant rectangular gram-positive rods in the absence of inflammatory cells (resulting from lysis by clostridial toxins). The clostridial toxins characteristically cause extensive hemolysis and bleeding.

Clostridial food poisoning (Clinical Case 30-2), a relatively common but underappreciated intoxication, is characterized by (1) a short incubation period (8 to 12 hours), (2) a clinical presentation that includes abdominal cramps and watery diarrhea but no fever, nausea, or vomiting, and (3) a clinical course lasting less than 24 hours. Disease results from ingestion of meat products (e.g., beef, chicken, turkey, gravy) contaminated with large numbers (10^8 to 10^9 organisms) of enterotoxin-producing type A *C. perfringens.* Holding contaminated foods at temperatures less than 60° C (46° C is optimal) allows spores that survived the cooking process to germinate and multiply to high numbers. Rapid

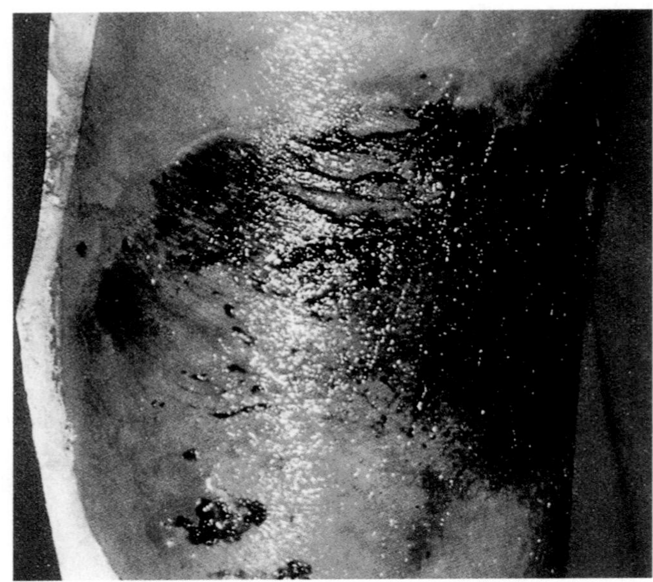

FIGURE 30-5 Clostridial cellulitis. Clostridia can be introduced into tissue during surgery or by a traumatic injury. This patient suffered a compound fracture of the tibia. Five days after the injury, the skin became discolored, and bullae and necrosis developed. A serosanguineous exudate and subcutaneous gas were present, but there was no evidence of muscle necrosis. The patient had an uneventful recovery. (From Lambert H, Farrar W, editors: *Infectious diseases illustrated,* London, 1982, Gower.)

Clinical Case 30-2 *Clostridium perfringens* Gastroenteritis

The Centers for Disease Control and Prevention reported two outbreaks of *C. perfringens* gastroenteritis associated with corned beef served at St. Patrick's Day celebrations (*MMWR Morb Mortal Wkly Rep* 43:137, 1994). On March 18, 1993, the Cleveland City Health Department received telephone calls from 15 persons who became ill after eating corned beef purchased from one delicatessen. After publicizing the outbreak, 156 persons contacted the Health Department with a similar history. In addition to a history of diarrhea, 88% complained of abdominal cramps and 13% had vomiting, which developed an average of 12 hours after eating the implicated meat. An investigation revealed the delicatessen had purchased 1400 pounds of raw, salt-cured meat, and beginning on March 12, portions of the corned beef were boiled for 3 hours, allowed to cool at room temperature, and then refrigerated. On March 16 and 17, the meat was removed from the refrigerator, heated to 48.8° C, and served. Cultures of the meat yielded greater than 10^5 colonies of *C. perfringens* per gram. The Health Department recommended that if the meat could not be served immediately after cooking, it should be rapidly cooled in ice and refrigerated. Before it is served, it should be warmed to at least 74° C to destroy the heat-sensitive enterotoxin.

refrigeration of food after preparation prevents this bacterial growth. Alternatively, reheating the food to 74° C can destroy the heat-labile enterotoxin.

Necrotizing enteritis (also called **enteritis necroticans** or **pig-bel**) is a rare necrotizing process in the jejunum characterized by acute abdominal pain, vomiting, bloody diarrhea, ulceration of the small intestine, and perforation of the intestinal wall, leading to peritonitis and shock. Mortality in patients with this infection approaches 50%. Beta toxin produced by *C. perfringens* type C is responsible for this disease. Necrotizing enteritis is most common in Papua New Guinea, with sporadic cases reported from other countries. This results from the dietary habits of the population, where disease can follow consumption of both undercooked contaminated pork and sweet potatoes. Sweet potatoes contain a heat-resistant trypsin inhibitor that protects the beta toxin from inactivation by trypsin. Other risk factors for the disease are exposure to large numbers of organisms and malnutrition (with loss of the proteolytic activity that inactivates the toxin).

Isolation of *C. perfringens* or other clostridial species in blood cultures can be alarming; however, more than half of the isolates are clinically insignificant, representing a transient bacteremia or, more likely, contamination of the culture with clostridia colonizing the skin. Patients with clinically significant **septicemia** complicating other infections (e.g., myonecrosis, necrotizing enteritis) will typically present dramatically with massive hemolysis and overwhelming septic shock.

Laboratory Diagnosis

The laboratory performs a confirmatory role in the diagnosis of clostridial soft-tissue diseases, because therapy must be initiated immediately. The microscopic detection of gram-positive rods in clinical specimens, usually in the absence of leukocytes, can be a very useful finding because these organisms have a characteristic morphology. It is also relatively simple to culture these anaerobes. Under appropriate conditions, *C. perfringens* divides every 8 to 10 minutes, so growth on agar media or in blood culture broths can be detected after incubation for only a few hours. The role of *C. perfringens* in food poisoning is documented by recovery of more than 10^5 organisms per gram of food or more than 10^6 bacteria per gram of feces collected within 1 day of the onset of disease. Immunoassays have also been developed for detection of the enterotoxin in fecal specimens; however, clostridial food poisoning is a clinical diagnosis, and culture or immunoassays are not commonly used.

Treatment, Prevention, and Control

C. perfringens soft-tissue infections, such as suppurative myositis and myonecrosis, must be treated aggressively with **surgical debridement** and **high-dose penicillin therapy.** Hyperbaric oxygen treatment has been used to manage these infections; however, the results are inconclusive. Despite all therapeutic efforts, the prognosis in patients with these diseases is poor, with mortality reported from 40% to almost 100%. Less serious, localized soft-tissue infections can be successfully treated with debridement and penicillin.

Clostridial food poisoning is managed by oral rehydration and in severe cases intravenous fluids and electrolytes. Antibiotic therapy is not recommended because this is a self-limiting disease (i.e., the diarrhea washes the bacteria out of the intestines, and the normal intestinal flora reestablishes itself).

Exposure to *C. perfringens* is difficult to avoid because the organisms are ubiquitous. Disease requires introduction of the organism into devitalized tissues and maintenance of an anaerobic environment favorable for bacterial growth. Thus proper wound care and the judicious use of prophylactic antibiotics can do much to prevent most infections.

• *Clostridium tetani*

Physiology and Structure

C. tetani is a large (0.5 to 2 × 2 to 18 μm), motile, spore-forming rod. The organism produces round, terminal spores that give it the appearance of a drumstick. Unlike *C. perfringens, C. tetani* is difficult to grow because the organism is extremely sensitive to oxygen toxicity; when growth is detected on agar media, it typically appears as a film over the surface of the agar rather than discrete colonies. The bacteria are proteolytic but unable to ferment carbohydrates.

Pathogenesis and Immunity

Although the vegetative cells of *C. tetani* die rapidly when exposed to oxygen, spore formation allows the organism to survive in the most adverse conditions. Of greater significance is the fact that *C. tetani* produces two toxins, an oxygen-labile hemolysin **(tetanolysin)** and a plasmid-encoded, heat-labile neurotoxin **(tetanospasmin).** The plasmid carrying the gene for tetanospasmin is nonconjugative, so a nontoxic *C. tetani* strain cannot be converted to a toxigenic strain. Tetanolysin is serologically related to streptolysin O and the hemolysins produced by *C. perfringens* and *Listeria monocytogenes;* however, the clinical significance of tetanolysin is unknown because it is inhibited by oxygen and serum cholesterol.

Tetanospasmin is produced during the stationary phase of growth, released when the cell is lysed, and responsible for the clinical manifestations of tetanus. Tetanospasmin (an **A-B toxin**) is synthesized as a single 150,000-Da peptide that is cleaved into a light (A-chain) subunit and a heavy (B-chain) subunit by an endogenous protease when the cell releases the neurotoxin. A disulfide bond and noncovalent forces hold the two chains together. The carbohydrate-binding domain of the carboxyl-terminal portion of the heavy (100,000-Da) chain binds to specific sialic acid receptors (e.g., polysialogangliosides) and adjacent glycoproteins on the surface of motor neurons. The intact toxin molecules are internalized in endosomal vesicles and transported in the neuron axon to motor neuron soma located in the spinal cord. In this location, the endosome becomes acidified, resulting in a conformational change in the N-terminus domain of the heavy chain, insertion into the endosome membrane, and passage of the toxin light chain into the cytosol of the cell. The light chain is a **zinc endopeptidase** that cleaves core proteins involved in the trafficking and release of neurotransmitters. Specifically, tetanospasmin **inactivates proteins that regulate release of the inhibitory neurotransmitters** glycine and gamma-aminobutyric acid (GABA). This leads to unregulated excitatory synaptic activity in the motor neurons, resulting in **spastic paralysis.** The toxin binding is irreversible, so recovery depends on whether new axonal terminals form.

Epidemiology

C. tetani is **ubiquitous.** It is found in fertile soil and transiently colonizes the GI tracts of many animals, including humans. The vegetative forms of *C. tetani* are extremely susceptible to oxygen toxicity, but the organisms sporulate readily and can survive in nature for a long time. Disease is relatively rare in the United States because of the high incidence of vaccine-induced immunity. Only 36 cases were reported in 2011, and the disease occurs primarily in elderly patients with waning immunity. However, tetanus is still responsible for many deaths in developing countries where vaccination is unavailable or medical practices are lax. It is estimated that more than 1 million cases occur worldwide, with a mortality rate ranging from 30% to 50%. At least half the deaths occur in neonates.

Clinical Diseases (Clinical Case 30-3; see Box 30-1)

The incubation period for tetanus varies from a few days to weeks. The duration of the incubation period is directly related to the distance of the primary wound infection from the central nervous system.

Generalized tetanus is the most common form. Involvement of the masseter muscles (trismus or lockjaw) is the presenting sign in most patients. The characteristic sardonic smile that results from the sustained contraction of the facial muscles is known as *risus sardonicus* (Figure 30-6). Other early signs are drooling, sweating, irritability, and persistent back spasms *(opisthotonos)* (Figure 30-7). The autonomic nervous system is involved in patients with more severe disease; the signs and symptoms include cardiac arrhythmias, fluctuations in blood pressure, profound sweating, and dehydration.

Another form of *C. tetani* disease is **localized tetanus,** in which the disease remains confined to the musculature at the site of primary infection. A variant is **cephalic tetanus,** in which the primary site of infection is the head. In contrast to the prognosis for patients with localized tetanus, the prognosis for patients with cephalic tetanus is very poor.

Neonatal tetanus (tetanus neonatorum) is typically associated with an initial infection of the umbilical stump that progresses to become generalized. The mortality in infants exceeds 90%, and developmental defects are present in survivors. This is almost exclusively a disease in developing countries.

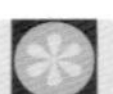

Clinical Case 30-3 Tetanus

The following is a typical history of a patient with tetanus (CDC, *MMWR Morb Mortal Wkly Rep* 51:613–615, 2002). An 86-year-old man saw a physician for care of a splinter wound in his right hand, acquired 3 days earlier while gardening. He was not treated with either a tetanus toxoid vaccine or tetanus immune globulin. Seven days later he developed pharyngitis, and after an additional 3 days, he presented to the local hospital with difficulty talking, swallowing, and breathing, and with chest pain and disorientation. He was admitted to the hospital with the diagnosis of stroke. On his fourth hospital day, he had developed neck rigidity and respiratory failure, requiring tracheostomy and mechanical ventilation. He was transferred to the medical intensive care unit, where the clinical diagnosis of tetanus was made. Despite treatment with tetanus toxoid and immune globulin, the patient died 1 month after admission to the hospital. This case illustrates that *Clostridium tetani* is ubiquitous in soil and can contaminate relatively minor wounds; it also illustrates the unrelenting progression of neurologic disease in untreated patients.

Laboratory Diagnosis

The diagnosis of tetanus, as with that of most other clostridial diseases, is made on the basis of the clinical presentation. The microscopic detection of *C. tetani* or recovery in culture is useful but frequently unsuccessful. Culture results are positive in only approximately 30% of patients with tetanus, because disease can be caused by relatively few organisms and the slow-growing bacteria are killed rapidly when exposed to air. Neither tetanus toxin nor antibodies to the toxin are detectable in the patient because the toxin is rapidly bound to motor neurons and internalized. If the organism is recovered in culture, production of toxin by the isolate can be confirmed with the tetanus antitoxin neutralization test in mice (a procedure performed only in public health reference laboratories).

Treatment, Prevention, and Control

The mortality associated with tetanus has steadily decreased during the past century, resulting in large part from the

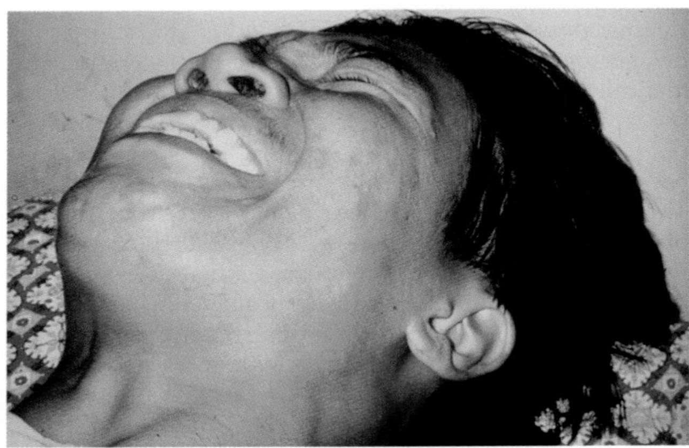

FIGURE 30-6 Facial spasm and risus sardonicus in a patient with tetanus. (From Cohen J, Powderly WG, Opal SM: *Infectious diseases,* ed 3, Philadelphia, 2010, Mosby.)

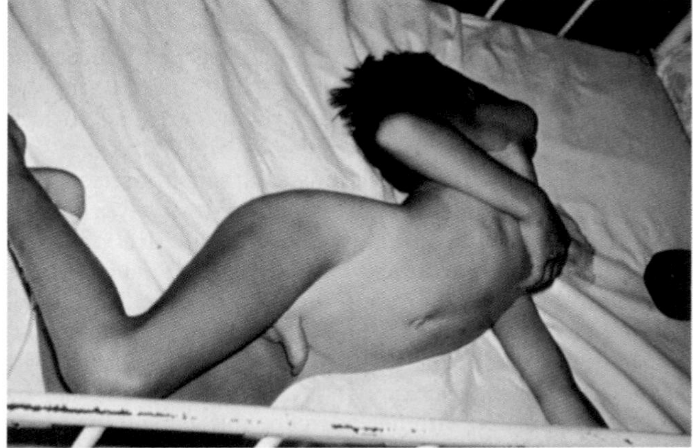

FIGURE 30-7 A child with tetanus and opisthotonos resulting from persistent spasms of the back muscles. (From Emond RT, Rowland HAK, Welsby P: *Colour atlas of infectious diseases,* ed 3, London, 1995, Wolfe.)

decreased incidence of tetanus in the United States. The highest mortality is in newborns and in patients in whom the incubation period is shorter than 1 week.

Treatment of tetanus requires **debridement** of the primary wound (which may appear innocuous), use of **penicillin** or **metronidazole** to kill the bacteria and reduce toxin production, **passive immunization** with human tetanus immunoglobulin to neutralize unbound toxin, and **vaccination** with tetanus toxoid (because infection does not confer immunity). Metronidazole and penicillin have equivalent activity against *C. tetani;* however, some have recommended metronidazole treatment because penicillin, like tetanospasmin, inhibits GABA activity, which can produce central nervous system excitability. Toxin bound to nerve endings is protected from antibiotics, thus the toxic effects must be controlled symptomatically until the normal regulation of synaptic transmission is restored. Vaccination with a series of three doses of tetanus toxoid, followed by booster doses every 10 years, is highly effective in preventing tetanus.

Clostridium botulinum

Physiology and Structure

The etiologic agents of botulism are a heterogeneous collection of large (0.6 to 1.4 × 3.0 to 20.2 μm), fastidious, spore-forming, anaerobic rods. These bacteria are subdivided into four groups based on phenotypic and genetic properties and certainly represent four separate species, although they have been historically classified within a single species, *C. botulinum.* Seven antigenically distinct botulinum toxins (A to G) have been described; human disease is associated with types A, B, E, and F. Other species of clostridia produce botulinum toxins, including *C. butyricum* (type E toxin), *C. baratii* (type F toxin), and *Clostridium argentinense* (type G toxin). Human disease has only rarely been associated with *C. butyricum* and *C. baratii* and not definitively demonstrated with *C. argentinense.*

Pathogenesis and Immunity

Similar to tetanus toxin, *C. botulinum* toxin is a 150,000-Da progenitor protein (A-B toxin) consisting of a small subunit (light, or A chain) with **zinc-endopeptidase** activity and a large, nontoxic subunit (B, or heavy chain). In contrast with the tetanus neurotoxin, the *C. botulinum* toxin is complexed with nontoxic proteins that protect the neurotoxin during passage through the digestive tract (this is unnecessary for tetanus neurotoxin). The carboxyl-terminal portion of the botulinum heavy chain binds specific sialic acid receptors and glycoproteins (different from those targeted by tetanospasmin) on the surface of motor neurons and stimulates endocytosis of the toxin molecule. Also, in contrast with tetanospasmin, the botulinum neurotoxin remains at the neuromuscular junction. Acidification of the endosome stimulates N-terminal, heavy-chain–mediated release of the light chain. The botulinum endopeptidase then **inactivates the proteins that regulate release of acetylcholine,** blocking neurotransmission at peripheral cholinergic synapses. Because acetylcholine is required for excitation of muscle, the resulting clinical presentation of botulism is a **flaccid paralysis.** As with tetanus, recovery of function after botulism requires regeneration of the nerve endings.

Epidemiology

C. botulinum is commonly isolated in soil and water samples throughout the world. In the United States, type A strains are found mainly in neutral or alkaline soil west of the Mississippi River, type B strains are found primarily in the eastern part of the country in rich organic soil, and type E strains are found only in wet soil. Although *C. botulinum* is commonly found in soil, disease is uncommon in the United States.

Four forms of botulism have been identified: (1) classic or foodborne botulism, (2) infant botulism, (3) wound botulism, and (4) inhalation botulism. In the United States, fewer than 25 cases of **foodborne botulism** are seen annually; most are associated with consumption of home-canned foods (types A and B toxins) and occasionally with consumption of preserved fish (type E toxin). The food may not appear spoiled, but even a small taste can cause full-blown clinical disease. **Infant botulism** is more common (although <100 cases are reported annually) and has been associated with consumption of foods (e.g., honey, infant milk powder) contaminated with botulinum spores and ingestion of spore-contaminated soil and dust (now the most common source of infant exposure). The incidence of **wound botulism** is unknown, but the disease is very rare. **Inhalation botulism** is a major concern in this era of bioterrorism. Botulinum toxin has been concentrated for purposes of aerosolization as a biological weapon. When administered in this manner, inhalation disease has a rapid onset and potentially high mortality.

Clinical Diseases (see Box 30-1)

Patients with **foodborne botulism** (Clinical Case 30-4) typically become weak and dizzy 1 to 3 days after consuming the contaminated food. Initial signs include blurred vision with fixed dilated pupils, dry mouth (indicative of the anticholinergic effects of the toxin), constipation, and abdominal pain. Fever is absent. Bilateral descending weakness of the peripheral muscles develops in patients with progressive disease (flaccid paralysis), and death is most commonly attributed to respiratory paralysis. Patients maintain a clear sensorium throughout the disease. Despite aggressive management of the patient's condition, the disease may continue to progress because the neurotoxin is irreversibly bound and inhibits the

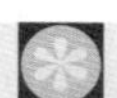

Clinical Case 30-4 Foodborne Botulism with Commercial Carrot Juice

The Centers for Disease Control and Prevention reported an outbreak of foodborne botulism associated with contaminated carrot juice (*MMWR Morb Mortal Wkly Rep* 55:1098, 2006). On September 8, 2006, three patients went to a hospital in Washington County, Georgia, with cranial nerve palsies and progressive descending flaccid paralysis resulting in respiratory failure. The patients had shared meals on the previous day. Because botulism was suspected, the patients were treated with botulinum antitoxin. The patients had no progression of their neurologic symptoms, but they remained hospitalized and on ventilators. An investigation determined that the patients had consumed contaminated carrot juice produced by a commercial vendor. Botulinum toxin type A was detected in the serum and stool of all three patients and in leftover carrot juice. An additional patient in Florida was also hospitalized with respiratory failure and descending paralysis after drinking carrot juice sold in Florida. Because carrot juice has a low acid content (pH 6.0), *Clostridium botulinum* spores can germinate and produce toxin if contaminated juice is left at room temperature.

release of excitatory neurotransmitters for a prolonged period. Complete recovery in patients often requires many months to years, or until the affected nerve endings regrow. Mortality in patients with foodborne botulism, which once approached 70%, has been reduced to 5% to 10% through the use of better supportive care, particularly in the management of respiratory complications.

Infant botulism (Clinical Case 30-5) was first recognized in 1976 and is now the most common form of botulism in the United States. In contrast with foodborne botulism, this disease is caused by neurotoxin produced in vivo by *C. botulinum* colonizing the GI tracts of infants. Although adults are exposed to the organism in their diet, *C. botulinum* cannot survive and proliferate in their intestines. However, in the absence of competitive bowel microbes, the organism can become established in the GI tracts of infants. The disease typically affects infants younger than 1 year (most between 1 and 6 months), and the symptoms are initially nonspecific (e.g., constipation, weak cry, or "failure to thrive"). Progressive disease with flaccid paralysis and respiratory arrest can develop; however, mortality in documented cases of infant botulism is very low (1% to 2%). Some infant deaths attributed to other conditions (e.g., sudden infant death syndrome) may actually be caused by botulism.

Wound botulism develops from toxin production by *C. botulinum* in contaminated wounds. Although the symptoms of disease are identical to those of foodborne disease, the incubation period is generally longer (4 days or more), and the GI tract symptoms are less prominent.

Laboratory Diagnosis

The clinical diagnosis of foodborne botulism is confirmed if toxin activity is demonstrated in the implicated food or in the patient's serum, feces, or gastric fluid. Infant botulism is confirmed if toxin is detected in the infant's feces or serum, or the organism cultured from feces. Wound botulism is confirmed if toxin is detected in the patient's serum or wound, or if the organism is cultured from the wound. Toxin activity is most likely to be found early in the disease. No single test for foodborne botulism has sensitivity greater than 60%; in contrast, toxin is detected in the serum of more than 90% of infants with botulism.

Isolation of *C. botulinum* from specimens contaminated with other organisms (e.g., feces, wounds) can be improved by heating the specimen for 10 minutes at 80° C to kill all non–spore-forming bacteria. Culture of the heated specimen on nutritionally enriched anaerobic media allows the heat-resistant *C. botulinum* spores to germinate. Demonstration of toxin production (typically performed at public health laboratories) must be done with a mouse bioassay. This procedure consists of the preparation of two aliquots of the isolate, mixing of one aliquot with antitoxin, and intraperitoneal inoculation of each aliquot into mice. If the antitoxin treatment protects the mice, toxin activity is confirmed. Samples of the implicated food, stool specimen, and patient's serum should also be tested for toxin activity.

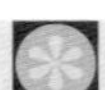

Clinical Case 30-5 Infant Botulism

In January 2003, four children with infant botulism were reported by the Centers for Disease Control and Prevention (*MMWR Morb Mortal Wkly Rep* 52:24, 2003). The following is the description of one of the children. A 10-week-old infant with a history of constipation in the first month of life was admitted to a hospital after having difficulty in sucking and swallowing for 2 days. The infant was irritable and had loss of facial expression, generalized muscle weakness, and constipation. Mechanical ventilation was required for 10 days because of respiratory failure. A diagnosis of infant botulism was established 29 days after onset of symptoms by detection of *C. botulinum* producing toxin type B in stool enrichment cultures. The patient was treated with Botulism Immune Globulin Intravenous (BIG-IV) and discharged fully recovered after 20 days. In contrast with foodborne botulism, diagnosis of infant botulism can be made by detecting the organism in the baby's stools.

Treatment, Prevention, and Control

Patients with botulism require the following treatment measures: (1) adequate **ventilatory support**, (2) elimination of the organism from the GI tract through the judicious use of gastric lavage and **metronidazole or penicillin** therapy, and (3) use of **trivalent botulinum antitoxin** versus toxins A, B, and E to inactivate unbound toxin circulating in the bloodstream. Ventilatory support is extremely important in reducing mortality. Protective levels of antibodies do not develop after disease, so patients remain susceptible to botulism.

Disease is prevented by destroying the spores in food (virtually impossible for practical reasons), preventing spore germination (by maintaining the food in an acid pH or storage at 4° C or colder), or destroying the preformed toxin (all botulinum toxins are inactivated by heating at 60° C to 100° C for 10 minutes). Infant botulism has been associated with consumption of honey contaminated with *C. botulinum* spores, so children younger than 1 year should not eat honey.

Other Clostridial Species

Many other clostridia have been associated with clinically significant disease. Their virulence is a result of their ability to survive exposure to oxygen by forming spores and producing many diverse toxins and enzymes. ***C. septicum*** (Figures 30-8 and 30-9) is a particularly important pathogen because it is a cause of nontraumatic myonecrosis and often

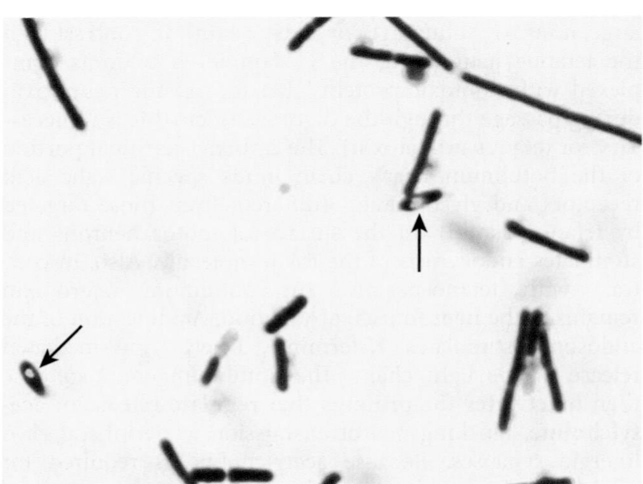

FIGURE 30-8 *Clostridium septicum:* note the spores *(arrows)* within the rods.

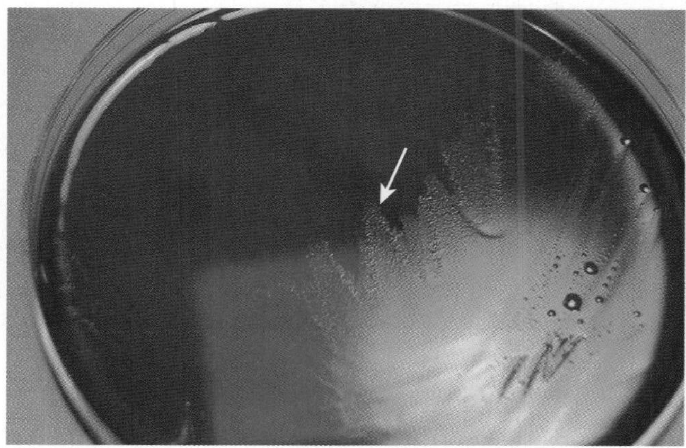

FIGURE 30-9 *Clostridium septicum:* note how the growth "swarms" *(arrow)* across the surface of the blood agar plate. This rapid spreading growth is also characteristic of rapid progression of disease in an infected patient.

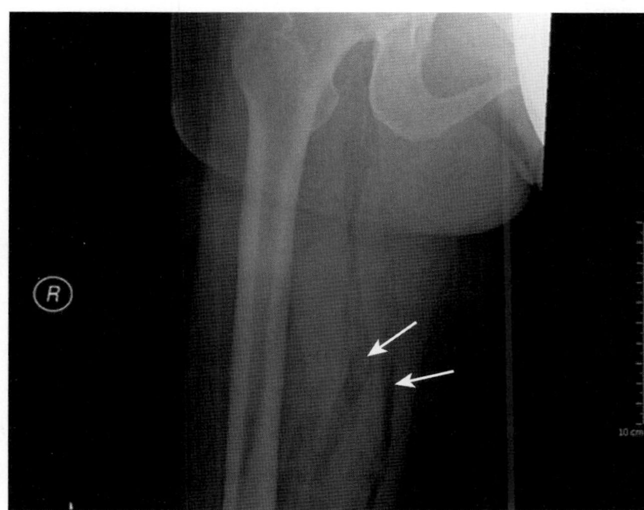

FIGURE 30-10 Radiograph of the leg of a patient with myonecrosis caused by *Clostridium septicum*. Note the gas *(arrows)* in the tissue.

exists in patients with occult colon cancer, acute leukemia, or diabetes. If the integrity of the bowel mucosa is compromised and the patient's body is less able to mount an effective response to the organism, *C. septicum* can spread into tissue and rapidly proliferate, producing gas and tissue destruction (Figure 30-10). Most patients have a fulminant course, dying within 1 to 2 days after initial presentation. ***C. sordellii*** is implicated in a fatal toxic shock syndrome associated with natural childbirth or medically-induced abortions (Clinical Case 30-6). ***C. tertium*** is another important clostridium that is commonly isolated in soil samples. It has primarily been associated with traumatic wound infections (e.g., war wounds, a fall producing a soil-contaminated wound). This organism can pose a diagnostic challenge because it can grow on aerobically incubated agar media. Correct identification can be made once spores are observed and it is determined that the organism grows better anaerobically.

Clinical Case 30-6 *Clostridium sordellii* Toxic Shock Syndrome Associated with Medical Abortions

A fatal toxic shock syndrome caused by *C. sordellii* has been associated with medical abortions. This is a description of this disease (Fischer et al, *N Engl J Med* 353:2352–2360, 2005). A previously healthy 22-year-old woman underwent a medically induced abortion with 200 mg of oral mifepristone followed by 800 μg of vaginal misoprostol. Five days later she presented to a local emergency department with nausea, vomiting, diarrhea, and severe abdominal pain. She was afebrile, tachycardic, and normotensive. The next day, her tachycardia (130 to 140 beats/min) remained persistent, she became hypotensive (blood pressure, 80/40 mm Hg), and her urine output decreased. Laboratory findings demonstrated hemoconcentration with elevated neutrophil count (leukomoid reaction) and severe metabolic acidosis. An emergency laparotomy was performed and revealed generalized edema of the abdominal and pelvic organs and 1 liter of serous peritoneal fluid. The patient died during the procedure, 23 hours after her initial presentation. Histopathologic examination of the uterus showed extensive inflammation, abscess formation, edema, necrosis, and hemorrhage. Numerous gram-positive rods were seen in the endometrium, and *C. sordellii* DNA was demonstrated in the uterine tissue by specific polymerase chain reaction (PCR) assays. Endometritis and toxic shock syndrome caused by *C. sordelli* is an uncommon but well-described complication of natural childbirth and medically induced abortions. Characteristic of this disease are the fulminant course, afebrile presentation, and hemoconcentration.

Bibliography

Aronoff D: *Clostridium novyi, sordellii,* and *tetani:* mechanisms of disease, *Anaerobe* 24:98–101, 2013.

Bauer M, Kuijper E, van Dissel J: European Society of Clinical Microbiology and Infectious Diseases (ESCMID): treatment guidance document for *Clostridium difficile* infection, *Clin Microbiol Infect* 15:1067–1079, 2009.

Cohen SH, Gerding DN, Johnson S, et al: Clinical practice guidelines for *Clostridium difficile* infection in adults: 2010 update by the Society for Healthcare Epidemiology of America (SHEA) and the Infectious Diseases Society of America (IDSA), *Infect Contr Hosp Epidemiol* 31:431–455, 2010.

Curry S: *Clostridium difficile, Clin Lab Med* 30:329–342, 2010.

Fischer M, Bhatnagar J, Guarner J, et al: Fatal toxic shock syndrome associated with *Clostridium sordellii* after medical abortion, *N Engl J Med* 353:2352–2360, 2005.

Grass J, Gould L, Mahon B: Epidemiology of foodborne disease outbreaks caused by *Clostridium perfringens,* United States, 1998–2010, *Foodborne Pathog Dis* 10:131–136, 2013.

Kennedy CL, Smith DJ, Lyras D, et al: Programmed cellular necrosis mediated by the pore-forming α-toxin from *Clostridium septicum, PLoS Pathogens* 5:e1000516, 2009.

Lalli G, Bohnert S, Deinhardt K, et al: The journey of tetanus and botulinum neurotoxins in neurons, *Trends Microbiol* 11:431–437, 2003.

Lessa F, Mu Y, Bamberg W, et al: Burden of *Clostridium difficile* infection in the United States, *N Engl J Med* 372:825–834, 2015.

Lindstrom M, Korkeala H: Laboratory diagnostics of botulism, *Clin Microbiol Rev* 19:298–314, 2006.

McCune V, Struthers J, Hawkey P: Faecal transplantation for the treatment of *Clostridium difficile* infection: a review, *Int J Antimicrob Agents* 43:201–206, 2014.

Schwan C, Stecher B, Tzivelekidis T, et al: *Clostridium difficile* toxin CDT induces formation of microtubule-based protrusions and increases adherence of bacteria, *PLoS Pathogens* 5:e1000626, 2009.

Stevens DL, Bryant AE: The role of clostridial toxins in the pathogenesis of gas gangrene, *Clin Infect Dis* 35(Suppl 1):S93–S100, 2002.

Voth DE, Ballard JD: *Clostridium difficile* toxins: mechanism of action and role in disease, *Clin Microbiol Rev* 18:247–263, 2005.

Ziakas P, Zacharioudakis I, Zervou F, et al: Asymptomatic carriers of toxigenic *C. difficile* in long-term care facilities: a meta-analysis of prevalence and risk factors, *PLoS ONE* 10(2):e0117195, 2015.

CHAPTER

NON–SPORE-FORMING ANAEROBIC BACTERIA

A 36-year-old woman with urinary retention, pelvic pain, and fever presented to the emergency department 6 days after transvaginal oocyte retrieval and embryo transfer for male infertility. The computed tomography scan revealed large multiloculated pelvic and tuboovarian abscesses. The woman improved following drainage of the abscesses and antibiotic therapy. Gram stain of the abscess material revealed a polymicrobic mixture of gram-positive and gram-negative bacteria, and both aerobic and anaerobic bacteria were recovered in culture.

1. What are the most likely anaerobic bacteria in this infection?
2. What is characteristic about most infections with *Actinomyces?*
3. What infections are typically caused by *Bacteroides fragilis?*
4. What antibiotics are usually active against *B. fragilis?*

Answers to these questions are available on StudentConsult.com.

• SUMMARIES CLINICALLY SIGNIFICANT ORGANISMS

Bacteroides fragilis

Trigger Words

Pleomorphic rod, capsule, abscess formation, drug resistance

Biology and Virulence

- Anaerobic, pleomorphic, gram-negative rod
- Surrounded by polysaccharide capsule
- Lipopolysaccharide major cell wall component but without endotoxin activity
- Polysaccharide capsule major virulence factor
- Heat-labile metalloprotease toxin responsible for diarrheal disease

Epidemiology

- Colonizes the gastrointestinal tract of animals and humans as a minor member of the microbiome; rare or absent from the oropharynx or genital tract of healthy individuals
- Endogenous infections

Diseases

- Associated with pleuropulmonary, intraabdominal, genital, and skin and soft-tissue infections characterized by abscess formation; bacteremia

Diagnosis

- Characteristic Gram stain from clinical specimens
- Grows rapidly in cultures incubated anaerobically
- Easily identified by biochemical tests, gene sequencing, and MALDI mass spectrometry

Treatment, Prevention, and Control

- Resistant to penicillin and 25% of isolates resistant to clindamycin; uniformly susceptible to metronidazole, and most strains to carbapenems and piperacillin-tazobactam

The non–spore-forming anaerobic cocci and rods are a heterogeneous group of bacteria that form the predominant bacterial population on the skin and mucosal surfaces (Table 31-1). The organisms are primarily opportunistic pathogens, typically responsible for endogenous infections, and are usually recovered in mixtures of aerobic and anaerobic bacteria. Many of these anaerobes have fastidious nutritional requirements and grow slowly on laboratory media. Fortunately, the appropriate management and treatment of most infections with these organisms can be based on the knowledge that a mixture of aerobic and anaerobic organisms is present in the clinical specimen and does not require isolation and identification of the individual organisms. An exception to these general rules is infections caused by *Bacteroides fragilis,* a rapidly growing gram-negative rod that can produce life-threatening disease.

• Anaerobic Gram-Positive Cocci

At one time, all clinically significant anaerobic cocci were included in the genus *Peptostreptococcus.* Unfortunately, it

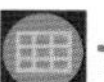
Table 31-1 Important Non–Spore-Forming Anaerobic Bacteria

Organism	Historical Derivation
Anaerobic Gram-Positive Cocci	
Anaerococcus	*an,* without; *aer,* air; *coccus,* berry or coccus (anaerobic coccus)
Atopobium	*atopos,* uncommon; *bios,* life
Finegoldia	Named after the American microbiologist Sid Finegold
Micromonas	*micro,* tiny; *monas,* cell (tiny cell)
Peptoniphilus	*peptonum,* peptone; *philus,* loving (loving peptones, major source of energy)
Peptostreptococcus	*pepto,* cook or digest (the digesting streptococcus)
Schleiferella	Named after the German microbiologist K.H. Schleifer
Anaerobic Gram-Positive Rods	
Actinomyces	*aktinos,* ray; *mykes,* fungus (ray fungus, referring to the radial arrangement of filaments in granules)
Bifidobacterium	*bifidus,* cleft; *bakterion,* small rod (a small clefted or bifurcated rod)
Eubacterium	*eu,* good or beneficial (a beneficial rod, that is, a rod normally present)
Lactobacillus	*lacto,* milk (milk bacillus; organism originally recovered in milk; also, lactic acid is the primary metabolic product of fermentation)
Mobiluncus	*mobilis,* capable of movement or being active; *uncus,* hook (motile curved rod)
Propionibacterium	*propionicum,* propionic acid (propionic acid is the primary metabolic product of fermentation)
Anaerobic Gram-Negative Cocci	
Veillonella	Named after A. Veillon, the French bacteriologist who isolated the type species
Anaerobic Gram-Negative Rods	
Bacteroides	*bacter,* staff or rod; *idus,* shape (rod-shaped)
Fusobacterium	*fusus,* a spindle; *bakterion,* a small rod (a small, spindle-shaped rod)
Parabacteroides	*para,* related to (related to *Bacteroides*)
Porphyromonas	*porphyreos,* purple; *monas,* unit (pigmented rods)
Prevotella	Named after the French microbiologist A.R. Prevot, a pioneer in anaerobic microbiology

was recognized that these organisms were organized in a single genus based primarily on their Gram-stain morphology and inability to grow aerobically. More sophisticated methods have since been used to reclassify many of these species into new genera. Although some anaerobic cocci are more virulent than others and some are associated with specific diseases, specific identification of the different genera is generally unnecessary, and knowledge that anaerobic cocci are associated with an infection is typically sufficient.

The anaerobic gram-positive cocci normally colonize the oral cavity, gastrointestinal (GI) tract, genitourinary tract, and skin. They produce infections when they spread from these sites to normally sterile sites. For example, bacteria colonizing the upper airways can cause sinusitis and pleuropulmonary infections; bacteria in the intestines can cause intraabdominal infections; bacteria in the genitourinary tract can cause endometritis, pelvic abscesses, and salpingitis; bacteria on the skin can cause cellulitis and soft-tissue infections; and bacteria that invade the blood can produce infections in bones and solid organs (Figure 31-1).

Laboratory confirmation of infections with anaerobic bacteria is complicated by the following three factors: (1) care must be taken to prevent contamination of the clinical specimen with the anaerobes that normally colonize the skin and mucosal surfaces, (2) the collected specimen must be transported in an oxygen-free container to prevent loss of the organisms, and (3) specimens should be cultured on nutritionally enriched media for a prolonged period (i.e., 5 to 7 days). In addition, some species of staphylococci and streptococci grow initially in an anaerobic atmosphere only and may be mistaken for anaerobic cocci. However, these organisms eventually grow well in air supplemented with 10% carbon dioxide (CO_2), so they cannot be classified as anaerobes.

Anaerobic cocci are usually susceptible to **penicillins** and **carbapenems** (e.g., imipenem, meropenem, ertapenem); have intermediate susceptibility to broad-spectrum cephalosporins, clindamycin, erythromycin, and the tetracyclines; and are resistant to the aminoglycosides (as are all anaerobes). Specific therapy is generally indicated in monomicrobic infections; however, because most infections with these organisms are polymicrobic, broad-spectrum therapy against aerobic and anaerobic bacteria is usually selected.

Anaerobic Gram-Positive Rods

The non–spore-forming gram-positive rods are a diverse collection of facultatively anaerobic or strictly anaerobic bacteria that colonize the skin and mucosal surfaces (Table 31-2;

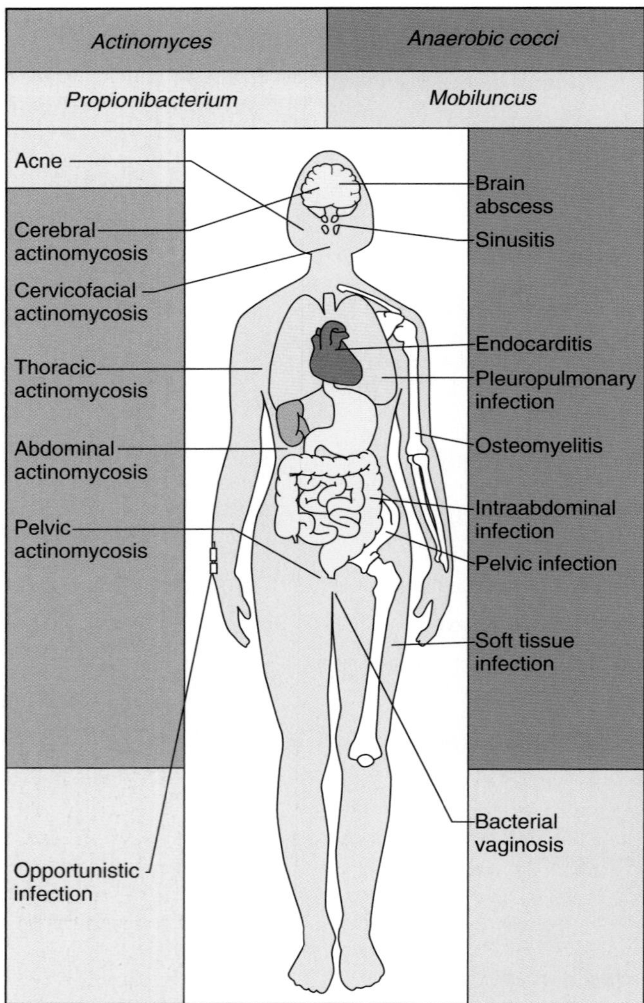

FIGURE 31-1 Diseases associated with anaerobic cocci and *Actinomyces, Propionibacterium,* and *Mobiluncus*—the latter three being anaerobic, non–spore-forming, gram-positive rods.

also see Table 31-1). *Actinomyces, Mobiluncus, Lactobacillus,* and *Propionibacterium* are well-recognized opportunistic pathogens, whereas other genera such as *Bifidobacterium* and *Eubacterium* can be isolated in clinical specimens but rarely cause human disease.

Actinomyces

Actinomyces organisms are facultatively anaerobic or strictly anaerobic gram-positive rods. They are not acid-fast (in contrast to the morphologically similar *Nocardia* species), they grow slowly in culture, and they tend to produce **chronic, slowly developing infections.** They typically develop delicate filamentous forms or hyphae (resembling fungi) in clinical specimens or when isolated in culture (Figure 31-2). However, these organisms are true bacteria in that they lack mitochondria and a nuclear membrane, reproduce by fission, and are inhibited by penicillin but not antifungal antibiotics. Almost 50 species have been described, and many have been implicated in human disease; however, many isolates were likely misidentified before gene sequencing and mass

 Table 31-2 **Anaerobic, Non–Spore-Forming, Gram-Positive Rods**

Organism	Human Disease
Actinomyces spp.	Localized oral infections, actinomycosis (cervicofacial, thoracic, abdominal, pelvic, central nervous system)
Propionibacterium spp.	Acne, lacrimal canaliculitis, opportunistic infections
Mobiluncus spp.	Bacterial vaginosis, opportunistic infections
Lactobacillus spp.	Endocarditis, opportunistic infections
Eubacterium spp.	Opportunistic infections
Bifidobacterium spp.	Opportunistic infections

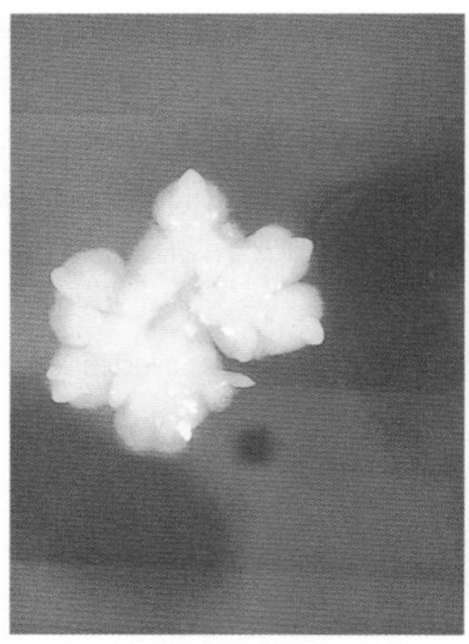

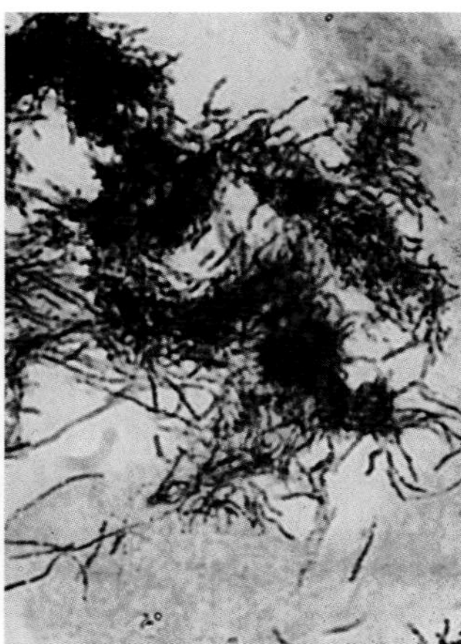

FIGURE 31-2 Macroscopic colony *(left)* and Gram stain *(right)* of *Actinomyces.*

spectrometry techniques were available. Regardless, identification at the genus level is generally sufficient.

Actinomyces organisms colonize the upper respiratory, GI, and female genital tracts but are not normally present on the skin surface. The organisms have a low virulence potential and cause disease only when the normal mucosal barriers are disrupted by trauma, surgery, or infection. Infections caused by actinomycetes are **endogenous,** with no evidence of person-to-person spread or disease originating from an exogenous source.

Classic disease caused by *Actinomyces* is termed **actinomycosis** (in keeping with the original idea that these organisms were fungi or "mycoses"). Actinomycosis is characterized by the development of chronic granulomatous lesions that become suppurative and form abscesses connected by sinus tracts. Macroscopic colonies of organisms resembling grains of sand can frequently be seen in the abscesses and sinus tracts. These colonies, called **sulfur granules** because they may appear yellow or orange, are masses of filamentous organisms bound together by calcium phosphate (Figure 31-3). The areas of suppuration are surrounded by fibrosing granulation tissue, which gives the surface overlying the involved tissues a hard or woody consistency.

Most actinomycetes infections are **cervicofacial,** developing in patients who have poor oral hygiene or have

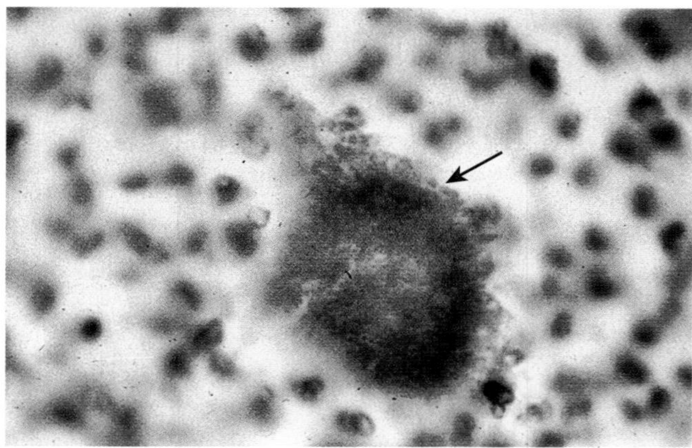

FIGURE 31-3 Sulfur granule collected from the sinus tract in a patient with actinomycosis. Delicate filamentous rods *(arrow)* are seen at the periphery of the crushed granule.

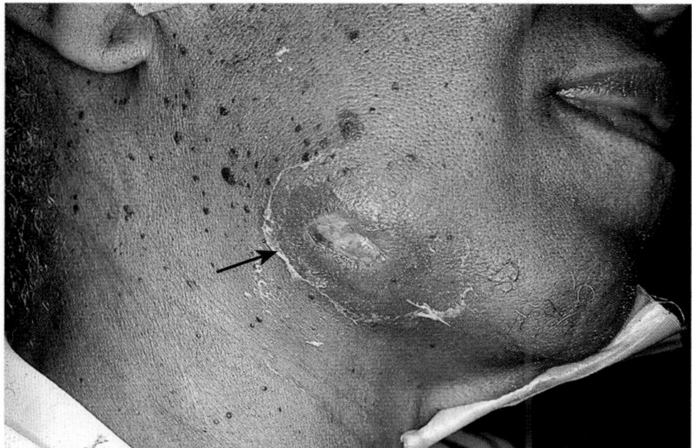

FIGURE 31-4 Patient suffering from cervicofacial actinomycosis. Note the draining sinus tract *(arrow)*.

undergone an invasive dental procedure or oral trauma (Figure 31-4). In these patients, the *Actinomyces* present in the mouth invade into the diseased tissue and initiate the infectious process. The disease may occur as an acute pyogenic infection or as a slowly evolving, relatively painless process. The finding of tissue swelling with fibrosis and scarring, as well as draining sinus tracts along the angle of the jaw and neck, should alert the physician to the possibility of actinomycosis. Symptoms of **thoracic actinomycosis** are nonspecific. Abscesses may form in the lung tissue early in the disease and then spread into adjoining tissues as the disease progresses. **Abdominal actinomycosis** can spread throughout the abdomen, potentially involving virtually every organ system. **Pelvic actinomycosis** can occur as a relatively benign form of vaginitis or, more commonly, there can be extensive tissue destruction, including development of tuboovarian abscesses or ureteral obstruction (Figure 31-5; Clinical Case 31-1). The most common manifestation of **central nervous system actinomycosis** is a solitary brain abscess, but meningitis, subdural empyema, and epidural abscess are also seen. Actinomycosis in patients with chronic granulomatous disease, presenting as a nonspecific febrile illness, has recently been described.

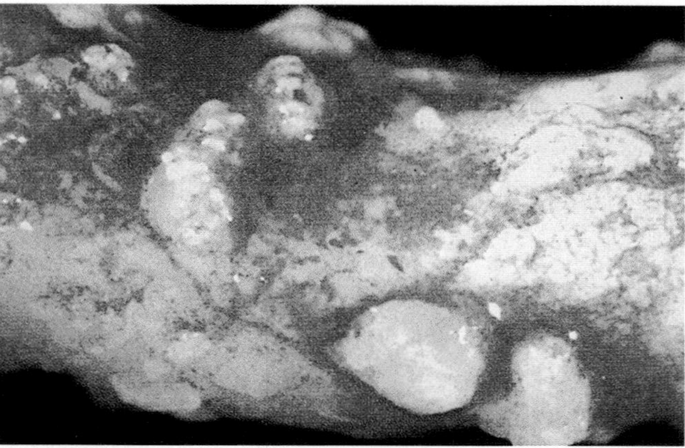

FIGURE 31-5 *Actinomyces* species can colonize the surface of foreign bodies, such as this intrauterine device, leading to the development of pelvic actinomycosis. (From Smith E. In Lambert H, Farrar W, editors: *Infectious diseases illustrated,* London, 1982, Gower.)

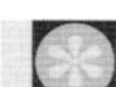

Clinical Case 31-1 Pelvic Actinomycosis

Quercia and associates (*Med Mal Infect* 36:393–395, 2006) described a classic presentation of pelvic actinomycosis associated with an intrauterine contraceptive device (IUD). The patient was a 41-year-old woman who presented with a 5-month history of abdominal and pelvic pain, weight loss, malaise, and a yellow vaginal discharge. Since 1994 she had used an IUD, which was removed in June 2004. Her symptoms began soon after removal of the IUD. A computed tomography scan revealed a large pelvic mass involving the fallopian tubes, as well as numerous hepatic abscesses. A surgical biopsy was performed, and *Actinomyces* was recovered in culture. She underwent surgical debridement and received oral therapy with a penicillin antibiotic for 1 year. This episode illustrates the chronic nature of actinomycosis and the need for surgical drainage and long-term antibiotic therapy.

Laboratory confirmation of actinomycosis is often difficult. Care must be used during collection of clinical specimens that they not become contaminated with *Actinomyces* that are part of the normal bacterial population on mucosal surfaces. Because the organisms are concentrated in sulfur granules and are sparse in involved tissues, a large amount of tissue or pus should be collected. If sulfur granules are detected in a sinus tract or in tissue, the granule should be crushed between two glass slides, stained, and examined microscopically. Thin, gram-positive, branching rods can be seen along the periphery of the granules (see Figure 31-3). *Actinomyces* are fastidious and grow slowly under anaerobic conditions; it can take 2 weeks or more for the organisms to be isolated. Colonies appear white and have a domed surface that can become irregular after incubation for a week or more, resembling the top of a molar (Figure 31-6). Recovery of *Actinomyces* in blood cultures should be evaluated carefully because most isolates represent transient, insignificant bacteremia from the oropharynx or GI tract.

Treatment for actinomycosis involves the combination of drainage of a localized abscess or **surgical debridement** of

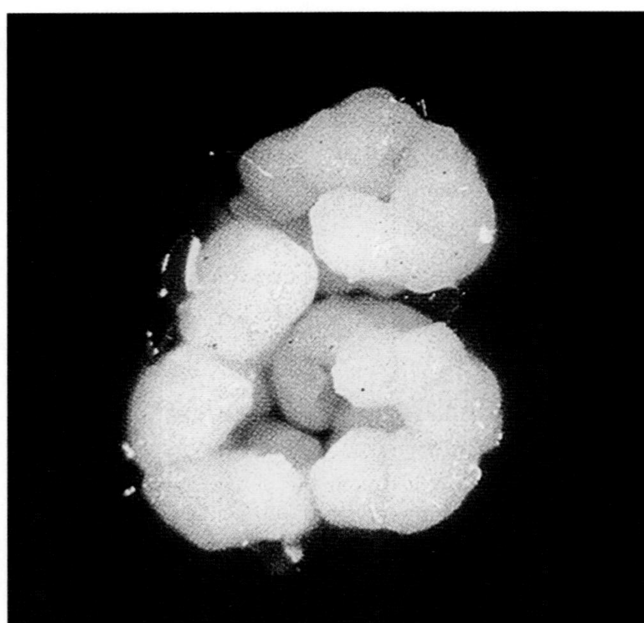

FIGURE 31-6 Molar tooth appearance of *Actinomyces israelii* after incubation for 1 week. This colonial morphology serves as a reminder that the bacteria are normally found in the mouth.

the involved tissues, and prolonged administration of antibiotics. *Actinomyces* are uniformly susceptible to **penicillin** (considered the antibiotic of choice), carbapenems, macrolides, and clindamycin. Most species are resistant to metronidazole, and the tetracyclines have variable activity. An undrained focus should be suspected in patients with infections that do not appear to respond to prolonged therapy (e.g., 4 to 12 months). The clinical response is generally good even in patients who have suffered extensive tissue destruction. Maintenance of good oral hygiene and the use of appropriate antibiotic prophylaxis when the mouth or GI tract is penetrated can lower the risk of these infections.

Lactobacillus

Lactobacillus species are facultatively anaerobic or strictly anaerobic rods. They are found as part of the normal flora of the mouth, stomach, intestines, and genitourinary tract. The organisms are most commonly isolated in urine specimens and blood cultures. Because lactobacilli are the most common organism in the urethra, their recovery in urine cultures usually is a result of contamination of the specimen, even when large numbers of the organisms are present. The reason lactobacilli rarely cause infections of the urinary tract is their inability to grow in urine. Invasion into blood occurs in one of the following three settings: (1) **transient bacteremia** from a genitourinary source (e.g., after childbirth or a gynecologic procedure), (2) **endocarditis** (Clinical Case 31-2), and (3) **opportunistic septicemia** in an immunocompromised patient. Strains of lactobacilli used as probiotics have occasionally been associated with human infections, most commonly in immunocompromised patients.

Treatment of endocarditis and opportunistic infections is difficult because lactobacilli are resistant to vancomycin (an antibiotic commonly active against gram-positive bacteria) and are inhibited but not killed by other antibiotics. A combination of **penicillin with an aminoglycoside** is required for bactericidal activity.

Clinical Case 31-2 *Lactobacillus* Endocarditis

The following is a classical description of endocarditis caused by *Lactobacillus* (Salvana and Frank, *J Infect* 53:5–10, 2006). A 62-year-old woman was admitted for atrial fibrillation and a 2-week history of flulike symptoms. The patient had had dental work performed 4 weeks before this admission and did not take antibiotic prophylaxis despite a history of rheumatic fever in childhood, with resultant mitral valve prolapse and regurgitation. On examination, the patient was afebrile, tachycardic, and mildly tachypneic. Cardiac examination was significant for a systolic murmur. Three blood cultures were collected, all of which yielded *Lactobacillus acidophilus* upon culture. The patient was treated with the combination of penicillin and gentamicin for a total of 6 weeks, resulting in complete recovery. This case illustrates the need for antibiotic prophylaxis during dental procedures for patients with underlying damaged heart valves, and the requirement for combined antibiotic therapy for successful treatment of serious infections caused by lactobacilli.

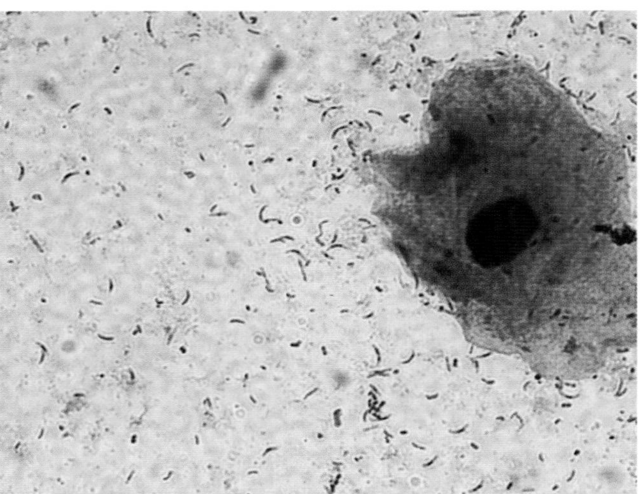

FIGURE 31-7 Gram stain of *Mobiluncus*. The bacterial cells are curved and have pointed ends.

Mobiluncus

Members of the genus *Mobiluncus* are obligate anaerobic, gram-variable or gram-negative, curved rods with tapered ends. Despite their appearance in Gram-stained specimens (Figure 31-7), they are classified as gram-positive rods because they (1) have a gram-positive cell wall, (2) lack endotoxin, and (3) are susceptible to vancomycin, clindamycin, erythromycin, and ampicillin but resistant to colistin. The organisms are fastidious, growing slowly even on enriched media supplemented with rabbit or horse serum. Of the two species of *Mobiluncus*, ***M. curtisii*** is rarely found in the vaginas of healthy women but is abundant in women with **bacterial vaginosis** (vaginitis). Their microscopic appearance is a useful marker for this disease, but the precise role of these organisms in the pathogenesis of bacterial vaginosis is unclear.

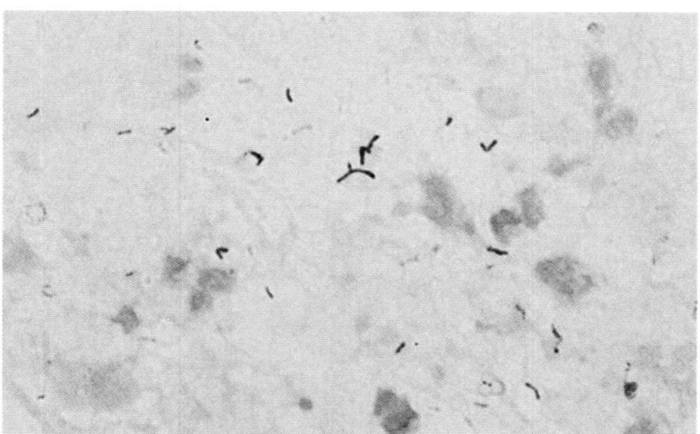

FIGURE 31-8 Gram stain of *Propionibacterium* in a blood culture.

Clinical Case 31-3 *Propionibacterium* Shunt Infection

Chu and associates (*Neurosurgery* 49:717–720, 2001) reported three patients with central nervous system infections with *Propionibacterium acnes*. The following patient illustrates the problems with this organism. A 38-year-old woman with congenital hydrocephalus presented with a 1-week history of decreased level of consciousness, headaches, and emesis. She had undergone numerous ventriculoperitoneal shunt placements in the past, with the last one placed 5 years before this presentation. The patient was afebrile and had no meningeal signs, but she was somnolent and arousable only by deep stimuli. Cerebrospinal fluid (CSF) collected from the shunt contained no erythrocytes but had 55 WBCs; protein levels were high and glucose slightly low. Pleomorphic gram-positive rods were observed on Gram stain, and *P. acnes* grew in the anaerobic culture of the CSF. After 1 week of therapy with high-dose penicillin, the CSF remained positive by Gram stain and culture. The patient was taken to surgery, where all foreign material was removed, and she was treated with penicillin for an additional 10 weeks. This patient illustrates the chronic, relatively asymptomatic nature of this disease, the need to remove the shunt and other foreign bodies, and the need to treat for a prolonged period of time.

Propionibacterium

Propionibacteria are small gram-positive rods often arranged in short chains or clumps (Figure 31-8). They are commonly found on the skin (in contrast with the *Actinomyces*), conjunctiva, and external ear, and in the oropharynx and female genital tract. The most commonly isolated species is ***Propionibacterium acnes***. *P. acnes* is responsible for two types of infections: (1) **acne vulgaris** (as the name implies) in teenagers and young adults and (2) **opportunistic infections** (Clinical Case 31-3) in patients with prosthetic devices (e.g., artificial heart valves or joints) or intravascular lines (e.g., catheters, cerebrospinal fluid shunts). Propionibacteria are also commonly isolated in blood cultures, but this finding usually represents contamination with bacteria on the skin at the phlebotomy site.

The central role of *P. acnes* in acne is to stimulate an inflammatory response. Production of a low-molecular-weight peptide by the bacteria residing in sebaceous follicles attracts leukocytes. The bacteria are phagocytized and, after release of bacterial hydrolytic enzymes (lipases, proteases, neuraminidase, and hyaluronidase), stimulate a localized inflammatory response. *P. propionicum* is associated with endodontic abscesses and lacrimal canaliculitis (inflammation of the tear duct).

Propionibacteria can grow on most common media, although it may take 2 to 5 days for growth to appear. Care must be taken to avoid contamination of the specimen with the organisms normally found on the skin. The significance of the recovery of an isolate must also be interpreted in light of the clinical presentation (e.g., a catheter or other foreign body can serve as a focus for these opportunistic pathogens).

Acne is unrelated to the effectiveness of skin cleansing, because the lesion develops within the sebaceous follicles. For this reason, acne is managed primarily through topical application of benzoyl peroxide and antibiotics. Antibiotics such as erythromycin and clindamycin have proved effective for treatment.

Bifidobacterium and *Eubacterium*

Bifidobacterium and *Eubacterium* species are commonly found in the oropharynx, large intestine, and vagina. These bacteria can be isolated in clinical specimens but have a very low virulence potential and usually represent clinically insignificant contaminants. Confirmation of their etiologic role in an infection requires their repeated isolation in large numbers from multiple specimens and the absence of other pathogenic organisms.

Anaerobic Gram-Negative Cocci

The anaerobic gram-negative cocci are rarely isolated in clinical specimens except when present as contaminants. Members of the genus *Veillonella* are the predominant anaerobes in the oropharynx, but they represent less than 1% of all anaerobes isolated in clinical specimens. The other anaerobic cocci are rarely isolated.

Anaerobic Gram-Negative Rods

The most important anaerobic gram-negative rods are in the genera *Bacteroides, Fusobacterium, Parabacteroides, Porphyromonas,* and *Prevotella* (see Table 31-1). These anaerobes are the predominant bacteria on most mucosal surfaces, outnumbering aerobic bacteria 10- to 1000-fold. Despite the abundance and diversity of these bacteria, most infections are caused by relatively few species (Table 31-3).

The genus *Bacteroides* is composed of more than 90 species and subspecies, with *Bacteroides fragilis* the most important member of this genus. A characteristic common to most species in the genus *Bacteroides* is that their growth is stimulated by bile. *Bacteroides* species are pleomorphic in size and shape and resemble a mixed population of organisms in a casually examined Gram stain (Figure 31-9). Other anaerobic gram-negative rods can be very small (e.g., *Porphyromonas, Prevotella*) or elongated (e.g., *Fusobacterium;* Figure 31-10). Most gram-negative anaerobes respond weakly to Gram stain, so stained specimens must be carefully examined. Although *Bacteroides* species grow rapidly in culture, the other anaerobic gram-negative rods are fastidious, and cultures may have to be incubated for 3 days or longer before the bacteria can be detected.

Table 31-3 Predominant Anaerobic Gram-Negative Bacteria Responsible for Human Disease

Infection	Bacteria
Head and neck	*Bacteroides ureolyticus*
	Fusobacterium nucleatum
	Fusobacterium necrophorum
	Porphyromonas asaccharolytica
	Porphyromonas gingivalis
	Prevotella intermedia
	Prevotella melaninogenica
Intraabdominal	*Bacteroides fragilis*
	Bacteroides thetaiotaomicron
	P. melaninogenica
Gynecologic	*B. fragilis*
	Prevotella bivia
	Prevotella disiens
Skin and soft tissue	*B. fragilis*
Bacteremia	*B. fragilis*
	B. thetaiotaomicron
	Fusobacterium spp.

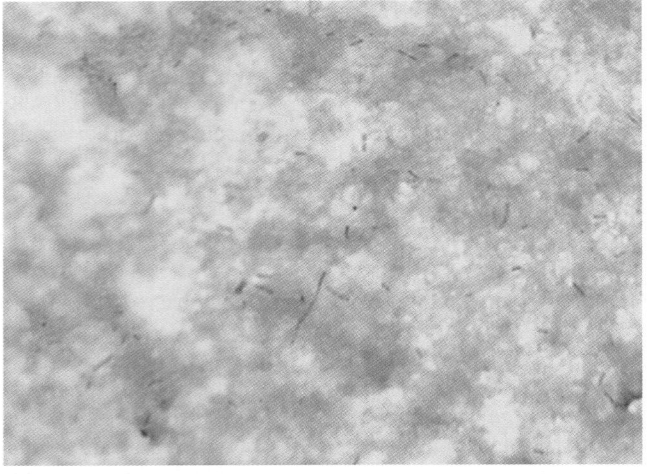

FIGURE 31-9 *Bacteroides fragilis.* Organisms appear as faintly staining, pleomorphic, gram-negative rods.

Physiology and Structure

Bacteroides have a typical gram-negative cell wall structure, which can be surrounded by a **polysaccharide capsule.** A major component of the cell wall is a surface lipopolysaccharide (LPS). In contrast to the LPS molecules in the aerobic gram-negative rods, the *Bacteroides* LPS has little or no endotoxin activity. This is because the lipid A component of LPS lacks phosphate groups on the glucosamine residues, and the number of fatty acids linked to the amino sugars is reduced; both factors are correlated with the loss of pyrogenic activity.

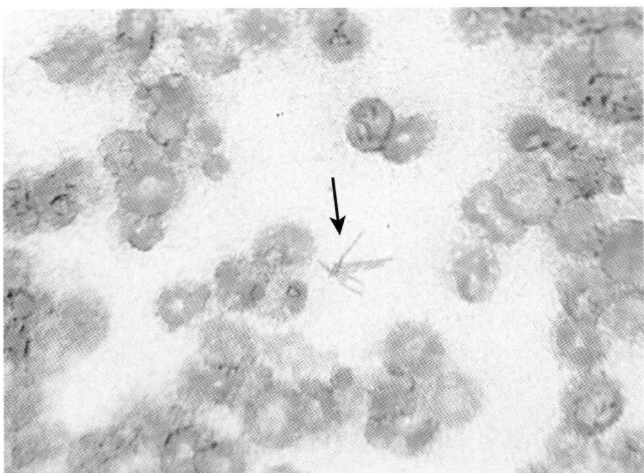

FIGURE 31-10 *Fusobacterium nucleatum.* Organisms *(arrow)* are thin, faintly staining, and elongated with tapered ends (e.g., fusiform).

Pathogenesis and Immunity

B. fragilis, other *Bacteroides* species, and *Porphyromonas gingivalis* can adhere to epithelial cells and extracellular molecules (e.g., fibrinogen, fibronectin, lactoferrin) by means of fimbriae. The fimbriae of *P. gingivalis* are also important for inducing expression of proinflammatory cytokines such as tumor necrosis factor (TNF)-α and interleukin (IL)-1β. *B. fragilis* and *Prevotella melaninogenica* strains can also adhere to peritoneal surfaces more effectively than other anaerobes because their surface is covered with a polysaccharide capsule. This capsule is also antiphagocytic, similar to other bacterial capsules, and it is the major virulence factor in *B. fragilis*. The short-chain fatty acids (e.g., succinic acid) produced during anaerobic metabolism inhibit phagocytosis and intracellular killing. Finally, proteases are produced by some *Porphyromonas* and *Prevotella* species that degrade immunoglobulins.

In general, anaerobes capable of causing disease can tolerate exposure to oxygen. Catalase and superoxide dismutase, which inactivate hydrogen peroxide and the superoxide free radicals (O_2^-), respectively, are present in many pathogenic strains.

Strains of enterotoxigenic *B. fragilis* that cause diarrheal disease produce a **heat-labile zinc metalloprotease toxin (*B. fragilis* toxin).** This toxin causes morphologic changes of the intestinal epithelium via F-actin rearrangement, with the resultant stimulation of chloride secretion and fluid loss. The enterotoxin also induces IL-8 secretion by intestinal epithelial cells, thus contributing to inflammatory damage to the epithelium.

Epidemiology

As already stated, anaerobes colonize the human body in large numbers (functioning to stabilize the resident bacterial flora), prevent colonization by pathogenic organisms from exogenous sources, aid in the digestion of food, and stimulate host immunity. These normal protective organisms produce disease only when they move from their endogenous homes to normally sterile sites. Thus the organisms in the resident flora are able to spread by trauma or disease from the normally colonized mucosal surfaces to sterile tissues or fluids.

As expected, endogenous infections are characterized by the presence of a polymicrobial mixture of organisms. It is important to realize, however, that the mixture of organisms that appear on healthy mucosal surfaces differs from the mixture in diseased tissues. Studies of the microbial population, or **microbiome,** of healthy mucosal surfaces show a complex mixture of many species of bacteria. In the disease state, the mixture changes to less diversity (i.e., fewer species are represented) and predominance of the most clinically significant organisms. For example, *B. fragilis* is commonly associated with pleuropulmonary, intraabdominal, and genital infections. However, the organism constitutes less than 1% of the colonic flora and is rarely isolated from the oropharynx or genital tract of healthy people unless highly selective techniques are used.

Clinical Diseases

Respiratory Tract Infections

Nearly half of the chronic infections of the sinuses and ears, and virtually all periodontal infections, involve mixtures of gram-negative anaerobes, with *Prevotella, Porphyromonas, Fusobacterium,* and non-*fragilis Bacteroides* the most commonly isolated. Anaerobes are less commonly associated with infections of the lower respiratory tract unless there is a history of aspiration of oral secretions.

Brain Abscess

Anaerobic infections of the brain are typically associated with a history of chronic sinusitis or otitis. Such history is confirmed by radiologic evidence of direct extension into the brain. A less common cause of such infections is bacteremic spread from a pulmonary source. In this case, multiple abscesses are present. The most common anaerobes in these polymicrobial infections are species of *Prevotella, Porphyromonas,* and *Fusobacterium* (as well as *Peptostreptococcus* and other anaerobic and aerobic cocci).

Intraabdominal Infections

Despite the diverse population of bacteria that colonize the GI tract, relatively few species are associated with intraabdominal infections. Anaerobes are recovered in virtually all of these infections, with *B. fragilis* the most common organism (Figure 31-11). Other important anaerobes are *B. thetaiotaomicron* and *P. melaninogenica,* as well as the anaerobic and aerobic gram-positive cocci.

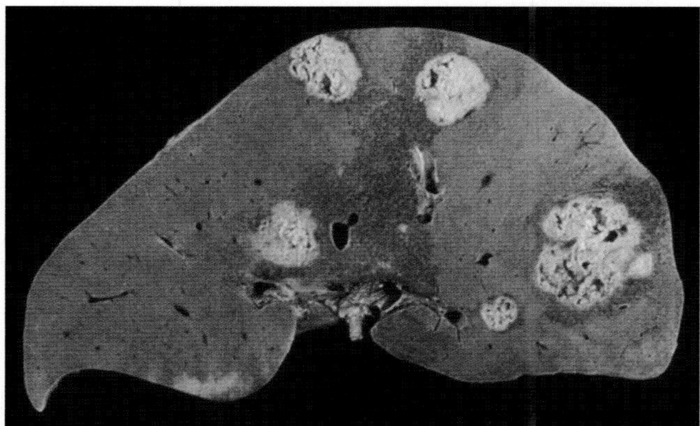

FIGURE 31-11 Liver abscesses caused by *Bacteroides fragilis.*

Gynecologic Infections

Mixtures of anaerobes are often responsible for causing infections of the female genital tract (e.g., pelvic inflammatory disease, abscesses, endometritis, surgical wound infections). Although a variety of anaerobes can be isolated in patients with these infections, *Prevotella bivia* and *Prevotella disiens* are the most important; *B. fragilis* is commonly responsible for abscess formation.

Skin and Soft-Tissue Infections (Clinical Case 31-4)

Although anaerobic gram-negative bacteria are not part of the normal flora of the skin (in contrast to *Peptostreptococcus* and *Propionibacterium* organisms), they can be introduced by a bite or through contamination of a traumatized surface. In some cases, the organisms may simply colonize a wound without producing disease; in other cases, colonization may quickly progress to life-threatening disease such as myonecrosis (Figure 31-12). *B. fragilis* is the organism most commonly associated with significant disease.

Bacteremia

Anaerobes were at one time responsible for more than 20% of all clinically significant cases of bacteremia; however, these organisms now cause 3% to 10% of such infections. The reduced incidence of disease is not completely understood but probably can be attributed to the widespread use of broad-spectrum antibiotics. *B. fragilis* is the anaerobe most commonly isolated in blood cultures.

Gastroenteritis

Strains of enterotoxin-producing *B. fragilis* can produce a self-limited watery diarrhea. The majority of infections have been observed in children younger than 5 years, although disease has also been reported in adults.

Laboratory Diagnosis

Microscopy

Microscopic examination of specimens from patients with suspected anaerobic infections can be useful. Although the

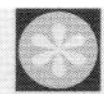

Clinical Case 31-4 Retroperitoneal Necrotizing Fasciitis

Pryor and associates (*Crit Care Med* 29:1071–1073, 2001) described an unfortunate patient with a polymicrobic fasciitis. A 38-year-old man with a 10-year history of human immunodeficiency virus infection underwent an uncomplicated hemorrhoidectomy. Over the next 5 days, thigh and buttock pain developed, as well as nausea and vomiting. At the time this patient presented to the hospital, he had a heart rate of 120 beats/min, blood pressure of 120/60 mm Hg, respiratory rate of 22 respirations/min, and temperature of 38.5° C. Physical examination revealed extensive erythema around the surgical site, flank, thighs, and abdominal wall. Gas was observed in the tissues underlying the areas of erythema and extended to his upper chest. At surgery, extensive areas of tissue necrosis and foul-smelling brownish exudates were found. Multiple surgeries to aggressively debride the involved tissues were necessary. Cultures obtained at surgery grew a mixture of aerobic and anaerobic organisms, with *Escherichia coli*, β-hemolytic streptococci, and *Bacteroides fragilis* predominating. This clinical case illustrates the potential complications of rectal surgery: aggressive destruction of tissue, polymicrobic etiology with *B. fragilis* as a prominent organism, and foul-smelling necrotic tissue with gas production.

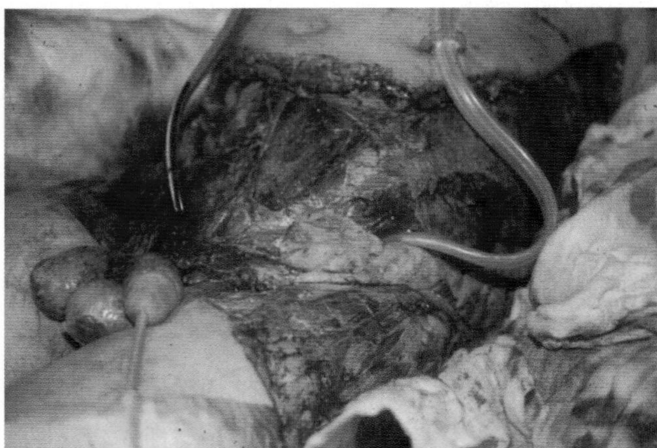

FIGURE 31-12 Synergistic polymicrobial infection involving *Bacteroides fragilis* and other anaerobes. The infection started at the scrotum and rapidly spread up the trunk and down the thighs, with extensive myonecrosis.

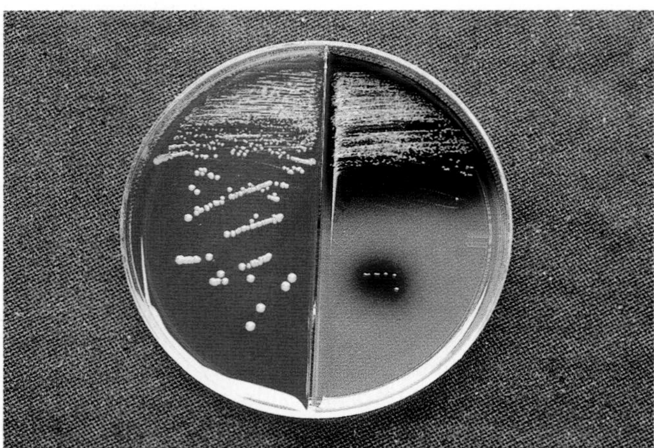

FIGURE 31-13 Growth of *Bacteroides fragilis* on *Bacteroides* bile-esculin agar. Most aerobic and anaerobic bacteria are inhibited by bile and gentamicin in this medium, whereas the *B. fragilis* group of organisms is stimulated by bile, resistant to gentamicin, and able to hydrolyze esculin, producing a black precipitate.

bacteria may stain faintly and irregularly, the finding of pleomorphic gram-negative rods can serve as useful preliminary information.

Culture

Specimens should be collected and transported to the laboratory in an oxygen-free system, promptly inoculated onto specific media for the recovery of anaerobes, and incubated in an anaerobic environment. Because most anaerobic infections are endogenous, it is important to collect specimens so that they are not contaminated with the normal bacterial population present on the adjacent mucosal surface. Specimens should also be kept in a moist environment, because drying causes significant bacterial loss.

Most *Bacteroides* grow rapidly and should be detected within 2 days; however, recovery of other gram-negative anaerobes may require longer incubation. In addition, it is sometimes difficult to recover all clinically significant bacteria because of the different organisms present in polymicrobial infections. The use of selective media, such as media supplemented with bile, has facilitated the recovery of most important anaerobes (Figure 31-13).

Biochemical Identification

Although identification of gram-negative anaerobes has traditionally been performed by biochemical tests, the proliferation of newly recognized species has made this approach unreliable. Sequence analysis of species-specific genes (e.g., 16S ribosomal RNA gene) is a reliable but time-consuming and expensive approach. More recently, proteomic tools (i.e., mass spectrometry for spectral analysis of species-specific protein profiles) have been used for organism identification.

Treatment, Prevention, and Control

Antibiotic therapy combined with surgical intervention is the main approach for managing serious anaerobic infections. Virtually all members of the *B. fragilis* group, many *Prevotella* and *Porphyromonas* species, and some *Fusobacterium* isolates produce β-lactamases. This enzyme renders the bacteria resistant to penicillin and many cephalosporins. Antibiotics with the best activity against gram-negative anaerobic rods are **metronidazole**, **carbapenems** (e.g., imipenem, meropenem), and **β-lactam–β-lactamase inhibitors** (e.g., piperacillin-tazobactam). Clindamycin resistance in *Bacteroides,* which is plasmid mediated, has become more prevalent; an average of 20% to 25% of the isolates in the United States are now resistant.

Because *Bacteroides* species constitute an important part of the normal microbial flora, and because infections result from endogenous spread of the organisms, disease is virtually impossible to control. It is important to recognize, however, that disruption of the natural barriers around the mucosal surfaces by diagnostic or surgical procedures can introduce these organisms into normally sterile sites. If the barriers are invaded, prophylactic treatment with antibiotics may be indicated.

Bibliography

Aldridge KE, O'Brien M: In vitro susceptibilities of the *Bacteroides fragilis* group species: change in isolation rates significantly affects overall susceptibility data, *J Clin Microbiol* 40:4349–4352, 2002.

Brook I, Frazier EH: Infections caused by *Propionibacterium* species, *Rev Infect Dis* 3:819–822, 1991.

Cannon JP, Lee TA, Bolanos JT, et al: Pathogenic relevance of *Lactobacillus:* a retrospective review of over 200 cases, *Eur J Clin Microbiol Infect Dis* 24:31–40, 2005.

Kononen E, Wade WG: Actinomyces and related organisms in human infections, *Clin Microbiol Rev* 28:419–442, 2015.

Murdoch D: Gram-positive anaerobic cocci, *Clin Microbiol Rev* 11:81–120, 1998.

Reichenbach J, Lopatin U, Mahlaoui N, et al: *Actinomyces* in chronic granulomatous disease: an emerging and unanticipated pathogen, *Clin Infect Dis* 49:1703–1710, 2009.

Sears C: Enterotoxigenic *Bacteroides fragilis:* a rogue among symbiotes, *Clin Microbiol Rev* 22:349–369, 2009.

Tiveljung A, Forsum U, Monstein H-J: Classification of the genus *Mobiluncus* based on comparative partial 16S rRNA gene analysis, *Int J Syst Bacteriol* 46:332–336, 1996.

Wexler H: *Bacteroides*: the good, the bad, and the nitty-gritty, *Clin Microbiol Rev* 20:593–621, 2007.

CHAPTER

TREPONEMA, BORRELIA, AND LEPTOSPIRA

A 23-year-old homosexual man **presented to the emergency department with a painless ulcer on the shaft of his penis. Primary syphilis was suspected and later confirmed by serologic tests. It is a very rare student who is not familiar with the diseases caused by the spirochetes discussed in this chapter: syphilis, Lyme disease, relapsing fever, and leptospirosis.**

1. Why do many patients with syphilis develop chronic infections even though penicillin is uniformly active against *Treponema pallidum?*
2. What reservoir and vector are most important for the transmission of *Borrelia burgdorferi* infections in humans?
3. What diagnostic test is most useful for early localized Lyme disease and for patients who develop arthritis or neurologic complications?
4. What specimens are optimum for recovering *Leptospira* in culture?

Answers to these questions are available on StudentConsult.com.

• SUMMARIES CLINICALLY SIGNIFICANT ORGANISMS

Treponema pallidum

Trigger Words

Thin coiled spirochete, not cultured, darkfield microscopy, STD and congenital infections, person-to-person, painless ulcer (chancre)

Biology and Virulence

- Coiled spirochete (0.1 to 0.2 × 6 to 20 μm) too thin to be seen with Gram or Giemsa stains; observed by darkfield microscopy
- Outer membrane proteins promote adherence to host cells
- Hyaluronidase facilitates perivascular infiltration
- Coating of fibronectin protects against phagocytosis
- Tissue destruction primarily results from host's immune response to infection

Epidemiology

- Humans are the only natural host
- Venereal syphilis transmitted by sexual contact or congenitally
- Syphilis occurs worldwide, with no seasonal incidence

Diseases

- Syphilis presents as primary disease (painless ulcer or chancre at site of infection, with regional lymphadenopathy and bacteremia), secondary syphilis (flulike syndrome with generalized mucocutaneous rash and bacteremia), and late-stage disease (diffuse chronic inflammation and destruction of any organ or tissue); congenital (latent multiorgan malformations, fetal death)

Diagnosis

- Darkfield or direct fluorescent antibody microscopy useful if mucosal ulcers are observed in primary or secondary stages of syphilis
- Serology is very sensitive in secondary and late stages of syphilis

Treatment, Prevention, and Control

- Penicillin is drug of choice; doxycycline is administered if patient is allergic to penicillin
- Safe sex practices should be emphasized, and sexual partners of infected patients should be treated
- No vaccine is available

Borrelia

Trigger Words

Large spirochetes, erythema migrans, Lyme disease, relapsing fever, hard and soft ticks, body louse

Biology and Virulence

- Borreliae are large (0.2 to 0.5 × 8 to 30 μm) and can be seen when stained with aniline dyes (e.g., Giemsa, Wright stains)
- Immune reactivity against Lyme disease agents may be responsible for clinical disease

Epidemiology

Lyme Disease

- *Borrelia burgdorferi* causes disease in the United States and Europe; *Borrelia garinii* and *Borrelia afzelii* cause disease in Europe and Asia
- Transmitted by hard ticks from mice to humans; reservoirs—mice, deer, ticks; vectors include *Ixodes scapularis* in eastern and midwestern United States, *Ixodes pacificus* in western United States, *Ixodes ricinus* in Europe, and *Ixodes persulcatus* in Eastern Europe and Asia

- 95% of Lyme disease cases in the United States are from two principal foci: the Northeast and Mid-Atlantic states (Maine to Virginia) and the Upper Midwest (Minnesota, Wisconsin)
- Individuals at risk for Lyme disease include people exposed to ticks in areas of high endemicity
- Worldwide distribution
- Seasonal incidence corresponds to feeding patterns of vectors; most cases of Lyme disease in the United States occur in late spring and early summer (feeding pattern of nymph stage of ticks); peak in June and July

Epidemic Relapsing Fever
- Etiologic agent is *Borrelia recurrentis*
- Person-to-person transmission; reservoir—humans; vector—human body louse
- Individuals at risk are people exposed to lice (epidemic disease) in crowded or unsanitary conditions
- Occurs in Ethiopia, Rwanda, and the Andean foothills

Endemic Relapsing Fever
- Many *Borrelia* species are responsible
- Transmitted from rodents to humans; reservoirs—rodents, small mammals, soft ticks; vector—soft ticks
- Individuals at risk are people exposed to ticks (endemic disease) in rural areas
- Worldwide distribution and is in the western part of the United States

Diseases

- Borreliae are responsible for two human diseases: Lyme disease and relapsing fever (epidemic and endemic)
- *Borrelia* species responsible for relapsing fever are able to undergo antigenic shift and escape immune clearance; periodic febrile and afebrile periods result from antigenic variation

Diagnosis

- Serology is test of choice for Lyme disease
- Polymerase chain reaction tests available for Lyme disease but relatively insensitive
- Microscopy is the test of choice for diagnosis of relapsing fever

Treatment, Prevention, and Control

- For early localized or disseminated Lyme disease, treatment is with amoxicillin, tetracycline, cefuroxime; late manifestations are treated with intravenous penicillin or ceftriaxone
- For relapsing fever, treatment is with tetracycline or erythromycin
- Improved sanitary conditions to decrease risk of epidemic relapsing fever
- Reduced exposure to hard ticks (Lyme disease) and soft ticks (relapsing fever) through use of insecticides, application of insect repellents to clothing, and wearing protective clothing that reduces exposure of skin to insects

Leptospira

Trigger Words

Thin, coiled spirochetes, flulike disease, aseptic meningitis, Weil disease, zoonotic, contaminated water exposure

Biology and Virulence

- Thin, coiled spirochetes (0.1×6 to 20 μm) that grow slowly in specialized cultures
- Able to directly invade and replicate in tissues, inducing an inflammatory response
- Immune complex produces renal disease (glomerulonephritis)
- Most disease is a mild virus-like syndrome
- Systemic leptospirosis presents most commonly as aseptic meningitis
- Overwhelming disease (Weil disease) is characterized by vascular collapse, thrombocytopenia, hemorrhage, and hepatic and renal dysfunction

Epidemiology

- U.S. reservoirs: rodents (particularly rats), dogs, farm animals, and wild animals
- Humans: accidental end-stage host
- Organism can penetrate the skin through minor breaks in the epidermis
- People are infected with leptospires through exposure to water contaminated with urine from an infected animal or handling of tissues from an infected animal
- People at risk are those exposed to urine-contaminated streams, rivers, and standing water; occupational exposure to infected animals for farmers, meat handlers, and veterinarians
- Infection is rare in the United States but has worldwide distribution
- Disease is more common during warm months (recreational exposure)

Diagnosis

- Microscopy not useful because too few organisms are generally present in fluids or tissues
- Culture blood or cerebrospinal fluid in the first 7 to 10 days of illness; urine after the first week
- Serology using the microscopic agglutination test is relatively sensitive and specific but not widely available in resource-limited countries; enzyme-linked immunosorbent assay tests are less accurate but can be used to screen patients

Treatment, Prevention, and Control

- Treatment with penicillin or doxycycline
- Doxycycline but not penicillin is used for prophylaxis
- Herds and domestic pets should be vaccinated
- Rats should be controlled

The bacteria in the order Spirochaetales have been grouped together on the basis of their common morphologic properties (Table 32-1). These spirochetes are thin, helical (0.1 to 0.5×5 to 20 μm), gram-negative bacteria. The order Spirochaetales is subdivided into 4 families and 14 genera, of which 3 genera (*Treponema* and *Borrelia* in the family Spirochaetaceae, and *Leptospira* in the family Leptospiraceae) are responsible for human disease (Table 32-2).

Treponema

The most important treponemal species that causes human disease is *Treponema pallidum,* with three subspecies. The subspecies are distinguished by their epidemiologic characteristics, clinical presentation, and host range in experimental animals. *T. pallidum* subspecies *pallidum* (referred to as *T. pallidum* in this chapter) is the etiologic agent of the

Table 32-1 Medically Important Genera in the Order Spirochaetales

Spirochaetales	Human Disease	Etiologic Agent
Family Spirochaetaceae		
Genus *Borrelia*	Epidemic relapsing fever	*B. recurrentis*
	Endemic relapsing fever	Many *Borrelia* species
	Lyme borreliosis	*B. burgdorferi, B. garinii, B. afzelii*
Genus *Treponema*	Venereal syphilis	*T. pallidum* subsp. *pallidum*
	Endemic syphilis (bejel)	*T. pallidum* subsp. *endemicum*
	Yaws	*T. pallidum* subsp. *pertenue*
Family Leptospiraceae		
Genus *Leptospira*	Leptospirosis	*Leptospira* spp.

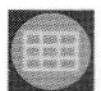
Table 32-2 Important Spirochetes

Organism	Historical Derivation
Treponema	*trepo,* turn; *nema,* a thread (a turning thread; refers to the morphology of the bacteria)
T. pallidum	*pallidum,* pale (refers to the fact that these organisms are not stained with traditional dyes)
Borrelia	Named after A. Borrel
B. recurrentis	*recurrens,* recurring (reference to relapsing fever)
B. hermsii	*hermsii,* of hermsi (named after the tick vector *Ornithodoros hermsii*)
B. burgdorferi	Named after W. Burgdorfer
Leptospira	*lepto,* thin; *spira,* a coil (a thin coil; refers to the morphology of the bacteria)

venereal disease **syphilis;** *T. pallidum* subspecies *endemicum* causes endemic syphilis **(bejel);** and *T. pallidum* subspecies *pertenue* causes **yaws.** Bejel and yaws are nonvenereal diseases.

Physiology and Structure

T. pallidum and related pathogenic treponemes are thin, tightly coiled spirochetes (0.1 to 0.2 × 6 to 20 μm) with pointed, straight ends. Traditional diagnostic tests such as microscopy and culture are of little value because the spirochetes are too thin to be seen with light microscopy in specimens stained with Gram or Giemsa stains, and these spirochetes do not grow in cell-free cultures. Limited growth of the organisms has been achieved in cultured rabbit epithelial cells, but replication is slow (doubling time is 30 hours) and can be maintained for only a few generations. The reason for this failure to grow *T. pallidum* in vitro is because the tricarboxylic acid cycle is missing in the bacteria and they are dependent on host cells for all purines, pyrimidines, and most amino acids. In addition, spirochetes are microaerophilic or anaerobic and extremely sensitive to oxygen, consistent with the discovery the bacteria have no genes for catalase or superoxide dismutase to protect them from oxygen toxicity.

Pathogenesis and Immunity

The inability to grow *T. pallidum* to high concentrations in vitro has limited detection of specific virulence factors in this organism. However, analysis of the entire genome sequence and the unique structural properties of this spirochete have revealed some insights. Although a number of lipoproteins are anchored in the bacterial cytoplasmic membrane, most or all are not exposed on the surface of the outer membrane. Thus the lack of species-specific antigens on the cell surface allows the spirochete to evade the immune system. Although the bacteria are able to resist phagocytosis, they can adhere to host fibronectin, allowing direct interaction with the host tissues. Analysis of the genome sequence demonstrates the presence of at least five hemolysins, but it is unclear if they mediate tissue damage. Likewise, it has been proposed that production of hyaluronidase facilitates perivascular infiltration, but this remains to be demonstrated. Most investigators believe that the tissue destruction and lesions observed in syphilis are primarily the consequence of the patient's immune response to infection.

Epidemiology

Syphilis is found worldwide and is the third most common sexually transmitted bacterial disease in the United States (after *Chlamydia trachomatis* and *Neisseria gonorrhoeae* infections). Overall, the incidence of disease has decreased since the advent of penicillin therapy in the early 1940s, although periodic increases have been observed that correspond to changes in sexual practices (e.g., use of birth control pills in the 1960s, gay bath houses in the 1970s, increased prostitution related to crack cocaine use in the 1990s). A troubling trend is evolving now. Between 2000 and 2012, the incidence of newly acquired disease has increased each year. In 2012 the Centers for Disease Control and Prevention (CDC) reported that there were almost 50,000 reported new cases of syphilis, with 15,667 primary and secondary stage disease, the most infectious forms of syphilis. The increase in syphilis is primarily in homosexual males. This likely reflects the mistaken perception that sexually acquired diseases, including human immunodeficiency virus (HIV) infections, can be controlled effectively with antibiotics, so unprotected sex is incorrectly considered a low-risk activity. Unfortunately, patients infected with syphilis are at increased risk for transmitting and acquiring HIV when genital lesions are present. Thus, despite a concerted public health effort to eliminate syphilis, this disease remains a serious problem in sexually active populations.

Natural syphilis is exclusive to humans and has no other known natural hosts. *T. pallidum* is extremely labile, unable to survive exposure to drying or disinfectants. Thus syphilis cannot be spread through contact with inanimate objects such as toilet seats. The most common route of spread is by direct sexual contact. The disease can also be acquired congenitally or by transfusion with contaminated blood. Syphilis is not highly contagious; the risk of contracting the disease after a single sexual contact is estimated to be 30%. However, contagiousness is influenced by the stage of disease in the infectious person. *T. pallidum* is transferred primarily during

Clinical Case 32-1 History of Syphilis

The origins of syphilis have been debated for decades. Examination of skeletal remains recovered in the Americas, Europe, Asia, and Africa may have resolved this debate. The disease we know as syphilis is likely to have evolved from yaws and, more recently, bejel. Each disease produces distinctive bone alterations. The earliest evidence of treponemal disease was in Africa and appeared to have spread to the Americas through an Asian route. At the time Columbus sailed to the Americas, syphilis was well established throughout the New World, including the Dominican Republic, where he landed. In contrast, there is no evidence of syphilis in pre-Columbian Europe, Africa, or Asia. Thus it is likely that Columbus' crew acquired this New World disease and introduced it into the Old World population upon their return home.

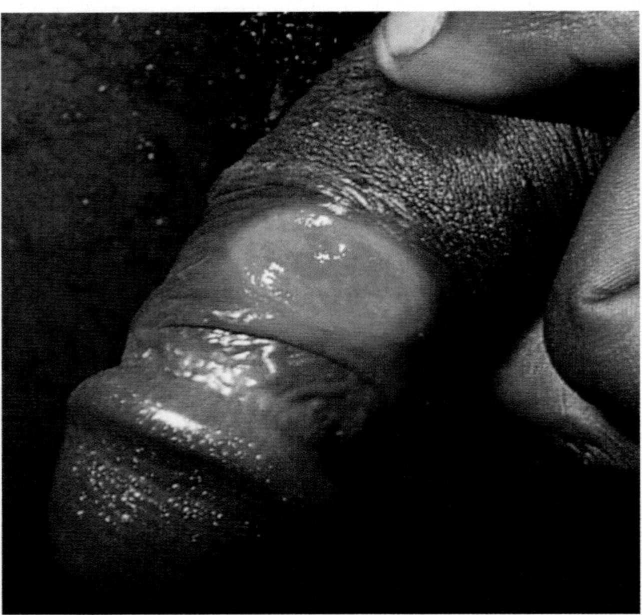

FIGURE 32-1 Primary chancre of the penile shaft. Typically the lesion is painless unless secondary bacterial infection is present. Large numbers of spirochetes are present in the lesion. (From Morse SA, Ballard RC, Holmes KK, et al: *Atlas of sexually transmitted diseases and AIDS,* ed 4, London, 2010, Saunders.)

the early stages of disease when many organisms are present in moist cutaneous or mucosal lesions. During the early stages of disease, the patient becomes bacteremic, and if the disease is untreated, intermittent bacteremia can persist for as long as 8 years. Congenital transmission from mother to fetus can occur at any time during this period. Even after bacteremia ceases, the disease can remain active.

Clinical Diseases (Clinical Case 32-1)

The clinical course of syphilis evolves through three phases. The initial or **primary phase** is characterized by one or more skin lesions **(chancres)** at the site where the spirochete penetrated (Figure 32-1). The lesion develops 10 to 90 days after the initial infection and starts as a papule but then erodes to become a **painless ulcer** with raised borders. Histologic examination of the lesion reveals endarteritis and periarteritis (characteristic of syphilitic lesions at all stages) and infiltration of the ulcer with polymorphonuclear leukocytes and macrophages. Phagocytic cells ingest spirochetes, but the organisms often survive, with abundant organisms present in the chancre. In most patients, a painless regional lymphadenopathy develops 1 to 2 weeks after the appearance of the chancre, which represents a local focus for the proliferation of spirochetes and dissemination in the blood. The fact that this ulcer heals spontaneously within 2 months gives the patient a false sense of relief.

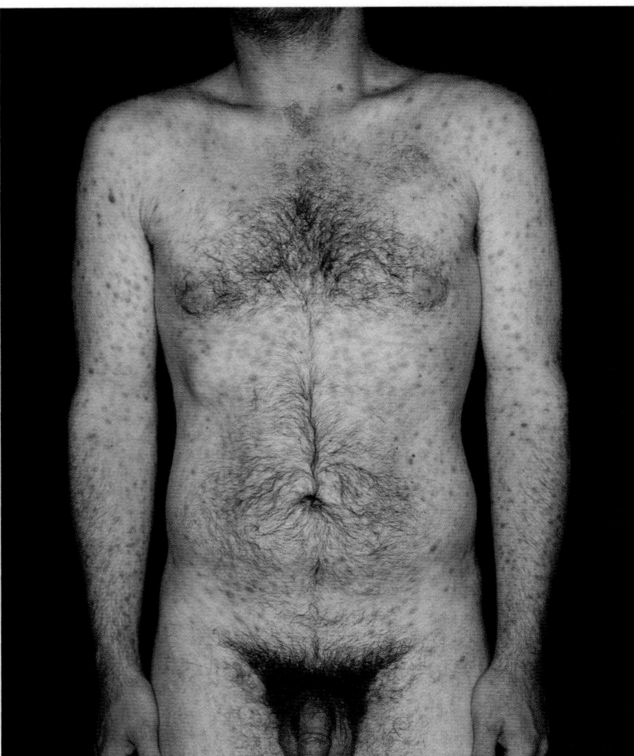

FIGURE 32-2 Disseminated rash in secondary syphilis. (From Habif TP: *Clinical dermatology: a color guide to diagnosis and therapy,* ed 5, London, 2010, Mosby.)

In the **secondary phase,** the clinical signs of disseminated disease appear, with prominent skin lesions dispersed over the entire body surface (Figure 32-2). In this stage, patients typically experience a flulike syndrome with sore throat, headache, fever, myalgias (muscle aches), anorexia, lymphadenopathy (swollen lymph nodes), and a generalized mucocutaneous rash. The flulike syndrome and lymphadenopathy generally appear first and then are followed a few days later by the disseminated rash. The rash can be variable (macular, papular, pustular) and cover the entire skin surface (including the palms and soles). Raised lesions called **condylomata lata** may occur in moist skinfolds, and erosions may develop in the mouth and on other mucosal surfaces. As with the primary chancre, these lesions are highly infectious. The rash and symptoms resolve spontaneously within a few weeks, and patients may undergo spontaneous remission, enter the latent or clinically inactive stage of disease, or progress to the **late phase** of disease.

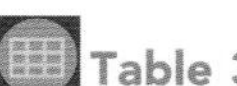

Table 32-3 Diagnostic Tests for Syphilis

Diagnostic Test	Method or Examination
Microscopy	Darkfield
	Direct fluorescent antibody staining
Culture	Not available
Serology	Nontreponemal tests: Venereal Disease Research Laboratory (VDRL) test Rapid plasma reagin (RPR) test Unheated serum reagin (USR) test Toluidine red unheated serum test (TRUST)
	Treponemal tests: Fluorescent treponemal antibody-absorption (FTA-ABS) *Treponema pallidum* particle agglutination (TP-PA) test Enzyme immunoassay (EIA)

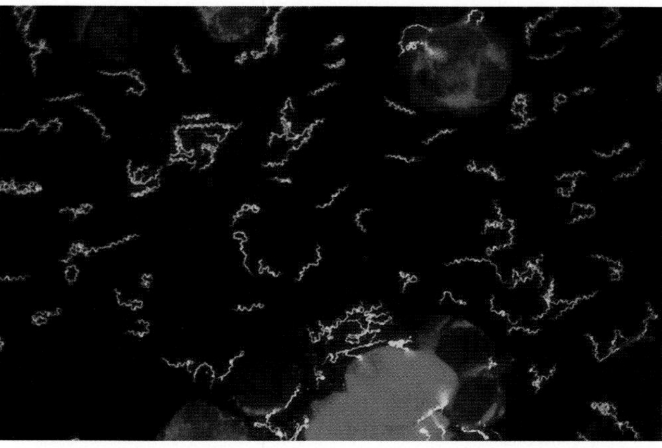

FIGURE 32-3 *Treponema pallidum* in the direct fluorescent antibody test for *T. pallidum*. (From Morse SA, Ballard RC, Holmes KK, et al: *Atlas of sexually transmitted diseases and AIDS*, ed 4, London, 2010, Saunders.)

Approximately one third of untreated patients progress to the tertiary stage of syphilis. Clinical symptoms of the diffuse chronic inflammation characteristic of late syphilis develop after an asymptomatic period of a few years to decades and can cause devastating destruction of virtually any organ or tissue (e.g., arteritis, dementia, blindness). Granulomatous lesions **(gummas)** may be found in bone, skin, and other tissues. The nomenclature of late syphilis reflects the organs of primary involvement (e.g., neurosyphilis, cardiovascular syphilis). An increased incidence of neurosyphilis despite adequate therapy for early syphilis has been documented in patients with acquired immunodeficiency syndrome (AIDS). In addition, spirochetes are introduced into the central nervous system during the early stages of disease, and neurologic symptoms (e.g., meningitis) can develop within the first few months of disease. Thus neurosyphilis is not exclusively a late manifestation.

In utero infections (congenital syphilis) can lead to serious fetal disease, resulting in latent infections, multiorgan malformations, or death of the fetus. Most infected infants are born without clinical evidence of the disease, but rhinitis then develops and is followed by a widespread desquamating maculopapular rash. Teeth and bone malformation, blindness, deafness, and cardiovascular syphilis are common in untreated infants who survive the initial phase of disease.

Laboratory Diagnosis (Table 32-3)

Microscopy

Because *T. pallidum* is too thin to be seen by light microscopy, **darkfield microscopy** or **special fluorescent stains** must be used. The diagnosis of primary, secondary, or congenital syphilis can be made rapidly by darkfield examination of the exudate from skin lesions; however, the test is reliable only when an experienced microscopist examines the clinical material immediately, when actively motile spirochetes can be observed. The spirochetes do not survive transport to the laboratory, and tissue debris can be mistaken for nonviable spirochetes. Material collected from oral and rectal lesions should not be examined, because nonpathogenic spirochetes can be routinely observed in those specimens. Because of the limitations of darkfield microscopy, a more useful test for detecting *T. pallidum* is the **direct fluorescent antibody test.** Fluorescein-labeled antitreponemal antibodies are used to stain the bacteria (Figure 32-3). A monoclonal antibody reagent is available that is specific for pathogenic treponemes, so oral and rectal specimens can be examined. In addition, nonviable spirochetes will also stain, so specimens do not need to be examined immediately after collection.

Culture

Efforts to culture *T. pallidum* in vitro should not be attempted, because the organism does not grow in artificial cultures.

Nucleic Acid–Based Tests

Nucleic acid amplification tests (i.e., polymerase chain reaction [PCR]) have been developed for detecting *T. pallidum* in genital lesions, infant blood, and cerebrospinal fluid (CSF) but are currently not widely available.

Antibody Detection

Syphilis is diagnosed in most patients on the basis of serologic tests. The two general types of tests used are biologically nonspecific (nontreponemal) tests and specific treponemal tests. The nontreponemal tests are used as screening tests because they are rapid to perform and inexpensive. Positive reactivity with one of these tests is confirmed with a treponemal test.

Nontreponemal tests measure immunoglobulin (Ig)G and IgM antibodies (also called **reaginic antibodies**) developed against lipids released from damaged cells during the early stage of disease and that appear on the cell surface of treponemes. The antigen used for the nontreponemal tests is **cardiolipin,** which is derived from beef heart. The two tests used most commonly are the **Venereal Disease Research Laboratory (VDRL) test** and the **rapid plasma reagin (RPR) test.** Both tests measure the flocculation of cardiolipin antigen by the patient's serum. Only the VDRL test should be used to test CSF from patients with suspected neurosyphilis. Other nontreponemal tests in use include the unheated serum reagin (USR) test and the toluidine red unheated serum test (TRUST). All nontreponemal tests have essentially the same sensitivity (70% to 85% for primary disease, 100% for secondary disease, 70% to 75% for late syphilis) and specificity (98% to 99%).

Treponemal tests use *T. pallidum* as the antigen and detect specific anti–*T. pallidum* antibodies. The treponemal test results can be positive before the nontreponemal test results become positive in early syphilis, and they can remain positive when the nonspecific test results revert to negative in some patients who have late syphilis. Historically, the most commonly used treponemal test was the **fluorescent treponemal antibody–absorption (FTA-ABS) test.** The FTA-ABS test is an indirect fluorescent antibody test. *T. pallidum* immobilized on glass slides is used as the antigen. The slide is overlayed with the patient's serum, which has been mixed with an extract of nonpathogenic treponemes. The fluorescein-labeled antihuman antibodies are then added to detect the presence of specific antibodies in the patient's serum. Because these tests are technically difficult to interpret, most laboratories now use either the ***Treponema pallidum*** **particle agglutination (TP-PA) test** or one of a number of specific **enzyme immunoassays (EIAs).** The TP-PA test is a microtiter agglutination test. Gelatin particles sensitized with *T. pallidum* antigens are mixed with dilutions of the patient's serum. If antibodies are present, the particles agglutinate. A variety of specific EIAs have been developed and appear to have sensitivities (80% to 95% for primary disease, 100% for secondary and late syphilis) and specificities (96% to 99%) similar to the FTA-ABS and TP-PA tests. These immunoassays are widely used in resource-limited countries where screening with traditional nontreponemal tests and use of more sensitive treponemal tests such as FTA-ABS is impractical.

Because positive reactions with the nontreponemal tests develop late during the first phase of disease, the serologic findings are negative in some patients who present with chancres. However, serologic results are positive within 3 months in all patients and remain positive in untreated patients with secondary syphilis. The antibody titers decrease slowly in patients with untreated syphilis, and serologic results are negative in approximately 25% to 30% of patients with late syphilis. Thus the limitation of the nontreponemal tests is reduced sensitivity in early primary disease and late syphilis. Although the results of treponemal tests generally remain positive for the life of the person who has syphilis, a negative test is unreliable in patients with AIDS.

Successful treatment of primary or secondary syphilis and, to a lesser extent, late syphilis leads to reduced titers measured in the VDRL and RPR tests. Thus these tests can be used to monitor the effectiveness of therapy, although seroreversion is slowed in patients in an advanced stage of disease, those with high initial titers, and those who have previously had syphilis. The treponemal tests are influenced less by therapy than are the VDRL and RPR tests, with seroreversion observed in less than 25% of patients successfully treated during the primary stage of the disease.

Transient false-positive reactions with the nontreponemal tests are seen in patients with acute febrile diseases, after immunizations, and in pregnant women. Long-term false-positive reactions occur most often in patients with chronic autoimmune diseases or infections that involve the liver or that cause extensive tissue destruction. Most false-positive reactions with the treponemal tests are observed in patients with elevated immunoglobulin levels and autoimmune diseases (Box 32-1).

Box 32-1 Conditions Associated with False-Positive Serologic Test Results for Syphilis

Nontreponemal Tests
Viral infection
Rheumatoid arthritis
Systemic lupus erythematosus
Acute or chronic illness
Pregnancy
Recent immunization
Drug addiction
Leprosy
Malaria
Multiple blood transfusions

Treponemal Tests
Pyoderma
Rheumatoid arthritis
Systemic lupus erythematosus
Psoriasis
Crural ulceration
Skin neoplasm
Drug addiction
Mycoses
Lyme disease
Acne vulgaris

Diagnosis of neurosyphilis and congenital syphilis can be problematic. The diagnosis of neurosyphilis is based on clinical symptoms and laboratory findings. A VDRL test on CSF is highly specific but not sensitive. Thus a positive VDRL confirms the diagnosis, but a negative test does not rule out neurosyphilis. In contrast, the FTA-ABS CSF test has high sensitivity but low specificity because of passive transfer of antitreponemal antibodies from blood to CSF. In this case, a positive FTA-ABS CSF test is consistent with neurosyphilis but is not diagnostic, and a negative test would essentially rule out the diagnosis. Positive serologic test results in infants of infected mothers can represent a passive transfer of antibodies or a specific immunologic response to a congenital infection. These two possibilities are distinguished by measuring the antibody titers in the sera of the infant during a 6-month period. The antibody titers in noninfected infants decrease to undetectable levels within 3 months of birth but remain elevated in infants who have congenital syphilis.

Treatment, Prevention, and Control

Penicillin is the drug of choice for treating *T. pallidum* infections. A single intramuscular dose of long-acting benzathine **penicillin G** is used for the early stages of syphilis, and three doses at weekly intervals is recommended for congenital and late syphilis. **Doxycycline** or **azithromycin** can be used as alternative antibiotics for patients allergic to penicillin. Only penicillin can be used for the treatment of neurosyphilis; thus penicillin-allergic patients must undergo desensitization. This is also true for pregnant women, who should not be treated with tetracyclines. Treatment failures with macrolides have been observed, so patients treated with azithromycin should be closely monitored.

Because protective vaccines are not available, syphilis can be controlled only through the practice of safe-sex techniques and adequate contact and treatment of the sex partners of patients who have been documented with infection. The control of syphilis and other venereal diseases has been complicated by an increase in prostitution among drug abusers and high-risk sexual practices in homosexual males.

Borrelia

Members of the genus *Borrelia* cause two important human diseases: **Lyme disease** and **relapsing fever.** The recorded history of Lyme disease began in 1977 when an unusual cluster of children with arthritis was noted in Lyme, Connecticut. Five years later, W. Burgdorfer discovered the spirochete responsible for this disease. Lyme disease is a tick-borne disease with protean manifestations, including dermatologic, rheumatologic, neurologic, and cardiac abnormalities. Initially it was believed that all cases of Lyme disease (or Lyme borreliosis) were caused by one organism, ***B. burgdorferi.*** However, subsequent studies have determined that a complex of at least 10 *Borrelia* species is responsible for Lyme disease in animals and humans. Three species—*B. burgdorferi, B. garinii,* and *Borrelia afzelii*—cause human disease, with *B. burgdorferi* found in the United States and Europe and *B. garinii* and *B. afzelii* found in Europe and central to eastern Asia. This chapter focuses on *B. burgdorferi* infections.

Relapsing fever is a febrile illness characterized by recurrent episodes of fever and septicemia separated by afebrile periods. Two forms of the disease are recognized. *Borrelia recurrentis* is the etiologic agent of **epidemic** or **louse-borne relapsing fever** and is spread person to person by the **human body louse** *(Pediculus humanus).* **Endemic relapsing fever** is caused by as many as 15 species of borreliae and is spread by infected **soft ticks** of the genus *Ornithodoros.*

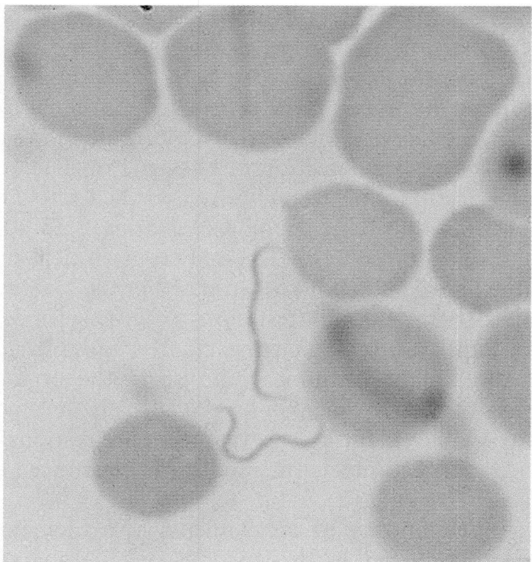

FIGURE 32-4 *Borrelia* organisms are present in the blood of this patient with endemic relapsing fever (Giemsa stain).

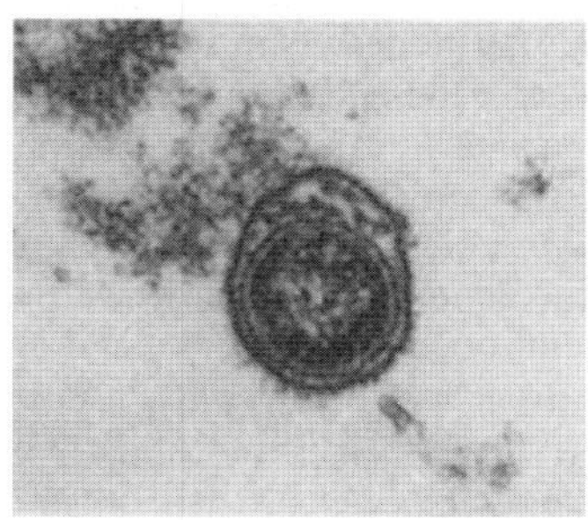

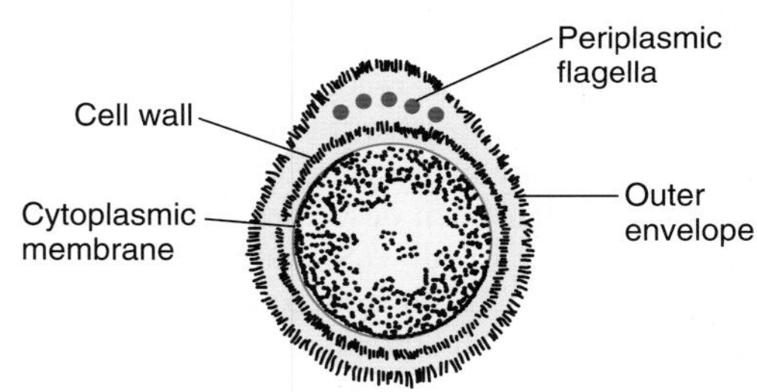

FIGURE 32-5 Electron micrograph and drawing of a cross-section through *Borrelia burgdorferi,* the agent that causes Lyme borreliosis. The protoplasmic core of the bacterium is enclosed in a cytoplasmic membrane and conventional cell wall. This in turn is surrounded by an outer envelope, or sheath. Between the protoplasmic core and outer sheath are periplasmic flagella (also called *axial fibrils*), which are anchored at either end of the bacterium and wrap around the protoplasmic core. (From Steere AC, Grodzicki RL, Kornblatt AN, et al: The spirochetal etiology of Lyme disease, *N Engl J Med* 308:733–740, 1983.)

Physiology and Structure

Members of the genus *Borrelia* stain poorly with the Gram stain reagents and are considered neither gram-positive nor gram-negative, even though they have an outer membrane similar to gram-negative bacteria. They are larger than other spirochetes (0.2 to 0.5 × 8 to 30 μm), stain well with aniline dyes (e.g., Giemsa or Wright stain), and can be easily seen by light microscopy when present in smears of peripheral blood from patients with relapsing fever but not those with Lyme disease (too few organisms to be observed) (Figures 32-4 and 32-5). Borreliae are microaerophilic and have complex nutritional needs (i.e., requiring *N*-acetylglucosamine, long-chain saturated and unsaturated fatty acids, glucose, and amino acids), which makes them difficult to grow in the lab. The species that have been successfully cultured have generation times of 18 hours or longer. Because culture is generally unsuccessful, diagnosis of diseases caused by borreliae is by serology (Lyme disease) or microscopy (relapsing fever).

Pathogenesis and Immunity

The growth of borreliae in both arthropod vectors and mammalian hosts is regulated by differential gene expression with up-regulation or down-regulation of outer surface proteins. For example, outer surface protein A (OspA) is expressed on the surface of *B. burgdorferi* residing in the midgut of unfed ticks. This protein binds specifically to gut proteins. Upon feeding, expression of this protein is repressed, allowing the spirochete to migrate to the salivary glands, and outer surface protein C (OspC) expression, which appears critical for transmission from ticks to mammals, is up-regulated.

Unfortunately, knowledge of the complete genome sequence of *B. burgdorferi* has not led to a clear understanding of how these organisms cause disease. *B. burgdorferi* organisms are present in low numbers in the skin when erythema migrans develops. This has been shown by culture of the organism from skin lesions or detection of bacterial nucleic acids by PCR amplification; however, culture and PCR tests are relatively insensitive in the early phase of disease. In addition, spirochetes are infrequently isolated from clinical material late in the disease. It is not known whether the viable organisms cause these late manifestations of disease or whether they represent immunologic cross-reactivity to *Borrelia* antigens. Although the immune response to the organism is depressed at the time that skin lesions initially develop, antibodies develop over months to years and are responsible for producing the complement-mediated clearance of the borreliae.

Our understanding of mechanisms by which borreliae cause relapsing fever is also incomplete. Members of the genus do not produce recognized toxins and are removed rapidly when a specific antibody response is mounted. The periodic febrile and afebrile cycles of relapsing fever result from the ability of the borreliae to undergo antigenic variation. These spirochetes carry a large number of genes homologous to the OspC gene, but only one gene is expressed at a time. When specific antibodies are formed, agglutination with complement-mediated lysis occurs, and the borreliae are cleared rapidly from the blood. However, switching of the expression of the gene family occurs at a frequency of 10^{-3} to 10^{-4} per generation. Thus a new population of spirochetes with a new lipoprotein coat will appear in the blood, heralding a new febrile episode. These antigenic shifts are the reason serology tests are not used to diagnose relapsing fever.

Epidemiology

Despite the relatively recent recognition of Lyme disease in the United States, retrospective studies have shown that the disease was present for many years in this and other countries. Lyme disease has been described on six continents, in many countries, and in all U.S. states. The incidence of disease has risen dramatically between 1982 (497 cases were reported) and 2012 (>30,000 cases were reported). **Lyme disease is the leading vector-borne disease in the United States.** In 2012, 95% of Lyme disease cases were reported from two U.S. foci: the Northeast and Mid-Atlantic states (Maine to Virginia) and the Upper Midwest (Minnesota and Wisconsin). In recent years the prevalence of Lyme disease in the Pacific West has decreased to low levels. **Hard ticks are the major vectors** of Lyme disease: *Ixodes scapularis* in the Northeast, Mid-Atlantic, and Midwest, and *Ixodes pacificus* on the West Coast. *Ixodes ricinus* is the major tick vector in Europe, and *Ixodes persulcatus* is the major tick vector in Eastern Europe and Asia. The major reservoir hosts in the United States are the white-footed mouse and the white-tailed deer. The **white-footed mouse** is the primary host of larval and nymph forms of *Ixodes* species, and the adult *Ixodes* species infest the **white-tailed deer.** Because the nymph stage causes more than 90% of the cases of documented disease, the mouse host is more relevant for human disease.

Ixodes larvae become infected when they feed on the mouse reservoir. The larva molts to a nymph in late spring and takes a second blood meal; in this case, humans can be accidental hosts. Although the borreliae are transmitted in the tick's saliva during a prolonged period of feeding (≥48 hours), most patients do not remember having had a specific tick bite, because the nymph is the size of a poppy seed. The nymphs mature into adults in the late summer and take a third feeding. Although the white-tailed deer is the natural host, humans can also be infected at this stage. Most infected patients are identified in June and July, although disease can be encountered throughout the year.

Infection	Reservoir	Vector
Relapsing fever epidemic (louse-borne)	Humans	Body louse 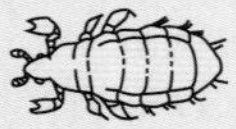
Relapsing fever endemic (tick-borne)	Rodents, soft ticks	Soft tick 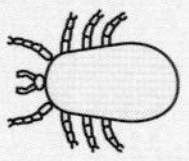
Lyme disease	Rodents, deer, domestic pets, hard ticks	Hard tick 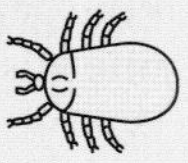

FIGURE 32-6 Epidemiology of *Borrelia* infections.

As previously mentioned, the etiologic agent of louse-borne epidemic relapsing fever is *B. recurrentis,* the vector is the human body louse, and humans are the only reservoir (Figure 32-6). Lice become infected after feeding on an infected person. The organisms are ingested, pass through the wall of the gut, and multiply in hemolymph. Disseminated disease is not believed to occur in lice; thus human infection occurs when the lice are crushed during feeding. Because infected lice do not survive for more than a few months, maintenance of the disease requires crowded, unsanitary conditions (e.g., wars, natural disasters) that permit frequent human contact with infected lice. Although epidemics of louse-borne relapsing fever swept from Eastern to Western Europe in the past century, the disease now appears to be restricted to Ethiopia, Eritrea, Somalia, and Sudan.

Several features distinguish **endemic relapsing fever** from epidemic disease. Tick-borne endemic relapsing fever is a **zoonotic disease,** with rodents, small mammals, and soft ticks (*Ornithodoros* species) the main reservoirs and **many species of *Borrelia*** responsible for the disease. Unlike the louse-borne infections, the borreliae that cause endemic disease produce a disseminated infection in ticks. In addition, the arthropods can survive and maintain an endemic reservoir of infection by transovarian transmission. Furthermore, ticks can survive for months between feedings. A history of a tick bite may not be elicited, because soft ticks are primarily nocturnal feeders and remain attached for only a few minutes. The ticks contaminate the bite wound with borreliae present in saliva or feces. Tick-borne disease is found worldwide, corresponding to the distribution of the *Ornithodoros* tick. In the United States, disease is primarily found in the western states, with Washington and California

 **Clinical Case 32-2 Lyme Disease in Lyme, Connecticut**

In 1977, Steere and associates (*Arthritis Rheum* 20:7–17, 1977) reported an epidemic of arthritis in eastern Connecticut. The authors studied a group of 39 children and 12 adults who developed an illness characterized by recurrent attacks of swelling and pain in a few large joints. Most attacks were for a week or less, but some attacks lasted for months. Twenty-five percent of the patients remembered they had an erythematous cutaneous lesion 4 weeks before the onset of their arthritis. This was the first report of Lyme disease, named after the town in Connecticut where the disease was first recognized. We now know the erythematous lesion (erythema migrans) is the characteristic presentation of early Lyme disease. A few years after this report, the *Borrelia* responsible for Lyme disease, *B. burgdorferi,* was isolated.

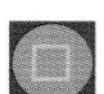 **Box 32-2 Definition of Lyme Disease**

Clinical Case Definition

Either of the Following:

Erythema migrans (≈5 cm in diameter)

At least one late manifestation (i.e., musculoskeletal, nervous system, or cardiovascular involvement) and laboratory confirmation of infection

Laboratory Criteria for Diagnosis

At Least One of the Following:

Isolation of *Borrelia burgdorferi*

Demonstration of diagnostic levels of immunoglobulin (Ig)M or IgG antibodies to the spirochetes

Significant increase in antibody titer between acute and convalescent serum samples

the most common. Worldwide, disease is found in Mexico, Central and South America, the Mediterranean, Central Asia, and much of Africa.

Clinical Diseases

Lyme Disease (Clinical Case 32-2)

Clinical diagnosis of Lyme disease is complicated by the varied manifestations of disease caused by *B. burgdorferi* and other *Borrelia* species, as well as the lack of reliable diagnostic tests. The clinical and laboratory definitions of Lyme disease recommended by the CDC are summarized in Box 32-2. The following paragraph is a description of Lyme disease in the United States. The frequency of the skin lesions and late manifestations differ in disease observed in other countries.

Lyme disease begins as an early localized infection, progresses to an early disseminated stage, and, if untreated, can progress to a late manifestation stage. After an incubation period of 3 to 30 days, one or more skin lesions typically develop at the site of the tick bite. The lesion **(erythema migrans)** begins as a small macule or papule and then enlarges over the next few weeks, ultimately covering an area ranging from 5 cm to more than 50 cm in diameter (Figure 32-7). The lesion typically has a flat, red border and central clearing as it develops; however, erythema, vesicle formation, and central necrosis can also be seen. The lesion fades and disappears within weeks, although new transient lesions may subsequently appear. Although the skin lesion is characteristic of Lyme disease, it is not pathognomonic. A similar skin lesion associated with disease of unknown etiology (STARI, or *s*outhern *t*ick-*a*ssociated *r*ash *i*llness) occurs after the bite of the *Amblyomma americanum* tick (lone star tick). These ticks, found in the southeast and south central regions of the United States, are not infected with *B. burgdorferi.* Other early signs and symptoms of Lyme disease include malaise, severe fatigue, headache, fever, chills, musculoskeletal pains, myalgias, and lymphadenopathy. These symptoms last for an average of 4 weeks.

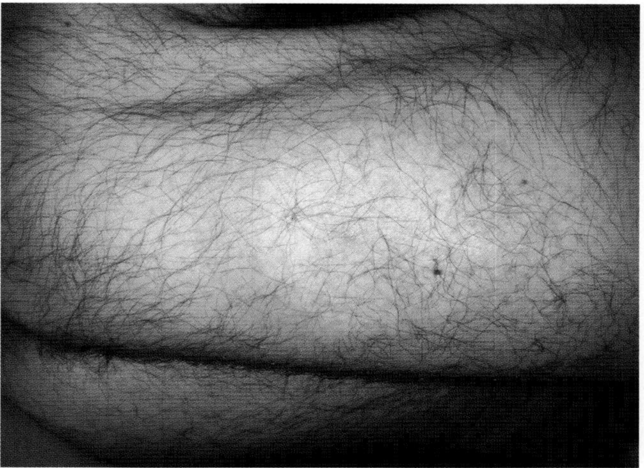

FIGURE 32-7 Erythema migrans rash on the thigh of the author's son (PRM). An engorged nymph stage of an *Ixodes* tick was found 3 days after exposure. Twelve days later, the rash appeared with accompanying localized pain and progressed to 5 cm in diameter with central clearing. The rash faded over the next week with doxycycline treatment, and the infection, confirmed by culture of the biopsy, resolved with no secondary complications.

Hematogenous dissemination will occur in untreated patients within days to weeks of the primary infection. This stage is characterized by systemic signs of disease (e.g., severe fatigue, headache, fever, malaise), arthritis and arthralgia, myalgia, erythematous skin lesions, cardiac dysfunction, and neurologic signs. Approximately 60% of patients with untreated Lyme disease will develop **arthritis,** typically involving the knee; approximately 10% to 20% will develop **neurologic manifestations** (most commonly facial nerve palsy); and 5% will have **cardiac complications** (usually varying degrees of atrioventricular block).

Late-stage manifestations of Lyme disease in untreated patients can develop months to years after the initial infection. Arthritis can involve one or more joints intermittently. Chronic skin involvement with discoloration and swelling (**acrodermatitis chronica atrophicans**; Figure 32-8) is more common in Lyme disease seen in Europe. The existence of chronic, symptomatic Lyme disease in appropriately treated patients has not been demonstrated definitively.

Relapsing Fever (Clinical Case 32-3)

The clinical presentations of epidemic louse-borne and endemic tick-borne relapsing fever are essentially the same, although a small pruritic eschar may develop at the site of the tick bite. After a 1-week incubation period, the disease

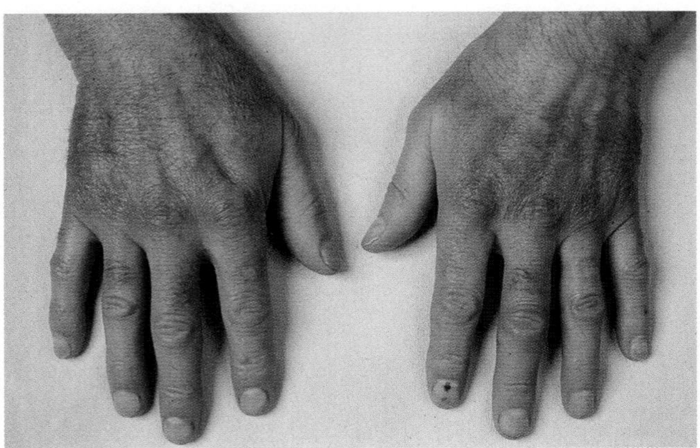

FIGURE 32-8 Acrodermatitis chronica atrophicans. Bluish-red skin lesions characteristic of late disseminated manifestations of Lyme borreliosis. (From Cohen J, Powderly WG, Opal SM: *Infectious diseases,* ed 3, Philadelphia, 2010, Mosby.)

Clinical Case 32-3 Outbreak of Tick-Borne Relapsing Fever

In August 2002, the New Mexico Department of Health was notified of an outbreak of tick-borne relapsing fever (*MMWR Morb Mortal Wkly Rep* 52:809–812, 2003). Approximately 40 people attended a family gathering held in a cabin in the mountains of northern New Mexico. Half of the family members slept overnight in the cabin. Some of the family arrived 3 days before the event to clean the unoccupied cabin. Four days after the event, one of the individuals who arrived early sought care at a local hospital with a 2-day history of fever, chills, myalgia, and a raised pruritic rash on the forearms. Spirochetes were observed on a peripheral blood smear. As many as 14 individuals who attended the family gathering developed symptoms consistent with relapsing fever and had either positive serology or spirochetes observed in blood smears. The majority had a history of fever, headache, arthralgia, and myalgia. Rodent nesting material was found inside the interior walls of the cabin. This outbreak of endemic relapsing fever illustrates the risks associated with exposure to ticks that feed on infected rodents, the fact that tick bites are generally not remembered because the feeding is for a short duration at night, and the relapsing nature of this febrile illness.

is heralded by the abrupt onset of shaking chills, fever, muscle aches, and headache. Splenomegaly and hepatomegaly are common. These symptoms correspond to the bacteremic phase of the disease and resolve after 3 to 7 days, when the borreliae are cleared from the blood. Bacteremia and fever return after a 1-week afebrile period. The clinical symptoms are generally milder and last a shorter time during this and subsequent **febrile episodes.** A single relapse is characteristic of epidemic louse-borne disease, and as many as 10 relapses occur in endemic tick-borne disease. The clinical course and outcome of epidemic relapsing fever tend to be more severe than they are in those with endemic disease, but this may be related to the patients' underlying poor state of health. Mortality with endemic disease is less than 5% but can be as high as 70% in louse-borne epidemic disease. Deaths are caused by cardiac failure, hepatic necrosis, or cerebral hemorrhage.

Laboratory Diagnosis

Microscopy

Microscopic examination of blood or tissues from patients with Lyme disease is not recommended, because *B. burgdorferi* is rarely seen in clinical specimens. Borreliae that cause relapsing fever can be observed during the febrile period on Giemsa- or Wright-stained preparation of blood. This is the most sensitive method for diagnosing relapsing fever, with smears positive for organisms in more than 70% of patients.

Culture

Some borreliae, including *B. recurrentis* and *Borrelia hermsii* (a common cause of endemic relapsing fever in the United States), can be cultured in vitro on specialized media. The cultures are rarely performed in most clinical laboratories because the media are not readily available and the organisms grow slowly on them. There has been limited success with the culture of *B. burgdorferi,* although isolation of the organism has been improved through the use of specialized media. However, the sensitivity of culture is low for all specimens except the initial skin lesion.

Nucleic Acid–Based Tests

Nucleic acid amplification techniques have a sensitivity of approximately 65% to 75% with skin biopsies, 50% to 85% with synovial fluid, and 25% with CSF specimens from patients with documented Lyme disease. These tests are generally restricted to research and reference laboratories, and the test results should be confirmed by culture or serology.

Antibody Detection

Serologic tests are not useful in the diagnosis of relapsing fever, because the borreliae that cause this condition undergo antigenic phase variation. In contrast, serologic testing is the diagnostic test of choice for patients with suspected Lyme disease. The tests most commonly used are the **immunofluorescence assay (IFA)** and **EIA.** The U.S. Food and Drug Administration has cleared more than 70 serologic assays for the diagnosis of Lyme disease. Unfortunately, all serologic tests are relatively insensitive during the early acute stage of disease. IgM antibodies appear 2 to 4 weeks after the onset of erythema migrans in untreated patients; the levels peak after 6 to 8 weeks of illness and then decline to a normal range after 4 to 6 months. The IgM level may remain elevated in some patients with a persistent infection. The IgG antibodies appear later. Their levels peak after 4 to 6 months of illness and persist during the late manifestations of the disease. Thus most patients with late complications of Lyme disease have detectable antibodies to *B. burgdorferi,* although the antibody level may be ablated in patients treated with antibiotics. Detection of antibodies in CSF is strong evidence for neuroborreliosis.

Although cross-reactions are uncommon, positive serologic results must be interpreted carefully, particularly if the titers are low (Box 32-3). Most false-positive reactions occur in patients with syphilis. These false results can be excluded by performing a nontreponemal test for syphilis; the result is negative in patients with Lyme disease. Western blot analysis has been used to confirm the specificity of a positive

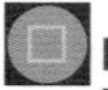

Box 32-3 Bacteria and Diseases Associated with Cross-Reactions in Serologic Tests for Lyme Borreliosis

Treponema pallidum
Oral spirochetes
Other *Borrelia* species
Juvenile rheumatoid arthritis
Rheumatoid arthritis
Systemic lupus erythematosus
Infectious mononucleosis
Subacute bacterial endocarditis

EIA or IFA reaction. A specimen with a negative EIA or IFA reaction does not require further testing. Guidelines for interpretation of Western immunoblots are available on the CDC website (www.cdc.gov). Antigenic heterogeneity in *B. burgdorferi* and other *Borrelia* species that cause Lyme disease affects the test sensitivity. The magnitude of this problem in the United States is unknown, but it should be significant in Europe and Asia, where multiple *Borrelia* species are found to cause Lyme disease. At present, serologic tests should be considered confirmatory and should not be performed in the absence of an appropriate history and clinical symptoms of Lyme disease.

Treatment, Prevention, and Control

The early manifestations of **Lyme disease** are managed effectively with orally administered **amoxicillin, doxycycline,** or **cefuroxime.** Antibiotic treatment lessens the likelihood and severity of late complications. Despite this intervention, Lyme arthritis and acrodermatitis chronica atrophicans occur in a small number of patients. Oral cefuroxime, doxycycline, or amoxicillin has been used for the treatment of these manifestations. Patients with recurrent arthritis or central or peripheral nervous system disease typically require parenteral treatment with intravenous ceftriaxone, cefotaxime, or penicillin G. Previously treated patients with chronic symptoms ("post–Lyme disease syndrome") should be treated symptomatically because there is no evidence that multiple courses of oral or parenteral antibiotics relieve the symptoms.

Relapsing fever has been treated most effectively with **tetracyclines** or **penicillins.** Tetracyclines are the drugs of choice but are contraindicated for pregnant women and young children. A Jarisch-Herxheimer reaction (shock-like profile with rigors, leukopenia, an increase in temperature, and a decrease in blood pressure) can occur in patients within a few hours after therapy is started and must be carefully managed. This reaction corresponds to the rapid killing of borreliae and the possible release of toxic products.

Prevention of tick-borne *Borrelia* diseases includes avoiding ticks and their natural habitats, wearing protective clothing (e.g., long pants tucked into socks), and applying insect repellents. Rodent control is also important in the prevention of endemic relapsing fever. Epidemic louse-borne disease is controlled through the use of delousing sprays and improvements in hygienic conditions.

Vaccines are not available for relapsing fever. A recombinant vaccine directed against the OspA antigen of *B. burgdorferi* was removed from the market in 2002.

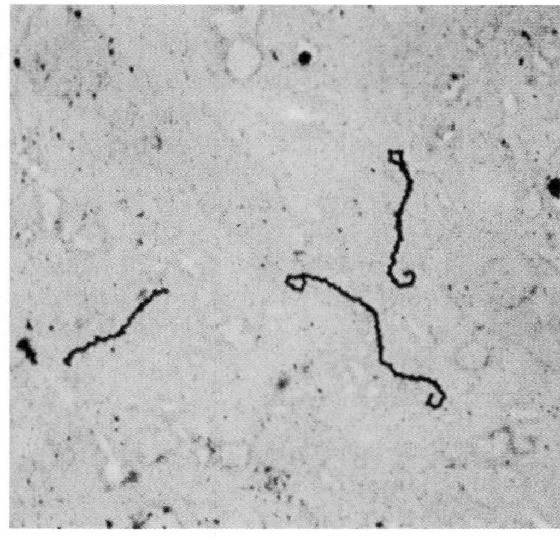

FIGURE 32-9 Silver staining of leptospires grown in culture. Notice the tightly coiled body with hooked ends. (From Emond R, Rowland H: *Color atlas of infectious diseases,* ed 3, London, 1995, Wolfe.)

• *Leptospira*

The taxonomy of the genus *Leptospira* is a source of great confusion. Traditionally the genus has been grouped by phenotypic properties, serologic relationships, and pathogenicity. Pathogenic strains were placed in the species *Leptospira interrogans,* and nonpathogenic strains were placed in the species *Leptospira biflexa*. Each of the two species contained many serovars (i.e., serologically distinct groups). Although this classification scheme exists in the literature, it is not consistent with nucleic acid analysis that supports subdividing the genus into three genera with 17 species in the genus *Leptospira*. To avoid confusion, leptospires will be referred to as pathogenic (for humans) or nonpathogenic without reference to either specific species or serovars.

Physiology and Structure

Leptospires **are thin, coiled spirochetes** (0.1 × 6.0 to 20.0 µm) with a hook at one or both pointed ends (Figure 32-9). Motility is by means of two periplasmic flagella extending the length of the bacteria and anchored at opposite ends. Leptospires are obligate aerobes with optimum growth at 28° C to 30° C in media supplemented with vitamins, long-chain fatty acids, and ammonium salts. The practical significance of this is that these organisms can be cultured in a specialized medium from clinical specimens collected from infected patients, although this is not commonly done.

Pathogenesis and Immunity

Pathogenic leptospires can cause subclinical infection, a mild influenza-like febrile illness, or severe systemic disease **(Weil disease)** with renal and hepatic failure, extensive vasculitis, myocarditis, and death. The number of infecting organisms, the host's immunologic defenses, and the virulence of the infecting strain influence the severity of the disease.

Because leptospires are thin and highly motile, they can **penetrate intact mucous membranes or skin through small cuts or abrasions.** They can then spread in the blood to all tissues, including the central nervous system. *L. interrogans* multiplies rapidly and damages the endothelium of small blood vessels, resulting in the major clinical manifestations of disease (e.g., meningitis, hepatic and renal dysfunction, hemorrhage). Organisms can be **found in blood and CSF early in the disease and in urine during the later stages.** Clearance of leptospires occurs when humoral immunity develops. However, some clinical manifestations may stem from immunologic reactions with the organisms. For example, meningitis develops after the organisms have been removed from the CSF and immune complexes have been detected in renal lesions.

Epidemiology

Leptospirosis has a worldwide distribution. Between 100 and 200 human infections occur in the United States each year, with more than half the cases reported in Hawaii. However, the incidence of disease is significantly underestimated because most infections are mild and misdiagnosed as a "viral syndrome" or viral aseptic meningitis. Because many states failed to report this disease to the public health service, mandatory reporting was discontinued in 1995; however, leptospirosis was reinstated as a nationally notifiable disease in 2013.

Leptospires infect two types of hosts: reservoir hosts and incidental hosts. Endemic, chronic infections are established in **reservoir hosts,** which serve as a permanent reservoir for maintaining the bacteria. Different species and serovars of leptospires are associated with specific reservoir hosts (important for epidemiologic investigations). The **most common reservoirs are rodents and other small mammals.** Leptospires usually cause asymptomatic infections in their reservoir host, in which the spirochetes colonize the renal tubules and are shed in urine in large numbers. Streams, rivers, standing water, and moist soil can be contaminated with urine from infected animals, with organisms surviving for as long as 6 weeks in such sites. Contaminated water or direct exposure to infected animals can serve as a source for infection in **incidental hosts** (e.g., dogs, farm animals, rodents, humans). Most human infections result from recreational exposure to contaminated water (e.g., lakes) or occupational exposure to infected animals (farmers, slaughterhouse workers, veterinarians). Most human infections occur during the warm months, when recreational exposure is greatest. Person-to-person spread has not been documented. By definition, chronic carriage is not established in incidental hosts.

Clinical Diseases (Clinical Case 32-4)

Most human infections with leptospires are clinically inapparent and detected only through the demonstration of specific antibodies. Infection is introduced through skin abrasions or the conjunctiva. Symptomatic infections develop after a 1- to 2-week incubation period and in two phases. The initial phase is similar to an influenza-like illness, with fever, myalgia (muscle pain), chills, headache, vomiting, or diarrhea. During this phase, the patient is bacteremic with the leptospires, and the organisms can frequently be isolated in CSF even though no meningeal symptoms are present. The symptoms may remit after 1 week or the patient may progress to the second phase that is characterized by more severe disease, with the sudden onset of headache, myalgia, chills, abdominal pain, and conjunctival suffusion (i.e., reddening of the eye). Severe disease can progress to vascular collapse, thrombocytopenia, hemorrhage, and hepatic and renal dysfunction.

Leptospirosis confined to the central nervous system can be mistaken for viral **aseptic meningitis,** because the course of the disease is generally uncomplicated and has a very low mortality rate. Culture of CSF is usually negative at this stage. In contrast, the icteric form of generalized disease (≈10% of all symptomatic infections) is more severe and associated with a mortality approaching 10% to 15%. Although hepatic involvement with jaundice (icteric disease, or **Weil disease**) is striking in patients with severe leptospirosis, hepatic necrosis is not seen and surviving patients do not suffer permanent hepatic damage. Similarly, most patients recover full renal function. Congenital leptospirosis can also occur. This disease is characterized by the sudden onset of headache, fever, myalgias, and a diffuse rash.

Clinical Case 32-4 Leptospirosis in Triathlon Participants

There are a number of reports of leptospirosis in athletes participating in water sport events. In 1998, public health officials reported leptospirosis in triathlon participants in Illinois and Wisconsin (*MMWR Morb Mortal Wkly Rep* 47:673–676, 1998). A total of 866 athletes participated in the Illinois event on June 21, 1998, and 648 participated in the Wisconsin event on July 5, 1998. The case definition of leptospirosis used for this investigation was onset of fever, followed by at least two of the following symptoms or signs: chills, headache, myalgia, diarrhea, eye pain, or red eyes. Nine percent of the participants met this case definition; two thirds sought medical care, including one third who were hospitalized. Leptospirosis was confirmed in a portion of these patients by serologic tests. These outbreaks illustrate the potential danger of swimming in contaminated water, the presentation of leptospirosis in a previously healthy population, and the severity of disease that can be experienced.

Laboratory Diagnosis

Microscopy

Because leptospires are thin, they are at the limit of the resolving power of a light microscope and thus cannot be seen by conventional light microscopy. Neither Gram stain nor silver stain is reliable in the detection of leptospires. Darkfield microscopy is also relatively insensitive, capable of yielding nonspecific findings.

Culture

Leptospires can be cultured on specially formulated media (e.g., Fletcher, EMJH [Ellinghausen-McCullough-Johnson-Harris], Tween 80-albumin). They grow slowly (generation time, 6 to 16 hours), requiring incubation at 28° C to 30° C for as long as 4 months; however, most cultures are positive within 2 weeks. Consistent with the two phases of illness, leptospires are present in blood or CSF during the first 10 days of infection and in urine after the first week and for as long as 3 months. Because the concentration of organisms in blood, CSF, and urine may be low, several specimens should be collected if leptospirosis is suspected. In addition, inhibitors present in blood and urine may delay or prevent recovery of leptospires. Likewise, urine must be treated to neutralize the pH and concentrated by centrifugation. A few drops of the sediment are then inoculated into the culture medium. Growth of the bacteria in culture is detected by darkfield microscopy.

Nucleic Acid–Based Tests

Preliminary work with the detection of leptospires using nucleic acid probes has had limited success. Techniques using nucleic acid amplification (e.g., PCR) are more sensitive than culture. Unfortunately, this technique is not widely available at this time, particularly in resource-limited countries where disease is common.

Antibody Detection

Because of the need for specialized media and prolonged incubation, most laboratories do not attempt to culture leptospires and thus rely on serologic techniques. The reference method for all serologic tests is the **microscopic agglutination test (MAT).** This test measures the ability of the patient's serum to agglutinate live leptospires. Because the test is directed against specific serotypes, it is necessary to use pools of leptospiral antigens. In this test, serial dilutions of the patient's serum are mixed with the test antigens and then examined microscopically for agglutination. Agglutinins appear in the blood of untreated patients after 5 to 7 days of illness, although this response may be delayed for as long as several months. Infected patients have a titer of at least 200 (i.e., agglutinins are detected in a 1:200 dilution of the patient's serum), and it may be 25,000 or higher. Patients treated with antibiotics may have a diminished antibody response or nondiagnostic titers. Agglutinating antibodies are detectable for many years after the acute illness; thus their presence may represent either a blunted antibody response in a treated patient with acute disease or residual antibodies in a person with a distant unrecognized infection with leptospires. Because the microscopic agglutination test uses live organisms, it is performed only in reference laboratories. Alternative tests, such as indirect hemagglutination, slide agglutination, and enzyme-linked immunosorbent assay (ELISA) are less sensitive and specific. These tests can be used to screen a patient, but positive reactions must be confirmed with the MAT or culture. Serologic cross-reactions occur with other spirochetal infections (i.e., syphilis, relapsing fever, Lyme disease) and legionellosis.

Treatment, Prevention, and Control

Leptospirosis is usually not fatal, particularly in the absence of icteric disease. Patients should be treated with either intravenously administered **penicillin** or **doxycycline.** Doxycycline, but not penicillin, can be used to prevent disease in persons exposed to infected animals or water contaminated with urine. It is difficult to eradicate leptospirosis because the disease is widespread in wild and domestic animals. However, vaccination of livestock and pets has proved successful in reducing the incidence of disease in these populations and therefore subsequent human exposure. Rodent control is also effective in eliminating leptospirosis in communities.

Bibliography

Aguero-Rosenfeld ME, Wang G, Schwartz I, et al: Diagnosis of Lyme borreliosis, *Clin Microbiol Rev* 18:484–509, 2005.

Antal GM, Lukehart SA, Meheus AZ: The endemic treponematoses, *Microbes Infect* 4:83–94, 2002.

Centers for Disease Control and Prevention: *Sexually transmitted disease surveillance 2012*, Atlanta, 2013, U.S. Department of Health and Human Services.

Feder HM Jr, Johnson BJ, O'Connell S, et al: Review article: a critical appraisal of "chronic Lyme disease," *N Engl J Med* 357:1422–1430, 2007.

Gayet-Ageron A, Lautenschlager S, Ninet B, et al: Sensitivity, specificity and likelihood rations of PCR in the diagnosis of syphilis: a systematic review and meta-analysis, *Sex Transm Infect* 89:251–256, 2013.

Jafari Y, Peeling RW, Shivkumar S, et al: Are *Treponema pallidum*–specific rapid and point-of-care tests for syphilis accurate enough for screening in resource limited settings? Evidence from a meta-analysis, *PLoS ONE* 8:e54695, 2013.

LaFond RE, Lukehart SA: Biological basis for syphilis, *Clin Microbiol Rev* 19:29–49, 2006.

Levitt PN: Leptospirosis, *Clin Microbiol Rev* 14:296–326, 2001.

Mitja O, Asiedu K, Mabey D: Yaws, *Lancet* 381:763–773, 2013.

Rothschild BM: History of syphilis, *Clin Infect Dis* 40:1454–1463, 2005.

Shapiro E: Lyme disease, *N Engl J Med* 370:1724–1731, 2014.

Steere AC, McHugh G, Damle N, et al: Prospective study of serologic tests for Lyme disease, *Clin Infect Dis* 47:188–195, 2008.

Toner B: Current controversies in the management of adult syphilis, *Clin Infect Dis* 44:S130–S146, 2007.

Wormser GP: Early Lyme disease, *N Engl J Med* 354:2794–2801, 2006.

Wormser GP, Dattwyler RJ, Shapiro ED, et al: The clinical assessment, treatment, and prevention of Lyme disease, human granulocytic anaplasmosis, and babesiosis: clinical practice guidelines by the Infectious Diseases Society of America, *Clin Infect Dis* 43:1089–1134, 2006.

CHAPTER 33

MYCOPLASMA AND UREAPLASMA

A 13-year-old girl was admitted to the hospital with a 5-day history of fever and a nonproductive cough. She had received 3 days of treatment with a cephalosporin as an outpatient, with no relief of symptoms. Upon admission, examination of the chest revealed bilateral crackling rales, dullness to percussion, and a chest radiograph that showed a right lower lobe infiltrate. Bacterial stains and cultures were negative, but a polymerase chain reaction (PCR) test for *Mycoplasma pneumoniae* was positive.

1. What is unique about the cellular structure of mycoplasmas? How does this affect their susceptibility to antibiotics?
2. What infections are attributed to *Mycoplasma pneumoniae*? *M. genitalium*? *M. hominis*?
3. What is the most sensitive test for the diagnosis of *M. pneumoniae* infection?

Answers to these questions are available on StudentConsult.com.

• SUMMARIES CLINICALLY SIGNIFICANT ORGANISMS

Mycoplasma pneumoniae

Trigger Words

No cell wall, person-to-person, tracheobronchitis

Biology and Virulence

- The smallest free-living bacterium; able to pass through 0.45-μm pore filters
- Absence of cell wall and a cell membrane containing sterols are unique among bacteria
- Slow rate of growth (generation time, 6 hours); strict aerobe
- P1 adhesin protein binds to base of cilia on epithelial cells, leading to eventual loss of ciliated epithelial cells
- Stimulates migration of inflammatory cells and release of cytokines

Epidemiology

- Worldwide disease with no seasonal incidence (in contrast to disease caused by most respiratory pathogens)
- Primarily infects children between ages 5 and 15 years, but all populations susceptible to disease
- Transmitted by inhalation of aerosolized droplet

Diseases

- Strict human pathogen
- Refer to Table 33-1 for disease

Diagnosis

- Refer to Table 33-2

Treatment, Prevention, and Control

- Drug of choice is erythromycin, doxycycline, or newer fluoroquinolones
- Immunity to reinfection is not lifelong, and vaccines have proved ineffective

The order Mycoplasmatales is subdivided into four genera: *Eperythrozoon, Haemobartonella, Mycoplasma,* and *Ureaplasma*. The most clinically significant genera are *Mycoplasma* (124 species) and *Ureaplasma* (7 species), and the most important species is *Mycoplasma pneumoniae* (also called **Eaton agent** after the investigator who originally isolated it). *M. pneumoniae* causes respiratory tract diseases such as tracheobronchitis and pneumonia. Other commonly isolated pathogens include *Mycoplasma genitalium, Mycoplasma hominis,* and *Ureaplasma urealyticum* (Table 33-1).

• Physiology and Structure

Mycoplasma and *Ureaplasma* organisms are the **smallest free-living bacteria.** They are unique among bacteria because they **do not have a cell wall** and their cell membrane contains **sterols.** In contrast, other cell wall–deficient bacteria (called **L forms**) do not have sterols in their cell membrane and can form cell walls under the appropriate growth conditions. Absence of the cell wall renders the mycoplasmas resistant to penicillins, cephalosporins, vancomycin, and other antibiotics that interfere with synthesis of the cell wall.

Table 33-1 **Important Mycoplasmataceae**

Organism	Site	Human Disease
Mycoplasma pneumoniae	Respiratory tract	Tracheobronchitis, pharyngitis, pneumonia, secondary complications (neurologic, pericarditis, hemolytic anemia, arthritis, mucocutaneous lesions)
Mycoplasma genitalium	Genitourinary tract	Nongonococcal urethritis, pelvic inflammatory disease
Mycoplasma hominis	Respiratory tract, genitourinary tract	Pyelonephritis, postpartum fever, systemic infections in immunocompromised patients
Ureaplasma urealyticum	Respiratory tract, genitourinary tract	Nongonococcal urethritis, pyelonephritis, spontaneous abortion, premature birth

The mycoplasmas form pleomorphic shapes varying from 0.2 to 0.3 µm coccoid forms to rods 0.1 to 0.2 µm in width and 1 to 2 µm long. Many can pass through the 0.45-µm filters used to remove bacteria from solutions, which was why the mycoplasmas were originally thought to be viruses. However, the organisms divide by binary fission (typical of all bacteria), grow on artificial cell-free media, and contain both ribonucleic acid (RNA) and deoxyribonucleic acid (DNA). Mycoplasmas are facultatively anaerobic (except *M. pneumoniae,* which is a **strict aerobe**), and require exogenous sterols supplied by animal serum added to the growth medium. The mycoplasmas **grow slowly,** with a generation time of 1 to 16 hours, and most form small colonies that are difficult to detect without extended incubation.

Pathogenesis and Immunity

M. pneumoniae is an extracellular pathogen that adheres to the respiratory epithelium by means of a specialized attachment structure that forms at one end of the cell. The structure consists of a complex of adhesion proteins, with the **P1 adhesin** the most important. The adhesions interact specifically with sialated glycoprotein receptors at the base of cilia on the epithelial cell surface (and on the surface of erythrocytes). Ciliostasis then occurs, after which first the cilia, then the ciliated epithelial cells, are destroyed. Loss of these cells interferes with the normal clearance of the upper airways and permits the bacteria to spread to the lower respiratory tract. This process is responsible for the persistent cough present in patients with symptomatic disease. *M. pneumoniae* functions as a superantigen, stimulating inflammatory cells to migrate to the site of infection and release cytokines, initially tumor necrosis factor-α and interleukin (IL)-1 and later IL-6. This process contributes to both the clearance of the bacteria and the observed disease.

A number of *Mycoplasma* species are able to rapidly change expression of surface lipoproteins, which is believed to be important for evading the host immune response and establishing persistent or chronic infections.

Epidemiology

M. pneumoniae is a strict human pathogen. Respiratory disease (e.g., tracheobronchitis, pneumonia) caused by *M. pneumoniae* occurs worldwide throughout the year, with no consistent increase in seasonal activity. Epidemic disease occurs every 4 to 8 years. Disease is most common in school-age children and young adults (ages 5 to 15 years), although all age groups are susceptible.

It has been estimated that 2 million cases of *M. pneumoniae* pneumonia and 100,000 pneumonia-related hospitalizations occur annually in the United States. However, *M. pneumoniae* disease is not a reportable disease, and reliable diagnostic tests are not widely available, so the true incidence is not known.

M. pneumoniae colonizes the nose, throat, trachea, and lower airways of infected individuals and is spread via large respiratory droplets during coughing episodes. Infection usually spreads among classmates, family members, or other close contacts. The attack rate is higher in children than in adults (overall average, ≈60%), presumably because most adults are partially immune from previous exposure. The incubation period and time of infectivity are prolonged, so disease can persist for months. *M. pneumoniae* is not part of the normal mucosa flora of humans; however, prolonged carriage can occur following symptomatic disease.

Infants, particularly females, are colonized with *M. hominis, M. genitalium,* and *Ureaplasma* species, with *Ureaplasma* organisms being isolated most often. Although carriage of these mycoplasmas usually does not persist, a small proportion of prepubertal children remains colonized. The incidence of genital mycoplasmas rises after puberty, corresponding to sexual activity. Approximately 15% of sexually active men and women are colonized with *M. hominis,* and 45% to 75% are colonized with *Ureaplasma.* The incidence of carriage in adults who are sexually inactive is no greater than that in prepubertal children.

Clinical Diseases (Clinical Case 33-1)

Exposure to *M. pneumoniae* typically results in **asymptomatic carriage.** The most common clinical presentation of *M. pneumoniae* infection is **tracheobronchitis.** Low-grade fever, malaise, headache, and a dry, nonproductive cough develop 2 to 3 weeks after exposure. Acute **pharyngitis** may also be present. Symptoms gradually worsen over the next few days and can persist for 2 weeks or longer. The bronchial passages primarily become infiltrated with lymphocytes and plasma cells. Pneumonia (referred to as primary **atypical pneumonia** or walking pneumonia) can also develop, with a patchy bronchopneumonia seen on chest radiographs that is typically more impressive than the physical findings. Myalgias and gastrointestinal tract symptoms are uncommon. Secondary complications include neurologic abnormalities (e.g., meningoencephalitis, paralysis, myelitis), pericarditis, hemolytic anemia, arthritis, and mucocutaneous lesions.

Because the genitourinary tract is colonized with other *Mycoplasma* species and *Ureaplasma,* it is difficult to determine the role of these organisms in disease in individual patients. However, it is generally accepted that *M. genitalium*

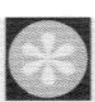

Clinical Case 33-1 *Mycoplasma pneumoniae* Pneumonia in a Young Adult

Caxboeck and associates (*Wien Klin Wochenschr* 119:379–384, 2007) described an unusual case of fatal *M. pneumoniae* pneumonia in a previously healthy 18-year-old woman. Before admission to the hospital, she had seen her physician with respiratory complaints and a chest radiograph consistent with pneumonia. A fluoroquinolone antibiotic was prescribed, but she failed to respond. Upon admission to the hospital, she had a temperature of 40° C and a productive cough. Her antibiotic was changed to a macrolide and cephalosporin; however, she continued to deteriorate, with progression of the pulmonary infiltrates, development of bilateral pleural effusions, and evidence of liver failure. Despite aggressive antibiotic therapy and respiratory support, her disease progressed to hemorrhagic pneumonia with multiorgan failure, and she died on hospital day 35. Diagnosis of *M. pneumoniae* infection was based on positive serology and the lack of other respiratory pathogens by microscopy, culture, and antigen testing. Although diagnosis by culture or polymerase chain reaction would be more convincing, the case illustrates the susceptibility of adults to mycoplasma infections and the uncommon but well-recognized occurrence of serious complications in susceptible patients. It should also be noted that this patient most likely had an undiagnosed immune defect that increased her susceptibility to this pathogen.

Table 33-2 Diagnostic Tests for *Mycoplasma pneumoniae* Infections

Test	Assessment
Microscopy	Test is not useful because organisms do not have a cell wall and do not stain with conventional reagents
Culture	Test is slow (2 to 6 weeks before positive diagnosis) and insensitive; it is not available in most laboratories
Molecular diagnosis	Polymerase chain reaction–based amplification assays, with excellent sensitivity; specificity is not well defined
Serology	
Complement fixation	Antibody titers versus glycolipid antigens peak in 4 weeks and persist for 6 to 12 months; poor sensitivity and specificity; rarely used today
Enzyme immunoassays	Multiple assays available, with varying sensitivity and specificity; assays directed versus P1 adhesin protein may be most specific
Cold agglutinin	Sensitivity and specificity poor, with cross-reactions with other respiratory pathogens (e.g., Epstein-Barr virus, cytomegalovirus, adenovirus); test commonly used but not recommended

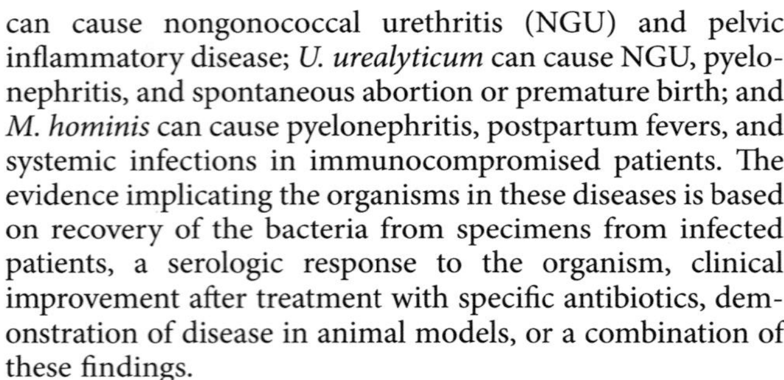

can cause nongonococcal urethritis (NGU) and pelvic inflammatory disease; *U. urealyticum* can cause NGU, pyelonephritis, and spontaneous abortion or premature birth; and *M. hominis* can cause pyelonephritis, postpartum fevers, and systemic infections in immunocompromised patients. The evidence implicating the organisms in these diseases is based on recovery of the bacteria from specimens from infected patients, a serologic response to the organism, clinical improvement after treatment with specific antibiotics, demonstration of disease in animal models, or a combination of these findings.

Laboratory Diagnosis (Table 33-2)

Microscopy is of no diagnostic value because mycoplasmas stain poorly with the Gram stain. Likewise, antigen tests have poor sensitivity and specificity and are not recommended. The most sensitive diagnostic tests are PCR amplification tests of species-specific gene targets, although the specificity for pathogenic mycoplasmas has not been established. *M. pneumoniae* can be isolated in culture from throat washings, bronchial washings, and expectorated sputum; however, the organisms grow slowly (generation time, 6 hours) and require special media supplemented with serum (provides sterols), yeast extract (for nucleic acid precursors), glucose, a pH indicator, and penicillin (to inhibit other bacteria). A positive culture result is definitive evidence of disease, but it is relatively **insensitive.** *M. hominis* is a facultative anaerobe that grows within 1 to 4 days. The colonies have a typical large, fried-egg appearance, and inhibition of their growth with specific antisera is used to differentiate them from other genital mycoplasmas. *Ureaplasma* requires urea for growth but is inhibited by the higher alkalinity resulting from the metabolism of urea. Thus the growth medium must be supplemented with urea and be highly buffered. Even if these steps are taken, ureaplasmas die rapidly after initial isolation. Serology tests are available for *M. pneumoniae.* Detection of antibodies directed against *M. pneumoniae* by complement fixation is the traditional serologic reference standard, but the test has poor sensitivity and antibodies directed against the target glycolipid antigen are also elicited by other *Mycoplasma* species and by host tissues. A number of enzyme immunoassays for the detection of immunoglobulin (Ig)M and IgG antibodies are available. In general, the tests are more sensitive than complement fixation tests and culture. The disadvantage with these tests is that sera have to be collected early in the course of disease and then after 3 to 4 weeks to demonstrate a rise in antibody levels. Historically, it was also possible to measure nonspecific reactions to the outer membrane glycolipids of *M. pneumoniae.* The most popular of these reactions is the production of **cold agglutinins** (e.g., IgM antibodies that bind to antigens on the surface of human erythrocytes at 4° C). This test is insensitive and nonspecific, so it should not be performed.

Treatment, Prevention, and Control

Erythromycin, tetracyclines (particularly doxycycline), and fluoroquinolones are equally effective in treating *M. pneumoniae* infections, although the tetracyclines and fluoroquinolones are reserved for use in adults. Tetracyclines have the advantage of also being active against most other mycoplasmas and chlamydia, a common cause of NGU. Erythromycin is used to treat *Ureaplasma* infections, because these organisms are resistant to tetracycline. Unlike the other mycoplasmas, *M. hominis* is resistant to erythromycin and occasionally to the tetracyclines. Clindamycin has been used to treat infections caused by these resistant strains.

The prevention of *Mycoplasma* disease is problematic. *M. pneumoniae* infections are spread by close contact; thus the isolation of infected people could theoretically reduce the risk of infection. Isolation is impractical, however, because patients are typically infectious for a prolonged period, even while receiving appropriate antibiotics. Inactivated vaccines and attenuated live vaccines have also proved disappointing. The protective immunity conferred by infection has been low. Infections with *M. hominis, M. genitalium,* and *Ureaplasma* are transmitted by sexual contact. Therefore these diseases can be prevented by avoidance of unprotected sexual activity.

Bibliography

Capoccia R, Greub G, Baud D: *Ureaplasma urealyticum, Mycoplasma hominis* and adverse pregnancy outcome, *Curr Opin Infect Dis* 26:2321–240, 2013.

Citti C, Nouvel L, Baranowski E: Phase and antigenic variation in mycoplasmas, *Future Microbiol* 5:1073–1085, 2010.

Daley G, Russell D, Tabrizi S, et al: *Mycoplasma genitalium:* a review, *Int J STD AIDS* 25:475–487, 2014.

Loens K, Ursi D, Goossens H, et al: Molecular diagnosis of *Mycoplasma pneumoniae* respiratory tract infections, *J Clin Microbiol* 41:4915–4923, 2003.

McGowin C, Anderson-Smits C: *Mycoplasma genitalium:* an emerging cause of sexually transmitted disease in women, *PLoS Pathog* 7:e1001324, 2011.

Meyer P, van Rossum A, Vink C: *Mycoplasma pneumoniae* in children: carriage, pathogenesis, and antibiotic resistance, *Curr Opin Infect Dis* 27:220–227, 2014.

Waites K, Katz B, Schelonka R: *Mycoplasmas* and *Ureaplasmas* as neonatal pathogens, *Clin Microbiol Rev* 18:757–789, 2005.

Waites K, Talkington D: *Mycoplasma pneumoniae* and its role as a human pathogen, *Clin Microbiol Rev* 17:697–728, 2004.

CHAPTER

RICKETTSIA, EHRLICHIA, AND RELATED BACTERIA

A 24-year-old man living in North Carolina came to the local emergency department because of fever, arthralgias, myalgias, and malaise. He was well until 4 days before admission, when he developed a fever reaching 40° C, chills, severe headache, and muscle aches. Physical examination revealed a critically ill man with a temperature of 39.7° C, pulse of 110 beats/min, respiratory rate of 28 breaths/min, blood pressure of 100/60 mm Hg, and a rash over his extremities, including his palms and soles. The patient recalled having had numerous tick bites 10 days before the onset of symptoms. Rocky Mountain spotted fever was considered in the diagnosis, and serologic tests for *Rickettsia* species confirmed this diagnosis.

1. What antibiotics can be used to treat this infection? Which antibiotics should not be used?
2. Which rickettsiae are associated with the following vectors: ticks, lice, mites, and fleas?
3. Why is use of the Gram stain inappropriate for the diagnosis of rickettsial infections?
4. *Ehrlichia* and *Anaplasma* have been historically associated with *Rickettsia*. Compare clinical disease caused by *Ehrlichia chaffeensis* and *Anaplasma phagocytophilum*.
5. What clinical diseases are caused by *Coxiella burnetii*?

Answers to these questions are available on StudentConsult.com.

• SUMMARIES CLINICALLY SIGNIFICANT ORGANISMS

Rickettsia rickettsii

Trigger Words

Intracellular bacteria, Rocky Mountain spotted fever, vasculitis, tick, microimmunofluorescence test

Biology and Virulence

- Small intracellular bacteria
- Stain poorly with Gram stain; best with Giemsa or Gimenez stains
- Replication occurs in cytoplasm and nucleus of endothelial cells, with resulting vasculitis
- Intracellular growth protects the bacteria from immune clearance

Epidemiology

- *R. rickettsii* is most common rickettsial pathogen in United States
- Hard ticks (e.g., dog tick, wood tick) are the primary reservoirs and vectors
- Transmission requires prolonged contact
- Distribution in Western Hemisphere; in United States, the majority of infections reported in five states: North Carolina, Oklahoma, Arkansas, Tennessee, and Missouri
- Disease is most common April through September

Diseases

- Rocky Mountain spotted fever characterized by high fever, severe headache, myalgias, and rash; complications common in untreated patients or where diagnosis is delayed

Diagnosis

- Serology (e.g., microimmunofluorescence test) is used most commonly for diagnosis

Treatment, Prevention, and Control

- Doxycycline is the drug of choice
- People should avoid tick-infested areas, wear protective clothing, and use effective insecticides
- People should remove attached ticks immediately
- No vaccine is currently available

Rickettsia prowazekii

Trigger Words

Intracellular bacteria, louse-borne typhus, Brill-Zinsser disease, vasculitis, human reservoir, microimmunofluorescence test

Biology and Virulence

- Small intracellular bacteria
- Stain poorly with Gram stain; best with Giemsa or Gimenez stains
- Replicate in cytoplasm of endothelial cells, with resulting vasculitis
- Intracellular growth protects the bacteria from immune clearance

Epidemiology

- Humans are the primary reservoir, with person-to-person transmission by louse vector
- It is believed that sporadic disease is spread from squirrels to humans via squirrel fleas
- Recrudescent disease can develop years after initial infection
- People at greatest risk are those living in crowded, unsanitary conditions

- Disease is worldwide, with most infections in Central and South America and Africa
- Sporadic disease is seen in the eastern United States

Diseases

- Epidemic typhus (louse-borne typhus) characterized by high fever, severe headache, and myalgias
- Recrudescent typhus (Brill-Zinsser disease) is a milder form of the disease

Diagnosis

- The microimmunofluorescence test is the test of choice

Treatment, Prevention, and Control

- Doxycycline is the drug of choice
- Controlled through improvements in living conditions and reduction of the lice population through use of insecticides
- Inactivated vaccine is available for high-risk populations

Ehrlichia and Anaplasma

Trigger Words

- Intracellular bacteria, monocytic and granulocytic disease, ticks

Biology and Virulence

- Small intracellular bacteria that stain poorly with Gram stain; best with Giemsa or Gimenez stains
- Replicates in phagosome of infected cells
- Intracellular growth protects bacteria from immune clearance
- Able to prevent fusion of phagosome with lysosome of monocytes or granulocytes
- Initiates inflammatory response that contributes to pathology

Epidemiology

- Depending on the species of *Ehrlichia,* important reservoirs are white-tailed deer, white-footed mouse, chipmunks, voles, and canines
- Ticks are important vectors, but transovarian transmission in inefficient
- Disease in United States is most common in the southeastern, Mid-Atlantic, midwestern, and south central states
- People at greatest risk are those exposed to ticks in the endemic areas
- Disease is most common April to October

Diseases

- Diseases are human monocytic ehrlichiosis and human anaplasmosis (formerly called *human granulocytic ehrlichiosis*)

Diagnosis

- Microscopy of limited value
- Serology and nucleic acid amplification tests are methods of choice

Treatment, Prevention, and Control

- Doxycycline is the drug of choice; rifampin is an acceptable alternative
- Prevention involves avoidance of tick-infested areas, use of protective clothing and insect repellents, and prompt removal of embedded ticks
- Vaccines are not available

Coxiella burnetii

Trigger Words

Intracellular bacteria, flulike acute disease, subacute endocarditis chronic disease, inhalation exposure, phase I and II antigens

Biology and Virulence

- Small intracellular bacteria that stain poorly with Gram stain; best with Giemsa or Gimenez stains
- Replicate in phagosomes of infected cells
- Exists in two forms: small cell variant infectious, extremely stable to environmental factors; large cell variant is the metabolically active form
- Phase transition occurs during infection: phase I with intact lipopolysaccharide (LPS), phase II with truncated LPS (O-antigen sugars missing)
- Intracellular growth protects the bacteria from immune clearance
- Able to replicate in acidic environment of phagosomes
- Extracellular form extremely stable; can survive in nature for a prolonged period

Epidemiology

- Many reservoirs, including mammals, birds, and ticks
- Most human infections associated with contact with infected cattle, sheep, goats, dogs, and cats
- Most disease acquired through inhalation; possible disease from consumption of contaminated milk; ticks are not an important vector for human disease
- Worldwide distribution
- No seasonal incidence

Diseases

- Most infections are asymptomatic; most common acute presentation is nonspecific influenza-like syndrome; less than 5% develop significant acute disease (pneumonia, hepatitis, pericarditis, fever)
- Endocarditis most common form of chronic disease

Diagnosis

- Detection of antibody response to phase I and phase II antigens is test of choice

Treatment, Prevention, and Control

- Doxycycline is the drug of choice for acute infections; hydroxychloroquine combined with doxycycline is used to treat chronic infections
- Phase I antigen vaccines are protective and safe if administered in a single dose before the animal or human has been exposed to *Coxiella;* not available in the United States for animals or humans

All of the bacteria discussed in this chapter were at one time classified in the family Rickettsiaceae, based on the observation that they were obligate aerobic, intracellular, gram-negative rods. Analysis of their deoxyribonucleic acid (DNA) sequences revealed that this classification was invalid, so three separate families were created: Rickettsiaceae with two genera, ***Rickettsia*** and ***Orientia;*** Anaplasmataceae with two genera, ***Ehrlichia*** and ***Anaplasma;*** and Coxiellaceae with **Coxiella** (Table 34-1).

Rickettsiaceae

The family Rickettsiaceae consists of two genera, *Rickettsia* and *Orientia,* and the genus *Rickettsia* is subdivided into the **spotted fever group** and the **typhus group.** Many species of *Rickettsia* in the spotted fever group are associated with human disease; however, only ***Rickettsia rickettsii*** (Rocky Mountain spotted fever) and ***Rickettsia akari*** (rickettsialpox) are discussed in this chapter. Two species of *Rickettsia*

Table 34-1 ***Rickettsia, Orientia, Ehrlichia, Anaplasma,* and *Coxiella***

Organism	Historical Derivation
Rickettsia rickettsii	Named after Howard Ricketts, who implicated the wood tick as the vector of Rocky Mountain spotted fever
R. akari	*akari,* mite; the vector of rickettsialpox
R. prowazekii	Named after Stanislav von Prowazek, an early investigator of typhus who was a victim of this disease
R. typhi	*typhi,* typhus or fever
Orientia tsutsugamushi	*Orientia,* Orient; *tsutsugamushi,* "mite disease," the popular name of this disease in the Orient
Ehrlichia	Named after the German microbiologist Paul Ehrlich
E. chaffeensis	First isolated in an Army reservist at Fort Chaffee, Arkansas
E. ewingii	Named after the American microbiologist William Ewing
Anaplasma	*an,* without; *plasma,* anything formed (a thing without form; referring to the intracytoplasmic inclusions)
A. phagocytophilum	*phago,* to eat; *kytos,* a vessel or enclosure; *philein,* to love (found in phagocytes)
Coxiella burnetii	Named after Herald Cox and F.M. Burnet, who isolated the bacterium from ticks in Montana and patients in Australia, respectively

are members of the typhus group: *R. prowazekii* and *R. typhi.* A single species is in the genus *Orientia,* ***Orientia tsutsugamushi,*** the organism responsible for the disease scrub typhus.

Physiology and Structure

The organisms of the family Rickettsiaceae are small (0.3 × 1 to 2 μm), structurally similar to gram-negative rods, and grow only in the cytoplasm of eukaryotic cells. The cell wall structures of *Rickettsia* are typical of gram-negative rods, with a peptidoglycan layer and lipopolysaccharide (LPS); however, the peptidoglycan layer is minimal (stains poorly with the Gram stain), and the LPS has only weak endotoxin activity. *Orientia* lacks both the peptidoglycan layer and LPS. Both groups of organisms are seen best with Giemsa or Gimenez stains (Figure 34-1).

Rickettsia and *Orientia* are strict intracellular parasites found free in the cytoplasm of infected cells. The bacteria enter eukaryotic cells by attaching to host cell surface receptors and stimulating phagocytosis. After engulfment, *Rickettsia* and *Orientia* degrade the phagosome membrane by producing a phospholipase and must be released into the cytoplasm or they will not survive. Multiplication in the host cell by binary fission is slow (generation time, 9 to 12 hours). The spotted fever group of *Rickettsia* and *Orientia* grow in the cytoplasm and nucleus of infected cells and are continually released from cells through long cytoplasmic projections. In contrast, the typhus group accumulates in the cell cytoplasm until the cell membranes lyse, signaling cell death and bacterial release. It is believed that the fundamental difference is caused by intracellular motility—the spotted fever group is able to polymerize host cell actin, whereas the typhus group lacks the required gene. Once these bacteria are released from the host cell, they are unstable and die quickly.

The genome of *R. prowazekii* has been sequenced, providing insight about the parasitic nature of these bacteria. The bacteria depend on their host cell for many functions: carbohydrate metabolism, lipid biosynthesis, nucleotide synthesis, and amino acid synthesis. Additionally, the bacteria are able to produce adenosine triphosphate (ATP) by means of the tricarboxylic acid cycle, or they can act as energy parasites using the host cell ATP as long as it is available.

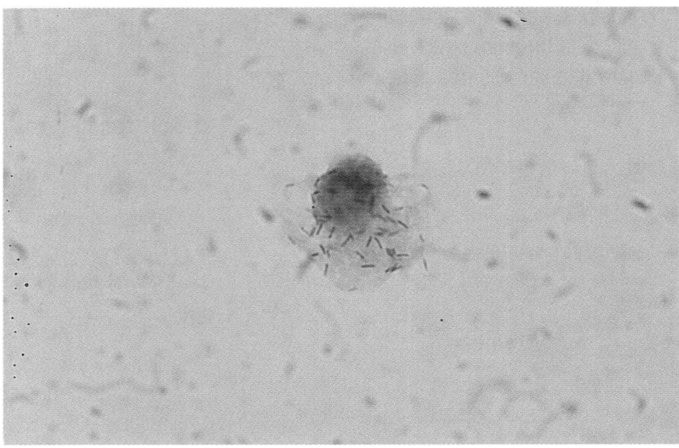

FIGURE 34-1 Gimenez stain of tissue culture cells infected with spotted fever group *Rickettsia.* (From Cohen J, Powderly WG: *Infectious diseases,* ed 2, St Louis, 2004, Mosby.)

Pathogenesis and Immunity

A good model for rickettsial infections is *R. rickettsii,* the agent responsible for **Rocky Mountain spotted fever** and the most common rickettsia causing human disease in the United States. There is no evidence that *R. rickettsii* produces toxins or that the host's immune response is responsible for the pathologic manifestations of Rocky Mountain spotted fever. The **outer membrane protein A (OmpA)** expressed on the surface of *R. rickettsii* is responsible for the ability of the bacteria to adhere to endothelial cells. After the bacteria penetrate into the cell, they are released from the phagosome, freely multiply in both the cytoplasm and nucleus, and move from cell to adjacent cell. The primary clinical manifestations appear to result from the replication of bacteria in endothelial cells, with subsequent damage to the cells and leakage of the blood vessels. Hypovolemia and hypoproteinemia caused by the loss of plasma into tissues can lead to reduced perfusion of various organs and organ failure. The host immune response to infection is based on cytokine-mediated intracellular killing and clearance by cytotoxic CD8 lymphocytes. Antibody response to rickettsial outer membrane proteins may also be important.

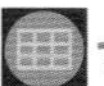 Table 34-2 **Epidemiology of Infections Caused by *Rickettsia* and Related Bacteria**

Organism	Disease	Reservoir	Vector	Distribution
Rickettsia rickettsii	Rocky Mountain spotted fever	Ticks, wild rodents	Hard ticks (dog tick, wood tick)	Western Canada, continental US, Mexico, Panama, Argentina, Brazil, Bolivia, Colombia, Costa Rica
R. akari	Rickettsialpox	Mites (chiggers), wild rodents	Mites	North America (particularly urban areas of Northeastern US), Mexico, Europe (e.g., Croatia, Ukraine, Turkey), Asia (e.g., Korea), Africa
R. prowazekii	Epidemic (louse-borne) typhus	Humans	Human body louse	Mountainous regions of Central and Eastern Africa (Burundi, Rwanda, Ethiopia), Central and South America, Asia
	Recrudescent typhus	Humans	Relapse disease	Worldwide
	Sporadic typhus	Flying squirrels, squirrel fleas and lice	Possibly squirrel fleas	United States
R. typhi	Endemic (murine) typhus	Cats, opossums, raccoons, skunks, wild rodents	Cat flea, rat flea	Worldwide
Orientia tsutsugamushi	Scrub typhus	Mites (chiggers), wild rodents	Mites	Japan, Eastern Asia, Northern Australia, Western and Southwestern Pacific
Ehrlichia chaffeensis	Human monocytic ehrlichiosis	Deer, dogs, foxes, coyotes, and wolves	Soft ticks (Lone Star tick	North and South America, Asia
E. ewingii	Human granulocytic ehrlichiosis	Dogs, deer	Soft ticks (Lone Star tick	North America (uncommon, Missouri)
Anaplasma phagocytophilum	Human granulocytic anaplasmosis	Small mammals (rodents, chipmunks, voles), deer, sheep	Soft ticks (Blacklegged tick)	North America (Upper Midwest and Northeast), Europe, Asia
Coxiella burnetii	Q fever	Mammals, birds, ticks	Ticks incidental (most infections following inhalation)	Worldwide

US, United States.

Epidemiology

The pathogenic species of *Rickettsia* and *Orientia* are maintained in animal and arthropod reservoirs and are transmitted by arthropod vectors (e.g., ticks, mites, lice, fleas; Table 34-2). Humans are accidental hosts. Rickettsiae are maintained in reservoir hosts (primarily rodents) and their arthropod vectors (e.g., ticks, mites, fleas). Because **transovarian transmission** occurs in arthropods, they can serve as both vector and host. The exception to this is *R. prowazekii,* for which humans are the primary host and the arthropod vector is the human body louse. The bacteria kill the louse, so transovarian transmission is not important.

The distribution of rickettsial diseases is determined by the distribution of the arthropod host/vector. Most infections with tick vectors (e.g., spotted fevers) have a restricted geographic distribution, whereas rickettsial infections with other vectors, such as lice *(R. prowazekii),* fleas *(R. typhi),* and mites *(R. akari, O. tsutsugamushi),* have worldwide distribution (see Table 34-2).

In 2011, more than 2800 cases of Rocky Mountain spotted fever were reported in the United States. More than 90% of the infections occurred from **April to September,** corresponding to the period of greatest tick activity, with the majority of infections reported in five states: North Carolina, Oklahoma, Arkansas, Tennessee, and Missouri. The principal reservoir and vector for *R. rickettsia* are **hard ticks** in the family Ixodidae. The three hard ticks most commonly associated with disease in the United States are the **American dog tick *(Dermacentor variabilis)*** in the southeastern states and on the West Coast, **brown dog tick (*Rhipicephalus sanguineus*)** in Arizona, and **wood tick *(Dermacentor andersoni)*** in the Rocky Mountain States and southwestern Canada. Other tick vectors have been identified in Central and South America. A person must be exposed to the tick for a lengthy period (e.g., ≥6 hours) before transmission occurs. The dormant avirulent rickettsiae are activated by the warm blood meal and then released from the tick salivary glands into the blood of the human host.

R. akari, the agent responsible for causing **rickettsialpox,** is one of the few rickettsiae in the spotted fever group that have a **cosmopolitan** distribution and are transmitted by infected **mites.** Culture-confirmed disease has been reported from Ukraine, Croatia, Korea, and the United States, primarily in the New York City area. A cluster of cases was documented in New York City following the release of *Bacillus anthracis* in 2001, when biopsies of eschars from city residents were demonstrated to contain *R. akari* and not *B. anthracis.* Based on this experience, it is likely that rickettsialpox is underdiagnosed in endemic areas. Infections with *R. akari* are maintained in the rodent population through the bite of mouse ectoparasites (e.g., mites) and in mites by transovarian transmission. Humans become accidental hosts when bitten by infected mites.

R. prowazekii, one of two members of the typhus group of rickettsiae, is the etiologic agent of **epidemic** or **louse-borne typhus. Humans** are the principal reservoir of this disease, and the vector is the **human body louse,** *Pediculus humanus.* Epidemic typhus occurs among people living in crowded, unsanitary conditions that favor the spread of body lice—conditions such as those that arise during wars, famines, and natural disasters. Lice die from their infection within 2 to 3 weeks, preventing transovarian transmission of *R. prowazekii.* The disease is present in Central and South America, Africa, and less commonly in the United States.

The incidence of the disease in the United States is unknown because it is not a disease reportable to public health departments. Sporadic disease in the United States is primarily restricted to rural areas of the eastern states. In this area, **flying squirrels** as well as squirrel fleas and lice are infected with *R. prowazekii.* Squirrel lice do not feed on humans, but the fleas are less discriminating and may be responsible for transmitting the *Rickettsia* from squirrels to humans. Epidemiologic and serologic evidence supports this hypothesis.

Recrudescent disease with *R. prowazekii* **(Brill-Zinsser disease)** can occur in people years after their initial infection. Such people in the United States are primarily Eastern European immigrants who were exposed to epidemic typhus during World War II.

Endemic or murine typhus is caused by *R. typhi.* Disease is distributed worldwide primarily in warm, humid areas. In the United States, 50 to 100 cases are reported annually, with most cases in the Gulf States (especially Texas) and Southern California. Endemic disease continues to be reported in people living in the temperate and subtropical coastal areas of Africa, Asia, Australia, Europe, and South America. **Rodents** are the primary reservoir, and the **rat flea** *(Xenopsylla cheopis)* is the principal vector. However, the **cat flea** *(Ctenocephalides felis),* which infests cats, opossums, raccoons, and skunks, is considered an important vector for disease in the United States. Most cases occur during the warm months.

O. tsutsugamushi is the etiologic agent for **scrub typhus,** a disease transmitted to humans by **mites** (chiggers, red mites). The reservoir is the mite population, in which the bacteria are transmitted by transovarian means. Infection is also present in the **rodent** population, which can serve as a reservoir for mite infections. Rodents are not believed to be an important reservoir for human disease, because mites feed only once during their life, so they cannot transmit infection from rodents to humans. Scrub typhus is present in people living in eastern Asia, Australia, and Japan and other Western Pacific islands. It can also be imported into the United States.

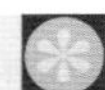

Clinical Case 34-1 Rocky Mountain Spotted Fever

Oster and associates (*N Engl J Med* 297:859–863, 1977) described a series of patients who acquired Rocky Mountain spotted fever after working with *Rickettsia rickettsii* in the laboratory. One patient, a 21-year-old veterinary technician, presented to a clinic with complaints of myalgia and a nonproductive cough. He was treated with penicillin and discharged. Over the next few days, he developed chills and a headache. When he returned to the hospital, he had a temperature of 40.0° C and a macular rash on his extremities and trunk. Intramuscular tetracycline was started, but he remained febrile, and the rash evolved to petechiae on his truck, his extremities, and the soles of his feet. Bilateral pleural effusions developed, and intravenous tetracycline was begun. Over the next 2 weeks, the effusions resolved and the patient made a slow but uneventful recovery. Although this patient was not working directly with *R. rickettsiae,* he had visited a laboratory that was processing the bacterium. This patient illustrates the characteristic presentation of Rocky Mountain spotted fever—headache, fever, myalgias, and a macular rash that can evolve into a petechial or spotted rash.

Clinical Diseases

Symptomatic Rocky Mountain spotted fever (Clinical Case 34-1) develops 7 days (range, 2 to 14 days) after the tick bite (Table 34-3), although the patient may not recall the painless tick bite. The onset of disease is heralded by a high fever and headache that may be associated with malaise, myalgias, nausea, vomiting, abdominal pain, and diarrhea. A macular rash develops in 90% of patients after 3 days, initially on the wrists, arms, and ankles and then spreading to the trunk. The palms and soles can also be involved. The rash can evolve to the "spotted" or petechial form, which is a harbinger of more severe disease. Complications of Rocky Mountain spotted fever include neurologic manifestations, pulmonary and renal failure, and cardiac abnormalities. A delay in diagnosis, either because the clinical presentation is not characteristic or the physician does not recognize the disease, is associated with a worse prognosis. The fatality rate in untreated disease is 10% to 25%.

Clinical infection with *R. akari* (rickettsialpox) is biphasic. First a papule develops at the site where the mite bites the host. The papule appears approximately 1 week after the bite and quickly progresses to ulceration and then **eschar formation.** During this period, the rickettsiae spread systemically. After an incubation period of 7 to 24 days (average, 9 to 14 days), the second phase of the disease develops abruptly, with high **fever,** severe headache, chills, sweats, myalgias, and photophobia. A generalized **papulovesicular rash** forms within 2 to 3 days. A poxlike progression of the rash is then seen in which vesicles form and then crust over. Presence of the rash distinguishes this disease from anthrax and, in a patient with a high fever and eschar, should raise suspicion of rickettsialpox. Despite the appearance of the disseminated rash, rickettsialpox is usually mild and uncomplicated, and complete healing is seen within 2 to 3 weeks without treatment (Clinical Case 34-2).

In one study of epidemic typhus in Africa, clinical disease developed an average of 8 days after exposure (range, 2 to 30 days). Most of the patients initially had nonspecific symptoms, then within 1 to 3 days, high **fever,** severe **headache,** and **myalgias.** Other symptoms can include pneumonia, arthralgia, and neurologic involvement (stupor, confusion, coma). A petechial or macular rash develops in many patients, but this may be obscured in darkly pigmented individuals. The mortality rate in the absence of treatment is 20% to 30% but may be much higher in populations with poor general health and nutrition and lacking proper supportive medical care. In patients

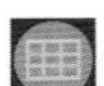 Table 34-3 **Human Diseases Caused by *Rickettsia* and Related Bacteria**

Disease	Average Incubation Period (Days)	Clinical Presentation	Rash	Eschar	Mortality without Treatment (%)
Rocky Mountain spotted fever	7	Abrupt onset; fever, headache, malaise, myalgias, nausea, vomiting, abdominal pain	>90%; macular; centripetal spread	No	10-25
Rickettsialpox	9-14	Abrupt onset; fever, headache, chills, myalgias, photophobia	100%; papulovesicular; generalized	Yes	Low
Epidemic typhus	8	Abrupt onset; fever, headache, chills, myalgias, arthralgia	20%-80%; macular; centrifugal spread	No	20
Endemic typhus	7-14	Gradual onset; fever, headache, myalgias, cough	50%; maculopapular rash on trunk	No	Low
Scrub typhus	10-12	Abrupt onset; fever, headache, myalgias	<50%; maculopapular rash; centrifugal	No	1-15
Human monocytic ehrlichiosis	7-14	High fever, headache malaise, myalgias; leukopenia, thrombocytopenia, elevated serum transaminases	Rash (more common in children than in adults)	No	2-3
Human granulocytic ehrlichiosis	7-14	High fever, headache malaise, myalgias	Rash	No	Insufficient data
Human granulocytic anaplasmosis	5-10	High fever, headache, malaise, myalgias, leukopenia, thrombocytopenia, elevated serum transaminases	Rash in < 10% of patients	No	<1
Q fever	10-14	Abrupt onset; high fever, headache, malaise, myalgias; may progress to hepatitis, pneumonia, or subacute endocarditis (chronic Q fever)	No	No	<5

 Clinical Case 34-2 **Rickettsialpox in New York City**

Koss and associates (*Arch Dermatol* 139:1545–1552, 2003) described 18 patients with rickettsialpox who were diagnosed at Columbia Presbyterian Medical Center in New York City during a 20-month period after the anthrax bioterrorism attack in the fall of 2001. The patients presented to the hospital because they had a necrotic eschar and were thought to have cutaneous anthrax. The patients also had fever, headache, and a papulovesicular rash. Many patients also complained of myalgias, sore throat, arthralgias, and gastrointestinal symptoms. Immunohistochemical staining of eschar and skin biopsies confirmed the diagnosis of rickettsialpox and not cutaneous anthrax. These patients illustrate the diagnostic difficulties of recognizing uncommon diseases even when the clinical presentation is characteristic.

with uncomplicated disease, the body temperature returns to normal within 2 weeks, but complete convalescence may take 3 months or longer. The rickettsiae may remain dormant for years and then reactivate to cause recrudescent epidemic typhus or Brill-Zinsser disease. At the time symptoms develop, bacteremia occurs and the patient is potentially infectious for lice. The course of this form of disease is generally milder and a rash is frequently absent, thus making diagnosis more difficult.

The incubation period for *R. typhi* disease (murine typhus) is 7 to 14 days. The symptoms appear abruptly, with fever, severe headache, chills, myalgias, and nausea most common. A rash develops in approximately half of infected patients, most commonly late in the illness. It is typically restricted to the chest and abdomen. The course of disease is generally uncomplicated, lasting less than 3 weeks even in untreated patients.

O. tsutsugamushi disease (scrub typhus) develops suddenly after a 6- to 18-day incubation period (average, 10 to 12 days), with severe **headache, fever,** and **myalgias.** A macular to papular rash develops on the trunk in less than half of patients and spreads centrifugally to the extremities. Generalized lymphadenopathy, splenomegaly, central nervous system complications, and heart failure can occur. Fever in untreated patients disappears after 2 to 3 weeks.

Laboratory Diagnosis

Microscopy

Although rickettsiae stain poorly with Gram stain, they can be stained with Giemsa or Gimenez stains. Specific fluorescein-labeled antibodies can also be used to stain the intracellular bacteria in biopsy tissue specimens. This direct detection of *R. rickettsiae* antigens is a rapid, specific method for confirming the clinical diagnosis of Rocky Mountain spotted fever but is primarily available only through reference laboratories.

Nucleic Acid–Based Tests

Specific nucleic acid amplification tests are now used in many reference laboratories for the diagnosis of rickettsial diseases. Unfortunately, these assays are relatively insensitive when blood samples are used.

Culture

Although isolation of rickettsiae in tissue culture systems or embryonated eggs is relatively easy, only reference laboratories with extensive experience with rickettsiae routinely perform these cultures. If culture is attempted, buffy coat preparations of blood or skin biopsy specimens should be processed.

Antibody Detection

Although the **Weil-Felix test** (which involves the differential agglutination of cross-reacting *Proteus* antigens) has been used historically for the diagnosis of rickettsial infections, it is no longer recommended, because it is insensitive and nonspecific. Unfortunately, this test is still used in laboratories with limited resources. The serology test that is considered the reference method is the microimmunofluorescence (MIF) test. The test detects antibodies directed against outer membrane proteins (species-specific) and the LPS antigen. Because the LPS antigen is shared among rickettsial species, the Western blot immunoassay must be performed to define the individual species. The sensitivity and specificity of MIF is high, with diagnostic levels of antibodies generally detected in the second week of illness. Commercially prepared enzyme immunoassays are also available but generally have a lower sensitivity and specificity when compared with MIF.

Treatment, Prevention, and Control

The drug of choice for treating all rickettsial infections is **doxycycline.** Although tetracyclines are generally contraindicated for pregnant women and young children, this antibiotic is recommended for all patients with suspected rickettsial disease, because it is the most effective antibiotic and inadequately treated disease is associated with a high morbidity and mortality. Fluoroquinolones (e.g., ciprofloxacin) have good in vitro activity, but clinical experience is inadequate to recommend this for primary therapy. Chloramphenicol also has activity in vitro against rickettsiae, but its use for treatment of infections is associated with a higher incidence of relapse. Prompt diagnosis and institution of appropriate therapy usually result in a satisfactory prognosis; unfortunately, this scenario may not occur if key clinical signs (e.g., rash) develop late or not at all. In addition, the serologic findings often are not available until 2 or more weeks after the onset of disease, also delaying the start of treatment. Therefore it is recommended that empirical therapy with doxycycline be started as soon as the diagnosis is considered.

Vaccines are not available for rickettsial disease except for louse-borne typhus. Prevention of disease involves avoiding tick-infested areas, use of protective clothing and insect repellents, and prompt removal of attached ticks. Rodent control is important for diseases where these represent an important reservoir. Effective louse-control measures are used to manage epidemic typhus.

Anaplasmataceae

The genera *Ehrlichia* and *Anaplasma* consist of intracellular bacteria that parasitize granulocytes, monocytes, erythrocytes, and platelets. Three species of these genera are important human pathogens: *Ehrlichia chaffeensis,* responsible for **human monocytic ehrlichiosis;** *Ehrlichia ewingii,* the etiologic agent of **human granulocytic ehrlichiosis;** and *Anaplasma phagocytophilum,* the agent for **human granulocytic anaplasmosis.**

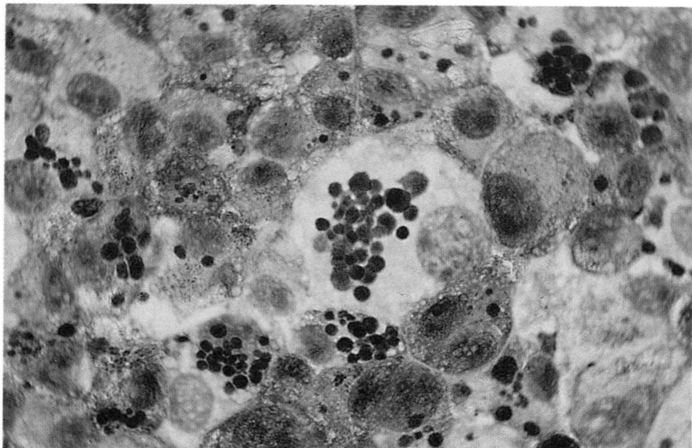

FIGURE 34-2 Multiple morulae of *Ehrlichia canis (E. chaffeensis)* in DH82 tissue culture cells. (From Cohen J, Powderly WG: *Infectious diseases,* ed 2, St Louis, 2004, Mosby.)

Physiology and Structure

In contrast with *Rickettsia* and *Orientia, Ehrlichia* and *Anaplasma* remain in the phagocytic vacuole after entry into the host cell. Fusion with lysosomes is prevented because expression of appropriate receptors on the phagocytic vacuole surface is interrupted. Thus the bacteria can multiple by binary fission in the phagosome without exposure to the hydrolytic lysosome enzymes. Two morphologic forms of the bacteria exist: small (0.2 to 0.4 µm) **elementary bodies** and larger (0.8 to 1.5 µm) **reticulate bodies.** A few days after the cell is infected, the replicating elementary bodies assemble into membrane-enclosed masses called **morulae** (Figure 34-2). Progressive infection leads to lysis of the infected cell, release of bacteria, and subsequent infection of new cells. Detection of morulae when the cells are stained with **Giemsa** or **Wright stains** is a rapid, specific diagnostic test; however, relatively few infected cells may be seen, so a negative test is not helpful.

The cell wall structure of *Ehrlichia* and *Anaplasma* is similar to that of gram-negative bacteria; however, the bacteria lack genes for synthesis of peptidoglycan or LPS. In addition, many of the genes of the glycolytic pathway are also absent. A number of protein antigens are shared among species in these genera, as well as with species of other genera. For this reason, cross-reactive antibodies are commonly observed in serologic assays.

Pathogenesis and Immunity

The intracellular location of the organisms protects them from the host's antibody response. However, bacterial stimulation of proinflammatory cytokine production is believed to play an important role in activating macrophages that act either directly on infected cells or on antibody-opsonized bacteria during their extracellular phase.

Epidemiology (see Table 34-2)

The first human infection in the United States with these organisms was reported in 1986. In 2011, approximately 2575 cases of ehrlichiosis and anaplasmosis were reported in the United States. The prevalence of this disease is underestimated because serologic studies have shown that antibodies to *E. chaffeensis* are at least as common as antibodies to *R. rickettsii,* which has a similar geographic distribution. *E. chaffeensis* disease in the United States is found predominantly in the Midwest (Missouri, Arkansas, Oklahoma) and coastal Atlantic (Maryland, Virginia, New Jersey, New York) states. This area corresponds to the geographic distribution of *Amblyomma americanum* (Lone Star tick), the primary vector responsible for transmitting the organism, and of white-tailed deer, an important reservoir for *E. chaffeensis*. Other animals that can serve as hosts include domestic dogs, foxes, coyotes, and wolves. *E. ewingii* is relatively uncommon and has been primarily reported in Missouri.

Disease caused by *A. phagocytophilum* is found primarily in the upper midwestern states (Minnesota, Wisconsin) and northeast Atlantic states (Massachusetts, Connecticut, New York, New Jersey). The reservoirs are small mammals (e.g., white-footed mouse, chipmunks, voles), and the vectors are *Ixodes* ticks. More than 90% of all disease caused by *Ehrlichia* and *Anaplasma* in the United States occurs between mid-April and late October.

Transovarian transmission of *Ehrlichia* and *Anaplasma* in ticks does not occur (in contrast with *Rickettsia* and *Orientia*), so these bacteria must be maintained in reservoir vertebrate hosts. Ticks become infected when an immature stage (e.g., larva, nymph) ingests blood from a naturally infected host and then transmits the bacteria to another mammalian host (e.g., human) during the next blood meal. Humans are accidental hosts and thus transmission terminates at this stage.

Clinical Diseases

Human Monocytic Ehrlichiosis

Human monocytic ehrlichiosis is caused by *E. chaffeensis* after infection of blood monocytes and mononuclear phagocytes in tissues and organs. Approximately 1 to 2 weeks after a tick bite, patients develop a flulike illness with **high fever,** headache, malaise, and myalgias. A late-onset **rash** develops in 30% to 40% of patients (more common in children than in adults). **Leukopenia, thrombocytopenia,** and **elevated serum transaminases** develop in the majority of patients and can range from mild to severe. Although mortality is low (2% to 3%), more than half the infected patients require hospitalization and experience a prolonged recovery period. A fulminant septic syndrome can develop, particularly in immunocompromised patients. The pathology of this infection is disproportionate to the number of infected cells or microbial burden present in tissue. It is believed that *E. chaffeensis* disturbs mononuclear phagocytic function and regulation of the inflammatory response. Thus the immune response both eliminates the pathogen and produces much of the tissue damage.

Human (Canine) Granulocytic Ehrlichiosis

E. ewingii primarily causes disease in canines, with humans the accidental hosts. Because there is serologic cross-reactivity between *E. ewingii* and *E. chaffeensis,* the incidence of infections with this organism is likely to be underestimated. The clinical presentation is similar to that of *E. chaffeensis,* with fever, headaches, and myalgias. Leukopenia, thrombocytopenia, and elevated serum transaminases are also seen.

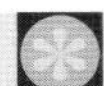

Clinical Case 34-3 Human Anaplasmosis

Heller and associates (*N Engl J Med* 352:1358–1364, 2005) described a 73-year-old man who presented to their hospital with fever, weakness, and leg myalgias. Six days before his admission, he had traveled to South Carolina, and 3 days later, he developed intense leg pains, a high fever, and generalized weakness. Upon admission, he was febrile, tachycardic, and hypertensive; the liver and spleen could not be palpated, and no cutaneous rash was noted. Cultures for bacteria, fungi, and viruses were negative. A peripheral blood smear showed rare intracytoplasmic inclusions in the granulocytes, suggestive of morulae. Polymerase chain reaction analysis of blood samples collected on the second and third hospital days were positive for *Anaplasma phagocytophilum* DNA, confirming the diagnosis of anaplasmosis. The patient was treated successfully with a 14-day course of doxycycline, although residual muscle weakness and pain persisted. Serum collected during the convalescent period was positive for *Anaplasma.* It is noteworthy that the patient did not remember a tick bite during his South Carolina trip, consistent with the observation that the early tick stages, larva and nymphs, are most commonly associated with human disease.

Human Anaplasmosis (Clinical Case 34-3)

Human granulocytic anaplasmosis is caused by *A. phagocytophilum*. Granulocytes (i.e., neutrophils, eosinophils, basophils) are primarily infected. The disease presents 5 to 10 days after exposure as a flulike illness with a high fever, headache, malaise, and myalgias; a rash is observed in less than 10% of patients. As with human monocytic ehrlichiosis, leukopenia, thrombocytopenia, and serum transaminase elevation are observed in most patients. More than half the infected patients require hospitalization, and severe complications, particularly peripheral neuropathies (e.g., demyelinating polyneuropathy, facial palsy) can occur. Despite the potential severity of this disease, mortality is less than 1%. As with *E. chaffeensis* infections, the pathology of this disease appears related to macrophage activation.

Laboratory Diagnosis

The clinical presentation of *Ehrlichia* and *Anaplasma* infections is not distinctive, and although the geographic distribution of disease has limited overlap, laboratory testing is required for a definitive diagnosis. Microscopy has limited value because the bacteria stain poorly with the Gram stain, and detection of intracytoplasmic inclusions (clumps or organisms, morulae) in Giemsa-stained preparations of peripheral blood is only useful during the first week of illness. Morulae are detected in less than 10% of patients with monocytic ehrlichiosis and in 25% to 75% of patients with granulocytic anaplasmosis. Likewise, although *Ehrlichia* organisms have been cultured in vitro in established cell lines, this procedure is not performed in most clinical laboratories. The most common methods for laboratory diagnosis of ehrlichiosis are nucleic acid amplification (NAA) tests and serology. Species-specific DNA amplification tests are available in some reference laboratories and can provide a sensitive, specific diagnostic test for acute disease. An increase in the antibody titer is typically observed 3 to 6 weeks after the initial presentation, so these serologic tests are primarily confirmatory. Sensitivity of the NAA tests and serology is reduced in patients receiving effective therapy. *E.*

chaffeensis and *E. ewingii* are closely related and cannot be differentiated by serology. The specificity of the serology tests is compromised by cross-reactions with organisms responsible for Rocky Mountain spotted fever, Q fever, Lyme disease, brucellosis, and Epstein-Barr virus infections.

Treatment, Prevention, and Control

Patients with suspected ehrlichiosis and anaplasmosis should be treated with **doxycycline.** Therapy should not be delayed to wait for laboratory confirmation of the disease. Rifampin has been used to treat patients who are unable to tolerate doxycycline. Fluoroquinolones, penicillins, cephalosporins, chloramphenicol, aminoglycosides, and macrolides are ineffective. Infection is prevented by avoidance of tick-infested areas, wearing protective clothing, and use of insect repellents. Embedded ticks should be removed promptly. Vaccines are not available.

• Coxiellaceae

Coxiella burnetii

Coxiella burnetii are gram-negative bacteria that stain weakly with the Gram stain, grow intracellularly in eukaryotic cells, and are associated with arthropods (e.g., **ticks**). The disease caused by *C. burnetii* is **Q (query) fever,** so named because the initial investigation of an outbreak in Australian abattoir workers did not identify the causal organism.

Physiology and Structure

Two structural forms of *C. burnetii* are recognized: **small cell variants** that are resistant to environmental stress (e.g., heat, desiccation, chemical agents) and **large cell variants** that are the metabolically active form. Additionally, *C. burnetii* undergoes a phase transition similar to what is observed in some other gram-negative bacteria. In the phase observed in nature **(phase I),** *C. burnetii* has an intact LPS; however, mutations can occur in the LPS genes, resulting in a molecule with lipid A and core sugars but missing the outermost O-antigen sugars **(phase II).** This phase variation is important for understanding the progression of disease and for diagnostic purposes.

Small cell variants attach to macrophages and monocytes and are internalized in a phagocytic vacuole. The normal progression after phagocytosis of most organisms is fusion of the phagosome with a series of endosomes (intracellular vesicles), resulting in a drop in intracellular pH, followed by fusion with lysosomes containing hydrolytic enzymes and resultant bacterial death. This occurs with *C. burnetii* if phase II organisms are ingested; however, phase I *Coxiella* is able to arrest this process before lysosomal fusion. In addition, the organisms require acid pH for their metabolic activities, which in turn protects them from the killing activities of most antibiotics.

Pathogenesis and Immunity

Slowly replicating intracellular pathogens must avoid programmed cell death (apoptosis), which is an important component of intrinsic immunity. *Coxiella* is able to regulate the cell signaling pathways in its phagocytic home so that cell death is delayed. The ability of *C. burnetii* to cause either acute or chronic disease is determined in part by the organism's ability to survive intracellularly. In the presence of interferon-γ, phagosome-lysosome fusion occurs, leading to bacterial death; however, in chronic infections, interleukin-10 is overproduced by the host cell, which interferes with fusion and allows intracellular survival of *C. burnetii*.

Epidemiology (see Table 34-2)

C. burnetii is extremely stable in harsh environmental conditions and **can survive in soil and milk for months to years.** The range of hosts for *C. burnetii* is wide, with infections being found in mammals, birds, and numerous species of ticks. Farm animals, such as sheep, cattle, and goats, and recently infected cats, dogs, and rabbits, are the **primary reservoirs** for human disease. The bacteria can reach high concentrations in the placenta of infected livestock. Dried placentas left on the ground after parturition and feces, urine, and tick feces can contaminate soil, which in turn can serve as a focus for infection if these bacteria become airborne and are inhaled. Human infections occur after the **inhalation of airborne particles** from a contaminated environmental source or, less commonly, after ingestion of contaminated **unpasteurized milk** or other dairy products. Ticks do not transmit disease to humans.

Q fever has a worldwide distribution. Although fewer than 150 infections are reported annually in the United States, this figure is certainly an underestimation of the actual prevalence of the disease. Infection is common in livestock in the United States, but symptomatic disease in livestock is rare. Human exposure—particularly for ranchers, veterinarians, and food handlers—is frequent, and experimental studies have shown that the infectious dose of *C. burnetii* is small (≤10 bacteria). Thus most human infections are asymptomatic or mild, a finding confirmed by serologic studies that have shown that most persons with detectable antibodies do not have a history of disease. Infections also go undetected because diagnostic tests for *C. burnetii* are often not considered.

Clinical Diseases (Clinical Case 34-4)

The majority of individuals exposed to *C. burnetii* have an **asymptomatic infection,** and most symptomatic infections are mild, presenting with nonspecific **flulike symptoms** with an abrupt onset, high-grade fever, fatigue, headache, and myalgias. Less than 5% of infected persons develop symptoms severe enough to require hospitalization, with the most common presentations being **hepatitis, pneumonia,** or isolated **fevers.** Hepatitis is usually asymptomatic or presents with fever and increase in serum transaminases. Most cases of pneumonia are mild with a nonproductive cough, fever, and nonspecific findings on chest radiograph. Histologically, diffuse granulomas are typically seen in the involved organs. Chronic Q fever (symptoms lasting >6 months) can develop months to years after the initial exposure and occurs almost exclusively in patients with predisposing conditions such as underlying valvular heart disease or immunosuppression. **Subacute endocarditis** is the most common presentation and can be difficult to diagnose because of the lack of specific signs and symptoms. However, chronic Q fever is a serious illness with significant mortality and morbidity, even in patients with rapid diagnosis and appropriate treatment.

 **Clinical Case 34-4 *Coxiella burnetii* Endocarditis**

Karakousis and associates (*J Clin Microbiol* 44:2283–2287, 2006) described a 31-year-old man from West Virginia who developed chronic endocarditis caused by *C. burnetii.* At the time the patient was admitted to the hospital, he described an 11-month history of fevers, night sweats, paroxysmal coughing, fatigue, and weight loss. He had received various antibiotic treatments for bronchitis, with no relief. His past medical history was significant for congenital heart disease, with placement of a shunt as an infant. He lived on a farm and participated in birthing his calves. His cardiac examination upon admission revealed a murmur; no hepatosplenomegaly or peripheral stigmata of endocarditis were noted, and his liver enzymes were elevated. All bacterial and fungal blood cultures were negative; however, serology for *Coxiella* phase I and phase II antibodies were markedly elevated. Treatment with doxycycline and rifampin was initiated, and the patient rapidly defervesced. Although prolonged treatment was recommended, the patient was unreliable, and he rapidly became symptomatic every time he discontinued one or both antibiotics. He also refused to take hydroxychloroquine because of his concerns about retinal toxicity. This patient typifies the risk for patients with underlying heart disease and the difficulties in treating this infection.

Laboratory Diagnosis

Q fever can be diagnosed by culture (not commonly performed), serology, or the polymerase chain reaction (PCR). Culture can be performed in tissue culture cells and recently in a cell-free medium; however, culture is rarely performed except in research laboratories licensed to work with these highly contagious organisms. **Serology** is the most commonly used diagnostic test. As previously mentioned, *C. burnetii* undergoes phase variation characterized by the development of phase I and II antigens. The phase I antigens are only weakly antigenic. A variety of methods are used to measure antibody production: the microagglutination tests, indirect immunofluorescence antibody (IFA) test, and enzyme-linked immunosorbent assay (ELISA). IFA is the test of choice, although ELISA is used in many laboratories and appears to be as sensitive. Cross-reactions occur with *Bartonella,* which can cause a similar disease, so all serologic tests should include an assay for both organisms. In acute Q fever, immunoglobulin (Ig)M and IgG antibodies are developed primarily against **phase II antigens.** A diagnosis of chronic Q fever is confirmed by the demonstration of antibodies against both **phase I and II antigens,** with the titers to the phase I antigen typically higher. NAA techniques such as PCR have been developed in reference laboratories but are generally not available for routine diagnosis. In addition, although the tests are sensitive when tissue samples are examined, the sensitivity is poor with serum. PCR-based tests are not required for the diagnosis of chronic *C. burnetii* infections, because these patients characteristically have high levels of antibodies present.

Treatment, Prevention, and Control

Treatment of acute and chronic *C. burnetii* infections is guided by clinical experience, not in vitro susceptibility tests. Currently, it is recommended that acute infections be treated for 14 days with **doxycycline.** Chronic disease should be treated for a prolonged period with a bactericidal combination of drugs, **doxycycline and the alkalinizing agent hydroxychloroquine.** Fluoroquinolones (e.g., ofloxacin, pefloxacin) have been used as an alternative to doxycycline but are contraindicated in children and pregnant women.

Inactivated whole-cell vaccines and partially purified antigen vaccines for Q fever have been developed, and the vaccines prepared from phase I organisms have been shown to provide the best protection. Vaccination of animal herds appears efficacious unless the animals have been previously infected naturally. Vaccination does not eradicate *Coxiella* in infected animals or decrease asymptomatic shedding. Likewise, vaccination of humans with phase I vaccines is protective if the vaccinees are uninfected. Vaccination of previously infected individuals is contraindicated because immune stimulation can lead to an increase in adverse reactions. For this reason, a single-dose vaccine with no booster immunizations is recommended.

Bibliography

Angelakis E, Raoult D: Review: Q fever, *Vet Microbiol* 140:297–309, 2010.

Bakken J, Dumler S: Human granulocytic anaplasmosis, *Infect Dis Clin North Am* 22:433–448, 2008.

Dumler JS, Madigan JE, Pusterla N, et al: Ehrlichioses in humans: epidemiology, clinical presentation, diagnosis, and treatment, *Clin Infect Dis* 45:S45–S51, 2007.

Dumler JS, Walker D: Rocky Mountain spotted fever—changing ecology and persisting virulence, *N Engl J Med* 353:551–553, 2005.

Ghigo E, Pretat L, Desnues B, et al: Intracellular life of *Coxiella burnetii* in macrophages: an update, *Ann N Y Acad Sci* 1166:55–66, 2009.

Gürtler L, Bauerfeind U, Blümel J, et al: *Coxiella burnetii*—pathogenic agent of Q (Query) fever, *Transfus Med Hemother* 41:60–72, 2014.

Ismail N, Bloch K, McBride J: Human ehrlichiosis and anaplasmosis, *Clin Lab Med* 30:261–292, 2010.

Koss T, Carter EL, Grossman ME, et al: Increased detection of rickettsialpox in a New York City hospital following the anthrax outbreak of 2001, *Arch Dermatol* 139:1545–1552, 2003.

Paddock CD, Koss T, Eremeeva ME, et al: Isolation of *Rickettsia akari* from eschars of patients with rickettsialpox, *Am J Trop Med Hyg* 75:732–738, 2006.

Parola P, Paddock C, Raoult D: Tick-borne rickettsioses around the world: emerging diseases challenging old concepts, *Clin Microbiol Rev* 18:719–756, 2005.

Richards A: Rickettsial vaccines: the old and the new, *Expert Rev Vaccines* 3:541–555, 2004.

Rikihisa Y: *Anaplasma phagocytophilum* and *Ehrlichia chaffeensis*: subversive manipulators of host cells, *Nat Rev Microbiol* 8:328–339, 2010.

Shannon J, Heinzen R: Adaptive immunity to the obligate intracellular pathogen *Coxiella burnetii*, *Immunol Res* 43:138–148, 2009.

CHAPTER

CHLAMYDIA AND CHLAMYDOPHILA

A 14-day-old girl was readmitted to the pediatric intensive care unit with respiratory distress, dyspnea, fever, and a dry, unproductive, staccato cough. Chest radiographs demonstrated right bronchopneumonia. The preliminary diagnosis of chlamydial infant pneumonia was made and confirmed by nucleic acid amplification tests. Although *Chlamydia trachomatis* is the best known member of the family Chlamydiaceae, *Chlamydophila psittaci* and *Chlamydophila pneumoniae* also cause significant human disease.

1. Which members of the Chlamydiaceae family cause respiratory disease? Ocular disease? Genital disease?

2. Why is it significant that *C. trachomatis* serotype A does not induce immunity?

3. What laboratory tests are useful for confirming the diagnosis of infections with *Chlamydia* and *Chlamydophila?*

Answers to these questions are available on StudentConsult.com.

• SUMMARIES CLINICALLY SIGNIFICANT ORGANISMS

Chlamydia trachomatis

Trigger Words

Intracellular bacteria, elementary and reticulate bodies, trachoma, infant pneumonia, urethritis, lymphogranuloma venereum (LGV), person-to-person

Biology and Virulence

- Small gram-negative rods
- Strict intracellular parasite of humans
- Two distinct forms: infectious elementary bodies and noninfectious reticulate bodies
- Lipopolysaccharide antigen shared by *Chlamydia* and *Chlamydophila* species
- Major outer membrane proteins are species specific
- Two biovars associated with human disease: trachoma and LGV
- Infects nonciliated columnar, cuboidal, and transitional epithelial cells
- Prevents fusion of phagosome with cellular lysosomes

Epidemiology

- Most common sexually transmitted bacteria in United States
- Ocular trachoma primarily in North and sub-Saharan Africa, the Middle East, South Asia, South America
- LGV highly prevalent in Africa, Asia, and South America

Diseases

- Pathologic effects of trachoma caused by repeated infections
- Diseases—refer to Box 35-1

Diagnosis

- Culture is highly specific but relatively insensitive
- Antigen tests (direct fluorescent antibody, enzyme-linked immunosorbent assay) are relatively insensitive
- Molecular amplification tests are the most sensitive and specific tests currently available

Treatment, Prevention, and Control

- Treat LGV with doxycycline or erythromycin
- Treat ocular or genital infections with azithromycin or doxycycline
- Treat newborn conjunctivitis or pneumonia with erythromycin
- Safe sex practices and prompt treatment of patient and sexual partners help control infections

The family Chlamydiaceae consists of two clinically important genera, *Chlamydia* and *Chlamydophila,* with three species responsible for human disease: ***Chlamydia trachomatis, Chlamydophila psittaci,*** and ***Chlamydophila pneumoniae*** (Table 35-1). Other species have been placed into the two genera, but they are uncommon human pathogens and are not discussed in this chapter.

The Chlamydiaceae are **obligate intracellular parasites** that were once considered viruses because they are small enough to pass through 0.45 µm filters; however, the organisms have the following properties of bacteria: they (1) possess inner and outer membranes similar to those of gram-negative bacteria, (2) contain both deoxyribonucleic acid (DNA) and ribonucleic acid (RNA), (3) possess prokaryotic ribosomes, (4) synthesize their own proteins, nucleic acids, and lipids, and (5) are susceptible to numerous antibacterial antibiotics.

Unlike other bacteria, the Chlamydiaceae have a unique developmental cycle, forming metabolically inactive infectious forms **(elementary bodies [EBs])** and metabolically active noninfectious forms **(reticulate bodies [RBs])**. Properties that differentiate the three important human pathogens in this family are summarized in Table 35-2.

Box 35-1 Chlamydiaceae: Clinical Summaries

Chlamydia trachomatis

Trachoma: chronic inflammatory granulomatous process of eye surface, leading to corneal ulceration, scarring, pannus formation, and blindness

Adult inclusion conjunctivitis: acute process with mucopurulent discharge, dermatitis, corneal infiltrates, and corneal vascularization in chronic disease

Neonatal conjunctivitis: acute process characterized by a mucopurulent discharge

Infant pneumonia: after a 2- to 3-week incubation period, the infant develops rhinitis, followed by bronchitis with a characteristic dry cough

Urogenital infections: acute process involving the genitourinary tract with characteristic mucopurulent discharge; asymptomatic infections common in women

Lymphogranuloma venereum: a painless ulcer develops at the site of infection that spontaneously heals, followed by inflammation and swelling of lymph nodes draining the area, then progression to systemic symptoms

Chlamydophila pneumoniae

Respiratory infections: can range from asymptomatic or mild disease to severe atypical pneumonia requiring hospitalization

Atherosclerosis: *C. pneumoniae* has been associated with inflammatory plaques in blood vessels; the etiologic role in this disease is controversial

Chlamydophila psittaci

Respiratory infections: can range from asymptomatic colonization to severe bronchopneumonia with localized infiltration of inflammatory cells, necrosis, and hemorrhage

Family Chlamydiaceae

Physiology and Structure

Much like a spore, EBs are resistant to many harsh environmental factors. Although recent evidence has demonstrated a peptidoglycan layer in the cell wall of replicating RBs, this has not been demonstrated in EBs. Even though the peptidoglycan layer may be absent in EBs, they possess a central dense core surrounded by a cytoplasmic membrane and a double-layer outer membrane. The cell wall contains a **lipopolysaccharide (LPS)** that is common to all members of the family. The LPS has only **weak endotoxin activity.** The **major outer membrane protein (MOMP)** in the cell wall is an important structural component of the outer membrane and is unique for each species. Variable regions in the gene encoding this protein are found in *C. trachomatis* and are responsible for 18 serologic variants (called **serovars**). Similar variable regions are found in *C. psittaci* MOMP; in contrast, the *C. pneumoniae* MOMP is homogenous, and only a single serovar has been described. A second highly conserved outer membrane protein, **OMP 2,** is shared by all

Table 35-1 Important Chlamydiaceae

Organism	Historical Derivation
Chlamydia	*chlamydis,* a cloak
C. trachomatis	*trachomatis,* of trachoma or rough (the disease trachoma is characterized by rough granulations on the conjunctival surfaces that lead to chronic inflammation and blindness)
Chlamydophila	*chlamydis,* a cloak; *phila,* dear (dear to the cloak; related to *Chlamydia*)
C. pneumoniae	*pneumoniae,* pneumonia
C. psittaci	*psittacus,* a parrot (disease associated with birds)

Table 35-2 Differentiation of Chlamydiaceae That Cause Human Disease

Property	*Chlamydia trachomatis*	*Chlamydophila pneumoniae*	*Chlamydophila psittaci*
Host range	Primarily human pathogen	Primarily human pathogen	Primarily animal pathogen; occasionally infects humans
Biovars	LGV and trachoma	TWAR	Many
Diseases	LGV; ocular trachoma, oculogenital disease, infant pneumonia	Bronchitis, pneumonia, sinusitis, pharyngitis, coronary artery disease (?)	Pneumonia (psittacosis)
Elementary body morphology	Round, narrow periplasmic space	Pear-shaped, large periplasmic space	Round, narrow periplasmic space
Inclusion body morphology	Single round inclusion per cell	Multiple uniform inclusions per cell	Multiple variably sized inclusions per cell
Plasmid DNA	Yes	No	Yes
Iodine-staining glycogen in inclusions	Yes	No	No
Susceptibility to sulfonamides	Yes	No	No

DNA, Deoxyribonucleic acid; *LGV,* lymphogranuloma venereum.

members of the family Chlamydiaceae. This cysteine-rich protein is responsible for the extensive disulfide cross-links that provide the stability in the EBs.

The EBs cannot replicate but are infectious; that is, they can bind to receptors on host cells and stimulate uptake by the infected cell. In this intracellular location, the EBs convert into RBs, the metabolically active replicating chlamydial form. Because the extensive cross-linked proteins are absent in RBs, this form is osmotically fragile; however, they are protected by their intracellular location.

The Chlamydiaceae replicate by means of a unique growth cycle that occurs within susceptible host cells (Figure 35-1). The cycle is initiated when the small (300 to 400 nm), infectious EBs become attached to the microvilli of susceptible cells, followed by active penetration into the host cell. After they are internalized, the bacteria remain within cytoplasmic phagosomes, where the replicative cycle proceeds. If the outer membrane of the EB is intact, fusion of cellular lysosomes with the EB-containing phagosome is inhibited, thus preventing intracellular killing. If the outer membrane is damaged or the bacteria are inactivated by heat or coated with antibodies, phagolysosomal fusion occurs, with subsequent bacterial killing. Within 6 to 8 hours after entering the cell, the EBs reorganize into the larger (800 to 1000 nm), metabolically active RBs. The Chlamydiaceae are **energy parasites** because they use host cell adenosine triphosphate for their energy requirements. Some strains may also depend on the host to provide specific amino acids. The RBs replicate by binary fission, similar to other bacteria, and histologic stains can readily detect the phagosome with accumulated RBs, called an **inclusion.** Approximately 18 to 24 hours after infection, the RBs begin reorganizing into the smaller EBs, and between 48 and 72 hours, the cell ruptures and then releases the infectious bacteria.

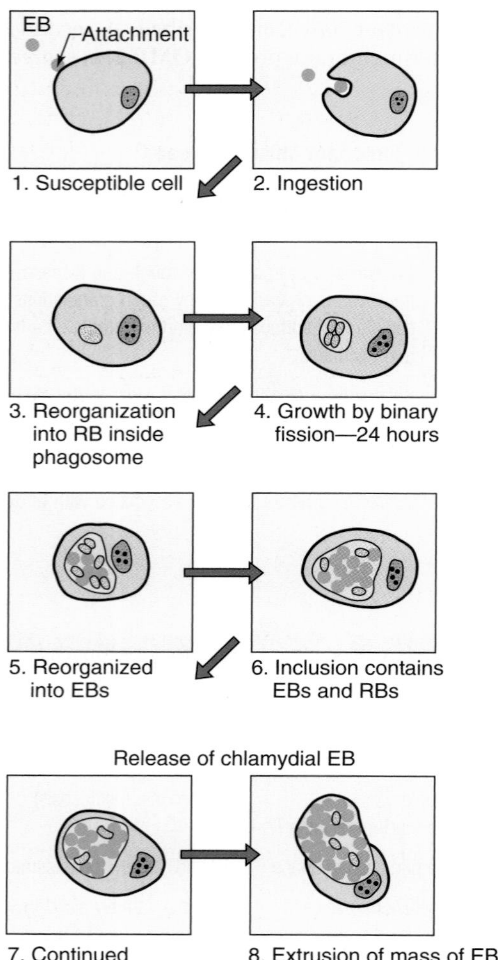

FIGURE 35-1 The growth cycle of *Chlamydia trachomatis. EB,* Elementary body; *RB,* reticulate body. (Modified from Batteiger B, Jones R: Chlamydial infections, *Infect Dis Clin North Am* 1:55–81, 1987.)

Chlamydia trachomatis

C. trachomatis has a limited host range, with infections restricted to humans (Box 35-1). The species responsible for human disease are subdivided into two **biovars: trachoma** and **lymphogranuloma venereum (LGV).** The biovars have been further divided into **serovars** based on antigenic differences in the MOMP. Specific serovars are associated with specific diseases (Table 35-3).

Pathogenesis and Immunity

The range of cells that *C. trachomatis* can infect is limited. Receptors for EBs are primarily restricted to nonciliated columnar, cuboidal, and transitional epithelial cells, which are found on the mucous membranes of the urethra, endocervix, endometrium, fallopian tubes, anorectum, respiratory tract, and conjunctivae. The LGV serovars are more invasive than the other serovars because they replicate in mononuclear phagocytes. The clinical manifestations of chlamydial infections are caused by (1) the direct destruction of cells during replication and (2) the proinflammatory cytokine response they stimulate.

Chlamydiae gain access through minute abrasions or lacerations. In LGV, the lesions form in the lymph nodes draining the site of primary infection (Figure 35-2). Granuloma formation is characteristic. The lesions may become necrotic, attract polymorphonuclear leukocytes, and cause the inflammatory process to spread to surrounding tissues. Subsequent rupture of the lymph node leads to formation of abscesses or sinus tracts. Infection with non-LGV serovars of *C. trachomatis* stimulates a severe inflammatory response consisting of neutrophils, lymphocytes, and plasma cells.

Infection does not confer long-lasting immunity; rather, reinfection characteristically induces a vigorous inflammatory response with subsequent tissue damage. This response produces the vision loss in patients with chronic ocular infections, and scarring with sterility and sexual dysfunction in patients with genital infections.

Table 35-3 Clinical Spectrum of *Chlamydia trachomatis* Infections

Serovars	Disease
A, B, Ba, C	Trachoma
D-K	Urogenital tract disease
L1, L2, L2a, L2b, L3	Lymphogranuloma venereum

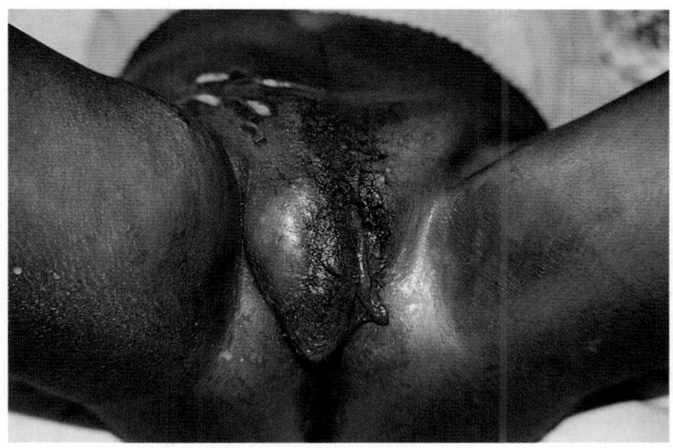

FIGURE 35-2 Patient with lymphogranuloma venereum causing unilateral vulvar lymphedema and inguinal buboes. (From Cohen J, Powderly WG, Opal SM: *Infectious diseases,* ed 3, Philadelphia, 2010, Mosby.)

Epidemiology

C. trachomatis is found worldwide and causes trachoma (chronic keratoconjunctivitis), oculogenital disease, pneumonia, and LGV. Trachoma is endemic in North and sub-Saharan Africa, the Middle East, South Asia, and South America. The World Health Organization estimates six million people are blind due to trachoma, and more than 150 million people are in need of treatment. Trachoma is the **leading cause of preventable blindness.** Infections occur predominantly in children, who are the chief reservoir of *C. trachomatis* in endemic areas. The incidence of infection is lower in older children and adolescents; however, the incidence of blindness continues to rise through adulthood as the disease progresses. Eye-to-eye transmission of trachoma is by droplet, hands, contaminated clothing, and flies that transmit ocular discharges from the eyes of infected children to the eyes of uninfected children. Because a high percentage of children in endemic areas harbor *C. trachomatis* in their respiratory and gastrointestinal tracts, the pathogen may also be transmitted by respiratory droplet or through fecal contamination. Trachoma generally is endemic in communities where the living conditions are crowded, sanitation is poor, and the personal hygiene of the people is poor—all risk factors that promote the transmission of infections.

Most cases of *C. trachomatis* **adult inclusion conjunctivitis** occur in people who are 18 to 30 years of age, and genital infection probably precedes eye involvement. Autoinoculation and oral-genital contact are believed to be the routes of transmission. A third form of *C. trachomatis* eye infection is **newborn inclusion conjunctivitis,** an infection acquired during passage of the infant through an infected birth canal. *C. trachomatis* conjunctivitis develops in approximately 25% of infants whose mothers have active genital infections.

Pulmonary infection with *C. trachomatis* also occurs in newborns. A diffuse **interstitial pneumonia** develops in 10% to 20% of infants exposed to the pathogen at birth.

C. trachomatis is thought to be the most common **sexually transmitted bacterial disease** in the United States. More than 1.4 million infections were reported in the United States in 2012; however, this figure is believed to be an underestimate because most infected patients either do not seek medical treatment or are treated without a specific diagnosis. It is estimated that almost 3 million Americans are infected each year, and as many as 50 million new infections occur annually worldwide. Most genital tract infections are caused by serotypes D to K.

LGV is a chronic sexually transmitted disease caused by *C. trachomatis* serotypes L1, L2, L2a, L2b, and L3. It occurs sporadically in the United States and other industrialized countries but is highly prevalent in Africa, Asia, and South America. Acute LGV is seen more frequently in men, primarily because symptomatic infection is less common in women.

Clinical Diseases

Trachoma

Trachoma is a **chronic disease** caused by serovars A, B, Ba, and C. Initially, patients have a **follicular conjunctivitis** with diffuse inflammation that involves the entire conjunctiva. The conjunctivae become scarred as the disease progresses, causing the patient's eyelids to turn inward. The turned-in eyelashes abrade the cornea, eventually resulting in corneal ulceration, scarring, pannus formation (invasion of vessels into the cornea), and loss of vision. It is common for trachoma to recur after apparent healing, most likely a result of subclinical infections that have been documented in children in endemic areas and in immigrants to the United States who acquired trachoma during childhood in their native countries.

Adult Inclusion Conjunctivitis

An acute follicular conjunctivitis caused by the *C. trachomatis* strains associated with genital infections (serovars A, B, Ba, D to K) has been documented in sexually active adults. The infection is characterized by mucopurulent discharge, keratitis, corneal infiltrates, and occasionally some corneal vascularization. Corneal scarring has been observed in patients with chronic infection.

Neonatal Conjunctivitis

Eye infections can also develop in **infants exposed to *C. trachomatis* at birth.** After an incubation of 5 to 12 days, the infant's eyelids swell, hyperemia occurs, and copious purulent discharge appears. Untreated infections may run a course as long as 12 months, during which time conjunctival scarring and corneal vascularization occur. Infants who are untreated or are treated with topical therapy only are at risk for *C. trachomatis* pneumonia.

Infant Pneumonia (Clinical Case 35-1)

The incubation period for infant pneumonia is variable, but the onset generally occurs 2 to 3 weeks after birth. Rhinitis is initially observed in such infants, after which a **distinctive staccato cough** develops. The child remains afebrile throughout the clinical illness, which can last for several weeks. Radiographic signs of infection can persist for months.

Ocular Lymphogranuloma Venereum

The LGV serotypes of *C. trachomatis* have been implicated in Parinaud oculoglandular conjunctivitis, a conjunctival

Clinical Case 35-1 *Chlamydia trachomatis* Pneumonia in Newborn Infants

Niida and associates (*Eur J Pediatr* 157:950–951, 1998) described two infant girls with *C. trachomatis* pneumonia. The first infant was born by vaginal delivery after 39 weeks' gestation and the second by caesarean section (because of fetal distress) at 40 weeks' gestation. The infants were in good condition until fever and tachypnea developed at 3 and 13 days, respectively. Chest radiographs showed infiltrates over the whole lungs. Cultures of blood, urine, throat, feces, and cerebrospinal fluid were negative, but antigen tests for *C. trachomatis* were positive from conjunctival and nasopharyngeal swabs. These cases illustrate the presentation of pneumonia in infants infected with *C. trachomatis* at or near birth, although the characteristic staccato cough was not described.

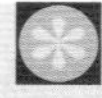

Clinical Case 35-2 Reiter Syndrome and Pelvic Inflammatory Disease

Serwin and associates (*J Eur Acad Derm Vener* 20:735–736, 2006) described a 30-year-old man who presented to a university hospital with complaints of dysuria for a 3-year duration, penile inflammation, joint swelling, and fever. Skin lesions and nail changes were also noted. High levels of *Chlamydia* antibodies were present, but antigen tests and nucleic acid amplification tests of the urethral exudates and conjunctiva were negative for *Chlamydia trachomatis*. A diagnosis of Reiter syndrome was made, and treatment with ofloxacin was initiated. Complete remission of the skin lesions and urethral symptoms was achieved. The patient's wife was also admitted to the hospital with a history of 2 years of lower abdominal pain and vaginal bleeding and discharge. The diagnosis of pelvic inflammatory disease (PID) was made, and *C. trachomatis* infection was confirmed by positive cervical and urethral antigen tests (direct fluorescent antibody). The vaginal smear was also positive for *Trichomonas vaginalis*. These patients illustrate two complications of *C. trachomatis* urogenital infections: Reiter syndrome and PID.

inflammation associated with preauricular, submandibular, and cervical lymphadenopathy.

Urogenital Infections (Clinical Case 35-2)

Most genital tract infections in women are asymptomatic (as many as 80%) but can nevertheless become symptomatic. The clinical manifestations include bartholinitis, cervicitis, endometritis, perihepatitis, salpingitis, and urethritis. Asymptomatic patients with chlamydial infection are an important reservoir for the spread of *C. trachomatis*. A mucopurulent discharge (Figure 35-3) is seen in patients with symptomatic infection, whose specimens generally yield more organisms on cultures than specimens from patients with asymptomatic infections. Urethritis caused by *C. trachomatis* may occur with or without a concurrent cervical infection.

Although most *C. trachomatis* genital infections in men are symptomatic, as many as 25% of the infections will be inapparent. Approximately 35% to 50% of cases of nongonococcal urethritis are caused by *C. trachomatis;* dual infections with both *C. trachomatis* and *Neisseria gonorrhoeae* are not uncommon. Symptoms of the chlamydial infection develop after successful treatment of the gonorrhea, because the

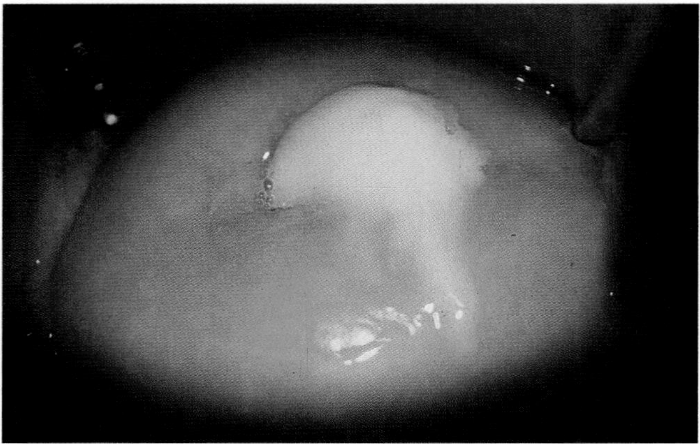

FIGURE 35-3 Mucopurulent cervicitis caused by *Chlamydia trachomatis.* (From Cohen J, Powderly W: *Infectious diseases,* ed 2, St Louis, 2004, Mosby. Photo by J. Paavonen.)

incubation period is longer and the use of β-lactam antibiotics to treat gonorrhea would be ineffective against *C. trachomatis*. Although there is less purulent exudate in patients with chlamydial urethral infections, such infections cannot be differentiated reliably from gonorrhea, so specific diagnostic tests for both organisms should be performed.

It is believed that **Reiter syndrome** (urethritis, conjunctivitis, polyarthritis, and mucocutaneous lesions) is initiated by genital infection with *C. trachomatis*. Although chlamydiae have not been isolated from the synovial fluid of such patients, chlamydial EBs have been observed in synovial fluid or tissue specimens from men with sexually acquired reactive arthritis. The disease usually occurs in young white men. Approximately 50% to 65% of patients with Reiter syndrome have a chlamydial genital infection at the onset of arthritis, and serologic studies indicate that more than 80% of men with Reiter syndrome have evidence of a preceding or concurrent infection with *C. trachomatis*.

Lymphogranuloma Venereum

After an incubation of 1 to 4 weeks, a primary lesion appears at the site of infection (e.g., penis, urethra, glans, scrotum, vaginal wall, cervix, vulva) in patients with LGV. The lesion (either a papule or an ulcer) is often overlooked because it is small, is painless, and heals rapidly. The absence of pain differentiates these ulcers from those observed in herpes simplex virus infections. The patient may experience fever, headache, and myalgia when the lesion is present.

The second stage of infection is marked by inflammation and swelling of the lymph nodes draining the site of initial infection. The inguinal nodes are most commonly involved, becoming painful, fluctuant **buboes** that gradually enlarge and can rupture, forming draining fistulas. Systemic manifestations include fever, chills, anorexia, headache, meningismus, myalgias, and arthralgia.

Proctitis is common in women with LGV, resulting from lymphatic spread from the cervix or the vagina. Proctitis develops in men after anal intercourse or as the result of lymphatic spread from the urethra. Untreated LGV may resolve at this stage or may progress to a chronic ulcerative phase in which genital ulcers, fistulas, strictures, or genital elephantiasis develop.

Laboratory Diagnosis

C. trachomatis infection can be diagnosed (1) on the basis of cytologic, serologic, or culture findings, (2) through the direct detection of antigen in clinical specimens, and (3) through the use of nucleic acid–based tests. The sensitivity of each method depends on the patient population examined, the site where the specimen is obtained, and the nature of the disease. For example, symptomatic infections are generally easier to diagnose than asymptomatic infections because more chlamydiae are present in the specimen. The quality of the specimen is also important. Although it may seem obvious, specimens must be obtained from the involved site (e.g., urethra, cervix, rectum, oropharynx, conjunctiva) and not from pus or a vaginal exudate, where relatively few organisms may be present. Chlamydiae infect columnar or squamocolumnar cells; therefore, endocervical and not vaginal specimens should be collected. It has been estimated that one third of the specimens submitted for study in patients with suspected *Chlamydia* infection are inappropriate.

Antigen Detection

Two general approaches have been used to detect chlamydial antigens in clinical specimens: **direct immunofluorescence staining** with fluorescein-conjugated monoclonal antibodies (Figure 35-4) and **enzyme-linked immunosorbent assays.** In both assays, antibodies are used that have been prepared against either the chlamydial MOMP or the cell wall LPS. Because antigenic determinants on LPS may be shared with other bacteria, particularly those in fecal specimens, tests that target the LPS antigen are less specific. The sensitivity of each assay method has been reported to vary enormously, but neither is considered as sensitive as culture or nucleic acid–based tests, particularly if male urethral specimens or specimens from asymptomatic patients are used. The latter pose a problem because they may contain relatively few chlamydiae.

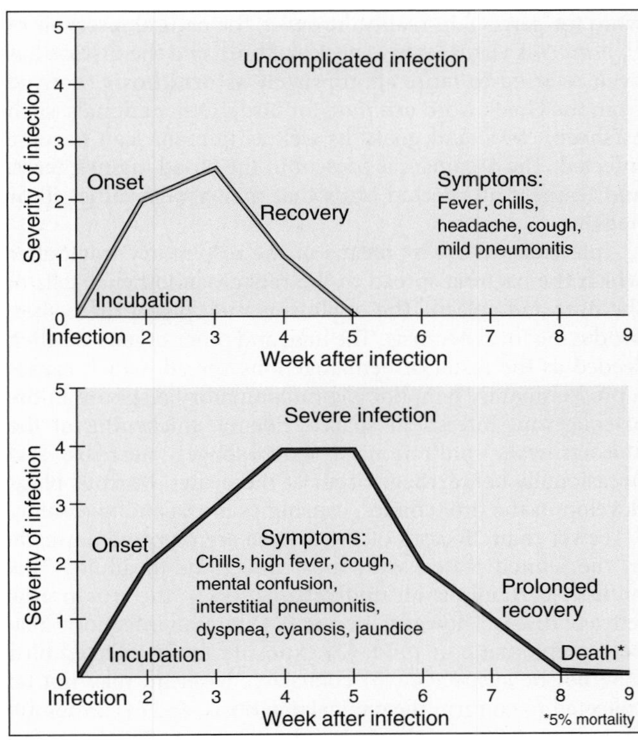

FIGURE 35-4 Time course of *Chlamydophila psittaci* infection.

Nucleic Acid–Based Tests

Nucleic acid amplification tests (NAATs) are the test of choice for the diagnosis of chlamydia infections (generally reported to be 90% to 98% sensitive and very specific). First-voided urine from a patient with urethritis can be used as well as urethral discharge. Care must be used to monitor for the presence of inhibitors (e.g., urine) to the amplification reaction and to prevent cross-contamination of specimens.

Culture

The isolation of *C. trachomatis* in cell culture remains the most **specific** method of diagnosing *C. trachomatis* infections but is **relatively insensitive** compared with NAA techniques. The bacteria infect a restricted range of cell lines in vitro, similar to the narrow range of cells they infect in vivo. The sensitivity of culture is compromised if inadequate specimens are used and if chlamydial viability has been lost during transport of the specimen. It has been estimated that the sensitivity of the findings yielded by a single endocervical specimen may be only 70% to 85%.

Antibody Detection

Serologic testing is of limited value in the diagnosis of *C. trachomatis* urogenital infections in adults because the test cannot differentiate between current and past infections. Demonstration of a significant increase in antibody levels can be useful; however, this increase may not be demonstrated for a month or longer, particularly in patients who receive antibiotic treatment. Testing for immunoglobulin (Ig)M antibodies is also usually not helpful because these antibodies may not be detected in adolescents and adults. An exception is the detection of IgM antibodies in infants with chlamydial pneumonitis.

Antibody tests for the diagnosis of LGV can be helpful. Infected patients produce a vigorous antibody response that can be detected by complement fixation (CF), microimmunofluorescence (MIF), or enzyme immunoassay (EIA). The CF test is directed against the genus-specific LPS antigen. Thus a positive result (i.e., fourfold increase in titer or a single titer ≥ 1:256) is highly suggestive of LGV. Confirmation is determined by the MIF test, which is directed against species- and serovar-specific antigens (the chlamydial MOMPs). Similar to the CF test, EIAs are genus specific. The advantage of these tests is that they are less technically cumbersome; however, the results must be confirmed by MIF.

Treatment, Prevention, and Control

It is recommended that patients with LGV be treated with doxycycline for 21 days. Treatment with erythromycin is recommended for children younger than 9 years, pregnant women, and patients unable to tolerate doxycycline. Ocular and genital infections in adults should be treated with one dose of azithromycin or doxycycline for 7 days. Newborn conjunctivitis and pneumonia should be treated with erythromycin for 10 to 14 days.

It is difficult to prevent trachoma, because the population with endemic disease commonly has limited access to medical care. The blindness associated with advanced stages of trachoma can be prevented only by prompt treatment of early disease and prevention of reexposure. Although treatment can be successful in individuals living in areas where the disease is endemic, it is difficult to eradicate the disease within a population and to prevent reinfections unless sanitary conditions are improved. *Chlamydia* conjunctivitis and genital infections are prevented through the use of safe sex practices and the prompt treatment of symptomatic patients and their sexual partners.

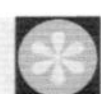

Clinical Case 35-3 Psittacosis in a Previously Healthy Man

Scully and associates (*N Engl J Med* 338:1527–1535, 1998) described a 24-year-old man who was admitted into a local hospital in acute respiratory distress. Several days before his hospitalization, he developed nasal congestion, myalgia, dry cough, mild dyspnea, and a headache. Immediately before admission, the cough became productive and he developed pleuritic pain, fever, chills, and diarrhea. Radiographs demonstrated consolidation of the right upper lobe of the lungs and patchy infiltrates in the left lower lobe. Despite the fact that his antibiotic treatment included erythromycin, doxycycline, ceftriaxone, and vancomycin, his pulmonary status did not begin to improve for 7 days, and he was not discharged from the hospital until a month after his admission. A careful history revealed the man had been exposed to parrots in a hotel lobby while vacationing. The diagnosis of *Chlamydophila psittaci* pneumonia was made by growing the organism in cell culture and serologic tests.

Chlamydophila pneumoniae

C. pneumoniae was first isolated from the conjunctiva of a child in Taiwan. It was initially considered a psittacosis strain because the morphology of the inclusions produced in cell culture was similar. However, it was subsequently shown that the Taiwan isolate (TW-183) was related serologically to a pharyngeal isolate designated AR-39 and was unrelated to psittacosis strains. This new organism was initially called TWAR (from the two original isolates), then classified as *Chlamydia pneumoniae,* and finally placed in the new genus *Chlamydophila.* Only a single serotype (TWAR) has been identified. Respiratory secretions transmit infection; no animal reservoir has been identified.

C. pneumoniae is a **human pathogen** that causes sinusitis, pharyngitis, bronchitis, and pneumonia. Infections are believed to be transmitted person to person by respiratory secretions. The prevalence of infections is very controversial, with wide variations reported in the literature, in large part because of significant variation in diagnostic test methods. It is believed that most *C. pneumoniae* infections are asymptomatic or mild, causing a persistent cough and malaise; most patients do not require hospitalization. More severe respiratory tract infections typically involve a single lobe of the lungs. These infections cannot be differentiated from other atypical pneumonias such as those caused by *Mycoplasma pneumoniae, Legionella pneumophila,* and respiratory viruses.

The role of *C. pneumoniae* in the pathogenesis of atherosclerosis remains to be defined. It is known that *C. pneumoniae* can infect and grow in smooth muscle cells, endothelial cells of the coronary artery, and macrophages. The organism has also been demonstrated in biopsy specimens of atherosclerotic lesions by means of culture, polymerase chain reaction amplification, immunohistologic staining, electron microscopy, and in situ hybridization. Thus the association of *C. pneumoniae* with atherosclerotic lesions is clear. What is not clear is the role of the organism in the development of atherosclerosis. It has been proposed that the disease results from an inflammatory response to chronic infection; however, this remains to be proven.

Diagnosis of *C. pneumoniae* infections is difficult. The organisms do not grow in the cell lines used for the isolation of *C. trachomatis,* and although *C. pneumoniae* will grow in the HEp-2 cell line, this cell line is not used in most clinical laboratories. Detection of *C. pneumoniae* by NAATs has been successful; however, significant interlaboratory variation has been reported among laboratories with experience in the use of these assays. The MIF test is the only acceptable test for serodiagnosis. The criteria for the diagnosis of acute *C. pneumoniae* infection is a single IgM titer of greater than 16 or a fourfold increase in IgG titer. A single elevated IgG titer cannot be used. Because IgG antibodies do not appear for 6 to 8 weeks after infection, serologic testing has limited value for the diagnosis of an acute infection.

Macrolides (erythromycin, azithromycin, clarithromycin), doxycycline, or levofloxacin is recommended for treatment of *C. pneumoniae* infections, although evidence supporting their use is limited. Control of exposure to *C. pneumoniae* is likely to be difficult because the bacterium is ubiquitous.

Chlamydophila psittaci (Clinical Case 35-3)

C. psittaci is the cause of psittacosis (parrot fever), which can be transmitted to humans. The disease was first observed in parrots, thus the name **psittacosis** (*psittakos* is the Greek word for parrot). In reality, however, the natural reservoir of *C. psittaci* is virtually any species of bird, and the disease has been referred to more appropriately as **ornithosis** (derived from the Greek word *ornithos,* for bird). Other animals, such as sheep, cows, and goats, as well as humans, can become infected. The organism is present in the blood, tissues, feces, and feathers of infected birds that may appear either ill or healthy.

Infection occurs by means of the respiratory tract, after which the bacteria spread to the reticuloendothelial cells of the liver and spleen. The organisms multiply in these sites, producing focal necrosis. The lung and other organs are then seeded as the result of hematogenous spread, which causes a predominantly lymphocytic inflammatory response in the alveolar and interstitial spaces. Edema, thickening of the alveolar wall, infiltration of macrophages, necrosis, and occasionally hemorrhage occur at these sites. Mucous plugs develop in the bronchioles, causing cyanosis and anoxia.

Fewer than 25 cases of the disease are reported annually in the United States, with most infections in adults. This number certainly is an underestimation of the true prevalence of disease, however, because (1) human infections may be asymptomatic or mild, (2) exposure to an infected bird may not be suspected, (3) convalescent serum may not be collected to confirm the clinical diagnosis, and (4) antibiotic therapy may blunt the antibody response. Furthermore, because of the serologic cross-reactions with *C. pneumoniae,* specific estimates of the prevalence of disease will remain unreliable until a definitive diagnostic test is developed.

The bacterium is usually transmitted to humans through the inhalation of dried excrement, urine, or respiratory secretions from psittacine birds (e.g., parrots, parakeets, macaws, cockatiels). Person-to-person transmission is rare. Veterinarians, zookeepers, pet shop workers, and employees of poultry-processing plants are at increased risk for this infection.

The illness develops after an incubation of 5 to 14 days and usually manifests as headache, high fever, chills, malaise, and myalgias (see Figure 35-4). Pulmonary signs include a nonproductive cough, rales, and consolidation. Central nervous system involvement is common, usually consisting of headache, but encephalitis, convulsions, coma, and death may occur in severe untreated cases. Patients may suffer gastrointestinal tract symptoms such as nausea, vomiting, and diarrhea. Other systemic symptoms include carditis, hepatomegaly, splenomegaly, and follicular keratoconjunctivitis.

Psittacosis is usually diagnosed on the basis of serologic findings. A fourfold increase in titer, shown by the CF testing of paired acute and convalescent phase sera, is suggestive of *C. psittaci* infection, but the species-specific MIF test must be performed to confirm the diagnosis. *C. psittaci* can be isolated in cell culture (e.g., with L cells) after 5 to 10 days of incubation, although this procedure is rarely performed in clinical laboratories.

Infections can be treated successfully with doxycycline or macrolides. Person-to-person transmission rarely occurs, so isolation of the patient and prophylactic treatment of contacts are not necessary. Psittacosis can be prevented only through the control of infections in domestic and imported pet birds. Such control can be achieved by treating birds with chlortetracycline hydrochloride for 45 days. No vaccine currently exists for this disease.

Bibliography

Arcari CM, Gaydos CA, Nieto FJ, et al: Association between *Chlamydia pneumoniae* and acute myocardial infarction in young men in the United States military: the importance of timing of exposure measurement, *Clin Infect Dis* 40:1123–1130, 2005.

Bebear C, de Barbeyrac B: Genital *Chlamydia trachomatis* infections, *Clin Microbiol Infect* 15:4–10, 2009.

Beeckman D, Vanrompay D: Zoonotic *Chlamydophila psittaci* infections from a clinical perspective, *Clin Microbiol Infect* 15:11–17, 2009.

Byrne G: *Chlamydia trachomatis* strains and virulence: rethinking links to infection prevalence and disease severity, *J Infect Dis* 201:S126–S133, 2010.

Centers for Disease Control and Prevention: Recommendations for the laboratory-based detection of *Chlamydia trachomatis* and *Neisseria gonorrhoeae*—2014, *MMWR Recomm Rep* 63(RR-02):1–19, 2014.

Gambhir M, Basáñez MG, Turner F, et al: Trachoma: transmission, infection, and control, *Lancet Infect Dis* 7:420–427, 2007.

Kern J, Maass V, Maass M: Molecular pathogenesis of chronic *Chlamydia pneumoniae* infections: a brief overview, *Clin Microbiol Infect* 15:36–41, 2009.

Kumar S, Hammerschlag M: Acute respiratory infection due to *Chlamydia pneumoniae*: current status of diagnostic methods, *Clin Infect Dis* 44:568–576, 2007.

Liechti GW, Kuru E, Hall E, et al: A new metabolic cell-wall labeling method reveals peptidoglycan in *Chlamydia trachomatis*, *Nature* 506:507–510, 2014.

Morré SA, Rozendaal L, van Valkengoed IG, et al: Urogenital *Chlamydia trachomatis* serovars in men and women with a symptomatic or asymptomatic infection: an association with clinical manifestations? *J Clin Microbiol* 38:2292–2296, 2000.

Nunes A, Gomes J: Evolution, phylogeny, and molecular epidemiology of *Chlamydia*, *Infect Genet Evol* 23:49–64, 2014.

Van der Bij AK, Spaargaren J, Morré SA, et al: Diagnostic and clinical implications of anorectal lymphogranuloma venereum in men who have sex with men: a retrospective case-control study, *Clin Infect Dis* 42:186–194, 2006.

Vasilevsky S, Greub G, Nardelli-Haefliger D, et al: Genital *Chlamydia trachomatis*: understanding the roles of innate and adaptive immunity in vaccine research, *Clin Microbiol Rev* 27:346–370, 2014.

SECTION

5

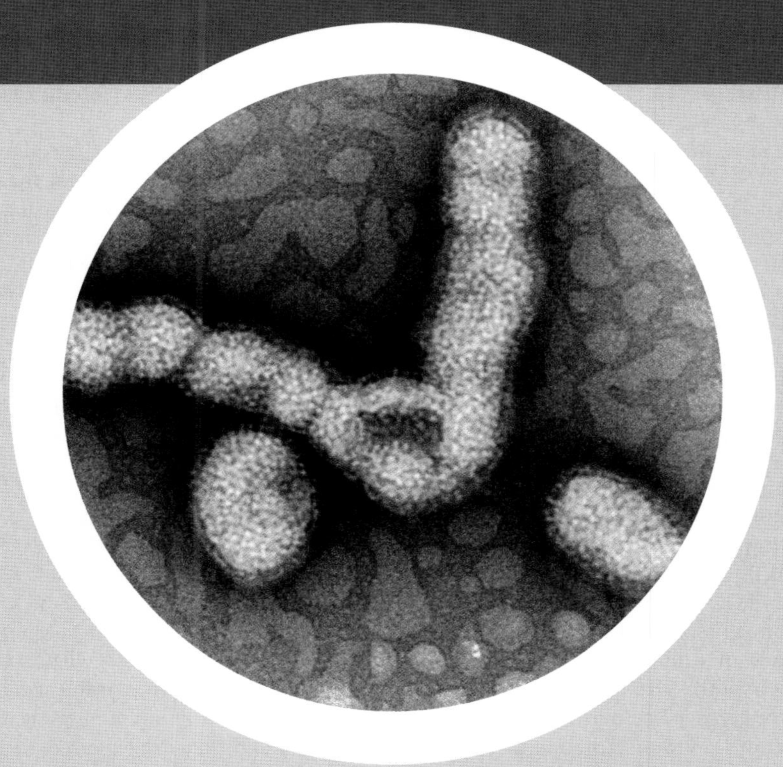

VIROLOGY

CHAPTER

36

VIRAL CLASSIFICATION, STRUCTURE, AND REPLICATION

Viruses were first described as "filterable agents." Their small size allows them to pass through filters designed to retain bacteria. Unlike most bacteria, fungi, and parasites, **viruses are obligate intracellular parasites** that depend on the biochemical machinery of the host cell for replication. In addition, *reproduction of viruses occurs by assembly of the individual components rather than by binary fission* (Boxes 36-1 and 36-2).

The simplest viruses consist of a genome of deoxyribonucleic acid (DNA) or ribonucleic acid (RNA) packaged in a protective shell of protein and, for some viruses, a membrane (Figure 36-1). Viruses lack the capacity to make energy or substrates, cannot make their own proteins, and cannot replicate their genome independently of the host cell. To use the cell's biosynthetic machinery, the virus must be adapted to the biochemical rules of the cell.

The physical structure and genetics of viruses have been optimized by mutation and selection to infect humans and other hosts. To do this, the virus must be capable of transmission between hosts, must traverse the skin or other protective barriers of the host, must be adapted to the biochemical machinery of the host cell for replication, and must escape elimination by the host immune response.

Knowledge of the structural **(size and morphology)** and genetic **(type and structure of nucleic acid)** features of a virus provides insight into how the virus replicates, spreads, and causes disease. The concepts presented in this chapter are repeated in greater detail in the discussions of specific viruses in later chapters.

• Classification

Viruses range from the structurally simple and small parvoviruses and picornaviruses to the large and complex poxviruses and herpesviruses. Their names may describe viral characteristics, the diseases they are associated with, or even the tissue or geographic locale where they were first identified. Names such as **picornavirus** (*pico,* "small"; *rna,* "ribonucleic acid") or **togavirus** (*toga,* Greek for "mantle," referring to a membrane envelope surrounding the virus) describe the structure of the virus. The name **retrovirus** (*retro,* "reverse") refers to the virus-directed synthesis of DNA from an RNA template, whereas the *poxviruses* are named for the disease smallpox, caused by one of its members. The **adenoviruses** (*adeno*ids) and the **reoviruses** (*r*espiratory, *e*nteric, *o*rphan) are named for the body site from which they were first isolated. Reovirus was discovered before it was associated with a specific disease, and thus it was designated an "orphan" virus. Norwalk virus is named for Norwalk, Ohio; coxsackievirus is named for Coxsackie, New York; and many of the togaviruses, arenaviruses, and bunyaviruses are named after African places where they were first isolated.

Viruses can be grouped by characteristics such as disease (e.g., hepatitis), target tissue, means of transmission (e.g., enteric, respiratory), or vector (e.g., arboviruses; arthropod-borne virus) (Box 36-3). *The most consistent and current means of classification is by physical and biochemical characteristics, such as size, morphology (e.g., presence or absence of a membrane envelope), type of genome, and means of replication* (Figures 36-2 and 36-3). DNA viruses associated with human disease are divided into seven families (Tables 36-1 and 36-2). The RNA viruses may be divided into at least 13 families (Tables 36-3 and 36-4).

• Virion Structure

The units for measurement of virion size are nanometers (nm). The clinically important viruses range from 18 nm (parvoviruses) to 300 nm (poxviruses) (Figure 36-4). The latter are almost visible with a light microscope and are approximately one fourth the size of staphylococcal bacteria. *Larger virions can hold a larger genome that can encode more proteins, and they are generally more complex.*

The **virion** (the virus particle) consists of a nucleic acid **genome** packaged into a protein coat **(capsid)** or a membrane **(envelope)** (see Figure 36-4). The virion may also contain certain essential or accessory enzymes or other proteins to facilitate initial replication in the cell. Capsid or nucleic acid–binding proteins may associate with the genome to form a **nucleocapsid,** which may be the same as the virion or surrounded by an envelope.

The genome of the virus consists either of DNA or RNA. The DNA can be single or double stranded, linear or circular. The RNA can be either positive sense (+) (like messenger RNA [mRNA]) or negative sense (−) (analogous to a photographic negative), double stranded (+/−), or ambisense (containing + and − regions of RNA attached end to end). The RNA genome may also be segmented into pieces, with each piece encoding one or more genes. Just as there are many different types of computer memory devices, all of these forms of nucleic acid can maintain and transmit the genetic information of the virus. Similarly, the larger the genome, the more information (genes) it can carry and the

Box 36-1 Definition and Properties of a Virus

Viruses are filterable agents.
Viruses are obligate intracellular parasites.
Viruses cannot make energy or proteins independently of a host cell.
Viral genomes may be RNA or DNA but not both.
Viruses have a naked capsid or an envelope morphology.
Viral components are assembled and do not replicate by "division."

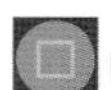

Box 36-2 Consequences of Viral Properties

Viruses are not living.
Viruses must be infectious to endure in nature.
Viruses must be able to use host cell processes to produce their components (viral messenger RNA, protein, and identical copies of the genome).
Viruses must encode any required processes not provided by the cell.
Viral components must self-assemble.

Box 36-3 Means of Classification and Naming of Viruses

Structure: size, morphology, and nucleic acid (e.g., picornavirus [small RNA], togavirus)
Biochemical characteristics: structure and mode of replication*
Disease: encephalitis and hepatitis viruses, for example
Means of transmission: arbovirus spread by insects, for example
Host cell (host range): animal (human, mouse, bird), plant, bacteria
Tissue or organ (tropism): adenovirus and enterovirus, for example

*This is the current means of taxonomic classification of viruses.

larger the capsid or envelope structure required to contain the genome.

The outer layer of the virion is the **capsid** or **envelope.** These structures are the package, protection, and delivery vehicle during transmission of the virus from one host to another and for spread within the host to the target cell. The surface structures of the capsid and envelope mediate the interaction of the virus with the target cell through a **viral attachment protein (VAP)** or structure. *Removal or disruption of the outer package inactivates the virus. Antibodies generated against the VAP prevent virus infection.* The influence of virion structure on viral properties is summarized in Boxes 36-4 and 36-5.

The **capsid** is a rigid structure able to withstand harsh environmental conditions. Like a soccer ball, naked capsid viruses also have a tough exterior and are generally resistant to drying, acid, and detergents, including the acid and bile of the enteric tract. Many of these viruses are transmitted by the fecal-oral route and can endure transmission even in sewage.

The **envelope** is a membrane composed of lipids, proteins, and glycoproteins. The membranous structure of the envelope can be maintained only in aqueous solutions. It is readily disrupted by drying, acidic conditions, detergents, and solvents such as ether, which results in inactivation of the virus. *As a result, enveloped viruses must remain wet and are generally transmitted in fluids, respiratory droplets, blood,*

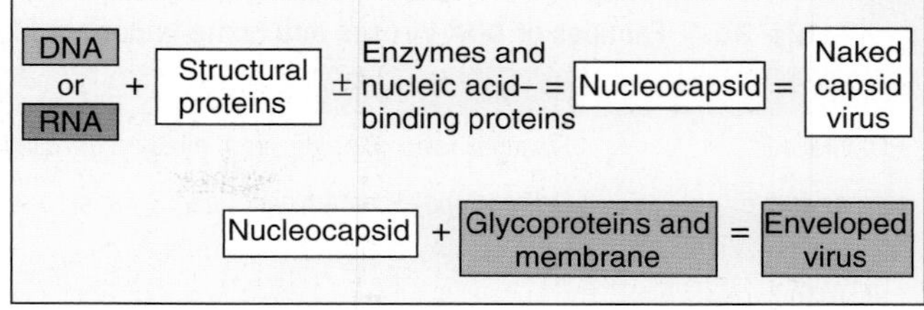

FIGURE 36-1 Components of the basic virion.

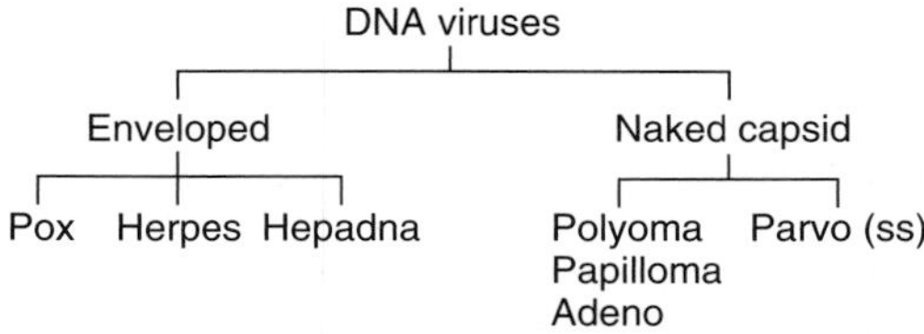

FIGURE 36-2 The DNA viruses and their morphology. The viral families are determined by the structure of the genome and the morphology of the virion. *ss,* Single-stranded genome.

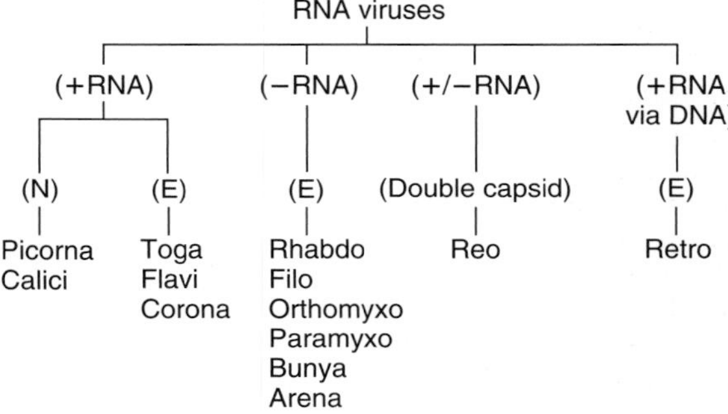

FIGURE 36-3 The RNA viruses, their genome structure, and their morphology. The viral families are determined by the structure of the genome and the morphology of the virion. *E,* Enveloped; *N,* naked capsid.

and tissue. Most cannot survive the harsh conditions of the gastrointestinal tract.

Capsid Viruses

The viral capsid is assembled from individual proteins associated into progressively larger units. All of the components of the capsid have chemical features that allow them to fit together and to assemble into a larger unit. Individual structural proteins associate into **subunits,** which associate into **protomers, capsomeres** (distinguishable in electron micrographs), and finally, a recognizable **procapsid** or **capsid** (Figure 36-5). A procapsid requires further processing to the final, transmissible capsid. For some viruses, the capsid forms around the genome; for others the capsid forms as an empty shell (procapsid) to be filled by the genome.

The simplest viral structures that can be built stepwise are symmetric and include **helical** and **icosahedral** structures. Helical structures appear as rods, whereas the icosahedron is an approximation of a sphere assembled from symmetric subunits (Figure 36-6). Nonsymmetric capsids are complex forms and are associated with certain bacterial viruses (phages).

Table 36-1 Families of DNA Viruses and Some Important Members

Family*	Members†
POXVIRIDAE	*Smallpox virus,* vaccinia virus, monkeypox, canarypox, molluscum contagiosum
Herpesviridae	*Herpes simplex virus types 1 and 2,* varicella-zoster virus, Epstein-Barr virus, cytomegalovirus, human herpesviruses 6, 7, and 8
Adenoviridae	*Adenovirus*
Papillomaviridae	*Papillomavirus*
Polyomaviridae	*JC virus,* BK virus, SV40
Parvoviridae	*Parvovirus B19,* adeno-associated virus
Hepadnaviridae	*Hepatitis B virus*

*The size of type is indicative of the relative size of the virus.
†The italicized virus is the prototype virus for the family.

Table 36-2 Properties of Virions of Human DNA Viruses

	Genome*		Virion		
Family	Molecular Mass × 10^6 Daltons	Nature	Shape	Size (nm)	Encodes Polymerase?†
Poxviridae	85-140	ds, linear	Brick-shaped, enveloped	300 × 240 × 100	+‡ǁ
Herpesviridae	100-150	ds, linear	Icosadeltahedral, enveloped	Capsid, 100-110 Envelope, 120-200	+
Adenoviridae	20-25	ds, linear	Icosadeltahedral with fibers	70-90	+
Hepadnaviridae	1.8	ds, circular§	Spherical, enveloped	42	+‡¶
Polyoma- and papillomaviridae	3-5	ds, circular	Icosadeltahedral	45-55	–
Parvoviridae	1.5-2.0	ss, linear	Icosahedral	18-26	–

ds, Double-stranded; *ss,* single-stranded.
*Genome invariably a single molecule.
†DNA-dependent DNA polymerase (unless otherwise noted).
‡Polymerase carried in the virion.
§Circular molecule is double stranded for most of its length but contains a single-stranded region.
ǁPoxviruses also encode a DNA-dependent RNA polymerase.
¶DNA-dependent RNA polymerase (reverse transcriptase).

Table 36-3 Families of RNA Viruses and Some Important Members

Family*	Members†
PARAMYXOVIRIDAE	Parainfluenza virus, Sendai virus, *measles virus,* mumps virus, respiratory syncytial virus, metapneumovirus
ORTHOMYXOVIRIDAE	*Influenza virus* types A, B, C and thogotoviruses
CORONAVIRIDAE	*Coronavirus,* severe acute respiratory syndrome (SARS) virus, Middle East respiratory syndrome (MERS) virus
Arenaviridae	*Lassa fever virus,* Tacaribe virus complex (Junin and Machupo viruses), lymphocytic choriomeningitis virus
Rhabdoviridae	*Rabies virus,* vesicular stomatitis virus
Filoviridae	*Ebola virus,* Marburg virus
Bunyaviridae	*California encephalitis virus,* La Crosse virus, sandfly fever virus, hemorrhagic fever virus, Hanta virus
Retroviridae	Human T-cell leukemia virus types I and II, *human immunodeficiency virus,* animal oncoviruses
Reoviridae	*Rotavirus,* Colorado tick fever virus
Togaviridae	Rubella virus; *western, eastern, and Venezuelan equine encephalitis virus;* Ross River virus; Sindbis virus; Semliki Forest virus; chikungunya virus
Flaviviridae	*Yellow fever virus,* dengue virus, St. Louis encephalitis virus, West Nile virus, hepatitis C virus
Caliciviridae	*Norwalk virus,* calicivirus
Picornaviridae	Rhinoviruses, *poliovirus,* echoviruses, coxsackievirus, hepatitis A virus
Delta	Delta agent

*The size of the type is indicative of the relative size of the virus.
†The italicized virus is the prototype virus for the family.

Table 36-4 Properties of Virions of Human RNA Viruses

	Genome*		Virion			
Family	**Molecular Mass × 10^6 Daltons**	**Nature**	**Shape***	**Size (nm)**	**Polymerase in Virion**	**Envelope**
Paramyxoviridae	5-7	ss, –	Spherical	150-300	+	+
Orthomyxoviridae	5-7	ss, –, seg	Spherical	80-120	+	+
Coronaviridae	6-7	ss, +	Spherical	80-130	–	+[†]
Arenaviridae	3-5	ss, –, seg	Spherical	50-300	+	+[†]
Rhabdoviridae	4-7	ss, –	Bullet-shaped	180 × 75	+	+
Filoviridae	4-7	ss, –	Filamentous	800 × 80	+	+
Bunyaviridae	4-7	ss, –	Spherical	90-100	+	+[†]
Retroviridae	2 × (2-3)[‡]	ss, +	Spherical	80-110	+[§]	+
Reoviridae	11-15	ds, seg	Icosahedral	60-80	+	–
Picornaviridae	2.5	ss, +	Icosahedral	25-30	–	–
Togaviridae	4-5	ss, +	Icosahedral	60-70	–	+
Flaviviridae	4-7	ss, +	Spherical	40-50	–	+
Caliciviridae	2.6	ss, +	Icosahedral	35-40	–	–

ds, Double-stranded; *seg,* segmented; *ss,* single-stranded; + *or* –, polarity of single-stranded nucleic acid.
*Some enveloped viruses are very pleomorphic (sometimes filamentous).
[†]No matrix protein.
[‡]Genome has two identical single-stranded RNA molecules.
[§]Reverse transcriptase.

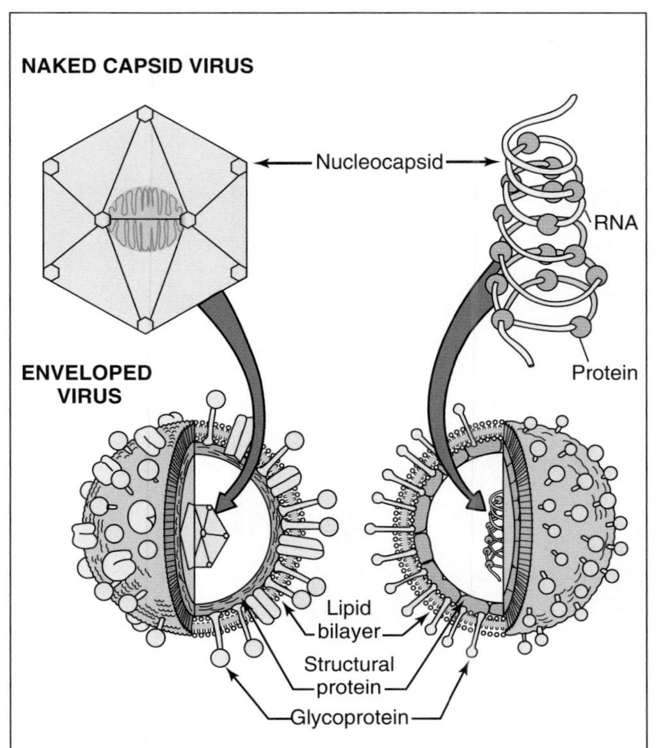

FIGURE 36-4 The structures of a naked icosahedral capsid virus *(top left)* and enveloped viruses *(bottom)* with an icosahedral *(left)* nucleocapsid or a helical *(right)* ribonucleocapsid. Helical nucleocapsids are always enveloped for human viruses.

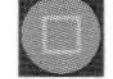

Box 36-4 Virion Structure: Naked Capsid

Component
Protein

Properties*
Is environmentally stable to the following:
- Temperature
- Acid
- Proteases
- Detergents
- Drying

Is released from cell by lysis

Consequences*
Can be spread easily (on fomites, from hand to hand, by dust, by small droplets)
Can dry out and retain infectivity
Can survive the adverse conditions of the gut
Can be resistant to detergents and poor sewage treatment
Antibody may be sufficient for immunoprotection

*Exceptions exist.

Box 36-5 Virion Structure: Envelope

Components
Membrane
Lipids
Proteins
Glycoproteins

Properties*
Is environmentally labile—disrupted by the following:
- Acid
- Detergents
- Drying
- Heat

Modifies cell membrane during replication
Is released by budding and cell lysis

Consequences*
Must stay wet
Cannot survive the gastrointestinal tract
Spreads in large droplets, secretions, organ transplants, and blood transfusions
Does not need to kill the cell to spread
May need antibody and cell-mediated immune response for protection and control
Elicits hypersensitivity and inflammation to cause immunopathogenesis

*Exceptions exist.

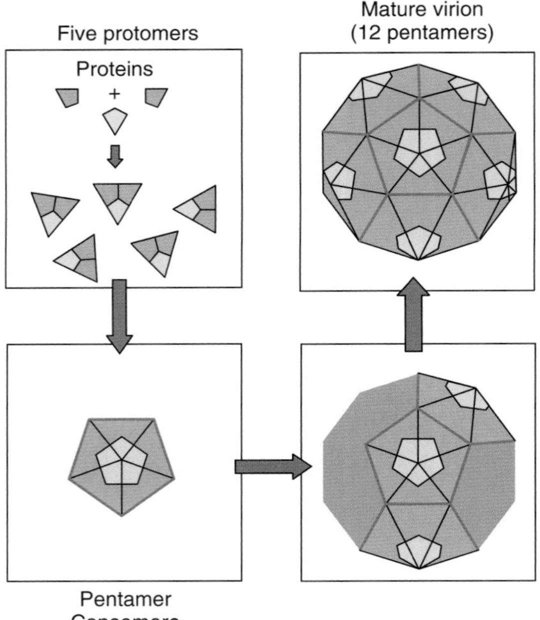

FIGURE 36-5 Capsid assembly of the icosahedral capsid of a picornavirus. Individual proteins associate into subunits, which associate into protomers, capsomeres, and an empty procapsid. Inclusion of the (+) RNA genome triggers its conversion to the final capsid form.

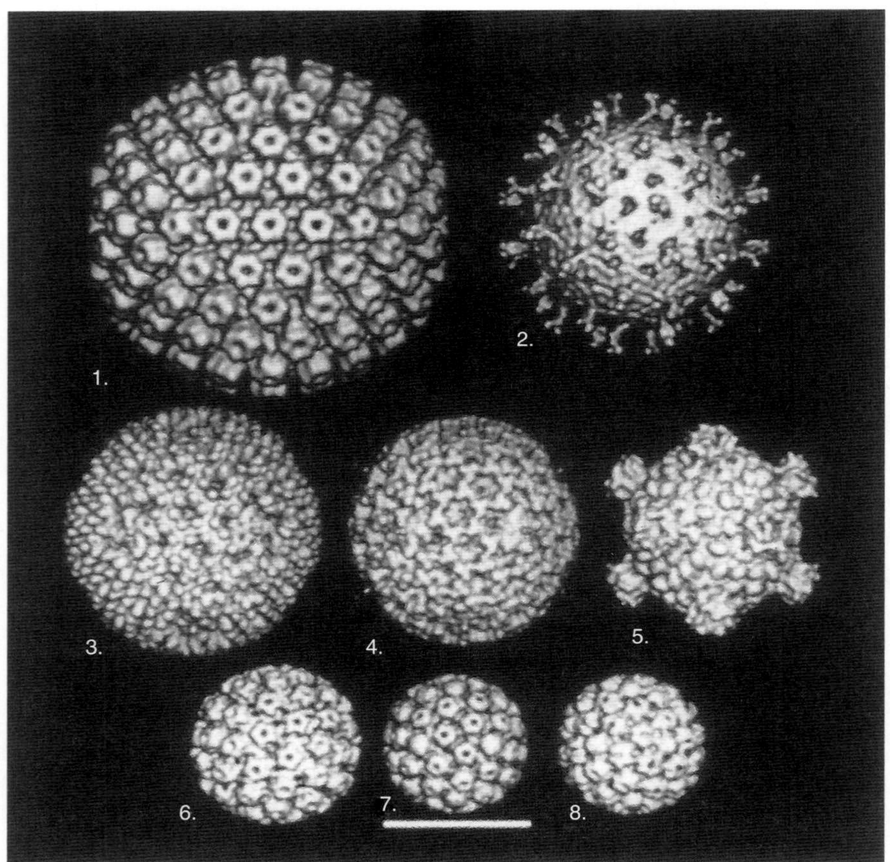

FIGURE 36-6 Cryoelectron microscopy and computer-generated three-dimensional image reconstructions of several icosahedral capsids. These images show the symmetry of capsids and the individual capsomeres. During assembly, the genome may fill the capsid through the holes in the herpesvirus, polyomavirus, and papillomavirus capsomeres. *1,* Equine herpesvirus nucleocapsid; *2,* simian rotavirus; *3,* reovirus type 1 (Lang) virion; *4,* intermediate subviral particle (reovirus); *5,* core (inner capsid) particle (reovirus); *6,* human papillomavirus type 19; *7,* mouse polyomavirus; *8,* cauliflower mosaic virus. Bar = 50 nm. (Courtesy Dr. Tim Baker, Purdue University, West Lafayette, Ind.)

The classic example of a virus with helical symmetry is the tobacco mosaic plant virus. Its capsomeres self-assemble on the RNA genome into rods that extend the length of the genome. The capsomeres cover and protect the RNA. Helical nucleocapsids are observed within the envelope of most negative-strand RNA viruses (see Figure 48-1).

Simple **icosahedrons** are used by small viruses such as the picornaviruses and parvoviruses. The icosahedron is made of 12 capsomeres, each with fivefold symmetry **(pentamer** or **penton).** For the picornaviruses, every pentamer is made up of five protomers, each of which is composed of three subunits of four separate proteins (see Figure 36-5). X-ray crystallography and image analysis of cryoelectron microscopy have defined the structure of the picornavirus capsid to the molecular level. These studies have depicted a canyon-like cleft, which is a "docking site" to bind to the receptor on the surface of the target cell (see Figure 46-2).

Larger capsid virions are constructed by inserting structurally distinct capsomeres between the pentons at the vertices. These capsomeres have six nearest neighbors **(hexons).** This extends the icosahedron and is called an **icosadeltahedron,** and its size is determined by the number of hexons inserted along the edges and within the surfaces between the pentons. *Older soccer balls were icosadeltahedrons.* For example, the herpesvirus nucleocapsid has 12 pentons and 150 hexons. The herpesvirus nucleocapsid is also surrounded by an envelope. The adenovirus capsid is composed of 252 capsomeres, with 12 pentons and 240 hexons. A long fiber is attached to each penton of adenovirus to serve as the VAP to bind to target cells, and it also contains the type-specific antigen (see Figure 42-1). The reoviruses have an icosahedral double capsid with fiber-like proteins partially extended from each vertex. The outer capsid protects the virus and promotes its uptake across the gastrointestinal tract and into target cells, whereas the inner capsid contains enzymes for the synthesis of RNA (see Figures 36-6 and 51-2).

Enveloped Viruses

The virion envelope is composed of lipids, proteins, and glycoproteins (see Figure 36-4 and Box 36-5). It has a membrane structure similar to cellular membranes. Cellular proteins are rarely found in the viral envelope, even though the envelope is obtained from cellular membranes. Most enveloped viruses are round or pleomorphic (see Figures 36-2 and 36-3 for the complete listing of enveloped viruses). Two exceptions are the poxvirus, which has a complex internal and a bricklike external structure, and the rhabdovirus, which is bullet shaped.

Most viral glycoproteins have asparagine-linked (*N*-linked) carbohydrates and extend through the envelope and away from the surface of the virion. For many viruses, these can be observed as spikes (Figure 36-7). Some glycoproteins act as **VAPs,** capable of binding to structures on target cells. VAPs that also bind to erythrocytes are termed **hemagglutinins (HAs).** Some glycoproteins have other functions, such as the neuraminidase (NA) of orthomyxoviruses (influenza) and the Fc receptor and the C3b receptor associated with herpes simplex virus (HSV) glycoproteins, or the fusion glycoproteins of paramyxoviruses. Glycoproteins, especially the VAPs, are also major antigens that elicit protective immunity.

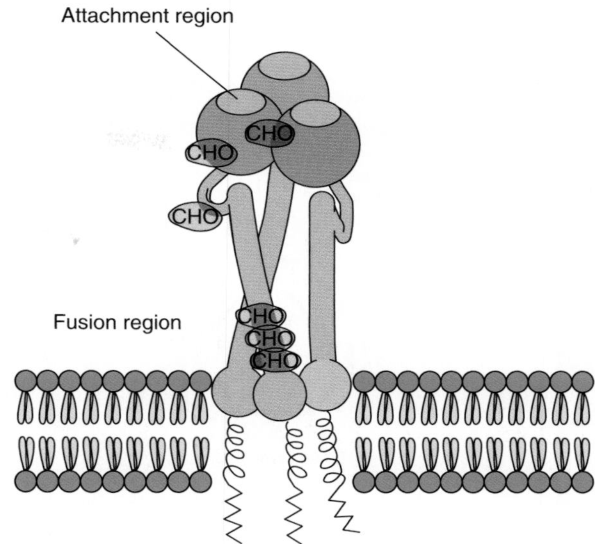

FIGURE 36-7 Diagram of the hemagglutinin glycoprotein trimer of influenza A virus, a representative spike protein. The region for attachment to the cellular receptor is exposed on the spike protein's surface. Under mild acidic conditions, the hemagglutinin folds over to bring the virion envelope and cellular membrane together and exposes a hydrophobic sequence to promote fusion. *CHO, N*-linked carbohydrate attachment sites. (Modified from Schlesinger MJ, Schlesinger S: Domains of virus glycoproteins, *Adv Virus Res* 33:1–44, 1987.)

The envelope of the togaviruses surrounds an icosahedral nucleocapsid containing a positive-strand RNA genome. The envelope contains spikes consisting of two or three glycoprotein subunits anchored to the virion's icosahedral capsid. This causes the envelope to adhere tightly and conform (shrink-wrap) to an icosahedral structure discernible by cryoelectron microscopy.

All of the negative-strand RNA viruses are enveloped. Components of the viral RNA-dependent RNA polymerase associate with the (–) RNA genome of the orthomyxoviruses, paramyxoviruses, and rhabdoviruses to form helical nucleocapsids. These enzymes are required to initiate virus replication, and their association with the genome ensures their delivery into the cell. **Matrix proteins** lining the inside of the envelope facilitate the assembly of the ribonucleocapsid into the virion. Influenza A (orthomyxovirus) is an example of a (–) RNA virus with a segmented genome. Its envelope is lined with matrix proteins and has two glycoproteins: the HA, which is the VAP, and an NA (see Figure 49-1). Bunyaviruses do not have matrix proteins.

The herpesvirus envelope is a baglike structure that encloses the icosadeltahedral nucleocapsid (see Figure 43-1). Depending on the specific herpesvirus, the envelope may contain as many as 11 glycoproteins. The interstitial space between the nucleocapsid and the envelope is called the **tegument,** and it contains enzymes, other proteins, and even RNA that facilitate the viral infection.

The poxviruses are enveloped viruses with large, complex, bricklike shapes (see Figure 44-1). The envelope encloses a dumbbell-shaped, DNA-containing nucleoid structure; lateral bodies; fibrils; and many enzymes and proteins,

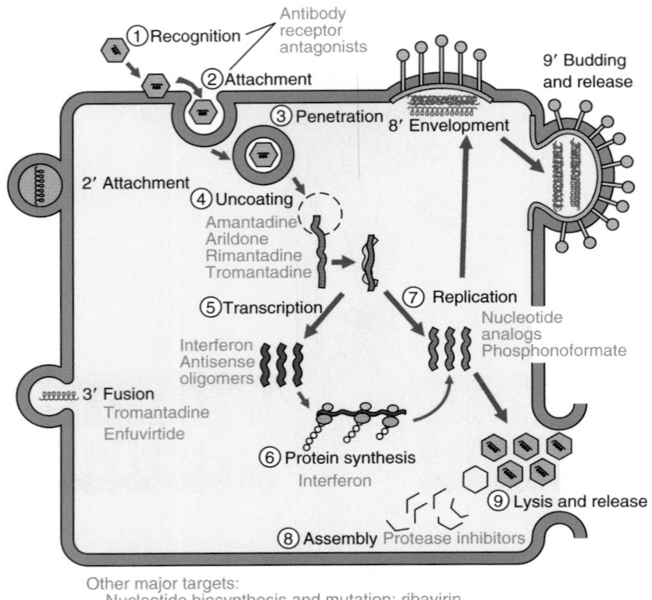

FIGURE 36-8 A general scheme of viral replication. Enveloped viruses may also enter by steps 2′ and 3′ and assemble and exit from the cell by steps 8′ and 9′. The antiviral drugs for susceptible steps in viral replication are listed in magenta.

including the enzymes and transcriptional factors required for mRNA synthesis.

• Viral Replication

The major steps in viral replication are the same for all viruses (Figure 36-8; Box 36-6). The cell acts as a factory, providing the substrates, energy, and machinery necessary for the synthesis of viral proteins and replication of the genome. Processes not provided by the cell must be encoded in the genome of the virus. The manner in which each virus accomplishes these steps and overcomes the cell's biochemical limitations is different for different structures of the genome and of the virion (whether it is enveloped or has a naked capsid). This is illustrated in the examples in Figures 36-11 to 36-13 (see later).

A single round of the viral replication cycle can be separated into several phases. During the **early phase** of infection, the virus must recognize an appropriate target cell, attach to the cell, penetrate the plasma membrane and be taken up by the cell, release (uncoat) its genome into the cytoplasm, and if necessary, deliver the genome to the nucleus. The **late phase** begins with the start of genome replication and viral macromolecular synthesis and proceeds through viral assembly and release. Uncoating of the genome from the capsid or envelope during the early phase abolishes its infectivity and identifiable structure, thus initiating the eclipse period. The **eclipse period,** like a solar eclipse, ends with the appearance of new virions after virus assembly. The **latent period** (not to be confused with latent infection), during which extracellular infectious virus is not detected, includes the eclipse period and ends with the release of new viruses (Figure 36-9). Each infected cell may produce as many as 100,000 particles; however, only 1% to 10% of these particles may be infectious. The noninfectious particles **(defective particles)** result from mutations and errors in the manufacture and assembly of the virion. The yield of infectious virus per cell, or **burst size,** and the time required for a single cycle of virus reproduction are determined by the properties of the virus and the target cell. Although it may seem wasteful to produce so many defective particles, the virus uses this mechanism to generate mutants that may have a selective advantage, and 1% of 100,000 viruses is still a lot of virus.

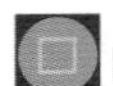

Box 36-6 Steps in Viral Replication

1. Recognition of the target cell
2. Attachment
3. Penetration
4. Uncoating
5. Macromolecular synthesis
   a. Early messenger RNA (mRNA) and nonstructural protein synthesis: genes for enzymes and nucleic acid–binding proteins
   b. Replication of genome
   c. Late mRNA and structural protein synthesis
   d. Posttranslational modification of protein
6. Assembly of virus
7. Budding of enveloped viruses
8. Release of virus

Recognition of and Attachment to the Target Cell

The binding of the **VAPs** or structures on the surface of the virion capsid (Table 36-5) to **receptors on the cell** (Table 36-6) initially determines which cells can be infected by a virus. *The receptors for the virus on the cell may be proteins or carbohydrates on glycoproteins or glycolipids.* Viruses that bind to receptors expressed on specific cell types may be restricted to certain species **(host range)** (e.g., human, mouse) or specific cell types. The susceptible target cell defines the **tissue tropism** (e.g., neurotropic, lymphotropic). Epstein-Barr virus (EBV), a herpesvirus, has a very limited host range and tropism because it binds to the C3d receptor (CR2) expressed on human B cells. The B19 parvovirus binds to globoside (blood group P antigen) expressed on erythroid precursor cells.

The viral attachment structure for a capsid virus may be part of the capsid or a protein that extends from the capsid. A canyon on the surface of picornaviruses, such as the rhinovirus 14, serves as a "keyhole" for the insertion of a portion of the intercellular adhesion molecule (ICAM-1) from the cell surface (see Figure 46-2). The fibers of the adenoviruses and the σ-1 proteins of the reoviruses at the vertices of the capsid interact with receptors expressed on specific target cells.

Specific glycoproteins are the VAPs of enveloped viruses. The HA of influenza A virus binds to specific sialic acid carbohydrates expressed on many but not all cells of different species. Similarly, the α-togaviruses and the flaviviruses are able to bind to receptors expressed on cells of many animal species, including arthropods, reptiles, amphibians, birds, and mammals. This allows them to infect animals, mosquitoes, and other insects and to be spread by them.

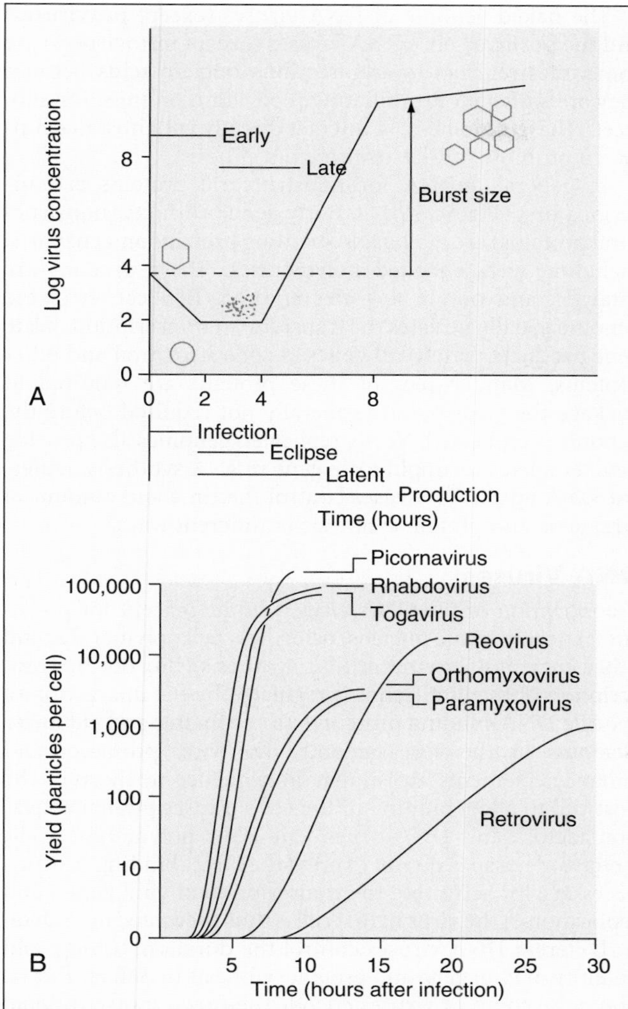

FIGURE 36-9 **A,** Single-cycle growth curve for a virus that is released by cell lysis. The different stages are defined by the absence of visible viral components (eclipse period) or infectious virus in the media (latent period), or the presence of macromolecular synthesis (early/late phases). **B,** Growth curve and burst size (yield) of representative viruses. (**A,** Modified from Davis BD, Dulbecco R, Eisen HN, et al: *Microbiology,* ed 4, Philadelphia, 1990, Lippincott; **B,** modified from White DO, Fenner F: *Medical virology,* ed 3, New York, 1986, Academic.)

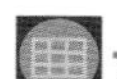 **Table 36-5 Examples of Viral Attachment Proteins**

Virus Family	Virus	Viral Attachment Protein
Picornaviridae	Rhinovirus	VP1-VP2-VP3 complex
Adenoviridae	Adenovirus	Fiber protein
Reoviridae	Reovirus	σ-1
	Rotavirus	VP7
Togaviridae	Semliki Forest virus	E1-E2-E3 complex gp
Rhabdoviridae	Rabies virus	G protein gp
Orthomyxoviridae	Influenza A virus	HA gp
Paramyxoviridae	Measles virus	HA gp
Herpesviridae	Epstein-Barr virus	gp350 and gp220
Retroviridae	Murine leukemia virus	gp70
	Human immunodeficiency virus	gp120

gp, Glycoprotein; *HA,* hemagglutinin.

 **Table 36-6 Examples of Viral Receptors**

Virus	Target Cell	Receptor*
Epstein-Barr virus	B cell	C3d complement receptor CR2 (CD21)
Human immunodeficiency virus	Helper T cell	CD4 molecule and chemokine coreceptor
Rhinovirus	Epithelial cells	ICAM-1 (immunoglobulin superfamily protein)
Poliovirus	Epithelial cells	Immunoglobulin superfamily protein
Herpes simplex virus	Many cells	Herpesvirus entry mediator (HVEM), nectin-1
Rabies virus	Neuron	Acetylcholine receptor, NCAM
Influenza A virus	Epithelial cells	Sialic acid
B19 parvovirus	Erythroid precursors	Erythrocyte P antigen (globoside)

CD, Cluster of differentiation; *ICAM-1,* intercellular adhesion molecule; *NCAM,* neural cell adhesion molecule.

*Other receptors for these viruses may also exist.

Penetration

Interactions between multiple VAPs and cellular receptors initiate the internalization of the virus into the cell. The mechanism of internalization depends on the virion structure and cell type. Most nonenveloped viruses enter the cell by receptor-mediated endocytosis or by viropexis. **Endocytosis** is a normal process used by the cell for the uptake of receptor-bound molecules such as hormones, low-density lipoproteins, and transferrin. Picornaviruses, papillomaviruses, and polyomaviruses may enter by **viropexis.** Hydrophobic structures of capsid proteins may be exposed after viral binding to the cells, and these structures help the virus or the viral genome slip through (direct penetration) the membrane.

Enveloped viruses fuse their membranes with cellular membranes to deliver the nucleocapsid or genome directly into the cytoplasm. The optimum pH for fusion determines whether penetration occurs at the cell surface at neutral pH or whether the virus must be internalized by endocytosis, and fusion occurs in an endosome at acidic pH. The fusion activity may be provided by the VAP or another protein. The HA of influenza A (see Figure 36-7) binds to sialic acid receptors on the target cell. Under the mild acidic conditions of the endosome, the HA undergoes a dramatic conformational change to expose hydrophobic portions capable of promoting membrane fusion. Paramyxoviruses have a fusion protein that is active at neutral pH to promote virus-to-cell fusion. Paramyxoviruses can also promote cell-to-cell fusion to form multinucleated giant cells **(syncytia).** Some herpesviruses and retroviruses fuse with cells at a neutral pH and induce syncytia after replication.

Uncoating

Once internalized, the nucleocapsid must be delivered to the site of replication within the cell and the capsid or envelope removed. The genome of DNA viruses, except for poxviruses, must be delivered to the nucleus, whereas most RNA viruses remain in the cytoplasm. The uncoating process may be initiated by attachment to the receptor or promoted by the acidic environment or proteases found in an endosome or lysosome. Picornavirus capsids are weakened by the release of the VP4 capsid protein to allow uncoating. VP4 is released by insertion of the receptor into the keyhole-like canyon attachment site of the capsid. Enveloped viruses are uncoated on fusion with cell membranes. Fusion of the herpesvirus envelope with the plasma membrane releases its nucleocapsid, which then "docks" with the nuclear membrane to deliver its DNA genome directly to the site of replication. The release of the influenza nucleocapsid from its matrix and envelope is facilitated by the passage of protons from inside the endosome through the ion pore formed by the influenza M2 membrane protein to acidify the virion.

The reovirus and poxvirus are only partially uncoated on entry. The outer capsid of reovirus is removed, but the genome remains in an inner capsid, which contains the polymerases necessary for RNA synthesis. The initial uncoating of the poxviruses exposes a subviral particle to the cytoplasm, allowing synthesis of mRNA by virion-contained enzymes. An uncoating enzyme can then be synthesized to release the DNA-containing core into the cytoplasm.

Macromolecular Synthesis

Once inside the cell, the genome must direct the synthesis of viral mRNA and protein and generate identical copies of itself. The genome is useless unless it can be transcribed into functional mRNAs capable of binding to ribosomes and being translated into proteins. The means by which each virus accomplishes these steps depends on the structure of the genome (Figure 36-10) and the site of replication.

The cell's machinery for transcription and mRNA processing is found in the nucleus. Most DNA viruses use the cell's DNA-dependent RNA polymerase II and other enzymes to make mRNA. (The names of the polymerases describe what they do—first the template and then the product [e.g., the polymerase that makes mRNA in the cell is a DNA-dependent RNA polymerase, and the enzyme that copies DNA is a DNA-dependent DNA polymerase]). In addition, the viral mRNAs acquire a 3′ polyadenylated (polyA) tail and a 5′ methylated cap (for binding to the ribosome) and are processed to remove introns before being exported to the cytoplasm like eukaryotic mRNA. Viruses that replicate in the cytoplasm must provide these functions or an alternative. Although poxviruses are DNA viruses, they replicate in the cytoplasm and therefore must encode enzymes for all these functions. Most RNA viruses replicate and produce mRNA in the cytoplasm, except for orthomyxoviruses and retroviruses. RNA viruses must encode the necessary enzymes for transcription and replication, because the cell has no means of replicating RNA. The mRNAs for RNA viruses may or may not acquire a 5′ cap or polyA tail.

The naked genome of DNA viruses (except poxviruses) and the positive-sense RNA viruses (except retroviruses) are sometimes referred to as **infectious nucleic acids** because they are sufficient for initiating replication on injection into a cell. These genomes can interact directly with host machinery to promote mRNA or protein synthesis.

In general, mRNA for nonstructural proteins is transcribed first (Figure 36-11). **Early gene products** (nonstructural proteins) are often DNA-binding proteins and enzymes, including virus-encoded polymerases. These proteins are catalytic, and only a few are required. Replication of the genome usually initiates the transition to transcription of late gene products. **Late viral genes** encode structural and other proteins. Many copies of these proteins are required to package the virus but are generally not required before the genome is replicated. Newly replicated genomes also provide new templates to amplify late gene mRNA synthesis. Different DNA and RNA viruses control the time and amount of viral gene and protein synthesis in different ways.

DNA Viruses

Transcription of the DNA virus genome (except for poxviruses) occurs in the nucleus, using host cell polymerases and other enzymes for viral mRNA synthesis (Box 36-7). Transcription of the viral genes is regulated by the interaction of specific DNA-binding proteins with promoter and enhancer elements in the viral genome. The viral promoter and enhancer elements are similar in sequence to those of the host cell to allow binding of the cell's transcriptional activation factors and DNA-dependent RNA polymerase. Cells from some tissues do not express the DNA-binding proteins necessary for activating the transcription of viral genes, and replication of the virus in that cell is thus prevented or limited.

Different DNA viruses control the duration, timing, and quantity of viral gene and protein synthesis in different ways. The more complex viruses encode their own transcriptional activators, which enhance or regulate the expression of viral genes. For example, HSV encodes many proteins that regulate the kinetics of viral gene expression, including the VMW 65 (α-TIF protein, VP16). VMW 65 is carried in the virion, binds to the host cell transcription-activating complex (Oct-1), and enhances its ability to stimulate transcription of the immediate early genes of the virus.

Genes may be transcribed from either DNA strand of the genome and in opposite directions. For example, the early and late genes of the SV40 polyomavirus are on opposite, nonoverlapping DNA strands. Viral genes may have introns requiring posttranscriptional processing of the mRNA by the cell's nuclear machinery (splicing). The late genes of papilloma- and polyomaviruses and adenoviruses are initially transcribed as a large RNA from a single promoter and then processed to produce several different mRNAs after removal of different intervening sequences (introns).

Replication of viral DNA follows the same biochemical rules as for cellular DNA and requires a DNA-dependent DNA polymerase, other enzymes, and deoxyribonucleotide triphosphates, especially thymidine. Replication is initiated at a unique DNA sequence of the genome called the **origin (ori).** This is a site recognized by cellular or viral nuclear factors and the **DNA-dependent DNA polymerase.** Viral DNA synthesis is semiconservative, and viral and cellular *DNA polymerases require a primer* to initiate synthesis of the

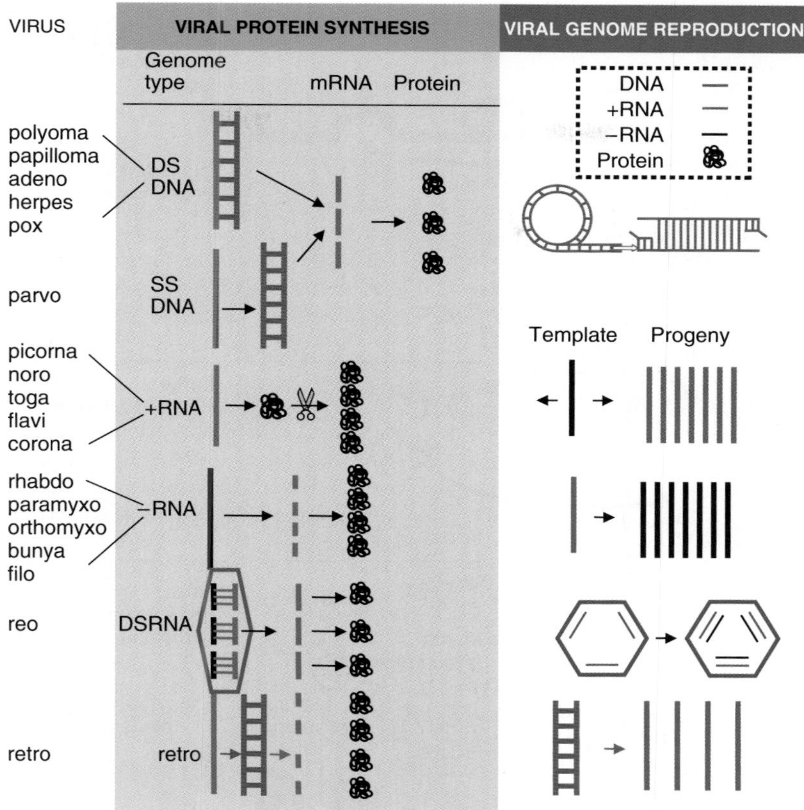

FIGURE 36-10 Viral macromolecular synthesis steps: the structure of the genome determines the mechanism of viral mRNA and protein synthesis and also genome replication. (1) Double-stranded DNA *(DS DNA)* uses host machinery in the nucleus (except poxviruses) to make mRNA, which is translated by host cell ribosomes into proteins. Replication of viral DNA occurs by semiconservative means, by rolling circle, linear, and in other ways. (2) Single-stranded DNA *(SS DNA)* is converted into DS DNA and replicates like DS DNA. (3) (+) RNA resembles an mRNA that binds to ribosomes to make a polyprotein that is cleaved into individual proteins. One of the viral proteins is an RNA polymerase that makes a (−) RNA template and then more (+) RNA genome progeny and mRNAs. (4) (−) RNA is transcribed into mRNAs and a full-length (+) RNA template by the RNA polymerase carried in the virion. The (+) RNA template is used to make (−) RNA genome progeny. (5) DS RNA acts like (−) RNA. The (−) strands are transcribed into mRNAs by an RNA polymerase in the capsid. New (+) RNAs get encapsidated and (−) RNAs are made in the inner capsid. (6) Retroviruses have (+) RNA that is converted to complementary DNA (cDNA) by reverse transcriptase carried in the virion. cDNA integrates into the host chromosome, and the host makes mRNAs, proteins, and full-length RNA genome copies.

DNA chain. The parvoviruses have DNA sequences that are inverted and repeated to allow the DNA to fold back and hybridize with itself to provide a primer. Replication of the adenovirus genome is primed by deoxycytidine monophosphate attached to a terminal protein. A cellular enzyme (primase) synthesizes an RNA primer to start the replication of the papilloma- and polyomavirus genomes, whereas the herpesviruses encode a primase.

Replication of the genome of the simple DNA viruses (e.g., parvoviruses, polyomaviruses, papillomaviruses) uses the host DNA-dependent DNA polymerases, whereas the larger, more complex viruses (e.g., adenoviruses, herpesviruses, poxviruses) encode their own polymerases *(Puny Parvo, Polyoma, and Papilloma viruses require cell Polymerases)*. Viral polymerases are usually faster but less precise than host cell polymerases, causing a higher mutation rate in viruses and providing a target for nucleotide analogs as antiviral drugs.

Hepadnavirus replication is unique in that a larger than genome positive-strand RNA copy is first synthesized by the cell's DNA-dependent RNA polymerase and circularizes. Viral proteins surround the RNA, a viral-encoded RNA-dependent DNA polymerase (reverse transcriptase) in this virion core makes a negative-strand DNA, and then the RNA is degraded. Positive-strand DNA synthesis is initiated but stops when the genome and core are enveloped, yielding a partially double-stranded, circular DNA genome.

Major limitations for replication of a DNA virus include availability of the DNA polymerase and deoxyribonucleotide substrates. Most cells in the resting phase of growth are not undergoing DNA synthesis, because the necessary enzymes are not present and deoxythymidine pools are limited. *The smaller the DNA virus, the more dependent the virus is on the host cell* to provide these functions (see Box 36-7). The parvoviruses are the smallest DNA viruses and replicate only in growing cells, such as erythroid precursor cells or fetal tissue. Speeding up the growth of the cell can enhance viral DNA and mRNA synthesis. The T antigen of SV40, the E6 and E7 of papillomavirus, and the E1a and E1b proteins of adenovirus bind to and prevent the function of growth-inhibitory

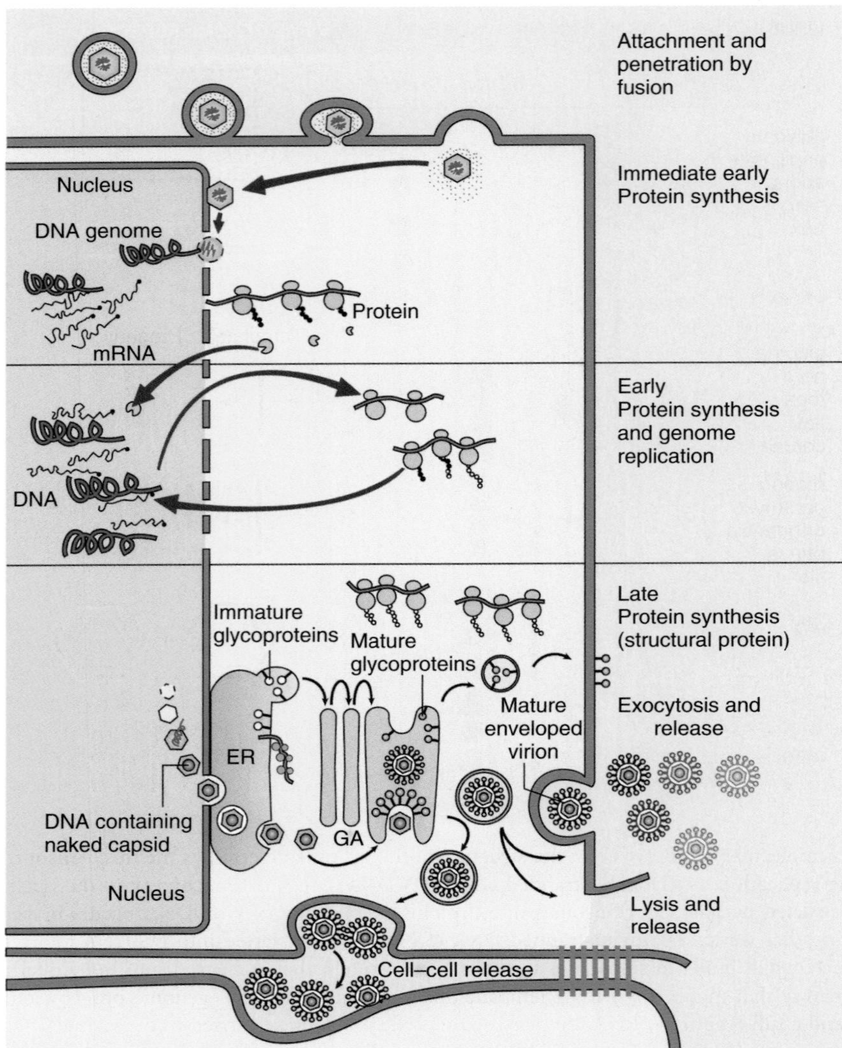

FIGURE 36-11 Replication of herpes simplex virus, a complex enveloped DNA virus. The virus binds to specific receptors and fuses with the plasma membrane. The nucleocapsid then delivers the DNA genome to the nucleus. Transcription and translation occur in three phases: immediate early, early, and late. Immediate early proteins promote the takeover of the cell; early proteins consist of enzymes, including the DNA-dependent DNA polymerase; and the late proteins are structural and other proteins, including the viral capsid and glycoproteins. The genome is replicated before transcription of the late genes. Capsid proteins migrate into the nucleus, assemble into icosadeltahedral capsids, and are filled with the DNA genome. The capsids filled with genomes bud through the nuclear and endoplasmic reticulum *(ER)* membranes into the cytoplasm, acquire tegument proteins, and then acquire their envelope as they bud through the viral glycoprotein-modified membranes of the trans-Golgi network. The virus is released by exocytosis or cell lysis. *GA,* Golgi apparatus.

proteins (p53 and the retinoblastoma gene product), resulting in cell growth, which also promotes virus replication. HSV is an example of a large DNA virus that encodes a DNA polymerase and scavenging enzymes (e.g., deoxyribonuclease, ribonucleotide reductase, thymidine kinase) to generate the necessary deoxyribonucleotide substrates for replication of its genome. Larger DNA viruses can replicate in growing and nongrowing cells.

RNA Viruses

Replication and transcription of RNA viruses are similar processes because the viral genomes are usually either an mRNA (positive-strand RNA) (Figure 36-12) or a template for mRNA (negative-strand RNA) (Figure 36-13; Box 36-8). During replication and transcription, a double-stranded RNA replicative intermediate is formed. Double-stranded RNA is not normally found in uninfected cells and is a strong inducer of innate host protections.

The RNA virus genome must code for **RNA-dependent RNA polymerases (replicases and transcriptases)** because the cell has no means of replicating RNA. Unlike DNA viruses, the RNA viruses must also provide the enzymes for synthesis and processing of the viral mRNA. This may be as simple as adding a terminal protein for the picornaviruses or like eukaryotic mRNA, the addition of a 5′methylguanosine cap and 3′polyadenosine. RNA viruses must also bring the machinery for these processes together with the genome or template.

Box 36-7 Properties of DNA Viruses

DNA is not transient or labile.
Many DNA viruses establish persistent infections (e.g., latent, immortalizing).
DNA genomes reside in the nucleus (except for poxviruses).
Viral DNA resembles host DNA for transcription and replication.
Viral genes must interact with host transcriptional machinery (except for poxviruses).
Viral gene transcription is temporally regulated.
Early genes encode DNA-binding proteins and enzymes.
Late genes encode structural and other proteins.
DNA polymerases require a primer to replicate the viral genome.
The larger DNA viruses encode means to promote efficient replication of their genome.
Parvovirus: requires cells undergoing DNA synthesis to replicate.
Papillomavirus: stimulates cell growth and DNA synthesis.
Polyomavirus: stimulates cell growth and DNA synthesis.
Hepadnavirus: stimulates cell growth, cell makes RNA intermediate, encodes a reverse transcriptase.
Adenovirus: stimulates cellular DNA synthesis and encodes its own polymerase.
Herpesvirus: stimulates cell growth, encodes its own polymerase and enzymes to provide deoxyribonucleotides for DNA synthesis, establishes latent infection in host.
Poxvirus: encodes its own polymerases and enzymes to provide deoxyribonucleotides for DNA synthesis, replication machinery, and transcription machinery in the cytoplasm.

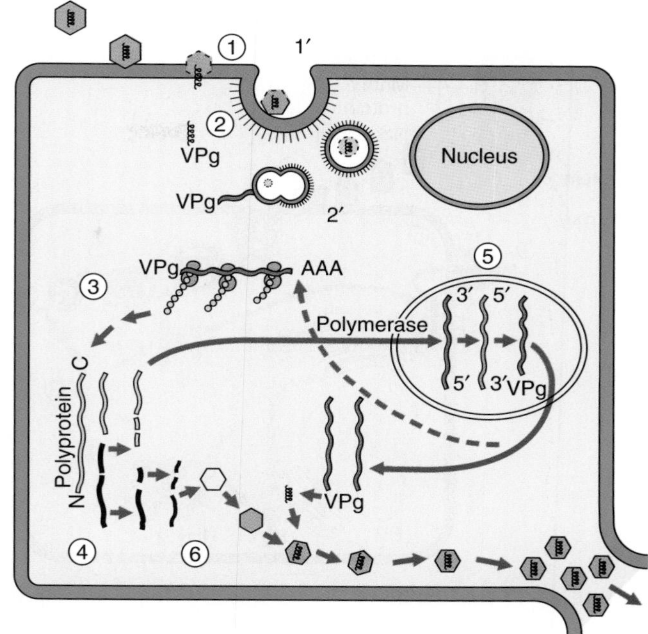

FIGURE 36-12 Replication of picornaviruses: a simple (+) RNA virus. *1,* Interaction of the picornaviruses with receptors on the cell surface defines the target cell and weakens the capsid. *2,* The genome is injected through the virion and across the cell membrane. *2′,* Alternatively, the virion is endocytosed, and then the genome is released. *3,* The genome is used as mRNA for protein synthesis. One large polyprotein is translated from the virion genome. *4,* Then the polyprotein is proteolytically cleaved into individual proteins, including an RNA-dependent RNA polymerase. *5,* Macromolecular synthesis proceeds in a vesicle. The polymerase makes a (−) strand template from the genome and replicates the genome. A protein *(VPg)* is covalently attached to the 5′ end of the viral genome. *6,* The structural proteins associate into the capsid structure, the genome is inserted, and the virions are released on cell lysis.

Because RNA is degraded relatively quickly, the RNA-dependent RNA polymerase must be provided or synthesized soon after uncoating to generate more viral RNA, or the infection will be aborted. Most viral RNA polymerases work at a fast pace but are also error prone, causing mutations. Replication of the genome provides new templates for production of more mRNA and genomes, which amplifies and accelerates virus replication.

The **positive-strand RNA viral genomes** of the picornaviruses, caliciviruses, coronaviruses, flaviviruses, and togaviruses act as mRNA, bind to ribosomes, and direct protein synthesis. *The naked positive-strand RNA viral genome is sufficient to initiate infection by itself.* Viral proteins are translated from the genome as a polyprotein that is cleaved by viral and cellular proteases into active proteins. The genome and enzymes necessary for virus replication assemble on a membrane scaffold or within a vesicle. The virus-encoded RNA-dependent RNA polymerase produces a negative-strand RNA template (antigenome), and this template is used to generate more mRNA and to replicate the genome. For picornaviruses and flaviviruses, the genome and negative-sense template RNA and mRNA are the same size. For the togaviruses, coronaviruses, and caliciviruses, a full-length template and mRNA is produced, and later smaller mRNAs for structural and other proteins (late genes) are generated from the template. The mRNAs for picornaviruses are not capped at the 5′ end, but RNA for other viruses have 5′ caps and polyA tails. Transcription and replication of coronaviruses share many of these aspects but are more complex.

The **negative-strand RNA virus genomes** of the rhabdoviruses, orthomyxoviruses, paramyxoviruses, filoviruses, and bunyaviruses are the templates for production of mRNA. The negative-strand RNA genome is not infectious by itself, and *a polymerase must be carried into the cell with the genome* (associated with the genome as part of the nucleocapsid) to make individual mRNA for the different viral proteins. As a result, a full-length positive-strand RNA must also be produced by the viral polymerase to act as a template to generate more copies of the genome. The (−) RNA genome is like the negatives from a roll of movie film: each frame encodes a photo/mRNA, but a full-length positive is required for replicating the roll. *Except for influenza viruses, transcription and replication of negative-strand RNA viruses occur in the cytoplasm.* The influenza transcriptase requires a primer to produce mRNA. It uses the 5′ ends of cellular mRNA in the nucleus as primers for its polymerase and, in the process, steals the 5′ cap from the cellular mRNA. The influenza genome is also replicated in the nucleus.

The reoviruses have a **segmented, double-stranded RNA genome** and undergo a more complex means of replication and transcription. The reovirus RNA polymerase is part of the inner capsid core; individual mRNA units are transcribed from each of the 10 or more segments of the genome while they are still in the core. The negative strands of the genome

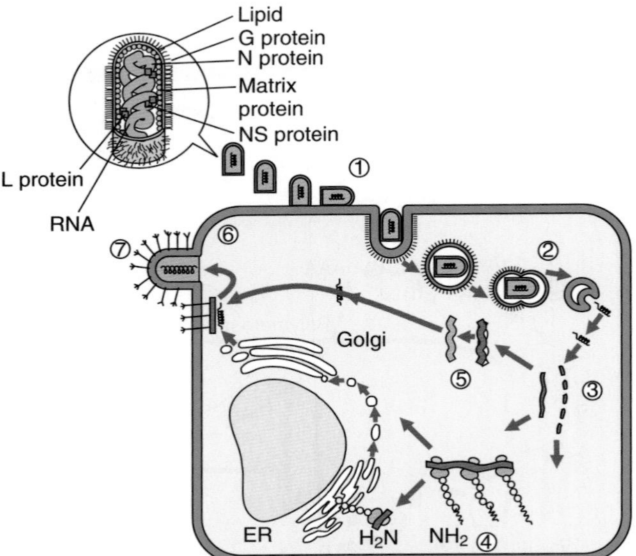

FIGURE 36-13 Replication of rhabdoviruses: a simple enveloped (−) RNA virus. *1,* Rhabdoviruses bind to the cell surface and are *(2)* endocytosed. The envelope fuses with the endosome vesicle membrane to deliver the nucleocapsid to the cytoplasm. The virion must carry a polymerase, which *(3)* produces five individual messenger RNAs (mRNAs) and a full-length (+) RNA template. *4,* Proteins are translated from the mRNAs, including one glycoprotein (G) which is co-translationally glycosylated in the endoplasmic reticulum *(ER),* processed in the Golgi apparatus, and delivered to the cell membrane. *5,* The genome is replicated from the (+) RNA template, and N, L, and NS proteins associate with the genome to form the nucleocapsid. *6,* The matrix protein associates with the G protein–modified membrane, which is followed by assembly of the nucleocapsid. *7,* The virus buds from the cell in a bullet-shaped virion.

 **Box 36-8 Properties of RNA Viruses**

RNA is labile and transient.
Most RNA viruses replicate in the cytoplasm.
Cells cannot replicate RNA. RNA viruses must encode an RNA-dependent RNA polymerase.
The genome structure determines the mechanism of transcription and replication.
RNA viruses are prone to mutation.
The genome structure and polarity determine how viral messenger RNA (mRNA) is generated and proteins are processed.
RNA viruses, except for (+) RNA genome, must carry polymerases.
All (−) RNA viruses are enveloped.

Picornaviruses, Togaviruses, Flaviviruses, Caliciviruses, and Coronaviruses

(+) RNA genome resembles mRNA and is translated into a polyprotein, which is proteolyzed. A (−) RNA template is used for replication. For togaviruses, coronaviruses, and caliciviruses, early proteins are translated from the genome and late proteins from smaller mRNAs transcribed from template.

Orthomyxoviruses, Paramyxoviruses, Rhabdoviruses, Filoviruses, and Bunyaviruses

(−) RNA genome is a template for individual mRNAs, but full-length (+) RNA template is required for replication. Orthomyxoviruses replicate and transcribe in the nucleus, and each segment of the genome encodes one mRNA and is a template.

Reoviruses

(+/−) Segmented RNA genome is a template for mRNA (+RNA). (+) RNA may also be encapsidated to generate the (+/−) RNA and then more mRNA.

Retroviruses

(+) Retrovirus RNA genome is converted into DNA, which is integrated into the host chromatin and transcribed as a cellular gene

segments are used as templates for mRNA in a manner similar to that of the negative-strand RNA viruses. Reovirus-encoded enzymes contained in the inner capsid core add the 5′ cap to viral mRNA. The mRNA does not have polyA. The mRNAs are released into the cytoplasm, where they direct protein synthesis or are sequestered into new cores. The positive-strand RNA in the new cores acts as a template for negative-strand RNA, and the core polymerase produces the progeny double-stranded RNA.

The arenaviruses have an **ambisense genome** with (−) sequences adjacent to (+) sequences. The early mRNAs of the virus are transcribed from the negative-sense portion of the genome, a full-length replicative intermediate is produced to generate a new genome, and the late mRNAs of the virus are transcribed from the region of the replicative intermediate that is complementary to the (+) sequences.

Although the **retroviruses** have a positive-strand RNA genome, the virus provides no means for replication of the RNA in the cytoplasm. Instead, the retroviruses carry two copies of the genome, two transfer RNA (tRNA) molecules, and an RNA-dependent DNA polymerase **(reverse transcriptase)** in the virion. The tRNA is used as a primer for synthesis of a circular complementary DNA **(cDNA)** copy of the genome. The cDNA is synthesized in the cytoplasm, travels to the nucleus, and is then integrated into the host chromatin. The viral genome becomes a cellular gene. Promoters at the end of the integrated viral genome enhance the transcription of the viral DNA sequences by the cell. Full-length RNA transcripts are used as new genomes, and individual mRNAs are generated by differential splicing of this RNA.

The most unusual mode of replication is reserved for the **deltavirus.** The deltavirus resembles a viroid. The genome is a circular, rod-shaped, single-stranded RNA, which is extensively hybridized to itself. As the exception, the deltavirus RNA genome is replicated by the host cell DNA-dependent RNA polymerase II in the nucleus. A portion of the genome forms an RNA structure called a ribozyme, which cleaves the RNA circle to produce an mRNA.

Viral Protein Synthesis

All viruses depend on the host cell ribosomes, tRNA, and mechanisms for posttranslational modification to produce their proteins. The binding of mRNA to the ribosome is mediated by a 5′ cap structure of methylated guanosine or a special RNA loop structure (internal ribosome entry sequence [IRES]), which binds within the ribosome to initiate protein synthesis. The cap structure, if used, is acquired in different ways by different viruses. The IRES structure was discovered first in the picornavirus genome and then in selected cellular mRNAs. Most but not all viral mRNA have a polyadenosine (polyA) tail, like eukaryotic mRNAs.

Unlike bacterial ribosomes, which can bind to a polycistronic mRNA and translate several gene sequences into separate proteins, the eukaryotic ribosome binds to mRNA and can make only one continuous protein, and then it falls off the mRNA. Each virus deals with this limitation differently, depending on the structure of the genome. For example, the entire genome of a positive-strand RNA virus is read by the ribosome and translated into one giant **polyprotein.** The polyprotein is subsequently cleaved by cellular and viral proteases into functional proteins. DNA viruses, retroviruses, and most negative-strand RNA viruses transcribe separate mRNA for smaller polyproteins or individual proteins. The orthomyxovirus and reovirus genomes are segmented, and most of the segments code for single proteins for this reason.

Viruses use different tactics to promote preferential translation of their viral mRNA instead of cellular mRNA. In many cases, the concentration of viral mRNA in the cell is so large it occupies most of the ribosomes, preventing translation of cellular mRNA. Adenovirus infection blocks the egress of cellular mRNA from the nucleus. HSV and other viruses inhibit cellular macromolecular synthesis and induce degradation of the cell's DNA and mRNA. To promote selective translation of its mRNA, poliovirus uses a virus-encoded protease to inactivate the 200,000-Da cap-binding protein of the ribosome to prevent binding and translation of the cell's 5′-capped cellular mRNA. Togaviruses and many other viruses increase the permeability of the cell's membrane; thus the ribosomal affinity for most cellular mRNA is decreased. All these actions also contribute to the cytopathology of the virus infection. The pathogenic consequences of these actions are discussed further in Chapter 37.

Some viral proteins require **posttranslational modifications** such as phosphorylation, glycosylation, acylation, or sulfation. Protein phosphorylation is accomplished by cellular or viral protein kinases and is a means of modulating, activating, or inactivating proteins. Several herpesviruses and other viruses encode their own protein kinases. *Viral glycoproteins are synthesized on membrane-bound ribosomes and have the amino acid sequences to allow insertion into the rough endoplasmic reticulum and N-linked glycosylation.* The high-mannose precursor form of the glycoproteins progresses from the endoplasmic reticulum through the vesicular transport system of the cell and is processed through the Golgi apparatus. The sialic acid–containing mature glycoprotein is expressed on the plasma membrane of the cell unless the glycoprotein expresses protein sequences for retention in an intracellular organelle. The presence of the glycoproteins determines where the virion will assemble within the cell. Other modifications, such as *O*-glycosylation, acylation, and sulfation of the proteins, can also occur during progression through the Golgi apparatus.

Assembly

Virion assembly is analogous to a three-dimensional interlocking puzzle that puts itself together in the box. The virion is built from small, easily manufactured parts that enclose the genome in a functional package. Each part of the virion has recognition structures that allow the virus to form the appropriate protein-protein, protein–nucleic acid, and (for enveloped viruses) protein-membrane interactions needed to assemble into the final structure. The assembly process begins when the necessary pieces are synthesized, and the concentration of structural proteins in the cell is sufficient to drive the process thermodynamically, much like a crystallization reaction. The assembly process may be facilitated by scaffolding proteins or other proteins, some of which are activated or release energy on proteolysis. For example, cleavage of the VP0 protein of poliovirus releases the VP4 peptide, which solidifies the capsid.

The site and mechanism of virion assembly in the cell depend on where genome replication occurs and whether the final structure is a naked capsid or an enveloped virus. Assembly of the DNA nucleocapsid for viruses other than poxviruses occurs in the nucleus and requires transport of the virion proteins into the nucleus. RNA virus and poxvirus assembly occurs in the cytoplasm.

Capsid viruses may be assembled as empty structures (procapsids) to be filled with the genome (e.g., picornaviruses), or they may be assembled around the genome. Nucleocapsids of the retroviruses, togaviruses, and the negative-strand RNA viruses assemble around the genome and are subsequently enclosed in an envelope. The helical nucleocapsid of negative-strand RNA viruses includes the RNA-dependent RNA polymerase necessary for mRNA synthesis in the target cell.

For enveloped viruses, newly synthesized and processed viral glycoproteins are delivered to cellular membranes by vesicular transport. Acquisition of an envelope occurs after association of the nucleocapsid with the viral glycoprotein-containing regions of host cell membranes in a process called **budding.** Matrix proteins for some negative-strand RNA viruses line and promote the adhesion of nucleocapsids with the glycoprotein-modified membrane. As more interactions occur, the membrane surrounds the nucleocapsid, and the virus buds from the membrane.

The type of genome and the protein sequence of the glycoproteins determine the site of budding. Most RNA viruses bud from the plasma membrane, and the virus is released from the cell at the same time without killing the cell. The flaviviruses, coronaviruses, and bunyaviruses acquire their envelope by budding into the endoplasmic reticulum and Golgi membranes and may remain cell associated in these organelles. The HSV nucleocapsid assembles in the nucleus and buds into and then out of the endoplasmic reticulum. The nucleocapsid is dumped into the cytoplasm, viral proteins associate with the capsid, and then the envelope is acquired by budding into a trans-Golgi network membrane decorated with the 10 viral glycoproteins. The virion is transported to the cell surface and released by exocytosis, on cell lysis, or transmitted through cell-to-cell bridges.

Viruses use different tricks to ensure that all the parts of the virus are assembled into complete virions. The RNA polymerase required for infection by negative-strand RNA viruses is carried on the genome as part of a helical nucleocapsid. The human immunodeficiency virus (HIV) and other retrovirus genomes are packaged in a procapsid consisting of a polyprotein containing the protease, polymerase, integrase, and structural proteins. This procapsid binds to viral glycoprotein-modified membranes, and the virion buds from the membrane. The virus-encoded protease is activated within the virion and cleaves the polyprotein to produce the final infectious nucleocapsid and the required proteins within the envelope.

Assembly of viruses with segmented genomes, such as influenza or reovirus, requires accumulation of one copy of each gene segment. The segments nest within structures created by the viral proteins.

Errors are made by the viral polymerase and during viral assembly. Empty virions and virions containing defective genomes are produced. As a result, the particle-to-infectious virus ratio, also called *particle-to-plaque-forming unit ratio,* is high, usually greater than 10, and during rapid viral replication can even be 10^4. Defective viruses can occupy the machinery (e.g., bind to the receptor) required for normal virus replication to prevent (interfere with) virus production **(defective interfering particles).**

Release

Viruses can be released from cells after lysis of the cell, by exocytosis, or by budding from the plasma membrane. Naked capsid viruses are generally released after lysis of the cell. Release of most enveloped viruses occurs after budding from the plasma membrane without killing the cell. Survival of the cell allows continual production and release of virus from the factory. Lysis and plasma membrane budding are efficient means of release. Viruses that bud or acquire their membrane in the cytoplasm (e.g., flaviviruses, poxviruses) remain cell associated and are released by exocytosis or cell lysis. Viruses that bind to sialic acid receptors (e.g., orthomyxoviruses, certain paramyxoviruses) may also have a neuraminidase (NA). The NA removes potential sialic acid receptors on the glycoproteins of the virion and the host cell to prevent clumping and facilitate release.

Reinitiation of the Replication

Spread of the infection occurs from virus released to the extracellular medium, but alternatively the virus, nucleocapsid, or genome can be transmitted *through cell-to-cell bridges, upon cell-to-cell fusion, or vertically to daughter cells.* These alternate routes allow the virus to escape antibody detection. Some herpesviruses, retroviruses, and paramyxoviruses can induce cell-to-cell fusion to merge the cells into multinucleated giant cells **(syncytia),** which become huge virus factories. The retroviruses and some DNA viruses can transmit their integrated copy of the genome vertically to daughter cells on cell division.

• Viral Genetics

Mutations spontaneously and readily occur in viral genomes, creating new virus strains with properties differing from the **parental,** or **wild-type, virus.** These variants can be identified by their nucleotide sequences, antigenic differences (serotypes), or differences in functional or structural properties. Most mutations have no effect or are detrimental to the virus. Mutations in essential genes can inactivate the virus. Mutations in other genes may produce antiviral drug resistance or alter the antigenicity or pathogenicity of the virus.

Errors in copying the viral genome during virus replication produce many mutations. This is because of the poor fidelity of the viral polymerase and the rapid rate of genome replication. In addition, RNA viruses do not have a genetic error-checking mechanism. As a result, the rates of mutation for RNA viruses are usually greater than for DNA viruses.

Mutations that inactivate essential genes are termed **lethal mutations.** These mutants are difficult to isolate because the virus cannot replicate. A **deletion mutant** results from loss or selective removal of a portion of the genome and the function it encodes. Other mutations may produce **plaque mutants,** which differ from the wild type in the size or appearance of the infected cells; **host range mutants,** which differ in the tissue type or species of target cell that can be infected; or **attenuated mutants,** which are variants that cause less serious disease in animals or humans. **Conditional mutants,** such as **temperature-sensitive (ts)** or **cold-sensitive mutants,** have a mutation in a gene for an essential protein that allows virus production only at certain temperatures. Whereas ts mutants generally grow well or relatively better at 30° C to 35° C, the encoded protein is inactive at elevated temperatures of 38° C to 40° C, preventing virus production. Live virus vaccines are often conditional or host range mutants and attenuated for human disease.

New virus strains can also arise by genetic interactions between viruses or between the virus and the cell (Figure 36-14). Intramolecular genetic exchange between viruses or the virus and the host is termed **recombination.** Recombination can occur readily between two related DNA viruses. For example, co-infection of a cell with the two closely related herpesviruses (HSV types 1 and 2) yields intertypic recombinant strains. These new hybrid strains have genes from types 1 and 2. Integration of retroviruses into host cell chromatin is a form of recombination. Recombination of two related RNA viruses, Sindbis and eastern equine encephalitis virus, resulted in creation of another togavirus, western equine encephalitis (WEE) virus.

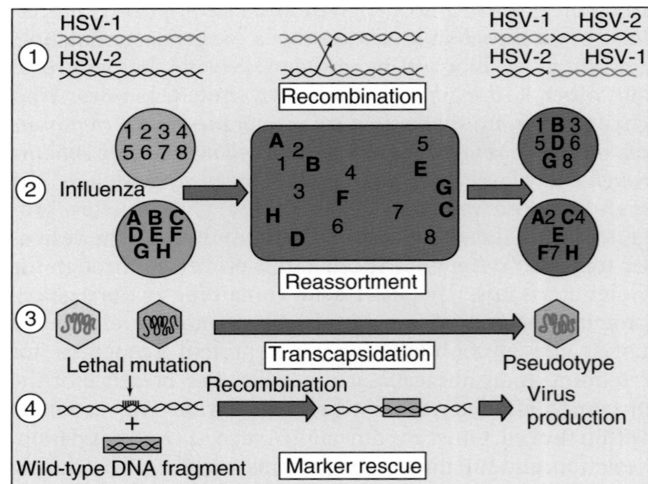

FIGURE 36-14 Genetic exchange between viral particles can give rise to new viral types, as illustrated. Representative viruses include the following: *1,* intertypic recombination of herpes simplex virus type 1 *(HSV-1)* and type 2 *(HSV-2); 2,* reassortment of two strains of influenza virus; *3,* rescue of a polyomavirus defective in assembly by a complementary defective virus (transcapsidation); and *4,* marker rescue of a lethal or conditional mutation.

Viruses with segmented genomes (e.g., influenza viruses and reoviruses) form hybrid strains on infection of one cell with more than one virus strain. This process, termed **reassortment,** is analogous to picking 10 marbles out of a box containing 10 black and 10 white marbles. Very different strains of influenza A virus are created on co-infection with a virus from different species (see Figure 49-5).

In some cases, a defective viral strain can be rescued by the replication of another mutant, by the wild-type virus, or by a cell line bearing a replacement viral gene. Replication of the other virus or expression of the gene in the cell provides the missing function required by the mutant **(complementation),** allowing replication to occur. An experimental disabled infectious single-cycle HSV (DISC-HSV) vaccine lacks an essential gene and is grown in a cell line that expresses that gene product to "complement" the virus. The vaccine virus can infect the normal cells of the individual, but the virions that are produced lack the function necessary for replication in other cells and cannot spread. Rescue of a lethal or conditional-lethal mutant with a defined genetic sequence, such as a restriction endonuclease DNA fragment, is called **marker rescue.** Marker rescue is used to map the genomes of viruses such as HSV. Virus produced from cells infected with different virus strains may be phenotypically mixed and have the proteins of one strain but the genome of the other **(transcapsidation). Pseudotypes** are generated when transcapsidation occurs between different types of viruses, but this is rare.

Individual virus strains or mutants are **selected** by their ability to use the host cell machinery and to withstand the conditions of the body and the environment. Cellular properties that can act as **selection pressures** include the growth rate of the cell and tissue-specific expression of certain proteins required by the virus (e.g., enzymes, glycoproteins, transcription factors) and proteins that prevent essential virus functions. The conditions of the body, its elevated temperature, innate and immune defenses, and tissue structure are also selection pressures for viruses. The viruses that cannot endure these conditions or evade the host defenses are eliminated. A small selective advantage in a mutant virus can shortly lead to its becoming the predominant viral strain. The high mutation rate of HIV promotes a switch in target cell tropism to include different types of T cells, the development of antiviral drug-resistant strains, and the generation of antigenic variants during a patient's course of infection.

The growth of virus under benign laboratory conditions allows weaker strains to survive because of the absence of the selective pressures of the human body. This process is used to select attenuated virus strains for use in vaccines.

• Viral Vectors for Therapy

Genetically manipulated viruses can be excellent delivery systems for foreign genes. Viruses can provide gene replacement therapy, can be used as vaccines to promote immunity to other agents or tumors, and can act as targeted killers of tumors. The advantages of using viruses are that they can be readily amplified by replication in appropriate cells, and they target specific tissues and deliver the DNA or RNA into the cell. Viruses that are being developed as vectors include retroviruses, adenoviruses, HSV, adeno-associated virus (parvovirus), poxviruses (e.g., vaccinia and canarypox) (see Figure 44-7), and even some togaviruses. The viral vectors are usually defective or attenuated viruses in which the foreign DNA replaces a virulence or unessential gene. The foreign gene may be under the control of a viral promoter or even a tissue-specific promoter. Defective virus vectors are grown in cell lines that express the missing viral functions "complementing" the virus. The progeny can deliver their nucleic acid but not produce infectious virus. Retroviruses and adeno-associated viruses can integrate into cells and permanently deliver a gene into the cell's chromosome. Adenovirus and HSV promote targeted delivery of the foreign gene to receptor-bearing cells. Genetically attenuated HSVs are being developed to specifically kill the growing cells of glioblastomas while sparing the surrounding neurons. Adenovirus and canarypox virus are being used to carry and express HIV and other genes as vaccines. Vaccinia virus carrying a gene for the rabies glycoprotein is already being used successfully to immunize raccoons, foxes, and skunks in the wild. Someday, virus vectors may be routinely used to treat cystic fibrosis, Duchenne muscular dystrophy, lysosomal storage diseases, and immunologic disorders.

Bibliography

Cann AJ: *Principles of molecular virology*, ed 4, San Diego, 2005, Academic.

Cohen J, Powderly WG: *Infectious diseases*, ed 2, St Louis, 2004, Mosby.

Flint SJ, Enquist LW, Racaniello VR, et al: *Principles of virology: molecular biology, pathogenesis, and control of animal viruses*, ed 3, Washington, DC, 2009, American Society for Microbiology Press.

Knipe DM, Howley PM, Griffin DE, et al: *Fields virology*, ed 5, Philadelphia, 2006, Lippincott Williams & Wilkins.

Richman DD, Whitley RJ, Hayden FG: *Clinical virology*, ed 3, Washington, DC, 2009, American Society for Microbiology Press.

Rosenthal KS: Viruses: microbial spies and saboteurs, *Infect Dis Clin Pract* 14:97–106, 2006.

Specter SC, Hodinka RL, Wiedbrauk DL, et al: *Clinical virology manual*, ed 4, Washington, DC, 2009, American Society for Microbiology Press.

Strauss JM, Strauss EG: *Viruses and human disease*, ed 2, San Diego, 2007, Academic.

Websites

All the virology on the WWW. www.virology.net/garryfavweb.html. Accessed August 7, 2015.

The big picture book of viruses. www.virology.net/Big_Virology/BVHomePage.html. Accessed August 7, 2015.

Stannard L: Virological methods slideset. http://virology-online.com/general/Test1.htm. Accessed August 7, 2015.

Stannard L: Virus ultra structure: electron micrograph images. http://web.uct.ac.za/depts/mmi/stannard/emimages.html. Accessed June 10, 2012.

CHAPTER

37 MECHANISMS OF VIRAL PATHOGENESIS

Viruses cause disease after they break through the natural protective barriers of the body, evade immune control, and either kill cells of an important tissue (e.g., brain) or trigger a destructive immune and inflammatory response. The outcome of a viral infection is determined by the nature of the virus-host interaction and the host's response to the infection (Box 37-1). The immune response is the best treatment, but it often contributes to the pathogenesis of a viral infection. The tissue targeted by the virus defines the nature of the disease and its symptoms. Viral and host factors govern the severity of the disease; they include the strain of virus, the inoculum size, and the general health of the infected person. The ability of the infected person's immune response to control the infection determines the severity and duration of the disease. A particular disease may be caused by several viruses that have a common tissue **tropism** (preference), such as hepatitis—liver, common cold—upper respiratory tract, encephalitis—central nervous system. On the other hand, a particular virus may cause several different diseases or no observable symptoms. For example, herpes simplex virus type 1 (HSV-1) can cause gingivostomatitis, pharyngitis, herpes labialis (cold sores), genital herpes, encephalitis, or keratoconjunctivitis, depending on the affected tissue, or it can cause no apparent disease at all. Although relatively benign, this virus can be life threatening in a newborn or an immunocompromised person.

Viruses encode activities **(virulence factors)** that promote the efficiency of viral replication, viral transmission, access and binding of the virus to target tissue, or escape of the virus from host defenses and immune resolution (see Chapter 10). These activities may not be essential for viral growth in tissue culture but are necessary for the pathogenicity or survival of the virus in the host. Loss of these virulence factors results in **attenuation** of the virus. Many live-virus vaccines are attenuated virus strains.

The discussion in this chapter focuses on viral disease at the cellular level (cytopathogenesis), the host level (mechanisms of disease), and the population level (epidemiology and control). The antiviral immune response is discussed here and in Chapter 10.

• Basic Steps in Viral Disease

Viral disease in the body progresses through defined steps, just like viral replication in the cell (Figure 37-1A). These steps are noted in Box 37-2.

The incubation period may proceed without symptoms **(asymptomatic)** or may produce nonspecific early symptoms such as fever, head or body aches, or chills, termed the **prodrome.** Often the viral infection is resolved by innate host protections, without symptoms. The symptoms of the disease are caused by tissue damage and systemic effects caused by the virus and the immune system. These symptoms may continue through **convalescence** while the body repairs the damage. The individual usually develops a memory immune response for future protection against a similar challenge with this virus.

• Infection of the Target Tissue

The virus gains **entry into the body** through breaks in the skin (cuts, bites, injections) or across the mucoepithelial membranes that line the orifices of the body (eyes, respiratory tract, mouth, genitalia, and gastrointestinal tract). The skin is an excellent barrier to infection. Tears, mucus, ciliated epithelium, stomach acid, bile, and immunoglobulin (Ig)A protect the orifices. *Inhalation is probably the most common route of viral infection.*

On entry into the body, the virus replicates in cells that express viral receptors and have the appropriate biosynthetic machinery. Many viruses initiate infection in the oral mucosa or upper respiratory tract. Disease signs may accompany viral replication at the primary site. The virus may replicate and remain at the primary site, disseminate to other tissues via the bloodstream or within mononuclear phagocytes and lymphocytes, or disseminate through neurons (see Figure 37-1B).

The bloodstream and lymphatic system are the predominant means of viral transfer in the body. The virus may gain access to them after tissue damage, upon uptake by macrophages, or on transport past the mucoepithelial cells of the oropharynx, gastrointestinal tract, vagina, or anus. Several enteric viruses (picornaviruses and reoviruses) bind to receptors on M cells, which translocate the virus to the underlying Peyer patches of the lymphatic system.

The transport of virus in the blood is termed **viremia.** The virus may either be free in the plasma or be cell associated in lymphocytes or macrophages. Viruses taken up by phagocytic macrophages may be inactivated, replicate, or be delivered to other tissues. Replication of a virus in macrophages, the endothelial lining of blood vessels, or the liver can cause the infection to be amplified and initiate development of a **secondary viremia.** In many cases, a secondary viremia precedes

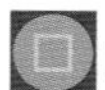 **Box 37-1 Determinants of Viral Disease**

Nature of the Disease
Target tissue
Portal of entry of virus
Access of virus to target tissue
Tissue tropism of virus
Permissiveness of cells for viral replication
Pathogenic activity (strain)

Severity of Disease
Cytopathic ability of virus
Immune status (naïve or immunized)
Competence of the immune system
Prior immunity to the virus
Immunopathology
Virus inoculum size
Length of time before resolution of infection
General health of the person
Nutrition
Other diseases influencing immune status
Genetic makeup of the person
Age

delivery of the virus to the **target tissue** (e.g., liver, brain, skin) and the manifestation of characteristic symptoms.

Viruses can gain access to the central nervous system or brain (1) from the bloodstream (e.g., arboencephalitis viruses), (2) from infected meninges or cerebrospinal fluid, (3) by means of the migration of infected macrophages, or (4) by infection of peripheral and sensory (olfactory) neurons. The meninges are accessible to many of the viruses spread by viremia, which may also provide access to neurons. Herpes simplex, varicella-zoster, and rabies viruses initially infect mucoepithelium, skin, or muscle, and then the peripheral innervating neuron, which transports the virus to the central nervous system or brain.

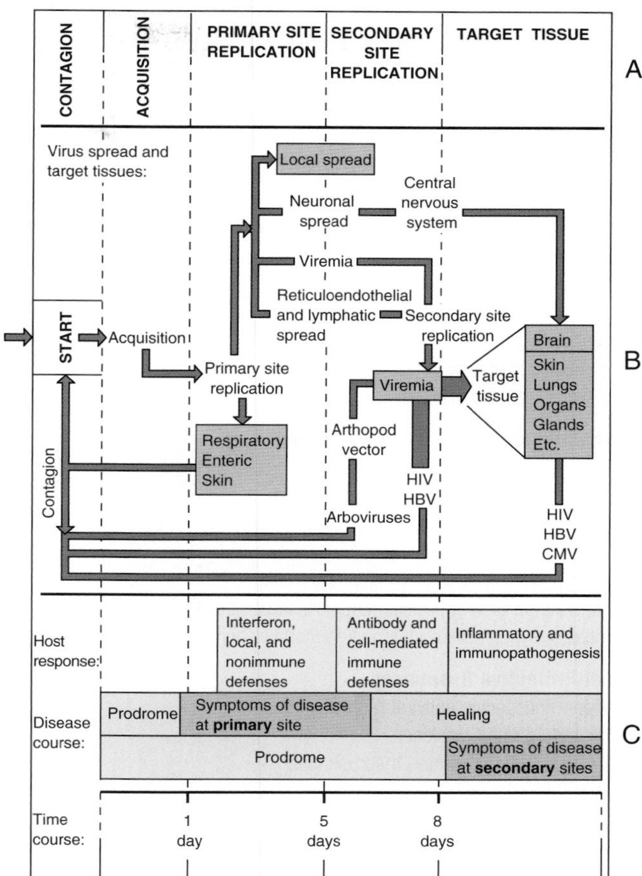

FIGURE 37-1 **A,** The stages of viral infection. The virus is released from one person, is acquired by another, replicates, and initiates a primary infection at the site of acquisition. Depending on the virus, it may then spread to other body sites and finally to a target tissue characteristic of the disease. **B,** The cycle starts with acquisition, as indicated, and proceeds until the release of new virus. The thickness of the arrow denotes the degree to which the original virus inoculum is amplified on replication. The boxes indicate a site or cause of symptoms. **C,** Time course of viral infection. The time course of symptoms and the immune response correlate with the stage of viral infection and depend on whether the virus causes symptoms at the primary site or only after dissemination to another (secondary) site. *CMV,* Cytomegalovirus; *HBV,* hepatitis B virus; *HIV,* human immunodeficiency virus.

• Viral Pathogenesis

Cytopathogenesis

The four potential outcomes of a viral infection of a cell are as follows (Box 37-3; Table 37-1):

1. Failed infection (abortive infection)
2. Cell death (lytic infection)
3. Replication without cell death (persistent infection)
4. Presence of virus without virus production but with potential for reactivation (latent-recurrent infection)

Viral mutants, which cause abortive infections, do not multiply and therefore disappear. Persistent infections may be (1) **chronic** (nonlytic, productive), (2) **latent** (limited viral macromolecular but no virus synthesis), (3) **recurrent** (periods of latency then virus production), or (4) **transforming** (immortalizing).

The nature of the infection is determined by the characteristics of the virus and the target cell. A **nonpermissive cell** may lack a receptor, important enzyme pathway, or transcriptional activator or express an antiviral mechanism that will not allow replication of a particular type or strain of

 **Box 37-2 Progression of Viral Disease**

1. **Acquisition** (entry into the body)
2. Initiation of infection at a primary site
3. Activation of innate protections
4. An **incubation period,** when the virus is amplified and may spread to a secondary site
5. Replication in the **target tissue,** which causes the characteristic disease signs
6. **Host responses** that limit and contribute (immunopathogenesis) to the disease
7. Virus production in a tissue that releases the virus to other people for **contagion**
8. **Resolution** or **persistent infection/chronic disease**

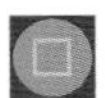 **Box 37-3 Determinants of Viral Pathogenesis**

Interaction of Virus with Target Tissue

Access of virus to target tissue
Stability of virus in the body
- Temperature and dryness
- Acid and bile of the gastrointestinal tract

Ability to cross skin or mucosal epithelial cells (e.g., cross the gastrointestinal tract into the bloodstream)
Ability to establish viremia
Ability to spread through the reticuloendothelial system
Target tissue
- Specificity of viral attachment proteins
- Tissue-specific expression of receptors

Cytopathologic Activity of the Virus

Efficiency of viral replication in the cell
- Optimum temperature for replication
- Permissiveness of cell for replication

Cytotoxic viral proteins
Inhibition of cell's macromolecular synthesis
Accumulation of viral proteins and structures (inclusion bodies)
Altered cell metabolism (e.g., cell immortalization)

Host Protective Responses

Antigen-nonspecific antiviral responses
- Interferon and cytokines
- Natural killer cells and macrophages

Antigen-specific immune responses
- T-cell responses
- Antibody responses

Viral mechanisms of escape of immune responses

Immunopathology

Interferon: flulike systemic symptoms
T-cell responses: cell killing, inflammation
Antibody: complement, antibody-dependent cellular cytotoxicity, immune complexes
Other inflammatory responses

 **Table 37-1 Types of Viral Infections at the Cellular Level**

Type	Virus Production	Fate of Cell
Abortive	–	No effect
Cytolytic	+	Death
Persistent		
Productive	+	Senescence
Latent	–	No effect
Transforming		
DNA viruses	–	Immortalization
RNA viruses	+	Immortalization

virus. For example, neurons and nongrowing cells lack the machinery and substrates for replication of some DNA viruses. These cells can also limit the amount of protein synthesis within the cells by phosphorylating elongation initiation factor-2α (eIF-2α) to prevent the assembly of ribosomes on 5′-capped mRNA, which shuts down most protein synthesis. This protection can be triggered by the large amount of protein synthesis required for virus production or the activation of the interferon (IFN)-α– or IFN-β–induced antiviral state. Herpesviruses and some other viruses prevent this by inhibiting the phosphorylating enzyme (protein kinase R) or by activating a cellular protein phosphatase to remove the phosphate on eIF-2α. Another example is APOBEC3, an enzyme that causes hypermutation inactivation of the cDNA of retroviruses. This is a mechanism for restricting the growth of the numerous endogenous retroviruses that are part of the human chromosome. The viral infectivity factor (Vif) protein of human immunodeficiency virus (HIV) overcomes this block by promoting the degradation of APOBEC3.

A **permissive cell** provides the biosynthetic machinery to support the complete replicative cycle of the virus. Replication of the virus in a **semipermissive cell** may be very inefficient, or the cell may support some but not all the steps in viral replication.

Replication of the virus can initiate changes in cells that lead to cytolysis or to alterations in the cell's appearance, functional properties, or antigenicity. The effects on the cell may result from viral takeover of macromolecular synthesis, accumulation of viral proteins or particles, modification or disruption of cellular structures, or manipulation of cellular functions (Table 37-2).

 **Table 37-2 Mechanisms of Viral Cytopathogenesis**

Mechanism	Examples
Inhibition of cellular protein synthesis	Poliovirus, herpes simplex virus (HSV), togaviruses, poxviruses
Inhibition and degradation of cellular DNA	Herpesviruses
Alteration of cell membrane structure	Enveloped viruses
Viral glycoprotein insertion	All enveloped viruses
Syncytia formation	HSV, varicella-zoster virus, paramyxoviruses, human immunodeficiency virus
Disruption of cytoskeleton	Nonenveloped viruses (accumulation), HSV
Permeability	Togaviruses, herpesviruses
Toxicity of virion components	Adenovirus fibers, reovirus NSP4 protein
Inclusion Bodies	**Examples**
Negri bodies (intracytoplasmic)	Rabies
Intranuclear basophilic (Owl's eye)	Cytomegalovirus (enlarged cells), adenoviruses
Cowdry type A (intranuclear)	HSV, subacute sclerosing panencephalitis (measles) virus
Intracytoplasmic acidophilic	Poxviruses
Perinuclear cytoplasmic acidophilic	Reoviruses

Lytic Infections

Lytic infection results when virus replication kills the target cell. Some viruses damage the cell and prevent repair by inhibiting the synthesis of cellular macromolecules or by producing degradative enzymes and toxic proteins. For example, HSV and other viruses produce proteins that inhibit the synthesis of cellular DNA and mRNA and synthesize other proteins that degrade host DNA to provide substrates for viral genome replication. Cellular protein synthesis may be actively blocked (e.g., poliovirus inhibits translation of 5′-capped cellular mRNA) or passively blocked (e.g., through production of much viral mRNA that successfully competes for ribosomes) (see Chapter 36).

Replication of the virus and accumulation of viral components and progeny within the cell can disrupt the structure and function of the cell or disrupt lysosomes, causing cell death. Expression of viral antigens on the cell surface and disruption of the cytoskeleton can change cell-to-cell interactions and the cell's appearance, making the cell a target for immune cytolysis. Viral nucleic acids in the cytoplasm can activate pathogen-associated molecular pattern (PAMP) receptors to activate the inflammasome, cytokine, and interferon responses that can limit virus replication.

Viral infection or cytolytic immune responses may induce **apoptosis** in the infected cell. Apoptosis is a preset cascade of events that, when triggered, leads to cellular suicide. This process may facilitate release of the virus from the cell, but it also limits the amount of virus that is produced by destroying the viral "factory." As a result, *many viruses (e.g., herpesviruses, adenoviruses, hepatitis C virus) encode methods for inhibiting apoptosis.*

Cell surface expression of the glycoproteins of some paramyxoviruses, herpesviruses, and retroviruses triggers the fusion of neighboring cells into **multinucleated giant cells** called **syncytia.** Cell-to-cell fusion may occur in the absence of new protein synthesis (fusion from without), as occurs in infections with paramyxoviruses, or it may require new protein synthesis (fusion from within), as occurs in infection with HSV. Syncytia formation allows the viral infection to spread from cell to cell and escape antibody detection. Syncytia may be fragile and susceptible to lysis. The syncytia that occurs in infection with HIV also causes death of the cells.

Some viral infections cause characteristic changes in the appearance and properties of the target cells. For example, chromosomal aberrations and degradation may occur and can be detected with histologic staining (e.g., marginated chromatin ringing the nuclear membrane in HSV- and adenovirus-infected cells). In addition, new stainable structures called **inclusion bodies** may appear within the nucleus or cytoplasm. These structures may result from virus-induced changes in the membrane or chromosomal structure or may represent the sites of viral replication or accumulations of viral capsids. Because the nature and location of these inclusion bodies are characteristic of particular viral infections, their presence facilitates laboratory diagnosis (see Table 37-2). Viral infection may also cause vacuolization, rounding of the cells, and other nonspecific histologic changes that are characteristics of sick cells.

Nonlytic Infections

A **persistent infection** occurs in an infected cell that is not killed by the virus. Some viruses cause a persistent productive infection because the virus is released gently from the cell through exocytosis or through budding (many enveloped viruses) from the plasma membrane. Thinking like a parasite, the virus does not want to kill the cell because the longer a cell is alive, the longer the virus remains in the body and the more virus is produced to spread to other cells or individuals.

A **latent infection** may result from DNA virus infection of a cell that restricts or lacks the machinery for transcribing all the viral genes, or the virus may encode functions that suppress virus replication (e.g., cytomegalovirus) to extend its parasitism. The specific transcription factors required by such a virus may be expressed only in specific tissues, in growing but not resting cells, or after hormone or cytokine induction. For example, HSV establishes a latent infection in neurons that do not express the nuclear factors required to transcribe the immediate early viral genes, but stress and other stimuli can activate the cells to allow viral replication.

Oncogenic Viruses

Some DNA viruses and retroviruses establish persistent infections that can also stimulate uncontrolled cell growth, causing **transformation** or **immortalization** of the cell (Figure 37-2). Characteristics of transformed cells include continued growth without senescence, alterations in cell morphology and metabolism, increased cell growth rate and sugar transport, loss of cell-contact inhibition of growth, and

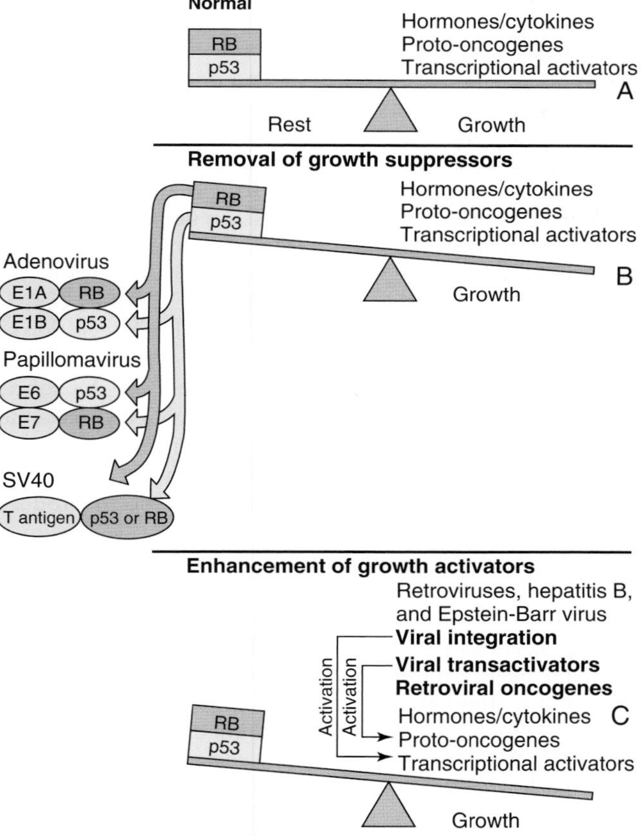

FIGURE 37-2 Mechanisms of viral transformation and immortalization. Cell growth is controlled **(A)** by the maintenance of a balance in the external and internal growth activators (accelerators) and by growth suppressors such as p53 and the retinoblastoma *(RB)* gene product (brakes). Oncogenic viruses alter the balance by removing the brakes **(B)** or by enhancing the effects of the accelerators **(C)**.

ability to grow in a suspension or pile up into foci when grown in a semisolid agar.

Different **oncogenic** viruses have different mechanisms for immortalizing cells. Viruses immortalize cells by (1) activating or providing growth-stimulating genes, (2) removing the inherent braking mechanisms that limit DNA synthesis and cell growth, (3) preventing apoptosis, or (4) providing or inducing growth-stimulating cytokines. Immortalization by DNA viruses occurs in semipermissive cells, which express only selected viral genes but do not produce virus. Synthesis of viral DNA, late mRNA, late proteins, or virus leads to cell death, which precludes immortalization. Several oncogenic DNA viruses integrate into the host cell chromosome. Papillomavirus, SV40 virus, and adenovirus encode proteins that bind and inactivate cell growth–regulatory proteins, such as p53 and the retinoblastoma gene product, thus releasing the brakes on cell growth. Loss of p53 also makes the cell more susceptible to mutation. Epstein-Barr virus immortalizes B cells by stimulating cell growth (as a B-cell mitogen) and by preventing programmed cell death (apoptosis).

Retroviruses (RNA viruses) use two approaches to oncogenesis. Some oncoviruses encode **oncogene** proteins (e.g., SIS, RAS, SRC, MOS, MYC, JUN, FOS) that are almost identical to the cellular proteins involved in cellular growth control (e.g., components of a growth-factor signal cascade [receptors, G proteins, protein kinases], or growth-regulating transcription factors). The overproduction or altered function of these oncogene products stimulates cell growth. These oncogenic viruses *rapidly* cause tumors to form. *However, no human retrovirus of this type has been identified.*

Human T-cell lymphotropic virus 1, the only human oncogenic retrovirus identified, uses more subtle mechanisms of leukemogenesis. It encodes a protein **(TAX)** that **transactivates** gene expression, including genes for growth-stimulating cytokines (e.g., interleukin [IL]-2). This constitutes the second approach to oncogenesis. The integration of the DNA copy of HTLV-1 near a cellular growth-stimulating gene can also cause the gene to be activated by the strong viral enhancer and promoter sequences encoded at each end of the viral genome (long terminal repeat [LTR] sequences). *HTLV-1–associated leukemias* ***develop slowly,*** *occurring 20 to 30 years after infection.* Retroviruses continue to produce virus in immortalized or transformed cells.

Some viruses may initiate tumor formation indirectly. Hepatitis B virus (HBV) and hepatitis C virus (HCV) may have mechanisms for direct oncogenesis; however, both viruses establish persistent infections that cause inflammation and require significant tissue repair. Inflammation and continuous stimulation of liver cell growth and repair may promote mutations that lead to tumor formation. Human herpesvirus 8 (HHV-8) promotes the development of Kaposi sarcoma by means of growth-promoting cytokines encoded by the virus; this disease occurs most often in immunosuppressed patients, such as those with acquired immunodeficiency syndrome (AIDS).

Viral transformation is the first step but is generally not sufficient to cause oncogenesis and tumor formation. Instead, over time, immortalized cells are more likely than normal cells to accumulate other mutations or chromosomal rearrangements that promote development of tumor cells. Immortalized cells may also be more susceptible to cofactors and tumor promoters (e.g., phorbol esters, butyrate) that enhance tumor formation. Approximately 15% of human cancers can be related to oncogenic viruses such as HTLV-1, HBV, HCV, papillomaviruses 16 and 18, HHV-8, and Epstein-Barr virus. HSV-2 may be a cofactor for human cervical cancer.

Host Defenses Against Viral Infection

The ultimate goals of the host antiviral innate and immune responses are to prevent entry, prevent spread, and eliminate the virus and the cells harboring or replicating the virus **(resolution).** The immune response is the best and in most cases the only means of controlling a viral infection. Innate humoral and cellular immune responses are important for antiviral immunity. The longer the virus replicates in the body, the greater the dissemination of the infection, the more rigorous the immune response necessary to control the infection, and the greater the potential for immunopathogenesis. Interferon and cytotoxic T-cell responses may have evolved primarily as antiviral defense mechanisms. A detailed description of the antiviral immune response is presented in Chapter 10.

The skin is the best barrier to infection. The orifices of the body (e.g., mouth, eyes, nose, ears, and anus) are protected by mucus, ciliated epithelium, tears, the gastric acid and bile of the gastrointestinal tract, and secreted IgA. After the virus penetrates these natural barriers, it activates the **antigen-nonspecific (innate) host defenses** (e.g., fever, interferon, macrophages, dendritic cells, natural killer [NK] cells), which attempt to limit and control local viral replication and spread. Unlike for bacteria, the innate response is triggered by infected cells or against infected cells, and the initial response is more likely to be mediated by interferon and cytokines (flulike symptoms) rather than inflammation mediated by complement and neutrophils. Viral molecules, including double-stranded RNA (which is the replicative intermediate of RNA viruses), certain forms of DNA and single-stranded RNA, and some viral glycoproteins, activate type I interferon production and innate cellular responses through interaction with cytoplasmic receptors or the Toll-like receptors (TLRs) in endosomes. *Innate responses prevent most viral infections from causing disease.*

Antigen-specific immune responses take several days to be activated and become effective. The goal of these protective responses is to resolve the infection by eliminating all infectious virus and virus-infected cells from the body. **Antibody** is effective against extracellular virus and may be sufficient to control cytolytic viruses because viral replication will eliminate the virion factory within the infected cell. Antibody is essential to control virus spread to target tissues by viremia. **Cell-mediated immunity** is required for lysis of cells infected with a **noncytolytic virus** (e.g., hepatitis A virus) and infections caused by **enveloped viruses.**

Prior immunity delivers antigen-specific immunity much sooner and more effectively than during a primary infection. It may not prevent the initial stages of infection but, in most cases, does prevent disease progression. On rechallenge, cell-mediated responses are more effective at limiting the local spread of virus, and serum antibody can prevent viremic spread of the virus. Memory immune responses can be generated by prior infection or vaccination.

Many viruses, especially the larger viruses, have the means to escape one or more aspects of immune control (see Chapter 10, Table 10-3). These mechanisms include preventing interferon action, changing viral antigens, spreading by cell-to-cell transmission to escape antibody, and suppressing antigen presentation and lymphocyte function. By preventing the consequences of the antiviral state induced by IFN-α and IFN-β, HSV protein synthesis and replication can continue. Inhibition of major histocompatibility complex (MHC) I expression by cytomegalovirus and adenoviruses prevents T-cell killing of the infected cell. Antigenic variation over the course of several years (antigenic shift and drift) by influenza or during the lifetime of the infected individual by HIV limits the antiviral efficacy of antibody. Failure to resolve the infection may lead to persistent infection, chronic disease, or death of the patient.

Immunopathology

The hypersensitivity and inflammatory reactions initiated by antiviral immunity can be the major cause of the pathologic manifestations and symptoms of viral disease (Table 37-3). Early responses to the virus and viral infection (e.g., interferon, cytokines) can initiate local inflammatory and systemic responses. For example, interferon and cytokines stimulate the **flulike systemic symptoms** (e.g., fever, malaise, headache) usually associated with *respiratory viral infections and viremias* (e.g., arboencephalitis viruses). These symptoms often precede **(prodrome)** the characteristic symptoms of the viral infection during the viremic stage. Some viral infections induce a large cytokine response (cytokine storm), and this can dysregulate immune responses and may trigger autoimmune diseases in genetically predisposed individuals. Later, immune complexes and complement activation (classic pathway), CD4 T-cell–induced type IV hypersensitivity, and CD8 cytolytic T-cell action may induce tissue damage. These actions often promote neutrophil infiltration and more cell damage.

The inflammatory response initiated by cell-mediated immunity is difficult to control and damages tissue. Infections by enveloped viruses, in particular, induce cell-mediated immune responses that usually produce more extensive immunopathologic conditions. For example, the classic symptoms of measles and mumps result from the **T-cell–induced inflammatory responses** rather than from cytopathologic effects of the virus. The presence of large amounts of antigen and antibody in blood during viremias or chronic infections (e.g., HBV infection) can initiate the **classic type III immune complex hypersensitivity reactions.** These **immune complexes** can activate the complement system, triggering inflammatory responses and tissue destruction. These immune complexes often accumulate in the kidney and cause glomerulonephritis.

In the case of dengue and measles viruses, partial immunity to a related or inactivated virus can result in a more severe host response and disease on subsequent challenge with a related or virulent virus. This is because antigen-specific T-cell and antibody responses are enhanced and induce significant inflammatory and hypersensitivity damage to infected endothelial cells **(dengue hemorrhagic fever)** or skin and the lung **(atypical measles).** In addition, a non-neutralizing antibody can facilitate the uptake of dengue and yellow fever viruses into macrophages through Fc receptors, where they can replicate.

Children generally have a less active cell-mediated immune response (e.g., NK or natural killer T [NKT] cells) than adults and therefore usually have milder symptoms during infections by some viruses (e.g., measles, mumps, Epstein-Barr, and varicella-zoster viruses). However, in the case of HBV, mild or no symptoms correlate with an inability to resolve the infection, resulting in chronic disease.

Table 37-3 Viral Immunopathogenesis

Immunopathogenesis	Immune Mediators	Examples
Flulike symptoms	Interferon, cytokines	Respiratory viruses, arboviruses (viremia-inducing viruses)
Type IV hypersensitivity and inflammation	T cells, macrophages, and polymorphonuclear leukocytes	Enveloped viruses
Immune complex disease	Antibody, complement	Hepatitis B virus, rubella
Hemorrhagic disease	T cell, antibody, complement	Yellow fever, dengue, Lassa fever, Ebola viruses
Postinfection cytolysis	T cells	Enveloped viruses (e.g., postmeasles encephalitis)
Cytokine storm	Antigen-presenting cells, T cells, cytokines	Enveloped and other viruses
Immunosuppression	T cells, macrophages, dendritic cells	Human immunodeficiency virus, cytomegalovirus, measles virus, influenza virus

• Viral Disease

The relative **susceptibility** of a person and the **severity** of the disease depend on the following factors:

1. The mechanism of exposure and site of infection
2. The immune status, age, and general health of the person
3. The viral dose
4. The genetics of the virus and the host

Once the host is infected, however, the host's immune status and competence are probably the major factors that determine whether a viral infection causes a life-threatening disease, a benign outcome, or no symptoms at all.

The stages of viral disease are shown in Figure 37-1C. During the **incubation period,** the virus is replicating but has not reached the target tissue or induced sufficient damage to cause the disease. *The incubation period is relatively short if the primary site of infection is the target tissue and produces the characteristic symptoms of the disease. Longer incubation periods occur when the virus must spread to other sites and be amplified before reaching the target tissue, or the symptoms are caused by immunopathology.* Nonspecific or flulike symptoms may precede the characteristic symptoms during the **prodrome.** The incubation periods for many common

Table 37-4 Incubation Periods of Common Viral Infections

Disease	Incubation Period (Days)*
Influenza	1-2
Common cold	1-3
Herpes simplex	2-8
Bronchiolitis, croup	3-5
Acute respiratory disease (adenoviruses)	5-7
Dengue	5-8
Enteroviruses	6-12
Poliomyelitis	5-20
Measles	9-12
Smallpox	12-14
Chickenpox	13-17
Mumps	16-20
Rubella	17-20
Mononucleosis	30-50
Hepatitis A	15-40
Hepatitis B	50-150
Rabies	30-100+
Papilloma (warts)	50-150
Human immunodeficiency virus	1-15 years
AIDS	1-10 years

Modified from White DO, Fenner F: *Medical virology,* ed 3, New York, 1986, Academic.

*Until first appearance of prodromal symptoms. Diagnostic signs (e.g., rash, paralysis) may not appear until 2 to 4 days later.

viral infections are listed in Table 37-4. Specific viral diseases are discussed in subsequent chapters and reviewed in Chapter 38.

The nature and severity of the symptoms of a viral disease are related to the function of the infected target tissue (e.g., liver, hepatitis; brain, encephalitis) and the extent of the immunopathologic responses triggered by the infection. **Inapparent infections** result if (1) the infected tissue is undamaged, (2) the infection is controlled before the virus reaches its target tissue, (3) the target tissue is expendable, (4) the damaged tissue is rapidly repaired, or (5) the extent of damage is below a functional threshold for that particular tissue. For example, many infections of the brain are inapparent or are below the threshold of severe loss of function, but encephalitis results if the loss of function becomes significant. Despite the lack of symptoms, virus-specific antibody will be produced. *Inapparent or asymptomatic infections are major sources of contagion.*

Viral infections may cause **acute** or **chronic disease (persistent infection).** The ability and speed with which a person's immune system controls and resolves a viral infection usually determine whether acute or chronic disease ensues, as well as the severity of the symptoms (Figure 37-3). The acute episode of a persistent infection may be asymptomatic (JC polyomavirus) or may later in life cause symptoms

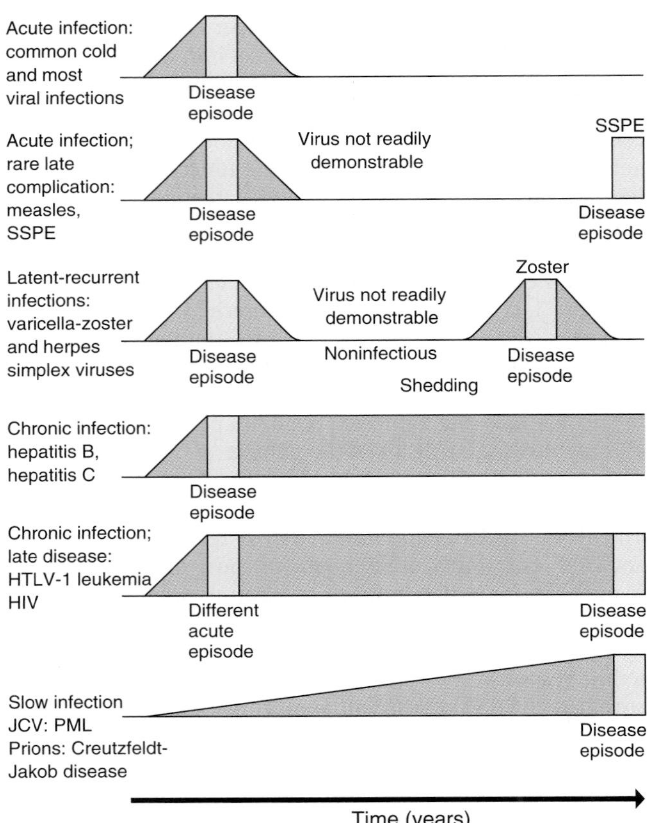

FIGURE 37-3 Acute infection and various types of persistent infection, as illustrated by the diseases indicated in the column at the left. *Blue* represents presence of virus; *green* indicates episode of disease. *HIV,* Human immunodeficiency virus; *HTLV-1,* human T-cell lymphotropic virus 1; *JCV,* JC virus; *PML,* progressive multifocal leukoencephalopathy; *SSPE,* subacute sclerosing panencephalitis. (Modified from White DO, Fenner FJ: *Medical virology,* ed 3, New York, 1986, Academic.)

similar to (varicella and zoster) or different from (HIV: acute versus AIDS) those of the acute disease. **Slow viruses and prions** have long incubation periods during which sufficient virus or tissue destruction accumulates before a rapid progression of symptoms.

Epidemiology

Epidemiology studies the spread of disease through a population. Infection of a population is similar to infection of a person in that the virus must spread through the population and is controlled by immunization of the population (Box 37-4). To endure, viruses must continue to infect new, immunologically naïve, susceptible hosts.

Exposure

People are exposed to viruses throughout their lives. However, some situations, vocations, lifestyles, and living arrangements increase the likelihood that a person will come in contact with certain viruses. In contrast, many viruses are ubiquitous. Previous exposure to HSV-1, HHV-6, varicella-zoster virus, parvovirus B19, Epstein-Barr virus,

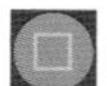

Box 37-4 Viral Epidemiology*

Mechanisms of Viral Transmission†
Aerosols
Food, water
Fomites (e.g., tissues, clothes)
Direct contact with secretions (e.g., saliva, semen)
Sexual contact, birth
Blood transfusion or organ transplant
Zoonoses (animals, insects [arboviruses])
Genetic (vertical) (e.g., retroviruses)

Disease and Viral Factors That Promote Transmission
Stability of virion in response to environment (e.g., drying, detergents, temperature)
Replication and secretion of virus into transmissible aerosols and secretions (e.g., saliva, semen)
Asymptomatic transmission
Transience or ineffectiveness of immune response to control reinfection or recurrence

Risk Factors
Age
Health
Immune status
Occupation: contact with agent or vector
Travel history
Lifestyle
Children in day-care centers
Sexual activity

Critical Community Size
Seronegative, susceptible people

Geography and Season
Presence of cofactors or vectors in the environment
Habitat and season for arthropod vectors (mosquitoes)
School session: close proximity and crowding
Home-heating season

Modes of Control
Quarantine
Elimination of the vector
Immunization
Vaccination
Treatment
Education

*Infection of a population instead of a person.

†See also Table 37-5.

and many respiratory and enteric viruses can be detected in most young children or by early adulthood by the presence of antibodies to the virus.

Poor hygiene and crowded living, school, and job conditions promote exposure to respiratory and enteric viruses. Day-care centers are consistent sources of viral infections, especially viruses spread by the respiratory and fecal-oral routes. Travel, summer camp, and vocations that bring people in contact with a virus vector (e.g., mosquitoes) put them at particular risk for infection by arboviruses and other zoonoses. Sexual promiscuity also promotes the spread and acquisition of several viruses. Health care workers, such as physicians, dentists, nurses, and technicians, are frequently exposed to respiratory and other viruses but are uniquely at risk for acquiring viruses from contaminated blood (HBV, HIV) or vesicle fluid (HSV).

Transmission of Viruses

Viruses are transmitted by direct contact (including sexual contact), injection with contaminated fluids or blood, transplantation of organs, and the respiratory and fecal-oral routes (Table 37-5). *The route of transmission depends on the source of the virus (the tissue site of viral replication and secretion) and the ability of the virus to endure the hazards and barriers of the environment and the body en route to the target tissue.* For example, viruses that replicate in the respiratory tract (e.g., influenza A virus) are released in aerosol droplets, whereas enteric viruses (e.g., picornaviruses and reoviruses) are passed by the fecal-oral route. Cytomegalovirus is transmitted in most bodily secretions because it infects mucoepithelial, secretory, and other cells found in the skin, secretory glands, lungs, liver, and other organs.

The presence or absence of an envelope is the major structural determinant of the mode of viral transmission. **Nonenveloped viruses** (naked capsid viruses) can withstand drying, the effects of detergents, and extremes of pH and temperature, whereas enveloped viruses generally cannot (see Chapter 36, Box 36-4). Specifically, most nonenveloped viruses can withstand the acidic environment of the stomach and the detergent-like bile of the intestines and mild disinfection and insufficient sewage treatment. These viruses are generally transmitted by the respiratory and fecal-oral routes and can often be acquired from contaminated objects **(fomites).** For example, hepatitis A virus, a picornavirus, is a nonenveloped virus that is transmitted by the fecal-oral route and acquired from contaminated water, shellfish, and food. Adenoviruses and many other nonenveloped viruses can be spread by contact with fomites such as handkerchiefs and toys.

Unlike the sturdy nonenveloped viruses, most **enveloped viruses** are comparatively fragile (see Chapter 36, Box 36-5). They require an intact envelope for infectivity. These viruses must remain wet and are spread (1) in respiratory droplets, blood, mucus, saliva, and semen, (2) by injection, or (3) in organ transplants. Most enveloped viruses are also labile to treatment with acid and detergents, a feature that precludes their being transmitted by the fecal-oral route. Exceptions are HBV and coronaviruses.

Animals and insects can also act as **vectors** that spread viral disease to other animals and humans and even to other locales. They can also be **reservoirs** for the virus, maintaining and amplifying the virus in the environment. Viral diseases that are shared by animals or insects and humans are called **zoonoses.** For example, raccoons, foxes, bats, dogs, and cats are reservoirs and vectors for the rabies virus. Arthropods (e.g., mosquitoes, ticks, sandflies) can act as vectors for togaviruses, flaviviruses, bunyaviruses, or reoviruses. These viruses are often referred to as **arboviruses** because they are *ar*thropod *bo*rne. A more detailed discussion of arboviruses is presented in Chapter 52. Most arboviruses have a very broad host range, capable of replicating in specific insects, birds, amphibians, and mammals, in addition to humans. Also, the arboviruses must establish a sufficient viremia in the animal reservoir so that the insect can acquire the virus during its blood meal.

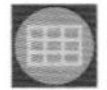 Table 37-5 **Viral Transmission**

Mode	Examples
Respiratory transmission	Paramyxoviruses, influenza viruses, picornaviruses, rhinoviruses, varicella-zoster virus, B19 virus
Fecal-oral transmission	Picornaviruses, rotavirus, reovirus, noroviruses, adenovirus
Contact (lesions, fomites)	HSV, rhinoviruses, poxviruses, adenovirus
Zoonoses (animals, insects)	Togaviruses (alpha), flaviviruses, bunyaviruses, orbiviruses, arenaviruses, hantaviruses, rabies virus, influenza A virus, orf (pox)
Transmission via blood	HIV, HTLV-1, HBV, HCV, hepatitis delta virus, cytomegalovirus
Sexual contact	Blood-borne viruses, HSV, human papillomavirus, molluscum contagiosum, HIV, HTLV-1, HBV, HCV
Maternal-neonatal transmission	Rubella virus, cytomegalovirus, B19 virus, echovirus, HSV, varicella-zoster virus, HIV
Genetic	Prions, retroviruses

HBV, Hepatitis B virus; *HCV,* hepatitis C virus; *HIV,* human immunodeficiency virus; *HSV,* herpes simplex virus; *HTLV-1,* human T-cell lymphotropic virus 1.

Other factors that can promote transmission of viruses are the potential for asymptomatic infection, crowded living conditions, certain occupations, certain lifestyles, day-care centers, and travel. Viral transmission during an asymptomatic infection (e.g., HIV, varicella-zoster virus) occurs unknowingly and is difficult to restrict. This is an important characteristic of **sexually transmitted diseases.** Viruses that cause persistent productive infections (e.g., cytomegalovirus, HIV) are a particular problem because the infected person is a continual source of virus that can be spread to immunologically naïve people. Viruses with many different serotypes (rhinoviruses) or viruses capable of changing their antigenicity (influenza and HIV) also readily find immunologically naïve populations.

Maintenance of a Virus in the Population

The persistence of a virus in a community depends on the availability of a critical number of immunologically naïve (seronegative), susceptible people. The efficiency of virus transmission determines the size of the susceptible population necessary for maintenance of the virus in the population. Immunization produced by natural means or by vaccination is the best way of reducing the number of such susceptible people.

Age

A person's age is an important factor in determining his or her susceptibility to viral infections. Infants, children, adults, and elderly persons are susceptible to different viruses and have different symptomatic responses to the infection. These differences may result from variations in body size, recuperative abilities, and most important, immune status in people in these age groups. Differences in lifestyles, habits, school environments, and job settings at different ages also determine when people are exposed to viruses.

Infants and children acquire a series of respiratory and exanthematous viral diseases at first exposure because they are immunologically naïve. Infants are especially prone to more serious presentations of paramyxovirus respiratory infections and viral gastroenteritis because of their small size and physiologic requirements (e.g., nutrients, water, electrolytes). However, children generally do not mount as severe an immunopathologic response as adults, and some diseases (herpesviruses) are more benign in children.

Elderly persons are especially susceptible to new viral infections and the reactivation of latent viruses. Because they are less able to initiate a new immune response, repair damaged tissue, and recover, elderly persons are therefore more susceptible to complications after infection and outbreaks of the new strains of the influenza A and B viruses. Elderly persons are also more prone to zoster (shingles), a recurrence of varicella-zoster virus, as a result of a decline in this specific immune response with age.

Immune Status

The competence of a person's immune response and immune history determine how quickly and efficiently the infection is resolved and can also determine the severity of the symptoms. The rechallenge of a person with prior immunity usually results in asymptomatic or mild disease without transmission. People who are in an immunosuppressed state as a result of AIDS, cancer, or immunosuppressive therapy are at greater risk of suffering more serious disease on primary infection (measles, vaccinia) and are more prone to suffer recurrences of infections with latent viruses (e.g., herpesviruses, papovaviruses).

Other Host Factors

General health plays an important role in determining the competence and nature of the immune response and ability to repair diseased tissue. Poor nutrition can compromise a person's immune system and decrease his or her tissue regenerative capacity. Measles becomes much more deadly for individuals deficient in vitamin A, possibly owing to an anti-inflammatory action of vitamin A. Immunosuppressive diseases and therapies may allow viral replication or recurrence to proceed unchecked. Genetic makeup also plays an important role in determining the response of the immune system to viral infection. Specifically, genetic differences in immune response genes, genes for viral receptors, and other genetic loci affect susceptibility to a viral infection and severity of disease.

Geographic and Seasonal Considerations

The geographic distribution of a virus is usually determined by whether the requisite cofactors or vectors are present or whether there is an immunologically naïve, susceptible population. For example, many of the arboviruses are limited to the ecologic niche of their arthropod vectors. Extensive global transportation is eliminating many of the geographically determined restrictions to virus distribution.

Seasonal differences in the occurrence of viral disease correspond with behaviors that promote spread of the virus. For example, respiratory viruses are more prevalent in the winter because crowding facilitates the spread of such viruses, and the temperature and humid conditions stabilize them. Enteric viruses, on the other hand, are more prevalent during the summer, possibly because hygiene is more lax during this season. The seasonal differences in arboviral diseases reflect the life cycle of the arthropod vector or its reservoir (e.g., birds).

Outbreaks, Epidemics, and Pandemics

Outbreaks of a viral infection often result from the introduction of a virus (e.g., hepatitis A) into a new location. The outbreak originates from a **common source** (e.g., food preparation) and often can be stopped once the source is identified. Norovirus outbreaks on cruise ships or from restaurants can often be traced to the dirty hands of an employee. **Epidemics** occur over a larger geographic area and generally result from the introduction of a new strain of virus into an immunologically naïve population. **Pandemics** are worldwide epidemics, usually resulting from the introduction of a new virus (e.g., HIV). Pandemics of influenza A used to occur approximately every 10 years as the result of the introduction of new strains of the virus.

• Control of Viral Spread

The spread of a virus can be controlled by quarantine, good hygiene, changes in lifestyle, elimination of the vector, or immunization of the population. **Quarantine** was once the only means of limiting epidemics of viral infections and is most effective for limiting the spread of viruses that always cause symptomatic disease (e.g., smallpox). It is now used in hospitals to limit the **nosocomial spread** of viruses, especially to high-risk patients (e.g., immunosuppressed people). Proper sanitation of contaminated items and disinfection of the water supply are means of limiting the spread of enteric viruses. Education and resultant changes in lifestyle have made a difference in the spread of sexually transmitted viruses such as HIV, HBV, and HSV. Elimination of an arthropod or its ecologic niche (e.g., drainage of the swamps it inhabits) has proved effective for controlling arboviruses.

The **best way to limit viral spread, however, is to immunize the population.** Immunization, whether produced by natural infection or by vaccination, protects individuals and reduces the size of the immunologically naïve, susceptible population necessary to promote the spread and maintenance of the virus.

Bibliography

Cann AJ: *Principles of molecular virology*, San Diego, 2005, Academic.

Carter J, Saunders V: *Virology: principles and applications*, Chichester, England, 2007, Wiley.

Cohen J, Powderly WG: *Infectious diseases*, ed 2, St Louis, 2004, Mosby.

Collier L, Oxford J: *Human virology*, ed 3, Oxford, England, 2006, Oxford University Press.

Emond RT, Welsby PD, Rowland HAK: *Color atlas of infectious diseases*, ed 4, St Louis, 2003, Mosby.

Evans AS, Kaslow RA: *Viral infections of humans: epidemiology and control*, ed 4, New York, 1997, Plenum.

Flint SJ, Enquist LW, Racaniello VR, et al: *Principles of virology: molecular biology, pathogenesis and control of animal viruses*, ed 3, Washington, DC, 2009, American Society for Microbiology Press.

Gershon AA, Hotez PJ, Katz SL: *Krugman's infectious diseases of children*, ed 11, St Louis, 2004, Mosby.

Goering R, Dockrell H, Zuckerman M, et al: *Mims' medical microbiology*, ed 4, Edinburgh, 2008, Mosby.

Haller O, Kochs G, Weber F: The interferon response circuit: induction and suppression by pathogenic viruses, *Virology* 344:119–130, 2006.

Hart CA, Broadhead RL: *Color atlas of pediatric infectious diseases*, St Louis, 1992, Mosby.

Hart CA, Shears P: *Color atlas of medical microbiology*, London, 2004, Mosby.

Knipe DM, Howley PM, Griffin DE, et al: *Fields virology*, ed 5, Philadelphia, 2006, Lippincott Williams & Wilkins.

Mandell GL, Bennet JE, Dolin R: *Principles and practice of infectious diseases*, ed 6, Philadelphia, 2005, Churchill Livingstone.

Mims CA, White DO: *Viral pathogenesis and immunology*, Oxford, England, 1984, Blackwell.

Richman DD, Whitley RJ, Hayden FG: *Clinical virology*, ed 3, Washington, DC, 2009, American Society Microbiology Press.

Rosenthal KS: Viruses: microbial spies and saboteurs, *Infect Dis Clin Pract* 14:97–106, 2006.

Sampayrac L: *How pathogenic viruses work*, Mississauga, Ontario, 2001, Jones and Bartlett.

Shulman ST, Phair JP, Peterson LR, et al: *The biological and clinical basis of infectious diseases*, ed 5, Philadelphia, 1997, WB Saunders.

Stark GR, Kerr IM, Williams BR, et al: How cells respond to interferons, *Ann Rev Biochem* 67:227–264, 1998.

Strauss JM, Strauss EG: *Viruses and human disease*, ed 2, San Diego, 2007, Academic.

Voyles BA: *The biology of viruses*, ed 2, Boston, 2002, McGraw-Hill.

White DO, Fenner FJ: *Medical virology*, ed 4, San Diego, 1994, Academic.

Zuckerman AJ, Banatvala JE, Pattison JR: *Principles and practice of clinical virology*, ed 5, Chichester, England, 2004, Wiley.

Websites

All the virology on the WWW. www.virology.net/garryfavweb.html. Accessed August 7, 2015.

The big picture book of viruses. www.virology.net/Big_Virology/BVHomePage.html. Accessed August 7, 2015.

Centers for Disease Control and Prevention: CDC A-Z index. www.cdc.gov/health/diseases.htm. Accessed August 7, 2015.

Centers for Disease Control and Prevention: Traveler's health. www.cdc.gov/travel/diseases.htm. Accessed August 7, 2015.

National Center for Infectious Diseases: Infectious disease information A-Z index. www.cdc.gov/ncidod/diseases/index.htm. Accessed August 7, 2015.

National Foundation for Infectious Diseases: Fact sheets on diseases. www.nfid.org/factsheets/Default.html. Accessed August 7, 2015.

Stannard L: Virus ultra structure. www.uct.ac.za/depts/mmi/stannard/linda.html. Accessed May 14, 2012.

World Health Organization: Immunization service delivery. www.who.int/immunization_delivery/en/. Accessed August 7, 2015.

World Health Organization: Infectious diseases. www.who.int/topics/infectious_diseases/en/. Accessed August 7, 2015.

CHAPTER

38 ROLE OF VIRUSES IN DISEASE

Viruses are obligate intracellular parasites and must replicate in an appropriate host cell to continue to exist. The virus uses the cell's biochemical machinery to make its components, and then these parts are assembled into new viruses. In many cases, this is lethal to the cell. The cell and innate and immune responses attempt to block viral replication or kill the infected cell to prevent spread of the virus to other sites in the body. Most viral infections cause mild or no symptoms and do not require extensive treatment. When disease occurs, it often results from the spread of the virus to important tissues and the killing of their cells by either virus replication, inflammation, or other host protections. In addition, viruses are excellent inducers of interferon and cytokine production, which results in systemic symptoms, including flulike symptoms.

The common cold, influenza, flulike syndromes, and gastroenteritis are common viral diseases. Other viral infections that target essential tissues and organs can cause serious and even life-threatening disease. In general, the symptoms and severity of a viral infection are determined by (1) the patient's ability to prevent the spread or rapidly resolve the infection before the virus can reach important organs or cause significant damage, (2) the importance of the target tissue, (3) the virulence of the virus, (4) the extent of immunopathology induced in response to the infection, and (5) the ability of the body to repair the damage.

Immunization by prior infection or vaccination is the best means of protection against viral disease. Unlike bacteria, there are relatively few targets for the development of antiviral drugs, but drugs are available for certain viruses.

In this chapter, viral diseases are discussed with respect to their symptoms, the organ system they target, and the host factors that influence their presentation. Subsequent chapters will discuss the characteristics of the members of specific viral families and the diseases they cause. **A return to this chapter will provide a good review of the viruses.**

• Viral Diseases

The major sites of viral disease are the respiratory tract; the gastrointestinal tract; the epithelial, mucosal, and endothelial linings of the skin, mouth, and genitalia; the lymphoid tissue; the liver and other organs; and the central nervous system (CNS) (Figure 38-1). The examples given in this chapter represent the more common viral causes of disease.

Oral and Respiratory Tract Infections

The oropharynx and respiratory tract are the **most common sites** of viral infection and disease (Table 38-1). The viruses are spread in respiratory droplets, aerosols, food, water, and saliva, as well as by close contact and on hands. Similar respiratory symptoms can be caused by several different viruses. For example, bronchiolitis may be caused by respiratory syncytial or parainfluenza virus. Alternatively, one virus may cause different symptoms in different people. Influenza virus can cause a mild upper respiratory tract infection in one person and life-threatening pneumonia in another. Vaccines and antiviral drugs are available for influenza.

Many viral infections start in the oropharynx or respiratory tract, infect the lung, and spread without causing significant respiratory symptoms. Varicella-zoster virus (VZV) and the measles virus initiate infection in the lung and can cause pneumonia but generally cause systemic infections, resulting in an exanthem (rash). Other viruses that establish primary infection of the oropharynx or respiratory tract and then progress to other sites include rubella, mumps, enteroviruses, and several human herpesviruses.

The symptoms and severity of a respiratory viral disease depend on the nature of the virus, the site of infection (upper or lower respiratory tract), and the immune status and age of the person. Conditions such as cystic fibrosis and smoking, which compromise the ciliated and mucoepithelial barriers to infection, increase the risk of serious disease.

Pharyngitis and oral disease are common viral presentations. Most enteroviruses (picornaviruses) infect the oropharynx and then progress by way of a viremia to other target tissues. For example, symptoms such as acute-onset pharyngitis, fever, and oral vesicular lesions are characteristic of coxsackievirus A infections (herpangina, hand-foot-and-mouth disease) and some coxsackievirus B and echovirus infections. Adenovirus and the early stages of Epstein-Barr virus (EBV) disease are characterized by sore throat and tonsillitis with exudative membranes; EBV goes on to cause infectious mononucleosis. Herpes simplex virus (HSV) causes local primary infections of the oral mucosa and face (gingivostomatitis) and then establishes a latent neuronal infection that can recur in the form of herpes labialis (cold sores, fever blisters). HSV is also a common cause of pharyngitis. HSV and coxsackievirus A may also involve the tonsils, but with vesicular lesions. Vesicular lesions on the buccal mucosa (Koplik spots) are an early diagnostic feature of measles infection.

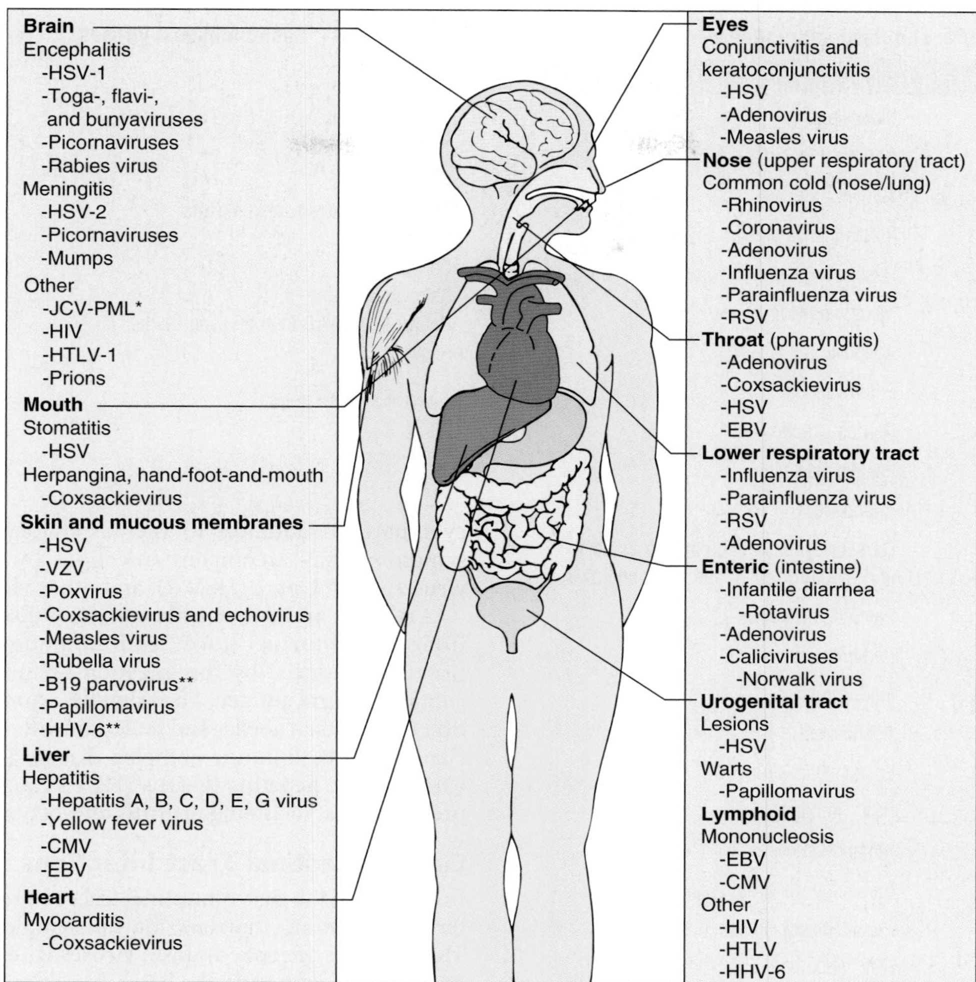

FIGURE 38-1 Major target tissues of viral disease. Asterisk *(*)* indicates progressive multifocal leukoencephalopathy *(PML).* Infection by viruses indicated by double asterisks *(**)* results in an immune-mediated rash. *CMV,* Cytomegalovirus; *EBV,* Epstein-Barr virus; *HHV-6,* human herpesvirus 6; *HIV,* human immunodeficiency virus; *HSV,* herpes simplex virus; *HTLV,* human T-cell lymphotropic virus; *JCV,* JC virus; *RSV,* respiratory syncytial virus; *VZV,* varicella-zoster virus.

Upper respiratory tract viral infections, including the common cold and pharyngitis, account for at least 50% of absenteeism from schools and the workplace, despite being generally benign. Rhinoviruses and coronaviruses are the predominant causes of upper respiratory tract infections. A runny nose (rhinitis) followed by congestion, cough, sneezing, conjunctivitis, headache, and sore throat are typical symptoms of the common cold. Other causes of the common cold or pharyngitis are specific serotypes of echoviruses and coxsackieviruses, adenoviruses, influenza viruses, parainfluenza viruses, metapneumovirus, and respiratory syncytial virus (RSV).

Tonsillitis, laryngitis, and **croup** (laryngotracheobronchitis) may accompany certain respiratory tract viral infections. Inflammatory responses to viral infection cause the trachea to narrow below the vocal cords (subglottic area), resulting in laryngitis (adults) and croup (children). This narrowing causes loss of voice; a hoarse, barking cough; and the risk, especially in young children, for a blocked airway and choking. Children infected with parainfluenza viruses are especially at risk for croup.

Lower respiratory tract viral infections can result in more serious disease. Symptoms of such infections include bronchiolitis (inflammation of the bronchioles), pneumonia, pneumonitis, and related diseases. Parainfluenza virus, metapneumovirus, and RSVs are major problems for infants and children but cause only asymptomatic infections or common cold symptoms in adults. Parainfluenza 3 virus, and especially RSV infections, are major causes of life-threatening pneumonia or bronchiolitis in infants younger than 6 months. Infection with these viruses does not provide lifelong immunity.

Influenza virus is probably the best known and most feared of the common respiratory viruses, with the annual introduction of new strains of virus ensuring the presence of immunologically naïve victims. Children are universally susceptible to new strains of virus, whereas older people may have been immunized during a prior outbreak of the annual strain. Despite such immunization, the elderly are especially susceptible to pneumonia caused by new strains of virus because they may not be able to mount a sufficient primary immune response to the new strain of influenza virus or to

 Table 38-1 **Oral and Respiratory Diseases**

Disease	Etiologic Agent
Common Cold	Rhinovirus*
	Coronavirus*
	Influenza viruses
	Parainfluenza viruses
	Respiratory syncytial virus (RSV)
	Metapneumovirus
	Adenovirus
	Enteroviruses
Pharyngitis	Herpes simplex virus
	Epstein-Barr virus
	Adenovirus*
	Coxsackievirus A* (herpangina, hand-foot-and-mouth disease) and other enteroviruses
Croup, Tonsillitis, Laryngitis, and Bronchitis (Children < 2 Years)	Parainfluenza virus 1*
	Parainfluenza virus 2
	Influenza virus
	Adenovirus
	Epstein-Barr virus
Bronchiolitis	RSV* (infants)
	Metapneumovirus
	Parainfluenza virus 3* (infants and children)
	Parainfluenza viruses 1 and 2
Pneumonia	RSV* (infants)
	Metapneumovirus
	Parainfluenza virus* (infants)
	Influenza virus*
	Adenovirus
	Varicella-zoster virus (primary infection of adults or immunocompromised hosts)
	Cytomegalovirus (infection of immunocompromised host)
	Measles

*Most common causal agents.

repair the tissue damage caused by the disease. Influenza infection also increases risk for life-threatening pneumonia by *Staphylococcus aureus* or streptococcal co-infections. Other possible viral agents of pneumonia are adenovirus, paramyxoviruses, and primary VZV infections of adults.

Flulike and Systemic Symptoms

Many viral infections cause classic **flulike symptoms** (e.g., fever, malaise, anorexia, headache, body aches), side effects caused by host responses to the infection. During the viremic phase, many viruses induce the release of interferon and cytokines. In addition to the respiratory viruses, flulike symptoms may accompany infections by arboencephalitis viruses, HSV type 2 (HSV-2), and other viruses.

Arthritis and other inflammatory diseases may result from the cytokine storm and immune hypersensitivity responses induced by the infection or immune complexes containing viral antigen. For example, parvovirus B19 infection (of adults), rubella, and infection with some togaviruses elicit arthritis. Immune complex disease that is associated with chronic hepatitis B virus (HBV) can result in various presentations, including arthritis and nephritis.

 Box 38-1 **Gastrointestinal Viruses**

Infants
Rotavirus A*
Adenovirus 40, 41
Coxsackievirus A24

Infants, Children, and Adults
Norwalk virus*
Calicivirus
Astrovirus
Rotavirus A and B (outbreaks in China)
Reovirus

*Most common causal agents.

Gastrointestinal Tract Infections

Infections of the gastrointestinal tract can result in gastroenteritis, vomiting, diarrhea, or no symptoms (Box 38-1). These viruses are naked capsid viruses with a physical structure that can withstand the harsh conditions of the gastrointestinal tract. Norwalk virus, caliciviruses, astroviruses, adenoviruses, reoviruses, and rotaviruses infect the small intestine but not the colon, altering the function or damaging the epithelial lining and the absorptive villi. This leads to malabsorption of water and an electrolyte imbalance. The resultant diarrhea in older children and adults is generally self-limited and can be treated with rehydration and restoration of the electrolyte balance. These viruses, especially rotavirus, are major problems for adults and children in regions where there is drought and starvation.

Viral gastroenteritis has a more significant effect on infants and may necessitate hospitalization. The extent of tissue damage and consequent loss of fluids and electrolytes may be life threatening. Rotavirus and adenovirus serotypes 40 and 41 are the major causes of infantile gastroenteritis. Vaccines are available for rotavirus.

Fecal-oral spread of the enteric viruses is promoted by poor hygiene and is especially prevalent in day-care centers. Norwalk virus and calicivirus outbreaks affecting older children and adults are generally linked to a common contaminated food or water source. Vomiting usually accompanies diarrhea in patients infected with the Norwalk virus and rotavirus. Although enteroviruses (picornaviruses) are spread by the fecal-oral route, they usually cause only mild or no gastrointestinal symptoms. Instead, these viruses establish a viremia, spread to other target organs, and then cause clinical disease.

Exanthems, Hemorrhagic Fevers, and Arthritides

Virus-induced skin disease (Table 38-2) can result from infection through the mucosa or small cuts or abrasions in the skin (HSV), as a secondary infection after establishment of a viremia (VZV and smallpox), or as a result of the inflammatory response mounted against viral antigens (parvovirus B19). The major classifications of viral rashes are maculopapular, vesicular, nodular, and hemorrhagic. **Macules** are flat, colored spots. **Papules** are slightly raised areas of the skin that may result from immune or inflammatory responses rather than the direct effects of the virus. **Nodules** are larger raised areas of the skin. **Vesicular lesions** are blisters and are likely to contain virus. Human papillomaviruses (HPV) cause warts, and molluscum contagiosum causes wartlike growths (nodules) by stimulating the growth of skin cells. There are vaccines for HPV.

The classic childhood exanthems are roseola infantum (exanthem subitum [HHV-6]), fifth disease (erythema infectiosum [parvovirus B19]), and (in unvaccinated children) varicella, measles, and rubella. The rash follows a viremia and is accompanied by fever. Rashes are also caused by enterovirus, alphavirus, and dengue and other flavivirus infections. They also are occasionally seen in patients with infectious mononucleosis. Vaccines are available for varicella-zoster, measles, mumps, and rubella.

The yellow fever virus, dengue virus, Ebola virus, Lassa fever, Sin Nombre virus, and other hemorrhagic fever viruses establish a viremia and infect the endothelial cell lining of the vasculature, possibly compromising the structure of the blood vessel. Viral or immune cytolysis can then lead to greater permeability or rupture of the vessel, producing a hemorrhagic rash with petechiae (pinpoint hemorrhages under the skin) and ecchymoses (massive bruises) and hence internal bleeding, loss of electrolytes, and shock.

Arthritis can be a consequence of direct infection of the joint or immune responses to viruses such as the togaviruses (e.g., Chikungunya, rubella), parvovirus B19, flaviviruses (e.g., dengue and hepatitis C virus [HCV]), HBV, human immunodeficiency virus (HIV), and human T-cell lymphotropic virus 1 (HTLV-1). Immune complexes containing viral antigen may trigger inflammatory responses, or the virus infection may trigger autoimmune responses, but most viral arthritis is temporary.

Table 38-2 Viral Exanthems

Condition	Etiologic Agent
Rash	
Rubeola	Measles virus
German measles	Rubella virus
Roseola infantum	Human herpesvirus 6*
Erythema infectiosum	Human parvovirus B19*
Boston exanthem	Echovirus 16
Infectious mononucleosis	Epstein-Barr virus, cytomegalovirus
Vesicles	
Oral or genital herpes	Herpes simplex virus*
Chickenpox/shingles	Varicella-zoster virus*
Hand-foot-and-mouth disease, herpangina	Coxsackievirus A*
Papillomas, etc.	
Warts	Papillomavirus*
Molluscum	Molluscum contagiosum*

*Most common causal agents.

Infections of the Eye

Infections of the eye result from direct contact with a virus or from viremic spread (Box 38-2). Conjunctivitis (pinkeye) is a normal feature of many childhood infections and is a characteristic of infections caused by specific adenovirus serotypes (3, 4a, and 7), measles virus, and rubella virus. Keratoconjunctivitis, caused by adenovirus (8, 19a, and 37), HSV, or VZV, involves the cornea and can cause severe damage. HSV disease can recur, causing scarring and blindness. Enterovirus 70 and coxsackievirus A24 can cause an acute hemorrhagic conjunctivitis. Cataracts are classic features of babies born with congenital rubella syndrome. Chorioretinitis is associated with cytomegalovirus (CMV) infection in newborns (congenital) as well as in immunosuppressed people (e.g., those with acquired immunodeficiency syndrome [AIDS]).

Box 38-2 Infections of Organs and Tissues

Liver
Hepatitis A,* B,* C,* G, D, and E viruses
Yellow fever virus
Epstein-Barr virus
Hepatitis in the neonate or immunocompromised person:
- Cytomegalovirus
- Herpes simplex virus
- Varicella-zoster virus
- Rubella virus (congenital rubella syndrome)

Heart
Coxsackievirus B

Kidney
Cytomegalovirus

Muscle
Coxsackievirus B (pleurodynia)

Glands
Cytomegalovirus
Mumps virus
Coxsackievirus B

Eye
Herpes simplex virus*
Adenovirus*
Measles virus
Rubella virus
Enterovirus 70
Coxsackievirus A24

*Most common causal agents.

Infections of the Organs and Tissues

Infection of the major organs may cause significant disease or result in further spread or secretion of the virus (see Box 38-2). The symptoms may arise from tissue damage or inflammatory responses.

The liver is a prominent target for many viruses that reach the liver by means of a viremia or the mononuclear phagocyte (reticuloendothelial) system. The liver acts as a source for a secondary viremia but can also be damaged by the infection. The classic symptoms of hepatitis result from infections with hepatitis A, B, C, G, D, and E viruses and yellow fever virus, and they are often associated with EBV infectious mononucleosis and CMV infections. The liver is also a major target in disseminated HSV infection of neonates and infants. Vaccines are available for hepatitis A and B and antiviral drugs for hepatitis B and C.

The heart and other muscles are also susceptible to viral infection and damage. Coxsackievirus can cause myocarditis or pericarditis in newborns, children, and adults. Coxsackievirus B can infect muscle and cause pleurodynia (Bornholm disease). Other viruses (e.g., influenza virus, CMV) can also infect the heart.

Infection of the secretory glands, accessory sexual organs, and mammary glands results in contagious spread of CMV. An inflammatory response to the infection, as occurs in **mumps** (parotitis, orchitis), may be the cause of the symptoms. Coxsackievirus B infection of islet cells can initiate autoimmune responses that cause type 1 diabetes. CMV infection of the kidney and reactivation are problems for immunosuppressed people and a predominant reason for kidney transplant failure.

Infections of the Central Nervous System

Viral infections of the brain and CNS may cause the most serious viral diseases because of the importance of the CNS and its very limited capacity to repair damage (Box 38-3). Tissue damage is usually caused by a combination of viral pathogenesis and immunopathogenesis. Most neurotropic viral infections are asymptomatic, however, because the virus does not reach the brain or does not cause sufficient tissue damage to produce symptoms.

Virus may spread to the CNS in blood (arboviruses) or in macrophages (HIV); it may spread from a peripheral infection of the neurons (olfactory), or it may first infect skin (HSV) or muscle (polio, rabies) and then progress to the innervating neurons. The virus may have a predilection for certain sites in the brain. For example, the temporal lobe is targeted in HSV encephalitis, the Ammon horn in rabies, and the anterior horn of the spinal cord and motor neurons in polio.

Viral infections of the CNS are usually distinguished from bacterial infections by the finding of mononuclear cells, low numbers of polymorphonuclear leukocytes, and normal or slightly reduced levels of glucose in the cerebrospinal fluid. Immunoassay detection of specific antigen, polymerase chain reaction detection of viral genomes or messenger RNA, or isolation of the virus from a cerebrospinal fluid or biopsy specimen confirms the diagnosis and identifies the viral agent. The season of the year also facilitates the diagnosis, in that enteroviral and arboviral diseases generally occur during the summer, whereas HSV encephalitis and other viral syndromes may be observed year-round.

 **Box 38-3 Central Nervous System Infections**

Meningitis

Enteroviruses
- Echoviruses
- Coxsackievirus*
- Poliovirus

Herpes simplex virus 2*
Adenovirus
Mumps virus
Lymphocytic choriomeningitis virus
Arboencephalitis viruses

Paralysis

Poliovirus
Enteroviruses 70 and 71
Coxsackievirus A7

Encephalitis

Herpes simplex virus 1*
Varicella-zoster virus
Arboencephalitis viruses*
Rabies virus
Coxsackieviruses A and B
Polioviruses

Postinfectious Encephalitis (Immune Mediated)

Measles virus
Mumps virus
Rubella virus
Varicella-zoster virus
Influenza viruses

Other

JC virus (progressive multifocal leukoencephalopathy [in immunosuppressed people])
Measles variant (subacute sclerosing panencephalitis)
Prions (encephalopathy)
Human immunodeficiency virus (AIDS dementia)
Human T-cell lymphotropic virus 1 (tropical spastic paraparesis)

AIDS, Acquired immunodeficiency syndrome.

*Most common causal agents.

Aseptic meningitis is caused by an inflammation and swelling of the meninges that envelopes the brain and spinal cord in response to infection with enteroviruses (especially echoviruses and coxsackieviruses), HSV-2, the mumps virus, or the lymphocytic choriomeningitis virus. The disease is usually self-limited and, unlike bacterial meningitis, resolves without sequelae unless the virus gains access to and infects neurons or the brain **(meningoencephalitis).** The viruses gain access to the meninges by means of a viremia.

Encephalitis and **myelitis** result from a combination of viral pathogenesis and immunopathogenesis in brain tissue and neurons and are either fatal or cause significant damage and permanent neurologic sequelae. HSV, VZV, rabies virus, California encephalitis viruses, West Nile and St. Louis encephalitis viruses, mumps, and measles virus are potential causes of encephalitis. Poliovirus and several other enteroviruses cause paralytic disease (myelitis).

HSV and VZV are ubiquitous and usually cause asymptomatic latent infections of the CNS but can also cause encephalitis. Most arboencephalitis virus infections result in flulike symptoms rather than encephalitis. Postmeasles encephalitis and subacute sclerosing panencephalitis were rare sequelae of measles in the prevaccine era.

Other virus-induced neurologic syndromes are HIV dementia, HTLV-1 tropical spastic paraparesis, JC papovavirus–induced progressive multifocal leukoencephalopathy (PML) in immunodeficient people, and the prion-associated spongiform encephalopathies (kuru, Creutzfeldt-Jakob disease, Gerstmann-Sträussler-Scheinker disease). PML and the spongiform encephalopathies have long incubation periods.

Hematologic Diseases

Lymphocytes and macrophages are not very permissive for viral replication but are targets for several viruses that establish persistent infections. These cells are also antigen-presenting cells, and during the acute phase of infection, viral replication of EBV, HIV, or CMV elicits a large T-cell response, resulting in **mononucleosis-like syndromes.** In addition, CMV, measles virus, and HIV infections of T cells are immunosuppressive. HIV reduces the numbers of CD4 helper T cells, further compromising the immune system. HTLV-1 infection causes little disease on infection but may lead to **adult T-cell leukemia** or tropical spastic paraparesis much later in life (Box 38-4).

Macrophages and cells of the macrophage lineage can be infected by many viruses. Macrophages act as vehicles for spreading the virus throughout the body because viruses replicate inefficiently in them, and the cells are generally not lysed by the infection. This process promotes persistent and chronic infections. The macrophage is the primary target cell for the dengue virus. Nonneutralizing antibody can promote uptake of dengue virus and HIV into the cell through Fc receptors. Macrophages and cells of the myeloid lineage are the initial cells infected with HIV and provide a reservoir for the virus and access to the brain. AIDS dementia is thought to result from the actions of HIV-infected macrophages and microglial cells in the brain. Antiviral drugs are available for HIV.

Sexually Transmitted Viral Diseases

Sexual transmission is a major route for the spread of papillomavirus, HSV, CMV, HIV, HTLV-1, HBV, HCV, and hepatitis D virus (HDV) (Box 38-5). Such viruses establish chronic and latent recurrent infections, with asymptomatic shedding into semen and vaginal secretions. These viral properties foster dissemination via a route of transmission that is used relatively infrequently and might be avoided during symptomatic disease. The viruses can also be transmitted neonatally or perinatally to infants. Papillomaviruses and HSV establish local primary infections, with recurrent disease at the initial site. Lesions and asymptomatic shedding are sources for sexual transmission and for perinatal transmission to the newborn. CMV and HIV infect myeloid and lymphoid cells under the mucosal lining, whereas the hepatitis viruses are delivered to the liver. CMV, HIV, and the hepatitis viruses are present in blood, semen, and vaginal secretions, which can transmit the virus to sexual partners and neonates.

Viruses Spread by Transfusion and Transplantation

HBV, HCV, HDV, HIV, HTLV-1, and CMV are transmitted by blood and organ transplants. These viruses are also present in semen and therefore are sexually transmitted. The chronic nature of the infection, the persistent asymptomatic release of the virus, or the infection of macrophages and lymphocytes promotes transmission by these routes. West Nile encephalitis virus establishes a sufficient viremia for a long enough period that transmission by transfusion has occurred. Screening of the blood supply for HBV, HCV, HIV, and HTLV has controlled transmission of these viruses in blood transfusions (Box 38-6). Blood for babies and organs are screened for CMV, but screening the general blood supply for CMV and other viruses has not been implemented, so the risk for infection remains.

Viruses Spread by Arthropods and Animals

Arthropod-borne viruses **(arboviruses)** include many of the togaviruses, flaviviruses, and bunyaviruses and the Colorado tick fever reovirus. These viruses establish sufficient viremia in birds or animals (host) to allow their acquisition by mosquitos or ticks (vector) and subsequent transmission to humans when humans enter the habitat of the vector and host. If a virus can establish a sufficient viremia in humans, then the virus—like yellow fever virus, West Nile, or St. Louis

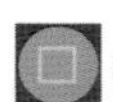

Box 38-4 Viruses Transmitted in Blood

Hepatitis B, C, G, D
Human immunodeficiency virus
Human T-cell lymphotropic virus 1
Cytomegalovirus
Epstein-Barr virus
West Nile encephalitis virus

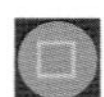

Box 38-5 Sexually Transmitted Viruses

Human papillomavirus 6, 11, 42
Human papillomavirus 16, 18, 31, 45, and others (high risk for human cervical carcinoma)
Herpes simplex virus (HSV-1 and HSV-2)
Cytomegalovirus
Hepatitis B, C, and D viruses
Human immunodeficiency virus
Human T-cell lymphotropic virus 1

Box 38-6 Screening of the Blood Supply

Human immunodeficiency syndrome
Hepatitis B
Hepatitis C
Human T-cell lymphotropic virus 1 and 2
West Nile encephalitis virus*
Syphilis

*Trial initiated in 2003 on 6 million units, with 818 positive units excluded from usage.

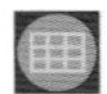 Table 38-3 **Arboviruses and Zoonoses**

Virus	Family	Reservoir/Vector
Eastern equine encephalitis	Togaviridae	Birds/*Aedes* mosquito
Western equine encephalitis	Togaviridae	Birds/*Culex* mosquito
West Nile encephalitis	Flaviviridae	Birds/*Culex* mosquito
St. Louis encephalitis	Flaviviridae	Birds/*Culex* mosquito
Chikungunya	Togaviridae	Birds, mammals/*Aedes* mosquito
California encephalitis	Bunyaviridae	Small mammals/*Aedes* mosquito
La Crosse encephalitis	Bunyaviridae	Small mammals/*Aedes* mosquito
Yellow fever	Flaviviridae	Birds/*Aedes* mosquito
Dengue	Flaviviridae	Monkeys/*Aedes* mosquito
Colorado tick fever	Reoviridae	Tick
Lymphocytic choriomeningitis	Arenaviridae	Rodents
Lassa fever	Arenaviridae	Rodents
Sin Nombre hantavirus	Bunyaviridae	Deer mice
Ebola	Filoviridae	Unknown
Rabies	Rhabdoviridae	Bats, foxes, raccoons, etc.
Influenza A	Orthomyxoviridae	Birds, swine, etc.

encephalitis virus—will be spread from people in an urban setting. Arena-, hanta-, and rhabdoviruses are transmitted to humans in saliva, urine, or feces or through the bite of an infected animal (Table 38-3). Rabies vaccines are available for individuals whose jobs put them at risk or who are suspected to have been infected with rabies.

Syndromes of Possible Viral Etiology

Several diseases either produce symptoms or have epidemiologic or other characteristics that resemble those of viral infections or may be the sequelae of viral infections (e.g., inflammatory responses to a persistent viral infection). They include **multiple sclerosis, Kawasaki disease, arthritis, diabetes,** and **chronic fatigue syndrome.** Also, the strong cytokine response to many virus infections may trigger a loss of tolerance to self-antigens to initiate autoimmune diseases.

• Chronic and Potentially Oncogenic Infections

Chronic infections occur when the immune system has difficulty resolving the infection. The DNA viruses (except parvovirus and poxvirus) and the retroviruses cause latent infections with the potential for recurrence. CMV and other herpesviruses; hepatitis viruses B, C, G, and D; and retroviruses cause chronic productive infections. These "passengers" may influence the health of the individual in subtle ways.

HBV, HCV, EBV, HHV-8, HPV, and HTLV-1 are associated with **human cancers.** EBV, HPV, and HTLV-1 can immortalize cells; after immortalization, cofactors, chromosomal aberrations, or both enable a clone of virus-containing cells to grow into a cancer. EBV normally causes infectious mononucleosis but is also associated with African Burkitt lymphoma, Hodgkin lymphoma, lymphomas in immunosuppressed individuals, and nasopharyngeal carcinoma; HTLV-1 is associated with human adult T-cell leukemia. Many papillomaviruses induce a simple hyperplasia characterized by the development of a wart; however, several other strains of HPV have been associated with human cancers (e.g., types 16, 18, 33, 35, 58, and 68 are associated with cervical carcinoma). Direct viral action or the inflammation and chronic cell damage and repair in livers infected by HBV or HCV can result in a tumorigenic event leading to hepatocellular carcinoma. HSV-2 has been associated with human cervical carcinoma, most likely as a cofactor. Immunosuppression in patients who have AIDS, patients undergoing cancer chemotherapy, or transplant recipients also allows the production of lymphoma by EBV. HHV-8 infection produces many cytokines to stimulate cell growth, and this growth can progress to Kaposi sarcoma, especially in persons with AIDS.

Vaccines are now available for HBV and high-risk HPV strains. Development of a worldwide vaccine program for HBV not only would reduce the spread of viral hepatitis but also would prevent the occurrence of primary hepatocellular carcinoma. Similarly, the HPV vaccines should also reduce the incidence of cervical carcinoma.

• Infections in Immunocompromised Patients

Patients with **deficient cell-mediated immunity** are generally more susceptible to serious disease from enveloped viruses (especially the herpesviruses, measles virus, and even the vaccinia virus used for smallpox vaccinations) and to recurrences of infections with latent viruses (herpesviruses and papovaviruses). Severe T-cell deficiencies also affect the antiviral antibody response. Cell-mediated immunodeficiencies can be congenital or acquired. They may result from genetic defects (e.g., Duncan disease, DiGeorge syndrome, Wiskott-Aldrich syndrome), leukemia or lymphoma, infections (e.g., AIDS), or immunosuppressive therapy.

Viruses cause atypical and more severe presentations in immunosuppressed people. For example, infections with herpesviruses (e.g., HSV, CMV, VZV) or the vaccinia smallpox vaccine, which are normally benign and localized, can progress locally or may disseminate and cause visceral and neurologic infections that can be life threatening. A measles infection might cause a giant cell (syncytial) pneumonia rather than the characteristic rash.

People with immunoglobulin A deficiency or hypogammaglobulinemia (antibody deficiency) have more problems with respiratory and gastrointestinal viruses. Hypogammaglobulinemic people are more likely to suffer significant disease after infection by viruses that progress by viremia, which also include the live polio vaccine, echovirus, and VZV.

• Congenital, Neonatal, and Perinatal Infections

The development and growth of the fetus are so ordered and rapid that a viral infection can damage or prevent appropriate formation of important tissues, leading to miscarriage or congenital abnormalities. Infection can occur in utero (prenatal—e.g., rubella, parvovirus B19, CMV, HIV), during transit through the birth canal by contact with lesions or blood (neonatal—e.g., HSV, HBV, CMV, HPV), or soon after birth (postnatal—e.g., HIV, CMV, HBV, HSV, coxsackievirus B, echovirus).

Neonates depend on the mother's immunity to protect them from viral infections. They receive maternal antibodies through the placenta and then in the mother's milk. This type of passive immunity can remain effective for 6 months to a year after birth. Maternal antibodies can (1) protect against spread of virus to the fetus during a viremia (e.g., rubella, B19), (2) protect against many enteric and respiratory tract viral infections, and (3) reduce the severity of other viral diseases after birth. Nevertheless, because the cell-mediated immune system is not mature at birth, newborns are susceptible to viruses that spread by cell-to-cell contact (e.g., RSV, HSV, VZV, CMV, HIV).

Rubella virus and CMV are examples of **teratogenic viruses** that can cause congenital infection and severe congenital abnormalities. HIV infection acquired in utero or from mother's milk initiates a chronic infection, leading to lymphadenopathy, failure to thrive, or encephalopathy within 2 years of birth. HSV can be acquired during passage through an infected birth canal and can result in life-threatening disseminated disease. Nosocomial infection of newborns can result in a similar outcome. If parvovirus B19 is acquired in utero, it can cause spontaneous abortion.

Bibliography

Atkinson W, Wolfe S, Hamborsky J, editors: *Epidemiology and prevention of vaccine-preventable diseases*, ed 12, Washington, DC, 2011, Public Health Foundation.

Centers for Disease Control and Prevention: Guidelines for prevention of transmission of human immunodeficiency virus and hepatitis B virus to health-care and public-safety workers, *MMWR Morb Mortal Wkly Rep* 38(Suppl 6):1–37, 1989.

Cohen J, Powderly WG: *Infectious diseases*, ed 2, St Louis, 2004, Mosby.

Ellner Emond RTD, Rowland HAK, Welsby P: *Colour atlas of infectious diseases*, ed 4, London, 2003, Mosby.

Gershon AA, Hotez PJ, Katz SL: *Krugman's infectious diseases of children*, ed 11, St Louis, 2004, Mosby.

Goering R, Dockrell H, Zuckerman M, et al: *Mim's medical microbiology*, ed 4, Edinburgh, 2008, Mosby.

Gorbach SL, Bartlett JG, Blacklow NR: *Infectious diseases*, ed 3, Philadelphia, 2004, WB Saunders.

Hart CA, Broadhead RL: *Color atlas of pediatric infectious diseases*, St Louis, 1992, Mosby.

Haukenes G, Haaheim LR, Pattison JR: *A practical guide to clinical virology*, New York, 1989, Wiley.

Knipe DM, Howley PM, Griffin DE, et al: *Fields virology*, ed 5, Philadelphia, 2006, Lippincott Williams & Wilkins.

Logan SAE, MacMahon E: Viral meningitis, *BMJ* 336:36–40, 2008.

Mandell GL, Bennet JE, Dolin R: *Principles and practice of infectious diseases*, ed 6, Philadelphia, 2005, Churchill Livingstone.

Outhred AC, Kok J, Dwyer DE: Viral arthritides, *Expert Rev Antiinfect Ther* 9:545–554, 2011.

Strauss JM, Strauss EG: *Viruses and human disease*, ed 2, San Diego, 2007, Academic.

White DO, Fenner FJ: *Medical virology*, ed 4, Orlando, Fla, 1994, Academic.

Websites

All the virology on the WWW. www.virology.net/garryfavweb.html. Accessed August 7, 2015.

The big picture book of viruses. www.virology.net/Big_Virology/BVHomePage.html. Accessed August 7, 2015.

Centers for Disease Control and Prevention: CDC A-Z index. www.cdc.gov/health/diseases.htm. Accessed August 7, 2015.

Centers for Disease Control and Prevention: Traveler's health. www.cdc.gov/travel/diseases.htm. Accessed August 7, 2015.

National Center for Infectious Diseases: Infectious disease information A-Z index. www.cdc.gov/ncidod/diseases/index.htm. Accessed August 7, 2015.

National Foundation for Infectious Diseases: Fact sheets on diseases. www.nfid.org/factsheets/Default.html. Accessed August 7, 2015.

Stannard L: Virus ultra structure. www.uct.ac.za/depts/mmi/stannard/linda.html. Accessed May 14, 2012.

World Health Organization: Immunization service delivery. www.who.int/immunization_delivery/en/. Accessed August 7, 2015.

World Health Organization: Infectious diseases. www.who.int/topics/infectious_diseases/en/. Accessed August 7, 2015.

CHAPTER

39 LABORATORY DIAGNOSIS OF VIRAL DISEASES

There have been many new developments in laboratory viral diagnosis that provide more rapid and sensitive viral identification from clinical samples. These include better antibody reagents and more sensitive assays for direct analysis of samples, molecular genetics techniques and genomic sequencing for direct identification of the virus, and assays that can identify multiple viruses (multiplex) and be automated. Often, isolation of the organism is unnecessary and avoided to minimize the risk to laboratory and other personnel. The quicker turnaround allows a more rapid choice of the appropriate antiviral therapy.

Viral laboratory studies are performed to (1) confirm the diagnosis by identifying the viral agent of infection, (2) determine appropriate antimicrobial therapy, (3) check on the compliance of the patient taking antiviral drugs, (4) define the course of the disease, (5) monitor the disease epidemiologically, and (6) educate physicians and patients.

The laboratory methods accomplish the following results:

1. Description of virus-induced **cytopathologic effects (CPEs)** on cells
2. Detection of viral particles
3. Isolation and growth of the virus
4. Detection and analysis of viral components (e.g., proteins [antigens], enzymes, genomes)
5. Evaluation of the patient's immune response to the virus **(serology)**

The molecular and immunologic techniques used for many of these procedures are described in Chapters 5 and 6. Viruses, viral antigens, viral genomes, and CPEs can be detected by means of direct analysis of clinical specimens and, for some viruses, after growth of the virus on tissue culture cells in the laboratory (Box 39-1).

• Specimen Collection

The patient's symptoms and history, including recent travel, the season of the year, and a presumptive diagnosis, help determine the appropriate procedures to be used to identify a viral agent (Table 39-1). Selection of the appropriate specimen for analysis is often complicated because several viruses may cause the same clinical disease. For example, the development of meningitis symptoms during the summer suggests an arbovirus, in which case cerebrospinal fluid (CSF) and blood should be collected, or an enterovirus, in which case CSF, a throat swab, and stool specimens should be collected for genome analysis and possible virus isolation. A focal encephalitis with a temporal lobe localization preceded by headaches and disorientation suggests herpes simplex virus (HSV) infection, for which CSF can be relatively quickly analyzed for viral deoxyribonucleic acid (DNA) sequences by polymerase chain reaction (PCR) amplification.

Specimens should be collected early in the acute phase of infection, before the virus ceases to be shed. For example, respiratory viruses may be shed for only 3 to 7 days, and shedding may lapse before the symptoms cease. HSV and varicella-zoster virus (VZV) may not be recoverable from lesions more than 5 days after the onset of symptoms. It may be possible to isolate an enterovirus from the CSF for only 2 to 3 days after the onset of the central nervous system manifestations. In addition, antibody produced in response to the infection may block the detection of virus.

The shorter the interval between the collection of a specimen and its delivery to the laboratory, the greater the potential for isolating a virus. The reasons are that many viruses are labile, and the samples are susceptible to bacterial and fungal overgrowth. Viruses are best transported and stored on ice and in special media that contain antibiotics and proteins, such as serum albumin or gelatin. Significant losses in infectious titers occur when enveloped viruses (e.g., HSV, VZV, influenza virus) are kept at room temperature or frozen at −20° C. This is not a risk for nonenveloped viruses (e.g., adenoviruses, enteroviruses).

• Cytology

Many viruses produce a characteristic CPE. Characteristic CPEs in the tissue sample or in cell culture include changes in cell morphology, cell lysis, vacuolation, syncytia (Figure 39-1), and inclusion bodies. **Syncytia** are multinucleated giant cells formed by viral fusion of individual cells. *Paramyxoviruses, HSV, VZV, and human immunodeficiency virus (HIV) promote syncytia formation.* **Inclusion bodies** are either histologic changes in the cells caused by viral components or virus-induced changes in cell structures. For example, intranuclear basophilic (owl's-eye) inclusion bodies found in large cells of tissues with cytomegalovirus (CMV) (see Chapter 43, Figure 43-17) or in the sediment of urine from patients with the infection are readily identifiable. Cowdry type A nuclear inclusions in single cells or in large syncytia (multiple cells fused together) are a characteristic finding in cells infected with HSV or VZV (Figure 39-2). Rabies may be detected through the finding of cytoplasmic Negri bodies (rabies virus inclusions) in brain tissue (Figure 39-3).

Box 39-1 Laboratory Procedures for Diagnosing Viral Infections

Cytologic examination
Electron microscopy
Virus isolation and growth
Detection of viral proteins (antigens and enzymes)
Detection of viral genomes
Serology

Table 39-1 Specimens for Viral Diagnosis

Common Pathogenic Viruses	Specimens for Culture	Procedures and Comments
Respiratory Tract		
Influenza virus, paramyxoviruses, coronavirus, rhinovirus, enterovirus (picornavirus)	Nasal washing, throat swab, nasal swab, sputum	RT-PCR, ELISA, multiplex assays detect several agents; cell culture
Gastrointestinal Tract		
Reovirus, rotavirus, adenovirus, Norwalk virus, other calicivirus	Stool, rectal swab	RT-PCR, ELISA; viruses are not cultured
Maculopapular Rash		
Adenovirus, enterovirus (picornavirus)	Throat swab, rectal swab	PCR, RT-PCR
Rubella virus, measles virus	Urine	RT-PCR, ELISA
Vesicular Rash		
Coxsackievirus, echovirus, HSV, VZV	Vesicle fluid, scraping, or swab, enterovirus in stool	HSV and VZV: vesicle scraping (Tzanck smear), cell culture, PCR, IF
Central Nervous System (Aseptic Meningitis, Encephalitis)		
Enterovirus (picornavirus)	Stool, CSF	RT-PCR
Arboviruses (e.g., togaviruses, bunyavirus)	Blood, CSF; rarely cultured	RT-PCR, serology; multiplex assays detect several agents
Rabies virus	Tissue, saliva, brain biopsy, CSF	IF of biopsy, RT-PCR
HSV, CMV, mumps virus, measles virus	CSF	PCR or RT-PCR, virus isolation, and antigen are assayed
Urinary Tract		
Adenovirus, CMV	Urine	PCR; CMV may be shed without apparent disease
Blood		
HIV, human T-cell leukemia virus, hepatitis B, C, and D viruses, EBV, CMV, HHV-6	Blood	ELISA for antigen or antibody, PCR, RT-PCR, multiplex assays

CMV, Cytomegalovirus; *CSF,* cerebrospinal fluid; *EBV,* Epstein-Barr virus; *ELISA,* enzyme-linked immunosorbent assay; *HHV-6,* human herpes virus 6; *HIV,* human immunodeficiency virus; *HSV,* herpes simplex virus; *IF,* immunofluorescence; *PCR,* polymerase chain reaction; *RT-PCR,* reverse transcriptase polymerase chain reaction; *VZV,* varicella-zoster virus.

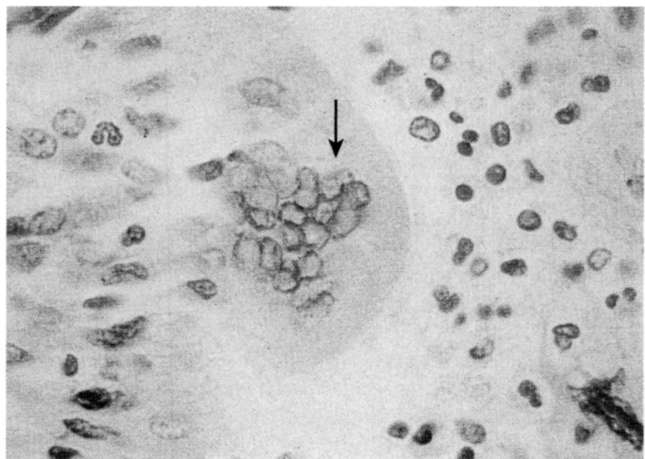

FIGURE 39-1 Syncytium formation by measles virus. Multinucleated giant cell *(arrow)* visible in a histologic section of lung biopsy tissue from a measles virus–induced giant cell pneumonia in an immunocompromised child. (From Hart C, Broadhead RL: *A color atlas of pediatric infectious diseases,* London, 1992, Wolfe.)

Often the cytologic specimens will be examined for the presence of specific viral antigens by immunofluorescence or viral genomes by in situ hybridization or PCR for a rapid, definitive identification. These tests are specific for individual viruses and must be chosen based on the differential diagnosis. These methods are discussed later.

• Electron Microscopy

Electron microscopy is not a standard clinical laboratory technique, but it can be used to detect and identify some viruses if sufficient viral particles are present. The addition of virus-specific antibody to a sample can cause viral particles to clump, thereby facilitating the detection and simultaneous identification of the virus (immunoelectron microscopy). Enteric viruses (e.g., rotavirus) that are produced in abundance and have a characteristic morphology can be detected in stool by these methods. Appropriately processed tissue from a biopsy or clinical specimen can also be examined for the presence of viral structures.

• Viral Isolation and Growth

Isolation of the virus allows subsequent analysis and archiving of samples but may put individuals at risk to infection. A virus can be grown in tissue culture, embryonated eggs, and experimental animals (Box 39-2). Although embryonated eggs are still used for the growth of virus for some vaccines (e.g., influenza), they have been replaced by cell cultures for routine virus isolation in clinical laboratories. Experimental animals are rarely used in clinical laboratories for the purpose of isolating viruses.

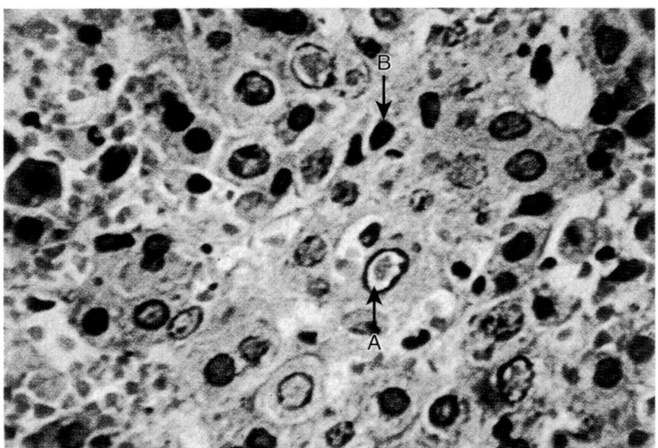

FIGURE 39-2 Herpes simplex virus (HSV)-induced cytopathologic effect. A biopsy specimen of an HSV-infected liver shows an eosinophilic Cowdry type A intranuclear inclusion body *(A)* surrounded by a halo and a ring of marginated chromatin at the nuclear membrane. An infected cell *(B)* exhibits a smaller condensed nucleus (pyknotic). (Courtesy Dr. JI Pugh, St Albans City Hospital, Hertfordshire, England; from Emond RT, Rowland HAK: *A color atlas of infectious diseases,* ed 3, London, 1995, Mosby.)

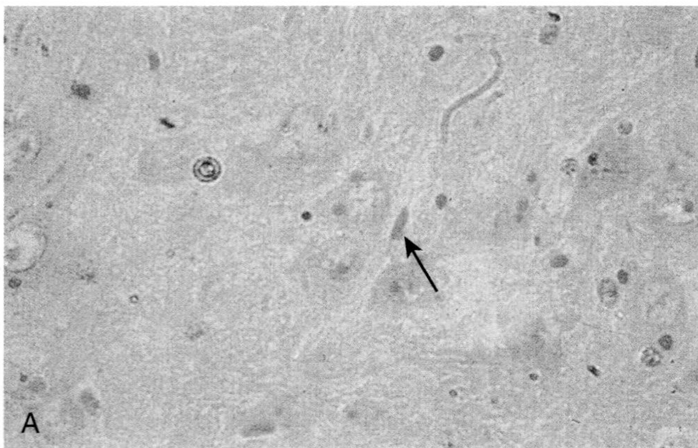

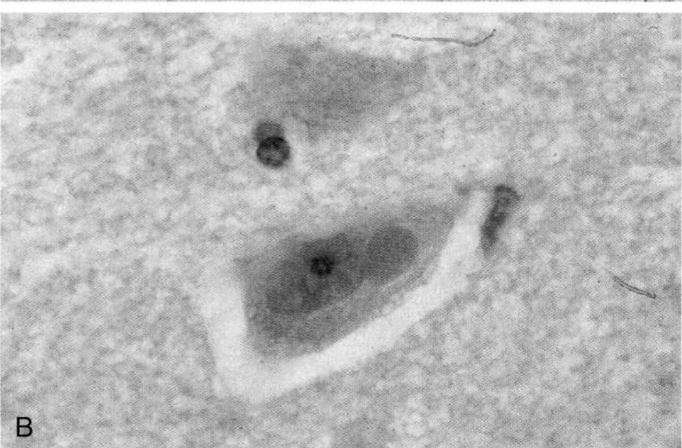

FIGURE 39-3 Negri bodies caused by rabies. **A,** A section of brain from a patient with rabies shows Negri bodies *(arrow).* **B,** Higher magnification from another biopsy specimen. (**A,** From Hart C, Broadhead RL: *A color atlas of pediatric infectious diseases,* London, 1992, Wolfe.)

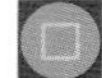

Box 39-2 Systems for Propagation of Viruses

- People
- Animals: cows (e.g., Jenner cowpox vaccine), chickens, mice, rats, suckling mice
- Embryonated eggs
- Organ culture
- Tissue culture
  - Primary
  - Diploid cell line
  - Tumor or immortalized cell line

Cell Culture

Specific types of tissue culture cells are used to grow viruses. **Primary cell cultures** are obtained by dissociating specific animal organs with trypsin or collagenase. The cells obtained by this method are then grown as monolayers (fibroblast or epithelial) or in suspension (lymphocyte) in artificial media supplemented with bovine serum or another source of growth factors. Primary cells can be dissociated with trypsin, diluted, and allowed to grow into new monolayers *(passed)* to become secondary cell cultures. **Diploid cell lines** are cultures of a single cell type that are capable of being passed a large but finite number of times before they senesce or undergo a significant change in their characteristics. **Tumor cell lines** and **immortalized cell lines,** usually initiated from human or animal tumors or by treatment of primary cells with oncogenic viruses or chemicals, consist of single cell types that can be passed continuously without senescing.

Primary monkey kidney cells are excellent for the recovery of influenza viruses, paramyxoviruses, many enteroviruses, and some adenoviruses. Human fetal diploid cells, which are generally fibroblastic cells, support the growth of a broad spectrum of viruses (e.g., HSV, VZV, CMV, adenoviruses, picornaviruses). HeLa cells, a continuous line of epithelial cells derived from a human cancer, are excellent for the recovery of respiratory syncytial virus, adenoviruses, and HSV. Many clinically significant viruses can be recovered in at least one of these cell cultures.

Viral Detection

A virus can be detected and initially identified through observation of the virus-induced CPE in the cell monolayer (Figure 39-4; Box 39-3), by immunofluorescence, or by genome analysis of the infected cell culture. For example, a single virus infects, spreads, and kills surrounding cells **(plaque).** The type of cell culture, characteristics of the CPE, and rapidity of viral growth can be used to initially identify many clinically important viruses. This approach to identifying viruses is similar to that used in the identification of bacteria, which is based on the growth and morphology of colonies on selective differential media.

Some viruses grow slowly or not at all or do not readily cause a CPE in cell lines typically used in clinical virology laboratories. Some cause diseases that are hazardous to personnel. These viruses are most frequently diagnosed on the basis of serologic findings or through detection of viral genomes or proteins.

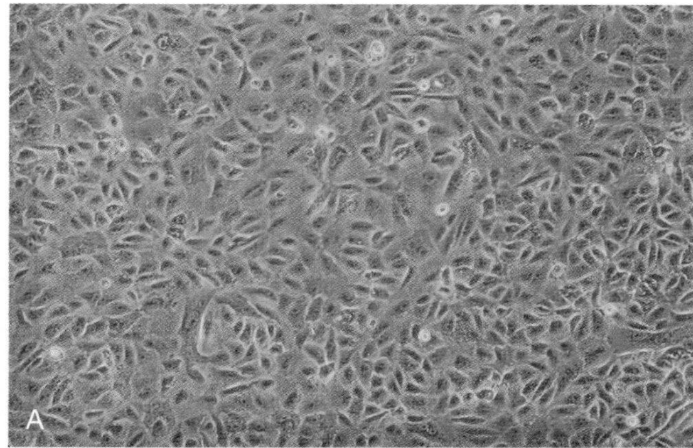

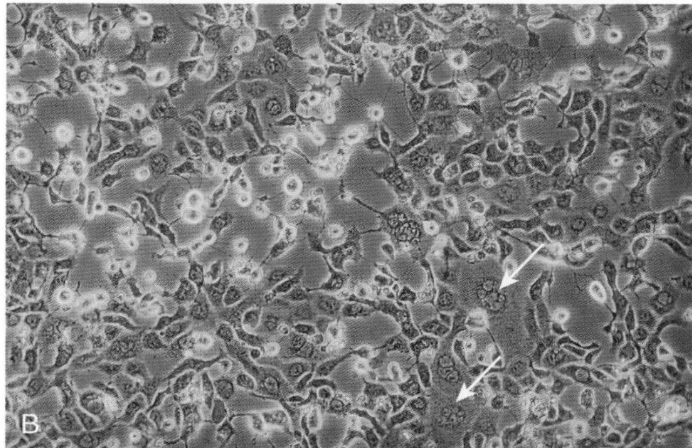

FIGURE 39-4 Cytopathologic effect of herpes simplex virus (HSV) infection. **A,** Uninfected Vero cells, an African green monkey kidney cell line. **B,** HSV-1–infected Vero cells showing rounded cells, multinucleated cells, and loss of the monolayer. *Arrows* point to syncytia.

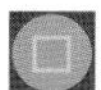

Box 39-3 Viral Cytopathologic Effects*

- Cell death
  - Cell rounding
  - Degeneration
  - Aggregation
  - Loss of attachments to culture dish
- Characteristic histologic changes: inclusion bodies in the nucleus or cytoplasm, margination of chromatin
- Syncytia: multinucleated giant cells caused by virus-induced cell-to-cell fusion
- Cell surface changes
  - Viral antigen expression
  - Hemadsorption (hemagglutinin expression)

*The effects may be characteristics of specific viruses.

Characteristic viral properties can also be used to identify viruses that do not have a classic CPE. For example, the rubella virus may not cause a CPE, but it does prevent (interfere with) the replication of picornaviruses in a process known as **heterologous interference,** which can be used to detect the rubella virus. Cells infected with the influenza virus, parainfluenza virus, mumps virus, and togavirus express a viral glycoprotein (hemagglutinin) that binds erythrocytes of defined animal species to the infected cell surface **(hemadsorption)** (Figure 39-5). When released into the cell culture medium, such viruses can be detected from the agglutination of erythrocytes, a process termed **hemagglutination.** The virus can then be identified from the specific antibody that blocks the hemagglutination, a process called **hemagglutination inhibition (HI).** An innovative approach to detection of HSV infection uses genetically modified tissue culture cells that express the β-galactosidase gene and can be stained blue when infected with HSV (enzyme-linked virus-inducible system [ELVIS]).

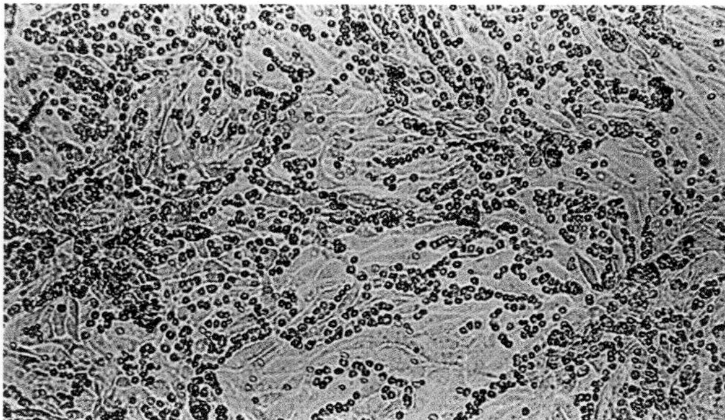

FIGURE 39-5 Hemadsorption of erythrocytes to cells infected with influenza viruses, mumps virus, parainfluenza viruses, or togaviruses. These viruses express a hemagglutinin on their surfaces, which binds to erythrocytes of selected animal species.

One can quantitate a virus by determining the greatest dilution that retains the following properties **(titer):**

1. **Tissue culture dose (TCD_{50}):** titer of virus that causes cytopathologic effects in half the tissue culture cells
2. **Lethal dose (LD_{50}):** titer of virus that kills 50% of a set of test animals
3. **Infectious dose (ID_{50}):** titer of virus that initiates a detectable symptom, antibody, or other response in 50% of a set of test animals

The number of infectious viruses can also be evaluated with a count of the plaques produced by 10-fold dilutions of sample **(plaque-forming units).** The ratio of viral particles (from electron microscopy) to plaque-forming units is always much greater than 1 because numerous defective viral particles are produced during viral replication.

Interpretation of Culture Results

In general, the detection of any virus in host tissues, CSF, blood, or vesicular fluid can be considered a highly significant finding. However, viral shedding may occur and be unrelated to the disease symptoms. Certain viruses can be intermittently shed without causing symptoms in the affected person for periods ranging from weeks (enteroviruses in feces) to many months or years (HSV or CMV in the oropharynx and vagina; adenoviruses in the oropharynx and intestinal tract). Similarly, a negative result cannot be conclusive, because the sample may have been improperly handled, contain neutralizing antibody, or be acquired before or after viral shedding.

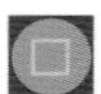 **Box 39-4 Assays for Viral Proteins and Nucleic Acids**

Proteins

Protein patterns (electrophoresis)
Enzyme activities (e.g., reverse transcriptase)
Hemagglutination and hemadsorption
Antigen detection (e.g., direct and indirect immunofluorescence, enzyme-linked immunosorbent assay, Western blot)

Nucleic Acids

Restriction endonuclease cleavage patterns
Size of RNA for segmented RNA viruses (electrophoresis)
DNA genome hybridization in situ (cytochemistry)
Southern, Northern, and dot blots
PCR (DNA)
Reverse transcriptase PCR (RNA)
Real-time quantitative PCR
Branched-chain DNA and related tests (DNA, RNA)
Genome sequencing

DNA, Deoxyribonucleic acid; *PCR,* polymerase chain reaction; *RNA,* ribonucleic acid.

• Detection of Viral Proteins

Enzymes and other proteins are produced during viral replication and can be detected by biochemical, immunologic, and molecular biological means (Box 39-4). The viral proteins can be separated by electrophoresis and their patterns used to identify and distinguish different viruses. For example, the electrophoretically separated HSV-infected cell proteins and virion proteins exhibit different patterns for different types and strains of HSV-1 and HSV-2.

The detection and assay of characteristic enzymes or activities can identify and quantitate specific viruses. For example, the presence of reverse transcriptase in serum or cell culture indicates the presence of a retrovirus or hepadnavirus. Antibodies can be used as sensitive and specific tools to detect, identify, and quantitate the virus and viral antigen in clinical specimens or cell cultures (immunohistochemistry). Specifically, monoclonal or monospecific antibodies are useful for distinguishing viruses. Viral antigens on the cell surface or within the cell can be detected by **immunofluorescence** and **enzyme immunoassay (EIA)** (see Chapter 6, Figures 6-2 and 6-3). Virus or antigen released from infected cells can be detected by **enzyme-linked immunosorbent assay (ELISA), radioimmunoassay (RIA),** and **latex agglutination (LA)** (see Chapter 6 for definitions). Test kits for single and multiple (multiplex) viral agents are commercially available. Multiplex kits for respiratory viruses can help determine whether antiviral therapy is available. Rapid ELISA-like detection kits, similar to pregnancy tests, are available for influenza and HIV.

The detection of CMV and other viruses can be enhanced through the use of a combination of cell culture and immunologic means. In this method, the clinical sample is centrifuged onto cells grown on a coverslip on the bottom of a **shell vial** (glass tube). This step increases the efficiency and accelerates the progression of infection of the cells on the coverslip. The cells can then be analyzed with immunofluorescence **(direct fluorescence)** or EIA for early viral antigens, which are detectable within 24 hours instead of the 7 to 14 days it takes for a CPE to become evident.

• Detection of Viral Genetic Material

The genetic sequence of a virus is a major distinguishing characteristic of the family, type, and strain of virus (see Box 39-4). The electrophoretic patterns of ribonucleic acid (RNA) (influenza, reovirus) or restriction endonuclease fragment lengths from DNA viral genomes are like genetic fingerprints for these viruses. Different strains of HSV-1 and HSV-2 can be distinguished in this way by **restriction fragment length polymorphism**. Newer methods for viral genome detection use sequence-specific genetic probes and PCR-like DNA and RNA amplification approaches that allow more rapid analysis and quantitation with a minimum of risk from infectious virus. Methods for sequencing genomes or portions of viruses have become rapid and inexpensive enough to become a routine viral identification method.

DNA probes, with sequences complementary to specific regions of a viral genome, can be used like antibodies as sensitive and specific tools for detecting a virus. These probes can detect the virus even in the absence of viral replication. DNA probe analysis is especially useful for detecting slowly replicating or nonproductive viruses, such as CMV and human papillomavirus, or when the viral antigen cannot be detected using immunologic tests (see Chapter 5, Figure 5-3). Specific viral genetic sequences in fixed, permeabilized tissue biopsy specimens can be detected by **in situ hybridization** (e.g., **fluorescence in situ hybridization [FISH]**).

Viral genomes can also be detected in clinical samples with the use of **dot blot** or **Southern blot analysis.** For the latter method, the viral genome or electrophoretically separated restriction endonuclease cleavage fragments of the genome are blotted onto nitrocellulose filters and then detected on the filter by their hybridization to DNA probes. Electrophoretically separated viral RNA (**Northern blot**–RNA:DNA probe hybridization) blotted onto a nitrocellulose filter can be detected in a similar manner. The DNA probes are detected with autoradiography or with fluorescent or EIA-like methods. Many viral probes and kits for detecting viruses are now commercially available.

For many laboratories, the method of choice for detection, quantification, and identification of viruses uses genome amplification techniques, including **PCR** for DNA genomes **and reverse transcriptase PCR (RT-PCR)** for RNA genomes. Use of the appropriate primers for PCR can promote a millionfold amplification of a target sequence in a few hours. This technique is especially useful for detecting latent and integrated sequences of viruses, such as retroviruses, herpesviruses, papillomaviruses, and other papovaviruses, as well as evidence of viruses present in low concentrations and viruses that are difficult or too dangerous to isolate in cell culture. RT-PCR uses the retroviral reverse transcriptase to convert viral RNA to DNA and allow PCR amplification of the viral nucleic acid sequences. RT-PCR was very useful for identifying and distinguishing the hantaviruses that caused the outbreak in New Mexico in 1993. These techniques are readily automated to analyze multiple samples and for different viruses (multiplex) and combined with rapid techniques for detection and sequencing the DNA products of the PCR. Analysis of the amplified viral nucleic acids is also being performed using matrix-assisted laser desorption ionization time-of-flight mass spectrometry (MALDI-TOF MS).

Real-time PCR is a rapid means of quantifying the amount of genomes within a patient (virus load). The concentration of the viral genome (RNA genomes would be converted to DNA) is proportional to the initial rate of the PCR amplification of the genomic DNA. This test is especially important for following the course of HIV infection.

PCR is the prototype for several other HIV genome amplification techniques. **Transcription-based amplification** uses reverse transcriptase and viral sequence–specific primers to make a complementary DNA (cDNA) and attaches a sequence recognized by the DNA-dependent RNA polymerase from the T7 bacteriophage. The DNA is transcribed to RNA by the T7 RNA polymerase, and the new RNA sequences are then cycled back into the reaction to amplify the relevant sequence. Unlike PCR, these reactions do not require special equipment.

Some other genome amplification and detection approaches are similar in concept to ELISA. These approaches use immobilized DNA sequences complementary to the relevant viral genomic sequence to capture the viral genome. This is followed by the binding of another complementary sequence that contains a detection system. The genome probe sequence may be attached to an extensively **branched chain of DNA** in which each of the branches elicits a reaction that amplifies the signal to detectable levels. Another variation of the theme uses an antibody that recognizes DNA-RNA complexes to capture viral DNA-RNA probe hybrids in the well of a plate, followed by an enzyme-labeled antibody and ELISA methods to detect the presence of the genome. Like ELISA, these methods can be automated and set up to analyze a panel of viruses.

• Viral Serology

The humoral immune response provides a history of a patient's infections. Serologic studies are used for the identification of viruses that are difficult to isolate and grow in cell culture, as well as viruses that cause diseases of long duration (e.g., EBV, HBV, HIV) (see Box 6-2). Serology can be used to identify the virus and its strain or serotype, whether it is an acute or chronic disease, and determine whether it is a primary infection or a reinfection. The detection of **virus-specific immunoglobulin (Ig)M antibody,** which is present during the first 2 or 3 weeks of a primary infection, generally indicates a recent primary infection. **Seroconversion** is indicated by at least **a fourfold increase in the antibody titer** between the serum obtained during the acute phase of disease and that obtained at least 2 to 3 weeks later during the convalescent phase. Reinfection or recurrence later in life causes an anamnestic (secondary or booster) response. Antibody titers may remain high in patients who suffer frequent recurrence of a disease (e.g., herpesviruses).

Because of the inherent imprecision of serologic assays based on twofold serial dilutions, a fourfold increase in the antibody titer between acute and convalescent sera is required to indicate seroconversion. For example, samples with 512 and 1023 units of antibody would both give a signal on a 512-fold dilution but not on a 1024-fold dilution, and the titers of both would be reported as 512. On the other hand, samples with 1020 and 1030 units are not significantly different but would be reported as titers of 512 and 1024, respectively.

The presence of antibodies to several key viral antigens and their titers can be used to identify the stage of disease caused by certain viruses. This approach is especially useful for the diagnosis of viral diseases with slow courses (e.g., hepatitis B, infectious mononucleosis caused by Epstein-Barr virus [EBV]) (see Chapters 43 and 55). In general, the first antibodies to be detected are directed against the antigens most available to the immune system (e.g., expressed on the virion or infected-cell surfaces). Later in the infection, when the infecting virus or the cellular immune response has lysed the cells, antibodies directed against the intracellular viral proteins and enzymes are detected. For example, antibodies to the envelope and capsid antigens of EBV are detected first. Then during convalescence, antibodies to nuclear antigens, such as the EBV nuclear antigen, are detected.

A **serologic battery or panel** consisting of assays for several viruses may be used for the diagnosis of certain diseases. Local epidemiologic factors, time of year, and patient factors such as immunocompetence, travel history, and age influence the choice of virus assays to be included in a panel. For example, HSV and the viruses of mumps, western and eastern equine encephalitides, and St. Louis, West Nile, and California encephalitides might be included in a panel of tests for central nervous system diseases.

Serologic Test Methods

The serologic tests used in virology are listed in Chapter 6, Box 6-1. **Neutralization** and **HI tests** assay antibody on the basis of its recognition of and binding to virus. The antibody coating of the virus blocks its binding to indicator cells (Figure 39-6). Antibody neutralization of virus inhibits infection and subsequent cytopathologic effects in tissue culture cells. For HI, antibody in serum prevents a standardized amount of virus from binding to and agglutinating erythrocytes.

The indirect fluorescent antibody test and solid-phase immunoassays, such as latex agglutination and **ELISA,** are commonly used to detect and quantitate viral antigen and antiviral antibody. The ELISA test is used to screen the blood supply to exclude individuals who are seropositive for hepatitis B and C viruses and HIV. **Western blot** analysis has become very important to confirm seroconversion and hence infection with HIV. The ability of the patient's antibody to recognize specific viral proteins separated by electrophoresis, transferred (blotted) onto a filter paper (e.g., nitrocellulose, nylon), and visualized with an enzyme-conjugated antihuman antibody confirms the ELISA-indicated diagnosis of HIV infection (Figure 39-7).

Limitations of Serologic Methods

The presence of an antiviral antibody indicates previous infection but is not sufficient to indicate when the infection occurred. The finding of virus-specific IgM, a fourfold increase in the antibody titer between acute and convalescent sera, or specific antibody profiles is indicative of recent infection. False-positive or false-negative test results may confuse the diagnosis. In addition, patient antibody may be bound with viral antigen (as occurs in patients with hepatitis B) in immune complexes, thereby preventing antibody

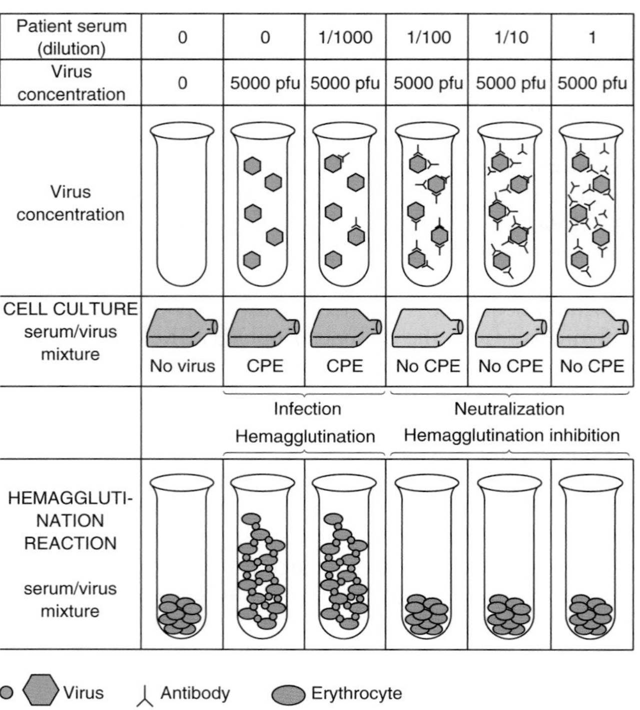

FIGURE 39-6 Neutralization, hemagglutination, and hemagglutination inhibition assays. In the assay shown, 10-fold dilutions of serum were incubated with virus. Aliquots of the mixture were then added to cell cultures or erythrocytes. In the absence of antibody, the virus infected the monolayer (indicated by cytopathologic effect *[CPE]*) or caused hemagglutination (i.e., formed a gel-like suspension of erythrocytes). In the presence of the antibody, infection was blocked, preventing CPE (neutralization), or hemagglutination was inhibited, allowing the erythrocytes to pellet. The titer of antibody of this serum would be 100. *pfu,* Plaque-forming units.

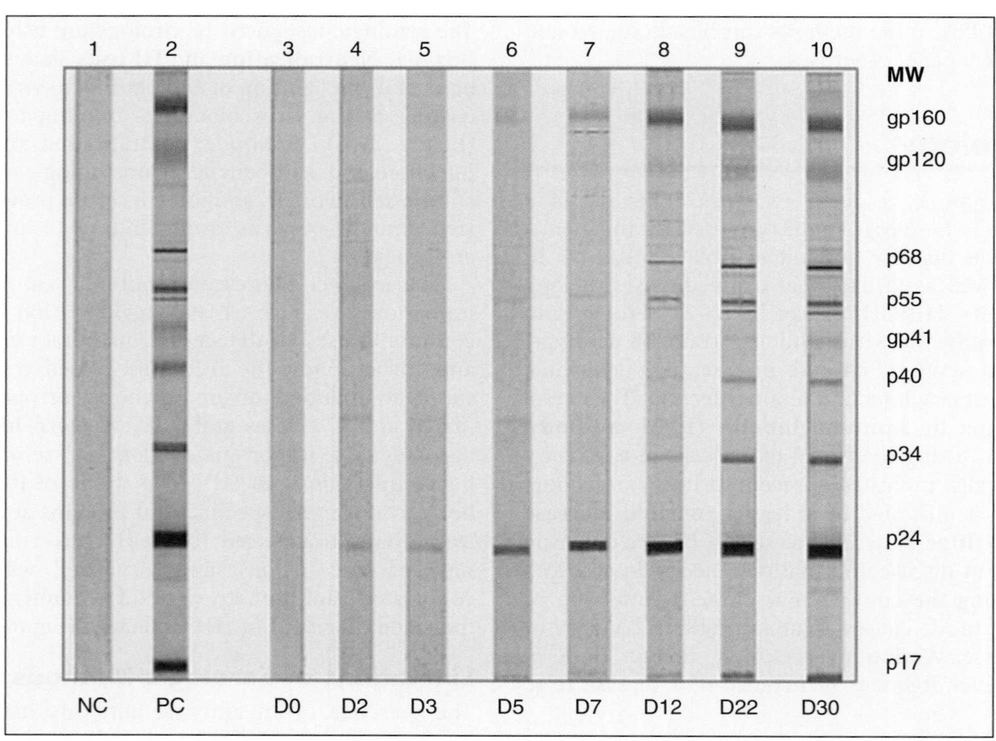

FIGURE 39-7 Western blot analysis of human immunodeficiency virus (HIV) antigens and antibody. HIV protein antigens are separated by electrophoresis and blotted onto nitrocellulose paper strips. Each strip is incubated with patient antibody, washed to remove the unbound antibody, and then reacted with enzyme-conjugated antihuman antibody and chromophoric substrate. Serum from an HIV-infected person binds and identifies the major antigenic proteins of HIV. These data demonstrate the seroconversion of one HIV-infected individual with sera collected on day 0 *(D0)* to day 30 *(D30)* compared to a known positive control *(PC)* and negative control *(NC)*. *MW,* molecular weight. (From Kuritzkes DR: Diagnostic tests for HIV infection and resistance assays. In Cohen J, Powderly WG: *Infectious diseases,* ed 2, St Louis, 2004, Mosby.)

detection. Serologic cross-reactions between different viruses may also confuse the identity of the infecting agent (e.g., parainfluenza and mumps express related antigens). Conversely, the antibody used in the assay may be too specific (many monoclonal antibodies) and may not recognize strains of virus from the same family, giving a false-negative result (e.g., rhinovirus). A good understanding of the clinical symptoms and knowledge of the limitations and potential problems with serologic assays aid the diagnosis.

Bibliography

Caliendo AM: Multiplex PCR and emerging technologies for the detection of respiratory pathogens, *Clin Infect Dis* 52(Suppl 4):S326–S330, 2011.

Carter J, Saunders V: *Virology: principles and applications*, Chichester, England, 2007, Wiley.

Cohen J, Powderly WG: *Infectious diseases*, ed 2, St Louis, 2004, Mosby.

Collier L, Oxford J: *Human virology*, ed 3, Oxford, England, 2006, Oxford University Press.

Forbes BA, Sahm DF, Weissfeld AS: *Bailey and Scott's diagnostic microbiology*, ed 12, St Louis, 2007, Mosby.

Hsiung GD: *Diagnostic virology*, ed 3, New Haven, Conn, 1982, Yale University Press.

Knipe DM, Howley PM, Griffin DE, et al: *Fields virology*, ed 5, Philadelphia, 2006, Lippincott Williams & Wilkins.

Leland DS, Ginocchio CC: Role of cell culture for virus detection in the age of technology, *Clin Microbiol Rev* 20:49–78, 2007.

Lennette EH: *Laboratory diagnosis of viral infections*, ed 3, New York, 1999, Marcel Dekker.

Menegus MA: Diagnostic virology. In Belshe RB, editor: *Textbook of human virology*, ed 2, St Louis, 1991, Mosby.

Murray PR: *Pocket guide to clinical microbiology*, ed 3, Washington, DC, 2004, American Society for Microbiology Press.

Persing DH, Tenover FC, Tang Y-W, et al: *Molecular microbiology: diagnostic principles and practice*, ed 2, Washington, DC, 2011, American Society for Microbiology Press.

Richman DD, Whitley RJ, Hayden FG: *Clinical virology*, ed 3, Washington, DC, 2009, American Society for Microbiology Press.

Specter S, Hodinka RL, Wiedbrauk DL, et al: *Clinical virology manual*, ed 4, Washington, DC, 2009, American Society for Microbiology Press.

Strauss JM, Strauss EG: *Viruses and human disease*, ed 2, San Diego, 2007, Academic.

Versalovic J: *Manual of clinical microbiology*, ed 10, Washington, DC, 2011, American Society for Microbiology Press.

Voyles BA: *The biology of viruses*, ed 2, Boston, 2002, McGraw-Hill.

Websites

Leland DS, Ginocchio CC: Role of cell culture for virus detection in the age of technology. www.ncbi.nlm.nih.gov/pmc/articles/PMC1797634/. Accessed April 16, 2015.

Stannard L: Viruses in cell culture. http://virology-online.com/general/Tests.htm. Accessed May 28, 2015.

CHAPTER

40 ANTIVIRAL AGENTS AND INFECTION CONTROL

Unlike bacteria, viruses are obligate intracellular parasites that use the host cell's biosynthetic machinery and enzymes for replication (see Chapter 36). Hence it is more difficult to inhibit viral replication without also being toxic to the host. Most antiviral drugs are targeted toward viral-encoded enzymes or structures of the virus that are important for replication. Most of these compounds are classic biochemical inhibitors of viral-encoded enzymes. Some antiviral drugs are actually stimulators of host innate immune protective responses.

Antiviral drugs are available for viruses that cause significant morbidity and mortality and also provide reasonable targets for drug action (Box 40-1), but unlike antibacterial drugs, the activity of most antiviral drugs is limited to a specific virus. Many antiviral drugs cause serious side effects owing to their toxicity. As has occurred with antibacterial drugs, resistance to antiviral drugs is becoming more of a problem because of the high rate of mutation for viruses and the long-term treatment of some patients, especially those who are immunocompromised (e.g., patients with acquired immunodeficiency syndrome [AIDS]).

• Targets for Antiviral Drugs

The different targets for antiviral drugs (e.g., structures, enzymes, or processes important or essential for virus production) are discussed with respect to the steps of the viral replication cycle they inhibit. These targets and their respective antiviral agents are listed in Table 40-1 (see also Chapter 36, Figure 36-8).

Virion Disruption

Enveloped viruses are susceptible to certain lipid and detergent-like molecules that disperse or disrupt the envelope membrane, thereby preventing acquisition of the virus. Rhinoviruses are susceptible to acid, and citric acid can be incorporated into facial tissues as a means of blocking viral transmission.

Attachment

The first step in viral replication is mediated by the interaction of a viral attachment protein with its cell surface receptor. This interaction can be blocked by **neutralizing antibodies,** which bind to the viral attachment protein, or by **receptor antagonists.** The administration of specific antibodies **(passive immunization)** is the oldest form of antiviral therapy. Receptor antagonists include peptide or sugar analogs of the cell receptor or the viral attachment protein that competitively blocks interaction of the virus with the cell. Compounds that bind to the C-C chemokine receptor 5 (CCR5) molecule block binding of human immunodeficiency virus (HIV) to macrophages and some CD4 T cells to prevent the initial infection. Acidic polysaccharides (e.g., heparan, dextran sulfate) interfere with viral binding and have been suggested for the treatment of infection with HIV, herpes simplex virus (HSV), and other viruses.

Penetration and Uncoating

Penetration and uncoating of the virus are required to deliver the viral genome into the cytoplasm of the host cell. Arildone, disoxaril, **pleconaril,** and other **methylisoxazole** compounds block uncoating of picornaviruses by fitting into a cleft in the receptor-binding canyon of the capsid and preventing disassembly of the capsid. For viruses that enter through endocytic vesicles, uncoating may be triggered by conformational changes in attachment proteins that promote fusion or by membrane disruption resulting from the acidic environment of the vesicle. **Amantadine, rimantadine,** and other hydrophobic amines (weak organic bases) are antiviral agents that can neutralize the pH of these compartments and inhibit virion uncoating. Amantadine and rimantadine only have activity against influenza A. These compounds bind to and block the hydrogen ion (H^+) channel formed by the viral M_2 protein. Without the influx of H^+, the M_1 matrix proteins do not dissociate from the nucleocapsid (uncoating), so movement of the nucleocapsid to the nucleus, transcription, and replication are prevented. Blockage of this proton pore also disrupts proper processing of the hemagglutinin protein late in the replication cycle. In the absence of a functional M_2 proton pore, the hemagglutinin inopportunely changes its conformation into its "fusion form" and is inactivated as it traverses the normally acidic Golgi environment. **Docosanol** inhibits the fusion of enveloped viruses, including HSV, with cellular membranes. **Tromantadine,** a derivative of amantadine, also inhibits penetration of HSV. Penetration and uncoating of HIV are blocked by a 33–amino acid peptide, T20 **(enfuvirtide [Fuzeon]),** which inhibits the action of the viral fusion protein gp41.

RNA Synthesis

Although messenger ribonucleic acid (mRNA) synthesis is essential for the production of virus, it is not a good target for antiviral drugs. It would be difficult to inhibit viral mRNA synthesis without affecting cellular mRNA synthesis. Deoxyribonucleic acid (DNA) viruses use the host cell's

 **Box 40-1 Viruses Treatable with Antiviral Drugs**

Herpes simplex virus
Varicella-zoster virus
Cytomegalovirus
Human immunodeficiency virus
Influenza A and B viruses
Respiratory syncytial virus
Hepatitis B and C viruses
Papillomavirus
Picornavirus

 **Table 40-1 Examples of Targets for Antiviral Drugs**

Replication Step or Target	Agent	Targeted Virus
Attachment	Peptide analogs of attachment protein	HIV (CCR5 co-receptor antagonist)
	Neutralizing antibodies	Most viruses
	Heparan and dextran sulfate	HIV, HSV
Penetration and uncoating	Amantadine, rimantadine	Influenza A virus
	Tromantadine, docosanol	HSV
	Arildone, disoxaril, pleconaril	Picornaviruses
Transcription	Interferon	HCVs, papillomavirus
	RNA polymerase	HCV
	Antisense oligonucleotides	—
Hypermutation/ guanosine analog	Ribavirin	HCV, respiratory syncytial virus, Lassa fever virus
Protein synthesis	Interferon	HCV, papillomavirus
DNA replication (polymerase)	Nucleoside analogs	Herpesviruses, HIV, hepatitis B virus, poxviruses, etc.
	Phosphonoformate, phosphonoacetic acid	Herpesviruses
Nucleoside scavenging (thymidine kinase)	Nucleoside analogs	HSV, varicella-zoster virus
Assembly (protease)	Hydrophobic substrate analogs	HIV, HCV
Assembly (neuraminidase)	Oseltamivir, zanamivir	Influenza A, B virus

CCR5, C-C chemokine receptor 5; *DNA,* deoxyribonucleic acid; *HCV,* hepatitis C virus; *HIV,* human immunodeficiency virus; *HSV,* herpes simplex virus.

transcriptases for mRNA synthesis. Most of the RNA polymerases encoded by RNA viruses may not be sufficiently different from host cell transcriptases to selectively inhibit this activity, and the high rate at which RNA viruses mutate results in the generation of many drug-resistant strains. **Sofosbuvir,** a prodrug for a nucleoside analog, was recently approved as an inhibitor of the hepatitis C virus polymerase. **Guanidine** and **2-hydroxybenzylbenzimidine** are two compounds that can block picornavirus RNA synthesis by binding to the 2C picornavirus protein, which is essential for RNA synthesis. **Ribavirin** resembles riboguanosine and promotes hypermutation and inhibits nucleoside biosynthesis, mRNA capping, and other processes (cellular and viral) important to the replication of many viruses.

The proper processing (splicing) and translation of viral mRNA can be inhibited by interferon and antisense oligonucleotides. **Isatin-β-thiosemicarbazone** induces mRNA degradation in poxvirus-infected cells and was used as a treatment for smallpox. Viral infection of an **interferon**-treated cell triggers a cascade of biochemical events that block viral replication. Specifically, the degradation of viral and cellular mRNA is enhanced, and ribosomal assembly is blocked, preventing protein synthesis and viral replication. Interferon is described further in Chapter 10. Interferon and artificial interferon inducers **(Ampligen, poly rI : rC)** have been approved for clinical use (papilloma, hepatitis B and C) or are in clinical trials.

Genome Replication

Most antiviral drugs are **nucleoside analogs,** which are compounds with modifications of the base, sugar, or both (Figure 40-1). The viral **DNA polymerases** of the herpesviruses and the **reverse transcriptases** of HIV and hepatitis B virus (HBV) *are the prime targets for most antiviral drugs because they are essential for virus replication and are different from host enzymes.* Before being used by the polymerase, the nucleoside analogs must be phosphorylated to the triphosphate form by viral enzymes (e.g., HSV thymidine kinase), cellular enzymes, or both. For example, the thymidine kinase of HSV and varicella-zoster virus (VZV) applies the first phosphate to **acyclovir (ACV),** and cellular enzymes apply the rest. HSV mutants lacking thymidine kinase activity are resistant to ACV. Cellular enzymes phosphorylate **azidothymidine (AZT)** and many other nucleoside analogs.

Nucleoside analogs selectively inhibit viral polymerases, because these enzymes are less accurate than host cell enzymes. The viral enzyme binds nucleoside analogs with modifications of the base, sugar, or both several hundred times better than the host cell enzyme. These drugs either **prevent chain elongation,** as a result of the absence of a 3′-hydroxyl on the sugar, or **alter recognition and base pairing,** as a result of a base modification, and induce inactivating mutations (see Figure 40-1). Hypermutation of a viral genome by an antiviral drug (like ribavirin) is the equivalent of replacing every fourth letter in an essay with a random letter. Antiviral drugs that cause termination of the DNA chain by means of modified nucleoside sugar residues include ACV, ganciclovir (GCV), valacyclovir, penciclovir, famciclovir, adefovir, cidofovir, adenosine arabinoside (vidarabine, ara-A), zidovudine (AZT), lamivudine (3TC), dideoxycytidine, and dideoxyinosine. Antiviral drugs that become incorporated into the viral genome and cause errors in replication (mutation) and transcription (inactive mRNA and proteins) because of modified nucleoside bases include **ribavirin, 5-iododeoxyuridine (idoxuridine),** and **trifluorothymidine (trifluridine).** The rapid rate and large extent of nucleotide incorporation by HIV- and herpesvirus-encoded

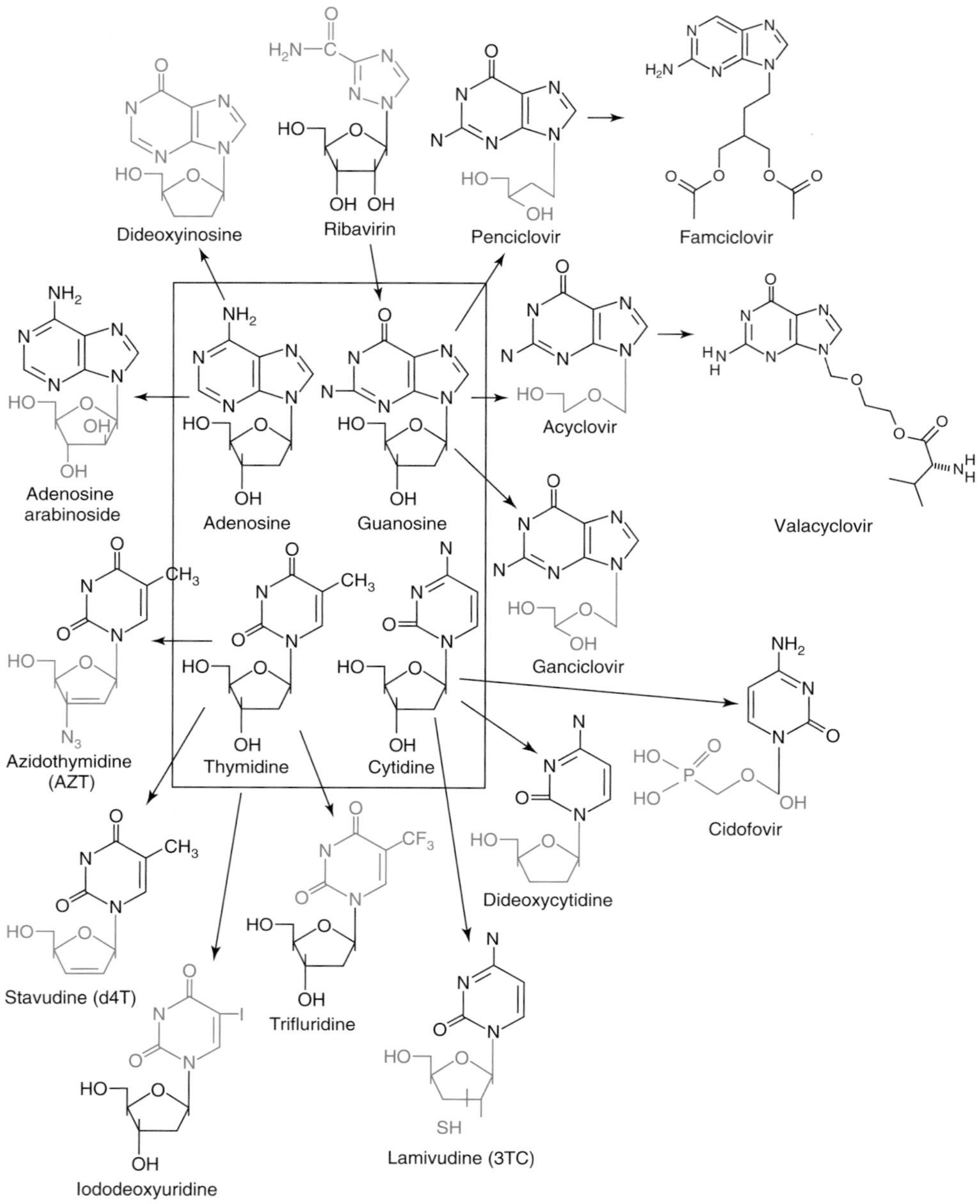

FIGURE 40-1 Structure of the most common nucleoside analogs that are antiviral drugs. The chemical distinctions between the natural deoxynucleoside and the antiviral drug analogs are highlighted. *Arrows* indicate related drugs. Valacyclovir is the L-valyl ester of acyclovir. Famciclovir is the diacetyl 6-deoxyanalog of penciclovir. Both of these drugs are metabolized to the active drug in the liver or intestinal wall.

polymerases make these viruses especially susceptible to these drugs. A variety of other nucleoside analogs are also being developed as antiviral drugs.

Pyrophosphate analogs resembling the byproduct of the polymerase reaction, such as **phosphonoformic acid (foscarnet, PFA)** and **phosphonoacetic acid,** are classic inhibitors of the herpesvirus polymerases. **Nevirapine, delavirdine,** and other nonnucleoside reverse transcriptase inhibitors bind, as noncompetitive inhibitors of the enzyme, to sites on the enzyme other than the substrate site.

Deoxyribonucleotide scavenging enzymes (e.g., the thymidine kinase and ribonucleoside reductase of the herpesviruses) are also enzyme targets of antiviral drugs. Inhibition of these enzymes reduces the levels of deoxyribonucleotides necessary for the replication of the DNA virus genome, preventing virus replication.

Integration of the cDNA of HIV into the host chromosome catalyzed by the viral integrase enzyme is essential for virus replication. An inhibitor of the integrase is now approved for anti-HIV therapy.

Protein Synthesis

Although bacterial protein synthesis is the target for several antibacterial compounds, viral protein synthesis is a poor target for antiviral drugs. The virus uses host cell ribosomes and synthetic mechanisms for replication, so selective inhibition is not possible. **Interferon (IFN)-α** and **IFN-β** stop a virus by promoting the inhibition of protein synthesis in the virus-infected cell. Inhibition of the posttranslational modification of proteins, such as the proteolysis of a viral polyprotein **(protease inhibitors)** or glycoprotein processing (castanospermine, deoxynojirimycin), can also inhibit virus replication. **Boceprevir** and **telaprevir** are two new protease inhibitors for treatment of hepatitis C virus (HCV). Proteases of other viruses, especially HIV (see later), are also targets for antiviral drugs.

Virion Assembly and Release

The **HIV protease** is unique and **essential** to the assembly of virions and the production of infectious virions. Computer-assisted molecular modeling was used to design inhibitors of the HIV protease, such as **saquinavir, ritonavir,** and **indinavir** (*navir,* "no virus"), that would fit into the active site of the enzyme. The enzyme structures were defined by x-ray crystallography and molecular biology studies.

The **neuraminidase of influenza** is essential to prevent aggregation of viral glycoproteins and allow their incorporation into the envelope. **Zanamivir (Relenza)** and **oseltamivir (Tamiflu)** act as enzyme inhibitors and, unlike amantadine and rimantadine, can inhibit influenza A and B. Amantadine and rimantadine also inhibit release of influenza A.

Stimulators of Host Innate Immune Protective Responses

Stimulation or supplementation of the natural response is an effective approach to limit or treat viral infections. Innate responses of dendritic cells, macrophages, and other cells can be stimulated by **imiquimod, resiquimod, and CpG oligodeoxynucleotides,** which bind to Toll-like receptors to stimulate release of protective cytokines, activation of natural killer cells, and subsequent cell-mediated immune responses. **Interferon** and interferon inducers, including mismatched polynucleotides and double-stranded RNA (e.g., **Ampligen, poly rI:rC**), facilitate the treatment of chronic diseases of hepatitis C and papillomaviruses. **Antibodies,** acquired naturally or by passive immunization (see Chapters 10 and 11), prevent both acquisition and spread of the virus. For example, passive immunization is administered after exposure to rabies and hepatitis A virus (HAV) and HBV.

• Nucleoside Analogs

Most of the antiviral drugs approved by the U.S. Food and Drug Administration (FDA) (Table 40-2) are nucleoside analogs that inhibit viral polymerases. Resistance to the drug is usually caused by a mutation of the polymerase.

Acyclovir, Valacyclovir, Penciclovir, and Famciclovir

ACV (acycloguanosine) and its valyl derivative, valacyclovir, differ in pharmacologic ways. ACV differs from the nucleoside guanosine by having an acyclic (hydroxyethoxymethyl) side chain instead of a ribose or deoxyribose sugar. *ACV has selective action against HSV and VZV, the herpesviruses that encode a thymidine kinase* (Figure 40-2). The viral thymidine kinase is required to activate the drug by phosphorylation, and host cell enzymes complete the progression to the diphosphate form and finally to the triphosphate form. Because there is no initial phosphorylation in uninfected

Table 40-2 Some Antiviral Drug Therapies Approved by the U.S. Food and Drug Administration

Virus	Antiviral Drug	Trade Name
Herpes Simplex and Varicella-Zoster Viruses	Acyclovir*	Zovirax
	Valacyclovir*	Valtrex
	Penciclovir	Denavir
	Famciclovir*	Famvir
	Trifluridine	Viroptic
Cytomegalovirus	Ganciclovir	Cytovene
	Valganciclovir	Valcyte
	Cidofovir	Vistide
	Phosphonoformate (foscarnet)	Foscavir
Influenza A Virus	Amantadine	Symmetrel
	Rimantadine	Flumadine
Influenza A and B Viruses	Zanamivir	Relenza
	Oseltamivir	Tamiflu
Chronic Hepatitis B Virus	Lamivudine	Epivir
	Adefovir dipivoxil	Hepsera
Hepatitis C Virus	Interferon-α, ribavirin	Various
	Boceprevir	Victrelis
	Telaprevir	Incivek
	Sofosbuvir	Sovaldi
Papillomavirus	Interferon-α	Various
Respiratory Syncytial Virus and Lassa Virus	Ribavirin	Virazole
Picornaviruses	Pleconaril	Picovir
Human Immunodeficiency Virus†		
Nucleoside analog reverse transcriptase inhibitors	Azidothymidine (zidovudine)	Retrovir
	Dideoxyinosine (didanosine)	Videx
	Dideoxycytidine (zalcitabine)	Hivid
	Stavudine (d4T)	Zerit
	Lamivudine (3TC)	Epivir
Nonnucleoside reverse transcriptase inhibitors	Nevirapine	Viramune
	Delavirdine	Rescriptor
Protease inhibitors	Saquinavir	Invirase
	Ritonavir	Norvir
	Indinavir	Crixivan
	Nelfinavir	Viracept
Integrase inhibitor	Raltegravir	Isentriss
CCR5 co-receptor antagonist	Maraviroc	Selzentry
Fusion inhibitor	Enfuvirtide	Fuzeon

CCR5, C-C chemokine receptor 5.
*Also active against varicella-zoster virus.
†A more complete list is found in Chapter 54.

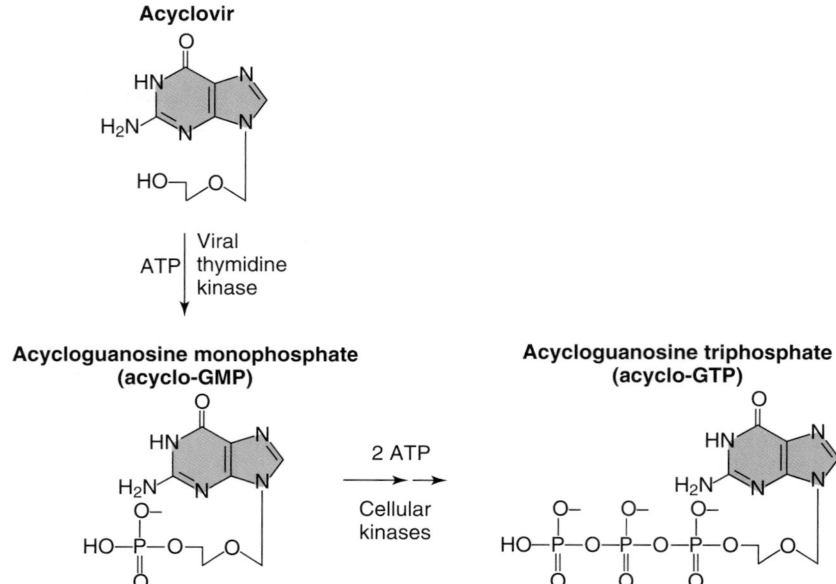

FIGURE 40-2 Activation of acyclovir (ACV) (acycloguanosine) in herpes simplex virus–infected cells. ACV is converted to acycloguanosine monophosphate *(acyclo-GMP)* by herpes-specific viral thymidine kinase and then to acycloguanosine triphosphate *(acyclo-GTP)* by cellular kinases. *ATP,* Adenosine triphosphate.

cells, there is no active drug to inhibit cellular DNA synthesis or cause toxicity. The ACV triphosphate causes termination of the growing viral DNA chain because there is no 3′-hydroxyl group on the ACV molecule to allow chain elongation. The minimal toxicity of ACV is also a result of a 100-fold or greater use by the viral DNA polymerase than by cellular DNA polymerases. **Resistance to ACV** develops by mutation of *either* the thymidine kinase, so that activation of ACV cannot occur, or the DNA polymerase, to prevent ACV binding.

ACV is effective against all HSV infections, including encephalitis, disseminated herpes, and other serious herpes diseases. The fact that it is not toxic to uninfected cells allows use of it and its analogs as a prophylactic treatment to prevent recurrent outbreaks, especially in immunosuppressed people. A recurrent episode may be prevented if it is treated before or soon after the triggering event. ACV inhibits the replication of HSV but cannot resolve the latent HSV infection.

Valacyclovir, the valyl ester derivative of ACV, is more efficiently absorbed after oral administration and rapidly converted into ACV, increasing the bioavailability of ACV for the treatment of HSV and serious VZV. ACV and valacyclovir can also be used for the treatment of VZV infection, although higher doses are required. VZV is less sensitive to the agent in part because ACV is phosphorylated less efficiently by the VZV thymidine kinase.

Penciclovir inhibits HSV and VZV in the same way ACV does but is concentrated and persists in the infected cells to a greater extent than ACV. Penciclovir also has some activity against the Epstein-Barr virus and cytomegalovirus (CMV). **Famciclovir** is a prodrug derivative of penciclovir that is well absorbed orally and then is converted to penciclovir in the liver or intestinal lining. Resistance to penciclovir and famciclovir develops in the same manner as for ACV.

Ganciclovir

GCV (dihydroxypropoxymethyl guanine) differs from ACV in having a single hydroxymethyl group in the acyclic side chain (see Figure 40-1). The remarkable result of this addition is that it confers considerable activity against CMV. CMV does not encode a thymidine kinase, but a viral-encoded protein kinase phosphorylates GCV. Once activated by phosphorylation, GCV inhibits all herpesvirus DNA polymerases. The viral DNA polymerases have nearly 30 times greater affinity for the drug than the cellular DNA polymerase. Similar to ACV, a valyl ester of GCV **(valganciclovir)** was developed to improve the pharmacologic properties of GCV.

GCV is effective in the treatment of CMV retinitis and shows some efficacy in the treatment of CMV esophagitis, colitis, and pneumonia in patients with AIDS. The potential for bone marrow and other toxicity limits its use. Of interest, this potential toxicity has been used as the basis for the development of an antitumor therapy. In one application, an HSV thymidine kinase gene was incorporated into the cells of a brain tumor with the use of a retrovirus vector. The retrovirus replicated only in the growing cells of the tumor, and the thymidine kinase was expressed only in the tumor cells, making the tumor cells susceptible to GCV.

Cidofovir and Adefovir

Cidofovir and **adefovir** are both nucleotide analogs and contain a phosphate attached to the sugar analog. This obviates the need for the initial phosphorylation by a viral enzyme. Compounds with this type of sugar analog are substrates for DNA polymerases or reverse transcriptases and have an expanded spectrum of susceptible viruses. Cidofovir, a cytidine analog, is approved for CMV infections in AIDS patients but can also inhibit replication of polyomavirus and papillomaviruses and inhibit the polymerases of herpesviruses, adenoviruses, and poxvirus. Adefovir and adefovir dipivoxil (a diester prodrug) are analogs of adenosine and are approved for treatment of HBV.

Azidothymidine

Originally developed as an anticancer drug, **AZT** was the first useful therapy for HIV infection. AZT (Retrovir), a nucleoside analog of thymidine, inhibits the reverse transcriptase of HIV (see Figure 40-1). Similar to other nucleosides, AZT must be phosphorylated by host cell enzymes. It lacks the 3′-hydroxyl necessary for DNA chain elongation and prevents complementary DNA synthesis. The selective therapeutic effect of AZT stems from the 100-fold lower sensitivity of the host cell DNA polymerase in comparison with the HIV reverse transcriptase.

Continuous oral AZT treatment is administered to HIV-infected people with depleted CD4 T-cell counts to prevent progression of disease. AZT treatment of pregnant HIV-infected women can reduce the likelihood of or prevent transmission of the virus to the baby. Side effects of AZT range from nausea to life-threatening bone marrow toxicity.

The high error rate of the HIV polymerase creates extensive mutations and promotes the development of antiviral drug-resistant strains. This problem is being addressed by the administration of multidrug therapy as initial therapy **(highly active antiretroviral therapy [HAART]).** It is more difficult for the HIV to develop resistance to multiple drugs with multiple target enzymes. Multidrug-resistant HIV strains are likely to be much weaker than the parent strains.

Dideoxyinosine, Dideoxycytidine, Stavudine, and Lamivudine

Several other nucleoside analogs have been approved as anti-HIV agents. **Dideoxyinosine** (didanosine) is a nucleoside analog that is converted to dideoxyadenosine triphosphate (see Figure 40-1). Similar to AZT, dideoxyinosine, **dideoxycytidine,** and **stavudine** (d4T) lack a 3′-hydroxyl group. The modified sugar attached to **lamivudine** (2′-deoxy-3′-thiacytidine [3TC]) also inhibits the HIV reverse transcriptase by preventing DNA chain elongation and HIV replication. These drugs are available for the treatment of AIDS that is unresponsive to AZT therapy, or they can be given in combination with AZT. Lamivudine is also active on the reverse transcriptase polymerase of HBV. Most of the anti-HIV agents have potential toxic side effects.

Ribavirin

Ribavirin is an analog of the nucleoside guanosine (see Figure 40-1) but differs from guanosine in that its base ring is incomplete and open. Similar to other nucleoside analogs, ribavirin must be phosphorylated. The drug is active in vitro against a broad range of viruses.

Ribavirin monophosphate resembles guanosine monophosphate and inhibits nucleoside biosynthesis, mRNA capping, and other processes important to the replication of many viruses. Ribavirin depletes the cellular stores of guanine by inhibiting inosine monophosphate dehydrogenase, an enzyme important in the synthetic pathway of guanosine. It also prevents the synthesis of the mRNA 5′ cap by interfering with the guanylation and methylation of the nucleic acid base. In addition, ribavirin triphosphate inhibits RNA polymerases and promotes hypermutation of the viral genome. Its multiple sites of action may explain the lack of ribavirin-resistant mutants.

Ribavirin is administered in an aerosol to children with severe respiratory syncytial virus bronchopneumonia and potentially to adults with severe influenza or measles. The drug may be effective for the treatment of influenza B, as well as Lassa, Rift Valley, Crimean-Congo, Korean, and Argentine hemorrhagic fevers, for which it is administered orally or intravenously. Ribavirin is approved for use against HCV in combination with IFN-α and protease inhibitors. Treatment can have serious side effects.

Other Nucleoside Analogs

Idoxuridine, trifluorothymidine (see Figure 40-1), and **fluorouracil** are analogs of thymidine. These drugs either (1) inhibit the biosynthesis of thymidine, a nucleotide essential for DNA synthesis, or (2) replace thymidine and become incorporated into the viral DNA. These actions inhibit further synthesis of the virus or cause extensive misreading of the genome, leading to mutation and inactivation of the virus. These drugs target cells in which extensive DNA replication is taking place, such as those infected with HSV, and spare the nongrowing cells from harm.

Idoxuridine was the first anti-HSV drug approved for human use but has been replaced by **trifluridine** and other more effective, less toxic agents. **Fluorouracil** is an antineoplastic drug that kills rapidly growing cells but has also been used for topical treatment of warts caused by human papillomaviruses.

Adenine arabinoside was the principal anti-HSV drug until ACV was introduced but is no longer used owing to difficulties in administration and toxicity. Ara-A is an adenosine nucleoside analog with an arabinose substituted for deoxyribose as the sugar moiety (see Figure 40-1). Many other nucleoside analogs that have antiviral activity are being investigated for clinical use against the herpesviruses, HBV, and HIV.

• Nonnucleoside Polymerase Inhibitors

Foscarnet (PFA) and the related phosphonoacetic acid (PAA) are simple compounds that resemble pyrophosphate (Figure 40-3). These drugs inhibit viral replication by binding

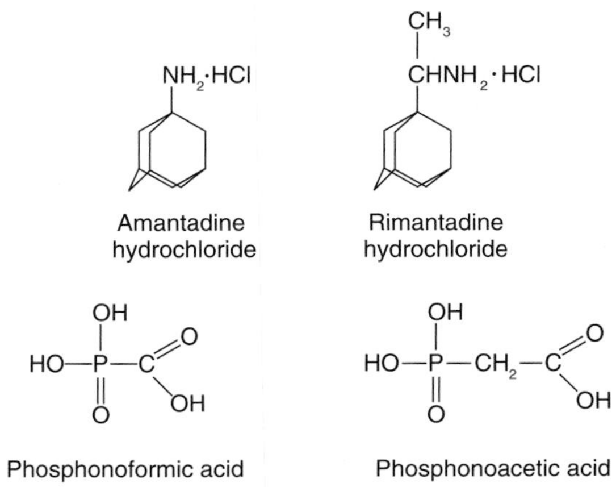

Amantadine hydrochloride

Rimantadine hydrochloride

Phosphonoformic acid

Phosphonoacetic acid

FIGURE 40-3 Structures of antiviral drugs.

to the pyrophosphate-binding site of the DNA polymerase to block nucleotide binding. PFA and PAA can cause renal and other problems because of their ability to chelate divalent metal ions (e.g., calcium) and become incorporated into bone. PFA inhibits the DNA polymerase of all herpesviruses and the HIV reverse transcriptase without having to be phosphorylated by nucleoside kinases (e.g., thymidine kinase). PFA has been approved for the treatment of CMV retinitis in patients with AIDS.

Nevirapine, delavirdine, efavirenz, and other nonnucleoside reverse transcriptase inhibitors bind to sites on the enzyme different from the substrate. Because these drugs' mechanisms of action differ from those of the nucleoside analogs, the mechanism of HIV resistance to the agents is also different. As a result, these drugs are very useful in combination with nucleoside analogs for the treatment of HIV infection.

• Protease Inhibitors

The unique structure of the HIV protease and its essential role in the production of a functional virion have made this enzyme a good target for antiviral drugs. **Saquinavir, indinavir, ritonavir, nelfinavir,** and other agents work by slipping into the hydrophobic active site of the enzyme to inhibit its action. Drug-resistant strains arise through mutation of the protease. Use of protease inhibitors significantly improved the outcomes for HIV patients. The combination of a protease inhibitor with AZT and a second nucleoside analog (HAART) can reduce blood levels of HIV to undetectable levels.

Protease inhibitors **(boceprevir, telaprevir, simeprevir)** are also improving the outlook for treating patients with chronic hepatitis C.

• Antiinfluenza Drugs

Amantadine and **rimantadine** are amphipathic amine compounds with clinical efficacy against the influenza A but not the influenza B virus (see Figure 40-3). These drugs have several effects on influenza A replication. Both compounds are acidotrophic and concentrate in and buffer the contents of the endosomal vesicles involved in the uptake of the influenza virus. This effect can inhibit the acid-mediated change in conformation in the hemagglutinin protein that promotes fusion of the viral envelope with cell membranes. However, the specificity for influenza A is a result of its ability to bind to and block the proton channel formed by the M_2 membrane protein of the influenza A virus. Resistance is the result of an altered M_2 or hemagglutinin protein.

Amantadine and rimantadine may be useful in ameliorating an influenza A infection if either agent is taken within 48 hours of exposure. They are also useful as a prophylactic treatment in lieu of vaccination. In addition, amantadine is an alternative therapy for Parkinson disease. The principal toxic effect is on the central nervous system, with patients experiencing nervousness, irritability, and insomnia.

Zanamivir (Relenza) and **oseltamivir (Tamiflu)** inhibit influenza A and B as enzyme inhibitors of the neuraminidase of influenza. Without the neuraminidase to cleave sialic acid, the hemagglutinin of the virus binds to these sugars on other glycoproteins, forming clumps and preventing assembly and virus release. These drugs can be taken prophylactically as an alternative to vaccination or, if taken within the first 48 hours of infection, to reduce the length of illness. Mutations in the neuraminidase cause resistance.

• Immunomodulators

Genetically engineered forms of IFN-α have been approved for human use. Interferons work by binding to cell surface receptors and initiating a cellular antiviral response. In addition, interferons stimulate the immune response and promote the immune clearance of viral infection.

IFN-α is active against many viral infections, including hepatitis A, B, and C; HSV; papillomavirus; and rhinovirus. It has been approved for the treatment of condyloma acuminatum (genital warts, a presentation of papillomavirus) and hepatitis C (in combination therapy). Attachment of polyethylene glycol to IFN-α (pegylated IFN-α) increases its potency. Pegylated IFN-α is used with ribavirin to treat hepatitis C infections. Natural interferon causes the influenza-like symptoms observed during many viremic and respiratory tract infections, and the synthetic agent has similar side effects during treatment. Interferon is discussed further in Chapters 10 and 37.

Imiquimod, a Toll-like receptor ligand, stimulates innate responses to attack the virus infection. This therapeutic approach can activate local protective responses against papillomas, which generally escape immune control.

• Infection Control

Infection control is essential in hospital and health care settings. The spread of respiratory viruses is the most difficult to prevent. Viral spread can be controlled in the following ways:

1. Limiting personnel contact with sources of infection (e.g., wearing gloves, mask, goggles; using quarantine)
2. Improving hygiene, sanitation, and disinfection
3. Ensuring that all personnel are immunized against common diseases
4. Educating all personnel regarding points 1, 2, and 3 and in the ways to decrease high-risk behaviors

Methods for disinfection differ for each virus and depend on its structure. Most viruses are inactivated by 70% ethanol, 15% chlorine bleach, 2% glutaraldehyde, 4% formaldehyde, or autoclaving (as described in *Guidelines for Prevention of Transmission of Human Immunodeficiency Virus and Hepatitis B Virus to Health-Care and Public-Safety Workers,* issued in 1989 by the U.S. Centers for Disease Control and Prevention [CDC]). Most enveloped viruses do not require such rigorous treatment and are inactivated by soap and detergents. Other means of disinfection are also available.

Special "universal" precautions are required for the handling of human blood; that is, all blood should be assumed to be contaminated with HIV or HBV and should be handled with caution. In addition to these procedures, special care must be taken with syringe needles and surgical tools contaminated with blood. Specific guidelines are available from the CDC.

Control of an outbreak usually requires identification of the source or reservoir of the virus, followed by cleanup, quarantine, immunization, or a combination of these measures. The first step in controlling an outbreak of gastroenteritis or hepatitis A is identification of the food, water, or possibly the day-care center that is the source of the outbreak.

Education programs can promote compliance with immunization programs and help people change lifestyles associated with viral transmission. Such programs have had a significant impact in reducing the prevalence of vaccine-preventable diseases such as smallpox, polio, measles, mumps, and rubella. It is hoped that educational programs will also promote changes in lifestyles and habits, to restrict the spread of the blood-borne and sexually transmitted HBV and HIV.

Bibliography

Carter J, Saunders V: *Virology: principles and applications*, Chichester, England, 2007, Wiley.

Cohen J, Powderly WG: *Infectious diseases*, ed 2, St Louis, 2004, Mosby.

Collier L, Oxford J: *Human virology*, ed 3, Oxford, England, 2006, Oxford University Press.

De Clercq E: A 40-year journey in search of selective antiviral chemotherapy, *Ann Rev Pharmacol Toxicol* 51:1–24, 2011.

Flint SJ, Enquist LW, Racaniello VR, et al: *Principles of virology: molecular biology, pathogenesis and control of animal viruses*, ed 3, Washington, DC, 2009, American Society for Microbiology Press.

Knipe DM, Howley PM, Griffin DE, et al: *Fields virology*, ed 5, Philadelphia, 2006, Lippincott Williams & Wilkins.

Richman DD: Antiviral drug resistance, *Antiviral Res* 71:117–121, 2006.

Richman DD, Whitley RJ, Hayden FG: *Clinical virology*, ed 3, Washington, DC, 2009, American Society for Microbiology Press.

Strauss JM, Strauss EG: *Viruses and human diseases*, ed 2, San Diego, 2007, Academic.

Websites

New Medical Information and Health Information: Antiviral drugs: Antiviral agents, antiviral medications. http://drugs.nmihi.com/antivirals.htm. Accessed April 20, 2015.

U.S. Food and Drug Administration: HBV and HCV. www.fda.gov/ForPatients/Illness/HepatitisBC/default.htm. Accessed April 20, 2015.

U.S. Food and Drug Administration: HIV drugs. www.fda.gov/ForPatients/Illness/HIVAIDS/default.htm. Accessed April 20, 2015.

U.S. Food and Drug Administration: Influenza (flu) antiviral drugs and related information. www.fda.gov/Drugs/DrugSafety/InformationbyDrugClass/ucm100228.htm. Accessed April 20, 2015.

CHAPTER

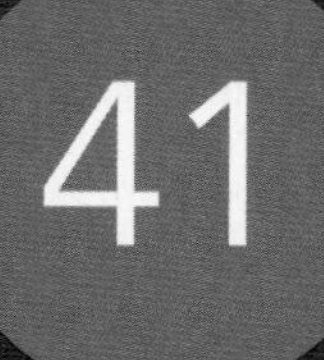

PAPILLOMAVIRUSES AND POLYOMAVIRUSES

A 47-year-old divorced, sexually active woman is seen for a routine gynecologic exam. She is a pack-a-day smoker. A Papanicolaou (Pap) smear is performed, and the report indicates high-grade squamous intraepithelial lesion (SIL) corresponding to a moderate dysplasia and cervical intraepithelial neoplasia (CIN) score of 2. Polymerase chain reaction (PCR) analysis indicates that cells in the lesion are infected with human papillomavirus 16 (HPV-16).

1. What properties of HPV-16 promote the development of cervical cancer?
2. How is the virus transmitted?
3. What is the nature of the immune response to the virus?
4. How can transmission and disease be prevented?

A 42-year-old man comes to his physician 9 months after a lung transplant, complaining that he has double vision, difficulty speaking, feels that his muscles do not work right, has difficulty with balance, has tingling of his hands and feet, and keeps forgetting things. A month later, he has difficulty speaking and needs assistance with normal daily functions. His mental and physical functions become progressively worse. He is treated with cidofovir, and his immunosuppressive therapy is eased, but his disease progresses to paralysis and he dies. A biopsy of the brain shows lesions with sites of demyelination, astrocytosis with atypical nuclei, and many histiocytes. PCR analysis demonstrates the presence of JC polyomavirus in the lesion, confirming a diagnosis of progressive multifocal leukoencephalopathy (PML).

5. What properties of JC virus promote the development of PML?
6. Why is this disease also prevalent in individuals with acquired immunodeficiency syndrome (AIDS)? Who else is at risk for this disease and why?

Answers to these questions are available on StudentConsult.com.

• SUMMARIES CLINICALLY SIGNIFICANT ORGANISMS

Papillomaviruses

Trigger Words

HPV, warts, koilocytes, cervical cancer, STD, CIN

Biology, Virulence, and Disease

- Small naked capsid, DNA genome
- E6 and E7 proteins inactivate p53 and RB to promote cell growth.
- Virus is acquired by close contact and infects the epithelial cells of the skin or mucous membranes.
- Tissue tropism and disease presentation depend on the papillomavirus type.
- Virus persists in the basal layer and then produces virus in terminally differentiated keratinocytes.
- Viruses cause benign outgrowth of cells into warts.
- HPV infection is hidden from immune responses and persists.
- Warts resolve slowly but spontaneously, possibly as a result of immune response.
- Certain types (HPV-16, HPV-18, etc.) associated with cervical carcinoma

Epidemiology

- Transmitted by direct contact, sexual contact (sexually transmitted disease), fomites, passage through infected birth canal for laryngeal papillomas (types 6 and 11)
- Warts common; STD
- Asymptomatic transmission, found worldwide, no seasonal incidence

Diagnosis

- PCR genome analysis of cervical swabs and tissue specimens

Treatment, Prevention, and Control

- Vaccines for HPV types 16, 18; or 6, 11, 16, 18, 31, 33, 45, 52, and 58

Polyomaviruses

Trigger Words

JCV: PML, opportunistic disease, abnormal oligodendrocytes, demyelination; BKV: kidney

Biology, Virulence, and Disease

- Small naked capsid, DNA genome
- T antigen inactivates p53 and RB to promote cell growth
- Virus is probably acquired through respiratory or oral route, infects tonsils and lymphocytes, and spreads by viremia to the kidneys early in life.
- Virus is ubiquitous and infections are asymptomatic.
- Virus establishes persistent and latent infection in organs such as kidneys and lungs.
- In immunocompromised people, JC virus (JCV) is activated, spreads to the brain, and causes progressive multifocal leukoencephalopathy (PML), a conventional slow virus disease.
- In PML, JCV partially transforms astrocytes and kills oligodendrocytes, causing characteristic lesions and sites of demyelination.
- PML lesions are demyelinated, with unusual large astrocytes and oligodendroglial cells with very large nuclei. BK virus is benign but may cause kidney disease in immunocompromised patients.

Epidemiology

- Transmitted by inhalation or contact with contaminated water or saliva
- Ubiquitous; immunocompromised people at risk for PML
- Found worldwide; no seasonal incidence

Diagnosis

- Presence of PCR-amplified viral DNA in cerebrospinal fluid and MRI or CT evidence of lesions

Treatment, Prevention, and Control

- No modes of control

What used to be called the **papovavirus family** (Papovaviridae) has been divided into two families, Papillomaviridae and Polyomaviridae (Table 41-1). These viruses are capable of causing lytic, chronic, latent, and transforming infections, depending on the host cell. Human papillomaviruses (HPVs) cause **warts,** and several genotypes are associated with human cancer (e.g., **cervical carcinoma**). **BK virus (BKV)** and **JC virus (JCV)**, members of the **Polyomaviridae,** usually cause asymptomatic infection but are associated with renal disease and **progressive multifocal leukoencephalopathy (PML),** respectively, in immunosuppressed people. **Simian virus 40 (SV40)** is the prototype polyomavirus.

The papillomaviruses and polyomaviruses are small, nonenveloped, icosahedral capsid viruses with double-stranded circular deoxyribonucleic acid (DNA) genomes (Box 41-1). They encode proteins that promote cell growth. The promotion of cell growth facilitates lytic viral replication in a permissive cell type but **may oncogenically transform a cell that is nonpermissive.** The polyomaviruses, especially SV40, have been studied extensively as model oncogenic viruses.

• Human Papillomaviruses

Structure and Replication

HPVs are distinguished and typed by DNA sequence homology. At least 100 types have been identified and classified into 16 (A through P) groups. HPV can be distinguished further as **cutaneous HPV** or **mucosal HPV** on the basis of the susceptible tissue. Within the mucosal HPV, there is a group associated with cervical cancer. Viruses in a group cause similar types of warts.

The **icosahedral capsid** of HPV is 50 to 55 nm in diameter and consists of two structural proteins that form 72 capsomeres (Figure 41-1). The HPV genome is **circular** and has approximately 8000 base pairs. The HPV DNA encodes seven or eight early genes (*E1* to *E8*), depending on the virus, and two late or structural genes (*L1* and *L2*). An upstream regulatory region contains the control sequences for transcription, the shared N-terminal sequence for the early proteins, and the origin of replication. All the genes are located on one strand (the plus strand) (Figure 41-2).

The replication cycle of HPV is linked to the life cycle of the keratinocyte and epithelial cell of the skin and mucosa. The virus accesses the basal cell layer through breaks in the skin (Figure 41-3). The L1 protein of HPV is the viral attachment protein and initiates replication by binding to heparin proteoglycans and integrin α6 and other receptors on the cell surface. The early genes of the virus stimulate cell growth, which facilitates replication of the viral genome by the host cell DNA polymerase when the cells divide. The virus-induced increase in cell number causes the basal and the prickle cell layer (stratum spinosum) to thicken (wart, condyloma, or papilloma). As the basal cell differentiates, the specific nuclear factors expressed in the different layers and types of skin and mucosa promote transcription of different viral genes. Expression of the viral genes correlates with the expression of specific keratins. The late genes encoding the structural proteins are expressed only in the terminally differentiated upper layer, and the virus assembles in the nucleus. As the infected skin cell matures and works its way to the surface, the virus matures and is shed with the dead cells of the upper layer.

Pathogenesis

Papillomaviruses infect and replicate in the squamous epithelium of skin **(warts)** and mucous membranes **(genital, oral, and conjunctival papillomas)** to induce epithelial proliferation. The HPV types are very tissue specific, causing different disease presentations. The wart develops because of virus stimulation of cell growth and thickening of the basal and prickle layers (stratum spinosum), as well as the stratum granulosum. **Koilocytes,** characteristic of papillomavirus infection, are enlarged keratinocytes with clear halos around shrunken nuclei. It usually takes 3 to 4 months for the wart to develop (Figure 41-4). The viral infection remains local and generally regresses spontaneously but can recur. The HPV pathogenic mechanisms are summarized in Box 41-2.

Innate and cell-mediated immunity are important for control and resolution of HPV infections. HPV can suppress or hide from protective immune responses. In addition to very low levels of antigen expression (except in the "near-dead" terminally differentiated skin cell), the keratinocyte is

Table 41-1 Human Papillomaviruses and Polyomaviruses and Their Diseases

Virus	Disease
Papillomavirus	Warts, condylomas, papillomas; cervical, penile, and anal cancer*
Polyomavirus	
BK virus	Renal disease†
JC virus	Progressive multifocal leukoencephalopathy†
Merkel cell virus	Merkel cell carcinoma

*High-risk genotypes are present in 99.7% of carcinomas.

†Disease occurs in immunosuppressed patients.

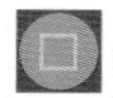

Box 41-1 Unique Properties of Polyomaviruses and Papillomaviruses

Papillomavirus: HPV types 1 to 100+ (as determined by genotype; types defined by DNA homology, tissue tropism, and association with oncogenesis)

Polyomavirus: SV40, **JC virus, BK virus,** KI, WU, Merkel cell polyomavirus (MCV)

Small icosahedral capsid virion

Double-stranded circular DNA genome replicated and assembled in nucleus

Viruses have defined tissue tropisms determined by receptor interactions and transcriptional machinery of cell

Viruses encode proteins that promote cell growth by binding to cellular growth-suppressor proteins p53 and p105RB (p105 retinoblastoma gene product); polyoma T antigen binds to p105RB and p53; high-risk **papillomavirus E6 protein binds to p53, activates telomerase, and suppresses apoptosis, and E7 protein binds to p105RB**

Viruses can cause lytic infections in permissive cells but cause abortive, persistent, or latent infections or **immortalize (transform)** nonpermissive cells

an immunologically privileged site for replication. Inflammatory responses are required to activate protective cytolytic responses and promote resolution of warts. Immunosuppressed persons have recurrences and more severe presentations of papillomavirus infections. Antibody to the L1 protein neutralizes the virus. Immunoglobulin (Ig)G produced by vaccination is secreted into the vagina and can protect against infection.

High-risk HPV types (e.g., HPV-16, HPV-18; see Table 41-2) can initiate the development of cervical carcinoma and oropharyngeal, esophageal, penile, and anal cancers. Viral DNA is found in benign and malignant tumors, especially mucosal papillomas. **Almost all cervical carcinomas contain integrated HPV DNA, with 70% from HPV-16 or HPV-18.** Breaking of the circular genome within the *E1* or *E2* genes to promote integration causes these genes to be inactivated, thereby preventing viral replication without preventing expression of other HPV genes, including the *E5, E6,* and *E7* genes (Figure 41-5). The E5, E6, and E7 proteins of HPV-16 and HPV-18 have been identified as **oncogenes.** The E5 protein enhances cell growth by stabilizing the epidermal growth factor receptor to make the cell more sensitive to growth signals, while the E6 and E7 proteins bind and prevent function of the cellular growth-suppressor (transformation-suppressor) proteins, p53 and the *p105* retinoblastoma gene product (RB). E6 binds the p53 protein and targets it for degradation, and E7 binds and inactivates p105. Enhanced cell growth and inactivation of p53 makes the cell more susceptible to mutation, chromosomal aberrations, or the action of a cofactor and thereby develops into cancer.

Epidemiology

HPV resists inactivation and can be transmitted on fomites such as the surfaces of countertops or furniture, bathroom floors, and towels (Box 41-3). Asymptomatic shedding may promote transmission. HPV infection is acquired (1) by direct contact through small breaks in the skin or mucosa,

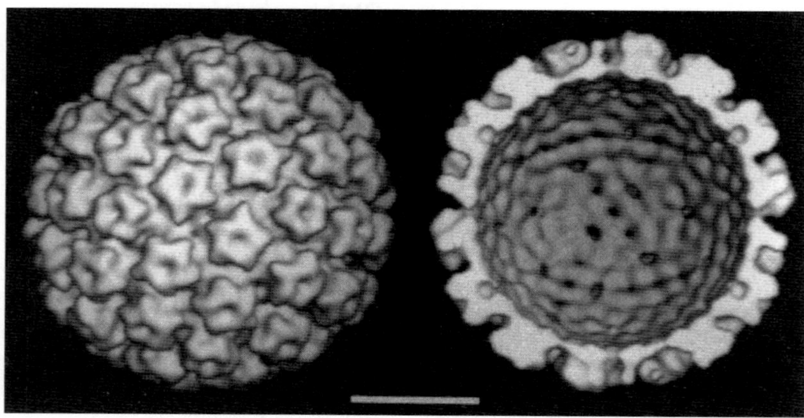

FIGURE 41-1 Computer reconstruction of cryoelectron micrographs of human papillomavirus (HPV). *Left,* View of the surface of HPV shows 72 capsomeres arranged in an icosadeltahedron. All the capsomeres appear to form a regular five-point star shape. *Right,* Computer cross-section of the capsid shows the interaction of the capsomeres and channels in the capsid. (From Baker TS, Newcomb WW, Olson NH, et al: Structures of bovine and human papillomaviruses. Analysis by cryoelectron microscopy and three-dimensional image reconstruction, *Biophys J* 60:1445–1456, 1991.)

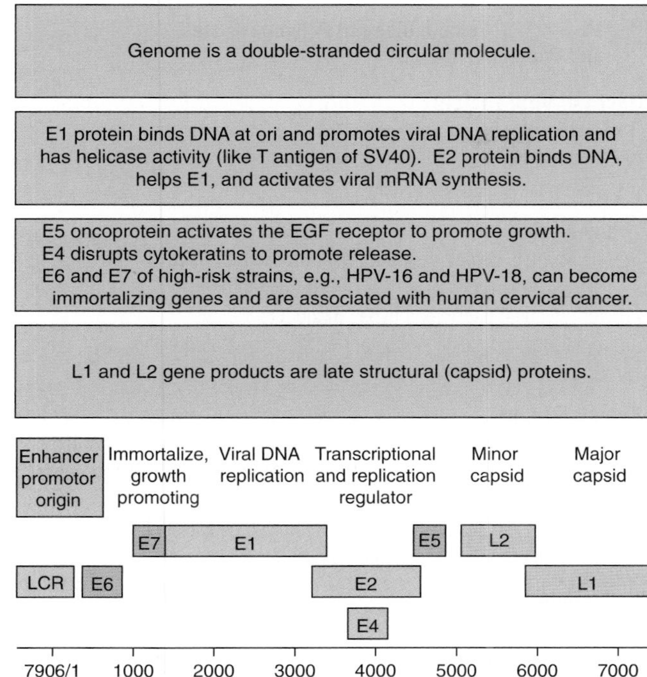

FIGURE 41-2 Genome of human papillomavirus type 16 (HPV-16). DNA is normally a double-stranded circular molecule, but it is shown here in a linear form. *E5,* Oncogene protein that enhances cell growth by stabilizing and activating the epidermal growth factor receptor; *E6,* oncogene protein that binds p53 and promotes its degradation; *E7,* oncogene protein that binds p105RB (p105 retinoblastoma gene product); *EGF,* epidermal growth factor; *L1,* major capsid protein; *L2,* minor capsid protein; *LCR* (URR), long control region (upstream regulatory region); *ori,* origin of replication. (Courtesy Tom Broker, Baltimore.)

(2) during sexual intercourse, or (3) while an infant is passing through an infected birth canal.

Common, plantar, and flat warts are most common in children and young adults. Laryngeal papillomas occur in young children and middle-aged adults.

HPV is possibly the most prevalent sexually transmitted infection in the world, with certain HPV types common among sexually active men and women. At least 20 million people in the United States are infected with HPV, with approximately 6 million new genital cases per year. HPV is present in 99.7% of all cervical cancers, with HPV-16 and HPV-18 in 70% of them. Other high-risk genotypes are more prevalent in different socioethnic groups. A recent study indicates that the most common high-risk HPV types for African American women are types 33, 35, 58, and 68. Other high-risk strains are listed in Table 41-2. High-risk HPV types are also present in oropharyngeal, penile, and anal cancers. HPV-6 and HPV-11 are low-risk HPV types for cervical carcinoma but cause condyloma acuminatum and oral and laryngeal papillomas. Cervical cancer is the second leading cause of cancer death in women (≈12,000 cases and 4000 deaths per year in the United States). Approximately 5% of all Pap smears contain HPV-infected cells, and 10% of women infected with the high-risk HPV types will develop cervical **dysplasia,** a precancerous state. Multiple sexual partners, smoking, a family history of cervical cancer, and immunosuppression are the major risk factors for infection and progression to cancer.

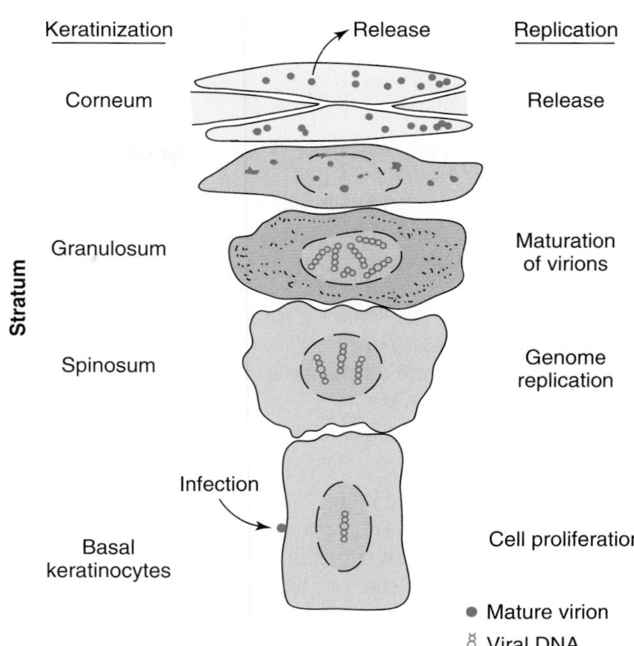

FIGURE 41-3 Development of papilloma (wart). Human papillomavirus infection promotes the outgrowth of the basal layer, increasing the number of prickle cells of the stratum spinosum (acanthosis). These changes cause the skin to thicken and promote the production of keratin (hyperkeratosis), thereby causing epithelial spikes to form (papillomatosis). Virus is produced in the granular cells close to the final keratin layer.

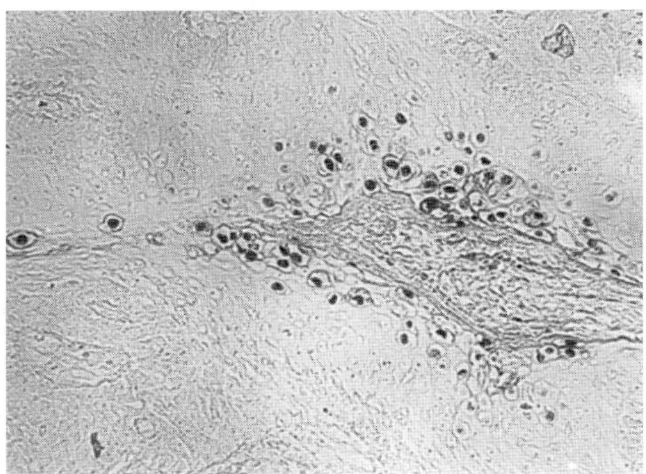

FIGURE 41-4 DNA probe analysis of a human papillomavirus-6–induced anogenital condyloma. A biotin-labeled DNA probe was localized by horseradish peroxidase–conjugated avidin conversion of a substrate to a chromogen precipitate. Dark staining is seen over the nuclei of koilocytotic cells. (From Belshe RB: *Textbook of human virology,* ed 2, St Louis, 1991, Mosby.)

Clinical Syndromes

The clinical syndromes and the HPV types that cause them are summarized in Table 41-2.

Box 41-2 Disease Mechanisms of Papillomaviruses and Polyomaviruses

Papillomaviruses

Virus is acquired by **close contact** and infects the epithelial cells of the skin or mucous membranes.

Tissue tropism and disease presentation depend on the papillomavirus type.

Virus persists in the basal layer and then produces virus in terminally differentiated keratinocytes.

Viruses cause benign outgrowth of cells into **warts.**

HPV infection is hidden from immune responses and persists.

Warts resolve spontaneously as a result of immune response.

Certain types are associated with **dysplasia** that may become **cancerous** with the action of cofactors.

DNA of specific HPV types is present (integrated) in the tumor cell chromosomes.

Polyomaviruses (JCV and BKV)

Virus is acquired through the respiratory or oral route, infects tonsils and lymphocytes, and spreads by viremia to the kidneys early in life.

Virus is ubiquitous, and infections are **asymptomatic.**

Virus establishes **persistent** and **latent** infection in organs such as the kidneys and lungs.

In **immunocompromised** people, JCV is activated, spreads to the brain, and causes **PML,** a conventional slow virus disease.

In PML, JCV partially transforms astrocytes and kills oligodendrocytes, causing characteristic lesions and sites of demyelination.

PML lesions are demyelinated, with unusual large astrocytes and oligodendroglial cells with very large nuclei. BKV is benign but may cause kidney disease in immunocompromised patients.

BKV, BK virus; *HPV,* human papillomavirus; *JCV,* JC virus; *PML,* progressive multifocal leukoencephalopathy.

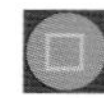

Box 41-3 Epidemiology of Polyomaviruses and Papillomaviruses

Disease/Viral Factors

Capsid virus is resistant to inactivation.

Virus persists in host.

Asymptomatic shedding is likely.

Transmission

Papillomavirus: **direct contact, sexual contact** (sexually transmitted disease) for certain virus types, or passage through infected birth canal for laryngeal papillomas (types 6 and 11)

Polyomavirus: inhalation or contact with contaminated water, stool, urine or saliva

Who Is at Risk?

Papillomavirus: warts are common; sexually active people at risk for infection with human papillomavirus types correlated with oral and genital cancers

Polyomavirus: ubiquitous; immunocompromised people at risk for progressive multifocal leukoencephalopathy

Geography/Season

Viruses are found worldwide.

There is no seasonal incidence.

Modes of Control

Vaccines for HPV types 6, 11, 16, 18

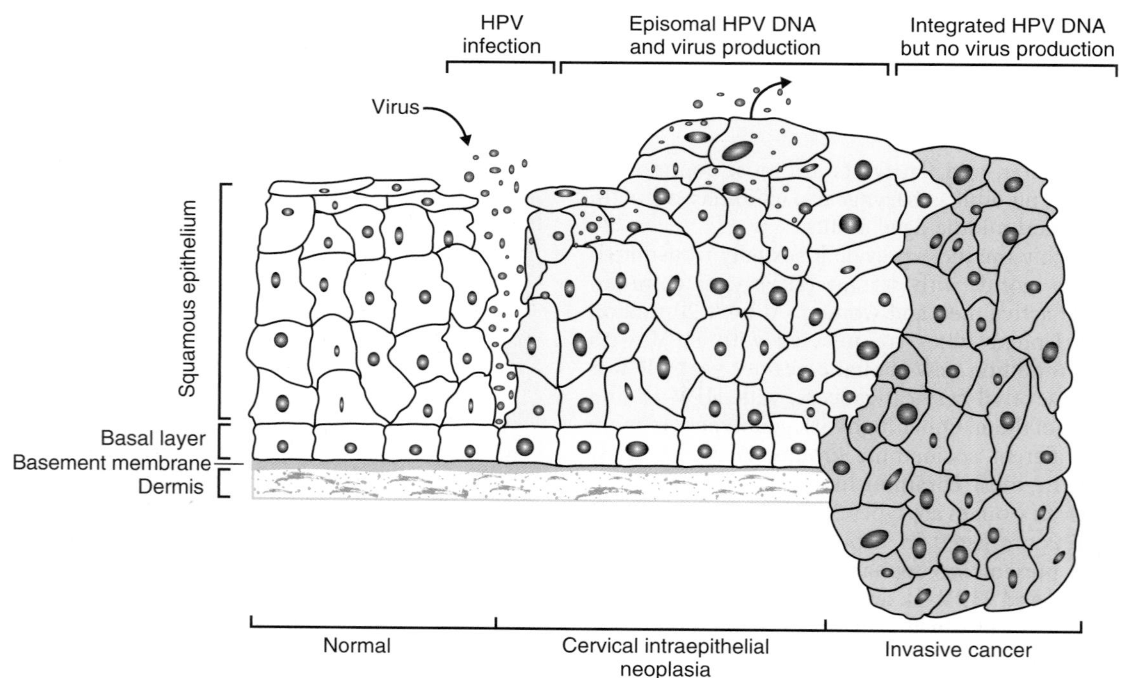

FIGURE 41-5 Progression of human papillomavirus *(HPV)*–mediated cervical carcinoma. HPV infects and replicates in the epithelial cells of the cervix, maturing and releasing virus as the epithelial cells progress through terminal differentiation. Growth stimulation of the basal cells produces a wart. In some cells, the circular genome integrates into host chromosomes, inactivating the *E2* gene, which is necessary for replication. Expression of the other genes without virus production stimulates growth of the cells and possible progression to neoplasia. (Adapted from Woodman CBJ, Collins SI, Young LS: The natural history of cervical HPV infection: unresolved issues, *Nat Rev Cancer* 7:11–22, 2007.)

Table 41-2 Clinical Syndromes Associated with Papillomaviruses

	Human Papillomavirus Types	
Syndrome	**Common**	**Less Common**
Cutaneous Syndromes		
Skin Warts		
Plantar wart	1	2, 4
Common wart	2, 4	1, 7, 26, 29
Flat wart	3, 10	27, 28, 41
Epidermodysplasia verruciformis	5, 8, 17, 20, 36	9, 12, 14, 15, 19, 21-25, 38, 46
Mucosal Syndromes		
Benign Head and Neck Tumors		
Laryngeal papilloma	6, 11	—
Oral papilloma	6, 11	2, 16
Conjunctival papilloma	11	—
Anogenital Warts		
Condyloma acuminatum	6, 11	1, 2, 10, 16, 30, 44, 45
Cervical intraepithelial neoplasia, cancer (high-risk types)	16, 18	31, 33, 35, 39, 45, 51, 52, 56, 58, 59, 66, 68, 69, 73, 82

Modified from Balows A, Hausler WJ Jr, Lennette EH, editors: *Laboratory diagnosis of infectious diseases: principles and practice,* vol 2, New York, 1988, Springer-Verlag. Data from Centers for Disease Control and Prevention: *Epidemiology and prevention of vaccine-preventable diseases,* ed 12, Washington, DC, 2001, Public Health Foundation.

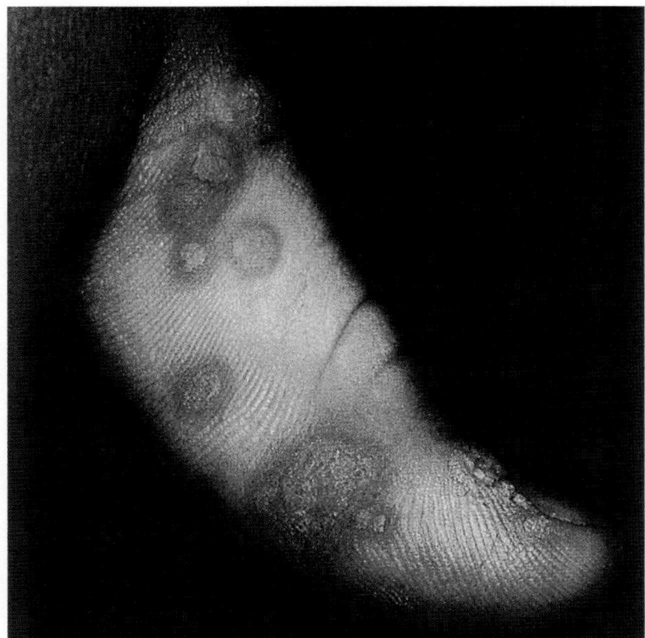

FIGURE 41-6 Common warts. (From Habif TP: *Clinical dermatology: a color guide to diagnosis and therapy,* St Louis, 1985, Mosby.)

Warts

A **wart** is a benign self-limited proliferation of skin that regresses with time. Most people with HPV infection have the common types of the virus (HPV-1 through HPV-4), which infect keratinized surfaces, usually on the hands and feet (Figure 41-6). Initial infection occurs in childhood or early adolescence. The incubation period before a wart develops may be as long as 3 to 4 months. The appearance of the wart (dome shaped, flat, or plantar) depends on the HPV type and the infected site.

Head and Neck Tumors

Single oral papillomas are the most benign epithelial tumors of the oral cavity. They are pedunculated with a fibrovascular stalk, and their surface usually has a rough, papillary appearance. They can occur in people of any age group, are usually solitary, and rarely recur after surgical excision. **Laryngeal papillomas** are commonly associated with HPV-6 and HPV-11 and are the most common benign epithelial tumors of the larynx. Infection of children probably occurs at birth and can be life threatening if the papillomas obstruct the airway. Occasionally, papillomas may be found farther down in the trachea and into the bronchi. As many as 80% of **oropharyngeal carcinomas** contain high-risk HPV DNA.

Anogenital Warts

Anogenital warts **(condylomata acuminata)** occur almost exclusively on the squamous epithelium of the external genitalia and perianal areas and are common for promiscuous individuals. Approximately 90% are caused by HPV-6 and HPV-11. Anogenital lesions infected with these types of HPV can be problematic but rarely become malignant in otherwise healthy people. Anal and penile warts can progress to cancer if caused by high-risk oncogenic strains of HPV.

Cervical Dysplasia and Neoplasia

HPV infection of the genital tract is a very common sexually transmitted disease. Infection is usually asymptomatic but may result in slight itching. Genital warts may appear as soft, flesh-colored warts that are flat, raised, and sometimes cauliflower shaped. The warts can appear within weeks or months of sexual contact with an infected person. Cytologic changes indicating HPV infection **(koilocytotic cells)** are detected in **Papanicolaou-stained cervical smears** (Pap smears) (Figure 41-7). Infection of the female genital tract by high-risk HPV types is associated with intraepithelial cervical neoplasia and cancer. The first neoplastic changes noted on light microscopy are termed **dysplasia.** Approximately 40% to 70% of the mild dysplasias spontaneously regress.

Cervical cancer is thought to develop through a continuum of progressive cellular changes from mild (cervical intraepithelial neoplasia [CIN I]) to moderate neoplasia (CIN II) to severe neoplasia or carcinoma in situ (see Figure 41-5). This sequence of events can occur over 1 to 4 years. Routine and regular Pap smears can promote early detection, treatment, and cure of cervical cancer.

Laboratory Diagnosis

A wart can be confirmed microscopically on the basis of its characteristic histologic appearance, which consists of

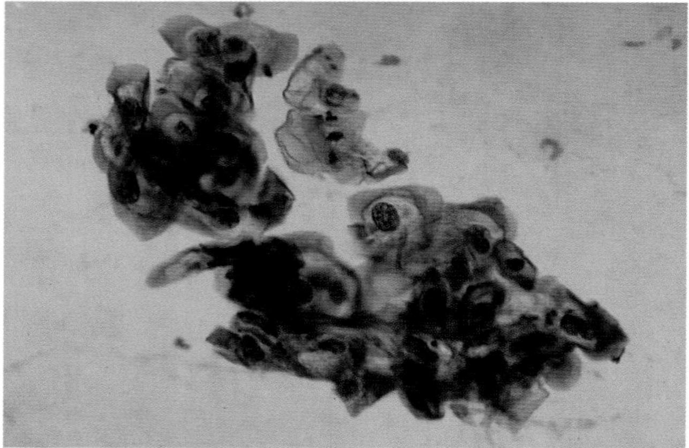

FIGURE 41-7 Papanicolaou stain of exfoliated cervicovaginal squamous epithelial cells, showing the perinuclear cytoplasmic vacuolization termed *koilocytosis* (vacuolated cytoplasm), which is characteristic of human papillomavirus infection (400× magnification).

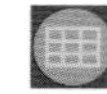

Table 41-3 Laboratory Diagnosis of Papillomavirus Infections

Test	Detects
Cytology	Koilocytotic cells
In situ DNA probe analysis*	Viral nucleic acid
Polymerase chain reaction*	Viral nucleic acid
Real-time PCR	Viral nucleic acid
Southern blot hybridization	Viral nucleic acid
Culture	Not useful

*Method of choice.

hyperplasia of the **prickle cells** and an excess production of keratin **(hyperkeratosis)** (see Figure 41-7). Papillomavirus infection can be detected in Pap smears by the presence of koilocytotic (vacuolated cytoplasm) squamous epithelial cells, which are rounded and occur in clumps (Table 41-3; see Figure 41-4). **DNA molecular probe, polymerase chain reaction (PCR), and real-time PCR** analysis of cervical swabs and tissue specimens are the methods of choice for establishing the diagnosis and typing of the HPV infection. Papillomaviruses do not grow in cell cultures, and tests for HPV antibodies are rarely used except in research studies.

Treatment, Prevention, and Control

Warts spontaneously regress, but the regression may take many months to years. Warts are removed because of pain and discomfort, for cosmetic reasons, and to prevent spread to other parts of the body or to other people. They are removed through the use of surgical cryotherapy, electrocautery, or chemical means (e.g., 10% to 25% solution of podophyllin), although recurrences are common. Surgery may be necessary for the removal of laryngeal papillomas.

Stimulators of innate and inflammatory responses, such as **imiquimod** (Aldara), **interferon,** and even stripping off duct tape, can promote more rapid healing. Topical or intralesional delivery of **cidofovir** can treat warts by selectively killing the HPV-infected cells. Cidofovir induces apoptosis by inhibiting the host cell DNA polymerase.

Immunization with a tetravalent (Gardasil: HPV-6, -11, -16, and -18), a nine-valent (Gardasil 9: 6, 11, 16, 18, 31, 33, 45, 52, and 58), or divalent (Cervarix: HPV-16 and -18) HPV vaccine is recommended for girls and boys starting at age 11 years—before sexual activity—to prevent cervical cancer and penile and anogenital warts. The vaccines consist of the L1 major capsid protein assembled into virus-like particles. Vaccinated women are not protected against all possible HPV strains. The HPV vaccine **is not a replacement for a Pap smear,** and women should continue to be tested. At present, the best way to prevent transmission of warts is to avoid coming in direct contact with infected tissue. Proper precautions (e.g., use of condoms) can prevent sexual transmission of HPV.

• Polyomaviridae

The human polyomaviruses, **BKV** and **JCV,** are ubiquitous but usually do not cause disease. Less prevalent human polyomaviruses include the KI, WU, and Merkel cell polyomaviruses. The human viruses are difficult to grow in cell culture. SV40 (a simian polyomavirus) and murine polyomaviruses, in particular, have been studied extensively as models of tumor-causing viruses, but only recently has a polyomavirus been associated with human cancers.

Structure and Replication

The polyomaviruses are smaller (45 nm in diameter), contain less nucleic acid (5000 base pairs), and are less complex than the papillomaviruses (see Box 41-1). The genomes of BKV, JCV, and SV40 are closely related and are divided into early, late, and noncoding regions (Figure 41-8). The early region on one strand codes for nonstructural **T (transformation) proteins** (including **large T, T′, and small t antigens**), and the late region, which is on the other strand, codes for **three viral capsid proteins (VP1, VP2,** and **VP3)** (Box 41-4). The noncoding region contains the origin of DNA replication and transcriptional control sequences for both early and late genes.

For JCV infection of glial cells, the virus binds to sialylated carbohydrates and serotonin receptors and then enters the cell by endocytosis. The DNA genome is uncoated and delivered to the nucleus. The early genes encode the large T and small t antigens, proteins that promote cell growth. Viral replication requires the transcriptional and DNA replication machinery provided by a growing cell. The large T antigens of SV40, BKV, and JCV have several functions. For example, the T antigen of SV40 binds to DNA and controls early and late gene transcription, as well as viral DNA replication. In addition, the T antigen binds to and inactivates the two major cellular growth-suppressor proteins, p53 and p105RB, promoting cell growth.

Similar to replication of the HPVs, replication of polyomavirus is highly dependent on host cell factors. Permissive cells allow the transcription of late viral messenger ribonucleic acid (mRNA) and viral replication, which results in cell

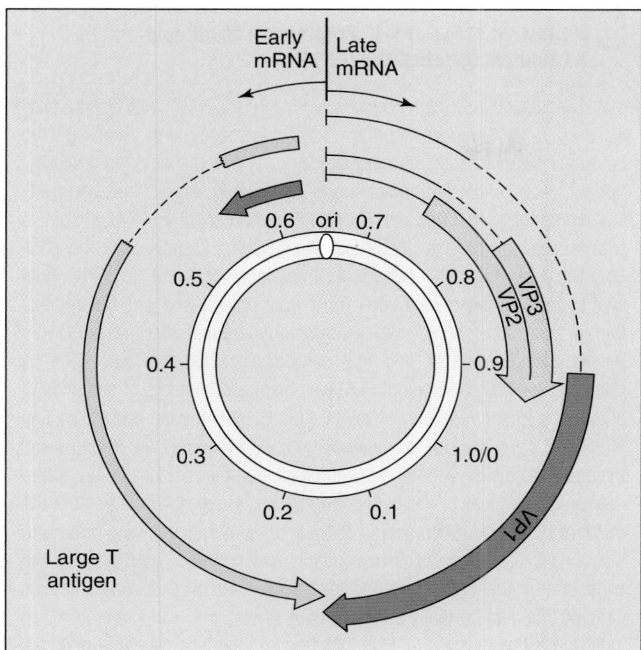

FIGURE 41-8 Genome of the SV40 virus. The genome is a prototype of other polyomaviruses and contains early, late, and noncoding regions. The noncoding region contains the start sequence for the early and late genes and for DNA replication *(ori)*. The individual early and late mRNAs are processed from the larger nested transcripts. (Modified from Butel JS, Jarvis DL: The plasma-membrane-associated form of SV40 large tumor antigen: biochemical and biological properties, *Biochim Biophys Acta* 865:171–195, 1986.)

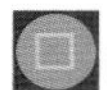 **Box 41-4 Polyomavirus Proteins**

Early

Large T: regulation of early and late messenger RNA transcription; DNA replication; cell growth promotion and transformation

Small t: viral DNA replication

Late

VP1: major capsid protein and viral attachment protein

VP2: minor capsid protein

VP3: minor capsid protein

death. The virus establishes latency in non-permissive cells (replication blocked by immune factors). Some animal cells allow only the early genes, including the T antigen, to be expressed, promoting cell growth and potentially leading to oncogenic transformation of the cell.

The polyomavirus genome is used very efficiently. The noncoding region of the genome contains the initiation sites for the early and late mRNAs and the origin of DNA replication. The three late proteins are produced from mRNAs, which have the same initiation site and then are processed into three unique mRNAs.

The circular viral DNA is maintained and replicated bidirectionally, similar to the way a bacterial plasmid is maintained and replicated. DNA replication precedes late mRNA transcription and protein synthesis. The virus is assembled in the nucleus, and virus is released by cell lysis.

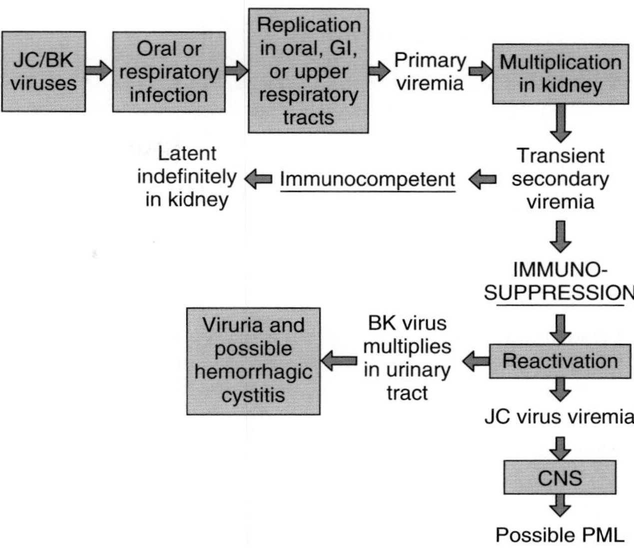

FIGURE 41-9 Mechanisms of spread of polyomaviruses within the body. *CNS,* Central nervous system; *GI,* gastrointestinal; *PML,* progressive multifocal leukoencephalopathy.

Pathogenesis

Each polyomavirus is limited to specific hosts and cell types within that host. For example, JCV and BKV are human viruses that probably enter the respiratory tract or tonsils, after which they infect lymphocytes and then the kidney with a minimal cytopathologic effect. BKV establishes latent infection in the kidney, and JCV establishes infection in the kidneys, B cells, monocyte-lineage cells, and other cells. Replication is blocked in immunocompetent persons.

In T-cell–deficient patients, such as those with the acquired immunodeficiency syndrome (AIDS), reactivation of the virus in the kidney leads to viral shedding in the urine and potentially severe urinary tract infections (BKV) or viremia and central nervous system infection (JCV) (Figure 41-9). JCV crosses the blood-brain barrier by replicating in the endothelial cells of capillaries. An abortive infection of astrocytes results in partial transformation, yielding enlarged cells with abnormal nuclei resembling glioblastomas. Productive lytic infections of oligodendrocytes cause demyelination (see Box 41-3). Although SV40, BKV, and JCV can cause tumors in hamsters, these viruses are not associated with any human tumors. Integration and inactivation of a function of the T antigen of the Merkel cell polyomavirus allows this virus to convert the Merkel cell into a tumor.

Epidemiology

Polyomavirus infections are ubiquitous, and most people are infected with both JCV and BKV by the age of 15 years (see Box 41-3). The viruses are spread in urine, in feces, and potentially in aerosols. Latent infections can be reactivated in people whose immune systems are suppressed because of AIDS, organ transplantation, or pregnancy. Approximately 10% of people with AIDS develop PML, and the disease is fatal in approximately 90% of all cases. The incidence has

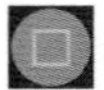 **Box 41-5 Clinical Summaries**

Wart: A 22-year-old patient develops a conical, flesh-colored, hard, scaly round area (papule) over the index finger. It has a rough surface and is nontender. Otherwise, the patient is healthy and has no other complaints. The wart is treated topically on a daily basis with salicylic acid to kill the cells harboring the virus and remove the wart.

Cervical papilloma: On cervical examination, a large, flat papule was observed, which turned white with application of 4% acetic acid. The Pap smear from this 25-year-old sexually active woman had koilocytotic cells.

Cervical carcinoma: A 32-year-old woman comes in for her routine Pap smear, which shows evidence of abnormal cells. A biopsy shows squamous cell carcinoma. PCR analysis of cellular DNA yields HPV-16 DNA.

Progressive multifocal leukoencephalopathy (PML): A 42-year-old AIDS patient has become forgetful and has difficulty speaking, seeing, and keeping his balance, which is suggestive of lesions in many sites in the brain. The condition progresses to paralysis and death. Autopsy shows foci of demyelination, with oligodendrocytes containing inclusion bodies only in the white matter.

A 37-year-old woman with multiple sclerosis was treated with natalizumab and interferon-β and developed PML.

AIDS, Acquired immunodeficiency syndrome; *Pap,* Papanicolaou; *PCR,* polymerase chain reaction.

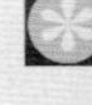 **Clinical Case 41-1 Progressive Multifocal Leukoencephalopathy (PML)**

Liptai and associates (*Neuropediatrics* 38:32–35, 2007) described a case in which a 15½-year-old human immunodeficiency virus (HIV)–infected boy presented with fatigue and depression. Symptoms included dizziness, double vision, and loss of motor coordination, as indicated in his handwriting, computer usage, and unsteady gait. He had acquired HIV by injection with an unclean syringe needle as an infant in a Transylvanian hospital. Over the years, his CD4 T-cell count slowly decreased, and his HIV genome load increased, most likely because of poor compliance with his anti-HIV therapy and a refusal of highly active antiretroviral therapy. A 30-mm nonenhancing lesion of the right cerebellar hemisphere was seen by magnetic resonance imaging. PML was diagnosed, based on detection of JC virus sequences in cerebrospinal fluid by polymerase chain reaction. Within 10 days, the boy lost the ability to walk and developed facial and hypoglossal palsies, with further neurologic deterioration, including severe depression and loss of ability to communicate. He died 4 months after the onset of symptoms. Microscopic analysis of the cerebellum and brainstem indicated broad areas of demyelination and necrosis, astrocytosis, and oligodendrocytes with nuclear inclusion bodies. Although JC virus infection is ubiquitous and normally benign, it causes PML in immunocompromised individuals. Previously rare, PML has become more prevalent in acquired immunodeficiency syndrome patients who are not on or are not compliant with anti-HIV therapy or for whom anti-HIV therapy is ineffective.

decreased with the success of the highly active antiretroviral therapy (HAART).

Early batches of live attenuated polio vaccine were contaminated with SV40 that was undetected in the primary monkey cell cultures used to prepare the vaccine. Although many people were vaccinated with the contaminated vaccines, no SV40-related tumors have been reported.

Clinical Syndromes (Box 41-5)

Primary infection is almost always asymptomatic. BKV and JCV are activated in immunocompromised patients, as indicated by the presence of virus in the urine of as many as 40% of these patients. The viruses are also reactivated during pregnancy, but no effects on the fetus have been noted. During pregnancy, cell-mediated immunity, including those activities that restrict the replication of polyomaviruses, are suppressed so that the fetus (a tissue graft) is not rejected.

The ureteral stenosis observed in renal transplant recipients appears to be associated with BKV, as is the hemorrhagic cystitis observed in bone marrow transplant recipients. **PML** caused by **JCV** is a subacute demyelinating disease that occurs in immunocompromised patients, including those with AIDS (Clinical Case 41-1). Immunotherapy that inhibits the α4-integrin adhesion protein (natalizumab) also increases risk for PML. Although rare, the incidence of PML has increased because of the increased numbers of people with AIDS and immunosuppressive therapy. As the name implies, patients may have multiple neurologic symptoms unattributable to a single anatomic lesion. Speech, vision, coordination, mentation, or a combination of these functions is impaired, followed by paralysis of the arms and legs and finally death. People who are diagnosed with PML live 1 to 4 months, and most die within 2 years.

The genome of a new polyomavirus, Merkel cell polyomavirus (MCV or MCPyV), was recently discovered integrated into the chromatin of Merkel cell carcinomas, a highly aggressive type of skin cancer. This is the first example of a polyomavirus associated with a human cancer.

Laboratory Diagnosis

The diagnosis of PML is confirmed by the presence of PCR-amplified viral DNA in cerebrospinal fluid and magnetic resonance imaging or computed tomographic evidence of lesions. Histologic examination of brain tissue obtained by biopsy or at autopsy will show foci of demyelination surrounded by oligodendrocytes with inclusions adjacent to areas of demyelination. The term *leukoencephalopathy* refers to the presence of lesions in only the white matter. There is little if any inflammatory cell response. In situ immunofluorescence, immunoperoxidase, DNA probe analysis, and PCR analysis of cerebrospinal fluid, urine, or biopsy material for the particular genetic sequences can also be used to detect virus. Urine cytologic tests can reveal the presence of JCV or BKV infection by revealing the existence of enlarged cells with dense basophilic intranuclear inclusions resembling those induced by cytomegalovirus. It is difficult to isolate BKV and JCV in tissue cultures; therefore this procedure is not attempted.

Treatment, Prevention, and Control

As for papillomaviruses, cidofovir can be used to treat polyomavirus infections. Decreasing the immunosuppression responsible for allowing the polyomavirus to be reactivated is also helpful. The ubiquitous nature of polyomaviruses and the lack of understanding of their modes of transmission make it unlikely that the primary infection can be prevented.

Bibliography

Arthur RR, Shah KV, Baust SJ, et al: Association of BK viruria with hemorrhagic cystitis in recipients of bone marrow transplants, *N Engl J Med* 315:230–234, 1986.

Carter J, Saunders V: *Virology: principles and applications*, Chichester, England, 2007, Wiley.

Chow LT, Broker TR: Human papillomavirus infections: warts or cancer? *Cold Spring Harb Perspect Biol* 5(7):a012997, 2013.

Cohen J, Powderly WG: *Infectious diseases*, ed 2, St Louis, 2004, Mosby.

Collier L, Oxford J: *Human virology*, ed 3, Oxford, 2006, Oxford University Press.

de Villiers EM, Fauquet C, Broker TR, et al: Classification of papillomaviruses, *Virology* 324:17–24, 2004.

Feng H, Shuda M, Chang Y, et al: Clonal integration of a polyomavirus in human Merkel cell carcinoma, *Science* 319:1096–1100, 2008.

Ferenczy A, Franco EL: Prophylactic human papillomavirus vaccines: potential for sea change, *Expert Rev Vaccines* 6:511–525, 2007.

Flint SJ, Enquist LW, Racaniello VR, et al: *Principles of virology: molecular biology, pathogenesis, and control of animal viruses*, ed 3, Washington, DC, 2009, American Society for Microbiology Press.

Franco EL, Harper DM: Vaccination against human papillomavirus infection: a new paradigm in cervical cancer control, *Vaccine* 23:2388–2394, 2005.

Gorbach SL, Bartlett JG, Blacklow NR: *Infectious diseases*, ed 3, Philadelphia, 2004, WB Saunders.

Howley PM: Role of the human papillomaviruses in human cancer, *Cancer Res* 51(Suppl 18):5019S–5022S, 1991.

Hseuh C, Reyes CV: Progressive multifocal leukoencephalopathy, *Am Fam Physician* 37:129–132, 1988.

Knipe DM, Howley PM, Griffin DE, et al: *Fields virology*, ed 5, Philadelphia, 2006, Lippincott Williams & Wilkins.

Major EO: Progressive multifocal leukoencephalopathy in patients on immunomodulatory therapies, *Annu Rev Med* 61:35–47, 2010.

Major EO, Amemiya K, Tornatore CS, et al: Pathogenesis and molecular biology of progressive multifocal leukoencephalopathy, *Clin Microbiol Rev* 5:49–73, 1992.

Mandell GL, Bennet JE, Dolin R: *Principles and practice of infectious diseases*, ed 6, Philadelphia, 2005, Churchill Livingstone.

Miller DM, Brodell RT: Human papillomavirus infection: treatment options for warts, *Am Fam Physician* 53:135–143, 1996.

Morrison EA: Natural history of cervical infection with human papillomavirus, *Clin Infect Dis* 18:172–180, 1994.

Raff AB, Woodham AW, Raff LM, et al: The evolving field of human papillomavirus receptor research: a review of binding and entry, *J Virol* 87(11):6062–6072, 2013.

Siddiqui MA, Perry CM: Human papillomavirus quadrivalent (types 6, 11, 16, 18) recombinant vaccine (Gardasil), *Drugs* 66:1263–1271, 2006.

Spence AR, Franco EL, Fetenczy A: The role of human papillomaviruses in cancer, *Am J Cancer* 4:49–64, 2005.

Strauss JM, Strauss EG: *Viruses and human disease*, ed 2, San Diego, 2007, Academic.

Voyles BA: *The biology of viruses*, ed 2, Boston, 2002, McGraw-Hill.

White DO, Fenner FJ: *Medical virology*, ed 4, New York, 1994, Academic.

Woodman CBJ, Collins SI, Young LS: The natural history of cervical HPV infection: unresolved issues, *Nat Rev Cancer* 7:11–22, 2007.

Zhi-Ming Zheng Z-M, Baker CC: Papillomavirus genome structure, expression, and post-transcriptional regulation, *Front Biosci* 11:2286–2302, 2006.

zür-Hausen H: Viruses in human cancers, *Science* 254:1167–1173, 1991.

Websites

National Cancer Institute: Pap test results. www.cancer.gov/cancertopics/understanding-cervical-changes/test-results. Accessed June 10, 2015.

Centers for Disease Control and Prevention: Human papillomavirus (HPV). www.cdc.gov/std/HPV/. Accessed June 10, 2015.

Centers for Disease Control and Prevention: Human papillomavirus (HPV). www.cdc.gov/hpv/. Accessed June 10, 2015.

Gearhart PA, Randall TC, Buckley RM, et al: Human papillomavirus. http://emedicine.medscape.com/article/219110-overview. Accessed June 10, 2015.

Merck: Gardasil. www.gardasil.com/. Accessed June 10, 2015.

Merck: Gardasil 9. www.gardasil9.com/. Accessed June 10, 2015.

National Institute of Allergy and Infectious Diseases: Human papillomavirus (HPV) and genital warts. www.niaid.nih.gov/topics/genitalwarts/pages/default.aspx. Accessed June 10, 2015.

CHAPTER

42 ADENOVIRUSES

A 19-year-old army recruit complained that he had a high fever, chills, cough, runny nose, and sore throat. Several other members of his unit complained of similar symptoms.

1. How is adenovirus transmitted?
2. Which adenovirus types are most likely to cause acute respiratory distress syndrome?
3. What other diseases can adenoviruses cause?
4. What type of immune response would protect against infection?
5. Why did the military develop an attenuated vaccine for adenovirus strains 4 and 7?

Answers to these questions are available on StudentConsult.com.

• SUMMARIES CLINICALLY SIGNIFICANT ORGANISMS

Adenoviruses

Trigger Words

Pharyngitis, conjunctivitis, atypical pneumonia, icosadeltahedral capsid

Biology, Virulence, and Disease

- Medium-sized icosadeltahedral capsid with fibers, linear DNA genome with terminal proteins
- E1A and E1B proteins inactivate E6 and E7 to promote growth
- Virus encodes polymerase
- Capsid virus resistant to inactivation
- Lytic virus
- Causes pharyngitis, conjunctivitis, atypical pneumonia, infantile gastroenteritis, acute respiratory disease
- Can be used as vector for making vaccines

Epidemiology

- Transmitted by aerosols, direct contact, fecal-oral, contaminated swimming pools

Diagnosis

- Immunological assays and PCR genome analysis

Treatment, Prevention, and Control

- Adenovirus types 4 and 7 vaccine only for military

Adenoviruses were first isolated in 1953 in a human adenoid cell culture. Since then, approximately 100 serotypes have been recognized, at least 52 of which infect humans. All human serotypes are included in a single genus within the family Adenoviridae. There are 7 subgroups for human adenoviruses (A through G) (Table 42-1). The viruses in each subgroup share many properties.

The first human adenoviruses to be identified, numbered 1 to 7, are the most common. Common disorders caused by the adenoviruses include **respiratory tract infection, pharyngoconjunctivitis (pinkeye), hemorrhagic cystitis,** and **gastroenteritis.** Several adenoviruses have oncogenic potential in animals but not humans, and for this reason have been extensively studied by molecular biologists. These studies have elucidated many viral and eukaryotic cellular processes. For example, analysis of the gene for the adenovirus hexon protein led to the discovery of introns and the splicing of eukaryotic messenger ribonucleic acid (mRNA). Adenovirus is also being used in genetic therapies to deliver deoxyribonucleic acid (DNA) for gene replacement and modification therapy (e.g., cystic fibrosis), to express genes for other viruses (e.g., human immunodeficiency virus [HIV]) as a vaccine, and as oncolytic therapy.

• Structure and Replication

Adenoviruses are double-stranded DNA viruses with a genome of approximately 36,000 base pairs, large enough to encode 30 to 40 genes. The adenovirus genome is a **linear double-stranded DNA** with a **terminal protein** (molecular mass, 55 kDa) covalently attached at each 5′ end. The virions

Table 42-1 Illnesses Associated with Adenoviruses

Disease	Types	Patient Population
Respiratory Diseases		
Febrile, undifferentiated upper respiratory tract infection	1, 3, 5, 7, 14, 21, etc.	Infants, young children
Pharyngoconjunctival fever	1, 2, 3, 4, 5, 7	Children, adults
Acute respiratory disease	1, 2, 4, 5, 6, 7, 14, 21	Infants, young children, military recruits
Pertussis-like syndrome	5	Infants, young children
Pneumonia	3, 4, 7, 14, 21, 30	Infants, young children, military recruits, immunocompromised patients
Other Diseases		
Acute hemorrhagic cystitis/nephritis	11, 21	Children, immunocompromised patients
Epidemic keratoconjunctivitis	8, 9, 11, 19, 35, 37	Any age
Gastroenteritis	40, 41	Infants, young children, immunocompromised patients
Hepatitis	1-5, 7, 31	Immunocompromised patients
Meningoencephalitis	2, 7	Children, immunocompromised patients

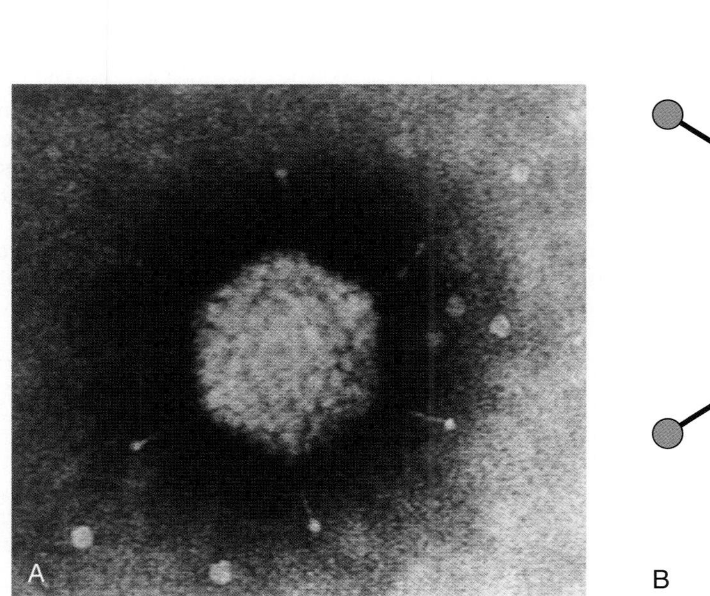

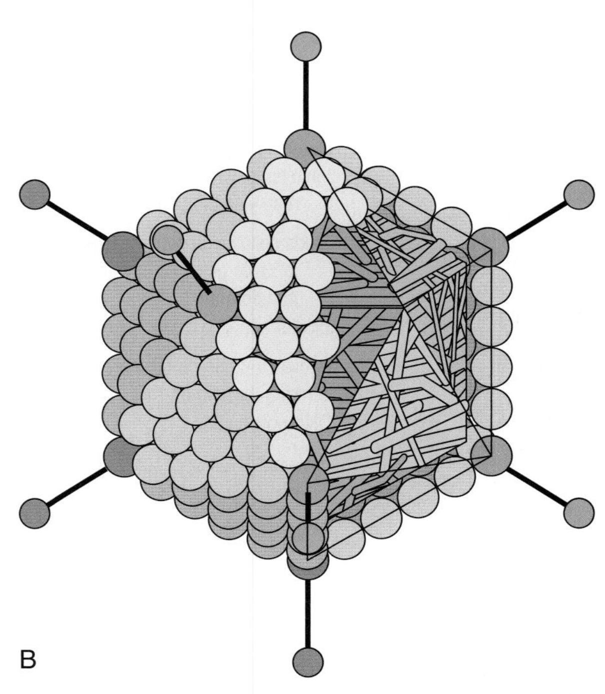

FIGURE 42-1 **A,** Electron micrograph of adenovirus virion with fibers. **B,** Model of adenovirus virion with fibers. (**A,** From Valentine RC, Pereira HG: Antigens and structure of the adenovirus, *J Mol Biol* 13:13–20, 1965. **B,** From Cohen J, Powderly WG, Opal SM: *Infectious diseases,* ed 3, Philadelphia, 2010, Mosby.)

have a unique structure. The **nonenveloped icosadeltahedral capsid** comprises 240 capsomeres that consist of hexons and pentons and has a diameter of 70 to 90 nm (Figure 42-1 and Box 42-1). The 12 pentons, which are located at each of the vertices, have a penton base and a fiber. The **fiber** contains the **viral attachment proteins.** The penton base and fiber are toxic to cells. The pentons and fibers also carry type-specific antigens.

The core complex within the capsid includes viral DNA and at least two major proteins. There are at least 11 proteins in the adenovirus virion, 9 of which have an identified structural function (Table 42-2).

The virus replication cycle takes approximately 32 to 36 hours and produces approximately 10,000 virions. Attachment of the viral fiber proteins to a glycoprotein member of the immunoglobulin superfamily of proteins (≈100,000 fiber receptors are present on each cell) initiates infection for most adenoviruses. This same receptor is used by many coxsackievirus B viruses; thus it is given the name **coxsackie adenovirus receptor.** Some adenoviruses use the class I major

Box 42-1 Unique Features of Adenovirus

Naked icosadeltahedral capsid has **fibers** (viral attachment proteins) at vertices.
Linear double-stranded genome has 5′ terminal proteins.
Synthesis of viral DNA polymerase activates a switch from early to late genes.
Virus encodes its own **DNA polymerase** and other proteins to facilitate growth and immune escape.
Human adenoviruses are grouped A through G by DNA homologies and by serotype (>55 human types).
Serotype is mainly a result of differences in the penton base and fiber protein, which determine the nature of tissue tropism and disease.
Virus causes **lytic, persistent,** and **latent** infections in humans, and some strains can **immortalize certain animal cells.**

Table 42-2 Major Adenovirus Proteins

Gene	Number	Molecular Mass (kDa)	Functions of Proteins
*E1A**			Activates viral gene transcription Binds cellular growth suppressor (p105RB) to promote cell growth and transformation Deregulates cell growth Inhibits activation of interferon response elements
E1B			Binds cellular growth suppressor (p53) to promote cell growth and transformation Blocks apoptosis
E2			Activates some promoters Terminal protein on DNA DNA polymerase
E3			Prevents TNF-α action; MHC I expression
E4			Limits viral cytopathologic effect
VA RNAs			Inhibits interferon response
Capsid	II	120	Contains family antigen and some serotyping antigens
	III	85	Penton base protein Toxic to tissue culture cells
	IV	62	Fiber Responsible for attachment; contains some serotyping antigens
	VI	24	Hexon-associated proteins
	VIII	13	Penton-associated proteins
	IX	12	"Capsid cement" nonessential
	IIIa	66	"Facilitates assembly"
Core	V	48	Core protein 1: DNA-binding protein
	VII	18	Core protein 2: DNA-binding protein

E, Early; *MHC I,* major histocompatibility complex I; *RB,* retinoblastoma gene product; *TNF-α,* tumor necrosis factor-α; *VA,* virus-associated.

*Early genes encode several messenger RNAs and proteins by alternative splicing patterns.

histocompatibility complex (MHC I) molecule as a receptor. Internalization is initiated by interaction of the penton base with an α_v integrin followed by receptor-mediated endocytosis in a clathrin-coated vesicle. The virus lyses the endosomal vesicle, and the capsid delivers the DNA genome to the nucleus. The penton and fiber proteins of the capsid are toxic to the cell and can inhibit cellular macromolecular synthesis.

A map of the adenovirus genome shows the locations of the viral genes (Figure 42-2). The genes are transcribed from both DNA strands and in both directions at different times during the replication cycle. Genes for related functions are clustered together. Most of the RNA transcribed from the adenovirus genome is processed into several individual mRNAs in the nucleus. Adenovirus encodes its own DNA polymerase and proteins that promote cell growth and suppress apoptosis and host immune and inflammatory responses.

Transcription of mRNA occurs in two phases. Early proteins promote cell growth and include a DNA polymerase that is involved in the replication of the genome. As for the papovaviruses, several adenovirus mRNAs are transcribed from the same promoter and share initial sequences but are produced through the splicing out of different introns. Transcription of the early *E1* gene, processing of the primary transcript (splicing out of introns to yield three mRNAs), and translation of the immediate early **E1A transactivator** protein are required for transcription of the early proteins. The early proteins include more DNA-binding proteins, the DNA polymerase, and proteins to help the virus escape the immune response. The **E1A** protein is also an oncogene, and together with the **E1B** protein, it can stimulate cell growth by binding to the cellular growth-suppressor proteins **p105RB** (*p105RB* retinoblastoma gene product) (E1A) and **p53** (E1B). In permissive cells, stimulation of cell division facilitates transcription and replication of the genome, with cell death resulting from virus replication. In nonpermissive cells, the virus

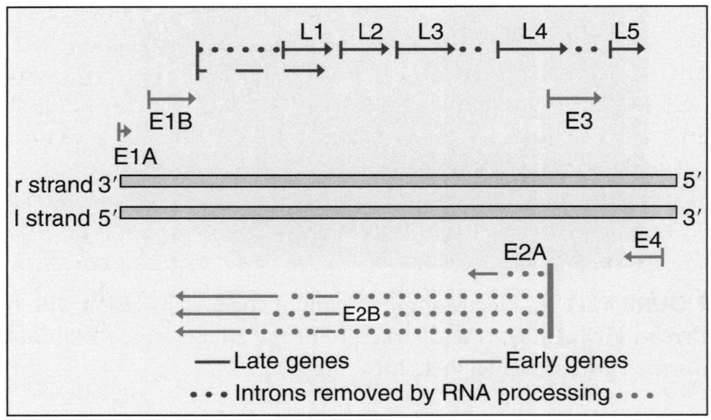

FIGURE 42-2 Simplified genome map of adenovirus type 2. Genes are transcribed from both strands (*l* and *r*) in opposite directions. The early genes are transcribed from four promoter sequences, and each generates several messenger RNAs by processing the primary RNA transcripts. This produces the full repertoire of viral proteins. The splicing pattern for only the E2 transcript is shown as an example. All of the late genes are transcribed from one promoter sequence. *E,* Early protein; *L,* late protein. (Modified from Jawetz E, Adelberg EA, Melnick JL: *Review of medical microbiology,* ed 17, Norwalk, Conn, 1987, Appleton & Lange.)

establishes latency, and the genome remains in the nucleus. For rodent, not human, cells, the E1A and E1B proteins may promote cell growth but without cell death, and therefore the virus oncogenically transforms the cell.

Viral DNA replication occurs in the nucleus and is mediated by the **viral-encoded DNA polymerase.** The polymerase uses the 55-kDa viral protein (terminal protein) with an attached cytosine monophosphate as a primer to replicate both strands of the DNA. The terminal protein remains attached to the DNA.

Late gene transcription starts after DNA replication. Most of the individual late mRNAs are generated from a large (83% of the genome) primary RNA transcript that is processed into individual mRNAs.

Capsid proteins are produced in the cytoplasm and then transported to the nucleus for viral assembly. Empty procapsids first assemble, and then the viral DNA and core proteins enter the capsid through an opening at one of the vertices. The replication and assembly processes are inefficient and prone to error, producing as few as one infectious unit per 2300 particles. DNA, protein, and numerous defective particles accumulate in nuclear inclusion bodies. The virus remains in the cell and is released when the cell degenerates and lyses.

• Pathogenesis and Immunity

Adenoviruses are capable of causing **lytic** (e.g., mucoepithelial cells), **latent** (e.g., lymphoid and adenoid cells), and **transforming** (hamster, not human) infections. These viruses initially infect epithelial cells lining the oropharynx, as well as the respiratory and enteric organs (Box 42-2). The viral fiber proteins determine the target cell specificity. The toxic activity of the penton base protein can result in inhibition of cellular mRNA transport and protein synthesis, cell rounding, and tissue damage.

The histologic hallmark of adenovirus infection is a dense, central intranuclear inclusion (that consists of viral DNA and protein) within an infected epithelial cell (Figure 42-3). These inclusions may resemble those seen in cells infected with cytomegalovirus, but adenovirus does not cause cellular enlargement (cytomegaly). Mononuclear cell infiltrates and epithelial cell necrosis are seen at the site of infection.

Viremia may occur after local replication of the virus, with subsequent spread to visceral organs (Figure 42-4). This dissemination is more likely to occur in immunocompromised patients than in immunocompetent ones. The virus has a propensity to become **latent and persist** in lymphoid and other tissue such as adenoids, tonsils, and Peyer patches and can be reactivated in immunosuppressed patients. Although certain adenoviruses (groups A and B) are **oncogenic in certain rodents,** adenovirus transformation of human cells has not been observed.

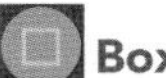

Box 42-2 Disease Mechanisms of Adenoviruses

- Virus is spread in **aerosols, in fecal matter,** and by **close contact.** Fingers spread virus to eyes.
- Virus infects **mucoepithelial cells** in the respiratory tract, gastrointestinal tract, and conjunctiva or cornea, causing cell damage directly.
- Disease is determined by the tissue tropism of the specific group or serotype of the virus strain.
- Virus **persists** in lymphoid tissue (e.g., tonsils, adenoids, Peyer patches).
- **Antibody** is important for prophylaxis and resolution, but cell-mediated immunity is also important.

Antibody is important for resolving lytic adenovirus infections and protects the person from reinfection with the same serotype but not other serotypes. Neutralizing antibody is directed at the fiber proteins. Cell-mediated immunity is important in limiting virus outgrowth, and immunosuppressed people suffer more serious and recurrent disease. Adenoviruses have several mechanisms to evade host defenses and help them persist in the host. They encode small virus-associated RNAs (VA RNAs) that prevent activation of the interferon-induced protein kinase R–mediated inhibition of viral protein synthesis. The viral E3 and E1A proteins block apoptosis induced by cellular responses to the virus or by T-cell or cytokine (e.g., tumor necrosis factor [TNF]-α) actions. Some strains of adenoviruses can inhibit $CD8^+$ cytotoxic T-cell action by preventing

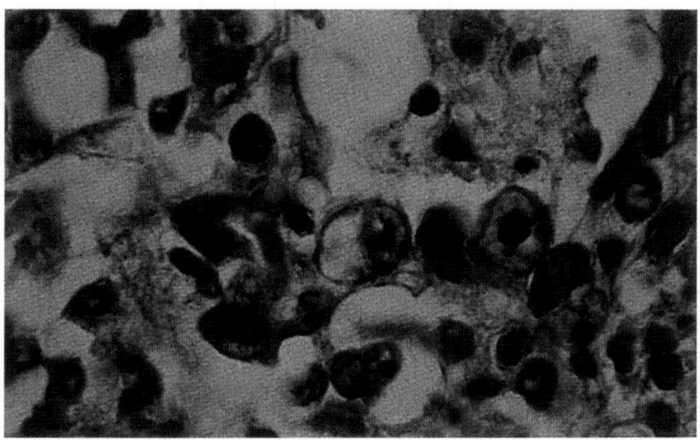

FIGURE 42-3 Histologic appearance of adenovirus-infected cells. Inefficient assembly of virions yields dark basophilic nuclear inclusion bodies containing DNA, proteins, and capsids.

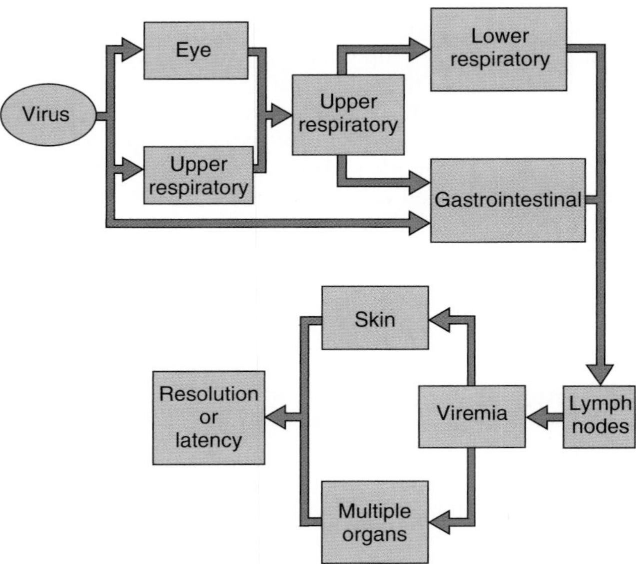

FIGURE 42-4 Mechanism of adenovirus spread within the body.

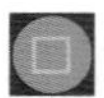

Box 42-3 Epidemiology of Adenoviruses

Disease/Viral Factors

Capsid virus is resistant to inactivation by gastrointestinal tract, drying, and detergents.

Disease symptoms may resemble those of other respiratory virus infections.

Virus may cause asymptomatic shedding.

Transmission

Direct contact, respiratory droplets and fecal matter on hands and fomites (e.g., towels, contaminated medical instruments), and inadequately chlorinated swimming pools and ponds

Who Is at Risk?

Children < 14 years of age

People in crowded areas (e.g., day-care centers, military training camps, swimming clubs)

Geography/Season

Virus is found worldwide.

There is no seasonal incidence.

Modes of Control

Live vaccine for serotypes 4 and 7 is available for military use.

proper expression of MHC I molecules and therefore antigen presentation.

• Epidemiology

Adenovirus virions resist drying, detergents, gastrointestinal tract secretions (acid, protease, and bile), and even mild chlorine treatment (Box 42-3). These virions are spread in aerosols and by the fecal-oral route, by fingers, by fomites (including towels and medical instruments), and in ponds or poorly chlorinated swimming pools. Crowds and close proximity, as occurs in classrooms and military barracks, promotes spread of the virus. Adenoviruses may be shed intermittently and over long periods from the pharynx and especially in feces. Most infections are asymptomatic, a feature that greatly facilitates their spread in the community.

Adenoviruses 1 through 7 are the most prevalent serotypes. From 5% to 10% of cases of pediatric respiratory tract disease are caused by adenovirus types 1, 2, 5, and 6, and the infected children shed virus for months after infection. Adenovirus causes 15% of the cases of gastroenteritis requiring hospitalization. Serotypes 4 and 7 seem especially able to spread among military recruits because of their close proximity and rigorous lifestyle.

• Clinical Syndromes (Box 42-4)

Adenoviruses primarily infect children and less commonly adults. Disease from reactivated virus occurs in immunocompromised children and adults. Specific clinical syndromes are associated with specific adenovirus types (see Table 42-1). The time course of adenovirus respiratory infection is shown in Figure 42-5.

Box 42-4 Clinical Summaries

Pharyngoconjunctival fever: A 7-year-old student develops sudden onset of red eyes, sore throat, and a fever of 38.9° C (102° F). Several children in the local elementary school have similar symptoms.

Gastroenteritis: An infant has diarrhea and is vomiting. Adenovirus serotype 41 is identified by polymerase chain reaction analysis of stool for epidemiologic reasons.

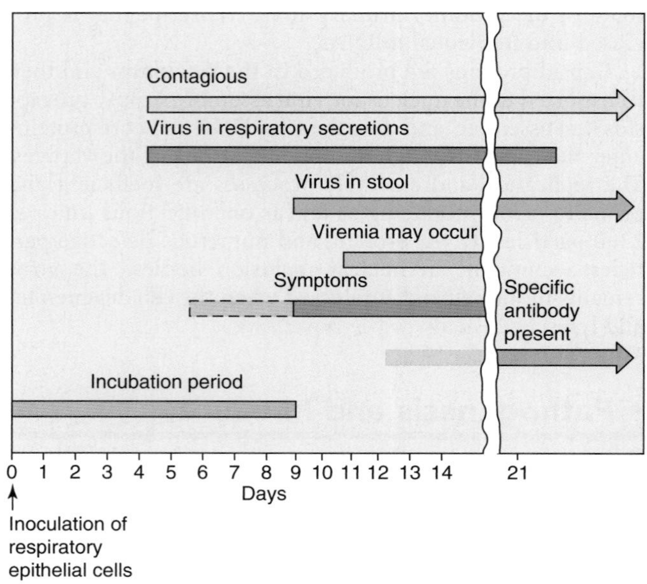

FIGURE 42-5 Time course of adenovirus respiratory infection.

Acute Febrile Pharyngitis and Pharyngoconjunctival Fever

Adenovirus causes **pharyngitis,** which is often accompanied by **conjunctivitis (pharyngoconjunctival fever).** Pharyngitis alone occurs in young children, particularly those younger than 3 years, and may mimic streptococcal infection. Affected patients have mild, flulike symptoms (including nasal congestion, cough, coryza, malaise, fever, chills, myalgia, and headache) that may last 3 to 5 days. Pharyngoconjunctival fever occurs more often in outbreaks involving older children.

Acute Respiratory Disease

Acute respiratory disease is a syndrome consisting of fever, runny nose, cough, pharyngitis, and possible conjunctivitis (Clinical Case 42-1). The high incidence of infection of military recruits stimulated the development and use of a vaccine for these serotypes.

Other Respiratory Tract Diseases

Adenoviruses cause coldlike symptoms, laryngitis, croup, and bronchiolitis. They can also cause a pertussis-like illness in children and adults that consists of a prolonged clinical course and true viral pneumonia.

Clinical Case 42-1 Pathogenic Adenovirus 14

The Centers for Disease Control and Prevention (*MMWR Morb Mortal Wkly Rep* 56:1181–1184, 2007) reported that analysis of isolates from trainees during an outbreak of febrile respiratory infection at Lackland Air Force Base showed 63% resulting from adenovirus, and 90% of these were adenovirus 14. Of the 423 cases, 27 were hospitalized with pneumonia, 5 required admission to the intensive care unit, and 1 patient died. In an analogous case reported by CNN (www.cnn.com/2007/HEALTH/conditions/12/19/killer.cold/index.html), an 18-year-old high school athlete complained of flulike symptoms with vomiting, chills, and fever of 104° F that progressed to life-threatening pneumonia within days. The adenovirus causing these infections is a mutant of the adenovirus 14 that was first identified in 1955. The adenovirus 14 mutant has spread around the United States, putting adults at risk for severe disease. Adenovirus 14 infection usually causes a benign respiratory infection in adults, with newborns and the elderly at higher risk for severe outcomes. Although most virus mutations produce a weaker virus, occasionally a more virulent antibody-escape or antiviral drug–resistant virus may occur.

Conjunctivitis and Epidemic Keratoconjunctivitis

Adenoviruses cause a follicular conjunctivitis (pinkeye) in which the mucosa of the palpebral conjunctiva becomes pebbled or nodular, and both conjunctivae (palpebral and bulbar) become inflamed (Figure 42-6). Such conjunctivitis may occur sporadically or in outbreaks that can be traced to a common source. Swimming pool conjunctivitis is a familiar example of a common-source adenovirus infection. Epidemic keratoconjunctivitis may be an occupational hazard for industrial workers. The most striking such epidemic occurred in people working in the naval shipyards of Pearl Harbor in Hawaii, where it caused more than 10,000 cases during 1941 and 1942. Irritation of the eye by a foreign body, dust, debris, and so forth is a risk factor for acquisition of this infection.

Gastroenteritis and Diarrhea

Adenovirus is a major cause of acute viral gastroenteritis, especially in infants. The enteric adenoviruses (types 40 to 42) do not replicate in the same tissue culture cells as do other adenoviruses and rarely cause fever or respiratory tract symptoms.

Other Manifestations

Adenovirus has also been associated with intussusception in young children, acute hemorrhagic cystitis with dysuria and hematuria in young boys, musculoskeletal disorders, and genital and skin infections. Adenovirus (type 36) is also associated with obesity.

Systemic Infection in Immunocompromised Patients

Immunocompromised patients are at risk for serious adenovirus infections, although not as much as they are for infections caused by herpesviruses. Adenoviral disease in immunocompromised patients includes pneumonia and hepatitis. Infection can originate from exogenous or endogenous (reactivation) sources.

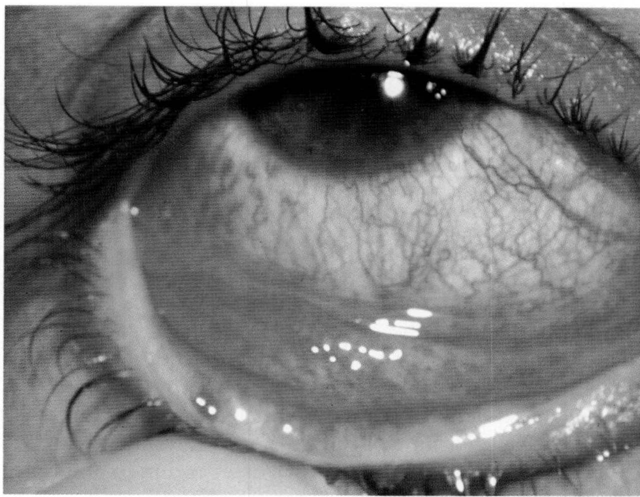

FIGURE 42-6 Conjunctivitis caused by adenovirus.

• Laboratory Diagnosis

For the results of virus isolation to be significant, the isolate should be obtained from a site or secretion relevant to the disease symptoms. The presence of adenovirus in the throat of a patient with pharyngitis is usually diagnostic if laboratory findings eliminate other common causes of pharyngitis, such as *Streptococcus pyogenes*.

Direct analysis of the clinical sample without virus isolation can be used for rapid detection and identification of adenoviruses. Immunoassays (e.g., fluorescent antibody and enzyme-linked immunosorbent assay) and genome assays (e.g., different variations of polymerase chain reaction [PCR] and DNA probe analysis) can be used to detect, type, and group the virus in clinical samples and tissue cultures. These approaches must be used for enteric adenovirus serotypes 40 to 42, which do not grow readily in available cell cultures. Serologic testing is rarely used except for epidemiologic purposes.

The isolation of most adenovirus types is best accomplished in cell cultures derived from epithelial cells (e.g., primary human embryonic kidney cells, continuous [transformed] lines, such as HeLa and human epidermal carcinoma cells). Within 2 to 20 days, the virus causes a lytic infection with characteristic inclusion bodies and cell death. Recovery of virus from cell culture requires an average of 6 days. The characteristic intranuclear inclusions can be seen in infected tissue during histologic examination. However, such inclusions are rare and must be distinguished from those produced by cytomegalovirus.

• Treatment, Prevention, and Control

Careful handwashing and chlorination of swimming pools can reduce transmission of adenovirus. There is no approved treatment for adenovirus infection, but cidofovir and ribavirin have been used to treat adenovirus-infected immunosuppressed individuals. Live oral vaccines have been used to prevent infections with adenovirus types 4 and 7 in military recruits but are not used in civilian populations.

Therapeutic Adenoviruses

Adenoviruses have been used and are being considered for gene delivery for correction of human diseases, including immune deficiencies (e.g., adenosine deaminase deficiency), cystic fibrosis, and lysosomal storage diseases. The virus is inactivated by deletion or mutation of the *E1* and other viral genes (e.g., *E2, E4*). The appropriate gene is inserted into the viral genome, replacing this DNA, and is controlled by an appropriate promoter. The resultant virus vector must be grown in a cell that expresses the missing viral functions (E1, E4) to complement the deficiency and allow production of virus. Types 4 and 7 and replication defective mutants of types 5, 26, and 35 are being developed to carry genes of HIV, Ebola, and other viruses as attenuated vaccines for these deadly viruses. For one of the latest innovations, T lymphocytes are infected with an adenovirus-encoding membrane-bound antibody to a surface cancer protein (chimeric antigen receptor [CAR]) to allow the T cells to recognize and attack the cancer. Adenoviruses lacking a functional *E1B* gene create a virus that selectively grows and kills tumor cells that lack p53 providing oncolytic therapy. Despite the genetically engineered attenuation, these viruses still may cause serious disease in immunocompromised individuals.

Bibliography

Balows A, Hausler WJ, Lennette EH: *Laboratory diagnosis of infectious diseases: principles and practice*, New York, 1988, Springer-Verlag.

Benihoud K, Yeh P, Perricaudet M: Adenovirus vectors for gene delivery, *Curr Opin Biotechnol* 10:440–447, 1999.

Cohen J, Powderly WG: *Infectious diseases*, ed 3, St Louis, 2004, Mosby.

Collier L, Oxford J: *Human virology*, ed 3, Oxford, 2006, Oxford University Press.

Doerfler W, Böhm P: Adenoviruses: model and vectors in virus-host interactions, *Curr Top Microbiol Immunol* (vol 272-273), New York, 2003, Springer-Verlag.

Flint SJ, Enquist LW, Racaniello VR, et al: *Principles of virology: molecular biology, pathogenesis, and control of animal viruses*, ed 3, Washington, DC, 2009, American Society for Microbiology Press.

Ginsberg HS: *The adenoviruses*, New York, 1984, Plenum.

Gorbach SL, Bartlett JG, Blacklow NR: *Infectious diseases*, ed 3, Philadelphia, 2004, WB Saunders.

Knipe DM, Howley PM: *Fields virology*, ed 6, Philadelphia, 2013, Lippincott Williams & Wilkins.

Kolavic-Gray SA, Binn LN, Sanchez JL, et al: Large epidemic of adenovirus type 4 infection among military trainees: epidemiological, clinical, and laboratory studies, *Clin Infect Dis* 35:808–818, 2002.

Lenaerts L, De Clercq E, Naesens L: Clinical features and treatment of adenovirus infections, *Rev Med Virol* 18:357–374, 2008.

Mandell GL, Bennet JE, Dolin R: *Principles and practice of infectious diseases*, ed 7, Philadelphia, 2010, Churchill Livingstone.

Robbins PD, Ghivizzani SC: Viral vectors for gene therapy, *Pharmacol Ther* 80:35–47, 1998.

Strauss JM, Strauss EG: *Viruses and human disease*, ed 2, San Diego, 2007, Academic.

Websites

National Cancer Institute: CAR T-cell therapy: engineering patients' immune cells to treat their cancers. www.cancer.gov/cancertopics/research-updates/2013/CAR-T-Cells. Accessed June 10, 2015.

Gompf SG, Kelkar D, Oehler R: Adenoviruses, 2014. http://emedicine.medscape.com/article/211738-overview. Accessed June 10, 2015.

CHAPTER

43 HUMAN HERPESVIRUSES

(a) A vesicular lesion erupts at the corner of a 27-year-old man's mouth 3 days after returning from a skiing trip.

(b) A 26-year-old pediatric medical resident develops serious pneumonia, and then vesicular lesions erupt in crops on his head, trunk, and elsewhere.

(c) Several high school cheerleaders developed a sore throat, fever, swollen glands, and were very tired. They shared a water bottle at a football game three weeks earlier.

(d) A 57-year-old heart transplant recipient had an outbreak of herpes simplex virus lesions, cytomegalovirus pneumonitis, and subsequently an Epstein-Barr virus–related lymphoma. The lymphoma resolved after immunosuppressive therapy was decreased.

1. Which viruses cause these diseases?
2. What features are similar/different for these viruses?
3. How were each of these infections obtained?
4. What are the risk factors for serious herpes disease?
5. Which of the infections can be prevented by vaccine or treated with antiviral drugs?

Answers to these questions are available on StudentConsult.com.

• SUMMARIES CLINICALLY SIGNIFICANT ORGANISMS

Herpesviruses

Trigger Words

HSV 1 and 2: neurotropic Cowdry type A inclusion bodies, syncytia, vesicle, Tzanck smear

VZV: neurotropic, (V) all stages of lesions, (Z) lesions along entire dermatome

EBV: B cell, heterophile-positive mononucleosis, Burkitt lymphoma

CMV: large cell and owl's eye inclusion body, opportunistic, mononucleosis, congenital disease

HHV-6: roseola

HHV-8: Kaposi sarcoma, AIDS-related disease

Biology, Virulence, and Disease

- Large, enveloped, containing icosadeltahedral capsid, DNA genome
- Encodes polymerase and other proteins (HSV and VZV: thymidine kinase)
- Cell-mediated immune response essential for control
- Lytic, latent, recurrent viruses; EBV and HHV-8 also associated with cancers
- HSV: oral/genital, encephalitis, keratoconjunctivitis, neonatal HSV; recurs from neurons
- VZV: pneumonia in adults, varicella, zoster; recurs from neurons
- EBV: heterophile-positive mononucleosis, B-cell lymphomas; recurs from memory B cell
- CMV: opportunistic disease, congenital CMV, retinitis
- HHV-6: roseola
- HHV-8: Kaposi sarcoma

Epidemiology

- Ubiquitous viruses
- Transmitted by direct contact, bodily fluids
- VZV transmitted by aerosol and direct contact

Diagnosis

- Culture, immunologic tests (EBV serology), PCR genome analysis

Treatment, Prevention, and Control

- Vaccine for VZV
- Antiviral drugs for HSV, VZV, and CMV

The herpesviruses are an important group of large deoxyribonucleic acid (DNA)–enveloped viruses with the following features in common: virion morphology, basic mode of replication, and capacity to establish latent and recurrent infections. Cell-mediated immunity is important for causing symptoms and controlling infection with these viruses. Herpesviruses encode proteins and enzymes that facilitate replication and interaction of the virus with the host. Epstein-Barr virus (EBV) and human herpesvirus 8 (HHV-8) are associated with human cancers (Box 43-1).

The human herpesviruses are grouped into three subfamilies on the basis of differences in viral characteristics (genome structure, tissue tropism, cytopathologic effect, and site of latent infection), as well as the pathogenesis of the disease and disease manifestation (Table 43-1). The human herpesviruses are herpes simplex viruses types 1 and 2 (HSV-1 and HSV-2), varicella-zoster virus (VZV), Epstein-Barr virus, cytomegalovirus (CMV), human herpesviruses 6 and 7 (HHV-6 and HHV-7), and the more recently discovered HHV-8, associated with Kaposi sarcoma.

Herpesvirus infections are common, and the viruses, except HHV-8, are **ubiquitous.** Although these viruses usually cause benign disease, especially in children, they can also cause significant morbidity and mortality, especially in immunosuppressed people. Fortunately, some herpesviruses encode targets for antiviral agents, and there is a live-virus vaccine for VZV.

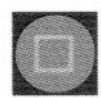

Box 43-1 Unique Features of Herpesviruses

- Herpesviruses have large, enveloped, icosadeltahedral capsids containing double-stranded DNA genomes.
- Herpesviruses encode many proteins that manipulate the host cell and immune response.
- Herpesviruses encode enzymes (DNA polymerase) that promote viral DNA replication and are good targets for antiviral drugs.
- DNA replication and capsid assembly occurs in the nucleus.
- Virus is released by exocytosis, by cell lysis, and through cell-to-cell bridges.
- Herpesviruses can cause lytic, persistent, latent, and (for Epstein-Barr virus) immortalizing infections.
- Herpesviruses are ubiquitous.
- Cell-mediated immunity is required for control.

Structure of Herpesviruses

The herpesviruses are **large, enveloped** viruses that contain **double-stranded DNA.** The virion is approximately 150 nm in diameter and has the characteristic morphology shown in Figure 43-1. The DNA core is surrounded by an **icosadeltahedral capsid** containing 162 capsomeres. This capsid is enclosed by a glycoprotein-containing envelope. Herpesviruses encode several glycoproteins for viral attachment, fusion, and escaping immune control. Attached to the capsid and in the space between the envelope and the capsid (the **tegument**) are viral proteins and enzymes that help initiate replication. As enveloped viruses, the herpesviruses are sensitive to acid, solvents, detergents, and drying.

Herpesviral genomes are linear, double-stranded DNA, but they differ in size and gene orientation (Figure 43-2). Direct or inverted repeat sequences bracket unique regions of the genome (unique long [U_L], unique short [U_S]), allowing circularization and recombination within the genome. Recombination among inverted repeats of HSV, CMV, and VZV allows large portions of the genome to flip the orientation of their U_L and U_S gene segments with respect to each other to form isomeric genomes.

Herpesvirus Replication

Herpesvirus replication is initiated by the interaction of viral glycoproteins with cell surface receptors (see Chapter 36, Figure 36-11). The tropism of some herpesviruses (e.g., EBV) is highly restricted because of the species and tissue-specific

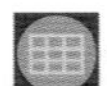

Table 43-1 Properties Distinguishing the Herpesviruses

Subfamily	Virus	Primary Target Cell	Site of Latency	Means of Spread
Alphaherpesvirinae				
HHV-1	Herpes simplex type 1	Mucoepithelial cells	Neuron	Close contact (STD)
HHV-2	Herpes simplex type 2	Mucoepithelial cells	Neuron	Close contact (STD)
HHV-3	Varicella-zoster virus	Mucoepithelial and T cells	Neuron	Respiratory and close contact
Gammaherpesvirinae				
HHV-4	Epstein-Barr virus	B cells and epithelial cells	B cell	Saliva (kissing disease)
HHV-8	Kaposi sarcoma–related virus	Lymphocytes and other cells	B cell	Close contact (sexual), saliva?
Betaherpesvirinae				
HHV-5	Cytomegalovirus	Monocytes, granulocytes, lymphocytes, and epithelial cells	Monocyte, myeloid stem cell, and ?	Close contact (STD), transfusions, tissue transplant, and congenital
HHV-6	Herpes lymphotropic virus	Lymphocytes and ?	T cell and ?	Saliva
HHV-7	HHV-7	Like HHV-6	T cell and ?	Saliva

HHV, Human herpesvirus; *STD,* sexually transmitted disease.
?, Indicates that other cells may also be the primary target or site of latency.

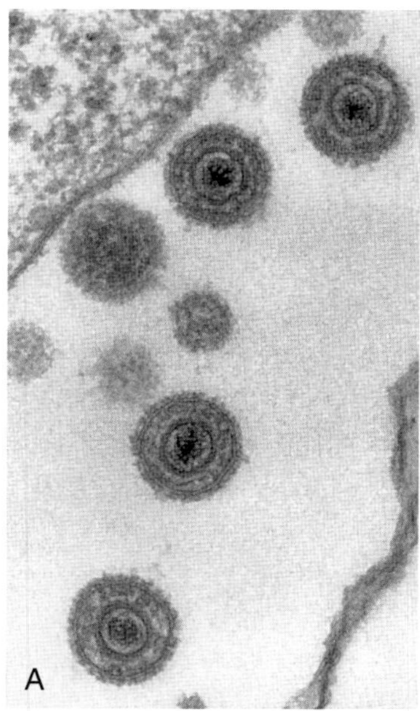

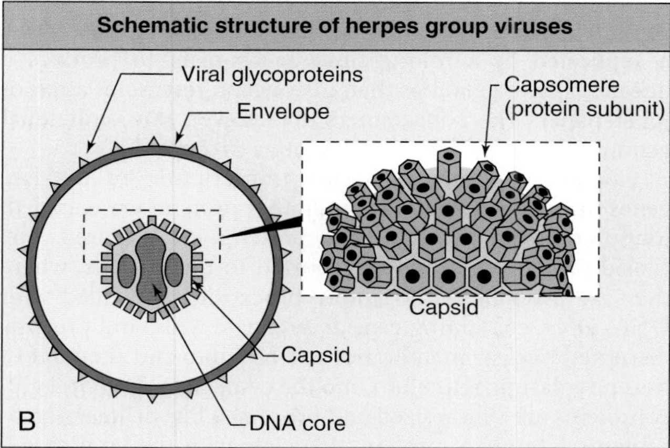

FIGURE 43-1 Electron micrograph (**A**) and general structure (**B**) of the herpesviruses. The DNA genome of the herpesvirus in the core is surrounded by an icosadeltahedral capsid and an envelope. Glycoproteins are inserted into the envelope. (**A,** From Cohen J, Powderly WG, Opal SM: *Infectious diseases,* ed 3, Philadelphia, 2010, Mosby.)

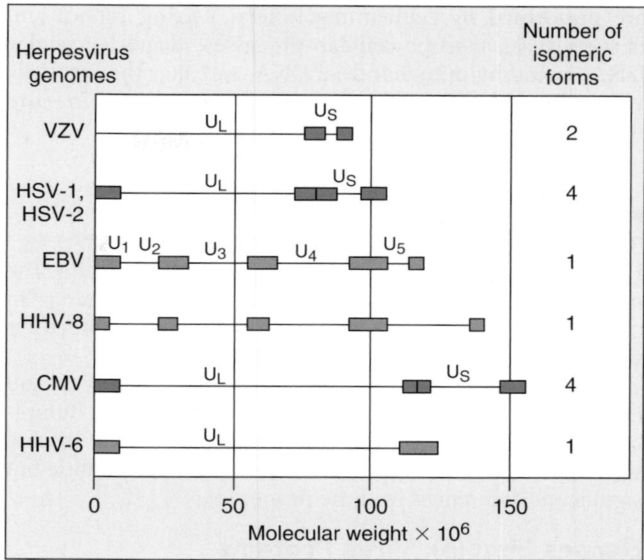

FIGURE 43-2 Herpesvirus genomes. The genomes of herpesviruses are doubled-stranded DNA. The length and complexity of the genome differ for each virus. Inverted repeats in herpes simplex virus *(HSV),* varicella-zoster virus *(VZV),* and cytomegalovirus *(CMV)* allow the genome to recombine with itself to form isomers. Large genetic repeat sequences are boxed. The genomes of HSV and CMV have two sections, the unique long *(U_L)* and the unique short *(U_S),* each of which is bracketed by two sets of inverted repeats of DNA. The inverted repeats facilitate the replication of the genome but also allow the U_L and U_S regions to invert independently of each other to yield four different genomic configurations, or isomers. VZV has only one set of inverted repeats and can form two isomers. Epstein-Barr virus *(EBV)* exists in only one configuration, with several unique regions surrounded by direct repeats. *Blue bars* indicate direct repeat DNA sequences; *green bars* indicate inverted repeated DNA sequences. *HHV-6,* Human herpesvirus 6; *HHV-8,* human herpesvirus 8.

expression of their receptors. The virus can fuse its envelope with the plasma membrane, releasing the nucleocapsid into the cytoplasm. Enzymes and transcription factors are carried into the cell in the tegument of the virion. The nucleocapsid docks with the nuclear membrane and delivers the genome into the nucleus, where the genome is transcribed and replicated.

Transcription of the viral genome and viral protein synthesis proceeds in a coordinated and regulated manner in three phases:

1. **Immediate early proteins (α),** consisting of proteins important for the regulation of gene transcription and takeover of the cell
2. **Early proteins (β),** consisting of more transcription factors and enzymes, including the DNA polymerase
3. **Late proteins (γ),** consisting mainly of structural proteins, which are generated after viral genome replication has begun

The viral genome is transcribed by the cellular DNA-dependent ribonucleic acid (RNA) polymerase and is regulated by viral-encoded and cellular nuclear factors. The interplay of these factors determines whether a lytic, persistent, or latent infection occurs. Cells that promote latent infection transcribe a special set of viral genes without genome replication. *Progression to early and late gene expression results in cell death and lytic infection.*

The **viral-encoded DNA polymerase,** which is a target of antiviral drugs, replicates the viral genome. **Viral-encoded scavenging enzymes** provide deoxyribonucleotide substrates for the polymerase. These and other viral enzymes facilitate replication of the virus in nongrowing cells that lack sufficient deoxyribonucleotides and enzymes for viral DNA synthesis (e.g., neurons). Other proteins manipulate cellular machinery to optimize replication, inhibit immune responses, and inhibit apoptosis or establish latency.

Empty procapsids assemble in the nucleus, are filled with DNA, bud into and out of the endoplasmic reticulum, acquire tegument-associated proteins and then an envelope at the Golgi membrane, and exit the cell by exocytosis or by lysis of the cell. Transcription, protein synthesis, glycoprotein processing, and exocytotic release from the cell are performed by cellular machinery. During replication, herpesviruses disrupt cellular processes, degrade cellular DNA, including mitochondrial DNA, and alter the cytoskeleton of the cells. The replication of HSV is discussed in more detail as the prototype of the herpesviruses.

• Herpes Simplex Virus

HSV was the first human herpesvirus to be recognized. The name *herpes* is derived from a Greek word meaning "to creep." "Cold sores" were described in antiquity, and their viral etiology was established in 1919.

The two types of herpes simplex viruses, HSV-1 and HSV-2, share many characteristics, including DNA homology, antigenic determinants, tissue tropism, and disease signs. However, they can still be distinguished by subtle but significant differences in these properties.

Herpes Simplex Virus Proteins

The HSV genome is large enough to encode approximately 80 proteins. Only half the proteins are required for viral replication; the others facilitate HSV's interaction with different host cells and the immune response. The HSV genome encodes enzymes that include a DNA-dependent DNA polymerase and scavenging enzymes such as deoxyribonuclease, thymidine kinase, ribonucleotide reductase, and protease. Ribonucleotide reductase converts ribonucleotides to deoxyribonucleotides, and thymidine kinase phosphorylates the deoxyribonucleosides to provide substrates for replication of the viral genome. The substrate specificities of these enzymes and the DNA polymerase differ significantly from those of their cellular analogs and thus represent potentially good targets for antiviral chemotherapy.

HSV encodes at least 10 glycoproteins that serve as viral attachment proteins (gB, gC, gD, gE/gI), fusion proteins (gB, gH/gL), structural proteins, immune escape proteins (gC, gE, gI), and other functions. For example, the C3 component of the complement system binds to gC and is depleted from serum. The Fc portion of immunoglobulin (Ig)G binds to a gE/gI complex, thereby camouflaging the virus and virus-infected cells. These actions reduce the antiviral effectiveness of antibody.

Replication

HSV can infect most types of human cells and even cells of other species. The virus generally causes lytic infections of fibroblasts and epithelial cells and latent infections of neurons (see Chapter 36, Figure 36-11, for a diagram).

HSV-1 binds quickly and efficiently to cells through an initial interaction with heparan sulfate, a proteoglycan found on the outside of many cell types, and then through a tighter interaction with receptor proteins at the cell surface. Penetration into the cell requires interaction with nectin-1 (herpesvirus entry mediator C), an intercellular adhesion molecule that is a member of the immunoglobulin protein family and similar to the poliovirus receptor. Nectin-1 is found on most cells and neurons. Another receptor is HveA, a member of the tumor necrosis factor receptor family that is expressed on activated T cells, neurons, and other cells. HSV can penetrate the host cell by fusion of its envelope with the cell surface membrane. On fusion, the virion releases its capsid into the cytoplasm, along with a protein that promotes the initiation of viral gene transcription, a viral-encoded protein kinase, and cytotoxic proteins. The capsid docks with a nuclear pore and delivers the genome into the nucleus.

The **immediate early gene products** include DNA-binding proteins that stimulate DNA synthesis and promote transcription of the early viral genes. During a latent infection of neurons, the only region of the genome to be transcribed generates the **latency-associated transcripts (LATs).** These RNAs are not translated into protein but encode micro-RNAs that inhibit expression of important immediate early and other genes.

The **early proteins** include the DNA-dependent DNA polymerase and a thymidine kinase. As catalytic proteins, relatively few copies of these enzymes are required to promote replication. Other early proteins inhibit production and initiate degradation of cellular messenger RNA (mRNA) and DNA. Expression of the early and late genes generally leads to cell death.

The genome is replicated as soon as the polymerase is synthesized. Circular end-to-end concatameric forms of the genome are made initially. Later in the infection, the DNA is replicated by a rolling-circle mechanism to produce a linear string of genomes that, in concept, resembles a roll of toilet paper. The concatamers are cleaved into individual genomes as the DNA is sucked into a procapsid.

Genome replication triggers transcription of the late genes from which structural and other proteins are encoded. Many copies of the structural proteins are required. The capsid proteins are then transported to the nucleus, where they are assembled into empty procapsids and filled with DNA. DNA-containing capsids associate with viral protein-disrupted nuclear membranes and bud into and then out of the endoplasmic reticulum into the cytoplasm. The viral glycoproteins are synthesized and processed like cellular glycoproteins. Tegument proteins associate with the viral capsid in the cytoplasm, and then the capsid buds into a portion of the trans-Golgi network to acquire their glycoprotein-containing envelope. The virus is released by exocytosis or cell lysis. Virus can also spread between cells through intracellular bridges, which allows the virus to escape antibody detection. Virus-induced syncytia formation also spreads the infection.

HSV infection of neurons may result in virus replication or establishment of latency, depending on which viral genes the neuron is capable of transcribing. Transcription of the LAT and no other viral gene will result in latency. As for other alphaherpesviruses, HSV encodes a thymidine kinase (scavenging enzyme) to facilitate replication in nondividing cells such as neurons. HSV also encodes ICP34.5, a unique protein that has multiple functions to facilitate virus growth in neurons. ICP34.5 removes a cellular block to protein synthesis activated in response to virus infection or as part of the response to interferon (IFN)-α.

Pathogenesis and Immunity

The mechanisms involved in the pathogenesis of HSV-1 and HSV-2 are very similar (Box 43-2). Both viruses initially infect, replicate in mucoepithelial cells, cause disease at the site of infection, and then establish latent infection of the innervating neurons. HSV-1 and HSV-2 differ in growth

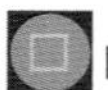 **Box 43-2 Disease Mechanisms for Herpes Simplex Viruses**

Disease is initiated by direct contact and depends on infected tissue (e.g., oral, genital, brain).
Virus causes direct cytopathologic effects.
Virus avoids antibody by cell-to-cell spread and syncytia.
Virus establishes latency in neurons (hides from immune response).
Virus is reactivated from latency by stress or immune suppression.
Cell-mediated immunity is required for resolution, with a limited role for antibody.
Cell-mediated immunopathologic effects contribute to symptoms.

 **Box 43-3 Triggers of Herpes Simplex Virus Recurrences**

Ultraviolet B radiation (skiing, tanning)
Fever (hence the name "fever blister")
Emotional stress (e.g., final examinations, big date)
Physical stress (irritation)
Menstruation
Foods: spicy, acidic, allergies
Immunosuppression:
- Transient (stress related)
- Chemotherapy, radiotherapy
- Human immunodeficiency virus

characteristics and antigenicity, and HSV-2 has a greater potential to cause viremia with associated systemic flulike symptoms.

HSV can cause **lytic** infections of most cells and **latent** infection of neurons. Cytolysis generally results from the virus-induced inhibition of cellular macromolecular synthesis, the degradation of host cell DNA, membrane permeation, cytoskeletal disruption, and senescence of the cell. Visible changes in the nuclear structure and margination of the chromatin occur, and **Cowdry type A acidophilic intranuclear inclusion bodies** are produced. Many strains of HSV also initiate **syncytia** formation. In tissue culture, HSV rapidly kills cells, causing them to appear rounded.

HSV initiates infection through mucosal membranes or breaks in the skin. The virus replicates in the cells at the base of the lesion and infects the innervating neuron, traveling by retrograde transport to the ganglion (the trigeminal ganglia for oral HSV and the sacral ganglia for genital HSV) (see Figure 43-5). CD8 T cells and IFN-γ are important to maintain HSV in latency. Upon reactivation, the virus then returns to the initial site of infection, and the infection may be inapparent or may produce **vesicular lesions.** The vesicle fluid contains infectious virions. Tissue damage is caused by a combination of viral pathology and immunopathology. The lesion generally heals without producing a scar.

Innate protections, including interferon and natural killer (NK) cells, may be sufficient to limit the initial progression of the infection. *T-helper 1 (TH1)–associated and CD8 cytotoxic killer T-cell responses are required to kill infected cells and resolve acute disease.* The immunopathologic effects of the cell-mediated and inflammatory responses are also a major cause of the disease signs. Antibody directed against the glycoproteins of the virus neutralizes extracellular virus, limiting its spread, but is not sufficient to resolve the infection. In the absence of functional cell-mediated immunity, HSV infection is likely to recur and be more severe, and may disseminate to the vital organs and the brain.

HSV has several ways to escape host protective responses. The virus blocks the interferon-induced inhibition of viral protein synthesis and encodes a protein to plug the transporter-associated-with-processing (TAP) channel, preventing delivery of peptides into the endoplasmic reticulum (ER), which blocks their association with class I major histocompatibility complex (MHC I) molecules and prevents CD8 T-cell recognition of infected cells. The virus can escape antibody neutralization and clearance by direct cell-to-cell spread and by going into hiding during latent infection of the neuron. In addition, the virion and virus-infected cells express antibody (Fc) and complement receptors that weaken these humoral defenses.

Latent infection occurs in neurons and results in no detectable damage. A **recurrence** can be activated by various stimuli (e.g., stress, trauma, fever, sunlight [ultraviolet B]) (Box 43-3). These events trigger virus replication in an individual nerve cell within the bundle and allow the virus to travel back down the nerve to cause lesions to develop at the same dermatome and location each time. The stress triggers reactivation by promoting replication of the virus in the nerve, by transiently depressing cell-mediated immunity, or by inducing both processes. The virus can be reactivated despite the presence of antibody. However, recurrent infections are generally less severe, more localized, and of shorter duration than the primary episodes because of the nature of the spread and the existence of memory immune responses.

Epidemiology

Because HSV can establish latency with the potential for asymptomatic recurrence, the infected person is a lifelong source of contagion (Box 43-4). HSV is transmitted in secretions and by close contact. As an enveloped virus, HSV is very labile and is readily inactivated by drying, detergents, and the conditions of the gastrointestinal tract. Although HSV can infect animal cells, HSV infection is exclusively a human disease.

HSV is transmitted in vesicle fluid, saliva, and vaginal secretions (the **"mixing and matching of mucous membranes"**). The site of infection, and hence the disease, is determined primarily by which mucous membranes are mixed. *Both types of HSV can cause oral and genital lesions.*

HSV-1 is usually spread by oral contact (kissing) or through the sharing of drinking glasses, toothbrushes, or other saliva-contaminated items. HSV-1 can infect the fingers or body through a cut or abraded skin. Autoinoculation may also cause infection of the eyes or fingers.

HSV-1 infection is common. More than 90% of people living in underdeveloped areas have the antibody to HSV-1 by 2 years of age.

HSV-2 is spread mainly by sexual contact or autoinoculation or from an infected mother to her infant at birth. Depending on a person's sexual practices and hygiene, HSV-2 may infect the genitalia, anorectal tissues, or oropharynx. The incidence of HSV-1 genital infection is approaching that of HSV-2. HSV may cause symptomatic or asymptomatic primary genital infection or recurrences. Neonatal infection usually results from the excretion of

Box 43-4 Epidemiology of Herpes Simplex Virus (HSV)

Disease/Viral Factors

Virus causes lifelong infection.

Recurrent disease is a source of contagion.

Virus may cause asymptomatic shedding.

Transmission

Virus is transmitted in saliva, in vaginal secretions, and by contact with lesion fluid (mixing and matching of mucous membranes).

Virus is transmitted orally and sexually and by placement into eyes and breaks in skin.

HSV-1 is generally transmitted orally; HSV-2 is generally transmitted sexually, but not exclusively.

Who Is at Risk?

Children and sexually active people are at risk for primary disease of HSV-1 and HSV-2, respectively.

Physicians, nurses, dentists, and others in contact with oral and genital secretions are at risk for infections of fingers (herpetic whitlow).

Immunocompromised people and neonates are at risk for disseminated life-threatening disease.

Geography/Season

Virus is found worldwide.

There is no seasonal incidence.

Modes of Control

Antiviral drugs are available for treatment and prophylaxis.

No vaccine is available.

Health care workers should wear gloves to prevent herpetic whitlow.

People with active genital lesions should refrain from intercourse until lesions are completely reepithelialized.

Clinical Case 43-1 Neonatal Herpes Simplex Virus (HSV)

Parvey and Ch'ien (*Pediatrics* 65:1150–1153, 1980) reported a case of neonatal HSV contracted during birth. During a breech presentation, a fetal monitor was placed on the buttocks of the baby, and because of the greatly prolonged labor, the baby was delivered by cesarean section. The 5-pound boy had minor difficulties that were successfully treated, but on the sixth day, vesicles with an erythematous base appeared at the site where the fetal monitor had been placed. HSV was grown from the vesicle fluid and from spinal fluid, cornea, saliva, and blood. The baby became moribund, with frequent apneic episodes and seizures. Intravenous treatment with adenosine arabinoside (ara-A; vidarabine) was initiated. The baby also developed bradycardia and occasional vomiting. The vesicles spread to cover the lower extremities and were also on the back, palm, nares, and right eyelid. Within 72 hours of ara-A treatment, the baby's condition started to improve. Treatment was continued for 11 days but discontinued because of a low platelet count. The baby was discharged on the 45th day after his birthday, and normal development was reported at 1 and 2 years of age. At 6 weeks after the birth, a herpes lesion was found on the mother's vulva. This baby was successfully treated with ara-A and was able to overcome the damage caused by the infection. The virus, most likely HSV-2, was probably acquired through an abrasion caused by the fetal monitor while the neonate was in the birth canal. Ara-A has since been replaced with antiviral drugs that are better, less toxic, and easier to administer: acyclovir, valacyclovir, and famciclovir.

HSV-2 from the cervix during vaginal delivery (Clinical Case 43-1) but can occur from an ascending in utero infection during a primary infection of the mother. Neonatal infection results in disseminated and neurologic disease with severe consequences.

Initial infection with HSV-2 occurs later in life than infection with HSV-1 and correlates with increased sexual activity. The current statistics indicate that 25% of adults in the United States are infected with HSV-2, which amounts to approximately 45 million people, with up to 1 million newly infected people per year.

Clinical Syndromes

HSV-1 and HSV-2 are common human pathogens that can cause painful but benign manifestations and recurrent disease (Figure 43-3). The HSV diseases may be caused by either HSV-1 or HSV-2, unless noted. *HSV can cause significant morbidity and mortality on infection of the eye or brain and on disseminated infection of an immunosuppressed person or a neonate.* In the classic manifestation, the lesion is a clear vesicle on an erythematous base ("dewdrop on a rose petal") and then progresses to pustular lesions, ulcers, and crusted lesions (Figure 43-4).

Oral herpes can be caused by HSV-1 or HSV-2. The lesions of herpes labialis or gingivostomatitis begin as clear vesicles that rapidly ulcerate. The vesicles may be widely distributed around or throughout the mouth, involving the palate, pharynx, gingivae, buccal mucosa, and tongue

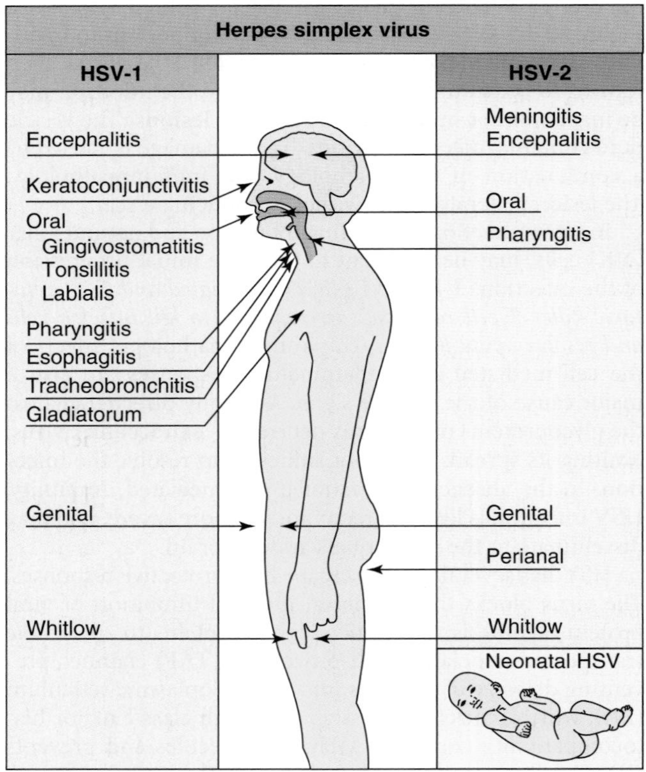

FIGURE 43-3 Disease syndromes of herpes simplex virus *(HSV)*. HSV-1 and HSV-2 can infect the same tissues and cause similar diseases but have a predilection for the sites and diseases indicated.

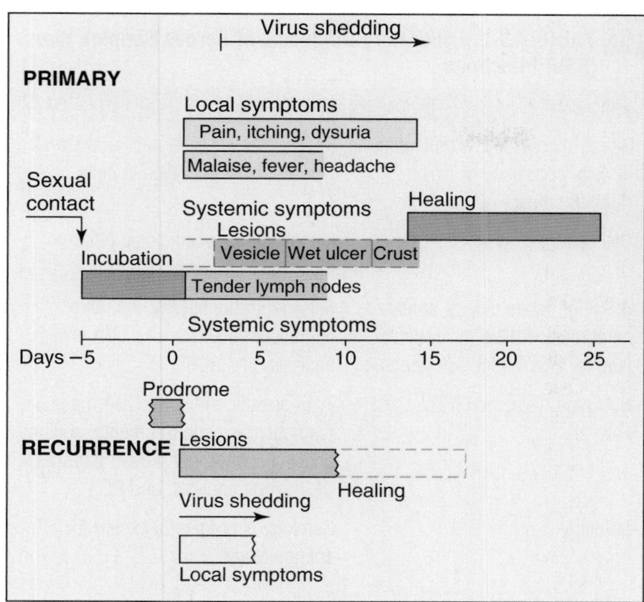

FIGURE 43-4 Clinical course of genital herpes infection. The time course and symptoms of primary and recurrent genital infection with herpes simplex virus type 2 are compared. *Top,* Primary infection; *bottom,* recurrent disease. (Data from Corey L, Adams HG, Brown ZA, et al: Genital herpes simplex virus infection: clinical manifestations, course and complications, *Ann Intern Med* 98:958–972, 1983.)

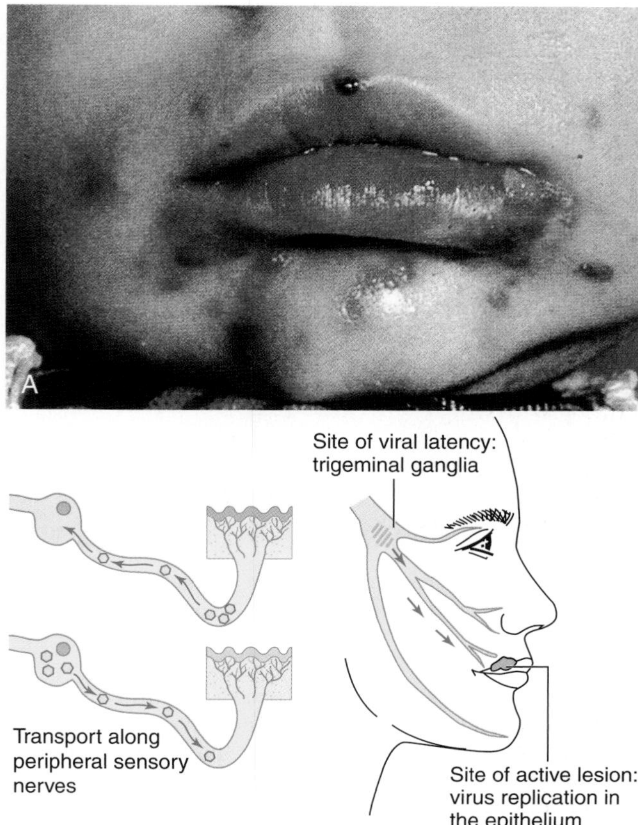

FIGURE 43-5 A, Primary herpes gingivostomatitis. **B,** Herpes simplex virus establishes latent infection and can recur from the trigeminal ganglia. (**A,** From Hart CA, Broadhead RL: *A color atlas of pediatric infectious diseases,* London, 1992, Wolfe. **B,** Modified from Straus SE: Herpes simplex virus and its relatives. In Schaechter M, Eisenstein BI, Medoff G, editors: *Mechanisms of microbial disease,* ed 2, Baltimore, 1993, Williams & Wilkins.)

(Figure 43-5). Many other conditions (e.g., coxsackievirus lesions, canker sores, acne) may resemble HSV lesions.

Infected people may experience recurrent mucocutaneous HSV infection **(cold sores, fever blisters)** (Figure 43-6) even though they never had a clinically apparent primary infection. The lesions usually occur at the corners of the mouth or next to the lips. Recurrent facial herpes infections are generally activated from the trigeminal ganglia. As noted earlier, the symptoms of a recurrent episode are less severe, more localized, and of shorter duration than those of a primary episode. **Herpes pharyngitis** is becoming a prevalent diagnosis in young adults with sore throats.

Herpetic keratitis is almost always limited to one eye. It can cause recurrent disease, leading to permanent scarring, corneal damage, and blindness. TH17 immune responses are more important for control of eye infections than other HSV infections.

Herpetic whitlow is an infection of the finger, and **herpes gladiatorum** is an infection of the body. The virus establishes infection through cuts or abrasions in the skin. Herpetic whitlow often occurs in nurses or physicians who attend patients with HSV infections, in thumb-sucking children (Figure 43-7), and in people who have genital HSV infections. Herpes gladiatorum is often acquired during wrestling or rugby.

Eczema herpeticum is acquired by children with active eczema. The underlying disease promotes the spread of the infection along the skin and potentially to the adrenal glands, liver, and other organs.

Genital herpes can be caused by HSV-1 or HSV-2. In male patients, the lesions typically develop on the glans or

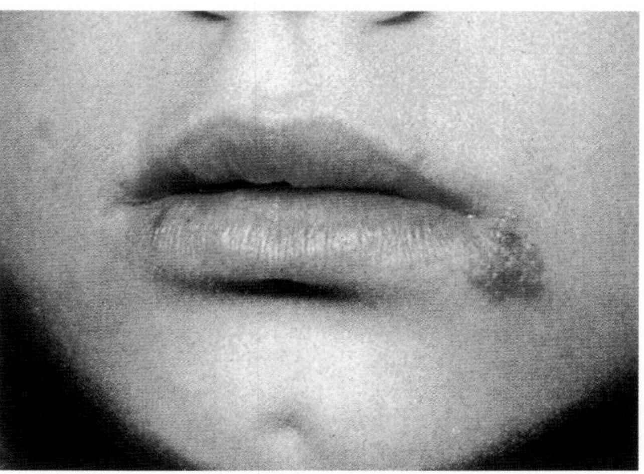

FIGURE 43-6 Cold sore of recurrent herpes labialis. It is less severe than that of primary disease. (From Hart CA, Broadhead RL: *A color atlas of pediatric infectious diseases,* London, 1992, Wolfe.)

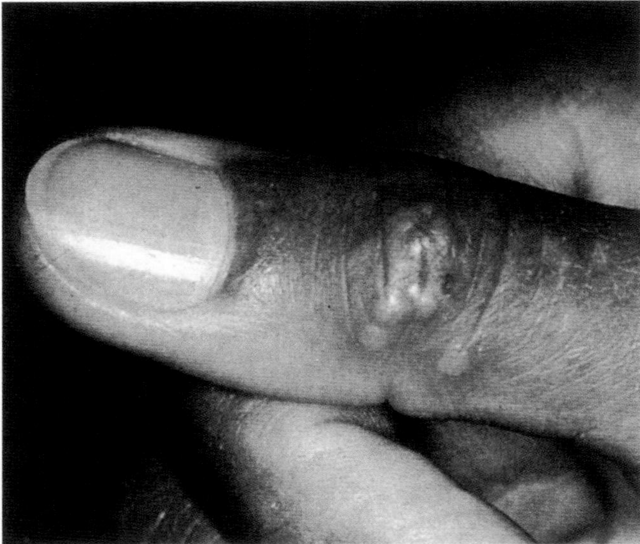

FIGURE 43-7 Herpetic whitlow. (From Emond RTD, Rowland HAK: *A color atlas of infectious diseases,* ed 3, London, 1995, Mosby.)

Table 43-2 **Laboratory Diagnosis of Herpes Simplex Virus (HSV) Infections**

Approach	Test/Comment
Direct microscopic examination of cells from base of lesion (Tzanck smear)	Multinucleated giant cells and Cowdry type A inclusion bodies in cells
Cell culture	Identifiable cytopathologic effect in most cell cultures
Assay of tissue biopsy, smear, cerebrospinal fluid, or vesicular fluid for HSV antigen or genome	Enzyme immunoassay, immunofluorescent stain, in situ DNA probe analysis, and PCR
HSV type distinction (HSV-1 vs. HSV-2)	Type-specific antibody, DNA maps of restriction enzyme fragments, sodium dodecyl sulfate–gel protein patterns, DNA probe analysis, and PCR
Serology	Serology is not useful except for epidemiology

DNA, Deoxyribonucleic acid; *PCR,* polymerase chain reaction.

shaft of the penis and occasionally in the urethra. In female patients, the lesions may be seen on the vulva, vagina, cervix, perianal area, or inner thigh and are frequently accompanied by itching and a mucoid vaginal discharge. Anal sex can lead to HSV proctitis, a condition in which the lesions are found in the lower rectum and anus. The lesions are usually painful. In patients of both sexes, a primary infection may be accompanied by fever, malaise, and myalgia, which are symptoms related to a transient viremia. The symptoms and time course of primary and recurrent genital herpes are compared in Figure 43-4.

Recurrent genital HSV disease is shorter in duration and less severe than the primary episode. In approximately 50% of patients, recurrences are preceded by a characteristic prodrome of burning or tingling in the area in which the lesions eventually erupt. Episodes of recurrence may be as frequent as every 2 to 3 weeks or may be infrequent. Unfortunately, any infected person may shed virus asymptomatically. Such individuals may be important vectors for spread of this virus.

Herpes encephalitis is usually caused by HSV-1. The lesions are generally limited to one of the temporal lobes. The viral pathology and immunopathology cause destruction of the temporal lobe and give rise to erythrocytes in the cerebrospinal fluid, seizures, focal neurologic abnormalities, and other characteristics of viral encephalitis. HSV is the most common viral cause of sporadic encephalitis and results in significant morbidity and mortality, even in patients who receive appropriate treatment. The disease occurs at all ages and at any time of the year. **HSV meningitis** may be a complication of genital HSV-2 infection, and if so, symptoms resolve by themselves.

HSV infection in the neonate is a devastating and often fatal disease caused most often by HSV-2. It may be acquired in utero, but more commonly it is contracted either during passage of the infant through the vaginal canal (possibly at the baby's scalp-monitor site) because the mother is shedding herpesvirus at the time of delivery, or it is acquired postnatally from family members or hospital personnel. The baby initially appears septic, and vesicular lesions may or may not be present. Because the cell-mediated immune response is not yet developed in the neonate, HSV disseminates to the liver, lung, and other organs, as well as to the central nervous system (CNS). Progression of the infection to the CNS results in death, mental retardation, or neurologic disability, even with treatment.

Laboratory Diagnosis

Direct Analysis of a Clinical Sample

Characteristic cytopathologic effects (CPEs) can be identified in a **Tzanck smear** (a scraping of the base of a lesion), Papanicolaou (Pap) smear, or biopsy specimen (Table 43-2). CPEs include syncytia, "ballooning" cytoplasm, and Cowdry type A intranuclear inclusions (see Chapter 39, Figure 39-2). A definitive diagnosis can be made by demonstrating viral antigen (using immunofluorescence or the immunoperoxidase method) or DNA (using in situ hybridization or polymerase chain reaction [PCR]) in the tissue sample or vesicle fluid.

Virus Isolation

Virus isolation is the most definitive assay for the diagnosis of HSV infection. Virus can be obtained from vesicles but not crusted lesions. Specimens are collected by aspiration of the lesion fluid or by application of a cotton swab to the vesicles and direct inoculation of the sample into cell cultures.

HSV produces CPEs within 1 to 3 days in HeLa cells, human embryonic fibroblasts, and other cells. Infected cells become enlarged and appear ballooned (see Chapter 39, Figure 39-4). Some isolates induce fusion of neighboring cells, giving rise to multinucleated giant cells (syncytia). A new, sensitive approach to isolation and identification uses a cell line that expresses β-galactosidase upon HSV infection of cells (enzyme-linked viral-inducible system [ELVIS]). Addition of the appropriate substrate produces color and allows detection of the enzyme in the infected cells.

Genome Detection

HSV type-specific DNA probes, specific DNA primers for PCR and quantitative PCR, are used to detect and differentiate HSV-1 and HSV-2. **PCR analysis** of cerebrospinal fluid has replaced immunofluorescence analysis of a brain biopsy in the diagnosis for herpes encephalitis. The distinction between HSV-1 or HSV-2 and different strains of either virus can also be made by restriction endonuclease cleavage patterns of the viral DNA.

Serology

Serologic procedures are useful only for diagnosing a primary HSV infection and for epidemiologic studies. They are not useful for diagnosing recurrent disease, because a significant rise in antibody titers does not usually accompany recurrent disease.

Treatment, Prevention, and Control

HSV encodes several target enzymes for antiviral drugs (Box 43-5) (see Chapter 40). Most antiherpes drugs are nucleoside analogs that are activated by the viral thymidine kinase and inhibit the viral DNA polymerase, an enzyme essential for viral replication and the best antiviral drug target. Treatment prevents or shortens the course of primary or recurrent disease. None of the drug treatments can eliminate latent infection.

The prototype anti-HSV drug is **acyclovir (ACV). Valacyclovir** (the valyl ester of ACV), **penciclovir,** and **famciclovir** (a derivative of penciclovir) are related to ACV in their mechanisms of action but have different pharmacologic properties. Vidarabine (adenosine arabinoside [Ara A]), idoxuridine (iododeoxyuridine), and trifluridine, also U.S. Food and Drug Administration (FDA) approved for treatment of HSV, are less effective. Although **cidofovir** and **adefovir** are active against HSV, cidofovir is only approved for treatment of CMV.

ACV is the most prescribed anti-HSV drug. Phosphorylation of ACV and penciclovir by the viral **thymidine kinase** and cellular enzymes activates the drug as a substrate for the viral **DNA polymerase.** These drugs are then incorporated into and **prevent elongation of the viral DNA** (see Chapter 40, Figure 40-2). ACV, valacyclovir, penciclovir, and famciclovir are relatively nontoxic, effective in treating serious presentations of HSV disease and first episodes of genital herpes, and also used for prophylactic treatment.

The most prevalent form of resistance to these drugs results from mutations that inactivate the thymidine kinase, thereby preventing conversion of the drug to its active form. Mutation of the viral DNA polymerase also produces resistance. Fortunately, resistant strains appear to be less virulent.

Ara-A is less soluble, less potent, and more toxic than ACV. Trifluridine, penciclovir, and ACV have replaced iododeoxyuridine as topical agents for the treatment of herpetic keratitis. Tromantadine, an amantadine derivative, is approved for topical use in countries other than the United States. It works by inhibiting penetration and syncytia formation. Docosonal inhibits entry of the virus, and other nonprescription treatments may be effective for specific individuals.

Avoidance of direct contact with lesions reduces the risk of infection. Unfortunately, the symptoms may be inapparent, and thus the virus can be transmitted unknowingly. Physicians, nurses, dentists, and technicians must be especially careful when handling potentially infected tissue or fluids. Wearing gloves can prevent acquisition of infections of the fingers (herpetic whitlow). People with recurrent herpetic whitlow disease are very contagious and can spread the infection to patients.

HSV is readily inactivated by soap, disinfectants, bleach, and 70% ethanol. Washing with soap readily disinfects the virus.

Patients who have a history of genital HSV infection must be instructed to refrain from sexual intercourse while they have prodromal symptoms or lesions and to resume sexual intercourse only after lesions are completely reepithelialized, because virus may be transmitted from lesions that have crusted over. Condoms may be useful and are undoubtedly better than nothing but may not be fully protective.

A pregnant woman who has active genital HSV infection or who is asymptomatically shedding the virus in the vagina at term may transmit HSV to the neonate if the infant is delivered vaginally. Such transmission can be prevented by cesarean section.

No vaccine is currently available for HSV. However, killed, subunit, vaccinia hybrid, genetically attenuated, and DNA vaccines are being developed to prevent acquisition of the virus or to treat infected people. The glycoprotein D is being used in several of these experimental vaccines.

Box 43-5 FDA-Approved Antiviral Treatments for Herpesvirus Infections

Herpes Simplex 1 and 2
Acyclovir
Penciclovir
Valacyclovir
Famciclovir
Trifluridine

Varicella-Zoster Virus
Acyclovir
Famciclovir
Valacyclovir
Varicella-zoster immune globulin
Zoster immune plasma
Live vaccine

Epstein-Barr Virus
None

Cytomegalovirus
Ganciclovir*
Valganciclovir*
Foscarnet*
Trifluridine
Cidofovir*

FDA, U.S. Food and Drug Administration.

*Also inhibits herpes simplex and varicella-zoster viruses.

• Varicella-Zoster Virus

VZV causes **chickenpox (varicella)** and, upon recurrence, causes herpes **zoster, or shingles.** As an alphaherpesvirus, VZV shares many characteristics with HSV, including (1) the ability to establish latent infection of neurons and recurrent disease, (2) the importance of cell-mediated immunity in controlling and preventing serious disease, and (3) the characteristic blister-like lesions. Like HSV, VZV encodes a **thymidine kinase** and is susceptible to the same **antiviral drugs.** Unlike HSV, VZV spreads predominantly by the **respiratory route** and, after local replication of the virus in the respiratory tract, by **viremia** to form skin lesions over the entire body.

Structure and Replication

VZV has the smallest genome of the human herpesviruses. VZV replicates in a similar manner but slower and in fewer types of cells than HSV. Human diploid fibroblasts in vitro and activated T cells, epithelial cells, and epidermal cells in vivo support productive VZV replication. New VZV is sequestered into lysosomes and degraded in most cells because of its binding to the mannose-6-phosphate receptor but is released from terminally differentiated skin cells that lack this protein. As such, it spreads within the body by cell-cell contact. Like HSV, VZV establishes a latent infection of neurons, but unlike HSV, several viral RNAs and specific viral proteins can be detected in the latently infected cells.

Pathogenesis and Immunity

VZV is generally acquired by inhalation, and primary infection begins in the tonsils and mucosa of the respiratory tract. The virus then progresses via the bloodstream and lymphatic system to the cells of the reticuloendothelial system (Figures 43-8 and 43-9; Box 43-6). A secondary viremia occurs after and spreads the virus throughout the body and to the skin. The virus infects T cells, and these cells can home to the skin and transfer virus to skin epithelial cells. The virus overcomes inhibition by IFN-α, and vesicles are produced in the skin. The virus remains cell associated and is transmitted on cell-to-cell interaction, except for terminally differentiated epithelial cells in the lungs and keratinocytes of skin lesions, which can release infectious virus. Virus replication in the lung is a major source of contagion. The virus causes a dermal vesiculopustular rash that develops over time in successive crops. Fever and systemic symptoms occur with the rash.

The virus becomes latent in the dorsal root or cranial nerve ganglia after the primary infection. The virus can be reactivated in older adults when immunity wanes or in patients with impaired cellular immunity. On reactivation, the virus replicates and is released along the entire neural pathway to infect the skin, causing a vesicular rash along the entire dermatome, known as **herpes zoster,** or **shingles.** This damages the neuron and may result in very painful postherpetic neuralgia.

IFN-α, interferon-stimulated protections, and NK and T cells limit the spread of the virus in tissue, but **antibody** is important for limiting the viremic spread of VZV. Passive immunization with **varicella-zoster immune globulin (VZIG)** within 4 days of exposure is protective. Cell-mediated immunity is essential for resolving the acute

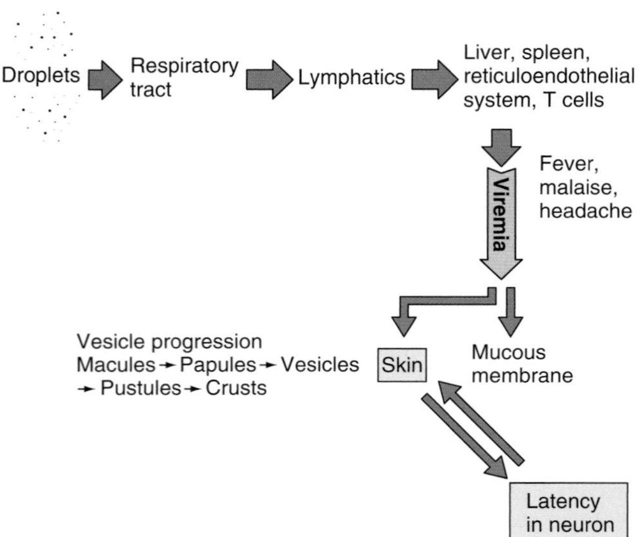

FIGURE 43-8 Mechanism of spread of varicella-zoster virus (VZV) within the body. VZV initially infects the respiratory tract and is spread to the reticuloendothelial system and T cells and then by cell-associated viremia to the skin.

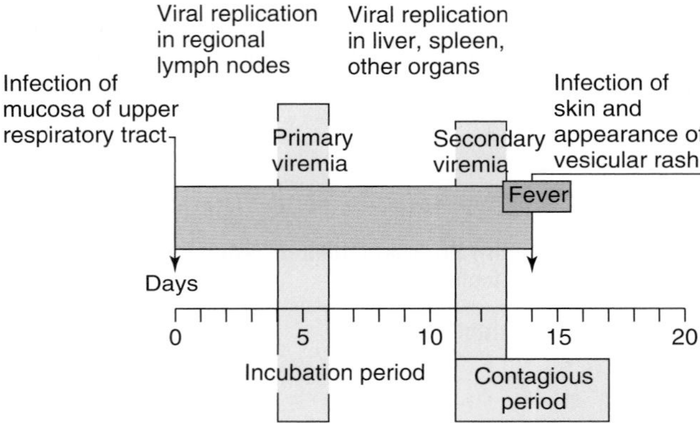

FIGURE 43-9 Time course of varicella (chickenpox). The course in young children, as presented in this figure, is generally shorter and less severe than that in adults.

Box 43-6 Disease Mechanisms of Varicella-Zoster Virus (VZV)

- Initial replication is in the respiratory tract.
- VZV infects epithelial cells, fibroblasts, T cells, and neurons.
- VZV can form syncytia and spread directly from cell to cell.
- Virus is spread by viremia in T cells to skin and causes lesions in successive crops.
- VZV can evade antibody clearance, and cell-mediated immune response is essential to control infection. Disseminated life-threatening disease can occur in immunocompromised people.
- Virus establishes latent infection of neurons, usually dorsal root and cranial nerve ganglia.
- Herpes zoster is a recurrent disease; it results from virus replication along the entire dermatome.
- Herpes zoster results from depression of cell-mediated immunity.

disease and controlling the latent infection. The virus causes more disseminated and more serious disease in the absence of cell-mediated immunity (e.g., in children with leukemia) and may recur on immunosuppression. Although important for protection, cell-mediated immune responses contribute to the symptomatology. An overzealous response in adults is responsible for causing more extensive cell damage and a more severe manifestation (especially in the lung) in primary infection than that seen in children. T-cell and antibody levels decrease later in life, allowing VZV recurrence and herpes zoster disease.

Epidemiology

VZV is extremely communicable, with rates of infection exceeding 90% among susceptible household contacts (Box 43-7). The disease is spread principally by the respiratory route but may also be spread through contact with skin vesicles. Patients are contagious before and during symptoms. More than 90% of adults in developed countries have the VZV antibody. Herpes zoster results from the reactivation of a patient's latent virus. The disease develops in approximately 10% to 20% of the population infected with VZV, and the incidence rises with age. Herpes zoster lesions contain viable virus and therefore may be a source of varicella infection in a nonimmune person (child).

Clinical Syndromes

Varicella (chickenpox) is one of the five **classic childhood exanthems** (along with rubella, roseola, fifth disease, and measles). The disease results from a primary infection with VZV; it is usually a mild disease of childhood and is normally symptomatic, although asymptomatic infection can occur (see Figure 43-9). Varicella characteristics include fever and a maculopapular rash that appear after an incubation period of approximately 14 days (Figure 43-10). Within hours, each maculopapular lesion forms a thin-walled vesicle on an erythematous base ("dewdrop on a rose petal") that measures approximately 2 to 4 mm in diameter. This vesicle is the hallmark of varicella. Within 12 hours, the vesicle becomes pustular and begins to crust, after which scabbed lesions appear. Successive crops of lesions appear for 3 to 5 days, and at any given time, all stages of skin lesions can be observed.

The rash spreads across the entire body but is more prevalent on the trunk and head than on the extremities. Its presence on the scalp distinguishes it from many other rashes. The lesions itch and cause scratching, which may lead to bacterial superinfection and scarring. Lesions on the mucous membrane typically occur in the mouth, conjunctivae, and vagina.

Primary infection is usually more severe in adults than in children. **Interstitial pneumonia** may occur in 20% to 30% of adult patients and may be fatal. The pneumonia results from inflammatory reactions at this primary site of infection.

As noted earlier, **herpes zoster** (*zoster* means "belt" or "girdle") is a recurrence of a latent varicella infection acquired earlier in the patient's life. Severe pain in the area innervated by the nerve usually precedes the appearance of the chickenpox-like lesions. The rash is limited to a dermatome and resembles varicella (Figure 43-11). A chronic pain syndrome called **postherpetic neuralgia,** which can persist for months to years, occurs in as many as 30% of patients in whom herpes zoster develops.

VZV infection in immunocompromised patients or neonates can result in serious, progressive, and potentially fatal disease. Defects of cell-mediated immunity in such patients increase the risk for dissemination of the virus to the lungs, brain, and liver, which may be fatal. The disease may occur in response to a primary exposure to varicella or because of recurrent disease.

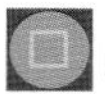

Box 43-7 Epidemiology of Varicella-Zoster Virus

Disease/Viral Factors

Virus causes lifelong infection.

Recurrent disease is a source of contagion.

Transmission

Virus is transmitted mainly by respiratory droplets but also by direct contact.

Who Is at Risk?

Children (ages 5 to 9) experience mild classic disease.

Teenagers and adults are at risk for more severe disease with potential pneumonia.

Immunocompromised people and newborns are at risk for life-threatening pneumonia, encephalitis, and progressive disseminated varicella.

Elderly and immunocompromised people are at risk for recurrent disease (herpes zoster [shingles]).

Geography/Season

Virus is found worldwide.

There is no seasonal incidence.

Modes of Control

Antiviral drugs are available.

Immunity may wane in the elderly population.

Varicella-zoster immunoglobulin is available for immunocompromised people and staff exposed to virus, as well as newborns of mothers showing symptoms within 5 days of birth.

Live vaccine (Oka strain) is available for children (varicella) and adults (zoster).

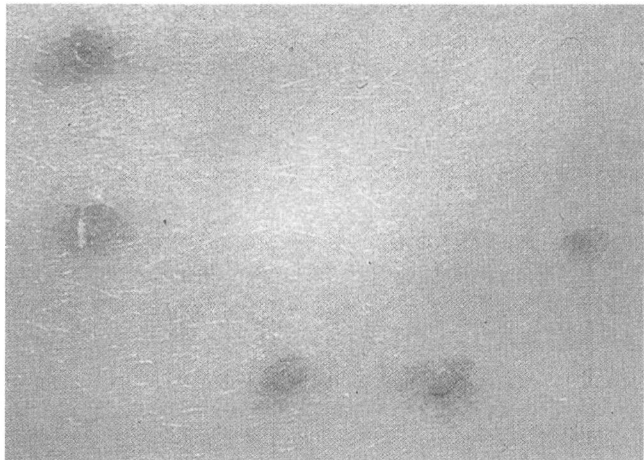

FIGURE 43-10 Characteristic rash of varicella in all stages of its evolution. (From Hart CA, Broadhead RL: *A color atlas of pediatric infectious diseases,* London, 1992, Wolfe.)

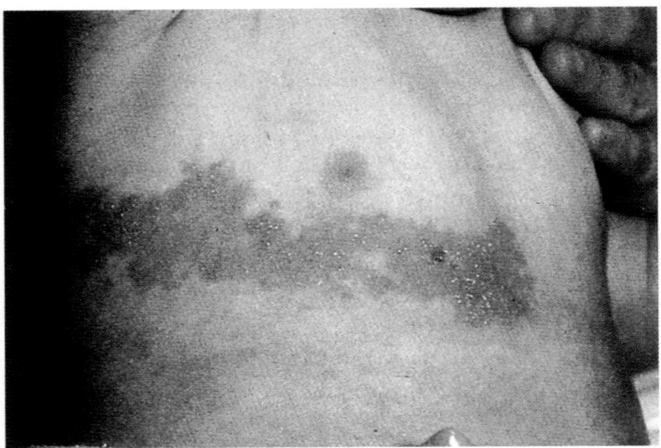

FIGURE 43-11 Herpes zoster ("shingles") in a thoracic dermatome.

Laboratory Diagnosis

The CPEs in VZV-infected cells are similar to those seen in HSV-infected cells and Cowdry type A intranuclear inclusions and syncytia. A direct fluorescent antibody to membrane antigen (FAMA) test can also be used to examine skin lesion scrapings or biopsy specimens. Antigen and genome detection are sensitive means of diagnosing VZV infection. PCR and genome detection techniques are especially useful for systemic and neuronal disease.

Isolation of VZV is not routinely done because the virus is labile during transport to the laboratory and replicates poorly in vitro.

Serologic tests that detect antibodies to VZV are used to screen populations for immunity to VZV. However, antibody levels are normally low, so sensitive tests such as immunofluorescence and enzyme-linked immunosorbent assay (ELISA) must be performed to detect the antibody. A significant increase in antibody level can be detected in people experiencing herpes zoster.

Treatment, Prevention, and Control

Treatment may be appropriate for adults and immunocompromised patients with VZV infections and for people with shingles, but no treatment is usually necessary for children with varicella. **ACV, famciclovir,** and **valacyclovir** have been approved for the treatment of VZV infections. The VZV DNA polymerase is much less sensitive to ACV treatment than the HSV enzyme, requiring larger doses of ACV or the improved pharmacodynamics of famciclovir and valacyclovir (see Box 43-5). There is no good treatment, but analgesics and other painkillers, topical anesthetics, or capsaicin cream may provide some relief from the postherpetic neuralgia that follows zoster.

As with other respiratory viruses, it is difficult to limit transmission of VZV. Because VZV infection in children is generally mild and induces lifelong immunity, exposure of children to VZV early in life is often encouraged. However, high-risk people (e.g., immunosuppressed children) should be protected from exposure to VZV.

Immunosuppressed patients susceptible to severe disease may be protected from serious disease through the administration of **VZIG.** VZIG is prepared through the pooling of plasma from seropositive people. VZIG prophylaxis can prevent viremic spread leading to disease but is ineffective as a therapy for patients already suffering from active varicella or herpes zoster disease.

A **live attenuated vaccine** for VZV (Oka strain) has been licensed for use in the United States and elsewhere and is administered after 2 years of age on the same schedule as the measles, mumps, and rubella vaccine. The vaccine induces production of protective antibody and cell-mediated immunity. A stronger version of this vaccine is available for adults older than 60 years; it boosts antiviral responses to limit the onset of zoster.

• Epstein-Barr Virus

EBV is the ultimate B-lymphocyte parasite, and the diseases it causes reflect this association. EBV was discovered by electron-microscopic observation of characteristic herpes virions in biopsy specimens of a B-cell neoplasm, African Burkitt lymphoma (AfBL). Its association with infectious mononucleosis was discovered accidentally when serum collected from a laboratory technician convalescing from infectious mononucleosis was found to contain the antibody that recognized AfBL cells. This finding was later confirmed in a large serologic study performed on college students.

EBV causes *heterophile antibody–positive infectious mononucleosis* and *stimulates the growth and immortalizes B cells* in tissue culture. EBV has been causally associated with **AfBL (endemic Burkitt lymphoma), Hodgkin disease,** and **nasopharyngeal carcinoma.** EBV has also been associated with B-cell lymphomas in patients with acquired or congenital immunodeficiencies.

Structure and Replication

EBV is a member of the subfamily Gammaherpesvirinae, with a very limited host range and a **tissue tropism** defined by the limited cellular expression of its receptor. The primary receptor for EBV is also *the receptor for the C3d component of the complement system (also called CR2 or CD21)*. It is expressed on B cells of humans and New World monkeys and on some epithelial cells of the oropharynx and nasopharynx. EBV also binds to MHC II.

EBV infection has the following three potential outcomes:

1. EBV can replicate in B cells or epithelial cells permissive for EBV replication and produce virus.
2. EBV can cause latent infection of memory B cells in the presence of competent T cells.
3. EBV can stimulate and immortalize B cells.

EBV encodes more than 70 proteins, different groups of which are expressed for the different types of infections.

EBV in saliva infects epithelial cells and then naïve resting B cells in the tonsils. The growth of the B cells is stimulated first by virus binding to the C3d receptor, a B-cell growth-stimulating receptor, and then by expression of the transformation and latency proteins. These include **Epstein-Barr nuclear antigens (EBNAs)** 1, 2, 3A, 3B, and 3C; latent proteins **(LPs); latent membrane proteins (LMPs) 1 and 2;** and two small Epstein-Barr–encoded RNA (EBER) molecules, EBER-1 and EBER-2. The EBNAs and LPs are DNA-binding proteins that are essential for establishing and maintaining

Table 43-3 **Markers of Epstein-Barr Virus (EBV) Infection**

Name	Abbreviation	Characteristics	Biological Association	Clinical Association
EBV nuclear antigens	EBNAs	Nuclear	EBNAs are nonstructural antigens and first antigens to appear; EBNAs seen in all infected and transformed cells	Anti-EBNA develops after resolution of infection
Early antigen	EA-R	Only cytoplasmic	EA-R appears before EA-D; appearance is first sign that infected cell has entered lytic cycle	
	EA-D	Diffuse in cytoplasm and nucleus	—	Anti-EA-D seen in infectious mononucleosis
Viral capsid antigen	VCA	Cytoplasmic	VCA are late proteins; found in virus-producing cells	Anti-VCA IgM is transient; anti-VCA IgG is persistent
Membrane antigen	MA	Cell surface	MAs are envelope glycoproteins	Same as VCA
Heterophile antibody		Recognition of Paul-Bunnell antigen on sheep, horse, or bovine erythrocytes	EBV-induced B-cell proliferation promotes production of heterophile antibody	Early symptom occurs in more than 50% of patients

EA, Early antigen; *EBNA,* Epstein-Barr nuclear antigen; *Ig,* immunoglobulin; *MA,* membrane antigen; *VCA,* viral capsid antigen.

the infection (EBNA-1), immortalization (EBNA-2), and other purposes. The LMPs are membrane proteins with oncoprotein-like activity. The genome becomes circularized; the cells proceed to follicles that become germinal centers in the lymph node, where the infected cells differentiate into memory cells. EBV protein synthesis ceases, and the virus establishes latency in these memory B cells. EBNA-1 will be expressed only at cell division to hold onto and retain the genome in the cells.

Antigen stimulation of the B cells and infection of certain epithelial cells allow transcription and translation of the ZEBRA (peptide encoded by the *Z*-gene region) transcriptional activator protein, which activates the immediate early genes of the virus and the lytic cycle. After synthesis of the DNA polymerase and replication of DNA, the structural and other late proteins are synthesized. They include gp350/220 (related glycoproteins of 350,000 and 220,000 Da), which is the viral attachment protein, and other glycoproteins. These glycoproteins bind to CD21 and MHC II molecules, receptors on B cells and epithelial cells, and also promote fusion of the envelope with cell membranes.

The viral proteins produced during a productive infection are serologically defined and grouped as **early antigen (EA), viral capsid antigen (VCA),** and the glycoproteins of the **membrane antigen (MA)** (Table 43-3). An early protein mimics a cellular inhibitor of apoptosis, and a late protein mimics the activity of human interleukin (IL)-10 (BCRF-1), which enhances B-cell growth and inhibits TH1 immune responses to facilitate virus replication.

Pathogenesis and Immunity

EBV has adapted to the human B cell and manipulates and uses the different phases of B-cell development to establish a lifelong infection. The diseases of EBV result from either an overactive immune response (infectious mononucleosis) or the lack of effective immune control (lymphoproliferative disease and hairy cell leukoplakia).

The productive infection of B cells and epithelial cells of the oropharynx, such as in the tonsils (Figure 43-12 and Box 43-8), promotes virus shedding into saliva to transmit the virus to other hosts and establishes a viremia to spread the virus to other B cells in lymphatic tissue and blood.

EBV proteins replace host factors that normally activate B-cell growth and development. In the absence of T cells (e.g., in tissue culture), EBV can immortalize B cells and promote the development of B-lymphoblastoid cell lines. In vivo, B-cell activation and proliferation occurs and is indicated by the spurious production of an IgM antibody to the Paul-Bunnell antigen, termed the **heterophile antibody** (see later discussion of serology).

The outgrowth of the B cell is controlled by a normal T-cell response to B-cell proliferation and to EBV antigenic peptides. B cells are excellent antigen-presenting cells and present EBV antigens on both MHC I and MHC II molecules. The activated T cells appear as **atypical lymphocytes** (also called **Downey cells**) (Figure 43-13). They increase in number in the peripheral blood during the second week of infection, accounting for 10% to 80% of the total white blood cell count at this time (hence the "mononucleosis").

Infectious mononucleosis is essentially *a "civil war" between the EBV-infected B cells and the protective T cells.* The classic **lymphocytosis** (increase in mononuclear cells), swelling of lymphoid organs (lymph nodes, spleen, and liver), and malaise associated with infectious mononucleosis results mainly from the activation and proliferation of T cells. A large amount of energy is required to power the T-cell response, leading to great fatigue. The sore throat of infectious mononucleosis is a response to EBV-infected epithelium and B cells in the tonsils and throat. Children have a less active immune response to EBV infection and therefore have very mild disease.

During productive infection, antibody is first developed against the components of the virion, VCA, and MA, and later against the EA. After resolution of the infection (lysis of the productively infected cells), antibody against the nuclear antigens (EBNAs) is produced. T cells are essential for limiting the proliferation of EBV-infected B cells and controlling the disease (Figure 43-14). EBV counteracts some of the protective action of TH1 CD4 T-cell responses during productive infection by producing an IL-10 analog

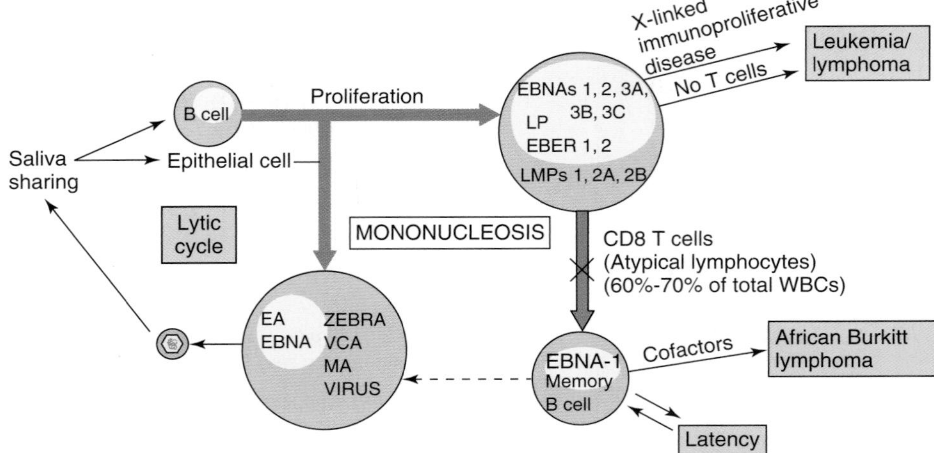

FIGURE 43-12 Progression of Epstein-Barr virus (EBV) infection. Infection may result in lytic, latent, or immortalizing infection, which can be distinguished on the basis of production of virus and expression of different viral proteins and antigens. T cells limit the outgrowth of the EBV-infected cells and maintain the latent infection. *CD,* Cluster of differentiation; *EA,* early antigen; *EBER,* Epstein-Barr–encoded RNA; *EBNA,* Epstein-Barr nuclear antigen; *LMPs,* latent membrane proteins; *LP,* latent protein; *MA,* membrane antigen; *VCA,* viral capsid antigen; *WBCs,* white blood cells; *ZEBRA,* peptide encoded by the *Z* gene region.

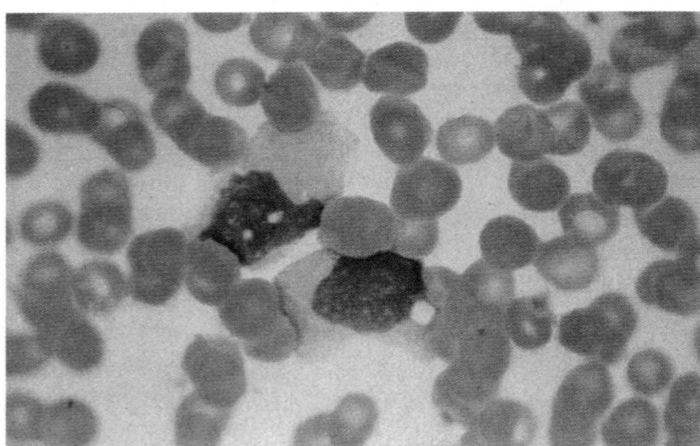

FIGURE 43-13 Atypical T-cell (Downey cell) characteristic of infectious mononucleosis. The cells have a more basophilic and vacuolated cytoplasm than normal lymphocytes, and the nucleus may be oval, kidney shaped, or lobulated. The cell margin may seem to be indented by neighboring red blood cells.

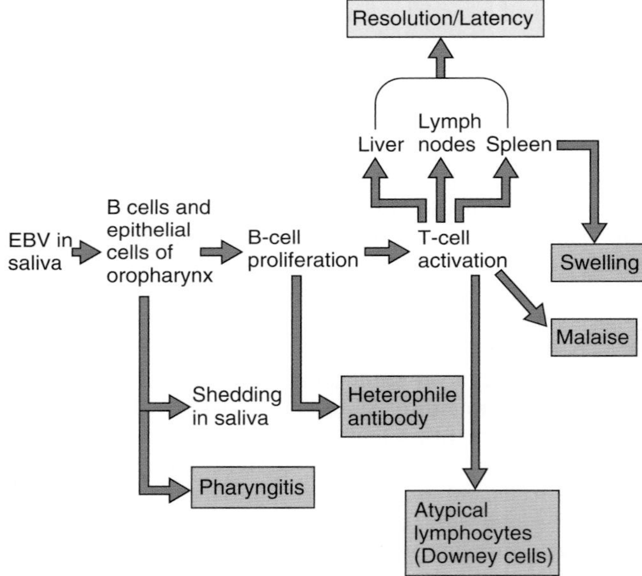

FIGURE 43-14 Pathogenesis of Epstein-Barr virus *(EBV).* EBV is acquired by close contact between persons through saliva and infects B cells. Resolution of the EBV infection and many of the symptoms of infectious mononucleosis result from activation of T cells in response to the infection.

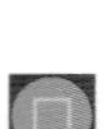 **Box 43-8 Disease Mechanisms of Epstein-Barr Virus (EBV)**

Virus in saliva initiates infection of oral epithelia and tonsillar B cells.
There is productive infection of epithelial and B cells.
Virus promotes growth of B cells (immortalizes).
T cells are stimulated by infected B cells; they kill and limit B-cell outgrowth. T cells are required for controlling infection. Antibody role is limited.
EBV establishes latency in memory B cells and is reactivated when the B cell is activated.
T-cell response (lymphocytosis) contributes to symptoms of **infectious mononucleosis.**
There is causative association with lymphoma in immunosuppressed people and African children living in malarial regions (African Burkitt lymphoma) and with nasopharyngeal carcinoma in China.

(BCRF-1) that inhibits the protective TH1 CD4 T-cell responses and also stimulates B-cell growth.

The virus persists in at least one memory B cell per milliliter of blood for the infected person's lifetime. EBV may be reactivated when the memory B cell is activated (especially in the tonsils or oropharynx) and may be shed in saliva.

Epidemiology

At least 70% of the population of the United States is infected by age 30. EBV is transmitted in saliva (Box 43-9). More than 90% of EBV-infected people intermittently shed the virus for

Box 43-9 Epidemiology of Epstein-Barr Virus

Disease/Viral Factors

Virus causes lifelong infection.
Recurrent disease is cause of contagion.
Virus may cause asymptomatic shedding.

Transmission

Transmission occurs via saliva, close oral contact ("kissing disease"), or sharing of items such as toothbrushes and cups.

Who Is at Risk?

Children experience asymptomatic disease or mild symptoms.
Teenagers and adults are at risk for infectious mononucleosis.
Immunocompromised people are at highest risk for life-threatening neoplastic disease.

Geography/Season

Infectious mononucleosis has worldwide distribution.
There is causative association with African Burkitt lymphoma in malarial belt of Africa.
There is no seasonal incidence.

Modes of Control

There are no modes of control.

Clinical Case 43-2 Epstein-Barr Virus (EBV) in the Immunocompromised Individual

Purtilo and associates (*Ann Intern Med* 101:180–186, 1984) reported on a boy with Duncan disease who presented with reduced levels of immunoglobulin (Ig)A, a history of thrush, and recurrent episodes of otitis media. This member of the Duncan family had an X-linked recessive, progressive, combined, variable immunodeficiency disease caused by a mutation in the SH2D1A protein, which prevents proper communication between B and T cells. After exposure to EBV at age 11 years, the boy did not develop antibodies to EBV, but generic serum IgM levels increased, and EBNA-positive immortalized B-cell lines readily grew from his peripheral blood. Establishment of the B-cell lines is indicative of aberrant T-cell control of the virus-induced B-cell proliferation. At age 18 years, he was treated with packed red cells for red cell aplasia, and then 9 weeks later, he developed infectious mononucleosis with fever, generalized lymphadenomegaly, tender liver and swollen spleen, lymphocytosis with a predominance of atypical lymphocytes, and a positive monospot test. Within another 6 months, he was agammaglobulinemic with no detectable B cells and suffered from *Haemophilus influenzae* and *Mycobacterium tuberculosis* pneumonias. After an additional 5 months, B cells were again detected. The onset of infectious mononucleosis at age 18 years may have resulted from new infection or a reactivation of the earlier infection. This case illustrates the unusual nature of EBV and other virus infections when the immune response is compromised.

life, even when totally asymptomatic. Children can acquire the virus at an early age by sharing contaminated drinking glasses. *Children generally have subclinical disease.* Saliva sharing between adolescents and young adults often occurs during kissing; thus EBV mononucleosis has earned the nickname "the kissing disease." Disease in these people may go unnoticed or may manifest in varying degrees of severity.

The geographic distribution of some EBV-associated neoplasms indicates a possible association with cofactors. Malaria appears to be a cofactor in the progression of chronic or latent EBV infection to AfBL. The restriction of nasopharyngeal carcinoma to people living in certain regions of China indicates a possible genetic predisposition to the cancer or the presence of cofactors in the food or environment. More subtle mechanisms may facilitate the role of EBV in 30% to 50% of cases of Hodgkin disease and other cancers.

Transplant recipients, patients with the acquired immunodeficiency syndrome (AIDS), and genetically immunodeficient people are at high risk for lymphoproliferative disorders initiated by EBV. These disorders may appear as polyclonal and monoclonal B-cell lymphomas. Such people are also at high risk for a productive EBV infection in the form of **hairy oral leukoplakia.**

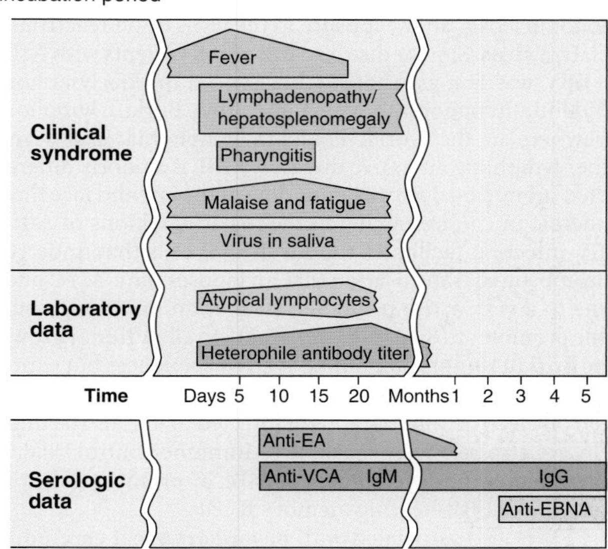

FIGURE 43-15 Clinical course of infectious mononucleosis and laboratory findings of those with the infection. Epstein-Barr virus infection may be asymptomatic or may produce the symptoms of mononucleosis. The incubation period can last as long as 2 months. *EA,* Early antigen; *EBNA,* Epstein-Barr nuclear antigen; *Ig,* immunoglobulin; *VCA,* viral capsid antigen.

Clinical Syndromes (Clinical Case 43-2)

Heterophile Antibody–Positive Infectious Mononucleosis

The triad of classic symptoms for infectious mononucleosis is **lymphadenopathy** (swollen glands), **splenomegaly** (large spleen), and **exudative pharyngitis** accompanied by high fever, malaise, and often hepatosplenomegaly (large liver and spleen). A rash may occur, especially after ampicillin treatment (for the sore throat). The major complaint of people with infectious mononucleosis is fatigue (Figure 43-15). The disease is rarely fatal in healthy people but can cause serious complications resulting from neurologic disorders, laryngeal obstruction, or rupture of the spleen. Neurologic complications include meningoencephalitis and Guillain-Barré syndrome. Mononucleosis-like syndromes can also be caused by CMV, HHV-6, *Toxoplasma gondii,* and human immunodeficiency virus (HIV). As for EBV, mononucleosis syndrome is due to T-cell proliferation in response to infection of an antigen-presenting cell, a B cell, a macrophage, or a dendritic cell, which stimulates CD4 and CD8 T cells with antigenic peptides on MHC II and MHC I. Similar to infections caused by other herpesviruses, EBV infection in a child is much milder than infection in an adolescent or adult. In fact, infection in children is usually subclinical.

Chronic Disease

EBV can cause cyclic recurrent disease in some people. These patients experience chronic tiredness and may also have low-grade fever, headaches, and a sore throat. This disorder is different from chronic fatigue syndrome, which has an unknown etiology.

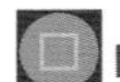

Box 43-10 Diagnosis of Epstein-Barr Virus (EBV)

1. Symptoms
   a. Mild headache, fatigue, fever
   b. Triad: lymphadenopathy, splenomegaly, exudative pharyngitis
   c. Other: hepatitis, ampicillin-induced rash
2. Complete blood cell count
   a. Hyperplasia
   b. Atypical lymphocytes (Downey cells, T cells)
3. **Heterophile antibody (transient)**
4. **EBV–antigen-specific antibody**

Epstein-Barr Virus–Induced Lymphoproliferative Diseases

On infection with EBV, people lacking T-cell immunity are likely to suffer life-threatening polyclonal leukemia-like B-cell proliferative disease and lymphoma instead of infectious mononucleosis. Men with congenital deficiencies of T-cell function are likely to suffer life-threatening X-linked lymphoproliferative disease. One such X-linked genetic defect in a T-cell gene (SLAM [signaling lymphocyte activation molecule]–associated protein) prevents the T cell from controlling B-cell growth during a normal immune response to antigen or because of EBV. Transplant recipients undergoing immunosuppressive treatment are at high risk for **post-transplant lymphoproliferative** disease, instead of infectious mononucleosis, after exposure to the virus or on reactivation of latent virus. Similar diseases are seen in patients with AIDS.

EBV was first associated with African Burkitt lymphoma (endemic lymphoma) (AfBL) and then Burkitt lymphoma elsewhere in the world, Hodgkin lymphoma, and several other lymphoproliferative diseases. AfBL is a poorly differentiated monoclonal B-cell lymphoma of the jaw and face that is endemic in children living in the malarial regions of Africa. EBV infection facilitates the survival of cells that undergo a chromosomal translocation that juxtaposes the *c-MYC* oncogene to a very active promoter, such as an immunoglobulin gene promoter [t(8;14), t(8;22), t(8;2)], to allow tumor growth. The Burkitt tumors contain EBV DNA sequences but express only the EBNA-1 viral antigen. Virions can occasionally be seen on electron micrographs of infected material. The tumor cells are also relatively invisible to immune control. Malaria may enhance the development of AfBL by promoting the proliferation of EBV-bearing memory B cells.

EBV is also associated with **nasopharyngeal carcinoma,** which is endemic in adults in Asia. The tumor cells contain EBV DNA, but unlike Burkitt lymphoma, in which the tumor cells are derived from lymphocytes, the tumor cells of nasopharyngeal carcinoma are of epithelial origin.

Hairy Oral Leukoplakia

Hairy oral leukoplakia is an unusual manifestation of a productive EBV infection of epithelial cells characterized by lesions of the tongue and mouth. It is an opportunistic manifestation that occurs in patients with AIDS.

Laboratory Diagnosis

EBV-induced infectious mononucleosis is diagnosed on the basis of the **symptoms** (Box 43-10), the finding of atypical lymphocytes, the presence of **lymphocytosis** (mononuclear cells constituting 60% to 70% of the white blood cell count, with 30% atypical lymphocytes), **heterophile antibody,** antibody to viral antigens, and viral DNA. Virus isolation is not practical. PCR and DNA probe analysis for the viral genome and amount of virus (virus load) and immunofluorescent identification of viral antigens are used to detect and follow the course of infection.

Atypical lymphocytes are probably the earliest detectable indication of an EBV infection. These cells appear with the onset of symptoms and disappear with resolution of the disease.

Heterophile antibody results from the nonspecific, mitogen-like activation of B cells by EBV and the production of a wide repertoire of antibodies. These antibodies include an IgM heterophile antibody that recognizes the Paul-Bunnell antigen on sheep, horse, and bovine erythrocytes but not that on guinea pig kidney cells. The heterophile antibody response can usually be detected by the end of the first week of illness and lasts for as long as several months. It is an excellent indication of EBV infection in adults but is not as reliable in children or infants. The horse cell (Monospot) test and ELISA are rapid and widely used for detection of the heterophile antibody.

Serologic tests for antibody to viral antigens are a more dependable method than heterophile antibody to confirm the diagnosis of EBV mononucleosis (Table 43-4; see Figure 43-15). EBV infection is indicated by the finding of any of the following: (1) IgM antibody to the VCA, (2) the presence of VCA antibody and the absence of EBNA antibody, or (3) elevation of antibodies to VCA and early antigen. The finding of both VCA and EBNA antibodies in serum indicates that the person had a previous infection. Generation of antibody to EBNA requires lysis of the infected cell and usually indicates T-cell control of active disease.

Treatment, Prevention, and Control

No effective treatment or vaccine is available for EBV disease (see Box 43-5). The ubiquitous nature of the virus and the potential for asymptomatic shedding make control of infection difficult. However, infection elicits lifelong immunity. Therefore, the best means of preventing infectious mononucleosis is exposure to the virus early in life because the disease is more benign in children.

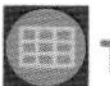
Table 43-4 Serologic Profile for Epstein-Barr Virus (EBV) Infection

	Patient's Clinical Status	Heterophile Antibodies	EBV-Specific Antibodies				Comment
			VCA-IgM	VCA-IgG	EA	EBNA	
Susceptible	–	–	–	–	–	–	Heterophile antibody present early in disease, anti-VCA and anti-MA present during disease, and anti-EBNA only present during convalescence
Acute primary infection	+	+	+	+	±	–	
Chronic primary infection	–	–	–	+	+	–	
Past infection	–	–	–	+	–	+	
Reactivation infection	–	–	–	+	+	+	
Burkitt lymphoma	–	–	–	+	+	+	
Nasopharyngeal carcinoma	–	–	–	+	+	+	

Modified from Balows A, Hausler WJ, Lennette EH, editors: *Laboratory diagnosis of infectious diseases: principles and practices,* New York, 1988, Springer-Verlag.
EA, Early antigen; *EBNA,* Epstein-Barr nuclear antigen; *IgG,* immunoglobulin G; *IgM,* immunoglobulin M; *VCA,* viral capsid antigen.

• Cytomegalovirus

CMV is a common human pathogen, infecting approximately 1% of all newborns and at least 50% to 80% of adults by age 40. It is the most common viral cause of **congenital defects.** Although usually causing mild or asymptomatic disease in children and adults, CMV is particularly important as an **opportunistic pathogen in immunocompromised patients.**

Structure and Replication

CMV is a member of the subfamily Betaherpesvirinae. It has the largest genome of the human herpesviruses. In contrast to the traditional definition of a virus, which states that a virion particle contains DNA or RNA, CMV carries specific mRNAs into the cell in the virion particle to facilitate infection. Human CMV replicates only in human cells. Fibroblasts, epithelial cells, granulocytes, macrophages, and other cells are permissive for CMV replication. Virus replication is much slower than for HSV, and CPE may not be seen for 7 to 14 days. This may facilitate the establishment of latent infection in myeloid stem cells, monocytes, lymphocytes, the stromal cells of the bone marrow, or other cells.

Pathogenesis and Immunity

The pathogenesis of CMV is similar to that of other herpesviruses in many respects (Box 43-11). CMV is an excellent parasite and readily establishes persistent and latent infections rather than an extensive lytic infection. CMV is highly cell associated and is spread throughout the body within infected cells, especially lymphocytes and leukocytes. The virus is reactivated by immunosuppression (e.g., corticosteroids, infection with HIV) and possibly by allogeneic stimulation (i.e., the host response to transfused or transplanted cells).

Cell-mediated immunity is essential for resolving and controlling the outgrowth of CMV infection. However, CMV is an expert at immune evasion and has several means for evading innate and immune responses. The virus prevents antigen presentation to both CD8 cytotoxic T cells and CD4 T cells by preventing the expression of MHC I molecules on the cell surface and by interfering with cytokine-induced expression of MHC II molecules on antigen-presenting cells (including the infected cells). A viral protein also blocks NK-cell attack of CMV-infected cells. Similar to EBV, CMV also encodes an IL-10 analog that would inhibit TH1 protective immune responses.

Box 43-11 Disease Mechanisms of Cytomegalovirus (CMV)

CMV is acquired from blood, tissue, and most body secretions.
CMV causes productive infection of epithelial and other cells.
CMV establishes latency in T cells, macrophages, and other cells.
Cell-mediated immunity is required for resolution and maintenance of latency and contributes to symptoms.
The role of antibody is limited.
Suppression of cell-mediated immunity allows recurrence and severe disease.
CMV generally causes subclinical infection.

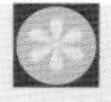
Clinical Case 43-3 A Role for Cytomegalovirus in Medulloblastoma

Cytomegalovirus (CMV) is present in a large percentage of medulloblastomas, the most common malignant brain tumor in children. In a study of these tumors by Baryawno and associates (*J Clin Invest* 121:4043–4055, 2011), CMV induced inflammation and promoted the production of interleukin 6, vascular endothelial growth factor, and prostaglandin E_2, which promoted the growth of the medulloblastoma cells. Treatment with ganciclovir and a non-steroid anti-inflammatory drug stopped the growth of these cells.

CMV is a common passenger in many children and adults and may reactivate throughout life to cause transient immune responses and inflammation and influence the health of the individual. CMV has been implicated as a cofactor for medulloblastoma, leukemia, and other diseases (Clinical Case 43-3).

Epidemiology and Clinical Syndromes

In most cases, CMV replicates and is shed without causing symptoms (Table 43-5). Activation and replication of CMV in the kidney and secretory glands promote its secretion in

Table 43-5 Sources of Cytomegalovirus Infection

Age Group	Source
Neonate	Transplacental transmission, intrauterine infections, cervical secretions
Baby or child	Body secretions: breast milk, saliva, tears, urine
Adult	Sexual transmission (semen), blood transfusion, organ graft

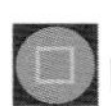

Box 43-12 Epidemiology of Cytomegalovirus Infection

Disease/Viral Factors
Virus causes lifelong infection.
Recurrent disease is source of contagion.
Virus causes asymptomatic shedding.

Transmission
Transmission occurs via blood, organ transplants, and all secretions (urine, saliva, semen, cervical secretions, breast milk, and tears).
Virus is transmitted orally and sexually, in blood transfusions, in tissue transplants, in utero, at birth, and by nursing.

Who Is at Risk?
Babies
Babies of mothers who experience seroconversion during term are at high risk for congenital defects
Sexually active people
Blood and organ recipients
Burn victims
Immunocompromised people: symptomatic and recurrent disease

Geography/Season
Virus is found worldwide.
There is no seasonal incidence.

Modes of Control
Antiviral drugs are available for serious disease.
Screening potential blood and organ donors for cytomegalovirus reduces transmission of virus.

Table 43-6 Cytomegalovirus Syndromes

Tissue	Children/Adults	Immunosuppressed Patients
Predominant presentation	Asymptomatic	Disseminated disease, severe disease
Eyes	—	Chorioretinitis
Lungs	—	Pneumonia, pneumonitis
Gastrointestinal tract	—	Esophagitis, colitis
Nervous system	Polyneuritis, myelitis	Meningitis and encephalitis, myelitis
Lymphoid system	Mononucleosis syndrome, posttransfusion syndrome	Leukopenia, lymphocytosis
Major organs	Carditis,* hepatitis*	Hepatitis
Neonates	Deafness, intracerebral calcification, microcephaly, mental retardation	—

*Complication of mononucleosis or posttransfusion syndrome.

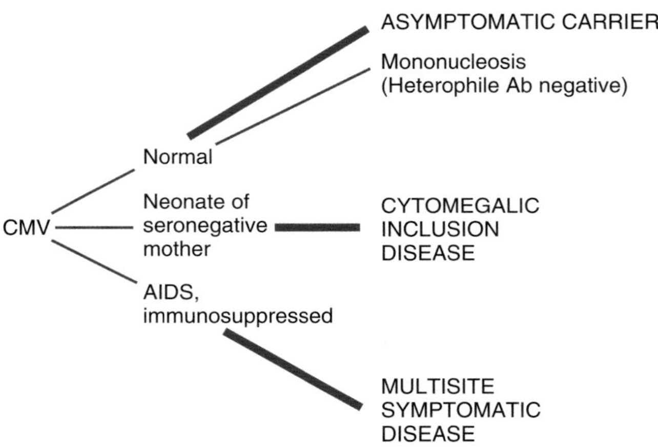

FIGURE 43-16 Outcomes of cytomegalovirus *(CMV)* infections. The outcome of CMV infection depends very heavily on the immune status of the patient. *Ab,* Antibody; *AIDS,* acquired immunodeficiency syndrome.

urine and bodily secretions. CMV can be isolated from urine, blood, throat washings, saliva, tears, breast milk, semen, stool, amniotic fluid, vaginal and cervical secretions, and tissues obtained for transplantation (Box 43-12 and Table 43-6). Virus can be transmitted to other individuals by means of blood transfusions and organ transplants. The congenital, oral, and sexual routes, blood transfusion, and tissue transplantation are the major means by which CMV is transmitted. CMV disease is an opportunistic disease, rarely causing symptoms in the immunocompetent host but causing serious disease in an immunosuppressed or immunodeficient person, such as a patient with AIDS or a neonate (Figure 43-16).

Congenital Infection

CMV is the most prevalent viral cause of congenital disease. Approximately 15% of stillborn babies are infected with CMV. Almost 1% of all newborns in the United States are infected with CMV before birth, and a large percentage of babies are infected within the first months of life. Of these, 80% may shed virus for long periods but will be asymptomatic, and 0.1% will have permanent CMV-related problems. Disease signs include small size, thrombocytopenia, microcephaly, intracerebral calcification, jaundice, hepatosplenomegaly, and rash **(cytomegalic inclusion disease).** Vision or hearing loss and mental retardation are common consequences of congenital CMV infection. The risk for serious birth defects is extremely high for infants born to mothers who had primary CMV infections during their pregnancies.

Fetuses are infected by virus in the mother's blood (primary infection) or by virus ascending from the cervix (after a recurrence). The symptoms of congenital infection are less severe or can be prevented by the immune response of a seropositive mother. Congenital CMV infection is best documented by isolation of the virus from the infant's urine during the first week of life.

Perinatal Infection

In the United States, approximately 60% of pregnant women are infected with CMV at term and are likely to experience reactivation of the virus during pregnancy. Approximately half the neonates born from an infected mother acquire CMV infection and become excreters of the virus at 3 to 4 weeks of age. Neonates may also acquire CMV from maternal milk or colostrum. Perinatal infection causes no clinically evident disease in healthy full-term infants. Significant clinical infection may occur in premature infants who acquire CMV from transfused blood, usually resulting in pneumonia and hepatitis.

Infection in Children and Adults

Approximately 40% of adolescents are infected with CMV, but this number increases to 70% to 85% of adults in the United States by the age of 40. CMV is more prevalent among people in low socioeconomic brackets living in crowded conditions and in people living in developing countries. CMV is a **sexually transmitted disease,** and 90% to 100% of patients attending sexually transmitted disease clinics are infected**.** The titer of the CMV in semen is the highest of that in any body secretion.

Although most CMV infections acquired in young adulthood are asymptomatic, patients may show a **heterophile-negative mononucleosis syndrome.** The symptoms of CMV disease are similar to those of EBV infection but with less severe pharyngitis and lymphadenopathy (see Figure 43-16). Although the presence of CMV-infected cells promotes a T-cell outgrowth (atypical lymphocytosis) similar to that seen in EBV infection, heterophile antibody is not present. Since CMV does not infect the B cell, nor does it stimulate or activate the B cell, there is no heterophile antibody. CMV disease should be suspected in a patient who has heterophile-negative mononucleosis or in whom there are signs of hepatitis but results of tests for hepatitis A, B, and C are negative.

Transmission via Transfusion and Transplantation

Transmission of CMV by blood most often results in an asymptomatic infection; if symptoms are present, they typically resemble those of mononucleosis. Fever, splenomegaly, and atypical lymphocytosis usually begin 3 to 5 weeks after transfusion. Pneumonia and mild hepatitis may also occur. CMV may also be transmitted by organ transplantation (e.g., kidneys, bone marrow), and CMV infection is often reactivated in transplant recipients during periods of intense immunosuppression.

Infection in the Immunocompromised Host

CMV is a prominent opportunistic infectious agent. In immunocompromised people, it causes symptomatic primary or recurrent disease (see Table 43-6).

CMV disease of the lung **(pneumonia and pneumonitis)** is a common outcome in immunosuppressed patients and can be fatal if not treated. CMV often causes **retinitis, colitis, or esophagitis** in patients who are severely immunodeficient (e.g., patients with AIDS). Interstitial pneumonia and encephalitis may also be caused by CMV but may be difficult to distinguish from infections caused by other opportunistic agents. CMV esophagitis may mimic candidal esophagitis. A smaller percentage of immunocompromised patients may experience CMV infection of the gastrointestinal tract. Patients with CMV colitis usually have diarrhea, weight loss, anorexia, and fever. Effective anti-HIV therapy has reduced the incidence of these diseases.

CMV is also responsible for the **failure of many kidney transplants.** This may be the result of virus replication in the graft after reactivation in the transplanted kidney or infection from the host.

Laboratory Diagnosis

Histology

The histologic hallmark of CMV infection is the **cytomegalic cell,** which is an **enlarged cell** (25 to 35 mm in diameter) that contains a dense, **central, "owl's eye," basophilic intranuclear inclusion body** (Figure 43-17 and Table 43-7). Such infected cells may be found in any tissue of the body and in urine and are thought to be epithelial in origin. The inclusions are readily seen with Papanicolaou or hematoxylin-eosin staining.

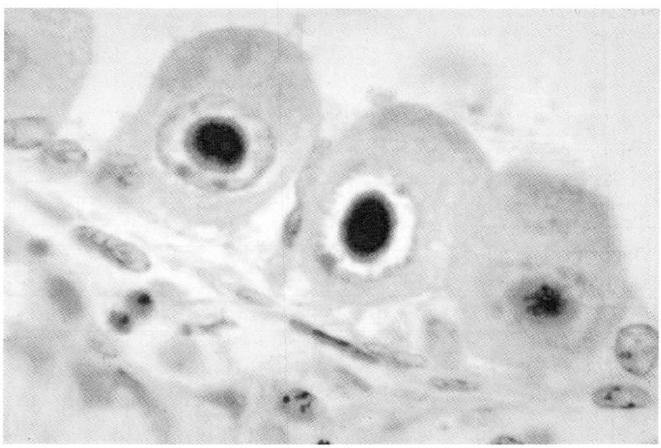

FIGURE 43-17 Cytomegalovirus-infected cell with basophilic nuclear inclusion body.

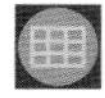

Table 43-7 Laboratory Tests for Diagnosing Cytomegalovirus Infection

Test	Finding
Cytology and histology*	"Owl's-eye" basophilic nuclear inclusion body Antigen detection
	In situ DNA probe hybridization
	PCR
Cell culture	Cytologic effect in human diploid fibroblasts (slow)
	Immunofluorescence detection of early antigens (faster)
	PCR (faster)
Serology	Primary infection

PCR, Polymerase chain reaction.

*Samples taken for analysis include urine, saliva, blood, bronchoalveolar lavage specimens, and tissue biopsy specimens.

Antigen and Genome Detection

A rapid, sensitive diagnosis can be obtained by detection of viral antigen, using immunofluorescence or an ELISA, or the viral genome, using PCR and related techniques in cells of a biopsy, blood, bronchoalveolar lavage, or urine sample (see Chapter 5, Figure 5-3).

Culture

CMV is grown in diploid fibroblast cell cultures and normally must be maintained for at least 4 to 6 weeks because the characteristic CPE develops very slowly in specimens with very low titers of the virus. Isolation of CMV is especially reliable in immunocompromised patients, who often have high titers of virus in their secretions. For example, in the semen of patients with AIDS, titers of viable virus may be greater than 10^6.

More rapid results are achieved by centrifuging a patient's sample onto cells grown on a coverslip within a shell vial. Specimens are examined after 1 to 2 days of incubation by indirect immunofluorescence for the presence of one or more of the immediate early viral antigens.

Serology

Seroconversion is usually an excellent marker for primary CMV infection. Titers of CMV-specific IgM antibody may be very high in patients with AIDS. However, CMV-specific IgM antibody may also develop during the reactivation of CMV and is therefore not a dependable indicator of primary infection.

Treatment, Prevention, and Control

Ganciclovir (dihydroxypropoxymethyl guanine), **valganciclovir** (valyl ester of ganciclovir), **cidofovir,** and **foscarnet** (phosphonoformic acid) have been approved by the FDA for the treatment of specific diseases resulting from CMV infections of immunosuppressed patients (see Box 43-5). Ganciclovir is structurally similar to ACV; it is phosphorylated and activated by a CMV-encoded protein kinase, inhibits the viral DNA polymerase, and causes DNA termination (see Chapter 40). Ganciclovir is more toxic than ACV. Ganciclovir can be used to treat severe CMV infections in immunocompromised patients. Valganciclovir is a prodrug of ganciclovir that can be taken orally, is converted to ganciclovir in the liver, and has better bioavailability than ganciclovir. Cidofovir is a phosphorylated cytidine nucleoside analog that does not require a viral enzyme for activation. Foscarnet is a simple molecule that inhibits the viral DNA polymerase by mimicking the pyrophosphate portion of nucleotide triphosphates.

CMV spreads mainly by the sexual, tissue transplantation, and transfusion routes, and spread by these means is preventable. Semen is a major vector for the sexual spread of CMV to both heterosexual and homosexual contacts. The use of condoms or abstinence would limit viral spread. Transmission of the virus can also be reduced through the screening of potential blood and organ donors for CMV seronegativity. Screening is especially important for donors of blood transfusions to be given to infants. Although congenital and perinatal transmission of CMV cannot effectively be prevented, a seropositive mother is least likely to produce a baby with symptomatic CMV disease. No vaccine for CMV is available.

• Human Herpesviruses 6 and 7

The two variants of HHV-6, HHV-6A and HHV-6B, and HHV-7, are members of the genus *Roseolovirus* of the subfamily Betaherpesvirinae. HHV-6 was first isolated from the blood of patients with AIDS and grown in T-cell cultures. It was identified as a herpesvirus because of its characteristic morphology within infected cells. Similar to CMV, HHV-6 is lymphotropic and ubiquitous. At least 45% of the population is seropositive for HHV-6 by age 2 years, and almost 100% by adulthood. In 1988, HHV-6 was serologically associated with a common disease of children, **exanthem subitum,** commonly known as **roseola.** HHV-7 was isolated in a similar manner from the T cells of a patient with AIDS who was also infected with HHV-6, and later it was also shown to cause exanthem subitum.

Pathogenesis and Immunity

HHV-6 infection occurs very early in life. The virus replicates in the salivary gland, is shed, and is transmitted in saliva.

HHV-6 primarily infects lymphocytes, especially CD4 T cells. HHV-6 establishes a latent infection in T cells and monocytes but may replicate on activation of the cells. Cells in which the virus is replicating appear large and refractile and have occasional intranuclear and intracytoplasmic inclusion bodies. Similar to the replication of CMV, the replication of HHV-6 is controlled by cell-mediated immunity. Similar to CMV, the virus is likely to become activated in patients with AIDS or other lymphoproliferative and immunosuppressive disorders and cause opportunistic disease.

Clinical Syndromes (Box 43-13)

Exanthem subitum, or roseola, is caused by either HHV-6B or HHV-7 and is one of the five classic childhood exanthems previously mentioned (Figure 43-18). It is characterized by the rapid onset of high fever of a few days' duration, which is followed by a rash on the trunk and face, and then it spreads and lasts only 24 to 48 hours. The presence of infected T cells or the activation of delayed-type hypersensitivity T cells in the skin may be the cause of the rash. The disease is effectively controlled and resolved by cell-mediated immunity, but the virus establishes a lifelong latent infection of T cells. Although usually benign, HHV-6 is the most common cause of febrile seizures in childhood (age 6 to 24 months).

HHV-6 may also cause a mononucleosis syndrome and lymphadenopathy in adults and may be a cofactor in the pathogenesis of AIDS. Similar to CMV, HHV-6 may reactivate in transplant patients and contribute to the failure of the graft. HHV-6 has also been associated with multiple sclerosis and chronic fatigue syndrome.

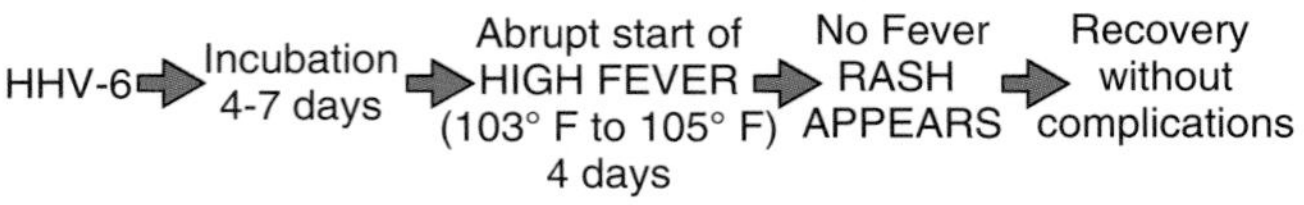

FIGURE 43-18 Time course of symptoms of exanthem subitum (roseola) caused by human herpesvirus 6 *(HHV-6)*. Compare these symptoms and this time course with those of fifth disease, which is caused by parvovirus B19 (see Chapter 45).

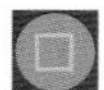 **Box 43-13 Clinical Summaries**

Herpes Simplex Virus (HSV)

Primary oral herpes: A 5-year-old boy has an ulcerative rash with vesicles around the mouth. Vesicles and ulcers are also present within the mouth. Results of a Tzanck smear show multinucleated giant cells (syncytia) and Cowdry type A inclusion bodies. The lesions resolve after 18 days.

Recurrent oral HSV: A 22-year-old medical student studying for examinations feels a twinge at the crimson border of his lip and 24 hours later has a single vesicular lesion at the site.

Recurrent genital HSV: A sexually active 32-year-old woman has a recurrence of ulcerative vaginal lesions with pain, itching, dysuria, and systemic symptoms 48 hours after being exposed to ultraviolet B light while skiing. The lesions resolve within 8 days. Results of a Papanicolaou smear show multinucleated giant cells (syncytia) and Cowdry type A inclusion bodies.

Encephalitis HSV: A patient has focal neurologic symptoms and seizures. Magnetic resonance imaging results show destruction of a temporal lobe. Erythrocytes are present in the cerebrospinal fluid, and polymerase chain reaction is positive for viral DNA.

Varicella-Zoster Virus

Varicella (chickenpox): A 5-year-old boy develops a fever and a maculopapular rash on his abdomen 14 days after meeting with his cousin, who also developed the rash. Successive crops of lesions appear for 3 to 5 days, and the rash spreads peripherally.

Zoster (shingles): A 65-year-old woman has a belt of vesicles along the thoracic dermatome and experiences severe pain localized to the region.

Epstein-Barr Virus

Infectious mononucleosis: A 23-year-old college student develops malaise, fatigue, fever, swollen glands, and pharyngitis. After empirical treatment with ampicillin for a sore throat, a rash appears. Heterophile antibody and atypical lymphocytes are detected from blood.

Cytomegalovirus (CMV)

Congenital CMV disease: A neonate exhibits microcephaly, hepatosplenomegaly, and rash. Intracerebral calcification is noted on a radiograph. The mother had symptoms similar to mononucleosis during the third trimester of her pregnancy.

Human Herpesvirus 6

Roseola (exanthem subitum): A 4-year-old child experiences a rapid onset of high fever that lasts for 3 days and then suddenly returns to normal. Two days later, a maculopapular rash appears on the trunk and spreads to other parts of the body.

In approximately 1% of individuals in the United States and the United Kingdom, HHV-6 is integrated into the telomeres of every chromosome and can be genetically transmitted to offspring. The virus may be reactivated by certain drugs (including antibiotics and steroids), produce virus, and may cause fatigue, cognitive dysfunction, and other problems.

• Other Human Herpesviruses

Human Herpesvirus 8 (Kaposi Sarcoma–Associated Herpesvirus)

HHV-8 DNA sequences were discovered in biopsy specimens of **Kaposi sarcoma, primary effusion lymphoma** (a rare type of B-cell lymphoma), **and multicentric Castleman disease** through the use of PCR analysis. Kaposi sarcoma is one of the characteristic opportunistic diseases associated with AIDS. Genome sequence analysis showed that the virus was unique and a member of the subfamily Gammaherpesvirinae. Similar to EBV, the B cell is the primary target cell for HHV-8, but the virus also infects a limited number of endothelial cells, monocytes, and epithelial and sensory nerve cells. Within the Kaposi sarcoma tumors, endothelial spindle cells contain the virus.

HHV-8 encodes several proteins that resemble human proteins and promote the growth and prevent apoptosis of the infected and surrounding cells. These proteins include an IL-6 homolog (growth and antiapoptosis), a Bcl-2 analog (antiapoptosis), chemokines, and a chemokine receptor. These proteins can promote growth and development of polyclonal Kaposi sarcoma cells in AIDS patients and others. HHV-8 DNA is present and is associated with peripheral blood lymphocytes, most likely B cells, in approximately 10% of immunocompetent people. HHV-8 is more prevalent in certain geographic areas (Italy, Greece, Africa) and in patients with AIDS. Kaposi sarcoma is the most common cancer in sub-Saharan Africa. The virus is most likely a sexually transmitted disease but may be spread by other means.

Herpesvirus simiae (B virus) (subfamily Alphaherpesvirinae, the simian counterpart of HSV) is indigenous to Asian monkeys. The virus is transmitted to humans by monkey bites or saliva, or even by tissues and cells widely used in virology laboratories. Once infected, a human may have pain, localized redness, and vesicles at the site where the virus entered. An encephalopathy develops and is often fatal; most people who survive have serious brain damage. PCR or serologic tests can be used to establish the diagnosis of B-virus infections. Virus isolation requires special facilities.

Bibliography

Boshoff C, Weiss RA: Kaposi sarcoma herpesvirus: new perspectives, *Curr Top Microbiol Immunol* (vol 312), New York, 2007, Springer-Verlag.

Cann AJ: *Principles of molecular virology*, San Diego, 2005, Academic.

Carter J, Saunders V: *Virology: principles and applications*, Chichester, England, 2007, Wiley.

Cohen J, Powderly WG: *Infectious diseases*, ed 2, St Louis, 2004, Mosby.

Collier L, Oxford J: *Human virology*, ed 3, Oxford, 2006, Oxford University Press.

Flint SJ, Enquist LW, Racaniello VR, et al: *Principles of virology: molecular biology, pathogenesis and control of animal viruses*, ed 3, Washington, DC, 2009, American Society for Microbiology Press.

Gorbach SL, Bartlett JG, Blacklow NR: *Infectious diseases*, ed 3, Philadelphia, 2004, WB Saunders.

Knipe DM, Howley PM, Griffin DE, et al: *Fields virology*, ed 5, Philadelphia, 2006, Lippincott Williams & Wilkins.

Mandell GL, Bennet JE, Dolin R: *Principles and practice of infectious diseases*, ed 6, Philadelphia, 2004, Churchill Livingstone.

McGeoch DJ: The genomes of the human herpesviruses: contents, relationships, and evolution, *Annu Rev Microbiol* 43:235–265, 1989.

Richman DD, Whitley RJ, Hayden FG: *Clinical virology*, ed 3, Washington, DC, 2009, American Society for Microbiology Press.

Strauss JH, Strauss EG: *Viruses and human disease*, ed 2, San Diego, 2007, Academic.

Voyles BA: *The biology of viruses*, ed 2, Boston, 2002, McGraw-Hill.

White DO, Fenner FJ: *Medical virology*, ed 4, New York, 1994, Academic.

Herpes Simplex Virus

Animations of steps of HSV infection and replication (website): www.dbc.uci.edu/~faculty/wagner/movieindex.html. Accessed May 14, 2012.

Arbesfeld DM, Thomas I: Cutaneous herpes simplex infections, *Am Fam Physician* 43:1655–1664, 1991.

Arduino PG, Porter SR: Herpes simplex virus type 1 infection: overview on relevant clinico-pathological features, *J Oral Pathol Med* 37:107–121, 2008.

Beauman JG: Genital herpes: a review, *Am Fam Physician* 72:1527–1534, 2005.

Cunningham AL, Diefenbach RJ, Miranda-Saksena M, et al: The cycle of human herpes simplex virus infection: virus transport and immune control, *J Infect Dis* 194(S1):S11–S18, 2006.

Dawkins BJ: Genital herpes simplex infections, *Prim Care* 17:95–113, 1990.

Kimberlin DW: Neonatal herpes simplex virus infection, *Clin Microbiol Rev* 17:1–13, 2004.

Landy HJ, Grossman JH: Herpes simplex virus, *Obstet Gynecol Clin North Am* 16:495–515, 1989.

National Institute of Allergy and Infectious Diseases: Genital herpes (website). www.niaid.nih.gov/topics/genitalherpes/Pages/default.aspx. Accessed August 7, 2015.

Rouse BT: Herpes simplex virus: pathogenesis, immunobiology and control, *Curr Top Microbiol Immunol* (vol 179), Berlin, New York, 1992, Springer-Verlag.

Whitley RJ, Kimberlin DW, Roizman B: Herpes simplex virus: state of the art clinical article, *Clin Infect Dis* 26:541–555, 1998.

Varicella-Zoster Virus

Abendroth A, et al: Varicella-zoster virus infections, *Curr Top Microbiol Immunol* (vol 342), Berlin, Heidelberg, 2010, Springer-Verlag.

Chia-Chi Ku V, Besser J, Abendroth A: Varicella-zoster virus pathogenesis and immunobiology: new concepts emerging from investigations with the SCIDhu mouse model, *J Virol* 79:2651–2658, 2005.

Gnann JW, Whitley RJ: Herpes zoster, *N Engl J Med* 347:340–346, 2002.

Ostrove JM: Molecular biology of varicella zoster virus, *Adv Virus Res* 38:45–98, 1990.

White CJ: Varicella-zoster virus vaccine, *Clin Infect Dis* 24:753–761, quiz 762–763, 1997.

Epstein-Barr Virus

Basgoz N, Preiksaitis JK: Post-transplant lymphoproliferative disorder, *Infect Dis Clin North Am* 9:901–923, 1995.

Cohen JI: The biology of Epstein-Barr virus: lessons learned from the virus and the host, *Curr Opin Immunol* 11:365–370, 1999.

Faulkner GC, Krajewski AS, Crawford DH: The ins and outs of EBV infection, *Trends Microbiol* 8:185–189, 2000.

Hutt-Fletcher L: Epstein Barr virus entry, *J Virol* 81:7825–7832, 2007.

Sugden B: EBV's open sesame, *Trends Biochem Sci* 17:239–240, 1992.

Takada K: Epstein-Barr virus and human cancer, *Curr Top Microbiol Immunol* (vol 258), New York, 2001, Springer-Verlag.

Thorley-Lawson DA: Epstein-Barr virus and the B cell: that's all it takes, *Trends Microbiol* 4:204–208, 1996.

Thorley-Lawson DA, Babcock GJ: A model for persistent infection with Epstein-Barr virus: the stealth virus of human B cells, *Life Sci* 65:1433–1453, 1999.

Cytomegalovirus and Human Herpesviruses 6, 7, and 8

Bigoni B, Dolcetti R, de Lellis L, et al: Human herpesvirus 8 is present in the lymphoid system of healthy persons and can reactivate in the course of AIDS, *J Infect Dis* 173:542–549, 1996.

Campadelli-Fiume G, Mirandoa P, Menotti L: Human herpesvirus 6: an emerging pathogen, *Emerg Infect Dis* 5:353–366, 1999. Website: www.cdc.gov/ncidod/eid/vol5no3/campadelli. Accessed May 14, 2012.

CDC home page on CMV (website): www.cdc.gov/cmv/index.html. Accessed August 7, 2015.

De Bolle L, Naesens L, De Clercq E: Update on human herpesvirus 6 biology, clinical features, and therapy, *Clin Microbiol Rev* 18:217–245, 2005.

Edelman DC: Human herpesvirus 8—a novel human pathogen, *Virol J* 2:78–110, 2005.

Flamand L, Komaroff AL, Arbuckle JH, et al: Review, part 1: human herpesvirus-6—basic biology, diagnostic testing, and antiviral efficacy, *J Med Virol* 82:1560–1568, 2010.

Gnann JW, Pellett PE, Jaffe HW: Human herpesvirus 8 and Kaposi sarcoma in persons infected with human immunodeficiency virus, *Clin Infect Dis* 30:S72–S76, 2000.

HHV-6 Foundation (website): http://hhv-6foundation.org/. Accessed March 20, 2014.

Integrated HHV-6 (website): http://hhv-6foundation.org/wp-content/uploads/2011/12/Pellett-2011-CIHHV-6-Q-A.pdf. Accessed March 20, 2014.

McDougall JK: Cytomegalovirus, *Curr Top Microbiol Immunol* (vol 154), Berlin, New York, 1990, Springer-Verlag.

Pellet PE, Black JB, Yamamoto Y: Human herpesvirus 6: the virus and the search for its role as a human pathogen, *Adv Virus Res* 41:1–52, 1992.

Plachter B, Sinzger C, Jahn G: Cell types involved in replication and distribution of human cytomegalovirus, *Adv Virus Res* 46:197–264, 1996.

Proceedings of a conference on pathogenesis of cytomegalovirus diseases, April 5–7, 1990, Irvine, California, *Transplant Proc* 23(Suppl 3):1–182, 1991.

Salvaggio MR: Human herpesvirus type 6 (website). www.emedicine.com/MED/topic1035.htm. Accessed August 7, 2015.

Shenk TE, Stinski MF: *Human cytomegalovirus*, New York, 2008, Springer-Verlag.

Stoeckle MY: The spectrum of human herpesvirus 6 infection: from roseola infantum to adult disease, *Annu Rev Med* 51:423–430, 2000.

Wyatt LS, Frenkel N: Human herpesvirus 7 is a constitutive inhabitant of adult human saliva, *J Virol* 66:3206–3209, 1992.

Yamanishi K, Okuno T, Shiraki K, et al: Identification of human herpesvirus-6 as a causal agent for exanthema subitum, *Lancet* 1:1065–1067, 1988.

CHAPTER

44

POXVIRUSES

A goat herder has a large vesicular lesion on his index finger.

1. How does the orf virus infecting this individual resemble smallpox?
2. What was the source, and how was it acquired?
3. How is replication of this virus different from other DNA viruses?
4. Why was it possible to eradicate wild-type smallpox virus?

A 57-year-old woman with rheumatoid arthritis and treated with a tumor necrosis factor antagonist notices a large number of umbilicated papules on the skin of her upper thighs.

5. How does the molluscum contagiosum virus resemble and differ from other poxviruses?
6. What was the source, and how was it acquired?
7. What other conditions increase susceptibility to this infection and presentation?

Answers to these questions are available on StudentConsult.com.

• SUMMARIES CLINICALLY SIGNIFICANT ORGANISMS

Poxviruses

Trigger Words

Molluscum, smallpox, zoonosis, vaccinia vaccine, cytoplasmic replication

Biology, Virulence, and Disease

- Very large, enveloped with complex morphology, linear DNA genome fused at ends, virus encodes DNA-dependent RNA and DNA-dependent DNA polymerases
- Cell-mediated immunity essential for control
- Molluscum contagiosum stimulates cell growth to cause wart-like growth; only infects humans
- Smallpox: lytic, only infects humans, vesicles appear all at once, bioterror agent
- Vaccinia, orf: lytic viruses, zoonotic

Epidemiology

- Smallpox transmitted by aerosols, direct contact. All others only by contact.

Diagnosis

- PCR genome analysis of lesion fluid

Treatment, Prevention, and Control

- Vaccinia virus as vaccine for smallpox
- Quarantine

The poxviruses include the human viruses **variola (smallpox)** (genus *Orthopoxvirus*) and **molluscum contagiosum** (genus *Molluscipoxvirus*) as well as some viruses that naturally infect animals but can cause incidental infection in humans **(zoonoses).** Many of these viruses share antigenic determinants with smallpox, allowing the use of an animal poxvirus for a human vaccine.

In 18th century England, smallpox accounted for 7% to 12% of all deaths and the deaths of one third of children. However, the development of the first live vaccine in 1796 and the later worldwide distribution of this vaccine led to eradication of smallpox by 1980. As a result, reference stocks of smallpox virus in two World Health Organization (WHO) laboratories were destroyed in 1996 after an international agreement to do so was reached. Unfortunately, smallpox did not disappear. Stocks of the virus still exist in the United States and Russia. While the world was successfully eliminating natural smallpox, the former Union of Soviet Socialist Republics (U.S.S.R.) was stockpiling immense amounts of weaponized smallpox virus for biowarfare. Smallpox is considered a *category A agent* by the U.S. Centers for Disease Control and Prevention (CDC), along with anthrax, plague, botulism, tularemia, and viral hemorrhagic fevers, because of their great potential as bioterrorism-biowarfare agents capable of large-scale dissemination and serious disease. The potential for these stocks of smallpox to be acquired and used by a terrorist has been the impetus to renew interest in developing new smallpox vaccine programs and antiviral drugs.

On a positive note, the vaccinia and canarypox viruses have found a beneficial use as gene delivery vectors and for the development of hybrid vaccines. These hybrid viruses contain and express the genes of other infectious agents, and infection results in immunization against both agents.

• Structure and Replication

Poxviruses are the largest viruses, almost visible on light microscopy (Box 44-1). They measure 230 × 300 nm and are ovoid to brick shaped with a complex morphology. The poxvirus virion particle must carry many enzymes, including a deoxyribonucleic acid (DNA)-dependent ribonucleic acid (RNA) polymerase, to allow viral messenger RNA (mRNA) synthesis to occur in the cytoplasm. The viral genome consists of a large, double-stranded, linear DNA that is fused at both ends. The structure and replication of vaccinia virus is representative of the other poxviruses (Figure 44-1). The genome of vaccinia virus consists of approximately 189,000 base pairs.

The replication of poxviruses is unique among the DNA-containing viruses in that the entire multiplication cycle takes place within the host cell cytoplasm (Figure 44-2). Thus poxviruses must encode the enzymes required for mRNA and DNA synthesis as well as activities other DNA viruses normally obtain from the host cell.

After binding to a cell surface receptor, the poxvirus outer envelope fuses with cellular membranes, either at the cell surface or within the cell. Early gene transcription is initiated on removal of the outer membrane. The virion core contains a specific transcriptional activator and all the enzymes necessary for transcription, including a multisubunit RNA polymerase, as well as enzymes for polyadenylate addition and capping mRNA. Among the early proteins produced is an uncoating protein (uncoatase) that removes the core membrane, thereby liberating viral DNA into the cell cytoplasm. Viral DNA then replicates in electron-dense cytoplasmic inclusions (Guarnieri inclusion bodies), referred to as **factories.** Late viral mRNA for structural, virion, and other proteins is produced after DNA replication. In poxviruses, unlike other viruses, the membranes assemble around the core factories. Approximately 10,000 viral particles are produced per infected cell. Different forms of viruses are released by exocytosis or upon cell lysis, but both are infectious.

Molluscum contagiosum virus infection proceeds similarly to the other poxviruses but is restricted to keratinocytes, stimulates the growth of the cell, prevents apoptosis, inhibits inflammation, and is not cytolytic. Like human papillomaviruses, the virus is released when the keratinocyte matures and senesces.

Box 44-1 Unique Properties of Poxviruses

- Poxviruses are the largest, most complex viruses.
- Poxviruses have complex, oval to brick-shaped morphology with internal structure.
- Poxviruses have a linear, double-stranded DNA genome with fused ends.
- Poxviruses are **DNA viruses that replicate in the cytoplasm.**
- Virus encodes and carries all proteins necessary for mRNA synthesis.
- Virus also encodes proteins for functions such as DNA synthesis, nucleotide scavenging, and immune escape mechanisms.
- Virus is assembled in inclusion bodies (Guarnieri bodies; factories), where it acquires its outer membranes.

• Pathogenesis and Immunity

After being inhaled, smallpox virus replicates in the upper respiratory tract (Figure 44-3). Dissemination occurs via lymphatic and cell-associated viremic spread. Internal and dermal tissues are inoculated after a second, more intense viremia, causing simultaneous eruption of the characteristic "pocks." Molluscum contagiosum and the other poxviruses, however, are acquired through direct contact with lesions and do not spread extensively. Molluscum contagiosum stimulates cell growth and causes a wartlike lesion rather than a lytic infection.

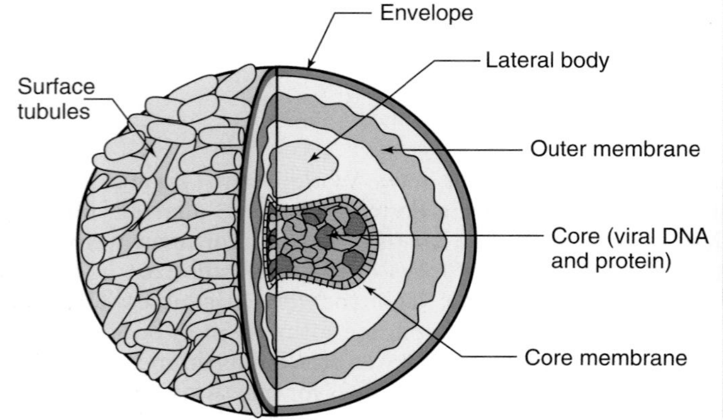

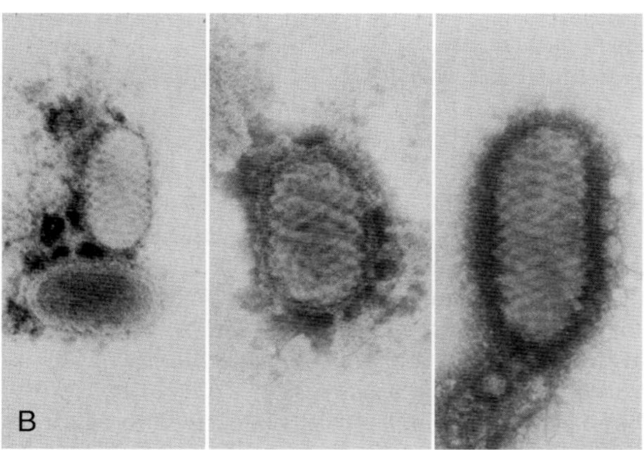

FIGURE 44-1 **A,** Structure of the vaccinia virus. Within the virion, the core assumes the shape of a dumbbell because of the large lateral bodies. Virions have a double membrane; the "outer membrane" assembles around the core in the cytoplasm, and the virus leaves the cell by exocytosis or upon cell lysis. **B,** Electron micrographs of orf virus. Note its complex structure.

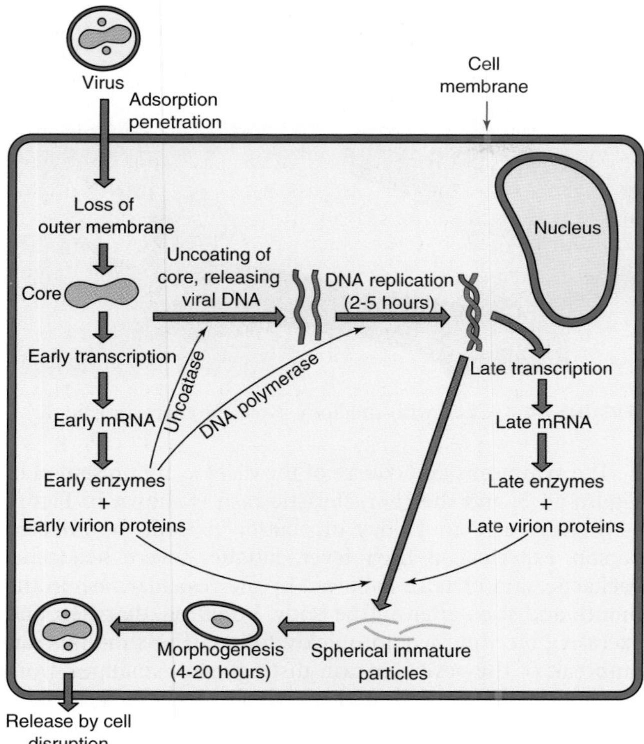

FIGURE 44-2 Replication of vaccinia virus. The core is released into the cytoplasm, where virion enzymes initiate transcription of early genes. A viral-encoded "uncoatase" enzyme then causes the release of DNA. Viral polymerase replicates the genome, and late transcription occurs. DNA and protein are assembled into cores with the core membrane. An outer membrane shrouds the core containing the lateral bodies and the enzymes required for infectivity. The virion is exocytosed or is released by cell lysis.

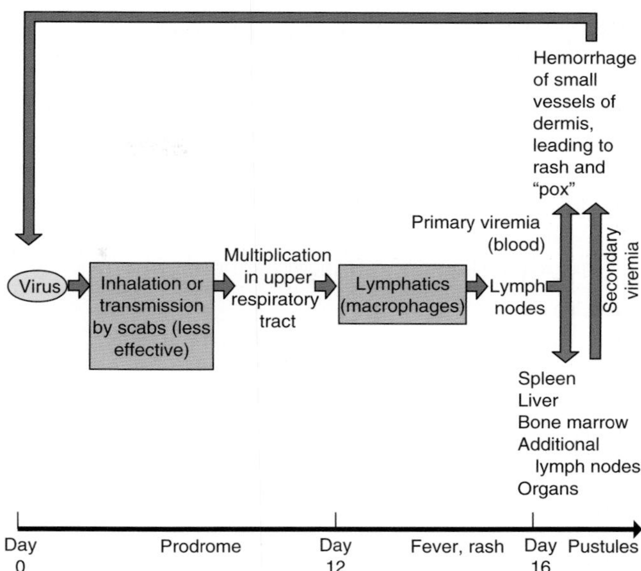

FIGURE 44-3 Spread of smallpox within the body. The virus enters and replicates in the respiratory tract without causing symptoms or contagion. The virus infects macrophages, which enter the lymphatic system and carry the virus to regional lymph nodes. The virus then replicates and initiates a viremia, causing the infection to spread to the spleen, bone marrow, lymph nodes, liver, and all organs, followed by the skin (rash). A secondary viremia causes the development of additional lesions throughout the host, followed by death or recovery with or without sequelae. Recovery from smallpox was associated with prolonged immunity and lifelong protection.

Box 44-2 Disease Mechanisms of Poxvirus

Smallpox is initiated by respiratory tract infection and is spread mainly by the lymphatic system and cell-associated viremia.

Molluscum contagiosum and other poxviruses are transmitted by contact.

Virus may cause initial stimulation of cell growth and then cell lysis.

Virus encodes immune evasion mechanisms.

Cell-mediated immunity and humoral immunity are important for resolution.

Most poxviruses share antigenic determinants, allowing preparation of "safe" live vaccines from animal poxviruses.

The poxviruses encode many proteins that facilitate their replication and pathogenesis in the host. They include proteins that initially stimulate host cell growth and then lead to cell lysis and viral spread.

Cell-mediated immunity is essential for resolving a poxvirus infection. However, up to 30% of the genome of poxviruses is devoted to activities that help the virus evade immune control, including proteins that impede the interferon, complement, inflammatory, antibody, and cell-mediated protective responses. In addition, these viruses can spread cell to cell and avoid antibody. The disease mechanisms of poxviruses are summarized in Box 44-2.

• Epidemiology

Smallpox and molluscum contagiosum are strictly human viruses. Smallpox is transmitted by aerosols and by contact with lesion material or by a fomite. Molluscum contagiosum is spread by direct contact (e.g., sexual contact, wrestling, self-inoculation) or by fomites (e.g., towels). In contrast, the natural hosts for the other poxviruses are vertebrates other than humans (e.g., cow, sheep, goats), and they infect humans only through accidental or occupational exposure (zoonosis). A recent outbreak of monkeypox in the United States is such an example. The infected individuals had purchased prairie dog pets that had been in contact with Gambian giant rats, which were the probable source of the virus. The revival of smallpox vaccination of military personnel has brought with it incidence of vaccine-mediated (vaccinia) disease in contacts.

Smallpox (variola) was very contagious and, as just noted, was spread primarily by the respiratory route. It was also spread less efficiently through close contact with dried virus on clothes or other materials. Despite the severity of the disease and its tendency to spread, several factors contributed to its elimination, as listed in Box 44-3.

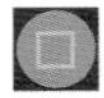

Box 44-3 Properties of Natural Smallpox That Led to Its Eradication

Viral Characteristics

Exclusive human host range (no animal reservoirs or vectors)
Single serotype (immunization protected against all infections)

Disease Characteristics

Consistent disease presentation with visible pustules (identification of sources of contagion allowed quarantine and vaccination of contacts)

Vaccine

Immunization with animal poxviruses protects against smallpox
Stable, inexpensive, and easy-to-administer vaccine
Presence of scar, indicating successful vaccination

Public Health Service

Successful worldwide World Health Organization program combining vaccination and quarantine

Table 44-1 Diseases Associated with Poxviruses

Virus	Disease	Source	Location
Variola	Smallpox (now extinct)	Humans	Extinct
Vaccinia	Used for smallpox vaccination	Laboratory product	—
Orf	Localized lesion	Zoonosis: sheep, goats	Worldwide
Cowpox	Localized lesion	Zoonosis: rodents, cats, cows	Europe
Pseudocowpox	Milker's nodule	Zoonosis: dairy cows	Worldwide
Monkeypox	Generalized disease	Zoonosis: monkeys, squirrels	Africa
Bovine papular stomatitis virus	Localized lesion	Zoonosis: calves, beef cattle	Worldwide
Tanapox	Localized lesion	Rare zoonosis: monkeys	Africa
Yabapox	Localized lesion	Rare zoonosis: monkeys, baboons	Africa
Molluscum contagiosum	Many skin lesions	Humans	Worldwide

Modified from Balows A, Hausler WJ, Lennette EH, editors: *Laboratory diagnosis of infectious diseases: principles and practice,* vol 2, New York, 1988, Springer-Verlag.

• Clinical Syndromes

The diseases associated with poxviruses are listed in Table 44-1.

Smallpox

The two variants of smallpox were variola major, which was associated with a mortality of 15% to 40%, and variola minor, which was associated with a mortality of 1%. Smallpox was usually initiated by infection of the respiratory tract, with subsequent involvement of local lymph glands, which in turn led to viremia.

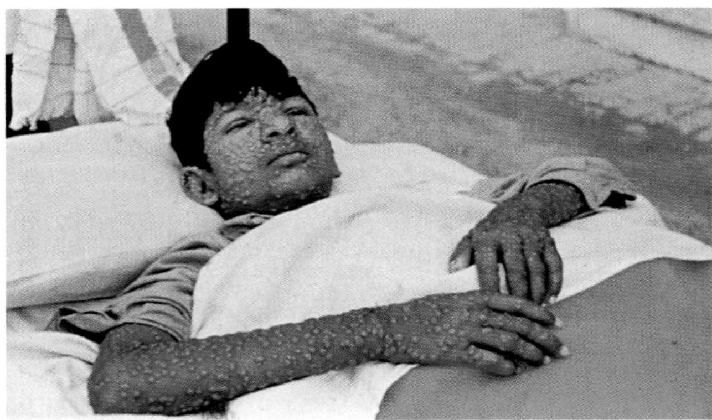

FIGURE 44-4 Child with smallpox. Note the characteristic rash.

The symptoms and course of the disease are presented in Figure 44-3, and the characteristic rash is shown in Figure 44-4. After a 5- to 17-day incubation period, the infected person experienced high fever, fatigue, severe headache, backache, and malaise, followed by the vesicular rash in the mouth and soon after on the body. Vomiting, diarrhea, and excessive bleeding would quickly follow. The simultaneous outbreak of the vesicular rash distinguishes smallpox from the vesicles of varicella-zoster, which erupt in successive crops.

Smallpox was the first disease to be controlled by immunization, and its eradication is one of the greatest triumphs of medical epidemiology. Eradication resulted from a massive WHO campaign to vaccinate all susceptible people, especially those exposed to anyone with the disease, and thereby interrupt the chain of human-to-human transmission. The campaign began in 1967 and succeeded. The last case of naturally acquired infection was reported in 1977, and eradication of the disease was acknowledged in 1980.

Variolation, an early approach to immunization, involved inoculation of susceptible people with the virulent smallpox pus. It was first performed in the Far East and later in England. Cotton Mather introduced the practice to America. Variolation was associated with a fatality rate of approximately 1%, a better risk than that associated with smallpox itself. In 1796, Jenner developed and then popularized a vaccine using the less virulent cowpox virus, which shares antigenic determinants with smallpox.

Renewed interest is being paid to antiviral drugs that are effective against smallpox and other poxviruses. Cidofovir, a nucleotide analog capable of inhibiting the viral DNA polymerase, is effective and approved for treatment of poxvirus infections. Newer, safer vaccines are being stockpiled in response to concerns regarding the use of smallpox in biowarfare.

Vaccinia and Vaccine-Related Disease (Clinical Case 44-1)

Vaccinia is the virus used for the smallpox vaccine. Although thought to be derived from cowpox, it may be a hybrid or other poxvirus. The vaccination procedure consisted of scratching live virus into the patient's skin with a bifurcated needle and then observing for the development of vesicles and pustules to confirm a "take." As the incidence of smallpox waned, however, it became apparent that there were more complications related to vaccination than cases of

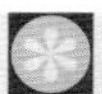

Clinical Case 44-1 Vaccinia Infection in Vaccinated Contacts

The Centers for Disease Control and Prevention (CDC) (*MMWR Morb Mortal Wkly Rep* 56:417–419, 2007) described the case of a woman who visited the public health clinic in Alaska because the pain from vaginal tears had increased over the course of 10 days. There was no fever, itching, or dysuria. Clinical examination showed two shallow ulcers, redness, and vaginal discharge. There was no inguinal lymphadenopathy. A viral specimen from the lesion was identified by the CDC as the vaccine strain of vaccinia virus. Presence of the virus was identified by a variation of a polymerase chain reaction test, which produces characteristic vaccinia DNA fragments from the genome. Although the woman routinely insisted on using condoms during sex, a condom broke during vaginal intercourse with a new male sex partner. The male partner was in the U.S. Military and had been vaccinated for smallpox 3 days before initiating his relationship with the woman. Virus from the lesion was placed on the condom or into the site. Military and other personnel are receiving vaccinia immunization for protection against weaponized smallpox. This increases the potential for unintentional transmission of the vaccinia vaccine virus. Other cases of vaccine-related vaccinia infection have included infants and individuals with atopic dermatitis, who had more severe consequences.

smallpox. Several of these complications were severe and even fatal. Therefore, routine smallpox vaccination began to be discontinued in the 1970s and was totally discontinued after 1980, but it has been reintroduced for military personnel and first responders in case of biowarfare.

Complications from vaccination included encephalitis and progressive infection (vaccinia necrosum), the latter occurring occasionally in immunocompromised patients who were inadvertently vaccinated. Recent cases of vaccine-related disease have been noted in family members and contacts of immunized military personnel (see Clinical Case 44-1). The virus was transmitted to these individuals by contact with vesicular fluid. They can be treated with vaccinia immune globulin and antiviral drugs.

Orf, Cowpox, and Monkeypox

Human infection with the orf (poxvirus of sheep and goat) or cowpox (vaccinia) virus is usually an occupational hazard resulting from direct contact with lesions on the animal. A single nodular lesion usually forms on the point of contact, such as the fingers, hand, or forearm, and is hemorrhagic (cowpox) or granulomatous (orf or pseudocowpox) (Figure 44-5). Vesicular lesions frequently develop and then regress in 25 to 35 days, generally without scar formation. The lesions may be mistaken for anthrax. The virus can be grown in culture or seen directly with electron microscopy but is usually diagnosed from the symptoms and patient history.

The more than 100 cases of illnesses resembling smallpox have been attributed to the monkeypox virus. Except for the outbreak in Illinois, Indiana, and Wisconsin in 2003, they all have occurred in western and central Africa, especially Zaire. Monkeypox causes a milder version of smallpox disease, including the pocklike rash.

Molluscum Contagiosum (Box 44-4)

Molluscum contagiosum is a common disease affecting 3% to 20% of the population. The lesions of molluscum

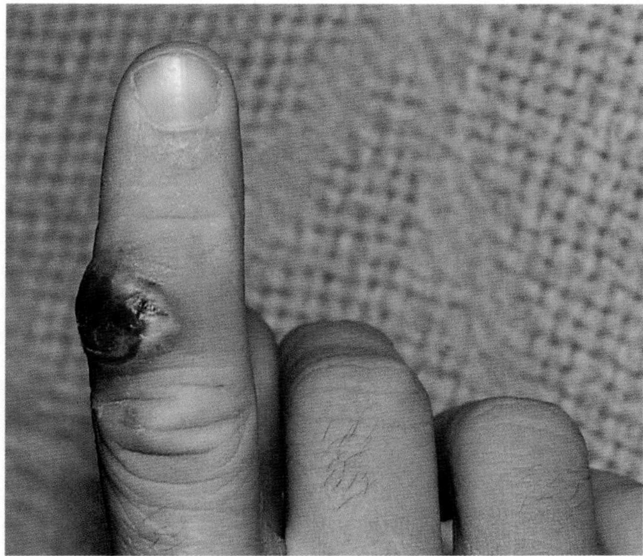

FIGURE 44-5 Orf lesion on the finger of a taxidermist. (Courtesy Joe Meyers, MD, Akron, Ohio.)

Box 44-4 Clinical Summary

Molluscum contagiosum: A 5-year-old girl has a group of wartlike growths on her arm that exude white material on squeezing.

contagiosum differ significantly from other pox lesions in being nodular to wartlike (Figure 44-6A). They begin as papules and then become pearl-like umbilicated nodules that are 2 to 10 mm in diameter and have a central caseous plug that can be squeezed out. They are most common on the trunk, genitalia, and proximal extremities and usually occur in a cluster of 5 to 20 nodules. The incubation period for molluscum contagiosum is 2 to 8 weeks. The disease is more common in children than adults, but its incidence is increasing in sexually active and immunocompromised individuals.

The diagnosis of molluscum contagiosum is confirmed histologically by the finding of characteristic large, eosinophilic, cytoplasmic inclusions (molluscum bodies) in epithelial cells (see Figure 44-6B). These bodies can be seen in biopsy specimens or in the expressed caseous core of a nodule. The molluscum contagiosum virus cannot be grown in tissue culture or animal models.

Lesions of molluscum contagiosum usually disappear within 2 to 12 months, presumably as a result of immune responses. The nodules can be removed by curettage (scraping) or application of liquid nitrogen or iodine solutions.

Hybrid Poxviruses for Gene Delivery and Vaccines

The vaccinia and canarypox viruses are being used as expression vectors to produce live recombinant/hybrid vaccines for more virulent infectious agents (Figure 44-7). For this process, a plasmid is constructed to contain the foreign gene that encodes the immunizing protein, and this gene is flanked by specific poxvirus gene sequences to promote recombination. This plasmid is inserted into a host cell, which is then infected with the poxvirus. The foreign gene is incorporated into the

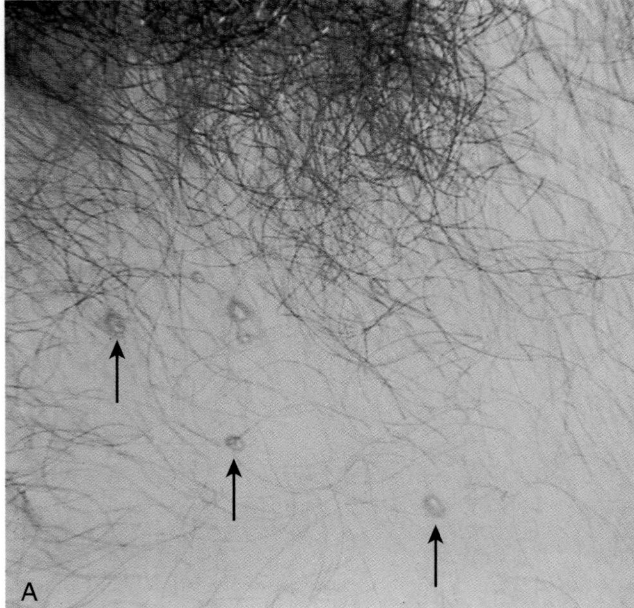

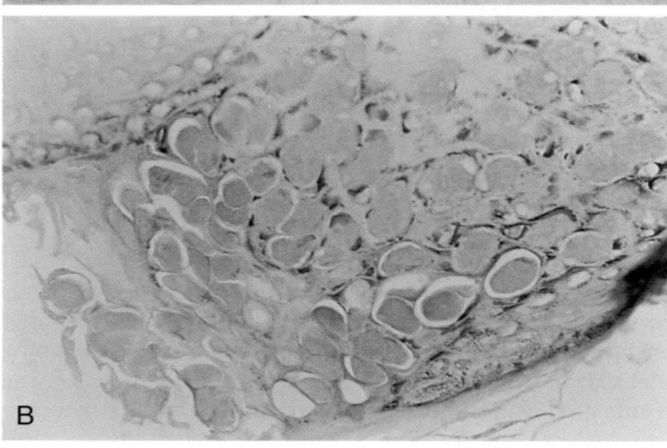

FIGURE 44-6 Molluscum contagiosum. **A,** Skin lesions *(arrows)*. **B,** Microscopic view; epidermis is filled with molluscum bodies (magnification 100×).

"rescuing" poxvirus genome because of the homologous viral sequences included on the plasmid. Immunization with the recombinant poxvirus results from expression of the foreign gene and its presentation to the immune response, almost as if by infection with the other agent. A vaccinia hybrid virus containing the G protein of rabies virus soaked onto a bait food and dropped into forests has been used successfully to immunize raccoons, foxes, and other mammals. Experimental vaccines for human immunodeficiency virus, hepatitis B, influenza, and other viruses have also been prepared using these techniques. The potential for producing other vaccines in this manner is unlimited.

Hybrid vaccinia viruses are also being used for oncolytic agents to selectively kill tumors and for gene replacement therapy.

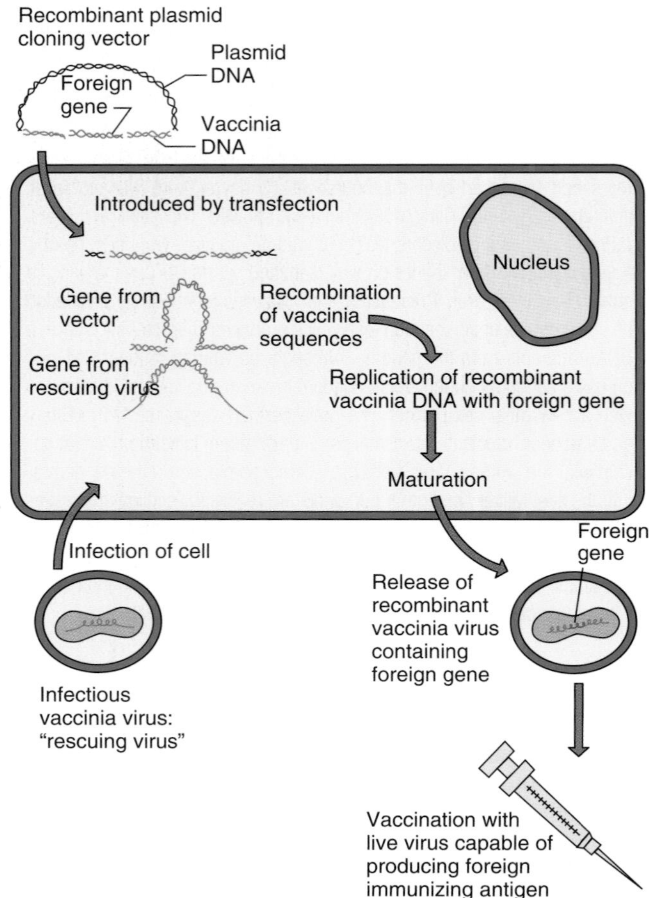

FIGURE 44-7 Vaccinia virus as an expression vector for the production of live recombinant vaccines. (Modified from Piccini A, Paoletti E: Vaccinia: virus, vector, vaccine, *Adv Virus Res* 34:43–64, 1988.)

Bibliography

Breman JG, Henderson DA: Diagnosis and management of smallpox, *N Engl J Med* 346:1300–1308, 2002.

Cann AJ: *Principles of molecular virology*, San Diego, 2005, Academic.

Carter J, Saunders V: *Virology: principles and applications*, Chichester, England, 2007, Wiley.

Cohen J, Powderly WG: *Infectious diseases*, ed 2, St Louis, 2004, Mosby.

Collier L, Oxford J: *Human virology*, ed 4, Oxford, 2011, Oxford University Press.

Fenner F: A successful eradication campaign: global eradication of smallpox, *Rev Infect Dis* 4:916–930, 1982.

Flint SJ, Enquist LW, Racaniello VR, et al: *Principles of virology: molecular biology, pathogenesis, and control of animal viruses*, ed 3, Washington, DC, 2009, American Society for Microbiology Press.

Gorbach SL, Bartlett JG, Blacklow NR: *Infectious diseases*, ed 3, Philadelphia, 2004, WB Saunders.

Knipe DM, Howley PM, Griffin DE, et al: *Fields virology*, ed 5, Philadelphia, 2006, Lippincott Williams & Wilkins.

Mandell GL, Bennet JE, Dolin R: *Principles and practice of infectious diseases*, ed 7, Philadelphia, 2010, Elsevier.

Moyer RW, Turner PC: Poxviruses, *Curr Top Microbiol Immunol* (vol 163), New York, 1990, Springer-Verlag.

Patel NA, Diven D: Vaccinia, 2014. http://emedicine.medscape.com/article/231773-overview. Accessed May 5, 2015.

Piccini A, Paoletti E: Vaccinia: virus, vector, vaccine, *Adv Virus Res* 34:43–64, 1988.

Randall CMH, Shisler JL: Molluscum contagiosum virus, *Future Virol* 8:561–573, 2013. Website: www.medscape.com/viewarticle/805709_print. Accessed May 5, 2015.

Richman DD, Whitley RJ, Hayden FG: *Clinical virology*, ed 3, Washington, DC, 2009, American Society for Microbiology Press.

Strauss JM, Strauss EG: *Viruses and human disease*, San Diego, 2002, Academic.

Voyles BA: *Biology of viruses*, ed 2, Boston, 2002, McGraw-Hill.

White DO, Fenner FJ: *Medical virology*, ed 4, New York, 1994, Academic.

CHAPTER

45 PARVOVIRUSES

A 6-year-old girl had a viral respiratory infection and then became very pale, weak, and tired and became severely anemic because of a transient aplastic crisis.

1. What predisposing condition exacerbated the relatively benign disease in this child?
2. What cell type is the host for this virus, and what determines this tropism?
3. What disease signs occur following infection of an adult? Of a fetus?

Answers to these questions are available on StudentConsult.com.

• SUMMARIES CLINICALLY SIGNIFICANT ORGANISMS

Parvoviruses

Trigger Words

B19, fifth disease, slapped cheeks, aplastic crisis, sickle crisis, spontaneous abortions

Biology, Virulence, and Disease

- Small, icosahedral capsid, single-strand DNA genome
- Must replicate in growing cell: erythroid precursor cells
- Children: erythema infectiosum (fifth disease); high fever during viremia followed later by rash
- Individuals with chronic anemia: aplastic crisis
- Adults: arthralgia and arthritis
- Fetus: anemia-related disease and death (hydrops fetalis)

Epidemiology

- Transmitted by aerosols, direct contact

Diagnosis

- Symptomatology, confirmation by PCR genome analysis of blood

Treatment, Prevention, and Control

- No modes of control or treatment

The Parvoviridae are the smallest of the deoxyribonucleic acid (DNA) viruses. Their small size and limited genetic repertoire make them more dependent than any other DNA virus on the host cell, or they require the presence of a helper virus to replicate. **B19** and **bocavirus** are the only parvoviruses known to cause human disease.

B19 normally causes **erythema infectiosum,** or **fifth disease,** a mild febrile exanthematous disease that occurs in children. It goes by the latter name because it was counted as one of five classic childhood exanthems (the first four being varicella, rubella, roseola, and measles). B19 is also responsible for episodes of **aplastic crisis in patients with chronic hemolytic anemia** and is associated with **acute polyarthritis** in adults. Infection of the fetus during pregnancy can result in hydrops fetalis and abortion. **Bocavirus** is a recently discovered virus that can cause acute respiratory disease, which may become severe in young children.

Other parvoviruses, such as RA-1 (isolated from a person with rheumatoid arthritis) and fecal parvoviruses, have not been shown to cause human disease. Feline and canine parvoviruses do not cause human disease and are preventable with vaccination of the pet.

Adeno-associated viruses (AAVs) are members of the genus *Dependovirus.* They commonly infect humans but replicate only in association with a second "helper" virus, usually an adenovirus. Dependoviruses neither cause illness nor modify infection by their helper viruses. These properties and the propensity of AAVs to integrate into the host chromosome have made genetically modified AAVs candidates for use in **gene-replacement therapy.** A third genus of the family, *Densovirus,* infects only insects.

• Structure and Replication

The parvoviruses are extremely small (18 to 26 nm in diameter) and have a nonenveloped icosahedral capsid (Figure 45-1 and Box 45-1). The B19 virus genome contains one

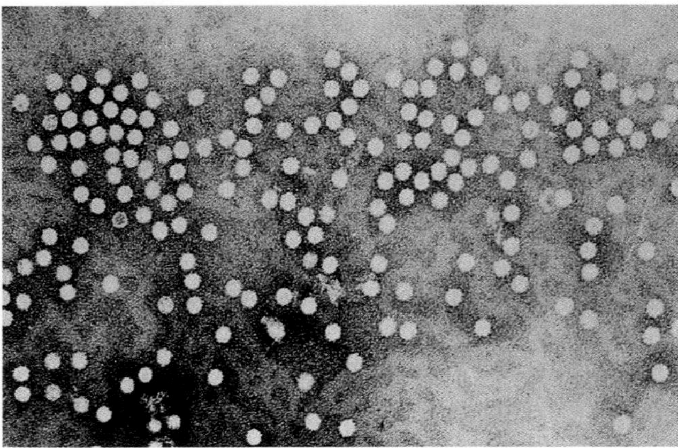

FIGURE 45-1 Electron micrograph of parvovirus. Parvoviruses are small (18 to 26 nm), nonenveloped viruses with single-stranded DNA. (Courtesy Centers for Disease Control and Prevention, Atlanta.)

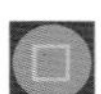

Box 45-1 Unique Properties of Parvoviruses

Smallest DNA virus
Naked icosahedral capsid
Single-stranded (+ or – sense) DNA genome
Requirement of growing cells (B19) or helper virus (dependovirus) for replication

Box 45-2 Parvovirus Genome

Single-stranded linear DNA genome
Approximately 5.5 kilobases in length
Plus and minus strands packaged into separate B19 virions
Ends of the genome have inverted repeats that hybridize to form hairpin loops and a primer for DNA synthesis
Separate coding regions for nonstructural (NS) and structural proteins (VP)

linear, single-stranded DNA molecule with a molecular mass of 1.5 to 1.8×10^6 Da (5500 bases in length) (Box 45-2). Plus or minus DNA strands are packaged separately into virions. The genome encodes three structural and two major nonstructural proteins. Unlike larger DNA viruses, the parvoviruses must infect mitotically active cells because they do not encode the means to stimulate cell growth or a polymerase. Only one serotype of B19 is known to exist.

B19 virus replicates in mitotically active cells and prefers cells of the erythroid lineage, such as fresh human bone marrow cells, erythroid cells from fetal liver, and erythroid leukemia cells (Figure 45-2). After binding to the erythrocyte blood group P antigen (globoside) and its internalization, the virion is uncoated, and the single-stranded DNA genome is delivered to the nucleus. Factors available only during the S phase of the cell's growth cycle and cellular DNA polymerases are required to generate a complementary DNA strand.

The single-stranded DNA virion genome is converted to a double-stranded DNA version, which is required for transcription and replication. Inverted repeat sequences of DNA at both ends of the genome fold back and hybridize with the genome to create a primer for the cell's DNA polymerase.

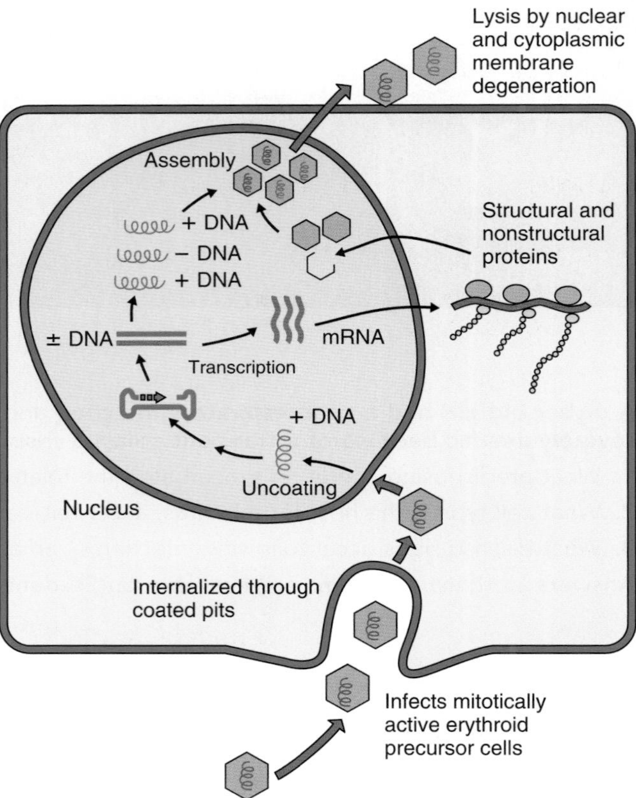

FIGURE 45-2 Postulated replication of parvovirus (B19) based on information from related viruses (minute virus of mice). The internalized parvovirus delivers its genome to the nucleus, where the single-stranded (plus or minus) DNA is converted to double-stranded DNA by host factors and DNA polymerases present only in growing cells. Transcription, replication, and assembly occur in the nucleus. Virus is released by cell lysis.

This creates the complementary strand and replicates the genome. The two major nonstructural proteins and the VP1 and VP2 structural capsid proteins are synthesized in the cytoplasm, and the structural proteins go to the nucleus, where the virion is assembled. The VP2 protein is cleaved later to produce VP3. The nuclear and cytoplasmic membrane degenerates, and the virus is released on cell lysis.

• Pathogenesis and Immunity

B19 targets and is cytolytic for erythroid precursor cells (Box 45-3). B19 disease is determined by the direct killing of these cells and the subsequent immune response to the infection (rash and arthralgia). The immunopathogenesis for B19 and rubella are similar; both are caused by immune complexes with virions, hence both cause rash and arthralgia in adults.

Studies performed in volunteers suggest that B19 virus first replicates in the nasopharynx or upper respiratory tract and then spreads by viremia to the bone marrow and elsewhere, where it replicates and kills erythroid precursor cells (Figure 45-3). Bocavirus also initiates infection in the respiratory tract, replicates in the respiratory epithelium, and causes disease.

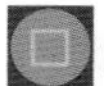

Box 45-3 Disease Mechanisms of B19 Parvovirus

Virus spreads by **respiratory** and **oral** secretions.
Virus **infects mitotically active erythroid precursor cells** in bone marrow and establishes lytic infection.
Virus establishes large **viremia** and can **cross the placenta.**
Antibody is important for resolution and prophylaxis.
Virus causes biphasic disease.
- Initial phase is related to viremia:
  - Flulike symptoms and viral shedding
- Later phase is related to immune response:
  - Circulating immune complexes of antibody and virions that do not fix complement
  - Erythematous maculopapular rash, arthralgia, and arthritis

Depletion of erythroid precursor cells and destabilization of erythrocytes initiate **aplastic crisis in persons with chronic anemia.**

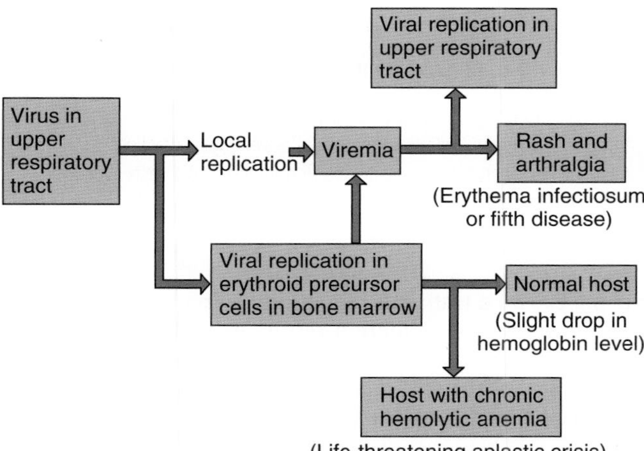

FIGURE 45-3 Mechanism of spread of parvovirus within the body.

B19 viral disease has a **biphasic course.** The *initial febrile stage is the infectious stage.* During this time, erythrocyte production is stopped for approximately 1 week because of the viral killing of erythroid precursor cells. A large viremia occurs within 8 days of infection and is accompanied by nonspecific flulike symptoms. Large numbers of viruses are also released into oral and respiratory secretions. Antibody stops the viremia and is important for resolution of the disease but contributes to the symptoms.

The *second, symptomatic, stage is immune mediated.* The rash and arthralgia seen in this stage coincide with the appearance of virus-specific antibody, the disappearance of detectable B19 virus, and the formation of immune complexes.

Hosts with chronic hemolytic anemia (e.g., sickle cell anemia) who are infected with B19 are at risk for a life-threatening reticulocytopenia that is referred to as **aplastic crisis.** The reticulocytopenia results from the combination of B19 depletion of red blood cell precursors and the shortened lifespan of erythrocytes caused by the underlying anemia.

Box 45-4 Epidemiology of B19 Parvovirus Infection

Disease/Viral Factors
Capsid virus resistant to inactivation
Contagious period precedes symptoms
Virus crosses placenta and infects fetus

Transmission
Transmitted via respiratory droplets

Who Is at Risk?
Children, especially those in elementary school: erythema infectiosum (fifth disease)
Parents of children with B19 infection
Pregnant women: fetal infection and disease
Persons with chronic anemia: aplastic crisis

Geography/Season
Virus found worldwide
Fifth disease more common in late winter and spring

Modes of Control
No modes of control

• Epidemiology

Approximately 65% of the adult population has been infected with B19 by age 40 (Box 45-4). Erythema infectiosum is most common in children and adolescents aged 4 to 15 years, who are a source of contagion. Arthralgia and arthritis are likely to occur in adults. Respiratory droplets and oral secretions most probably transmit the virus. Disease usually occurs in late winter and spring. Parenteral transmission of the virus by a blood-clotting–factor concentrate has also been described.

Bocavirus is found worldwide and causes disease in children younger than 2 years. The virus is transmitted in respiratory secretions but can also be isolated from stool.

• Clinical Syndromes (Clinical Case 45-1)

B19 virus, as stated earlier, is the cause of erythema infectiosum (fifth disease) (Box 45-5). Infection starts with an unremarkable prodromal period of 7 to 10 days during which the person is contagious. Infection of a normal host may cause either no noticeable symptoms or fever and nonspecific symptoms (e.g., sore throat, chills, malaise, myalgia), as well as a slight decrease in hemoglobin levels (Figure 45-4). This period is followed by a distinctive rash on the cheeks, which appear to have been slapped. The rash then usually spreads, especially to exposed skin such as the arms and legs (Figure 45-5), and then subsides over 1 to 2 weeks.

B19 infection in adults causes polyarthritis (with or without a rash) that can last for weeks, months, or longer. Arthritis of the hands, wrists, knees, and ankles predominates. The rash may precede the arthritis but often does not occur. B19 infection of immunocompromised people may result in chronic disease.

The most serious complication of parvovirus infection is the aplastic crisis that occurs in patients with chronic hemolytic anemia (e.g., sickle cell anemia). Infection in these

Clinical Case 45-1 B19 Infection of a Transplant Recipient

Persistent, rather than transient, anemia occurs upon human parvovirus B19 infection of immunosuppressed individuals. One such case was reported by Pamidi and associates (*Transplantation* 69:2666–2669, 2000). After 1 year of immunosuppressive therapy (mycophenolate mofetil, prednisone, and tacrolimus) after a kidney transplant, a 46-year-old man complained of dyspnea, lightheadedness, and fatigue upon exercise. Laboratory tests confirmed a diagnosis of anemia. Bone marrow analysis indicated erythroid hyperplasia with a predominance of immature erythroblasts. Proerythroblasts could be found, with deep basophilic cytoplasm and intranuclear inclusions that immunohistologically stained for B19 antigen. The patient received 16 units of packed red blood cells over 6 weeks, with continued anemia. Serology indicated the presence of IgM (1 : 10) but insignificant IgG anti-B19 antibody. Treatment with intravenous IgG for 5 days resulted in a dramatic improvement. Immunosuppressive therapy of this patient prevented expansion and class switch to an IgG antibody response because of the lack of helper T cells. Resolution of the encapsidated parvovirus is dependent upon a robust antibody response, and in its absence, the normal transient anemia resulting from virus replication in erythroid precursors cannot be resolved.

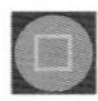

Box 45-5 Clinical Consequences of Parvovirus (B19) Infection

Mild flulike illness (fever, headache, chills, myalgia, malaise)
Erythema infectiosum (fifth disease)
Aplastic crisis in persons with chronic anemia
Arthropathy (polyarthritis: symptoms in many joints)
Risk of fetal loss as a result of B19 virus crossing the placenta, causing anemia-related disease but not congenital anomalies

FIGURE 45-4 Time course of parvovirus (B19) infection. B19 causes biphasic disease: first, an initial lytic infection phase characterized by febrile flulike symptoms, and then a noninfectious immunologic phase characterized by a rash and arthralgia. *IgG,* Immunoglobulin G.

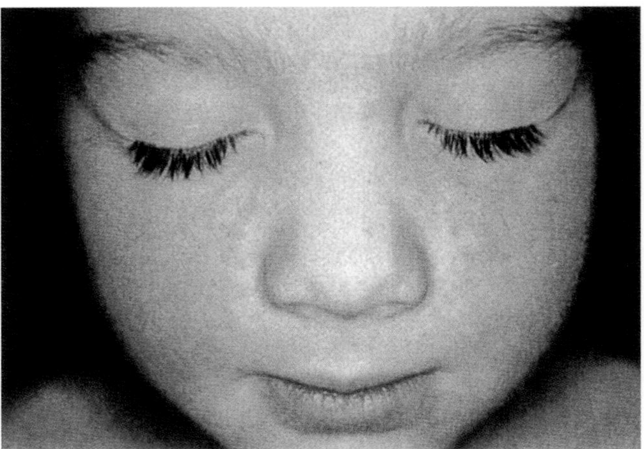

FIGURE 45-5 A "slapped-cheek" appearance is typical of the rash for erythema infectiosum. (From Hart CA, Broadhead RL: *A color atlas of pediatric infectious diseases,* London, 1992, Wolfe.)

Box 45-6 Clinical Summary

A 10-year-old patient has a 5-day history of a flulike illness (headache, fever, muscle pain, feels tired) and then a week later develops an intensely red rash over the cheeks and a fainter "lacy" rash over the trunk and extremities.

people causes a transient reduction in erythropoiesis in the bone marrow. The reduction results in a transient reticulocytopenia that lasts 7 to 10 days and a decrease in hemoglobin level. An aplastic crisis is accompanied by fever and nonspecific symptoms such as malaise, myalgia, chills, and itching. A maculopapular rash with arthralgia and some joint swelling may also be present.

B19 infection of a seronegative mother increases the risk for fetal death. The virus can infect the fetus and kill erythrocyte precursors, causing anemia, edema, hypoxia, and congestive heart failure **(hydrops fetalis).** Infection of seropositive pregnant women often has no adverse effect on the fetus. There is no evidence that B19 causes congenital abnormalities (Box 45-6; see Box 45-5).

Bocavirus may cause mild or severe acute respiratory disease. The more severe disease occurs in children younger than age 2, who may have bronchiolitis with wheezing and a viremia that extends long beyond the disease. A fatal case of bocavirus bronchiolitis has been reported.

• Laboratory Diagnosis

The diagnosis of erythema infectiosum is usually based on the clinical presentation. For B19 disease to be definitively diagnosed, however, specific immunoglobulin (Ig)M or viral DNA must be detected (i.e., to distinguish the rash of B19 from that of rubella in a pregnant woman). Enzyme-linked immunosorbent assays for B19 IgM and IgG are available. The polymerase chain reaction test is a very sensitive method for detecting the B19 and bocavirus genomes in clinical samples. Virus isolation is not performed.

• Treatment, Prevention, and Control

No specific antiviral treatment or means of control is available. Vaccines are available for dog and cat parvoviruses.

Bibliography

Allander T: Human bocavirus, *J Clin Virol* 41:29–33, 2008.

Anderson LJ: Human parvoviruses, *J Infect Dis* 161:603–608, 1990.

Anderson MJ: Parvoviruses. In Belshe RB, editor: *Textbook of human virology*, ed 2, St Louis, 1991, Mosby.

Berns KI: Parvovirus replication, *Microbiol Rev* 54:316–329, 1990.

Berns KI: *The parvoviruses*, New York, 1994, Plenum.

Brown KE: The expanding range of parvoviruses which infect humans, *Rev Med Virol* 20:231–244, 2010.

Brown KE, Young NS: Parvovirus B19 in human disease, *Annu Rev Med* 48:59–67, 1997.

Cann AJ: *Principles of molecular virology*, San Diego, 2005, Academic.

Carter J, Saunders V: *Virology: principles and applications*, Chichester, England, 2007, Wiley.

Cennimo DJ, Dieudonne A: Parvovirus B19 infection. http://emedicine.medscape.com/article/961063-overview. Accessed November 4, 2014.

Chorba T, Coccia P, Holman RC, et al: The role of parvovirus B19 in aplastic crisis and erythema infectiosum (fifth disease), *J Infect Dis* 154:383–393, 1986.

Cohen J, Powderly WG: *Infectious diseases*, ed 2, St Louis, 2004, Mosby.

Collier L, Oxford J: *Human virology*, ed 4, Oxford, 2011, Oxford University Press.

Flint SJ, Enquist LW, Racaniello VR, et al: *Principles of virology: molecular biology, pathogenesis and control of animal viruses*, ed 3, Washington, DC, 2009, American Society for Microbiology Press.

Gorbach SL, Bartlett JG, Blacklow NR: *Infectious diseases*, ed 3, Philadelphia, 2004, WB Saunders.

Knipe DM, Howley PM: *Fields virology*, ed 6, Philadelphia, 2013, Lippincott Williams & Wilkins.

Mandell GL, Bennet JE, Dolin R: *Principles and practice of infectious diseases*, ed 7, Philadelphia, 2010, Elsevier.

Naides SJ, Scharosch LL, Foto F, et al: Rheumatologic manifestations of human parvovirus B19 infection in adults, *Arthritis Rheum* 33:1297–1309, 1990.

Richman DD, Whitley RJ, Hayden FG: *Clinical virology*, ed 3, Washington, DC, 2009, American Society for Microbiology Press.

Török TJ: Parvovirus B19 and human disease, *Adv Intern Med* 37:431–455, 1992.

Ursic T, et al: Human bocavirus as the cause of a life-threatening infection, *J Clin Microbiol* 49:1179–1181, 2011.

Voyles BA: *The biology of viruses*, ed 2, Boston, 2002, McGraw-Hill.

Ware RE: Parvovirus infections. In Katz SL, Gershon AA, Hotez PJ, editors: *Krugman's infectious diseases of children*, ed 10, St Louis, 1998, Mosby.

Young NS, Brown KE: Parvovirus B19, *N Engl J Med* 350:586–597, 2004.

CHAPTER

46 PICORNAVIRUSES

A 9-day-old infant with a fever and appearing septic progressed to multisystem organ syndrome with a combination of hepatitis, meningoencephalitis, myocarditis, and pneumonia. The cerebrospinal fluid (CSF) had normal glucose levels and lacked neutrophil infiltrate. The infant was started on acyclovir therapy for a suspected congenital herpes simplex virus (HSV) infection. Genome analysis (polymerase chain reaction [PCR] and reverse transcriptase [RT]-PCR) of the CSF did not detect HSV but did detect an enterovirus that was subsequently identified as echovirus 11 and not coxsackievirus B. Several days earlier, the mother had a slight fever and a cold.

1. How did the baby become infected?
2. How does the viral structure facilitate virus spread in the body and transmission to others?
3. What type of immunity is protective for this virus, and why was the baby not protected?

Answers to these questions are available on StudentConsult.com.

• SUMMARIES CLINICALLY SIGNIFICANT ORGANISMS

Picornaviruses

Trigger Words

Polio: flaccid paralysis, major and minor disease, fecal-oral

Coxsackievirus A: vesicular diseases, meningitis; coxsackievirus B (body): pleurodynia, myocarditis

Other echovirus and enteroviruses: like coxsackievirus

Rhinoviruses: common cold, acid labile, does not replicate above 33° C

Biology, Virulence, and Disease

- Small size, icosahedral capsid, positive RNA genome with terminal protein
- Genome is sufficient for infection
- Encodes RNA-dependent RNA polymerase, replicates in cytoplasm

Enteroviruses

- Capsid virus resistant to inactivation
- Disease due to lytic infection of important target tissue
- Polio: cytolytic infection of motor neurons of anterior horn and brainstem, paralysis
- Coxsackievirus A: herpangina, hand-foot-and-mouth disease, common cold, meningitis
- Coxsackievirus B: pleurodynia, neonatal myocarditis, type 1 diabetes

Rhinoviruses

- Acid labile and cannot replicate at body temperature
- Restricted to upper respiratory tract
- Common cold

Epidemiology

- Enteroviruses transmitted by fecal-oral route and aerosols
- Rhinoviruses transmitted by aerosols and contact

Diagnosis

- Immune assays (ELISA) or RT-PCR genome analysis of blood, CSF, or other relevant sample

Treatment, Prevention, and Control

- OPV and IPV polio vaccines

Picornaviridae is one of the largest families of viruses and includes some of the most important human and animal viruses (Box 46-1). As the name indicates, these viruses are **small *(pico)*** ribonucleic acid **(RNA)** viruses that have a **naked capsid** structure. The family has more than 230 members divided into nine genera, including *Enterovirus, Rhinovirus, Hepatovirus* (hepatitis A virus; discussed in Chapter 55), *Cardiovirus*, and *Aphthovirus*. The enteroviruses are distinguished from the rhinoviruses by the stability of the capsid at pH 3, the optimum temperature for growth, the mode of transmission, and their diseases (Box 46-2).

Box 46-1 Picornaviridae

Enterovirus
- Poliovirus types 1, 2, and 3
- Coxsackievirus A types 1 to 22 and 24
- Coxsackievirus B types 1 to 6
- Echovirus* types 1 to 9, 11 to 27, and 29 to 34
- Enterovirus 68 to 71+

Rhinovirus types 1 to 100+
Cardiovirus
Aphthovirus
Hepatovirus
- Hepatitis A virus

*Enteric, cytopathic, human, orphan + virus.

Box 46-2 Unique Properties of Human Picornaviruses

Virion is a **naked, small** (25 to 30 nm), **icosahedral** capsid enclosing a single-stranded positive RNA genome.
Enteroviruses are resistant to pH 3 to pH 9, detergents, mild sewage treatment, and heat.
Rhinoviruses are labile at acidic pH; optimum growth temperature is 33° C.
Genome is a messenger ribonucleic acid (mRNA).
Naked genome is sufficient for infection.
Virus replicates in cytoplasm.
Viral RNA is translated into **polyprotein,** which is then cleaved into enzymatic and structural proteins.
Most viruses are **cytolytic.**

At least 90 serotypes of human enteroviruses exist and are classified as polioviruses, coxsackieviruses A and B, echoviruses, or for the more recently discovered viruses, as numbered enteroviruses (e.g., enterovirus 68). Several different disease syndromes may be caused by a specific serotype of enterovirus. Likewise, several different serotypes may cause the same disease, depending on the target tissue affected.

The capsids of enteroviruses are *very resistant to harsh environmental conditions* (sewage systems) and the conditions in the gastrointestinal tract, which facilitates their transmission by the fecal-oral route. Although they may initiate infection in the gastrointestinal tract, the enteroviruses rarely cause enteric disease. In fact, most infections are usually asymptomatic. The best-known and most-studied picornavirus is poliovirus, of which there are three serotypes.

Coxsackieviruses are named after the town of Coxsackie, New York, where they were first isolated. They are divided into two groups, A and B, on the basis of certain biological and antigenic differences and are further subdivided into numeric serotypes on the basis of additional antigenic differences.

The name **echovirus** is derived from ***e****nteric* ***c****ytopathic* ***h****uman* ***o****rphan* because the disease associated with these agents was not initially known. Since 1967, newly isolated enteroviruses have been distinguished numerically.

The human **rhinoviruses** consist of at least 100 serotypes and are the major cause of the common cold. They are *sensitive to acidic pH and replicate poorly at temperatures above 33° C.* These properties usually limit rhinoviruses to causing upper respiratory tract infections.

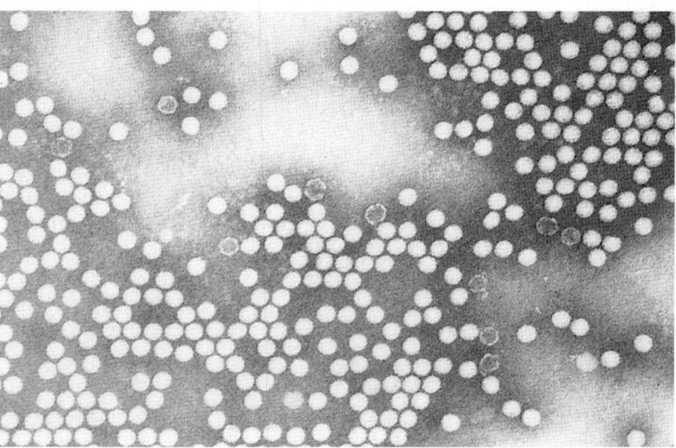

FIGURE 46-1 Electron micrograph of poliovirus. (Courtesy Centers for Disease Control and Prevention, Atlanta.)

• Structure

The plus-strand RNA of the picornaviruses is surrounded by an **icosahedral capsid** that is approximately 30 nm in diameter. The icosahedral capsid has 12 pentameric vertices, each of which is composed of five protomeric units of proteins. The protomers are made of four virion polypeptides (VP1 to VP4). VP2 and VP4 are generated by the cleavage of a precursor, VP0. VP4 in the virion solidifies the structure, but it is not generated until the genome is incorporated into the capsid. This protein is released on binding of the virus to the cellular receptor. The capsids are stable in the presence of heat, acid, and detergent, with the exception of the rhinoviruses, which are labile to acid. The capsid structure is so regular that paracrystals of virions often form in infected cells (Figures 46-1 and 46-2).

The **genome of the picornaviruses resembles a messenger RNA (mRNA)** (Figure 46-3). It is a single strand of plus-sense RNA of approximately 7200 to 8450 bases. It has a polyA (polyadenosine) sequence at the 3′ end and a small protein, VPg (viral protein genome-linked; 22 to 24 amino acids), attached to the 5′ end. The polyA sequence enhances the infectivity of the RNA, and the VPg is important in packaging the genome into the capsid and initiating viral RNA synthesis. *The naked picornavirus genome is sufficient for infection if microinjected into a cell.*

The genome encodes a polyprotein that is proteolytically cleaved by viral-encoded proteases to produce the enzymatic and structural proteins of the virus. In addition to the capsid proteins and VPg, the picornaviruses encode at least two proteases and an RNA-dependent RNA polymerase.

• Replication

The specificity of the picornavirus interaction for cellular receptors is the major determinant of the target tissue tropism and disease (see Chapter 36, Figure 36-12). The VP1 proteins at the vertices of the virion contain a canyon structure to which the receptor binds. Pleconaril and related antiviral compounds contain a 3-methylisoxazole group that binds to the floor of this canyon and alters its conformation to prevent the uncoating of the virus.

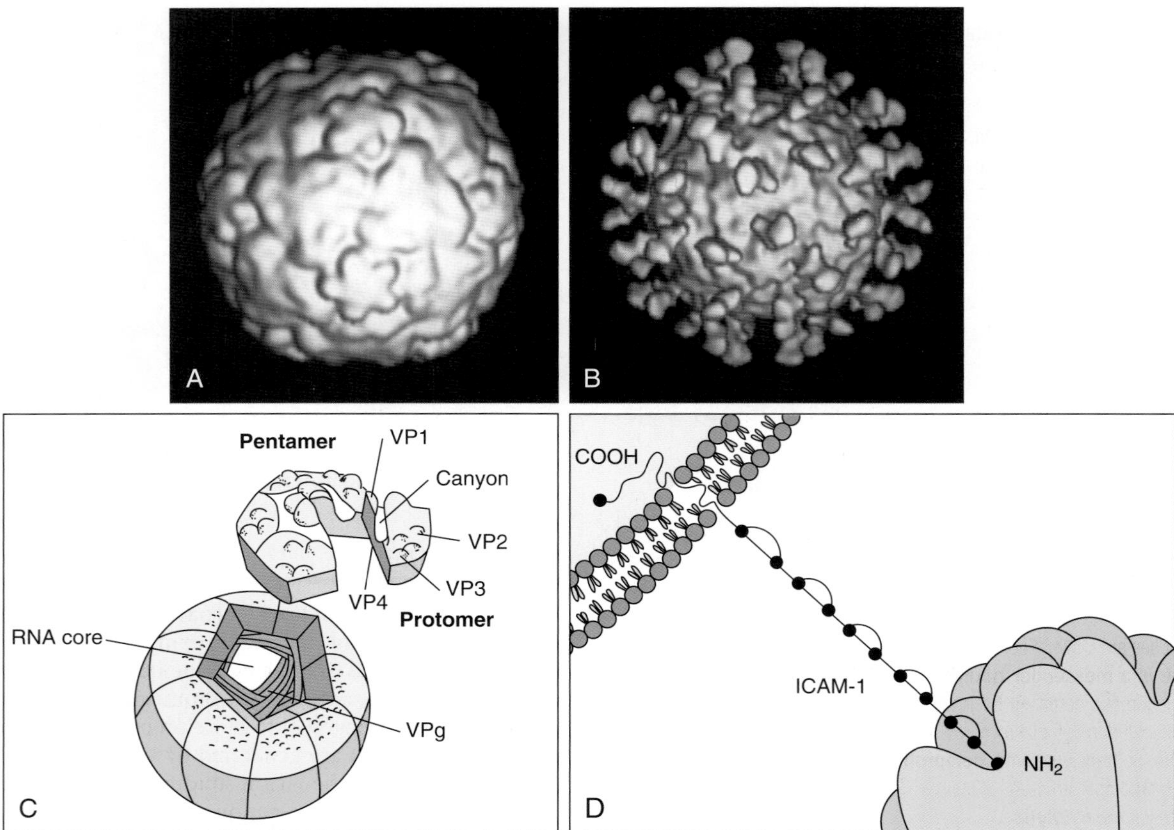

FIGURE 46-2 **A,** Cryoelectron microscopy computer-generated reconstruction of human rhinovirus 16. **B,** Cryoelectron microscopy reconstruction of the interaction of a soluble form of intercellular adhesion molecule-1 *(ICAM-1)* with human rhinovirus 16. Note: There is one ICAM-1 per capsomere. **C,** Structure of the human rhinovirus and its interaction with ICAM-1 on the target cell. **D,** Binding of the ICAM-1 molecule within the canyon of the virion triggers the opening of the capsid for release of the genome into the cell. *RNA,* Ribonucleic acid; *VP1, 2, 3, 4,* viral protein 1, 2, 3, 4; *VPg,* viral protein genome-linked. (**A** and **B**, Courtesy Tim Baker, Purdue University, West Lafayette, Ind.)

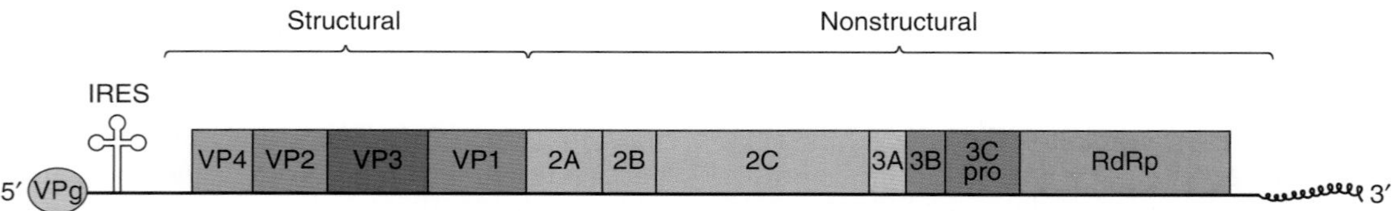

FIGURE 46-3 Structure of the picornavirus genome. The genome (7200 to 8400 bases) is translated as a polyprotein that is cleaved by viral-encoded proteases into individual proteins. *Viral genes*: *VP1, 2, 3, 4,* capsid proteins 1, 2, 3, 4; *2A* cleaves eIF4g to inhibit host protein synthesis; *2B, 2C, 3A, 3B* generate membrane-binding, vesicle-forming proteins that facilitate replication; *3B* also encodes VPg genome-binding protein; *3Cpro,* protease; *RdRp,* RNA-dependent RNA polymerase. (Redrawn from Whitton JL, Cornell CT, Feuer R: Host and virus determinants of picornavirus pathogenesis and tropism, *Nat Rev Microbiol* 3:765–776, 2005.)

The picornaviruses can be categorized according to their cell surface receptor specificity. The receptors for polioviruses, some coxsackieviruses, and rhinoviruses are members of the immunoglobulin superfamily of proteins. At least 80% of the rhinoviruses and several serotypes of coxsackievirus bind to the intercellular adhesion molecule-1 (ICAM-1) expressed on epithelial cells, fibroblasts, and endothelial cells. Several coxsackieviruses, echoviruses, and other enteroviruses bind to decay accelerating factor (CD55), and coxsackievirus B shares a receptor with adenovirus. Poliovirus binds to a different molecule (PVR/CD155) that is similar to the receptor for HSV. The poliovirus receptor is present on many different human cells, but not all of these cells will replicate the virus.

On binding to the receptor, the VP4 is released and the capsid weakened. The genome is then injected directly across the membrane through a channel created by the VP1 protein at one of the vertices of the virion. The genome binds directly to ribosomes, despite the lack of a 5′-cap structure. The ribosomes recognize a unique internal RNA loop (internal ribosome entry site [IRES]) in the genome that is also present in some cellular mRNAs. A **polyprotein** containing all the viral protein sequences is synthesized within 10 to 15 minutes of infection. This polyprotein is cleaved by viral proteases encoded in it. Viral proteins tether the genome to endoplasmic reticulum membranes, and the machinery for replication of the genome is collected into a vesicle. The viral RNA-dependent RNA polymerase generates a negative-strand RNA template from which the new mRNA/genome can be synthesized. The amount of viral mRNA increases rapidly in the cell, with the number of viral RNA molecules reaching as many as 400,000 per cell.

Most picornaviruses inhibit cellular RNA and protein synthesis during infection. For example, cleavage of the cell's cap-binding protein (eIF4-G) of the ribosome by a poliovirus protease prevents most cellular mRNA from binding to the ribosome. Inhibition of transcription factors decreases cellular mRNA synthesis, and permeability changes induced by picornaviruses reduce the ability of cellular mRNA to bind to the ribosome. In addition, viral mRNA can outcompete cellular mRNA for the factors required in protein synthesis. These activities contribute to the cytopathologic effect of the virus on the target cell.

As the viral genome is being replicated and translated, the structural proteins VP0, VP1, and VP3 are cleaved from the polyprotein by a viral-encoded protease and assembled into subunits. Five **subunits** associate into **pentamers,** and 12 **pentamers** associate to form the **procapsid.** After insertion of the genome, VP0 is cleaved into VP2 and VP4 to complete the **capsid.** As many as 100,000 virions per cell may be produced and released on cell lysis. The entire replication cycle may be as short as 3 to 4 hours.

• Enteroviruses

Pathogenesis and Immunity

Contrary to their name, enteroviruses do not usually cause enteric disease, but they do replicate within and are transmitted by the fecal-oral route. The diseases produced by the enteroviruses are determined mainly by differences in tissue tropism and the cytolytic capacity of the virus (Figure 46-4; Box 46-3). The virions are impervious to stomach acid, proteases, and bile. Enteroviruses are acquired through the upper respiratory tract and mouth. Viral replication is initiated in the mucosa and lymphoid tissue of the tonsils and pharynx, and the virus later infects M cells and lymphocytes of the Peyer patches and enterocytes in the intestinal mucosa. Primary viremia spreads the virus to receptor-bearing target tissues, including the reticuloendothelial cells of the lymph nodes, spleen, and liver, to initiate a second phase of viral replication, resulting in a secondary viremia and symptoms.

Most enteroviruses are cytolytic, replicating rapidly and causing direct damage to the target cell.

In the case of poliovirus, the virus gains access to the brain by infecting skeletal muscle and traveling up the innervating nerves to the brain, similar to the rabies virus (see Chapter 50). The virus is cytolytic for the motor neurons of the anterior horn and brainstem. The location and number of nerve cells destroyed by the virus govern the extent of paralysis and whether and when other neurons can reenervate the muscle and restore activity. The combined loss of neurons to polio and to old age may result in paralysis later in life, termed **postpolio syndrome.**

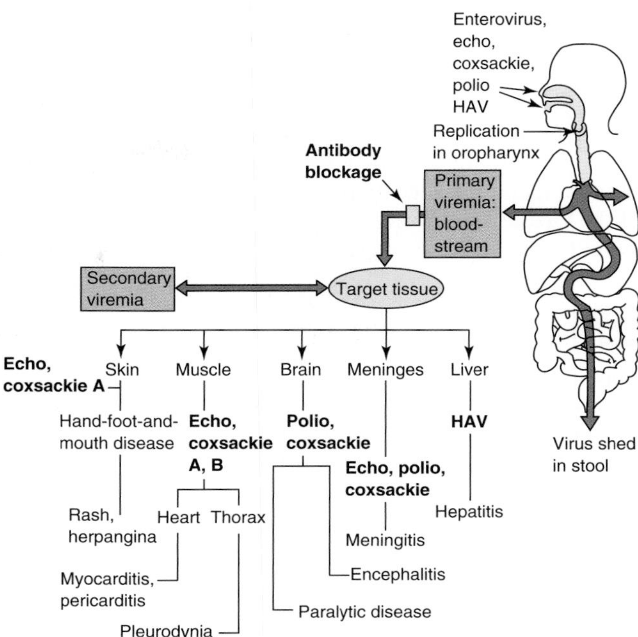

FIGURE 46-4 Pathogenesis of enterovirus infection. The target tissue infected by the enterovirus determines the predominant disease caused by the virus. *Coxsackie,* Coxsackievirus; *echo,* echovirus; *HAV,* hepatitis A virus; *polio,* poliovirus.

Box 46-3 Disease Mechanisms of Picornaviruses

Enteroviruses enter via the oropharynx, intestinal mucosa, or upper respiratory tract and infect the underlying lymphatic tissue; rhinoviruses are restricted to the upper respiratory tract.
In the absence of serum antibody, enterovirus spreads by viremia to cells of a receptor-bearing target tissue.
Different picornaviruses bind to different receptors, many of which are members of the immunoglobulin superfamily (i.e., intercellular adhesion molecule-1).
The infected target tissue determines the subsequent disease.
Viral, rather than immune, pathologic effects are usually responsible for causing disease.
The secretory antibody response is transitory but can prevent the initiation of infection.
Serum antibody blocks viremic spread to target tissue, preventing disease.
Enterovirus is shed in feces for long periods.
Infection is often asymptomatic or causes mild, flulike, or upper respiratory tract disease.

Viral shedding from the oropharynx can be detected for a short time before symptoms begin, whereas viral production and shedding from the intestine may last for 30 days or longer, even in the presence of a humoral immune response.

Antibody is the major protective immune response to the enteroviruses. Secretory antibody can prevent the initial establishment of infection in the oropharynx and gastrointestinal tract, and serum antibody prevents viremic spread to the target tissue and therefore disease. The time course for antibody development after infection with a live vaccine is presented in Figure 46-10 (see later). Cell-mediated immunity is not usually involved in protection but may play a role in resolution and pathogenesis.

Epidemiology

The enteroviruses are exclusively human pathogens (Box 46-4). As the name implies, these viruses primarily spread via the **fecal-oral** route. **Asymptomatic shedding** can occur for up to a month, putting virus into the environment. Poor sanitation and crowded living conditions foster transmission of the viruses (Figure 46-5). Sewage contamination of water supplies can result in enterovirus epidemics. Outbreaks of enterovirus disease are seen in schools and day-care settings, and summer is the major season for such disease. The coxsackieviruses and echoviruses may also be spread in aerosol droplets and cause respiratory tract infections.

With the success of the polio vaccines, the wild-type poliovirus has been eliminated from the Western Hemisphere (Figure 46-6) and most, but not all, of the world. Paralytic polio was never eliminated from Nigeria, Afghanistan, and Pakistan, and the viruses are spreading from these countries to others, including Somalia, Kenya, Ethiopia, Cameroon, Syria, and Israel. A small but significant number of vaccine-related cases of polio result from mutation of one of the three strains in the live vaccine virus, which reestablishes neurovirulence. Change in the receptor-binding VP1 protein gene has occurred by recombination with another enterovirus. This development has prompted a preference for use of the inactivated polio vaccine. Polioviruses are spread most often during the summer and autumn.

Paralytic polio was once considered a middle class disease because good hygiene would delay exposure of a person to the virus until late childhood, the adolescent years, or adulthood, when infection would produce the most severe symptoms. Infection during early childhood is more likely to be asymptomatic or cause very mild disease.

Similar to poliovirus infection, coxsackievirus A disease is generally more severe in adults than in children. Coxsackievirus B and some of the echoviruses (especially echovirus 11) can be particularly harmful to infants.

Box 46-4 Epidemiology of Enterovirus Infections

Disease/Viral Factors

Nature of disease correlates with specific enterovirus
Severity of disease correlates with age of person
Infection often asymptomatic, with viral shedding
Virion resistant to environmental conditions (detergents, acid, drying, mild sewage treatment, and heat)

Transmission

Fecal-oral route: poor hygiene, dirty diapers (especially in day-care settings)
Ingestion via contaminated food and water
Contact with infected hands and fomites
Inhalation of infectious aerosols

Who Is at Risk?

Young children: at risk for polio (asymptomatic or mild disease)
Older children and adults: at risk for polio (asymptomatic to paralytic disease)
Newborns and neonates: at highest risk for serious coxsackievirus, echovirus, and enterovirus disease

Geography/Season

Viruses have worldwide distribution; wild-type polio virtually eradicated in most countries because of vaccination programs
Disease more common in summer

Modes of Control

For polio, live oral polio vaccine (trivalent OPV) or inactivated trivalent polio vaccine (IPV) is administered
For other enteroviruses, no vaccine; good hygiene limits spread

Clinical Syndromes

The clinical syndromes produced by the enteroviruses are determined by several factors, including (1) viral serotype, (2) infecting dose, (3) tissue tropism, (4) portal of entry, (5) patient's age, gender, and state of health, and (6) pregnancy (Table 46-1). The incubation period for enterovirus disease varies from 1 to 35 days, depending on the virus, the target tissue, and the person's age. Viruses that affect oral and respiratory sites have the shortest incubation periods.

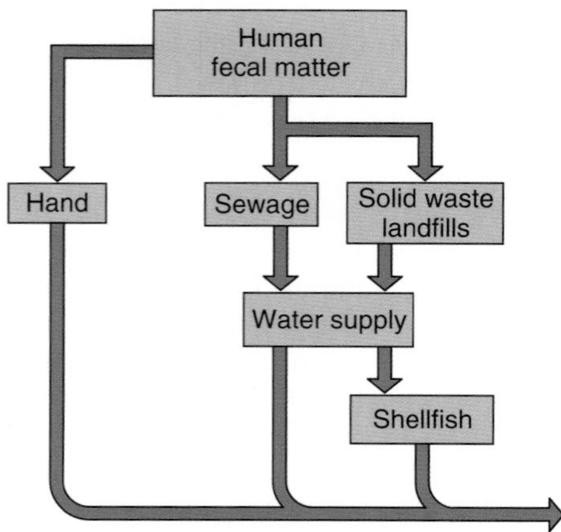

FIGURE 46-5 Transmission of enteroviruses. The capsid structure is resistant to mild sewage treatment, salt water, detergents, and temperature changes, allowing these viruses to be transmitted by fecal-oral routes, by fomites, and on hands.

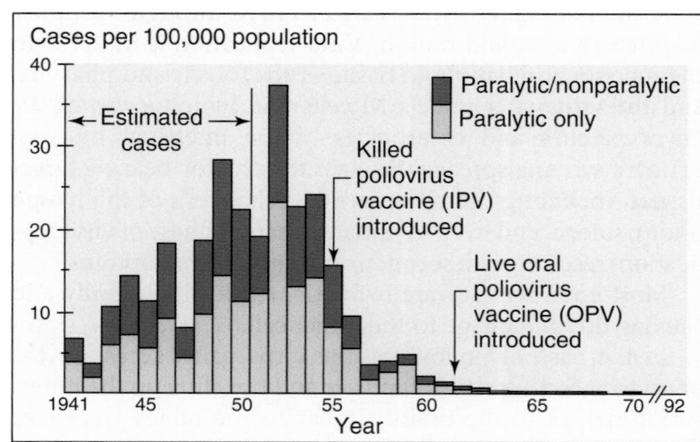

FIGURE 46-6 Incidence of polio in the United States. Killed (inactivated) polio vaccine (IPV) was introduced in 1955, and live oral polio vaccine (OPV) was introduced in 1961 and 1962. Wild-type polio has been eradicated in the United States. (Courtesy Centers for Disease Control and Prevention: *Immunization against disease: 1972,* Washington, DC, 1973, U.S. Government Printing Office.)

Table 46-1 Summary of Clinical Syndromes Associated with Major Enterovirus Groups*

Syndrome	Occurrence	Polioviruses	Coxsackievirus A	Coxsackievirus B	Echo-/Enteroviruses[†]
Asymptomatic	Frequent	+	+	+	+
Paralytic disease	Sporadic	+	+	+	+ (entero68)
Encephalitis, meningitis	Outbreaks	+	+	+	+
Carditis	Sporadic		+	+	+
Neonatal disease	Outbreaks			+	+
Pleurodynia	Outbreaks			+	
Herpangina	Common		+		
Hand-foot-and-mouth disease	Common		+		
Rash disease	Common		+	+	+
Acute hemorrhagic conjunctivitis	Epidemics		+		+ (entero70)
Respiratory tract infections	Common	+	+	+	+
Undifferentiated fever	Common	+	+	+	+
Diarrhea, gastrointestinal disease	Uncommon				+
Diabetes, pancreatitis	Uncommon			+	
Orchitis	Uncommon			+	

*A member(s) of this family cause(s) this disease.
[†]Enteroviruses 68 to 71+.

Poliovirus Infections

There are three poliovirus types, with 85% of the cases of paralytic polio caused by type 1. Reversion of the attenuated vaccine virus types 2 and 3 to virulence can cause vaccine-associated disease. Wild-type polio infections are rare because of the success of polio vaccines (see Figure 46-6). As noted earlier, however, vaccine-associated cases of polio do occur, and some populations remain unvaccinated, putting them at risk for infection. Poliovirus may cause one of the following four outcomes in unvaccinated people, depending on the progression of the infection (Figure 46-7):

1. **Asymptomatic illness** results if the viral infection is limited to the oropharynx and the gut. At least 90% of poliovirus infections are asymptomatic.
2. **Abortive poliomyelitis, the minor illness,** is a nonspecific febrile illness occurring in approximately 5% of infected people. Fever, headache, malaise, sore throat, and vomiting occur in such persons within 3 to 4 days of exposure.
3. **Nonparalytic poliomyelitis or aseptic meningitis** occurs in 1% to 2% of patients with poliovirus infections. In this disease, the virus progresses into the central nervous system and the meninges, causing back pain and muscle spasms in addition to the symptoms of the minor illness.
4. **Paralytic polio, the major illness,** occurs in 0.1% to 2.0% of persons with poliovirus infections and is the most severe outcome. It appears 3 to 4 days after the minor illness has subsided, thereby producing a biphasic illness. In this disease, the virus spreads from the blood to the anterior horn cells of the spinal cord and to the motor cortex of the brain. The severity of paralysis is determined by the extent of the neuronal infection and by which neurons are affected. Spinal paralysis may involve one or more limbs, whereas bulbar (cranial) paralysis may involve a combination of cranial nerves and even the medullary respiratory center.

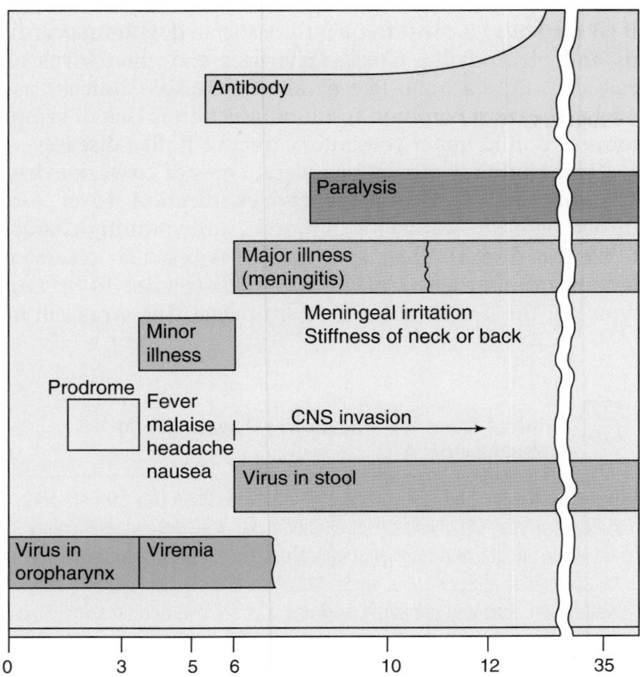

FIGURE 46-7 Progression of poliovirus infection. Infection may be asymptomatic or may progress to minor or major disease. *CNS,* Central nervous system.

Paralytic poliomyelitis is characterized by an asymmetric flaccid paralysis with no sensory loss. The degree of paralysis varies in that it may involve only a few muscle groups (e.g., one leg) or there may be complete flaccid paralysis of all four extremities. The paralysis may then progress over the first few days and may result in complete recovery, residual paralysis, or death. Most recoveries occur within 6 months, but as long as 2 years may be required for complete remission.

Bulbar poliomyelitis can be more severe, may involve the muscles of the pharynx, vocal cords, and respiration, and may result in death in 75% of patients. Iron lungs, chambers that provided external respiratory compression, were used during the 1950s to assist the breathing of patients with such polio disease. Before vaccination programs, iron lungs filled the wards of children's hospitals.

Postpolio syndrome is a sequela of poliomyelitis that may occur much later in life (30 to 40 years later) in 20% to 80% of the original victims. Affected persons suffer a deterioration of the originally affected muscles. Poliovirus is not present, but the syndrome is believed to result from a loss of neurons in the initially affected nerves.

Coxsackievirus and Echovirus Infections

Several clinical syndromes may be caused by either a coxsackievirus or an echovirus (e.g., aseptic meningitis), but certain illnesses are specifically associated with coxsackieviruses. Coxsackievirus A is associated with diseases involving vesicular lesions (e.g., herpangina), whereas coxsackievirus B ***(B* for *body)*** is most frequently associated with myocarditis and pleurodynia. Coxsackieviruses and enterovirus 68 can also cause a polio-like paralytic disease (Clinical Case 46-1). The most common result of infection is lack of symptoms or a mild upper respiratory tract or flulike disease.

Herpangina is caused by several types of coxsackievirus A and is not related to a herpesvirus infection. Fever, sore throat, pain on swallowing, anorexia, and vomiting characterize this disease. The classic finding is vesicular ulcerated lesions around the soft palate and uvula (Figure 46-8). Less typically, the lesions affect the hard palate. The virus can be recovered from the lesions or from feces. The disease is self-limited and requires only symptomatic management.

Hand-foot-and-mouth disease is a vesicular exanthem usually caused by coxsackievirus A16. The name is descriptive because the main features of this infection consist of vesicular lesions on the hands, feet, mouth, and tongue (Figure 46-9). The patient is mildly febrile, and the illness subsides in a few days.

Pleurodynia (Bornholm disease), also known as the **devil's grip,** is an acute illness in which patients have a

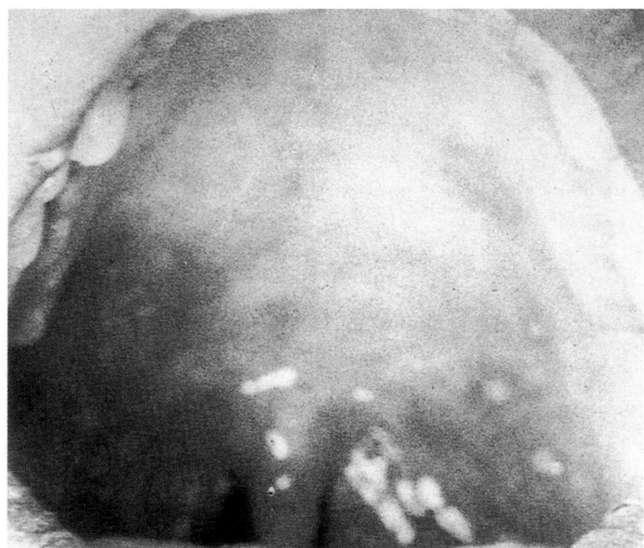

FIGURE 46-8 Herpangina. Characteristic discrete vesicles are seen on the anterior tonsillar pillars. (Courtesy Dr. GDW McKendrick; from Lambert HP et al: *Infectious diseases illustrated,* London, 1982, Gower.)

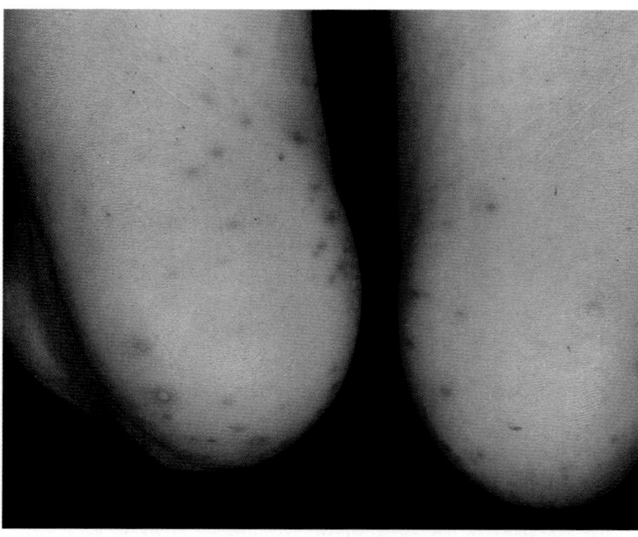

FIGURE 46-9 Hand-foot-and-mouth disease caused by coxsackievirus A. Lesions initially appear in the oral cavity and then develop within 1 day on the palms and, as seen here, the soles. (From Habif TP: *Clinical dermatology: a color guide to diagnosis and therapy,* ed 3, St Louis, 1996, Mosby.)

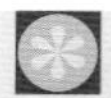

Clinical Case 46-1 Polio-like Disease due to Coxsackievirus A

In a case reported by Yoshimura and Kurashige (*Brain Dev* 20:540–542, 1998), a 4-year-old child's onset of abdominal pain, distended abdomen, inability to urinate, and inability to walk prompted admission to the hospital. All abdominal reflexes were gone, accompanied by bladder and rectal dysfunction. Pain and temperature sense was normal. Cerebrospinal fluid (CSF) showed an increase in cell count, with 393 cells/mm^3 and with 95% neutrophils and 5% lymphocytes. CSF protein and glucose were within normal values. Serologic analysis was negative for poliovirus, echovirus, and coxsackievirus types A4, A7, A9, B1, and B5, viruses reported to cause polio-like paralytic disease. Antibody for coxsackievirus A10 was detected during the acute phase (titer = 32) and after 4 weeks (titer = 128). Three weeks after admission, the child was able to walk again, but mild dysfunction of the bladder and rectum remained, even 3 months after admission. Although routine immunization has eliminated polio-induced paralysis in most parts of the world, polio-like disease can still be caused by other picornaviruses and revertants of the vaccine-related strains of polio.

sudden onset of fever and unilateral low thoracic, pleuritic chest pain that may be excruciating. Abdominal pain and even vomiting may also occur, and muscles on the involved side may be extremely tender. Pleurodynia lasts an average of 4 days but may relapse after the condition has been asymptomatic for several days. Coxsackievirus B is the causative agent.

Myocardial and **pericardial infections** caused by coxsackievirus B occur sporadically in older children and adults but are most threatening in newborns. Neonates with these infections have febrile illnesses and sudden and unexplained onset of heart failure. Cyanosis, tachycardia, cardiomegaly, and hepatomegaly occur. The mortality associated with the infection is high, and autopsy typically reveals involvement of other organ systems, including the brain, liver, and pancreas. Acute benign pericarditis affects young adults but may be seen in older persons. The symptoms resemble those of myocardial infarction with fever.

Viral (aseptic) meningitis is an acute febrile illness accompanied by headache and signs of meningeal irritation, including nuchal rigidity. Petechiae or a rash may occur in patients with enteroviral meningitis. Recovery is usually uneventful unless the illness is associated with encephalitis (meningoencephalitis) or occurs in children younger than 1 year. Outbreaks of picornavirus meningitis (echovirus 11) occur each year during the summer and autumn.

Fever, rash, and **common coldlike symptoms** may occur in patients infected with echoviruses or coxsackieviruses. The rash is usually maculopapular but may occasionally be petechial or even vesicular. The petechial type of eruption can be confused with the rash of meningococcemia, which is life threatening and must be treated. Enteroviral disease is usually less intense for the child than meningococcemia. Coxsackieviruses A21 and A24 and echoviruses 11 and 20 can cause rhinovirus-like symptoms resembling the common cold.

Other Enterovirus Diseases

Enterovirus 70 and a variant of coxsackievirus A24 have been associated with an extremely contagious ocular disease, **acute hemorrhagic conjunctivitis.** The infection causes subconjunctival hemorrhages and conjunctivitis. The disease has a 24-hour incubation period and resolves within 1 or 2 weeks. Some strains of coxsackievirus B and echovirus can be transmitted transplacentally to the fetus. Infection of the fetus or an infant by this or another route may produce severe disseminated disease. Coxsackievirus B infections of the beta cells of the pancreas are a major cause of **type 1 insulin-dependent diabetes** as a result of immune destruction of the islets of Langerhans.

Laboratory Diagnosis

Clinical Chemistry

Cerebrospinal fluid (CSF) from enterovirus aseptic meningitis can be distinguished from bacterial meningitis. The CSF lacks neutrophils, and the glucose level is usually normal or slightly low. The CSF protein level is normal to slightly elevated. The CSF is rarely positive for the virus.

Culture

Polioviruses may be isolated from the patient's pharynx during the first few days of illness, from the feces for as long as 30 days, but only rarely from CSF. The virus grows well in monkey kidney tissue culture. Coxsackieviruses and echoviruses can usually be isolated from the throat and stool during infection and often from CSF in patients with meningitis. Virus is rarely isolated in patients with myocarditis, because the symptoms occur several weeks after the initial infection. Coxsackievirus B can be grown on primary monkey or human embryo kidney cells. Many strains of coxsackievirus A do not grow in tissue culture but can be grown in suckling mice.

Genome and Serology Studies

The exact type of enterovirus can be determined through the use of specific antibody and antigen assays (e.g., neutralization, immunofluorescence, enzyme-linked immunosorbent assay) or reverse transcriptase polymerase chain reaction (RT-PCR) detection of viral RNA. RT-PCR of clinical samples has become a rapid and routine method to detect the presence of an enterovirus or distinguish a specific enterovirus, depending upon the primers used. RT-PCR has become especially important for confirming a diagnosis of echovirus 11 meningitis in an infant.

Serology can be used to confirm an enterovirus infection through detection of specific immunoglobulin (Ig)M or the finding of a fourfold increase in the antibody titer between the time of the acute illness and the period of convalescence. Because of their many serotypes, this approach may not be practical for detection of echovirus and coxsackievirus unless a specific virus is suspected.

Treatment, Prevention, and Control

Pleconaril is available on a limited basis. The drug inhibits penetration of picornaviruses into the cell. It must be administered early in the course of the infection.

Prevention of paralytic poliomyelitis is one of the triumphs of modern medicine. By 1979, infections with the wild-type poliovirus disappeared from the United States, with the number of cases of polio decreasing from 21,000 per year in the prevaccine era to 18 in unvaccinated patients in 1977. Similar to smallpox, polio has been targeted for elimination. Health care delivery to underdeveloped countries is more difficult, and for this reason, wild-type viral disease still exists in Africa, the Middle East, and Asia. Misinformation, misunderstanding, and political unrest in Africa and other parts of the world have also limited acceptance of polio vaccination. New worldwide vaccination programs have been developed to reach the goal.

The two types of poliovirus vaccine are (1) **inactivated polio vaccine (IPV),** developed by Jonas Salk, and (2) **live attenuated oral polio vaccine (OPV),** developed by Albert Sabin. Both vaccines incorporate the three strains of polio, are stable, are relatively inexpensive, and induce a protective antibody response (Figure 46-10). The IPV was proven effective in 1955, but the oral vaccine took its place because it is less expensive, easy to administer, limits production of virus and virus transmission, and elicits lifelong and mucosal immunity (Table 46-2).

In the absence of wild-type poliovirus, IPV has less potential for vaccine-related disease and is the vaccine of choice for routine vaccination. Children should receive the IPV at 2 months, 4 months, and 15 months and then at 4 to 6 years of age.

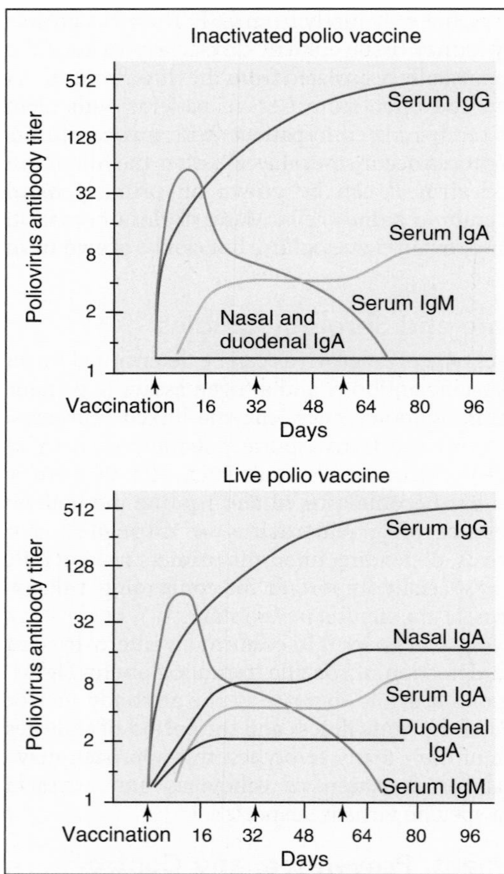

FIGURE 46-10 Serum and secretory antibody response to intramuscular inoculation of inactivated polio vaccine (IPV) and to oral live attenuated polio vaccine (OPV). Note the presence of secretory IgA induced by the OPV. *Ig,* Immunoglobulin. (Modified from Ogra P, Fishaut M, Gallagher MR: Viral vaccination via the mucosal routes, *Rev Infect Dis* 2:352–369, 1980. Copyright 1980, University of Chicago Press.)

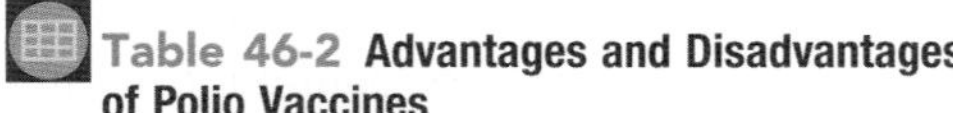
Table 46-2 Advantages and Disadvantages of Polio Vaccines

Vaccine	Advantages	Disadvantages
Live oral polio vaccine (OPV)	Effective Lifelong immunity Induction of secretory antibody response similar to that of natural infection Prevents spread of virus in feces Spread of attenuated virus to contacts promotes indirect immunization Inexpensive and easy to administer No need for repeated booster vaccine Herd immunity	Risk of vaccine-associated poliomyelitis in vaccine recipients or contacts; spread of vaccine to contacts without their consent Not safe for administration to immunodeficient patients
Inactivated polio vaccine (IPV)	Effective Good stability during transport and in storage Safe administration in immunodeficient patients No risk of vaccine-related disease	Lack of induction of secretory antibody Booster vaccine needed for lifelong immunity Requires sterile syringes and needles Injection more painful than oral administration Higher community immunization levels needed than with live vaccine Does not prevent replication and spread of virus from gastrointestinal tract

The OPV was **attenuated** (i.e., rendered less virulent) by passage in human or monkey cell cultures. Attenuation yielded a virus that can replicate in the oropharynx and intestinal tract but cannot infect neuronal cells. The vaccine elicits IgA and IgG that can stop virus spread in and from the gut as well as spread within the body. A mixed blessing of the live vaccine strain is that it is shed in feces for weeks and may be spread to close contacts. The spread will immunize or reimmunize close contacts, thus promoting mass immunization. In response to detection of wild-type poliovirus in sewage in 2013, Israel reinstituted OPV immunizations to ensure that polio transmission is also prevented. The major drawbacks of the live vaccine are that (1) the vaccine virus may infect an immunologically compromised person, and (2) there is a remote potential for the virus to revert to its virulent form and cause paralytic disease (1 per 4 million doses administered versus 1 in 100 persons infected with the wild-type poliovirus).

There are no vaccines for coxsackieviruses or echoviruses. Transmission of these viruses can presumably be reduced by improvements in hygiene and living conditions. Enteroviruses are impervious to most common disinfectants and detergents but can be inactivated by formaldehyde, hypochlorite, and chlorine.

• Rhinoviruses

Rhinoviruses are the most important cause of the **common cold** and upper respiratory tract infections. Such infections are self-limited, however, and do not cause serious disease. More than 100 serotypes of rhinovirus have been identified. At least 80% of the rhinoviruses have a common receptor that is also used by some of the coxsackieviruses. This receptor has been identified as ICAM-1, a member of the immunoglobulin superfamily, which is expressed on epithelial, fibroblast, and B-lymphoblastoid cells.

Pathogenesis and Immunity

Unlike the enteroviruses, rhinoviruses are **unable to replicate in the gastrointestinal tract** (see Box 46-3). The rhinoviruses are **labile to acidic pH.** Also, they **grow best at 33° C,** a feature that contributes to their preference for the cooler environment of the nasal mucosa. Infection can be initiated by as little as one infectious viral particle. During the peak of illness, nasal secretions contain concentrations of 500 to 1000 infectious virions per milliliter. The virus enters through the nose, mouth, or eyes and initiates infection of the upper respiratory tract, including the throat. Most viral replication occurs in the nose, and the onset and severity of the symptoms correlate with the time of viral shedding and quantity (titer) of virus shed. Infected cells release bradykinin and histamine, which cause a "runny nose."

Interferon, which is generated in response to the infection, may limit progression of the infection and contribute to the symptoms. Interestingly, the release of cytokines during inflammation can promote the spread of the virus by enhancing expression of ICAM-1 viral receptors.

Immunity to rhinoviruses is transient and unlikely to prevent subsequent infection (because of the numerous serotypes of the virus). Both nasal secretory IgA and serum IgG antibody are induced by a primary rhinovirus infection and can be detected within a week of infection. The secretory IgA response dissipates quickly, and immunity begins to wane approximately 18 months after infection. Cell-mediated immunity is not likely to play an important role in controlling rhinovirus infections.

Epidemiology

Rhinoviruses cause at least half of all upper respiratory tract infections (Box 46-5). Other agents likely to cause the symptoms of the common cold are enteroviruses, coronaviruses, adenoviruses, and parainfluenza viruses. Rhinoviruses can be transmitted by two mechanisms: as aerosols and on fomites (e.g., by hands or on contaminated inanimate objects). Hands appear to be the major vector, and direct person-to-person contact is the predominant mode of spread. These nonenveloped viruses are extremely stable and can survive on such objects for many hours.

Rhinoviruses produce clinical illness in only half of the persons infected. Asymptomatic persons are also capable of spreading the virus, even though they may produce less of it.

Rhinovirus "colds" occur most often in early autumn and late spring in persons living in temperate climates. This may reflect social patterns (e.g., return to school and day care) rather than any change in the virus itself.

Rates of infection are highest in infants and children. Children younger than 2 years "share" their colds with their families. Secondary infections occur in approximately 50% of family members, especially other children.

Many different rhinovirus serotypes may be found in a given community during a specific cold season, but the predominant strains are usually the newly categorized serotypes. This pattern indicates the existence of a gradual antigenic drift (mutation) similar to that seen for the influenza virus.

Box 46-5 Epidemiology of Rhinovirus Infections

Disease/Viral Factors
Virion is resistant to drying and detergents
Multiple serotypes preclude prior immunity
Replication occurs at optimum temperature of 33° C and cooler temperatures

Transmission
Direct contact via infected hands and fomites
Inhalation of infectious droplets

Who Is at Risk?
Persons of all ages

Geography/Season
Virus found worldwide
Disease more common in early autumn and late spring

Modes of Control
Washing hands and disinfecting contaminated objects help prevent spread

Clinical Syndromes (Box 46-6)

Common cold symptoms caused by rhinoviruses cannot readily be distinguished from those caused by other viral respiratory pathogens (e.g., enteroviruses, paramyxoviruses, coronaviruses). An upper respiratory tract infection usually begins with sneezing, which is soon followed by rhinorrhea (runny nose). The rhinorrhea increases and is then accompanied by symptoms of nasal obstruction. Mild sore throat also occurs, along with headache and malaise but usually without fever. The illness peaks in 3 to 4 days, but the cough and nasal symptoms may persist for 7 to 10 days or longer.

Laboratory Diagnosis

The clinical syndrome of the common cold is usually so characteristic that laboratory diagnosis is unnecessary. Virus can be obtained from nasal washings. Rhinoviruses are grown in human diploid fibroblast cells (e.g., WI-38) at 33° C. Virus is identified by the typical cytopathologic effect and the demonstration of acid lability. Serotyping is rarely necessary but can be performed with the use of pools of specific neutralizing sera. Identification can also be made by

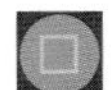

Box 46-6 Clinical Summaries

Poliovirus
Polio: A 12-year-old girl from Nigeria has headache, fever, nausea, and stiff neck. Symptoms improve and then recur several days later, with weakness and paralysis of her legs. She has no history of polio immunization.

Coxsackievirus A
Herpangina: Vesicular lesions on the tongue and roof of the mouth of a 7-year-old patient accompany fever, sore throat, and pain on swallowing.

Coxsackievirus B *(B* for *body)*
Pleurodynia: A 13-year-old boy has fever and severe chest pain with headache, fatigue, and aching muscles lasting for 4 days.

Coxsackievirus or Echovirus
Aseptic meningitis: A 7-month-old infant with fever and rash appears listless, with a stiff neck. A sample of his cerebrospinal fluid contains lymphocytes but has normal glucose and no bacteria. Full recovery occurs within 1 week.

Rhinovirus
Common cold: A 25-year-old office worker develops a runny nose, mild cough, and malaise with a low-grade fever. A coworker has had similar symptoms for the past few days.

genome analysis by RT-PCR. The performance of serologic testing to document rhinovirus infection is not practical.

Treatment, Prevention, and Control

There are many over-the-counter remedies for the common cold. Nasal vasoconstrictors may provide relief, but their use may be followed by rebound congestion and a worsening of symptoms. Inhaling hot, humidified air, and even the steam from hot chicken soup, may actually help by increasing nasal drainage.

No antiviral drugs are effective. Pleconaril and similar experimental antiviral drugs (e.g., arildone, rhodanine, disoxaril) contain a 3-methylisoxazole group that inserts into the base of the receptor-binding canyon and blocks uncoating of the virus. Enviroxime inhibits the viral RNA-dependent RNA polymerase. A polypeptide receptor analog based on the ICAM-1 protein structure has also been evaluated as an antiviral drug. Intranasal administration of interferon can block infection for a short time after a known exposure, but its long-term use (e.g., throughout the "cold season") could cause flulike symptoms that are at least as bad as those of the rhinovirus infection.

Rhinovirus is not a good candidate for a vaccine program. The multiple serotypes, the apparent antigenic drift in rhinoviral antigens, the requirement for secretory IgA production, and the transience of the antibody response pose major problems for vaccine development. In addition, the benefit-to-risk ratio would be very low because rhinoviruses do not cause significant disease.

Handwashing and disinfection of contaminated objects are the best means of preventing viral spread. Virucidal facial tissues impregnated with citric acid may also limit rhinovirus spread.

Bibliography

Ansardi DC, Porter DC, Anderson MJ, et al: Poliovirus assembly and encapsidation of genomic RNA, *Adv Virus Res* 46:1–68, 1996.

Buenz EJ, Howe CL: Picornaviruses and cell death, *Trends Microbiol* 14:28–38, 2006.

Cann AJ: *Principles of molecular virology*, San Diego, 2005, Academic.

Carter J, Saunders V: *Virology: principles and applications*, Chichester, England, 2007, Wiley.

Cohen J, Powderly WG: *Infectious diseases*, ed 2, St Louis, 2004, Mosby.

Collier L, Oxford J: *Human virology*, ed 4, Oxford, England, 2011, Oxford University Press.

Flint SJ, Enquist LW, Racaniello VR, et al: *Principles of virology: molecular biology, pathogenesis and control of animal viruses*, ed 3, Washington, DC, 2009, American Society for Microbiology Press.

Knipe DM, Howley PM: *Fields virology*, ed 6, Philadelphia, 2013, Lippincott Williams & Wilkins.

Levandowski RA: Rhinoviruses. In Belshe RB, editor: *Textbook of human virology*, ed 2, St Louis, 1991, Mosby.

McKinlay MA, Pevear DC, Rossmann MG: Treatment of the picornavirus common cold by inhibitors of viral uncoating and attachment, *Annu Rev Microbiol* 46:635–654, 1992.

Moore M, Morens DM: Enteroviruses including polioviruses. In Belshe RB, editor: *Textbook of human virology*, ed 2, St Louis, 1991, Mosby.

Plotkin SA, Vidor E: Poliovirus vaccine—inactive. In Plotkin SA, Orenstein WA, editors: *Vaccines*, ed 4, Philadelphia, 2004, WB Saunders.

Racaniello VR: One hundred years of poliovirus pathogenesis, *Virology* 344:9–16, 2006.

Richman DD, Whitley RJ, Hayden FG: *Clinical virology*, ed 3, Washington, DC, 2009, American Society for Microbiology Press.

Robbins FC: The history of polio vaccine development. In Plotkin SA, Orenstein WA, editors: *Vaccines*, ed 4, Philadelphia, 2004, WB Saunders.

Strauss JM, Strauss EG: *Viruses and human disease*, San Diego, 2002, Academic.

Sutter RW, Kew OM, Cochi SL: Poliovirus vaccine—live. In Plotkin SA, Orenstein WA, editors: *Vaccines*, ed 4, Philadelphia, 2004, WB Saunders.

Tracy S, Chapman NM, Mahy BWJ: Coxsackie B viruses, *Curr Top Microbiol Immunol* 223:153–167, 1997.

Voyles BA: *The biology of viruses*, ed 2, Boston, 2002, McGraw-Hill.

Whitton JL, Cornell CT, Feuer R: Host and virus determinants of picornavirus pathogenesis and tropism, *Nat Rev Microbiol* 3:765–776, 2005.

Websites

Alsina-Gilbert M, Sloan SB: Dermatologic manifestations of enteroviral infections. www.emedicine.com/derm/topic875.htm. Accessed April 4, 2015.

Lutwick LI: Picornavirus—overview. www.emedicine.com/med/topic1831.htm. Accessed April 4, 2015.

Manor Y, Shulman LM, Kaliner E, et al: Intensified environmental surveillance supporting the response to wild poliovirus type 1 silent circulation in Israel, 2013, *Euro Surveill* 19:20708, 2014. www.eurosurveillance.org/ViewArticle.aspx?ArticleId=20708. Accessed April 4, 2015.

Picornaviridae online. www.picornaviridae.com. Accessed April 4, 2015.

Porter KA, Ousmane MD, Burns CC, et al: Tracking progress toward polio eradication—worldwide, 2013–2014, *MMWR Morb Mortal Wkly Rep* 64(15):415–420, 2015. www.cdc.gov/mmwr/preview/mmwrhtml/mm6119a6.htm. Accessed May 8, 2015.

Rajnik M: Rhinovirus infection. www.emedicine.com/ped/topic2707.htm. Accessed April 4, 2015.

CHAPTER

47 CORONAVIRUSES AND NOROVIRUSES

A 17-year-old student complains that he has a cold.

1. What are the possible causes?
2. What properties of the virus restrict the infection to the upper respiratory tract?
3. How is it transmitted and acquired?

A day after eating burritos at a fast food restaurant, several medical students complained of serious diarrhea, nausea, vomiting, and a mild fever for 2 days. Other patrons also had gastroenteritis.

4. What are the likely causes of the gastroenteritis? How does the 24-hour incubation period help narrow the diagnosis?
5. How does this agent cause diarrhea?
6. What is the best means of detecting the agent?

Answers to these questions are available on StudentConsult.com.

• SUMMARIES CLINICALLY SIGNIFICANT ORGANISMS

Coronaviruses

Trigger Words

Common cold, SARS, MERS

Biology, Virulence, and Disease

- Medium size, enveloped, (+) RNA genome
- Detergent resistant due to glycoprotein corona (exception to the rule for enveloped viruses)
- Encodes RNA-dependent RNA polymerase, replicates in cytoplasm
- Most coronaviruses cannot replicate at body temperature, restricted to upper respiratory tract
- Most coronaviruses cause common cold
- MERS and SARS can replicate at 37° C
- Severe pneumonias

Epidemiology

- Transmitted by aerosols, direct contact, fecal oral, contaminated swimming pools

Diagnosis

- Symptomatology, RT-PCR genome analysis, or respiratory secretions

Treatment, Prevention, and Control

- Quarantine for SARS, MERS

Noroviruses (Caliciviridae)

Trigger Words

Outbreaks of diarrhea, cruise ships, watery diarrhea, vomiting

Biology, Virulence, and Disease

- Small size, capsid, (+) RNA genome
- Very resistant to environment, including detergents and other disinfectants
- Encodes RNA-dependent RNA polymerase, replicates in cytoplasm
- Damages intestinal brush border
- Diarrhea with nausea and vomiting

Epidemiology

- Transmitted by fecal-oral route, in contaminated foods and water; very resistant to inactivation

Diagnosis

- Symptomatology, RT-PCR genome analysis, or respiratory secretions

Treatment, Prevention, and Control

- Supportive care

• Coronaviruses

Coronaviruses are named for the solar corona–like appearance (the surface projections) of their virions when viewed with an electron microscope (Figure 47-1). Coronaviruses are the second most prevalent cause of the **common cold** (rhinoviruses are the first). Coronaviruses have caused outbreaks of **severe acute respiratory syndrome (SARS-CoV)** in China and the Middle East (Middle East respiratory syndrome [**MERS-CoV**]). Electron microscopic findings have also linked coronaviruses to gastroenteritis in children and adults.

Structure and Replication

Coronaviruses are **enveloped virions** with the longest **positive (+) ribonucleic acid (RNA)** genome. Virions measure 80 to 160 nm in diameter (Box 47-1). The glycoproteins on the surface of the envelope appear as club-shaped projections that appear as a halo (corona) around the virus. Unlike most enveloped viruses, the "corona" formed by the glycoproteins allows the virus to endure the conditions in the gastrointestinal tract and be spread by the fecal-oral route.

The large plus-stranded RNA genome (27,000 to 30,000 bases) associates with the N protein to form a helical

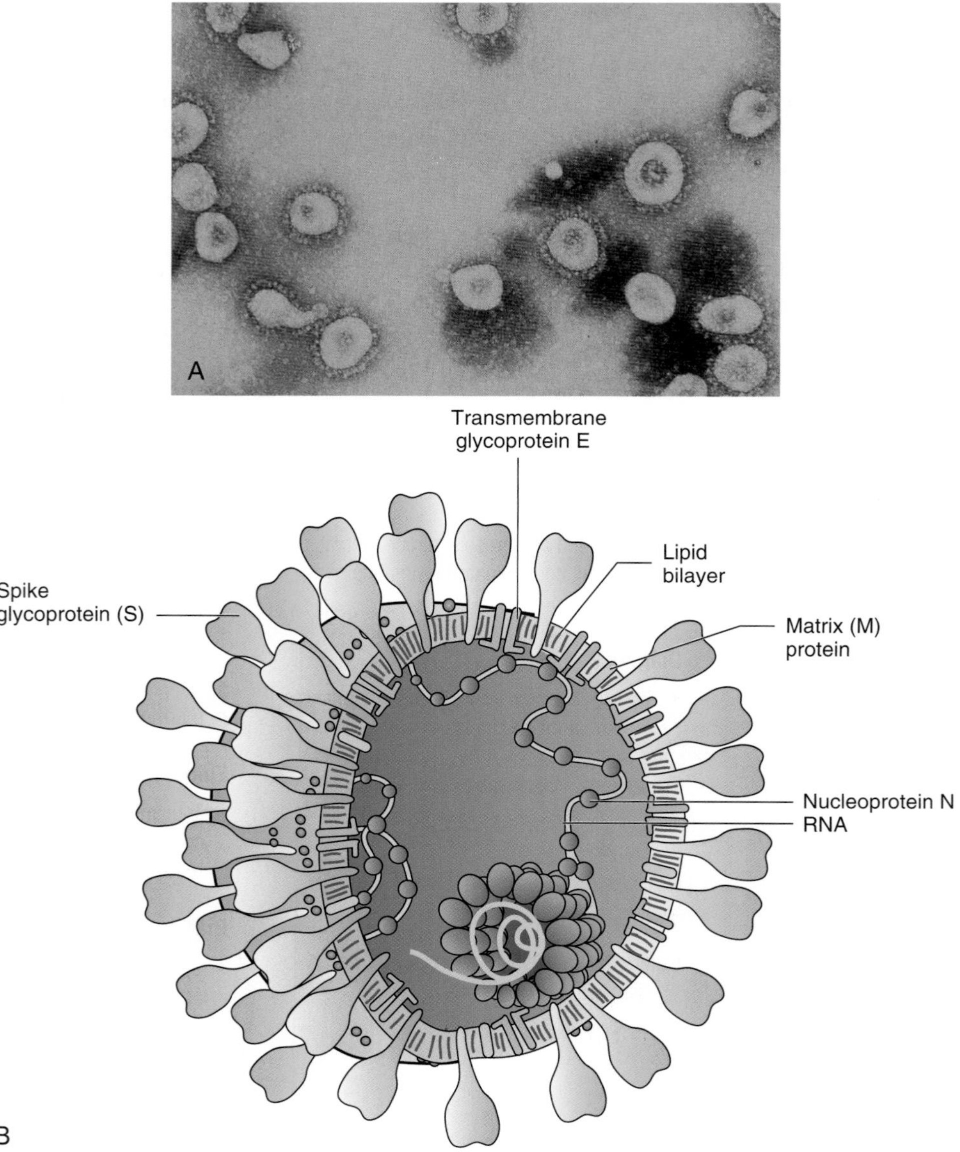

FIGURE 47-1 **A,** Electron micrograph of the human respiratory coronavirus (magnification 90,000×). **B,** Model of a coronavirus. The viral nucleocapsid is a long, flexible helix composed of the positive-strand genomic RNA and many molecules of the phosphorylated nucleocapsid protein N. The viral envelope consists of a lipid bilayer derived from the intracellular membranes of the host cell, two or three viral glycoproteins (Spike [S], E, possibly hemagglutinin-esterase [HE]), and a matrix protein. (**A,** Courtesy Centers for Disease Control and Prevention, Atlanta; **B,** Modified from Fields BF, Knipe DM: *Virology,* New York, 1985, Raven.)

nucleocapsid. Protein synthesis occurs in two phases, similar to that of the togaviruses. On infection, the genome is translated to produce a polyprotein that is cleaved to produce an RNA-dependent RNA polymerase (L [225,000 Da]) and other proteins. Transcription and replication of the genome occurs within membrane vesicles created by viral proteins. The L protein produces and then uses a negative-sense template RNA to replicate new genomes and produce five to seven **individual messenger ribonucleic acids (mRNAs)** for the individual viral proteins.

Virions contain the glycoproteins E1 (20,000 to 30,000 Da) and E2 (160,000 to 200,000 Da) and a core nucleoprotein (N [47,000 to 55,000 Da]); some strains also contain a hemagglutinin neuraminidase (E3 [120,000 to 140,000 Da]) (Table 47-1). The E2 glycoprotein is responsible for mediating viral attachment and membrane fusion and is the target of neutralizing antibodies. The E1 glycoprotein is a transmembrane matrix protein. The replication scheme for coronaviruses is shown in Figure 47-2.

Pathogenesis and Clinical Syndromes

Most human coronaviruses have an *optimum temperature for viral growth of 33° C to 35° C,* and therefore infection remains localized to the upper respiratory tract. Animal coronaviruses, including SARS-CoV and MERS-CoV, can replicate at 37° C and cause systemic disease. Coronaviruses cause cytolytic infections and when inoculated into the respiratory tracts of human volunteers, they infect and disrupt the function of ciliated epithelial cells (Box 47-2). The virus is most likely spread by aerosols. Most human coronaviruses cause an upper respiratory tract infection, accounting for approximately 10% to 15% of upper respiratory tract infections in humans. The disease is similar to the common cold caused by rhinoviruses but with a longer incubation period (average, 3 days). The infection may exacerbate a preexisting chronic pulmonary disease, such as asthma or bronchitis, and on rare occasions may cause pneumonia.

Infections occur mainly in infants and children. Coronavirus disease appears either sporadically or in outbreaks in the winter and spring. Usually, one strain predominates in an outbreak. Antibodies to coronaviruses are uniformly present by adulthood, but reinfections are common, despite the preexisting serum antibodies.

Coronavirus-like particles have also been seen in electron micrographs of stool specimens obtained from adults and children with diarrhea and gastroenteritis and in infants with neonatal necrotizing enterocolitis.

SARS-CoV and MERS-CoV are zoonoses. The outbreaks of these viral diseases have occurred when the animal reservoir has come in contact with man. SARS-CoV and MERS-CoV are cytolytic viruses that can replicate at body temperatures in epithelial cells, lymphocytes, and leukocytes. A combination of viral pathogenesis and immunopathogenesis causes significant lung, kidney, liver, and gastrointestinal tissue damage and depletion of immune cells.

SARS is a form of atypical pneumonia characterized by high fever (>38° C), chills, rigors, headache, dizziness, malaise, myalgia, cough, or breathing difficulty, leading to acute respiratory distress syndrome. Up to 20% of patients will also develop diarrhea. Persons with SARS were exposed within the previous 10 days. Mortality is at least 10% of symptomatic people. Although SARS-CoV is most likely transmitted in respiratory droplets, it is also present in sweat, urine, and feces.

The outbreak of SARS started in November 2002 in South China's Guangdong Province, was brought to Hong Kong by a physician working within the original outbreak, and then was brought to Vietnam, Toronto, and other places by travelers. The virus was shown to be a coronavirus by its electron microscopic morphology and by reverse transcriptase polymerase chain reaction (RT-PCR). The virus apparently jumped to man from animals (masked-palm civets, raccoon dogs, and Chinese ferret badgers) raised for food. A World Health Organization (WHO) global alert prompted containment measures to control the spread of the virus and limited the outbreak to 8000 known diseased individuals but with at least 784 deaths. Travel restrictions and public concern resulted in a loss of hundreds of millions of dollars in travel and other business.

MERS-CoV also causes acute respiratory distress syndrome, with a 50% mortality of those identified as infected with MERS. Most of the cases of MERS have occurred in the Arabian peninsula. Bats and camels are the natural reservoirs of MERS-CoV.

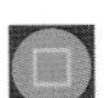

Box 47-1 Unique Features of Coronaviruses

Virus has medium-sized virions with a solar corona–like appearance.

Single-stranded, positive-sense RNA genome is enclosed in an envelope containing the E2 viral attachment protein, E1 matrix protein, and N nucleocapsid protein.

Translation of genome occurs in two phases: (1) the early phase produces an RNA polymerase (L), and (2) the late phase, from a negative-sense RNA template, yields structural and nonstructural proteins.

Virus assembles at the rough endoplasmic reticulum.

Virus is difficult to isolate and grow in routine cell culture.

Table 47-1 Major Human Coronavirus Proteins

Proteins	Molecular Weight (kDa)	Location	Functions
E2 (peplomeric glycoprotein)	160-200	Envelope spikes (peplomer)	Binding to host cells; fusion activity
H1 (hemagglutinin protein)	60-66	Peplomer	Hemagglutination
N (nucleoprotein)	47-55	Core	Ribonucleoprotein
E1 (matrix glycoprotein)	20-30	Envelope	Transmembrane protein
L (polymerase)	225	Infected cell	Polymerase activity

Modified from Balows A, Hausler WJ, Lennette EH, et al: *Laboratory diagnosis of infectious diseases: principles and practice,* New York, 1988, Springer-Verlag.

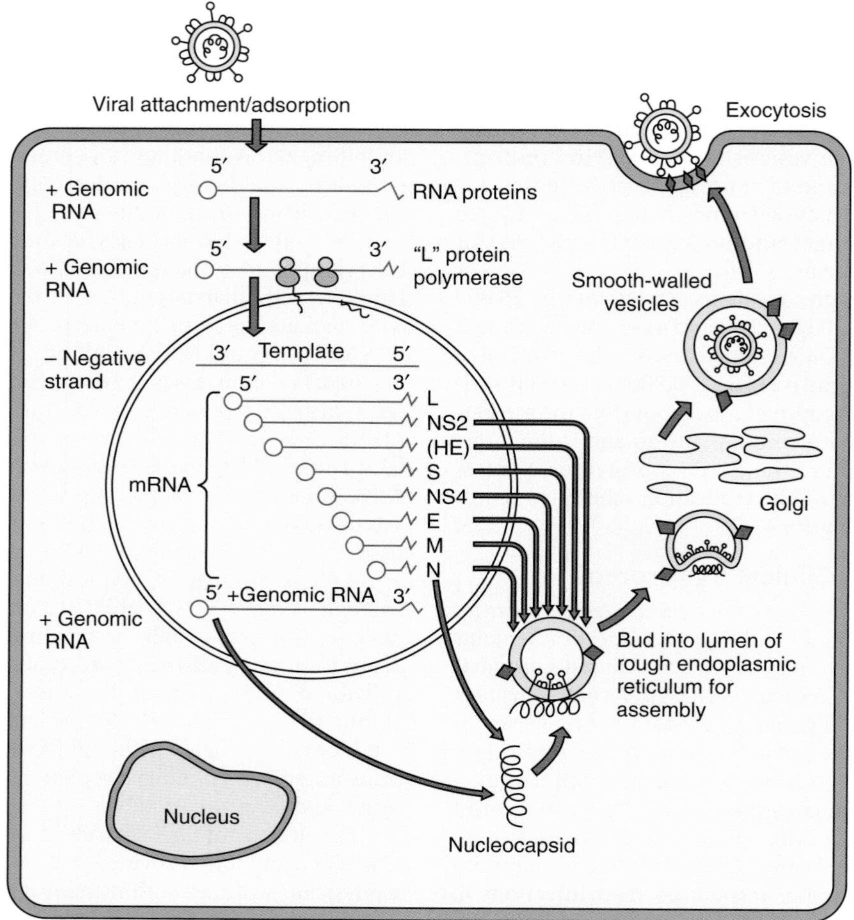

FIGURE 47-2 Replication of human coronaviruses. The E2 glycoprotein interacts with receptors on epithelial cells, the virus fuses or is endocytosed into the cell, and the genome is released into the cytoplasm. Protein synthesis is divided into early and late phases, similar to that in the togaviruses. The genome binds to ribosomes, and an RNA-dependent RNA polymerase is translated. This enzyme generates a full-length, negative-sense RNA template for the production of new virion genomes and six individual mRNAs for the other coronavirus proteins. The genome associates with rough endoplasmic reticulum membranes modified by virion proteins and buds into the lumen of the rough endoplasmic reticulum. Vesicles that contain virus migrate to the cell membrane, and virus is released by exocytosis. (Modified from Balows A, Hausler WJ, Lennette EH, et al: *Laboratory diagnosis of infectious diseases: principles and practice,* New York, 1988, Springer-Verlag.)

 **Box 47-2 Disease Mechanisms of Human Coronaviruses**

Virus infects epithelial cells of upper respiratory tract.

Virus replicates best at 33° C to 35° C; therefore it prefers the upper respiratory tract.

Reinfection occurs in the presence of serum antibodies.

The glycoprotein "corona" helps this enveloped virus survive the gastrointestinal tract.

Severe acute respiratory syndrome infection is exacerbated by inflammatory responses.

Laboratory Diagnosis

Laboratory tests are not routinely performed to diagnose coronavirus infections other than for SARS and MERS. RT-PCR is the method of choice for detection of the viral RNA genome in respiratory and stool samples. Virus isolation of the coronaviruses is difficult and for SARS-CoV and MERS-CoV requires stringent biosafety level 3 (BSL-3) conditions.

Treatment, Prevention, and Control

Control of respiratory transmission of the common cold form of coronavirus would be difficult and is probably unnecessary because of the mildness of the infection. Strict quarantine of infected individuals and screening for fever in travelers from a region with an outbreak of SARS-CoV and MERS-CoV limit the spread of these viruses. No vaccine or specific antiviral therapy is available.

• Noroviruses

Norovirus is the most common cause of foodborne disease outbreaks in the United States. The noroviruses are members of the Caliciviridae family, which also includes astroviruses and other small, round gastroenteritis viruses. Norwalk virus, the prototypical norovirus, was discovered during an epidemic of acute gastroenteritis in Norwalk, Ohio, in 1968 upon electron microscopic examination of stool samples from adults. Many of the other viruses in this family also bear the names of the geographic locations where they were identified (Box 47-3).

Structure and Replication

Noroviruses resemble and are approximately the same size as the picornaviruses. Their **positive-sense RNA genome** (≈7500 bases) has a VPg protein (viral protein genome-linked) and a 3′ terminal polyadenylate sequence similar to picornaviruses. The genome is contained in a 27-nm **naked capsid** consisting of 60,000-Da capsid proteins. Norwalk virions are round with a ragged outline, whereas other calicivirion capsomeres have cup-shaped indentations or a six-point star shape. The virions of the astroviruses have a five- or six-point star shape on the surface but no indentations. Antibodies from seropositive people can also be used to distinguish these viruses.

Most caliciviruses and astroviruses can be grown in cell culture, but the Norwalk viruses cannot. Expression of the structural protein genes of different Norwalk viruses in tissue culture cells produces Norwalk virus–like particles. These particles were used to show that Norwalk viruses bind to the carbohydrate of either the A, B, or O blood group antigen on the cell surface. The noroviruses enter and exit cells similar to the picornaviruses but transcribe an early and late mRNA similar to the togaviruses and coronaviruses. The early mRNA encodes a polyprotein containing the RNA polymerase and other enzymes. The late mRNA encodes the capsid proteins.

Pathogenesis

The norovirus strains that infect humans can only infect humans. As few as 10 virions will initiate disease in humans. The virus infects and damages the small intestine, preventing proper absorption of water and nutrients and causing a watery diarrhea. Gastric emptying may be delayed, causing vomiting. Shedding of the virus may continue for 2 weeks after symptoms have ceased. Immunity is generally short lived at best and may not be protective. The large number of strains and high rate of mutation allows reinfection despite antibodies from a previous exposure.

Epidemiology

Norwalk and related viruses typically cause outbreaks of gastroenteritis from a common source of contamination (e.g., water, shellfish, salad, raspberries, food service). These viruses are transmitted mainly by the fecal-oral route in stool and vomitus. The virus is resistant to drying and heat and can remain on surfaces for long periods. Infected individuals shed the largest amounts of virus when sick and for 3 days after recovery but continue to shed virus for up to 4 weeks. During peak shedding, 100 billion virions are released per gram of feces. Up to 30% of infected individuals are asymptomatic but can spread the infection.

Outbreaks in developed countries may occur year-round and have been described in schools, resorts, hospitals, nursing homes, restaurants, and cruise ships. Common-source outbreaks can often be traced to a careless, infected food handler. The Centers for Disease Control and Prevention estimates that nearly 50% (23 million U.S. cases per year) of all foodborne outbreaks of gastroenteritis can be attributed to noroviruses, which is a tribute to the importance of this virus. As many as 70% of children in the United States have antibodies to noroviruses by the age of 7 years.

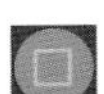

Box 47-3 Characteristics of Noroviruses

Viruses are small capsid viruses distinguishable by capsid morphology.
Viruses are resistant to environmental pressure: detergents, drying, and acid.
Viruses are transmitted by fecal-oral route in contaminated water and food.
Viruses cause outbreaks of gastroenteritis.
Disease resolves after 48 hours, without serious consequences.

Clinical Syndromes (Clinical Case 47-1; Box 47-4)

Norwalk and related viruses cause symptoms similar to those caused by the rotaviruses but in adults and children. Infection causes an acute onset of **diarrhea, nausea,**

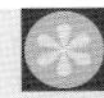

Clinical Case 47-1 Norwalk Virus Outbreak

Brummer-Korvenkontio and associates (*Epidemiol Infect* 129:335–360, 2002) described an outbreak of gastroenteritis in children who had attended a concert; infection was traced back to contamination of a specific seating area, bathrooms, and other areas visited by one individual. A male concert attendee was ill prior to attending a concert and then vomited four times in the concert hall: in a waste bin in the corridor, into the toilets, onto the floor of the fire escape, and on a carpeted area in the walkway. His family members showed symptoms within 24 hours. A children's concert for several schools was held the next day. Children sitting in the same section as the incident case and those who traversed the contaminated carpet had the highest incidence of disease, characterized by watery diarrhea and vomiting for approximately 2 days. RT-PCR analysis of fecal samples from two ill children detected Norwalk virus genomic RNA. Infected vomit may have up to a million viruses per milliliter, and only 10 to 100 viruses are required to transmit the disease. Contact with contaminated shoes, hands, clothing, or aerosols may have infected the children. The encapsidated nature of the Norwalk virus makes it resistant to routine cleansers; disinfection usually requires freshly prepared hypochlorite bleach–containing solutions or steam cleaning.

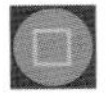

Box 47-4 Clinical Summaries

Coronaviruses

Common cold: A 25-year-old office worker develops a runny nose, mild cough, malaise, and a low-grade fever. A coworker has had similar symptoms for the past few days.

SARS: A 45-year-old businessman returned from a 2-week trip to China. Five days after returning home to the United States, he developed a fever of 101.5° F (38.6° C) and cough. Now he observes that it is harder to catch his breath.

Norovirus

Norwalk virus: On the third day of a cruise (incubation period of 24 to 60 hours), a group of 45 passengers on a cruise ship experienced watery diarrhea, nausea, and vomiting for 12 to 60 hours, depending on the individual.

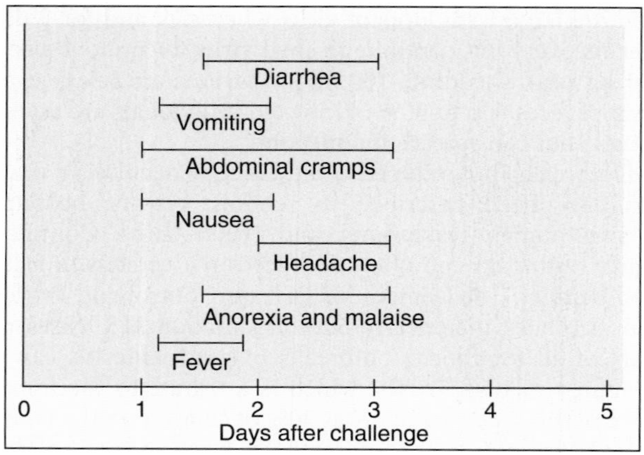

FIGURE 47-3 Response to ingestion of Norwalk virus. Symptoms vary in severity.

vomiting, and abdominal cramps, especially in children (Figure 47-3). Bloody stools do not occur. Fever may occur in as many as a third of patients. The incubation period is usually 12 to 48 hours, and the illness usually resolves within 1 to 3 days without problems but can last up to 6 days.

Laboratory Diagnosis

The use of RT-PCR for detection of the Norovirus genome in stool or emesis samples has enhanced the speed and detection of the virus during outbreaks. Immunoelectron microscopy can be used to concentrate and identify the virus from stool. Addition of an antibody directed against the suspected agent causes the virus to aggregate, thereby facilitating recognition. Enzyme-linked immunosorbent assay (ELISA) tests have been developed to detect the virus, viral antigen, and antibody to the virus. The other calicivirus-like agents are more difficult to detect.

Treatment, Prevention, and Control

There is no specific treatment for the diarrhea caused by caliciviruses or other small, round gastroenteritis viruses other than oral rehydration therapy. Outbreaks may be minimized by handling food carefully and by maintaining the purity of the water supply. Careful hand washing is also important. More resistant to environmental pressures than polioviruses or rotaviruses, Norwalk virus is resistant to heat (60° C), pH 3, detergent, and even the chlorine levels of drinking water. Contaminated surfaces can be cleaned with a 1:50 to 1:10 dilution of household bleach.

Bibliography

Balows A, Hausler WJ, Lennette EH: *Laboratory diagnosis of infectious diseases: principles and practice*, New York, 1988, Springer-Verlag.

Blacklow NR, Greenberg HB: Viral gastroenteritis, *N Engl J Med* 325:252–264, 1991.

Cann AJ: *Principles of molecular virology*, San Diego, 2005, Academic.

Carter J, Saunders V: *Virology: principles and applications*, Chichester, England, 2007, Wiley.

Christensen ML: Human viral gastroenteritis, *Clin Microbiol Rev* 2:51–89, 1989.

Cohen J, Powderly WG: *Infectious diseases*, ed 2, St Louis, 2004, Mosby.

Collier L, Oxford J: *Human virology*, ed 4, Oxford, England, 2011, Oxford University Press.

Flint SJ, Enquist LW, Racaniello VR, et al: *Principles of virology: molecular biology, pathogenesis and control of animal viruses*, ed 3, Washington, DC, 2009, American Society for Microbiology Press.

Graham RL, Donaldson EF, Baric RS: A decade after SARS: strategies for controlling emerging coronaviruses, *Nat Rev Microbiol* 11:836–848, 2013.

Gu J, Korteweg C: Pathology and pathogenesis of severe acute respiratory syndrome, *Am J Pathol* 170:1136–1147, 2007.

Hall AJ, Vinje J, Lopman B, et al: Updated norovirus outbreak management and disease prevention guidelines, *MMWR Morb Mortal Wkly Rep* 60:1–15, 2011.

Knipe DM, Howley PM: *Fields virology*, ed 6, Philadelphia, 2013, Lippincott Williams & Wilkins.

Meulen V, Siddell S, Wege H: *Biochemistry and biology of coronaviruses*, New York, 1981, Plenum.

Patel MM, Hall AJ, Vinje J, et al: Noroviruses: a comprehensive review, *J Clin Virol* 44:1–8, 2009.

Perlman S, Netland J: Coronaviruses post-SARS: update on replication and pathogenesis, *Nat Rev Microbiol* 7:439–450, 2009.

Richman DD, Whitley RJ, Hayden FG: *Clinical virology*, ed 3, Washington, DC, 2009, American Society for Microbiology Press.

Strauss JM, Strauss EG: *Viruses and human disease*, ed 2, San Diego, 2007, Academic.

Tan M, Huang P, Meller J, et al: Mutations within the P2 domain of norovirus capsid affect binding to human histo-blood group antigens: evidence for a binding pocket, *J Virol* 77:12562–12571, 2003.

Voyles BA: *The biology of viruses*, ed 2, Boston, 2002, McGraw-Hill.

Xi JN, Graham DY, Wang KN, et al: Norwalk virus genome cloning and characterization, *Science* 250:1580–1583, 1990.

Websites

Centers for Disease Control and Prevention: Norovirus. www.cdc.gov/ncidod/dvrd/revb/gastro/norovirus.htm. Accessed April 4, 2015.

Hall AJ, Wikswo ME, Pringle K, et al: Vital signs: foodborne norovirus outbreaks—United States, 2009-2012, *MMWR* 63:1–5, 2014. www.cdc.gov/mmwr/preview/mmwrhtml/mm63e0603a1.htm?s_cid=mm63e0603a1_e. Accessed April 4, 2015.

Kamps BS, Hoffmann C: SARS reference, 2003. www.sarsreference.com/sarsref/preface.htm. Accessed April 4, 2015.

National Institute of Allergy and Infectious Diseases: Severe acute respiratory syndrome. www.niaid.nih.gov/topics/sars/Pages/default.aspx. Accessed April 4, 2015.

Trivedi MN, Malhotra P: Severe acute respiratory syndrome (SARS), 2013. http://emedicine.medscape.com/article/237755-overview. Accessed April 4, 2015.

Vital Signs: Foodborne norovirus outbreaks—United States, 2009-2012. www.cdc.gov/mmwr/preview/mmwrhtml/mm63e0603a1.htm?s_cid=mm63e0603a1_e. Accessed April 4, 2015.

CHAPTER

48 PARAMYXOVIRUSES

A 10-year-old boy presented with cough, conjunctivitis, and coryza plus fever and lymphadenopathy, which progressed to a rash that spread from the hairline down his face and then his body. Within 10 days, the disease appeared to run its course, but a week after the start of the rash, an abrupt onset of headache, vomiting, and confusion progressed to coma, consistent with encephalitis.

1. How does measles replicate?
2. What are the characteristic signs of measles?
3. How is it transmitted?
4. Why was the boy susceptible to measles?
5. What other complications are associated with measles?

Answers to these questions are available on StudentConsult.com.

• SUMMARIES CLINICALLY SIGNIFICANT ORGANISMS

Paramyxoviruses

Trigger Words

Fusion, syncytia, aerosols, envelope
Measles: cough, conjunctivitis, coryza, photophobia, Koplik spots, rash, fever, SSPE, postmeasles encephalitis
Mumps: parotitis, orchitis, aseptic meningitis
Parainfluenza: croup, barking seal, pneumonia
Respiratory syncytial virus: infant, pneumonia

Biology, Virulence, and Disease

- Large size, enveloped, (–) RNA genome, fusion protein
- Encodes RNA-dependent RNA polymerase, replicates in cytoplasm
- Parainfluenza and mumps bind to sialic acid and encode neuraminidase activity (HN glycoprotein); measles and RSV glycoprotein bind to proteins
- Fusion protein promotes entry and cell-cell fusion (syncytia)
- Cell-mediated immune response essential for control but causes pathogenesis
- Measles: maculopapular rash, high fever with cough, conjunctivitis, coryza, Koplik spots (small gray lesions in mouth); giant cell pneumonia if T-cell deficient, postmeasles encephalitis, SSPE 5-7 years later due to measles variant
- Mumps: parotitis, orchitis, aseptic meningitis
- Parainfluenza: common cold, croup, bronchitis
- Respiratory syncytial virus (RSV): common cold, pneumonia, bronchiolitis, life threatening for premature infants

Epidemiology

- Transmitted by aerosols

Diagnosis

- Symptomatology, RT-PCR genome analysis of respiratory secretions

Treatment, Prevention, and Control

- Live attenuated vaccine for measles and mumps; RSV: passive immunization for premature infants at high risk; aerosolized ribavirin

The Paramyxoviridae include the genera *Morbillivirus, Paramyxovirus,* and *Pneumovirus* (Table 48-1). Human pathogens within the morbilliviruses include the measles virus; within the paramyxoviruses, the **parainfluenza** and **mumps** viruses; and within the pneumoviruses, the **respiratory syncytial virus (RSV)** and **metapneumovirus.** A new group of highly pathogenic paramyxoviruses, including two zoonosis-causing viruses, Nipah virus and Hendra virus, was identified in 1998 after an outbreak of severe encephalitis in Malaysia and Singapore. Their virions have

Table 48-1 Paramyxoviridae

Genus	Human Pathogen
Morbillivirus	Measles virus
Paramyxovirus	Parainfluenza viruses 1 to 4 Mumps virus
Pneumovirus	Respiratory syncytial virus Metapneumovirus

similar morphologies and protein components. Importantly, paramyxoviruses induce **cell-to-cell fusion** (syncytia formation and multinucleated giant cells).

These agents cause some well-known major diseases. Measles virus causes a potentially serious generalized infection characterized by a maculopapular rash **(rubeola).** Parainfluenza and metapneumoviruses cause upper and lower respiratory tract infections, primarily in children, including the common cold, pharyngitis, croup, bronchitis, bronchiolitis, and pneumonia. Mumps virus causes a systemic infection whose most prominent clinical manifestation is parotitis. RSV causes mild upper respiratory tract infections in children and adults but can cause life-threatening pneumonia in infants.

Measles and mumps viruses have only **one serotype,** and protection is provided by effective **live vaccines.** In the United States and other developed countries, successful vaccination programs using the live attenuated measles and mumps vaccines have made measles and mumps rare. In particular, these programs have led to the virtual elimination of the serious sequelae of measles in these countries.

• Structure and Replication

Paramyxoviruses are relatively large viruses with a **negative-sense, single-stranded ribonucleic acid (RNA)** (5 to 8×10^6 Da) genome in a helical nucleocapsid surrounded by a pleomorphic **envelope** of approximately 156 to 300 nm (Figure 48-1). They are similar in many respects to orthomyxoviruses but are larger and do not have the segmented genome of the influenza viruses (Box 48-1). Although there are similarities in paramyxovirus genomes, the order of the protein-coding regions differs for each genus. The paramyxovirus proteins are listed in Table 48-2.

The nucleocapsid consists of the negative-sense, single-stranded RNA associated with the nucleoprotein **(N),** polymerase phosphoprotein **(P),** and large **(L)** protein. The L protein is the RNA polymerase, the P protein facilitates RNA synthesis, and the N protein helps maintain genomic structure. The nucleocapsid associates with the matrix **(M)** protein lining the inside of the virion envelope. The envelope contains two glycoproteins, a fusion **(F)** protein, and a viral attachment protein (hemagglutinin-neuraminidase **[HN],** hemagglutinin **[H]**, or glycoprotein **[G]** protein) (see Box 48-1). To express membrane-fusing activity, the F protein must be activated by proteolytic cleavage, which produces F_1 and F_2 glycopeptides held together by a disulfide bond. Additional proteins (V, C, and W) result from alternative transcripts of the P gene and facilitate escape from innate host protections.

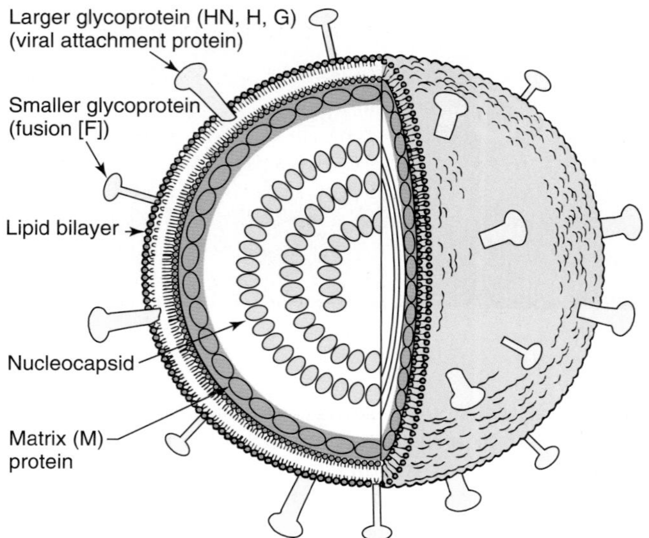

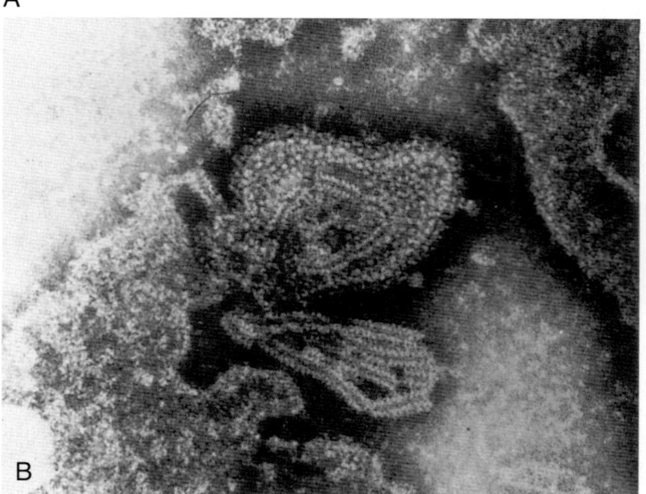

FIGURE 48-1 **A,** Model of paramyxovirus. The helical nucleocapsid—consisting of negative-sense, single-stranded RNA and the polymerase *(P),* nucleoprotein *(N),* and large protein *(L)*—associates with the matrix *(M)* protein at the envelope membrane surface. The nucleocapsid contains RNA transcriptase activity. The envelope contains the viral attachment glycoprotein (hemagglutinin-neuraminidase *[HN],* hemagglutinin *[H],* or G protein *[G],* depending upon the virus) and the fusion *(F)* protein. **B,** Electron micrograph of a disrupted paramyxovirus, showing the helical nucleocapsid. (**A,** Modified from Jawetz E, Melnick JL, Adelberg EA: *Review of medical microbiology,* ed 17, Norwalk, Conn, 1987, Appleton & Lange. **B,** Courtesy Centers for Disease Control and Prevention, Atlanta.)

Replication of the paramyxoviruses is initiated by the binding of the HN, H, or G glycoprotein on the virion envelope to their receptors. The HN of parainfluenza viruses bind to sialic acid on cell surface glycolipids and glycoproteins. Like influenza, they use the neuraminidase activity to cleave sialic acid on viral and cellular glycoproteins, prevent binding to itself, and facilitate exit from the cell. The other paramyxoviruses bind to protein receptors and do not need a neuraminidase activity. The F protein promotes fusion of the

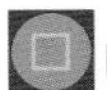

Box 48-1 Unique Features of the Paramyxoviridae

Large virion consists of a negative-sense RNA genome in a helical nucleocapsid surrounded by an envelope.

The three genera can be distinguished by the activities of the viral attachment protein: HN of parainfluenza virus and mumps virus binds to sialic acid and red blood cells (hemagglutinin) and neuraminidase activity, H of measles virus binds protein receptors and is also a hemagglutinin, but G of RSV binds to cells but is not a hemagglutinin.

Virus replicates in the cytoplasm.

Virions penetrate the cell by fusion with the plasma membrane and exit by budding from the plasma membrane without killing the cell.

Viruses induce cell-to-cell fusion, causing multinucleated giant cells **(syncytia).**

Cell-mediated immunity causes many of the symptoms but is essential for control of the infection.

Paramyxoviridae are transmitted in **respiratory droplets** and initiate infection in the respiratory tract.

Table 48-2 Major Viral-Encoded Proteins of Paramyxoviruses

Gene and Proteins*†	Virion Location	Protein Function
N: nucleoprotein	Major internal protein	Protection of viral RNA
P: phosphoprotein and C and V proteins	Association with nucleoprotein	Part of transcription complex; C and V are antagonists of innate responses
M: matrix	Inside virion envelope	Assembly of virions
F: fusion protein	Transmembranous envelope glycoprotein	Protein promotes fusion of cells, hemolysis, and viral entry
G: glycoprotein (HN, H, G)	Transmembranous envelope glycoprotein	Viral attachment protein
L: polymerase (large)	Association with nucleoprotein	Polymerase

*In order on the genome.

†Pneumoviruses also encode an SH and M2 protein.

envelope with the plasma membrane. Paramyxoviruses are also able to induce cell-to-cell fusion, thereby creating multinucleated giant cells (syncytia).

Replication of the genome occurs in a manner similar to that of other negative-strand RNA viruses (i.e., rhabdoviruses). The RNA polymerase is carried into the cell as part of the nucleocapsid. Transcription, protein synthesis, and replication of the genome all occur in the host cell's cytoplasm. The genome is transcribed into individual messenger RNAs (mRNAs) and a full-length positive-sense RNA template. New genomes associate with the L, N, and N proteins to form helical nucleocapsids that associate with the M proteins on viral glycoprotein-modified plasma membranes. The glycoproteins are synthesized and processed like cellular glycoproteins. Mature virions then bud from the host cell plasma membrane and exit without killing the cell. Replication of the paramyxoviruses is represented by the RSV infectious cycle shown in Figure 48-2.

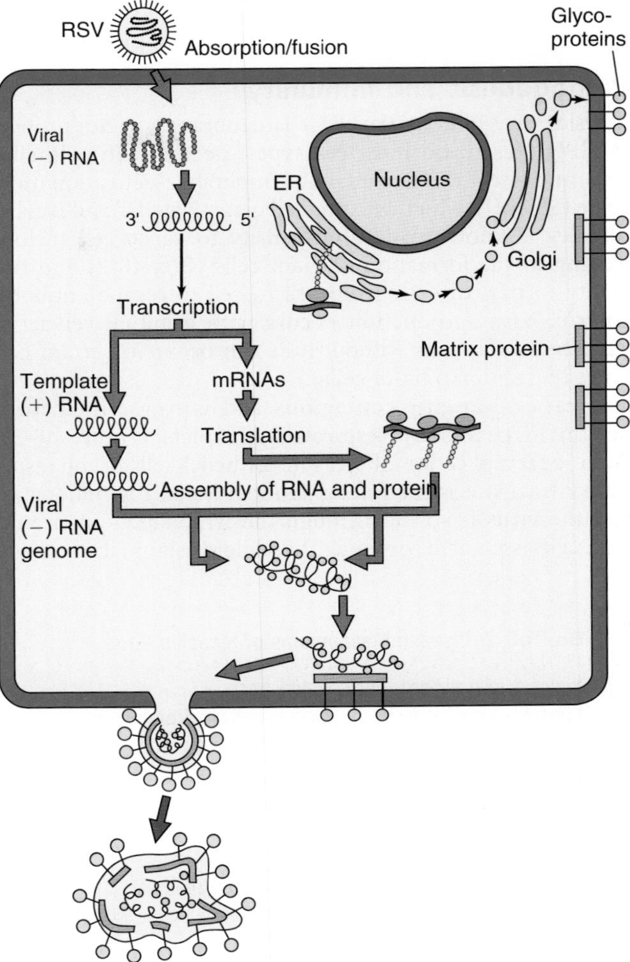

FIGURE 48-2 Replication of paramyxoviruses. The virus binds to glycolipids or proteins and fuses with the cell surface. Individual messenger RNAs *(mRNAs)* for each protein and a full-length template are transcribed from the genome. Replication occurs in the cytoplasm. Proteins associate with the new genome, and the nucleocapsid associates with matrix and glycoprotein-modified plasma membranes. The virus leaves the cell by budding. *(−)*, Negative sense; *(+)*, positive sense; *ER*, endoplasmic reticulum; *RSV*, respiratory syncytial virus. (Modified from Balows A et al: *Laboratory diagnosis of infectious diseases: principles and practice*, New York, 1988, Springer-Verlag.)

• Measles Virus

Measles, also known as rubeola, is one of the five classic childhood exanthems, along with rubella, roseola, fifth disease, and chickenpox. Historically, measles was one of the most common and unpleasant viral infections, with serious potential sequelae. Before 1960, more than 90% of the population younger than 20 years had experienced the rash, high fever, cough, conjunctivitis, and coryza of measles. Measles is still one of the most prominent causes of disease (>10 million cases per year) and death (120,000 deaths in 2012) worldwide in unvaccinated populations. The development of effective vaccine programs has made measles a rare disease in developed countries, but children remain unvaccinated or do not receive their boosters and outbreaks of measles occur.

Pathogenesis and Immunity

Measles virus binds to the CD46 (membrane cofactor protein [MCP]) present on most cell types, nectin 4 on epithelial cells, and also CD150 (signaling lymphocyte-activation molecule [SLAM]), which is expressed on activated T and B cells. Measles is known for its propensity to cause cell fusion, leading to the formation of giant cells (Box 48-2) and the ability to pass directly from cell to cell to escape antibody control. Virus production occurs with eventual cell lysis. Persistent infections without lysis can occur in certain cell types (e.g., human brain cells).

Measles is **highly contagious** and is transmitted from person to person by **respiratory droplets** (Figure 48-3). After local replication of virus in epithelial cells of the respiratory tract, the virus infects monocytes and lymphocytes, and the virus is spread through the lymphatic system and by a cell-associated viremia. The wide dissemination of the virus causes infection of the conjunctiva, respiratory tract, urinary tract, small blood vessels, lymphatic system, and central nervous system. The characteristic **maculopapular** measles rash is caused by immune T cells targeted to measles-infected endothelial cells lining small blood vessels. Recovery follows the rash in most patients, who then have **lifelong immunity** to the virus. Death due to pneumonia, diarrhea, or encephalitis can occur. The time course of measles infection is shown in Figure 48-4.

Measles can cause encephalitis in three ways: (1) direct infection of neurons, (2) a postinfectious encephalitis that is believed to be immune mediated, and (3) subacute sclerosing panencephalitis (SSPE) caused by a defective variant of measles generated during the acute disease. The SSPE virus replicates poorly, stays cell associated, and causes symptoms and cytopathologic effect in neurons many years after acute disease.

Measles and other paramyxoviruses are excellent inducers of interferon (IFN)-α and IFN-β but also have mechanisms to antagonize their action. Cell-mediated immunity is responsible for most of the symptoms and is essential for control of measles infection. T-cell–deficient children who are infected with measles have an atypical presentation consisting of **giant cell pneumonia without a rash.** Measles is more severe for people deficient in vitamin A. Vitamin A is important for optimal effector T-cell function and resolution of measles infection. Antibody, including maternal antibody and passive immunization, can block the viremic but not cell-cell spread of the virus to prevent or lessen disease. Protection from reinfection is lifelong.

Measles infection is immunosuppressive. The virus depresses the immune response by (1) directly infecting

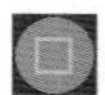 **Box 48-2 Disease Mechanisms of Measles Virus**

Virus infects epithelial cells of respiratory tract.
Virus spreads systemically in lymphocytes and by **viremia.**
Virus replicates in cells of conjunctivae, respiratory tract, urinary tract, lymphatic system, blood vessels, and central nervous system (CNS).
Rash is caused by T-cell response to virus-infected epithelial cells lining capillaries.
Virus causes immunosuppression.
Cell-mediated immunity is essential to control infection.
Sequelae in the CNS may result from immunopathogenesis (postinfectious measles encephalitis) or development of defective mutants (subacute sclerosing panencephalitis).

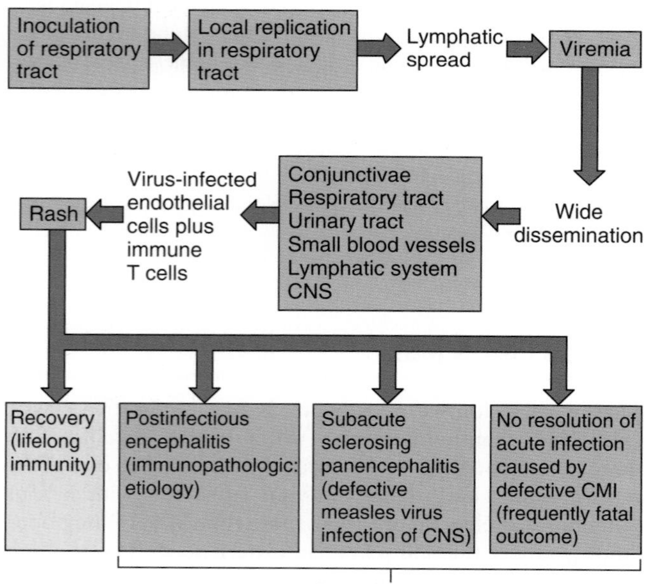

FIGURE 48-3 Mechanisms of spread of the measles virus within the body and the pathogenesis of measles. *CMI,* Cell-mediated immunity; *CNS,* central nervous system.

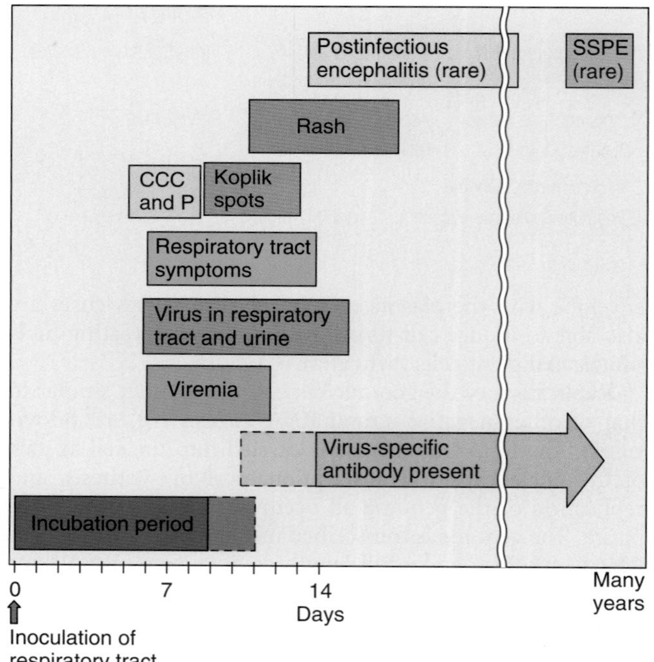

FIGURE 48-4 Time course of measles virus infection. Characteristic prodrome symptoms are cough, conjunctivitis, coryza, and photophobia *(CCC and P),* followed by the appearance of Koplik spots and rash. *SSPE,* Subacute sclerosing panencephalitis.

monocytes and T and B cells and (2) depressing interleukin (IL)-12 production and TH1-type T-cell helper responses. Depression of cell-mediated immune and delayed-type hypersensitivity (DTH) responses increases risk to concurrent opportunistic and other infections. This immunosuppression lasts for weeks or months after the disease.

Epidemiology

The development of effective vaccine programs has made measles a rare disease in the United States. In areas without a vaccine program, epidemics tend to occur in 1- to 3-year cycles, when a sufficient number of susceptible people have accumulated. Many of these cases occur in preschool-aged children who have not been vaccinated and live in large urban areas. The incidence of infection peaks in the winter and spring. Measles is still common in people living in developing countries, especially in individuals who refuse immunization or have not received a booster in their teenage years. Immunocompromised, malnourished, and vitamin A–deficient people with measles may not be able to resolve the infection, resulting in death. It is the most significant cause of death in children aged 1 to 5 years in several countries.

Measles, which can be spread in respiratory secretions before and after the onset of characteristic symptoms, is one of the most contagious infections known (Box 48-3). In a household, approximately 90% of exposed susceptible people become infected, and 95% of these people develop clinical disease.

The measles virus has only one serotype and infects only humans, and infection usually manifests with symptoms. These properties facilitated development of an effective vaccine program. Once vaccination was introduced, the yearly incidence of measles dropped dramatically in the United States, from 300 to 1.3 per 100,000 (U.S. statistics for 1981-1988). This change represented a 99.5% reduction in the incidence of infection from the prevaccination years of 1955 to 1962. Incidence of measles must be reported to state and federal health departments.

Despite the effectiveness of vaccination programs, poor compliance and the prevaccinated population (children < 2 years) continue to provide susceptible individuals. The virus may surface from within the community or can be imported by immigration from areas of the world lacking an effective vaccine program. Once again, outbreaks of measles are occurring more often in the United States, France, and England. In 2011, most of the cases in the United States were imported from other countries, and most of the patients were unvaccinated. An outbreak of measles in a day-care center (10 infants too young to have been vaccinated and two adults) was traced to an infant from the Philippines.

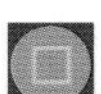

Box 48-3 Epidemiology of Measles

Disease/Viral Factors

Virus has large enveloped virion that is easily inactivated by dryness and acid.

Contagion period precedes symptoms.

Host range is limited to humans.

Only one serotype exists.

Immunity is lifelong.

Transmission

Inhalation of large-droplet aerosols

Who Is at Risk?

Unvaccinated people

Malnourished people, who have more serious outcomes

Immunocompromised people, who have more serious outcomes

Geography/Season

Virus found worldwide

Virus endemic from autumn to spring, possibly because of crowding indoors

Modes of Control

Live attenuated vaccine (Schwartz or Moraten variants of Edmonston B strain) can be administered.

Immune serum globulin can be administered after exposure.

Clinical Syndromes

Measles is a serious febrile illness (Table 48-3). The incubation period lasts 7 to 13 days, and the prodrome starts with **high fever** and **"CCC and P"—cough, coryza, conjunctivitis**, and **photophobia.** The disease is most infectious during this time.

After 2 days of prodromal illness, the typical mucous membrane lesions known as **Koplik spots** (Figure 48-5) appear. They are seen most commonly on the buccal mucosa across from the molars, but they may appear on other mucous membranes as well, including the conjunctivae and the vagina. The vesicular lesions, which last 24 to 48 hours, are usually small (1 to 2 mm) and are best described as grains of salt surrounded by a red halo. Their appearance with the other disease signs establishes with certainty the diagnosis of measles.

Within 12 to 24 hours of the appearance of Koplik spots, the **exanthem** of measles starts below the ears and spreads over the body. The **rash is maculopapular** and is usually very extensive, and often the lesions become confluent. The rash, which takes 1 or 2 days to cover the body, fades in the same order in which it appeared. The fever is highest and the patient is sickest on the day the rash appears (Figure 48-6).

Pneumonia, which can also be a serious complication, accounts for 60% of the deaths caused by measles. Similar to the incidence of the other complications associated with

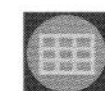

Table 48-3 Clinical Consequences of Measles Virus Infection

Disorder	Symptoms
Measles	Characteristic maculopapular rash, cough, conjunctivitis, coryza, photophobia, Koplik spots *Complications*: otitis media, croup, pneumonia, blindness, encephalitis
Atypical measles	More intense rash (most prominent in distal areas); possible vesicles, petechiae, purpura, or urticaria
Postmeasles encephalitis	Acute onset of headache, confusion, vomiting, possible coma after rash dissipates
Subacute sclerosing panencephalitis	Central nervous system manifestations (e.g., personality, behavior, and memory changes; myoclonic jerks; spasticity; blindness)

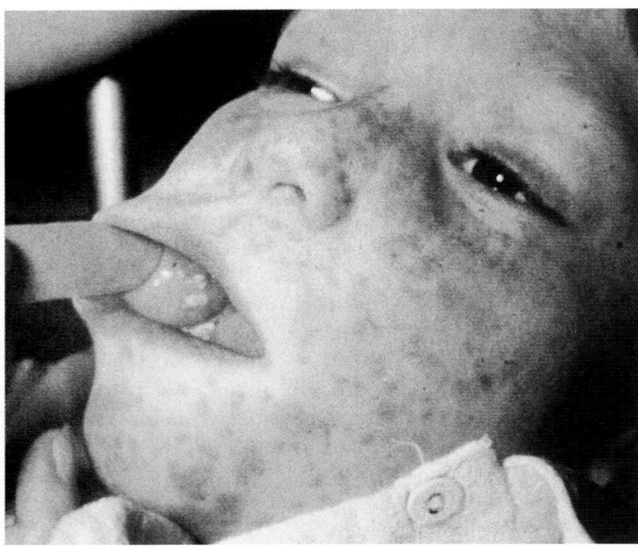

FIGURE 48-5 Koplik spots in the mouth and exanthem. Koplik spots usually precede the measles rash and may be seen for the first day or two after the rash appears. (Courtesy Dr. JI Pugh, St Albans City Hospital, West Hertfordshire, England; from Emond RTD, Rowland HAK: *A color atlas of infectious diseases,* ed 3, London, 1995, Mosby.)

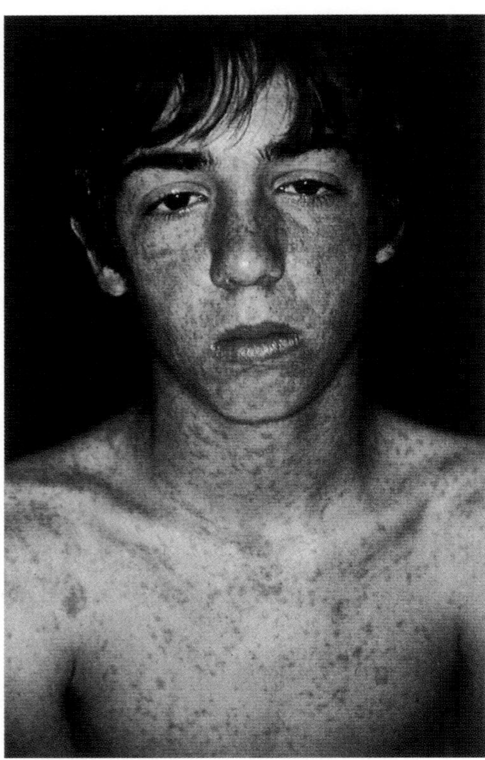

FIGURE 48-6 Measles rash. (From Habif TP: *Clinical dermatology: color guide to diagnosis and therapy,* St Louis, 1985, Mosby.)

measles, the mortality associated with pneumonia is higher in the malnourished and for the extremes of age. **Bacterial superinfection** is common in patients with pneumonia caused by the measles virus.

One of the most feared complications of measles is **encephalitis,** which occurs in as few as 0.5% of those infected but carries a fatality rate of 15%. Encephalitis may rarely occur during acute disease but usually begins 7 to 10 days after the onset of illness. This **postinfectious encephalitis** is caused by immunopathologic reactions, is associated with demyelination of neurons, and occurs more often in older children and adults.

Atypical measles occurred in people who received the older inactivated measles vaccine and were subsequently exposed to the wild-type measles virus. It may also rarely occur in those vaccinated with the attenuated virus vaccine. Prior sensitization with insufficient protection can enhance the immunopathologic response to the challenge by wild-type measles virus. The illness begins abruptly and is a more intense presentation of measles.

Subacute sclerosing panencephalitis (SSPE) is an extremely serious, very late neurologic sequela of measles that afflicts approximately seven of every one million patients. The incidence of SSPE has decreased markedly because of measles vaccination programs.

This disease occurs when a defective measles virus persists in the brain, affects multiple loci in the brain (panencephalitis), and acts as a slow virus. The virus can replicate and spread directly from cell to cell but is not released. SSPE is most prevalent in children who were initially infected when younger than 2 years and occurs approximately 7 years after clinical measles. The patient demonstrates changes in personality, behavior, cognition, and memory, followed by myoclonic jerks, blindness, and spasticity, and progresses to coma and death. Unusually high levels of measles antibodies are found in the blood and cerebrospinal fluid of patients with SSPE. Measles antigen and genome can be detected in neurons as well as Cowdry type A inclusion bodies (these inclusion bodies are usually a marker for herpes simplex virus but are also seen in SSPE).

The immunocompromised and malnourished child is at highest risk for severe outcome of measles (Clinical Case 48-1). **Giant cell pneumonia without rash** occurs in children lacking T-cell immunity. Whereas the death rate of measles in the United States is only 0.1%, complications, severe bacterial superinfection, and pneumonia in malnourished children result in up to 60% mortality.

Laboratory Diagnosis

The clinical manifestations of measles are usually so characteristic that it is rarely necessary to perform laboratory tests to establish the diagnosis. The measles virus should not be isolated. Respiratory tract secretions, urine, blood, and brain tissue are the recommended specimens. It is best to collect respiratory and blood specimens during the prodromal stage and until 1 to 2 days after the appearance of the rash. Measles antigen can be detected with immunofluorescence in pharyngeal cells or urinary sediment; the measles genome can be identified by reverse transcriptase polymerase chain reaction (RT-PCR) in respiratory tract secretions, urine, blood, and brain tissue. Characteristic cytopathologic effects, including multinucleated giant cells with cytoplasmic inclusion bodies, can be seen in Giemsa-stained cells taken from the upper respiratory tract and urinary sediment.

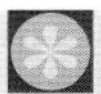

Clinical Case 48-1 Measles in the Immunocompromised Child

The lack of cell-mediated immune responses allows measles infection of immunocompromised individuals to progress to serious outcomes. In a case reported by Pullan and associates (*Br Med J* 1:1562–1565, 1976), within 3 days of exposure to measles, a child on chemotherapy for acute lymphoblastic leukemia (ALL) received pooled immunoglobulin. Despite the IgG therapy, 23 days after exposure, she developed an extensive measles rash that became hemorrhagic. She had a fever of 39.5° C and bronchopneumonia. Measles was grown from nasopharyngeal secretions, and immunohistochemistry identified giant cells (syncytia) containing measles antigen within the secretions. Her chemotherapy was stopped, and she received several massive doses of immunoglobulin. She started to improve 1 month after the onset of the rash.

In another case, during the 2.5 years that a boy was under treatment for ALL, he suffered severe herpes simplex virus infections around the mouth and herpes zoster on his trunk. During the third year on therapy, he was exposed to measles from his sister and received pooled IgG. After 19 days, he developed mild respiratory symptoms but no rash. After 29 days, he refused to go to school and misbehaved; behavioral changes progressed. After 9 weeks, he developed focal motor seizures, increased drowsiness, slurring of speech, and confusion, which progressed to coma and death within 8 days of the onset of seizures. Serology indicated a lack of measles antibody. Autopsy indicated the presence of cytomegalovirus but not measles in the lungs. The brain showed extensive degeneration, but no virus was isolated from the samples. Brain sections indicated large intranuclear and cytoplasmic inclusion bodies with tubular structures that resembled measles nucleocapsids in the cytoplasm. Immunofluorescence with antibody from individuals with **subacute sclerosing panencephalitis (SSPE)** or antimeasles antibody indicated the presence of measles antigen. These cases illustrate the excessive pathology measles can cause in the absence of a competent T-cell response. The lack of immune control allowed progression of the virus to the brain, where it or a variant (SSPE) caused pathology leading to encephalitis.

Antibody, especially immunoglobulin (Ig)M, can be detected when the rash is present.

Treatment, Prevention, and Control

As stated previously, a live attenuated measles vaccine, in use in the United States since 1963, has been responsible for significant reduction in the incidence of measles. The Schwartz or Moraten attenuated strains of the original Edmonston B vaccine are currently being used. Live attenuated vaccine is given to all children after 12 months of age, in combination with mumps and rubella **(measles-mumps-rubella [MMR] vaccine)** and the varicella vaccines (Box 48-4). Although early childhood immunization is successful in more than 95% of vaccinees, revaccination before grade school or junior high school is required in many states. Owing to the very contagious nature of measles, vaccine-induced herd immunity is very important to prevent spread of the virus in the population. A decrease to 93% immunized within the population creates a risk of a measles outbreak. Complacency or misinformation regarding immunization risks causes many parents to refrain from vaccinating their children, putting them at risk of infection, disease, and becoming sources of contagion to others.

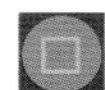

Box 48-4 Measles-Mumps-Rubella Vaccine

Composition: live attenuated viruses
Measles: Schwartz or Moraten substrains of Edmonston B strain
Mumps: Jeryl Lynn strain
Rubella: RA/27-3 strain
Vaccination schedule: after 12 months of age and at age 4 to 6 years or before junior high school (12 years of age)
Efficiency: 95% lifelong immunization with a single dose

Data from Update on adult immunization. Recommendations of the Immunization Practices Advisory Committee (ACIP), *MMWR Recomm Rep* 40(RR-12):1–94, 1991.

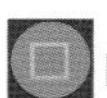

Box 48-5 Disease Mechanisms of Parainfluenza Viruses

There are four serotypes of viruses.
Infection is **limited to the respiratory tract;** upper respiratory tract disease is most common, but significant disease can occur with lower respiratory tract infection.
Parainfluenza viruses do *not* cause viremia or become systemic.
Diseases include **coldlike** symptoms, **bronchitis** (inflammation of bronchial tubes), and **croup** (laryngotracheobronchitis).
Infection induces protective immunity of short duration.

Because measles is strictly a human virus with only one serotype, it is a good candidate for eradication, but this is prevented by difficulties in distributing the vaccine to regions that lack proper refrigeration facilities (e.g., Africa) and distribution networks.

Hospitals in areas experiencing endemic measles may wish to vaccinate or check the immune status of their employees to decrease the risk of nosocomial transmission. Pregnant women, immunocompromised individuals, and people with allergies to gelatin or neomycin (components of the vaccine) should not receive the MMR vaccine. Exposed susceptible people who are immunocompromised should be given immune globulin to lessen the risk and severity of clinical illness. This product is most effective if given within 6 days of exposure. High-dose vitamin A treatment reduces the risk of measles mortality and is recommended by the World Health Organization. No specific antiviral treatment is available for measles.

• Parainfluenza Viruses

Parainfluenza viruses, which were discovered in the late 1950s, are respiratory viruses that usually cause **mild coldlike symptoms** but can also cause **serious respiratory tract disease.** Four serologic types within the parainfluenza genus are human pathogens. Types 1, 2, and 3 are second only to RSV as important causes of severe lower respiratory tract infection in infants and young children. They are especially associated with **laryngotracheobronchitis (croup).** Type 4 causes only mild upper respiratory tract infection in children and adults.

Pathogenesis and Immunity

Parainfluenza viruses infect epithelial cells of the upper respiratory tract (Box 48-5). The virus replicates more rapidly than measles and mumps viruses and can cause giant cell formation and cell lysis. Unlike measles and mumps viruses, the parainfluenza viruses rarely cause viremia. The viruses generally stay in the upper respiratory tract, causing only coldlike symptoms. In approximately 25% of cases, the virus spreads to the lower respiratory tract, and in 2% to 3%, disease may take the severe form of laryngotracheobronchitis.

The cell-mediated immune response both causes cell damage and confers protection. IgA responses are protective but short lived. Parainfluenza viruses manipulate cell-mediated immunity to limit development of memory. Multiple serotypes and the short duration of immunity after natural infection make reinfection common, but the reinfection disease is milder, suggesting at least partial immunity.

Epidemiology

Parainfluenza viruses are ubiquitous, and infection is common (Box 48-6). The virus is transmitted by person-to-person contact and respiratory droplets. Primary infections usually occur in infants and children younger than 5 years. Reinfections occur throughout life, indicating short-lived immunity. Infections with parainfluenza viruses 1 and 2, the major causes of croup, tend to occur in the autumn, whereas parainfluenza virus 3 infections occur throughout the year. All these viruses spread readily within hospitals and can cause outbreaks in nurseries and pediatric wards.

Clinical Syndromes

Parainfluenza viruses 1, 2, and 3 may cause respiratory tract syndromes ranging from a **mild coldlike upper respiratory tract infection** (coryza, pharyngitis, mild bronchitis, wheezing, and fever) to **bronchiolitis** and **pneumonia.** Older children and adults generally experience milder infections than those seen in young children, although pneumonia may occur in the elderly.

A parainfluenza virus infection in infants may be more severe than infections in adults, causing bronchiolitis, pneumonia, and most notably croup (laryngotracheobronchitis).

Box 48-6 Epidemiology of Parainfluenza Virus Infections

Disease/Viral Factors

Virus has a large enveloped virion that is easily inactivated by dryness and acid.

Contagion period precedes symptoms and may occur in absence of symptoms.

Host range is limited to humans.

Reinfection can occur later in life.

Transmission

Inhalation of large-droplet aerosols

Who Is at Risk?

Children: at risk for mild disease or croup

Adults: at risk for reinfection with milder symptoms

Geography/Season

Virus is ubiquitous and worldwide.

Incidence is seasonal.

Modes of Control

There are no modes of control.

Croup results in subglottal swelling that may close the airway. Hoarseness, a "seal bark" cough, tachypnea, tachycardia, and suprasternal retraction develop in infected patients after a 2- to 6-day incubation period. Most children recover within 48 hours. The principal differential diagnosis is epiglottitis caused by *Haemophilus influenzae.*

Laboratory Diagnosis

Parainfluenza virus is isolated from nasal washings and respiratory secretions and grows well in primary monkey kidney cells. Similar to other paramyxoviruses, the virions are labile during transit to the laboratory. The presence of virus-infected cells in aspirates or in cell culture is indicated by the finding of syncytia and is identified with immunofluorescence. Similar to the hemagglutinin of the influenza viruses, the hemagglutinin of the parainfluenza viruses promotes hemadsorption and hemagglutination. The serotype of the virus can be determined through the use of specific antibody to block hemadsorption or hemagglutination (hemagglutination inhibition). Rapid RT-PCR techniques are the method of choice to detect and identify parainfluenza viruses from respiratory secretions.

Treatment, Prevention, and Control

Treatment of croup consists of the administration of nebulized cold or hot steam and careful monitoring of the upper airway. On rare occasions, intubation may become necessary. No specific antiviral agents are available.

Vaccination with killed vaccines is ineffective, possibly because they fail to induce local secretory antibody and appropriate cellular immunity. No live attenuated vaccine is available.

• Mumps Virus

Mumps virus is the cause of acute, benign viral **parotitis** (painful swelling of the salivary glands). Mumps is rarely seen in countries that promote use of the live vaccine, which is administered with the measles and rubella live vaccines, but outbreaks have occurred recently.

Mumps virus was isolated in embryonated eggs in 1945 and in cell culture in 1955. The virus is most closely related to parainfluenza virus 2, but there is no cross-immunity with the parainfluenza viruses.

Pathogenesis and Immunity

The mumps virus, of which only one serotype is known, causes a lytic infection of cells (Box 48-7). The virus initiates

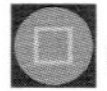

Box 48-7 Disease Mechanisms of Mumps Virus

Virus infects epithelial cells of respiratory tract.

Virus spreads systemically by viremia.

Infection of parotid gland, testes, and central nervous system occurs.

Principal symptom is swelling of parotid and other glands caused by inflammation.

Cell-mediated immunity is essential for control of infection and responsible for causing some of the symptoms. Antibody is not sufficient because of virus's ability to spread cell to cell.

infection in the epithelial cells of the upper respiratory tract and infects the parotid gland, either by way of the Stensen duct or by means of a viremia. The virus is spread by the viremia throughout the body to the testes, ovary, pancreas, thyroid, and other organs. Infection of the central nervous system, especially the meninges, occurs in as many as 50% of those infected (Figure 48-7). Inflammatory responses cause swelling of glands and are mainly responsible for the symptoms. The time course of human infection is shown in Figure 48-8. Immunity is lifelong.

Epidemiology

Mumps, like measles, is a very communicable disease with only one serotype, and it infects only humans (Box 48-8). In the absence of vaccination programs, infection occurs in 90% of people by the age of 15 years. The virus spreads by direct person-to-person contact and respiratory droplets. The virus is released in respiratory secretions from patients who are asymptomatic and during the 7-day period before clinical illness, so it is virtually impossible to control the spread of the virus. Living or working in close quarters promotes the spread of the virus, and the incidence of the infection is greatest in the winter and spring.

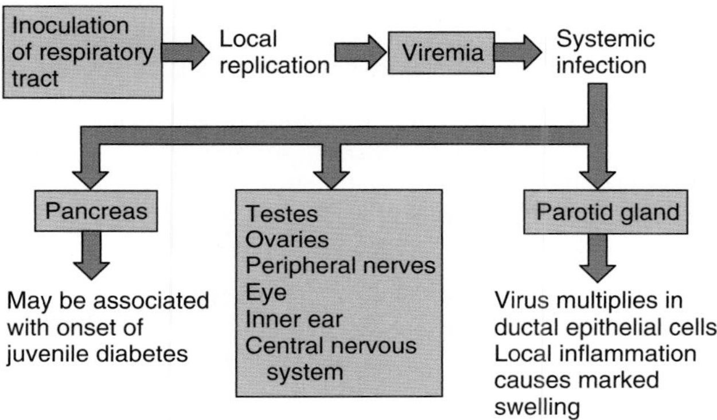

FIGURE 48-7 Mechanism of spread of mumps virus within the body.

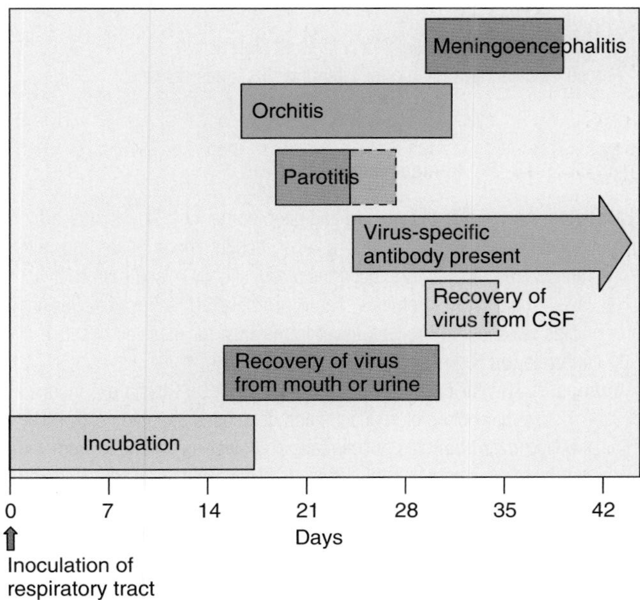

FIGURE 48-8 Time course of mumps virus infection. *CSF,* Cerebrospinal fluid.

Clinical Syndromes

Mumps infections are often asymptomatic. Clinical illness usually manifests as a parotitis that is almost always bilateral and accompanied by fever. Onset is sudden. Oral examination reveals redness and swelling of the ostium of the Stensen (parotid) duct. The swelling of other glands (epididymo-orchitis, oophoritis, mastitis, pancreatitis, and thyroiditis) and meningoencephalitis may occur a few days after the onset of the viral infection but can occur in the absence of parotitis. The swelling that results from mumps orchitis may cause sterility. Mumps virus involves the central nervous system in approximately 50% of patients; 10% of those affected may exhibit mild meningitis, with 5 per 1000 cases of encephalitis.

Laboratory Diagnosis

Virus can be recovered from saliva, urine, the pharynx, secretions from the Stensen duct, and cerebrospinal fluid. Virus is present in saliva for approximately 5 days after the onset of symptoms and in urine for as long as 2 weeks. Mumps virus grows well in monkey kidney cells, causing the formation of multinucleated giant cells. Hemadsorption of guinea pig erythrocytes also occurs on virus-infected cells because of the viral hemagglutinin.

A clinical diagnosis can be confirmed by RT-PCR detection of viral genomes or by ELISA, immunofluorescence, and hemagglutination inhibition tests to detect mumps virus, antigen, or antibody.

Treatment, Prevention, and Control

Vaccines provide the only effective means for preventing the spread of mumps infection. Since the introduction of the live

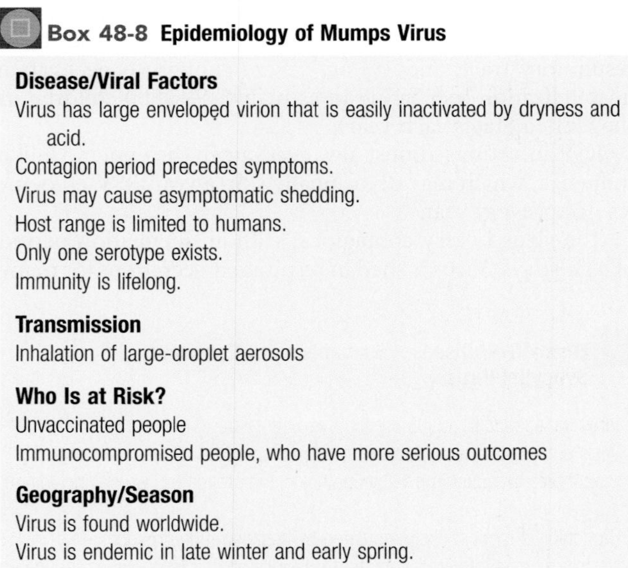

Box 48-8 Epidemiology of Mumps Virus

Disease/Viral Factors

Virus has large enveloped virion that is easily inactivated by dryness and acid.
Contagion period precedes symptoms.
Virus may cause asymptomatic shedding.
Host range is limited to humans.
Only one serotype exists.
Immunity is lifelong.

Transmission

Inhalation of large-droplet aerosols

Who Is at Risk?

Unvaccinated people
Immunocompromised people, who have more serious outcomes

Geography/Season

Virus is found worldwide.
Virus is endemic in late winter and early spring.

Modes of Control

Live attenuated vaccine (Jeryl Lynn strain) is part of measles-mumps-rubella vaccine.

attenuated vaccine (Jeryl Lynn vaccine) in the United States in 1967 and its administration as part of the MMR vaccine, the yearly incidence of the infection has declined from 76 to less than 1 per 100,000 until recently. As with measles, outbreaks due to increasing numbers of individuals who are unvaccinated or did not receive a booster immunization have occurred. In 2014, there was an outbreak in Columbus, Ohio, in schools and universities, with more than 230 reported cases. Antiviral agents are not available.

• Respiratory Syncytial Virus

RSV, first isolated from a chimpanzee in 1956, is a member of the *Pneumovirus* genus. The glycoprotein of RSV does not bind to sialic acid or red blood cells, and therefore the virus does not need or have a neuraminidase. It is the most common cause of **fatal acute respiratory tract infection** in infants and young children. It infects virtually everyone by 2 years of age, and reinfections occur throughout life, even among elderly persons.

Pathogenesis and Immunity

RSV produces an infection that is localized to the respiratory tract (Box 48-9). As the name suggests, RSV induces syncytia. The pathologic effect of RSV is mainly caused by direct viral invasion of the respiratory epithelium, which is followed by immunologically mediated cell injury. Necrosis of the bronchi and bronchioles leads to the formation of "plugs" of mucus, fibrin, and necrotic material within smaller airways. The narrow airways of young infants are readily obstructed by such plugs. Natural immunity does not prevent reinfection, and vaccination with killed vaccine appears to enhance the severity of subsequent disease.

Epidemiology

RSV is very prevalent in young children; almost all children have been infected by 2 years of age (Box 48-10), with global annual infection rates of 64 million and mortality of 160,000. As many as 25% to 40% of these cases involve the lower respiratory tract, and 1% are severe enough to necessitate hospitalization (occurring in as many as 95,000 children in the United States each year).

RSV infections almost always occur in the winter. Unlike influenza, which may occasionally skip a year, RSV epidemics occur every year.

The virus is very contagious, with an incubation period of 4 to 5 days. Virus is shed in respiratory secretions for many days after infection, especially by infants. The virus is transmitted in aerosols but also on hands and by fomites.

Introduction of the virus into a nursery, especially into an intensive care nursery, can be devastating. Virtually every infant becomes infected, and the infection is associated with considerable morbidity and occasionally death. Infants born prematurely and children younger than 2 years with complicated congenital heart disease or chronic lung disease are at high risk to serious RSV disease. Outbreaks of serious disease may also occur among the elderly population (e.g., in nursing homes).

Clinical Syndromes (Box 48-11)

RSV can cause any respiratory tract illness, from a **common cold** to **pneumonia** (Table 48-4). Upper respiratory tract infection with prominent rhinorrhea (runny nose) is most

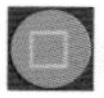

Box 48-9 Disease Mechanisms of Respiratory Syncytial Virus

Virus causes localized infection of respiratory tract.
Virus does not cause viremia or systemic spread.
Pneumonia results from cytopathologic spread of virus (including syncytia).
Bronchiolitis is most likely mediated by host's immune response.
Narrow airways of young infants are readily obstructed by virus-induced pathologic effects.
Maternal antibody is insufficient to protect infant from infection.
Natural infection does not prevent reinfection.

Box 48-10 Epidemiology of Respiratory Syncytial Virus

Disease/Viral Factors
Virus has a large enveloped virion that is easily inactivated by dryness and acid.
Contagion period precedes symptoms and may occur in the absence of symptoms.
Host range is limited to humans.

Transmission
Inhalation of large-droplet aerosols

Who Is at Risk?
Infants: lower respiratory tract infection (bronchiolitis and pneumonia)
Premature neonates: serious disease
Children: spectrum of disease from mild to pneumonia
Adults: reinfection with milder symptoms
Immunocompromised, chronic heart and lung problems: serious disease

Geography/Season
Virus is ubiquitous and found worldwide.
Incidence is seasonal.

Modes of Control
Immune globulin is available for infants at high risk.
Aerosol ribavirin is available for infants with serious disease.

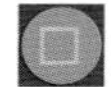

Box 48-11 Clinical Summaries

Measles: An 18-year-old woman had been home for 10 days after a trip to Haiti when she developed a fever, cough, runny nose, and mild redness of her eyes. She now has a red, slightly raised rash over her face, trunk, and extremities. There are several 1-mm white lesions inside her mouth. She was never immunized for measles because of an irrelevant "egg allergy."

Mumps: A 30-year-old man returning from a trip to Russia experienced a 1- to 2-day period of headache and decreased appetite, followed by swelling over both sides of his jaw. The swelling extended from the bottom of the jaw to in front of the ear. Five days after the jaw swelling appeared, the patient began complaining of nausea and lower abdominal and testicular pain.

Croup: An irritable 2-year-old toddler with little appetite has a sore throat, fever, and hoarse voice and coughs with the sound of a barking seal. A high-pitched noise (stridor) is heard on inhalation. Flaring of the nostrils indicates difficulty breathing.

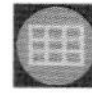

Table 48-4 Clinical Consequences of Respiratory Syncytial Virus Infection

Disorder	Age Group Affected
Bronchiolitis, pneumonia, or both	Fever, cough, dyspnea, and cyanosis in children < 1 year Pneumonia in elderly, or those with chronic heart disease, chronic lung disease, or immunocompromised
Febrile rhinitis and pharyngitis	Children
Common cold	Older children and adults

common in older children and adults. A more severe lower respiratory tract illness, **bronchiolitis,** may occur in infants. Because of inflammation at the level of the bronchiole, there is air trapping and decreased ventilation. Clinically, the patient usually has low-grade fever, tachypnea, tachycardia, and expiratory wheezes over the lungs. Bronchiolitis is usually self-limited, but it can be a frightening disease to observe in an infant. It may be fatal in premature infants, persons with underlying lung disease, and immunocompromised people.

Laboratory Diagnosis

RSV is difficult to isolate in cell culture. Presence of the viral genome in infected cells and nasal washings can be detected by RT-PCR techniques, and commercially available immunofluorescence and enzyme immunoassay tests are available for detection of the viral antigen.

Treatment, Prevention, and Control

In otherwise healthy infants, treatment is supportive, consisting of administration of oxygen, intravenous fluids, and nebulized cold steam. Aerosolized **ribavirin,** a guanosine analog, is approved for treatment of infants with severe disease, but its use is infrequent. **Prophylactic and therapeutic passive immunization** with anti-RSV immunoglobulin or monoclonal antibody (palivizumab) is available for young children at high risk to serious disease.

Infected children must be isolated. Infection-control measures are required for hospital staff caring for infected children to avoid transmitting the virus to uninfected patients. These measures include hand washing and wearing gowns, goggles, and masks.

No vaccine is currently available for RSV prophylaxis. A previously available vaccine containing inactivated RSV caused recipients to have more severe RSV disease when subsequently exposed to the live virus. This development is thought to be the result of a heightened immunologic response at the time of exposure to the wild virus.

• Human Metapneumovirus

Human metapneumovirus is a recently recognized member of the Pneumovirinae subfamily. Use of RT-PCR methods was and remains the means of detecting the pneumoviruses and distinguishing them from other respiratory disease viruses. Its identity was unknown until recently because it is difficult to grow in cell culture. The virus is ubiquitous, and almost all 5-year-old children have experienced a virus infection and are seropositive.

As with its close cousin RSV, infections by human metapneumovirus may be asymptomatic, cause common cold–type disease, or cause serious bronchiolitis and pneumonia. Seronegative children, the elderly, and immunocompromised people are at risk for disease. Human metapneumovirus probably causes 15% of common colds in children, especially those complicated by otitis media. Signs of disease usually include cough, sore throat, runny nose, and high fever. Approximately 10% of patients with metapneumovirus will experience wheezing, dyspnea, pneumonia, bronchitis, or bronchiolitis. As with other common cold agents, laboratory identification of the virus is not performed routinely but can be performed by RT-PCR. Supportive care is the only therapy available for these infections.

• Nipah and Hendra Viruses

A new paramyxovirus, Nipah virus, was isolated from patients after an outbreak of severe encephalitis in Malaysia and Singapore in 1998. Nipah virus is more closely related to the Hendra virus, discovered in 1994 in Australia, than to other paramyxoviruses. Both viruses have broad host ranges, including pigs, humans, dogs, horses, cats, and other mammals. For Nipah virus, the reservoir is a fruit bat (flying fox). The virus can be obtained from fruit contaminated by infected bats or amplified in pigs and then spread to humans. The human is an accidental host for these viruses, but the outcome of human infection is severe. Disease signs include flulike symptoms, seizures, and coma. Of the 269 cases occurring in 1999, 108 were fatal. Another epidemic in Bangladesh in 2004 had a higher mortality rate.

Bibliography

Cann AJ: *Principles of molecular virology*, San Diego, 2005, Academic.

Carter J, Saunders V: *Virology: principles and applications*, Chichester, England, 2007, Wiley.

Centers for Disease Control and Prevention: Public-sector vaccination efforts in response to the resurgence of measles among preschool-aged children: United States, 1989–1991, *MMWR Morb Mortal Wkly Rep* 41:522–525, 1992.

Cohen J, Powderly WG: *Infectious diseases*, ed 2, St Louis, 2004, Mosby.

Collier L, Oxford J: *Human virology*, ed 4, Oxford, 2011, Oxford University Press.

Flint SJ, Enquist LW, Racaniello VR, et al: *Principles of virology: molecular biology, pathogenesis and control of animal viruses*, ed 3, Washington, DC, 2009, American Society for Microbiology Press.

Galinski MS: Paramyxoviridae: transcription and replication, *Adv Virus Res* 40:129–163, 1991.

Gershon A, Hotez P, Katz S: *Krugman's infectious diseases of children*, ed 11, St Louis, 2004, Mosby.

Griffin DE, Oldstone MM: Measles: pathogenesis and control, *Curr Top Microbiol Immunol* 330:1, 2009.

Hart CA, Broadhead RL: *Color atlas of pediatric infectious diseases*, St Louis, 1992, Mosby.

Hinman AR: Potential candidates for eradication, *Rev Infect Dis* 4:933–939, 1982.

Knipe DM, Howley PM: *Fields virology*, ed 6, New York, 2013, Lippincott Williams & Wilkins.

Lennette EH: *Laboratory diagnosis of viral infections*, ed 3, New York, 1999, Marcel Dekker.

Meulen V, Billeter MA: Measles virus, *Curr Top Microbiol Immunol* 191:1–196, 1995.

Moss WJ, Griffen DE: Measles, *Lancet* 379:153–164, 2012.

Strauss JM, Strauss EG: *Viruses and human disease*, ed 2, San Diego, 2007, Academic.

Voyles BA: *The biology of viruses*, ed 2, Boston, 2002, McGraw-Hill.

Websites

Centers for Disease Control and Prevention: Human parainfluenza viruses (HPIVs). www.cdc.gov/parainfluenza/index.html. Accessed April 4, 2015.

Centers for Disease Control and Prevention: Measles (rubeola). www.cdc.gov/measles/index.html. Accessed April 4, 2015.

Centers for Disease Control and Prevention: Mumps. www.cdc.gov/mumps/index.html. Accessed April 4, 2015.

Centers for Disease Control and Prevention: Respiratory syncytial virus infection (RSV). www.cdc.gov/rsv/. Accessed April 4, 2015.

Chen SSP: Measles, 2014. http://emedicine.medscape.com/article/966220-overview. Accessed April 4, 2015.

Clinical case of SSPE. http://path.upmc.edu/cases/case595.html. April 4, 2015.

Defendi GL, Demirci CS, Abuhammour W: Mumps. http://emedicine.medscape.com/article/966678-overview. Accessed April 4, 2015.

Krilov LR: Respiratory syncytial virus (RSV) infection. http://emedicine.medscape.com/article/971488-overview. Accessed April 4, 2015.

CHAPTER

49 ORTHOMYXOVIRUSES

On April 15, 2009, a 33-year-old woman from California at 35 weeks' gestation had a 1-day history of myalgias, dry cough, and low-grade fever when examined by her obstetrician-gynecologist. The patient had not recently traveled to Mexico. Rapid influenza diagnostic testing performed in the physician's office was positive. On April 19, she was examined in a local emergency department, with worsening shortness of breath, fever, and productive cough. She experienced severe respiratory distress and was intubated and placed on mechanical ventilation. An emergency cesarean delivery was performed, resulting in a healthy female infant. On April 21, the patient developed acute respiratory distress syndrome (ARDS). The patient began receiving oseltamivir on April 28 and broad-spectrum antibiotics but died on May 4.*

1. How did the woman acquire the infection?
2. What is the normal presentation, and what is abnormal about this presentation of influenza?
3. What put the woman at higher risk and why?
4. How did this strain of influenza evolve?

Answers to these questions are available on StudentConsult.com.

• SUMMARIES CLINICALLY SIGNIFICANT ORGANISMS

Orthomyxoviruses

Trigger Words

Aerosols, envelope, segmented genome/reassortment, hemagglutinin, neuraminidase, antigenic drift (outbreaks), antigenic shift (pandemics), zoonosis

Biology, Virulence, and Disease

- Large size, enveloped, (–) segmented RNA genome
- Encodes RNA-dependent RNA polymerase, replicates in nucleus (exception to the rule)
- Each segment encodes one or two proteins
- Mixed infection results in genetic mixing of segments: reassortment
- Binds to sialic acid (HA glycoprotein) and encodes neuraminidase activity (NA glycoprotein)
- Antibody can block disease
- Cell-mediated immune response important for control but causes pathogenesis
- Influenza A, not influenza B, is a zoonosis
- Acute flulike symptoms due to large cytokine release
- Extensive destruction of ciliated epithelium
- Pneumonia by influenza or secondary bacterial infection

Epidemiology

- Transmitted by aerosols
- Annual epidemics due to mutations, pandemics due to reassortment of genome segments between human and animal viruses

Diagnosis

- Symptomatology, RT-PCR genome analysis of respiratory secretions, immunology tests (ELISA), hemagglutination and hemagglutination inhibition

Treatment, Prevention, and Control

- Annual vaccine contains two influenza A and one influenza B strain: inactivated vaccines contain HA and NA, live attenuated nasal vaccine (for 2- to 49-year-olds)
- Neuraminidase inhibitor and amantadine/rimantadine antiviral drugs

*Adapted from Centers for Disease Control and Prevention (CDC): Novel influenza A (H1N1) virus infections in three pregnant women—United States, April–May 2009, *MMWR Morb Mortal Wkly Rep* 58:497–500. www.cdc.gov/mmwr/preview/mmwrhtml/mm58d0512a1.htm.

Influenza A, B, and C viruses are the most important members of the Orthomyxoviridae family. Only influenza A and B viruses cause significant human disease, and only influenza A can be a zoonosis. Thogotoviruses are arboviruses including the tick-borne Bourbon virus. This virus caused a lethal infection in Bourbon, Kansas, in 2014. The orthomyxoviruses are **enveloped and have a segmented negative-sense ribonucleic acid (RNA) genome.** The segmented genome of these viruses facilitates development of new strains through mutation and reassortment of the gene segments among different human and animal (influenza A) strains of virus. This genetic instability is responsible for the annual **epidemics (mutation: drift)** and for influenza A **periodic pandemics (reassortment: shift)** of influenza infection worldwide.

Influenza is one of the most prevalent and significant viral infections. Probably the most famous influenza **pandemic (worldwide)** is the Spanish influenza that swept the world in 1918-1919, killing 20 to 40 million people. In fact, more people died of influenza during that time than in the battles of World War I. Pandemics caused by novel influenza viruses occurred in 1918, 1947, 1957, 1968, 1977, and 2009. Fortunately, prophylaxis with vaccines and antiviral drugs is available.

Influenza viruses cause respiratory symptoms and the classic flulike symptoms of fever, malaise, headache, and myalgias (body aches). The term **flu,** however, has been mistakenly used to refer to many other respiratory and viral infections (e.g., "intestinal flu").

• Structure and Replication

Influenza virions are pleomorphic, appearing spherical or tubular (Figure 49-1; Box 49-1) and ranging in diameter from 80 to 120 nm. The envelope contains two glycoproteins, **hemagglutinin (HA)** and **neuraminidase (NA),** and the **membrane (M_2) protein** and is internally lined by the **matrix (M_1) protein.** The genome of the influenza A and B viruses consists of **eight different helical nucleocapsid segments,** each of which contains a negative-sense RNA associated with the **nucleoprotein (NP)** and the **transcriptase (RNA polymerase components: PB1, PB2, PA)** (Table 49-1). Influenza C has only seven genomic segments.

The genomic segments in the influenza A virus range from 890 to 2340 bases. All the proteins are encoded on separate segments, with the exception of the nonstructural proteins (NS_1 and NS_2) and the M_1 and M_2 proteins, which are transcribed from one segment each.

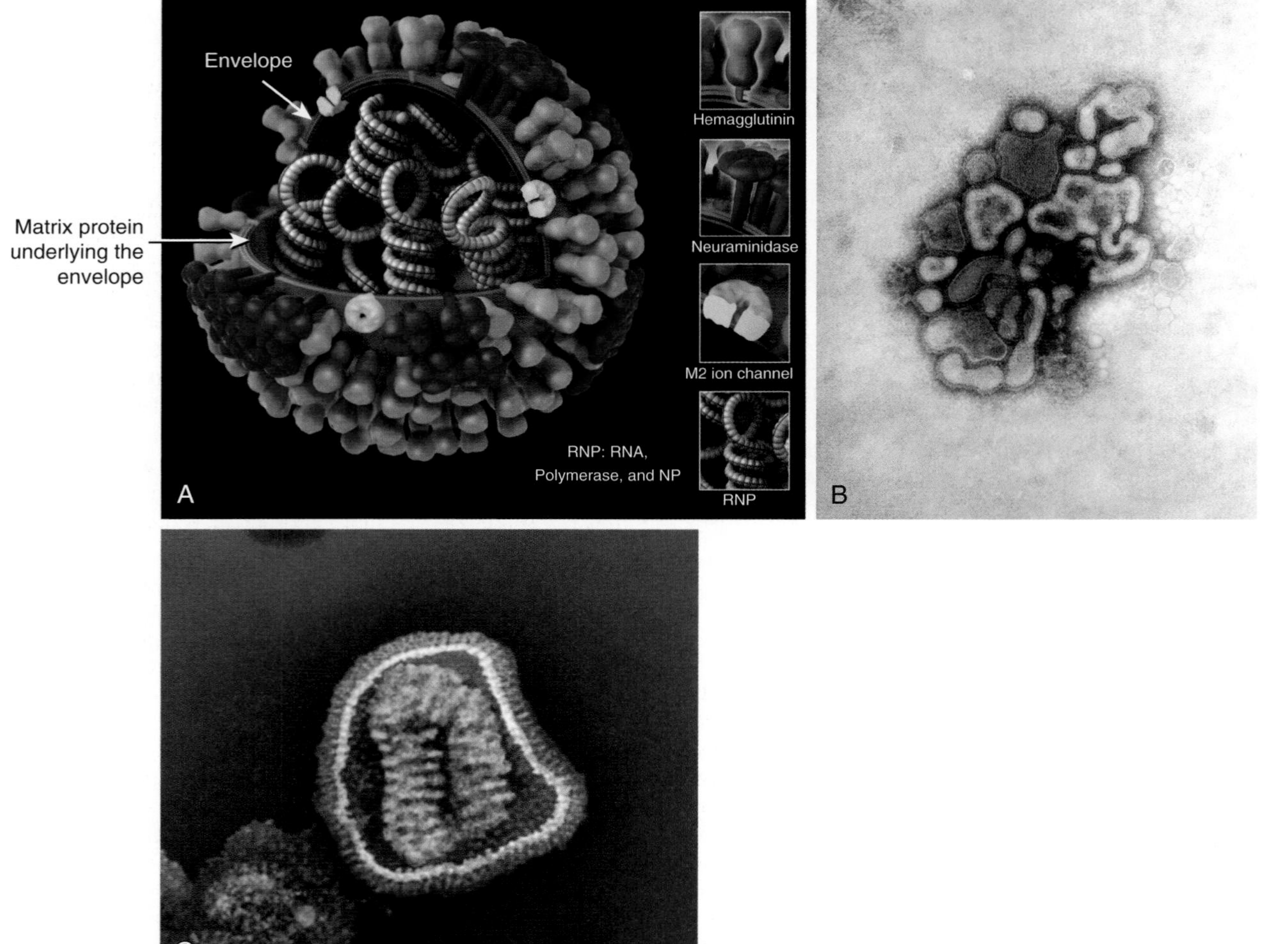

FIGURE 49-1 **A,** Model of influenza A virus. **B** and **C,** Electron micrographs of influenza A virus. *NP,* Nucleoprotein; *RNA,* ribonucleic acid; *RNP,* ribonucleoprotein complex. (Courtesy Centers for Disease Control and Prevention.)

Box 49-1 Unique Features of the Influenza A and B Viruses

The **enveloped virion** has a genome of **eight unique negative-sense RNA nucleocapsid segments.**

Hemagglutinin glycoprotein is the viral attachment protein and fusion protein; it elicits neutralizing, protective antibody responses.

Influenza transcribes and replicates its genome in the target cell nucleus but assembles and buds from the plasma membrane.

The antiviral drugs **amantadine and rimantadine** target the M_2 (membrane) protein for *influenza A only* to inhibit the uncoating step.

The antiviral drugs **zanamivir and oseltamivir** inhibit the neuraminidase protein of influenza A and B.

The segmented genome promotes **genetic diversity** caused by **mutation** and **reassortment** of segments on infection with two different strains.

Influenza A infects humans, mammals, and birds (zoonosis).

Table 49-1 Products of Influenza Gene Segments

Segment*	Protein	Function
1	PB2	Polymerase component
2	PB1	Polymerase component
3	PA	Polymerase component
4	HA	Hemagglutinin, viral attachment protein, fusion protein, target of neutralizing antibody
5	NP	Nucleocapsid protein
6	NA	Neuraminidase (cleaves sialic acid and promotes virus release)
7†	M_1	Matrix protein: viral structural protein (interacts with nucleocapsid and envelope, promotes assembly)
	M_2	Membrane protein (forms membrane channel and target for amantadine, facilitates uncoating and HA production)
8†	NS_1	Nonstructural protein (inhibits cellular messenger RNA translation)
	NS_2	Nonstructural protein (promotes export of nucleocapsid from nucleus)

*Listed in decreasing order of size.

†Encodes two messenger RNAs.

The **HA** forms a spike-shaped trimer; each unit is activated by a protease and is cleaved into two subunits held together by a disulfide bond (see Chapter 36, Figure 36-7). The HA has several functions. It is the viral attachment protein, binding to sialic acid on epithelial cell surface receptors; it promotes fusion of the envelope to the cell membrane at acidic pH; it hemagglutinates (binds and aggregates) human, chicken, and guinea pig red blood cells; and it elicits the protective neutralizing antibody response. Changes in HA undergo minor ("drift") and major ("shift") changes in receptor specificity and antigenicity. *Shifts occur only with influenza A virus, and the different HAs are designated H1, H2…H16.*

The **NA** glycoprotein forms a tetramer and has enzyme activity. The NA cleaves the sialic acid on glycoproteins,

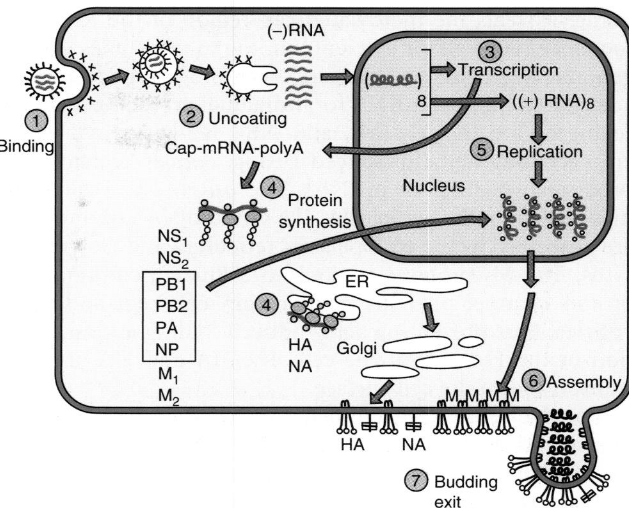

FIGURE 49-2 Replication of influenza A virus. After binding *(1)* to sialic acid–containing receptors, influenza is endocytosed and fuses *(2)* with the vesicle membrane. Unlike for most other ribonucleic acid *(RNA)* viruses, transcription *(3)* and replication *(5)* of the genome occur in the nucleus. Viral proteins are synthesized *(4)*, helical RNP nucleocapsid segments form and associate *(6)* with the M_1 protein–lined membranes containing M_2 and the hemagglutinin *(HA)* and neuraminidase *(NA)* glycoproteins. The virus buds *(7)* from the plasma membrane and eventually kills the cell. *(–)*, Negative sense; *(+)*, positive sense; *ER*, endoplasmic reticulum; *NP*, nucleocapsid; *NS_1*, *NS_2*, nonstructural proteins 1 and 2; *PA*, *PB1*, *PB2*, polymerase components; *polyA*, polyadenylate.

including the cell receptor. Cleavage of the sialic acid on virion HA prevents clumping and facilitates the release of virus from infected cells, making NA a target for two antiviral drugs, **zanamivir (Relenza)** and **oseltamivir (Tamiflu).** *The NA of influenza A virus also undergoes antigenic shift, and the different NAs are designated N1, N2…N9.*

The **M_1, M_2,** and **NP** proteins are type specific and are therefore used to differentiate influenza A from B or C viruses. The M_1 proteins line the inside of the virion and promote assembly. The M_2 protein forms a proton channel in membranes and promotes uncoating and viral release. The M_2 of influenza A is a target for the antiviral drugs **amantadine** and **rimantadine.**

Viral replication begins with the binding of HA to sialic acid on cell surface glycoproteins (Figure 49-2). The different HAs ($HA_{1\text{-}16}$) bind to different sialic acid structures, which determines the species and tissue that can be infected. The virus is then internalized into a coated vesicle and transferred to an endosome. Acidification of the endosome causes the HA to bend over and expose hydrophobic fusion-promoting regions of the protein. The viral envelope then fuses with the endosome membrane. The proton channel formed by the M_2 protein promotes acidification of the envelope contents to break the interaction between the M_1 protein and the NP, allowing uncoating and delivery of the nucleocapsid into the cytoplasm.

Unlike most RNA viruses, the influenza nucleocapsid travels to the nucleus, where it is transcribed into messenger RNA (mRNA). The transcriptase (PA, PB1, and PB2) uses host cell mRNA as a primer for viral mRNA synthesis. In so doing, it steals the methylated cap region of the RNA, the sequence required for efficient binding to ribosomes. All the genomic segments are transcribed into 5′-capped, 3′-polyadenylated (polyA) mRNA for individual proteins except the segments for the M_1, M_2, and NS_1, NS_2 proteins, which are each differentially spliced (using cellular enzymes) to produce two different mRNAs. The mRNAs are translated into protein in the cytoplasm. The HA and NA glycoproteins are processed by the endoplasmic reticulum and Golgi apparatus. The M_2 protein inserts into cellular membranes. Its proton channel prevents acidification of Golgi and other vesicles, thus preventing acid-induced folding and inactivation of the HA within the cell. The HA and NA are then transported to the cell surface.

Positive-sense RNA templates for each segment are produced, and the negative-sense RNA genome is replicated in the nucleus. The genomic segments associate with polymerase and NP proteins to form nucleocapsids, and the NS_2 protein facilitates the transport of ribonucleocapsids into the cytoplasm, where they interact with the M_1 protein–lined plasma membrane sections containing M_2, HA, and NA. The virus buds selectively from the apical (airway) surface of the cell as a result of the preferential insertion of the HA in this membrane. Virus is released approximately 8 hours after infection.

• Pathogenesis and Immunity

Influenza initially establishes a local upper respiratory tract infection (Figure 49-3; Box 49-2). To do so, the virus first targets and kills mucus-secreting, ciliated, and other epithelial cells, causing the loss of this primary defense system. With a lack of ciliated epithelium, swallowed oral and nasal bacteria (e.g., *Staphylococcus aureus*) cannot be expelled and may cause pneumonia. NA facilitates the development of the infection by cleaving sialic acid (neuraminic acid) residues of the mucus, thereby providing access to tissue. Preferential release of the virus at the apical surface of epithelial cells and into the lung promotes cell-to-cell spread and transmission to other hosts. In the lower respiratory tract, the infection can cause severe desquamation (shedding) of bronchial or alveolar epithelium down to a single-cell basal layer or to the basement membrane.

In addition to compromising the mucociliary defenses of the respiratory tract, influenza infection promotes bacterial adhesion to the epithelial cells. Pneumonia may result from a viral pathogenesis or from a secondary bacterial infection. Influenza may also cause a transient or low-level viremia but rarely involves tissues other than the lung.

Influenza infection is an excellent inducer of interferon. Systemic interferon and cytokine responses peak at 3 to 4 days post infection, almost the same time as virus in nasal washes, and are responsible for the systemic "flulike" symptoms. T-cell responses are important for effecting recovery and immunopathogenesis, but antibody, including vaccine-induced antibody, can prevent disease. As for measles, influenza infection depresses macrophage and T-cell function, hindering immune resolution. Of interest, recovery often precedes detection of antibody in serum or secretions.

Protection against reinfection is primarily associated with the development of antibodies to HA, but antibodies to NA are also protective. The antibody response is specific for each strain of influenza, whereas the cell-mediated immune response is more general and is capable of reacting to influenza strains of the same type (influenza A or B virus). Antigenic targets for T-cell responses include peptides from HA but also from the nucleocapsid proteins (NP, PB2) and M_1 protein. The NP, PB2, and M_1 proteins differ considerably for influenza A and B but minimally between strains of these viruses; hence T-cell memory may provide future protection against infection by a strain different from the immunizing strain.

The symptoms and time course of the disease are determined by the extent of viral and immune killing of epithelial tissue and cytokine action. Influenza is normally a self-limited disease that rarely involves organs other than the

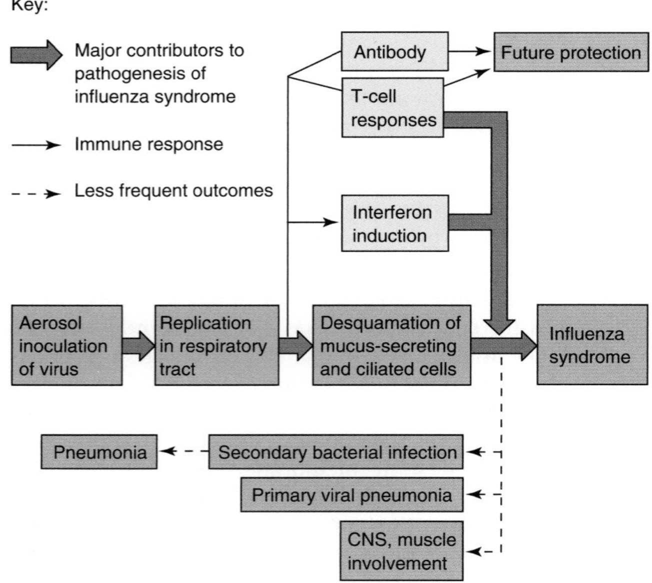

FIGURE 49-3 Pathogenesis of influenza A virus. The symptoms of influenza are caused by viral pathologic and immunopathologic effects, but the infection may promote secondary bacterial infection. *CNS*, Central nervous system.

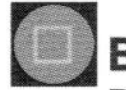

Box 49-2 Disease Mechanisms of Influenza A and B Viruses

Virus infects the upper and lower respiratory tract.

Systemic symptoms are caused by the interferon and cytokine response to the virus. Local symptoms result from epithelial cell damage, including ciliated and mucus-secreting cells.

Interferon and cell-mediated immune responses (natural killer and T cells) are important for immune resolution and immunopathogenesis.

Infected people are predisposed to bacterial superinfection because of the loss of natural barriers and exposure of binding sites on epithelial cells.

Antibody is important for future protection against infection and is specific for defined epitopes on hemagglutinin (HA) and neuraminidase (NA) proteins.

The HA and NA of influenza A virus can undergo **major (reassortment: shift)** and **minor (mutation: drift)** antigenic changes to ensure the presence of immunologically naïve susceptible people.

Influenza B virus undergoes only minor antigenic changes.

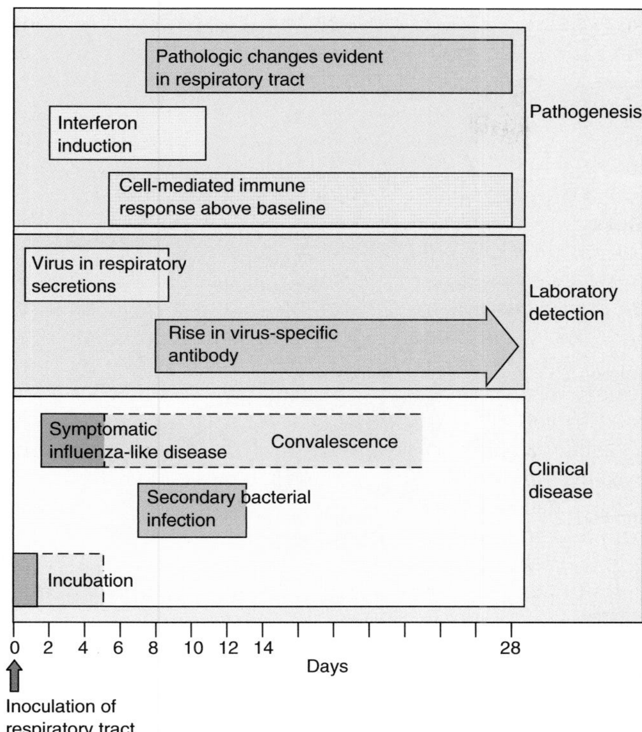

FIGURE 49-4 Time course of influenza A virus infection. The classic "flu syndrome" occurs early. Later, pneumonia may result from bacterial pathogenesis, viral pathogenesis, or immunopathogenesis.

lung. The acute onset of *many of the classic "flu" symptoms (e.g., fever, malaise, headache, and myalgia) is associated with interferon and cytokine induction.* Virus production may be controlled within 4 to 6 days post infection, but tissue damage due to innate and immune inflammatory responses continues. Repair of the compromised tissue is initiated within 3 to 5 days of the start of symptoms but may take as long as a month or more, especially for elderly people. The time course of influenza virus infection is illustrated in Figure 49-4.

• Epidemiology

Strains of influenza A virus are classified by the following characteristics:

1. Type (A)
2. Place of original isolation
3. Date of original isolation
4. HA and NA type

For example, a current strain of influenza virus might be designated A/Bangkok/1/79 (H3N2), meaning that it is an influenza A virus that was first isolated in Bangkok in January 1979 and contains HA (H3) and NA (N2) antigens.

Strains of influenza B are designated by (1) type, (2) geography, and (3) date of isolation (e.g., B/Singapore/3/64) but without specific mention of HA or NA antigens, because influenza B does not undergo antigenic shift or pandemics as does influenza A.

Minor antigenic changes resulting from mutation of the HA and NA genes are called **antigenic drift.** This process occurs every 2 to 3 years, causing local outbreaks of influenza A and B infection. **Major antigenic changes (antigenic shift)** result from reassortment of genomes among different strains, including animal strains. *This process occurs only with the influenza A virus.* Such changes are often associated with the occurrence of pandemics. *In contrast to influenza A, influenza B is predominantly a human virus and does not undergo antigenic shift.*

Table 49-2 Influenza Pandemics Resulting from Antigenic Shift

Year of Pandemic	Influenza A Subtype
1918	H1N1
1947	H1N1
1957	H2N2; Asian flu strain
1968	H3N2; Hong Kong flu strain
1977	H1N1; Russian
1997, 2003	H5N1: China, avian
2009	H1N1, swine flu

Antigenic shifts occur infrequently, but the pandemics they cause can be devastating (Table 49-2). For example, the prevalent influenza A virus in 1947 was the H1N1 subtype. In 1957, there was a shift in both antigens, resulting in an H2N2 subtype. H3N2 appeared in 1968, and H1N1 reappeared in 1977. The reappearance of H1N1 put the population younger than age 30 years at risk of disease. Prior exposure and an anamnestic antibody response protected members of the population older than 30 years.

The genetic diversity of influenza A is fostered by its segmented genomic structure and ability to infect and replicate in humans and many animal species **(zoonosis),** including birds and pigs. Hybrid viruses are created by coinfection of a cell with different strains of influenza A virus, allowing the genomic segments to randomly associate into new virions. An exchange of the HA glycoproteins may generate a new virus that can infect an immunologically naïve human population. Figure 49-5 depicts the origins of the pandemic A/California/04/2009/H1N1 virus through multiple reassortments of human, avian, and pig influenza viruses, resulting in a virus that was able to infect humans (Clinical Case 49-1).

Because of its high population density and proximity of humans, pigs, chickens, and ducks, China is often the breeding ground for new reassortant viruses and the source of many of the pandemic strains of influenza. In 1997, a highly pathogenic avian influenza virus (HPAIV) (H5N1) strain was isolated from at least 18 humans and caused six deaths in Hong Kong (Clinical Case 49-2). The virus was spread by domestic and wild water fowl in their feces and directly from bird to man, with cases occurring around the globe. Although primarily an avian virus, inhalation of large amounts of virus (shared living environments) can lead to infection and killing of cells of the lower human lung. Outbreaks of avian influenza require destruction of all potentially infected birds, such as for the 1.6 million chickens in Hong Kong, to destroy the potential source of the virus. Outbreaks in 2013 and 2014 of lethal H7N9 disease in China have been traced to chicken-to-human transmission in live poultry markets.

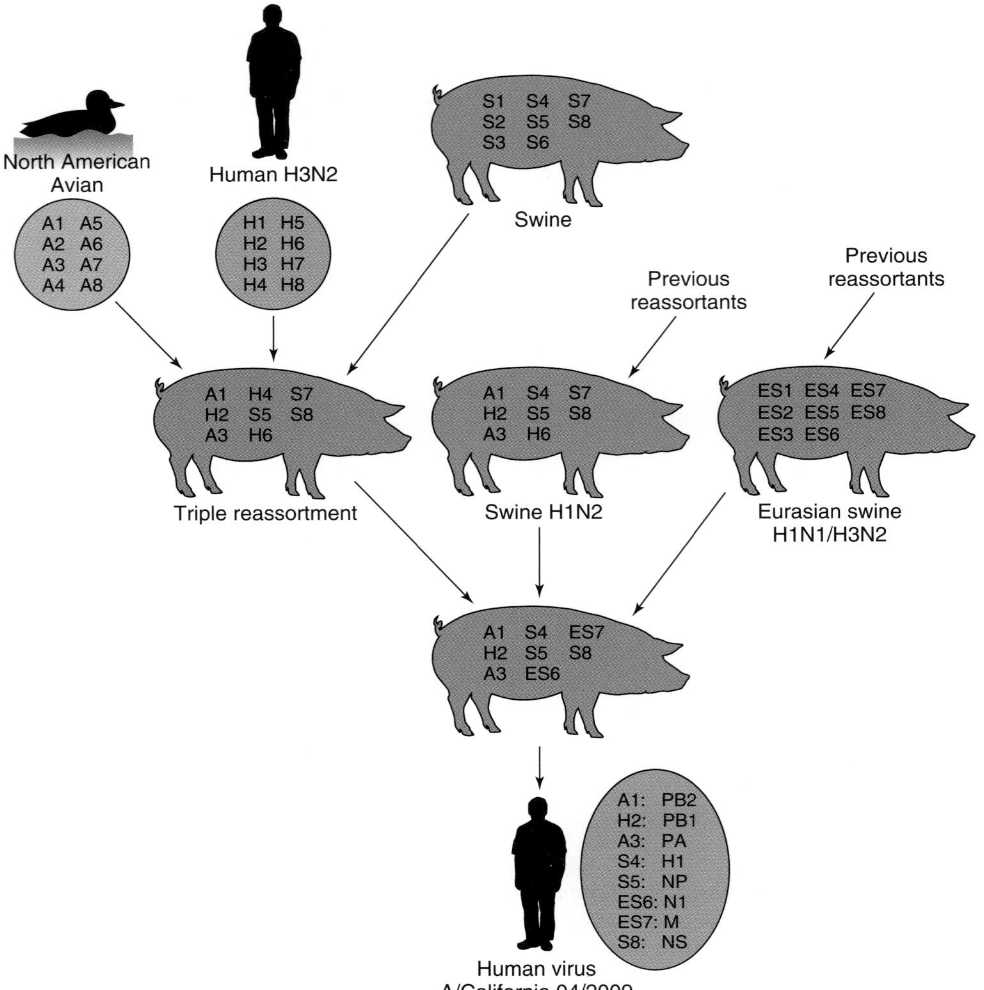

FIGURE 49-5 Generation of A/CALIFORNIA/04/2009 (H1N1) pandemic swine flu by multiple reassortments of genomic segments of influenza A virus. The pandemic H1N1 virus arose from the mixing of a triple reassortment of avian, human, and swine viruses with two other swine viruses, each of which were also generated by reassortment between swine, human, and other influenza viruses. This new virus emerged in the spring of 2009 (out of season) in Mexico but was first identified in California.

Clinical Case 49-1 Pandemic Influenza A/California/04/2009 (H1N1)

In the spring of 2009, a new amantadine- and rimantadine-resistant reassortant H1N1 virus was detected in a 10-year-old patient in California and proceeded to cause a pandemic. As indicated in Figure 49-5, the virus is a triple-triple reassortant of multiple swine, avian, and human influenza viruses. The virus originated in Mexico and rapidly spread as many cases went unrecognized because of the unseasonal nature of the outbreak. Up to 25,000 deaths have occurred worldwide, primarily in people between the ages of 22 months and 57 years. People with chronic medical conditions, especially pregnant women, were at greatest risk to complications, but unlike other outbreaks, this virus had a tendency to affect younger and healthier individuals. Of interest, many people older than 60 years had cross-reactive antibody resulting from prior exposure to an H1N1 influenza virus. Neuraminidase inhibitors were made available for prophylaxis, but detection of resistant strains became a concern. By September, a vaccine had been developed, approved, and manufactured and was available for distribution on a prioritized basis, and then it was administered with the seasonal influenza vaccine. The pandemic was declared over by August 2010, and the H1N1 virus joined H3N2 and influenza B as a seasonal virus.

The changing antigenic nature of influenza ensures a large proportion of immunologically naïve susceptible people (especially children) in the population each year (Box 49-3). An influenza outbreak can be readily detected from increased absenteeism in schools and at work and the number of emergency department visits. The influenza season for the Northern Hemisphere is usually from late fall to early spring.

Influenza infection is spread readily via small airborne droplets expelled during talking, breathing, and coughing. Low humidity and cool temperatures stabilize the virus, and close proximity during the winter months promotes its spread. The virus can also survive on countertops for as long as a day.

The most susceptible population is children, and school-aged children are most likely to spread the infection. Contagion precedes symptoms and lasts for a long time, especially in children. Children, immunosuppressed people (including pregnant women), the elderly, and people with heart and lung ailments (including smokers) are at highest risk for more serious disease, pneumonia, or other complications of

Clinical Case 49-2 H5N1 Avian Influenza

The first case of H5N1 avian influenza in a human was described by Ku and Chan (*J Paediatr Child Health* 35:207–208, 1999). After a 3-year-old boy from China developed a fever of 40° C and abdominal pain, he was given antibiotics and aspirin. On the third day, he was hospitalized with sore throat, and his chest radiograph demonstrated bronchial inflammation. Blood studies showed a left shift with 9% band forms. On the sixth day, the boy was still febrile and fully conscious, but on the seventh day, his fever increased, he was hyperventilating, and his blood oxygen levels decreased. A chest radiograph indicated severe pneumonia. The patient was intubated. On the eighth day, the boy was diagnosed with fulminant sepsis and acute respiratory distress syndrome (ARDS). Therapy for ARDS and other attempts to improve oxygen uptake were unsuccessful. He was treated empirically for sepsis, herpes simplex virus infection (acyclovir), methicillin-resistant *Staphylococcus aureus* (vancomycin), and fungal infection (amphotericin B), but his condition deteriorated further, with disseminated intravascular coagulation and liver and renal failure. He died on the 11th day. Laboratory results indicated elevated influenza A antibody on the eighth day, and influenza A was isolated from a tracheal isolate taken on the ninth day. The isolate was sent to the Centers for Disease Control and Prevention and elsewhere, where it was typed as H5N1 avian influenza and named *A/Hong Kong/156/97 (H5N1)*. The child may have contracted the virus while playing with pet ducklings and chickens at his kindergarten. Although the H5N1 virus still has difficulty infecting humans, this case demonstrates the speed and severity of the respiratory and systemic manifestations of avian influenza H5N1 disease.

infection. More than 90% of mortalities occur in patients who are older than 65 years, but rapidly progressing lethal bacterial pneumonias secondary to influenza can occur in young healthy individuals.

Extensive surveillance of influenza A and B outbreaks is conducted to identify new strains that should be incorporated into new vaccines. The prevalence of a particular strain of influenza A or B virus changes each year and reflects the particular immunologic naïveté of the population at that time. Surveillance also extends into the animal populations because of the possible presence of recombinant animal influenza A strains that can cause human pandemics.

• Clinical Syndromes (Box 49-4)

Depending on the degree of immunity to the infecting strain of virus and other factors, disease may range from asymptomatic to severe. Patients with underlying cardiorespiratory disease, people with immune deficiency (even that associated with pregnancy), the elderly, and smokers are more prone to have a severe case.

After an incubation period of 1 to 4 days, the "flu syndrome" begins with a brief prodrome of malaise and headache lasting a few hours. The prodrome is followed by the abrupt and intense onset of fever, chills, severe myalgias, loss of appetite, weakness and fatigue, sore throat, and usually a nonproductive cough. The fever persists for 3 to 8 days, and unless a complication occurs, recovery is complete within 7 to 10 days. Influenza in young children (<3 years) resembles other severe respiratory tract infections, potentially causing bronchiolitis, croup, otitis media, vomiting, and abdominal pain, accompanied rarely by febrile convulsions (Table 49-3). Complications of influenza include bacterial pneumonia, myositis, and Reye syndrome. The central nervous system can also be involved. Influenza B disease is similar to influenza A disease.

Influenza may directly cause pneumonia, but it more commonly promotes a secondary bacterial superinfection that leads to bronchitis or a rapidly progressing and potentially lethal pneumonia. The tissue damage caused by progressive influenza virus infection of alveoli can be extensive, leading to hypoxia and bilateral pneumonia. Secondary bacterial infection usually involves *Streptococcus pneumoniae, Haemophilus influenzae,* or *S. aureus.* In these infections, sputum usually is produced and becomes purulent.

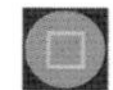

Box 49-3 Epidemiology of Influenza A and B Viruses

Disease/Viral Factors

Virus has a large, enveloped virion that is easily inactivated by dryness, acid, and detergents.

Segmented genome facilitates major genetic changes, especially on hemagglutinin and neuraminidase proteins.

Influenza A infects many vertebrate species, including other mammals and birds.

Co-infection with animal and human strains of influenza A can generate very different virus strains by genetic reassortment.

Transmission of virus often precedes symptoms.

Transmission

Virus is spread by inhalation of small aerosol droplets expelled during talking, breathing, and coughing.

Virus likes a cool, less humid atmosphere (e.g., winter heating season).

Virus is extensively spread by schoolchildren.

Who Is at Risk?

Seronegative people

Adults: classic flu syndrome

Children: asymptomatic to severe respiratory tract infections

High-risk groups: elderly and immunocompromised people, people in nursing homes or with underlying cardiac or respiratory problems (including asthma sufferers and smokers)

Geography/Season

Worldwide occurrence. Epidemics are local; pandemics are worldwide.

Disease is more common in winter.

Modes of Control

Amantadine, rimantadine, zanamivir, and oseltamivir have been approved for prophylaxis or early treatment.

Killed and live vaccines contain predicted yearly strains of influenza A and B viruses.

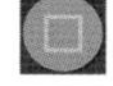

Box 49-4 Clinical Summary

Influenza A: A 70-year-old woman has rapid onset of fever with headache, myalgia, sore throat, and nonproductive cough. The disease progresses to pneumonia with bacterial involvement. There is no history of recent immunization with influenza A vaccine. Her husband is treated with amantadine or a neuraminidase inhibitor.

Table 49-3 **Diseases Associated with Influenza Virus Infection**

Disorder	Symptoms
Acute influenza infection in adults	Rapid onset of fever, malaise, myalgia, sore throat, and nonproductive cough
Acute influenza infection in children	Acute disease similar to that in adults but with higher fever, gastrointestinal tract symptoms (abdominal pain, vomiting), otitis media, myositis, and more frequent croup
Complications of influenza virus infection	Primary viral pneumonia Secondary bacterial pneumonia Myositis and cardiac involvement Neurologic syndromes: Guillain-Barré syndrome Encephalopathy Encephalitis Reye syndrome

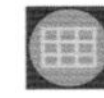

Table 49-4 **Laboratory Diagnosis of Influenza Virus Infection**

Test	Detects
Cell culture in primary monkey kidney or Madin-Darby canine kidney cells	Presence of virus; limited cytopathologic effects
Hemadsorption to infected cells	Presence of hemagglutinin protein on cell surface
Hemagglutination	Presence of virus in secretions
Hemagglutination inhibition	Type and strain of influenza virus or specificity of antibody
Antibody inhibition of hemadsorption	Identification of influenza type and strain
Immunofluorescence, ELISA	Influenza virus and antigens in respiratory secretions or tissue culture
Serology: hemagglutination inhibition, hemadsorption inhibition, ELISA, immunofluorescence, complement fixation	Seroepidemiology
Genomics: RT-PCR	Identification of influenza type and strain

ELISA, Enzyme-linked immunosorbent assay; *RT-PCR,* reverse transcriptase polymerase chain reaction.

Influenza disease may include other sites in certain people. For example, myositis (inflammation of muscle) may occur in children. Encephalopathy, although rare, may accompany an acute influenza illness and can be fatal. Postinfluenza encephalitis occurs 2 to 3 weeks after recovery from influenza. These diseases are thought to be autoimmune diseases triggered by influenza.

Reye syndrome is an acute encephalitis that affects children and occurs after a variety of acute febrile viral infections, including varicella and influenza B and A diseases. Children given salicylates (aspirin) are at increased risk for this syndrome. In addition to encephalopathy, hepatic dysfunction is present. The mortality rate may be as high as 40%.

• Laboratory Diagnosis

The diagnosis of influenza is usually based on the characteristic symptoms, the season, and the presence of the virus in the community. Laboratory methods that distinguish influenza from other respiratory viruses and identify its type and strain confirm the diagnosis (Table 49-4).

Influenza viruses are obtained from respiratory secretions taken early in the illness. The virus can be isolated in primary monkey kidney cell cultures or the Madin-Darby canine kidney cell line. Although cytolytic, the cytopathologic effects of the virus are often difficult to distinguish but may be noted within as few as 2 days (average, 4 days). Before the cytopathologic effects develop, the addition of guinea pig erythrocytes may reveal **hemadsorption** (adherence of these erythrocytes to HA-expressing infected cells) (see Chapter 39, Figure 39-5). Addition of influenza virus–containing fluids to erythrocytes promotes formation of a gel-like aggregate resulting from **hemagglutination.** Hemagglutination and hemadsorption are not specific to influenza viruses; parainfluenza and other viruses also exhibit these properties.

More rapid techniques detect and identify the influenza genome or antigens of the virus. Rapid antigen assays (<30 minutes) can detect and distinguish influenza A and B. Reverse transcriptase polymerase chain reaction (RT-PCR) and multiplex RT-PCR assays can detect and distinguish influenza A and B, different strains (e.g., H5N1), and other respiratory viruses. Enzyme immunoassay or immunofluorescence can be used to detect viral antigen in exfoliated cells, respiratory secretions, or cell culture. Immunofluorescence or inhibition of hemadsorption or hemagglutination (hemagglutination inhibition) with specific antibody (see Chapter 39, Figure 39-6) can also detect and distinguish different influenza strains.

• Treatment, Prevention, and Control

Hundreds of millions of dollars are spent on acetaminophen, antihistamines, and similar drugs to relieve the symptoms of influenza. The antiviral drug **amantadine** and its analog **rimantadine** inhibit an uncoating step of the influenza A virus but do not affect the influenza B and C viruses. The target for their action is the M_2 protein. **Zanamivir** and **oseltamivir** inhibit both influenza A and B as enzyme inhibitors of neuraminidase. Without neuraminidase, the hemagglutinin of the virus binds to sialic acid on other glycoproteins and viral particles to form clumps, thereby preventing virus release. Zanamivir is inhaled, whereas oseltamivir is taken orally as a pill. These drugs are effective for prophylaxis and for treatment during the first 24 to 48 hours after the onset of influenza A illness. Treatment cannot prevent the later host-induced immunopathogenic stages of the disease. Naturally resistant or mutant strains are selected when antiviral prophylaxis is used and are becoming more prevalent. Stockpiles of oseltamivir have been developed in many countries as a rapid response to an outbreak and an alternative to vaccines.

The airborne spread of influenza is almost impossible to limit. However, the best way to control the virus is through immunization. Natural immunization, which results from prior exposure, is protective for long periods. Vaccines representing the "strains of the year" and antiviral drug prophylaxis can also prevent infection.

The inactivated subunit influenza vaccines are a mixture of extracts or purified HA and NA proteins from three or four different strains of virus. HA and NA are purified from virus grown in embryonated eggs, from infected tissue culture cells, or by recombinant gene technology. Killed (formalin-inactivated) virion preparations are also used. Ideally, the vaccine incorporates antigens of the A and B influenza strains that will be prevalent in the community during the upcoming winter. For instance, the trivalent influenza vaccine for the Northern Hemisphere for the 2013-2014 season included an A/California/7/2009 (H1N1)–like virus, an A/Victoria/361/2011 (H3N2)–like virus, and a B/Massachusetts/2/2012-like virus. Vaccination is routinely recommended for all individuals and especially persons older than 50 years, health care workers, pregnant women who will be in their second or third trimester during flu season, people living in a nursing home, people with chronic pulmonary heart disease, and others at high risk. As of 2008, all children aged 5 to 18 years should also be vaccinated. Persons with serious allergies to eggs can get the recombinant or tissue culture–generated vaccines or the live vaccine.

A live attenuated influenza vaccine (LAIV) is also available for administration as a nasal spray instead of a "flu shot." The trivalent vaccine consists of reassortant viruses that contain the HA and NA gene segments of the desired influenza strains within a master donor virus that is cold adapted for optimum growth at 25° C. This vaccine is restricted to infecting the nasopharynx and will elicit a more natural protection, including cell-mediated, serum antibody, and mucosal-secretory immunoglobulin (Ig)A antibody. The vaccine is only recommended for people aged 2 to 50 years.

Thogotoviruses

Thogotoviruses have six or seven genomic segments and are arboviruses capable of infecting humans and other vertebrates. They are spread primarily by ticks but possibly by mosquitoes. In 2014, a previously healthy man died of a tick-borne disease that resembled Rocky Mountain spotted fever. It is named the Bourbon virus after Bourbon, Kansas, where it was isolated.

Bibliography

Cann AJ: *Principles of molecular virology*, San Diego, 2005, Academic.

Carr CM, Chaudhry C, Kim PS: Influenza hemagglutinin is spring-loaded by a metastable native conformation, *Proc Natl Acad Sci U S A* 94:14306–14313, 1997.

Carter J, Saunders V: *Virology: principles and applications*, Chichester, England, 2007, Wiley.

Cohen J, Powderly WG: *Infectious diseases*, ed 2, St Louis, 2004, Mosby.

Collier L, Oxford J: *Human virology*, ed 4, Oxford, 2011, Oxford University Press.

Cox NJ, Subbarao K: Global epidemiology of influenza: past and present, *Annu Rev Med* 51:407–421, 2000.

Das K, Aramini JM, Ma LC, et al: Structures of influenza A proteins and insights into antiviral drug targets, *Nat Struct Mol Biol* 17:530–538, 2010.

Flint SJ, Enquist LW, Racaniello VR, et al: *Principles of virology: molecular biology, pathogenesis and control of animal viruses*, ed 3, Washington, DC, 2009, American Society for Microbiology Press.

Knipe DM, Howley PM: *Fields virology*, ed 6, Philadelphia, 2013, Lippincott Williams & Wilkins.

Laver WG, Bischofberger N, Webster RG: The origin and control of pandemic influenza, *Perspect Biol Med* 43:173–192, 2000.

Poland GA, Jacobson RM, Targonski PV: Avian and pandemic influenza: an overview, *Vaccine* 25:3057–3061, 2007.

Richman DD, Whitley RJ, Hayden FG: *Clinical virology*, ed 3, Washington, DC, 2009, American Society for Microbiology Press.

Salomon R, Webster RG: The influenza virus enigma, *Cell* 136:402–410, 2009.

Strauss JM, Strauss EG: *Viruses and human disease*, ed 2, San Diego, 2007, Academic.

Voyles BA: *The biology of viruses*, ed 2, Boston, 2002, McGraw-Hill.

Webster RG, Govorkova EA: H5N1 Influenza, continuing evolution and spread, *N Engl J Med* 355:2174–2177, 2006.

Websites

Centers for Disease Control and Prevention: Bourbon virus. www.cdc.gov/ncezid/dvbd/bourbon/. Accessed May 10, 2015.

Centers for Disease Control and Prevention: The 2009 H1N1 pandemic: summary highlights, April 2009-2010, 2010. www.cdc.gov/h1n1flu/cdcresponse.htm. Accessed April 4, 2015.

Centers for Disease Control and Prevention: Seasonal influenza (flu). www.cdc.gov/flu/. Accessed April 4, 2015.

Derlet RW, Nguyen HH, Sandrock CE: Influenza, 2012. http://emedicine.medscape.com/article/219557-overview. Accessed April 4, 2015.

International Federation of Pharmaceutical Manufacturers and Associations: IFPMA influenza vaccine supply international task force. www.ifpma.org/resources/influenza-vaccines/ifpma-influenza-task-force/about-the-influenza-task-force/article/about-the-influenza-task-force.html. Accessed April 4, 2015.

National Institute of Allergy and Infectious Disease: Flu (influenza). www.niaid.nih.gov/topics/flu/Pages/default.aspx. Accessed May 11, 2015.

Webster RG: Influenza: an emerging disease, 1998. wwwnc.cdc.gov/eid/article/4/3/98-0325_article.htm. Accessed April 4, 2015.

CHAPTER

50 RHABDOVIRUSES, FILOVIRUSES, AND BORNAVIRUSES

A 15-year-old girl picked up a bat and was bitten on her hand. One month later, she developed double vision, nausea, and vomiting. Over the course of 4 days, her neurologic disease developed, and she had a fever of 38.9° C. Rabies was suspected, and rabies virus–specific antibodies were detected in the patient's serum and cerebrospinal fluid (1 : 32 titer). The patient was put into a drug-induced coma with ventilator support and treated with intravenous ribavirin for 7 days, when cerebrospinal fluid antibody titers rose to 1 : 2048. After 3 months, she was able to walk with assistance, ride a stationary cycle for 8 minutes, feed herself a soft solid diet, solve math puzzles, use sign language, and was regaining the ability to speak. This is the only example of a patient surviving without having received timely postexposure rabies immunization.*

1. How is rabies infection confirmed?
2. What is the usual disease progression following a bite from a rabid animal?
3. When is antirabies antibody detected in a normal rabies disease presentation?
4. What is postexposure rabies immunization, and why does it work?
5. How does ribavirin inhibit the replication of rabies and other viruses?

Answers to these questions are available on StudentConsult.com.

• SUMMARIES CLINICALLY SIGNIFICANT ORGANISMS

Rhabdoviruses

Trigger Words

Mad dog, hydrophobia, salivation, bullet-shaped virion, Negri bodies

Biology, Virulence, and Disease

- Medium size, bullet shaped, enveloped, (–) RNA genome
- Encodes RNA-dependent RNA polymerase, replicates in cytoplasm
- Antibody can block disease
- Virus spreads along neurons to salivary glands and brain
- Antibody produced after virus reaches brain
- Incubation period depends on proximity of bite to CNS and infectious dose

Epidemiology

- Zoonosis
- Reservoir in skunks, raccoons, foxes, badgers, bats (aerosols)

Diagnosis

- RT-PCR, antigen detection in biopsy, presence of Negri bodies in infected cells

Treatment, Prevention, and Control

- Immunization with killed vaccine AFTER bite and antirabies immunoglobulin
- Prophylaxis if job-related risk
- Inactivated vaccine for pets
- Vaccinia virus hybrid vaccine for wild animals

• Rhabdoviruses

Members of the family Rhabdoviridae (from the Greek word **rhabdos,** meaning "rod") include pathogens for a variety of mammals, fish, birds, and plants. The family contains *Vesiculovirus* (vesicular stomatitis viruses [VSVs]), *Lyssavirus* (Greek for "frenzy") (rabies and rabies-like viruses), an unnamed genus constituting the plant rhabdovirus group, and other ungrouped rhabdoviruses of mammals, birds, fish, and arthropods.

Rabies virus is the most significant pathogen of the rhabdoviruses. Until Louis Pasteur developed the killed-rabies vaccine, a bite from a "mad" dog always led to the characteristic symptoms of **hydrophobia** and certain death.

*Adapted from Centers for Disease Control and Prevention: Recovery of a patient from clinical rabies—Wisconsin, 2004, *MMWR Morb Mortal Wkly Rep* 53:1171–1173, 2004.

Physiology, Structure, and Replication

Rhabdoviruses are simple viruses encoding only five proteins and appearing as **bullet-shaped enveloped virions** with a diameter of 50 to 95 nm and length of 130 to 380 nm (Figure 50-1; Box 50-1). Spikes composed of a trimer of the glycoprotein (G) cover the surface of the virus. The viral attachment protein, G protein, generates neutralizing antibodies. The G protein of the vesicular stomatitis virus is a simple glycoprotein with N-linked glycan. This G protein was used as the prototype for studying eukaryotic glycoprotein processing.

Within the envelope, the **helical nucleocapsid** is coiled symmetrically into a cylindrical structure, giving it the appearance of striations (see Figure 50-1). The nucleocapsid is composed of one molecule of **single-stranded, negative-sense ribonucleic acid (RNA)** of approximately 12,000 bases and the nucleoprotein (N), large (L), and nonstructural (NS) proteins. The L and NS proteins constitute the RNA-dependent RNA polymerase. The N protein is the major structural protein of the virus. It protects the RNA from ribonuclease digestion and maintains the RNA in a configuration acceptable for transcription. The matrix (M) protein lies between the envelope and the nucleocapsid. The replicative cycle of VSV is the prototype for the rhabdoviruses and other negative-strand RNA viruses (see Chapter 36, Figure 36-13). The viral G protein attaches to the host cell and virions are internalized by endocytosis. Rabies virus binds to either the nicotinic acetylcholine receptor (AChR), neural cell adhesion molecule (NCAM), or other molecules. The viral envelope then fuses with the membrane of the endosome on acidification of the vesicle. This uncoats the nucleocapsid, releasing it into the cytoplasm, where replication takes place. Endosomal vesicles may deliver whole rabies virions along the axon to neuronal cell bodies, where its replication takes place.

The RNA-dependent RNA polymerase associated with the nucleocapsid transcribes the viral genomic RNA, producing five individual messenger RNAs (mRNAs). For rabies virus, this occurs in the Negri bodies. These mRNAs are then translated into the five viral proteins. The viral genomic RNA is also transcribed into a full-length, positive-sense RNA template that is used to generate new genomes. The G protein is synthesized by membrane-bound ribosomes, processed by the Golgi apparatus, and delivered to the cell surface in membrane vesicles. The M protein associates with the G protein–modified membranes.

Assembly of the virion occurs in two phases: (1) assembly of the nucleocapsid in the cytoplasm and (2) envelopment and release at the cell plasma membrane. The genome associates with the N protein and then with the polymerase proteins L and NS to form the nucleocapsid. Association of the nucleocapsid with the M protein at the plasma membrane induces coiling into its condensed form and the characteristic bullet shape of the virion. The virus then buds through the plasma membrane and is released when the entire nucleocapsid is enveloped. Cell death and lysis occur after infection. The time for a single cycle of replication depends upon the cell type and the inoculum size.

Pathogenesis and Immunity

Rabies infection usually results from the bite of a rabid animal (Box 50-2). Rabies infection of the animal causes secretion of the virus in the animal's saliva and promotes aggressive behavior ("mad" dog), which in turn promotes transmission of the virus. The virus can also be transmitted through inhalation of aerosolized virus (as may be found in bat caves), in transplanted infected tissue (e.g., cornea), and by inoculation through intact mucosal membranes.

The virus replicates quietly at the site for days to months (Figure 50-2) before progressing to the central nervous system (CNS). Rabies virus travels by retrograde axoplasmic

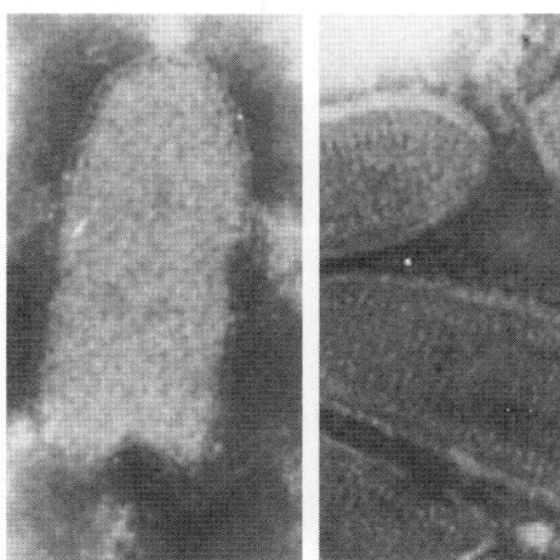
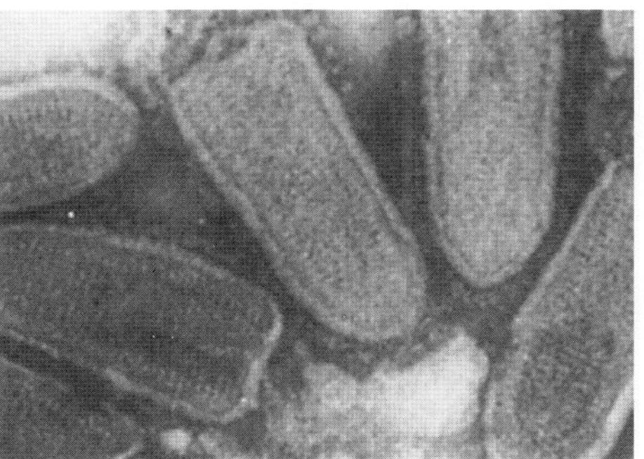

FIGURE 50-1 Rhabdoviridae seen by electron microscopy: rabies virus *(left)* and vesicular stomatitis virus *(right)*. (From Fields BN: *Virology*, New York, 1985, Raven.)

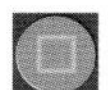

Box 50-1 Unique Features of Rhabdoviruses

Bullet-shaped, enveloped, negative-sense, single-stranded RNA viruses that encode five proteins
Prototype for replication of negative-strand enveloped viruses
Replication in cytoplasm

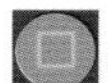

Box 50-2 Disease Mechanisms of Rabies Virus

Rabies is usually transmitted in saliva and acquired from the bite of a rabid animal.
Rabies virus is **not very cytolytic** and seems to remain cell associated.
Virus replicates in the muscle at the site of the bite, with minimal or no symptoms **(incubation phase).**
The length of the incubation phase is determined by the infectious dose and the proximity of the infection site to the central nervous system (CNS) and brain.
After weeks to months, the virus infects the peripheral nerves and travels up the CNS to the brain **(prodrome phase).**
Infection of the brain causes classic symptoms, coma, and death **(neurologic phase).**
During the neurologic phase, the virus spreads to the glands, skin, and other body parts, including the salivary glands, from where it is transmitted.
Rabies infection does not elicit an antibody response until the late stages of the disease, when the virus has spread from the CNS to other sites.
Administration of antibody can block progression of the virus and disease if given early enough.
The long incubation period allows active immunization as a postexposure treatment.

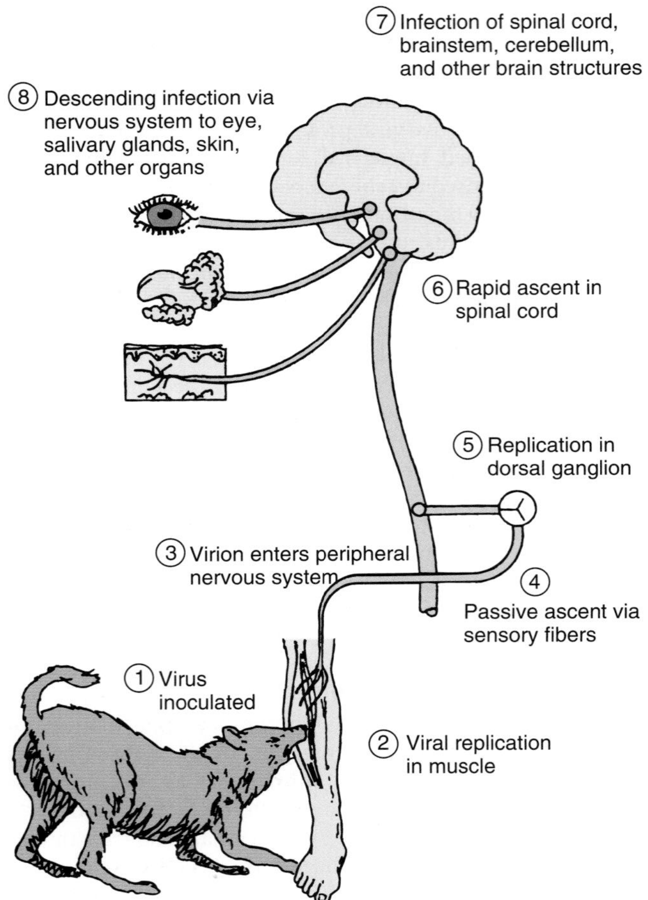

FIGURE 50-2 Pathogenesis of rabies virus infection. Numbered steps describe the sequence of events. (Modified from Belshe RB: *Textbook of human virology,* ed 2, St Louis, 1991, Mosby.)

transport to the dorsal root ganglia and the spinal cord. Once the virus gains access to the spinal cord, the brain becomes rapidly infected. The affected areas are the hippocampus, brainstem, ganglionic cells of the pontine nuclei, and Purkinje cells of the cerebellum. The virus then disseminates from the CNS via afferent neurons to highly innervated sites such as the skin of the head and neck, **salivary glands,** retina, cornea, nasal mucosa, adrenal medulla, renal parenchyma, and pancreatic acinar cells. After the virus invades the brain and spinal cord, encephalitis develops and neurons degenerate. Despite extensive CNS involvement and impairment of CNS function, little histopathologic change can be observed in the affected tissue, other than the presence of Negri bodies (see section on Laboratory Diagnosis).

Rabies is fatal once clinical disease is apparent. The length of the incubation period is determined by the (1) concentration of the virus in the inoculum, (2) proximity of the wound to the brain, (3) severity of the wound, (4) host's age, and (5) host's immune status.

In contrast to other viral encephalitis syndromes, rabies is minimally cytolytic and rarely causes inflammatory lesions. Viral proteins inhibit apoptosis and aspects of interferon action. Neutralizing antibodies are not apparent until after the clinical disease is well established. Little antigen is released, and the infection probably remains hidden from the immune response. Cell-mediated immunity appears to play little or no role in protection against rabies virus infection.

Antibody can block the spread of virus to the CNS and brain if administered or generated by vaccination during the incubation period. The incubation period is usually long enough to allow generation of a therapeutic protective antibody response after active immunization with the killed rabies vaccine.

Box 50-3 Epidemiology of Rabies Virus

Disease/Viral Factors

Virus-induced aggressive behavior in animals promotes virus spread.
Disease has long, asymptomatic incubation period.

Transmission

Zoonosis
- Reservoir: wild animals
- Vector: wild animals and unvaccinated dogs and cats

Source of virus
- Major: saliva in bite of rabid animal (including bats)
- Minor: aerosols in bat caves containing rabid bats

Who Is at Risk?

Veterinarians and animal handlers
Person bitten by a rabid animal
Inhabitants of countries with no pet vaccination program

Geography/Season

Virus found worldwide, except in some island nations
No seasonal incidence

Modes of Control

Vaccination program is available for pets.
Vaccination is available for at-risk personnel.
Vaccination programs have been implemented to control rabies in forest mammals.

Epidemiology

Rabies is the **classic zoonotic infection** spread from animals to humans (Box 50-3). It is endemic in a variety of animals worldwide, except in Australia. Rabies is maintained and spread in two ways. In urban rabies, dogs are the primary transmitter, and in sylvatic (forest) rabies, many species of wildlife can serve as transmitters. In the United States, rabies is more prevalent in cats because they are not vaccinated. Virus-containing aerosols, bites, and scratches from infected bats also spread the disease. The principal reservoir for rabies in most of the world, however, is the dog. In Latin America and Asia, this feature is a problem because of the existence of many stray unvaccinated dogs and the absence of rabies-control programs. Although rare, there are cases of rabies transmission via corneal and organ transplants.

Because of the excellent dog vaccination program in the United States, sylvatic rabies accounts for most of the cases of animal rabies in this country. Statistics for animal rabies are collected by the Centers for Disease Control and Prevention, which in 1999 recorded more than 8000 documented cases of rabies in raccoons, skunks, bats, and farm animals, in addition to dogs and cats (Figure 50-3). Badgers and foxes are also major carriers of rabies in Western Europe. In South America, vampire bats transmit rabies to cattle, resulting in losses of millions of dollars each year.

Although underreported, it is estimated that rabies accounts for 55,000 deaths (mostly children) annually worldwide, with at least 20,000 deaths in India, where the virus is transmitted by dogs in 96% of cases. In Latin America, cases of human rabies primarily result from contact with rabid dogs in urban areas. In Indonesia, an outbreak of more than 200 human cases of rabies in 1999 prompted the killing of more than 40,000 dogs on the islands. The incidence of human rabies in the United States is approximately one case per year, due in large part to effective dog vaccination programs and limited human contact with skunks, raccoons, and bats. Since 1990, human cases of rabies in the United States have been caused primarily by bat variants of the virus. The World Health Organization estimates that 10 million people per year receive treatment after exposure to animals suspected of being rabid.

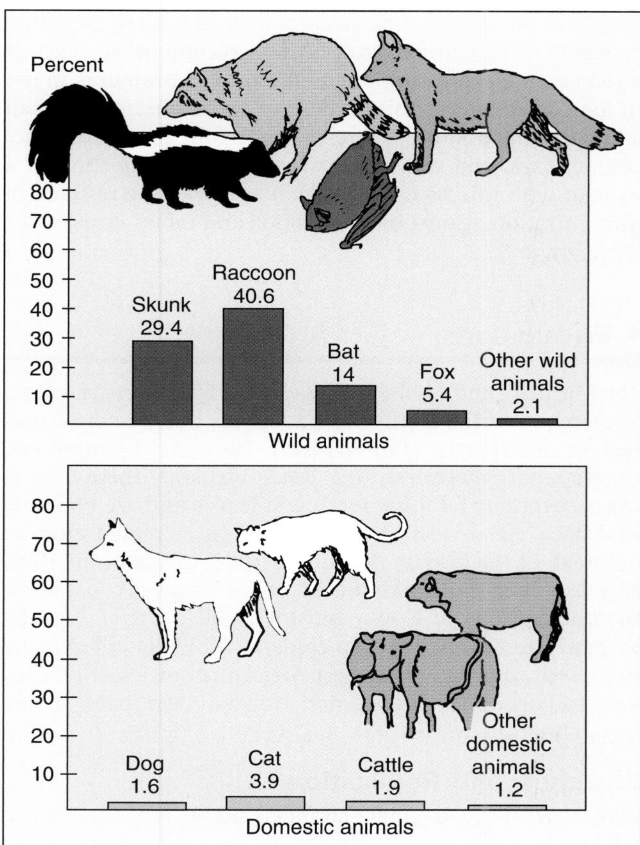

FIGURE 50-3 Distribution of animal rabies in the United States, 1999. Percentages relate to the total number of cases of animal rabies. (Data from Krebs JW, Rupprecht CE, Childs JE: Rabies surveillance in the United States during 1999, *J Am Vet Med Assoc* 217:1799–1811, 2000.)

Clinical Syndromes (Box 50-4)

Rabies is virtually always fatal unless treated by vaccination. After a long but highly variable incubation period, the prodrome phase of rabies ensues (Table 50-1). The patient has symptoms such as fever, malaise, headache, pain or paresthesia (itching) at the site of the bite, gastrointestinal symptoms, fatigue, and anorexia. The prodrome usually lasts 2 to 10 days, after which the neurologic symptoms specific to rabies appear. **Hydrophobia** (fear of water), the most characteristic symptom of rabies, occurs in 20% to 50% of patients. It is triggered by the pain associated with the patient's attempts to swallow water. Focal and generalized seizures, disorientation, and hallucinations are also common during the neurologic phase. Paralysis (15% to 60% of patients) may be the only manifestation of rabies and may lead to respiratory failure.

The patient becomes comatose after the neurologic phase, which lasts from 2 to 10 days. This phase almost universally

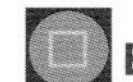 **Box 50-4 Clinical Summary**

Rabies: A 3-year-old girl was found to have a bat flying in her bedroom. The bat apparently was there all night. There was no evidence of any bite wound or contact, and the bat was caught and released. Three weeks later, the child developed a change in behavior, becoming irritable and agitated. This state quickly progressed to confusion, uncontrollable thrashing about, and inability to handle her secretions. She eventually became comatose and died from respiratory arrest.

 **Table 50-1 Progression of Rabies Disease**

Disease Phase	Symptoms	Time (Days)	Viral Status	Immunologic Status
Incubation phase	Asymptomatic	60-365 after bite	Low titer, virus in muscle	—
Prodrome phase	Fever, nausea, vomiting, loss of appetite, headache, lethargy, pain at site of bite	2-10	Low titer, virus in CNS and brain	—
Neurologic phase	Hydrophobia, pharyngeal spasms, hyperactivity, anxiety, depression CNS symptoms: loss of coordination, paralysis, confusion, delirium	2-7	High titer, virus in brain and other sites	Detectable antibody in serum and CNS
Coma	Coma, hypotension, hypoventilation, secondary infections, cardiac arrest	0-14	High titer, virus in brain and other sites	—
Death	—	—	—	—

CNS, Central nervous system.

leads to death resulting from neurologic and pulmonary complications.

Laboratory Diagnosis

The occurrence of neurologic symptoms in a person who has been bitten by an animal generally establishes the diagnosis of rabies. Unfortunately, *evidence of infection, including symptoms and the detection of antibody, does not occur until it is too late for intervention.* Laboratory tests are usually performed to confirm the diagnosis and determine whether a suspected individual or animal is rabid (postmortem).

Antigen detection using direct immunofluorescence or genome detection using reverse transcriptase polymerase chain reaction (RT-PCR) are relatively quick and sensitive assays that are the preferred methods for diagnosing rabies. Samples of saliva are easy to test, but serum, spinal fluid, skin biopsy material from the nape of the neck, brain biopsy or autopsy material, and impression smears of corneal epithelial cells can also be examined.

Infected cells will have intracytoplasmic inclusions consisting of aggregates of viral nucleocapsids **(Negri bodies)** in affected neurons (see Chapter 39, Figure 39-3). Although their finding is diagnostic of rabies, Negri bodies are seen in only 70% to 90% of brain tissue from infected humans.

Rabies antibody titers in serum and cerebrospinal fluid are usually measured by enzyme-linked immunosorbent assay (ELISA). Antibody usually is not detectable until late in the disease, however.

Treatment and Prophylaxis

Clinical rabies is almost always fatal unless treated with post-rabies immunization. Once the symptoms have appeared, little other than supportive care can be given. There is one case of successful cessation of disease progression by post-exposure ribavirin treatment (see introductory case study).

Postexposure prophylaxis is the only hope for preventing overt clinical illness in the affected person. Although human cases of rabies are rare, approximately 20,000 people receive rabies prophylaxis each year in the United States alone. Prophylaxis should be initiated for anyone exposed by bite or by contamination of an open wound or mucous membrane to the saliva or brain tissue of an animal suspected to be infected with the virus, unless the animal is tested and shown not to be rabid.

The first protective measure is local treatment of the wound. The wound should be washed immediately with soap and water or another substance that inactivates the virus. Antirabies immunoglobulin is injected near the wound.

Subsequently, four immunizations with rabies vaccine are administered within 2 weeks, with one initial dose of human rabies immunoglobulin (HRIG) or equine antirabies serum. Passive immunization with HRIG provides antibody until the patient produces antibody in response to the vaccine. The slow course of rabies disease allows active immunity to be generated in time to afford protection.

The rabies vaccine is a killed-virus vaccine prepared through chemical inactivation of rabies infected–tissue culture human diploid cells (HDCV) or chick embryo cells. These vaccines cause fewer negative reactions than the older vaccines (Semple and Fermi), which were prepared in the brains of adult or suckling animals. Serum monitoring and preexposure vaccination should be performed on animal workers, laboratory workers who handle potentially infected tissue, and people traveling to areas where rabies is endemic. HDCV is administered intramuscularly to these individuals and provides 2 years of protection.

Ultimately the prevention of human rabies hinges on effective control of rabies in domestic and wild animals. Its control in domestic animals depends on removal of stray and unwanted animals and vaccination of all dogs and cats. A variety of attenuated oral vaccines have also been used successfully to immunize foxes. A live recombinant vaccinia virus vaccine expressing the rabies virus G protein is in use in the United States. This vaccine, which is injected into bait and parachuted into the forest, successfully immunizes raccoons, foxes, and other animals. Accidental injection of a woman with this vaccinia-rabies hybrid vaccine resulted in immunization against both smallpox and rabies viruses (see Bibliography).

• Filoviruses

The **Marburg** and **Ebola** viruses (Figure 50-4) were classified as members of the family Rhabdoviridae but are now classified as **filoviruses (Filoviridae).** They are **filamentous, enveloped, negative-strand RNA viruses.** These agents cause **severe or fatal hemorrhagic fevers** and are **endemic in Africa.** Awareness of the Ebola virus increased after an outbreak of the disease in Zaire in 1995, in Gabon in 1996, and also after the release of the movie *Outbreak,* based on the book by Robin Cook, and the book *The Hot Zone* by Richard Preston. In 2014, an epidemic of Ebola killed many thousands, mostly in the West African countries of Liberia, Sierra Leone, and Guinea, and isolated cases have spread throughout the world.

Structure and Replication

Filoviruses have a single-stranded RNA genome (4.5×10^6 Da) that encodes seven proteins. The virions form enveloped filaments with a diameter of 80 nm but may also assume other shapes. They vary in length from 800 nm to as long as 1400 nm. The nucleocapsid is helical and enclosed in an envelope containing one glycoprotein. The glycoprotein

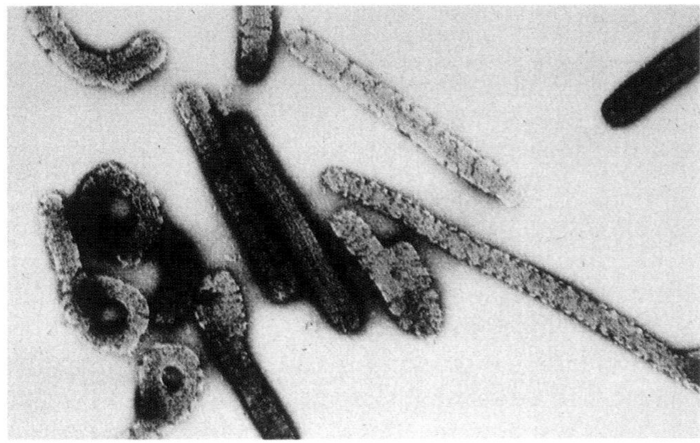

FIGURE 50-4 Electron micrograph of Ebola virus. (Courtesy Centers for Disease Control and Prevention, Atlanta.)

(GP) is cleaved into two components, and a shorter version is secreted. The Ebola virus binds to Niemann-Pick C1 (NPC1), a cholesterol transfer protein, and T-cell immunoglobulin and mucin domain 1 (TIM-1), which is also the hepatitis A virus receptor. The virus enters the cell and replicates in the cytoplasm like the rhabdoviruses.

Pathogenesis

The filoviruses replicate efficiently, producing large amounts of virus in endothelial cells, monocytes, macrophage, dendritic cells, and other cells. Replication in monocytes elicits a cytokine storm of proinflammatory cytokines similar to a superantigen-induced cytokine storm. Viral cytopathogenesis causes extensive tissue necrosis in parenchymal cells of the liver, spleen, lymph nodes, and lungs. Infection of endothelial cells interferes with binding, prevents production of cell adhesion proteins, and causes cytolysis, leading to vascular injury and leakage. Strains with mutations in the glycoprotein gene lack the hemorrhagic component of disease. The widespread hemorrhage that occurs in affected patients causes edema and hypovolemic shock. The virus can also evade host innate and immune responses. A small soluble glycoprotein is shed and can inhibit neutrophil activation and block antibody action. The viral proteins can also inhibit interferon production and action.

Epidemiology

Marburg virus infection was first detected among laboratory workers in Marburg, Germany, who had been exposed to tissues from apparently healthy African green monkeys. Rare cases of Marburg virus infection have been seen in Zimbabwe and Kenya.

Ebola virus was named for the river in the Democratic Republic of Congo (formerly Zaire) where it was discovered. Outbreaks of Ebola virus disease have occurred in the Democratic Republic of Congo, Sudan, and, most recently, Liberia, Sierra Leone, and Guinea. During an outbreak, the Ebola virus is so lethal it can eliminate the susceptible population before it can be spread from the region. In urban areas, spread of the virus is more difficult to control. In rural areas of central Africa, as much as 18% of the population has antibody to this virus, indicating that subclinical infections do occur.

These viruses may be endemic in bats or wild monkeys and can be spread to humans and between humans. Contact with the animal reservoir or direct contact with infected blood or secretions can spread the disease. These viruses have been transmitted by accidental injection and through the use of contaminated syringes. Health care workers tending to the sick and monkey handlers may be at risk. In response to the 2014 epidemic, screening similar to that for SARS coronavirus was initiated at major airports, and all patients in the United States with flulike symptoms are asked for their travel history.

Clinical Syndromes

Marburg and Ebola viruses (Clinical Case 50-1) are the most severe causes of viral hemorrhagic fevers. The illness usually begins with flulike symptoms such as headache and myalgia. Nausea, vomiting, and diarrhea occur within a few days; a rash also may develop. Subsequently, hemorrhage from multiple sites (especially the gastrointestinal tract) and death occur in as many as 90% of patients with clinically evident disease.

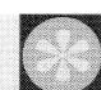

Clinical Case 50-1 Ebola

Emond and associates described the following case of Ebola infection (*Br Med J* 2:541–544, 1977). Within 6 days of a needle-stick accident while handling animal liver infected with Ebola virus, a scientist complained of abdominal pain and nausea. He was transferred to a high-security infectious disease unit and placed in an isolation room. At admission (day 1), he was experiencing fatigue, anorexia, nausea, and abdominal pain and had a fever of 38° C. Interferon was administered twice a day, and it appeared to have worked, except that the next morning his fever returned (39° C). He was given heat-inactivated convalescent serum with no immediate effect. On day 4, he sweated profusely, and his temperature dropped to normal, but he had a new rash on his chest. At midday of day 4, he experienced sudden violent shivering, fever of 40° C, nausea, vomiting, and diarrhea. These symptoms continued for 3 days, with spread of the rash across his body. On day 6, more convalescent serum and rehydration treatment were administered. The patient made a slow recovery over the next 10 weeks. Virus (detected by electron microscopy and inoculation of guinea pigs) was present in his blood from the first day of symptoms. (Currently, the analysis would be performed by reverse transcriptase polymerase chain reaction, with less risk to laboratory personnel.) Virus titers dropped by 1000-fold after interferon treatment and were undetectable by day 9. Treatment of the patient and handling of samples were performed under the strictest isolation conditions available at the time. Even though the scientist took precautions and soaked his hand in bleach as soon as possible, his fate was already sealed. Luckily, interferon therapy and convalescent serum were available to limit the extent of disease progression. In their absence, he would have died from a rapidly progressing hemorrhagic disease.

Laboratory Diagnosis

All specimens from patients with a suspected filovirus infection must be handled with extreme care to prevent accidental infection. Handling of these viruses requires **level 4 isolation** procedures that are not routinely available. Viral antigens can be detected in tissue by direct immunofluorescence analysis and in fluids by ELISA. RT-PCR amplification of the viral genome in secretions can be used to confirm the diagnosis and minimize handling of samples.

Treatment, Prevention, and Control

Antibody-containing serum, artificially produced antibody (ZMAPP), and interferon and ribavirin therapies have been tried in patients with filovirus infections. Infected patients should be quarantined, and contaminated animals should be sacrificed. Handling of the viruses, infected individuals, dead bodies, and contaminated materials requires very stringent (level 4) isolation procedures.

• Borna Disease Virus

Borna disease virus (BDV) is the only member of a family of enveloped, negative-strand RNA viruses. BDV was first associated with infection of horses in Germany. The virus has received considerable recent interest because of its association with specific neuropsychiatric diseases such as schizophrenia.

Structure and Replication

The 8910-nucleotide-long genome of BDV encodes five detectable proteins, including a polymerase (L), nucleoprotein (N), phosphoprotein (P), matrix protein (M), and envelope glycoprotein (G). Unlike most negative-strand viruses, BDV replicates in the nucleus. Although this is similar to the orthomyxoviruses, BDV differs in that its genome is unsegmented.

Pathogenesis

BDV is highly neurotropic and capable of spreading throughout the CNS. BDV also infects parenchymal cells of different organs and peripheral blood mononuclear cells. The virus is not very cytolytic and establishes a persistent infection in the infected individual. T-cell immune responses are important for controlling BDV infections but also contribute to tissue damage leading to disease.

Clinical Syndromes

Although there is limited understanding of the BDV disease in humans, infection of animals can result in subtle losses of learning and memory and in fatal immune-mediated meningoencephalitis. Many of the outcomes of BDV infection of laboratory animals resemble human neuropsychiatric diseases, including depression, bipolar disorder, schizophrenia, and autism. The presence of antibodies to the virus and/or infected peripheral blood mononuclear cells in higher-than-background numbers of patients with schizophrenia, autism, and other neuropsychiatric diseases suggests that BDV either causes or exacerbates these mental illnesses.

Epidemiology

BDV is capable of infecting many different mammalian species (zoonosis), including horses, sheep, and humans. Most outbreaks of the virus have occurred in central Europe, but it has also been detected in North America and Asia. Neither the reservoir nor the mode of transmission of BDV is known. Higher levels of infection of humans are present where outbreaks in horses have been observed.

Laboratory Diagnosis

Infection can be detected by direct analysis for the viral genome and mRNA in peripheral blood mononuclear cells using RT-PCR. Serologic analysis of antibody to the viral proteins continues to be used to identify an association of BDV with human diseases.

Treatment

Similar to many other RNA viruses, BDV is sensitive to ribavirin treatment. Ribavirin treatment may be a reasonable treatment approach for some psychoneurologic disorders if BDV is demonstrated as a cofactor.

Bibliography

Anderson LJ, Nicholson TG, Tauxe RV, et al: Human rabies in the United States, 1960–1979: epidemiology, diagnosis, and prevention, *Ann Intern Med* 100:728–735, 1984.

Centers for Disease Control and Prevention: Rabies vaccine, absorbed: a new rabies vaccine for use in humans, *MMWR Morb Mortal Wkly Rep* 37:217–223, 1988.

Cohen J, Powderly WG: *Infectious diseases*, ed 2, St Louis, 2004, Mosby.

Fishbein DB: Rabies, *Infect Dis Clin North Am* 5:53–71, 1991.

Flint SJ, Enquist LW, Racaniello VR, et al: *Principles of virology: molecular biology, pathogenesis and control of animal viruses*, ed 3, Washington, DC, 2009, American Society for Microbiology Press.

Knipe DM, Howley PM: *Fields virology*, ed 6, Philadelphia, 2013, Lippincott Williams & Wilkins.

Plotkin SA: Rabies: state of the art clinical article, *Clin Infect Dis* 30:4–12, 2000.

Richman DD, Whitley RJ, Hayden FG: *Clinical virology*, ed 3, Washington, DC, 2009, American Society for Microbiology Press.

Rupprecht CE: Human infection due to recombinant vaccinia-rabies glycoprotein virus, *N Engl J Med* 345:582–586, 2001.

Schnell MJ, McGettigan JP, Wirblich C, et al: The cell biology of rabies virus: using stealth to reach the brain, *Nat Rev Microbiol* 8:51–61, 2010.

Steele JH: Rabies in the Americas and remarks on the global aspects, *Rev Infect Dis* 10(Suppl 4):S585–S597, 1988.

Strauss JM, Strauss EG: *Viruses and human disease*, ed 2, San Diego, 2007, Academic.

Warrell DA, Warrell MJ: Human rabies and its prevention: an overview, *Rev Infect Dis* 10(Suppl 4):S726–S731, 1988.

Winkler WG, Bogel K: Control of rabies in wildlife, *Sci Am* 266:86–92, 1992.

Wunner WH, Larson JK, Dietzschold B, et al: The molecular biology of rabies viruses, *Rev Infect Dis* 10(Suppl 4):S771–S784, 1988.

Filoviruses

Centers for Disease Control and Prevention: Ebola (Ebola virus disease). www.cdc.gov/vhf/ebola/. Accessed October 14, 2014.

Groseth A, Feldmann H, Strong JE: The ecology of Ebola virus, *Trends Microbiol* 15:408–416, 2007.

King JW: Ebola, 2014. http://emedicine.medscape.com/article/216288-overview. Accessed October 14, 2014.

Klenk HD: Marburg and Ebola viruses, *Curr Top Microbiol Immunol* 235:225, 1999.

Mohamadzadeh M, Chen L, Schmaljon AL: How Ebola and Marburg viruses battle the immune system, *Nat Rev Immunol* 7:556–567, 2007.

Preston R: *The hot zone*, New York, 1994, Random House.

Sodhi A: Ebola virus disease, *Postgrad Med* 99:75–76, 1996.

Bornaviruses

Jordan I, Lipkin WI: Borna disease virus, *Rev Med Virol* 11:37–57, 2001.

Richt JA, Pfeuffer I, Christ M, et al: Borna disease virus infection in animals and humans, *Emerg Infect Dis* 3:343–352, 1997. www.cdc.gov/ncidod/eid/vol3no3/richt.htm.

Websites

Centers for Disease Control and Prevention: Ebola (Ebola virus disease). www.cdc.gov/vhf/ebola/outbreaks/guinea/. Accessed April 4, 2015.

Centers for Disease Control and Prevention: Ebola hemorrhagic fever. www.cdc.gov/vhf/ebola/index.html. Accessed May 11, 2015.

Centers for Disease Control and Prevention: Rabies. www.cdc.gov/rabies/. www.cdc.gov/features/dsRabies/index.html. Accessed April 4, 2015.

Gompf SG, Pham TM, Somboonwit C, et al: Rabies. http://emedicine.medscape.com/article/220967-overview. Accessed April 4, 2015.

Hatalski CG, Lewis AJ, Lipkin WI: Borna disease, *Emerg Infect Dis* 3:129–135, 1997. www.cdc.gov/ncidod/EID/vol3no2/hatalski.htm. Accessed April 4, 2015.

Kapitanyan R, Pryor PW II, Bertolini J, et al: Emergency treatment of rabies. http://emedicine.medscape.com/article/785543-overview. Accessed April 4, 2015.

King JW, Markanday A: Ebola virus. http://emedicine.medscape.com/article/216288-overview. Accessed April 4, 2015.

Richt JA, et al: Borna disease virus infection in animals and humans, *Emerg Infect Dis* 3:129–135, 1997. wwwnc.cdc.gov/eid/article/3/3/pdfs/97-0311.pdf. Accessed May 11, 2015.

WHO: Rabies. www.who.int/topics/rabies/en/. Accessed April 4, 2015.

CHAPTER

51 REOVIRUSES

In January, a 6-month-old boy was seen in the emergency department after 2 days of persistent watery diarrhea and vomiting accompanied by a low-grade fever and mild cough. The infant appeared dehydrated and required hospitalization. The patient attended a day-care center.

1. In addition to rotavirus, what other viral agents must be considered in the differential diagnosis of this infant's disease? What agents would need consideration if the patient were a teenager or an adult?
2. How would the diagnosis of rotavirus have been confirmed?
3. How was the virus transmitted? How long was the patient contagious?
4. Who was at risk for serious disease?

Answers to these questions are available on StudentConsult.com.

• SUMMARIES CLINICALLY SIGNIFICANT ORGANISMS

Reoviruses

Trigger Words

Fecal-oral, infantile diarrhea, double-double (capsid and double-stranded segmented RNA genome), oral vaccine

Biology, Virulence, and Disease

- Medium size, double capsid, double-stranded segmented RNA genome
- Capsid resistant to inactivation
- Encodes RNA-dependent RNA polymerase, replicates in cytoplasm
- Each segment encodes one or two proteins
- Mixed infection results in genetic mixing of segments: reassortment
- Rotavirus induces cholera-type diarrhea
- One of the most serious causes of diarrhea in young children
- Colorado tick fever, zoonosis, dengue-like disease with rash

Epidemiology

- Rotavirus
- Worldwide and ubiquitous, occurs year round
- Fecal-oral spread, very contagious, young children at risk for serious disease

Diagnosis

- ELISA for virus in stool

Treatment, Prevention, and Control

- Treatment: supportive rehydration
- Prevention: oral live vaccines administered 2, 4, 6 months of age
- Control: hand washing and good hygiene

The **Reoviridae** consist of the orthoreoviruses, rotaviruses, orbiviruses, and coltiviruses (Table 51-1). The name reovirus was proposed in 1959 by Albert Sabin for a group of respiratory and enteric viruses that were not associated with any known disease **(*r*espiratory, *e*nteric, *o*rphan)**. The Reoviridae are nonenveloped viruses with **double-layered protein capsids** containing **10 to 12 segments of the double-stranded ribonucleic acid (dsRNA) genomes.** These viruses are stable in detergents, over wide pH and temperature ranges, and in airborne aerosols. The orbiviruses and coltiviruses are spread by arthropods and are arboviruses.

The **orthoreoviruses,** also referred to as **mammalian reoviruses** or simply reoviruses, were first isolated in the 1950s from the stools of children. They are the prototype of this virus family, and the molecular basis of their pathogenesis has been studied extensively. In general, these viruses cause asymptomatic infections in humans.

Rotaviruses cause **human infantile gastroenteritis,** a very common disease. In fact, rotaviruses account for approximately 50% of all cases of diarrhea in children requiring hospitalization because of dehydration. Rotaviruses are even more of a problem in underdeveloped countries, where before the development of vaccines they were responsible for at least 1 million deaths each year from uncontrolled viral diarrhea in undernourished children. Fortunately, newer vaccines have lessened the incidence of this disease worldwide.

• Structure

Rotaviruses and reoviruses share many structural, replicative, and pathogenic features. Reoviruses and rotaviruses have an icosahedral morphology with a double-layered capsid (60 to 80 nm in diameter) (Figure 51-1; Box 51-1) and a double-stranded segmented genome **("double:double").** The name **rotavirus** is derived from the Latin word **rota,** meaning **"wheel,"** which refers to the virion's appearance in negative-stained electron micrographs (Figure 51-2). Proteolytic cleavage of the outer capsid (as occurs in the gastrointestinal tract) activates the virus for infection and produces an **intermediate/infectious subviral particle (ISVP).**

The outer capsid is composed of structural proteins (Figures 51-3 and 51-4) that surround a nucleocapsid core that includes enzymes for RNA synthesis and 10 (reovirus) or 11 (rotavirus) different double-stranded RNA genomic segments. For rotavirus, the outer capsid has two layers, an intermediate layer consisting of the major capsid protein (VP6) and an outer layer that contains the viral attachment protein (VP4) and glycoprotein (VP7). Of interest, rotaviruses resemble enveloped viruses in that they (1) have glycoproteins (VP7, NSP4) that are on the outside of the virion, (2) acquire but then lose an envelope during assembly, and (3) appear to have a fusion protein activity that promotes direct penetration of the target cell membrane.

The genomic segments of rotaviruses and reoviruses encode structural and nonstructural proteins. As for the influenza virus, reassortment of gene segments can occur and thus create hybrid viruses. The genomic segments of reovirus, the proteins they encode, and their functions are summarized in Table 51-2; those of rotavirus are summarized in Table 51-3. Core proteins include enzymatic activities required for the transcription of messenger RNA (mRNA). They include a 5′-methyl guanosine mRNA capping enzyme and an RNA polymerase. The σ1 protein (reovirus) and VP4 (rotavirus) are located at the vertices of the capsid and extend from the surface like spike proteins. They have several functions, including viral attachment and hemagglutination, and they elicit neutralizing antibodies. VP4 is activated by protease cleavage into VP5 and VP8 proteins, exposing a structure similar to that of the fusion proteins of paramyxoviruses. Its cleavage facilitates productive entry of the virus into cells.

Table 51-1 Reoviridae Responsible for Human Disease

Virus	Disease
Orthoreovirus*	Mild upper respiratory tract illness, gastrointestinal tract illness, biliary atresia
Orbivirus/coltivirus	Febrile illness with headache and myalgia (zoonosis)
Rotavirus	Gastrointestinal tract illness, respiratory tract illness (?)

*Reovirus is the common name for the family Reoviridae and for the specific genus *Orthoreovirus.*

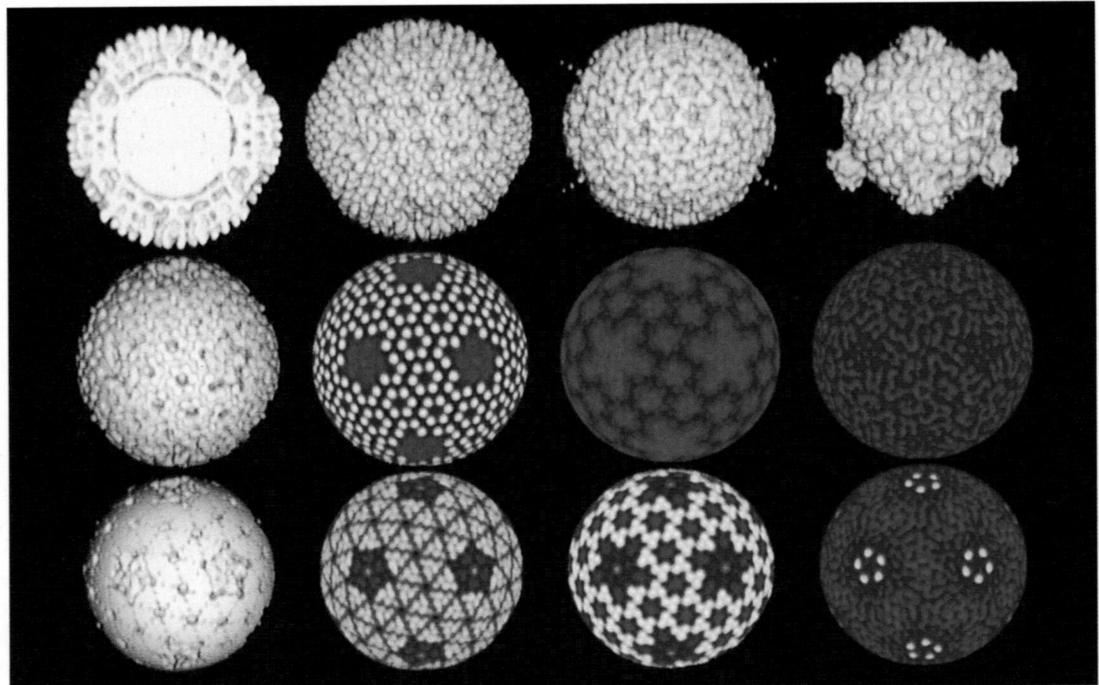

FIGURE 51-1 Computer reconstruction of cryoelectron micrographs of human reovirus type 1 (Lang). *Top, left to right:* Cross section of virion, intermediate/infectious subviral particle (ISVP), and core particle. The ISVP and core particles are generated by proteolysis of the virion and play important roles in the replication cycle. *Center and bottom:* Computer-generated images of the virions at different radii after the outer layers of features have been shaved off. The colors help one visualize the symmetry and molecular interactions within the capsid. (Courtesy Tim Baker, Purdue University, West Lafayette, Ind.)

Box 51-1 Unique Features of Reoviridae

Double-layered capsid virion (60 to 80 nm) has icosahedral symmetry containing 10 to 12 (depending on the virus) unique **double-stranded genomic segments** *(double:double virus).*

Virion is **resistant** to environmental and gastrointestinal conditions (e.g., detergents, acidic pH, drying).

Rotavirus and orthoreovirus virions are activated by mild proteolysis to intermediate/infectious subviral particles, increasing their infectivity.

Inner capsid contains a complete transcription system, including RNA-dependent RNA polymerase and enzymes for 5′ capping and polyadenylate addition.

Viral replication occurs in the cytoplasm. Double-stranded RNA remains in the inner core.

Inner capsid aggregates around (+) RNA and transcribes (–) RNA in the cytoplasm.

Rotavirus-filled inner capsid buds into the endoplasmic reticulum, acquiring its outer capsid and a membrane, which is then lost.

Virus is released by cell lysis.

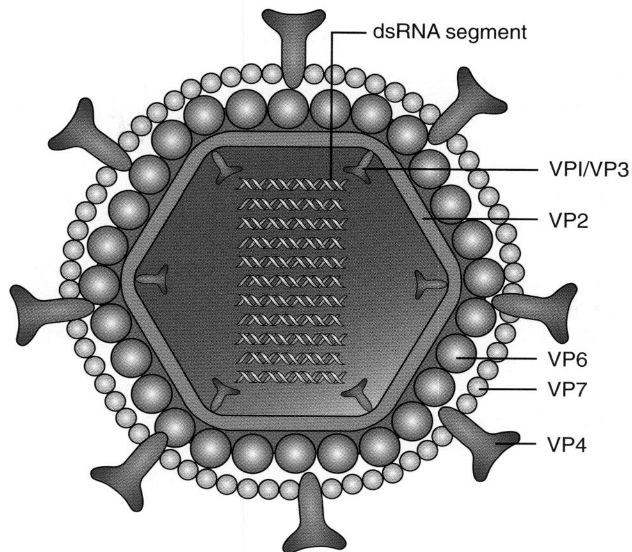

FIGURE 51-3 Schematic of rotavirus. See Table 51-3 for descriptions of the viral proteins. *dsRNA,* Double-stranded ribonucleic acid.

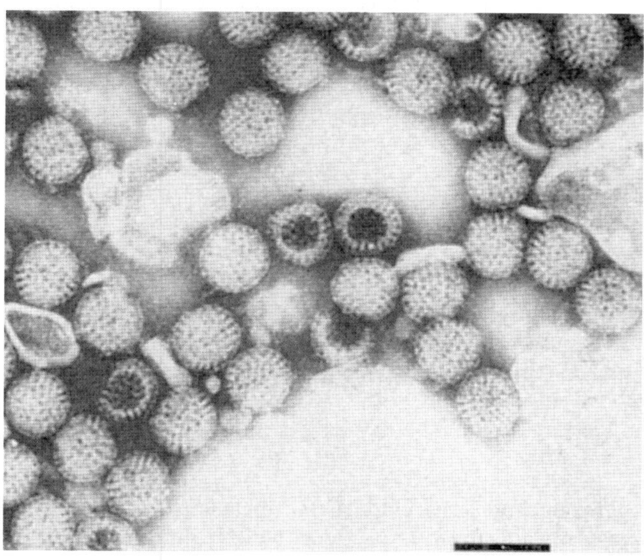

FIGURE 51-2 Electron micrograph of rotavirus. Bar = 100 nm. (From Fields BN, Knipe DM, Chanock RM, et al: *Virology,* New York, 1985, Raven.)

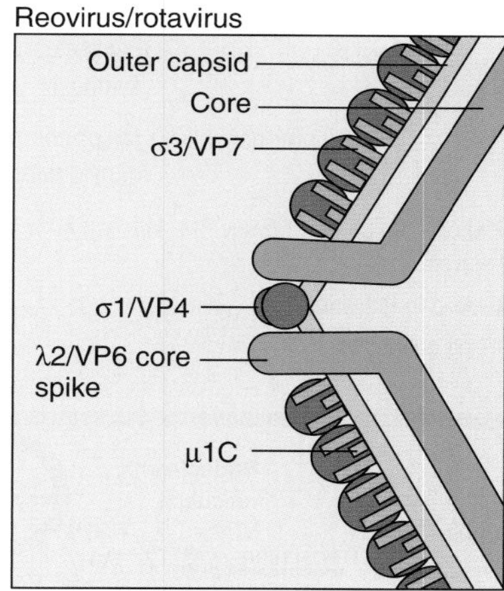

FIGURE 51-4 Structure of rotavirus core and outer proteins. See Tables 51-2 and 51-3 for descriptions of the viral proteins. (Modified from Sharpe AH, Fields BN: Pathogenesis of viral infections. Basic concepts derived from the reovirus model, *N Engl J Med* 312:486–497, 1985.)

Replication

Replication of reoviruses and rotaviruses starts with ingestion of the virus (Figure 51-5). The virion outer capsid protects the inner nucleocapsid and core from the environment, especially the acidic environment of the gastrointestinal tract. The complete virion is then partially digested in the gastrointestinal tract and activated by protease cleavage and loss of the external capsid proteins (σ3/VP7) and cleavage of the σ1/VP4 protein to produce the ISVP. The σ1/VP4 protein at the vertices of the ISVP binds to sialic acid–containing glycoproteins on epithelial and other cells. Additional receptors include the β-adrenergic receptor for reovirus and integrin molecules for rotavirus. The VP4 of rotavirus also promotes penetration of the virion into the cell. Whole virions of reovirus and rotavirus can also be taken up by receptor-mediated endocytosis.

The ISVP releases the core into the cytoplasm, and the enzymes in the core initiate mRNA production. The **dsRNA always remains in the core.** Transcription of the genome occurs in two phases, early and late. In a manner similar to a negative-sense RNA virus, each of the negative-sense (–) RNA strands is used as a template by virion core enzymes, which synthesize individual mRNAs. Virus-encoded enzymes within the core add a 5′-methyl guanosine cap and a 3′-polyadenylate tail. The 5′-methyl guanosine cap was first discovered for reovirus mRNA and then shown to occur for cellular mRNA. The mRNA then leaves the core and is translated. Later, virion proteins and positive-sense (+) RNA segments associate together into corelike structures that

Table 51-2 Functions of Reovirus Gene Products

Genomic Segments (Molecular Weight, Da)	Protein	Function (If Known)
Large Segments (2.8 × 106)		
1	λ3 (inner capsid)	Polymerase
2	λ2 (outer capsid)	Capping enzyme
3	λ1 (inner capsid)	Transcriptase component
Medium Segments (1.4 × 106)		
1	μ2 (inner capsid)	—
2	μ1C (outer capsid)	Cleaved from μ1, complexes with σ3, promotes entry
3	μNS	Promotes viral assembly*
Small Segments (0.7 × 106)		
1	σ1 (outer capsid)	Viral attachment protein, hemagglutinin, determines tissue tropism†
2	σ2 (inner capsid)	Facilitates viral RNA synthesis
3	σNS	Facilitates viral RNA synthesis
4	σ3 (outer capsid)	Major component of outer capsid with μ1C

Modified from Fields BN, Knipe DM, Howley PM: *Virology,* ed 3, New York, 1996, Lippincott-Raven.

*Proteins are not found in the virion.

†Target of neutralizing antibodies.

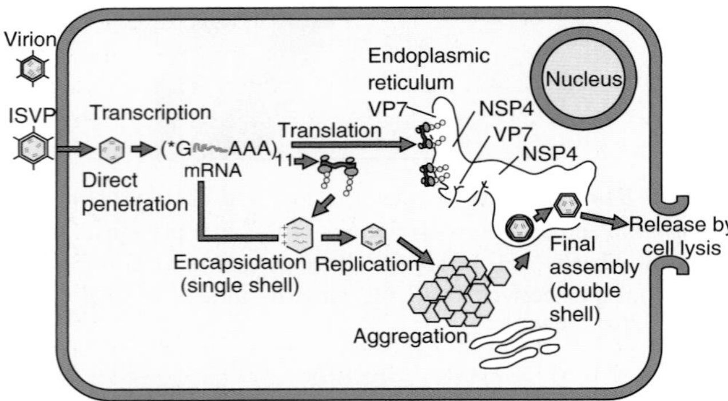

FIGURE 51-5 Replication of rotavirus. Rotavirus virions can be activated by protease (e.g., in the gastrointestinal tract) to produce an intermediate/infectious subviral particle *(ISVP).* The virion or ISVP binds, penetrates the cell, and loses its outer capsid. The inner capsid contains the enzymes for messenger ribonucleic acid *(mRNA)* transcription using the (±) strand as a template. Some mRNA segments are transcribed early, others are transcribed later. Enzymes in the virion cores attach 5′-methyl capped guanosine *(*G)* and 3′-polyadenylate sequence (poly A *[AAA]*) to mRNA. (+) RNA is mRNA and is also enclosed into inner capsids as a template to replicate the ± segmented genome. VP7 and NSP4 are synthesized as glycoproteins and expressed in the endoplasmic reticulum. The capsids aggregate and "dock" onto the NSP4 protein in the endoplasmic reticulum, acquiring VP7 and its outer capsid and an envelope. The virus loses the envelope and leaves the cell on cell lysis.

Table 51-3 Functions of Rotavirus Gene Products

Gene Segment	Protein (Location)	Function
1	VP1 (inner capsid)	Polymerase
2	VP2 (inner capsid)	Transcriptase component
3	VP3 (inner capsid)	mRNA capping
4	VP4 (outer capsid spike protein at vertices of virion)	Activation by protease to VP5 and VP8 in ISVP, hemagglutinin, viral attachment protein*
5	NSP1 (NS53)	RNA binding
6	VP6 (inner capsid)	Major structural protein of inner capsid, binding to NSP4 at ER to promote assembly of outer capsid
7	NSP3 (NS34)	RNA binding
8	NSP2 (NS35)	RNA binding, important for genome replication and packaging
9	VP7 (outer capsid)	Type-specific antigen, major outer capsid component that is glycosylated in ER and facilitates attachment and entry*
10	NSP4 (NS28)	Glycosylated protein in ER that promotes inner capsid binding to ER, transient envelopment, and addition of outer capsid; acts as enterotoxin to mobilize calcium and cause diarrhea
11	NSP5 (NS26)	RNA binding
11	NSP6	Binds to NSP5

ER, Endoplasmic reticulum; *ISVP,* intermediate/infectious subviral particle; *mRNA,* messenger ribonucleic acid.

*Target of neutralizing antibody.

aggregate into large cytoplasmic inclusions. The (+) RNA segments are copied to produce (−) RNAs in the new cores, replicating the double-stranded genome. The new cores either generate more (+) RNA or are assembled into virions.

The assembly processes for reovirus and rotavirus differ. In the assembly of reovirus, the outer capsid proteins associate with the core, and the virion leaves the cell upon cell lysis. Assembly of rotavirus resembles that of an enveloped virus in that the rotavirus cores associate with the NSP4 viral protein on the outside of the endoplasmic reticulum (ER); on budding into the ER, they acquire its VP7 outer capsid glycoprotein. The membrane is lost in the ER, and the virus leaves the cell during cell lysis. Cellular macromolecular synthesis is inhibited within 8 hours of infection.

• Orthoreoviruses (Mammalian Reoviruses)

The orthoreoviruses are ubiquitous. The virions are very stable and have been detected in sewage and river water. The mammalian reoviruses occur in three serotypes referred to as **reovirus types 1, 2, and 3;** these serotypes are based on neutralization and hemagglutination inhibition tests.

Pathogenesis and Immunity

Orthoreoviruses do not cause significant disease in humans. However, studies of reovirus disease in mice have advanced our understanding of the pathogenesis of viral infections in humans. Depending on the reovirus strain, the virus can be neurotropic or viscerotropic in mice. The functions and virulence properties of the reovirus proteins were identified through comparison of the activities of interstrain hybrid (reassortant) viruses that differ in only one genomic segment (encoding one protein). With this approach, the new activity is attributable to the genomic segment from the other virus strain.

After ingestion and proteolytic production of the ISVP, the orthoreoviruses bind to M cells in the small intestine, which then transfer the virus to the lymphoid tissue of Peyer patches lining the intestines. The viruses then replicate and initiate a viremia. Although the virus is cytolytic in vitro, it causes few if any symptoms before entering the circulation and producing infection at a distant site. In the mouse model, the viral attachment protein (σ1) facilitates viral spread to the mesenteric lymph nodes and determines whether the virus is neurotropic.

Mice, and presumably humans, mount protective humoral and cellular immune responses to outer capsid proteins. Although orthoreoviruses are normally lytic, they can also establish persistent infection in cell culture.

Epidemiology

The virus is primarily spread by the fecal-oral route and potentially in aerosols. As already mentioned, the orthoreoviruses have been found worldwide. Most people are infected during childhood.

Clinical Syndromes

Orthoreoviruses infect people of all ages; linking specific diseases to these agents has been difficult. Most infections are asymptomatic or so mild they go undetected. These viruses have been linked to common coldlike, mild upper respiratory tract illness (low-grade fever, rhinorrhea, and pharyngitis), gastrointestinal tract disease, and biliary atresia.

Laboratory Diagnosis

Human orthoreovirus infection can be detected through assay of the viral antigen or RNA in clinical material, virus isolation, or serologic assays for virus-specific antibody. Throat, nasopharyngeal, and stool specimens from patients with suspected upper respiratory tract or diarrheal disease are used as samples. Human orthoreoviruses can be isolated using mouse L-cell fibroblasts, primary monkey kidney cells, and HeLa cells. Serologic assays can be performed for epidemiologic purposes.

Treatment, Prevention, and Control

Orthoreovirus disease is mild and self-limited. For this reason, treatment has not been necessary, and prevention and control measures have not been developed.

• Rotaviruses

Rotaviruses are common agents of infantile diarrhea worldwide. The rotaviruses are a large group of gastroenteritis-causing viruses infecting many different mammals and birds.

Rotavirus virions are relatively stable to environmental abuse, including treatment with detergents, pH extremes of 3.5 to 10, and even repeated freezing and thawing. Within the intestine, proteolytic enzymes such as trypsin enhance infectivity.

Human and animal rotaviruses are divided into serotypes, groups, and subgroups. Serotypes are distinguished primarily by the VP7 (glycoprotein, G) and VP4 (protease-sensitive protein, P) outer capsid proteins. Groups are determined primarily on the basis of the antigenicity of VP6 and the electrophoretic mobility of the genomic segments. Seven groups (A to G) of human and animal rotaviruses have been identified on the basis of the VP6 inner capsid protein. Human disease is caused by group A rotavirus and occasionally group B and C rotaviruses.

Pathogenesis and Immunity

The rotavirus can survive the acidic environment in a buffered stomach or in a stomach after a meal and is converted to the ISVP by proteases (Box 51-2). Viral replication occurs after adsorption of the ISVP to columnar epithelial cells covering the villi of the small intestine. Approximately 8 hours after infection, cytoplasmic inclusions that contain newly synthesized proteins and RNA are seen. As many as 10^{10} viral particles per gram of stool may be released during disease. Studies of the small intestine, either of experimentally infected animals or in biopsy specimens from infants, show shortening and blunting of the microvilli and mononuclear cell infiltration into the lamina propria.

Similar to cholera, rotavirus infection prevents absorption of water, causing a net secretion of water and loss of ions, which together result in a watery diarrhea. The **NSP4 protein** of rotavirus acts in a **toxin-like manner** to promote calcium ion influx into enterocytes which disrupts the cytoskeleton and the tight junctions to cause leakage and also the release of cytokines and neuronal activators which alter water absorption. The loss of fluids and electrolytes can lead to severe dehydration and even death if therapy does not include electrolyte replacement. Of interest, the diarrhea also promotes spread and transmission of the virus.

Immunity to infection depends upon antibody, primarily immunoglobulin (Ig)A, in the lumen of the gut. Antibodies to the VP7 and VP4 neutralize the virus. Actively or passively acquired antibody (including antibody in colostrum and mothers' milk) can lessen the severity of disease but does not consistently prevent reinfection. In the absence of antibody, the inoculation of even small amounts of virus causes infection and diarrhea. Infection in infants and small children is generally symptomatic, whereas in adults it is usually asymptomatic.

 **Box 51-2 Disease Mechanisms of Rotavirus**

- Virus is spread by the **fecal-oral route** and possibly the respiratory route.
- Cytolytic and toxin-like action on the intestinal epithelium causes loss of electrolytes and prevents reabsorption of water.
- **Disease can be significant** in infants < 24 months, but it is asymptomatic in adults.
- Large amounts of virus are released during the diarrheal phase.

Epidemiology

Rotaviruses are ubiquitous worldwide, with 95% of children infected by 3 to 5 years of age (Box 51-3). Rotaviruses are passed from person to person by the **fecal-oral route.** Maximal shedding of the virus occurs 2 to 5 days after the start of diarrhea but can occur without symptoms. The virus survives well on fomites (e.g., furniture and toys) and on hands because it can withstand drying. Outbreaks occur in preschools and day-care centers and among hospitalized infants.

Rotaviruses are **one of the most common causes of serious diarrhea in young children** worldwide. Prior to the vaccines, 4 out of 5 children would get rotavirus diarrhea and 1 out of 7 of them required medical help, with 20 to 50 deaths per year in the United States and as many as 500,000 deaths worldwide. In North America, outbreaks occur during the autumn, winter, and spring. More severe disease occurs in severely malnourished children. In developing countries, rotavirus diarrhea is a very contagious, severe, life-threatening disease for infants and occurs year round. Several outbreaks of group B rotavirus have occurred in China because of contaminated water supplies that affected millions of people.

Clinical Syndromes (Clinical Case 51-1; Box 51-4)

Rotavirus is a major cause of gastroenteritis. The incubation period for rotavirus diarrheal illness is estimated to be 48 hours. The major clinical findings in hospitalized patients are **vomiting, diarrhea, fever,** and **dehydration.** Neither fecal leukocytes nor blood occurs in stool for this form of diarrhea. Rotavirus gastroenteritis is a self-limited disease, and recovery is generally complete and without sequelae. However, the infection may prove fatal in infants who are malnourished and dehydrated before the infection.

Laboratory Diagnosis

The clinical findings in patients with rotavirus infection resemble those of other viral diarrheas (e.g., Norwalk virus). Most patients have large quantities of virus in stool, making direct detection of viral antigen the method of choice for diagnosis. Enzyme-linked immunoassay and latex agglutination are quick, easy, and relatively inexpensive ways to detect rotavirus in stool. Viral particles in specimens can also be readily detected on electron microscopy or by immunoelectron microscopy. Reverse transcriptase polymerase chain reaction (RT-PCR) is useful to detect and distinguish the genotypes of rotavirus.

Cell culture of rotavirus requires pretreatment of the virus with trypsin to generate the ISVP for infection to occur but is not used for diagnostic purposes.

Treatment, Prevention, and Control

Rotaviruses are acquired very early in life. Their ubiquitous nature makes it difficult to limit the spread of the virus and infection. Hospitalized patients with disease must be isolated to limit spread of the infection to other susceptible patients.

No specific antiviral therapy is available for a rotavirus infection. The morbidity and mortality associated with rotavirus diarrhea result from dehydration and electrolyte imbalance. Similar to the therapy for cholera, rehydration therapy is necessary to replace fluids so that blood volume and electrolyte and acid-base imbalances are corrected.

Development of a safe rotavirus vaccine was a high priority for protecting children, especially those in underdeveloped countries, from potentially fatal disease. Animal rotaviruses, such as the rhesus monkey rotavirus and the

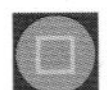 **Box 51-3 Epidemiology of Rotavirus**

Disease/Viral Factors

Capsid virus is resistant to environmental and gastrointestinal conditions.
Large amounts of virus are released in fecal matter.
Asymptomatic infection can result in release of virus.

Transmission

Virus is transmitted in fecal matter, especially in day-care settings.
Respiratory transmission may be possible.

Who Is at Risk?

Rotavirus Group A

Infants < 24 months of age: at risk for infantile gastroenteritis with potential dehydration
Older children and adults: at risk for mild diarrhea
Undernourished people in underdeveloped countries: at risk for diarrhea, dehydration, and death

Rotavirus Group B (Adult Diarrhea Rotavirus)

Infants, older children, and adults in China: at risk for severe gastroenteritis

Geography/Season

Virus is found worldwide.
Disease is more common in autumn, winter, and spring.

Modes of Control

Hand washing and isolation of known cases are modes of control.
Live vaccines use attenuated human or bovine reassorted rotavirus.

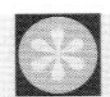 **Clinical Case 51-1 Rotavirus Infection of Adults**

Mikami and associates (*J Med Virol* 73:460–464, 2004) described an outbreak of acute gastroenteritis that occurred over a 5-day period in 45 of 107 children (aged 11 to 12 years) after a 3-day school trip. The source person for the outbreak was ill at the start of the trip. A case of rotavirus acute gastroenteritis is defined as three or more episodes of diarrhea and/or two or more episodes of vomiting per day. Other symptoms included fever, nausea, fatigue, abdominal pain, and headache. The rotavirus responsible for the outbreak was identified from stool of several individuals as serotype G2 group A rotavirus by comparison of the genomic ribonucleic acid migration pattern by electrophoresis, by reverse transcriptase polymerase chain reaction, and by enzyme-linked immunosorbent assay of virus obtained from stool samples. Although rotavirus is the most common cause of infantile diarrhea, this virus, especially the G2 strain, also causes gastroenteritis in adults. This article illustrated the different laboratory methods available for detection of a virus that is difficult to grow in tissue culture.

 **Box 51-4 Clinical Summary**

Rotavirus: A 1-year-old infant has watery diarrhea, vomiting, and fever for 4 days. Enzyme-linked immunosorbent assay analysis of stool confirms rotavirus. The baby is very dehydrated.

Nebraska calf diarrhea virus, share antigenic determinants with human rotaviruses and do not cause disease in humans. A human–rhesus monkey reassortant vaccine (Rotashield) was recalled in 1999 because of the incidence of intussusception (misfolding of the bowel possibly resulting from inflammatory reactions to the vaccine) in a small number of infants. Two new safer rotavirus vaccines have since been developed and are U.S. Food and Drug Administration approved in the United States and elsewhere. RotaTeq consists of five reassortant bovine rotaviruses containing the VP4 or VP7 of five different human rotaviruses. The RotaRix vaccine is a single-strain attenuated human rotavirus. The **vaccines are administered orally as young as possible,** at 2, 4, and 6 months of age.

• Coltiviruses and Orbiviruses

The coltiviruses and orbiviruses infect vertebrates and invertebrates. The coltiviruses cause Colorado tick fever and related human disease. The orbiviruses mainly cause disease in animals, including blue tongue disease of sheep, African horse sickness, and epizootic hemorrhagic disease of deer.

Colorado tick fever, an acute disease characterized by fever, headache, and severe myalgia, was originally described in the 19th century and is now believed to be one of the most common tick-borne viral diseases in the United States. Although hundreds of infections occur annually, the exact number is not known, because Colorado tick fever is not a reportable disease.

The structure and physiology of the coltiviruses and orbiviruses are similar to those of the other Reoviridae, with the following major exceptions:

1. The outer capsid of the orbiviruses has no discernible capsomeric structure, even though the inner capsid is icosahedral.
2. The virus causes viremia, infects erythrocyte precursors, and remains in the mature red blood cells, protected from the immune response.
3. The orbivirus life cycle includes vertebrates and invertebrates (insects).

Colorado tick fever viruses have 12 double-stranded RNA genomic segments, and orbiviruses have 10.

Pathogenesis

Colorado tick fever virus infects erythroid precursor cells without severely damaging them. The virus remains within the cells even after they mature into red blood cells; this factor protects the virus from clearance. The resulting viremia can persist for weeks or months even after cessation of symptoms. Both of these factors promote transmission of the virus to the tick vector.

Serious hemorrhagic disease can result from infection of vascular endothelial and vascular smooth muscle cells and pericytes, thereby weakening capillary structure. The weakness leads to leakage, hemorrhage, and potentially hypotension and shock. Neuronal infection can lead to meningitis and encephalitis.

Epidemiology

Colorado tick fever occurs in western and northwestern areas of the United States and western Canada at elevations of 4000 to 10,000 feet, the habitat of the wood tick *Dermacentor andersoni* (Figure 51-6). Ticks acquire the virus by feeding on a viremic host and subsequently transmit the virus in saliva when feeding on a new host. Natural hosts of this virus include many mammals, including squirrels, chipmunks, rabbits, and deer. Human disease is observed during the spring, summer, and autumn, seasons when humans are more likely to invade the habitat of the tick.

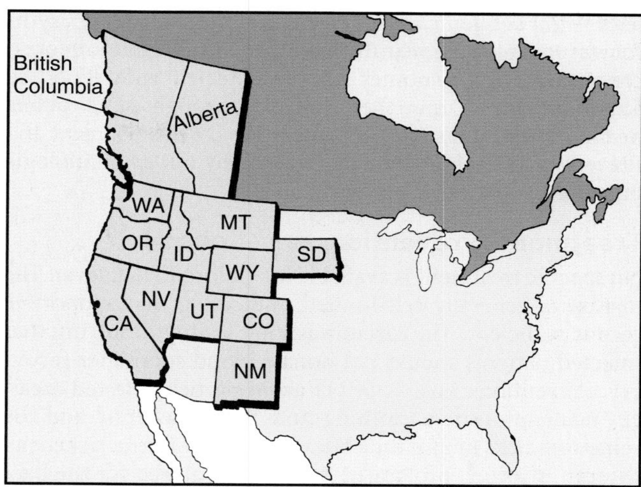

FIGURE 51-6 Geographic distribution of Colorado tick fever.

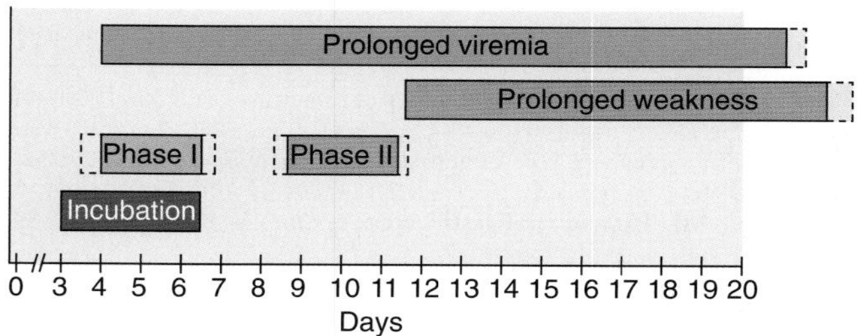

FIGURE 51-7 Time course of Colorado tick fever.

Clinical Syndromes

Colorado tick fever virus generally causes mild or subclinical infection. The symptoms of the acute disease resemble those of dengue fever. After a 3- to 6-day incubation period, symptomatic infections start with the sudden onset of fever, chills, headache, photophobia, myalgia, arthralgia, and lethargy (Figure 51-7). Characteristics of the infection include a biphasic fever, conjunctivitis, and possibly lymphadenopathy, hepatosplenomegaly, and a maculopapular or petechial rash. A leukopenia involving both neutrophils and lymphocytes is an important hallmark of the disease. Children occasionally have a more severe hemorrhagic disease. Colorado tick fever must be differentiated from Rocky Mountain spotted fever, a tick-borne rickettsial infection characterized by a rash, because the latter disease may require antibiotic treatment.

Laboratory Diagnosis

A diagnosis of Colorado tick fever can be established through direct detection of viral antigens, virus isolation, or serologic tests. Viral antigen can be detected on the surfaces of erythrocytes in a blood smear through the use of immunofluorescence, and viral genomes can be detected with RT-PCR. Laboratory tests may be available through state public health departments or the Centers for Disease Control and Prevention. Serology can be performed for epidemiologic purposes.

Treatment, Prevention, and Control

No specific treatment is available for Colorado tick fever. The disease is generally self-limited, indicating that supportive care is sufficient. The viremia is long lasting, implying that infected patients should not donate blood soon after recovery. Prevention consists of (1) avoiding tick-infested areas, (2) using protective clothing and tick repellents, and (3) removing ticks before they bite. Unlike tick-borne rickettsial disease, in which prolonged feeding is required for the bacteria to be transmitted, the coltivirus from the tick's saliva can enter the bloodstream rapidly.

Bibliography

Bellamy AR, Both GW: Molecular biology of rotaviruses, *Adv Virol* 38:1–44, 1990.

Blacklow NR, Greenberg HB: Viral gastroenteritis, *N Engl J Med* 325:252–264, 1991.

Christensen ML: Human viral gastroenteritis, *Clin Microbiol Rev* 2:51–89, 1989.

Cohen J, Powderly WG: *Infectious diseases*, ed 2, St Louis, 2004, Mosby.

Feigin RD, Cherry JD, Demmler GJ, et al: *Textbook of pediatric infectious disease*, ed 5, Philadelphia, 2004, Saunders.

Flint SJ, Enquist LW, Racaniello VR, et al: *Principles of virology: molecular biology, pathogenesis and control of animal viruses*, ed 3, Washington, DC, 2009, American Society for Microbiology Press.

Gershon AA, Hotez PJ, Katz SL: *Krugman's infectious diseases of children*, ed 11, St Louis, 2004, Mosby.

Glass RI: New hope for defeating rotavirus, *Sci Am* 294:47–55, 2006.

Greenberg HB, Estes MK: Rotaviruses: from pathogenesis to vaccination, *Gastroenterology* 136:1939–1951, 2009.

Joklik WK: *The Reoviridae*, New York, 1983, Plenum.

Knipe DM, Howley PM: *Fields virology*, ed 6, Philadelphia, 2013, Lippincott Williams & Wilkins.

Murray PR, Baron EJ, Jorgensen JH, et al: *Manual of clinical microbiology*, ed 9, Washington, DC, 2007, American Society for Microbiology Press.

Nibert ML, Furlong DB, Fields BN: Mechanisms of viral pathogenesis: distinct forms of reovirus and their roles during replication in cells and host, *J Clin Invest* 88:727–734, 1991.

Ramig RF: Rotaviruses, *Curr Top Microbiol Immunol* (vol 185), Berlin, 1994, Springer-Verlag.

Ramig RF: Systemic rotavirus infection, *Expert Rev Anti Infect Ther* 5:591–612, 2007.

Richman DD, Whitley RJ, Hayden FG: *Clinical virology*, ed 3, Washington, DC, 2009, American Society for Microbiology Press.

Roy P: Reoviruses: entry, assembly and morphogenesis, *Curr Top Microbiol Immunol* (vol 309), Heidelberg, Germany, 2006, Springer-Verlag.

Sharpe AH, Fields BN: Pathogenesis of viral infections: basic concepts derived from the reovirus model, *N Engl J Med* 312:486–497, 1985.

Strauss JM, Strauss EG: *Viruses and human disease*, ed 2, San Diego, 2007, Academic.

Tyler KL, Oldstone MBA: Reoviruses, *Curr Top Microbiol Immunol* (vol 233), Berlin, 1998, Springer-Verlag.

Websites

Centers for Disease Control and Prevention: Rotavirus. www.cdc.gov/rotavirus/. Accessed August 7, 2015.

Nguyen DD, Henin SS, King BR: Rotavirus. http://emedicine.medscape.com/article/803885-overview. Accessed August 7, 2015.

Rasouli G, King JW: Reoviruses. http://emedicine.medscape.com/article/227348-overview. Accessed August 7, 2015.

CHAPTER

TOGAVIRUSES AND FLAVIVIRUSES

A 5-year-old Indonesian girl died of hemorrhagic shock. The presence of dengue virus serotype 3 in her blood was confirmed by reverse transcriptase polymerase chain reaction (RT-PCR).

1. How was the child infected with dengue virus?
2. What are the diseases caused by dengue virus?
3. What types of immune responses are protective? Potentially harmful?
4. Where is dengue prevalent? Why?

Answers to these questions are available on StudentConsult.com.

• SUMMARIES CLINICALLY SIGNIFICANT ORGANISMS

Togaviruses

Trigger Words

Arboviruses: mosquito, encephalitis
Rubella: German measles, congenital disease, rash, vaccine

Biology, Virulence, and Disease

- Small size, envelope surrounds icosahedral nucleocapsid, (+) RNA genome
- Encodes RNA-dependent RNA polymerase, replicates in cytoplasm
- Early and late mRNA and proteins produced
- Antibody can block disease
- Virus spreads in blood to neurons and brain
- Prodrome of flulike symptoms due to interferon and cytokine response
- Arboviruses: equine encephalitis viruses (WEE, EEE, VEE)
- Rubella: benign childhood rash, swollen glands. Adult complications: arthritis, encephalitis. Congenital infection: teratogenic, cataracts, deafness, microcephaly, etc.

Epidemiology

- Arboviruses:
  Zoonosis
  Reservoir in birds
  Vectors are *Aedes* and *Culex* mosquitoes
- Rubella:
  Aerosol spread, only infects humans
  Unvaccinated individuals at risk
  Fetus at high risk

Diagnosis

- RT-PCR, ELISA

Treatment, Prevention, and Control

- Arboviruses: mosquito control
- Live attenuated rubella vaccine at 1 year of age in MMR; booster at 4-6 years

Flaviviruses

Trigger Words

Arboviruses: mosquito, encephalitis
Hepatitis C virus: see Chapter 55, Hepatitis Viruses

Biology, Virulence, and Disease

- Small size, envelope surrounds icosahedral nucleocapsid, (+) RNA genome
- Encodes RNA-dependent RNA polymerase, replicates in cytoplasm
- Neutralizing antibody can block disease
- Nonneutralizing antibody promotes dengue virus infection
- Virus spreads in blood to neurons and brain
- Prodrome of flulike symptoms due to interferon and cytokine response
- Arboviruses
- Encephalitis viruses: St. Louis, West Nile, Japanese encephalitis viruses
- Hemorrhagic disease:
  Yellow fever: jaundice, black vomit
  Dengue: hemorrhagic fever, breakbone fever, dengue shock syndrome

Epidemiology

- Endemic to habitat of mosquito
- Arboviruses:
  Zoonosis
  Reservoir in birds
  Vectors are *Aedes* or *Culex* mosquitoes

Diagnosis

- RT-PCR, ELISA

Treatment, Prevention, and Control

- Arboviruses: mosquito control
- Yellow fever virus: attenuated live vaccine

The members of the Togaviridae and Flaviviridae families are enveloped, positive-sense, single-stranded ribonucleic acid (RNA) viruses (Box 52-1). The *Alphavirus* genus of togaviruses and *Flavivirus* are discussed together because of similarities in the diseases they cause and in their epidemiology. Most are transmitted by arthropods and are therefore **arboviruses (*ar*thropod-*bo*rne viruses).** They differ in size, morphology, gene sequence, and replication.

The Togaviridae (togaviruses) can be classified into the following major genera (Table 52-1): *Alphavirus, Rubivirus,* and *Arterivirus.* No known arteriviruses cause disease in humans, so this genus is not discussed further. **Rubella** virus is the only member of the *Rubivirus* group; it is discussed separately because its disease manifestation **(German measles)** and its means of spread differ from those of the alphaviruses. The Flaviviridae include the flaviviruses, pestiviruses, and hepaciviruses (hepatitis C and G viruses). Hepatitis C and G are discussed in Chapter 55.

Box 52-1 Unique Features of Togaviruses and Flaviviruses

Viruses have enveloped, single-stranded, positive-sense RNA.
Togavirus replication includes early (nonstructural) and late (structural) protein synthesis.
Togaviruses replicate in the cytoplasm and bud at plasma membranes.
Flaviviruses replicate in the cytoplasm and bud at intracellular membranes.

• Alphaviruses and Flaviviruses

Alphaviruses and flaviviruses are classified as arboviruses because they are usually spread by arthropod vectors. These viruses have a very **broad host range,** including vertebrates (e.g., mammals, birds, amphibians, reptiles) and invertebrates (e.g., mosquitoes, ticks). Diseases spread by animals or with an animal reservoir are called **zoonoses.** Examples of pathogenic alphaviruses and flaviviruses are listed in Table 52-2.

Structure and Replication of Alphaviruses

The alphaviruses have an **icosahedral capsid** and a positive-sense, single-strand RNA genome that resembles messenger RNA (mRNA). They are slightly larger than picornaviruses (45 to 75 nm in diameter) and are surrounded by an

Table 52-1 Togaviruses and Flaviviruses

Virus Group	Human Pathogens
Togaviruses	
Alphavirus	Arboviruses
Rubivirus	Rubella virus
Arterivirus	None
Flaviviruses	Arboviruses
Hepaciviridae	Hepatitis C virus
Pestivirus	None

Table 52-2 Arboviruses

Virus	Vector	Host	Distribution	Disease
Alphaviruses				
Sindbis*	*Aedes* and other mosquitoes	Birds	Africa, Australia, India	Subclinical
Semliki Forest*	*Aedes* and other mosquitoes	Birds	East and West Africa	Subclinical
Venezuelan equine encephalitis	*Aedes, Culex*	Rodents, horses	North, South, and Central America	Mild systemic; severe encephalitis
Eastern equine encephalitis	*Aedes, Culiseta*	Birds	North and South America, Caribbean	Mild systemic; encephalitis
Western equine encephalitis	*Culex, Culiseta*	Birds	North and South America	Mild systemic; encephalitis
Chikungunya	*Aedes*	Humans, monkeys	Africa, Asia	Fever, arthralgia, arthritis
Flaviviruses				
Dengue*	*Aedes*	Humans, monkeys	Worldwide, especially tropics	Mild systemic; breakbone fever, dengue hemorrhagic fever, and dengue shock syndrome
Yellow fever*	*Aedes*	Humans, monkeys	Africa, South America	Hepatitis, hemorrhagic fever
Japanese encephalitis	*Culex*	Pigs, birds	Asia	Encephalitis
West Nile encephalitis	*Culex*	Birds	Africa, Europe, Central Asia, North America	Fever, encephalitis, hepatitis
St. Louis encephalitis	*Culex*	Birds	North America	Encephalitis
Russian spring-summer encephalitis	*Ixodes* and *Dermacentor* ticks	Birds	Russia	Encephalitis
Powassan encephalitis	*Ixodes* ticks	Small mammals	North America	Encephalitis

*Prototypical viruses.

envelope (Latin **toga,** "cloak"). The togavirus genome encodes **early** and **late proteins.**

Alphaviruses have two or three glycoproteins that associate to form a single spike. The carboxy (COOH) terminus of the glycoproteins is anchored in the capsid, forcing the envelope to wrap tightly ("shrink-wrap") and take on the shape of the capsid (Figure 52-1). The capsid proteins of all the alphaviruses are similar in structure and are antigenically cross-reactive. The viruses can be grouped (complexes) and also distinguished by different antigenic determinants on their envelope glycoproteins.

The alphaviruses attach to specific receptors expressed on many different cell types from many different species (Figure 52-2). The host range for these viruses includes vertebrates (e.g., humans, monkeys, horses, birds, reptiles, amphibians) and invertebrates (e.g., mosquitoes, ticks). However, the individual viruses have different tissue tropisms, accounting somewhat for the different disease presentations.

The virus enters the cell by means of receptor-mediated endocytosis (see Figure 52-2). The viral envelope then fuses with the membrane of the endosome on acidification of the vesicle to deliver the capsid and genome into the cytoplasm.

Once released into the cytoplasm, the alphavirus genomes bind to ribosomes as mRNA. The alphavirus genome is translated in early and late phases. The initial two thirds of the alphavirus RNA is translated into a polyprotein that is subsequently cleaved into four nonstructural early proteins (NSPs 1 through 4). The protease is part of the polyprotein and precedes the site of cleavage. Each of these proteins is a portion of the RNA-dependent RNA polymerase. The enzymes for replication of the genome assemble on a membrane scaffold, a full-length 42S negative-sense RNA is synthesized as a template for replication of the genome, and more 42S positive-sense mRNA is produced. In addition, a 26S late mRNA, corresponding to one third of the genome, is transcribed from the template. The 26S RNA encodes the capsid (C) and envelope (E1 through E3) proteins. Late in the replication cycle, viral mRNA can account for as much as 90% of the mRNA in the infected cell. The abundance of late mRNAs allows production of a large amount of the structural proteins required for packaging the virus.

The structural proteins are produced by protease cleavage of the late polyprotein that was produced from the 26S mRNA. The C protein is translated first and is cleaved from the polyprotein. A signal sequence is then made that associates the nascent polypeptide with the endoplasmic reticulum. Thereafter, envelope glycoproteins are translated, glycosylated, and cleaved from the remaining portion of the polyprotein to produce the E1, E2, and E3 glycoprotein

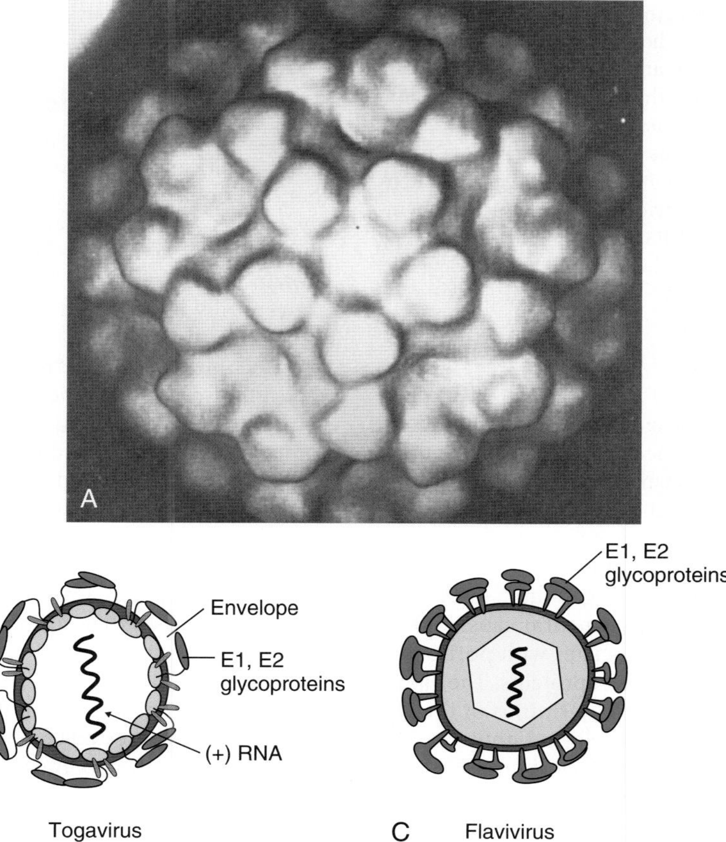

FIGURE 52-1 Alphavirus morphology. **A,** Morphology of the alphavirus virion obtained from cryoelectron microscopy and image processing of the micrographs to show that the envelope is held tightly and conforms to the icosahedral shape and symmetry of the capsid. **B,** Cross section of alpha-togavirus. The envelope is tightly associated with the capsid. **C,** Cross section of flavivirus. The envelope protein surrounds the membrane envelope, which encloses an icosahedral nucleocapsid. *RNA,* Ribonucleic acid. (**A,** From Fuller SD: The T = 4 envelope of Sindbis virus is organized by interactions with a complementary T = 3 capsid, *Cell* 48:923–934, 1987.)

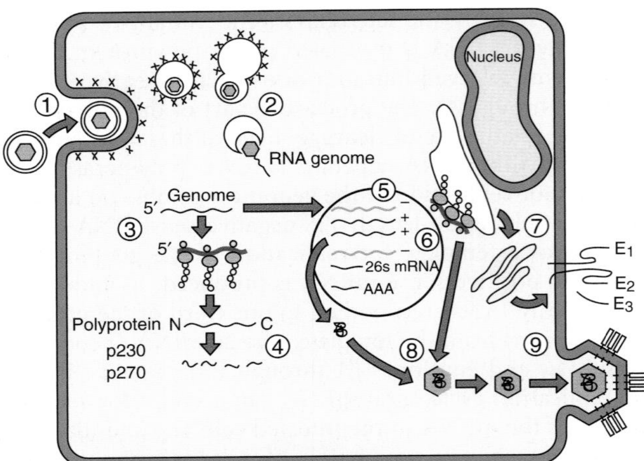

FIGURE 52-2 Replication of a togavirus. *1,* Togaviruses bind to cell receptors and are internalized in a coated vesicle. *2,* On acidification of the endosome, the viral envelope fuses with the endosomal membrane to release the nucleocapsid into the cytoplasm. *3,* Ribosomes bind to the positive-sense ribonucleic acid *(RNA)* genome, and the p230 or p270 (full-length) early polyproteins are made. *4,* The polyproteins are cleaved to produce nonstructural proteins 1 to 4 (NSP1 to NSP4), which include a polymerase to transcribe the genome into a negative-sense RNA template. *5,* The replication enzymes assemble onto cellular membrane scaffolds and the template is used to produce a full-length 42S positive-sense mRNA genome and a late 26S mRNA for the structural proteins. *6,* The capsid (C) protein is translated first and cleaved. A signal peptide is exposed, the peptide associates with the endoplasmic reticulum *7,* where the E glycoproteins are synthesized and glycosylated. They are transferred to the Golgi apparatus and then the plasma membrane. *8,* The capsid proteins assemble on the 42S genomic RNA and then associate with regions of cytoplasmic and plasma membranes containing the E1, E2, and E3 spike proteins. *9,* Budding from the plasma membrane releases the virus. *AAA,* Polyadenylate; *mRNA,* messenger ribonucleic acid.

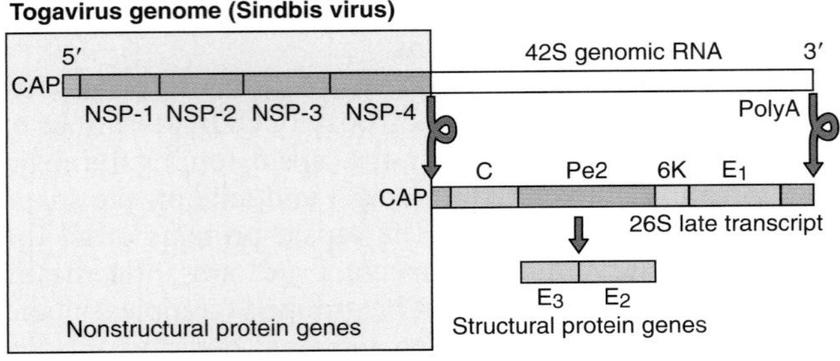

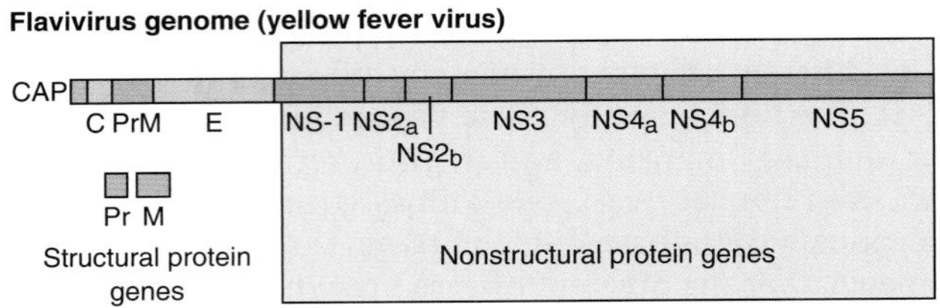

FIGURE 52-3 Comparison of the togavirus (alphavirus) and flavivirus genomes. *Alphavirus:* The enzymatic activities are translated from the 5′ end of the input genome, promoting their early rapid translation. The structural proteins are translated later from a smaller messenger ribonucleic acid (mRNA) transcribed from the genomic template. *Flavivirus:* The genes for the structural proteins of the flaviviruses are at the 5′ end of the genome/mRNA, and only one species of polyprotein is made, which represents the entire genome. *PolyA,* Polyadenylate.

spikes. The E3 is released from most alphavirus glycoprotein spikes. The glycoproteins are processed by the normal cellular machinery in the endoplasmic reticulum and Golgi apparatus and are also acetylated and acylated with long-chain fatty acids. Alphavirus glycoproteins are then transferred efficiently to the plasma membrane.

The C proteins associate with the genomic RNA soon after their synthesis and form an icosahedral capsid. Once this step is completed, the capsid associates with portions of the membrane expressing the viral glycoproteins. The alphavirus capsid has binding sites for the C-terminus of the glycoprotein spike, which pulls the envelope tightly around itself in a manner like shrink-wrapping (see Figures 52-1 and 52-2). Alphaviruses are released on budding from the plasma membrane.

Of interest, the western equine encephalitis virus (WEEV) was created by recombination of two alphaviruses, the eastern equine encephalitis virus (EEEV) and the Sindbis virus. The beginning of the WEEV genome is almost identical to EEEV, with similar glycoproteins and virulence genes, whereas the end of the genome resembles Sindbis.

Structure and Replication of Flaviviruses

The flaviviruses also have a positive-strand RNA genome, an icosahedral capsid, and an envelope but are slightly smaller than an alphavirus (40 to 65 nm in diameter). The E viral glycoprotein folds over, pairs up with another E glycoprotein, and lies flat across the surface of the virion to form an outer protein layer (see Figure 52-1). Most of the flaviviruses are antigenically related, and antibodies to one virus may neutralize another virus.

Attachment and penetration of the flaviviruses occur in the same way as described for the alphaviruses. Antibody can enhance infectivity and promote viral uptake into macrophages, monocytes, and other cells that have Fc receptors when the virus is coated with antibody. The major differences between alphaviruses and flaviviruses are in the organization of their genomes and their mechanisms of protein synthesis. The entire flavivirus genome is translated into a single polyprotein in a manner more similar to the process for picornaviruses than for alphaviruses (Figure 52-3). As a result, there is no temporal distinction in the translation of the different viral proteins. The polyprotein produced from the yellow fever genome contains five nonstructural proteins, including a protease and components of the RNA-dependent RNA polymerase, plus the capsid and envelope structural proteins.

Unlike in the alphavirus genome, the structural genes are at the 5′-end of the flavivirus genome. As a result, the portions of the polyprotein containing the structural (not the catalytic) proteins are synthesized first and with the greatest efficiency. This arrangement may allow production of more structural proteins, but it decreases the efficiency of nonstructural protein synthesis and the initiation of viral replication. This feature of flaviviruses may contribute to the lag before detection of their replication.

The entire flavivirus polyprotein associates with the endoplasmic reticulum membrane and then is cleaved into its components. Unlike the togaviruses, the flaviviruses acquire their envelope by budding into the endoplasmic reticulum rather than at the cell surface. The virus is then released by exocytosis or cell lysis mechanisms. This route is less efficient, and the virus may remain cell associated.

Pathogenesis and Immunity

Because the arboviruses are acquired from the bite of an arthropod such as a mosquito, knowledge of the course of infection in both the vertebrate host and the invertebrate vector is important for an understanding of the diseases. These viruses can cause lytic or persistent infections of both vertebrate and invertebrate hosts (Box 52-2). Infections of invertebrates are usually persistent, with continued virus production.

The death of an infected cell results from a combination of virus-induced insults. The large amount of viral RNA produced on the replication and transcription of the genome blocks cellular mRNA from binding to ribosomes. Increased permeability of the target cell membrane and changes in ion concentrations can alter enzyme activities and favor the translation of viral mRNA over cellular mRNA. The displacement of cellular mRNA from the protein synthesis machinery prevents rebuilding and maintenance of the cell and is a major cause of the death of the virus-infected cell.

Female mosquitoes acquire the alphaviruses and flaviviruses by taking a blood meal from a **viremic vertebrate host.** *A sufficient viremia must be maintained in the vertebrate host to allow acquisition of the virus by the mosquito.* The virus then infects the epithelial cells of the midgut of the mosquito, spreads through the basal lamina of the midgut to the circulation, and infects the salivary glands. The virus sets up a persistent infection and replicates to high titers in these cells. The salivary glands can then release virus into the saliva. Not all arthropod species support this type of infection, however. For example, the normal vector for WEEV is the *Culex tarsalis* mosquito, but certain strains of virus are limited to the midgut of this mosquito, cannot infect its salivary glands, and therefore cannot be transmitted to humans.

On biting a host, the female mosquito regurgitates virus-containing saliva into the victim's bloodstream. The virus then circulates freely in the host's plasma and comes into contact with susceptible target cells, such as the endothelial cells of the capillaries, monocytes, dendritic cells, and macrophages.

The ultimate nature of alphavirus and flavivirus disease is determined by (1) the specific tissue tropisms of the individual virus type, (2) the concentration of infecting virus, and (3) individual responses to the infection. These viruses are associated with **mild systemic disease, encephalitis, arthrogenic disease,** or **hemorrhagic disease.**

The initial viremia produces systemic symptoms such as fever, chills, headaches, backaches, and other flulike symptoms within 3 to 7 days of infection. Most of these symptoms can be attributed to the effects of the interferon and other cytokines produced in response to the viremia and infection of host cells. Most viral infections do not progress beyond the mild systemic disease associated with viremia. A secondary viremia can produce sufficient virus to infect target organs (e.g., brain, liver, skin, vasculature), depending on the tissue tropism of the virus (Figure 52-4). The virus gains access to the brain by infecting the endothelial cells lining the small vessels of the brain or the choroid plexus. Hemorrhagic disease and shock, as for dengue virus, results from viral and immune-induced cytolysis of infected vascular endothelial cells exacerbated by extensive cytokine production (cytokine storm), which induces vascular leakage.

The primary target cells of the flaviviruses are of the monocyte-macrophage lineage. Although these cells are found throughout the body and may have different characteristics, they express Fc receptors for antibody and release cytokines on challenge. Flavivirus infection is enhanced 200- to 1000-fold by nonneutralizing antiviral antibody that promotes binding of the virus to the Fc receptors and its uptake into the cell.

Immune Response

Replication of the alphaviruses and flaviviruses produces a double-stranded RNA replicative intermediate that is a good inducer of interferon (IFN)-α and IFN-β. The interferon limits replication of the virus and is also released into the bloodstream to stimulate innate and immune responses.

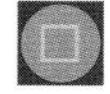

Box 52-2 Disease Mechanisms of Togaviruses and Flaviviruses

Viruses are cytolytic, except for rubella and hepatitis C.
Viruses establish viremia and systemic infection.
Viruses are good inducers of interferon and cytokines, which can account for the flulike symptoms during prodrome.
Viruses, except rubella and hepatitis C, are arboviruses.
Flaviviruses can infect cells of the monocyte-macrophage lineage. Nonneutralizing antibody can enhance flavivirus infection via Fc receptors on cells.

	Flulike Syndrome	Encephalitis	Hepatitis	Hemorrhage	Shock
Dengue	+		+	+	+
Yellow fever	+		+	+	+
St. Louis encephalitis	+	+			
West Nile encephalitis	+	+			
Venezuelan encephalitis	+	+			
Western equine encephalitis	+	+			
Eastern equine encephalitis	+	+			
Japanese encephalitis	+	+			

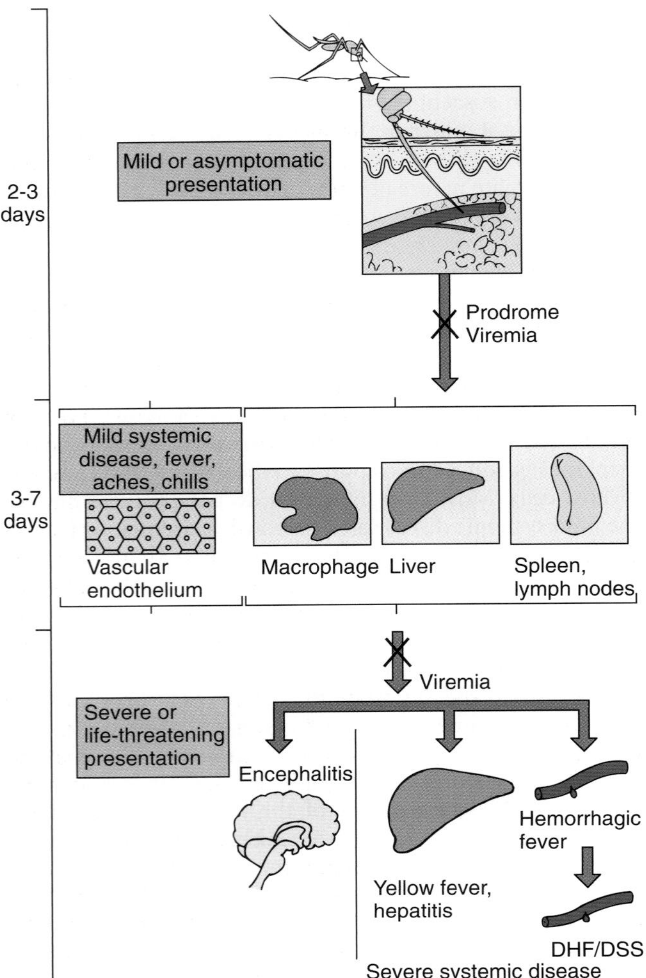

FIGURE 52-4 Disease syndromes of the alphaviruses and flaviviruses. Primary viremia may be associated with mild systemic disease. Most infections are limited to this. If sufficient virus is produced during the secondary viremia to escape innate and immune protection and to reach critical target tissues, severe systemic disease or encephalitis may result. If antibody is present *(X)*, viremia is blocked. For dengue virus, rechallenge with another strain can result in severe dengue hemorrhagic fever *(DHF)*, which can cause dengue shock syndrome *(DSS)* because of the loss of fluids from the vasculature.

Interferon and other cytokines are produced following infection of plasmacytoid dendritic and other cells in blood, causing rapid onset of the flulike symptoms characteristic of mild systemic disease.

Circulating immunoglobulin (Ig)M is produced within 6 days of infection, followed by production of IgG. Antibody to the viral attachment protein blocks viremic spread of the virus and subsequent infection of other tissues. Through recognition of the type-common antigens expressed on all viruses in the family, immunity to one flavivirus can provide some protection against infection with other flaviviruses. Cell-mediated immunity is also important in controlling the primary infection.

Immunity to these viruses is a double-edged sword. Inflammation resulting from the cell-mediated immune response can destroy tissues and significantly contribute to the pathogenesis of encephalitis. Hypersensitivity reactions (initiated by formation of immune complexes with virions and viral antigens) and the activation of complement can cause arthritides and contribute to hemorrhagic symptoms. An antibody to another flavivirus that does not neutralize the virus can enhance the uptake of flaviviruses into macrophages and other cells that express Fc receptors. Immune responses to a related strain of dengue virus that do not prevent infection can exacerbate immunopathogenesis, leading to dengue hemorrhagic fever or dengue shock syndrome.

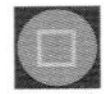

Box 52-3 Epidemiology of Alphavirus and Flavivirus Infection

Disease/Viral Factors

Enveloped virus must stay wet and can be inactivated by drying, soap, and detergents.

Virus can infect mammals, birds, reptiles, and insects.

Asymptomatic or nonspecific (flulike fever or chills), encephalitis, hemorrhagic fever, or arthritis

Transmission

Specific arthropods characteristic of each virus (zoonosis: arbovirus)

Who Is at Risk?

People who enter ecologic niche of arthropods infected by arboviruses

Geography/Season

Endemic regions for each arbovirus are determined by habitat of mosquito or other vector.

Aedes mosquito, which carries dengue and yellow fever, is found in urban areas and in pools of water.

Culex mosquito, which carries St. Louis encephalitis and West Nile encephalitis viruses, is found in forest and urban areas.

Disease is more common in summer.

Modes of Control

Mosquito breeding sites and mosquitoes should be eliminated.

Live attenuated yellow fever virus and inactivated Japanese encephalitis virus vaccines

Epidemiology

Alphaviruses and most flaviviruses are prototypical arboviruses (Box 52-3). To be an arbovirus, the virus must be able to (1) infect both vertebrates and invertebrates, (2) initiate a sufficient viremia in a vertebrate host for a sufficient time to allow acquisition of the virus by the invertebrate vector, and (3) initiate a persistent productive infection of the salivary gland of the invertebrate to provide virus for the infection of other host animals. **Humans are usually "dead-end" hosts** in that they cannot spread the virus back to the vector because they do not maintain a persistent viremia. *If the virus is not in the blood, the mosquito cannot acquire it.* A full cycle of infection occurs when the virus is transmitted by the arthropod vector and amplified in a susceptible, immunologically naïve host **(reservoir),** allowing reinfection of other arthropods (Figure 52-5). The vectors, natural hosts, and geographic distribution of representative alphaviruses and flaviviruses are listed in Table 52-2.

These viruses are usually restricted to a specific arthropod vector, its vertebrate host, and their ecologic niche. The most

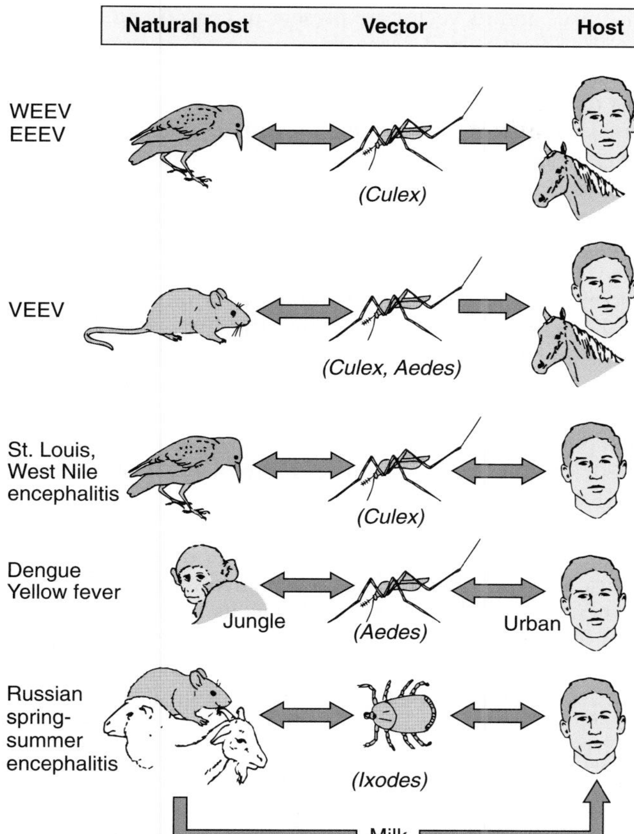

FIGURE 52-5 Patterns of alphavirus and flavivirus transmission. Birds and small mammals are the hosts that maintain and amplify an arbovirus, which is spread by the insect vector upon a blood meal. A *double arrow* indicates a cycle of replication in both host (including man) and vector. "Dead-end" infections with no transmission of the virus back to the vector are indicated by the single arrow. *EEEV,* Eastern equine encephalitis virus; *VEEV,* Venezuelan equine encephalitis virus; *WEEV,* western equine encephalitis virus.

common vector is the mosquito, but ticks and sandflies spread some arboviruses. Even in a tropical region overrun with mosquitoes, spread of these viruses is still restricted to a specific genus of mosquitoes. Not all arthropods can act as good vectors for each virus. For example, *Culex quinquefasciatus* is resistant to infection by WEEV (alphavirus) but is an excellent vector for St. Louis encephalitis virus (flavivirus).

Birds and small mammals are the usual reservoir hosts for the alphaviruses and flaviviruses, but reptiles and amphibians can also act as hosts. A large population of viremic animals can develop in these species to continue the infection cycle of the virus. For example, West Nile encephalitis virus (WNV) was first noted in 1999 as an outbreak in New York by the unusual deaths of captive birds at the Bronx Zoo. Reverse transcriptase polymerase chain reaction (RT-PCR) analysis identified the virus as WNV. The virus is transmitted by *Culex pipiens* mosquitoes, and crows, blue jays, and other wild birds are the reservoir. The virus spread throughout the United States, and by 2006, the virus and human disease had been noted in almost every state. WNV establishes a sufficient viremia in humans to be a risk factor for transmission through blood transfusions. Documentation of two such cases has led to screening blood donors for WNV and rejecting donors who have fever and headache during the week of blood donation.

Arbovirus diseases occur during the summer months and rainy seasons, when the arthropods breed, and the arboviruses are cycled among a host reservoir (birds), an arthropod (e.g., mosquitoes), and human hosts. This cycle maintains and increases the amount of virus in the environment. In the winter, the vector is not present to maintain the virus. The virus may either (1) persist in arthropod larvae or eggs or in reptiles or amphibians that remain in the locale or (2) migrate with the birds and then return during the summer.

When humans travel into the ecologic niche of the mosquito vector, they risk being infected by the virus. Pools of standing water, drainage ditches, and trash dumps in cities can also provide breeding grounds for mosquitoes such as *Aedes aegypti,* the vector for yellow fever, dengue, and chikungunya viruses. An increase in the population of these mosquitoes, as has occurred in the United States, puts the human population at risk for infection. Health departments in many areas monitor birds and mosquitoes caught in traps for arboviruses and initiate control measures such as insecticide spraying when necessary.

Urban outbreaks of arbovirus infections occur when the reservoirs for the virus are humans or urban animals. Humans can be reservoir hosts for yellow fever, dengue, and chikungunya viruses (see Figure 52-5). These viruses are maintained by *Aedes* mosquitoes in a **sylvatic** or **jungle cycle,** in which monkeys are the natural host, and also in an **urban cycle,** in which humans are the host. *A. aegypti,* a vector for each of these viruses, is a household mosquito. It breeds in pools of water, open sewers, and other accumulations of water in cities. St. Louis encephalitis and WNV are maintained in an urban environment because their vectors, *Culex* mosquitoes, breed in stagnant water, including puddles and sewage, and the reservoir group includes common city birds (e.g., crows). A large number of inapparent infections accompanies the incidence or an outbreak of arbovirus encephalitis.

Clinical Syndromes

More humans are infected with alphaviruses and flaviviruses than show significant characteristic symptoms. The incidence of arbovirus disease is sporadic. Alphavirus infections are usually asymptomatic or cause low-grade disease such as **flulike symptoms** (chills, fever, rash, aches) that correlate with systemic infection during the initial viremia. EEEV, WEEV, and Venezuelan equine encephalitis virus (VEEV) infections can progress to **encephalitis** in humans. The equine encephalitis viruses are usually more of a problem to livestock than to humans. An affected human may experience fever, headache, and decreased consciousness 3 to 10 days after infection. Unlike herpes simplex virus encephalitis, the disease generally resolves without significant sequelae, but there is the possibility of paralysis, mental disability, seizures, and death. The name **chikungunya** (Swahili for "that which bends up") refers to the crippling arthritis associated with serious disease caused by infection with these viruses. Like dengue virus, chikungunya virus is spread by *A. aegypti,* but a recently developed mutant virus can be spread by *A. albopictus* (the Asian tiger mosquito). The incidence of chikungunya has greatly increased since 2000. This disease is prevalent from western Africa across southern Asia to the Philippines and in South America and has spread to the Caribbean Islands and United States because of the return of the *A. aegypti* mosquito, its vector.

Most flavivirus infections are relatively benign, but serious **aseptic meningitis** and **encephalitic** or **hemorrhagic disease** can occur. The encephalitis viruses include **St. Louis, West Nile,** Japanese, Murray Valley, and Russian spring-summer viruses. Symptoms and outcomes are similar to those of the togavirus encephalitides. Hundreds to thousands of cases of St. Louis encephalitis virus disease are noted in the United States annually. Approximately 20% of individuals infected with WNV will develop West Nile fever, characterized by fever, headache, tiredness, and body aches, occasionally with a rash on the trunk of the body and swollen lymph glands usually lasting only a few days (Clinical Case 52-1). Encephalitis, meningitis, or meningoencephalitis occurs in approximately 1% of WNV-infected individuals. Individuals older than 50 years and the immunocompromised are at higher risk for serious disease.

The hemorrhagic viruses are dengue and yellow fever viruses. **Dengue virus** is a major worldwide problem, with at least 100 million cases of dengue fever and 300,000 cases of **dengue hemorrhagic fever (DHF)** occurring per year. The virus and its vector are present in central and northern South America, and cases have occurred in Puerto Rico, Texas, and Florida. The incidence of the more serious DHF has quadrupled since 1985. Dengue fever is also known as **breakbone fever;** the symptoms and signs consist of high fever, headache, rash, and back and bone pain that last 6 to 7 days. On rechallenge with another of the four related strains, dengue can also cause DHF and **dengue shock syndrome (DSS).** Nonneutralizing antibody promotes uptake of the virus into macrophages, which causes memory T cells to become activated, release cytokines, and initiate inflammatory reactions. These reactions and the virus result in weakening and rupture of the vasculature, internal bleeding, and loss of plasma, leading to shock symptoms and internal bleeding. In 1981 in Cuba, dengue-2 virus infected a population previously exposed to dengue-1 virus between 1977 and 1980, leading to an epidemic of more than 100,000 cases of DHF/DSS and 168 deaths.

Yellow fever infections are characterized by severe systemic disease, with degeneration of the liver, kidney, and heart, as well as hemorrhage. Liver involvement causes the jaundice from which the disease gets its name, but massive gastrointestinal hemorrhages ("black vomit") may also occur. The mortality rate associated with yellow fever during epidemics is as high as 50%.

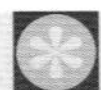

Clinical Case 52-1 West Nile Encephalitis Virus (WNV)

Hirsch and Warner (*N Engl J Med* 348:2239–2247, 2003) described the case of a 38-year-old Massachusetts woman who presented with a progressively worsening headache with photophobia and fever. Because it was August, she was on summer vacation and 10 days earlier (−10) had traveled to St. Louis and stayed for 8 days. While there, she walked in the woods and visited the zoo. A day before the onset of these symptoms (−1), she vacationed along the Atlantic shore and noted that she had been bitten by mosquitos and removed ticks from her dog. Four days later (+4), she was admitted with fever (40° C), chills, rapid heartbeat, confusion, lightheadedness, and lethargy. Although appearing alert, oriented, and only slightly ill, her neck was rigid and Kernig sign was present. The signs of meningitis prompted testing of cerebrospinal fluid, which contained immunoglobulin (Ig)M to WNV and low titers to St. Louis encephalitis (SLE) virus. Patient antibody neutralized WNV but not SLE virus infection of tissue culture cells, suggesting that the activity to SLE was due to cross-reactivity between flaviviruses. Tests for other organisms were negative. She was treated empirically for meningitis and for herpes simplex virus (HSV) (acyclovir). Antibacterial and anti-HSV treatment for meningitis and encephalitis were necessary until the laboratory results were available. On day 5 post onset, she became more lethargic and had difficulty answering questions. Magnetic resonance imaging (MRI) indicated subtle changes in the brain. On day 6, she could not distinguish her right from her left hand, but her headache lessened, and she could respond to commands. On day 7, she had a tremor in her right arm, but her mental status was improving, and by day 8, she was alert and lucid. On day 9, a cranial MRI was normal; on day 10, she was recovered; and on day 11, she was released from the hospital. The season of the year, exposure to insects, and travel by this woman were suggestive of several different arboviral encephalitis diseases in addition to WNV. Viruses in the differential diagnosis included eastern equine encephalitis, SLE, Powassan virus (tick-borne flavivirus), HSV, and WNV. Unlike HSV encephalitis, flavivirus meningoencephalitis usually resolves with limited sequelae.

Laboratory Diagnosis

Detection and characterization of the alphaviruses and flaviviruses is now performed by RT-PCR testing of viral mRNA in blood or other samples. Monoclonal antibodies to the individual viruses have become a useful tool for distinguishing the individual species and strains of viruses. The alphaviruses and flaviviruses can be grown in both vertebrate and mosquito cell lines, but most are difficult to isolate. A variety of serologic methods can be used to diagnose infections, but the serologic cross-reactivity among viruses limits distinction of the actual viral species in many cases.

Treatment, Prevention, and Control

No treatments exist for arbovirus diseases, other than supportive care. *The easiest means of preventing the spread of any arbovirus is elimination of its vector and breeding grounds.* After 1900, when Walter Reed and his colleagues discovered that yellow fever was spread by *A. aegypti,* the number of cases was reduced from 1400 to none within 2 years, purely through control of the mosquito population. Many public health departments monitor bird and mosquito populations in a region for arboviruses and periodically spray to reduce the mosquito population. Avoidance of the breeding grounds of a mosquito vector is also a good preventive measure.

A live vaccine against yellow fever virus and killed vaccines against EEEV, WEEV, Japanese encephalitis virus, and Russian spring-summer encephalitis virus are available. A live Japanese encephalitis virus vaccine is used in China. These vaccines are meant for people working with the virus or at risk for contact. A live vaccine against VEEV is available but only for use in domestic animals. Vaccines consisting of all four strains of dengue virus are being developed to ensure that immune enhancement of the disease on subsequent challenge does not occur. An interesting approach to the dengue virus vaccine consists of chimeric viruses in which the glycoprotein and other genes for each of the other dengue virus strains is inserted into either an attenuated dengue 2 virus or the 17D yellow fever virus.

The yellow fever vaccine is prepared from the 17D strain isolated from a patient in 1927 and grown for long periods in monkeys, mosquitoes, embryonic tissue culture, and embryonated eggs. The vaccine is administered intradermally and elicits lifelong immunity to yellow fever and possibly other cross-reacting flaviviruses.

• Rubella Virus

Rubella virus has the same structural properties and mode of replication as the other togaviruses. However, unlike the other togaviruses, rubella is a **respiratory virus** and **does not cause readily detectable cytopathologic effects.**

Rubella is one of the five **classic childhood exanthems,** along with measles, roseola, fifth disease, and chickenpox. Rubella, meaning "little red" in Latin, was first distinguished from measles and other exanthems by German physicians; thus the common name for the disease, **German measles.** In 1941, an astute Australian ophthalmologist, Norman McAlister Gregg, recognized that maternal rubella infection was the cause of congenital cataracts. Maternal rubella infection has since been correlated with several other **severe congenital defects.** This finding prompted the development of a unique program to vaccinate children to prevent infection of pregnant women and neonates.

Pathogenesis and Immunity

Rubella virus is not cytolytic, but the replication of rubella prevents (in a process known as **heterologous interference**) the replication of superinfecting picornaviruses. This property allowed the first isolations of rubella virus in 1962.

Rubella infects the upper respiratory tract and then spreads to local lymph nodes, which coincides with a period of lymphadenopathy (Figure 52-6). This stage is followed by establishment of viremia, which spreads the virus throughout the body. Infection of other tissues and the characteristic mild rash occur. The prodromal period lasts approximately 2 weeks (Figure 52-7). The infected person can shed virus in respiratory droplets during the prodromal period and for as long as 2 weeks after the onset of the rash.

Immune Response

Antibody is generated after the viremia, and its appearance correlates with the appearance of the rash. The antibody limits viremic spread, but cell-mediated immunity plays an important role in resolving the infection. Only one serotype of rubella exists, and natural infection produces lifelong protective immunity. Most important, serum antibody in a pregnant woman prevents spread of the virus to the fetus. *Immune complexes most likely cause the rash and arthralgia associated with rubella infection.*

Congenital Infection

Rubella infection in a pregnant woman can result in serious congenital abnormalities in the child. If the mother does not have antibody, the virus can replicate in the placenta and spread to the fetal blood supply and throughout the fetus. Rubella can replicate in most tissues of the fetus. The virus may not be cytolytic, but the normal growth, mitosis, and chromosomal structure of the cells of the fetus can be altered by the infection. The alterations can lead to improper development of the fetus, small size of the infected baby, and the **teratogenic effects** associated with congenital rubella infection. The nature of the disorder is determined by the (1) tissue affected and (2) stage of development disrupted. Since the vaccine era, cytomegalovirus has replaced rubella as the most common cause of congenital defects.

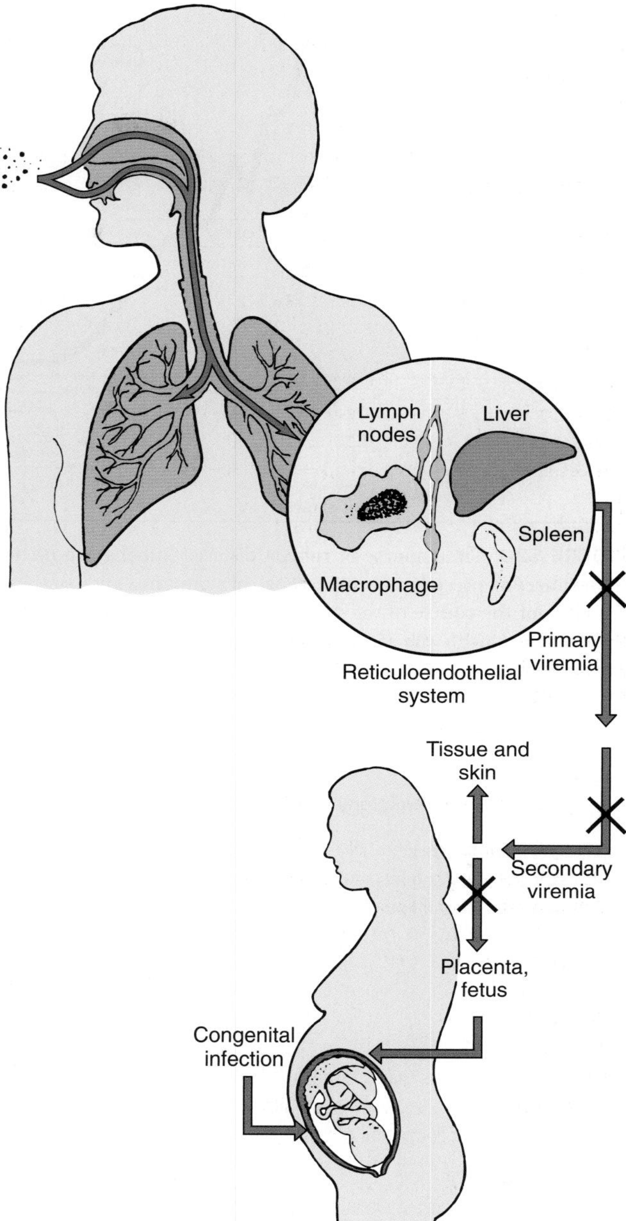

FIGURE 52-6 Spread of rubella virus within the host. Rubella enters and infects the nasopharynx and lung and then spreads to the lymph nodes and monocyte-macrophage system. The resulting viremia spreads the virus to other tissues and the skin. Circulating antibody can block the transfer of virus at the indicated points *(X)*. In an immunologically deficient pregnant woman, the virus can infect the placenta and spread to the fetus.

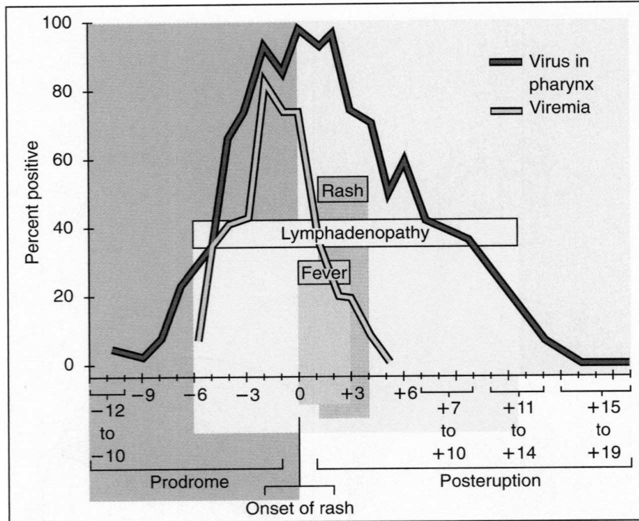

FIGURE 52-7 Time course of rubella disease. Rubella production in the pharynx precedes the appearance of symptoms and continues throughout the course of the disease. The onset of lymphadenopathy coincides with the viremia. Fever and rash occur later. The person is infectious as long as the virus is produced in the pharynx. (Modified from Plotkin SA, Orenstein WA, Offit PA: *Vaccines*, ed 5, Philadelphia, 2008, Saunders.)

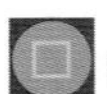

Box 52-4 Epidemiology of Rubella Virus

Disease/Viral Factors

Rubella infects only humans.
Virus can cause asymptomatic disease.
There is one serotype.

Transmission

Respiratory route

Who Is at Risk?

Children: mild exanthematous disease
Adults: more severe disease with arthritis or arthralgia
Fetus < 20 weeks: congenital defects

Modes of Control

Live attenuated vaccine administered as part of the measles-mumps-rubella vaccine

The virus may persist in tissues such as the lens of the eye for 3 to 4 years and may be shed up to a year after birth. Presence of the virus during the development of the baby's immune response may even have a tolerogenic effect on the system, preventing effective clearance of the virus after birth.

Epidemiology

Humans are the only host for rubella (Box 52-4). The virus is spread in respiratory secretions and is generally acquired during childhood. Spread of virus, before or in the absence of symptoms, and crowded conditions (e.g., day-care centers) promote contagion.

Approximately 20% of women of childbearing age escape infection during childhood and are susceptible to infection unless vaccinated. Programs in many U.S. states test expectant mothers for antibodies to rubella.

Table 52-3 Estimated Morbidity Associated with the 1964-1965 U.S. Rubella Epidemic

Clinical Events	Number Affected
Rubella cases	12,500,000
Arthritis-arthralgia	159,375
Encephalitis	2084
Deaths	
Excess neonatal deaths	2100
Other deaths	60
TOTAL DEATHS	2160
Excess fetal wastage	6250
Congenital rubella syndrome	
Deaf children	8055
Deaf/blind children	3580
Mentally retarded children	1790
Other congenital rubella syndrome symptoms	6575
TOTAL CONGENITAL RUBELLA SYNDROME	20,000
Therapeutic abortions	5000

From National Communicable Disease Center: *Rubella surveillance, Report No. 1,* Washington, DC, June 1969, U.S. Department of Health, Education, and Welfare.

FIGURE 52-8 Close-up of the rubella rash. Small erythematous macules are visible. (From Hart CA, Broadwell RL: *A color atlas of pediatric infectious disease,* London, 1992, Wolfe.)

Before the development and use of the rubella vaccine, cases of rubella in schoolchildren would be reported every spring, and major epidemics of rubella occurred at regular 6- to 9-year intervals. The severity of the 1964-1965 epidemic in the United States is shown in Table 52-3. Congenital rubella occurred in as many as 1% of all the children born in cities such as Philadelphia during this epidemic. The immunization program has succeeded in eliminating endemic rubella virus infection in the United States.

Clinical Syndromes

Rubella disease is normally benign in children. After a 14- to 21-day incubation period, the symptoms in children consist of a 3-day **maculopapular** or **macular rash** and swollen glands (Figure 52-8). Infection in adults, however, can be more severe and include problems such as bone and joint pain (arthralgia and arthritis) and (rarely) thrombocytopenia or postinfectious encephalopathy. Immunopathologic

Box 52-5 Prominent Clinical Findings in Congenital Rubella Syndrome

Cataracts and other ocular defects
Heart defects
Deafness
Intrauterine growth retardation
Failure to thrive
Mortality within the first year
Microcephaly
Mental retardation

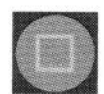

Box 52-6 Clinical Summaries

West Nile encephalitis: During August, a 70-year-old man from a swampy area of Louisiana develops fever, headache, muscle weakness, nausea, and vomiting. He has difficulty answering questions. He progresses into a coma. Magnetic resonance imaging results show no specific localization of lesions (unlike in herpes simplex virus encephalitis). His disease progresses to respiratory failure and death. His 25-year-old niece, living next door, complains of sudden onset of fever (39° C [102.2° F]), headache, and myalgias, with nausea and vomiting lasting 4 days. (See website: www.postgradmed.com/issues/2003/07_03/gelfand.shtml.)

Yellow fever: A 42-year-old man had fever (103° F), headache, vomiting, and backache that started 3 days after returning from a trip to Central America. He appeared normal for a short time, but then his gums started to bleed, he had bloody urine and vomited blood, and he developed petechiae, jaundice, and a slower and weakened pulse. He started to improve 10 days after the onset of disease.

Rubella: A 6-year-old girl from Romania developed a faint rash on her face, accompanied by mild fever and lymphadenopathy. Over the next 3 days, the rash progressed to other parts of the body. She had no history of rubella immunization.

effects resulting from cell-mediated immunity and hypersensitivity reactions are a major cause of the more severe forms of rubella in adults.

Congenital disease is the most serious outcome of rubella infection. The fetus is at major risk until the 20th week of pregnancy. Maternal immunity to the virus resulting from prior exposure or vaccination prevents spread of the virus to the fetus. The most common manifestations of congenital rubella infection are cataracts, mental retardation, cardiac abnormalities, and deafness (Boxes 52-5 and 52-6; see Table 52-3). The mortality in utero and within the first year after birth is high for affected babies.

Laboratory Diagnosis

Isolation of the rubella virus is difficult and rarely attempted. When isolation of the virus is necessary, the virus is usually obtained from urine. Presence of the virus can be detected by RT-PCR detection of viral RNA. The diagnosis is usually confirmed by the presence of antirubella-specific IgM. Antibodies to rubella are assayed early in pregnancy to determine the immune status of the woman; this test is required in many states.

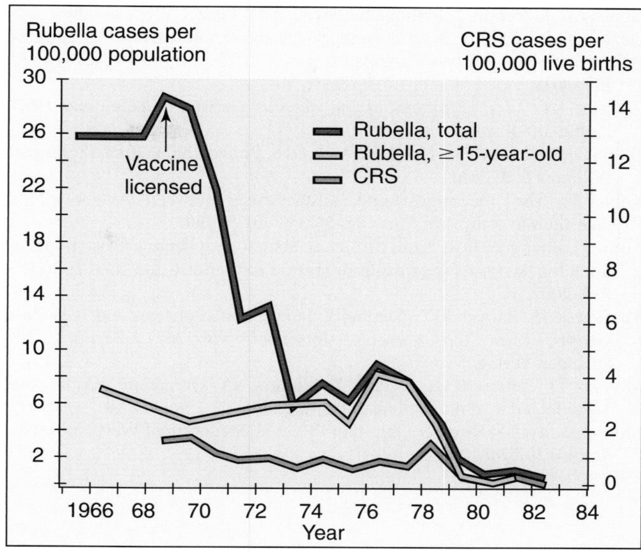

FIGURE 52-9 Effect of rubella virus vaccination on the incidence of rubella and congenital rubella syndrome *(CRS)*. (Modified from Williams MN, Preblud SR: Current trends: rubella and congenital rubella—United States, 1983, *MMWR Morb Mortal Wkly Rep* 33:237–247, 1984.)

Treatment, Prevention, and Control

No treatment is available for rubella. The best means of preventing rubella is vaccination with the live cold-adapted RA27/3 vaccine strain of virus (Figure 52-9). The live rubella vaccine is usually administered with the measles and mumps vaccines **(MMR vaccine)** after 12 months of age. The triple vaccine is included routinely in well-baby care. Vaccination promotes both humoral and cellular immunity.

The primary reason for the rubella vaccination program is to prevent congenital infection by decreasing the number of susceptible people in the population, especially children. As a result, there are fewer seronegative mothers and a smaller chance they will be exposed to the virus from contact with infectious children. Because only one serotype for rubella exists and humans are the only reservoir, vaccination of a large proportion of the population can significantly reduce the likelihood of exposure to the virus.

Bibliography

Chambers TJ, Hahn CS, Galler R, et al: Flavivirus genome organization, expression, and replication, *Annu Rev Microbiol* 44:649–688, 1990.

Chambers TJ, Monath TP: The flaviviruses: detection, diagnosis, and vaccine development, vol 61; The flaviviruses: pathogenesis and immunity, vol 60. In *Adv Virus Res*, San Diego, 2003, Elsevier Academic.

Cohen J, Powderly WG: *Infectious diseases*, ed 2, St Louis, 2004, Mosby.

Fernandez-Garcia MD, Mazzon M, Jacobs M, et al: Pathogenesis of flavivirus infections: using and abusing the host cell, *Cell Host Microbe* 5:318–328, 2009.

Flint SJ, Enquist LW, Racaniello VR, et al: *Principles of virology: molecular biology, pathogenesis and control of animal viruses*, ed 3, Washington, DC, 2009, American Society for Microbiology Press.

Gelfand MS: West Nile virus infection. What you need to know about this emerging threat, *Postgrad Med* 114:31–38, 2003.

Gorbach SL, Bartlett JG, Blacklow NR: *Infectious diseases*, ed 3, Philadelphia, 2004, Saunders.

Gould EA, Solomon T: Pathogenic flaviviruses, *Lancet* 371:500–509, 2008.
Guabiraba R, Ryffel B: Dengue virus infection: current concepts in immune mechanisms and lessons from murine models, *Immunology* 141:143–156, 2014.
Johnson RT: *Viral infections of the nervous system*, Philadelphia, 1998, Lippincott-Raven.
Knipe DM, Howley PM: *Fields virology*, ed 6, Philadelphia, 2013, Lippincott Williams & Wilkins.
Koblet H: The "merry-go-round": alphaviruses between vertebrate and invertebrate cells, *Adv Virus Res* 38:343–403, 1990.
Kuhn RJ, Zhang W, Rossmann MG, et al: Structure of dengue virus: implications for flavivirus organization, maturation, and fusion, *Cell* 108:717–725, 2002.
Mackenzie JS, Barrett ADT, Deubel V: Japanese encephalitis and West Nile viruses, *Curr Top Microbiol Immunol* (vol 267), Berlin, 2002, Springer-Verlag.
Monath TP: Yellow fever vaccine. In Plotkin SA, Orenstein WA, editors: *Vaccines*, ed 4, Philadelphia, 2004, Saunders.
Mukhopadhyay S, Kim BS, Chipman PR, et al: Structure of West Nile virus, *Science* 302:248, 2003.
Nash D, Mostashari F, Fine A, et al: The outbreak of West Nile virus infection in the New York City area in 1999, *N Engl J Med* 344:1807–1814, 2001.
Plotkin SA, Reef S: Rubella vaccine. In Plotkin SA, Orenstein WA, editors: *Vaccines*, ed 4, Philadelphia, 2004, Saunders.
Richman DD, Whitley RJ, Hayden FG: *Clinical virology*, ed 3, Washington, DC, 2009, American Society for Microbiology Press.
Strauss JM, Strauss EG: *Viruses and human disease*, ed 2, San Diego, 2007, Academic.
Tsai TF: Arboviral infections in the United States, *Infect Dis Clin North Am* 5:73–102, 1991.

Websites

Centers for Disease Control and Prevention: Arboviruses. www.cdc.gov/ncezid/dvbd/. Accessed May 13, 2015.
Centers for Disease Control and Prevention: Dengue. www.cdc.gov/dengue/. Accessed April 22, 2015.
Centers for Disease Control and Prevention: West Nile virus. www.cdc.gov/ncidod/dvbid/westnile/index.htm. Accessed April 22, 2015.
Dengue map. www.healthmap.org/dengue/index.php. Accessed April 22, 2015.

CHAPTER

53 BUNYAVIRIDAE AND ARENAVIRIDAE

A 50-year-old man was visiting family in Liberia and stayed in a house infested with rodents. He developed severe flulike symptoms, a sore throat, and red eyes and was treated with amoxicillin and chloroquine. His condition worsened, with increased fever, severe headache, and swollen lymph nodes, tonsils, and spleen. He began to cough up blood and then went into shock and died.

1. How was this individual infected with Lassa fever virus?

2. What are the unique characteristics of arenaviruses?

3. How are they similar to bunyaviruses? Different?

Answers to these questions are available on StudentConsult.com.

• SUMMARIES CLINICALLY SIGNIFICANT ORGANISMS

Bunyaviruses

Trigger Words

Arboviruses: mosquito, encephalitis
Hantaviruses: rodent, hemorrhagic disease

Biology, Virulence, and Disease

- Medium size, enveloped, (–) segmented RNA genome
- Encodes RNA-dependent RNA polymerase, replicates in cytoplasm
- Antibody can block disease
- Virus spreads in blood to tissues, neurons, and brain
- Prodrome of flulike symptoms due to interferon and cytokine response
- Encephalitis: La Crosse, California encephalitis
- Hantaviruses: pulmonary syndrome

Epidemiology

- Encephalitis viruses: zoonosis, reservoir in birds, vector is *Culex* mosquito
- Hantavirus: inhalation of aerosols from rodent urine or feces

Diagnosis

- RT-PCR, ELISA

Treatment, Prevention, and Control

- Arboviruses: mosquito control
- Hantaviruses: rodent control

Arenaviruses

Trigger Words

Rodent, Lassa fever: hemorrhagic disease, lymphocytic choriomeningitis virus: LCMV, meningitis

Biology, Virulence, and Disease

- Medium size, enveloped, (–) segmented RNA genome
- Encodes RNA-dependent RNA polymerase, replicates in cytoplasm
- Antibody can block disease
- Virus spreads in blood to tissues, neurons, and brain
- Prodrome of flulike symptoms due to interferon and cytokine response
- Lymphocytic choriomeningitis (LCMV): meningitis
- Lassa fever: hemorrhagic fever

Epidemiology

- Inhalation of aerosols from rodent urine or feces
- LCMV: worldwide
- Lassa fever: Africa

Diagnosis

- RT-PCR, ELISA

Treatment, Prevention, and Control

- Rodent control

The Bunyaviridae and Arenaviridae share several similarities. The viruses of these families are negative-strand ribonucleic acid (RNA)-enveloped viruses with similar modes of replication. Both are zoonoses; most of the Bunyaviridae are also arboviruses, but the Arenaviridae are not. Many of the viruses from these families cause encephalitis or hemorrhagic disease.

• Bunyaviridae

The Bunyaviridae constitute a "supergroup" of at least **200 enveloped, segmented, negative-strand RNA viruses.** The supergroup of mammalian viruses is further broken down into genera on the basis of structural and biochemical features: *Bunyavirus, Phlebovirus, Nairovirus,* and *Hantavirus* (Table 53-1). Most of the Bunyaviridae are **arboviruses** (*ar*thropod-*bo*rne) that are spread by mosquitoes, ticks, or flies and are endemic to the environment of the vector. The **hantaviruses** are the exception; they are carried by **rodents.** New viruses are still being discovered, including the tick-borne Heartland phlebovirus in the United States in 2012. In 2011, the tick-borne severe fever with thrombocytopenia syndrome virus (SFTSV) was discovered in China.

Structure

The bunyaviruses are roughly spherical particles 90 to 120 nm in diameter (Box 53-1). The envelope of the virus contains two glycoproteins (G1 and G2) and encloses three unique negative-strand RNAs, the large **(L),** medium **(M),** and small **(S)** RNAs that are associated with protein to form nucleocapsids (Table 53-2). The genome segments for the La Crosse and related California encephalitis viruses form circles. The nucleocapsids include the RNA-dependent RNA polymerase (L protein) and two nonstructural proteins (NS_s, NS_m) (Figure 53-1). Unlike other negative-strand RNA viruses, the Bunyaviridae **do not have a matrix protein.** The genera of Bunyaviridae are distinguished by differences in (1) the number and sizes of the virion proteins, (2) the lengths of the L, M, and S strands of the genome, and (3) how they are transcribed.

Replication

The Bunyaviridae replicate in the same way as other enveloped negative-strand RNA viruses. For most Bunyaviridae, the G1 glycoprotein interacts with β integrins on the cell surface, and the virus is internalized by endocytosis. After fusion of the envelope with endosomal membranes on acidification of the vesicle, the nucleocapsid is released into the cytoplasm, and messenger RNA (mRNA) and protein synthesis begin. Like influenza, the bunyaviruses steal the 5′-capped portion of mRNAs to prime the synthesis of viral mRNAs; but unlike influenza, this occurs in the cytoplasm.

The M strand encodes the NS_m nonstructural protein and the G1 (viral attachment) and G2 proteins, and the L strand encodes the L protein (polymerase) (see Table 53-2). The S strand of RNA encodes two nonstructural proteins, N and NS_s. For the *Phlebovirus* group, the S strand is ambisense, such that one mRNA is transcribed from the genome and the other from the (+) RNA template for replication.

The glycoproteins are synthesized and glycosylated in the endoplasmic reticulum, after which they are transferred to the Golgi apparatus but not translocated to the plasma membrane. Virions are assembled by budding into the Golgi apparatus and are released by cell lysis or exocytosis.

Pathogenesis

Most of the Bunyaviridae are arboviruses and possess many of the same pathogenic mechanisms as the togaviruses and flaviviruses (Box 53-2). For example, the viruses are spread by an arthropod vector and are injected into the blood to initiate a viremia. Progression past this stage to secondary viremia and further dissemination of the virus can deliver the virus to target sites such as the central nervous system, liver, kidney, and vascular endothelium to cause disease. Many Bunyaviridae cause encephalitis; others cause hepatic necrosis or hemorrhagic disease (e.g., Crimean-Congo hemorrhagic fever and Hantaan hemorrhagic disease) in ways similar to the toga and flaviviruses. In the latter infection, hemorrhagic necrosis of the kidney occurs often. Like togaviruses, flaviviruses, and arenaviruses, the bunyaviruses are good inducers of type 1 interferons. Bunyavirus disease is due to a combination of immune and viral pathogenesis.

Table 53-1 Notable Bunyaviridae Genera*

Genus	Members	Insect Vector	Pathologic Conditions	Vertebrate Hosts
Bunyavirus	Bunyamwera virus, California encephalitis virus, La Crosse virus, Oropouche virus; 150 members	Mosquito	Febrile illness, encephalitis, rash	Rodents, small mammals, primates, marsupials, birds
Phlebovirus	Rift Valley fever virus, sandfly fever virus, Heartland virus; 38 members	Fly, tick	Sandfly fever, hemorrhagic fever, encephalitis, conjunctivitis, myositis	Sheep, cattle, domestic animals
Nairovirus	Crimean-Congo hemorrhagic fever virus; 6 members	Tick	Hemorrhagic fever	Hares, cattle, goats, seabirds
Uukuvirus	Uukuniemi virus; 7 members	Tick	—	Birds
Hantavirus	Hantaan virus	None	Hemorrhagic fever with renal syndrome, adult respiratory distress syndrome	Rodents
	Sin Nombre	None	Hantavirus pulmonary syndrome, shock, pulmonary edema	Deer mouse

*Additional viruses possess several common properties with Bunyaviridae but are as yet unclassified.

Unlike the other bunyaviruses, rodents are the reservoir and vector for hantaviruses, and humans acquire the virus by breathing aerosols contaminated with infected urine. The virus initiates infection and remains in the lung, where it causes hemorrhagic tissue destruction and lethal pulmonary disease.

Epidemiology

Most bunyaviruses are transmitted by infected mosquitoes, ticks, or *Phlebotomus* flies to rodents, birds, and larger animals (Box 53-3). The animals then become the **reservoirs** for the virus, thereby continuing the cycle of infection. Humans are infected when they enter the environment of the insect vector (Figure 53-2) but are usually dead-end hosts. Transmission occurs during the summer, but unlike many other arboviruses, many of the Bunyaviridae can survive a winter in the mosquito eggs and remain in a locale.

Many of the members of this virus family are found in South America, southeastern Europe, Southeast Asia, and Africa and bear the exotic names of their ecologic niches.

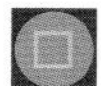

Box 53-1 Unique Features of Bunyaviruses

There are at least 200 related viruses in five genera that share a common morphology and basic components.
Virion is enveloped with three (L, M, S) negative-sense ribonucleic acid nucleocapsids but no matrix proteins.
Virus replicates in the cytoplasm.
Virus can infect humans, animals, and arthropods.
Virus in an arthropod can be transmitted to its eggs.

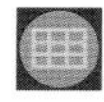

Table 53-2 Genome and Proteins of California Encephalitis Virus

Genome*	Proteins
L	RNA polymerase, 170 kDa
M	G1 glycoprotein, 75 kDa
	G2 glycoprotein, 65 kDa
	NS_m (nonstructural) protein, 15-17 kDa
S	N (nonstructural) protein, 25 kDa
	NS_s (nonstructural) protein, 10 kDa

*Negative-strand RNA.

Box 53-2 Disease Mechanisms for Bunyaviruses

Virus is acquired from an arthropod bite (e.g., mosquito).
For hantaviruses, the virus is acquired from rodent urine.
Initial viremia may cause flulike symptoms.
Establishment of secondary viremia may allow virus access to specific target tissues that define the disease, including the central nervous system, organs, and vascular endothelium.
Antibody is important in controlling viremia; interferon and cell-mediated immunity may prevent the outgrowth of infection and contribute to disease.

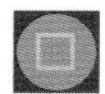

Box 53-3 Epidemiology of Bunyavirus Infections

Disease/Viral Factors

Virus is able to replicate in mammalian and arthropod cells.
Virus is able to pass into ovary and infect arthropod eggs, allowing virus to survive during winter.

Transmission

Via arthropods blood meal; California encephalitis group: *Aedes* mosquito
Aedes mosquitoes are aggressive daytime feeders and live in forests.
Aedes mosquitoes lay eggs in small pools of water trapped in places such as trees and tires.
Hantavirus is transmitted in aerosols from rodent urine and by close contact with infected rodents.

Who Is at Risk?

People in habitat of arthropod or rodent vector
California encephalitis group: campers, forest rangers, woodsmen

Geography/Season

Disease incidence correlates with distribution of vector.
Disease more common in summer

Modes of Control

Elimination of vector or vector's habitat
Avoidance of vector's habitat

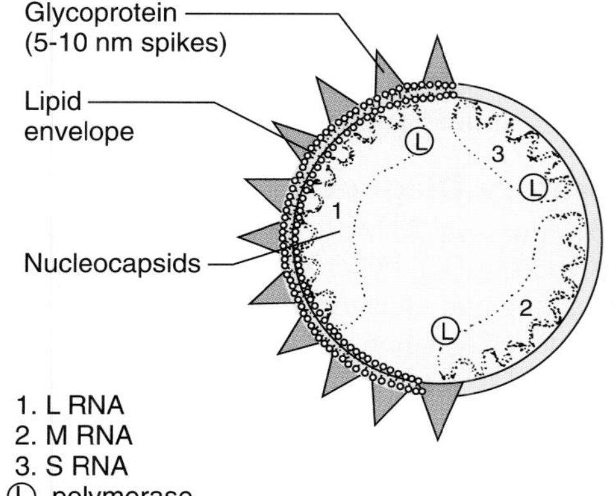

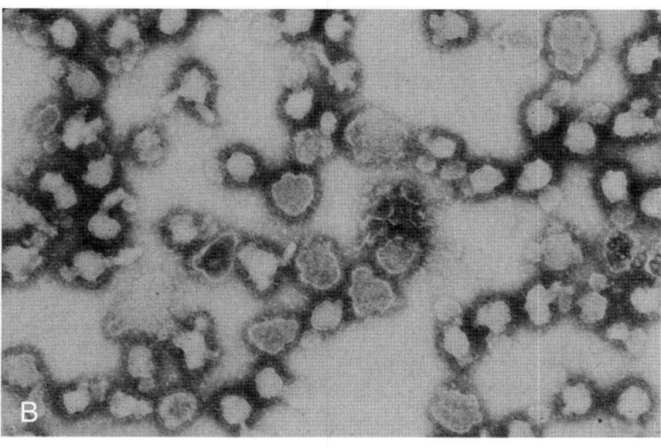

FIGURE 53-1 **A**, Model of the bunyavirus particle. **B**, Electron micrograph of La Crosse variant of bunyavirus. Note the spike proteins at the surface of the virion envelope. *RNA*, Ribonucleic acid. (**A**, Modified from Fraenkel-Conrat H, Wagner RR: *Comprehensive virology,* vol 14, New York, 1979, Plenum. **B**, Courtesy Centers for Disease Control and Prevention, Atlanta.)

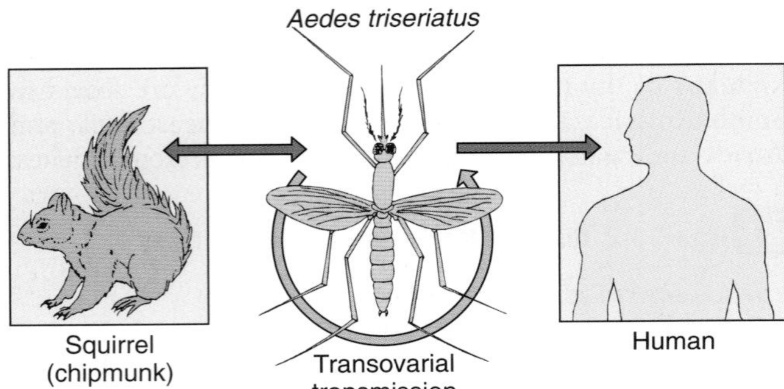

FIGURE 53-2 Transmission of La Crosse (California) encephalitis virus.

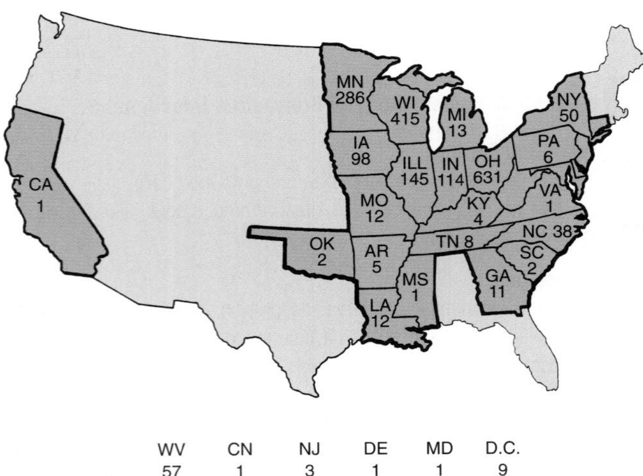

FIGURE 53-3 Distribution of California encephalitis, 1964 to 2010. (Courtesy Centers for Disease Control and Prevention, Atlanta.)

Viruses of the **California encephalitis virus group** (e.g., La Crosse virus) are spread by mosquitoes found in the forests of North America (Figure 53-3). Up to 150 cases of encephalitis occur during the summer each year in the United States, but most infections are asymptomatic. These viruses are spread mainly by aggressive day-biting *Aedes triseriatus,* which breeds in the water in tree holes and in discarded tires.

The hantaviruses do not have an arthropod vector but are maintained in a rodent species specific for each virus. Humans are infected by close contact with rodents or through inhalation of aerosolized rodent urine. In May 1993, a deadly outbreak of **hantavirus pulmonary syndrome** occurred in the Four Corners area of New Mexico. The outbreak is attributed to increased contact with the deer mouse vector during a season of unusually high rainfall, greater availability of food, and rise in the rodent population. Viruses of the Sin Nombre subfamily were isolated from the victims and rodents. Since this incident, viruses from this subfamily have been associated with outbreaks of respiratory tract disease in the eastern and western United States and Central and South America.

Clinical Syndromes (Clinical Case 53-1)

Bunyaviridae, even those that can cause serious disease, usually cause relatively mild nonspecific febrile, flulike, viremia-related illness (see Table 53-1) that is indistinguishable from illnesses caused by other viruses. The incubation period for these illnesses is approximately 48 hours, and the fevers typically last 3 days.

Encephalitis illnesses (e.g., La Crosse virus) are sudden in onset after an incubation period of approximately 1 week, and symptoms at this time consist of fever, headache, lethargy, and vomiting. Seizures occur in 50% of patients with encephalitis, usually early in the illness. Signs of meningitis may also be present. The illness lasts 10 to 14 days. Death occurs in less than 1% of patients, but seizure disorders may occur as sequelae in as many as 20%.

Hemorrhagic fevers such as Rift Valley fever are characterized by petechial hemorrhages, ecchymosis, epistaxis, hematemesis, melena, and bleeding of the gums. Death occurs in as many as half of patients with hemorrhagic disease. The **hantavirus pulmonary syndrome** is a terrible disease, manifesting initially as a prodrome of fever and muscle aches but followed rapidly by interstitial pulmonary edema, respiratory failure, and death within days.

Clinical Case 53-1 Hantavirus in Virginia

The Centers for Disease Control and Prevention (*Morb Mortal Wkly Rep* 53:1086–1089, 2004) reported a case of hantavirus in a 32-year-old wildlife sciences graduate student. The patient visited the emergency department (ED) in Blacksburg, Virginia, after experiencing fever, cough, and a "sore chest." The student had been trapping, handling, and studying mice during the previous month. Neither he nor his colleagues wore gloves while handling the mice or their excreta; they did not wash prior to eating and had numerous mouse bites on their hands. He had a fever of 39.3° C and normal lung function, but a chest radiograph indicated a faint right-sided pneumonia. The man started vomiting in the ED and was admitted. The pneumonia progressed, and he became more hypoxic, eventually requiring intubation and mechanical ventilation. On the next day, he was given activated protein C to prevent disseminated intravascular coagulation. The patient continued to fail and died on the third day after hospitalization. Serum specimens contained immunoglobulin (Ig)M and IgG antibody and genomic ribonucleic acid (determined by reverse transcriptase polymerase chain reaction) to hantavirus, and viral antigens were present in the spleen. Although the hantavirus received its greatest notoriety with the Sin Nombre virus outbreak in the southwestern United States in 1993, it can occur wherever people come in contact with the urine and feces of rodents carrying these viruses. Cases have been reported in 31 of the United States.

Laboratory Diagnosis

Detection of viral RNA by reverse transcriptase polymerase chain reaction (RT-PCR) has become the accepted method for detecting and identifying bunyaviruses. The Sin Nombre and Convict Creek hantaviruses were initially identified with the RT-PCR test, using primers with characteristic hantavirus sequences.

Serologic tests can be performed to confirm a diagnosis of bunyavirus infection. Enzyme-linked immunosorbent assay (ELISA) may detect antigen in clinical specimens from patients with an intense viremia (e.g., Rift Valley fever, hemorrhagic fever with renal syndrome, Crimean-Congo hemorrhagic fever) or from mosquitoes.

Treatment, Prevention, and Control

No specific therapy for infections of the Bunyaviridae is available. Human disease is prevented by interruption of the contact between humans and the vector, whether arthropod or mammal. Arthropod vectors are controlled by (1) eliminating the growth conditions for the vector, (2) spraying with insecticide, (3) installing netting or screening at windows and doors, (4) wearing protective clothing, and (5) controlling the tick infestation of animals. Rodent control minimizes the transmission of many viruses, especially hantaviruses.

• Arenaviruses

The arenaviruses include **lymphocytic choriomeningitis (LCMV)** and **hemorrhagic fever viruses** such as the **Lassa, Junin,** and **Machupo** viruses. These viruses cause persistent infections in specific rodents and can be transmitted to humans as **zoonoses.**

Structure and Replication

Arenaviruses are seen in electron micrographs as **pleomorphic enveloped viruses** (diameter, 120 nm) that have a **sandy appearance** (the name comes from the Greek word ***arenosa,*** meaning "sandy") because of the **ribosomes in the virion** (Box 53-4). Although functional, the ribosomes do not seem to serve a purpose. Virions contain a nucleocapsid with **two single-stranded RNA circles** (S, 3400 nucleotides; L, 7200 nucleotides) and a transcriptase. The L strand is a negative-sense RNA and encodes the polymerase. The S strand encodes the nucleoprotein (N protein), and the glycoproteins but is **ambisense.** Whereas the mRNA for the N protein is transcribed directly from the ambisense S strand, the mRNA for the glycoprotein is transcribed from a full-length template of the S strand. Like togaviruses, the glycoproteins are produced as late proteins after genome replication. Arenaviruses replicate in the cytoplasm and acquire their envelope by budding from the host cell plasma membrane.

Arenaviruses readily cause persistent infections. This may result from inefficient transcription of the glycoprotein genes and thus poor virion assembly.

Pathogenesis

Arenaviruses are able to infect macrophages, induce cytokine and interferon release, and promote cell and vascular damage. T-cell–induced immunopathologic effects significantly exacerbate tissue destruction. The incubation period for arenavirus infections averages 10 to 14 days.

Epidemiology

Most arenaviruses, except for the virus that causes LCM, are found in the tropics of Africa and South America. The arenaviruses, like the hantaviruses, infect specific rodents and are endemic to the rodents' habitats. Chronic asymptomatic infection is common in these animals and leads to long-term viral shedding in saliva, urine, and feces. Humans may become infected through inhalation of aerosols, consumption of contaminated food, or contact with fomites. Bites are not a usual mechanism of spread.

The virus that causes LCM infects hamsters and house mice *(Mus musculus)*. It was found in 20% of mice in Washington, DC. Lassa fever virus infects *Mastomys natalensis*, an African rodent. The Lassa fever virus is spread from human to human through contact with infected secretions or body fluids, but the viruses that cause LCM and other hemorrhagic fevers are rarely, if ever, spread in this way.

During 1999-2000, three cases of fatal hemorrhagic disease in California were found to be caused by the Whitewater Arroyo arenavirus. This virus is normally found in the white-throated wood rat, so its occurrence in humans constitutes a newly emergent disease. The disease association was made by a special RT-PCR assay.

Clinical Syndromes (Box 53-5)

Lymphocytic Choriomeningitis

The name of this virus, **lymphocytic choriomeningitis virus,** suggests that meningitis is a typical clinical event, but actually LCM usually causes a febrile illness with flulike myalgia. Only about 10% of infected persons progress to a central nervous system infection. The meningeal illness, if it occurs, will start 10 days after the initial phase of illness, with full recovery. Perivascular mononuclear infiltrates may be seen in neurons of all sections of the brain and in the meninges of an affected patient.

Lassa and Other Hemorrhagic Fevers

Lassa fever, which is endemic to West Africa, is the best known of the hemorrhagic fevers caused by an arenavirus. Other agents, however, such as the Junin and Machupo viruses, cause similar syndromes in the inhabitants of Argentina and Bolivia, respectively.

Clinical illness is characterized by fever, coagulopathy, petechiae, and occasional visceral hemorrhage, as well as liver and spleen necrosis, but not vasculitis. Hemorrhage and shock also occur, as does occasional cardiac and liver damage. In contrast to LCM, hemorrhagic fevers cause no lesions in the central nervous system. Pharyngitis, diarrhea, and vomiting may be prevalent, especially in patients with Lassa fever. Death occurs in as many as 50% of those with Lassa fever

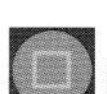
Box 53-4 Characteristics of Arenaviruses

Virus has **enveloped** virion with two **circular, negative-RNA** genome segments (L, S). Virion appears **sandy because of ribosomes.**

S genome segment is ambisense.

Arenaviruses are zoonoses, establishing persistent infections in rodents.

Pathogenesis of arenavirus infections is largely attributed to immunopathogenesis.

Box 53-5 Clinical Summary

Lassa fever: Approximately 10 days after returning from a trip to visit family in Nigeria, a 47-year-old man developed flulike symptoms with a higher-than-expected fever and malaise. The disease got progressively worse, and after 3 days, the patient developed abdominal pain, nausea, vomiting, diarrhea, pharyngitis, bleeding gums, and began vomiting blood. He developed shock and then died.

and in a smaller percentage of those infected with the other arenaviruses that cause hemorrhagic fevers. The diagnosis is suggested by recent travel to endemic areas.

Laboratory Diagnosis

An arenavirus infection is usually diagnosed on the basis of serologic and genomic (RT-PCR) findings. These viruses are too dangerous for isolation. Throat specimens can yield arenaviruses; urine is a source for the Lassa fever virus but not for the LCM virus. The risk of infection is substantial for laboratory workers handling body fluids. Therefore, if the diagnosis is suspected, laboratory personnel should be so warned and the specimens processed only in facilities that specialize in the isolation of contagious pathogens **(level 3 for LCM and level 4 for Lassa fever and other arenaviruses)**.

Treatment, Prevention, and Control

The antiviral drug **ribavirin** has limited activity against arenaviruses and can be used to treat Lassa fever. However, supportive therapy is usually all that is available for patients with arenavirus infections.

These rodent-borne infections can be prevented by limiting contact with the vector. For example, improved hygiene to limit contact with mice reduced the incidence of LCM in Washington, DC. In the geographic areas where hemorrhagic fever occurs, trapping rodents and carefully storing food may decrease exposure to the virus.

The incidence of laboratory-acquired cases can be reduced if samples submitted for arenavirus isolation are processed in at least level 3 or 4 biosafety facilities and not in the usual clinical virology laboratory.

Bibliography

Bishop DHL, Shope RE: *Bunyaviridae*, New York, 1979, Plenum.

Cohen J, Powderly WG: *Infectious diseases*, ed 2, St Louis, 2004, Mosby.

Flint SJ, Enquist LW, Racaniello VR, et al: *Principles of virology: molecular biology, pathogenesis and control of animal viruses*, ed 3, Washington, DC, 2009, American Society for Microbiology Press.

Gonzalez JP, et al: Arenaviruses, *Curr Top Microbiol Immunol* (vol 315), Berlin, 2007, Springer-Verlag, pp 253–288.

Gorbach SL, Bartlett JG, Blacklow NR: *Infectious diseases*, ed 3, Philadelphia, 2004, Saunders.

Knipe DM, Howley PM: *Fields virology*, ed 6, Philadelphia, 2013, Lippincott Williams & Wilkins.

Kolakofsky D: Bunyaviridae, *Curr Top Microbiol Immunol* (vol 169), Berlin, 1991, Springer-Verlag.

Oldstone MBA: Arenaviruses I and II, *Curr Top Microbiol Immunol* (vol 262-263), Berlin, 2002, Springer-Verlag.

Peters CJ, Simpson GL, Levy H: Spectrum of hantavirus infection: hemorrhagic fever with renal syndrome and hantavirus pulmonary syndrome, *Annu Rev Med* 50:531–545, 1999.

Schmaljohn CS, Nichol ST: Hantaviruses, *Curr Top Microbiol Immunol* (vol 256), Berlin, 2001, Springer-Verlag.

Strauss JM, Strauss EG: *Viruses and human disease*, ed 2, San Diego, 2007, Academic.

Tsai TF: Arboviral infections in the United States, *Infect Dis Clin North Am* 5:73–102, 1991.

Walter CT, Barr JN: Recent advances in the molecular and cellular biology of bunyaviruses, *J Gen Virol* 92:2467–2484, 2011. Available at http://vir.sgmjournals.org/content/early/2011/08/22/vir.0.035105-0.full.pdf+html.

Wrobel S: Serendipity, science, and a new hantavirus, *FASEB J* 9:1247–1254, 1995.

Websites

Anderson WE, Soliman E, Perez N: California encephalitis. http://emedicine.medscape.com/article/234159-overview. Accessed April 22, 2015.

Centers for Disease Control and Prevention: Hantavirus. www.cdc.gov/hantavirus/index.html. Accessed April 22, 2015.

Centers for Disease Control and Prevention: Heartland virus. www.cdc.gov/ncezid/dvbd/heartland/index.html. Accessed May 18, 2015.

Centers for Disease Control and Prevention: La Crosse encephalitis. www.cdc.gov/lac/. Accessed April 22, 2015.

Centers for Disease Control and Prevention: Lassa fever. www.cdc.gov/vhf/lassa/. Accessed May 14, 2015.

Centers for Disease Control and Prevention: Lymphocytic choriomeningitis (LCMV). www.cdc.gov/vhf/lcm/. Accessed May 14, 2015.

Gompf SG, Smith KM, Choe U: Arenaviruses. http://emedicine.medscape.com/article/212356-overview. Accessed April 22, 2015.

CHAPTER

54 RETROVIRUSES

A 63-year-old woman **has tuberculosis and a severe oral *Candida* yeast infection. Her CD4 T-cell level was 50/µl, and 200,000 human immunodeficiency virus (HIV) genomes/ml of blood were detected. Although monogamous, she finds out that her husband was not.**

1. What cell types does HIV infect, and why does this have such an impact on the patient's immune response?
2. How does the virus replicate?
3. To what other opportunistic infections is this woman susceptible?
4. What are risk factors for infection?
5. How can the infection be treated?

Answers to these questions are available on StudentConsult.com.

• SUMMARIES CLINICALLY SIGNIFICANT ORGANISMS

Retroviruses

Trigger Words

Reverse transcriptase, integration, syncytia
HIV: AIDS, CD4, chemokine co-receptor, opportunistic diseases
HTLV: leukemia, flower cell, CD4 T cell

Biology, Virulence, and Disease

- Medium size, envelope, nucleocapsid, (+) RNA genome
- Simple retroviruses have three genes: *gag, pol, env*
- Complex retroviruses (HIV, HTLV) have *gag, pol, env,* and other important genes
- Encodes RNA-dependent DNA polymerase (reverse transcriptase [RT]), replicates in nucleus
- Virion carries RT, integrase, and protease enzymes
- Replicates through DNA intermediate, integrates viral DNA into host chromosome
- Causes syncytia
- Incapacitates and escapes immune control
- Oncornaviruses may encode oncogene and have a short latency period before cancer
- HTLV-1, no oncogene, long latency period before leukemia
- HTLV: acute T-cell lymphocytic leukemia, tropical spastic paraparesis
- HIV: initially infects CD4/CCR5 macrophages, dendritic cells, and T cells; initial disease phase resembles mononucleosis followed by latent period; AIDS results when CD4 T cells drop below 200/µL
- Endogenous retroviruses: integrated and approximately 8% of human genome

Epidemiology

- Worldwide
- Transmitted in blood and semen
- High-risk groups: promiscuous individuals, IV drug users, infants of infected mothers

Diagnosis

- RT-PCR, ELISA

Treatment, Prevention, and Control

- HIV treatment with nucleoside analogs, protease inhibitors, and other antiviral drugs
- Prevention by screening of blood supply, safe sex, education

The retroviruses are probably the most studied group of viruses in molecular biology. These viruses are **enveloped positive-strand ribonucleic acid (RNA)** viruses with a unique morphology and means of replication. In 1970, Baltimore and Temin showed that the retroviruses encode an **RNA-dependent deoxyribonucleic acid (DNA) polymerase (reverse transcriptase [RT])** and replicate through a DNA intermediate. The DNA copy of the viral genome is then integrated into the host chromosome to become a cellular gene. This discovery, which earned Baltimore, Temin, and Dulbecco the 1975 Nobel Prize, contradicted what had been the central dogma of molecular biology—that genetic information passed from DNA to RNA and then to protein.

The first retrovirus to be isolated was the Rous sarcoma virus, shown by Peyton Rous to produce solid tumors (sarcomas) in chickens. Like most retroviruses, the Rous sarcoma virus proved to have a very limited host and species range. Cancer-causing retroviruses have since been isolated from other animal species and are classified as RNA tumor viruses or **oncornaviruses.** Many of these viruses alter cellular growth by expressing analogs of cellular growth-controlling genes **(oncogenes).** Not until 1981, however, when Robert Gallo and his associates isolated human T-cell lymphotropic virus 1 (HTLV-1) from a person with adult human T-cell leukemia, was a human retrovirus associated with human disease.

In the late 1970s and early 1980s, an unusual number of young homosexual men, Haitians, heroin addicts, and hemophiliacs in the United States (the initial "4H club" of risk groups) were noted to be dying of normally benign opportunistic infections. Their symptoms defined a new disease, the **acquired immunodeficiency syndrome (AIDS).** However, as is now known, AIDS is not limited to these groups but can occur in anyone exposed to the virus. Now approximately 34 million men, women, and children around the world are living with the virus that causes AIDS. Montagnier and associates in Paris, and Gallo and colleagues in the United States, reported the isolation of the human immunodeficiency virus (HIV-1) from patients with lymphadenopathy and AIDS. A closely related virus, designated **HIV-2,** was isolated later and is prevalent in West Africa. HIV appears to have been acquired by humans from chimpanzees and then rapidly spread through Africa and the world by an increasingly mobile population. Although a devastating disease that cannot be completely cured, the development of antiviral drug cocktails (highly active antiretroviral therapy [HAART]) has allowed many HIV patients to resume a normal life.

Endogenous retroviruses, the ultimate parasites, have integrated, are transmitted vertically, and may take up as much as 8% of the human chromosome. Although they may not produce virions, they may still contribute to or influence functions of the body.

Our understanding of the retroviruses has paralleled progress in molecular biology and immunology. In turn, the retroviruses have provided a major tool for molecular biology, the RT enzyme, and through the study of viral oncogenes have also provided a means of advancing our understanding of cell growth, differentiation, and oncogenesis.

The three subfamilies of human retroviruses are the **Oncovirinae** (HTLV-1, HTLV-2, HTLV-5), the **Lentivirinae** (HIV-1, HIV-2), and the **Spumavirinae** (Table 54-1). Although a spumavirus was the first human retrovirus to be isolated, no such virus has been associated with human disease.

Classification

The retroviruses are classified by the diseases they cause, tissue tropism and host range, virion morphology, and genetic complexity (see Table 54-1). The **oncoviruses** include the only retroviruses that can **immortalize or transform target cells.** These viruses are also categorized by the morphology of their core and capsid as type A, B, C, or D, as seen in electron micrographs (Figure 54-1; see Table 54-1). The **lentiviruses are slow viruses associated with neurologic and immunosuppressive diseases.** The spumaviruses, represented by a foamy virus, cause a distinct cytopathologic effect but, as already noted, do not seem to cause clinical disease.

Structure

The retroviruses are roughly spherical, enveloped, RNA viruses with a diameter of 80 to 120 nm (Figure 54-2 and Box 54-1). The envelope contains viral glycoproteins and is acquired by budding from the plasma membrane. The **envelope surrounds a capsid that contains two identical copies of the positive-strand RNA genome** inside an electron-dense core. The virion also contains 10 to 50 copies of the **reverse transcriptase and integrase enzymes** and **two cellular transfer RNA (tRNAs).** These tRNAs are base-paired to each copy of the genome to be used as a primer for the RT. The morphology of the core differs for different viruses

Table 54-1 Classification of Retroviruses

Subfamily	Characteristics	Examples
Oncovirinae	Are associated with cancer and neurologic disorders	—
B	Have eccentric nucleocapsid core in mature virion	Mouse mammary tumor virus
C	Have centrally located nucleocapsid core in mature virion	Human T-cell lymphotropic virus* (HTLV-1, HTLV-2, HTLV-5), Rous sarcoma virus (chickens)
D	Have nucleocapsid core with cylindrical form	Mason-Pfizer monkey virus
Lentivirinae	Have slow onset of disease, cause neurologic disorders and immunosuppression, are viruses with D-type cylindrical nucleocapsid core	Human immunodeficiency virus* (HIV-1, HIV-2), visna virus (sheep), caprine arthritis/encephalitis virus (goats)
Spumavirinae	Cause no known clinical disease but cause characteristic vacuolated "foamy" cytopathology	Human foamy virus*
Human endogenous retroviruses (HERVs)	Retrovirus sequences that are integrated into human genome	Human placental virus

*Also classified as complex retroviruses because of the requirement for accessory proteins for replication.

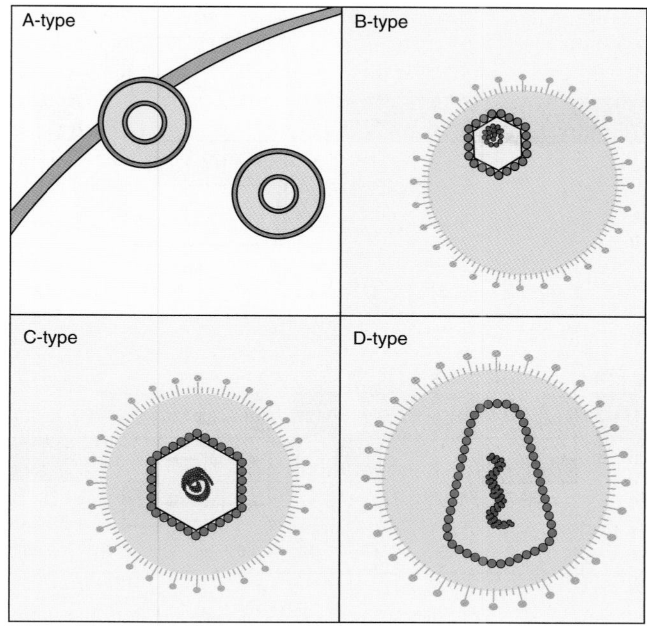

FIGURE 54-1 Morphologic distinction of retrovirions. The morphology and position of the nucleocapsid core are used to classify the viruses. A-type particles are immature intracytoplasmic forms that bud through the plasma membrane and mature into B-type, C-type, and D-type particles.

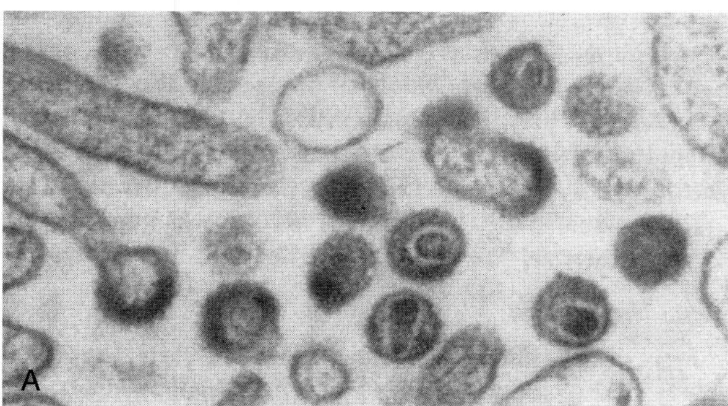

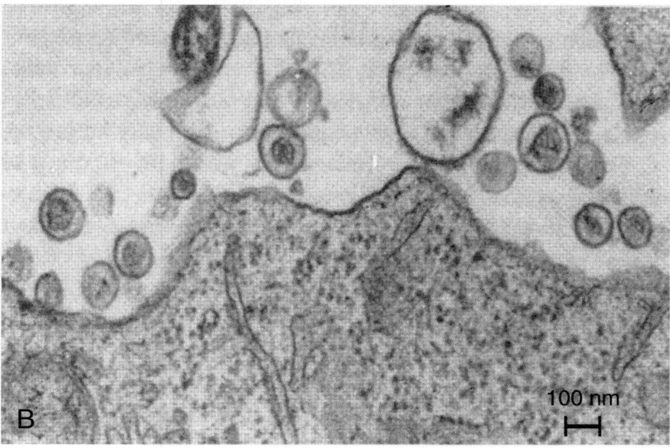

FIGURE 54-2 Electron micrographs of two retroviruses. **A,** Human immunodeficiency virus. Note the cone-shaped nucleocapsid in several of the virions. **B,** Human T-cell lymphotropic virus. Note the C-type morphology characterized by a central symmetric nucleocapsid. (From Belshe RB: *Textbook of human virology,* ed 2, St Louis, 1991, Mosby.)

Box 54-1 Unique Characteristics of Retroviruses

Virus has an **enveloped** spherical virion that is 80 to 120 nm in diameter and encloses a capsid containing **two** copies of the **positive-strand RNA** genome (≈9 kilobases for human immunodeficiency virus [HIV] and human T-cell lymphotropic virus).
RNA-dependent DNA polymerase **(reverse transcriptase),** two copies of tRNA, protease, and integrase enzymes are carried in the virion.
Virus receptor is the initial determinant of tissue tropism.
Replication proceeds through a DNA intermediate termed the *provirus.*
The provirus **integrates** randomly into the host chromosome and becomes a cellular gene.
Transcription of the genome is regulated by the interaction of host transcription factors with promoter and enhancer elements in the long terminal repeat portion of the genome.
Simple retroviruses encode *gag, pol,* and *env* genes. **Complex viruses** also encode accessory genes (e.g., *tat, rev, nef, vif,* and *vpu* for HIV).
Virus assembles and buds from the plasma membrane.
Final morphogenesis of HIV *requires* protease cleavage of Gag and Gag-Pol polypeptides after envelopment.

and is used as a means of classifying the retroviruses (see Figure 54-1). The HIV virion core resembles a truncated cone (Figure 54-3).

The retrovirus genome has a 5′-cap and is polyadenylated at the 3′-end (Figure 54-4 and Table 54-2). Although the genome resembles a messenger RNA (mRNA), it is not infectious because it does not encode a polymerase that can directly generate more mRNA.

The genome of the **simple retroviruses** *consists of three major genes that encode polyproteins* for the following enzymatic and structural proteins of the virus: **Gag** (group-specific antigen, *capsid, matrix,* and *nucleic acid–binding proteins*), **Pol** (*polymerase, protease,* and *integrase*), and **Env** (envelope, *glycoproteins*). At each end of the genome are **long terminal repeat (LTR)** sequences. The LTR sequences contain promoters, enhancers, and other gene sequences used for binding different cellular transcription factors. Oncogenic viruses may also contain a growth-promoting **oncogene.** The **complex retroviruses,** including HTLV and HIV and other lentiviruses, express early and late proteins and encode several virulence-enhancing proteins that require more complex transcriptional processing (splicing) than the simple retroviruses.

The viral glycoproteins are produced by proteolytic cleavage of the polyprotein encoded by the *env* gene. The size of the glycoproteins differs for each group of viruses. For example, the (glycoprotein) gp62 of HTLV-1 is cleaved into gp46 and p21, and the *gp160 of HIV is cleaved into gp41 and gp120.* These glycoproteins form lollipop-like trimer spikes that are visible on the surface of the virion. The larger of the HIV glycoproteins (gp120), which binds to cell surface receptors, initially determines the tissue tropism of the virus and is recognized by neutralizing antibody. The smaller subunit (gp41 in HIV) forms the lollipop stick and promotes cell-to-cell fusion. The gp120 of HIV is extensively glycosylated, and *its antigenicity can drift and receptor specificity can shift by mutations that occur during the course of a chronic HIV infection.* These factors impede antibody clearance of the virus.

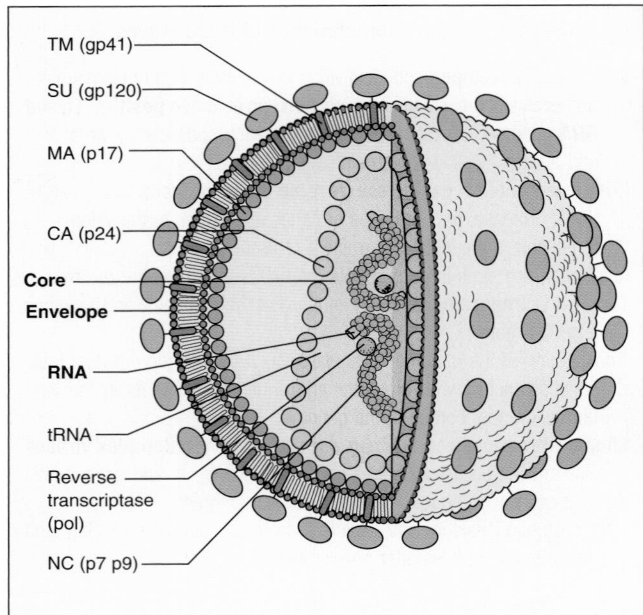

FIGURE 54-3 Cross section of human immunodeficiency virus. The enveloped virion contains two identical ribonucleic acid *(RNA)* strands, RNA polymerase, integrase, and two transfer RNAs *(tRNA)* base-paired to the genome within the protein core. This is surrounded by proteins and a lipid bilayer. The envelope spikes are the glycoprotein *(gp)*120 attachment protein and gp41 fusion protein. *CA,* Capsid; *MA,* matrix; *NC,* nucleocapsid; *SU,* surface component; *TM,* transmembrane component of envelope glycoprotein. (Modified from Gallo RC, Montagnier L: AIDS in 1988. *Sci Am* 259:41–48, 1988. Copyright George Kelvin.)

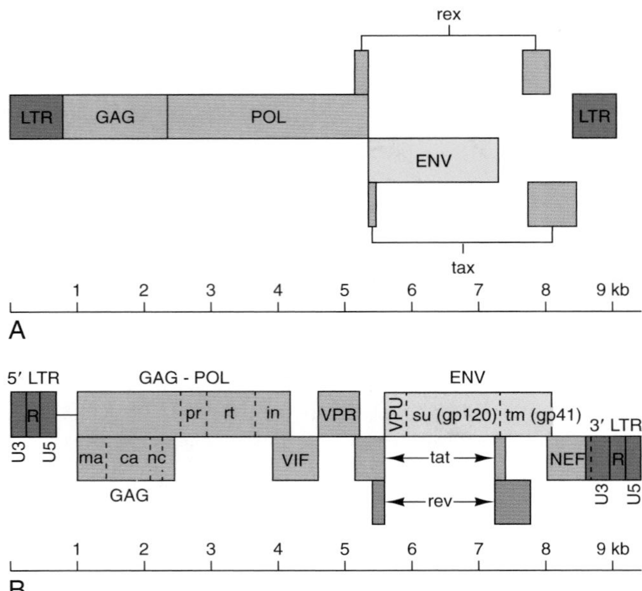

FIGURE 54-4 Genomic structure of human retroviruses. **A,** Human T-cell lymphotropic virus (HTLV-1). **B,** Human immunodeficiency virus (HIV-1). The genes are defined in Table 54-2 and Figure 54-3. Unlike the other genes of these viruses, production of the messenger RNA for *tax* and *rex* genes (HTLV-1) and *tat* and *rev* genes (HIV) requires excision of two intron units. HIV-2 has a similar genome map but has a vpx but not a vpu gene. *ENV,* Envelope glycoprotein gene; *GAG,* group antigen gene; *LTR,* long terminal repeat; *POL,* polymerase gene. Protein nomenclature for HIV: *ca,* Capsid protein; *in,* integrase; *ma,* matrix protein; *nc,* nucleocapsid protein; *pr,* protease; *rt,* reverse transcriptase; *su,* surface glycoprotein component; *tm,* transmembrane glycoprotein component. (Modified from Belshe RB: *Textbook of human virology,* ed 2, St Louis, 1991, Mosby.)

• Replication

Replication of HIV will serve as an example for the other retroviruses unless noted. Infection starts with binding of the viral glycoprotein spikes (trimer of gp120 and gp41 molecules) to the primary receptor, **the CD4 protein,** and then a second receptor, a 7-transmembrane G-protein–coupled chemokine receptor (Figure 54-5). *Binding to the receptor is the initial and major determinant of tissue tropism and host range for a retrovirus.* The co-receptor used upon initial infection by HIV is **CCR5,** which is expressed on **myeloid and peripheral, activated, central memory, intestinal, and other subsets of CD4 T cells (macrophages, [M]-tropic virus).** Later, during chronic infection of a person, the *env* gene mutates so that the gp120 binds to a different chemokine receptor **(CXCR4),** which is expressed primarily on T cells **(T-tropic virus)** (Figure 54-6). Binding to the chemokine receptor activates the cell and brings the viral envelope and cell plasma membrane close together, allowing the gp41 to interact with and promote fusion of the two membranes. Binding to CCR5 and gp41-mediated fusion are targets for antiviral drugs. HIV can also bind to a cellular adhesion molecule, α-4 β-7 integrin (also known as VLA-4 [very late antigen-4] and the gut homing receptor for T cells), and DC-SIGN (dendritic cell–specific intercellular adhesion molecule-3-grabbing nonintegrin) on dendritic and other cells.

Once the genome is released into the cytoplasm, the early phase of replication begins. The RT, encoded by the *pol* gene, uses the tRNA in the virion as a primer and synthesizes a **complementary** negative-strand DNA **(cDNA).** The RT also acts as a ribonuclease H, degrades the RNA genome, and then synthesizes the positive strand of DNA (Figure 54-7). The RT is the major target for antiviral drugs. During the synthesis of the virion DNA **(provirus),** sequences from each end of the genome (U3 and U5) are duplicated, thus attaching the LTRs to both ends. This process creates sequences necessary for integration and *creates enhancer and promoter sequences within the LTR for regulation of transcription.* The DNA copy of the genome is larger than the original RNA.

RT is very error prone. For example, the error rate for the RT from HIV is one error per 2000 bases, or approximately five errors per genome (HIV, 9000 base pairs), the equivalent of at least one typo on every page of this text but different errors for every book. This genetic instability of HIV is responsible for promoting the generation of new strains of virus during a person's disease, a property that may alter the pathogenicity of the virus and promote immune escape.

Unlike other retroviruses, the double-stranded cDNA of HIV and other lentiviruses can enter the nucleus through

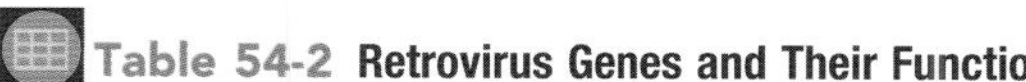

Table 54-2 Retrovirus Genes and Their Function

Gene	Virus	Function
gag	All	Group-specific antigen: core and capsid proteins
int	All	Integrase
pol	All	Polymerase: reverse transcriptase, protease, integrase
pro	All	Protease
env	All	Envelope: glycoproteins
tax	HTLV	Transactivation of viral and cellular genes
tat	HIV-1	Transactivation of viral and cellular genes
rex	HTLV	Regulation of RNA splicing and promotion of export to cytoplasm
rev	HIV-1	Regulation of RNA splicing and promotion of export to cytoplasm
nef	HIV-1	Decreases cell surface CD4; facilitates T-cell activation, progression to AIDS (essential)
vif	HIV-1	Virus infectivity, promotion of assembly, blocks a cellular antiviral protein
vpu	HIV-1	Facilitates virion assembly and release, induces degradation of CD4
vpr (vpx)*	HIV-1	Transport of complementary DNA to nucleus, arresting of cell growth; facilitates replication in macrophages
LTR	All	Promoter, enhancer elements

AIDS, Acquired immunodeficiency syndrome; *DNA,* deoxyribonucleic acid; *HIV,* human immunodeficiency virus; *HTLV,* human T-cell lymphotropic virus; *LTR,* long terminal repeat (sequence); *RNA,* ribonucleic acid.

*Only in HIV-2.

nuclear pores of resting T cells. Dissolution of the nuclear envelope upon cell division is required by other retroviruses. The cDNA is then spliced into the host chromosome with the aid of a virus-encoded, virion-carried enzyme, **integrase.** Integration requires cell growth, but the cDNA of HIV and other lentiviruses can remain in the nucleus and cytoplasm in a nonintegrated circular DNA form until the cell is activated. Integrase is a target for an antiviral drug.

Once integrated, the late phase begins and viral DNA **provirus** is transcribed as a cellular gene by the host RNA polymerase II. Transcription of the genome produces a full-length RNA, which for simple retroviruses is processed to produce several mRNAs that contain the *gag, gag-pol,* or *env* gene sequences. The full-length transcripts of the genome can also be assembled into new virions.

Because the provirus acts as a cellular gene, its replication depends on the extent of methylation of the viral DNA and on the cell's growth rate, but mostly on the ability of the cell to recognize the enhancers and promoter sequences encoded in the LTR region. Stimulation of the cell by cytokines or mitogens produced in response to other infections generates transcription factors that bind to the LTR and for HIV are required to activate transcription of the integrated genome. If the virus encodes viral oncogenes, these proteins promote cell growth and stimulate transcription and hence viral

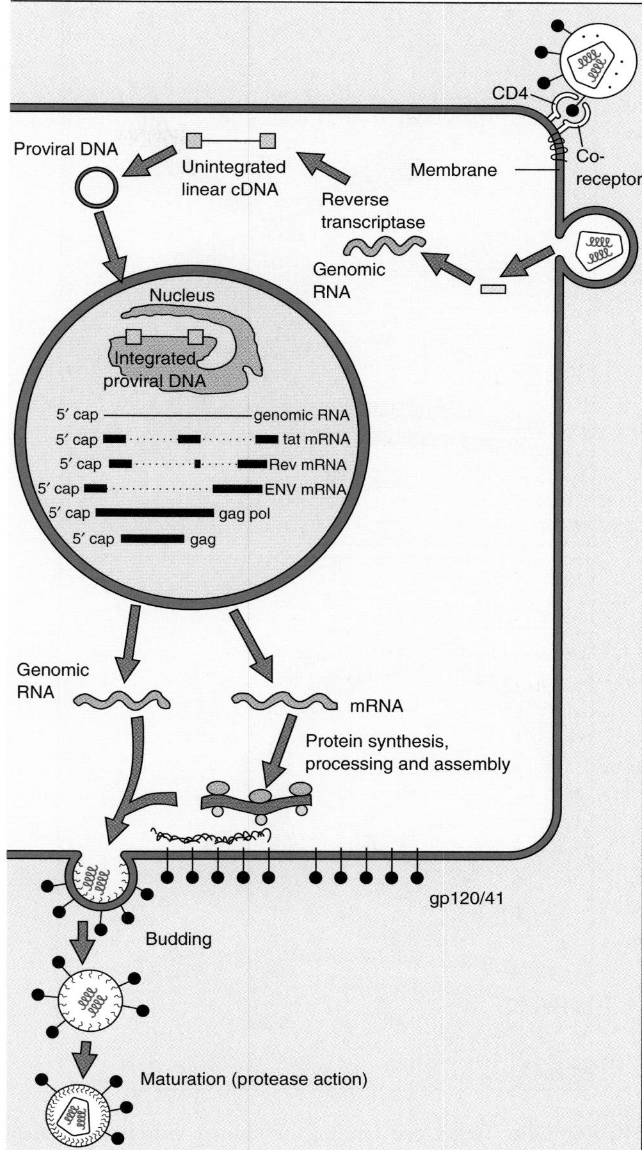

FIGURE 54-5 The life cycle of human immunodeficiency virus (HIV). HIV binds to CD4 and chemokine co-receptors and enters by fusion. The genome is reverse transcribed into deoxyribonucleic acid *(DNA)* in the cytoplasm, enters the nucleus, and is integrated into the nuclear DNA. Transcription and translation of the genome occur as a cellular gene in a fashion similar to that of human T-cell lymphotropic virus (see Figure 54-7). The virus assembles at the plasma membrane and matures after budding from the cell. *cDNA,* Complementary DNA; *mRNA,* messenger ribonucleic acid. (Modified from Fauci AS: The human immunodeficiency virus: infectivity and mechanisms of pathogenesis, *Science* 239:617–622, 1988.)

replication. *The ability of a cell to transcribe the retroviral genome is also a major determinant of tissue tropism and host range for a retrovirus.*

HTLV and HIV are **complex retroviruses** and undergo two phases of transcription. During the early phase, HTLV-1 expresses two proteins, **Tax** and **Rex,** which regulate viral replication. Unlike the other viral mRNAs, the mRNA for Tax and Rex requires more than one splicing step. The *rex*

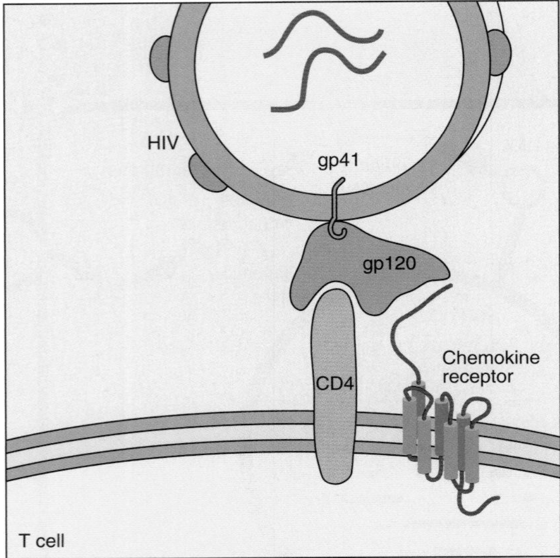

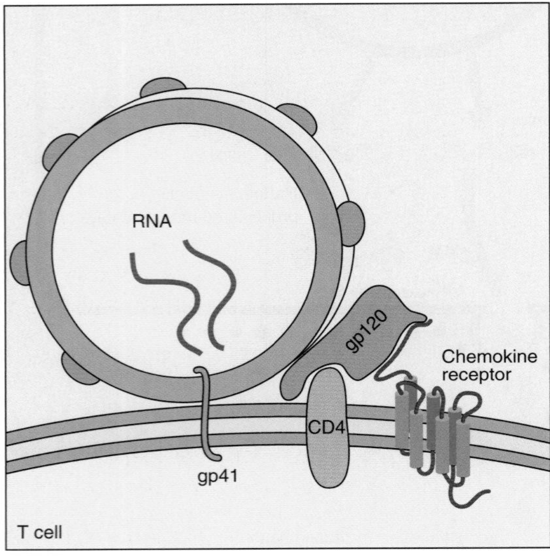

FIGURE 54-6 Target cell binding of human immunodeficiency virus *(HIV)*. The CCR5 chemokine receptor is co-receptor with CD4 upon initial infection of an individual, and after mutation of the *env* gene, the CXCR4 receptor is also used. *RNA,* Ribonucleic acid. (Modified from Balter M: New hope in HIV disease, *Science* 274:1988, 1996.)

gene encodes two proteins that bind to a structure on the viral mRNA and thereby prevents further splicing and promotes mRNA transport to the cytoplasm. The doubly spliced *tax/rex* mRNA is expressed early (at a low concentration of Rex), and structural proteins are expressed late (high concentration of Rex). Late in the infection, Rex selectively enhances expression of the singly spliced structural genes, which are required in abundance. The tax protein is a **transcriptional activator** and enhances transcription of the viral genome from the promoter gene sequence in the 5′ LTR. Tax also activates other genes, including those for interleukin (IL)-2, IL-3, granulocyte-macrophage colony-stimulating factor, and the receptor for IL-2. Activation of these genes promotes the growth of the infected T cell, which enhances virus replication.

HIV replication is regulated by as many as six **"accessory" gene products** (see Table 54-2). The **Tat** protein, like Tax, is a transactivator of the transcription of viral and cellular genes. The **Rev** protein acts like the Rex protein to regulate and promote transport of viral mRNA into the cytoplasm. The **Nef** protein reduces cell surface expression of CD4 and major histocompatibility class I (MHC I) molecules, alters T-cell signaling pathways, regulates the cytotoxicity of the virus, and is required to maintain high viral loads. The Nef protein appears to be essential for causing the infection to progress to AIDS. The **Vif** protein promotes assembly and maturation and binds to an antiviral cellular protein (APOBEC-3G) to prevent it from hypermutating the cDNA and helps the virus replicate in myeloid and other cells. The **Vpu protein** reduces cell surface CD4 expression and enhances virion release. The **Vpr protein** (Vpx in HIV-2) is important for transport of the cDNA into the nucleus. Vpr protein also arrests the cell in the G2 phase of the growth cycle, which is likely to be optimal for HIV replication. Vpx facilitates virus replication in dendritic cells and macrophages. Interestingly, this facilitates antigen presentation on MHC-1 antigens, which promotes CD8 cytotoxic T-cell production, which can limit HIV-2 disease progression.

The proteins translated from the *gag, gag-pol,* and *env* mRNAs are synthesized as polyproteins and are subsequently cleaved to functional proteins (see Figure 54-7). The viral glycoproteins are synthesized, glycosylated, and processed by the endoplasmic reticulum and Golgi apparatus. These glycoproteins are then cleaved, associate to form trimers, and migrate to the plasma membrane.

The Gag and Gag-Pol polyproteins are acylated and then bind to the plasma membrane containing the envelope glycoprotein. The association of two copies of the genome and cellular transfer RNA molecules promotes budding of the virion. After envelopment and release from the cell, the viral protease cleaves the Gag and Gag-Pol polyproteins to release the RT and form the virion core, thus ensuring inclusion of these components into the virion. The protease step is required for the production of infectious virions and is a target for antiviral drugs.

Envelopment and release of retroviruses occur at the cell surface. The HIV envelope picks up cellular proteins, including MHC molecules, upon budding. Replication and budding of the retrovirus does not necessarily kill the cell. HIV can also spread from cell to cell through the production of multinucleated giant cells, or syncytia. Syncytia are fragile, and their formation enhances the cytolytic activity of the virus.

• Human Immunodeficiency Virus

There are four genotypes of HIV-1, designated M (main), N, O, and P. Most HIV-1 is of the M subtype, and this is divided into 11 subtypes, or clades, designated A to K (for HIV-2, A to F). The designations are based on differences in the sequence of their *env* (7% to 12% difference) and *gag* genes and hence the antigenicity and immune recognition of the gp120 and capsid proteins of these viruses.

Pathogenesis and Immunity

The major determinant in the pathogenesis and disease caused by HIV is the **virus tropism for CD4-expressing T**

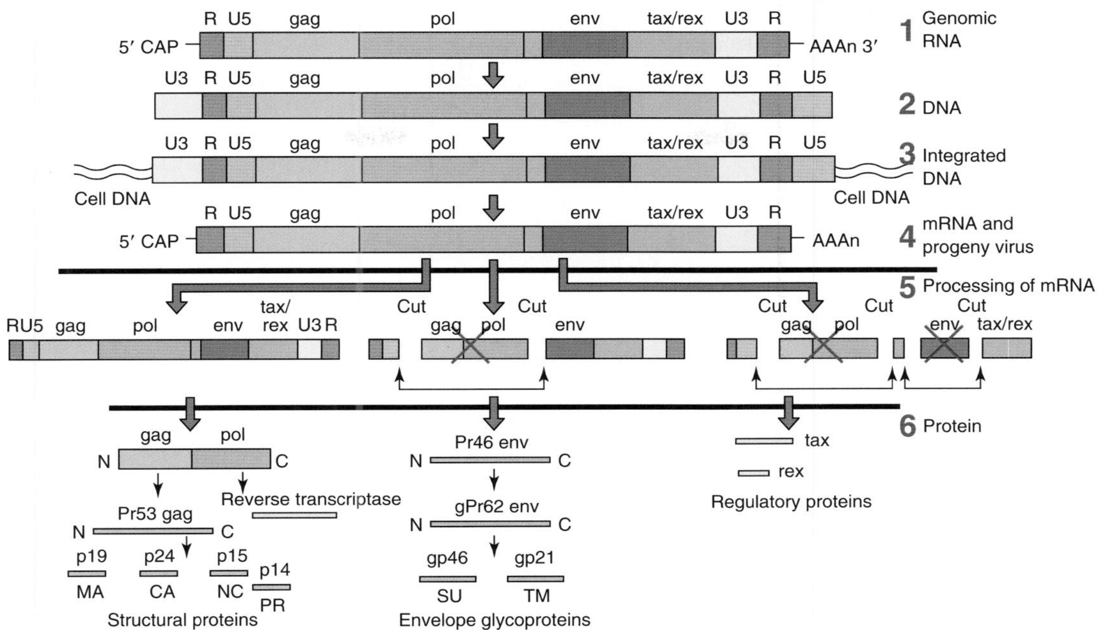

FIGURE 54-7 Transcription and translation of human T-cell lymphotropic virus. (A similar but more complex approach is used for human immunodeficiency virus.) *(1)* Genomic ribonucleic acid *(RNA)* is reverse transcribed and *(2)* circularized and then *(3)* integrated into the host chromatin. *(4)* A full-length RNA and *(5)* individual messenger RNAs *(mRNAs)* are processed from this RNA. The mRNA for *tax* and *rex* requires excision of two sequences *(red X),* the *gag-pol* and *env* sequences. The other mRNAs, including the *env* mRNA, require excision of one sequence. *(6)* Translation of these mRNAs produces polyproteins, which are subsequently cleaved. *AAAn,* Polyadenylate. Gene nomenclature: *env,* Envelope glycoprotein; *gag,* group antigen gene; *pol,* polymerase; *rex,* regulator of splicing; *tax,* transactivator. Protein nomenclature: *C,* Carboxyl terminus of peptide; *CA,* capsid; *MA,* matrix; *N,* amino terminus; *NC,* nucleocapsid; *PR,* protease; *SU,* surface component; *TM,* transmembrane component of envelope glycoprotein. Prefixes: *gp,* glycoprotein; *gPr,* glycosylated precursor polyprotein; *p,* protein; *PR,* precursor polyprotein.

cells and myeloid cells (Figure 54-8 and Box 54-2). HIV-induced immunosuppression (AIDS) results from a reduction in the number of CD4 T cells, which decimates the ability to activate and control innate and immune responses.

During sexual transmission, HIV infects a mucosal surface, enters, and rapidly infects cells of the mucosa-associated lymphoid tissue (MALT), including the intestine. The initial stages of infection are mediated by M-tropic viruses that bind to CD4 and the CCR5 chemokine receptors on dendritic and other monocyte-macrophage lineage cells, as well as memory, TH1, most intestine-associated T cells, and other CD4 T cells. Individuals who are deficient in the CCR5 receptor are also resistant to HIV infection, and CCR5 binding is a target for an antiviral drug. The CCR5-delta 32 mutation that prevents surface expression of this co-receptor is prevalent in northern Europeans (1% are homozygous and 10% to 15% are heterozygous for the mutation).

Targeting of CCR5 or α-4 β-7 integrin–expressing CD4 T cells rapidly depletes the intestinal lymphoid tissue of CD4 T cells. Depletion of the intestinal CD4 T-cell population wreaks havoc on immune regulation of normal gut flora and maintenance of the intestinal mucosal epithelium, leading to leakage and diarrhea.

Macrophages, DCs, memory T cells, and hematopoietic stem cells are persistently infected with HIV and are the major reservoirs and means of distribution of HIV (Trojan horse). HIV can bind to the DC-SIGN lectin molecule and remain on the surface of dendritic cells (including follicular DCs). CD4 T cells can be infected with the cell-bound HIV or by cell-to-cell transmission of virus upon binding to the DC. Late in the disease progression, mutation in the env gene for the gp120 occurs for some of the virus, and this shifts its tropism from M-tropic (R5) to T-tropic (X4 virus). The gp120 of the T-tropic virus binds to CD4 and the CXCR4 chemokine receptor. Some viruses may use both receptors (R5X4 viruses). This expands the viral target range to include almost all CD4 T cells.

Killing of CD4 T cells may result from direct HIV-induced cytolysis (including syncytia formation) (Table 54-3) and cytotoxic T-cell–induced immune cytolysis, but large numbers of nonpermissive resting T cells commit a type of inflammatory cell suicide (pyroptosis) induced by the presence of large amounts of nonintegrated circular DNA copies of the genome. Pyroptosis is an inflammatory form of cell death that may lure more unactivated T cells to the site to be infected and also succumb to pyroptosis.

The course of HIV disease parallels the reduction in CD4 T-cell numbers and the amount of virus in the blood (Figure 54-9). HIV infects and depletes the intestinal CCR5-expressing CD4 T cells very soon after infection. During the subsequent acute phase of the infection, there is a large burst of virus production (10^7 particles/ml of plasma). T-cell proliferation in response to antigen presentation by infected dendritic cells, macrophages, and even activated CD4 T cells

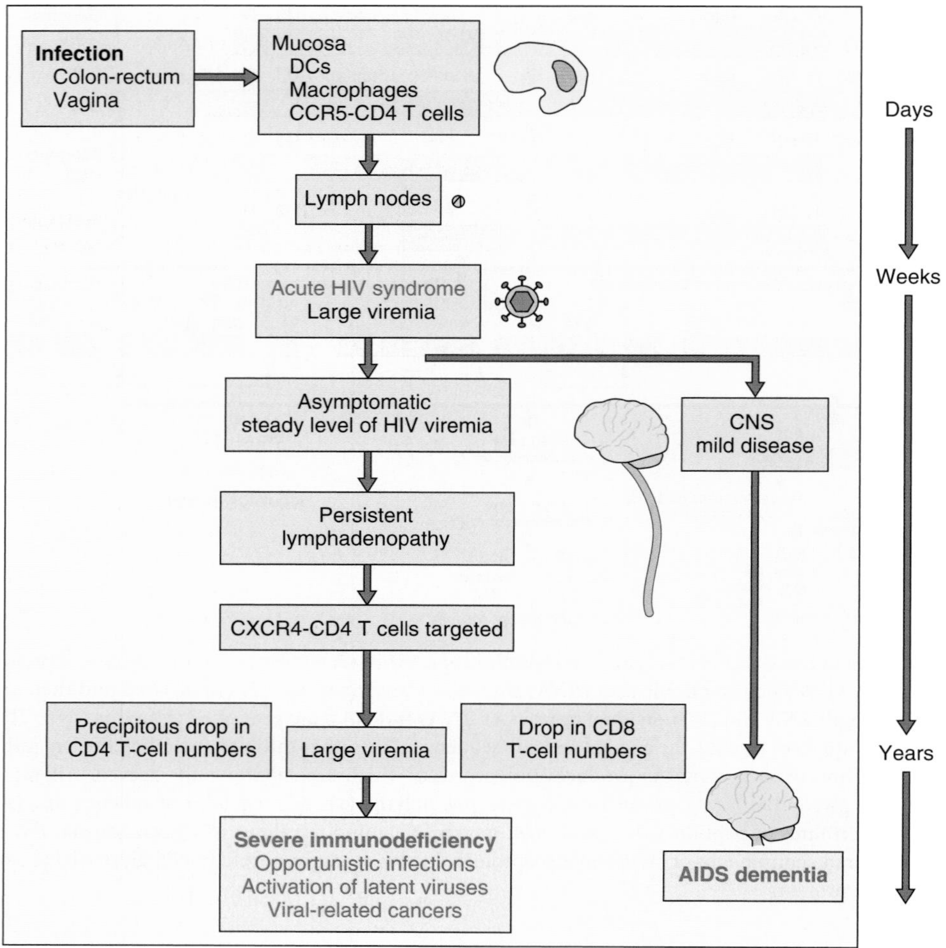

FIGURE 54-8 Pathogenesis of human immunodeficiency virus *(HIV).* HIV causes lytic and latent infection of macrophage, dendritic cells, and CD4 T cells and disrupts neuron function. The outcomes of these actions are immunodeficiency and acquired immunodeficiency syndrome *(AIDS)* dementia. *CNS,* Central nervous system. (Modified from Fauci AS: The human immunodeficiency virus: infectivity and mechanisms of pathogenesis, *Science* 239:617–622, 1988.)

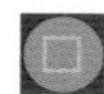

Box 54-2 Disease Mechanisms of Human Immunodeficiency Virus

Human immunodeficiency virus primarily infects CD4 T cells and cells of the myeloid lineage (e.g., monocytes, macrophages, alveolar macrophages of the lung, dendritic cells, and microglial cells of the brain).

Virus causes lytic infection of activated permissive CD4 T cells and induces apoptosis-like death of nonpermissive CD4 T cells.

Virus causes persistent low-level productive and latent infection of myeloid lineage cells and memory T cells.

Virus causes syncytia formation, with cells expressing large amounts of CD4 antigen (T cells); subsequent lysis of the cells occurs.

Virus alters T-cell, dendritic cell, and macrophage cell function.

Virus reduces CD4 T-cell numbers and helper-cell activation of CD8 T-cell, macrophage, and other cell functions.

CD8 T-cell numbers and macrophage function decrease.

Infected microglial cells disrupt neuronal function.

promotes a **mononucleosis-like syndrome.** CD8 T cells kill many infected cells and limit virus production. Virus levels in the blood decrease and the individual is asymptomatic (latent period), but viral replication continues in the lymph nodes, causing disruption of structure and function, and

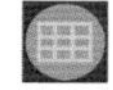

Table 54-3 Means of Human Immunodeficiency Virus Escape from the Immune System

Characteristic	Function
Infection of dendritic cells, macrophages, and CD4 T helper cells	Loss of activators and controllers of the immune system
Antigenic drift (via mutation) of gp120	Evasion of antibody detection
Heavy glycosylation of gp120	Evasion of antibody detection
Direct cell-to-cell spread and syncytia formation	Evasion of antibody detection

CD4 T-cell numbers continue to drop. Late in the disease, CD4 levels decrease to the point that they cannot maintain the antiviral action of CD8 T cells, and then virus levels in the blood increase greatly, T-tropic virus rises, CD4 T-cell numbers drop faster, the structure of the lymph nodes is destroyed, and the patient becomes immunodeficient.

The central role of the CD4 helper T cells in the initiation and control of innate and immune responses is indicated by the onset of opportunistic diseases after HIV infection (Figure 54-10). Activated CD4 T cells initiate immune responses by the release of cytokines required for the activation of epithelial cells, neutrophils, macrophages, other T cells, B cells, and natural killer cells. The CD4 TH17 responses that activate neutrophils and protect the mucoepithelium are the first to be depleted (CD4 numbers < 500/µl), increasing susceptibility to fungal and bacterial infections. As the CD4 T cells decrease (CD4 numbers < 200/µl), TH1 responses dissipate and cannot activate sufficient numbers of CD8 T cells and macrophages to control latent and new infections of intracellular bacteria and viruses (e.g., herpesviruses and JC polyomavirus progressive multifocal leukoencephalopathy [PML] and EBV and HHV8-associated cancers [Hodgkin and non-Hodgkin lymphomas, Kaposi sarcoma]).

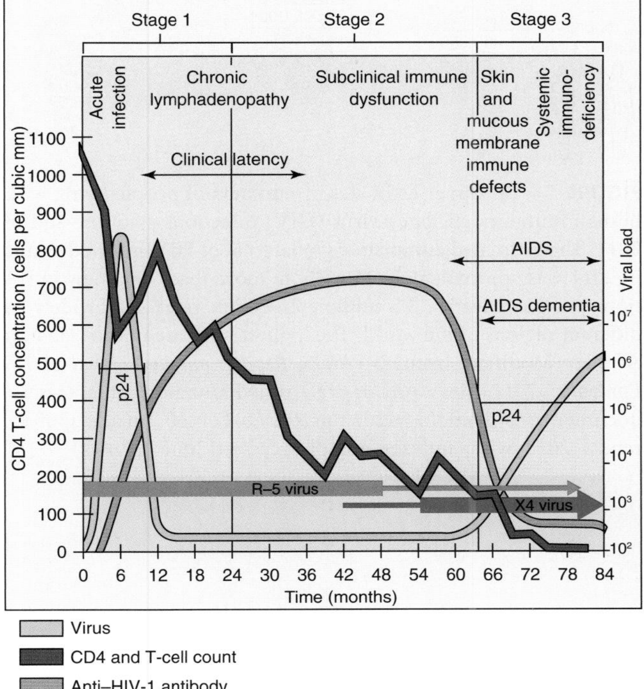

FIGURE 54-9 Time course and stages of human immunodeficiency virus *(HIV)*. A long clinical latency period follows the initial mononucleosis-like symptoms. Initial infection is with the R5–M-tropic virus, and later the X4–T-tropic virus arises. The progressive decrease in the number of CD4 T cells, even during the latency period, allows opportunistic infections to occur. The stages in HIV disease are defined by the CD4 T-cell levels and occurrence of opportunistic diseases. (Modified from Redfield RR, Burke DS: HIV infection: the clinical picture, *Sci Am* 259:90–98, 1988; updated 1996.)

In addition to immunodepression, HIV can also cause neurologic abnormalities. The microglial cell and macrophage are the predominant HIV-infected cell types in the brain. Infected monocytes and microglial cells release neurotoxic substances or chemotactic factors that promote inflammatory responses and neuronal death in the brain. Immunosuppression also puts the individual at risk of opportunistic infections of the brain.

The innate and immune response attempts to restrict viral infection but also contributes to pathogenesis. The infected cells have enzymes that restrict retrovirus replication (including endogenous retroviruses), but HIV can override their actions. The presence of unintegrated HIV cDNA triggers type 1 interferon production but also inflammatory cell suicide (pyroptosis). CD8 T cells are critical to limiting HIV disease progression. CD8 T cells can kill infected cells by direct cytotoxic action and can produce suppressive factors that restrict viral replication, including chemokines that also block the binding of virus to its co-receptor. Individuals with certain MHC types (human leukocyte antigen [HLA] B27 or B57) will preferentially bind HIV peptides rather than cellular peptides to make infected cells better targets for CD8 T-cell killing, and these individuals are more resistant to HIV disease. Neutralizing antibodies are generated against gp120. Antibody-coated virus can be infectious, however, and is taken up by macrophages.

HIV has several ways of escaping immune control. Most significant is the virus's ability to undergo mutation and hence alter its antigenicity and escape antibody clearance. Persistent infection of macrophages and resting CD4 T cells maintains the virus in an immune-privileged cell and cells in immune-privileged tissues (e.g., central nervous system and genital organs) (see Table 54-3). Ultimately, infection of CD4 T cells compromises the entire immune system.

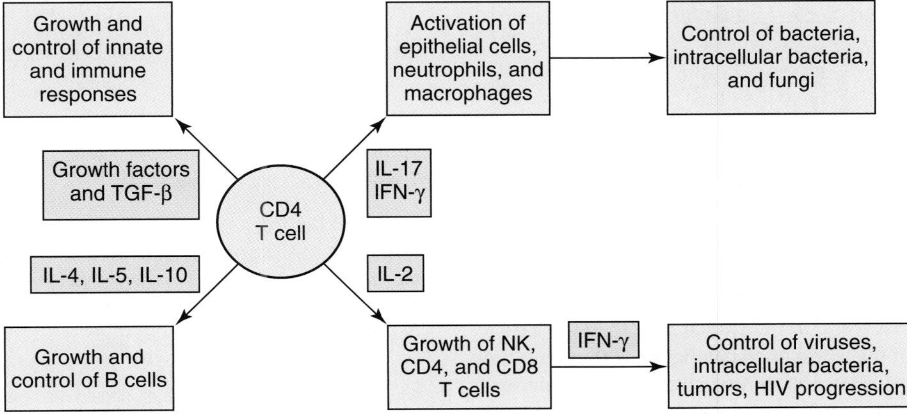

FIGURE 54-10 CD4 T cells have a critical role in activating and regulating cell-mediated immune responses, especially toward intracellular pathogens. Human immunodeficiency virus *(HIV)*–induced loss of CD4 T cells results in loss of the functions activated and regulated by the indicated cytokines. *IFN,* Interferon; *IL,* interleukin; *NK,* natural killer; *TGF-β,* transforming growth factor-*β*.

Epidemiology

AIDS was first noted in homosexual men in the United States but has spread in epidemic proportions throughout the population (Figures 54-11 and 54-12; Box 54-3). Although the numbers continue to rise, as of 2014, the rate of increase has stabilized because of prevention campaigns.

HIV-1 is genetically most similar to a chimpanzee immunodeficiency virus. HIV-2 is more similar to simian immunodeficiency virus. The initial human infection occurred in Africa before the 1930s but went unnoticed in rural areas. The migration of infected people to the cities and increased nonsterile use of syringes after the 1960s brought the virus into population centers, and cultural acceptance of prostitution promoted its transmission throughout the population.

Geographic Distribution

HIV-1 infections are spreading worldwide, with the largest number of AIDS cases in sub-Saharan Africa but with a growing number of cases in Asia, the United States, and the rest of the world (see Figure 54-12). HIV-2 is more prevalent in Africa (especially West Africa) than in the United States and other parts of the world. HIV-2 produces a disease similar to but less severe than AIDS. Heterosexual transmission is the major means of spread of HIV-1 and HIV-2 in

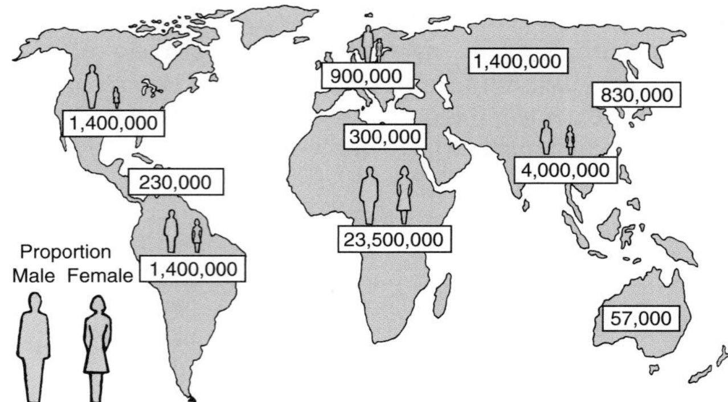

FIGURE 54-12 Upper estimates of numbers of people living with human immunodeficiency virus (HIV) infections as of the end of 2011. The estimated cumulative global total of HIV-infected adults in 2011 was approximately 34 million: more than 7000 new infections per day; deaths, 2.5 million. Infection rates vary widely in different regions of the world. The highest rates are in sub-Saharan Africa. (Modified from *UNAIDS Report on the global AIDS Epidemic 2012.* www.unaids.org/en/media/unaids/contentassets/documents/epidemiology/2012/gr2012/20121120_unaids_global_report_2012_with_annexes_en.pdf. Accessed June 3, 2014.)

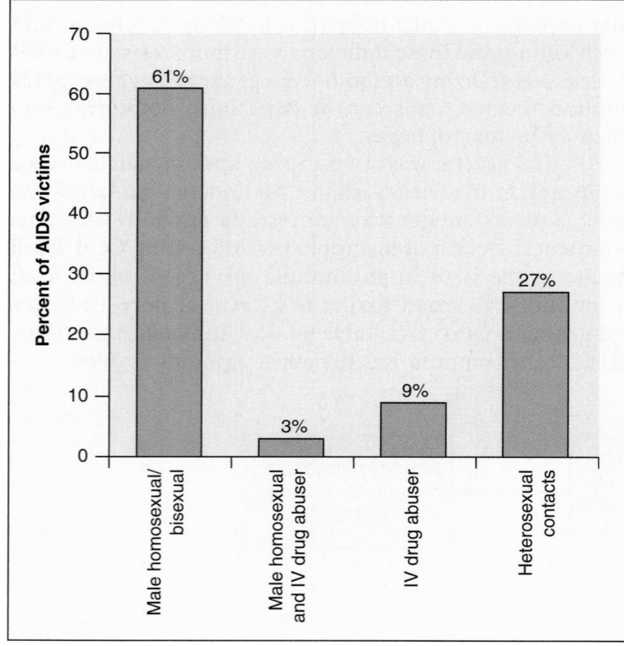

FIGURE 54-11 Acquired immunodeficiency syndrome *(AIDS)* statistics for the United States as of 2011. The percentages of AIDS cases are presented by exposure category for men, women, and children younger than 13 years. In the United States, unlike Africa and many other parts of the world, men having sex with men is the largest exposure category. However, intravenous *(IV)* drug abusers and heterosexual partners are becoming more prevalent. (From Centers for Disease Control and Prevention: HIV in the United States: at a glance. www.cdc.gov/hiv/resources/factsheets/us.htm. Accessed April 29, 2015.)

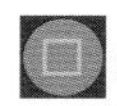

Box 54-3 Epidemiology of Human Immunodeficiency Virus (HIV) Infections

Disease Viral Factors

Enveloped virus is easily inactivated and must be transmitted in body fluids.

Disease has a long prodromal period.

Virus can be shed before development of identifiable symptoms.

Transmission

Virus is present in blood, semen, and vaginal secretions.

See Table 54-4 for modes of transmission.

Who Is at Risk?

Intravenous drug abusers, sexually active people with many partners (MSM and heterosexual), prostitutes, newborns of HIV-positive mothers, sexual partners of infected individuals

Blood and organ transplant recipients and hemophiliacs treated before 1985 (before prescreening programs)

Geography/Season

There is an expanding epidemic worldwide.

There is no seasonal incidence.

Modes of Control

Antiviral drugs limit progression of disease.

Vaccines for prevention and treatment are in trials.

Safe, monogamous sex helps limit spread.

Sterile injection needles should be used.

Circumcision

Large-scale screening programs should be established for blood for transfusions, organs for transplants, and clotting factors used by hemophiliacs.

MSM, Men who have sex with men.

Africa, with men and women equally affected by these viruses. The different clades of HIV-1 have different worldwide geographic distributions.

Although rare, there are cases of long-term survivors. Some of these result from infection with HIV strains that lack a functional Nef protein. The Nef protein is necessary to promote the progression of HIV infection to AIDS. Resistance to the virus also correlates with a lack of or mutation of the CCR5 chemokine co-receptor for the virus or specific HLA types that promote more vigorous cytotoxic T-cell responses.

Transmission

The presence of **HIV in the blood, semen, and vaginal secretions** of infected people and **the long asymptomatic period of infection** are factors that have promoted spread of the disease through sexual contact and exposure to contaminated blood and blood products (Table 54-4). The fetus and newborn are likely to acquire the virus from an infected mother. HIV is *not,* however, transmitted by casual contact, touching, hugging, kissing, coughing, sneezing, insect bites, water, food, utensils, toilets, swimming pools, or public baths.

Populations at Highest Risk

Sexually active people (men who have sex with men [MSM] and heterosexual men and women), intravenous drug abusers and their sexual partners, and the newborns of HIV-positive mothers are at highest risk for HIV infections, with black and Hispanic persons disproportionately represented in the HIV-positive population.

As already noted, AIDS was initially described in young, promiscuous, homosexual men and is still prevalent in the gay community. Anal intercourse is an efficient means of viral transmission. However, heterosexual transmission by vaginal intercourse and intravenous drug abuse have become the major routes by which HIV is being spread in the larger population. The prevalence of HIV in drug abusers stems from sharing contaminated syringe needles, a common practice in "shooting galleries." In New York alone, more than 80% of intravenous drug abusers are positive for the HIV antibody, and these people are now the major source of heterosexual and congenital transmission of the virus. Tattoo needles and contaminated inks are other potential means by which HIV can be transmitted.

Before 1985, people receiving blood transfusions or organ transplants and hemophiliacs receiving clotting factors from pooled blood were at high risk for HIV infection. HIV was spread in many countries by health care workers using shared or improperly sterilized syringe needles or instruments. Proper screening of the blood supply and transplant tissue in the United States and elsewhere has practically eliminated the danger of HIV being transmitted in blood transfusions (see Figure 54-12). Hemophiliacs who receive pooled clotting factors are protected further by proper handling of the factor (prolonged heating) to kill the virus or by the use of genetically engineered proteins.

Health care workers are at risk for HIV infection from accidental needlesticks or cuts or through the exposure of broken skin and mucosal membranes to contaminated blood. Fortunately, studies of needlestick victims have shown that seroconversion occurs in less than 1% of those exposed to HIV-positive blood.

Table 54-4 Transmission of Human Immunodeficiency Virus Infection

Routes	Specific Transmission
Known Routes of Transmission	
Inoculation in blood	Transfusion of blood and blood products
	Needle sharing among intravenous drug abusers
	Needlestick, open wound, and mucous membrane exposure in health care workers
	Tattoo needles
Sexual transmission	Anal and vaginal intercourse
Perinatal transmission	Intrauterine transmission
	Peripartum transmission
	Breast milk
Routes Not Involved in Transmission	
Close personal contact	Household members
	Health care workers not exposed to blood

Clinical Syndromes

AIDS is one of the most devastating epidemics ever recorded. Most HIV-infected people will become symptomatic, and the overwhelming majority of them will ultimately succumb to the disease without treatment. HIV disease progresses from an asymptomatic nonspecific disease to profound immunosuppression, referred to as **AIDS** (Clinical Case 54-1; see Figure 54-9). The diseases related to AIDS mainly consist of opportunistic infections, cancers, and the direct effects of HIV on the central nervous system (Table 54-5).

The initial symptoms following HIV infection (acute phase, 2 to 4 weeks after infection) may resemble those of influenza or infectious mononucleosis, with "aseptic" meningitis or a rash occurring up to 3 months after infection (Box 54-4). As in EBV mononucleosis, the symptoms stem from T-cell responses triggered by a widespread infection of antigen-presenting cells (macrophages). These symptoms subside spontaneously after 2 to 3 weeks and are followed by a period of asymptomatic infection or a persistent generalized lymphadenopathy that may last for several years. During this period, the virus is replicating in the lymph nodes.

Deterioration of the immune response is indicated by increased susceptibility to opportunistic pathogens. The onset of symptoms correlates with a reduction in the number of CD4 T cells to less than 500/μl and increased levels of virus (as determined by polymerase chain reaction [PCR]-related techniques) and protein p24 in the blood. Full-blown AIDS occurs when **CD4 T-cell counts are less than 200/μl** (oftentimes to 50/μl or undetectable) and **virus load is greater than 75,000 copies/ml** and involves the onset of more significant diseases, including HIV wasting syndrome (weight loss and diarrhea for > 1 month) and opportunistic infections, malignancies, and dementia (see Table 54-5).

AIDS may be manifested in several different ways, including lymphadenopathy and fever, opportunistic infections, malignancies, and AIDS-related dementia.

Clinical Case 54-1 An Early Case of HIV/AIDS

Elliott and associates (*Ann Int Med* 98:290–293, 1983) reported that in July 1981, a 27-year-old man complained of dysuria, fever, chills, night sweats, weakness, dyspnea, cough with white sputum, anorexia, and a 16-pound weight loss. For the past 7 years, he had been receiving up to 4 monthly infusions of factor VIII concentrate to correct his hemophilia. He did not have any other risk factors for HIV infection. In August, pulmonary infiltrates were visible by chest radiograph, and in September, blood test results were hemoglobin 10.7 g/dl, leukocytes 4200/μl with 50% polymorphonuclear leukocytes, 2% band forms, 36% lymphocytes, and 12% monocytes. Immunoglobulin G antibody was present to cytomegalovirus, Epstein-Barr virus, *Toxoplasma,* hepatitis B surface antigen, and hepatitis B core. An immune deficiency was suggested by a lack of response in tuberculin, mumps, and *Candida* skin tests. The presence of *Pneumocystis jirovecii* in a methenamine silver stain of a transbronchial lung biopsy specimen prompted oral treatment with trimethoprim/sulfamethoxazole. Episodes of thrush caused by *Candida albicans* prompted treatment with ketoconazole. In May of 1982, development of splenomegaly and lymphadenopathy prompted admission to the hospital, with a leukocyte count of 2100/μl and only 11% lymphocytes. At this time, *Mycobacterium avium-intracellulare* was detected in bone marrow, lymph nodes, and granulomas, and total lymphocyte counts were 448/μl, compared to a normal count of 2668/μl; levels were not responsive to mitogen stimulation. In July 1982, total lymphocyte count fell to 220/μl, with 45/μl CD3-positive T cells (normal 1725 and 64, respectively) and a CD4:CD8 ratio of 1:4 (normal 2.2:1). The patient continued to deteriorate and died at the end of September 1982. Cytomegalovirus was isolated from lung and liver and *M. avium-intracellulare* from most tissue samples. In 1981, AIDS was a newly described disease, and HIV had not been discovered. Monoclonal antibodies and immunophenotyping were new technologies. The patient acquired HIV infection from the factor VIII concentrate at a time before routine screening of the blood supply.

Box 54-4 Clinical Summary

A 32-year-old former heroin addict had a mononucleosis-like illness for 2 weeks. He recalled experiencing occasional night sweats and fever for 3 years and then presented with thrush, cytomegalovirus retinitis, and *Pneumocystis* pneumonia. His CD4 T-cell count was 50/μl. He was started on highly active antiretroviral therapy.

Lymphadenopathy and Fever

Lymphadenopathy and fever develop insidiously and may be accompanied by weight loss and malaise. These findings may persist indefinitely or progress. Symptoms may also include opportunistic infections, diarrhea, night sweats, and fatigue. The wasting disease is termed **slim disease** in Africa.

Opportunistic Infections

Normally benign infections caused by agents such as *Candida albicans* and other fungi, DNA viruses capable of recurrent disease, parasites, and intracellularly growing bacteria cause significant disease after HIV depletion of CD4 T cells and subsequent reduction of CD8 T cells (see Table 54-5). ***Pneumocystis jirovecii*–induced *Pneumocystis* pneumonia (PCP)** is a major sign of AIDS. Oral candidiasis (thrush), cerebral toxoplasmosis, and cryptococcal meningitis also often occur, as do prolonged and severe viral infections, including molluscum contagiosum poxvirus, papovaviruses (JC virus, causing progressive multifocal leukoencephalopathy), and recurrences of the herpesviruses (e.g., herpes simplex virus, varicella-zoster virus, Epstein-Barr virus [EBV; hairy leukoplakia of the mouth, EBV-associated lymphomas], cytomegalovirus [especially retinitis, pneumonia, and bowel disease]). Tuberculosis and other mycobacterial diseases and diarrhea caused by common pathogens (*Salmonella, Shigella,* and *Campylobacter* species) and uncommon agents (cryptosporidia, mycobacteria, and *Amoeba* species) are also common problems.

Table 54-5 Indicator Diseases of Acquired Immunodeficiency Syndrome*

Infection	Disease (Selected)
Opportunistic Infections	
Protozoal	Toxoplasmosis of the brain
	Cryptosporidiosis with diarrhea
	Isosporiasis with diarrhea
Fungal	Candidiasis of the esophagus, trachea, and lungs
	Pneumocystis jirovecii (previously called *Pneumocystis carinii*) pneumonia
	Cryptococcosis (extrapulmonary)
	Histoplasmosis (disseminated)
	Coccidioidomycosis (disseminated)
Viral	Cytomegalovirus disease
	Herpes simplex virus infection (persistent or disseminated)
	Progressive multifocal leukoencephalopathy (JC virus)
	Hairy leukoplakia caused by Epstein-Barr virus
Bacterial	*Mycobacterium avium-intracellulare* complex (disseminated)
	Any "atypical" mycobacterial disease
	Extrapulmonary tuberculosis
	Salmonella septicemia (recurrent)
	Pyogenic bacterial infections (multiple or recurrent)
Opportunistic Neoplasias	Kaposi sarcoma
	Primary lymphoma of the brain
	Hodgkin and non-Hodgkin lymphomas
	HPV-associated cancers
Others	HIV wasting syndrome
	HIV encephalopathy
	Lymphoid interstitial pneumonia

Modified from Belshe RB: *Textbook of human virology,* ed 2, St Louis, 1991, Mosby.

HIV, Human immunodeficiency virus; *HPV,* human papillomavirus.

*Manifestations of HIV infection—defining AIDS according to criteria of Centers for Disease Control and Prevention.

Malignancies

The most notable malignancy to develop in patients with AIDS is the HHV-8–associated Kaposi sarcoma, a rare and otherwise benign skin cancer that disseminates to involve visceral organs in immunodeficient patients. EBV-related lymphomas are also prevalent.

Dementia Related to AIDS

AIDS-related dementia may result from opportunistic infection or HIV infection of the macrophages and microglial cells of the brain. Patients with this condition may undergo a slow deterioration of their intellectual abilities and exhibit other signs of a neurologic disorder, similar to the signs of the early stages of Alzheimer disease. Neurologic deterioration could also result from infection with one of the many opportunistic infections.

Laboratory Diagnosis

Tests for HIV infection are performed for one of four reasons: (1) to identify those with the infection so that antiviral drug therapy can be initiated, (2) to identify carriers who may transmit infection to others (specifically blood or organ donors, pregnant women, and sex partners), (3) to follow the course of disease and confirm the diagnosis of AIDS, or (4) to evaluate the efficacy of treatment (Table 54-6).

The chronic nature of the disease allows use of serologic tests to document HIV infection, as supplemented by genome detection and quantitation with PCR-related techniques. Unfortunately, serologic tests cannot identify recently infected people. HIV is very difficult to grow in tissue culture, and virus isolation is not performed. Recent infection or late-stage disease are indicated by the presence of large quantities of viral RNA in blood samples, the p24 viral antigen, or the RT enzyme (see Figure 54-9).

Genomics

Newer methods for detection and quantitation of HIV genomes in blood have become a mainstay for following the course of an HIV infection and the efficacy and patient compliance with antiviral therapy. After converting viral RNA into DNA with a RT (laboratory provided), the cDNA of the genome can be detected by PCR and quantitated by real-time PCR, branched-chain DNA amplification, and other methods (see Chapter 5). Determination of the viral load (amount of genome in blood) is an excellent indicator of the course of disease and efficacy of therapy.

Table 54-6 Laboratory Analysis for Human Immunodeficiency Virus

Test	Purpose
Serology	
Enzyme-linked immunosorbent assay	Initial screening
Latex agglutination	Initial screening
Rapid oral antibody test	Initial screening
Western blot analysis (for antibody)	Confirmation test
Virion RNA RT-PCR	Detection of virus in blood
Real-time RT-PCR	Quantitation of virus in blood
Branched-chain DNA	Quantitation of virus in blood
p24 antigen	Early marker of infection
Isolation of virus	Test not readily available
CD4 T-cell counts, CD4:CD8 T-cell ratio	Indicators of HIV disease

DNA, Deoxyribonucleic acid; *HIV*, human immunodeficiency virus; *RNA*, ribonucleic acid; *RT-PCR*, reverse transcriptase polymerase chain reaction.

Serology

Screening of blood and organ donors is performed by serology, despite its inability to detect a recent infection. HIV antibody may develop slowly, taking 4 to 8 weeks in most patients; however, it may take 6 months or more in as many as 5% of those infected (see Figure 54-9). Enzyme-linked immunosorbent assays (ELISAs) or agglutination procedures are used for routine screening. The ELISA test, however, can yield false-positive results. Western blot analysis is used to confirm seropositive results. The Western blot assay (see Chapters 5 and 39, Figure 39-7) demonstrates the presence of antibody to the viral antigens (p24 or p31) and glycoproteins (gp41 and gp120/160). Rapid screening tests are available that detect the p24 antigen and/or anti-HIV antibodies in blood.

Immunologic Studies

The status of an HIV infection can be inferred from an analysis of the T-cell subsets. The absolute number of CD4 lymphocytes and the *ratio of CD4 to CD8 lymphocytes* are *abnormally low* in HIV-infected people. The particular concentration of CD4 lymphocytes identifies the stage of AIDS. The choice to initiate therapy is usually based on CD4 T-cell counts.

Treatment, Prevention, and Control

The principal (as of 2014) anti-HIV therapies are listed in Box 54-5. The anti-HIV drugs approved by the U.S. Food and Drug Administration can be classified as inhibitors of **binding, fusion-penetration, integrase or protease or nucleoside analog reverse transcriptase inhibitors, or nonnucleoside reverse transcriptase inhibitors.**

Inhibition of binding to the CCR5 co-receptor with a receptor agonist (maraviroc) or fusion of the viral envelope and cell membrane with a peptide (T-20: enfuvirtide) that blocks the action of the gp41 molecule will prevent the initial infection event. Inhibition of the integrase prevents all subsequent events in the replication of the virus. Inhibition of the RT prevents the initiation of virus replication by blocking cDNA synthesis. Azidothymidine (AZT) and the other nucleotide analogs are phosphorylated by cellular enzymes and incorporated into cDNA by the RT to cause DNA chain termination. Nonnucleoside RT inhibitors (nevirapine) inhibit the enzyme by other mechanisms. Protease inhibitors block the morphogenesis of the virion by inhibiting cleavage of the Gag and Gag-Pol polyproteins. The viral proteins and resulting virion are inactive. Most anti-HIV drugs have significant side effects, and the search continues for new anti-HIV drugs. Each of the replicative steps and all of the viral proteins are being targeted for development of new anti-HIV drugs.

AZT was the first successful anti-HIV therapy. Although still given to infants born to HIV-positive mothers for 6

Box 54-5 Potential Antiviral Therapies for Human Immunodeficiency Virus Infection

Nucleoside Analog Reverse Transcriptase Inhibitors (NRTIs)
Azidothymidine (AZT) (Zidovudine) [Retrovir]
Dideoxyinosine (ddI) (Didanosine) [Videx]
d4T (Stavudine) [Zerit]
3TC (Lamivudine) [Epivir]
Tenofovir disoproxil fumarate (adenosine class) [Viread]
ABC (Abacavir) [Ziagen]
FTC (Emtricitabine) [Emtriva]

Nonnucleoside Reverse Transcriptase Inhibitors (NNRTIs)
Nevirapine [Viramune]
Delavirdine [Rescriptor]
Efavirenz [Sustiva]
Etravirene [Intelence]
Rilpivirine [Edurant]

Protease Inhibitors (PIs)
Tipranavir [Aptivus]
Darunavir [Prezista]
Ritonavir [Norvir]
Indinavir [Crixivan]
Nelfinavir [Viracept]
Fosamprenavir [Lexia]
Atazanavir [Reyataz]

Binding and Fusion Inhibitors
CCR5 inhibitor (maraviroc) [Selzentry]
T-20 (enfuvirtide) [Fuzeon]

Integrase Inhibitor
Raltegravir [Isentress]

Examples of Highly Active Antiretroviral Therapy (HAART)
Efavirenz/tenofovir/emtricitabine (EFV/TDF/FTC) [Atripla]*
Abacavir/zidovudine/lamivudine [Trizivir]
Dolutegravir/abacavir/lamivudine [Triumeq]*
Emtricitabine, rilpivirine, and tenofovir disoproxil fumarate [Complera]*
Elvitegravir/cobicistat/tenofovir/emtricitabine [Stribild]*

Modified from www.fda.gov/ForConsumers/byAudience/ForPatientAdvocates/HIVandAIDSActivities/ucm118915.htm and http://aidsinfo.nih.gov/education-materials/fact-sheets/21/58/fda-approved-hiv-medicines.

*Complete one-pill, once-daily drug regimen.

weeks postpartum, single use of AZT or another nucleotide analog by itself is decreasing. Anti-HIV therapy is currently given as a cocktail of several antiviral drugs termed **highly active antiretroviral treatment (HAART)** (see Box 54-5). Use of a mixture of drugs with different mechanisms of action has less potential to select for resistance. Multidrug therapy can reduce blood levels of virus to nearly zero and reduce morbidity and mortality in many patients with advanced AIDS. These drugs are often difficult to tolerate, and each drug has its own side effects. Customization of HAART for each patient can minimize the drug side effects, ease the pill-taking regimen, and allow the patient to return to nearly normal health and lifestyle. Some HAARTs are taken once a day as a single pill, assisting compliance. Therapy should be initiated for individuals showing symptoms of AIDS, AIDS-defining illnesses, or if CD4 T cells drop to less than 350/µl. Therapy may also be considered if viral loads are high (>100,000), even if CD4 numbers are above 350/µl. Therapy is also suggested for postexposure prophylaxis (e.g., needlestick) if HIV is detected in the individual. HAART is expensive and may require taking many pills during the day.

Education

The principal way HIV infection can be controlled is by educating the population about the methods of transmission and the measures that may curtail viral spread. For instance, monogamous relationships, the practice of safe sex, and use of condoms reduce the possibility of exposure. Because contaminated needles are a major source of HIV infection in intravenous drug abusers, people must be taught that needles must not be shared. The reuse of contaminated needles in clinics was the source of outbreaks of AIDS in the former Soviet bloc and other countries. In some places, efforts have been launched to provide sterile equipment to intravenous drug abusers. A successful anti-HIV education campaign in Uganda has been cited as more effective than antiviral drugs for saving lives.

Blood, Blood Product, and Organ Screening

Potential blood and organ donors are screened before they donate blood, tissue, and blood products. People testing positive for HIV must not donate blood. People who anticipate a future need for blood, such as those awaiting elective surgery, should consider donating blood beforehand. To limit the worldwide epidemic, blood screening must be initiated in developing nations as well.

Infection Control

The infection-control procedures for HIV infection are the same as those for hepatitis B virus. They include use of universal blood and body fluid precautions, which are based on the assumption that all patients are infectious for HIV and other blood-borne pathogens. Precautions include wearing protective clothing (e.g., gloves, mask, gown) and using other barriers to prevent exposure to blood products. Syringes and surgical instruments should never be reused unless carefully disinfected. Contaminated surfaces should be disinfected with 10% household bleach, 70% ethanol or isopropanol, 2% glutaraldehyde, and 4% formaldehyde, or 6% hydrogen peroxide. Washing laundry in hot water with detergent should be sufficient to inactivate HIV.

Approaches to Prophylaxis

There are many difficulties in development of a vaccine against HIV. A successful vaccine must be able to block the initial infection and the movement of infected dendritic cells and T cells to lymph nodes. Otherwise, like herpesviruses, HIV infection rapidly establishes a chronic or latent infection. The vaccine must elicit neutralizing antibody and cell-mediated immunity. The primary target of neutralizing antibody, the gp120, is different for the different HIV clades and even within a clade; there are many antigenically distinct mutants that change during the infection of the individual. Cell-mediated immunity is necessary because the virus can be spread through cell-to-cell bridges and remains latent, thereby hiding from antibody. Finally, testing of the vaccine is difficult and expensive because large numbers of susceptible people must be evaluated, and long-term follow-up is required to monitor the efficacy of each formulation.

Several different approaches have been tried for developing an HIV vaccine. Live attenuated vaccines (e.g., deletion of the *nef* gene) were too dangerous because they still cause disease in infants and may establish chronic infection. Protein subunit vaccines with gp120 or its precursor, gp160, by themselves, elicit only antibody to a single strain of HIV and have not been successful. The most recent HIV vaccines prime T-cell responses with a vaccinia, canarypox, or defective adenovirus vector or with a DNA vaccine consisting of eukaryotic expression vectors (plasmids) containing the gene for gp160 *(env)* and other HIV genes. This is followed by a protein boost with gp120 or gp160 to activate B cells and develop neutralizing antibody. The gp120 and gp160 proteins are genetically engineered and expressed in different eukaryotic cell systems (e.g., yeast, baculovirus).

Incorporation of an anti-HIV drug into contraceptive creams has demonstrated some ability to reduce transmission of HIV. Circumcision of males reduces their risk of infection; circumcision eliminates a site of frequent infections and a unique microbiome that can cause breaks in the skin and inflammation, both of which may increase susceptibility to HIV infection.

• Human T-Cell Lymphotropic Virus and Other Oncogenic Retroviruses

The Oncovirinae were originally called the **RNA tumor viruses** and have been associated with the development of leukemias, sarcomas, and lymphomas in many animals. These viruses are not cytolytic. Members of this family are distinguished by their mechanism of cell transformation (immortalization) and thus the length of the latency period between infection and development of disease (Table 54-7).

The **sarcoma and acute leukemia viruses** have incorporated modified versions of cellular genes (proto-oncogenes) encoding growth-controlling factors into their genome ***(v-onc).*** These include genes that encode growth hormones, growth hormone receptors, protein kinases, guanosine triphosphate–binding proteins (G-proteins), and nuclear DNA–binding proteins. These viruses can cause transformation of cells relatively rapidly and are highly oncogenic. *No human virus of this type has been identified.*

At least 35 different viral oncogenes have been identified (Table 54-8). Transformation results from the overproduction or altered activity of the growth-stimulating protein encoded by the oncogene. Increased cell growth then promotes transcription, which also promotes viral replication. Incorporation of the oncogene into many of these viruses causes the coding sequences for the *gag, pol,* or *env* genes to be replaced, such that most of these viruses are defective and require helper viruses for replication. Many of these viruses become endogenous and then are transmitted vertically through the germline of the animal.

The **leukemia viruses,** including HTLV-1, are competent in terms of replication but cannot transform cells in vitro. They cause cancer after a **long latency period** of at least 30 years. The leukemia viruses promote cell growth in more indirect ways than the oncogene-encoding viruses. For HTLV-1, a transcriptional regulator, Tax, is produced and is capable of activating promoters in the LTR region and specific cellular genes (including growth-controlling and cytokine genes, such as those encoding IL-2 and granulocyte-macrophage colony-stimulating factor) to promote the outgrowth of that cell. Alternatively, by integrating near cellular growth–controlling genes, the enhancer and promoter gene sequences encoded in the viral LTR region can promote expression of growth-stimulating proteins. Neoplastic transformation to produce leukemia requires other genetic changes that are more likely to occur because of the stimulated growth of the infected cell. These viruses are also associated with nonneoplastic neurologic disorders and other diseases. For example, HTLV-1 causes **adult acute T-cell lymphocytic leukemia (ATLL)** and **HTLV-1–associated myelopathy (tropical spastic paraparesis),** a nononcogenic neurologic disease.

The human oncoviruses include HTLV-1, HTLV-2, and HTLV-5, but only HTLV-1 has been definitively associated with disease (i.e., ATLL). HTLV-2 was isolated from atypical forms of hairy cell leukemia, and HTLV-5 was isolated from a malignant cutaneous lymphoma. HTLV-1 and HTLV-2 share as much as 50% homology.

Table 54-7 Mechanisms of Retrovirus Oncogenesis

Disease	Speed	Effect
Acute leukemia or sarcoma	Fast: oncogene	Direct effect Provision of growth-enhancing proteins
Leukemia	Slow: transactivation	Indirect effect Transactivation protein (Tax) or long terminal repeat promoter sequences that enhance expression of cellular growth genes

Table 54-8 Representative Examples of Oncogenes

Function	Oncogene	Virus
Tyrosine kinase	*Src*	Rous sarcoma virus
	Abl	Abelson murine leukemia virus
	Fes	ST feline sarcoma virus
Growth factor receptors	*Erb*-B (EGF receptor)	Avian erythroblastosis virus
	Erb-A (thyroid hormone receptor)	Avian erythroblastosis virus
Guanosine triphosphate–binding proteins	Ha-*ras*	Harvey murine sarcoma virus
	Ki-*ras*	Kirsten murine sarcoma virus
Nuclear proteins	*Myc*	Avian myelocytomatosis virus
	Myb	Avian myeloblastosis virus
	Fos	Murine osteosarcoma virus FBJ
	Jun	Avian sarcoma virus 17

EGF, Epidermal growth factor; *FBJ,* Finkel-Biskis-Jinkins; *ST,* Snyder-Theilen.

Pathogenesis and Immunity

HTLV-1 is cell associated and is spread in cells after blood transfusion, sexual intercourse, or breastfeeding. The virus enters the bloodstream and infects the CD4 helper T cells. In addition to blood and lymphatic organs, these T cells have a tendency to reside in the skin, thus contributing to the symptoms of ATLL. Neurons also express a receptor for HTLV-1.

HTLV is competent for replication, with the *gag, pol,* and *env* genes transcribed, translated, and processed as described earlier. In addition to its action on viral genes, the Tax protein transactivates the cellular genes for the T-cell growth factor IL-2 and its receptor (IL-2R), which activates growth in the infected cell. A cellular protein, HBZ, limits Tax activity, promoting cell survival. The virus may remain latent or may replicate slowly for many years but may also induce the clonal outgrowth of particular T-cell clones.

There is a long latency period (≈30 years) before the onset of leukemia. Although the virus can induce a polyclonal outgrowth of T cells, HTLV-1–induced adult T-cell leukemia is usually monoclonal.

Antibodies are elicited to the gp46 and other proteins of HTLV-1. HTLV-1 infection also causes immunosuppression.

Epidemiology

HTLV-1 is transmitted and acquired by the same routes as HIV. It is endemic in southern Japan, the Caribbean, Central Africa, and among African Americans in the southeastern United States. In the endemic regions of Japan, the children acquire HTLV-1 at birth and in breast milk from their mothers, whereas the adults are infected sexually. The number of seropositive people in some regions of Japan may be as high as 35% (Okinawa), with twice the mortality rate from leukemia compared to other regions. Intravenous drug abuse and blood transfusion are becoming the most prominent means of transmitting the virus in the United States, where the high-risk groups for HTLV-1 infection are the same as those for HIV infection.

Clinical Syndromes

HTLV infection is usually asymptomatic but can progress to ATLL in approximately 1 in 20 persons over a 30- to 50-year period. ATLL caused by HTLV-1 is a neoplasia of the CD4 helper T cells that can be acute or chronic. The malignant cells have been termed "flower cells" because they are pleomorphic and contain lobulated nuclei. In addition to an elevated white blood cell count, this form of ATLL is characterized by skin lesions similar to those seen in another leukemia, Sézary syndrome. ATLL is usually fatal within a year of diagnosis, regardless of treatment. HTLV-1 can also cause other diseases, including uveitis, HTLV-associated infectious dermatitis, and other inflammatory disorders.

Laboratory Diagnosis

HTLV-1 infection is detected using ELISA to find virus-specific antigens in blood, using reverse transcriptase–polymerase chain reaction (RT-PCR) for viral RNA, or using ELISA to detect specific antiviral antibodies.

Treatment, Prevention, and Control

A combination of AZT and interferon-α has been effective in some patients with ATLL. However, no particular treatment has been approved for the management of HTLV-1 infection.

The measures used to limit the spread of HTLV-1 are the same as those used to limit transmission of HIV. Sexual precautions, screening of the blood supply, and increased awareness of the potential risks and diseases are ways to prevent transmission of the virus. Routine screening for HTLV-1, HIV, hepatitis B virus, and hepatitis C virus is performed to protect the blood supply. Maternal infection of children is very difficult to control, however.

• Endogenous Retroviruses

Different retroviruses have integrated into and become a part of the chromosomes of humans and animals. In fact, retrovirus sequences may make up at least 8% of the human genome. Complete and partial provirus sequences with gene sequences similar to those of HTLV, mouse mammary tumor virus, and other retroviruses can be detected in humans. These endogenous viruses generally lack the ability to replicate because of deletions or the insertion of termination codons or because they are poorly transcribed. One such retrovirus can be detected in placental tissue and is activated by pregnancy. This virus produces syncytin, necessary to facilitate placental function. Another endogenous retrovirus is associated with prostate cancer.

Bibliography

Caldwell JC, Caldwell P: The African AIDS epidemic, *Sci Am* 274:62–68, 1996.

Centers for Disease Control and Prevention: Updated U.S. Public Health Service guidelines for the management of exposures to HBV, HCV, and HIV and recommendations for postexposure prophylaxis, *MMWR Morb Mortal Recomm Rep* 50(RR–11):1–42, 2001.

Cohen J, Powderly WG: *Infectious diseases*, ed 2, St Louis, 2004, Mosby.

Doltch G, Cavrois M, Lassen KG, et al: Abortive HIV infection mediates CD4 T cell depletion and inflammation in human lymphoid tissue, *Cell* 143:789–801, 2010.

Flint SJ, Enquist LW, Racaniello VR, et al: *Principles of virology: molecular biology, pathogenesis and control of animal viruses*, ed 3, Washington, DC, 2009, American Society for Microbiology Press.

Knipe DM, Howley PM: *Fields virology*, ed 6, Philadelphia, 2013, Lippincott Williams & Wilkins.

Kräusslich HG: *Morphogenesis and maturation of retroviruses*, Berlin, 1996, Springer-Verlag.

Levy JA: *HIV and the pathogenesis of AIDS*, ed 7, Washington, DC, 2007, American Society for Microbiology Press.

Morse SA, Ballard RC, Holmes KK, et al: *Atlas of sexually transmitted diseases and AIDS*, ed 3, St Louis, 2003, Mosby.

Ng VL, McGrath MS: Human T-cell leukemia virus involvement in adult T-cell leukemia, *Cancer Bull* 40:276–280, 1988.

Oldstone MBA, Vitkovic L: *HIV and dementia*, Berlin, 1995, Springer-Verlag.

Ryan FP: Human endogenous retroviruses in health and disease: a symbiotic perspective, *J R Soc Med* 97:560–565, 2004.

Stine GJ: *AIDS update 2011*, New York, 2011, McGraw-Hill.

Strauss JM, Strauss EG: *Viruses and human disease*, ed 2, San Diego, 2007, Academic.

HIV/AIDS and HTLV Websites

About.com: AIDS/HIV. http://aids.about.com/. Accessed April 29, 2015.

AIDS Education Global Information System: Homepage. www.aegis.com. Accessed April 29, 2015.

Bennett NJ: HIV disease. http://emedicine.medscape.com/article/211316-overview. Accessed April 29, 2015.

Centers for Disease Control and Prevention: HIV/AIDS statistics and surveillance. www.cdc.gov/hiv/library/reports/surveillance/index.html. Accessed May 18, 2015.

National Institute of Allergy and Infectious Diseases: NIAID's HIV/AIDS research program. www.niaid.nih.gov/topics/hivaids/Pages/Default.aspx. Accessed April 29, 2015.

National Institutes of Health: http://aidsinfo.nih.gov/. Accessed April 29, 2015.

Szczypinska EM, Wallace MR, Wainscoat B, et al: Human T-cell lymphotropic viruses. http://emedicine.medscape.com/article/219285-overview. Accessed April 29, 2015.

UNAIDS: Data and analysis. www.unaids.org/en/dataanalysis/. Accessed May 18, 2015.

UNAIDS: Homepage. www.unaids.org/. Accessed April 29, 2015.

University of California, San Francisco: HIV InSite. http://hivinsite.ucsf.edu. Accessed April 29, 2015.

U.S. Department of Health and Human Services: Clinical guidelines portal: federally approved HIV/AIDS medical practice guidelines. http://aidsinfo.nih.gov/guidelines. Accessed April 29, 2015.

The White House: National HIV/AIDS strategy for the United States. www.whitehouse.gov/sites/default/files/uploads/NHAS.pdf. Accessed July 2, 2015.

HIV Therapy Websites

Panel on Antiretroviral Guidelines for Adults and Adolescents: Guidelines for the use of antiretroviral agents in HIV-1–infected adults and adolescents. Department of Health and Human Services. http://aidsinfo.nih.gov/contentfiles/AdultandAdolescentGL.pdf. Accessed April 29, 2015.

Panel on Antiretroviral Guidelines for Adults and Adolescents: Tables from *Guidelines for the use of antiretroviral agents in HIV-1–infected adults and adolescents*. Department of Health and Human Services. http://aidsinfo.nih.gov/contentfiles/AA_Tables.pdf. Accessed April 29, 2015.

World Health Organization: Rapid advice: antiretroviral therapy for HIV infection in adults and adolescents, November 2009. www.who.int/hiv/pub/arv/rapid_advice_art.pdf. Accessed April 29, 2015.

CHAPTER

55 HEPATITIS VIRUSES

A 43-year-old woman complained of fatigue, nausea, and abdominal discomfort. She had a slight fever, her urine was dark yellow, and her abdomen was distended and tender. Serologic assays demonstrated the presence of immunoglobulin (Ig)M antibody to the hepatitis B core antigen (HBcAg) and the presence of the hepatitis B surface antigen (HBsAg) and the hepatitis Be antigen (HBeAg). She also had IgG to hepatitis A virus.

1. Which aspects are common to hepatitis disease and which are specific to hepatitis B virus (HBV)?
2. How does serology define the course of this disease?
3. How is this infection transmitted?
4. How could this infection be prevented? Treated?

A 41-year-old intravenous drug abuser complained of fatigue, nausea, and abdominal discomfort. He had a slight fever, his urine was dark yellow, and his abdomen was distended and tender. Serologic assays demonstrated the presence of IgG antibody to the HBsAg but no hepatitis antigens or other anti-HBV antibodies. Reverse transcriptase polymerase chain reaction (RT-PCR) analysis of his serum detected the hepatitis C virus genome.

5. Is this person infected with HBV? Has this person ever been infected with HBV?
6. What is the most likely disease outcome for this patient? Other patients with this infection?
7. How can this infection be treated?

Answers to these questions are available on StudentConsult.com.

• SUMMARIES CLINICALLY SIGNIFICANT ORGANISMS

Hepatitis Viruses

Trigger Words

Hepatitis A: acute/sudden onset, picornavirus, fecal-oral

Hepatitis B: blood-borne, STD, hepadnavirus, reverse transcriptase, chronic, Dane particle, HBsAg

Hepatitis C: chronic, STD, flavivirus

Hepatitis D: defective, hepatitis B helper virus, fulminant disease

Hepatitis E: fecal-oral, acute/sudden onset, pregnant women

Biology, Virulence, and Disease

- Liver disease defines symptoms
- Non-lytic viruses: cell-mediated immunity causes symptoms
- Hepatitis A: non-lytic picornavirus, acute onset, no sequelae
- Hepatitis B: hepadnavirus, enveloped and encodes reverse transcriptase
  - Disease followed by serology
  - Chronic disease 5% of time, especially in children
  - Risk for primary hepatocellular carcinoma (PHC)
- Hepatitis C: flavivirus
  - Causes chronic disease in 70% of patients
  - Risk for PHC and cirrhosis after long period
- Hepatitis D: viroid-like, requires HBV as helper virus
- Hepatitis E: calici-like virus, acute onset, no sequelae, severe for pregnant women

Epidemiology

- HAV, HEV: fecal-oral transmission
- HBV, HCV, HDV: spread in blood, tissue, and semen; STDs

Diagnosis

- RT-PCR, ELISA

Treatment, Prevention, and Control

- HAV: inactivated vaccine, hygiene
- HEV: hygiene
- HBV: virus-like particle HBsAg vaccine, screening of blood supply, safe sex, antiviral drugs
- HCV: screening of blood supply, safe sex, antiviral drugs
- HDV: immunization for HBV

The hepatitis alphabet of viruses includes at least six viruses, A through E and G (Table 55-1; a fun summary is provided in Box 55-1). Although the target organ for each of these viruses is the liver and the basic hepatitis symptoms are similar, they differ greatly in their structure, mode of replication, mode of transmission, and in the time course and sequelae of the disease they cause. **Hepatitis A and hepatitis B viruses (HAV, HBV)** are the classic hepatitis viruses, and **hepatitis C, D, E, and G viruses (HCV, HDV [the delta agent], HEV, HGV)** are called **non-A, non-B hepatitis (NANBH) viruses.** Other viruses can also cause hepatitis.

Each of the hepatitis viruses infects and damages the liver, causing the classic **icteric symptoms of jaundice and the release of liver enzymes.** The specific virus causing the disease can be distinguished by the course, nature, and serology of the disease. These viruses are readily spread because infected people are contagious before, or even without, showing symptoms.

Hepatitis A, which is sometimes known as **infectious hepatitis,** (1) is caused by a picornavirus, a ribonucleic acid (RNA) virus; (2) is spread by the fecal-oral route; (3) has an incubation period of approximately 1 month, after which icteric symptoms start abruptly; (4) does not cause chronic liver disease; and (5) rarely causes fatal disease.

Hepatitis B, previously known as **serum hepatitis,** (1) is caused by a hepadnavirus with a deoxyribonucleic acid (DNA) genome; (2) is spread parenterally by blood or needles, by sexual contact, and perinatally; (3) has a median

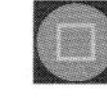

Box 55-1 Everything You Want to Know About Hepatitis Viruses à la Dr. Seuss; by K.S. Rosenthal

Hepatitis A, B, C
Hepatitis D, E, G
Liver is the target
But immune response hurts me
Liver suffers from A to G

Eat the virus, it won't stay
E and A go away
Poop, water, and shellfish dot dot A
That's the acute virus that goes away
Pregnant woman fears the E
It is deadly but not for me

B and C and also D
Blood, tissue, and semen can carry the three
B and C stay with me
PHC with C and B
For the baby, chronic B
HBsAg you will see

Anti-HBs no more sick
Vaccines do this, that's the trick
Treat the RT for the B
Immunize for A or B
Risky business A through G
Yellow eyes you will see

Table 55-1 Comparative Features of Hepatitis Viruses

Feature	Hepatitis A	Hepatitis B	Hepatitis C	Hepatitis D	Hepatitis E
Common name	"Infectious"	"Serum"	"Non-A, non-B posttransfusion"	"Delta agent"	"Enteric non-A, non-B"
Virus structure	Picornavirus; capsid, (+) RNA	Hepadnavirus; envelope, DNA	Flavivirus; envelope, (+) RNA	Viroid-like; envelope, circular RNA	Calicivirus-like; capsid, (+) RNA
Transmission	Fecal-oral	Parenteral, sexual	Parenteral, sexual	Parenteral, sexual	Fecal-oral
Onset	Abrupt	Insidious	Insidious	Abrupt	Abrupt
Incubation period (days)	15-50	45-160	14-180+	15-64	15-50
Severity	Mild	Occasionally severe	Usually subclinical; 70% chronicity	Co-infection with HBV occasionally severe; superinfection with HBV often severe	Normal patients, mild; pregnant women, severe
Mortality	<0.5%	1%-2%	≈4%	High to very high	Normal patients, 1%-2%; pregnant women, 20%
Chronicity/carrier state	No	Yes	Yes	Yes	No
Other disease associations	None	Primary hepatocellular carcinoma, cirrhosis	Primary hepatocellular carcinoma, cirrhosis	Cirrhosis, fulminant hepatitis	None
Laboratory diagnosis	Symptoms and anti-HAV IgM	Symptoms and serum levels of HBsAg, HBeAg, and anti-HBc IgM	Symptoms and anti-HCV ELISA, genome testing	Anti-HDV ELISA	—

DNA, Deoxyribonucleic acid; *ELISA,* enzyme-linked immunosorbent assay; *HAV,* hepatitis A virus; *HBc,* hepatitis B core; *HBeAg,* hepatitis Be antigen; *HBsAg,* hepatitis B surface antigen; *HBV,* hepatitis B virus; *HCV,* hepatitis C virus; *HDV,* hepatitis D virus; *IgM,* immunoglobulin M, *RNA,* ribonucleic acid.

incubation period of approximately 3 months, after which icteric symptoms start insidiously; (4) is followed by chronic hepatitis in 5% to 10% of patients; and (5) is causally associated with primary hepatocellular carcinoma (PHC). More than one third of the world's population has been infected with HBV, resulting in 1 to 2 million deaths per year. The incidence of HBV is decreasing, however, especially in infants, because of the development and use of the HBV subunit vaccine.

HCV is also widely prevalent, with more than 170 million chronically infected carriers of the disease. HCV is spread by the same routes as HBV but is more prone to cause chronic disease. HCV also increases risk for PHC. HCV is a flavivirus with an RNA genome. **HGV** is also a flavivirus and causes chronic infections. **HEV** is an enteric encapsidated virus with an RNA genome in its own family, and its disease resembles HAV.

Hepatitis D, or **delta hepatitis,** is unique in that it requires actively replicating HBV as a "helper virus" and occurs only in patients who have active HBV infection. HBV provides an envelope for HDV RNA and its antigens. HDV exacerbates the symptoms caused by HBV.

• Hepatitis A Virus

HAV causes infectious hepatitis and is spread by the fecal-oral route. HAV infections often result from consumption of contaminated water, shellfish, or other food. HAV is a **picornavirus** and was formerly called *enterovirus 72*, but it has been placed into a new genus, *Heparnavirus,* on the basis of its unique genome.

Structure

HAV has a 27-nm, **naked, icosahedral capsid** surrounding a **positive-sense single-stranded RNA** genome consisting of approximately 7470 nucleotides (Figure 55-1). As a picornavirus, the HAV genome has a VPg protein attached to the 5′ end and a polyadenylate sequence attached to the 3′ end. The capsid is even more stable than other picornaviruses to acid and other treatments (Box 55-2). There is only one serotype of HAV.

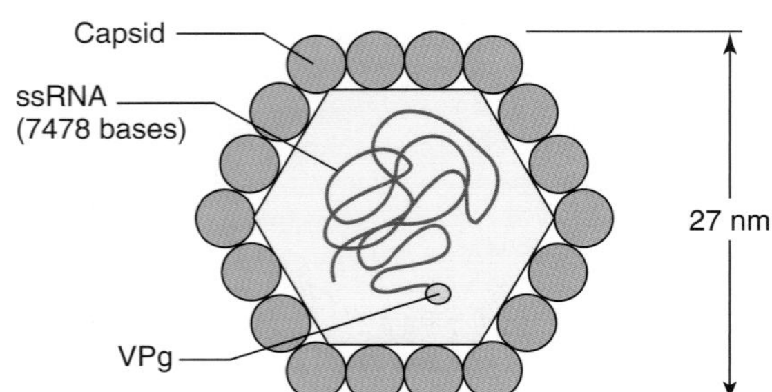

FIGURE 55-1 The picornavirus structure of hepatitis A virus. The icosahedral capsid is made up of four viral polypeptides (VP1 to VP4). Inside the capsid is a single-stranded positive-sense ribonucleic acid *(ssRNA)* that has a genomic viral protein *(VPg)* on the 5′ end.

Replication

HAV replicates like other picornaviruses (see Chapter 46). It interacts specifically with the HAV cell receptor 1 glycoprotein (HAVCR-1, also known as T-cell immunoglobulin and mucin domain protein [TIM-1]) expressed on liver cells and T cells. The structure of HAVCR-1 can vary for different individuals, and specific forms correlate with severity of disease. Unlike other picornaviruses, however, HAV is not cytolytic and is released by exocytosis. Laboratory isolates of HAV have been adapted to grow in primary and continuous monkey kidney cell lines, but clinical isolates are difficult to grow in cell culture.

Pathogenesis

HAV is ingested and probably enters the bloodstream through the epithelial lining of the oropharynx or the intestines to reach its target, the parenchymal cells of the liver (Figure 55-2). The virus replicates in hepatocytes and Kupffer cells. Virus is produced in these cells and is released into the bile and from there into the stool. Virus is shed in large

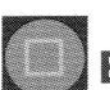 **Box 55-2 Characteristics of Hepatitis A Virus**

Stable to:
Acid at pH 1
Solvents (ether, chloroform)
Detergents
Saltwater, groundwater (months)
Drying (stable)

Temperature:
4° C for weeks: stable
56° C for 30 minutes: stable
61° C for 20 minutes: partial inactivation

Inactivated by:
Chlorine treatment of drinking water
Formalin (0.35%, 37° C, 72 hours)
Peracetic acid (2%, 4 hours)
β-Propiolactone (0.25%, 1 hour)
Ultraviolet radiation (2 μW/cm²/min)

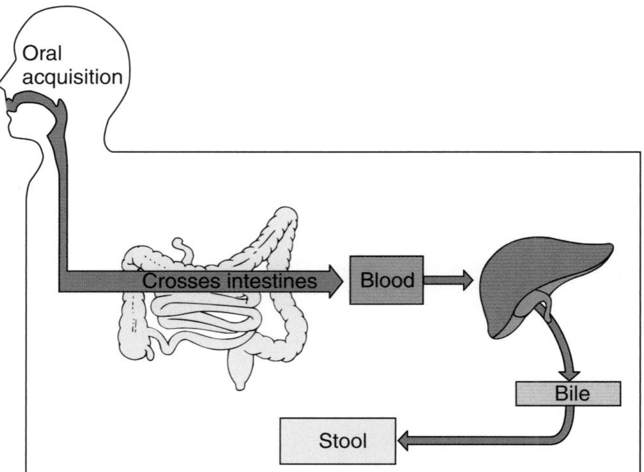

FIGURE 55-2 Spread of hepatitis A virus within the body.

quantity into the stool approximately 10 days before symptoms of jaundice appear or antibody can be detected.

HAV replicates slowly in the liver without producing apparent cytopathic effects. Although interferon limits viral replication, natural killer cells and cytotoxic T cells are required to eliminate infected cells. Antibody, complement, and antibody-dependent cellular cytotoxicity also facilitate clearance of the virus and induction of immunopathology. Icterus, resulting from damage to the liver, occurs when cell-mediated immune responses and antibody to the virus can be detected. Antibody protection against reinfection is lifelong.

The liver pathology caused by HAV infection is indistinguishable histologically from that caused by HBV. It is most likely caused by immunopathology and not virus-induced cytopathology. However, **unlike HBV, HAV cannot initiate a chronic infection** and is not associated with hepatic cancer.

Epidemiology

Approximately 40% of acute cases of hepatitis are caused by HAV (Box 55-3). The virus spreads readily in a community because most infected people are contagious 10 to 14 days before symptoms occur, and 90% of infected children and 25% to 50% of infected adults have **inapparent but productive** infections.

The virus is released into stool in high concentrations and is spread via the **fecal-oral** route. Virus is spread in contaminated water, in food, and by dirty hands. HAV is resistant to detergents, acid (pH of 1), and temperatures as high as 60° C, and it can survive for many months in fresh water and salt water. Raw or improperly treated sewage can taint the water supply and contaminate shellfish. Shellfish, especially clams, oysters, and mussels, are important sources of the virus because they are efficient filter feeders and can therefore concentrate the viral particles, even from dilute solutions. This is exemplified by an epidemic of HAV that occurred in Shanghai, China, in 1988, when 300,000 people were infected with the virus after eating clams obtained from a polluted river.

HAV outbreaks usually originate from a common source (e.g., water supply, restaurant, day-care center). Asymptomatic shedding and a long (15 to 40 days) incubation period make it difficult to identify the source. Day-care settings are a major source for spread of the virus among classmates and their parents. A further problem is posed by the fact that because the children and personnel in day-care centers may be transient, the number of contacts at risk for HAV infection from a single day-care center can be great.

HAV infections are relatively common, with greater incidence with poor hygienic conditions and overcrowding. Most people infected with HAV in developing countries are children who have mild illness and then lifelong immune protection against reinfection. In the United States, the incidence has dropped significantly with use of the vaccine.

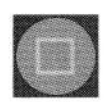

Box 55-3 Epidemiology of Hepatitis A Virus (HAV) and Hepatitis E Virus (HEV)

Disease/Viral Factors

Capsid viruses are strongly resistant to inactivation.
Contagious period extends from before to after symptoms.
Virus may cause asymptomatic shedding.

Transmission

Virus can be transmitted via fecal-oral route.
Ingestion of contaminated food and water can cause infection.
HAV in shellfish is from sewage-contaminated water.
Virus can be transmitted by food handlers, day-care workers, and children.

Who Is at Risk?

People in overcrowded, unsanitary areas
Travelers to high-risk regions
Children: mild disease, possibly asymptomatic; day-care centers are a major source of spread of HAV
Adults: abrupt-onset hepatitis
Pregnant women: high mortality associated with HEV

Geography/Season

Virus is found worldwide.
There is no seasonal incidence.

Means of Control

Good hygiene
HAV: passive antibody protection for contacts
- Killed vaccine
- Live vaccine in China

Clinical Syndromes

The symptoms caused by HAV are very similar to those caused by HBV and stem from immune-mediated damage to the liver. The **symptoms occur abruptly** 15 to 50 days after exposure, intensify for 4 to 6 days before the icteric (jaundice) phase, and can last for up to 2 months (Figure 55-3). Initial symptoms include fever, fatigue, nausea, loss of appetite, vomiting, and abdominal pain. Dark urine (bilirubinuria), pale stool, and then jaundice may be accompanied

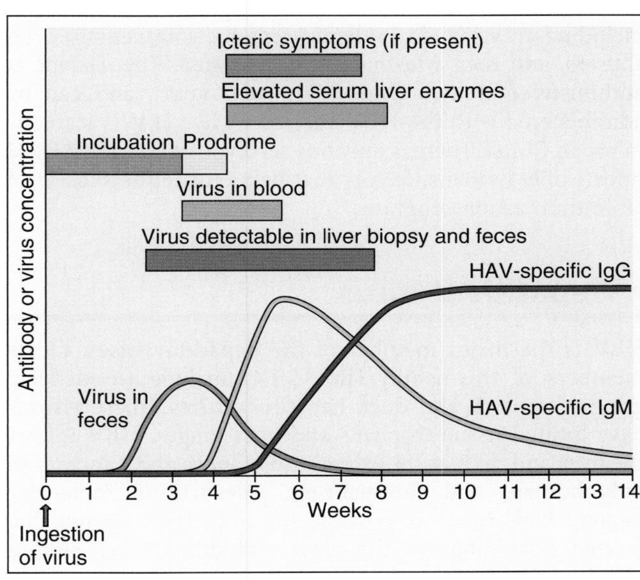

FIGURE 55-3 Time course of hepatitis A virus *(HAV)* infection. Note that the person is contagious prior to onset of symptoms and that symptoms correlate with the onset of immune responses. *Ig,* Immunoglobulin.

by abdominal pain and itch. As already noted, disease in children is generally milder than that in adults and is usually asymptomatic. Jaundice is observed in 70% to 80% of adults but in only 10% of children (<6 years of age). Symptoms generally wane during the jaundice period. Viral shedding in the stool precedes the onset of symptoms by approximately 14 days but stops before the cessation of symptoms. Complete recovery occurs 99% of the time within 2 to 4 weeks of onset.

Fulminant hepatitis in HAV infection occurs in one to three persons per 1000 and is associated with an 80% mortality rate. Unlike HBV, immune complex–related symptoms (e.g., arthritis, rash) rarely occur in people with HAV disease.

Laboratory Diagnosis

The diagnosis of HAV infection is generally made on the basis of the time course of the clinical symptoms, identification of a known infected source, and most reliably, results of specific serologic tests. The best way to demonstrate an acute HAV infection is by finding anti-HAV IgM, as measured by an enzyme-linked immunosorbent assay (ELISA) or radioimmunoassay. Virus isolation is not performed, because efficient tissue culture systems for growing the virus are not available.

Treatment, Prevention, and Control

The spread of HAV is reduced by interrupting the fecal-oral spread of the virus. This is accomplished by avoiding potentially contaminated water or food, especially uncooked shellfish. Proper hand washing, especially in day-care centers, mental hospitals, and other care facilities, is vitally important. Chlorine treatment of drinking water is generally sufficient to kill the virus.

Prophylaxis with immune serum globulin given before or early in the incubation period (i.e., <2 weeks after exposure) is 80% to 90% effective in preventing clinical illness.

Killed HAV vaccines are recommended for all children after 1 year of age and for adults at high risk for infection, including travelers to endemic regions, intravenous drug abusers, and men who have sex with men. The vaccine is administered in two doses, 6 months apart, and can be administered with the HBV vaccine. A live HAV vaccine is in use in China. There is only one serotype of HAV, and HAV infects only humans, factors that help ensure the success of an immunization program.

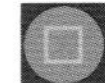

Box 55-4 Unique Features of Hepadnaviruses

Virus has enveloped virion containing partially double-stranded, circular DNA genome.
Replication is through an overlapping circular RNA intermediate.
Virus encodes and carries a reverse transcriptase.
Virus encodes several proteins (HBsAg [L, M, S]; HBe/HBc antigens) that share genetic sequences but with different in-frame start codons.
HBV has a strict tissue tropism to the liver.
HBV-infected cells produce and release large amounts of HBsAg particles lacking DNA.
The HBV genome can integrate into the host chromosome.

DNA, Deoxyribonucleic acid; *HBc,* hepatitis B core antigen; *HBe,* hepatitis Be antigen; *HBsAg,* hepatitis B surface antigen; *HBV,* hepatitis B virus; *RNA,* ribonucleic acid.

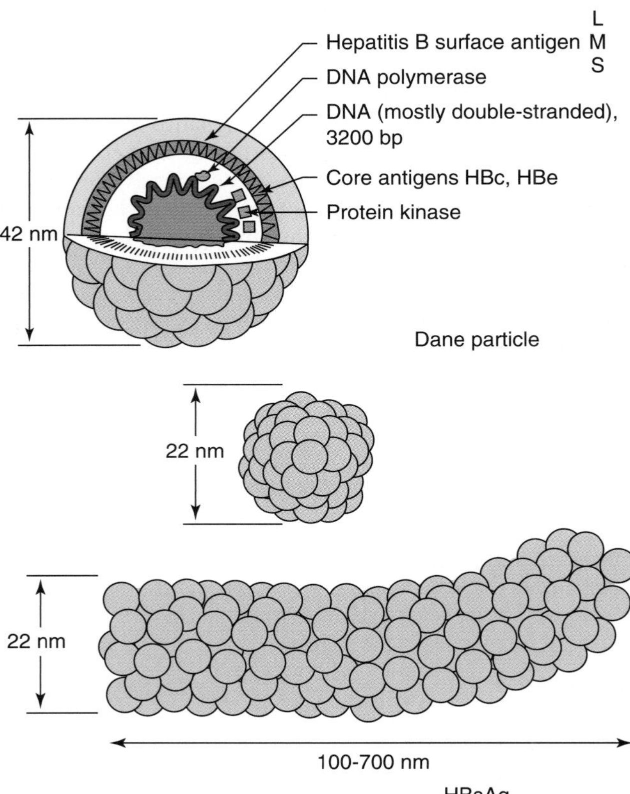

FIGURE 55-4 Hepatitis B virus (Dane particle) and hepatitis B surface antigen *(HBsAg)* particles. The spherical HBsAg consists mainly of the S form of HBsAg, with some M. The filamentous HBsAg has S, M, and L forms. *bp,* Base pair; *DNA,* deoxyribonucleic acid; *L,* gp42; *M,* gp36; *S,* gp27.

• Hepatitis B Virus

HBV is the major member of the **hepadnaviruses.** Other members of this family (Box 55-4) include woodchuck, ground squirrel, and duck hepatitis viruses. These viruses have limited tissue tropisms and host ranges. HBV infects the liver and, to a lesser extent, the kidneys and pancreas of only humans and chimpanzees. Advances in molecular biology have made it possible to study HBV despite the limited host range of the virus and difficult cell-culture systems in which to grow it.

Structure

HBV is a small enveloped DNA virus with several unusual properties (Figure 55-4). Specifically, the **genome is a small, circular, partly double-stranded DNA** of only 3200 bases. Although a DNA virus, it encodes a **reverse transcriptase** and replicates through an **RNA intermediate.**

The virion, also called the **Dane particle,** is 42 nm in diameter. The virions are unusually stable for an enveloped virus. They resist treatment with ether, low pH, freezing, and moderate heating. These characteristics assist transmission from one person to another and hamper disinfection.

The HBV **virion includes a protein kinase and a polymerase** with reverse transcriptase and ribonuclease H activity, as well as a P protein attached to the genome. All of this is surrounded by an icosahedral capsid formed by the **hepatitis B core antigen (HBcAg)** and an envelope containing three forms of the glycoprotein **hepatitis B surface antigen (HBsAg).** A **hepatitis Be antigen (HBeAg)** protein shares most of its protein sequence with HBcAg but is processed differently by the cell, is primarily secreted into serum, does not self-assemble (like a capsid antigen), and expresses different antigenic determinants.

HBsAg-containing particles are released into the serum of infected people and outnumber the actual virions. These particles can be spherical (but smaller than the Dane particle) or filamentous (see Figure 55-4). They are immunogenic and were processed into the first commercial vaccine against HBV.

HBsAg, originally termed the *Australia antigen,* includes three glycoproteins (L, M, and S) encoded by the same gene and read in the same frame but translated into protein from different AUG (adenine, uracil, guanine) start codons. The S (gp27; 24 to 27 kDa) glycoprotein is completely contained in the M (gp36; 33 to 36 kDa) glycoprotein, which is contained in the L (gp42; 39 to 42 kDa) glycoprotein; all share the same C-terminal amino acid sequences. All three forms of HBsAg are found in the virion. The S glycoprotein is the major component of HBsAg particles; it self-associates into 22-nm spherical particles that are released from the cells. The filamentous particles of HBsAg found in serum contain mostly S but also small amounts of the M and L glycoproteins and other proteins and lipids. The glycoproteins of HBsAg contain the group-specific (termed **a**) and type-specific determinants of HBV (termed **d** or **y** and **w** or **r**). Combinations of these antigens (e.g., adw, ayw, adr, ayr) result in eight subtypes of HBV that are useful epidemiologic markers.

Replication

The replication of HBV is unique for several reasons (see Box 55-4). First, HBV has a distinctly defined tropism for the liver. Its small genome also necessitates economy, as illustrated by the pattern of its transcription and translation. In addition, *HBV replicates through an RNA intermediate and produces and releases antigenic decoy particles (HBsAg)* (Figure 55-5).

The attachment of HBV to hepatocytes is mediated by the HBsAg glycoproteins. Several liver cell receptors have been suggested, including the transferrin receptor, the asialoglycoprotein receptor, and human liver annexin V. The mechanism of entry is not known, but HBsAg binds to polymerized human serum albumin and other serum proteins, and binding and uptake of these proteins may facilitate virus uptake by the liver.

On penetration into the cell, the nucleocapsid delivers the genome to the nucleus, where the partial DNA strand of the genome is completed to form a complete double-stranded DNA circle. Transcription of the genome is controlled by cellular transcription elements found in hepatocytes. The DNA is transcribed from different starting points on the circle but have the same 3′ end. There are three major classes (2100, 2400, and 3500 bases) and two minor classes (900 bases) of overlapping messenger RNAs (mRNAs) (Figure 55-6). The 3500-base mRNA is larger than the genome. It encodes the HBc and HBe antigens, the polymerase, and a protein primer for DNA replication and acts as the template

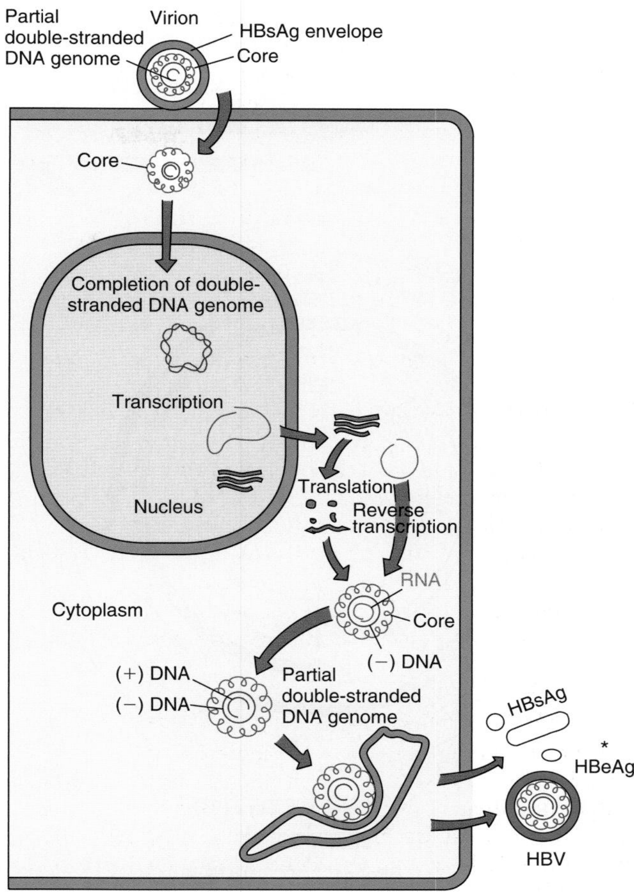

FIGURE 55-5 Replication of hepatitis B virus *(HBV).* After entry into the hepatocyte and uncoating of the nucleocapsid core, the partially double-stranded deoxyribonucleic acid *(DNA)* genome is delivered to the nucleus and completed. Transcription of the genome produces four messenger RNAs (mRNAs), including an mRNA larger than the genome (3500 bases). The mRNA then moves to the cytoplasm and is translated into protein. Core proteins assemble around the 3500-base mRNA, and negative-sense DNA is synthesized by a reverse transcriptase activity in the core. The ribonucleic acid *(RNA)* is then degraded while a positive-sense *(+)* DNA is synthesized. The filled core associates with HBsAg-containing endoplasmic reticulum membranes, is enveloped before completion of the positive-sense DNA, and is then released by exocytosis with HBsAg-containing particles. *HBeAg,* Hepatitis Be antigen; *HBsAg,* hepatitis B surface antigen.

for replication of the genome. The HBe and HBc are related proteins that are translated from different in-phase start codons of closely related mRNA. This causes differences in their processing and structure, **with shedding of the HBe and incorporation of HBc into the virion.** The HBe protein retains a signal sequence that targets it to the endoplasmic reticulum and the secretory pathway. Similarly, the 2100-base mRNA encodes the small and medium glycoproteins from different in-phase start codons. The 2400-base mRNA that encodes the large glycoprotein overlaps the 2100-base mRNA. The 900-base mRNA encodes the X protein, which promotes viral replication as a transactivator of transcription and as a protein kinase.

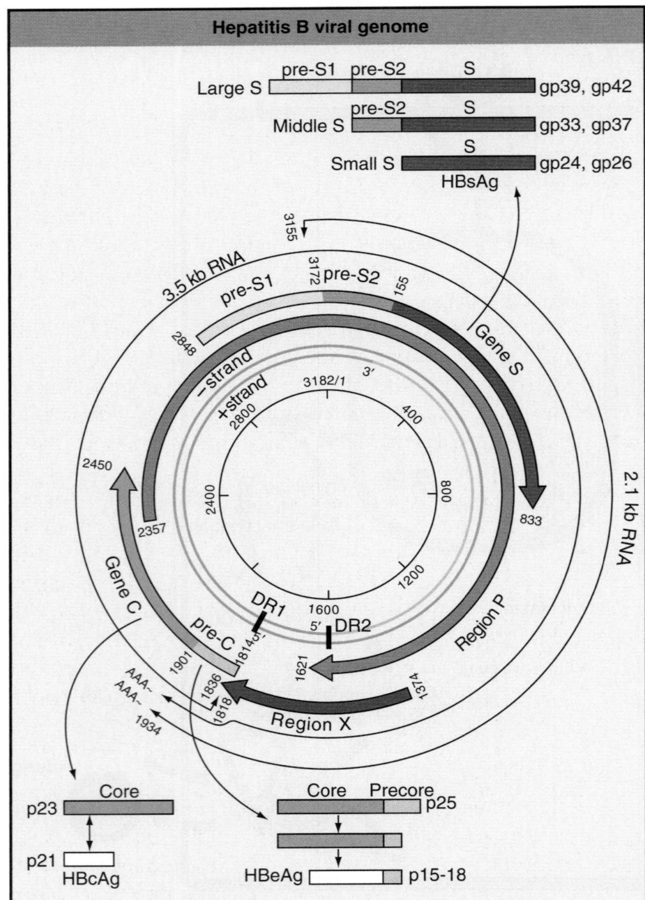

FIGURE 55-6 DNA, RNA, mRNA, and proteins of hepatitis B virus. The *inner green circles* represent the DNA genome, with the nucleotide number at the center. DR1 and DR2 are direct repeat sequences of DNA and are important for replication and integration of the genome. The 3500-base transcript *(outer black thin-line circle)* is larger than the genome and is the template for replication of the genome. Bold arcs represent mRNA for viral proteins. Note that several proteins are translated from the same mRNA but from different AUG codons and that different mRNAs overlap. *AAA,* 3′ PolyA (polyadenylate) at end of mRNA; *AUG,* adenine, uracil, guanine; *C,* C mRNA for hepatitis B core antigen (HBcAg); *HBsAg,* hepatitis B surface antigen; *l,* large glycoprotein; *m,* medium glycoprotein; *P,* polymerase-protein primer for replication; *s,* small glycoprotein; *S,* mRNA for HBs antigen; *X,* X mRNA. (From Cohen J, Powderly WG, Opal SM: *Infectious diseases,* ed 3, Philadelphia, 2010, Mosby.)

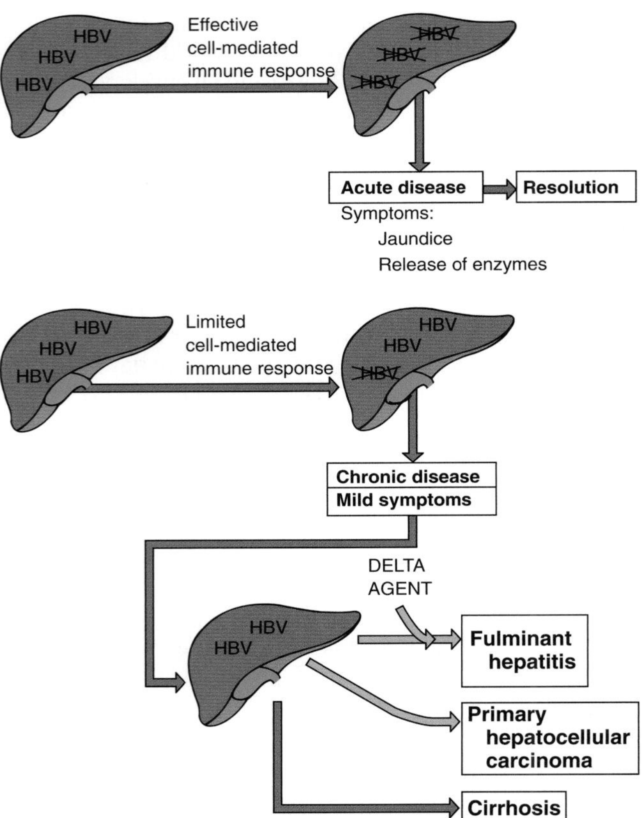

FIGURE 55-7 Major determinants of acute and chronic hepatitis B virus *(HBV)* infection. HBV infects the liver but does not cause direct cytopathology. Cell-mediated immune lysis of infected cells produces the symptoms and resolves the infection. Insufficient immunity can lead to chronic disease. Chronic HBV disease predisposes a person to more serious outcomes. *Purple arrows* indicate symptoms; *green arrows* indicate a possible outcome.

Replication of the genome utilizes the larger-than-genome 3500-base mRNA. This is packaged into the core nucleocapsid that contains the RNA-dependent DNA polymerase (P protein). This polymerase has **reverse transcriptase** and ribonuclease H activity, but HBV lacks the integrase activity of the retroviruses. The 3500-base RNA acts as a template, and negative-strand DNA is synthesized using a protein primer from the P protein, which remains covalently attached to the 5′ end. After this, the RNA is degraded by the ribonuclease H activity as the positive-strand DNA is synthesized from the negative-sense DNA template. However, this process is interrupted by envelopment of the nucleocapsid at the HBsAg-containing endoplasmic reticulum membrane, thereby capturing genomes containing a complete circular and incomplete DNA strand. The virion and HBsAg-containing particles are then released from the hepatocyte by exocytosis, without killing the cell.

The entire genome can also be integrated into the host cell chromatin. HBsAg, but not other proteins, can often be detected in the cytoplasm of cells containing integrated HBV DNA. The significance of the integrated DNA in viral replication is not known, but integrated viral DNA has been found in hepatocellular carcinomas.

Pathogenesis and Immunity

HBV can cause acute or chronic, symptomatic or asymptomatic disease. Which of these occurs seems to be determined by the person's immune response to the infection (Figure 55-7).

The major source of infectious virus is blood, but HBV can be found in semen, saliva, milk, vaginal and menstrual secretions, and amniotic fluid. The most efficient way to acquire HBV is through injection of the virus into the bloodstream (Figure 55-8). Common but less efficient routes of

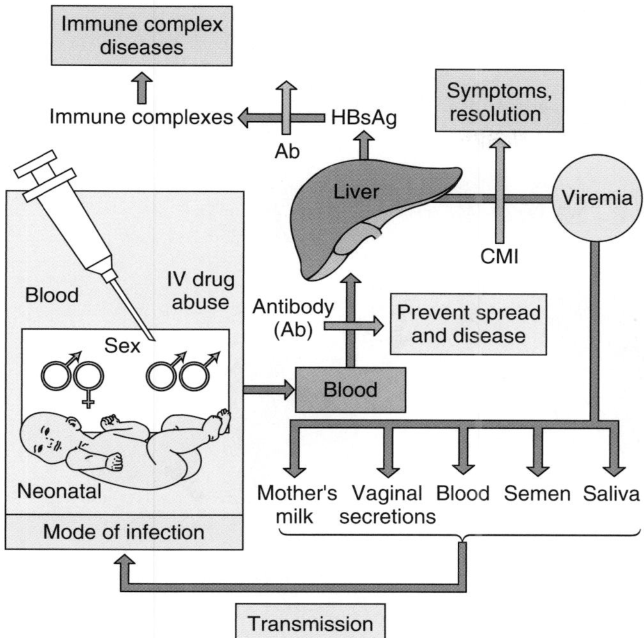

FIGURE 55-8 Spread of hepatitis B virus (HBV) in the body. Initial infection with HBV occurs through injection, unprotected sex, and birth. The virus then spreads to the liver, replicates, induces a viremia, and is transmitted in various body secretions in addition to blood to start the cycle again. Symptoms are caused by cell-mediated immunity *(CMI)* and immune complexes between antibody and hepatitis B surface antigen *(HBsAg)*. *IV,* Intravenous.

infection are sexual contact and birth. The virus starts to replicate in hepatocytes of the liver within 3 days of its acquisition, with minimal cytopathic effect. Symptoms may not be observed for 45 days or longer because they are primarily caused by immunopathology. The infectious dose, the route of infection, and the person determine the incubation period. Infection proceeds for a relatively long time without causing liver damage (i.e., elevation of liver enzyme levels) or symptoms. Copies of the HBV genome integrate into the hepatocyte chromatin and can remain latent. Intracellular buildup of filamentous forms of HBsAg can produce the ground-glass hepatocyte cytopathology characteristic of HBV infection. HBsAg particles continue to be released into the blood even after virion release has ended and until the infection is resolved. *An individual is infectious when both the HBsAg and the HBeAg components of the virion can be detected in the blood.*

Cell-mediated immunity and inflammation are responsible for causing the symptoms and effecting resolution of the HBV infection by eliminating the infected hepatocyte. An insufficient T-cell response to the infection generally results in the occurrence of mild symptoms, an inability to resolve the infection, and development of chronic hepatitis (see Figure 55-7). Chronic infection also exhausts CD8 T cells, preventing them from killing infected cells. Antibody (as generated by vaccination) can protect against initial infection by preventing delivery of the virus to the liver. Later in the infection, the large amount of HBsAg in serum binds to and blocks the action of neutralizing antibody, which limits the antibody's ability to resolve an infection. Immune complexes formed between HBsAg and anti-HBs contribute to the development of hypersensitivity reactions (type III), leading to problems such as vasculitis, arthralgia, rash, and renal damage.

Antibodies to HBc and HBe are present in serum but are nonprotective. The HBeAg protein, like HBsAg, is released into serum, and during its production, anti-HBe is bound to the antigen and undetectable. The HBc antigen is present in cells or virions and inaccessible to the antibody in blood. As a result, anti-HBc is detectable upon production, throughout and after the course of the infection.

Infants and young children have an immature cell-mediated immune response and are less able to resolve the infection, but they suffer less tissue damage and milder symptoms. As many as 90% of infants infected perinatally become chronic carriers. Viral replication persists in these people for long periods.

During the acute phase of infection, the liver parenchyma shows degenerative changes consisting of cellular swelling and necrosis, especially in hepatocytes surrounding the central vein of a hepatic lobule. The inflammatory cell infiltrate is mainly composed of lymphocytes. Resolution of the infection allows the parenchyma to regenerate. Fulminant infections, activation of chronic infections, or co-infection with the delta agent can lead to permanent liver damage and cirrhosis.

Epidemiology

In the United States, more than 12 million people have been infected with HBV (1 out of 20), with 5000 deaths per year. In the world, one out of three people have been infected with HBV, with approximately a million deaths per year. More than 350 million people worldwide have chronic HBV infection. In developing nations, as many as 15% of the population may be infected during birth or childhood. High rates of seropositivity are observed in Italy, Greece, Africa, and Southeast Asia (Figure 55-9). In some areas of the world (southern Africa and southeastern Asia), the seroconversion rate is as high as 50%. PHC, a long-term sequela of the infection, is also endemic in these regions.

The many asymptomatic chronic carriers with virus in blood and other body secretions foster spread of the virus. In the United States, 0.1% to 0.5% of the general population are chronic carriers, but this is very low in comparison with many areas of the world. Carrier status may be lifelong.

The virus is spread by sexual, parenteral, and perinatal routes. Transmission occurs through contaminated blood and blood components by transfusion, needle sharing, acupuncture, ear piercing, or tattooing and through very close personal contact involving the exchange of semen, saliva, and vaginal secretions (e.g., sex, childbirth) (see Figure 55-8). Medical personnel are at risk in accidents involving needlesticks or sharp instruments. People at particular risk are listed in Box 55-5. Sexual promiscuity and drug abuse are major risk factors for HBV infection. HBV can be transmitted to babies through contact with the mother's blood at birth and in the mother's milk. Babies born to chronic HBV-positive mothers are at highest risk for infection. Serologic screening of donor units in blood banks has greatly reduced the risk of acquisition of the virus from contaminated blood or blood products. Safer sex habits adopted to prevent human immunodeficiency virus (HIV) transmission and the administration of

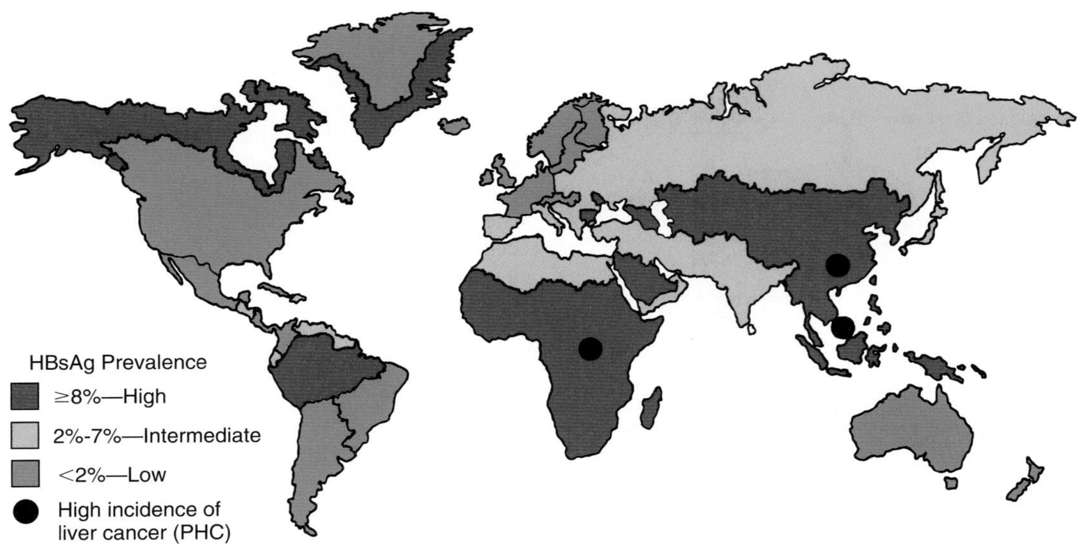

FIGURE 55-9 Worldwide prevalence of hepatitis B carriers and primary hepatocellular carcinoma *(PHC)*. *HBsAg*, Hepatitis B surface antigen. (Courtesy Centers for Disease Control and Prevention, Atlanta.)

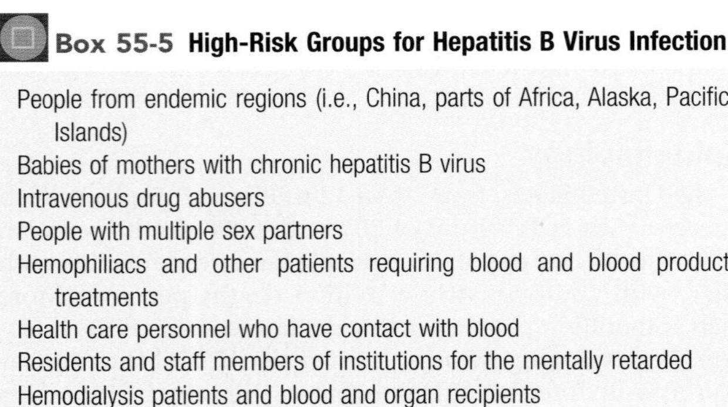

Box 55-5 High-Risk Groups for Hepatitis B Virus Infection

People from endemic regions (i.e., China, parts of Africa, Alaska, Pacific Islands)
Babies of mothers with chronic hepatitis B virus
Intravenous drug abusers
People with multiple sex partners
Hemophiliacs and other patients requiring blood and blood product treatments
Health care personnel who have contact with blood
Residents and staff members of institutions for the mentally retarded
Hemodialysis patients and blood and organ recipients

the HBV vaccine have also been responsible for decreasing the transmission and incidence of HBV.

One of the major concerns about HBV is its association with PHC. This type of carcinoma probably accounts for 250,000 to 1 million deaths per year worldwide; in the United States, approximately 5000 deaths per year are attributed to PHC.

Clinical Syndromes

Acute Infection

As already noted, the clinical presentation of HBV in children is less severe than that in adults, and infection may even be asymptomatic. Clinically apparent illness occurs in as many as 25% of those infected with HBV (Figures 55-10 to 55-12).

HBV infection is characterized by a **long incubation period and an insidious onset.** Symptoms during the prodromal period may include fever, malaise, and anorexia, followed by nausea, vomiting, abdominal discomfort, and chills. The classic icteric symptoms of liver damage (e.g., jaundice, dark urine, pale stools) follow soon thereafter. Recovery is indicated by a decline in the fever and renewed appetite.

Fulminant hepatitis occurs in approximately 1% of icteric patients and may be fatal. It is marked by more severe symptoms and indications of severe liver damage, such as ascites and bleeding.

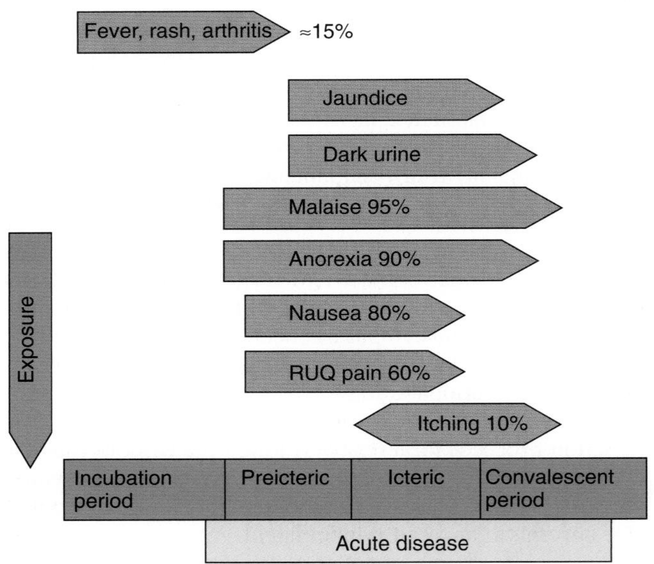

FIGURE 55-10 Symptoms of typical acute viral hepatitis B infection are correlated with the four clinical periods of this disease. *RUQ*, Right upper quadrant. (Modified from Hoofnagle JH: Type A and type B hepatitis, *Lab Med* 14:705–716, 1983.)

HBV infection can promote hypersensitivity reactions that are caused by immune complexes of HBsAg and antibody. These may produce rash, polyarthritis, fever, acute necrotizing vasculitis, and glomerulonephritis.

Chronic Infection

Chronic hepatitis occurs in 5% to 10% of people with HBV infections, usually after mild or inapparent initial disease. Approximately one third of these people have chronic active hepatitis, with continued destruction of the liver leading to scarring of the liver, cirrhosis, liver failure, or PHC. The

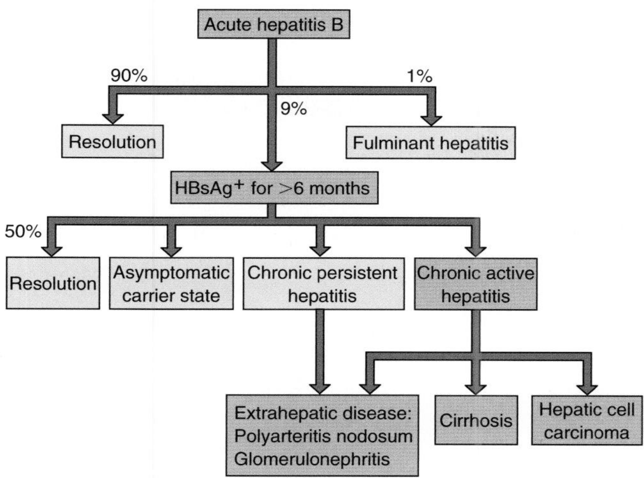

FIGURE 55-11 Clinical outcomes of acute hepatitis B infection. *HBsAg,* Hepatitis B surface antigen. (Modified from White DO, Fenner F: *Medical virology,* ed 3, New York, 1986, Academic.)

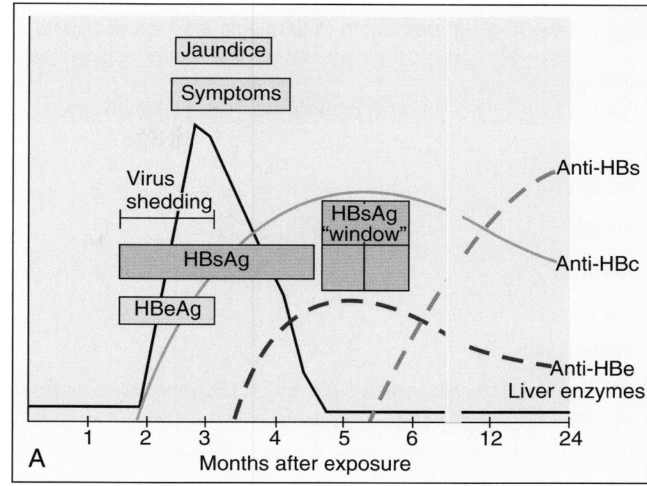

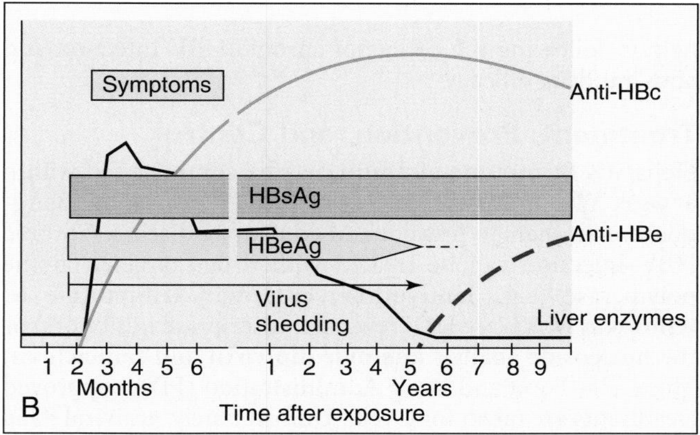

FIGURE 55-12 **A,** The serologic events associated with the typical course of acute hepatitis B disease. **B,** Development of the chronic hepatitis B virus carrier state. Routine serodiagnosis depends on detection of immunoglobulin M anti-HBc during the "hepatitis B surface antigen *(HBsAg)* window," when HBs and anti-HBs are undetectable. *Anti-HBc,* Antibody to hepatitis B core antigen [HBcAg]; *Anti-HBe,* antibody to hepatitis Be antigen [HBeAg]; *Anti-HBs,* antibody to HBsAg. (Modified from Hoofnagle JH: Serologic markers of hepatitis B virus infection, *Annu Rev Med* 32:1–11, 1981.)

other two thirds have chronic passive hepatitis and are less likely to have problems. Chronic hepatitis may be detected accidentally by finding elevated liver enzyme levels on a routine blood chemistry profile. Chronically infected people are the major source for spread of the virus and are at risk for fulminant disease if they become co-infected with HDV.

Primary Hepatocellular Carcinoma

The World Health Organization estimates that 80% of all cases of PHC can be attributed to chronic HBV infections. The HBV genome is integrated into these PHC cells, and the cells express HBV antigens. PHC is usually fatal and is one of the three most common causes of cancer mortality in the world. In Taiwan, at least 15% of the population are carriers of HBV, and nearly half die of PHC or cirrhosis. PHC, like cervical cancer, is a vaccine-preventable human cancer.

HBV may induce PHC by promoting continued liver repair and cell growth in response to inflammation and tissue damage or by integrating into the host chromosome and stimulating cell growth directly. Such integration could stimulate genetic rearrangements or juxtapose viral promoters next to cellular growth-controlling genes. Alternatively, a protein encoded by the HBV X gene may transactivate (turn on) the transcription of cellular proteins and stimulate cell growth. The presence of the HBV genome may allow a subsequent mutation to promote carcinogenesis. The latency period between HBV infection and PHC may be as short as 9 years or as long as 35 years.

Laboratory Diagnosis

The initial diagnosis of hepatitis can be made on the basis of the clinical symptoms and the presence of liver enzymes in the blood (see Figure 55-12). However, the serology of HBV infection describes the course and nature of the disease (Table 55-2). Acute and chronic HBV infections can be distinguished by the presence of HBsAg and HBeAg in the serum and the pattern of antibodies to the individual HBV antigens.

HBsAg and HBeAg are secreted into the blood during viral replication. Detection of HBeAg is the best correlate to the presence of infectious virus. **A chronic or unresolved infection can be distinguished by the continued finding of HBeAg, HBsAg, or both, and a lack of detectable antibody to these antigens.** Antibody to HBsAg indicates resolution of infection or vaccination. Immune complexes of HBeAg and HBsAg and antibody inhibit antibody production and obscure detection of the complexed antigen. Although for different reasons, HBsAg/anti-HBs and Clark Kent/Superman can never be seen together at the same time.

Antibody to HBcAg indicates current or prior infection by HBV, and IgM anti-HBc is the best way to diagnose a recent acute infection, especially while the infection is being resolved and when neither HBsAg nor anti-HBs can be detected (the window).

The amount of virus in blood can be determined by quantitative genome assays using polymerase chain reaction (PCR) and related techniques. Knowing the viral load can

Table 55-2 Interpretation of Serologic Markers of Hepatitis B Virus Infection

Serologic Reactivity	Disease State					Healthy State	
	Early (Presymptomatic)	Early Acute	Acute	Chronic	Late Acute	Resolved	Vaccinated
Anti-HBc	–	–	+*	+	+/–	+	–
Anti-HBe	–	–	–	–	+/–	+/–†	–
Anti-HBs	–	–	–	–	–	+	+
HBeAg	–	+	+	+	–	–	–
HBsAg	+	+	+	+	+	–	–
Infectious virus	+	+	+	+	+	–	–

HBc, Hepatitis B core; *HBeAg,* hepatitis Be antigen; *HBsAg,* hepatitis B surface antigen.
*Anti-HBc immunoglobulin M should be present.
†Anti-HBe may be negative after chronic disease.

help in following the course of chronic HBV infection and antiviral drug efficacy.

Treatment, Prevention, and Control

Hepatitis B immune globulin may be administered within a week of exposure and to newborn infants of HBsAg-positive mothers to prevent and ameliorate disease. Chronic HBV infection can be treated with drugs targeted at the polymerase (e.g., **lamivudine, entecavir, telbivudine or tenofovir,** which are HIV reverse transcriptase inhibitors) or the nucleoside analogs **adefovir dipivoxil and famciclovir.** These U.S. Food and Drug Administration (FDA)-approved treatments are taken for 1 year. Unfortunately, antiviral drug resistance can develop. **Pegylated interferon-α** can also be effective and is taken for at least 4 months.

Transmission of HBV in blood or blood products has been greatly reduced by screening donated blood for the presence of HBsAg and anti-HBc. Additional efforts to prevent transmission of HBV include safe sex and avoiding lifestyles that facilitate spread of the virus. Household contacts and sexual partners of HBV carriers are at increased risk, as are patients undergoing hemodialysis, recipients of pooled plasma products, health care workers exposed to blood, and babies born to HBV-carrier mothers.

Vaccination is recommended for infants, children, and especially people in high-risk groups (see Box 55-5). For newborns of HBsAg-positive mothers and people accidentally exposed either percutaneously or permucosally to blood or secretions from an HBsAg-positive person, vaccination is useful even after exposure. Immunization of mothers should decrease the incidence of transmission to babies and older children, also reducing the number of chronic HBV carriers. Prevention of chronic HBV will reduce the incidence of PHC.

The HBV vaccines form virus-like particles. The initial HBV vaccine was derived from the 22-nm HBsAg particles in human plasma obtained from chronically infected people. The current vaccine was genetically engineered by the insertion of a plasmid containing the S gene for HBsAg into a yeast, *Saccharomyces cerevisiae.* The protein self-assembles into particles, which enhances its immunogenicity.

The vaccine must be given in a series of three injections, with the second and third given 1 and 6 months after the first. The single serotype and limited host range (humans) help ensure the success of an immunization program.

Universal blood and body fluid precautions are used to limit exposure to HBV. It is assumed that all patients are infected. Gloves are required for handling blood and body fluids; wearing protective clothing and eye protection may also be necessary. Special care should be taken with needles and sharp instruments. HBV-contaminated materials can be disinfected with 10% bleach solutions, but unlike most enveloped viruses, HBV is not readily inactivated by detergents.

• Hepatitis C and G Viruses

HCV was identified in 1989 after isolation of a viral RNA from a chimpanzee infected with blood from a person with NANBH. The viral RNA obtained from blood was converted to DNA with reverse transcriptase, its proteins were expressed, and antibodies from people with NANBH were then used to detect the viral proteins. These studies led to the development of ELISA and genomic and other tests for detection of the virus, which still cannot be grown in tissue culture.

HCV is the predominant cause of NANBH viral infections and was the major cause of posttransfusion hepatitis before routine screening of the blood supply for HCV. There are more than 170 million carriers of HCV in the world—3% of the population—and more than 4 million in the United States. HCV is transmitted by means similar to HBV but has an even greater potential for establishing persistent chronic hepatitis. Many HCV-infected individuals are also infected with HBV or HIV. The chronic hepatitis often leads to cirrhosis and potentially to hepatocellular carcinoma.

Structure and Replication

HCV is the only member of the *Hepacivirus* genus of the **Flaviviridae** family. There are six major genotypes of HCV (clades), and between and within each genotype there is considerable genetic and antigenic diversity. HCV is 30 to 60 nm in diameter, has a **positive-sense RNA genome,** and is **enveloped.** The genome of HCV (9100 nucleotides) encodes 10 proteins, including two glycoproteins (E1, E2).

The viral RNA-dependent RNA polymerase is error prone and generates mutations in the glycoprotein and other genes. This generates antigenic variability. Such variability makes development of a vaccine very difficult.

HCV infects only humans and chimpanzees. HCV binds to multiple cell surface receptors expressed on hepatocytes and B lymphocytes that also facilitate its entry into the cell. The receptors include CD81 (tetraspanin) surface receptors, scavenger receptor class B type I (SRB1), and tight junction proteins claudin-1 and occludin. HCV can also coat itself with low-density lipoprotein or very-low-density lipoprotein and then use the lipoprotein receptor to facilitate uptake into hepatocytes. The virus replicates like other flaviviruses. The virion assembles at and buds into the endoplasmic reticulum, becoming cell associated. HCV proteins inhibit apoptosis and interferon-α action by binding to the tumor necrosis factor receptor and to protein kinase R. These actions prevent the death of the host cell and promote escape from host protections to promote persistent infection.

Pathogenesis

The ability of HCV to remain cell associated and prevent host cell death promotes persistent infection but results in liver disease later in life. Up to 10^{12} particles per day can be produced in chronically infected, potentially asymptomatic individuals. The virus's ability to evade interferon action and change its antigenicity help the virus establish chronic disease. Cell-mediated immune responses are necessary to resolve the infection but also cause tissue damage. Antibody to HCV is not protective. As for HBV, once established, the chronic infection can exhaust CD8 cytotoxic T cells so they cannot resolve the infection. The extent of lymphocytic infiltration, inflammation, portal and periportal fibrosis, and lobular necrosis in liver biopsies can be used to grade the severity of disease. It has been suggested that the cytokines of inflammation and continual liver repair and induction of cell growth occurring during chronic HCV infection are predisposing factors in the development of PHC.

Epidemiology

HCV is **transmitted primarily in infected blood** and sexually. Intravenous drug abusers and tattoo recipients are at highest risk to HCV infection. Screening procedures have led to a reduction in the levels of transmission by blood transfusion and organ donation (Box 55-6). Almost all (>90%) HIV-infected people who are or were intravenous drug users are infected with HCV. HCV is especially prevalent in southern Italy, Spain, central Europe, Japan, and parts of the Middle East (e.g., almost 20% of Egyptian blood donors are HCV positive). The **high incidence of chronic asymptomatic infections** promotes the spread of the virus in the population.

Box 55-6 Epidemiology of Hepatitis B, C, and D Viruses

Disease/Viral Factors

Enveloped virus is labile to drying. HBV is less sensitive to detergents than other enveloped viruses.
Virus is shed during asymptomatic periods.
HBV (10%) and HCV (70%) cause chronic infection with potential virus shedding.

Transmission

In blood, semen, and vaginal secretions (HBV: saliva and mother's milk)
Via transfusion, needlestick injury, shared drug paraphernalia, sexual intercourse, and breast-feeding

Who Is at Risk?

Children: mild asymptomatic disease with establishment of chronic infection
Adults: insidious onset of hepatitis
HBV-infected people co-infected or superinfected with HDV: abrupt, more severe symptoms with possible fulminant disease
Adults with chronic HBV or HCV: at high risk for cirrhosis and primary hepatocellular carcinoma

Geography/Season

Viruses are found worldwide.
There is no seasonal incidence.

Modes of Control

Avoidance of high-risk behavior
HBV: virus-like particle (HBsAg) vaccine
HBV and HCV screening of blood supply

HBV, Hepatitis B virus; *HCV,* hepatitis C virus; *HDV,* hepatitis D virus.

Clinical Syndromes (Clinical Case 55-1)

HCV causes three types of disease (Figure 55-13): (1) acute hepatitis with resolution of the infection and recovery in 15% of cases, (2) chronic persistent infection with possible progression to disease much later in life for 70% of infected persons, and (3) severe rapid progression to cirrhosis in 15% of patients. A viremia can be detected within 1 to 3 weeks of a transfusion of HCV-contaminated blood. The viremia lasts 4 to 6 months in people with an acute infection and longer

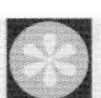

Clinical Case 55-1 Hepatitis C Virus (HCV)

In a case reported by Morsica and associates (*Scand J Infect Dis* 33:116–120, 2001), a 35-year-old woman was admitted with malaise and jaundice. Elevated blood levels of bilirubin (71.8 μmol/l; normal value < 17 μmol/l) and aspartate amino transferase (ALT) (410 IU/l; normal value < 30 IU/l) indicated liver damage. Serology was negative for antibodies to hepatitis A, hepatitis B, hepatitis C, Epstein-Barr virus, cytomegalovirus, and HIV-1. However, HCV genomic RNA sequences were detected by reverse transcriptase polymerase chain reaction analysis. ALT levels peaked on the third week after admission and returned to normal by the eighth week. HCV genomes in blood were undetectable by the eighth week. Anti-HCV antibody was also detected by the eighth week. It was suspected that she was infected by her sexual partner, and this was confirmed by genotyping virus obtained from both individuals. Confirmation was provided by partial sequence analysis of the *E2* gene from the two viral isolates. The 5% genetic divergence detected between the isolates was less than the ≈20% divergence expected for unrelated strains. Before the analysis, the sexual partner was unaware of his chronic HCV infection. Even more than HBV, which is also transmitted by sexual and parenteral means, HCV causes inapparent and chronic infections. Inapparent transmission of the virus, as in this case, enhances spread of the virus. The molecular analysis demonstrates the genetic instability of the HCV genome, a possible mechanism for facilitating its chronic infection by changing its antigenic appearance to promote escape from the immune response.

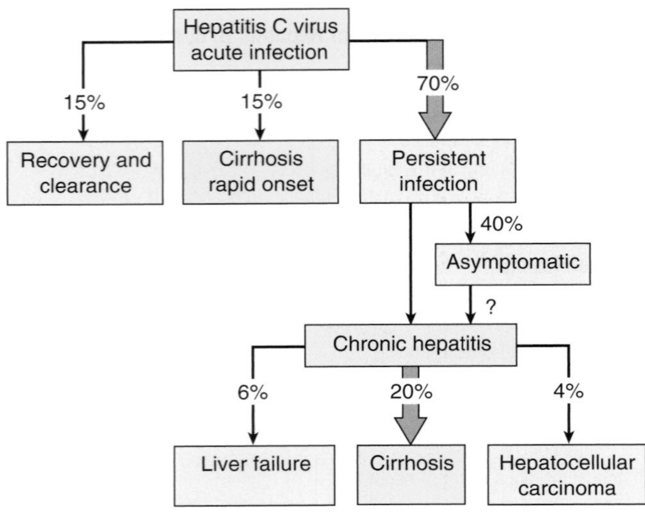

FIGURE 55-13 Outcomes of hepatitis C virus infection.

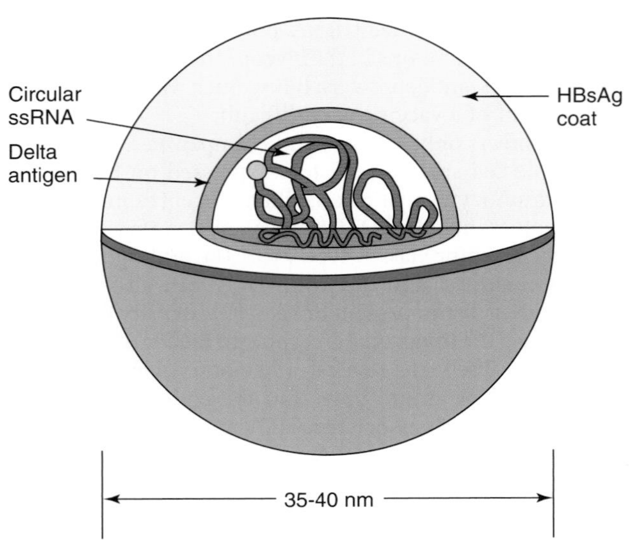

FIGURE 55-14 The delta hepatitis virion. *HBsAg,* Hepatitis B surface antigen; *ssRNA,* single-stranded RNA.

than 10 years in those with a persistent infection. In its acute form, HCV infection is similar to acute HAV and HBV infection, but the inflammatory response is less intense and the symptoms are usually milder. More commonly (>70% of cases), the initial disease is asymptomatic but establishes chronic persistent disease. The predominant symptom is chronic fatigue. Chronic persistent disease often progresses to chronic active hepatitis within 10 to 15 years and to cirrhosis (20% of chronic cases) and liver failure (20% of cirrhotic cases) after 20 years. HCV-induced liver damage may be exacerbated by alcohol, certain medications, and other hepatitis viruses to promote cirrhosis. HCV promotes the development of hepatocellular carcinoma after 30 years in up to 5% of chronically infected patients.

Laboratory Diagnosis

The diagnosis and detection of HCV infection are based on ELISA recognition of anti-HCV antibody or detection of the RNA genome. Seroconversion occurs within 7 to 31 weeks of infection. ELISA is used for screening the blood supply from normal donors. As for HIV, results can be confirmed by Western immunoblot procedures. Antibody is not always detectable in viremic people, immunocompromised patients, or those receiving hemodialysis. Genome detection and quantitation by RT-PCR, branched-chain DNA, and related techniques is the gold standard for confirming a diagnosis of HCV and for following the success of antiviral drug therapy. Genetic assays are less strain specific and can detect HCV RNA in seronegative people.

Treatment, Prevention, and Control

Recombinant interferon-α or pegylated interferon (treated with polyethylene glycol to enhance its biological lifetime), alone or with ribavirin, were the only available treatments for HCV until 2011, when two virus-specific protease inhibitors, boceprevir and telaprevir, and more recently ledipasvir, became approved. Sofosbuvir, an inhibitor of the polymerase, is also available. Other antiviral drugs and drug cocktails, without interferon, are in development. As for HIV, the addition of these HCV-specific inhibitors to the previous antiviral protocol is important to limit the evolution of drug resistance and has made a significant difference in therapeutic efficacy, with a reduction in treatment side effects.

Precautions for preventing transmission of HCV are similar to those for HBV and other blood-borne pathogens. The blood supply and organ donors are screened for HCV. Persons with HCV should not share any personal care items or syringe needles that may get contaminated with blood and should practice safe sex. Alcohol drinking should be limited because it exacerbates the liver damage caused by HCV.

• Hepatitis G Virus

HGV (also known as GB virus-C [GBV-C]) resembles HCV in many ways. HGV is a flavivirus, is transmitted in blood, and has a predilection for chronic hepatitis infection. It is identified by detection of the genome by RT-PCR or other RNA detection methods.

• Hepatitis D Virus

Approximately 15 million people in the world are infected with HDV (delta agent), and the virus is responsible for causing 40% of **fulminant hepatitis** infections. HDV is unique in that it uses HBV and target cell proteins to replicate and produce its one protein. It is a viral parasite, proving that "even fleas have fleas." **HBsAg is essential for packaging the virus.** The delta agent resembles plant virus satellite agents and viroids in its size, genomic structure, and requirement for a helper virus for replication (Figure 55-14).

Structure and Replication

The **HDV RNA genome is very small** (≈1700 nucleotides), and unlike other viruses, the single-stranded RNA is circular and forms a rod shape as a result of its extensive base pairing. The virion is approximately the same size as the HBV virion (35 to 37 nm in diameter). The genome is surrounded by the

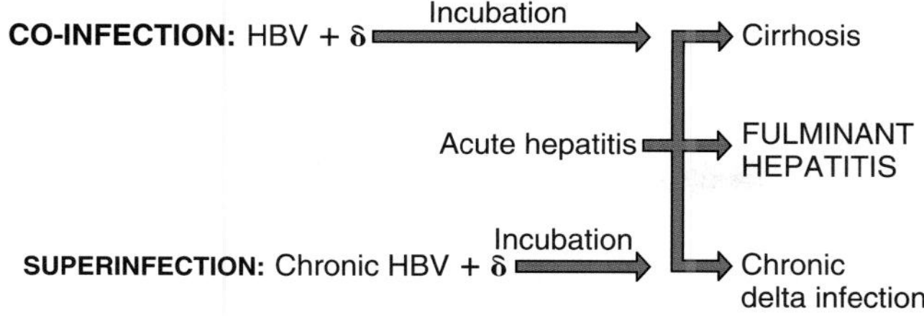

FIGURE 55-15 Consequences of delta virus infection. Delta virus (*δ*) requires the presence of hepatitis B virus *(HBV)* infection. Superinfection of a person already infected with HBV (carrier) causes more rapid, severe progression than co-infection *(shorter arrow)*.

delta antigen core, which in turn is surrounded by an HBsAg-containing envelope. The **delta antigen** exists as a small (24 kDa) or large (27 kDa) form; the small form is predominant.

The delta agent binds to and is internalized by hepatocytes in the same manner as HBV because it has HBsAg in its envelope. The transcription and replication processes of the HDV genome are unusual. The host cell's RNA polymerase II makes an RNA copy to replicate the genome. The genome then forms an RNA structure called a **ribozyme,** which cleaves the RNA circle to produce an mRNA for the small delta antigen. The gene for the delta antigen is mutated by a cellular enzyme (double-stranded RNA-activated adenosine deaminase) during infection, thereby allowing production of the large delta antigen. Production of this antigen limits replication of the virus but also promotes association of the genome with HBsAg to form a virion, and the virus is then released from the cell.

Pathogenesis

The delta agent can replicate and cause disease only in people with active HBV infections. Because the two agents are transmitted by the same routes, a person can be **co-infected** with HBV and the delta agent. A person with chronic HBV can also be **superinfected** with the delta agent. More rapid, severe progression occurs in HBV carriers superinfected with HDV than in people co-infected with HBV and the delta agent, because during co-infection, HBV must first establish its infection before HDV can replicate (Figure 55-15), whereas superinfection of an HBV-infected person allows the delta agent to replicate immediately.

Replication of the delta agent results in cytotoxicity and liver damage. Persistent delta agent infection is often established in HBV carriers. Antibodies are elicited against the delta agent, but protection is provided by antibodies to HBsAg, generated by vaccination or infection, because it is the external antigen and viral attachment protein for HDV. Unlike HBV disease, damage to the liver occurs as a result of the direct cytopathic effect of the delta agent combined with the underlying immunopathology of the HBV disease.

Epidemiology

The delta agent infects children and adults with underlying HBV infection (see Box 55-6), and people who are persistently infected with both HBV and HDV are a source for the virus. The agent has a worldwide distribution, infecting approximately 5% of the 3×10^8 HBV carriers, and is endemic in southern Italy, the Amazon Basin, parts of Africa, and the Middle East. Epidemics of HDV infection occur in North America and Western Europe, usually in illicit drug users. HDV is spread by the same routes as HBV, and the same groups are at risk for infection, with parenteral drug abusers, hemophiliacs, and others receiving blood products at highest risk. Screening of the blood supply has reduced the risk for recipients of blood products.

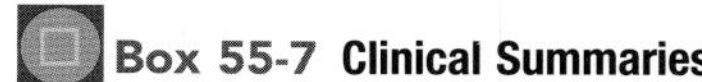

Box 55-7 Clinical Summaries

Hepatitis A: A 37-year-old man develops fever, chills, headache, and fatigue 4 weeks after eating at a greasy-spoon diner. Within 2 days, he develops anorexia, vomiting, and right upper quadrant abdominal pain followed by jaundice, dark-colored urine, and pale stools persisting for 12 days. Then symptoms decrease.

Hepatitis B: A 27-year-old intravenous (IV) drug user develops symptoms of hepatitis 60 days after using a dirty needle.

Hepatitis B and D: A different IV drug user develops symptoms of hepatitis, altered mental capacity, and massive hepatic necrosis and then dies.

Hepatitis C: Elevated liver enzymes were detected in an individual during a physical examination. Hepatitis C virus in the blood was detected by enzyme-linked immunosorbent assay. Ten years later, cirrhosis and liver failure developed, requiring a liver transplant.

Clinical Syndromes (Box 55-7)

The delta agent increases the severity of HBV infections. Fulminant hepatitis is more likely to develop in people infected with the delta agent than in those infected with the other hepatitis viruses. This very severe form of hepatitis causes altered brain function (hepatic encephalopathy), extensive jaundice, and massive hepatic necrosis, which is fatal in 80% of cases. Chronic infection with the delta agent can occur in people with chronic HBV.

Laboratory Diagnosis

The presence of the agent can be noted by detecting the RNA genome, the delta antigen, or anti-HDV antibodies. ELISA and radioimmunoassay procedures are available for detection. The delta antigen can be detected in the blood during the acute phase of disease in a detergent-treated serum sample. RT-PCR techniques can be used to detect the virion genome in blood.

Treatment, Prevention, and Control

There is no known specific treatment for HDV hepatitis. Because the delta agent depends on HBV for replication and is spread by the same routes, prevention of infection with HBV prevents HDV infection. Immunization with HBV vaccine protects against delta virus infection. If a person has already acquired HBV, delta agent infection may be prevented by halting illicit intravenous drug use and avoiding HDV-contaminated blood products.

• Hepatitis E Virus

HEV (E-NANBH) (the *E* stands for *enteric* or *epidemic*) is predominantly spread by the fecal-oral route, especially in contaminated water (see Box 55-3). HEV is unique but resembles the caliciviruses, based on its size (27 to 34 nm), RNA genome, and naked capsid structure. Although HEV is found throughout the world, it is most problematic in developing countries. Epidemics have been reported in India, Pakistan, Nepal, Burma, North Africa, and Mexico.

The symptoms and course of HEV disease are similar to those of HAV disease; it causes only acute disease. However, the symptoms for HEV may occur later than those of HAV disease. The mortality rate associated with HEV disease is 1% to 2%, approximately 10 times that associated with HAV disease. HEV infection is especially serious in pregnant women (mortality rate of ≈20%).

Bibliography

Blum HE, Gerok W, Vyas GN: The molecular biology of hepatitis B virus, *Trends Genet* 5:154–158, 1989.

Cann AJ: *Principles of molecular virology*, San Diego, 2005, Academic.

Carter J, Saunders V: *Virology: principles and applications*, Chichester, England, 2007, Wiley.

Casey JL: Hepatitis delta virus, *Curr Top Microbiol Immunol* (vol 307), Heidelberg, Germany, 2006, Springer-Verlag.

Catalina G, Navarro V: Hepatitis C: a challenge for the generalist, *Hosp Pract* 35:97–108, 2000.

Cohen J, Powderly WG: *Infectious diseases*, ed 2, St Louis, 2004, Mosby.

Collier L, Oxford J: *Human virology*, ed 4, Oxford, England, 2011, Oxford University Press.

Fallows DA, Goff AP: Hepadnaviruses: current models of RNA encapsidation and reverse transcription, *Adv Virus Res* 46:167–196, 1996.

Flint SJ, Enquist LW, Racaniello VR, et al: *Principles of virology: molecular biology, pathogenesis and control of animal viruses*, ed 3, Washington, DC, 2009, American Society for Microbiology Press.

Ganem D, Prince AM: Hepatitis B virus infection—natural history and clinical consequences, *N Engl J Med* 350:1118–1119, 2004.

Grimm D, Thimme R, Blum HE: HBV life cycle and novel drug targets, *Hepatol Int* 5:644–653, 2011.

Hagedorn CH, Rice CM: The hepatitis C viruses, *Curr Top Microbiol Immunol* (vol 242), Berlin, 2000, Springer-Verlag.

Hoofnagle JH: Type A and type B hepatitis, *Lab Med* 14:705–716, 1983.

Knipe DM, Howley PM: *Fields virology*, ed 6, Philadelphia, 2013, Lippincott Williams & Wilkins.

Lauer GM, Walker BD: Medical progress: hepatitis C virus infection, *N Engl J Med* 345:41–52, 2001.

Lok ASF: Chronic hepatitis B, *N Engl J Med* 346:1682–1683, 2002.

Mason WS, Seeger C: Hepadnaviruses: molecular biology and pathogenesis, *Curr Top Microbiol Immunol* (vol 162), Berlin, 1991, Springer-Verlag.

Murray PR, Baron EJ, Jorgensen JH, et al: *Manual of clinical microbiology*, ed 9, Washington, DC, 2007, American Society for Microbiology Press.

Plageman PGW: Hepatitis C virus, *Arch Virol* 120:165–180, 1991.

Robinson W, Koike K, Will H: *Hepadnavirus*, New York, 1987, Liss.

Strauss JM, Strauss EG: *Viruses and human disease*, ed 2, San Diego, 2007, Academic.

Tam AW, Smith MM, Guerra ME, et al: Hepatitis E virus: molecular cloning and sequencing of the full-length viral genome, *Virology* 185:120–131, 1991.

Taylor JM: Hepatitis delta virus, *Virology* 344:71–76, 2006.

Voyles BA: *The biology of viruses*, ed 2, Boston, 2002, McGraw-Hill.

Websites

Centers for Disease Control and Prevention: Viral hepatitis. www.cdc.gov/hepatitis/. Accessed April 29, 2015.

Cernescu C, Ruta S, Gheorghe L, et al: #4: Hepatitis C treatment, 2011 edition. www.flyingpublisher.com/0004.php. Accessed April 29, 2015.

Gilroy RK: Hepatitis A. http://emedicine.medscape.com/article/177484-overview. Accessed April 29, 2015.

Hepatitis B Foundation: Statistics. www.hepb.org/hepb/statistics.htm. Accessed April 29, 2015.

Mauss S, Berg T, Rockstroh J, et al: #11: The 2012 short guide to hepatitis C. www.flyingpublisher.com/0011.php. Accessed April 29, 2015.

Mukhrjee S, Dhawan VK: Hepatitis C. http://emedicine.medscape.com/article/177792-overview. Accessed April 29, 2015.

National Institute of Allergy and Infectious Diseases: Viral hepatitis. www.niaid.nih.gov/topics/hepatitis/Pages/default.aspx. Accessed April 29, 2015.

Nature: Hepatitis C. www.nature.com/nature/outlook/hepatitis-c/index.html. Accessed April 29, 2015.

Pascarella S, Negroa F: Hepatitis D virus: an update. http://onlinelibrary.wiley.com/doi/10.1111/j.1478-3231.2010.02320.x/pdf. Accessed May 20, 2015.

Sutphen SK: Hepatitis A and B vaccines. www.medscape.org/viewarticle/564225. Accessed May 20, 2015.

WHO Alert: Hepatitis A factsheet. www.who.int/csr/disease/hepatitis/whocdscsredc2007/en/index4.html. Accessed Accessed April 29, 2015.

WHO Alert: Hepatitis B factsheet. www.who.int/csr/disease/hepatitis/whocdscsrlyo20022/en/index4.html. Accessed April 29, 2015.

WHO Alert: Hepatitis C factsheet. www.who.int/mediacentre/factsheets/fs164/en/. Accessed April 29, 2015.

CHAPTER

56 PRION DISEASES

A 73-year-old man complained of weakness, forgetfulness, difficulty speaking, and involuntary movements of his right arm. After 3 months, myoclonus (muscle twitching) and other neurologic signs were noted and he was hospitalized. Protein 14-3-3 was detected in cerebrospinal fluid, but there was no evidence of an infection. The patient's condition continued to deteriorate, he slipped into a coma, and he died 4 months after the onset of symptoms. At autopsy, brain sections showed vacuolation and amyloid-containing plaques and fibrils, but there was no evidence of inflammatory cells.

1. Which disease signs indicate a prion disease?
2. Why are prions so resistant to disinfection?
3. Why was there not evidence of an immune response?

Answers to these questions are available on StudentConsult.com.

• SUMMARIES CLINICALLY SIGNIFICANT ORGANISMS

Prions

Trigger Words

Creutzfeldt-Jakob disease, spongiform encephalopathy, kuru, presenile dementia

Biology, Virulence, and Disease

- Prions are infectious protein aggregates resistant to inactivation
- Prions consist of subunits with an alternate conformation of normal host proteins (PrP)
- Prion binds to normal PrP, alters their conformation, and builds fibrils
- Collect in brain, where they cause spongiform vacuoles
- No immune response, no inflammation
- Acquired, genetic, and sporadic forms of prion disease
- Creutzfeldt-Jakob disease (presenile dementia), kuru, Gerstmann-Sträussler-Scheinker disease, fatal familial insomnia

Epidemiology

- Transmitted on contaminated surgical devices, by injection, in food, or genetic

Diagnosis

- Symptomatology, MRI, indirect assays

Treatment, Prevention, and Control

- Rigorous disinfection procedures
- No means of prevention or control

Spongiform encephalopathies, which are slow neurodegenerative diseases, are caused by proteinaceous infectious particles termed *prions.* Unlike conventional viruses, prions have no virion structure or genome, elicit no immune response, and are extremely resistant to inactivation by heat, disinfectants, and radiation (Table 56-1). **Prion diseases can be sporadic, genetic, or acquired.** After long incubation periods, these agents cause damage to the central nervous system, leading to a subacute spongiform encephalopathy. The long incubation period, which can last 30 years in humans, has made study of these agents difficult.

Acquired (by infection) human prion diseases include kuru, Creutzfeldt-Jakob disease (CJD), and variant CJD (vCJD). Genetic prion diseases include CJD, Gerstmann-Sträussler-Scheinker (GSS) syndrome, and fatal familial insomnia (FFI). Sporadic occurrences of CJD and FFI occur more commonly (85% to 90% of cases) than genetic (10% to 15%) or acquired (1% to 3%). The animal diseases include scrapie, bovine spongiform encephalopathy (BSE ["mad cow disease"]), chronic wasting disease (in mule, deer, and elk), and transmissible mink encephalopathy (Box 56-1).

Carlton Gajdusek won the Nobel Prize for showing that kuru has an infectious etiology and for developing a method for analyzing the agent. Stanley Prusiner won the Nobel Prize in 1997 for developing a hamster infection model for the scrapie agent. He and his coworkers were able to purify, characterize, and then clone the genes for the scrapie and other prion agents and show that the disease-related prion protein is sufficient to cause disease.

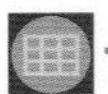

Table 56-1 Comparison of Classic Viruses and Prions

Characteristic	Virus	Prion
Filterable infectious agents	Yes	Yes
Presence of nucleic acid	Yes	No
Defined morphology (electron microscopy)	Yes	No
Presence of protein	Yes	Yes
Disinfection by:		
Formaldehyde	Yes	No
Proteases	Some	No
Heat (80° C)	Most	No
Ionizing and ultraviolet radiation	Yes	No
Disease		
Cytopathologic effect	Yes	No
Incubation period	Depends on virus	Long
Immune response	Yes	No
Interferon production	Yes	No
Inflammatory response	Yes	No

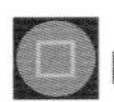

Box 56-1 Prion Diseases

Human
Kuru
Creutzfeldt-Jakob disease (CJD)
Variant CJD (vCJD)
Gerstmann-Sträussler-Scheinker (GSS) syndrome
Fatal familial insomnia (FFI)
Sporadic fatal insomnia

Animal
Scrapie (sheep and goats)
Transmissible mink encephalopathy
Bovine spongiform encephalopathy (BSE [mad cow disease])
Chronic wasting disease (mule, deer, and elk)

• Structure and Physiology

Unlike viruses, prions are resistant to a wide range of chemical and physical treatments, such as formaldehyde, ultraviolet radiation, and heat up to 80° C. The prion, which lacks detectable nucleic acids, consists of protease-resistant, hydrophobic, fibrillar aggregates of a normal cell surface glycoprotein. The normal protein is termed **PrP^C** (cellular prion protein) (27,000 to 30,000 Da), is protease sensitive, and is held in the cell membrane by a linkage between its terminal serine and a special lipid, glycophosphatidylinositol (GPI-linked protein). PrP^C interacts with and modulates the function of numerous membrane proteins in the brain, including potassium channels, NMDA receptors, and the neural cell adhesion molecule. Aggregation of the PrP^C changes the conformation of the protein from a primarily α-helical to a β-sheet enriched form to produce the aberrant protein termed **PrP^{Sc}** (scrapie-like prion protein) (Table 56-2). PrP^{Sc} is protease resistant, aggregates into amyloid rods (fibrils), and is cell free.

Table 56-2 Comparison of Scrapie Prion Protein (PrP^{Sc}) and (Normal) Cellular Prion Protein (PrP^C)

Characteristic	PrP^{Sc}	PrP^C
Structure	Multimeric	Monomeric
Protease resistance	Yes	No
Presence in scrapie fibrils	Yes	No
Location in or on cells	Cytoplasmic vesicles and extracellular milieu	Plasma membrane
Turnover	Days	Hours

The current theory to explain how an aberrant protein could cause disease is called *template-mediated protein refolding.* A linear aggregate of PrP^{Sc} binds to an anionic structure on the cell surface, such as a glycosaminoglycan, and the normal PrP^C on the cell surface. This causes the PrP^C to refold, acquire the structure of PrP^{Sc}, and join the chain. The α-helical structure of the PrP^C is changed to a more β-pleated sheet structure of the PrP^{Sc}. When the string of PrP^{Sc} breaks, it creates new primers upon which more prions can be built. The PrP^C continue to be made by the cell, and as they bind to the PrP^{Sc} primers, the cycle continues. The human version of the PrP^C is encoded on chromosome 20. The fact that these plaques consist of host protein may explain the lack of an immune response to these agents in patients with the spongiform encephalopathies.

Different strains of PrP^{Sc} occur because of mutations in the PrP^C (genetic) or because of self-perpetuating alternative folding patterns of the protein (sporadic or acquired). Specific mutations at codon 129 determine the severity of CJD. Conformational rather than genetic mutation is another property that distinguishes prions from viruses. When the PrP^{Sc} aggregates, the PrP^{Sc} acts as a template to transmit its conformation onto each new PrP^{Sc}, which can then perpetuate the change, analogous to a mutation in the genetic template (deoxyribonucleic acid [DNA] or ribonucleic acid [RNA]) of a virus. The different conformational strains can have different properties and varying disease aspects (e.g., incubation period).

Aggregation of other proteins into prions or prion-like structures may cause or contribute to human diseases such as Alzheimer disease, Huntington disease, and Parkinson disease.

• Pathogenesis

Prion infection can occur by ingestion, penetration through cuts in the skin, or by direct infection of the brain or neuronal tissue with prion-containing tissue. After ingestion, the prions accumulate in highly enervated secondary lymphoid tissue in follicular dendritic cells and B cells and then travel up neurons to the central nervous system and the brain.

Spongiform encephalopathy describes the appearance of the vacuolated neurons, as well as their loss of function and lack of an immune response or inflammation (Box 56-2). The formation of amyloid-containing plaques and fibrils, a proliferation and hypertrophy of astrocytes, and vacuolation of neurons and adjacent glial cells are observed

Box 56-2 Pathogenic Characteristics of Prions

No cytopathologic effect in vitro
Long doubling time of at least 5.2 days
Long incubation period
Cause vacuolation of neurons (spongiform), amyloid-like plaques, gliosis
Cause loss of muscle control, shivering, tremors, dementia
Lack of antigenicity
Lack of inflammation
Lack of immune response
Lack of interferon production

(Figure 56-1). The PrP^{Sc} reaches high concentrations in the brain and is taken up by neurons and phagocytic cells but is difficult to degrade, a feature that may contribute to the vacuolation of brain tissue. Prions can also be isolated from tissue other than the brain, but only the brain shows any pathologic changes. No inflammation or immune response to the agent is generated, distinguishing this disease from classic viral encephalitis. Protein markers (tau protein or 14-3-3 brain protein) can be detected in the cerebrospinal fluid of symptomatic persons, but this is not specific for prion disease.

The incubation period for CJD and kuru may be as long as 30 years, but once the symptoms become evident, disease progresses rapidly and death usually occurs within a year.

• Epidemiology

CJD is transmitted predominantly by (1) injection, (2) transplantation of contaminated tissue (e.g., corneas), (3) contact with contaminated medical devices (e.g., brain electrodes), and (4) food (Box 56-3). CJD usually affects persons older than 50 years. CJD, FFI, and GSS syndrome are also inheritable, and families with genetic histories of these diseases have been identified. The diseases are rare but occur worldwide.

Kuru was limited to a very small area of the New Guinea highlands. The name of the disease means "shivering" or "trembling," and the disease was related to the cannibalistic practices of the Fore tribe of New Guinea. Before Gajdusek intervened, it was the custom of these people to eat the bodies of their deceased kinsmen. When Gajdusek began his study, he noted that women and children, in particular, were the most susceptible to the disease, and he deduced that the reasons were that the women and children prepared the food, and they were given the less desirable viscera and brains to eat. Their risk for infection was higher because they handled the contaminated tissue, making it possible for the agent to be introduced through the conjunctiva or cuts in the skin. In addition, they ingested the neural tissue, which contains the highest concentrations of the kuru agent. Cessation of this cannibalistic custom has stopped the spread of kuru.

An epidemic of BSE (mad cow disease) in 1980 in the United Kingdom and the unusual incidence of a more rapidly progressing CJD in younger people (<45 years) in 1996 prompted concern that contaminated beef was the source of this new variant of CJD. Infection of cattle was most likely

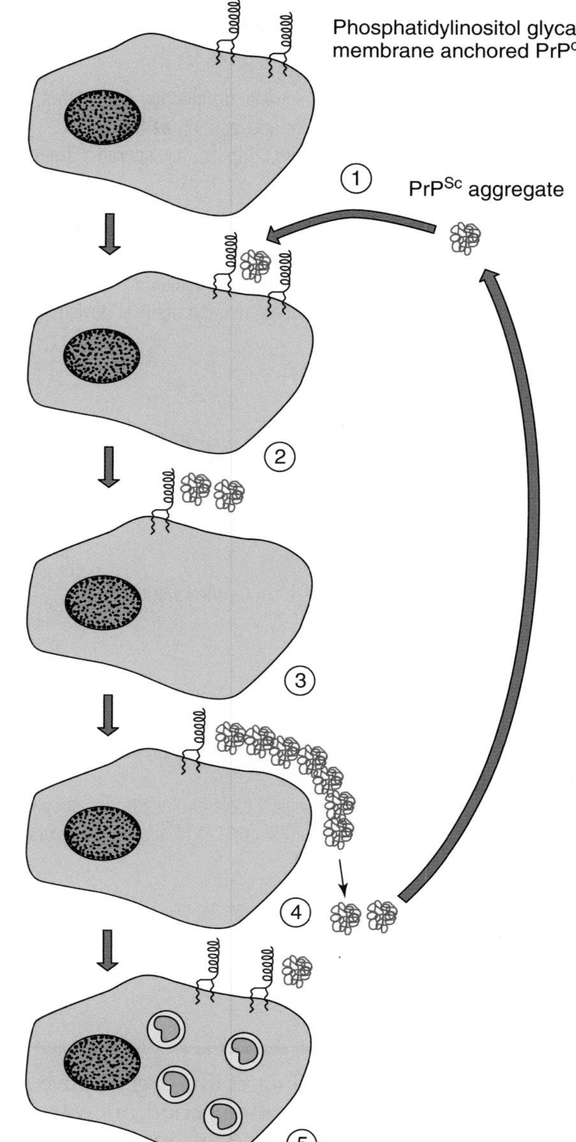

FIGURE 56-1 Template-mediated protein refolding model for proliferation of prions. PrP^C is a normal cellular protein that is anchored in the cell membrane by phosphatidylinositol glycan. PrP^{Sc} is a hydrophobic globular protein that aggregates with itself and with PrP^C on the cell surface *(1)*. PrP^C acquires the conformation of PrP^{Sc} *(2)*. The cell synthesizes new PrP^C *(3)*, and a chain is built along cell surface anionic glycosaminoglycans *(4)*. The chain breaks upon phagocytosis or from shear forces and releases PrP^{Sc} aggregates that act like seed crystals to start the cycle over. A form of PrP^{Sc} is internalized by neuronal cells and accumulates *(5)*. Other models have been proposed.

caused by the use of contaminated animal byproducts (e.g., sheep entrails, brains) as a protein supplement in cattle feed. Ingestion of contaminated beef is likely to be the cause of 153 cases of vCJD, more than 98% of which have occurred in the United Kingdom.

In addition to infection, prion diseases can also be familial (genetic) or sporadic, with no known history of exposure. GSS syndrome and FFI are familial prion diseases.

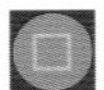 **Box 56-3 Epidemiology of Disease Caused by Prions**

Disease/Viral Factors

Agents are impervious to standard microbial disinfection procedures.

Diseases have very long incubation periods, as long as 30 years.

Disease acquisition may be infectious, genetic, or sporadic (random occurrence).

Transmission

Transmission is via **infected tissue,** or syndrome may be **inherited.**

Infection occurs through cuts in skin, transplantation of contaminated tissues (e.g., cornea), and use of contaminated medical devices (e.g., brain electrodes).

Infection by ingestion of infected tissue

Who Is at Risk?

Members (especially women and children) of the Fore tribe in New Guinea were at risk for kuru because of ritual cannibalism.

Surgeons, transplant and brain-surgery patients, and others are at risk for CJD and GSS syndrome.

Geography/Season

GSS syndrome and CJD have sporadic occurrence worldwide.

There is no seasonal incidence.

Modes of Control

No treatments are available.

Cessation of ritual cannibalism has led to the disappearance of kuru.

Elimination of animal products from livestock feed to prevent vCJD development and transmission

For GSS syndrome and CJD, neurosurgical tools and electrodes should be disinfected in 5% hypochlorite solution or 1.0 M sodium hydroxide or autoclaved at 15 psi for 1 hour.

CJD, Creutzfeldt-Jakob disease; *GSS,* Gerstmann-Sträussler-Scheinker; *vCJD,* variant Creutzfeldt-Jakob disease.

• Clinical Syndromes

The slow virus agents cause a progressive, degenerative neurologic disease with a long incubation period, but with rapid progression to death after the onset of symptoms (Figure 56-2; Clinical Case 56-1; Box 56-4). The spongiform encephalopathies are characterized by a loss of muscle control, shivering, myoclonic jerks and tremors, loss of coordination, rapidly progressive dementia, and death.

• Laboratory Diagnosis

There are no methods for directly detecting prions in tissue, and there is no serologic response. The initial diagnosis must be made on clinical grounds. Confirmation of the diagnosis can be made by magnetic resonance imaging, detection of elevated levels of 14-3-3 protein or tau protein in CSF, or a proteinase K–resistant form of PrP in a Western blot using antibody to PrP in a tonsil biopsy. At autopsy, the characteristic amyloid plaques, spongiform vacuoles, and immunohistologically detected PrP can be observed. The ability of PrP^{Sc} to initiate the polymerization of normal PrP is utilized in the protein-misfolding cyclic assay (PMCA) to amplify the number of PrP^{Sc} units and can be used to detect the presence of prions.

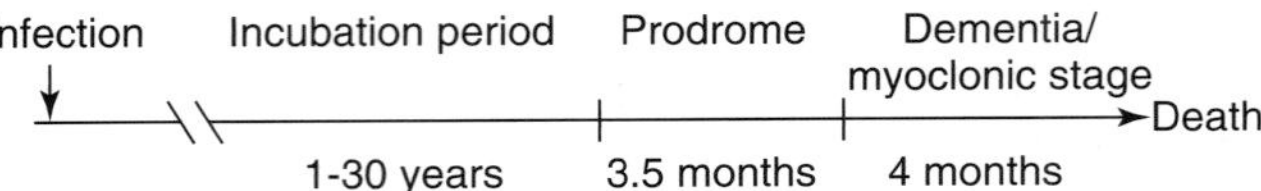

FIGURE 56-2 Progression of transmissible Creutzfeldt-Jakob disease.

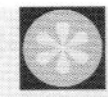 **Clinical Case 56-1 Transmission of Creutzfeldt-Jakob Disease (CJD) by Transfusion**

In a case reported by Wroe and associates (*Lancet* 368:2061–2067, 2006), a 30-year-old man consulted his family doctor because of fatigue and inability to concentrate. The symptoms were attributed to a respiratory tract infection. Neurologic exams for the patient at this time were normal. History was significant for the fact that during surgery 7 years earlier, the patient had received packed red cells, including blood from a donor who died 1 year later with variant CJD (vCJD). Within 6 months of his initial presentation, the patient had difficulty maintaining balance, a tendency to stagger, some memory problems, a tremor in his hands, and "searing pain" in his legs. At this time, there was no evidence of changes in vision or mental status. After another 6 weeks, his mental status and memory decreased, balance and walking became difficult and painful, magnetic resonance neuroimaging and electroencephalogram indicated changes, and a blood test showed the presence of the vCJD prion protein (PrP^{Sc}). The patient's mental status and physical ability continued to decline; he became mute, bedridden, poorly responsive, and he died 8 years and 8 months after the transfusion. Western immunoblot of autopsy samples from the brain and tonsils contained the PrP^{Sc} protein. PrP plaques and spongiform encephalopathy were noted in the brain.

Because of the long incubation period for prion diseases, prevention of transfusion transmission of CJD is difficult. vCJD has a more rapid onset of disease, and this case shows the classic progression through the five stages: (1) incubation (6 years), (2) prodromal fatigue and difficulty concentrating (18 months), (3) progressive neurologic decline (9 months), (4) late neurologic phase (4 months), and (5) terminal phase. Immunoblot analysis of treated prion protein can now distinguish the PrP^{Sc} from the normal protein in samples that can be taken from the patient's tonsils (or at autopsy, from the brain).

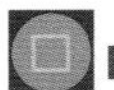 **Box 56-4 Clinical Summaries**

Creutzfeldt-Jakob disease: A 63-year-old man complained of poor memory and difficulty with vision and muscle coordination. Over the course of the next year, he developed senile dementia and irregular jerking movements, progressively lost muscle function, and then died.

Variant Creutzfeldt-Jakob disease: A 25-year-old is seen by a psychiatrist for anxiety and depression. After 2 months, he has problems with balance and muscle control and has difficulty remembering. He develops myoclonus and dies within 12 months of onset.

• Treatment, Prevention, and Control

No treatment exists for kuru or CJD. The causative agents are also impervious to the disinfection procedures used for other viruses, including formaldehyde, detergents, and ionizing radiation. Autoclaving at 15 psi for 1 hour (instead of 20 minutes) or treatment with 5% hypochlorite solution or 1.0 M sodium hydroxide can be used for decontamination.

Because these agents can be transmitted on instruments and brain electrodes, such items should be carefully disinfected before being reused.

The outbreak of BSE and vCJD in the United Kingdom promoted legislation to ban animal products in livestock feed and encouraged more careful monitoring of cattle. Prion disease has not been a problem in cattle in the United States. Cattle must be younger than 5 years old to minimize the possibility of accumulation of aberrant PrP and so that muscle tissue would have the lowest amount of PrP.

Bibliography

Aguzzi A, Nuvolone M, Zhu C: The immunobiology of prion diseases, *Nat Rev Immunol* 13:888–902, 2013.

Aguzzi A, Zhu C: Five questions on prion diseases, *PLoS Pathog* 8:e1002651, 2012.

Belay ED: Transmissible spongiform encephalopathies in humans, *Annu Rev Microbiol* 53:283–314, 1999.

Brown P, Coker-Vann M, Pomeroy K, et al: Diagnosis of Creutzfeldt-Jakob disease by Western blot identification, *N Engl J Med* 314:547–551, 1986.

Cohen J, Powderly WG: *Infectious diseases*, ed 2, St Louis, 2004, Mosby.

Flint SJ, Enquist LW, Racaniello VR, et al: *Principles of virology: molecular biology, pathogenesis and control of animal viruses*, ed 3, Washington, DC, 2009, American Society for Microbiology Press.

Halfmann R, Alberti S, Lindquist S: Prions, protein homeostasis, and phenotypic diversity, *Trends Cell Biol* 20:125–133, 2010.

Hsich G, Kenney K, Gibbs CJ, et al: The 14-3-3 brain protein in cerebrospinal fluid as a marker for transmissible spongiform encephalopathies, *N Engl J Med* 335:924–930, 1996.

Knipe DM, Howley PM: *Fields virology*, ed 6, Philadelphia, 2013, Lippincott Williams & Wilkins.

Lee KS, Caughey B: A simplified recipe for prions, *Proc Natl Acad Sci U S A* 104:9551–9552, 2007.

Manson JC: Understanding transmission of the prion diseases, *Trends Microbiol* 7:465–467, 1999.

Mercer RC, Ma L, Watts JC, et al: The prion protein modulates A-type K^+ currents mediated by Kv4.2 complexes through dipeptidyl aminopeptidase-like protein 6, *J Biol Chem* 288:37241–37255, 2013.

Prusiner SB: Molecular biology and genetics of neurodegenerative diseases caused by prions, *Adv Virus Res* 41:241–280, 1992.

Prusiner SB: Prions, prions, prions, *Curr Top Microbiol Immunol* (vol 207), Berlin, 1996, Springer-Verlag.

Prusiner SB: A unifying role for prions in neurodegenerative diseases, *Science* 336:1511–1512, 2012.

Richman DD, Whitley RJ, Hayden FG: *Clinical virology*, ed 3, Washington, DC, 2009, American Society for Microbiology Press.

Takada LT, Geschwind MD: Prion diseases, *Semin Neurol* 33:348–356, 2013.

Websites

Centers for Disease Control and Prevention: Prion diseases. www.cdc.gov/ncidod/dvrd/prions/. Accessed April 29, 2015.

Freudenrich CC: How mad cow disease works. http://science.howstuffworks.com/mad-cow-disease6.htm. Accessed April 29, 2015.

Genetics Home Reference: Prion disease. http://ghr.nlm.nih.gov/condition=priondisease. Accessed April 29, 2015.

National Prion Disease Pathology Surveillance Center: Homepage. www.cjdsurveillance.com/. Accessed May 20, 2015.

SECTION

6

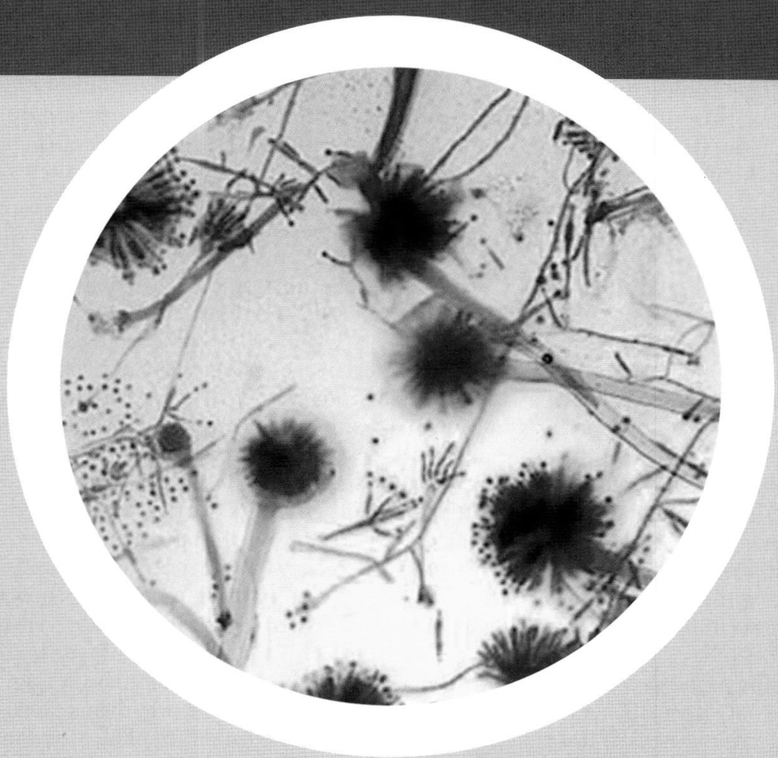

MYCOLOGY

CHAPTER

57 FUNGAL CLASSIFICATION, STRUCTURE, AND REPLICATION

This chapter provides an overview of fungal classification, structure, and reproduction. The very basic aspects of fungal cell organization and morphology are discussed, as well as the broad categories of human mycoses. We have purposely simplified the fungal taxonomy and use it to highlight the major phyla of fungi causing disease in humans: the Ascomycota (Ascomycetes), the Basidiomycota (Basidiomycetes), the Glomeromycota (Mucormycetes), and the Microspora (Microsporidia).

• The Importance of Fungi

The fungi represent a ubiquitous and diverse group of organisms, the main purpose of which is to degrade organic matter. All fungi lead a heterotrophic existence as **saprobes** (organisms that live on dead or decaying matter), **symbionts** (organisms that live together and in which the association is of mutual advantage), **commensals** (organisms living in a close relationship in which one benefits from the relationship and the other neither benefits nor is harmed), or as **parasites** (organisms that live on or within a host from which they derive benefits without making any useful contribution in return; in the case of pathogens, the relationship is harmful to the host).

Fungi have emerged in the past 2 decades as major causes of human disease (Table 57-1), especially among those individuals who are immunocompromised or hospitalized with serious underlying diseases. Among these patient groups, fungi serve as opportunistic pathogens, causing considerable morbidity and mortality. The overall incidence of specific invasive mycoses continues to increase with time, and the list of opportunistic fungal pathogens likewise increases each year. In short, *there are no nonpathogenic fungi!* This increase in fungal infections can be attributed to the ever-growing number of immunocompromised patients, including transplant patients, individuals with acquired immunodeficiency syndrome (AIDS), patients with cancer and undergoing chemotherapy, and those individuals who are hospitalized with other serious underlying conditions and who undergo a variety of invasive procedures.

• Fungal Taxonomy, Structure, and Replication

The fungi are classified in their own separate kingdom, Kingdom Fungi. They are eukaryotic organisms that are distinguished from other eukaryotes by a rigid cell wall composed of chitin and glucan and a cell membrane in which ergosterol is substituted for cholesterol as the major sterol component (Figure 57-1).

Classic fungal taxonomy relies heavily on morphology and mode of spore production. Increasingly, however, ultrastructural features, biochemical, and **molecular characteristics** are brought to bear, often resulting in changes in the original taxonomic designation. The advent of rapid DNA sequencing has resulted in a revolution in fungal taxonomy based on a phylogenetic approach to species recognition that relies on comparative analysis of variable nucleic acid characters to define a fungal species. Thus a species is defined as a group of organisms that share concordance of multiple gene genealogies (DNA sequences at different gene locations) rather than organisms that share a common morphology or that can mate together.

Fungi may be unicellular or multicellular. The most simple grouping, based on morphology, lumps fungi into either **yeasts** or **molds.** A yeast can be defined morphologically as a cell that reproduces by budding or fission (Figure 57-2), where a progenitor or "mother" cell pinches off a portion of itself to produce a progeny or "daughter" cell. The daughter cells may elongate to form sausage-like **pseudohyphae.** Yeasts are usually unicellular and produce round, pasty, or mucoid colonies on agar. Molds, on the other hand, are multicellular organisms consisting of threadlike tubular structures called **hyphae** (see Figure 57-2) that elongate at their tips by a process known as **apical extension.** Hyphae are either **coenocytic** (hollow and multinucleate) or **septate** (divided by partitions or crosswalls) (see Figure 57-2). The hyphae form together to produce a matlike structure called a **mycelium.** The colonies formed by molds are often described as **filamentous, hairy,** or **woolly.** When growing on agar or other solid surfaces, molds produce hyphae, termed **vegetative hyphae,** that grow on or beneath the surface of the culture medium, and also hyphae that project above the surface of the medium, so-called **aerial hyphae.** The aerial hyphae may produce specialized structures known as **conidia** (asexual reproductive elements) (Figure 57-3). The conidia may be produced by either a blastic (budding) process or a thallic process, where hyphal segments fragment into individual cells or **arthroconidia.** The conidia are easily airborne and serve to disseminate the fungus. The size, shape, and certain developmental features of conidia are used as a means of identifying fungi to genus and species. Many fungi of medical importance are termed **dimorphic** because they may exist in both a yeast and a mold form.

Table 57-1 Incidence and Mortality Rates of Selected Invasive Fungal Infections

Pathogen	Incidence (No. of Cases per Year)	Mortality Rates (% in Infected Populations)
Candida species	>400,000	46-75
Cryptococcus neoformans	>1,000,000	20-70
Aspergillus species	>200,000	30-95
Pneumocystis jirovecii	>400,000	20-80
Agents of endemic mycoses	>60,000	<1-70
Agents of mucormycosis	>10,000	30-90

Modified from Brown GD, Denning DW, Gow NA, et al: Hidden killers: human fungal infections, *Sci Transl Med* 4:165rv13, 2012.

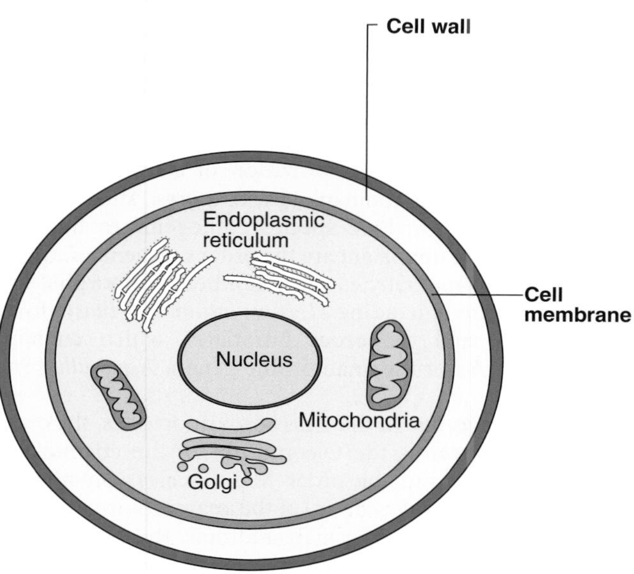

FIGURE 57-1 Diagram of a fungal cell.

Most fungi exhibit aerobic respiration, although some are facultatively anaerobic (fermentative) and others are strictly anaerobic. Metabolically fungi are heterotrophic and biochemically versatile, producing both primary (e.g., citric acid, ethanol, glycerol) and secondary (e.g., antibiotics [penicillin], amanitins, aflatoxins) metabolites. Relative to the bacteria, fungi are slow growing, with cell doubling times in terms of hours rather than minutes.

A simplified taxonomic scheme listing the four major taxa of fungi of medical importance is shown in Table 57-2. Of the estimated several hundred thousand different fungi, only about 200 are known to cause human disease, although this number appears to be increasing.

Fungi reproduce by formation of spores that may be sexual (involving meiosis, preceded by fusion of the protoplasm and nuclei of two compatible mating types) or asexual (involving mitosis only). The fungi in the Ascomycota, Basidiomycota, Glomeromycota, and Microspora produce both sexual and asexual spores (Table 57-3). The form of the fungus producing sexual spores is termed the **teleomorph,** and the form producing asexual spores is termed the **anamorph.** The fact that the teleomorph and anamorph of the

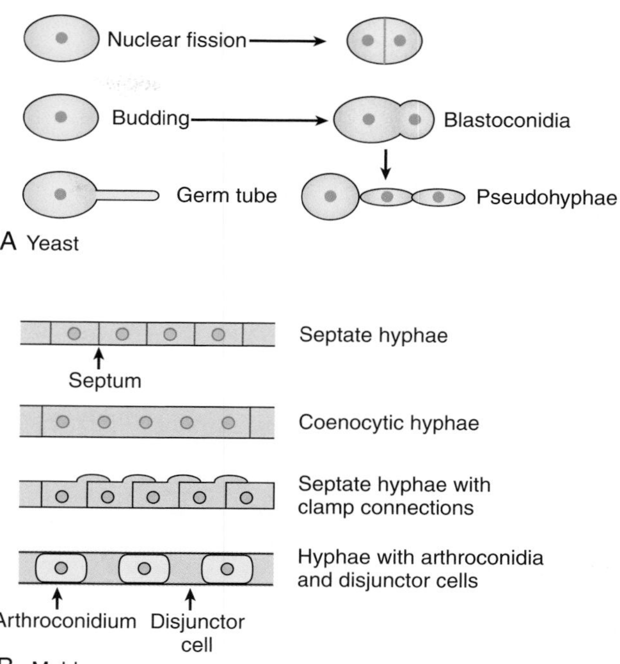

FIGURE 57-2 Fungal cell morphology. **A,** Yeast cells reproducing by nuclear fission and by blastoconidia formation. The elongation of budding yeast cells to form pseudohyphae is shown, as is the formation of a germ tube. **B,** Types of hyphae seen with various molds.

same fungus have different names (e.g., *Ajellomyces capsulatum* [teleomorph] and *Histoplasma capsulatum* [anamorph]) is a source of confusion for nonmycologists.

In light of this confusion and to recognize the impact of molecular taxonomy, the code of mycologic nomenclature was modified to apply a policy where a given fungus will have only one name; it will no longer be necessary to provide different names for different morphologies of the same fungus. All legitimate names proposed for a species can serve as the correct name for that species. At this time it is permissible to refer to a fungus by its asexual designation if that is the form usually obtained in culture. For example, *Histoplasma capsulatum* is the anamorph of the ascomycete *Ajellomyces capsulatum*. The anamorph is the stage that is most often encountered in culture, and only under special conditions is the sexual stage formed. Thus the clinical isolate is known as *Histoplasma capsulatum*.

Asexual spores consist of two general types: **sporangiospores** and **conidia.** Sporangiospores are asexual spores produced in a containing structure or **sporangia** (see Figure 57-3) and are characteristic of genera belonging to the Mucorales, such as *Rhizopus* and *Mucor* spp. Conidia are asexual spores that are borne naked on specialized structures as seen in *Aspergillus* spp. (see Figure 57-3), *Penicillium* spp., and the dermatophytes.

• Ascomycota (Ascomycetes)

The phylum Ascomycota contains almost 50% of all named fungal species and accounts for approximately 80% of fungi of medical importance. Sexual reproduction leads to the

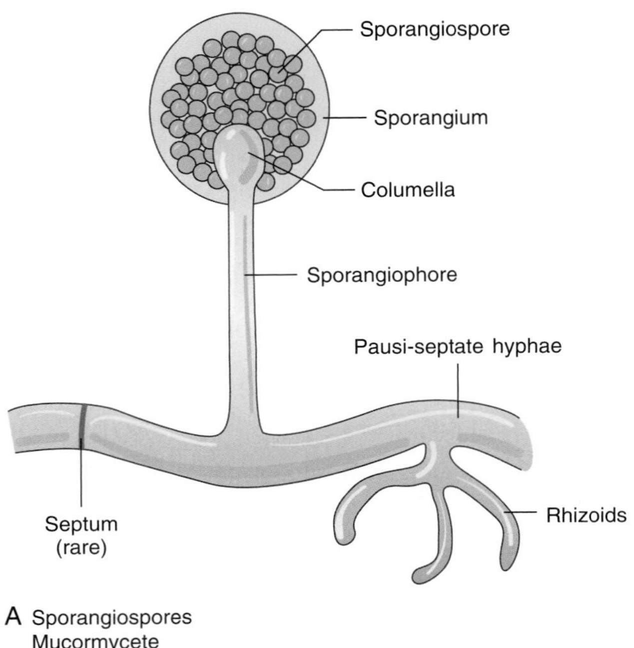

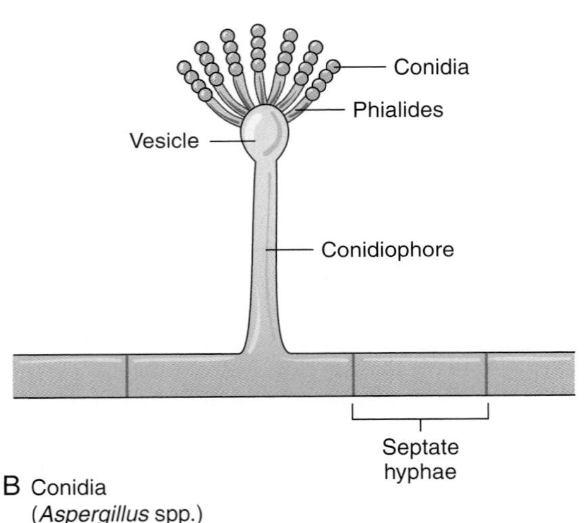

FIGURE 57-3 Examples of asexual spore formation and associated structures seen with a Mucorales **(A)** and an *Aspergillus* spp. **(B).**

development of ascospores, which are produced in a specialized saclike structure known as an ascus. Asexual reproduction consists of the production of conidia from a generative or conidiogenous cell.

The Ascomycota consists of four classes of medical importance: the Pneumocystidomycetes, Saccharomycetes, Eurotiomycetes, and Sordariomycetes. The class Pneumocystidomycetes contains the genus *Pneumocystis,* formerly classified as a protozoan but now reassigned to the Kingdom Fungi on the basis of gene sequence comparisons. Saccharomycetes contains the ascomycetous yeasts, whereas Eurotiomycetes and Sordariomycetes contain the filamentous ascomycetes.

Pneumocystidomycetes: Pneumocystidomycetes is a new class that was recently described to include an organism, *Pneumocystis carinii,* formerly considered to be a protozoan. The reclassification of *Pneumocystis* was based on molecular evidence that it was most closely related to the ascomycete *Schizosaccharomyces pombe.* Further molecular studies resulted in the naming of human-derived strains as *Pneumocystis jirovecii.* The organism exists in a vegetative trophic form that reproduces asexually by binary fission. Fusion of compatible mating types results in a spherical cyst or spore case, which on maturity contains eight spores.

Saccharomycetes: The class Saccharomycetes contains the ascomycetous yeasts (order Saccharomycetales), which are characterized by vegetative yeast cells that proliferate by budding or fission (see Figure 57-2A). Many members of the order Saccharomycetales have an anamorphic stage belonging to the genus *Candida* (see Table 57-2). This genus, which consists of approximately 200 anamorphic species, has teleomorphs in more than 10 different genera, including *Clavispora, Debaromyces, Issatchenkia, Kluyveromyces,* and *Pichia.* Under the "one fungus one name" concept, many of these will be renamed.

Eurotiomycetes: In the class Eurotiomycetes, sexual reproduction leads to the formation of a thin-walled sac (ascus) that contains the haploid ascospores. This class has seven orders that include species pathogenic to humans. Among the more important are the order Onygenales, which contains the dermatophytes and a number of dimorphic systemic pathogens (including *H. capsulatum* and *Blastomyces dermatitidis*), and the order Eurotiales, which contains the teleomorphs of the anamorphic genera *Aspergillus* and *Penicillium.*

Sordariomycetes: In the class Sordariomycetes, the order Hypocreales contains the teleomorphs of the anamorphic genus *Fusarium,* and the order Microascales contains the teleomorphs *(Pseudallescheria)* of the anamorphic genus *Scedosporium* (see Table 57-2). In addition, the teleomorphs of numerous melanized (dematiaceous) fungi of medical importance belong to orders in this class.

• Basidiomycota (Basidiomycetes)

Most members of the Basidiomycetes have a separate filamentous form, but some are typical yeasts. Sexual reproduction leads to the formation of haploid basidiospores on the outside of a generative cell termed a **basidium.** The most prominent human pathogens in the phylum Basidiomycetes are the basidiomycetous yeasts with anamorphic stages belonging to the genera *Cryptococcus, Malassezia,* and *Trichosporon.* The genus *Cryptococcus,* which contains more than 30 different species, has teleomorphs (sexual stages) that have been assigned to the genera *Filobasidium* and *Filobasidiella.*

The filamentous basidiomycetes are increasingly recognized as causes of opportunistic fungal infections. In culture these organisms often produce fast-growing, sterile, white colonies with **clamp connections** (see Figure 57-2B)—hyphal outgrowths that form a bypass around the septum to facilitate the migration of a nucleus. Whereas most filamentous basidiomycetes are wood-rotting fungi, the most frequently reported cause of human infection is *Schizophylum commune.*

Table 57-2 Medically Important Fungi (Kingdom Fungi)

Taxonomic Designation	Representative Genera	Human Disease
Phylum Glomeromycota (Mucormycetes)		
Order: Mucorales	*Rhizopus, Mucor, Lichtheimia, Saksenaea*	Mucormycosis: opportunistic in patients with diabetes, leukemia, severe burns, or malnutrition; rhinocerebral infections
Order: Entomophthorales	*Basidiobolus, Conidiobolus*	Entomophthoromycosis: subcutaneous and gastrointestinal infections
Phylum: Basidiomycota (Basidiomycetes)	Teleomorphs of *Cryptococcus, Malassezia,* and *Trichosporon* spp.	Cryptococcosis and numerous mycoses
Phylum: Ascomycota (Ascomycetes)		
Class: Pneumocystidomycetes	*Pneumocystis jirovecii*	*Pneumocystis* pneumonia
Class: Saccharomycetes	Teleomorphs of *Candida* spp.; *Saccharomyces*	Numerous mycoses
Class: Eurotiomycetes Order: Onygenales	*Arthroderma* (teleomorphs of *Trichophyton* and *Microsporum*); *Ajellomyces* (teleomorphs of *Blastomyces* and *Histoplasma* spp.)	Dermatophytoses, systemic mycoses
Order: Eurotiales	Teleomorphs of *Aspergillus* spp.	Aspergillosis
Class: Sordariomycetes Order: Hypocreales	Teleomorphs of *Fusarium* spp.	Keratitis and other invasive mycoses
Order: Microascales	*Pseudallescheria* (teleomorph of *Scedosporium* spp.)	Pneumonia, mycetoma, and invasive mycoses
Phylum: Microspora (Microsporidia)	*Encephalitozoon, Enterocytozoon, Nosema, Trachipleistophora*	Keratoconjunctivitis, sinusitis, pneumonitis, diarrhea, encephalitis, disseminated infection

Modified from Brandt ME, Warnock DW: Taxonomy and classification of fungi. In Versalovic J, et al, editors: *Manual of clinical microbiology,* ed 10, Washington, DC, 2011, American Society for Microbiology Press.

Table 57-3 Biological, Morphologic, and Reproductive Characteristics of Pathogenic Fungi

Organism Group	Representative Genera	Morphology	Reproduction
Mucormycetes	*Rhizopus, Mucor, Lichtheimia, Basidiobolus*	Broad, thin-walled, coenocytic hyphae, 6-25 μm with nonparallel sides; spores contained within sporangium; rootlike structures called *rhizoids* characteristic of some genera	Asexual: production of sporangiospores within sporangium. Sexual: production of zygospores formed by fusion of compatible mating types
Basidiomycetes	Anamorphic basidiomycetous yeasts *(Cryptococcus, Malassezia, Trichosporon)*	Budding yeasts, hyphae, and arthroconidia. Hyphae that produce basidiospores (not seen in nature or in patients). Hyphae with clamp connections	Asexual: production of conidia by budding from a mother cell or within a hyphal fragment. Sexual: fusion of compatible nuclei followed by meiosis to form basidiospores or not identified
Pneumocystidomycetes	*Pneumocystis jirovecii*	Trophic forms and cystlike structures	Asexual: binary fission. Sexual: fusion of compatible mating types to form zygote; compartmentalization of spores within cyst
Saccharomycetes	*Candida* and *Saccharomyces*	Budding yeasts and hyphae, pseudohyphae	Asexual: production of conidia by budding from a mother cell. Sexual: either not seen or by conjugation between two single cells or by "mother-bud" conjugation
Eurotiomycetes	Dermatophytes, *Blastomyces, Histoplasma, Aspergillus, Fusarium, Scedosporium* spp.	Budding yeasts, septate hyphae, asexual conidia borne on specialized structures	Asexual: production of conidia by budding from a mother cell. Sexual: ascospores produced in a specialized structure called an *ascus* or not seen

• Glomeromycota (Mucormycetes, formerly Zygomycetes)

The Glomeromycota (Mucormycetes) include molds with broad, sparsely septate, coenocytic hyphae. The subphylum Mucoromycotina has been proposed to accommodate the **Mucorales,** and the subphylum Entomophthoromycotina includes the **Entomophthorales.** These fungi produce **sexual zygospores** after the fusion of two compatible mating types. The asexual spores of the order Mucorales (see Figure 57-3) are contained within a sporangium (sporangiospores). The sporangia are borne at the tips of stalk like **sporangiophores** that terminate in a bulbous swelling called the **columella** (see Figure 57-3). The presence of rootlike structures called **rhizoids** is helpful in identifying specific genera within the Mucorales. The order Mucorales is the most clinically important and includes the genera *Lichtheimia* (formerly *Absidia*), *Mucor*, *Rhizopus,* and *Rhizomucor*. The other order, Entomophthorales, is less common and includes the genera *Basidiobolus* and *Conidiobolus*. These organisms cause tropical subcutaneous mucormycosis. The asexual spores are borne singly on short sporophores and are forcibly ejected when mature.

• Microspora (Microsporidia)

Microsporidia are obligate intracellular, unicellular, spore-forming eukaryotes. Previously categorized as protists, organisms of the phylum Microspora were recently assigned to the Kingdom Fungi on the basis of genetic studies indicating that these organisms were derived from an endoparasitic chytrid ancestor on the earliest diverging branch of the fungal phylogenetic tree. Furthermore, structural features of the organisms, such as the presence of chitin in the spore wall, diplokaryotic nuclei, and electron-dense spindle plaques associated with the nuclear envelope, suggest a possible relationship between fungi and microsporidia. Conversely, the life cycle of microsporidia is unique and unlike that of any other fungal species. More than 160 microsporidial genera and 1300 species that are pathogenic in every major animal group have been identified. Presently, human infections have been shown to involve nine different genera (*Anncaliia, Encephalitozoon, Endoreticulatus, Enterocytozoon, Nosema, Pleistophora, Vittaforma, Tubulinosema,* and *Trachipleistophora)* as well as unclassified microsporidia that have been assigned to the collective group *Microsporidium*.

• Classification of Human Mycoses

In addition to the formal taxonomic classification of fungi, fungal infections may be classified according to the tissues infected as well as by specific characteristics of organism groups. These classifications include the superficial, cutaneous, and subcutaneous mycoses, the endemic mycoses, and the opportunistic mycoses (Table 57-4).

Superficial Mycoses

Superficial mycoses are those infections that are limited to the very superficial surfaces of the skin and hair. They are nondestructive and of cosmetic importance only. The clinical infection termed **pityriasis versicolor** is characterized by discoloration or depigmentation and scaling of the skin. **Tinea nigra** refers to brown- or black-pigmented macular patches localized primarily to the palms. The clinical entities of black and white piedra involve the hair and are characterized by nodules composed of hyphae that encompass the hair shaft. The fungi associated with these superficial infections include *Malassezia furfur, Hortae werneckii, Piedraia hortae,* and *Trichosporon* spp.

Cutaneous Mycoses

Cutaneous mycoses are infections of the keratinized layer of skin, hair, and nails. These infections may elicit a host response and become symptomatic. Signs and symptoms include itching, scaling, broken hairs, ringlike patches of the skin, and thickened discolored nails. The Dermatophytes are fungi classified in the genera *Trichophyton, Epidermophyton,* and *Microsporum*. Infections of the skin involving these organisms are called **dermatophytoses. Tinea unguium** refers to infections of the toes involving these agents. Onychomycosis includes infections of the nails caused by the dermatophytes as well as nondermatophytic fungi (e.g., *Candida* and *Aspergillus* spp.).

Subcutaneous Mycoses

Subcutaneous mycoses involve the deeper layers of the skin, including the cornea, muscle, and connective tissue, and are caused by a broad spectrum of taxonomically diverse fungi. The fungi gain access to the deeper tissues usually by traumatic inoculation and remain localized, causing abscess formation, nonhealing ulcers, and draining sinus tracts. The host immune system recognizes the fungi, resulting in variable tissue destruction and frequently epitheliomatous hyperplasia. Infections may be caused by hyaline molds, such as *Acremonium* spp. and *Fusarium* spp., and by pigmented or dematiaceous fungi, such as *Alternaria* spp., *Cladosporium* spp., and *Exophiala* spp. (phaeohyphomycoses, chromoblastomycoses). Subcutaneous mycoses tend to remain localized and rarely disseminate systemically.

Endemic Mycoses

The endemic mycoses are fungal infections caused by the classic dimorphic fungal pathogens *H. capsulatum, B. dermatitidis, Emmonsia pasteuriana, Coccidioides immitis, Coccidioides posadasii, Paracoccidioides brasiliensis,* and *Talaromyces (Penicillium) marneffei*. These fungi exhibit thermal dimorphism (exist as yeasts or spherules at 37° C and molds at 25° C) and are generally confined to geographic regions where they occupy specific environmental or ecologic niches. The endemic mycoses are often referred to as **systemic mycoses** because these organisms are true pathogens and can cause infection in healthy individuals. All of these agents produce a primary infection in the lung, with subsequent dissemination to other organs and tissues.

Opportunistic Mycoses

The opportunistic mycoses are infections attributable to fungi that are normally found as human commensals or in the environment. With the exception of *Cryptococcus neoformans* and *Cryptococcus gattii,* these organisms exhibit inherently low or limited virulence and cause infection in

Table 57-4 Classification of Human Mycoses and Representative Etiologic Agents

Superficial Mycoses	Cutaneous and Subcutaneous Mycoses	Endemic Mycoses	Opportunistic Mycoses
Black piedra	Dermatophytoses	Blastomycosis	Aspergillosis
Piedraia hortae	*Microsporum* spp.	*Blastomyces dermatitidis*	*Aspergillus fumigatus*
Tinea nigra	*Trichophyton* spp.	Histoplasmosis	*A. flavus*
Hortae werneckii	*Epidermophyton floccosum*	*Histoplasma capsulatum*	*A. niger*
Pityriasis versicolor	Tinea unguium	Coccidioidomycosis	*A. terreus*
Malassezia furfur	*Trichophyton* spp.	*Coccidioides immitis/posadasii*	Candidiasis
White piedra	*E. floccosum*	Penicilliosis	*Candida albicans*
Trichosporon spp.	Onychomycosis	*Talaromyces (Penicillium) marneffei*	*C. glabrata*
	Candida spp.	Paracoccidioidomycosis	*C. parapsilosis*
	Aspergillus spp.	*Paracoccidioides brasiliensis*	*C. tropicalis*
	Trichosporon spp.	Emmonsiasis	Cryptococcosis
	Geotrichum spp.	*Emmonsia pasteuriana*	*Cryptococcus neoformans*
	Mycotic keratitis		Trichosporonosis
	Fusarium spp.		*Trichosporon* spp.
	Aspergillus spp.		Hyalohyphomycosis
	Candida spp.		*Acremonium* spp.
	Chromoblastomycosis		*Fusarium* spp.
	Fonsecaea spp.		*Paecilomyces* spp.
	Phialophora spp.		*Scedosporium* spp.
			Mucormycosis
			Rhizopus spp.
			Mucor spp.
			Lichtheimia corymbifera
			Phaeohyphomycosis
			Alternaria spp.
			Curvularia spp.
			Bipolaris spp.
			Wangiella spp.
			Pneumocystosis
			Pneumocystis jirovecii
			Microsporidiosis

individuals who are debilitated, immunosuppressed, or who carry implanted prosthetic devices or vascular catheters. Virtually any fungus can serve as an opportunistic pathogen, and the list of those identified as such becomes longer each year. The most common opportunistic fungal pathogens are the yeasts *Candida* spp. and *C. neoformans,* the mold *Aspergillus* spp., and *P. jirovecii*. Because of its inherent virulence, *C. neoformans* is often considered a "systemic" pathogen. Although this fungus may cause infection in immunologically normal individuals, it clearly is seen more frequently as an opportunistic pathogen in the immunocompromised population.

Summary

With the ever-increasing number of individuals at risk for fungal infection, it is imperative that physicians "think fungus" when confronting a suspected infection. The list of documented fungal pathogens is extensive, and one can no longer ignore or dismiss fungi as "contaminants" or clinically insignificant when isolated from clinical material. It is also apparent that the prognosis and response to therapy may vary with the type of fungus causing infection, as well as with the immunologic status of the host. Thus physicians must become familiar with the various fungi, their epidemiologic and pathogenic features, as well as the optimal approaches to diagnosis and therapy. These issues will be discussed in detail in subsequent chapters according to the classification scheme shown in Table 57-4.

Bibliography

Brandt ME, Warnock DW: Taxonomy and classification of fungi. In Versalovic J, et al, editors: *Manual of clinical microbiology*, ed 10, Washington, DC, 2011, American Society for Microbiology Press.

Brandt ME, Park BJ: Think fungus—prevention and control of fungal infections, *Emerg Infect Dis* 19:1688–1689, 2013.

Brown GD, Denning DW, Gow NAR, et al: Hidden killers: human fungal infections, *Sci Transl Med* 4:165rv13, 2012.

Hawksworth DL, Crous PW, Dianese JC, et al: The Amsterdam declaration on fungal nomenclature, *IMA Fungus* 2:105–112, 2011.

CHAPTER

58 PATHOGENESIS OF FUNGAL DISEASE

Although a great deal is known regarding the molecular and genetic basis for bacterial and viral pathogenesis, our understanding of the pathogenesis of fungal infections is limited. Relatively few fungi are sufficiently virulent to be considered **primary pathogens** (Table 58-1). Primary pathogens are capable of initiating infection in a normal, apparently immunocompetent host. They are able to colonize the host, find a suitable microenvironmental niche with sufficient nutritional substrates, avoid or subvert the normal host defense mechanisms, and then multiply within the microenvironmental niche. Among the acknowledged primary fungal pathogens are four ascomycetous fungi, the endemic dimorphic pathogens *Blastomyces dermatitidis, Coccidioides immitis* (and *Coccidioides posadasii*), *Histoplasma capsulatum,* and *Paracoccidioides brasiliensis.* Each of these organisms possesses putative virulence factors that allow them to actively breach host defenses that ordinarily restrict the invasive growth of other microbes (see Table 58-1). When large numbers of conidia of any of these four fungi are inhaled by humans—even if these individuals are healthy and immunocompetent—infection and colonization, tissue invasion, and systemic spread of the pathogen commonly occur. As with most primary microbial pathogens, these fungi may also serve as **opportunistic pathogens,** given that the more severe forms of each mycosis are seen most often in individuals who are compromised in their innate and/or acquired immune defenses.

In general, healthy immunocompetent individuals have a high innate resistance to fungal infection, despite the fact that they are constantly exposed to the infectious forms of various fungi present as part of the normal commensal flora (endogenous) or in the environment (exogenous). The opportunistic fungal pathogens, such as *Candida* spp., *Cryptococcus neoformans,* and *Aspergillus* spp., generally only cause infection when there are disruptions in the protective barriers of the skin and mucous membranes or when defects in the host immune system allow them to penetrate, colonize, and reproduce in the host (see Table 58-1). However, even with these opportunists, there are factors associated with the organism rather than the host that contribute to the ability of the fungus to cause disease (see Table 58-1).

• Primary Fungal Pathogens

All of the primary systemic fungal pathogens are agents of respiratory infections, and none is an obligate parasite. Each has a **saprobic phase** characterized by filamentous septate hyphae, typically found in soil or decaying vegetation, that produce the airborne infectious cells. Likewise, the **parasitic phase** of each fungus is adapted to grow at 37° C and to reproduce asexually in the alternative environmental niche of the host respiratory mucosa (see Chapter 64, Figure 64-1). This ability to exist in alternate morphogenic forms **(dimorphism)** is one of several special characteristics **(virulence factors)** that allow these fungi to cope with the hostile environmental conditions of the host (see Table 58-1).

Blastomyces dermatitidis

Like the other endemic dimorphic fungal pathogens, *B. dermatitidis* often causes a self-limited respiratory infection (see Chapter 64). However, blastomycosis is distinguished from the other endemic mycoses by the high incidence of clinical disease, compared with the mild or asymptomatic form among individuals infected in epidemics. The pathogenic potential of *B. dermatitidis* is underscored by the clinical severity of most sporadic cases of blastomycosis.

Important factors for the in vivo survival of *B. dermatitidis,* and any of the endemic dimorphic pathogens for that matter, are the ability of the inhaled pathogen to reach the alveoli, undergo transformation to an alternate phase (yeast or spherule) capable of replicating at 37° C, and colonize the respiratory mucosa. After inhalation of conidia or hyphal fragments of *B. dermatitidis,* the elements of the saprobic phase of the fungus presumably contact and adhere to the epithelial layer of the alveolus and then transform into the parasitic yeast phase in a process known as **thermal dimorphism.** This conversion from conidia (2 to 10 μm diameter) to the larger yeast form (8 to 30 μm diameter) provides an important survival advantage to the fungus. Whereas the conidia are small enough to be readily ingested and killed by human neutrophils, the yeast cells are able to resist the phagocytic attack of neutrophils and mononuclear cells during the early stages of the inflammatory response. Rather than adapting to the intracellular microenvironment of phagolysosomes, as does *H. capsulatum, B. dermatitidis* yeast cells shed their immunodominant antigen from the cell surface and subsequently modify their cell wall composition, allowing them to escape recognition by macrophages. Thus they are able to colonize tissue and disseminate through the bloodstream.

Modulation of Yeast and Host Immune System Interactions

The main immunoreactive moiety present on the surface of the yeast cells but not on the conidia of *B. dermatitidis* is a

 **Table 58-1 Characteristics of Primary and Opportunistic Fungal Pathogens**

	Habitat/Infection	Pathogenesis	Putative Virulence Factors	Clinical Forms of Mycosis
Primary Pathogens				
Blastomyces dermatitidis Saprobic phase • Septate mycelium and conidia Parasitic phase • Large, broad-based, budding yeast	Saprobic habitat • Soil and organic debris • Endemic area: southeastern United States and Ohio-Mississippi River Valley Mode of infection • Inhalation of conidia	Inhaled conidia convert to yeast; localized yeast invasion of host invokes inflammatory reaction; yeast escapes recognition by macrophages and disseminates via bloodstream	• Growth at 37° C • Thermal dimorphism • Modulation of yeast-host immune system interactions • Generation of TH2 response Shedding of WI-1	• Primary pulmonary blastomycosis • Chronic pulmonary blastomycosis • Disseminated blastomycosis • Cutaneous • Bone, genitourinary tract, and brain
Coccidioides immitis (posadasii) Saprobic phase • Septate hyphae and arthroconidia Parasitic phase • Spherules with endospores	Saprobic habitat • Desert soil: southwestern United States, Mexico, regions of Central and South America Mode of infection • Inhalation of arthroconidia • Percutaneous inoculation (rare)	Inhaled arthroconidia reach alveoli; convert to spherule that gives rise to endospores; endospores phagocytosed but survive; large (60-100 μm) spherules escape phagocytosis; alkaline environment allows survival within phagosome	• Growth at 37° C • Thermal dimorphism • Resistance of conidia to phagocytic killing • Stimulation of ineffective TH2 response • Urease production • Extracellular proteinase production • Molecular mimicry	• Initial pulmonary infection • Chronic pulmonary coccidioidomycosis • Disseminated coccidioidomycosis • Meningitis • Bone and joints • Genitourinary • Cutaneous • Ophthalmic
Histoplasma capsulatum Saprobic phase • Septate hyphae, microconidia, and tuberculate macroconidia Parasitic phase • Small, intracellular, budding yeast	Saprobic habitat • Soil enriched with bird/bat guano • Eastern half of United States, most of Latin America, parts of Asia, Europe, Middle East; var. *duboisii* occurs in Africa Mode of infection • Inhalation of conidia	Inhaled conidia convert to yeast; yeast ingested by macrophages; survive and proliferate within phagosome; some yeast forms remain dormant within macrophage, others proliferate and kill macrophages, releasing daughter cells	• Growth at 37° C • Thermal dimorphism • Survival in macrophages • Modulate pH of phagosome • Iron and calcium uptake • Alteration of cell wall composition	• Clinically asymptomatic pulmonary and "cryptic dissemination" • Acute pulmonary histoplasmosis • Mediastinitis and pericarditis • Chronic pulmonary histoplasmosis • Mucocutaneous • Disseminated
Paracoccidioides brasiliensis Saprobic phase • Septate hyphae, conidia Parasitic phase • Yeast with multiple buds	Saprobic habitat • Soil and vegetation • Central and South America Mode of infection • Inhalation of conidia	Inhaled conidia convert to large multipolar budding yeast; ingested but not cleared by macrophages; may be dormant for up to 40 years. Disseminate to oral and nasopharyngeal mucosa	• Growth at 37° C • Thermal dimorphism • Intracellular survival • Hormonal influences • Alteration of cell wall • Ineffective TH2 response to gp43	• Diverse clinical manifestations • Chronic single organ involvement • Chronic multifocal involvement (lungs, mouth, nose) • Juvenile progressive disease: lymph nodes, skin and visceral involvement
Opportunistic Pathogens				
Candida species Saprobic and parasitic phases are the same: budding yeast, hyphae, pseudohyphae	Saprobic habitat • Gastrointestinal mucosa, vaginal mucosa, skin, nails Mode of infection • Gastrointestinal translocation • Intravascular catheters	Mucosal overgrowth with subsequent invasion; usually impaired mucosal barrier; hematogenous dissemination. Transfer from hands of health care worker to catheter hub; catheter colonization and hematogenous dissemination	• Growth at 37° C • Bud-hyphae transition • Adherence • Cell surface hydrophobicity • Cell wall mannans • Proteases and phospholipases • Phenotypic switching	• Simple mucosal colonization • Mucocutaneous candidiasis • Oral/vaginal thrush • Hematogenous dissemination • Hepatosplenic candidiasis • Endophthalmitis

Continued

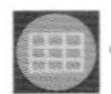

Table 58-1 Characteristics of Primary and Opportunistic Fungal Pathogens—cont'd

	Habitat/Infection	Pathogenesis	Putative Virulence Factors	Clinical Forms of Mycosis
Cryptococcus neoformans Saprobic and parasitic phases are the same: encapsulated budding yeast	Saprobic habitat • Soil enriched with bird (pigeon) guano Mode of infection • Inhalation of aerosolized yeast • Percutaneous inoculation	Inhaled yeast cells ingested by macrophages; survive intracellularly; capsule inhibits phagocytosis; capsule and melanin protect from oxidative injury; hematogenous and lymphatic dissemination to brain	• Growth at 37° C • Polysaccharide capsule • Melanin • Alpha-mating type	• Primary cryptococcal pneumonia • Meningitis • Hematogenous dissemination • Genitourinary (prostatic) cryptococcosis • Primary cutaneous cryptococcosis
Aspergillus species Saprobic phase • Septate mycelium, conidial heads, and conidia Parasitic phase • Septate mycelium; conidia, and conidial heads usually only seen in cavitary lesions	Saprobic habitat • Soil, plants, water, pepper, air Mode of infection • Inhalation of conidia • Transfer to wounds via contaminated tape/bandages	Inhaled conidia bind to fibrinogen and laminin in alveolus; conidia germinate, and hyphal forms secrete proteases and invade epithelium; vascular invasion results in thrombosis and infarction of tissue; hematogenous dissemination	• Growth at 37° C • Binding to fibrinogen and laminin • Secretion of elastase and proteases • Catalase • Gliotoxin (?)	• Allergic bronchopulmonary aspergillosis • Sinusitis • Aspergilloma • Invasive aspergillosis • Lung • Brain • Skin • Gastrointestinal • Heart

From Cole GT: Fungal pathogenesis. In Anaissie EJ, McGinnis MR, Pfaller MA, editors: *Clinical mycology,* New York, 2003, Churchill Livingstone.

120-kDa cell wall glycoprotein, WI-1. This glycoprotein appears to play a key role in the pathogenesis of *B. dermatitidis* in that it promotes adhesion of the yeast cell to macrophages and elicits a potent response of both the humoral and cellular immune systems. WI-1 is expressed by all virulent isolates of *B. dermatitidis* examined thus far.

It appears that avirulent mutant strains of *B. dermatitidis* with high levels of expression of WI-1 on their cell surface are recognized by macrophages, phagocytosed, and rapidly eliminated from the host. In contrast, virulent strains of this fungus shed copious amounts of WI-1 during growth and through this process are able to avoid recognition by macrophages. Presentation of WI-1, whether it remains associated with the cell surface or shed into the milieu apart from the cell, is a key aspect of the pathogenicity of this fungus.

It also appears that the carbohydrate composition of the yeast cell wall plays a role in the presentation and shedding of WI-1 and thus in pathogenicity. One of the major components of the yeast cell wall is 1,3-α-glucan. There is an inverse relationship between the amount of 1,3-α-glucan present in the cell wall of *B. dermatitidis* and the amount of detectable WI-1 at the cell surface. Virulent strains of *B. dermatitidis* produce yeast cells that have thickened walls containing large amounts of 1,3-α-glucan and, when mature, have little detectable WI-1 on their cell surface. Conversely, avirulent strains exhibit thin walls that lack 1,3-α-glucan but have abundant WI-1 on their surface. It is speculated that the incorporation of 1,3-α-glucan into the cell wall masks the WI-1 surface glycoprotein and plays a role in releasing a modified antigen (85-kDa component) into the microenvironment of the infection site. By masking the WI-1 antigen, the yeast is able to escape recognition by macrophages and disseminate hematogenously. Shedding the 85-kDa component of WI-1 may also facilitate immune evasion by binding or consuming antibody opsonins and complement away from the yeast cell surface. Likewise, the released WI-1 component may also saturate macrophage receptors and decrease the efficiency of binding and phagocytosis of yeast cells.

Presentation of Surface Antigen Modulates the T-Helper Pathway of Immune Response

Different subsets of CD4 T-helper (TH) cells exist that secrete different patterns of cytokines in response to an antigenic stimulus. After an initial encounter with an antigen, TH cells may become polarized, secreting predominantly interleukin (IL)-2 and interferon (IFN)-γ (TH1 pattern) or predominantly IL-4, IL-5, and IL-10 (TH2 pattern). IFN-γ and IL-2 activate macrophages and cytotoxic T and NK (natural killer) cells, respectively, for clearance of intracellular organisms, whereas TH2 cytokines favor B-cell growth and differentiation, isotype switching to immunoglobulin (Ig)E, and eosinophil differentiation and activation, responses that may lead to protection against some pathogens but that have also been implicated in allergy and hypersensitivity reactions.

T-cell–mediated immune response to *B. dermatitidis* is essential for immunoprotection against this pathogen. Mice immunized with WI-1 develop a robust TH2 response to the antigen. Of note, in a mouse infection model of blastomycosis, infected mice that developed features of a TH2 response died with a chronic, progressive infection, whereas those infected animals that developed a TH1 response restricted the spread of the pathogen and were able to respond to antifungal therapy and recover from the disease. Thus a robust TH2 response may not be helpful in clearing *B. dermatitidis* infection and may even retard its clearance. By releasing large amounts of the 85-kDa fragment of WI-1, the yeast cells of *B. dermatitidis* may be able to out-maneuver both arms of the immune response by evasion of the cellular response and the stimulation of a dominant but ineffective humoral response.

Coccidioides immitis

C. immitis and *C. posadasii* are primary pathogens capable of causing a wide range of disease states (see Chapter 64). These fungi are endemic to the Desert Southwest of the United States, and although they both demonstrate different morphologies in their saprobic and parasite phases, they are distinguished from the other endemic dimorphic fungi by the unique features of the parasitic phase (see Chapter 64, Figure 64-1). Among the various putative virulence factors that may contribute to the pathogenicity of this organism are the resistance of the infective conidia to phagocytic killing, the ability to stimulate an ineffective TH2 immune response (similar to *B. dermatitidis*), the production of urease and extracellular proteinases, and the capacity for molecular mimicry (see Table 58-1).

Resistance of Conidia to Phagocytic Killing

The saprobic phase of *C. immitis* (and *C. posadasii*) consists of septate filamentous hyphae that when mature produce barrel-shaped arthroconidia separated from one another by empty disjunctor cells (see Chapter 57, Figure 57-2B; Chapter 64, Figures 64-1D and 64-7). The arthroconidia are very hydrophobic and easily aerosolized. These conidia are small enough (3 to 5 µm × 2 to 4 µm) that, when inhaled, they can be carried deep into the respiratory tract, frequently to the level of the alveoli. The outer wall of the conidia is composed primarily of protein (50%), including small cysteine-rich polypeptides known as **hydrophobins** because of their distinct hydropathic profiles. The remainder of the wall composition includes lipids (25%), carbohydrates (12%), and an unidentified pigment. It is thought that this hydrophobic outer layer has antiphagocytic properties, because its removal resulted in increased phagocytosis of *C. immitis* arthroconidia by human polymorphonuclear neutrophils (PMNs), compared with their phagocytosis of intact arthroconidia. Of importance, neither the intact conidia nor the conidia with the outer wall layer removed were effectively killed after ingestion by PMNs. It appears that the infectious arthroconidia of *C. immitis* have both active and passive barriers against attack by the host's innate defenses in the lungs.

Stimulation of an Ineffective TH2 Immune Response by *Coccidioides immitis*

It is known that individuals with coccidioidal infections all produce antibody to a predominant glycoprotein (SOWgp) of an outer wall layer of the parasitic cells (spherules). Both arms of the T-helper immune pathway, TH1 and TH2, are stimulated by SOWgp. Activation of the TH1 pathway is known to be associated with spontaneous resolution of coccidioidal infection in mice. Furthermore, it has been shown that mice that are susceptible to infection with *C. immitis* show a TH2 response to infection, whereas resistant strains show more of a TH1 response. Thus, similar to that described for *B. dermatitidis*, TH2 responses to SOWgp may not contribute to clearance of *C. immitis* and may even be detrimental in control of the infection. The more severe forms of coccidioidomycosis are accompanied by depressed cell-mediated immunity and high serum levels of *C. immitis*–specific complement fixing antibody, consistent with a predominantly TH2 response. Although not much is known of the cytokine profile of humans during coccidioidal infections, it is reasonable to speculate that immunodominant antigens of *C. immitis* that elicit a profound increase in IL-10 and IL-4 may direct the immune response to a TH2 pathway. Such immunomodulation may contribute to increased severity of the mycotic infection.

Urease Production

The environmental niche for the saprobic form of *C. immitis* is alkaline desert soil. Both saprobic and parasitic phases of this organism have been shown to release ammonia and ammonium ions when grown in vitro, resulting in an alkalinization of the culture medium. The endospores of *C. immitis* release much more ammonia/ammonium ions than do spherules when grown in any acidic (pH 5.0) conditions. Newly released endospores have been shown to be surrounded by an alkaline halo produced by the ammonia/ammonium ions.

The endospores of *C. immitis* are readily phagocytosed by alveolar macrophages but once ingested are able to survive intracellularly. It has been shown that viable intracellular endospores are surrounded by an alkaline halo at their cell surface, suggesting that the production of ammonia/ammonium ions may contribute to survival of the pathogen within the phagosome of the activated macrophage.

The ability of *C. immitis* to generate an alkaline microenvironment and respond to acidification by increasing the amount of ammonia/ammonium ions released from its parasitic cells are features that may contribute to the pathogenesis of this fungus. Although the details of ammonia generation and how cell-surface alkalinity affects phagocyte function are poorly understood, it has been proposed that the major source of ammonia produced by *C. immitis* is due to urease activity. Urease is a metalloenzyme that is localized in the cytoplasmic fraction of microbial cells; it catalyzes the hydrolysis of urea to yield ammonia and carbamate. The carbamate subsequently hydrolyzes to yield another molecule of ammonia. The maximum amount of urease protein detected in *C. immitis* is in endosporulating spherules, which correlates with the developmental stage, where the highest amounts of ammonia/ammonium ion have been recorded. Taken together, this information suggests that urease activity contributes to the pathogenicity of *C. immitis.*

Extracellular Proteinases

Fungal pathogens produce an array of acid, neutral, and alkaline proteinases that are active over a wide pH range and exhibit broad substrate specificity. It has been suggested that certain extracellular enzymes secreted by fungi may play key roles in invasive growth that may ultimately lead to the death of the infected host. Secreted proteinases may permit the ingress of skin and mucosal barriers, partial neutralization of active host defenses, transmigration of endothelial layers, and subsequent hematogenous dissemination, leading to the establishment of infection in various anatomic sites.

C. immitis, as a primary fungal pathogen, is able to breach the respiratory mucosal barrier, enter the bloodstream and/or the lymphatic system, and disseminate to other organs of the body. Both the saprobic (conidial cell) and parasitic forms of the fungus express several proteinases during cell growth. The conidial cell produces a 36-kDa extracellular proteinase capable of breaking down human collagen, elastin, and hemoglobin, as well as IgG and IgA. Cleavage of secretory immunoglobulins by opportunistic fungal pathogens has been correlated with the ability of these organisms to colonize the host mucosa. A 66-kDa alkaline proteinase capable of digesting structural proteins, found in lung tissue, is thought to be secreted during the entire course of disease caused by *C. immitis.* All patients with coccidioidomycosis produce antibodies directed against this enzyme, and it is thought that this alkaline proteinase may play an important role in host tissue colonization and invasion by spherules and endospores of *C. immitis.*

Molecular Mimicry

When molecules produced by a pathogenic microbe are structurally, antigenically, and functionally similar to host molecules, this characteristic is termed **molecular mimicry.** In some instances, infection may result in the generation of antibodies by the host that cross-react with host tissues and produce an autoimmune-type pathology. Fungi have been shown to produce molecules that are functionally but not necessarily structurally similar to host molecules ("functional mimicry"). Fungal molecules have been identified that function similar to integrins, complement receptors, and sex hormones.

An estrogen-binding protein has been isolated from cytosolic fractions of *C. immitis.* It is known that physiologic concentrations of progesterone and 17-β-estradiol stimulate the rate of *C. immitis* growth and endospore release. This information coincides with the recognition of pregnancy, especially during the third trimester, as a major risk factor for disseminated coccidioidomycosis.

Histoplasma capsulatum

It is well known that most people infected with *H. capsulatum* recover without complications and without specific antifungal therapy (see Chapter 64). Nevertheless, reactivation of pulmonary and extrapulmonary histoplasmosis in immunocompromised patients who originally experienced cryptic dissemination of the fungus is documented throughout the literature. Inhalation of conidia from the environment, coupled with failure to evacuate the fungus by mucociliary mechanisms, provides the opportunity for the inhaled conidia to transform into yeasts, which are ingested by mononuclear phagocytes. *H. capsulatum* is found almost exclusively within host cells, where it may actively replicate or remain dormant.

Histoplasma capsulatum Resides in Host Macrophages

Conversion of inhaled conidia of *H. capsulatum* to yeast cells is critical for survival of the pathogen within the host and occurs within hours of infection. Although theoretically a single conidium may be sufficient to establish an infection, it is usually assumed that a very large conidial inoculum is necessary to establish disseminated disease in a healthy immunocompetent individual. The phagocytes that are mobilized to the site of infection are effective in killing ingested conidia but are less so against the yeast form.

It is known that the organism facilitates uptake by the host phagocytes by producing substances that contribute to the chemotaxis of alveolar macrophages; however, the details of how the pathogen resists the destructive efforts of the macrophages remain unclear. It is suggested that certain phosphoinositol-containing sphingolipids in the yeast cell wall may interfere with the oxidative response of the macrophage to the fungal pathogen. The fact that the macrophages are the primary host cells in which the yeast phase of *H. capsulatum* resides is thought to be an important strategy for survival and dissemination of the pathogen. There are several factors thought to be important in the ability of the fungus to persist within the phagolysosome of the macrophage and add significantly to the pathogenicity of the organism: pH modulation, iron and calcium uptake, and alteration of the yeast cell wall.

Modulation of the pH of the Phagolysosome

The yeast cells of *H. capsulatum* are rapidly ingested by alveolar macrophages. After ingestion, the pH of the phagolysosome containing one or more yeast cells is elevated (6.0 to 6.5) above that which is optimal for many of the lysosomal enzymes. This pH modulation not only interferes with enzyme activity but also influences antigen processing within the cell and contributes to survival of the pathogen in vivo. Although it is tempting to implicate *H. capsulatum* urease in this process, it is not considered to be a major factor, because the pH is only elevated in the phagosome containing the yeast cell. If the fungal urease was involved, the ammonia/ammonium ions produced would be expected to diffuse out of the phagosome and raise the pH in the rest of the host cell as well.

Iron and Calcium Uptake

Iron is an important cofactor of several different metalloenzymes and heme-containing proteins. Microorganisms obtain iron from the environment by producing siderophores that chelate ferric iron and form soluble iron complexes. *H. capsulatum* traps iron by virtue of a hydroxamic siderophore, although the role of this siderophore in survival of the fungus within the macrophage is unknown. The ability of the fungus to modulate the intraphagolysosomal pH between 6.0 and 6.5 is critical to the uptake of iron by yeast cells. A pH greater than 6.5 renders iron inaccessible to *H. capsulatum.*

As with iron, yeast cells within the phagolysosome must have an efficient mechanism for binding and transporting Ca^{2+}. Yeast cells, but not mycelial cells, release large amounts of a calcium-binding protein, CBP1, into the surrounding microenvironment. CBP1 has been suggested to be important in calcium acquisition during intracellular parasitism. The yeast phase–specific expression of CBP1 may provide *H. capsulatum* with another important adaptive mechanism for its survival within the phagolysosome of the macrophage.

Alteration of Yeast Cell Wall Composition

Similar to *B. dermatitidis,* most *H. capsulatum* strains have 1,3-α-glucan in their cell wall. Spontaneous mutants of *H. capsulatum* that have lost the 1,3-α-glucan component have been shown to infect and persist within macrophages without apparent harm to the host cell. In contrast, normal wild-type yeasts with 1,3-α-glucan can infect and survive within macrophages but also can proliferate within the phagolysosome and ultimately kill the phagocyte-releasing yeast cells that go on to infect new macrophages. Thus it appears that distinctive microenvironments found within host cells can influence the selection of variants that have the potential for long-term persistence within the host, as well as those that produce a more rapidly proliferative process.

Paracoccidioides brasiliensis

Infection caused by *P. brasiliensis* is initiated by the inhalation of conidia into the lungs, after which the fungus may disseminate hematogenously or lymphatically to virtually all parts of the body (see Chapter 64). A unique feature of paracoccidioidomycosis compared to the other endemic mycoses is that primary pulmonary infections that subsequently disseminate most often manifest as mucosal lesions of the mouth, nose, and occasionally the gastrointestinal tract.

The yeast cell wall of *P. brasiliensis* is rich in alkali-soluble glucans such as 1,3-α-glucan. As with several other of the endemic dimorphic fungal pathogens, it is thought that the presence of 1,3-α-glucan in the outermost layer of the yeast cell wall is essential for survival of the fungus in vivo. It appears that macrophages are key elements of the innate response to infection by *P. brasiliensis*. Macrophages are able to contain *P. brasiliensis* infection but usually do not eliminate the yeast cells. Despite an early clinical resolution of infection, residual lesions containing viable yeast cells may reactivate up to 40 years later, causing relapse and serious sequelae. Characteristics of *P. brasiliensis* that are considered important in the pathogenesis of infection include response to hormonal factors, expression of 1,3-α-glucan, and immune responses to an immunodominant antigen, gp43.

Hormonal Influences on Infection

Although skin test reactivity to paracoccidioidin is comparable among both males and females living in areas endemic for paracoccidioidomycosis, the male/female ratio of symptomatic disease is 78:1. Subclinical infection appears to occur at the same rate in both genders; however, progression to clinically overt disseminated disease is much more frequent in males. This observation has led to the hypothesis that hormonal factors play a very important role in the pathogenesis of paracoccidioidomycosis.

In contrast to *C. immitis,* where estrogen stimulates fungal growth and endosporulation, the transition from conidia to the yeast form of *P. brasiliensis* is inhibited by estrogen. This results in rapid clearance of the infection in females, whereas the infection is allowed to progress in males. An alternative explanation is that male sex hormones have an immunoinhibitory effect that facilitates establishment of infection. This remains an area of active investigation. Regardless, it appears that the early events of host-fungal interaction after natural infection are hormonally modulated and therefore are significantly different in males and females. These differences could account for the markedly higher susceptibility of males to paracoccidioidomycosis.

Role of Cell Wall Glucans in the Pathogenesis of *Paracoccidioides brasiliensis*

The cell wall of *P. brasiliensis* contains four main polysaccharides: galactomannan, 1,3-α-glucan, 1,3-β-glucan, and chitin. The 1,3-α-glucan component is only expressed in the yeast form of the organism, and its expression correlates with virulence. Mutant strains of *P. brasiliensis* that lack this glucan are avirulent and are much more susceptible to digestion by neutrophils.

The 1,3-β-glucan fraction of the cell wall acts as an important immunomodulator and when exposed on the fungal cell wall, elicits an intense inflammatory response. β-Glucans are unmasked when levels of 1,3-α-glucan are reduced, leading to the hypothesis that the ratio of 1,3-α-glucan to 1,3-β-glucan in the cell wall of *P. brasiliensis* may be more important in pathogenesis than the individual polysaccharide components. It is important to realize that the relationship between the α-/β-glucan ratio in the *P. brasiliensis* cell wall and the type of immune response are similar to those seen in both histoplasmosis and blastomycosis. In each case, a high 1,3-α-glucan content of the yeast cell is related to increased virulence, and absent or decreased levels of this component are related to reduced virulence. Alteration in the cell wall composition of the yeast cells of all three of these dimorphic pathogens is also related to their ability to become sequestered within cells and tissues and to persist as viable elements for years after infection.

Responses to an Immunodominant Antigen, gp43

The yeast phase of *P. brasiliensis* secretes an immunodominant 43-kDa glycoprotein (gp43) that is both an important serodiagnostic antigen and a putative virulence factor. The gp43 antigen is a receptor for laminin-1 and may be responsible for adhesion of the yeast cell to the host basement membrane. This antigen also binds to macrophages and elicits both a strong humoral response and a delayed-type hypersensitivity (DTH) response in humans.

The immunologic defense against infection with *P. brasiliensis* depends on cellular rather than humoral immunity. An impaired DTH response correlates with increased severity of disease. Mice immunized with gp43 develop both a TH1- and TH2-type immune response, whereas gp43 and a second antigen, gp70, are major contributors to a humoral response in humans. It is possible that patient immune reactivity to gp43 and gp70 is dominated by a TH2 pathway with inadequate T-cell response. If patient cell-mediated immunity to *P. brasiliensis* is actually compromised by such T-cell hyporesponsiveness, this could be a mechanism (as seen in histoplasmosis and coccidioidomycosis) underlying the immunopathogenesis of paracoccidioidomycosis.

• Opportunistic Pathogens

The state of the host is of primary importance in determining the pathogenicity of opportunistic fungal pathogens such as *Candida* spp., *C. neoformans,* and *Aspergillus* spp. In most instances, these organisms may exist as benign colonizers or as environmental saprobes and only cause serious infection when there is a breakdown of host defenses. There are factors associated with these organisms, however, that may be considered "virulence factors" in that they contribute to the disease process and in some instances may explain the differences in pathogenicity of the various organisms.

Candida Species

Candida spp. are the most common of the opportunistic fungal pathogens (see Chapter 65). It is now well established that *Candida* spp. colonize the gastrointestinal mucosa and reach the bloodstream through gastrointestinal translocation or via contaminated vascular catheters, interact with host defenses, and exit the intravascular compartment to invade deep tissues of target organs such as the liver, spleen, kidneys, heart, and brain. Characteristics of the organism that are thought to contribute to pathogenicity include the ability to adhere to tissues, the ability to exhibit yeast-hyphal dimorphism, cell-surface hydrophobicity, proteinase secretion, and phenotypic switching (see Table 58-1).

The ability of *Candida* spp. to adhere to a variety of tissues and inanimate surfaces is considered important in the early stages of infection. The adherence capability of the various species of *Candida* is directly related to their virulence ranking in various experimental models. Adherence is achieved by a combination of specific (ligand-receptor interaction) and nonspecific (electrostatic, van der Waals forces) mechanisms.

The ability to undergo the yeast-to-hypha transformation has long been considered to have some importance in pathogenicity. Most species of *Candida* are capable of such transformation, which has been shown to be regulated by both pH and temperature. The yeast-hyphal transformation is one way for *Candida* spp. to respond to changes in the microenvironment. The hyphae of *C. albicans* exhibit **thigmotropism** (a sense of touch), which allows them to grow along grooves and through pores and may aid in infiltration of epithelial surfaces.

The composition of the cell surface of *Candida* spp. may affect both the hydrophobicity of the cell and the immune response to the cell. The type and degree of glycosylation of the mannoproteins on the cell surface may affect the hydrophobicity of the cell and therefore adhesion to epithelial cells. The germ tubes of *C. albicans* are hydrophobic, whereas the buds or blastoconidia are hydrophilic. The various glycoproteins of *C. albicans* also suppress the immune response to the organism by mechanisms that are not well understood.

As discussed with the primary pathogens, the ability of *Candida* spp. to secrete various enzymes may also influence the pathogenicity of the organism. Several species of *Candida* secrete aspartyl proteinases that hydrolyze host proteins involved in defenses against infection, thus allowing the yeasts to breach connective tissue barriers. Likewise, phospholipases are produced by most species of *Candida* causing infection in humans. These enzymes damage host cells and are considered important in tissue invasion.

The ability of *Candida* spp. to rapidly switch from one morphotype to another has been termed **phenotypic switching.** Although originally applied to changes in gross colony morphology, it is now known that the different switch phenotypes observed on solid culture media represent differences in bud and hypha formation, expression of cell wall glycoproteins, proteolytic enzyme secretion, susceptibility to oxidative damage by neutrophils, and antifungal susceptibility and resistance. Phenotypic switching contributes to the virulence of *Candida* spp. by allowing the organism to rapidly adapt to changes in its microenvironment and thereby facilitate its ability to survive, invade tissues, and escape from host defenses.

Cryptococcus neoformans

C. neoformans is an encapsulated yeast that causes human infection throughout the world. Although this organism can infect apparently normal hosts, it causes disease much more frequently and with greater severity in immunocompromised hosts. In considering the pathogenesis of cryptococcosis, it is useful to consider both host defenses and putative virulence factors.

There are three main lines of defense against infection by *C. neoformans*: alveolar macrophages, inflammatory phagocytic cells, and T-cell and B-cell responses. Development of cryptococcosis largely depends on the competence of the host's cellular defenses and the number and virulence of the inhaled yeast cells.

The first line of defense is the alveolar macrophages. These cells are capable of ingesting the yeast cells but are limited in their ability to kill them. Macrophages that contain ingested yeast cells produce various cytokines for the recruitment of neutrophils, monocytes, NK cells, and cells from the bloodstream into the lung. They also act as antigen-presenting cells and induce the differentiation and proliferation of T and B lymphocytes that are specific for *C. neoformans.* The recruited cells are effective in killing *C. neoformans* by intracellular and extracellular mechanisms (both oxidative and nonoxidative).

The antibody response to this organism is nonprotective but serves to opsonize the yeast cells, thus enhancing cell-mediated cytotoxicity. Likewise, the complement system enhances the efficacy of the antibody response and provides opsonins and chemotactic factors for phagocytosis and recruitment of inflammatory cells.

An effective host response to *C. neoformans* is a complex interaction of cellular and humoral immune factors. When these factors are impaired, the infection disseminates, usually by migration of macrophages containing viable yeast cells, from the lung to the lymphatics and the bloodstream to the brain.

The main factors that are inherent in *C. neoformans* and that allow the yeast to evade the host defenses and establish infection include the ability to grow at 37° C, produce a thick polysaccharide capsule, synthesize melanin, and be an alpha-mating phenotype (MATalpha) (see Table 58-1).

The capsule of *C. neoformans* protects the cell from phagocytosis and from cytokines induced by the phagocytic process; it also suppresses both cellular and humoral immunity. The capsule can physically block the opsonic effect of complement and anticryptococcal antibodies, and the negative charge it confers produces an electrostatic repulsion between the yeast cells and the host effector cells. Furthermore, the capsular material interferes with antigen presentation and limits the production of nitric oxide (toxic for cryptococcal cells) by the host cells.

Melanin is produced by the fungus by virtue of a membrane-bound phenoloxidase enzyme and is deposited within the cell wall. It is thought that melanin enhances the integrity of the cell wall and increases the net negative charge of the cell, further protecting it from phagocytosis. Melanization is thought to be responsible for the neurotropism of *C. neoformans* and may protect the cell from oxidative stress, temperature extremes, iron reduction, and microbicidal peptides.

The alpha-mating phenotype is associated with the presence of the gene ***STE12alpha,*** which has been proven to modulate the expression of several other genes whose functions are important for the production of the capsule and melanin.

Aspergillus Species

Aspergillosis is the most common invasive mold infection worldwide. Aspergilli are ubiquitous saprobes in nature and may be found in soil, potted plants, decaying vegetation, pepper, and construction sites. *Aspergillus* spp. can cause disease in humans by airway colonization with subsequent allergic reactions, colonization of preexisting cavities (aspergilloma), or by tissue invasion.

The primary route of infection in aspergillosis is by inhalation of aerosolized conidia (2.5 to 3 μm) that settle in lungs, nasopharynx, or sinuses. In the lungs, alveolar macrophages and neutrophils play a major role in the host defense against *Aspergillus* spp. The macrophages ingest and kill the conidia, whereas the neutrophils adhere to and kill the hyphae that arise upon germination of the conidia. Those hyphal forms that are not killed may invade the pulmonary tissue and vasculature, leading to thrombosis and local tissue necrosis as well as to hematogenous dissemination to other target organs (brain).

Aspergilli secrete various metabolic products, such as gliotoxins, and a variety of enzymes, including elastase, phospholipase, various proteases, and catalase, which may play a role in virulence. Gliotoxin inhibits macrophage phagocytosis, as well as T-cell activation and proliferation; however, it is not known whether clinically significant amounts of gliotoxin are produced in human disease.

Aspergillus fumigatus conidia bind to human fibrinogen as well as to laminin in the alveolar basement membrane. It is thought that this could be an important first step that allows the fungus to establish residence in host tissues. Binding to fibrinogen and laminin could facilitate adherence of conidia, whereas secretion of elastase and acid proteases could assist with host cell invasion by the hyphae.

Invasive aspergillosis is highly associated with neutropenia and impaired neutrophil function. *Aspergillus* conidia are resistant to killing by neutrophils, but germinating conidia and hyphae are readily killed. In chronic granulomatous disease, neutrophils are unable to generate the respiratory burst to kill catalase-producing microorganisms. Aspergilli produce catalase, an enzyme that breaks down hydrogen peroxide. The strong association of aspergillosis with chronic granulomatous disease underscores the importance of neutrophil function in the host defense against aspergillosis and provides indirect evidence for catalase as a virulence factor. The increased risk of aspergillosis in individuals receiving high doses of corticosteroids is generally thought to be due to impairment of macrophage and perhaps T-cell function. In addition, corticosteroids have been shown to enhance the growth of *Aspergillus* spp. in culture. It is not known whether *Aspergillus* spp. have specific steroid-binding proteins analogous to those that have been found on other fungi.

Bibliography

Cole GT: Fungal pathogenesis. In Anaissie EJ, McGinnis MR, Pfaller MA, editors: *Clinical mycology*, New York, 2003, Churchill Livingstone.

Cramer RA Jr, Perfect JR: Recent advances in understanding human opportunistic fungal pathogenesis mechanisms. In Annaisie EJ, McGinnis MR, Pfaller MA, editors: *Clinical mycology*, ed 2, New York, 2009, Churchill Livingstone.

Dignani MC, Solomkin JS, Anaissie EJ: Candida. In Annaisie EJ, McGinnis MR, Pfaller MA, editors: *Clinical mycology*, ed 2, New York, 2009, Churchill Livingstone.

Heitman J, Filler SG, Edwards JE Jr, et al: *Molecular principles of fungal pathogenesis*, Washington, DC, 2006, American Society for Microbiology Press.

Nemecek JC, Wuthrich M, Klein BS: Global control of dimorphism and virulence in fungi, *Science* 312:583–588, 2006.

CHAPTER

59 ROLE OF FUNGI IN DISEASE

A summary of fungi (yeasts and molds) most commonly associated with human disease is presented in this chapter. Mycotic diseases in humans develop as pathogenic processes in one or more organ systems. The affected systems may be as superficial as the outer layers of the skin or as deep as the heart, central nervous system, or abdominal viscera. Although a single fungus may be more commonly associated with infection involving a single organ system (e.g., *Cryptococcus neoformans* and the central nervous system), more often, several different organisms may produce a similar disease syndrome. Because the management of a given infection may differ according to the etiologic agent, to guide subsequent diagnostic and therapeutic efforts, it is useful to develop a differential diagnosis that includes the most likely fungal pathogens.

Because the development of a fungal infection depends on factors that often outweigh the virulence potential of the infecting organism, one must take into account numerous factors such as the immune status of the host, the opportunity for interaction between host and fungus (e.g., Is the fungus **endogenous** to the patient or **exogenous?**), and the potential infectious dose (e.g., in the case of an endemic dimorphic fungus) in determining the possibility of a fungal infection, the significance of the microbiological data (e.g., culture results), and the necessity to treat and with what agent. Fungal infections often occur in very sick patients, and it is not possible to summarize here the incredibly complex interactions that ultimately lead to the establishment of infection and disease in each organ system. Instead, this chapter provides a very broad listing of the various fungi commonly associated with specific clinical manifestations and/or infections at specific body sites (Table 59-1). This information is meant to be used in conjunction with that in Chapter 60, Table 60-1, as an aid in establishing a differential diagnosis and for selection of the most likely clinical specimens that will help establish a specific etiologic diagnosis. Other factors that may be important in determining the relative frequency with which specific fungi cause disease (e.g., age, comorbidities, host immunity, epidemiologic exposures and risk factors) are covered in the individual chapters in this text or in the more comprehensive infectious disease texts cited in this and other chapters.

Table 59-1 Summary of Fungi Associated with Human Disease

System Affected	Pathogens
Upper Respiratory Infections	
Oropharyngeal	*Candida* spp., *Cryptococcus neoformans, Histoplasma capsulatum, Blastomyces dermatitidis, Paracoccidioides brasiliensis, Talaromyces (Penicillium) marneffei, Geotrichum candidum*
Sinusitis	*Aspergillus* spp., Mucormycetes, *Fusarium* spp., dematiaceous molds (e.g., *Alternaria, Bipolaris, Exophiala* spp.)
Laryngeal	*Histoplasma capsulatum, Sporothrix schenckii, Blastomyces dermatitidis*
Esophageal	*Candida* spp.
Ear Infections	
External otitis	*Aspergillus niger, Candida* spp.
Eye Infections	
Endophthalmitis	*Candida* spp., *Aspergillus* spp., *Blastomyces dermatitidis, Coccidioides immitis/posadasii, Fusarium* spp., *Histoplasma capsulatum, Cryptococcus neoformans*
Keratitis	*Candida* spp., *Fusarium* spp., dematiaceous molds, *Scedosporium* spp., *Purpureocillium lilacinum*
Sinoorbital	Mucormycetes, *Aspergillus* spp., dematiaceous molds
Dacryocystitis and canaliculitis	*Candida albicans, Aspergillus niger*

 Table 59-1 **Summary of Fungi Associated with Human Disease—cont'd**

System Affected	Pathogens
Pleuropulmonary and Bronchial Infections	
Bronchitis	*Aspergillus* spp., *Cryptococcus neoformans*
Pneumonia	*Aspergillus* spp., Mucormycetes, *Fusarium* spp., *Scedosporium apiospermum, Trichosporon* spp., dematiaceous molds, *Cryptococcus neoformans/gattii, Histoplasma capsulatum, Blastomyces dermatitidis, Coccidioides immitis/posadasii, Paracoccidioides brasiliensis, Talaromyces (Penicillium) marneffei, Pneumocystis jirovecii, Candida* spp. (rare)
Fungus ball	*Aspergillus* spp., Mucormycetes, *Scedosporium apiospermum, Fusarium* spp., *Candida* spp.
Empyema	*Aspergillus* spp., Mucormycetes, *Scedosporium apiospermum, Fusarium* spp., *Candida* spp., *Coccidioides immitis/posadasii*
Genitourinary Tract Infections	
Vulvovaginal	*Candida* spp., *Saccharomyces cerevisiae*
Cystitis and pyelonephritis	*Candida* spp. (most common), *Cryptococcus neoformans, Aspergillus* spp., *Coccidioides immitis/posadasii, Histoplasma capsulatum, Blastomyces dermatitidis* (rare), *Trichosporon* spp. (rare), *Blastoschizomyces capitatus* (rare), *Rhodotorula* spp. (rare)
Epididymitis and orchitis	*Candida* spp., *Cryptococcus neoformans, Aspergillus* spp., *Coccidioides immitis/posadasii, Histoplasma capsulatum, Blastomyces dermatitidis* (all rare)
Prostatitis	*Candida* spp. (common), *Cryptococcus neoformans* (common), *Blastomyces dermatitidis* (common), *Histoplasma capsulatum, Aspergillus* spp. (rare), *Coccidioides immitis/posadasii* (rare)
Intraabdominal Infections	
Peritonitis	*Candida* spp., *Rhodotorula* spp., *Trichosporon* spp., *Aspergillus* spp. (rare)
Visceral abscesses	*Candida* spp., *Trichosporon* spp., *Blastoschizomyces capitatus*
Cardiovascular Infections	
Endocarditis	*Candida* spp., *Trichosporon* spp., *Rhodotorula* spp., *Aspergillus* spp., other hyaline hyphomycetes (e.g., *Fusarium, Sarocladium [Acremonium]*), dematiaceous molds
Pericarditis	*Candida* spp., *Aspergillus* spp., *Histoplasma capsulatum, Coccidioides immitis/posadasii*
Central Nervous System	
Meningitis	*Candida* spp., *Cryptococcus neoformans/gattii, Aspergillus* spp., Mucormycetes (rare), *Coccidioides immitis/posadasii, Histoplasma capsulatum, Blastomyces dermatitidis* (rare), *Rhodotorula* spp., *Blastoschizomyces capitatus, Talaromyces (Penicillium) marneffei*
Brain abscess	*Candida* spp., *Cryptococcus neoformans/gattii, Aspergillus* spp., Mucormycetes, *Scedosporium apiospermum, Trichosporon* spp., *Trichoderma* spp., dematiaceous molds (especially *Cladophialophora bantiana* and *Bipolaris hawaiiensis*), endemic dimorphic fungi (rare)
Skin and Soft-Tissue Infections	
Superficial and cutaneous	Dermatophytes, *Candida* spp., *Neoscytalidium* spp., *Scopulariopsis* spp., *Aspergillus* spp., *Malassezia* spp., *Purpureocillium lilacinum*
Subcutaneous	Dematiaceous molds, *Fusarium* spp., *Acremonium* spp., *Scedosporium apiospermum, Sporothrix schenckii, Basidiobolus* sp., *Conidiobolus* sp.
Wounds (surgical or traumatic)	*Candida* spp., Mucormycetes, *Aspergillus* spp., *Fusarium* spp., *Trichosporon* spp., *Rhodotorula* spp., *Scedosporium prolificans*
Cutaneous nodules (hematogenous)	*Candida* spp., *Aspergillus* spp., Mucormycetes, *Cryptococcus neoformans, Trichosporon* spp., *Blastomyces dermatitidis, Coccidioides immitis/posadasii, Talaromyces (Penicillium) marneffei, Fusarium* spp., *Acremonium* spp., dematiaceous molds (rare), *Histoplasma capsulatum* var. *duboisii*
Bone and Joint Infections	
Osteomyelitis	*Blastomyces dermatitidis, Coccidioides immitis/posadasii, Candida* spp., *Cryptococcus neoformans, Aspergillus* spp., Mucormycetes, dematiaceous molds (mycetoma), other hyaline hyphomycetes (e.g., *Scedosporium* spp., *Trichosporon*), *Histoplasma capsulatum* var. *duboisii*
Arthritis	*Coccidioides immitis/posadasii, Blastomyces dermatitidis, Cryptococcus neoformans, Candida* spp., *Aspergillus* spp., dematiaceous molds (mycetoma; rare), *Histoplasma capsulatum* (rare), *Paracoccidioides brasiliensis* (rare), *Sporothrix schenckii* (rare)

Continued

Table 59-1 Summary of Fungi Associated with Human Disease—cont'd

System Affected	Pathogens
Other Infections	
Prosthetic joint	*Candida* spp., all others very rare
Hematogenous dissemination	*Candida* spp., *Histoplasma capsulatum, Blastomyces dermatitidis, Coccidioides immitis/posadasii, Cryptococcus neoformans/gattii, Paracoccidioides brasiliensis, Sporothrix schenckii, Aspergillus* spp., *Fusarium* spp., *Trichosporon* spp., *Malassezia* spp., *Blastoschizomyces capitatus, Talaromyces (Penicillium) marneffei,* others (e.g., *Rhodotorula, Acremonium, Saccharomyces* spp. in neutropenic or transplant patients)

Bibliography

Anaisse EJ, McGinnis MR, Pfaller MA: *Clinical mycology*, ed 2, New York, 2009, Churchill Livingstone.

Guarner J, Brandt ME: Histopathologic diagnosis of fungal infection in the 21st century, *Clin Microbiol Rev* 24:247–280, 2011.

Pfaller MA, Diekema DJ: Rare and emerging opportunistic fungal pathogens: concern for resistance beyond *Candida albicans* and *Aspergillus fumigatus*, *J Clin Microbiol* 42:4419–4431, 2004.

Pfaller MA, Diekema DJ: Epidemiology of invasive mycoses in North America, *Crit Rev Microbiol* 36:1–53, 2010.

Versalovic J, et al: *Manual of clinical microbiology*, ed 10, Washington, DC, 2011, American Society for Microbiology Press.

CHAPTER

60 LABORATORY DIAGNOSIS OF FUNGAL DISEASE

The spectrum of mycotic disease ranges from superficial cutaneous and mucosal infections that may be locally irritating to highly invasive processes associated with classic systemic and opportunistic pathogens. Serious infections are being reported with an ever-increasing array of pathogens, including well-known pathogenic fungi such as *Candida, Cryptococcus neoformans, Histoplasma capsulatum,* and *Aspergillus,* as well as lesser known hyaline and dematiaceous molds (see Chapter 57, Tables 57-1 and 57-2). Modern medical mycology has become the study of mycoses caused by a variety of taxonomically diverse fungi.

Opportunistic mycoses pose a significant diagnostic challenge to clinicians and mycologists alike because of the complexity of the patient population at risk and the increasing array of fungi that may infect these individuals. Successful diagnosis and treatment of mycotic infections in the compromised patient is highly dependent on a team approach involving clinicians, medical mycologists, and pathologists.

This chapter provides a general description of the principles of specimen collection and processing necessary for the diagnosis of most fungal infections. An overview of direct microscopy, culture, immunologic, and molecular diagnostic testing is also provided. Specific details of these and other procedures used in the diagnosis of fungal infections may be found in several reference texts listed in the Bibliography.

• Clinical Recognition of Fungal Infections

Prompt diagnosis of invasive mycoses requires a high index of suspicion and an appreciation of specific risk factors that may predispose a patient to such infections. Clinical suspicion, thorough history and physical examination, including a search for cutaneous and mucosal lesions, inspection of all implanted devices (catheters, etc.), a careful ophthalmologic examination, diagnostic imaging studies, and procurement of appropriate specimens for laboratory diagnosis are all essential steps that must be taken to optimize the diagnosis and treatment of fungal infections. Unfortunately, although specific fungi may be associated with "classic" case scenarios, such as onychomycosis and lower extremity skin lesions caused by *Fusarium* in a patient with neutropenia, or sinus infection caused by *Rhizopus* in a diabetic patient with ketoacidosis, clinical signs and symptoms are not specific for fungal infections and are often not helpful in distinguishing between bacterial and fungal infections in a patient at risk for both types of infection. To provide the best treatment and clinical support, it is also important to know not only that the patient is infected with a fungus but what the fungus is. Thus diagnosis of fungal infections depends on three basic laboratory approaches: (1) microbiological, (2) immunologic, and (3) histopathologic (Box 60-1). These approaches may be supplemented by molecular and biochemical methods of organism detection and identification. Use of the newer methods for detection of fungal antigens and nucleic acids offers great promise for rapid diagnosis of fungal infections.

• Conventional Laboratory Diagnosis

Specimen Collection and Processing

As with all types of infectious processes, laboratory diagnosis of fungal infection is directly dependent on proper collection of appropriate clinical material and prompt delivery of the specimens to the clinical laboratory. Selection of specimens for culture and microscopic examination is based not only on information obtained from clinical examination and radiographic studies but also on consideration of the most likely fungal pathogen that may cause a specific type of infection (Table 60-1). Specimens should be collected aseptically or after proper cleaning and decontamination of the site to be sampled. An adequate amount of clinical material must be submitted promptly for culture and microscopy. Unfortunately, many specimens submitted to the laboratory are of poor quality and insufficient amount and are not appropriate to make a diagnosis. Specimens should be submitted whenever possible in a sterile leak-proof container and be accompanied by a relevant clinical history. The laboratory depends on clinical information in making decisions as to the best way to process the specimen to ensure recovery of the etiologic agent. The clinical history is also useful in interpreting the results of culture and other laboratory testing, especially when dealing with specimens from nonsterile sites such as sputum and skin. Furthermore, clinical information alerts laboratory personnel that they may be dealing with a potentially dangerous pathogen such as *Coccidioides immitis/posadasii* or *H. capsulatum.*

Transportation of specimens to the laboratory should be prompt; however, delayed processing of specimens for fungal culture may not be as detrimental as with specimens for bacteriologic, virologic, or parasitologic examination. In general, if processing is delayed, the specimens for fungal

Box 60-1 Laboratory Methods for Diagnosing Fungal Disease

Conventional Microbiological Methods
Direct microscopy (Gram, Giemsa, and calcofluor white stains)
Culture
Identification
Susceptibility testing

Histopathologic Methods
Routine stains (H&E)
Special stains (GMS, PAS, mucicarmine)
Direct immunofluorescence
In situ hybridization

Immunologic Methods
Antibody
Antigen

Molecular Methods
Direct detection (nucleic acid amplification)
Identification
Strain typing

Biochemical Methods
Metabolites
Cell wall components
Enzymes

GMS, Gomori methenamine silver; *H&E,* hematoxylin and eosin; *PAS,* periodic acid–Schiff.

culture may be stored at 4° C for a short time without loss of organism viability.

Similar to specimens for bacteriologic examination, there are some specimens that are better than others for the diagnosis of fungal infections (see Table 60-1). Cultures of blood and other normally sterile body fluids should be done if clinical indications suggest a hematogenous process or involvement of a closed space such as the central nervous system. Skin lesions should be biopsied and material sent for both histopathologic examination and culture. Oral and vaginal mucosal infections are generally best diagnosed by clinical presentation and direct microscopic examination of secretions or mucosal scrapings because cultures often yield growth that represents normal flora or even contaminants. Similarly, diagnosis of gastrointestinal fungal infections is best made by biopsy and histopathologic examination rather than by culture. Twenty-four–hour collections of sputum or urine are not appropriate for mycologic examination because they typically become overgrown with both bacterial and fungal contaminants.

Stains and Direct Microscopic Examination

Direct microscopic examination of tissue sections and clinical specimens is generally considered to be among the most rapid and cost-effective means of diagnosing fungal infections. Microscopic detection of yeasts or hyphal structures in tissue may be accomplished in less than an hour, whereas culture results may not be available for days or even weeks. In certain instances, the fungus may not only be detected but identified by microscopy because it possesses a distinctive morphology. Specifically, detection of characteristic cysts, yeast cells, or spherules can provide an etiologic diagnosis of infections caused by *Pneumocystis jirovecii, H. capsulatum, Blastomyces dermatitidis,* or *C. immitis/posadasii,* respectively. Although the morphologic appearance of *Candida,* a Mucormycete, or *Trichosporon* in tissue may lead to the diagnosis of the type of infection (i.e., candidiasis, mucormycosis, trichosporonosis), the actual species of fungus causing the infection would remain unknown pending culture. Microscopic detection of fungi in tissue serves to guide the laboratory in selecting the most appropriate means to culture the specimen and also is helpful in determining the significance of culture results. The latter is especially true when the organism isolated in culture is a known component of the normal flora or is frequently found in the environment.

Direct microscopy is clearly useful in diagnosing fungal infection; however, both false-negative and false-positive results may occur. Microscopy is less sensitive than culture, and a negative direct examination does not rule out a fungal infection.

A number of different stains and microscopic techniques may be used to detect and characterize fungi directly in clinical material (Table 60-2). The approaches used most often in the clinical mycology laboratory include the fluorescent reagent calcofluor white or staining of smears and touch preparations with either Gram or Giemsa stains. Calcofluor white stains the cell walls of fungi, causing the fungi to fluoresce for easier and faster detection (Figure 60-1). The Gram stain is useful for detection of yeasts, such as species of *Candida* or *Cryptococcus* (Figure 60-2), and filamentous fungi such as *Aspergillus* (Figure 60-3). Fungi are typically gram-positive but may appear speckled or gram-negative (see Figures 60-2 and 60-3). The Giemsa stain is especially useful for detecting the intracellular yeast forms of *H. capsulatum* in peripheral blood smears, bone marrow, or touch preparations of tissue (Figure 60-4).

The respiratory pathogen *P. jirovecii* may be detected in induced sputum or specimens obtained by bronchoscopy. The cysts may be stained with Gomori methenamine silver (GMS) stain (Figure 60-5) or by a fluorescent monoclonal antibody, and the trophic and intracystic forms are stained with the Giemsa stain (Figure 60-6).

Stains such as hematoxylin and eosin (H&E), GMS, and periodic acid–Schiff (PAS) are performed in the cytology and/or histopathology laboratory and used for detection of fungi in cytologic preparations, fine-needle aspirates, tissues, body fluids, and exudates (see Tables 60-1 and 60-2). These stains can detect fungi such as *B. dermatitidis, H. capsulatum, C. immitis/posadasii, Candida* spp., *C. neoformans,* and the hyphae of Mucormycetes (Figure 60-7), *Aspergillus,* and other molds. Fungi may be visualized with the H&E stain, but small numbers of organisms may be missed. The more fungus-specific stains are the GMS and PAS stains. These stains are useful in detecting small numbers of organisms and for clearly defining characteristic features of fungal morphology. Histologic examination of fixed tissue provides the opportunity to determine whether the fungus is invading the tissue or merely present superficially, information that is helpful in distinguishing between infection and colonization. The microscopic morphologic features of several of the more common fungal pathogens are presented in Table 60-3.

 Table 60-1 **Body Sites, Specimen Collection, and Diagnostic Procedures for Selected Fungal Infections**

Infection Site and Infecting Organism	Specimen Options	Collection Methods	Diagnostic Procedure
Blood			
Candida, Cryptococcus neoformans, Histoplasma capsulatum, Fusarium, Aspergillus terreus, Talaromyces marneffei, Trichosporon	Whole blood	Venipuncture (sterile)	Culture, broth, culture, lysis-centrifugation, nucleic acid amplification
	Serum	Venipuncture (sterile)	Antigen (*Candida, Cryptococcus,* and *Histoplasma*), nucleic acid amplification, β-D-glucan
	Urine	Sterile	Antigen *(Histoplasma)*
Bone Marrow			
Histoplasma capsulatum, Talaromyces marneffei	Aspirate	Sterile	Microscopic examination, culture
	Serum	Venipuncture (sterile)	Serology, *(Histoplasma)* antigen, antibody
	Urine	Sterile	Antigen *(Histoplasma)*
Central Nervous System			
Candida, Cryptococcus neoformans/gattii, Aspergillus, Scedosporium, dematiaceous molds, *Mucormycetes, Histoplasma, Coccidioides*	Spinal fluid	Sterile	Microscopic examination, culture, antigen *(Cryptococcus)*
	Biopsy	Sterile, nonsterile to histopathology	Microscopic examination, culture (do not grind tissue)
	Serum	Sterile	Antigen (*Aspergillus, Cryptococcus,* and *Histoplasma*)
Bone and Joint			
Candida, Fusarium, Aspergillus, Histoplasma capsulatum, Coccidioides immitis/posadasii, Blastomyces dermatitidis, Talaromyces marneffei, Sporothrix schenckii	Aspirate	Sterile	Microscopic examination, culture
	Biopsy	Sterile, nonsterile to histopathology	Microscopic examination, culture (do not grind tissue)
	Serum	Venipuncture	Serology, antigen, antibody
Eye			
Fusarium, Candida, Cryptococcus neoformans, Aspergillus, Mucormycetes	Cornea	Scraping or biopsy	Microscopic examination, culture
	Vitreous fluid	Sterile aspirate	Microscopic examination, culture
Urogenital System			
Candida, Cryptococcus neoformans, Trichosporon, Rhodotorula	Urine	Sterile	Microscopic examination, culture
Rarely: *Histoplasma capsulatum, Blastomyces dermatitidis, Coccidioides immitis/posadasii*	Vaginal, urethral, prostatic secretions or discharge	Saline swab	Microscopic examination, wet mount, calcofluor white/KOH, culture
	Serum	Venipuncture	Serology (antibody)
	Biopsy	Sterile, nonsterile to histopathology	Microscopic examination, culture (do not grind tissue)
Respiratory Tract			
Cryptococcus neoformans/gattii, Aspergillus, Fusarium, Mucormycetes, Scedosporium apiospermum, dematiaceous molds, endemic dimorphic fungi, *Pneumocystis jirovecii*	Sputum	Induced, no preservative	Microscopic examination, culture nucleic acid amplification,

Continued

Table 60-1 **Body Sites, Specimen Collection, and Diagnostic Procedures for Selected Fungal Infections—cont'd**

Infection Site and Infecting Organism	Specimen Options	Collection Methods	Diagnostic Procedure
	Lavage	No preservative	Microscopic examination, culture, galactomannan *(Aspergillus)*, β-D-glucan, nucleic acid amplification
	Transbronchial	Aspirate or biopsy	Microscopic examination, culture
	Open lung biopsy	Sterile, nonsterile to histopathology	Microscopic examination, culture (do not grind tissue)
	Serum	Venipuncture	Serology, antigen, antibody, nucleic acid amplification, β-D-glucan
	Urine	Sterile	Antigen *(Histoplasma)*
Skin and Mucous Membranes			
Candida, Cryptococcus neoformans, Trichosporon, Aspergillus, Mucormycetes, Fusarium, dematiaceous molds, endemic dimorphic fungi, *Sporothrix schenckii*	Biopsy	Sterile, nonsterile to histopathology	Microscopic examination, culture (do not grind tissue)
	Mucosal	Saline swab	Microscopic examination, wet mount, calcofluor white/KOH, culture
	Skin scraping	Nonsterile	Calcofluor white/KOH
	Serum	Venipuncture	Serology, antigen, antibody, nucleic acid amplification
	Urine	Sterile	Antigen *(Histoplasma)*
Multiple Systemic Sites			
Candida, Cryptococcus neoformans/gattii, Trichosporon, hyaline molds, dematiaceous molds, endemic dimorphic fungi	Whole blood	Venipuncture (sterile)	Culture, broth, lysis-centrifugation, nucleic acid amplification
	Serum	Venipuncture (sterile)	Serology, antigen, antibody, nucleic acid amplification, β-D-glucan
	Urine	Sterile	Antigen *(Histoplasma)*
	Biopsy	Sterile, nonsterile to histopathology	Microscopic examination, culture (do not grind tissue)

KOH, Potassium hydroxide.

Culture

The most sensitive means of diagnosing a fungal infection is usually considered to be isolation of the fungus in culture. Culture is also necessary in most instances to identify the etiologic agents. Optimal recovery of fungi from clinical material depends on procurement of an adequate clinical specimen and then employing culture methods that will ensure recovery of organisms that are usually present in small amounts and are slow growing. No single culture medium is sufficient to isolate all medically important fungi, and it is generally accepted that at least two types of media, selective and nonselective, be used. The nonselective medium will permit the growth of rapidly growing yeasts and molds, as well as the more slowly growing fastidious fungi. Fungi will grow in most media used for bacteria; however, growth may be slow, and a more enriched medium, such as brain-heart infusion (BHI) agar or SABHI (Sabouraud dextrose and BHI) agar, is recommended. Fastidious dimorphic fungi, such as *H. capsulatum* and *B. dermatitidis,* usually require a blood-containing medium, such as BHI with 5% to 10% sheep blood, for optimal recovery from clinical material. Cycloheximide is often added to this medium to inhibit the more rapidly growing yeasts and molds that may contaminate the specimen. Although cycloheximide does not affect the endemic dimorphic pathogens, it will inhibit the growth of many opportunistic pathogens (e.g., *Candida, Aspergillus*) that might also be the etiologic agent of infection. For this reason, one should always pair cycloheximide-containing media with complementary media without cycloheximide. Specimens that may be contaminated with bacteria should be inoculated onto selective media, such as SABHI or BHI supplemented with antibiotics (penicillin plus streptomycin is often used). Specific fungi may require specialized media. For example, *Malassezia furfur,* an agent that causes superficial skin infections and infections of vascular catheters, requires a medium containing olive oil or another source of long-chain fatty acids for optimal recovery.

Media have been formulated to provide the presumptive identification of yeast based on colonial morphologic features. The addition of certain substrates or chromogens to

Table 60-2 Selected Methods and Stains Commonly Used for Direct Microscopic Detection of Fungal Elements in Clinical Specimens

Method/Stain	Use	Comments
Calcofluor white stain	Detection of all fungi, including *Pneumocystis jirovecii*	Rapid (1-2 min); detects fungal cell wall chitin by bright fluorescence. Used in combination with potassium hydroxide. Requires fluorescent microscope with proper filters. Background fluorescence may make examination of some specimens difficult.
Fluorescent monoclonal antibody treatment	Examination of respiratory specimen for *Pneumocystis jirovecii*	Sensitive and specific method for detecting the cysts of *Pneumocystis jirovecii*. Does not stain the extracystic (trophic) forms.
Giemsa stain	Examination of bone marrow, peripheral blood smears, touch preparations of tissue, and respiratory specimens	Detects intracellular *Histoplasma capsulatum* and both intracystic and trophic forms of *Pneumocystis jirovecii*. Does not stain the cyst wall of *Pneumocystis*. Does stain organisms other than *Histoplasma* and *Pneumocystis*.
Gram stain	Detection of bacteria and fungi	Commonly performed on clinical specimens. Will stain most yeasts and hyphal elements. Most fungi stain gram-positive, but some, such as *Cryptococcus neoformans*, exhibit stippling or appear gram-negative.
Hematoxylin and eosin (H&E) stain	General purpose histologic stain	Best stain to demonstrate host reaction in infected tissue. Stains most fungi, but small numbers of organisms may be difficult to differentiate from background. Useful in demonstrating natural pigment in dematiaceous fungi.
Gomori methenamine silver (GMS) stain	Detection of fungi in histologic sections and *Pneumocystis jirovecii* cysts in respiratory specimens	Best stain for detecting all fungi. Stains hyphae and yeast forms black against a green background. Usually performed in histopathology laboratory.
Mucicarmine stain	Histopathologic stain for mucin	Useful for demonstrating capsular material of *Cryptococcus neoformans*. May also stain the cell walls of *Blastomyces dermatitidis* and *Rhinosporidium seeberi*.
Periodic acid–Schiff (PAS) stain	Histologic stain for fungi	Stains both yeasts and hyphae in tissue. PAS-positive artifacts may resemble yeast cells.

Modified from Pfaller MA, McGinnis MR: The laboratory and clinical mycology. In Anaissie EJ, McGinnis MR, Pfaller MA, editors: *Clinical mycology,* ed 2, New York, 2009, Churchill Livingstone.

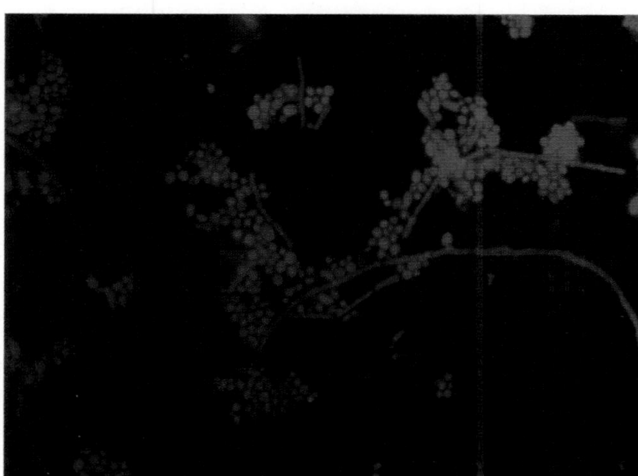

FIGURE 60-1 Calcofluor white stain demonstrating budding yeasts and pseudohyphae of *Candida albicans.*

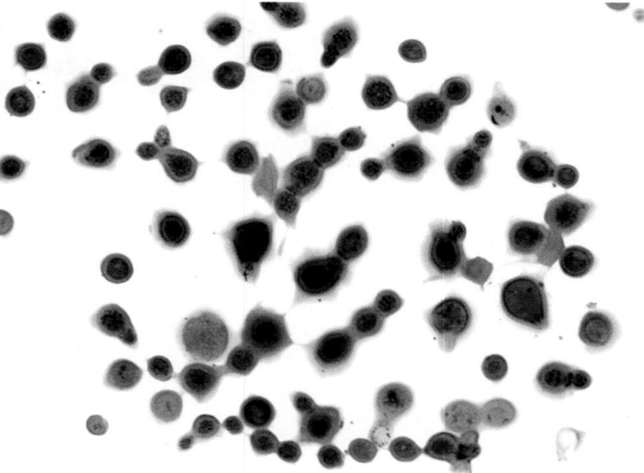

FIGURE 60-2 Gram stain of *Cryptococcus neoformans.* Variable-sized, encapsulated, budding yeasts showing a stippled pattern resulting from uneven retention of crystal violet stain.

the agar medium allows direct detection of specific enzymatic activities characteristic of selected species of yeast. CHROMagar Candida is one such medium that can be used for simultaneous isolation and presumptive identification of *Candida albicans, Candida tropicalis,* and *Candida krusei.* CHROMagar is selective for fungi, and use of this medium shortens the time to presumptive identification of the organisms and allows easier detection of multiple yeast species present in a specimen based on characteristic colors of colonies produced by different species of *Candida* (see Figure 65-5). CHROMagar may be coupled with the rapid trehalose test (RAT) for identification of *Candida glabrata* and has been shown to be useful in the rapid identification and determination of fluconazole susceptibility of *Candida* species

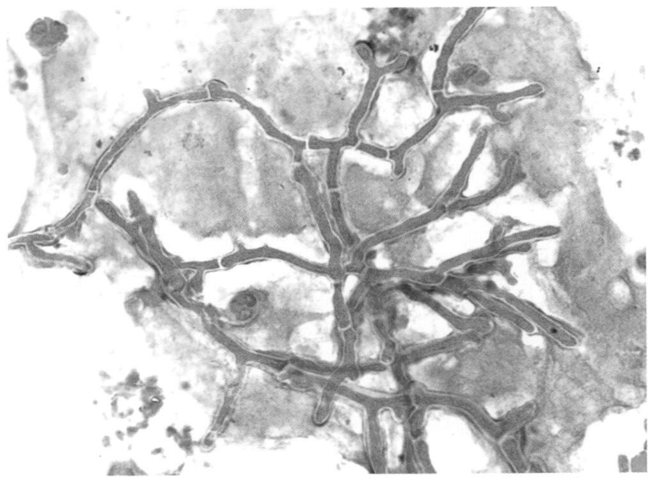

FIGURE 60-3 Gram stain of *Aspergillus.* This specimen did not retain the crystal violet stain and appears gram-negative.

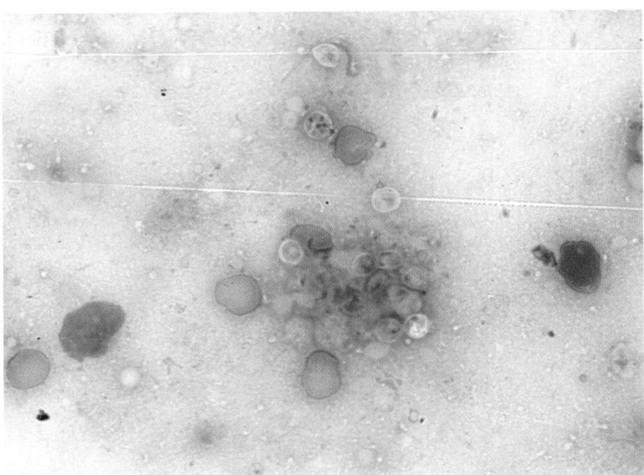

FIGURE 60-6 Giemsa stain showing intracystic and trophic forms of *Pneumocystis jirovecii.*

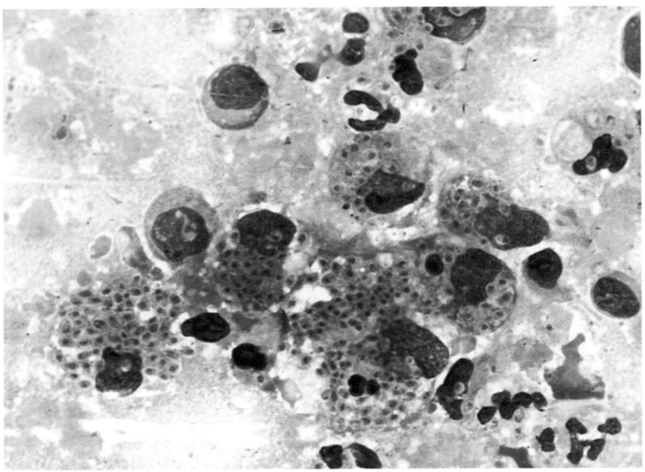

FIGURE 60-4 Giemsa stain showing intracellular yeast forms of *Histoplasma capsulatum.*

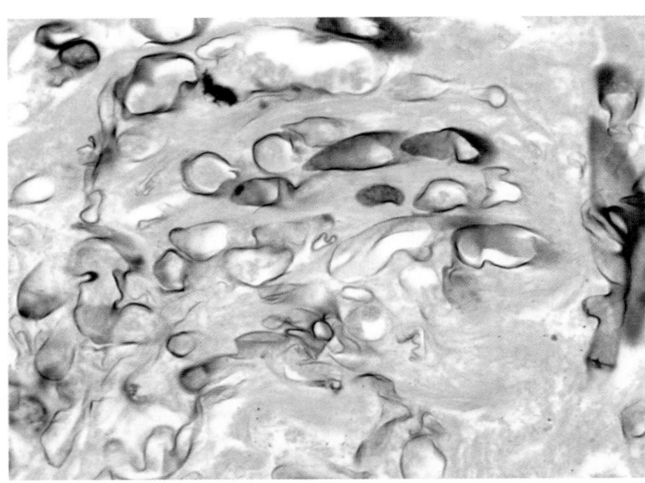

FIGURE 60-7 Silver stain of *Rhizopus.*

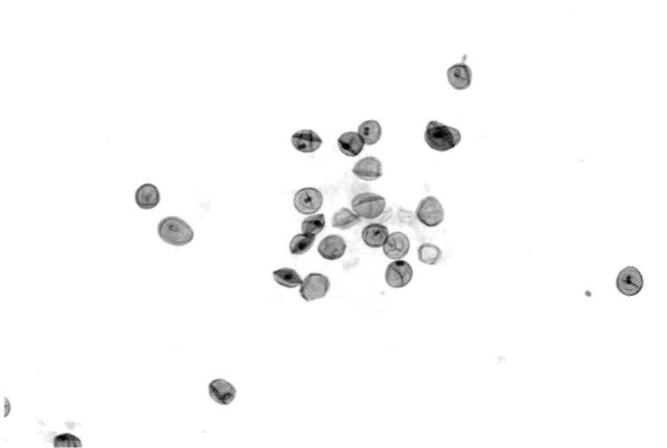

FIGURE 60-5 Silver stain of *Pneumocystis jirovecii* cysts.

directly from positive blood cultures. Other chromogenic media and a rapid colorimetric test based on the detection of L-proline aminopeptidase and beta-galactose-aminidase have been developed specifically for the rapid identification of *C. albicans.*

Detection of fungemia is an important measure in diagnosing invasive fungal infection. Although contamination of blood cultures with a fungus may take place, for the most part, blood cultures positive for fungi are significant. Unfortunately, blood cultures are often negative despite the presence of disseminated disease, especially when the infecting organism is a mold. Detection of fungemia has improved with the development of continuous-monitoring blood culture instruments and improved media formulations that take into account the growth requirements of fungi as well as bacteria. In addition to these broth-based systems, the agar-based lysis-centrifugation method provides a flexible and sensitive method for detection of fungemia caused by yeasts, molds, and dimorphic pathogens (see Table 60-1).

Table 60-3 Characteristic Features of Selected Opportunistic and Pathogenic Fungi in Clinical Specimens and Cultures

Fungus	Microscopic Morphologic Features in Clinical Specimens	Characteristic Morphologic Features in Culture		Additional Tests for Identification
		Macroscopic	Microscopic	
Candida	Oval budding yeasts 2-6 µm in diameter; hyphae and pseudohyphae may be present	Variable morphology; colonies usually pasty, white to tan and opaque; may have smooth or wrinkled morphology	Clusters of blastoconidia, pseudohyphae, and/or terminal chlamydospores in some species	Germ tube production by *C. albicans, C. dubliniensis,* and *C. stellatoidea* PNA-FISH, MALDI-TOF MS, gene sequencing Carbohydrate assimilation; morphology on corn meal agar, CHROMagar, rapid trehalose test
Cryptococcus neoformans	Spherical budding yeasts of variable size, 2-15 µm; capsule may be present; no hyphae or pseudohyphae	Colonies are shiny, mucoid, dome shaped, and cream to tan in color	Budding spherical cells of varying size; capsule present; no pseudohyphae; cells may have multiple narrow-based buds	Tests for urease (+), phenoloxidase (+), and nitrate reductase (–); latex agglutination or EIA test for polysaccharide antigen; mucicarmine and melanin stains in tissue
Aspergillus	Septate dichotomously branched hyphae of uniform width (3-6 µm)	Varies with species; *A. fumigatus:* blue-green to gray, *A. flavus:* yellow-green, *A. niger:* black	Varies with species; conidiophores with enlarged vesicles covered with flask-shaped metulae or phialides; hyphae are hyaline and septate	Identification based on microscopic and colonial morphology Gene sequencing
Mucormycetes	Broad, thin-walled, pauciseptate hyphae, 6-25 µm with nonparallel sides and random branches; hyphae stain poorly with GMS stain and often stain well with H&E stain	Colonies are rapid growing, wooly, and gray-brown to gray-black in color	Broad, ribbon-like hyphae with rare septa; sporangium or sporangiola produced from sporangiophore; rhizoids present in some species	Identification based on microscopic morphologic features Gene sequencing
Dematiaceous molds (see Chapter 57, Table 57-5)	Pigmented (brown, tan, or black) hyphae, 2-6 µm wide; may be branched or unbranched; often constricted at point of septation	Colonies are usually rapidly growing, wooly, and gray, olive, black, or brown in color	Varies depending on genus and species; hyphae are pigmented; conidia may be single or in chains, smooth or rough, and dematiaceous	Identification based on microscopic and colonial morphology Gene sequencing
Histoplasma capsulatum	Small (2-4 µm) budding yeasts within macrophages	Colonies are slow growing and white or buff-brown in color (25° C); yeast phase colonies (37° C) are smooth, white, and pasty	Thin septate hyphae that produce tuberculate macroconidia and smooth-walled microconidia (25° C); small, oval, budding yeasts produced at 37° C	Demonstration of temperature-regulated dimorphism by conversion from mold to yeast phase at 37° C; exoantigen and nucleic acid probe tests allow identification without phase conversion
Blastomyces dermatitidis	Large (8-15 µm), thick-walled, broad-based budding yeast	Colonies vary from membranous, yeastlike colonies to cottony, white, moldlike colonies at 25° C; when grown at 37° C, yeast phase colonies are wrinkled, folded, and glabrous	Hyaline septate hyphae with one-celled smooth conidia (25° C); large, thick-walled, budding yeast at 37° C	Demonstration of temperature-regulated dimorphism; exoantigen and nucleic acid probe tests
Coccidioides immitis/ posadasii	Spherical thick-walled spherules, 20-200 µm; mature spherules contain small 2-5 µm endospores	Colonies initially appear moist and glabrous, rapidly becoming downy and gray-white with a tan or brown reverse	Hyaline hyphae with rectangular arthroconidia separated by empty disjunctor cells	Exoantigen and nucleic acid probe tests
Sporothrix schenckii	Yeastlike cells of varying sizes; some may appear elongated or cigar shaped; tissue reaction forms asteroid bodies	Colonies initially smooth, moist, and yeastlike, becoming velvety as aerial hyphae develop (25° C); tan to brown pasty colonies at 37° C	Thin, branching, septate hyphae; conidia borne in rosette-shaped clusters at the end of the conidiophore (25° C); variable-sized budding yeasts produced at 37° C	Demonstration of thermal dimorphism; exoantigen and nucleic acid probe

Continued

Table 60-3 **Characteristic Features of Selected Opportunistic and Pathogenic Fungi in Clinical Specimens and Cultures—cont'd**

Fungus	Microscopic Morphologic Features in Clinical Specimens	Characteristic Morphologic Features in Culture		Additional Tests for Identification
		Macroscopic	Microscopic	
Talaromyces marneffei	Oval intracellular yeast cells with septum	Colonies produce diffusible red pigment at 25° C	Septate hyphae with metulae, phialides with chains of conidia in a "paint brush" distribution (25° C); yeast cells divide by fission (37° C)	Demonstration of thermal dimorphism
Pneumocystis jirovecii	Cysts are round, collapsed, or crescent shaped; trophic forms seen on special stains	(Not applicable)	(Not applicable)	Immunofluorescent stain, GMS, Giemsa, toluidine blue stains (see Table 60-2)

EIA, Enzyme immunoassay; *GMS,* Gomori methenamine silver; *H&E,* hematoxylin and eosin; *PNA-FISH,* peptide nucleic acid–fluorescent in situ hybridization; *MALDI-TOF MS,* matrix-assisted laser desorption–time of flight mass spectrometry.

Once inoculated, fungal cultures should be incubated in air at a proper temperature and for a sufficient period of time to ensure recovery of fungi from clinical specimens. Most fungi grow optimally at 25° C to 30° C, although most species of *Candida* can be recovered from blood cultures incubated at 35° C to 37° C. Culture dishes should be sealed with gas-permeable tape to prevent dehydration. Specimens submitted for fungal culture are generally incubated for 2 weeks; however, most blood cultures become positive within 5 to 7 days. Determination of the clinical significance of a fungal isolate must be made in consultation with the responsible clinician in the context of the clinical setting of the patient.

Identifying Characteristics of Various Fungi

Determination of the identity of the specific etiologic agent of mycotic disease may have a direct bearing on prognosis and therapeutic considerations. It is becoming clear that a single therapeutic approach (e.g., using amphotericin B) is inadequate for many fungal infections (see Chapter 61). Identification of fungal pathogens may have additional diagnostic and epidemiologic implications. Knowing the genus and species of the infecting agent can also provide access to fungal registries and to the literature where the experiences of others may serve as a guide to the clinical course of infection and response to therapy, especially for the more unusual opportunistic mycoses.

Distinguishing yeastlike fungi from molds is the first step in identifying a fungal isolate. Gross colony morphology usually provides a good clue: yeastlike fungi form pasty, opaque colonies, and molds form large, filamentous colonies that vary in texture, color, and topography. Microscopic examination provides further delineation and often is all that is required for identification of many fungi (see Table 60-3). Identification to genus and species, depending on the fungus, requires more detailed microscopic study to delineate characteristic structures. Yeast identification usually requires additional biochemical and physiologic testing, whereas identification of both yeasts and molds may be enhanced by specialized immunologic, molecular, and proteomic characterization (see Table 60-3).

Among the newer rapid methods for identification of *Candida* and other yeasts are the techniques of peptide nucleic acid (PNA)–fluorescence in situ hybridization (FISH) and matrix-assisted laser desorption/ionization time-of-flight (MALDI-TOF) mass spectrometry (MS). The PNA FISH tests (AdvanDx, Woburn, MA) are based on a fluorescein-labeled PNA probe that specifically detects *C. albicans, C. tropicalis,* or *C. glabrata* as individual species or detects a yeast species group (e.g., *C. albicans* and *C. parapsilosis* fluoresce green and *C. glabrata* and *C. krusei* fluoresce red with the Yeast Traffic Light PNA FISH kit) in blood cultures by targeting species-specific rRNA sequences. The probes are added to smears made directly from the contents of the blood culture bottle and are hybridized for 90 minutes. Recent modifications to the probes and reagents have resulted in a second-generation test (*Quick*FISH) that shortens the assay time to 30 minutes. Smears are subsequently examined by fluorescence microscopy. The test has been shown to have excellent sensitivity (99%), specificity (100%), positive predictive value (100%), and negative predictive value (99.3%). This approach may provide a time savings of 24 to 48 hours, compared with conventional laboratory methods used for identification. It allows physicians to be notified of the yeast's identity along with positive blood culture results. Rapid, accurate identification of *C. albicans, C. tropicalis, C. parapsilosis, C. glabrata,* and *C. krusei* should promote optimal antifungal therapy with the most cost-effective agents, resulting in improved outcomes and significant antifungal savings for hospitals.

MALDI-TOF MS uses species-specific patterns of peptides and protein masses to identify microorganisms. It has been shown to be highly accurate in identifying a broad array of bacteria and recently has been shown to provide a rapid and reliable tool for identification of yeasts, yeastlike fungi, and molds. The technique involves extraction of proteins from the fungal cells, spotting of the specimen on a grid, and overlaying the spot with a matrix. The spectrum is generated rapidly (≈10 minutes per specimen) and is compared to a reference database. In several studies, the method has been shown to be highly accurate and to provide a combination of the lowest expenditure of consumables, easy interpretation of results, and a fast turnaround time. Limitations to date include a lack of robust databases for the less common yeasts and relatively poor performance in identifying molds aside from *Aspergillus* species.

Identification of yeastlike fungi to the species level often requires determination of the biochemical and physiologic profile of the organism in addition to assessment of the microscopic morphology (see Table 60-3). Although nucleic acid sequencing and proteomic methods are rapidly becoming the standard methods for identification of molds, the classical method for identification of a mold is based almost entirely on its microscopic morphology. The important features include the shape, method of production, and arrangement of conidia or spores and the size and appearance of the hyphae. Preparation of material for microscopic examination must be done in such a way that it produces minimal disruption of the arrangement of the reproductive structures and their conidia or spores. Determination of the presence of melanin and thermal-regulated dimorphism are also important features. Immunologic and/or nucleic acid probe–based tests are often used to identify the endemic dimorphic pathogens, and nucleic acid sequencing is being applied as an aid in the identification of a variety of molds. The characteristic features of several of the commonly isolated filamentous and dimorphic pathogens are listed in Table 60-3.

Amplification-based molecular approaches are being developed to provide more rapid and objective identification of both yeasts and molds, compared with traditional phenotypic methods. Ribosomal targets and internal transcribed spacer (ITS) regions have shown particular promise for molecular identification of some fungi. Several recent studies have confirmed the tremendous potential of these approaches as powerful tools in the identification of clinically important yeasts and molds; however, the existing sequence databases are limited with regard to both the quality and accuracy of their entries. Presently, with the availability of improved sequencing techniques, broader and more reliable databases, and more readily available kits and software, this technology has become a competitive alternative to the classic mycologic identification techniques used for clinically important fungi.

• Immunologic, Molecular, and Biochemical Markers for Direct Detection of Invasive Fungal Infections

Rapid, sensitive, and specific diagnostic tests for serious fungal infections would allow more timely and focused application of specific therapeutic measures. As such, tests for the detection of antibodies and antigens, metabolites, and fungus-specific nucleic acids have great appeal. Considerable progress has been made in several of these areas in recent years (Table 60-4), although with few exceptions, such testing still remains confined to reference laboratories or the research setting.

Determination of antibody (Ab) and/or antigen (Ag) titers in serum may be useful in diagnosing fungal infections. When performed in a serial fashion, Ab/Ag titers also provide a means of monitoring the progression of disease and the patient's response to therapy. With the exception of antibody tests for histoplasmosis and coccidioidomycosis, however, most tests for antibodies lack both sensitivity and specificity for diagnosis of invasive fungal infections.

Detection of fungal cell wall and cytoplasmic antigens and metabolites in serum or other body fluids represents the most direct means of providing a serologic diagnosis of invasive fungal infection (see Table 60-4). The best examples of this approach are the commercially available tests for detection of the polysaccharide antigens of *C. neoformans* and *H. capsulatum*. These tests have proven to be of great value in the rapid diagnosis of cryptococcal meningitis and disseminated histoplasmosis, respectively. Immunoassays for detection of *Aspergillus* galactomannan and *Candida* mannan and antimannan are now commercially available.

Another fungal-specific cell wall component is 1,3-β-glucan. This material may be detected in the serum of patients infected with *Candida, Aspergillus,* and *P. jirovecii* through its interaction in the limulus lysate assay. Studies of this test for β-glucan, which indicates the presence of fungi but does not identify the genus causing the infection, have been promising in certain highly selective patient populations.

Detection of fungal metabolites has potential for the rapid diagnosis of both candidiasis and aspergillosis (see Table 60-4). Detection of D-arabinitol in serum appears to be an indication of hematogenously disseminated candidiasis, whereas detection of elevated levels of D-mannitol in bronchoalveolar lavage fluid may be useful in the diagnosis of pulmonary aspergillosis. Because of the lack of a commercially available test and problems with method-dependent variability in sensitivity and specificity, the diagnostic utility of metabolite detection remains uncertain.

Application of the polymerase chain reaction (PCR) to directly detect fungal-specific nucleic acids in clinical material offers great promise for the rapid diagnosis of fungal infections. A variety of target sequences have been investigated and found to be of potential diagnostic value for most of the more common opportunistic and systemic fungal pathogens (see Table 60-4). Recent developments, such as real-time gene chip technology and the coupling of nanotechnology with magnetic resonance detection, will facilitate the broad use of this technology, although it is not yet available in most mycology laboratories. A recent meta-analysis of PCR in the diagnosis of invasive candidiasis found that the use of whole blood as the test sample, multilocus panfungal targets (e.g., rRNA, P450 gene targets), and an in vitro detection limit no higher than 10 colony-forming units (CFU)/ml provided optimal sensitivity and specificity. Recent advances in technology promise to decrease the limit of detection of *Candida* in whole blood to as low as 1 CFU/ml.

In addition to detection of fungi in clinical material, immunologic, molecular, and proteomic methods have also proven useful in the identification of fungi in culture. Nucleic acid probes are useful in identifying the endemic dimorphic pathogens, and analysis of ribosomal deoxyribonucleic acid sequences is being applied to both common and uncommon opportunistic yeasts and molds. With the expansion of fungal databases, MALDI-TOF MS is rapidly becoming established as a rapid, accurate, and cost-effective approach to the identification of yeasts and molds from culture. Exoantigen immunodiffusion tests are widely applied to identify *H. capsulatum, B. dermatitidis,* and *C. immitis/posadasii,* obviating the need to demonstrate thermal dimorphism in the identification of these agents (see Table 60-3).

 Table 60-4 **Antigenic, Biochemical, and Molecular Markers for Direct Detection of Invasive Fungal Infections**

Organism	Cell Wall or Capsule Components	Cytoplasmic Antigens	Metabolites	Genomic DNA Sequences*
Candida	Mannans LA RIA EIA 1,3-β-glucans Limulus test Chitin Spectrophotometry	Enolase EIA Immunoblot Antienolase antibody EIA 47-kDa breakdown product of HSP-90 Enzyme-linked dot Immunobinding assay	D-Arabinitol Rapid enzymatic ClC/FID Mass spectroscopy/GLC	Actin Chitin synthase P450 ITS Ribosomal RNA genes
Cryptococcus neoformans	Capsular polysaccharide LA EIA		D-Mannitol Mass spectroscopy/GLC	Ribosomal RNA genes ITS *URA5* gene
Aspergillus	Galactomannan LA EIA RIA 1,3-β-glucans Limulus test Chitin Spectrophotometry		D-Mannitol GLC/FID Mass spectroscopy/GLC	P450 Ribosomal RNA genes ITS Alkaline protease Mitochondrial
Blastomyces dermatitidis	Cell wall RIA for 120-kDa cell wall adhesion protein EIA for galactomannan			Ribosomal RNA genes ITS
Histoplasma capsulatum	Cell wall RIA and EIA for polysaccharide antigen			Ribosomal RNA genes ITS
Talaromyces marneffei	Cell wall mannoprotein EIA			ITS
Coccidioides immitis	Cell wall galactomannan EIA			Ribosomal RNA genes

Modified from Mujeeb I, et al: Fungi and fungal infections. In McClatchey KD, editor: *Clinical laboratory medicine,* ed 2, Philadelphia, 2002, Lippincott Williams & Wilkins.

DNA, Deoxyribonucleic acid; *EIA,* enzyme immunoassay; *FID,* flame ionization detector; *GLC,* gas-liquid chromatography; *HSP-90,* heat shock protein-90; *ITS,* internal transcribed spacer region; *LA,* latex agglutination; *P450,* lanosterol 14-alpha-demethylase gene; *RIA,* radioimmunoassay; *RNA,* ribonucleic acid.

*All sequences detected by polymerase chain reaction.

Bibliography

Alexander BD, Pfaller MA: Contemporary tools for the diagnosis and management of invasive mycoses, *Clin Infect Dis* 43(Suppl 1):S15–S27, 2006.

Avni T, Leibovici L, Paul M: PCR diagnosis of invasive candidiasis: systematic review and meta-analysis, *J Clin Microbiol* 49:665–670, 2011.

Borman AM, Johnson EM: Genomics and proteomics as compared to conventional phenotypic approaches for the identification of the agents of invasive fungal infections, *Curr Fungal Infect Rep* 7:235–243, 2013.

Guarner J, Brandt ME: Histopathologic diagnosis of fungal infections in the 21st century, *Clin Microbiol Rev* 24:247–280, 2011.

Karageorgopoulos DE, Vouloumanou EK, Ntziora F, et al: β-D-glucan assay for the diagnosis of invasive fungal infections: a meta-analysis, *Clin Infect Dis* 52:750–770, 2011.

Neely LA, Audeh M, Phung NA, et al: T2 magnetic resonance enables nanoparticle-mediated rapid detection of candidemia in whole blood, *Sci Transl Med* 5:182ra54, 2013.

Pfaller MA, McGinnis MR: The laboratory and clinical mycology. In Anaissie EJ, McGinnis MR, Pfaller MA, editors: *Clinical mycology*, ed 2, New York, 2009, Churchill Livingstone.

CHAPTER

61 ANTIFUNGAL AGENTS

Antifungal therapy has undergone a tremendous transformation in recent years. Once the sole domain of the agents amphotericin B and 5-fluorocytosine, which were toxic and difficult to use, the treatment of mycotic disease has now been advanced by the availability of several new systemically active agents and new formulations of other older agents that provide comparable if not superior efficacy with significantly less toxicity.

In this chapter, we will review the antifungal agents, both systemic and topical (Table 61-1). We will discuss their spectrum, potency, mode of action, and clinical indications for use as therapeutic agents. We will also discuss the mechanisms of resistance to the various classes of antifungal agents and the in vitro methods for determining the susceptibility and resistance of fungi to the available agents.

The terminology appropriate for this discussion is summarized in Box 61-1, and the sites and modes of action of antifungals are seen in Figure 61-1.

• Systemically Active Antifungal Agents

Amphotericin B and its lipid formulations are polyene macrolide antifungals used in the treatment of serious life-threatening mycoses (see Table 61-1). Another polyene, nystatin, is a topical agent. A lipid formulation of nystatin has been developed for systemic use but remains investigational.

The basic structure of polyenes consists of a large lactone ring, a rigid lipophilic chain containing three to seven double bonds, and a flexible hydrophilic portion bearing several hydroxyl groups (Figure 61-2). Amphotericin B contains seven conjugated double bonds and may be inactivated by heat, light, and extremes of pH. It is poorly soluble in water and is not absorbed by the oral or intramuscular route of administration. The conventional formulation of amphotericin B for intravenous (IV) administration is amphotericin B deoxycholate. The lipid formulations of amphotericin B were developed in an effort to circumvent the nephrotoxic nature of conventional amphotericin B and in many instances have replaced the deoxycholate form.

Amphotericin B (and its lipid formulations) exerts its antifungal action by at least two different mechanisms. The primary mechanism involves the binding of amphotericin B to ergosterol, the principal membrane sterol of fungi. This binding produces ion channels that destroy the osmotic integrity of the fungal cell membrane and lead to leakage of intracellular constituents and cell death (Figure 61-3). Amphotericin B also binds to cholesterol, the main membrane sterol of mammalian cells, but does so less avidly than to ergosterol. The binding of amphotericin B to cholesterol accounts for most of the toxicity observed when amphotericin B is administered to humans. An additional mechanism of action of amphotericin B involves direct membrane damage resulting from the generation of a cascade of oxidative reactions triggered by the oxidation of amphotericin B itself. This process may be a major contributor to the rapid fungicidal activity of amphotericin B via the generation of toxic free radicals.

The spectrum of activity of amphotericin B is broad and includes most strains of *Candida, Cryptococcus neoformans, Aspergillus* spp., the Mucormycetes, and the endemic dimorphic pathogens *(Blastomyces dermatitidis, Coccidioides immitis, Histoplasma capsulatum, Paracoccidioides brasiliensis,* and *Talaromyces marneffei)* (Table 61-2). *Aspergillus terreus, Fusarium* spp., *Pseudallescheria boydii, Scedosporium prolificans, Trichosporon* spp., and certain dematiaceous fungi may be resistant to amphotericin B. Likewise, reduced susceptibility to amphotericin B has been noted among some strains of *Candida guilliermondii, Candida glabrata, Candida krusei, Candida lusitaniae,* and *Candida rugosa.* Resistance to amphotericin B has been associated with alterations in membrane sterols, usually a reduction in ergosterol.

Amphotericin B is widely distributed in various tissues and organs, including liver, spleen, kidney, bone marrow, and lung. Although negligible concentrations of amphotericin B can be found in cerebrospinal fluid, it is generally effective in treating fungal infections of the central nervous system. Amphotericin B is considered to be fungicidal against most fungi.

The primary clinical indications for amphotericin B include invasive candidiasis, cryptococcosis, aspergillosis, mucormycosis, blastomycosis, coccidioidomycosis, histoplasmosis, paracoccidioidomycosis, penicilliosis (talaromycosis) marneffei, and sporotrichosis. The lipid formulations of amphotericin B offer an improved efficacy-to-toxicity profile and are primarily recommended for the treatment of documented fungal infections in individuals failing conventional amphotericin B or with impaired renal function.

The main adverse effects of amphotericin B include nephrotoxicity and infusion-related side effects such as fever, chills, myalgias, hypotension, and bronchospasm. The major advantage of the lipid formulations of amphotericin B are the significantly reduced side effects, especially nephrotoxicity. Lipid formulations are not superior to conventional

Table 61-1 Systemic and Topical Antifungal Agents in Use and in Development

Antifungal Agents	Route	Mechanism of Action	Comments
Allylamines			
Naftifine Terbinafine	Topical Oral, topical	Inhibition of squalene epoxidase	Terbinafine has very broad spectrum and acts synergistically with other antifungals
Antimetabolite			
Flucytosine	Oral	Inhibition of DNA and RNA synthesis	Used in combination with amphotericin B and fluconazole; toxicity and secondary resistance are problems
Imidazoles			
Ketoconazole, bifonazole, clotrimazole, econazole, miconazole, oxiconazole, sulconazole, terconazole, tioconazole	Oral, topical	Inhibits lanosterol 14-α-demethylase cytochrome P450-dependent enzymes	Ketoconazole has modest broad-spectrum activity and toxicity problems
Triazoles			
Fluconazole	Oral, IV	Same as imidazoles but more specific binding to target	Limited spectrum (yeasts); good central nervous system penetration; good in vivo activity; primary and secondary resistance seen with *Candida krusei* and *Candida glabrata,* respectively
Itraconazole	Oral	Same as imidazoles but more specific binding to target enzyme	Broad-spectrum activity; erratic absorption; toxicity and drug interactions are problems
Voriconazole	Oral, IV	Same as imidazoles but more specific binding to target enzyme	Broad spectrum, including yeasts and molds; active vs. *Candida krusei;* many drug interactions
Posaconazole	Oral, IV	Same as imidazoles but more specific binding to target enzyme	Broad spectrum including activity vs. Mucormycetes
Isavuconazole	Oral, IV	Same as imidazoles but more specific binding to target enzyme	Broad spectrum, including yeasts and molds; FDA approved for treatment of invasive aspergillosis and invasive mucormycosis
Albaconazole, ravuconazole		Same as other azoles	Investigational; broad spectrum, including yeasts and molds
Echinocandins			
Caspofungin, anidulafungin, micafungin	IV	Inhibition of fungal cell wall glucan synthesis	Caspofungin is approved for treatment of invasive candidiasis and aspergillosis; anidulafungin is approved for treatment of invasive candidiasis; micafungin is approved for treatment of invasive candidiasis; fungicidal activity against *Candida*
Aminocandin		Same as other echinocandins	Investigational
Polyenes			
Amphotericin B	IV, topical	Binds to ergosterol, causing direct oxidative membrane damage	Established agent; broad spectrum; toxic
Lipid formulations (amphotericin B lipid complex or colloidal dispersion, liposomal amphotericin B)	IV	Same as amphotericin B	Broad spectrum; less toxic, expensive
Nystatin	Oral suspension, topical	Same as amphotericin B	Liposomal formulation (IV) under investigation
Other			
Nikkomycin Z	IV	Inhibition of fungal cell wall chitin synthesis	Investigational agent; possibly useful in combination with other antifungals
Sordarin and azasordarin derivatives		Inhibition of elongation factor 3	Investigational agent; broad-spectrum activity, including *Pneumocystis jirovecii*

 **Table 61-1 Systemic and Topical Antifungal Agents in Use and in Development—cont'd**

Antifungal Agents	Route	Mechanism of Action	Comments
Amorolfine	Topical	Miscellaneous, varied	
Butenafine HC	Topical		
Ciclopirox olamine	Topical		
Griseofulvin	Oral		
Haloprogin	Topical		
Tolnaftate	Topical		
Undecylenate	Topical		

IV, Intravenous.

 **Box 61-1 Terminology**

Antifungal spectrum: Range of activity of an antifungal agent against fungi. A broad-spectrum antifungal agent inhibits a wide variety of fungi, including both yeastlike fungi and molds, whereas a narrow-spectrum agent is active only against a limited number of fungi.

Fungistatic activity: Level of antifungal activity that **inhibits** the growth of an organism. This is determined in vitro by testing a standardized concentration of organisms against a series of antifungal dilutions. The lowest concentration of the drug that inhibits the growth of the organism is referred to as the **minimum inhibitory concentration (MIC).**

Fungicidal activity: The ability of an antifungal agent to **kill** an organism in vitro or in vivo. The lowest concentration of the drug that kills 99.9% of the test population is called the **minimum fungicidal concentration (MFC).**

Antifungal combinations: Combinations of antifungal agents that may be used to (1) enhance efficacy in the treatment of a refractory fungal infection, (2) broaden the spectrum of empirical antifungal therapy, (3) prevent the emergence of resistant organisms, and (4) achieve a synergistic killing effect.

Antifungal synergism: Combinations of antifungal agents that have enhanced antifungal activity when used together compared with the activity of each agent alone.

Antifungal antagonism: Combination of antifungal agents in which the activity of one of the agents interferes with the activity of the other agent.

Efflux pumps: Families of drug transporters that serve to actively pump antifungal agents out of the fungal cells, thus decreasing the amount of intracellular drug available to bind to its target.

amphotericin B in terms of efficacy and are much more expensive.

Azoles

The azole class of antifungals may be divided in terms of structure into the imidazoles (two nitrogens in the azole ring) and the triazoles (three nitrogens in the azole ring) (see Figure 61-2). Among the imidazoles, only ketoconazole has systemic activity. The triazoles all have systemic activity and include fluconazole, itraconazole, voriconazole, posaconazole, and isavuconazole (see Table 61-1). Ravuconazole and albaconazole are also triazoles and are currently investigational (see Table 61-1).

Both imidazoles and triazoles act by inhibiting the fungal cytochrome P450-dependent enzyme lanosterol 14-α-demethylase (Figure 61-4). This enzyme is involved in the conversion of lanosterol to ergosterol, and its inhibition disrupts membrane synthesis in the fungal cell. Depending on the organism and specific azole, inhibition of ergosterol synthesis results in inhibition of fungal cell growth (fungistatic) or cell death (fungicidal). In general, the azoles exhibit fungistatic activity against yeastlike fungi such as *Candida* spp. and *C. neoformans;* however, itraconazole, voriconazole, posaconazole, and isavuconazole appear to be fungicidal against *Aspergillus* spp.

Ketoconazole is an orally absorbed lipophilic member of the imidazole class of antifungal agents. Its spectrum of activity includes the endemic dimorphic pathogens, *Candida* spp., *C. neoformans,* and *Malassezia* spp., although it is generally less active than the triazole antifungal agents (see Table 61-2). It is variably active against *P. boydii* and has little or no useful clinical activity against the Mucormycetes, *Aspergillus* spp., *S. prolificans,* or *Fusarium* spp.

Absorption of ketoconazole by the oral route of administration is erratic and requires an acid gastric pH. Its lipophilicity ensures penetration and concentration into fatty tissues and purulent exudates; however, because it is highly (>99%) protein bound, it penetrates poorly into the central nervous system.

Ketoconazole may cause serious adverse effects, including gastric and hepatic toxicity, nausea, vomiting, and rash. At high doses, significant endocrine side effects have been observed secondary to suppression of testosterone and cortisol levels.

Because of the availability of more potent and less toxic agents, the clinical indications for use of ketoconazole are quite limited. It is at best a second-line agent for the treatment of non–life-threatening, nonmeningeal forms of histoplasmosis, blastomycosis, coccidioidomycosis, and paracoccidioidomycosis in immunocompetent individuals. Similarly, it may be used in the treatment of mucocutaneous candidiasis and lymphocutaneous sporotrichosis.

Fluconazole is a first-generation triazole with excellent oral bioavailability and low toxicity. Fluconazole is used extensively and is active against most species of *Candida, C. neoformans,* dermatophytes, *Trichosporon* spp., *H. capsulatum, C. immitis,* and *P. brasiliensis* (see Table 61-2). Among *Candida* spp., decreased susceptibility is seen with *C. krusei*

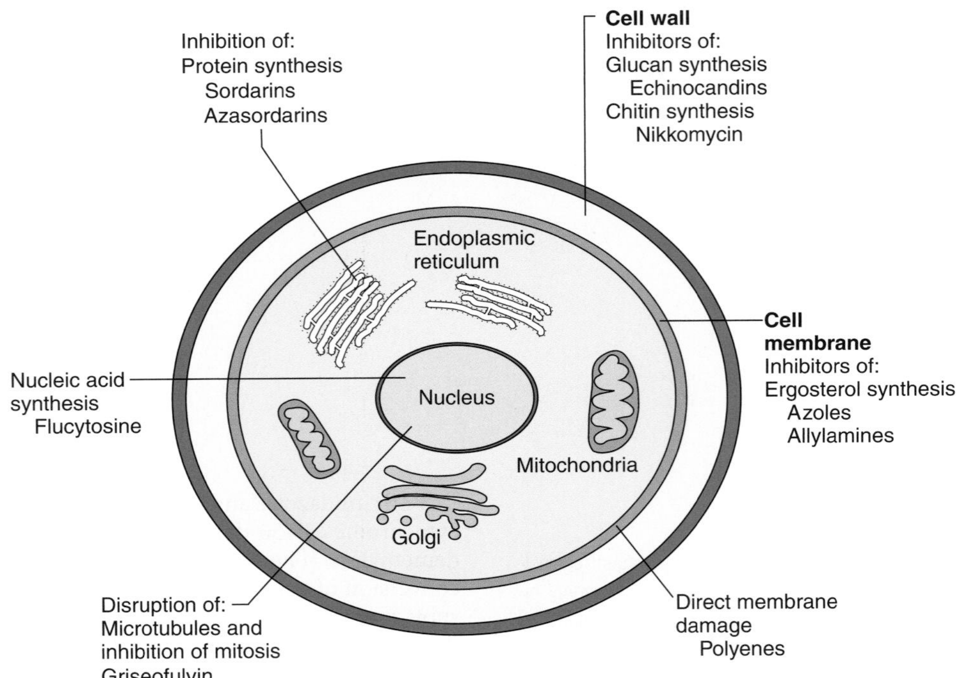

FIGURE 61-1 Sites of action of antifungals.

and *C. glabrata.* Whereas *C. krusei* must be considered intrinsically resistant to fluconazole, infections with *C. glabrata* may be treated successfully with high doses (e.g., 12 mg/kg/day) of fluconazole. Resistance may develop when fluconazole is used to treat histoplasmosis, and it has only limited activity against *B. dermatitidis.* Fluconazole is not active against the opportunistic molds, including *Aspergillus* spp., *Fusarium* spp., and the Mucormycetes.

Fluconazole is a water-soluble agent and may be administered orally or intravenously. Protein binding is low, and the drug is distributed to all organs and tissues, including the central nervous system. Severe side effects such as exfoliative dermatitis or liver failure are uncommon.

Because of its low toxicity, ease of administration, and fungistatic activity against most yeastlike fungi, fluconazole has an important role in the treatment of candidiasis, cryptococcosis, and coccidioidomycosis. It is used as primary therapy for candidemia and mucosal candidiasis and as prophylaxis in selected high-risk populations. It is used in maintenance therapy of cryptococcal meningitis in patients with acquired immunodeficiency syndrome (AIDS) and is the agent of choice in the treatment of meningitis caused by *C. immitis.* Fluconazole is a second-line agent in the treatment of histoplasmosis, blastomycosis, and sporotrichosis.

Itraconazole is a lipophilic triazole that may be administered orally in capsule or in solution. Itraconazole has a broad spectrum of antifungal activity, including against *Candida* spp., *C. neoformans, Aspergillus* spp., dermatophytes, dematiaceous molds, *P. boydii, Sporothrix schenckii,* and the endemic dimorphic pathogens (see Table 61-2). Itraconazole has activity against some but not all fluconazole-resistant strains of *C. glabrata* and *C. krusei.* Itraconazole-resistant strains of *Aspergillus fumigatus* have been reported but are uncommon. The Mucormycetes, *Fusarium,* and *S. prolificans* are resistant to itraconazole.

As with ketoconazole, oral absorption of itraconazole is erratic and requires an acid gastric pH. Absorption is enhanced with the oral solution when given in the fasting state. Itraconazole is highly protein bound and exhibits fungistatic activity against yeastlike fungi and fungicidal activity against *Aspergillus* spp.

The efficacy of itraconazole in the treatment of hematogenous candidiasis has not been adequately assessed, although it is useful in the treatment of cutaneous and mucosal forms of candidiasis. Itraconazole is often used in the treatment of dermatophytic infections and is the treatment of choice for lymphocutaneous sporotrichosis and non–life-threatening nonmeningeal forms of histoplasmosis, blastomycosis, and paracoccidioidomycosis. It may be useful in nonmeningeal coccidioidomycosis, for maintenance treatment of cryptococcal meningitis, and for some forms of phaeohyphomycosis (see Table 61-2). Itraconazole is considered a second-line agent for treatment of invasive aspergillosis; however, it is not useful in the treatment of infections caused by *Fusarium* spp., the Mucormycetes, or *S. prolificans.*

In contrast to fluconazole, drug interactions are common with itraconazole. Severe hepatotoxicity is rare, and other side effects, such as gastrointestinal intolerance, hypokalemia, edema, rash, and elevated transaminases, occur infrequently.

Voriconazole is a broad-spectrum triazole with activity against *Candida* spp., *C. neoformans, Trichosporon* spp., *Aspergillus* spp., *Fusarium* spp., dematiaceous fungi, and the endemic dimorphic pathogens (see Table 61-2). Among the *Candida* species, voriconazole is active against *C. krusei* and some but not all strains of *Candida albicans* and *C. glabrata* with reduced susceptibility to fluconazole. Although voriconazole has no activity against the Mucormycetes, it is active against fungi that are resistant to amphotericin B, including *A. terreus* and *P. boydii.*

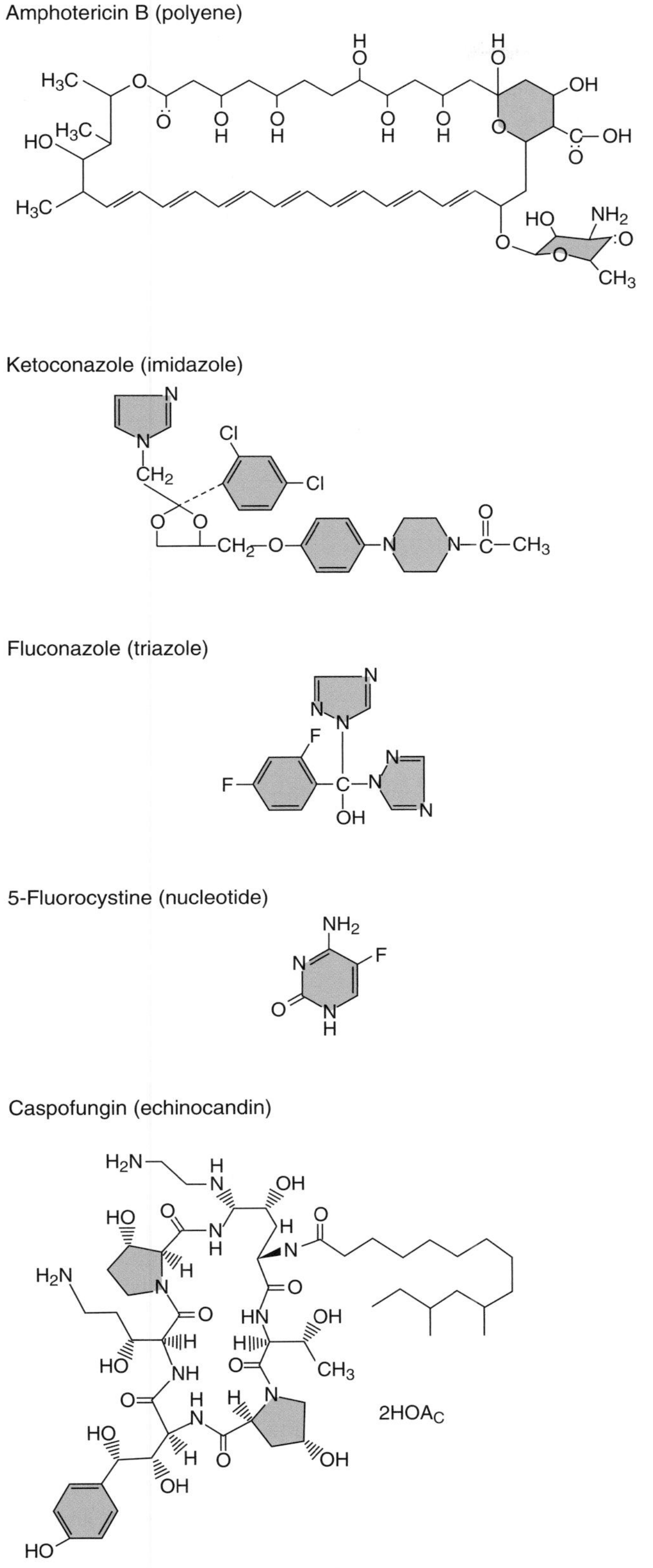

Amphotericin B (polyene)

Ketoconazole (imidazole)

Fluconazole (triazole)

5-Fluorocystine (nucleotide)

Caspofungin (echinocandin)

2HOAc

FIGURE 61-2 Chemical structures of antifungals representing five different classes.

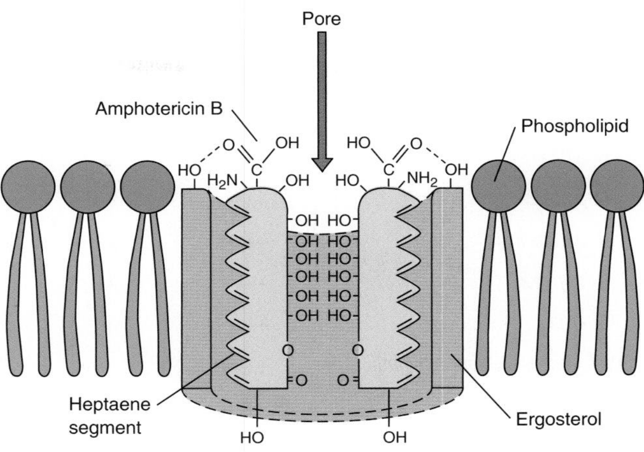

FIGURE 61-3 Mechanisms of action of amphotericin B.

Voriconazole is available in both oral and IV formulations. It has excellent penetration into the central nervous system as well as other tissues. Voriconazole exhibits fungistatic activity against yeastlike fungi and is fungicidal against *Aspergillus* spp.

Voriconazole has a primary indication for the treatment of invasive aspergillosis. It is also approved for treatment of infections caused by *P. boydii* and *Fusarium* spp. in patients intolerant of or with infections refractory to other antifungal agents. Voriconazole has proven efficacy in the treatment of various forms of candidiasis and has been used successfully in the treatment of a variety of infections caused by emerging or refractory pathogens, including brain abscesses caused by *Aspergillus* spp. and *P. boydii.*

Voriconazole is generally well tolerated, although approximately one third of patients experience transient visual disturbances. Other adverse effects include liver enzyme abnormalities, skin reactions, and hallucinations or confusion. Interactions with other drugs that are metabolized by the hepatic P450 enzyme system are common.

Posaconazole is a triazole derivative with a chemical structure similar to itraconazole. Posaconazole demonstrates potent activity against *Candida, Cryptococcus,* dimorphic fungi, and filamentous fungi, including *Aspergillus* as well as the Mucormycetes.

Posaconazole is available as an immediate-release oral suspension containing polysorbate 80 as an emulsifying agent and in an IV formulation. In contrast to voriconazole, posaconazole absorption is enhanced with food intake and is greatest with a concomitant fatty meal. There is a relatively wide patient-to-patient variability in peak serum concentrations, suggesting that posaconazole therapeutic drug monitoring may be important in optimizing the use of this agent. A new tablet with delayed release and absorption in the small bowel, leading to better bioavailability, has also been developed. Similar to voriconazole, posaconazole exhibits fungistatic activity against yeastlike fungi and is fungicidal against *Aspergillus* spp.

Posaconazole has U.S. Food and Drug Administration (FDA) approval for prophylaxis of invasive fungal infection in hematopoietic stem cell transplant (HSCT) recipients with graft-versus-host disease (GVHD) and patients with hematologic malignancies and prolonged neutropenia. It is also

Table 61-2 Spectrum and Relative Activity of Systemically Active Antifungal Agents

Organism	AMB	FC	KTZ	ITZ	FCZ	VCZ	ECH
Candida spp.							
C. albicans	++++	++++	+++	++++	++++	++++	++++
C. glabrata	+++	++++	++	++	++	+++	++++
C. parapsilosis	++++	++++	+++	++++	++++	++++	+++
C. tropicalis	+++	++++	+++	+++	++++	++++	++++
C. krusei	++	+	+	++	0	++++	++++
Cryptococcus neoformans/gattii	++++	+++	+	++	+++	++++	0
Aspergillus spp.	++++	0	+	++++	0	++++	+++
Fusarium spp.	+++	0	0	+	0	+++	0
Mucormycetes	++++	0	0	0	0	0	+
Endemic Dimorphic							
Blastomyces dermatitidis	++++	0	++	++++	+	++++	++
Coccidioides immitis	++++	0	++	++++	++++	++++	++
Histoplasma capsulatum	++++	0	++	++++	++	++++	++
Talaromyces marneffei	++++	0	++	++++	++	++++	
Sporothrix schenckii	++++	0	++	++++	++		
Dematiaceous molds	++++	+	++	++++	+	++++	0

AMB, Amphotericin B; *ECH,* echinocandins (anidulafungin, caspofungin, and micafungin); *FC,* flucytosine; *FCZ,* fluconazole; *ITZ,* itraconazole; *KTZ,* ketoconazole; *VCZ,* voriconazole.

0, Inactive or not recommended; +, occasional activity; ++, moderate activity with resistance noted; +++ reliable activity with occasional resistance; ++++ very active, resistance rare or not described.

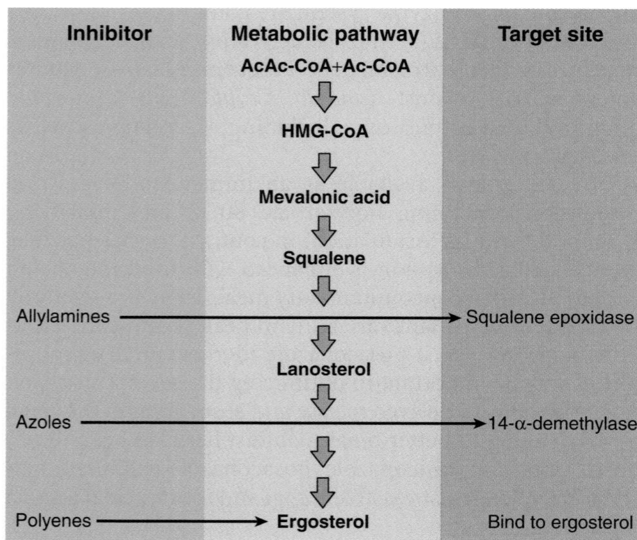

FIGURE 61-4 Metabolic pathway for the synthesis of ergosterol, showing sites of inhibition by allylamine, azole, and polyene antifungal agents. *Ac-CoA,* Acetyl coenzyme A; *HMG-CoA,* hydroxymethylglutaryl coenzyme A.

FDA approved for treatment of oropharyngeal candidiasis. In Europe, posaconazole is additionally approved for the following fungal infections refractory to amphotericin B and/or itraconazole: aspergillosis, fusariosis, chromoblastomycosis, mycetoma, and coccidioidomycosis.

Posaconazole is generally well tolerated. The most common adverse events are mild and include gastrointestinal complaints, rash, facial flushing, dry mouth, and headache. As with other azoles, hepatic toxicity has been described, and monitoring of liver function tests is recommended before and during treatment with posaconazole. Interactions with other drugs that are metabolized by the hepatic P450 enzyme system are common.

Isavuconazole (Astellas Pharma, Basilea Pharmaceutica) is a water-soluble triazole antifungal agent that can be administered orally or intravenously. Isavuconazole has predictable and dose-proportional pharmacokinetics and has completed clinical trials for the treatment of candidemia and invasive candidiasis, treatment of invasive aspergillosis, and treatment of rare mold infections. Isavuconazole has shown good in vitro activity against *Candida* and other yeast species as well as *Aspergillus* spp. other than *A. niger* and members of the Mucormycetes. It recently (in 2015) has been approved by the FDA for treatment of invasive aspergillosis and invasive mucormycosis.

Echinocandins

The echinocandins are a novel, highly selective class of semi-synthetic lipopeptides (see Figure 61-2) that inhibit the synthesis of 1,3-β-glucans, important constituents of the fungal cell wall (Figure 61-5; see Table 61-1 and Figure 61-1). Because mammalian cells do not contain 1,3-β-glucans, this class of agents is selective in its toxicity for fungi in which the glucans play an important role in maintaining the osmotic integrity of the fungal cell. Glucans are also important in cell division and cell growth. Inhibition of the glucan synthesis enzyme complex results in fungicidal activity against *Candida* spp. and fungistatic activity against *Aspergillus* spp. At present, there are three echinocandins (anidulafungin, caspofungin, micafungin) approved for use in treatment or prevention of various mycoses (see Table 61-1).

The spectrum of activity of the echinocandins is limited to those fungi in which 1,3-β-glucans constitute the dominant cell wall glucan component. As such, they are active against *Candida* and *Aspergillus* spp. and have variable activity against dematiaceous fungi and endemic dimorphic pathogens (see Table 61-2). They are inactive against *C. neoformans, Trichosporon* spp., *Fusarium* spp. and other hyaline molds, and the Mucormycetes. The echinocandins have excellent activity against fluconazole-resistant strains of *Candida* spp., although strains of *C. glabrata* with co-resistance to both azoles and echinocandins have been described in the United States and Europe. Primary or acquired resistance to this class of agents appears to be uncommon among clinical isolates of *Candida* and *Aspergillus* species.

The echinocandins must be administered intravenously and are highly (>95%) protein bound. They are distributed to all major organs, although concentrations in cerebrospinal fluid are low. All of the echinocandins are very well tolerated and have few drug-drug interactions.

Among the three echinocandins, all have similar spectrum and potency against *Candida* and *Aspergillus* species.

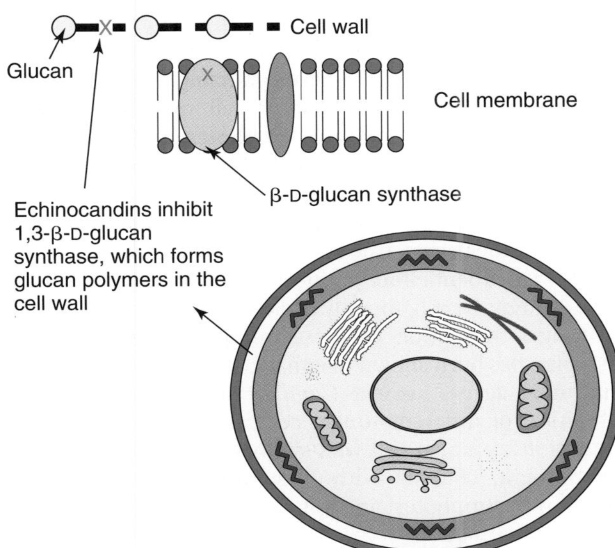

FIGURE 61-5 Mechanism of action of the echinocandins.

Caspofungin is approved for treatment of invasive candidiasis, including candidemia, and for treatment of patients with invasive aspergillosis refractory to or intolerant of other approved antifungal therapies. Anidulafungin is approved for treatment of esophageal candidiasis and candidemia, and micafungin is approved for treatment of esophageal candidiasis and candidemia and for prevention of invasive candidiasis.

Antimetabolites

Flucytosine (5-fluorocytosine [5-FC]) is the only available antifungal agent that functions as an antimetabolite. It is a fluorinated pyrimidine analog that exerts antifungal activity by interfering with the synthesis of deoxyribonucleic acid (DNA), ribonucleic acid (RNA), and proteins in the fungal cell (see Figure 61-1). Flucytosine enters the fungal cell via cytosine permease and is deaminated to 5-fluorouracil (5-FU) in the cytoplasm. The 5-FU is converted to 5-fluorouridylic acid, which then competes with uracil in the synthesis of RNA, with resultant RNA miscoding and inhibition of DNA and protein synthesis.

The antifungal spectrum of flucytosine is limited to *Candida* spp., *C. neoformans, Rhodotorula* spp., *Saccharomyces cerevisiae,* and selected dematiaceous molds (see Table 61-2). Although primary resistance to flucytosine is rare among isolates of *Candida* spp., resistance may develop among *Candida* and *C. neoformans* during flucytosine monotherapy. Flucytosine is not active against *Aspergillus* spp., the Mucormycetes, or other hyaline molds.

Flucytosine is water soluble and has excellent bioavailability when administered orally. High concentrations of flucytosine may be achieved in serum, cerebrospinal fluid, and other body fluids. Major toxicities are observed when flucytosine serum concentrations exceed 100 µg/ml and include bone marrow suppression, hepatotoxicity, and gastrointestinal intolerance. Monitoring of serum concentrations of flucytosine is important in avoiding toxicity.

Flucytosine is not used as monotherapy, because of the propensity for secondary resistance. Combinations of flucytosine with either amphotericin B or fluconazole have been shown to be efficacious in treating both cryptococcosis and candidiasis.

Allylamines

The allylamine class of antifungal agents includes terbinafine, which has systemic activity, and naftifine, which is a topical agent (see Table 61-1). These agents inhibit the enzyme squalene epoxidase, which results in a decrease in ergosterol and an increase in squalene within the fungal cell membrane (see Figures 61-1 and 61-4).

Terbinafine is a lipophilic antifungal agent with a broad spectrum of activity that includes dermatophytes, *Candida* spp., *Malassezia furfur, C. neoformans, Trichosporon* spp., *Aspergillus* spp., *S. schenckii,* and *T. marneffei* (see Table 61-2). It is available in oral and topical formulations and achieves high concentrations in fatty tissues, skin, hair, and nails.

Terbinafine is efficacious in the treatment of virtually all forms of dermatomycoses, including onychomycosis, and exhibits few side effects. It has shown clinical effectiveness in the treatment of sporotrichosis, aspergillosis, and chromoblastomycosis and has shown promise for the treatment of infections caused by fluconazole-resistant *Candida* spp. when used in combination with fluconazole.

Griseofulvin

Griseofulvin is an oral agent used in the treatment of infections caused by the dermatophytes. It is thought to inhibit fungal growth by interaction with microtubules within the fungal cell, resulting in inhibition of mitosis (see Table 61-1 and Figure 61-1).

Griseofulvin is considered a second-line agent in the treatment of dermatophytoses. Newer agents, such as itraconazole and terbinafine, are more rapid acting and provide greater efficacy. Griseofulvin is also associated with a number of mild side effects, including nausea, diarrhea, headache, hepatotoxicity, rash, and neurologic side effects.

• Topical Antifungal Agents

A wide variety of topical antifungal preparations are available for the treatment of superficial cutaneous and mucosal fungal infections (see Table 61-1). Topical preparations are available for most classes of antifungal agents, including polyenes (amphotericin B, nystatin, pimaricin), allylamines (naftifine and terbinafine), and numerous imidazoles and miscellaneous agents (see Table 61-1). Creams, lotions, ointments, powders, and sprays are available for use in the treatment of cutaneous infections and onychomycosis, whereas mucosal infections are best treated with suspensions, tablets, troches, or suppositories.

Whether one uses topical or systemic therapy for treatment of cutaneous or mucosal fungal infections usually depends on the status of the host and the type and extent of infection. Whereas most cutaneous dermatophytic infections and oral or vaginal candidiasis will respond to topical therapy, the refractory nature of infections such as onychomycosis or tinea capitis ("ringworm" of the scalp) usually calls for long-term systemic therapy.

• Investigational Antifungal Agents

At present, there are several antifungal agents in various stages of clinical evaluation. These investigational agents include some with established modes of action, as well as some novel classes of antifungal agents, such as a liposomal formulation of nystatin, novel triazole agents (albaconazole and ravuconazole), echinocandins (aminocandin) and non-echinocandin glucan synthase inhibitors (ML-3118), an inhibitor of chitin synthesis (nikkomycin Z), and sordarin and azasordarin derivatives (see Table 61-1). The mechanisms of action and spectra of activity of liposomal nystatin, the novel triazoles, and echinocandins are essentially the same as those of the currently available members of each class (see Tables 61-1 and 61-2). To a varying degree, the newer agents in each class offer the potential for more favorable pharmacokinetic and pharmacodynamic proprieties, decreased toxicities or drug-drug interactions, or possible improved activity against certain pathogens that are refractory to presently available agents. For example, the new agent MK-3118 shares the glucan synthase target with the echinocandins but interacts with the target at a different position and thus retains activity against strains of *Candida* with *fks* mutations that produce resistance to the echinocandins. Inhibition of chitin synthesis in the fungal cell wall by nikkomycin Z provides another novel approach that may be useful in concert with other inhibitors of cell wall or cell membrane synthesis. The development of agents with novel mechanisms of action is both necessary and promising for future advances in the area of antifungal therapy.

• Combinations of Antifungal Agents in the Treatment of Mycoses

The high mortality of opportunistic fungal infections has spurred the development of new antifungal agents, including some with novel mechanisms of action (see Table 61-1). In addition to aggressive use of new antifungal agents such as voriconazole and caspofungin as monotherapy, the use of azole-, echinocandin-, and polyene-based combinations for treatment of the more difficult-to-treat mycoses (e.g., opportunistic mold infections) is the focus of intense interest and discussion. The rationale behind combination therapy is that by using combinations of antifungal agents, one may achieve a better clinical outcome than with monotherapy. The push toward the use of combination antifungal therapy is especially strong for infections such as invasive aspergillosis, where the associated mortality is unacceptably high.

In considering combination therapy, one seeks to achieve **synergy** and avoid **antagonism. Synergy** is achieved when the outcome obtained with the combination of agents is significantly better than that obtained with either drug alone. Conversely, **antagonism** is when the combination is less active or efficacious than either drug alone. In the case of antifungal therapy, there are several mechanisms one may consider in developing an effective combination treatment strategy: (1) Different stages of the same biochemical pathway can be inhibited. This is a classic approach for achieving synergy with antiinfective agents. An example of this approach to antifungal therapy would be the combination of terbinafine with an azole, where both agents attack the sterol pathway at different points (see Figure 61-4), resulting in inhibition of ergosterol synthesis and disruption of the fungal cell membrane. (2) Increased penetration of one agent into the cell by virtue of the permeabilizing action of another agent on the fungal cell wall or cell membrane can be achieved. The combination of amphotericin B (cell membrane disruption) and flucytosine (inhibition of nucleic acid synthesis intracellularly) is a classic example of this interaction. (3) Inhibition of the transport of one agent out of the cell by another agent can be achieved. Many fungi employ energy-dependent efflux pumps to actively pump antifungal agents out of the cell, thereby avoiding the toxic effects of the antifungal. Inhibition of these pumps by agents such as reserpine has been shown to enhance the activity of the azole antifungal agents against *Candida* spp. (4) Simultaneous inhibition of different fungal cell targets can be achieved. Inhibition of fungal cell wall synthesis by an agent such as caspofungin, coupled with disruption of cell membrane function by amphotericin B or azoles, is an example of this type of combination.

Although the potential value of combination antifungal therapy is appealing, there are several possible downsides to this strategy that must be considered. Antagonism among antifungal agents when used in combination is also a distinct possibility and may occur via several different mechanisms: (1) The action of one agent results in a decrease in the target of another agent. The action of azole antifungal agents depletes the cell membrane of ergosterol, which is the primary target for amphotericin B. (2) The action of one antifungal agent results in the modification of the target of another agent. The inhibition of ergosterol synthesis by azole antifungal agents results in the accumulation of methylated sterols, to which amphotericin B binds less well. (3) Blocking of the target site of one agent by another may occur. Lipophilic agents such as itraconazole may adsorb to the fungal cell surface and inhibit the binding of amphotericin B to membrane sterols.

Despite these possible positive and negative scenarios, data supporting the achievement of synergy when various combinations are used clinically are limited. Likewise, antagonism may be demonstrated in the laboratory, but significant antagonism has not been observed clinically with antifungal combinations. By considering all the laboratory and clinical data for antifungal combination therapy, one arrives at a very limited number of instances where combination therapy has been shown to be beneficial in the treatment of invasive mycoses (Table 61-3).

The strongest data exist for the treatment of cryptococcosis, where the combination of amphotericin B and flucytosine has been shown to be beneficial in the treatment of cryptococcal meningitis. The data are less strong for the combination of flucytosine with fluconazole or amphotericin B with triazoles; however, these combinations appear to be beneficial in treating cryptococcosis as well.

Candidiasis is generally treated adequately with a single antifungal agent such as amphotericin B, caspofungin, or fluconazole; however, combination therapy may be useful in selected situations. The combination of amphotericin B and fluconazole has proven benefits in treating candidemia. Likewise, the combination of terbinafine plus an azole is promising in the treatment of refractory oropharyngeal candidiasis. Flucytosine in combination with either amphotericin B or triazoles has positive effects on survival and tissue burden of infection in animal models of candidiasis. Currently, combination therapy of candidiasis should be reserved for specific individual settings such as meningitis, endocarditis, hepatosplenic infection, and candidiasis that are recurrent or refractory to single-agent therapy.

Although the clinical setting of invasive aspergillosis is where combination therapy is most attractive, the data to support its use are limited. At present, there is a single randomized trial published that evaluates the use of combination therapy in the treatment of invasive aspergillosis. The results of this study provide compelling, but not definitive, conclusions that combination therapy (voriconazole plus anidulafungin) may be beneficial in treating invasive aspergillosis. Studies in vitro and in animals have produced variable results. Whereas amphotericin B plus rifampin appears synergistic, studies with flucytosine or rifampin plus amphotericin B or azoles have been inconsistent. Despite the desperate need for better treatment options for invasive aspergillosis, there is only modest evidence that combination therapy will improve clinical outcome. Combination therapy should be used with caution until more clinical data are available.

Table 61-3 Summary of Potentially Useful Antifungal Combinations for Treatment of Common Mycoses

Infection	Antifungal Combination	Comments
Candidiasis	AMB + FCZ	Good clinical success in humans with candidemia
	AMB + FC	Clinical success in humans with peritonitis
Cryptococcosis	AMB + FC	Good clinical success in humans with cryptococcal meningitis
	AMB + FCZ	Clinical success in humans with cryptococcal meningitis
	FC + FCZ	Clinical success in humans with cryptococcal meningitis
Aspergillosis	AMB + FC	In vivo benefit (animal model); minimal human data
	AMB + azoles	No benefit in animals
	AMB + echinocandins	In vivo benefit (animal model); minimal human data
	Triazoles + echinocandins	In vivo benefit (animal model); modest human data

AMB, Amphotericin B; *FC*, flucytosine; *FCZ*, fluconazole.

• Mechanisms of Resistance to Antifungal Agents

Given the prominent role of *Candida* spp. as etiologic agents of invasive mycoses, it is not surprising that most of our understanding of the mechanisms of resistance to antifungal agents comes from studies of *C. albicans* and other species of *Candida*. Much less is known of resistance mechanisms in *Aspergillus* spp. and *C. neoformans*, and almost no information on antifungal resistance mechanisms is available for other opportunistic fungal pathogens.

In contrast to mechanisms of resistance to antibacterial agents, there is no evidence that fungi are capable of destroying or modifying antifungal agents as a means of achieving resistance. Likewise, antifungal resistance genes are not transmissible from cell to cell in the manner that occurs with many bacterial resistance genes. It is apparent, however, that multidrug efflux pumps, target alterations, and reduced access to drug targets are important mechanisms of resistance to antifungal agents, just as they are for antibacterial resistance (Table 61-4). In contrast to the rapid emergence and spread of high-level multidrug resistance that occurs in bacteria, antifungal resistance usually develops slowly and involves the emergence of intrinsically resistant species or a gradual stepwise alteration of cellular structures or functions that results in resistance to an agent to which there has been prior exposure.

Polyenes

Resistance to polyenes, and amphotericin B in particular, remains uncommon despite extensive use over more than 30 years. Decreased susceptibility to amphotericin B has been

Table 61-4 Mechanisms Involved in Development of Resistance to Antifungal Agents in Pathogenic Fungi

Fungus	Amphotericin B	Flucytosine	Itraconazole	Fluconazole	Echinocandins
Aspergillus fumigatus			Altered target enzyme, 14-α-demethylase Decreased azole accumulation		
Candida albicans	Decrease in ergosterol Replacement of polyene-binding sterols Masking of ergosterol	Loss of permease activity Loss of cytosine deaminase activity Loss of uracil phosphoribosyl-transferase activity		Overexpression or mutation of 14-α-demethylase Overexpression of efflux pumps, *CDR* and *MDR* genes	Mutation in *fks1* gene
Candida glabrata	Alteration or decrease in ergosterol content	Loss of permease activity		Overexpression or mutation of 14-α-demethylase Overexpression of efflux pumps (*CgCDR* genes)	Mutation in *fks1* and/or *fks2* gene
Candida krusei	Alteration or decrease in ergosterol content			Active efflux Reduced affinity for target enzyme, 14-α-demethylase	Mutation in *fks1* gene
Candida lusitaniae	Alteration or decrease in ergosterol content Production of modified sterols				
Cryptococcus neoformans	Defects in sterol synthesis Decreased ergosterol Production of modified sterols			Alterations in target enzyme Overexpression of MDR efflux pump	

reported in isolates of *C. lusitaniae, C. glabrata, C. krusei,* and *C. guilliermondii.* Although primary resistance may be seen, most resistance to amphotericin B among *Candida* spp. is secondary to amphotericin B exposure during therapy. *Aspergillus* spp. are generally susceptible to amphotericin B; however, *A. terreus* is unique in that it appears to be resistant both in vitro and in vivo. Although secondary resistance to amphotericin B has been reported in *C. neoformans,* it is quite rare.

The mechanism of amphotericin B resistance appears to be the result of qualitative and quantitative alterations in the fungal cell. Amphotericin B–resistant mutants of *Candida* spp. and *C. neoformans* have been shown to have a reduced ergosterol content, replacement of polyene-binding sterols (ergosterol) by ones that bind polyenes less well (fecosterol), or masking of ergosterol in the cell membranes so that binding with polyenes is hindered because of steric or thermodynamic factors. The molecular mechanism of amphotericin B resistance has not been determined; however, sterol analysis of resistant strains of *Candida* spp. and *C. neoformans* suggests that they are defective in *ERG2, ERG3,* or *ERG6* genes encoding for the C-8 sterol isomerase, C-5 sterol desaturase enzymes, and C-24 sterol methyltransferase, respectively.

Azoles

The ubiquitous use of azoles, especially fluconazole, for the treatment and prevention of fungal infections has given rise to reports of emerging resistance to this class of antifungal agents. Fortunately, primary resistance to fluconazole is rare among most species of *Candida* causing bloodstream infection. Among the five most common species of *Candida* isolated from the blood of infected patients (*C. albicans, C. glabrata, Candida parapsilosis, Candida tropicalis,* and *C. krusei*), only *C. krusei* is considered intrinsically resistant to fluconazole. Among the remaining species, approximately 10% of *C. glabrata* exhibit primary resistance to fluconazole, and less than 2% of *C. albicans, C. parapsilosis,* and *C. tropicalis* are resistant to this agent. The new triazoles (voriconazole, posaconazole, ravuconazole) are more potent than fluconazole against *Candida* spp., including activity against *C. krusei* and some fluconazole-resistant strains of other *Candida* spp.; however, there is a strong positive correlation between the activity of fluconazole and that of the other triazoles, suggesting some degree of cross-resistance within the class.

Primary resistance to fluconazole is also rare among clinical isolates of *C. neoformans.* Secondary resistance has been described in isolates obtained from individuals with AIDS and relapsing cryptococcal meningitis.

Although resistance to the azoles is considered to be rare among *Aspergillus* spp., increased resistance has been noted in several geographic regions since 1999. Recent evidence from the Netherlands and Denmark suggests the possibility that azole resistance in *A. fumigatus* may be a side effect of environmental fungicide use. Cross-resistance between itraconazole, posaconazole, and voriconazole varies according to the mechanism of resistance.

Azole resistance in *Candida* spp. can be the result of the following mechanisms: a modification in the quantity or quality of the target enzymes, reduced access of the drug to the target, or some combination of these mechanisms. Thus point mutations in the gene *(ERG11)* encoding the target enzyme, lanosterol 14-α-demethylase, leads to an altered target with decreased affinity for azoles. Overexpression of *ERG11* results in overproduction of the target enzyme, creating the need for higher concentrations of the drug within the cell to inactivate all the target enzyme molecules. Up-regulation of genes encoding for multidrug efflux pumps results in active efflux of the azole antifungal agents out of the cell. Up-regulation of genes encoding the **major facilitator type efflux pump *(MDR)*** leads to fluconazole resistance, and up-regulation of genes encoding the **adenosine triphosphate (ATP)-binding cassette transporters *(CDR)*** leads to resistance to multiple azoles. These mechanisms may act individually, sequentially, or simultaneously, resulting in strains of *Candida* that exhibit progressively higher levels of azole resistance.

The mechanisms of azole resistance in *Aspergillus* spp. are now well characterized in *A. fumigatus* but not in other species of *Aspergillus*. It appears that both increased drug efflux and alterations in the 14-α-demethylase target enzyme serve as mechanisms for resistance to itraconazole, posaconazole, and voriconazole among isolates of *A. fumigatus*. Specific mutations in the *CYP51A* gene encoding the target enzyme may result in resistance to one, two, or all three triazoles. Additional and as yet undefined mechanisms of resistance may also contribute to azole resistance in *A. fumigatus* isolates from patients undergoing long-term azole therapy.

Similarly, secondary resistance to fluconazole among isolates of *C. neoformans* has been associated with overexpression of MDR efflux pumps and alteration of the target enzyme. *C. neoformans* has also been shown to have a CDR-type efflux pump.

Echinocandins

Caspofungin, anidulafungin, and micafungin all demonstrate potent fungicidal activity against *Candida* spp., including azole-resistant strains. Clinical isolates of *Candida* spp. with reduced susceptibility to the echinocandins are uncommon but increasingly recognized among patients undergoing long-term treatment with these agents. Efforts to produce caspofungin-resistant mutants of *C. albicans* in the laboratory have shown that the frequency with which these mutants arise is very low (1 in 10^8 cells), suggesting a low potential for the emergence of resistance in the clinical setting. Echinocandin resistance has likewise been rare among clinical isolates of *Aspergillus*; however, laboratory-derived echinocandin-resistant mutants have been selected.

The mechanism of resistance to the echinocandins that has been characterized in laboratory strains of *C. albicans* and clinical strains of *C. albicans, C. glabrata, C. tropicalis, C. krusei,* and *C. lusitaniae* is one of an altered glucan synthesis enzyme complex that shows a decreased sensitivity to inhibition by agents within the class. These strains have point mutations in the *fks1* or *fks2 (C. glabrata)* gene that encodes for an integral membrane protein (Fks1p, Fks2p), which is the catalytic subunit of the glucan synthesis enzyme complex. The *fks* mutation results in strains that are resistant to all of the echinocandins but retain susceptibility to polyene and azole antifungal agents. The *fks* gene is also essential in *Aspergillus* spp., and laboratory-derived *fks1* mutants of *A. fumigatus* have been shown to exhibit decreased susceptibility to all of the echinocandins in vitro and in vivo. The echinocandin-resistant strain of *A. fumigatus* was shown to have decreased fitness for causing infection relative to a wild-type strain, suggesting that this may account for the paucity of clinical strains expressing echinocandin resistance.

Flucytosine

Primary resistance to flucytosine is uncommon among clinical isolates of *Candida* spp. and *C. neoformans*. Secondary resistance, however, is well documented to occur among both *Candida* spp. and *C. neoformans* during monotherapy with this agent.

Flucytosine resistance may develop because of decreased uptake of the drug (loss of permease activity) or by loss of enzymatic activity necessary to convert flucytosine to 5-FU (cytosine deaminase) and 5-fluorouridylic acid (FUMP pyrophosphorylase). Uracil phosphoribosyltransferase, another enzyme in the pyrimidine salvage pathway, is also important in the formation of FUMP (5-fluorouracilmonophosphate), and loss of its activity is sufficient to confer resistance to flucytosine.

Allylamines

Although clinical failures can occur during treatment of fungal infections with terbinafine and naftifine, they have not been shown to be the result of resistance to these agents. It has been shown that the CDR1 multidrug efflux pump can use terbinafine as a substrate, suggesting that efflux-mediated resistance to allylamines is a possibility.

Clinical Factors Contributing to Resistance

Antifungal therapy may fail clinically despite the fact that the drug employed is active against the infecting fungus. The complex interaction of the host, drug, and fungal pathogen may be influenced by a wide variety of factors, including the immune status of the host, site and severity of the infection, presence of a foreign body (e.g., catheter, vascular graft), activity of the drug at the site of infection, dose and duration of therapy, and patient compliance with the antifungal regimen. It must be recognized that the presence of neutrophils, use of immunomodulating drugs, concomitant infections (e.g., human immunodeficiency virus), surgical procedures, age, and nutritional status of the host all may be more important in determining the outcome of the infection than the ability of the antifungal agent to inhibit or kill the infecting organism.

Antifungal Susceptibility Testing

In vitro susceptibility testing of antifungal agents is designed to determine the relative activity of one or more agents against the infecting pathogen in hopes of selecting the best option for treatment of the infection. Thus antifungal susceptibility tests are performed for the same reasons tests with antibacterial agents are performed. Antifungal susceptibility tests will (1) provide a reliable estimate of the relative activity of two or more antifungal agents against the tested organism, (2) correlate with in vivo antifungal activity and predict the likely outcome of therapy, (3) provide a means with which to monitor the development of resistance among a normally susceptible population of organisms, and (4) predict the therapeutic potential of newly developed investigational agents.

Standardized methods for performing antifungal susceptibility testing are reproducible, accurate, and available for use in clinical laboratories. Antifungal susceptibility testing is now increasingly and appropriately used as a routine adjunct to the treatment of fungal infections. Guidelines for the use of antifungal testing as a complement to other laboratory studies have been developed. Selective application of antifungal susceptibility testing, coupled with broader identification of fungi to the species level, is especially useful in difficult-to-manage fungal infections. One must keep in mind, however, that the in vitro susceptibility of an infecting organism to the antimicrobial agent is only one of several factors that may influence the likelihood that therapy for an infection will be successful (see Clinical Factors Contributing to Resistance).

Bibliography

Gubbins PO, Anaissie EJ: Antifungal therapy. In Anaissie EJ, McGinnis MR, Pfaller MA, editors: *Clinical mycology*, ed 2, New York, 2009, Churchill Livingstone.

Howard SJ, Arendrup MC: Acquired antifungal drug resistance in *Aspergillus fumigatus:* epidemiology and detection, *Med Mycol* 49(Suppl 1):S90–S95, 2011.

Johnson EM, Espinel-Ingroff AV, Pfaller MA: Susceptibility test methods: yeasts and filamentous fungi. In Versalovic J, et al, editors: *Manual of clinical microbiology*, ed 10, Washington, DC, 2011, American Society for Microbiology Press.

Johnson MD, MacDougall C, Ostrosky-Zeichner L, et al: Combination antifungal therapy, *Antimicrob Agents Chemother* 48:693–715, 2004.

Kanafani ZA, Perfect JR: Resistance to antifungal agents: mechanisms and clinical impact, *Clin Infect Dis* 46:120–128, 2008.

Perlin DS: Resistance to echinocandin-class antifungal drugs, *Drug Resist Updates* 10:121–130, 2007.

Pfaller MA: Antifungal drug resistance: mechanisms, epidemiology, and consequences for treatment, *Am J Med* 125:S3–S13, 2012.

CHAPTER

62 SUPERFICIAL AND CUTANEOUS MYCOSES

Darrell, a 24-year-old medical student, just loves his new bulldog puppy, Delbert. He recently purchased Delbert from a local "backyard" breeder. Darrell has taken to giving Delbert frequent "smooches" on his muzzle, which Delbert loves because he knows a treat is soon to follow. After about 3 months of proud puppy ownership and "smooching," Darrell noticed that his mustache began itching, and his upper lip was beginning to swell. Over a 1-week period, his upper lip became swollen and inflamed, and small pustular areas became apparent among the sparse hairs of his moustache. Similar changes were also becoming apparent on Delbert's muzzle. This concerned Darrell, so he promptly took Delbert to the veterinarian. The veterinarian took one look at the pair, wrote a prescription for Delbert, and told Darrell that he should make a visit to the dermatologist.

1. What was the likely cause of Darrell/Delbert's affliction? Be specific.
2. How would you go about making a diagnosis?
3. How would you go about treating this infection?
4. Who gave what to whom?

Answers to these questions are available on StudentConsult.com.

• SUMMARIES CLINICALLY SIGNIFICANT ORGANISMS

Dermatophytes

Trigger Words

Tinea, KOH preparation, ringworm, azoles, terbinafine, circular, scaling lesion with central clearing and hair loss

Biology, Virulence, and Disease

- Include filamentous fungi in the genera *Trichophyton, Epidermophyton,* and *Microsporum*
- Keratinophilic and keratinolytic; able to invade and break down skin, hair, and nails
- In infections of skin, hair, and nails, only outermost keratinized layers invaded
- Various forms of dermatophytosis (tineas or "ringworm") classified according to anatomic site or structure involved
- Clinical signs and symptoms vary

Epidemiology

- Classified into three categories based on natural habitat: geophilic, zoophilic, and anthropophilic
- Geophilic: live in soil, occasional pathogens of both animals and humans
- Zoophilic: parasitize hair and skin of animals but can be transmitted to humans
- Anthropophilic: infect humans, may be transmitted directly or indirectly from person to person
- Occur worldwide, especially in tropical and subtropical regions

Diagnosis

- Demonstration of fungal hyphae by direct microscopy of skin, hair, or nail samples
- Isolation of organisms in culture

Treatment, Prevention, and Control

- Localized infections that do not involve hair or nails may be treated effectively with topical antifungal agents (azoles, terbinafine, haloprogin)
- All others require oral therapy (griseofulvin, itraconazole, fluconazole, terbinafine)

Fungal infections of the skin and skin structures are extremely common. These infections are generally categorized by the structures the fungi colonize or invade:

1. Superficial mycoses, limited to the outmost layers of the skin and hair
2. Cutaneous mycoses, infections that involve the deeper layers of the epidermis and its integuments, the hair and nails
3. Subcutaneous mycoses, involving the dermis, subcutaneous tissues, muscle, and fascia. The subcutaneous mycoses

will be discussed separately in Chapter 63. This chapter will deal with the superficial and cutaneous mycoses.

• Superficial Mycoses

Agents of superficial mycoses are fungi that colonize the keratinized outer layers of the skin, hair, and nails. Infections caused by these organisms elicit little or no host immune response and are nondestructive and thus asymptomatic. They are usually of cosmetic concern only and are easy to diagnose and treat.

Pityriasis (Tinea) Versicolor

Pityriasis versicolor is a common superficial fungal infection seen worldwide. In certain tropical environments, it may affect up to 60% of the population. It is caused by the lipophilic yeast species of the *Malassezia furfur* complex: *M. furfur, M. sympodialis, M. globosa, M. restricta, M. slooffiae, M. obtusa, M. dermatis, M. japonica*, and *M. yamatoensis*. In routine clinical reporting, referring to these organisms as members of the *M. furfur* complex is usually sufficient.

Morphology

When viewed in skin scrapings, members of the *M. furfur* complex appear as clusters of spherical or oval, thick-walled yeastlike cells, 3 to 8 μm in diameter (Figure 62-1). The yeast cells may be mixed with short, infrequently branched hyphae that tend to orient end to end. The yeastlike cells represent phialoconidia and show polar bud formation with a "lip" or collarette around the point of bud initiation on the parent cell (Figure 62-2). In culture on standard media containing or overlaid with olive oil, species of the *M. furfur* complex grow as cream-colored to tan yeastlike colonies composed of budding yeastlike cells; hyphae are infrequently produced.

Epidemiology

Pityriasis versicolor is a disease of healthy persons that occurs worldwide, but it is most prevalent in tropical and subtropical regions. Young adults are most commonly affected. *M. furfur* and other members of the species complex are not found as saprophytes in nature, and pityriasis versicolor has not been documented in animals. Human infection is thought to result from direct or indirect transfer of infected keratinous material from one person to another.

Clinical Syndromes

The lesions of pityriasis versicolor are small hypopigmented or hyperpigmented macules. The upper trunk, arms, chest, shoulders, face, and neck are most often involved, but any part of the body may be affected (Figure 62-3). The lesions are irregular, well-demarcated patches of discoloration that may be raised and covered by a fine scale. Because species of the *M. furfur* complex tend to interfere with melanin production, lesions are hypopigmented in dark-skinned individuals. In light-skinned individuals, the lesions are pink to pale brown and become more obvious when they fail to tan after exposure to sunlight. Little or no host reaction occurs, and the lesions are asymptomatic, with the exception of mild pruritus in severe cases. The *M. furfur* complex has also been associated with folliculitis, obstructive dacryocystitis, systemic infections in patients receiving intravenous lipid infusions and seborrheic dermatitis, especially in patients with the acquired immunodeficiency syndrome (AIDS).

Laboratory Diagnosis

The laboratory diagnosis of pityriasis versicolor is made by direct visualization of the fungal elements on microscopic examination of epidermal scales in 10% potassium hydroxide (KOH) with or without calcofluor white. The organisms are usually numerous and may also be visualized with hematoxylin and eosin (H&E) or periodic acid–Schiff (PAS) stains (see Figure 62-1). The lesions will also fluoresce with a yellowish color upon exposure to a Wood lamp.

Although not usually necessary for establishing the diagnosis, culture may be performed using synthetic mycologic media supplemented with olive oil as a source of lipid. Growth of yeastlike colonies appear after incubation at 30° C for 5 to 7 days. Microscopically, the colonies are composed of budding yeastlike cells with occasional hyphae.

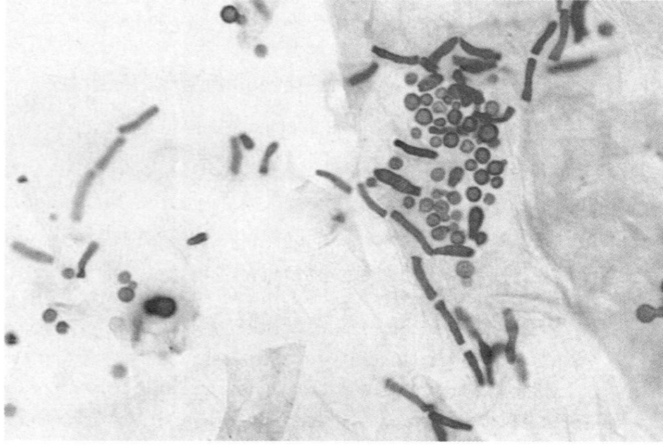

FIGURE 62-1 Pityriasis versicolor. Periodic acid–Schiff–stained skin scraping showing yeastlike cells and short, infrequently branched hyphae that are often oriented end to end (×100). (From Connor DH, Schwartz DA: *Pathology of infectious diseases,* Stamford, Conn, 1997, Appleton & Lange.)

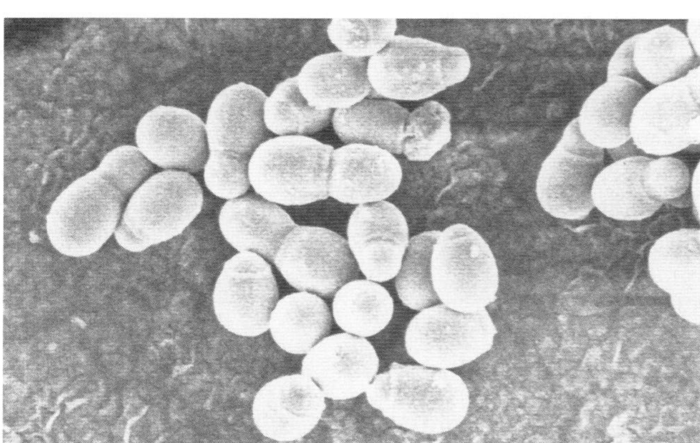

FIGURE 62-2 Scanning electron micrograph of *Malassezia furfur* demonstrating the liplike collarette around the point of bud initiation on the parent cell. (Courtesy S.A. Messer.)

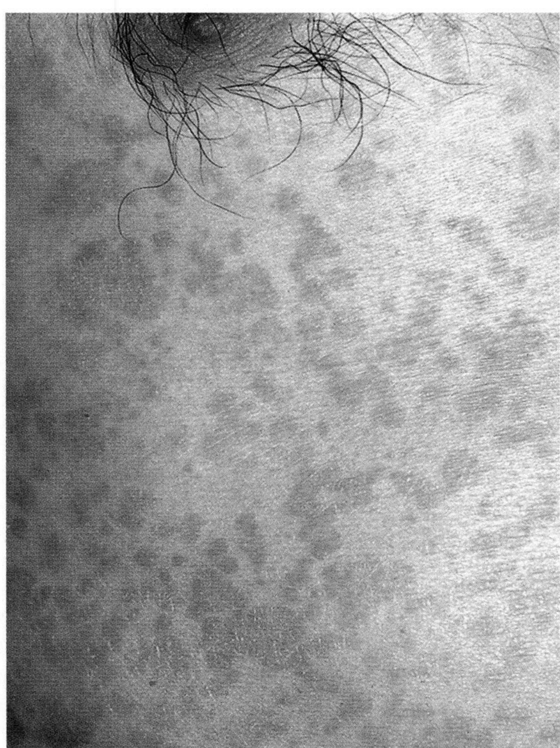

FIGURE 62-3 Pityriasis versicolor. Multiple pale brown, hyperpigmented patches on chest and shoulders. (From Gawkrodger D, Ardern-Jones M: *Dermatology: an illustrated colour text.* Edinburgh, 2012, Churchill-Livingstone, p 42, Fig. 2.)

Treatment

Although spontaneous cure has been reported, the disease is generally chronic and persistent. Treatment consists of the use of topical azoles or selenium sulfide shampoo. For more widespread infection, oral ketoconazole or itraconazole may be used.

Tinea Nigra

Tinea nigra is a superficial phaeohyphomycosis caused by the black fungus *Hortaea werneckii* (formerly *Exophiala werneckii*).

Morphology

Microscopically, *H. werneckii* appears as dematiaceous, frequently branched, septate hyphae, 1.5 to 3.0 µm wide. Arthroconidia and elongate budding cells are also present (Figure 62-4). *H. werneckii* also grows in culture on standard mycologic media at 25° C, where it is a black mold producing annelloconidia (conidia possessing annelids or rings), which often slide down the sides of the conidiophore.

Epidemiology

Tinea nigra is a tropical or subtropical condition. It is likely contracted by traumatic inoculation of the fungus into the superficial layers of the epidermis. It is most prevalent in Africa, Asia, and Central and South America. Children and young adults are most often affected, with a higher incidence in females.

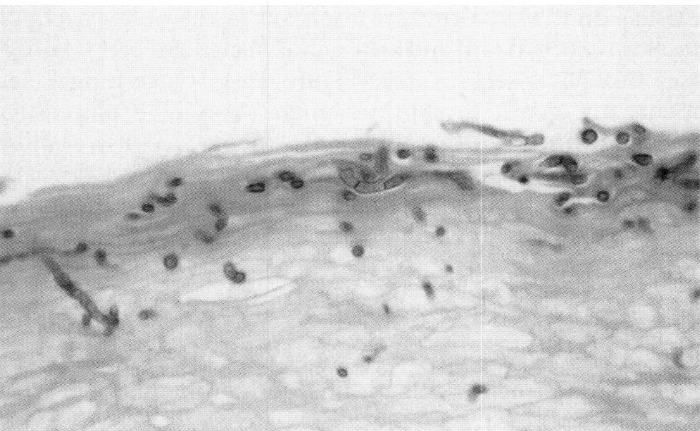

FIGURE 62-4 Tinea nigra. Dematiaceous hyphae of *Hortaea werneckii* (hematoxylin and eosin, ×100). (From Connor DH, Schwartz DA: *Pathology of infectious diseases,* Stamford, Conn, 1997, Appleton & Lange.)

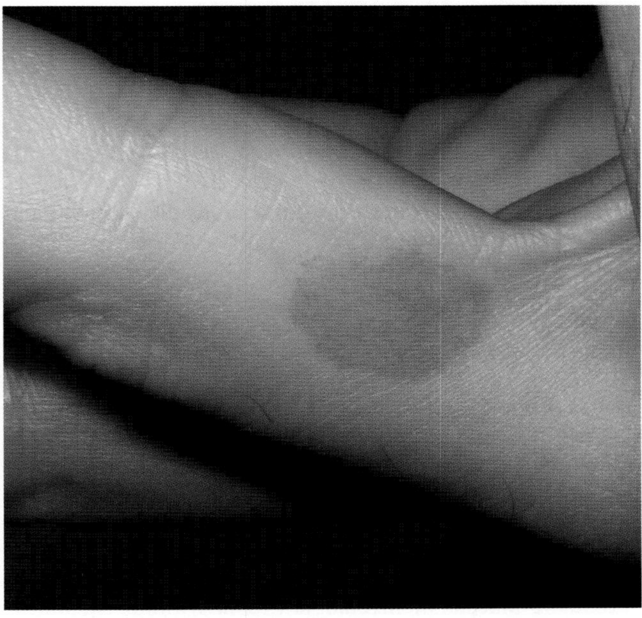

FIGURE 62-5 Tinea nigra. Darkly pigmented macules with irregular edges present on the palm. (From Bolognia J, Jorizzo JL, Schaffer JV: *Dermatology,* London, 2012, Saunders, Fig. 77-2; courtesy Frank Samarin, MD.)

Clinical Syndromes

Tinea nigra appears as a solitary, irregular, pigmented (brown to black) macule, usually on the palms or soles (Figure 62-5). There is no scaling or invasion of hair follicles, and the infection is not contagious. Because of its superficial location, there is little or no discomfort or host reaction. Because the lesion grossly may resemble a malignant melanoma, biopsy or local excision may be considered. Such invasive procedures may be avoided by a simple microscopic examination of skin scrapings of the affected area.

Laboratory Diagnosis

Tinea nigra is easily diagnosed by microscopic examination of skin scrapings placed in 10% to 20% KOH. The pigmented hyphae and yeast forms are confined to the outer layers of the stratum corneum and are easily detected on H&E-stained (see Box 60-1) sections (see Figure 62-4). Once fungal elements are detected, skin scrapings should be placed on mycologic media with antibiotics. A dematiaceous yeastlike colony should appear within 3 weeks, becoming velvety with age. Microscopic examination reveals two-celled, cylindrical, yeastlike cells and, depending upon the age of the colony, toruloid hyphae.

Treatment

The infection responds well to topical therapy, including Whitfield ointment, azole creams, and terbinafine.

White Piedra

White piedra is a superficial infection of hair caused by yeastlike fungi of the genus *Trichosporon: T. ovoides* (causes scalp hair white piedra), *T. inkin* (causes most cases of pubic white piedra), and *T. asahii.*

Morphology

Microscopic examination reveals hyphal elements, arthroconidia (rectangular cells resulting from the fragmentation of hyphal cells), and blastoconidia (budding yeast cells).

Epidemiology

This condition occurs in tropical and subtropical regions and is related to poor hygiene.

Clinical Syndromes

White piedra affects the hairs of the groin and axillae. The fungus surrounds the hair shaft and forms a white to brown swelling along the hair strand. The swellings are soft and pasty and may be easily removed by running a section of the hair between the thumb and forefinger. The infection does not damage the hair shaft.

Laboratory Diagnosis

When microscopic examination reveals hyphal elements, arthroconidia, and/or budding yeast cells, infected hair should be placed on mycologic media without cycloheximide (cycloheximide will inhibit *Trichosporon* spp.). *Trichosporon* spp. will form cream-colored, dry, wrinkled colonies within 48 to 72 hours upon incubation at room temperature. The various species of *Trichosporon* can be identified in the same manner as other yeast isolates. Sugar assimilations, potassium nitrate (KNO_3) assimilation (negative), urease production (positive), and morphology on cornmeal agar (both arthroconidia and blastoconidia are present) should be determined.

Treatment

Treatment may be accomplished by the use of topical azoles; however, improved hygiene and shaving of the infected hair are also effective and usually negate the necessity of medical treatment.

Black Piedra

Another condition affecting the hair, primarily the scalp, is black piedra. The causative agent of black piedra is *Piedraia hortae.*

Morphology

The organism grows as a pigmented (brown to reddish-black) mold. As the culture ages, spindle-shaped ascospores are formed within specialized structures (asci). These structures (asci and ascospores) are also produced within the rock-hard hyphal mass that surrounds the hair shaft.

Epidemiology

Black piedra is uncommon and has been reported from tropical areas in Latin America and Central Africa. It is thought to be a condition of poor hygiene.

Clinical Syndromes

Black piedra presents as small dark nodules that surround the hair shafts. It is asymptomatic and generally involves the scalp. The hyphal mass is held together by a cement-like substance and contains asci and ascospores, the sexual phase of the fungus.

Laboratory Diagnosis

Examination of the nodule reveals branched, pigmented, hyphae held together by a cement-like substance. *P. hortae* can be cultured on routine mycologic media. Very slow growth may be observed at 25° C and may begin as a yeast-like colony, later becoming velvety as hyphae develop. Asci may be observed microscopically, usually ranging from 4 to 30 µm and containing up to eight ascospores.

Treatment

Treatment of black piedra is easily accomplished by a haircut and proper regular washings.

• Cutaneous Mycoses

Cutaneous mycoses include infections caused by dermatophytic fungi (dermatophytosis) and nondermatophytic fungi (dermatomycosis) (Table 62-1). Because of the overwhelming importance of dermatophytes as etiologic agents of cutaneous mycoses, the majority of this section will deal with those fungi. The nondermatophytic fungi will be discussed regarding their role in onychomycosis. The superficial and cutaneous infections caused by *Candida* spp. will be discussed in Chapter 65.

Dermatophytoses (Clinical Cases 62-1 and 62-2)

The term **dermatophytosis** refers to a complex of diseases caused by any of several species of taxonomically related filamentous fungi in the genera *Trichophyton, Epidermophyton,* and *Microsporum* (Tables 62-1 through 62-3). These fungi are known collectively as the **dermatophytes,** and all possess the ability to cause disease in humans and/or animals. All have in common the ability to invade the skin, hair, or nails. In each case, these fungi are keratinophilic and keratinolytic and so are able to break down the keratin surfaces of these structures. In the case of skin infections, the dermatophytes invade only the upper outermost layer of the epidermis, the stratum corneum. Penetration below the granular layer of the epidermis is rare. Likewise with hair and nails, being part of the skin, only the keratinized layers are invaded. The

 **Table 62-1 Common and Uncommon Agents of Superficial and Cutaneous Dermatomycoses and Dermatophytoses**

	Type of Infection									
Fungus	**TP**	**TCO**	**TCR**	**TCA**	**TBA**	**TVR**	**O**	**TN**	**BP**	**WP**
Dermatophytic										
Trichophyton rubrum	X	X	X				X			
T. mentagrophytes complex	X	X	X	X			X			
T. tonsurans		X		X			X			
T. verrucosum		X		X	X					
T. equinum				X						
T. violaceum				X						
T. schoenleinii				X						
T. megnini							X			
Epidermophyton floccosum	X		X				X			
Microsporum canis		X		X						
M. audouinii				X						
Nondermatophytic										
Scopulariopsis brevicaulis							X			
Neoscytalidium spp. and *Scytalidium* spp.	X						X			
Malassezia spp.						X				
Candida albicans	X		X				X			
Aspergillus terreus							X			
Sarocladium (Acremonium) spp.							X			
Fusarium spp.							X			
Trichosporon spp.										X
Piedraia hortae									X	
Hortaea werneckii								X		

BP, Black piedra; *O,* onychomycosis; *TBA,* tinea barbae; *TCA,* tinea capitis; *TCO,* tinea corporis; *TCR,* tinea cruris; *TN,* tinea nigra; *TP,* tinea pedis; *TVR,* tinea versicolor; *WP,* white piedra; *X,* etiologic agents of dermatomycoses or dermatophycoses.

 **Clinical Case 62-1 Dermatophytosis in an Immunocompromised Host**

Squeo and associates (*J Am Acad Dermatol* 39:379–380, 1998) describe a case of a 55-year-old renal transplant recipient with onychomycosis and chronic tinea pedis who presented with tender nodules on his left medial heel. He then developed papules and nodules on his right foot and calf. A skin biopsy demonstrated periodic acid–Schiff–positive, thick-walled, round cells, 2 to 6 μm in diameter in the dermis. Skin biopsy culture grew *Trichophyton rubrum. T. rubrum* has been described as an invasive pathogen in immunocompromised hosts. The clinical presentation, histopathology, and early fungal culture growth suggested *Blastomyces dermatitidis* in the differential diagnosis before the final identification of *T. rubrum.*

 **Clinical Case 62-2 Tinea Capitis in an Adult Woman**

Martin and Elewski (*J Am Acad Dermatol* 49:S177–S179, 2003) describe an 87-year-old woman with a 2-year history of a pruritic, painful, scaling scalp eruption and hair loss. Her previous treatment for this condition included numerous courses of systemic antibiotics and prednisone without success. Of interest in her social history was that she had recently acquired several stray cats that she kept inside her home. On physical examination, there were numerous pustules throughout the scalp, with diffuse erythema, crusting, and scale extending to the neck. There was extremely sparse scalp hair and prominent posterior cervical lymphadenopathy. She had no nail pitting. A Wood light examination of the scalp produced negative findings. A skin biopsy specimen and fungal, bacterial, and viral cultures were obtained. Bacterial culture grew rare *Enterococcus* species, whereas viral cultures showed no growth. The scalp biopsy specimen revealed an endothrix dermatophyte infection. Fungal culture grew *Trichophyton tonsurans.* The patient was treated with griseofulvin and Selsun shampoo. When seen at a 2-week follow-up visit, the patient demonstrated new hair growth and a resolution of her pustular eruption. With the brisk clinical response and culture growth of *T. tonsurans,* treatment with griseofulvin was continued for 8 weeks. The scalp hair grew back normally without permanent alopecia. Adults with alopecia require an evaluation for tinea capitis, including fungal cultures.

Table 62-2 Characteristic In Vitro and In Vivo Features of Dermatophytes

	In Vitro		In Vivo Hair	
Genus	**Macroconidia**	**Microconidia**	**Invasion**	**Fluorescence***
Epidermophyton	Smooth walled, borne in clusters of two or three	Absent	NA	NA
Microsporum	Numerous, large, thick, and rough walled[†]	Rare	Ectothrix	+/–[‡]
Trichophyton	Rare, smooth, thin-walled	Numerous, spherical, teardrop or peg shaped[§]	Endothrix[‖]	+/–[¶]

NA, Not applicable.
*Fluorescence with a Wood lamp.
[†]Except *M. audouinii.*
[‡]*M. gypseum* not fluorescent.
[§]Except *T. schoenleinii.*
[‖]*T. verrucosum,* ectothrix; *T. schoenleinii,* favic.
[¶]*T. schoenleinii* is fluorescent.

Table 62-3 Classification of Dermatophytes According to Ecologic Niche

Ecologic Niche	Species	Principal Hosts	Geographic Distribution	Prevalence
Anthropophilic	*Epidermophyton floccosum*		Worldwide	Common
	Microsporum audouinii		Worldwide	Common
	M. ferrugineum		Africa, Asia	Endemic
	Trichophyton concentricum		Asia, Pacific Islands	Endemic Rare
	T. megnini		Europe, Africa	Endemic
	T. mentagrophytes var. *interdigitale*		Worldwide	Common
	T. rubrum		Worldwide	Common
	T. schoenleinii		Europe, Africa	Endemic
	T. soudanese		Africa	Endemic
	T. tonsurans		Worldwide	Common
	T. violaceum		Europe, Africa, Asia	Common
Zoophilic	*M. canis*	Cat, dog, horse	Worldwide	Common
	M. gallinae	Fowl	Worldwide	Rare
	M. nanum	Swine	Worldwide	Rare
	M. persicolor	Vole	Europe, United States	Rare
	T. equinum	Horse	Worldwide	Rare
	T. mentagrophytes var. *mentagrophytes*	Rodent	Worldwide	Common
	var. *erinacei*	Hedgehog	Europe, New Zealand, Africa	Occasional
	var. *quinckeanum*	Mouse	Worldwide	Rare
	T. simii	Monkey	India	Occasional
	T. verrucosum	Cow	Worldwide	Common
Geophilic	*M. gypseum* complex		Worldwide	Occasional
	T. vanbreuseghemii		Worldwide	Rare

From Hiruma M, Yamaguchi H: Dermatophytes. In Anaissie EJ, McGinnis MR, Pfaller MA, editors: *Clinical mycology,* New York, 2003, Churchill Livingstone.

various forms of dermatophytosis are referred to as tineas or "ringworm." Clinically, the tineas are classified according to the anatomic site or structure affected: (1) tinea capitis of the scalp, eyebrows, and eyelashes, (2) tinea barbae of the beard, (3) tinea corporis of the smooth or glabrous skin, (4) tinea cruris of the groin, (5) tinea pedis of the foot, and (6) tinea unguium of the nails (also known as **onychomycosis**). The clinical signs and symptoms of dermatophytosis vary according to the etiologic agents, host reaction, and site of infection.

Morphology

Each genus of dermatophytic mold is characterized by a specific pattern of growth in culture and by the production of macroconidia and microconidia (see Table 62-2). Further identification to species level requires consideration of colony morphology, spore production, and nutritional requirements in vitro.

Microscopically, the genus *Microsporum* is identified by observation of its macroconidia, whereas microconidia are the characteristic structures of the genus *Trichophyton* (see Table 62-2). *Epidermophyton floccosum* does not produce microconidia, but its smooth-walled macroconidia borne in clusters of two or three are quite distinctive (Figure 62-6). *Microsporum canis* produces characteristic large, multicellular (five to eight cells per conidium), thick- and rough-walled macroconidia (Figure 62-7). *Trichophyton rubrum* produces microconidia that are teardrop or peg shaped and borne along the sides of hyphae (Figure 62-8), whereas *Trichophyton mentagrophytes* produces both single cigar-shaped macroconidia and grapelike clusters of spherical microconidia (Figure 62-9). *T. tonsurans* produces variably sized and shaped microconidia, with relatively large spherical conidia often located right alongside small parallel-walled conidia and other microconidia of various sizes and shapes (Figure 62-10).

In skin biopsies, all dermatophytes are morphologically similar and appear as hyaline septate hyphae, chains of arthroconidia, or dissociated chains of arthroconidia that invade the stratum corneum, hair follicles, and hairs. When the hair is infected, the pattern of fungal invasion can be either **ectothrix, endothrix,** or **favic** depending on the dermatophytic species (Figure 62-11). Septate hyphae may be seen within the hair shaft in all three patterns. In the **ectothrix** pattern, **arthroconidia** are formed on the outside of

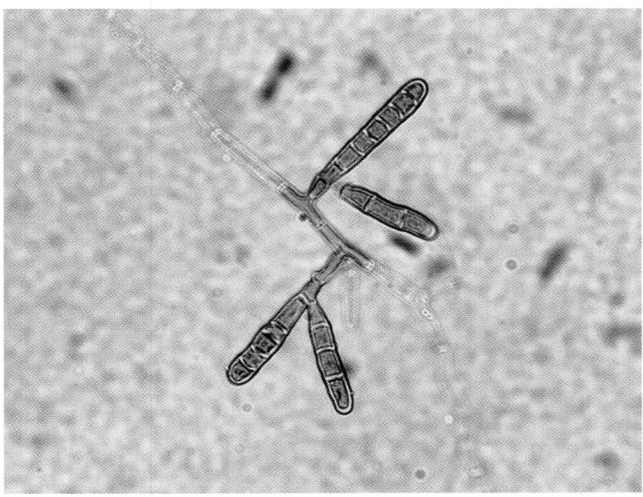

FIGURE 62-6 *Epidermophyton floccosum.* Lactophenol cotton blue showing smooth-walled macroconidia.

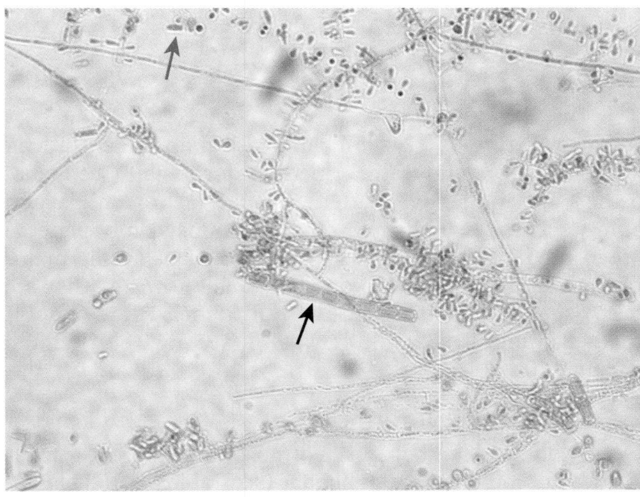

FIGURE 62-8 *Trichophyton rubrum.* Lactophenol cotton blue showing multicelled macroconidia *(black arrow)* and teardrop- and peg-shaped microconidia *(red arrow).*

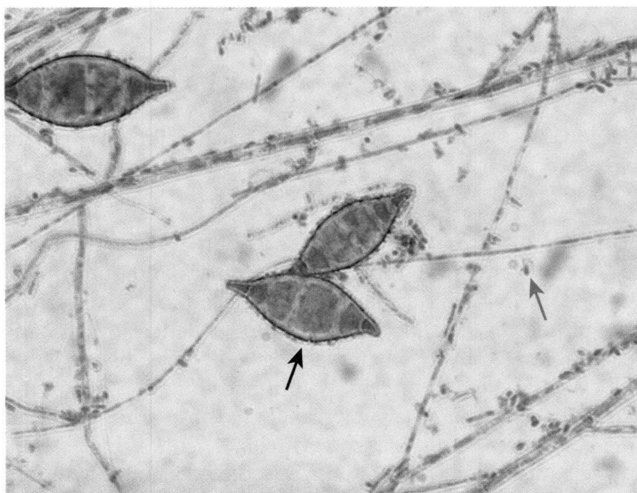

FIGURE 62-7 *Microsporum canis.* Lactophenol cotton blue showing rough-walled macroconidia *(black arrow)* and microconidia *(red arrow).*

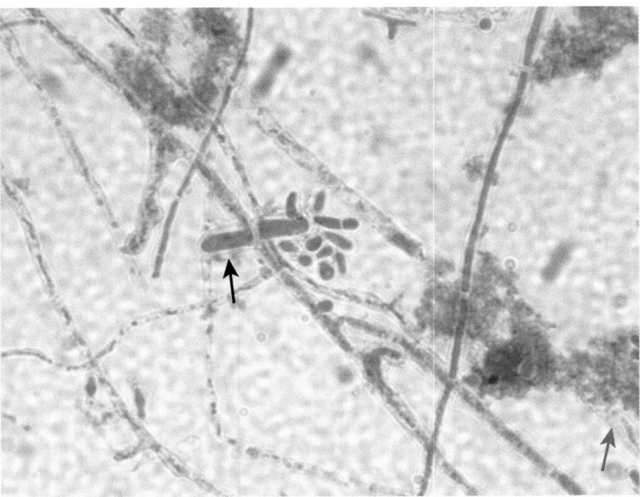

FIGURE 62-9 *Trichophyton mentagrophytes.* Lactophenol cotton blue showing cigar-shaped macroconidia *(black arrow)* and grapelike clusters of microconidia *(red arrow).*

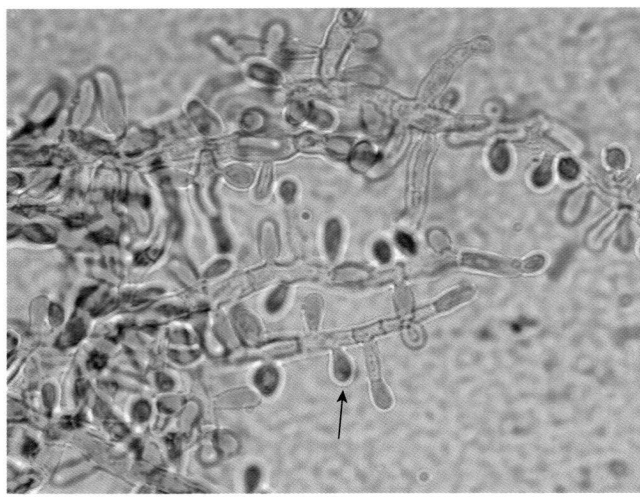

FIGURE 62-10 *Trichophyton tonsurans.* Lactophenol cotton blue showing microconidia *(black arrow).*

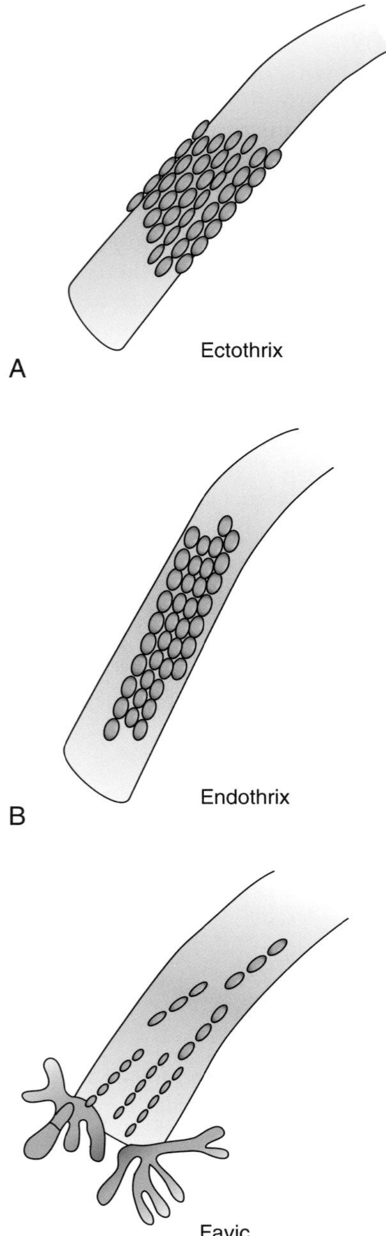

FIGURE 62-11 Schematic of **(A)** ectothrix hair infection, **(B)** endothrix hair infection, and **(C)** favic hair infection.

the hair (Figure 62-12; see Figure 62-11); in the **endothrix** pattern, arthroconidia are formed inside the hair (see Figure 62-11); and in the **favic** pattern, hyphae, arthroconidia, and empty spaces resembling air bubbles ("honeycomb" pattern) are formed inside the hair (see Figure 62-11). The dermatophytes can usually be seen on H&E stain; however, they are best visualized with special stains for fungi, such as Gomori methenamine silver (GMS) and PAS (see Figure 62-12 and Chapter 60).

Ecology and Epidemiology

Dermatophytes can be classified into three different categories based on their natural habitat (see Table 62-3): (1) **geophilic,** (2) **zoophilic,** and (3) **anthropophilic.** The geophilic dermatophytes live in the soil and are occasional pathogens of both animals and humans. Zoophilic dermatophytes normally parasitize the hair and skin of animals but can be transmitted to humans. Anthropophilic dermatophytes generally infect humans and may be transmitted directly or indirectly from person to person. This classification is quite useful prognostically and emphasizes the importance of identifying the etiologic agent of dermatophytoses. Species of dermatophytes that are considered anthropophilic tend to cause chronic, relatively noninflammatory infections that are difficult to cure. In contrast, the zoophilic and geophilic dermatophytes tend to elicit a profound host reaction, causing lesions that are highly inflammatory and respond well to therapy. In some instances, these infections may heal spontaneously.

The dermatophytes are worldwide in distribution (see Table 62-3), and infection may be acquired from the transfer of arthroconidia or hyphae, or keratinous material containing these elements, from an infected host to a susceptible uninfected host. Dermatophytes may remain viable in desquamated skin scales or hair for long periods, and infection may be either by direct contact or indirect via fomites. Individuals of both sexes and all ages are susceptible to dermatophytosis; however, tinea capitis is more common in prepubescent children, and tinea cruris and tinea pedis are primarily diseases of adult males. Although dermatophytoses occur worldwide, especially in tropical and subtropical regions, individual dermatophyte species may vary in their geographic distribution and in their virulence for humans (see Table 62-3). For example, *Trichophyton concentricum*, the cause of tinea imbricata, is confined to the islands of the South Pacific and Asia, whereas *T. tonsurans* has replaced *Microsporum audouinii* as the principal agent of tinea capitis in the United States. Infections caused by dermatophytes are generally endemic but may assume epidemic proportions in selected settings (e.g., tinea capitis in schoolchildren). On a worldwide scale, *T. rubrum* and *T. mentagrophytes* account for 80% to 90% of all dermatophytoses.

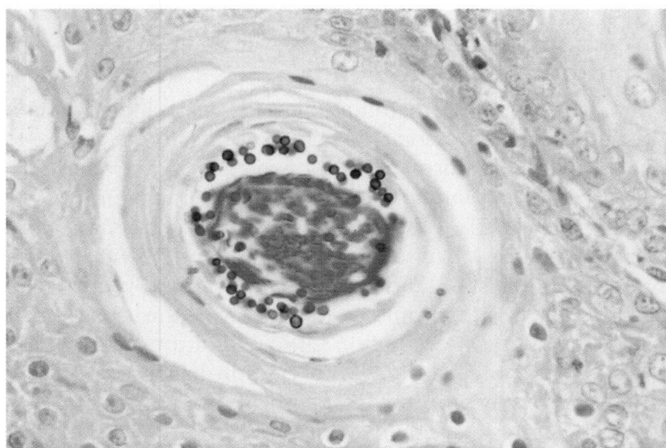

FIGURE 62-12 Arthroconidia surrounding a hair shaft. Ectothrix hair infection caused by *Microsporum canis* (Gomori methenamine silver–hematoxylin and eosin, ×160). (From Connor DH, Schwartz DA: *Pathology of infectious diseases,* Stamford, Conn, 1997, Appleton & Lange.)

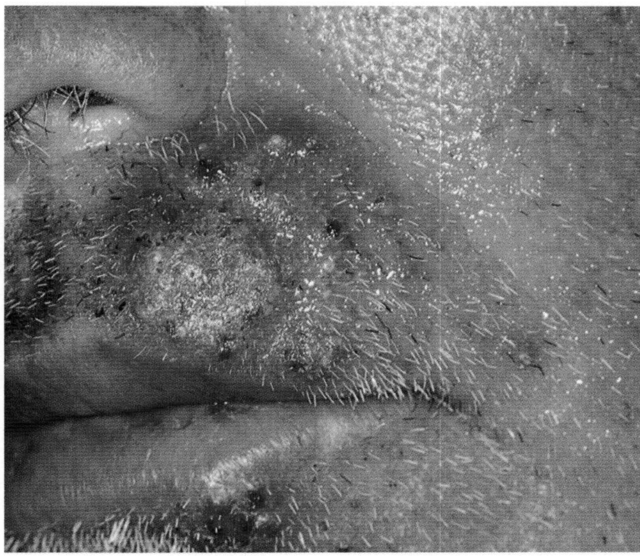

FIGURE 62-14 Tinea barbae caused by *Trichophyton verrucosum.* (From James W, Berger T, Elston D: *Andrews' diseases of the skin,* ed 11, London, 2011, Saunders, Fig. 15-3.)

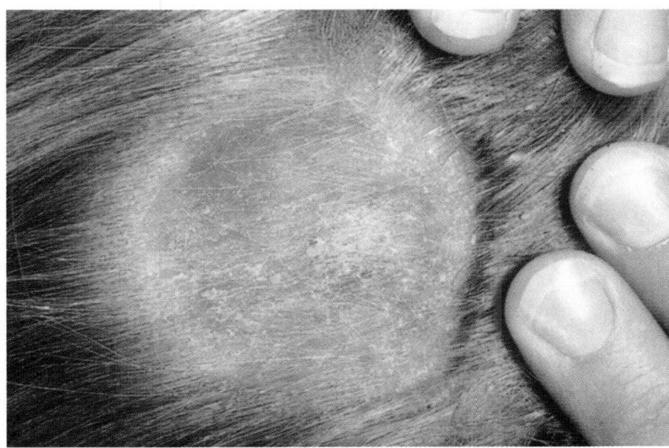

FIGURE 62-13 Tinea capitis caused by *Microsporum canis.* (From Hay RJ: Cutaneous and subcutaneous mycoses. In Anaissie EJ, McGinnis MR, Pfaller MA, editors: *Clinical mycology,* New York, 2003, Churchill Livingstone.)

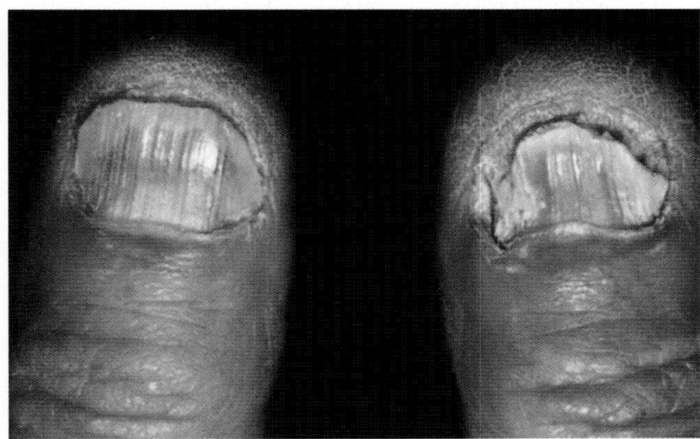

FIGURE 62-15 Onychomycosis caused by *Trichophyton rubrum.* (From Hay RJ: Cutaneous and subcutaneous mycoses. In Anaissie EJ, McGinnis MR, Pfaller MA, editors: *Clinical mycology,* New York, 2003, Churchill Livingstone.)

Clinical Syndromes

Dermatophytoses manifest a wide range of clinical presentations that may be affected by factors such as the species of dermatophytes, inoculum size, site of infection, and immune status of the host. Any given disease manifestation may result from several different species of dermatophytes, as shown in Table 62-1.

The classic pattern of dermatophytosis is the "ringworm" pattern of a ring of inflammatory scaling with diminution of inflammation toward the center of the lesion. Tineas of hair-bearing areas often present as raised circular or ring-shaped patches of alopecia with erythema and scaling (Figure 62-13) or as more diffusely scattered papules, pustules, vesicles, and kerions (severe inflammation involving the hair shaft) (Figure 62-14). Hairs infected with certain species (e.g., *M. canis, M. audouinii, Trichophyton schoenleinii*) often fluoresce yellow-green when exposed to a Wood light (see Table 62-2). Infections of smooth skin commonly present as erythematous and scaling patches that expand in a centripetal pattern with central clearing. Dermatophytoses of the foot and hand may often become complicated by onychomycosis (Figure 62-15), in which the nail plate is invaded and destroyed by the fungus. Onychomycosis (tinea unguium) is caused by a variety of dermatophytes (see Table 62-1) and is estimated to affect approximately 3% of the population in most temperate countries. It is a disease seen mostly in adults, with toenails affected more commonly than fingernails. The infection is usually chronic, and the nails become thickened, discolored, raised, friable, and deformed (see Figure 62-15). *T. rubrum* is the most common etiologic agent in most countries. A rapidly progressive form of onychomycosis that originates from the proximal nailfold and involves the upper and underside of the nail is seen in AIDS patients.

Laboratory Diagnosis

The laboratory diagnosis of dermatophytoses relies on the demonstration of fungal hyphae by direct microscopy of skin, hair, or nail samples and the isolation of organisms in culture. Specimens are mounted in a drop of 10% to 20% KOH on a glass slide and examined microscopically. Filamentous hyaline hyphal elements characteristic of dermatophytes may be seen in skin scrapings, nail scrapings, and hairs. In examining specimens for fungal elements, calcofluor white has been used with excellent results.

Cultures are always useful and can be obtained by scraping the affected areas and placing the skin, hair, or nail clippings onto standard mycologic media such as Sabouraud agar, with and without antibiotics, or dermatophyte test medium. Colonies develop within 7 to 28 days. Their gross and microscopic appearance and nutritional requirements can be used in identification. More recently, molecular and proteomic methods have been used to provide rapid and specific means of identifying those unusual isolates that are difficult to identify using conventional phenotypic approaches.

Treatment

Dermatophytic infections that are localized and do not affect hair or nails can usually be treated effectively with topical agents; all others require oral therapy. Topical agents include azoles (miconazole, clotrimazole, econazole, tioconazole, and itraconazole), terbinafine, and haloprogin. Whitfield ointment (benzoic and salicylic acids) is an optional agent for dermatophytosis, but responses are usually slower than those seen with agents with specific antifungal activity.

Oral antifungal agents with systemic activity against dermatophytes include griseofulvin, itraconazole, fluconazole, and terbinafine. The azoles and terbinafine are more rapidly and broadly efficacious than griseofulvin, especially for treatment of onychomycosis.

Onychomycosis Caused by Nondermatophytic Fungi

A number of nondermatophytic molds, as well as *Candida* species, have been associated with nail infections (see Table 62-1). These organisms include *Scopulariopsis brevicaulis, Neoscytalidium dimidiatum, Scytalidium hyalinum,* and a variety of others, including *Aspergillus, Fusarium,* and *Candida* species. Among these organisms, *S. brevicaulis, Neoscytalidium* spp., and *Scytalidium* spp. are proven nail pathogens. The other fungi certainly may be the cause of nail pathology, but interpretation of nail cultures with these organisms should be done with caution because they may simply represent saprophytic colonization of abnormal nail material. Criteria used to determine an etiologic role for these fungi include isolation on multiple occasions and the presence of abnormal hyphal or conidial structures on microscopic examination of nail material.

Infections caused by *S. brevicaulis, N. dimidiatum,* and *S. hyalinum* are notoriously difficult to treat because they are not usually susceptible to any antifungals. Partial surgical removal of infected nails, coupled with oral itraconazole or terbinafine or intensive treatment with 5% amorolfine nail lacquer or Whitfield ointment, may be useful in achieving a clinical response.

Bibliography

Chandler FW, Watts JC: *Pathologic diagnosis of fungal infections*, Chicago, 1987, American Society for Clinical Pathology Press.

Hay RJ: Cutaneous and subcutaneous mycoses. In Anaissie EJ, McGinnis MR, Pfaller MA, editors: *Clinical mycology*, New York, 2003, Churchill Livingstone.

Hiruma M, Yamaguchi H: Dermatophytes. In Anaissie EJ, McGinnis MR, Pfaller MA, editors: *Clinical mycology*, New York, 2003, Churchill Livingstone.

Summerbell RC: *Trichophyton, Microsporum, Epidermophyton*, and agents of superficial mycoses. In Versalovic J, et al, editors: *Manual of clinical microbiology*, ed 10, Washington, DC, 2011, American Society for Microbiology Press.

CHAPTER

63 SUBCUTANEOUS MYCOSES

A 40-year-old "ecotourist" was on an extended trip to the jungles of Costa Rica. During this time, she camped, climbed trees, waded in streams, slogged through mud, and endured drenching rains. She lost her shoes about 2 weeks into the "adventure" and continued to hike about barefoot for another 2 weeks, during which time she sustained minor cuts and abrasions to both feet. Approximately 6 months after returning home, somewhere in the midwestern United States, she noticed mild swelling of her right foot. There was no pain, inflammation, or drainage from the foot. She comes to you for medical advice.

1. What is the differential diagnosis of this process?
2. What types of fungi might cause this infection?
3. How will you proceed with establishing the diagnosis?
4. What are the therapeutic options and the likelihood they will be successful?

Answers to these questions are available on StudentConsult.com.

• SUMMARIES CLINICALLY SIGNIFICANT ORGANISMS

Sporothrix schenckii

Trigger Words

Thorn prick, rose handler's disease, sphagnum moss, lymphocutaneous nodules

Biology, Virulence, and Disease

- Thermally dimorphic fungus; grows as a mold at room temperature (e.g., 25° C) and as a pleomorphic yeast at 37° C and in tissue
- Infection is chronic; nodular and ulcerative lesions develop along lymphatics that drain primary site of inoculation

Epidemiology

- Sporadic, most common in warmer climates: Japan, North and South America
- Outbreaks related to forest work, mining, gardening
- Classic infection associated with traumatic inoculation of soil, vegetable, or organic matter contaminated with fungus
- Zoonotic transmission reported in armadillo hunters and in association with infected cats

Diagnosis

- Subcutaneous infection with lymphangitic spread
- Definitive diagnosis requires culture of infected pus or tissue
- In tissue, organism appears as a pleomorphic budding yeast

Treatment, Prevention, and Control

- Classic treatment: oral potassium iodide in saturated solution
- Itraconazole: safe, highly effective, treatment of choice
- Alternatives: terbinafine, fluconazole, posaconazole
- Local application of heat shown to be effective

Eumycotic Mycetoma (*Phaeoacremonium, Curvularia, Fusarium, Madurella, Mediacopsis, Biatrophia, Trematosphaeria, Exophiala, Falciformispora*, and *Scedosporium/Pseudallescheria* Species)

Trigger Words

Grains, sinus tract, dematiaceous, subcutaneous, mycetoma

Biology, Virulence, and Disease

- Caused by a wide array of true fungi (as opposed to actinomycotic mycetomas, which are caused by bacteria)
- Localized chronic granulomatous infectious process involving cutaneous and subcutaneous tissues
- Painless subcutaneous nodule; increases slowly but progressively in size
- Local spread may breach tissue planes, destroying muscle, fascia, bone
- Hematogenous or lymphatic spread rare

Epidemiology

- Primarily in tropical areas with low rainfall; most common in Africa and India
- Traumatic implantation into exposed body parts; foot and hand most common; back, shoulders, chest wall may also be involved
- Men more often affected than women
- Etiologic agent varies from country to country
- Mycetomas not contagious

Diagnosis

- Demonstration of grains or granules grossly visible in draining sinus tracts; may also be seen on tissue biopsy
- Microscopic examination of granules
- Culture usually needed for identification of organism

Treatment, Prevention, and Control

- Usually unsuccessful; poor response to most antifungal agents
- Specific antifungal therapy may slow progression: terbinafine, voriconazole, posaconazole
- Local excision usually ineffective; amputation is the only definitive treatment

Conidiobolus coronatus and *Basidiobolus ranarum (haptosporus)*

Trigger Words

Entomophthoromycosis, subcutaneous, Splendore-Hoeppli, mucormycotic

Biology, Virulence, and Disease

- Subcutaneous entomophthoromycosis caused by Mucormycetes of the order Entomophthorales: *Conidiobolus coronatus, Basidiobolus ranarum*
- Chronic subcutaneous form of mucormycosis
- Occurs sporadically as a result of subcutaneous implantation or inhalation of fungus present in plant debris
- *B. ranarum:* infection presents with disk-shaped, rubbery, moveable masses localized to shoulder, pelvis, hips, thighs; may become quite large and ulcerate
- *C. coronatus:* confined to rhinofacial area; facial deformity may be quite dramatic
- Angioinvasion does not occur; dissemination or involvement of deep structures rare

Epidemiology

- Both types seen most commonly in Africa, India
- Both fungi are saprophytes present in leaf and plant debris
- Rare diseases without known predisposing factors
- *B. ranarum:* infection occurs after traumatic implantation of fungus into subcutaneous tissues of thighs, buttocks, trunk; occurs mainly in children; male/female ratio 3:1
- *C. coronatus:* infection occurs after inhalation of fungal spores, with subsequent invasion of tissues of nasal cavity, paranasal sinuses, facial soft tissues; predominantly seen in young adults; male/female ratio 10:1

Diagnosis

- Clinical diagnosis usually evident based on gross physical appearance
- Both types of subcutaneous entomophthoromycosis require biopsy for definitive diagnosis

Treatment, Prevention, and Control

- Both types of infection may be treated with itraconazole; oral potassium iodide in saturated solution may be used
- Facial reconstructive surgery may be necessary in the case of *C. coronatus* infection

Many fungal pathogens can produce subcutaneous lesions as part of their disease process; however, certain fungi are commonly introduced traumatically through the skin and have a propensity to involve the deeper layers of the dermis, subcutaneous tissue, and bone. Although they may ultimately present clinically as lesions on the skin surface, they rarely spread to distant organs. In general, the clinical course is chronic and insidious; once established, the infections are refractory to most antifungal therapy. The main subcutaneous fungal infections include lymphocutaneous sporotrichosis, chromoblastomycosis, eumycotic mycetoma, subcutaneous entomophthoromycosis, and subcutaneous phaeohyphomycosis. Two additional subcutaneous fungal or fungal-like processes, lobomycosis and rhinosporidiosis, are discussed separately in Chapter 66.

Although lymphocutaneous sporotrichosis is caused by a single fungal pathogen, *Sporothrix schenckii,* the other subcutaneous mycoses are clinical syndromes caused by multiple fungal etiologies (Table 63-1). The causative agents of subcutaneous mycoses are generally considered to have low pathogenic potential and are commonly isolated from soil, wood, or decaying vegetation. Exposure is largely occupational or related to hobbies (e.g., gardening, wood gathering). Infected patients generally have no underlying immune defect.

• Lymphocutaneous Sporotrichosis

Lymphocutaneous sporotrichosis (Clinical Case 63-1) is caused by *Sporothrix schenckii,* a dimorphic fungus that is ubiquitous in soil and decaying vegetation. Infection with this organism is chronic and is characterized by nodular and ulcerative lesions that develop along lymphatics that drain the primary site of inoculation (Figure 63-1). Dissemination to other sites (e.g., bones, eyes, lungs, central nervous system) is extremely rare (<1% of all cases) and will not be discussed further. At room temperature, *S. schenckii* grows as a mold (Figure 63-2), and at 37° C and in tissue, it is a pleomorphic yeast (Figure 63-3; see Table 63-1).

Morphology

S. schenckii is thermally dimorphic. Mycelial-form cultures grow rapidly and have a wrinkled membranous surface that gradually becomes tan, brown, or black. Microscopically, the mold form consists of narrow, hyaline, septate hyphae that produce abundant oval conidia (2×3 µm to 3×6 µm) borne on delicate sterigmata or in a rosette or "daisy petal" formation on conidiophores (see Figure 63-2). The yeast form consists of spherical, oval, or elongated ("cigar-shaped") yeastlike cells, 2 to 10 µm in diameter, with single or (rarely) multiple buds (see Table 63-1 and Figure 63-3). Although this is the "tissue phase" of *S. schenckii,* yeast forms are rarely seen on histopathologic examination of tissue.

Epidemiology

Sporotrichosis is usually sporadic and is most common in warmer climates. The major known areas of current endemicity are in Japan and North and South America, especially Mexico, Brazil, Uruguay, Peru, and Colombia. Outbreaks of infection related to forest work, mining, and gardening have occurred. Classic infection is associated with traumatic

Table 63-1 Common Agents of Subcutaneous Mycoses

Disease	Etiologic Agent(s)	Typical Morphology in Tissue	Usual Host Reaction
Sporotrichosis	*Sporothrix schenckii*	Pleomorphic, spherical to oval or cigar-shaped yeasts, 2-10 μm diameter with single or multiple (rare) buds See Figure 63-3	Mixed suppurative and granulomatous Splendore-Hoeppli material surrounds fungus (asteroid body) See Figure 63-4
Chromoblastomycosis	*Cladophialophora (Cladosporium) carrionii* *Fonsecaea compacta* *Fonsecaea pedrosoi* *Phialophora verrucosa* *Rhinocladiella* spp. *Exophiala* spp.	Large, 6-12 μm diameter, spherical, thick-walled, brown muriform cells (sclerotic bodies) with septations along one or two planes; pigmented hyphae may be present See Figure 63-6	Mixed suppurative and granulomatous Pseudoepitheliomatous hyperplasia
Eumycotic mycetoma	*Phaeoacremonium* spp. *Fusarium* spp. *Aspergillus nidulans* *Scedosporium boydii* *Madurella* spp. *Exophiala jeanselmei* among others	Granules, 0.2 to several mm diameter, composed of broad (2-6 μm) hyaline (pale granules) or dematiaceous (black granules) septate hyphae that branch and form chlamydoconidia	Suppurative with multiple abscesses, fibrosis, and sinus tracts; Splendore-Hoeppli material
Subcutaneous entomophthoromycosis	*Basidiobolus ranarum (haptosporus)* *Conidiobolus coronatus*	Short, poorly stained hyphal fragments, 6-25 μm diameter, nonparallel sides, pauciseptate, random branches See Figure 63-10	Eosinophilic abscesses and granulation tissue, Splendore-Hoeppli material around hyphae
Subcutaneous phaeohyphomycosis	*Exophiala jeanselmei* *Exophiala dermatitidis* *Alternaria* spp. *Chaetomium* spp. *Curvularia* spp. *Phialophora* spp. among others	Pigmented (brown) hyphae, 2-6 μm diameter, branched or unbranched, often constricted at prominent septations; yeast forms and chlamydoconidia may be present See Figure 63-11	Subcutaneous cystic or solid granulomas; overlying epidermis rarely affected

Modified from Chandler FW, Watts JC: *Pathologic diagnosis of fungal infections,* Chicago, 1987, American Society for Clinical Pathology Press.

Clinical Case 63-1 Sporotrichosis

Haddad and colleagues (*Med Mycol* 40:425–427, 2002) described a case of lymphangitic sporotrichosis after injury with a fish spine. The patient was an 18-year-old male fisherman, resident in a rural area of São Paulo state in Brazil, who wounded his third left finger on the dorsal spines of a fish that was netted during his work. Subsequently, the area around the injury developed edema, ulceration, pain, and purulent secretion. The primary care physician interpreted the lesion as a pyogenic bacterial process and prescribed a 7-day course of oral tetracycline. No improvement was noted, and the therapy was changed to cephalexin, with similar results.

At examination 15 days after the accident, the patient presented with an oozing ulcer and nodules on the dorsum of the left hand and arm, forming an ascending nodular lymphangitic pattern. The diagnostic hypotheses considered were localized lymphangitic sporotrichosis, sporotrichoid leishmaniasis, and atypical mycobacteriosis *(Mycobacterium marinum).* A histopathologic examination of material from the lesion revealed a chronic ulcerated granulomatous pattern of inflammation with intraepidermal microabscesses. No acid-fast bacilli or fungal elements were found. Culture of biopsy material on Sabouraud agar grew a mold characterized by septate thin hyphae with conidia arranged in a rosette at the end of the conidiophores, consistent with *Sporothrix schenckii.* An intradermal reaction to sporotrichin was positive as well. The patient was treated with oral potassium iodide, with clinical resolution at 2 months of therapy.

The clinical presentation in this case was typical of sporotrichosis; however, the source of the infection (fish spine) was unusual. Despite the greater incidence of infection by *M. marinum* among fishermen and aquarists, sporotrichosis must be remembered when these workers show lesions in an ascending lymphangitic pattern after being injured by contact with fish.

inoculation of soil or vegetable or organic matter contaminated with the fungus. Zoonotic transmission has been reported in armadillo hunters and in association with infected cats. Between 1998 and 2001, a large outbreak of cat-transmitted sporotrichosis involving 178 patients was reported in Rio de Janeiro, Brazil.

Clinical Syndromes

Lymphangitic sporotrichosis classically appears after local trauma to an extremity. The initial site of infection appears as a small nodule that may ulcerate. Secondary lymphatic nodules appear about 2 weeks after the appearance of the primary lesion and consist of a linear chain of painless subcutaneous nodules that extend proximally along the course of lymphatic drainage of the primary lesion (see Figure 63-1). With time, the nodules may ulcerate and discharge pus. Primary cutaneous lesions may remain "fixed" without lymphangitic spread. Clinically, these lesions appear nodular, verrucous, or ulcerative and grossly may resemble a malignant process such as squamous cell carcinoma. Other infectious causes of lymphangitic and ulcerative lesions that must be ruled out include mycobacterial and nocardial infections.

Laboratory Diagnosis

Definitive diagnosis usually requires culture of infected pus or tissue. *S. schenckii* grows within 2 to 5 days on a variety of mycologic media and appears as a budding yeast at 35° C and as a mold at 25° C (see Figures 63-2 and 63-3). Laboratory confirmation may be established by converting the mycelial growth to the yeast form by subculture at 37° C or immunologically through the use of the exoantigen test. In tissue, the organism appears as a 2- to 10-µm pleomorphic budding yeast (see Figure 63-3) but is rarely observed in human lesions. The appearance of **Splendore-Hoeppli** material surrounding yeast cells (asteroid body) may be helpful (Figure 63-4) but is also seen in other types of infection (see Table 63-1). A serologic test is available commercially but is rarely used in the diagnosis of sporotrichosis.

Treatment

The classic treatment for lymphocutaneous sporotrichosis is oral potassium iodide in saturated solution. The efficacy and low cost of this medication make it a favored option, especially in resource-poor countries; however, it must be given daily over 3 to 4 weeks and has frequent adverse effects (nausea, salivary gland enlargement). Itraconazole has been shown to be safe and highly effective at low doses and is the current treatment of choice. Patients who do not respond may be given a higher dose of itraconazole, terbinafine, or potassium iodide. Fluconazole or posaconazole may be used if the patient cannot tolerate these other agents. Spontaneous

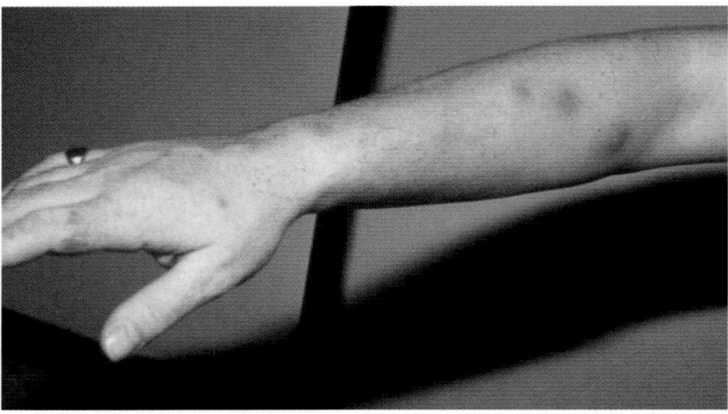

FIGURE 63-1 Classic lymphocutaneous form of sporotrichosis, demonstrating a chain of subcutaneous nodules along the lymphatic drainage of the arm. (From Kradin RL: *Diagnostic pathology of infectious disease,* Philadelphia, 2010, Saunders, Fig. 19-89.)

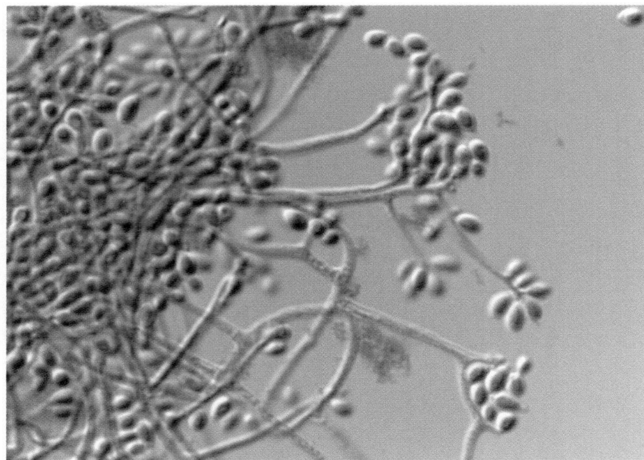

FIGURE 63-2 Mold phase of *Sporothrix schenckii.*

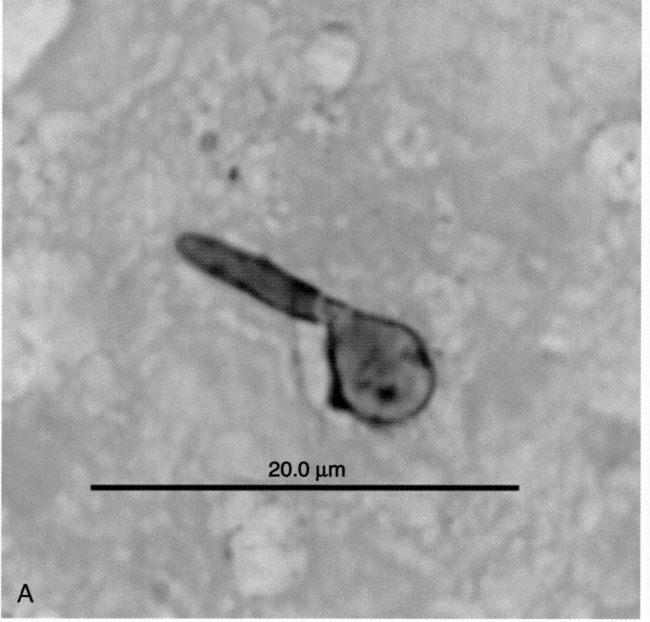

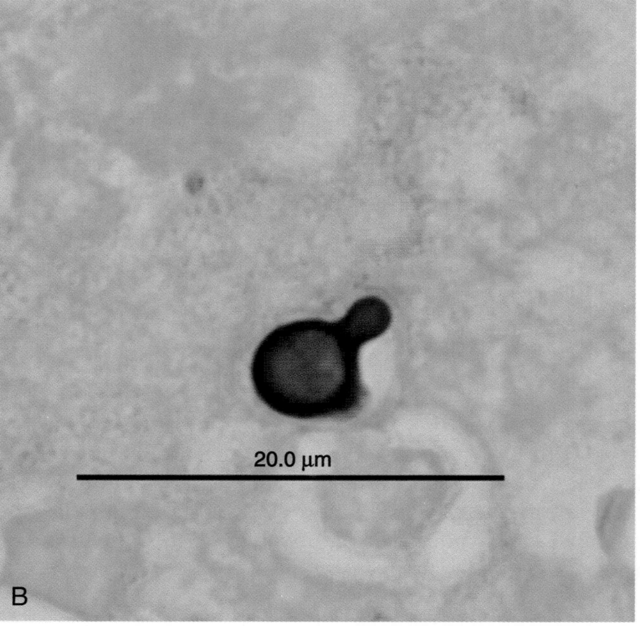

FIGURE 63-3 **A** and **B,** Lung biopsy from disseminated sporotrichosis. The yeast in **A** has a long cigar-shaped bud (Gomori methenamine silver). (From Anaissie EJ, McGinnis MR, Pfaller MA, editors: *Clinical mycology,* London, 2009, Churchill Livingstone.)

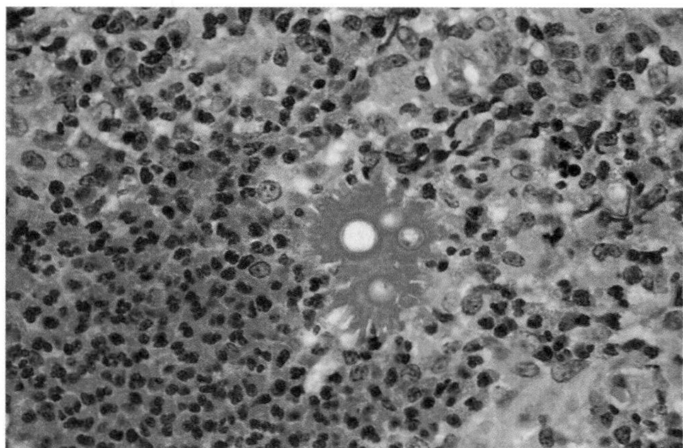

FIGURE 63-4 Asteroid body in sporotrichosis. The spherical yeastlike cells are surrounded by Splendore-Hoeppli material (hematoxylin and eosin, ×160). (From Connor DH, Schwartz DA: *Pathology of infectious diseases*, Stamford, Conn, 1997, Appleton & Lange.)

Clinical Case 63-2 Chromoblastomycosis

Marques and associates (*Med Mycol* 42:261–261, 2004) described a 52-year-old farmer from Brazil who presented with complaints of darkly pigmented pruritic skin lesions. The problem had appeared 2 years earlier and had progressed slowly since then. The patient was unaware of previous trauma but recalled an insect bite on his left arm. Initially, the lesion that developed at this site was a small, raised, erythematous papule. Later, a new crop of lesions appeared on the left leg and, more recently, on the forehead and left side of the face. Physical examination revealed extensive lesions in scaly plaques situated at different sites on the face, arm, and leg. Direct potassium hydroxide examination of biopsies of the lesions showed numerous pigmented, bilaterally dividing, rounded, sclerotic cells (Medlar bodies), thus confirming the clinical diagnosis of chromoblastomycosis. Cultures of the biopsies grew a darkly pigmented mold that was identified on the basis of characteristic conidiation as *Rhinocladiella aquaspersa*. The lesions improved with ketoconazole therapy, with decreasing pruritic symptoms. Unfortunately, the patient was lost to follow-up. Chromoblastomycosis caused by *R. aquaspersa* is relatively uncommon. Furthermore, this case is unusual in that the lesions were dispersed over three different anatomic regions. Of note, the occurrence of facial lesions is very unusual.

remission is rare but was seen in 13 of the 178 cases in Brazil. The local application of heat has also been shown to be effective.

• Chromoblastomycosis

Chromoblastomycosis (chromomycosis; Clinical Case 63-2) is a chronic fungal infection affecting skin and subcutaneous tissues. It is characterized by the development of slow-growing verrucous nodules or plaques (Figure 63-5). Chromoblastomycosis is most commonly seen in the tropics, where the warm, moist environment, coupled with the lack of protective footwear and clothing, predisposes individuals to direct inoculation with infected soil or organic matter. The organisms most often associated with chromoblastomycosis are pigmented (dematiaceous) fungi of the genera *Fonsecaea, Cladosporium, Exophiala, Cladophialophora, Rhinocladiella,* and *Phialophora* (see Table 63-1).

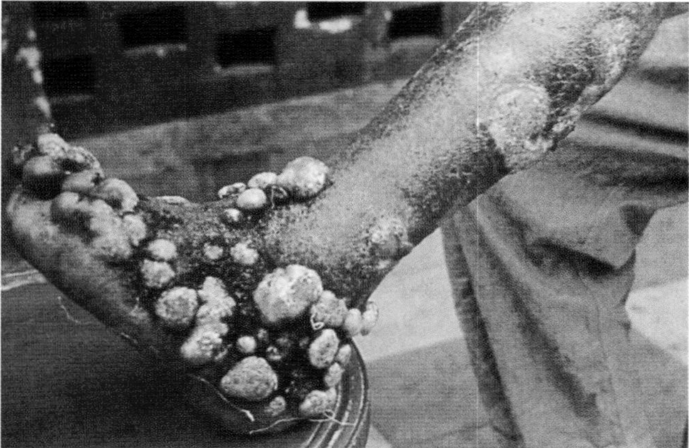

FIGURE 63-5 Chromoblastomycosis of the foot and leg. (From Connor DH, Schwartz DA: *Pathology of infectious diseases*, Stamford, Conn, 1997, Appleton & Lange.)

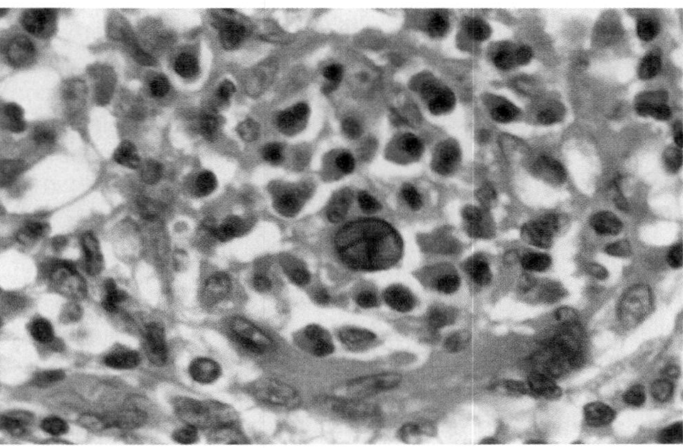

FIGURE 63-6 Brown-pigmented muriform cell, or Medlar body, of chromoblastomycosis (hematoxylin and eosin, ×250). (From Connor DH, Schwartz DA: *Pathology of infectious diseases*, Stamford, Conn, 1997, Appleton & Lange.)

Morphology

The fungi that cause chromoblastomycosis are all dematiaceous (naturally pigmented) molds but are morphologically diverse, and most are capable of producing several different forms when grown in culture. For example, *Exophiala* spp. may grow as a mold and produce conidia-bearing cells called **annelids** and also as a yeastlike form that may appear in freshly isolated colonies. Although the basic form of these organisms is a pigmented septate mold, the different mechanisms of sporulation produced in culture makes specific identification difficult. Specific identification may require nucleic acid sequence analysis.

In contrast to the diverse morphology seen in culture, in tissue the fungi that cause chromoblastomycosis all characteristically form muriform cells (sclerotic bodies, **Medlar**

bodies) that are chestnut brown because of the melanin in their cell walls (Figure 63-6; see Table 63-1). Muriform cells divide by internal septation and appear as cells with vertical and horizontal lines within the same or different planes (see Figure 63-6). In addition to muriform cells, pigmented hyphae may also be present. The fungal cells may be free within the tissue but most often are contained within macrophages or giant cells.

Epidemiology

Chromoblastomycosis generally affects individuals working in rural areas of the tropics. The etiologic agents grow on woody plants and in the soil. Most infections have been in men and involve legs and arms, likely the result of occupational exposure. Other body sites include shoulders, neck, trunk, buttocks, face, and ears. Local climatic factors may influence the distribution of different infections and different etiologic agents. For example, in Madagascar, infections caused by *Fonsecaea pedrosoi* are seen in areas of high rainfall (200 to 300 cm annually), whereas in the same island, infections caused by *Cladophialophora carrionii* occur in areas of low rainfall (50 to 60 cm annually). In the Americas, *F. pedrosoi* is the principal cause of chromoblastomycoses, and the lesions most often involve the lower extremities. In contrast, in Australia, the most common cause is *C. carrionii,* and the lesions are most frequently on the upper limbs, especially the hands. There are no reports of person-to-person transmission.

Clinical Syndromes

Chromoblastomycosis tends to be chronic, pruritic, progressive, indolent, and resistant to treatment. In most instances, patients do not present until the infection is well established. Early lesions are small, warty papules and usually enlarge only slowly. There are different morphologic forms of the disease, ranging from verrucous lesions to flat plaques. Established infections appear as multiple large, warty, "cauliflower-like" growths that are usually clustered within the same region (see Figure 63-5). Satellite lesions may occur secondary to autoinoculation. Plaquelike lesions often show central scarring as they enlarge. Ulceration and cyst formation may occur. Large lesions are hyperkeratotic, and the limb is grossly distorted because of fibrosis and secondary lymphedema (see Figure 63-5). Secondary bacterial infection may also occur and contribute to regional lymphadenitis, lymph stasis, and eventual elephantiasis.

Laboratory Diagnosis

The clinical presentation (see Figure 63-5), histopathologic findings of chestnut-brown muriform cells (see Figure 63-6), and isolation in culture of one of the causal fungi (see Table 63-1) confirm the diagnosis. Scrapings obtained from the surface of the warty lesions where small dark dots are observed may result in the demonstration of the characteristic cells when mounted in 20% potassium hydroxide (KOH). Biopsy specimens stained with hematoxylin and eosin (H&E) (see Chapter 60) will also show the organism present in the epidermis or in microabscesses containing macrophages and giant cells. The inflammatory reaction is both suppurative and granulomatous, with dermal fibrosis and **pseudoepitheliomatous hyperplasia.** The organisms are easily cultured from the lesions, although identification may be difficult. There are no serologic tests available for chromoblastomycosis.

Treatment

Treatment with specific antifungal therapy is often ineffective because of the advanced stage of infection upon presentation. The drugs that appear to be most effective are itraconazole and terbinafine. More recently, posaconazole has been used with modest success. These agents are often combined with flucytosine in refractory cases. In an effort to improve the response to treatment, attempts are often made to shrink larger lesions with local heat or cryotherapy before administering antifungal agents. Because of the risk of recurrences developing within the scar, surgery is not indicated. Squamous cell carcinomas may develop in long-standing lesions, and those with atypical areas or fleshy outgrowths should be biopsied to rule out this complication.

• Eumycotic Mycetoma

Eumycotic mycetomas are those caused by true fungi, as opposed to actinomycotic mycetomas, which are caused by aerobic actinomycetes (bacteria). This section will deal only with the eumycotic mycetomas.

As with chromoblastomycosis, most eumycotic mycetomas are seen in the tropics. A mycetoma is defined clinically as a localized, chronic, granulomatous, infectious process involving cutaneous and subcutaneous tissues. It is characterized by the formation of multiple granulomas and abscesses that contain large aggregates of fungal hyphae known as **granules** or **grains.** These grains contain cells that have marked modifications of internal and external structure, ranging from reduplications of the cell wall to the formation of a hard cement-like extracellular matrix. The abscesses drain externally through the skin, often with extrusion of granules. The process may be quite extensive and deforming, with destruction of muscle, fascia, and bone. The etiologic agents of eumycotic mycetoma encompass a wide range of fungi, including *Phaeoacremonium, Curvularia, Fusarium, Madurella, Mediacopsis, Biatrophia, Trematosphaeria, Exophiala, Falciformispora,* and *Scedosporium/Pseudallescheria* species (see Table 63-1).

Morphology

The granules of eumycotic mycetomas are composed of septate fungal hyphae that are 2 to 6 µm or greater in width and are either dematiaceous (black grain) or hyaline (pale or white grain), depending on the etiologic agent (Figure 63-7). The hyphae are frequently distorted and bizarre in form and size. Large, spherical, thick-walled chlamydoconidia are often present. The hyphae may be embedded in an amorphous cement-like substance. Splendore-Hoeppli material often interdigitates among the mycelial elements at the periphery of the granule. Eumycotic granules may be differentiated from actinomycotic granules based on morphologic (branched filaments versus septate hyphae and chlamydoconidia) and staining (gram-positive beaded rods versus periodic acid–Schiff [PAS]- and Gomori methenamine silver [GMS]-positive hyphae) characteristics (see Chapter 60). Culture is usually necessary for definitive identification of the fungus (or actinomycete) involved.

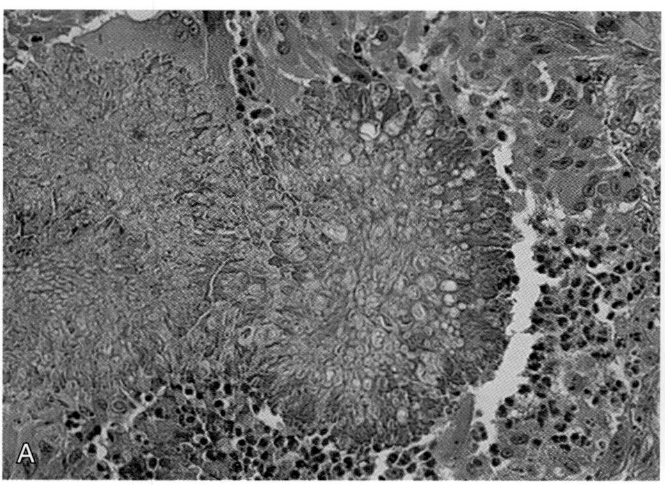

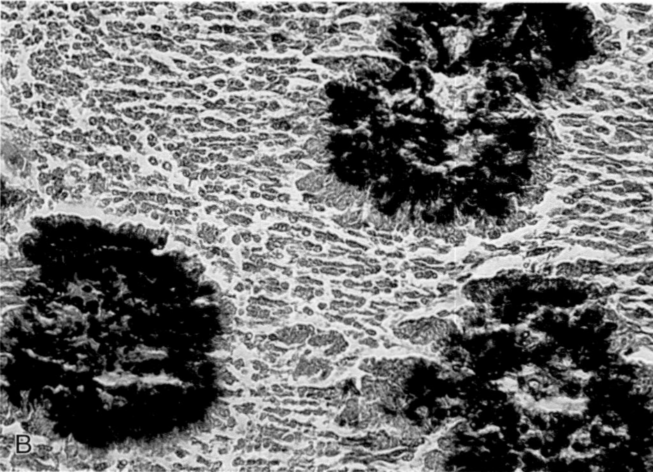

FIGURE 63-7 **A,** Mycetoma granule of *Curvularia geniculata.* **B,** Compact dematiaceous hyphae and chlamydoconidia embedded in cement-like substance.

Epidemiology

Mycetomas are primarily seen in tropical areas with low rainfall. Eumycotic mycetomas are more frequent in Africa and the Indian subcontinent but also may be seen in Brazil, Venezuela, and the Middle East. All patients are infected from sources in nature via traumatic percutaneous implantation of the etiologic agent into exposed parts of the body. The foot and hand are most common, but back, shoulders, and chest-wall infections are also seen. Men are more often affected than women. The fungi that cause eumycotic mycetomas differ from country to country, and the agents that are common in one region are rarely reported from others. Mycetomas are not contagious.

Clinical Syndromes

Similar to chromoblastomycosis, patients with eumycotic mycetoma most commonly present with long-standing infection. The earliest lesion is a small, painless, subcutaneous nodule or plaque that increases slowly but progressively in size. As the mycetoma develops, the affected area gradually enlarges and becomes disfigured as a result of chronic inflammation and fibrosis. With time, sinus tracts appear on the skin surface and drain serosanguineous fluid that often contains grossly visible granules. The infection commonly breaches tissue planes and destroys muscle and bone locally. Hematogenous or lymphatic spread from a primary focus to distant sites or viscera is extremely rare.

Laboratory Diagnosis

The key to the diagnosis of eumycotic mycetoma is the demonstration of grains or granules. Grains may be grossly visible in draining sinus tracts or may be expressed onto a glass slide. Material may also be obtained by deep surgical biopsy.

Grains can be visualized microscopically by mounting in 20% KOH. The hyphae are usually clearly visible, as is the presence or absence of pigmentation. Grains can be washed and then cultured or fixed and sectioned for histopathology.

Grains are easily visualized in tissue stained with H&E (see Figure 63-7). Special stains such as PAS and GMS may also be helpful. Although the color, shape, size, and microscopic morphology may be characteristic of a specific causal agent, culture is usually necessary for definitive identification of the organism. Most organisms will grow on standard mycologic medium; however, inclusion of an antibiotic such as penicillin may be useful to inhibit contaminating bacteria, which may overgrow the fungus.

Treatment

Treatment of eumycotic mycetoma is usually unsuccessful. Response of the various etiologic agents to amphotericin B, ketoconazole, or itraconazole is variable and often poor, although such therapy may slow the course of infection. Promising treatment responses have recently been reported for terbinafine, voriconazole, and posaconazole. Local excision is usually ineffective or not possible, and amputation is the only definitive treatment. Because these infections are usually slowly progressive and may be slowed further by specific antifungal therapy, the decision to amputate should take into account the rate of progression, symptomatology, availability of adequate prosthetics, and the patient's individual circumstances. For all these reasons, it is imperative to differentiate eumycotic mycetoma from actinomycotic mycetoma. Medical therapy is usually effective in cases of actinomycotic mycetoma.

• Subcutaneous Entomophthoromycosis

Subcutaneous **entomophthoromycosis,** also known as subcutaneous mucormycosis, is caused by Mucormycetes of the order Entomophthorales: *Conidiobolus coronatus* and *Basidiobolus ranarum (haptosporus)* (see Table 63-1). Both of these fungi cause a chronic subcutaneous form of mucormycosis that occurs sporadically as a result of traumatic implantation of the fungus present in plant debris in tropical environments. They differ in that they cause infections with different anatomic locations: *B. ranarum* causes subcutaneous infection of the proximal limbs in children, whereas *C. coronatus* infection is localized to the facial area, predominantly in adults (Figures 63-8 and 63-9).

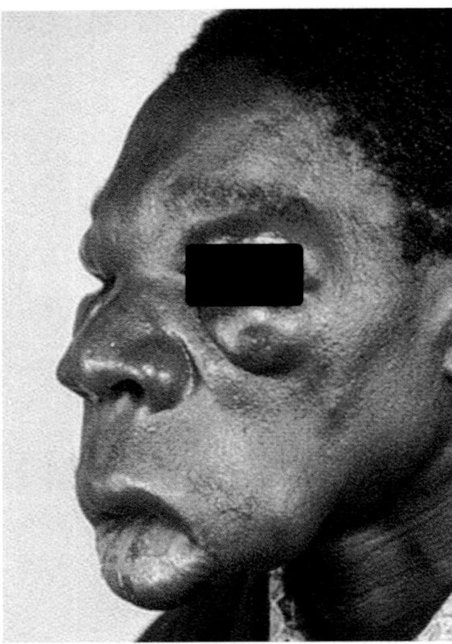

FIGURE 63-8 Subcutaneous entomophthoromycosis caused by *Conidiobolus coronatus.* (From Hay RJ: Fungal infections, *Clin Dermatol* 24(3):201–212, 2006, Fig. 6.)

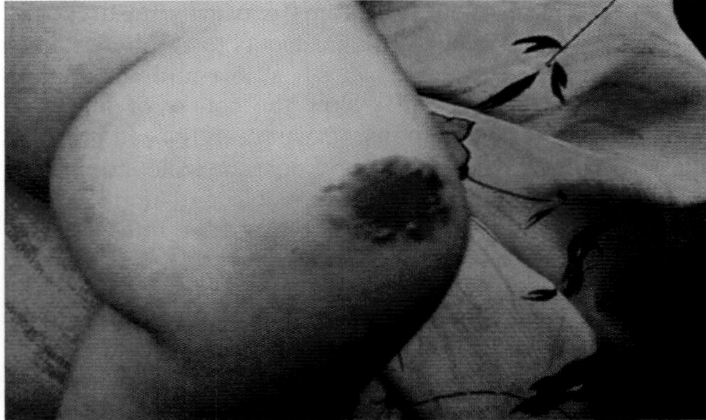

FIGURE 63-9 Subcutaneous entomophthoromycosis caused by *Basidiobolus ranarum.* The right thigh is extensively swollen and indurated. (From Anaparthy UR, Deepika G: A case of subcutaneous zygomycosis, *Indian Dermatol Online J* 5:51–54, 2014, Fig. 1.)

Morphology

The appearance of the agents of subcutaneous entomophthoromycosis in tissue differs from that of the mucoraceous Mucormycetes. Hyphal elements are sparse and often appear as hyphal fragments surrounded by intensely eosinophilic Splendore-Hoeppli material (Figure 63-10). The inflammatory response is granulomatous and rich in eosinophils. The hyphal fragments are thin walled and poorly staining. Although septae are infrequent, they are more prominent than those seen with Mucoraceae. The hyphae of the Entomophthoraceae are not angioinvasive.

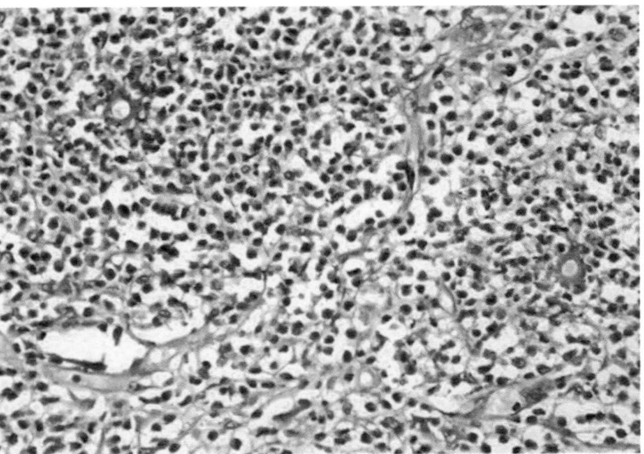

FIGURE 63-10 Subcutaneous entomophthoromycosis. Broad hyphal fragments surrounded by eosinophilic Splendore-Hoeppli material (hematoxylin and eosin, ×160). (From Anand M, Deshmukh SD, Pande DP, et al: Subcutaneous zygomycosis due to *Basidiobolus ranarum*: a case report from Maharastra, India, *J Trop Med* 2010:950390, 2010.)

Epidemiology

Both types of subcutaneous entomophthoromycosis are seen most commonly in Africa and, to a lesser extent, India. Infection caused by *B. ranarum* has also been reported from the Middle East, Asia, and Europe, whereas that caused by *C. coronatus* has been reported from Latin America as well as Africa and India. Both fungi are saprophytes that are present in leaf and plant debris. *B. ranarum* has also been found in the intestinal contents of small reptiles and amphibians. Both are rare diseases without known predisposing factors (e.g., acidosis or immunodeficiency). Infection caused by *B. ranarum* is thought to occur after traumatic implantation of the fungus into the subcutaneous tissues of the thighs, buttocks, and trunk. This form of subcutaneous entomophthoromycosis occurs mainly in children (80% < age 20), with a male/female ratio of 3 : 1. *C. coronatus* infections occur after inhalation of the fungal spores, which then invade the tissues of the nasal cavity, the paranasal sinuses, and facial soft tissues. There is a 10 : 1 male/female ratio, and the disease is seen predominantly among young adults. Infection among children is rare.

Clinical Syndromes

Patients infected with *B. ranarum* have disk-shaped, rubbery, movable masses that may be quite large and are localized to the shoulder, pelvis, hips, and thighs (see Figure 63-9). The masses may expand locally and eventually ulcerate. Dissemination or involvement of deeper structures is rare. Gastrointestinal basidiobolomycosis has recently been reported in the southwestern United States.

C. coronatus infection is confined to the rhinofacial area and often does not come to medical attention until there is a noticeable swelling of the upper lip or face (see Figure 63-8). The swelling is firm and painless and may progress slowly to involve the nasal bridge and the upper and lower face, including the orbit. The facial deformity can be quite dramatic; however, because of the lack of angioinvasion, intracranial extension does not occur.

Laboratory Diagnosis

Both types of subcutaneous entomophthoromycosis require biopsy for diagnosis, despite the characteristic clinical features of the infections. The histopathologic picture is the same for both organisms (see Figure 63-10) and is marked by focal clusters of inflammation, with eosinophils and typical mucormycotic hyphae often surrounded by eosinophilic Splendore-Hoeppli material. The organisms can be cultured from clinical material on standard mycologic medium.

Treatment

Both types of infection may be treated with itraconazole. Alternatively, oral potassium iodide in saturated solution has been used. Facial reconstructive surgery may be necessary in the case of *C. coronatus* infection; extensive fibrosis remains after eradication of the fungus.

• Subcutaneous Phaeohyphomycosis

Phaeohyphomycosis (Clinical Case 63-3) is a term used to describe a heterogeneous array of fungal infections caused by pigmented (dematiaceous) fungi that are present in tissue as irregular hyphae (Figure 63-11) rather than the sclerotic muriform cells seen in chromoblastomycosis (see Table 63-1 and Figure 63-6). These infections may be caused by a wide range of fungi, all of which exist in nature as saprophytes of soil, wood, and decaying vegetation. Phaeohyphomycotic processes may be superficial, subcutaneous, or deeply invasive or disseminated. The superficial (see Chapter 62) and deeply invasive (see Chapter 65) forms are discussed in their respective chapters. The subcutaneous form is discussed in this section.

Clinical Case 63-3 Phaeohyphomycosis in a Renal Transplant Patient

Marques and associates (*Med Mycol* 44:671–676, 2006) described a case of subcutaneous phaeohyphomycosis in a renal transplant recipient. The patient was a 49-year-old diabetic man who for 5 years had been given immunosuppressive therapy with prednisone and cyclosporine A after kidney transplantation. He presented with a 1-year history of draining foot lesions. The patient denied any history of local trauma but had been working in rural activities at the time of the initial complaint. He had been treated for presumed bacterial infection, without response. Dermatologic examination revealed two confluent erythematous cystic tumors on the dorsum of the left foot, with drainage points emitting a serosanguineous secretion. A local computed tomography scan showed only circumscribed hypodense lesions. A needle aspiration and a large biopsy were obtained to confirm the presumed diagnosis of phaeohyphomycosis. Histopathologic examination revealed intense inflammatory infiltrates and rare hyphal elements. Culture of the biopsy material revealed a slow-growing mold that eventually demonstrated a beige to gray-brown coloration. The organism was eventually identified as *Phaeoacremonium parasiticum* by a combination of morphology and molecular identification methods. The patient was treated with itraconazole coupled with local irrigation and a decrease in the dosing of cyclosporine A and achieved a satisfactory response.

This case illustrates an apparent trend for immunocompromised organ transplant patients with localized *P. parasiticum* infections to have acquired their infections without recognized trauma. It is unclear whether such infections are acquired via minor skin fissures or via inhalation or ingestion of an infectious particle, with subsequent translocation to subcutaneous capillary beds, where slightly diminished temperature or other local conditions may favor growth.

Morphology

The agents of subcutaneous phaeohyphomycosis are numerous and diverse (see Table 63-1), but all grow as black molds in culture and appear as dark-walled, irregular, hyphal, and yeastlike forms in tissue (see Figure 63-11). The hyphae vary from 2 to 6 µm wide and may be branched or septate and are often constricted at the point of septation. Bizarre thick-walled vesicular swellings that may be as large as 25 µm in diameter may be present, as well as budding yeastlike structures. Cell wall pigmentation ranges from light to dark and may require special stains (e.g., Fontana-Masson melanin stain) to confirm the dematiaceous nature of the fungus. In culture, the different fungi grow as black or brown molds and are identified by their characteristic mode of sporulation.

Epidemiology

More than 20 different dematiaceous fungi have been cited as causes of subcutaneous phaeohyphomycosis. The most frequent etiologic agents have been *Exophiala jeanselmei, Alternaria, Curvularia,* and *Phaeoacremonium* spp. (see Table 63-1). Because these fungi are found in soil and plant debris, the route of infection is thought to be secondary to traumatic implantation of the fungus. Indeed, wood splinters have been found in histopathologic material, suggesting the mode of inoculation and possibly that the formation of the characteristic phaeohyphomycotic cyst is a reaction to implantation. There is no explanation for why some organisms produce phaeohyphomycotic cysts and others develop into mycetomas.

Clinical Syndromes

Most commonly, subcutaneous phaeohyphomycosis presents as a solitary inflammatory cyst. The lesions generally

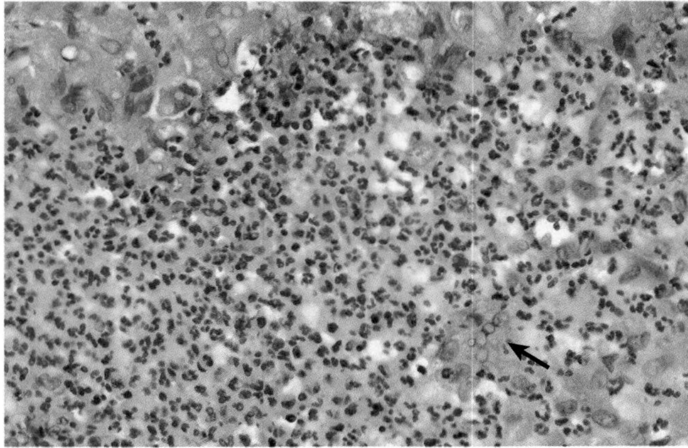

FIGURE 63-11 Subcutaneous phaeohyphomycosis. Dematiaceous yeastlike cells and septate hyphae of *Exophiala spinifera* with surrounding Splendore-Hoeppli material *(arrow)* (hematoxylin and eosin, ×250). (From Brinster N, Liu V, Diwan H, et al: *Dermatopathology: a volume in the high yield pathology series,* Philadelphia, 2011, Saunders, p 258, Fig. 5.)

occur on the feet and legs, although the hands and other body sites may be involved. The lesions grow slowly and expand over a period of months or years. They may be firm or fluctuant and are usually painless. If located near a joint, they may be mistaken for a synovial cyst and may become large enough to interfere with movement. Other manifestations include formation of pigmented plaquelike lesions that are indurated but nontender.

Laboratory Diagnosis

The diagnosis is made upon surgical excision of the cyst. On histopathologic examination, the appearance is of an inflammatory cyst with a fibrous capsule, granulomatous reaction, and central necrosis. Individual and clustered dematiaceous fungal elements are seen within giant cells and extracellularly amid the necrotic debris (see Figure 63-11). In general, the pigmentation is easily seen on examination of H&E-stained tissue. The organisms can be grown in culture and identified by their pattern of sporulation.

Treatment

The main treatment is surgical excision. Plaquelike lesions may not be amenable to this approach and generally respond to treatment with itraconazole with or without concomitant flucytosine. Posaconazole, voriconazole, and terbinafine may also be active against these groups of fungi.

Bibliography

Ahmed AOA, De Hoog GS: Fungi causing eumycotic mycetoma. In Versalovic J, et al, editors: *Manual of clinical microbiology*, ed 10, Washington, DC, 2011, American Society for Microbiology Press.

Barros MB, Schubach Ade O, do Valle AC, et al: Cat-transmitted sporotrichosis epidemic in Rio de Janeiro, Brazil: description of a series of cases, *Clin Infect Dis* 38:529–535, 2004.

Chandler FW, Watts JC: *Pathologic diagnosis of fungal infections*, Chicago, 1987, American Society for Clinical Pathology Press.

Connor DH, Schwartz DA: *Pathology of infectious diseases*, Stamford, Conn, 1997, Appleton & Lange.

Garcia-Hermoso D, et al: Agents of systemic and subcutaneous mucormycosis and entomophthoromycosis. In Versalovic J, et al, editors: *Manual of clinical microbiology*, ed 10, Washington, DC, 2011, American Society for Microbiology Press.

Guarro J, De Hoog GS: *Bipolaris, Exophiala, Scedosporium, Sporothrix*, and other melanized fungi. In Versalovic J, et al, editors: *Manual of clinical microbiology*, ed 10, Washington, DC, 2011, American Society for Microbiology Press.

Kauffman CA, Bustamante B, Chapman SW, et al: Clinical practice guidelines for the management of sporotrichosis: 2007 update by the Infectious Diseases Society of America, *Clin Infect Dis* 45:1255, 2007.

CHAPTER

64 SYSTEMIC MYCOSES CAUSED BY DIMORPHIC FUNGI

Jane and Joan were two avid "outdoors persons" in their mid-30s. In the past 5 years, they had been spelunking in southern Missouri, backpacking in northern Wisconsin, and camping in Arizona. Most recently, they had been renovating an old farmhouse in rural Iowa, and in the process had to tear down an old chicken coop that was attached to the back of the house. About 1 week into the process, they both suffered from a flulike illness, and Jane developed a cough and shortness of breath. They sought medical attention at the family practice clinic. At the clinic, Joan appeared fine, but Jane was noted to be quite short of breath and appeared ill. The doctor thought it would be a good idea to get a chest radiograph for Jane. Joan got one too, just in case. Jane's chest radiograph showed a diffuse bilateral pneumonia. Although Joan's radiograph did not show pneumonia, it was noted that she had a solitary nodule in the right upper lobe.

1. What dimorphic fungal pathogens were Jane and Joan exposed to?
2. What constitutes a dimorphic fungus?
3. Aside from dimorphism, what feature is common to all of the endemic mycoses?
4. Describe the life cycles of the dimorphic endemic pathogens.
5. What do you think is the cause of Jane's pneumonia? How would you make the diagnosis?
6. How would you treat her pneumonia?
7. What do you think accounts for Joan's lung nodule? How would you make the diagnosis? How would you treat her?

Answers to these questions are available on StudentConsult.com.

• SUMMARIES CLINICALLY SIGNIFICANT ORGANISMS

Blastomyces dermatitidis

Trigger Words

Mississippi River Valley, broad-based budding yeast, healthy and immunocompromised, granuloma

Biology, Virulence, and Disease

- Thermally dimorphic fungus: large nonencapsulated budding yeast cells in tissue and in culture at 37° C; mold colonies form in culture at 25° C
- Usual route of infection is inhalation of conidia
- Severity of symptoms and course of disease depends on extent of exposure and immune status of exposed individual; most are asymptomatic
- Classic form of blastomycosis: chronic cutaneous involvement

Epidemiology

- Ecologic niche: decaying organic matter
- Area of endemicity: southeastern and south central states, especially bordering Ohio and Mississippi river basins; Midwest states and Canadian provinces bordering Great Lakes; and an area in New York and Canada along the St. Lawrence River
- Outbreaks of infection have been associated with occupational or recreational contact with soil

Diagnosis

- Microscopic detection of fungus in tissue or other clinical material, with confirmation by culture
- Antigen detection and PCR

Treatment, Prevention, and Control

- Pulmonary blastomycosis in immunocompromised patients and those with progressive pulmonary disease should be treated
- All patients with evidence of hematogenous dissemination require antifungal therapy
- Lipid formulation of amphotericin B: treatment of choice for meningeal disease and other life-threatening presentations
- Mild or moderate disease: itraconazole; fluconazole, posaconazole, or voriconazole may be substituted for itraconazole

Coccidioides immitis and *C. posadasii*

Trigger Words

Valley fever, coccidioidal granuloma, arthroconidia, spherule, skin test, precipitin test

Biology, Virulence, and Disease

- Coccidioidomycosis caused by two indistinguishable species: *C. immitis* and *C. posadasii*
- *C. immitis* localized to California; *C. posadasii,* most infections outside California
- Disease caused by inhalation of infectious arthroconidia
- Asymptomatic or subclinical, self-limited flulike illness, acute and chronic pulmonary disease, single or multisystem dissemination
- Dimorphic fungi; endosporulating spherule in tissue, mold in culture at 25° C and in nature

Epidemiology

- Endemic to U.S. Desert Southwest, northern Mexico, scattered areas of Central and South America
- Organism found in soil; growth in environment enhanced by bat and rodent droppings; cycles of drought/rain enhance organism dispersion
- Persons ≥ 65 years and those with HIV infection disproportionately affected
- Risk of disseminated disease highest in certain ethnic groups (Filipino, African American, Native American, Hispanic), males (9:1), women in third trimester of pregnancy, individuals with cellular immune deficiency, persons at extremes of age

Diagnosis

- Histopathologic examination of tissue or other clinical material, isolation of fungus in culture, serology
- Histopathologic examination that reveals endosporulating spherules in sputum, exudates, or tissue is sufficient to establish the diagnosis
- Culture at 25° C takes days and poses risk to laboratory workers; all work with molds should be performed in suitable biosafety cabinet
- Serology (antigen and antibody) may be useful for initial screening, confirmation, or prognostic evaluation

Treatment, Prevention, and Control

- Most individuals with primary infection do not require therapy
- For those with concurrent risk factors or a more severe presentation: lipid formulation of amphotericin B followed by an oral azole as maintenance therapy (severe disease)
- Chronic cavitary pulmonary disease: azole for at least 1 year
- Nonmeningeal extrapulmonary disseminated infections: oral azole
- Meningeal coccidioidomycosis: fluconazole; itraconazole, posaconazole or voriconazole are secondary choices

Histoplasma capsulatum

Trigger Words

Intracellular yeasts, bird and bat droppings, chicken coop, caves, guano, granulomas

Biology, Virulence, and Disease

- Histoplasmosis caused by two varieties of *Histoplasma capsulatum*
- *H. capsulatum* var. *capsulatum:* causes pulmonary and disseminated infections
- *H. capsulatum* var. *duboisii:* causes predominantly skin and bone lesions
- Disease caused by inhalation of infectious microconidia
- Severity of symptoms and course of disease depend on extent of exposure and immune status of infected individual; most are asymptomatic, self-limited; flulike illness also occurs
- Thermically dimorphic fungus: hyaline mold in nature and in culture at 25° C, budding yeast in tissue (intracellular) and in culture at 37° C

Epidemiology

- *H. capsulatum* var. *capsulatum:* localized to Ohio and Mississippi river valleys; occurs throughout Mexico and Central and South America
- *H. capsulatum* var. *duboisii:* confined to tropical Africa (e.g., Gabon, Uganda, Kenya)
- Found in soil with high nitrogen content (e.g., areas contaminated with bird or bat droppings)
- Outbreaks of disease have been associated with exposure to bird roosts, caves, and decaying buildings or urban renewal projects involving excavation and demolition
- Immunocompromised individuals and children most prone to develop symptomatic disease
- Reactivation of disease and dissemination common among immunosuppressed individuals, especially those with AIDS

Diagnosis

- Direct microscopy, culture of clinical material, serology (antigen and antibody), β-D-glucan, and PCR have been useful
- Yeast phase of organism can be detected in sputum, bronchoalveolar lavage fluid, peripheral blood films, bone marrow, and tissue stained with Giemsa, GMS, or PAS stains
- Cultures should be handled in a biosafety cabinet
- Serologic diagnosis employs tests for antibody and antigen

Treatment, Prevention, and Control

- Severe acute infections: lipid formulation of amphotericin B followed by oral itraconazole
- Chronic pulmonary histoplasmosis: lipid formulation of amphotericin B followed by itraconazole
- Disseminated infection: lipid formulation of amphotericin B followed by itraconazole

Paracoccidioides brasiliensis

Trigger Words

Pilot's wheel, South American blastomycosis, ulcer, multiple buds

Biology, Virulence, and Disease

- Thermally dimorphic fungus: slowly growing mold phase in nature and at 25° C, yeast phase (variable sized with single or multiple buds) in tissue and in culture at 37° C
- Usual route of infection is inhalation or possible traumatic inoculation of conidia or hyphal fragments
- Paracoccidioidomycosis may be subclinical or progressive with acute or chronic pulmonary forms or acute, subacute, or chronic disseminated forms

Epidemiology

- Endemic throughout Latin America, areas of high humidity, rich vegetation, moderate temperatures, acid soil
- Ecologic niche not well established
- Overt disease uncommon among children and adolescents; in adults, disease more common in men aged 30 to 50 years
- Most patients with clinically apparent disease live in rural areas and have close contact with soil
- No reports of epidemics or person-to-person transmission

Diagnosis

- Demonstration of characteristic yeast forms on microscopic examination of clinical material: oval to round with double refractile walls and single or multiple buds; "pilot-wheel" morphology
- May be isolated in culture and should be handled in a biosafety cabinet
- Serology testing may help in suggesting diagnosis, evaluating response to therapy

Treatment, Prevention, and Control

- Itraconazole: treatment of choice for most forms of disease
- More severe or refractory forms: lipid formulation of amphotericin B followed by either itraconazole or sulfonamide therapy

The **dimorphic** fungal pathogens are organisms that exist in a mold form in nature or in the laboratory at 25° C to 30° C, and in a yeast or spherule form in tissues or when grown on enriched medium in the laboratory at 37° C (Figure 64-1). The majority of organisms in this group are considered primary **systemic** pathogens because of their ability to cause infection in both "normal" and immunocompromised hosts and for their propensity to involve the deep viscera after dissemination of the fungus from the lungs after its inhalation from nature. The dimorphic systemic pathogens include *Blastomyces dermatitidis, Coccidioides immitis* and *Coccidioides posadasii, Histoplasma capsulatum* var. *capsulatum* and *H. capsulatum* var. *duboisii, Paracoccidioides brasiliensis,* and *Talaromyces* (formerly *Penicillium*) *marneffei* (Table 64-1). These organisms are also known as **endemic** pathogens in that their natural habitat is delimited to specific geographic regions (Figure 64-2) and infection caused by a particular fungus is acquired by inhalation of spores from that specific environment and geographic location (see Table 64-1). *H. capsulatum, C. immitis (C. posadasii),* and *T. marneffei* have emerged as major opportunistic pathogens in individuals with acquired immunodeficiency syndrome (AIDS) and other forms of immunosuppression. Recognition of these endemic mycoses may be complicated by the fact that they may become manifest only after the patient has left the area of endemicity. Often the infection may be quiescent, only to reactivate when the individual becomes immunosuppressed and is living in an area where the fungus is not endemic. In addition to these dimorphic pathogens, a recent report from South Africa suggests that a new species of *Emmonsia* related to the dimorphic fungus *Emmonsia pasteuriana* may be an emerging dimorphic pathogen in individuals with late-stage HIV infection.

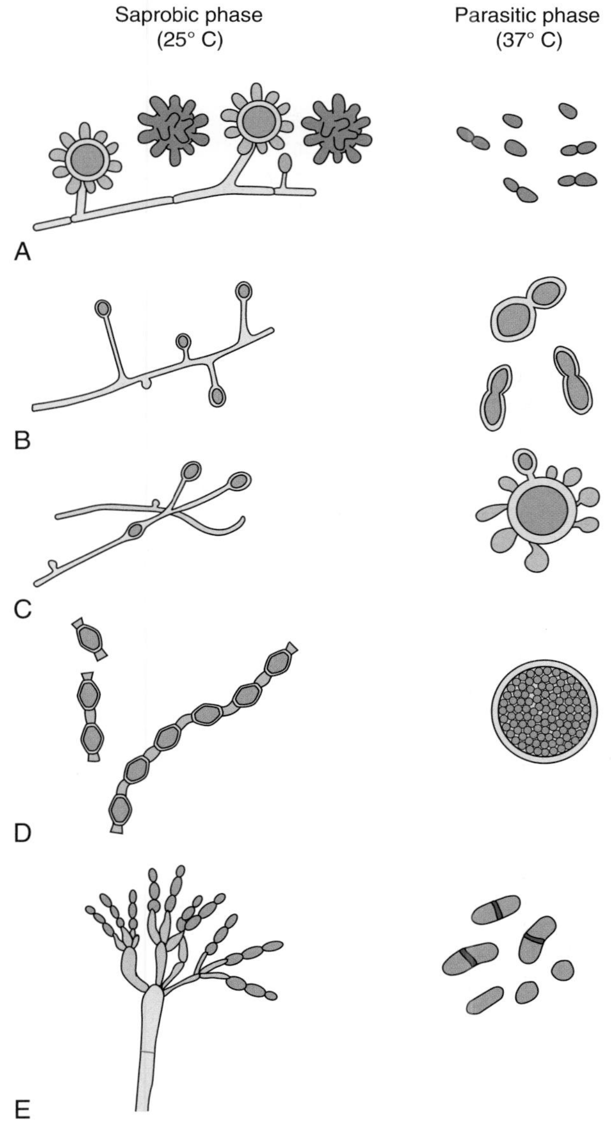

Saprobic phase (25° C)

Parasitic phase (37° C)

A

B

C

D

E

FIGURE 64-1 Saprobic and parasitic phases of endemic dimorphic fungi. **A,** *Histoplasma capsulatum.* **B,** *Blastomyces dermatitidis.* **C,** *Paracoccidioides brasiliensis.* **D,** *Coccidioides immitis.* **E,** *Talaromyces marneffei.*

• Blastomycosis

Blastomycosis (Clinical Case 64-1) is a systemic fungal infection caused by the dimorphic pathogen *Blastomyces dermatitidis.* Like other endemic mycoses, this infection is confined to specific geographic regions, with most infections originating in the Mississippi River basin, around the Great Lakes, and in the southeastern region of the United States (see Figure 64-2). Cases have also been diagnosed in other parts of the world, including Africa, Europe, and the Middle East.

Morphology

As a thermally dimorphic fungus, *B. dermatitidis* produces nonencapsulated yeastlike cells in tissue and in culture on enriched media at 37° C and white to tan, filamentous mold colonies on standard mycologic media at 25° C. The mold form produces round to oval or pear-shaped conidia (2 to 10 µm) located on long or short terminal hyphal branches (Figure 64-3). Older cultures may also produce 7- to 18-µm diameter thick-walled chlamydospores. This form of *B. dermatitidis* is not diagnostic and may not be distinguishable from the monomorphic *Chrysosporium* spp. or from an early culture of *H. capsulatum.*

The yeast form of *B. dermatitidis* is seen in tissue and in culture at 37° C. This form is quite distinctive (Figure 64-4). The yeast cells are spherical, hyaline, 8 to 15 µm in diameter, multinucleated, and have thick "double-contoured" walls. The cytoplasm is often retracted from the rigid cell wall as a result of shrinkage during the fixation process. The yeast cells reproduce by the formation of buds or **blastoconidia.** The buds are usually single and attached to the parent cell by broad bases (see Figure 64-4).

The yeast forms may be visualized in tissue stained with hematoxylin and eosin (H&E); however, the fungal stains Gomori methenamine silver (GMS) and periodic acid–Schiff (PAS) help locate the organisms and delineate their morphology.

Epidemiology

The ecologic niche of *B. dermatitidis* appears to be in decaying organic matter. Studies in humans and animals indicate that infection is acquired after inhalation of aerosolized conidia produced by the fungus growing in soil and leaf litter

Table 64-1 Characteristics of Endemic Dimorphic Mycoses

Mycosis	Etiology	Ecology	Geographic Distribution	Morphology in Tissue	Clinical Manifestation
Blastomycosis	*Blastomyces dermatitidis*	Decaying organic material	North America (Ohio and Mississippi river valleys) Africa	Broad-based budding yeasts (8-15 μm in diameter)	Pulmonary disease (<50%) Extrapulmonary: skin, bone, genitourinary, central nervous system Disseminated disease in immunocompromised patients
Coccidioidomycosis	*Coccidioides immitis* *Coccidioides posadasii*	Soil, dust	Southwestern United States, Mexico, Central and South America	Spherules (20-60 μm) containing endospores (2-4 μm)	Asymptomatic pulmonary infection (60%) in normal host Progressive pulmonary infection and dissemination (skin, bone, joints, meninges) in immunocompromised patients
Histoplasmosis capsulati	*Histoplasma capsulatum* var. *capsulatum*	Soil with high nitrogen content (bird/bat droppings)	North America (Ohio and Mississippi river valleys), Mexico, Central and South America	Small (2-4 μm), oval, narrow-based, budding yeasts (intracellular)	Asymptomatic pulmonary infection (90%) in normal host and low-intensity exposure Disseminated disease in immunocompromised host and in children
Histoplasmosis duboisii	*Histoplasma capsulatum* var. *duboisii*	Soil with high nitrogen content	Tropical areas of Africa	Larger (8-15 μm), thick-walled, budding yeast; prominent isthmus and bud scar	Low rate of pulmonary disease; higher frequency of skin and bone involvement
Paracoccidioidomycosis	*Paracoccidioides brasiliensis*	Likely soil associated	South and Central America	Thin to moderately thick-walled, multiply budding yeast (15-30 μm; pilot wheel)	Self-limited pulmonary disease; progressive pulmonary infection and dissemination (skin, mucosa, bones, lymph nodes, viscera, and meninges); more common in children and immunocompromised patients
Talaromycosis marneffei	*Talaromyces marneffei*	Soil Bamboo rat	Southeast Asia	Globose to elongated sausage-shaped yeasts (3-5 μm) that are intracellular and divide by fission	Disseminated infection (skin, soft tissues, viscera) more common in AIDS Resembles histoplasmosis, cryptococcosis, or tuberculosis

Modified from Anstead GM, Patterson TF: Endemic mycoses. In Anaissie EJ, McGinnis MR, Pfaller MA, editors: *Clinical mycology,* ed 2, New York, 2009, Churchill Livingstone.

AIDS, Acquired immunodeficiency syndrome.

(Figure 64-5). Outbreaks of infection have been associated with occupational or recreational contact with soil, and infected individuals include all ages and both genders. A recent large outbreak of blastomycosis in Wisconsin was marked by both geographic and ethnic clustering, with a disproportionate number of infections occurring in persons of Hmong ethnicity, suggesting a possible genetic predisposition to infection with this fungus. Blastomycosis is not transmitted from patient to patient; however, laboratory-acquired primary cutaneous and pulmonary blastomycosis has been reported.

In North America, the area of endemicity overlaps that of histoplasmosis (see Figure 64-2) and includes the southeastern and south central states, especially those bordering the Ohio and Mississippi river basins, the Midwest states and Canadian provinces bordering the Great Lakes, and an area in New York and Canada along the St. Lawrence River. Blastomycosis is also endemic in Africa. It is estimated that one to two cases of symptomatic blastomycosis requiring therapy occur per 100,000 population each year in areas with endemic disease. Among animals, dogs are most susceptible; the infection rate is estimated to be 10 times that for humans.

Clinical Syndromes

The usual route of infection in blastomycosis is inhalation of conidia (see Figure 64-5). As with most endemic mycoses, the severity of symptoms and course of the disease are dependent on the extent of exposure and immune status of the exposed individual. Based largely on studies of blastomycosis outbreaks, it appears that symptomatic disease occurs in less than half of infected individuals. Clinical illness caused by *B. dermatitidis* may present as pulmonary disease or an extrapulmonary disseminated disease. Among those patients with extrapulmonary dissemination, two thirds

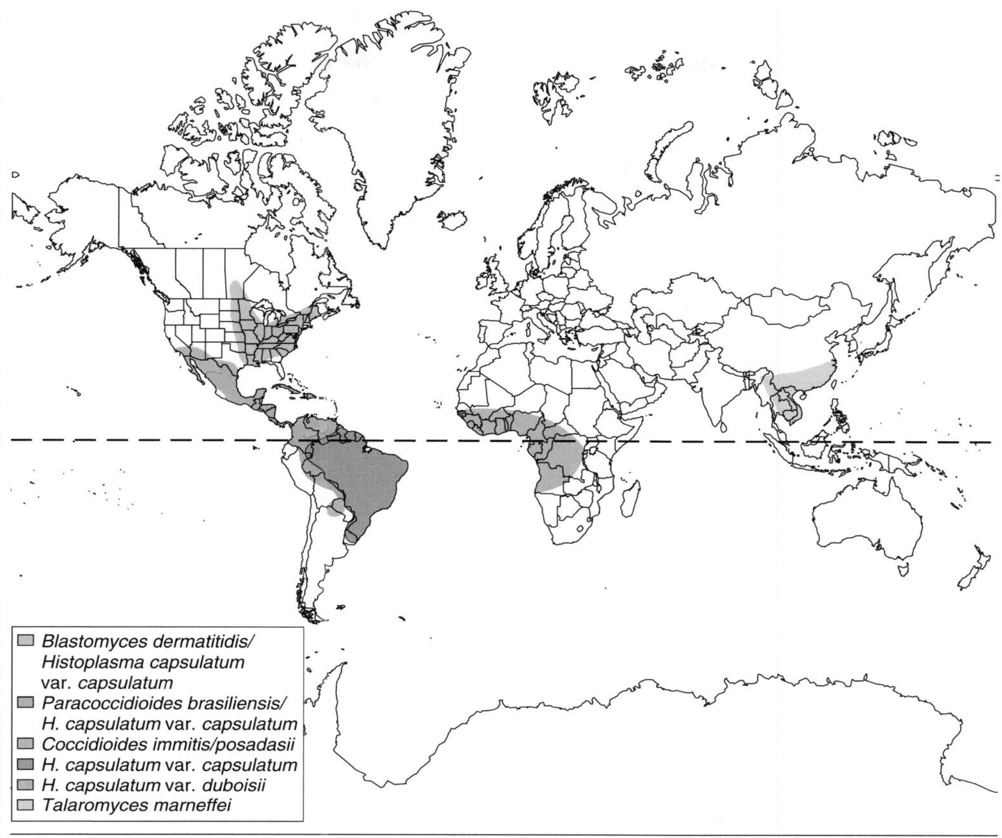

FIGURE 64-2 Major geographic regional distribution of the endemic mycoses.

Clinical Case 64-1 Central Nervous System (CNS) Blastomycosis

Buhari and colleagues (*Infect Med* 24[Suppl 8]:12–14, 2007) reported a case of CNS blastomycosis. The patient was a 56-year-old homeless man from Detroit who presented with a 2-week history of left hemiparesis, aphasia, and generalized headache. There was no history of rash, respiratory symptoms, or fever. His medical history was significant for a left craniotomy 30 years ago for intracranial hemorrhage caused by trauma. He lived in an abandoned building and was not taking any medications. On examination, he had expressive aphasia, new-onset left hemiparesis, and bilateral carotid bruits. The rest of the physical examination was unremarkable, as were routine serum chemistries and hematologic parameters. He was negative for antibodies to human immunodeficiency virus. A chest radiograph was unremarkable. A contrast-enhanced computed tomography scan of the head demonstrated multiple ring-enhancing lesions in the right cerebrum, with surrounding vasogenic edema and midline shift; significant encephalomalacia and generalized atrophy were present in the left cerebral hemisphere.

Serum and urine tests were negative for *Cryptococcus* (serum) and *Histoplasma* (serum and urine) antigens. Tuberculin skin tests were nonreactive, and imaging studies of the sinuses, chest, and abdomen were unremarkable. A brain biopsy was performed, and histopathologic examination revealed granulomatous inflammation and budding yeasts consistent with *Blastomyces dermatitidis.* Subsequent culture confirmed the diagnosis of CNS blastomycosis. The patient was treated with dexamethasone and amphotericin B but developed hypertension and bradycardia, with subsequent cardiopulmonary arrest and death.

This is an example of an unusual presentation of CNS blastomycosis without any other evidence of disseminated disease. The clinical syndrome of hypertension, bradycardia, and cardiopulmonary arrest suggest that the patient died of increased intracranial pressure, either as a complication of the infection or the diagnostic brain biopsy.

exhibit involvement of skin and bones. Other sites of hematogenous dissemination include prostate, liver, spleen, kidney, and central nervous system (CNS).

Pulmonary blastomycosis may be asymptomatic or present as a mild flulike illness. More severe infection resembles bacterial pneumonia with acute onset, high fever, lobar infiltrates, and cough. Progression to fulminant adult respiratory distress syndrome with high fever, diffuse infiltrates, and respiratory failure may occur. A more subacute or chronic respiratory form of blastomycosis may resemble tuberculosis or lung cancer, with radiographic presentation of pulmonary mass lesions or fibronodular infiltrates.

A classic form of blastomycosis is that of chronic cutaneous involvement. The cutaneous form of blastomycosis is almost always the result of hematogenous dissemination from the lung, in most instances without evident pulmonary lesions or systemic symptoms. The lesions may be papular, pustular, or indolent, ulcerative-nodular, and verrucous with

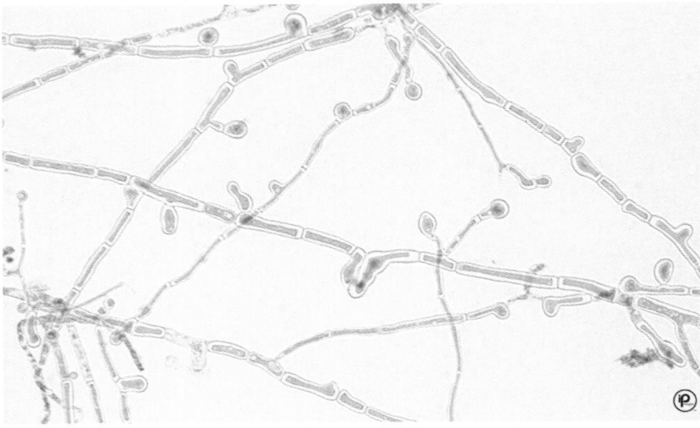

FIGURE 64-3 *Blastomyces dermatitidis* mold phase.

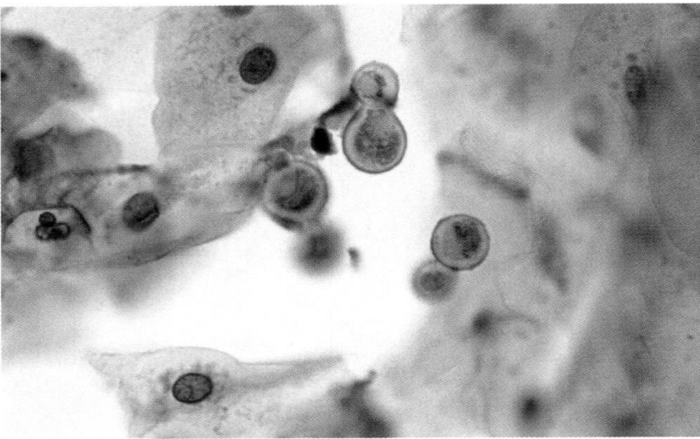

FIGURE 64-4 Giemsa stain of *Blastomyces dermatitidis* showing broad-based budding yeast.

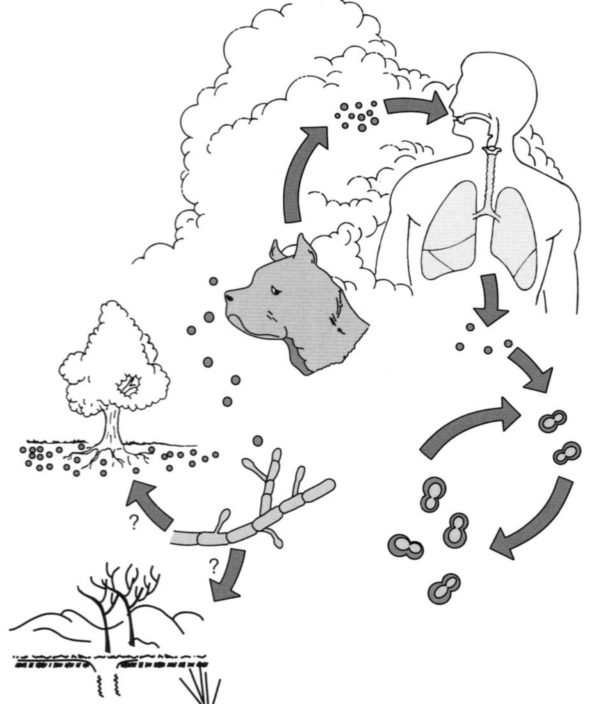

FIGURE 64-5 Natural history of the mold (saprobic) and yeast (parasitic) cycle of *Blastomyces dermatitidis*.

crusted surfaces and raised serpiginous borders. They are usually painless and localized to exposed areas such as the face, scalp, neck, and hands. They may be mistaken for squamous cell carcinoma. Left untreated, cutaneous blastomycosis takes on a chronic course with remissions and exacerbations and gradual increase in the size of lesions.

Blastomycosis is relatively uncommon among individuals with AIDS or other immunocompromising conditions. However, when it occurs in these individuals, it tends to be acute, involve the CNS, and have a much poorer prognosis.

Laboratory Diagnosis

The diagnosis of blastomycosis rests with microscopic detection of the fungus in tissue or other clinical material, with confirmation by culture (Table 64-2). The most useful specimens for the diagnosis of pulmonary blastomycosis include sputum, bronchoalveolar lavage, or lung biopsy. Direct examination of material stained with GMS, PAS, Papanicolaou, or Giemsa stains should be performed. Likewise, fresh wet preparations of sputum, cerebrospinal fluid, urine, pus, skin scrapings, and tissue impression smears may be examined directly using calcofluor white and fluorescence microscopy to detect the characteristic yeast forms. When typical broad-based budding yeast forms are present, a definitive diagnosis may be made.

Culture of clinical material on selective and nonselective mycologic media incubated at both 25° C to 30° C and at 37° C should be performed. The mycelial form of the fungus is easily cultured at 25° C to 30° C; however, growth is slow, often requiring 4 weeks or more. The mycelial form (see Figure 64-3) is not diagnostic, and the identity must be confirmed by conversion to the yeast form at 37° C, exoantigen testing (immunologic detection of cell-free antigen A), or nucleic acid probe hybridization. Care should be taken to handle the culture in an appropriate biosafety cabinet, because the conidia are infectious.

Although serologic tests to detect antibodies directed at *B. dermatitidis* antigens are available (see Table 64-2), they are neither sensitive nor specific and are of little use in diagnosis. A test to detect antigen in serum and urine is commercially available, but cross-reaction with other endemic mycoses is considerable, and it is unclear what role it will play in diagnosis. Detection of serum (1→3)-β-D-glucan (BDG) has not been shown to be useful in the diagnosis of blastomycosis, whereas real-time polymerase chain reaction (RT-PCR) has value when performed on blood, tissue, or respiratory specimens.

Treatment

The decision to treat patients with blastomycosis must take into consideration the clinical form and severity of disease, as well as the immune status of the patient and toxicity of antifungal agents. Clearly, pulmonary blastomycosis in immunocompromised patients and those with progressive pulmonary disease should be treated. Likewise, all patients with evidence of hematogenous dissemination (e.g., skin, bone, all nonpulmonary sites) require antifungal therapy. Amphotericin B, preferably a lipid formulation, is the agent of choice for the treatment of life-threatening or meningeal disease. Mild or moderate disease may be treated with itraconazole. Fluconazole, posaconazole, or voriconazole may be alternatives for those patients unable to tolerate

Table 64-2 Diagnosis of Endemic Dimorphic Mycoses

		Morphology in Culture			
Mycosis	**Culture**	**25° C**	**37° C**	**Histopathology**	**Serology**
Blastomycosis	Sputum, BAL, lung tissue, skin biopsy, CSF	Mold, round to oval or pear-shaped conidia (2-10 μm diameter)	Thick-walled, broad-based budding yeast (8-15 μm)	Broad-based budding yeast	Antibody: CF, ID, EIA (poor sensitivity and specificity) Antigen: serum and urine (performance undefined)
Coccidioidomycosis	Sputum, BAL, tissue, CSF	Mold with barrel-shaped arthroconidia (3-6 μm)	NA	Spherules (20-60 μm) containing endospores	Antibody: TP, CF, ID, LPA (diagnostic and prognostic) Antigen: urine (performance undefined)
Histoplasmosis capsulati	Sputum, BAL, blood, bone marrow, tissue, CSF	Mold with tuberculate macroconidia (8-15 μm) and small oval microconidia (2-4 μm)	Small (2-4 μm) budding yeast	Intracellular budding yeast	Antibody: CF, ID Antigen: serum and urine (92% sensitive in disseminated disease)
Paracoccidioidomycosis	Sputum, BAL, tissue	Mold, round microconidia (2-3 μm), and intercalary chlamydospores	Large (15-30 μm) multiple budding yeast	Large multiple budding yeast	Antibody: ID, CF (variable specificity; CF useful for monitoring response)
Talaromycosis marneffei	Blood, bone marrow, tissue, CSF	Mold with diffusible red pigment Conidiophores terminating in conspicuous, penicillus-bearing, ellipsoidal, smooth conidia	Pleomorphic elongated yeast (1-8 μm) with transverse septa	Intracellular elongated yeast with transverse septa	Under development

BAL, Bronchoalveolar lavage; *CF*, complement fixation; *CSF*, cerebrospinal fluid; *EIA*, enzyme immunoassay; *ID*, immunodiffusion; *LPA*, latex particle agglutination; *NA*, not applicable; *TP*, tube precipitin.

itraconazole. Depending upon disease severity and host status, therapeutic success rates with amphotericin B or azole therapy range from 70% to 95%. Survival for AIDS patients and other immunocompromised patients is about half this figure. The latter patients may require long-term suppressive therapy with itraconazole in an effort to avoid relapses of the infection.

• Coccidioidomycosis

Coccidioidomycosis (Clinical Case 64-2) is an endemic mycosis caused by either of two indistinguishable species, *Coccidioides immitis* and *C. posadasii*. The disease is caused by inhalation of infectious arthroconidia (Figure 64-6) and may range from asymptomatic infection (in most people) to progressive infection and death. The two species differ in geographic distribution and genotype: *C. immitis* is localized to California, and *C. posadasii* accounts for the majority of infections outside California. Aside from these differences, there appears to be no additional difference in phenotype or pathogenicity. As such, the more familiar name *C. immitis* will be used in this chapter.

Like syphilis and tuberculosis, coccidioidomycosis causes a wide variety of lesions and has been called "the great imitator." Synonyms for coccidioidomycosis include **coccidioidal granuloma** and **San Joaquin Valley fever** among others.

Morphology

C. immitis (C. posadasii) is a dimorphic fungus that exists as a mold in nature and when cultured in the laboratory at 25° C, and as an endosporulating spherule in tissue and under very specific conditions in vitro (Figures 64-7 and 64-8; see Table 64-2 and Figure 64-1). A variety of mold morphologies may be seen in culture at 25° C. Initial growth is white to gray, moist, and glabrous and occurs within 3 to 4 days. It rapidly develops abundant aerial mycelia, and the colony enlarges into a circular "bloom." Mature colonies usually become tan to brown or lavender.

Microscopically, the vegetative hyphae give rise to fertile hyphae that produce alternating (separated by disjunctor cells) hyaline arthroconidia (see Figure 64-7). When released, the infectious conidia are typically "barrel-shaped" and have an annular frill at both ends. As the culture ages, the vegetative hyphae also fragment into arthroconidia.

Upon inhalation, the arthroconidia (2.5 to 4 μm wide) become rounded as they convert to spherules in the lung (see Figure 64-8). At maturity, the spherules (20 to 60 μm in diameter) produce endospores by a process known as **progressive cleavage.** Rupture of the spherule walls releases the endospores, which in turn form new spherules (see Figure 64-6). In approximately 10% to 30% of pulmonary cavities associated with coccidioidomycosis, branched septate hyphae and arthroconidia may be produced.

Epidemiology

Coccidioidomycosis is endemic to the desert southwestern United States, northern Mexico, and scattered areas of Central and South America (see Figure 64-2). *C. immitis* is found in soil, and the growth of the fungus in the environment is enhanced by bat and rodent droppings. Exposure to the infectious arthroconidia is greatest in late summer and

Clinical Case 64-2 Coccidioidomycosis

Stafford and colleagues (*Infect Med* 24[Suppl 8]:23–25, 2007) describe a 31-year-old African American U.S. Army soldier who presented with fever, chills, night sweats, and a nonproductive cough of 4 weeks' duration. In addition, he had recently detected a painless right breast mass. His past medical history was unremarkable. He was stationed at Fort Irwin, California, where he was working as a telephone repairman. His physical exam was unremarkable except for a firm, nontender, 3-cm subcutaneous mass overlying the right breast. Multiple small (<1 cm) nontender lymph nodes were palpable in the axillae and groin. Laboratory studies revealed a white blood count of 11.9/μl, with 30% eosinophils. Serum chemistries were notable for an elevated alkaline phosphatase level. Results of blood cultures, tests for serum *Cryptococcus* antigen, urinary *Histoplasma* antigen, and human immunodeficiency virus antibody were negative, as was a tuberculin skin test. A chest radiograph showed bilateral interstitial micronodules in a miliary pattern, as well as a right-sided paratracheal fullness. A computed tomography (CT) scan of the chest confirmed the presence of diffuse 1- to 2-mm micronodules in all lobes. The CT scan also showed a lobular parenchymal mass lesion in the right middle lobe and a right chest wall mass. A fine-needle aspirate of the right breast mass revealed spherules filled with endospores, consistent with coccidioidomycosis. Culture of the material grew *Coccidioides immitis.* A serology panel for *C. immitis* was positive and revealed immunoglobulin G complement fixation titers at a dilution of greater than 1 : 256. Cerebrospinal fluid analysis was normal, but a bone scan revealed multiple regions of increased osteoblastic activity involving the left scapula, right anterior fifth rib, and midthoracic vertebral regions. Treatment was initiated with amphotericin B, but increasing neck pain prompted further imaging, which demonstrated a lytic lesion of the C1 vertebral body and a paravertebral mass. Despite antifungal therapy, progressive enlargement of the mass necessitated surgical debridement. The patient was continued on amphotericin B lipid formulation, with plans for long-term, perhaps lifelong, antifungal therapy.

This is an example of the serious problems posed by coccidioidomycosis. Clues to the diagnosis of disseminated coccidioidomycosis in this patient included an infectious prodrome, peripheral eosinophilia, hilar lymphadenopathy, characteristic pattern of organ involvement (lungs, bones, soft tissues), residence in an endemic area, and African American ethnicity (higher risk group for dissemination).

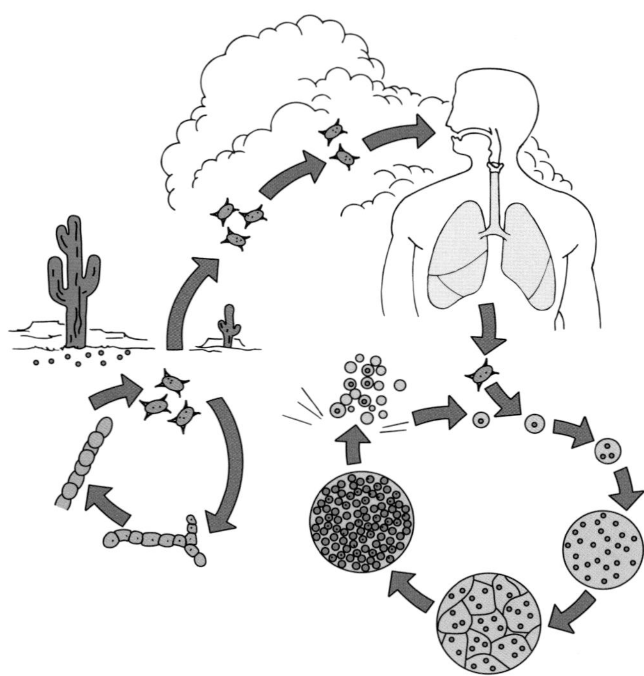

FIGURE 64-6 Natural history of the mold (saprobic) and spherule (parasitic) cycle of *Coccidioides immitis.*

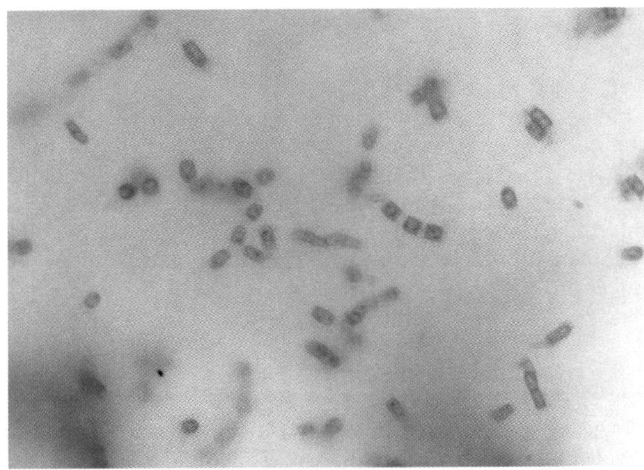

FIGURE 64-7 *Coccidioides immitis* mold phase.

fall when dusty conditions prevail. Cycles of drought and rain enhance dispersion of the organism because heavy rains facilitate the growth of the organism in the nitrogenous soil wastes, and subsequent drought and windy conditions favor aerosolization of arthroconidia (see Figure 64-6). Acquisition of coccidioidomycosis occurs principally by inhalation of arthroconidia, and in endemic areas, infection rates may be 16% to 42% by early adulthood. The incidence of coccidioidomycosis is approximately 15 cases per 100,000 population annually in the endemic area; however, it is known to disproportionately affect persons aged 65 and older (≈36 per 100,000) and those with human immunodeficiency virus (HIV) infection (≈20 per 100,000).

Clinical Syndromes

C. immitis is probably the most virulent of all human mycotic pathogens. Inhalation of only a few arthroconidia produces primary coccidioidomycosis, which may include asymptomatic pulmonary disease (≈60% of patients) or a self-limited flulike illness marked by fever, cough, chest pain, and weight loss. Patients with primary coccidioidomycosis may have a variety of allergic reactions (≈10%) as a result of immune complex formation, including an erythematous macular rash, erythema multiforme, and erythema nodosum.

Primary disease usually resolves without therapy and confers a strong, specific immunity to reinfection, which is detected by the coccidioidin skin test. In patients symptomatic for 6 weeks or longer, the disease progresses to secondary coccidioidomycosis, which may include nodules, cavitary disease, or progressive pulmonary disease (5% of cases); single or multisystem dissemination follows in approximately 1% of this population. Extrapulmonary sites of infection include skin, soft tissues, bones, joints, and meninges. Persons in certain ethnic groups (e.g., Filipino, African American, Native American, Hispanic) run the highest risk

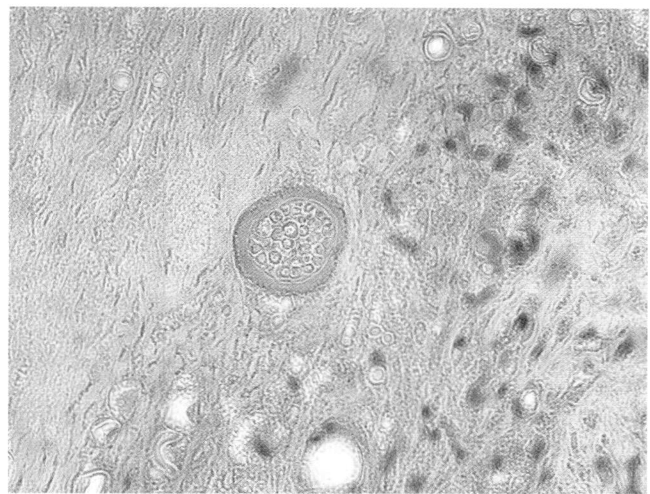

FIGURE 64-8 *Coccidioides immitis* spherule filled with endospores.

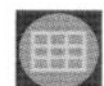

Table 64-3 Risk Factors for Disseminated Coccidioidomycosis

Risk Factor	Highest Risk
Age	Infants and elderly
Sex	Male
Genetics	Filipino > African American > Native American > Hispanic > Asian
Serum CF antibody titer	>1:32
Pregnancy	Late pregnancy and postpartum
Skin test	Negative
Depressed cell-mediated immunity	Malignancy, chemotherapy, steroid treatment, HIV infection

From Cohen J, Powderly WG, Opal SM: *Infectious diseases,* ed 3, Philadelphia, 2010, Mosby.

CF, Complement fixation; *HIV,* human immunodeficiency virus.

of dissemination, with meningeal involvement a common sequela (Table 64-3). In addition to ethnicity, males (9:1), women in the third trimester of pregnancy, individuals with a cellular immunodeficiency (e.g., AIDS, organ transplantation recipients, those treated with tumor necrosis factor antagonists), and persons at the extremes of age are at high risk for disseminated disease (see Table 64-3). The mortality in disseminated disease exceeds 90% without treatment, and chronic infection is common.

Laboratory Diagnosis

The diagnosis of coccidioidomycosis includes the use of histopathologic examination of tissue or other clinical material, isolation of the fungus in the culture, and serologic testing (see Table 64-2). Direct microscopic visualization of endosporulating spherules in sputum, exudates, or tissue is sufficient to establish the diagnosis (see Figure 64-8) and is preferred over culture because of the highly infectious nature of the mold when grown in culture. Clinical exudates should be examined directly in 10% to 20% potassium hydroxide (KOH) with calcofluor white, and tissue from biopsy can be stained with H&E or specific fungal stains such as GMS or PAS (see Figure 64-8).

Clinical specimens may be cultured on routine mycologic media at 25° C. Colonies of *C. immitis* develop within 3 to 5 days, and typical sporulation may be seen in 5 to 10 days. Because of the highly infectious nature of the fungus, all plates or tubes should be sealed using gas-permeable tape (plates) or screw caps (tubes) and only examined within a suitable biosafety cabinet. Identification of *C. immitis* from culture may be accomplished by using the exoantigen immunodiffusion (ID) test or nucleic acid hybridization. Conversion of the mold into spherules in vitro is not usually attempted outside of a research setting.

Several serologic procedures exist for initial screening, confirmation, or prognostic evaluation (see Table 64-2). For initial diagnosis, the combined use of the ID test and the latex particle agglutination (LPA) test detects approximately 93% of cases. The complement fixation (CF) and tube precipitin (TP) tests may also be used for diagnosis as well as prognosis. Prognostic studies frequently employ serial CF titers; rising titers are a bad prognostic sign, and falling titers indicate improvement. A coccidioidal urinary antigen test has been developed, but its relatively low sensitivity of 71% limits its clinical utility. Neither BDG nor PCR tests have been shown to be any more useful than culture for the diagnosis of coccidioidomycosis.

Treatment

Most individuals with primary coccidioidomycosis do not require specific antifungal therapy. For those with concurrent risk factors (see Table 64-3), such as organ transplant, HIV infection, high doses of corticosteroids, or when there is evidence of unusually severe infection, treatment is necessary. Primary coccidioidomycosis in the third trimester of pregnancy or during the immediate postpartum period requires treatment with a lipid formulation of amphotericin B.

Immunocompromised patients or others with diffuse pneumonia should be treated with a lipid formulation of amphotericin B followed by an azole (fluconazole, itraconazole, posaconazole, or voriconazole) as maintenance therapy. The total length of therapy should be at least 1 year. Immunocompromised patients should be maintained on an oral azole as secondary prophylaxis.

Chronic cavitary pneumonia should be treated with an oral azole for at least 1 year. In cases where the response is suboptimal, alternatives are to switch to another azole (e.g., from itraconazole to fluconazole), increase the dose of the azole in the case of fluconazole, or switch to lipid amphotericin B. Surgical treatment is required in the event of rupture of a cavity into the pleural space, hemoptysis, or for localized refractory lesions.

Treatment of nonmeningeal extrapulmonary disseminated infections is based on oral azole therapy with either fluconazole or itraconazole (posaconazole and voriconazole are also options). In the case of vertebral involvement or inadequate clinical response, treatment with lipid amphotericin B is recommended, along with appropriate surgical debridement and stabilization.

Meningeal coccidioidomycosis is managed with administration of fluconazole or itraconazole (secondary choice because of poor CNS penetration) indefinitely. Posaconazole and voriconazole are also alternative choices. Intrathecal administration of amphotericin B is recommended only in the event of failure of azole therapy, because of its toxicity when administered by this route.

• Emmonsiosis

The genus *Emmonsia* contains three species that have been associated with human disease. *Emmonsia crescens* and *E. parva* are the agents of adiaspiromycosis, a generally self-limited pulmonary disease described in Chapter 66. The thermally dimorphic species *E. pasteuriana* has been reported to have caused a single case of disseminated infection in an Italian patient with late-stage HIV infection. A second case of progressive pulmonary disease in a German farmer was due to a thermally dimorphic fungus that was identified only as an *Emmonsia* species. Most recently, a dimorphic fungal pathogen most closely related to *E. pasteuriana* was reported as causing disseminated infection in HIV-infected adults in South Africa.

Morphology

The species of *Emmonsia* isolated from patients in South Africa was a thermally dimorphic fungus that grew as a mold at 25° C and as a yeast at 37° C. At 25° C colonies grew at a slow to moderate rate, taking on a cerebriform appearance and becoming light brown with powdery segments over time. Light microscopy revealed septate hyaline hyphae (1 to 1.5 µm in diameter) with numerous smooth-walled oval conidia. The conidia were borne on short stalks that formed perpendicular to a swollen vesicle. The vesicles give rise to four to eight stalks or pedicles, each forming a terminal conidium, establishing a flower-shaped arrangement of four to eight conidia grouped together. When mature the conidia had distinctly tuberculated cell walls. No adiaspores were seen in any of the cultures incubated at 37° C or 40° C.

Upon incubation at 37° C for 10 to 14 days, the mycelial cultures were converted to the yeast phase. Yeast colonies were smooth and beige to light brown in color. The yeast cells were small (2 to 4 µm in diameter), thin-walled, globose to oval with single or multiple narrow-based budding. The macroscopic and microscopic features were indistinguishable from those of *E. pasteuriana.*

Epidemiology

Aside from cases of adiaspiromycosis, disseminated infection due to *Emmonsia* spp. occurred in Italy (1 case), Germany (1 case), and South Africa (13 cases). As such there is little in the way of information to document specific areas of endemicity. The South African cases were all diagnosed following the introduction of broad-range PCR for fungal diagnosis and identification in July 2008. Thus the apparent clustering of cases and the "emergence" of *Emmonsia* spp. in South Africa may simply represent improved detection of the causative organism rather than introduction of a new opportunistic pathogen. All the South African cases occurred in adults with late-stage HIV infection, and all cases had extensive cutaneous involvement. Although the African cases closely resembled *E. pasteuriana,* phylogenetic analysis suggested that these isolates represented a previously unidentified species of *Emmonsia.* Aside from the tight clustering of the cases and isolates, no additional epidemiologic details were provided. It is known that *Emmonsia* species may be found in the environment and that *E. crescens* and *E. parva* cause pulmonary disease in small mammals. The likely mode of infection with the "new" species of *Emmonsia* is by inhalation of fungal conidia from the environment, similar to that seen with adiaspiromycosis.

Clinical Syndromes

All reported cases of disseminated infection due to *Emmonsia* spp. occurred in immunocompromised adults, the vast majority of whom suffered from late-stage HIV infection. The South African patients all had very low $CD4^+$ T-cell counts (median, 16 cells/mm^3), were profoundly anemic, and had widespread skin lesions that varied from erythematous papules and plaques to ulcerated boggy and crusted plaques. The majority of cases (85%) had chest radiograph findings that mimicked tuberculosis. The infection was rapidly fatal in three patients, one of which had yeast cells detected by microscopic examination of peripheral blood. In eight of nine patients who underwent liver function studies, abnormalities in alkaline phosphatase and γ-glutamyltransferase levels suggested possible hepatic infiltration. Given that only individuals with cutaneous involvement were investigated by PCR and culture, it is possible that infected patients without skin lesions who had extracutaneous involvement such as pulmonary or hepatic disease were not identified.

Laboratory Diagnosis

The yeast cells of *Emmonsia* spp. were readily detected by histopathologic examination of skin biopsies and were isolated in culture from blood, bone marrow, and cutaneous tissue. Cultures of cerebrospinal fluid and sputum were negative. Phylogenetic analysis of five genes (large subunit rDNA [LSU], internal transcribed spacer rDNA regions [ITS 1-2], and genes encoding actin, β-tubulin, and interin PRP8) revealed that the fungus belonged to the genus *Emmonsia* and was most closely related to *E. pasteuriana.*

Treatment

Most of the South African patients responded rapidly to treatment with amphotericin B deoxycholate followed by itraconazole maintenance therapy. Three patients died shortly after the diagnosis was made.

• Histoplasmosis

Histoplasmosis (Clinical Case 64-3) is caused by two varieties of *Histoplasma capsulatum*: *H. capsulatum* var. *capsulatum* and *H. capsulatum* var. *duboisii* (see Table 64-1). *H. capsulatum* var. *capsulatum* causes pulmonary and disseminated infections in the eastern half of the United States and most of Latin America, whereas *H. capsulatum* var. *duboisii* causes predominantly skin and bone lesions and is restricted to the tropical areas of Africa (see Figure 64-2).

Morphology

Both varieties of *H. capsulatum* are thermally dimorphic fungi existing as a hyaline mold in nature and in culture at 25° C and as an intracellular budding yeast in tissue and in culture at 37° C (Figures 64-9, 64-10, and 64-11; see Table

Clinical Case 64-3 Disseminated Histoplasmosis

Mariani and Morris (*Infect Med* 24[Suppl 8]:17–19, 2007) describe a case of disseminated histoplasmosis in a patient with acquired immunodeficiency syndrome. The patient was a 42-year-old El Salvadoran woman who was admitted to the hospital for evaluation of progressive dermatosis involving the right nostril, cheek, and lip, despite antibiotic therapy. She was positive for human immunodeficiency virus (CD4 lymphocyte count 21/μl) and had lived in Miami for the past 18 years. The lesion first appeared on the right nostril 3 months before admission. The patient sought medical attention and was treated unsuccessfully with oral antibiotics. Over the following 2 months, the lesion increased in size, involving the right nares and malar region, and was accompanied by fever, malaise, and a 50-lb weight loss. A necrotic area developed on the superior aspect of the right nostril, extending to the upper lip. A presumptive diagnosis of leishmaniasis was entertained, based in part on the patient's country of origin and a possible exposure to a sandfly bite.

Laboratory studies revealed anemia and lymphopenia. A chest radiograph was normal, and a computed tomography scan of the head showed a soft-tissue mass in the right nasal cavity. Histopathologic evaluation of a skin biopsy showed chronic inflammation, with intracytoplasmic budding yeasts. Culture of the biopsy grew *Histoplasma capsulatum,* and results of a urine *Histoplasma* antigen test were positive. The patient was treated with amphotericin B followed by itraconazole with good results.

This case underscores the ability of *H. capsulatum* to remain clinically latent for many years, only to reactivate upon immunosuppression of the host. Cutaneous manifestations of histoplasmosis are usually a consequence of progression from primary (latent) to disseminated disease. Histoplasmosis is not endemic to southern Florida but is endemic to much of Latin America, where the patient had lived before moving to Miami. A high index of suspicion and confirmation with skin biopsies, cultures, and testing for urinary antigen are crucial for timely and appropriate treatment of disseminated histoplasmosis.

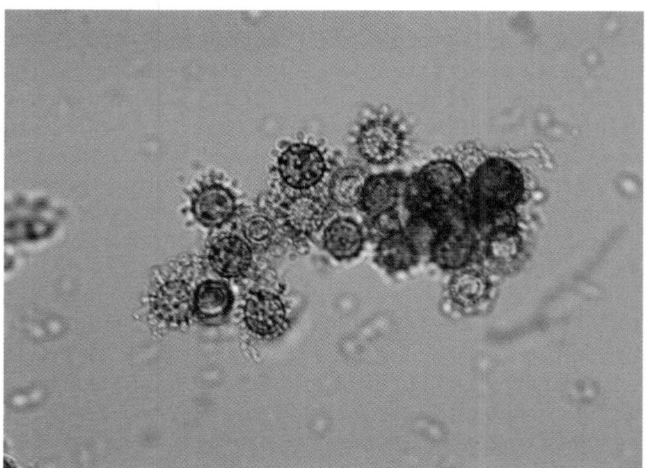

FIGURE 64-9 *Histoplasma capsulatum* mold phase showing tuberculate macroconidia.

64-2). In culture, the mold forms of *H. capsulatum* var. *capsulatum* and var. *duboisii* are indistinguishable macroscopically and microscopically. The mold colonies grow slowly and develop as white or brown hyphal colonies after several days to a week. The mold form produces two types of conidia: (1) large (8 to 15 μm), thick-walled, spherical macroconidia with spikelike projections (tuberculate macroconidia) that arise from short conidiophores (Figure 64-12; see Figure 64-1) and (2) small oval microconidia (2 to 4 μm) with smooth or slightly rough walls that are sessile or on short stalks (see Figures 64-1 and 64-12). The yeast cells are thin walled, oval, and measure 2 to 4 μm (var. *capsulatum*) (see Figure 64-10) or thicker walled and 8 to 15 μm (var. *duboisii*) (see Figure 64-11). The yeast cells of both varieties of *H. capsulatum* are intracellular in vivo and are uninucleated (see Figures 64-10 and 64-11).

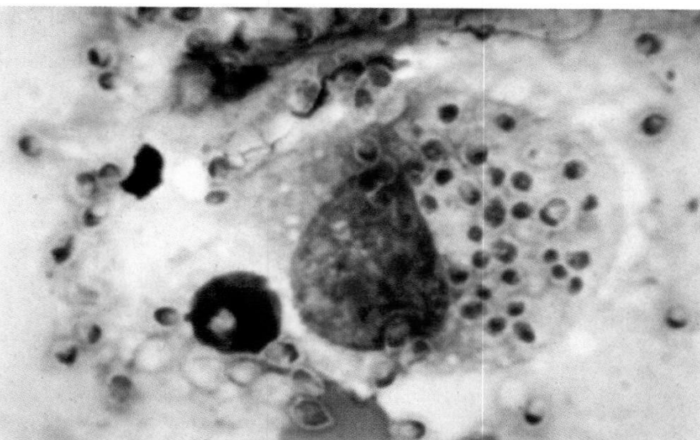

FIGURE 64-10 Giemsa-stained preparation showing intracellular yeast forms of *Histoplasma capsulatum* var. *capsulatum.*

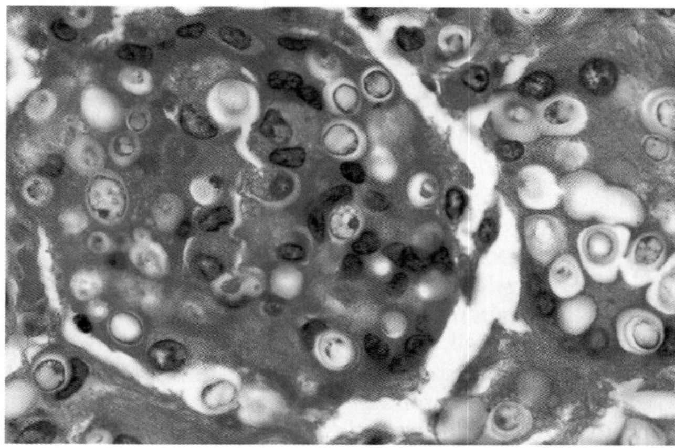

FIGURE 64-11 Hematoxylin and eosin–stained tissue section showing intracellular yeast forms of *Histoplasma capsulatum* var. *duboisii.* (From Connor DH, Schwartz DA: *Pathology of infectious diseases,* Stamford, Conn, 1997, Appleton & Lange.)

Epidemiology

Histoplasmosis capsulati is localized to the broad regions of the Ohio and Mississippi river valleys in the United States and occurs throughout Mexico and Central and South America (see Figure 64-2 and Table 64-1). Histoplasmosis duboisii, or African histoplasmosis, is confined to the tropical areas of Africa, including Gabon, Uganda, and Kenya (see Figure 64-2 and Table 64-1).

The natural habitat of the mycelial form of both varieties of *H. capsulatum* is soil with a high nitrogen content, such as that found in areas contaminated with bird or bat droppings. Outbreaks of histoplasmosis have been associated

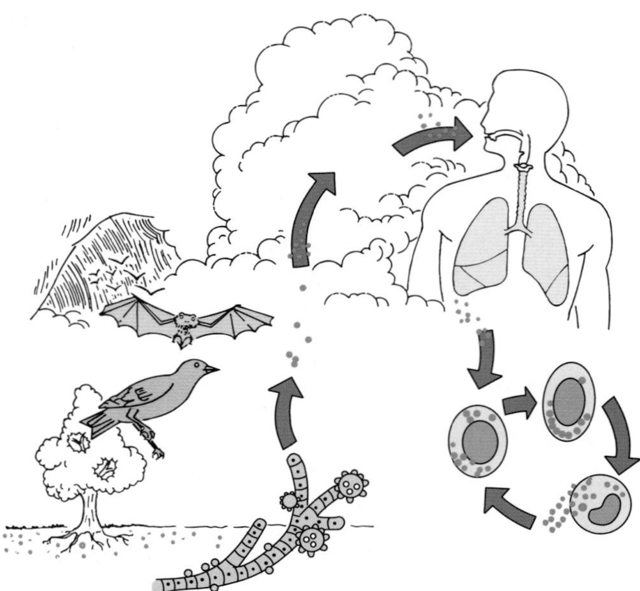

FIGURE 64-12 Natural history of the mold (saprobic) and yeast (parasitic) cycle of *Histoplasma capsulatum.*

with exposure to bird roosts, caves, and decaying buildings or urban renewal projects involving excavation and demolition. Aerosolization of microconidia and hyphal fragments in the disturbed soil, with subsequent inhalation by exposed individuals, is considered to be the basis for these outbreaks (see Figure 64-12). Although attack rates may reach 100% in certain of these exposures, most cases remain asymptomatic and are detected only by skin testing. Immunocompromised individuals and children are more prone to develop symptomatic disease with either variety of *Histoplasma.* Reactivation of the disease and dissemination is common among immunosuppressed individuals, especially those with AIDS.

Clinical Syndromes

The usual route of infection for both varieties of histoplasmosis is via inhalation of microconidia, which in turn germinate into yeasts within the lung and may remain localized or disseminate hematogenously or by the lymphatic system (see Figure 64-12). The microconidia are rapidly phagocytosed by pulmonary macrophages and neutrophils, and it is thought that conversion to the parasitic yeast form takes place intracellularly.

Histoplasmosis Capsulati

The clinical presentation of histoplasmosis caused by *H. capsulatum* var. *capsulatum* is dependent upon the intensity of exposure and immunologic status of the host. Asymptomatic infection occurs in 90% of individuals after a low-intensity exposure. In the event of an exposure to a heavy inoculum, however, most individuals exhibit some symptoms. The self-limited form of acute pulmonary histoplasmosis is marked by a flulike illness with fever, chills, headache, cough, myalgias, and chest pain. Radiographic evidence of hilar or mediastinal adenopathy and patchy pulmonary infiltrates may be seen. Most acute infections resolve with supportive care and do not require specific antifungal treatment. In rare instances, usually after very heavy exposure, acute respiratory distress syndrome may be seen. In approximately 10% of patients, inflammatory sequelae such as persistent lymphadenopathy with bronchial obstruction, arthritis, arthralgias, or pericarditis may be seen. Another rare complication of histoplasmosis is a condition known as **mediastinal fibrosis,** in which persistent host response to the organism may result in massive fibrosis and constriction of mediastinal structures, including the heart and great vessels.

Progressive pulmonary histoplasmosis may follow acute infection in approximately 1 in 100,000 cases per year. Chronic pulmonary symptoms are associated with apical cavities and fibrosis and are more likely to occur in patients with prior underlying pulmonary disease. These lesions generally do not heal spontaneously, and persistence of the organism leads to progressive destruction and fibrosis secondary to the immune response to the organism.

Disseminated histoplasmosis follows acute infection in 1 in 2000 adults and is much higher in children and immunocompromised adults. Disseminated disease may assume a chronic, subacute, or acute course. Chronic disseminated histoplasmosis is characterized by weight loss and fatigue, with or without fever. Oral ulcers and hepatosplenomegaly are common.

Subacute disseminated histoplasmosis is marked by fever, weight loss, and malaise. Oropharyngeal ulcers and hepatosplenomegaly are prominent. Bone marrow involvement may produce anemia, leukopenia, and thrombocytopenia. Other sites of involvement include the adrenals, cardiac valves, and CNS. Untreated subacute disseminated histoplasmosis will result in death in 2 to 24 months.

Acute disseminated histoplasmosis is a fulminant process most commonly seen in severely immunosuppressed individuals, including those with AIDS, organ transplant recipients, and those receiving steroids or other immunosuppressive chemotherapy. In addition, children younger than 1 year and adults with debilitating medical conditions are also at risk, given sufficient exposure to the fungus. In contrast to the other forms of histoplasmosis, acute disseminated disease may present with a septic shock–like picture, with fever, hypotension, pulmonary infiltrates, and acute respiratory distress. Oral and gastrointestinal ulcerations and bleeding, adrenal insufficiency, meningitis, and endocarditis may also be seen. If untreated, acute disseminated histoplasmosis is fatal within days to weeks.

Histoplasmosis Duboisii

In contrast to classic histoplasmosis, pulmonary lesions are uncommon in African histoplasmosis. The localized form of histoplasmosis duboisii is a chronic disease characterized by regional lymphadenopathy with lesions of skin and bone. Skin lesions are papular or nodular and eventually progress to abscesses, which then ulcerate. About one third of patients will exhibit osseous lesions characterized by osteolysis and involvement of contiguous joints. The cranium, sternum, ribs, vertebrae, and long bones are most frequently involved, often with overlying abscesses and draining sinuses.

A more fulminant disseminated form of histoplasmosis duboisii may be seen in profoundly immunodeficient individuals. Hematogenous and lymphatic dissemination to bone marrow, liver, spleen, and other organs occurs and is marked by fever, lymphadenopathy, anemia, weight loss, and

Table 64-4 Laboratory Tests for Histoplasmosis

Test	Sensitivity (% True Positives) in Disease States		
	Disseminated	Chronic Pulmonary	Self-Limited*
Antigen	92	21	39
Culture	85	85	15
Histopathology	43	17	9
Serology	71	100	98

From Cohen J, Powderly WG, Opal SM: *Infectious diseases,* ed 3, Philadelphia, 2010, Mosby.

*Includes acute pulmonary histoplasmosis, rheumatologic syndrome, and pericarditis.

organomegaly. This form of the disease is uniformly fatal unless promptly diagnosed and treated.

Laboratory Diagnosis

The diagnosis of histoplasmosis may be made by direct microscopy, culture of blood, bone marrow, or other clinical material, and by serology, including antigen detection in blood and urine (Table 64-4; see Table 64-2). The yeast phase of the organism can be detected in sputum, bronchoalveolar lavage fluid, peripheral blood films, bone marrow, and tissue stained with Giemsa, GMS, or PAS stains (see Figure 64-10). In tissue sections, cells of *H. capsulatum* var. *capsulatum* are yeastlike, hyaline, spherical to oval, 2 to 4 µm in diameter, and uninucleate and have single buds attached by a narrow base. The cells are usually intracellular and clustered together. The cells of *H. capsulatum* var. *duboisii* are also intracellular, yeastlike, and uninucleate but are much larger (8 to 15 µm) and have thick "double-contoured" walls. They are usually in macrophages and giant cells (see Figure 64-11).

Because of the high organism burden in patients with disseminated disease, cultures of respiratory specimens, blood, bone marrow, and tissue are of value. They are less useful in self-limited or localized disease (see Table 64-4). Growth of the mycelial form in culture is slow, and once isolated, the identification must be confirmed by conversion to the yeast phase or by use of exoantigen testing or nucleic acid hybridization. As with the other dimorphic pathogens, cultures of *Histoplasma* must be handled with care in a biosafety cabinet.

Serologic diagnosis of histoplasmosis employs tests for both antigen and antibody detection (see Table 64-2). Antibody detection assays include a CF assay and an ID test. These tests are usually used together to maximize sensitivity and specificity, but neither is useful in the acute setting; CF and ID are often negative in immunocompromised patients with disseminated infection.

Detection of *Histoplasma* antigen in serum and urine by enzyme immunoassay has become very useful, particularly in diagnosing disseminated disease (see Tables 64-2 and 64-4). The sensitivity of antigen detection is greater in urine specimens than in blood and ranges from 21% in chronic pulmonary disease to 92% in disseminated disease. Serial measurements of antigen may be used to assess response to therapy and for establishing relapse of the disease. Both BDG and PCR have been useful in the diagnosis of histoplasmosis. Whereas BDG has only modest sensitivity and specificity (87% and 65%, respectively), PCR has shown excellent sensitivity (100%) and specificity (95%) and has been applied to a wide range of clinical samples.

Treatment

Because most patients with histoplasmosis recover without therapy, the first decision must be whether specific antifungal therapy is necessary or not. Some immunocompetent patients with more severe infection may exhibit prolonged symptoms and may benefit from treatment with itraconazole. In cases of severe acute pulmonary histoplasmosis with hypoxemia and acute respiratory distress syndrome, a lipid formulation of amphotericin B should be administered acutely, followed by oral itraconazole to complete a 12-week course.

Chronic pulmonary histoplasmosis also warrants treatment because it is known to progress if left untreated. Treatment with lipid amphotericin B, followed by itraconazole for 12 to 24 months, is recommended.

Disseminated histoplasmosis usually responds well to lipid amphotericin B therapy. Once stabilized, the patient may be switched to oral itraconazole to be administered over 6 to 18 months. Patients with AIDS may require lifelong therapy with itraconazole. Alternative azole agents include posaconazole, voriconazole, or fluconazole; however, secondary resistance to fluconazole has been described in patients on long-term maintenance therapy.

Histoplasmosis of the CNS is universally fatal if not treated. The therapy of choice is lipid amphotericin B followed by fluconazole for 9 to 12 months.

Patients with severe obstructive mediastinal histoplasmosis require lipid amphotericin B therapy. Itraconazole may be used for outpatient therapy.

• Paracoccidioidomycosis

Paracoccidioidomycosis is a systemic fungal infection caused by the dimorphic pathogen *Paracoccidioides brasiliensis.* This infection is also known as **South American blastomycosis** and is the major dimorphic endemic fungal infection in Latin American countries. Primary paracoccidioidomycosis usually occurs in young people as a self-limited pulmonary process. At this stage, it rarely displays a progressive acute or subacute course. Reactivation of a primary quiescent lesion may occur years later, resulting in chronic progressive pulmonary disease with or without involvement of other organs.

Morphology

The mold phase of *P. brasiliensis* grows slowly in vitro at 25° C. White colonies become apparent in 3 to 4 weeks, eventually taking on a velvety appearance. Glabrous, wrinkled, brownish colonies may also be seen. The mycelial form is nondescript and nondiagnostic: hyaline septate hyphae with intercalated chlamydoconidia. Specific identification requires conversion to the yeast form or exoantigen testing.

The characteristic yeast form is seen in tissue and in culture at 37° C. Variable-sized (3 to 30 µm or more in diameter) oval to round yeastlike cells with double refractile walls and single or multiple buds (blastoconidia) are characteristic of this fungus (Figure 64-13). The blastoconidia are connected to the parent cell by a narrow isthmus, and six or

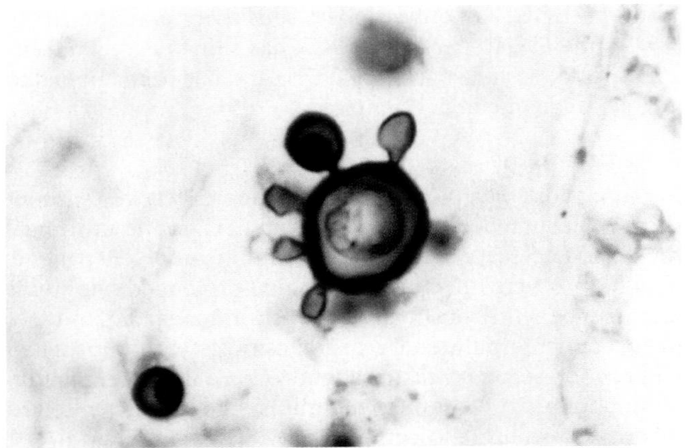

FIGURE 64-13 Gomori methenamine silver–stained yeast form of *Paracoccidioides brasiliensis* showing multiple budding "pilot wheel" morphology. (From Connor DH, Schwartz DA: *Pathology of infectious diseases,* Stamford, Conn, 1997, Appleton & Lange.)

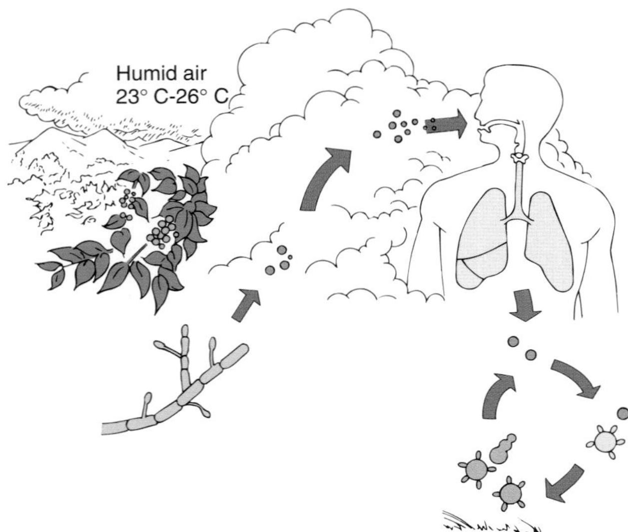

FIGURE 64-14 Natural history of the mold (saprobic) and yeast (parasitic) cycle of *Paracoccidioides brasiliensis.*

more of various sizes may be produced from a single cell ("mariner's wheel" or "pilot-wheel" morphology). The variability in size and number of blastoconidia and their connection to the parent cell are identifying features (see Figure 64-13). These features are best disclosed by GMS stain but may also be seen in H&E-stained tissues or in KOH mounts of clinical material.

Epidemiology

Paracoccidioidomycosis is endemic throughout Latin America but is more prevalent in South America than Central America (see Figure 64-2). The highest incidence is seen in Brazil, followed by Colombia, Venezuela, Ecuador, and Argentina. All patients diagnosed outside of Latin America previously had lived in Latin America. The ecology of the endemic areas includes high humidity, rich vegetation, moderate temperatures, and acid soil. These conditions are found along rivers from the Amazon jungle to small indigenous forests in Uruguay. *P. brasiliensis* has been recovered from soil in these areas; however, its ecologic niche is not well established. The portal of entry is thought to be either by inhalation or traumatic inoculation (Figure 64-14), although even this is poorly understood. Natural infection has only been documented in armadillos.

Although infection occurs in children (peak incidence 10 to 19 years), overt disease is uncommon in both children and adolescents. In adults, disease is more common in men aged 30 to 50 years. Estrogen-mediated inhibition of the mold-to-yeast transition may account for the 15:1 male/female ratio of clinical disease. Most patients with clinically apparent disease live in rural areas and have close contact with the soil. There are no reports of epidemics or human-to-human transmission. Depression of cell-mediated immunity correlates with the acute progressive form of the disease.

Clinical Syndromes

Paracoccidioidomycosis may be subclinical or progressive with acute or chronic pulmonary forms or acute, subacute, or chronic disseminated forms of the disease. Most primary infections are self-limited; however, the organism may become dormant for long periods of time and reactivate to cause clinical disease concomitant with impaired host defenses. A subacute disseminated form is seen in younger patients and immunocompromised individuals with marked lymphadenopathy, organomegaly, bone marrow involvement, and osteoarticular manifestations mimicking osteomyelitis. Recurrent fungemia results in dissemination and frequent skin lesions. Pulmonary and mucosal lesions are not seen in this form of the disease.

Adults most often present with a chronic pulmonary form of the disease marked by respiratory problems, often as the sole manifestation. The disease progresses slowly over months to years, with persistent cough, purulent sputum, chest pain, weight loss, dyspnea, and fever. Pulmonary lesions are nodular, infiltrative, fibrotic, and cavitary.

Although 25% of patients exhibit only pulmonary manifestations of the disease, the infection can disseminate to extrapulmonary sites in the absence of diagnosis and treatment. Prominent extrapulmonary locations include skin and mucosa, lymph nodes, adrenal glands, liver, spleen, CNS, and bones. The mucosal lesions are painful and ulcerated and usually confined to the mouth, lips, gums, and palate. More than 90% of these individuals are male.

Laboratory Diagnosis

The diagnosis is established by demonstration of the characteristic yeast forms on microscopic examination of sputum, bronchoalveolar lavage fluid, scrapings or biopsy of ulcers, pus draining from lymph nodes, cerebrospinal fluid, or tissue (see Table 64-2). The organism may be visualized by a variety of staining methods, including calcofluor white fluorescence, H&E, GMS, PAS, or Papanicolaou stains (see Figure 64-13). The presence of multiple buds distinguishes *P. brasiliensis* from *Cryptococcus neoformans* and *B. dermatitidis.*

Isolation of the organism in culture requires confirmation by demonstration of thermal dimorphism or exoantigen testing (detection of exoantigen 1, 2, and 3). Cultures should be manipulated in a biosafety cabinet.

Serologic testing using either ID or CF to demonstrate antibody may be helpful in suggesting the diagnosis and evaluating response to therapy (see Table 64-2). Application of both antigen detection and PCR-based diagnostic tests has been limited thus far.

Treatment

Itraconazole is the treatment of choice for most forms of the disease and generally must be given for at least 6 months. More severe or refractory infections may require lipid amphotericin B therapy followed by either itraconazole or sulfonamide therapy. Relapses are common with sulfonamide therapy, and both dose and duration require adjustment based on clinical and mycologic parameters. Fluconazole has some activity against this organism, although frequent relapses have limited its use for the treatment of this disease.

• Talaromycosis (Penicilliosis) Marneffei

Talaromycosis marneffei is a disseminated mycosis caused by the dimorphic fungus *Talaromyces* (formerly *Penicillium*) *marneffei*. This infection involves the mononuclear phagocytic system and occurs primarily in HIV-infected individuals in Thailand and southern China (see Figure 64-2).

Morphology

T. marneffei is the only species of *Talaromyces* that is a pathogenic dimorphic fungus. In its mold phase in culture at 25° C, it exhibits sporulating structures that are typical of the genus (see Figure 64-1). Identification is aided by the formation of a soluble red pigment that diffuses into the agar (see Table 64-3).

At 37° C in culture and in tissue, *T. marneffei* grows as a yeast-like organism that divides by fission and exhibits a transverse septum (Figure 64-15). The yeast form is intracellular in vivo and in this way resembles *H. capsulatum,* although it is somewhat more pleomorphic and elongated and does not bud (see Table 64-2 and Figures 64-10 and 64-15).

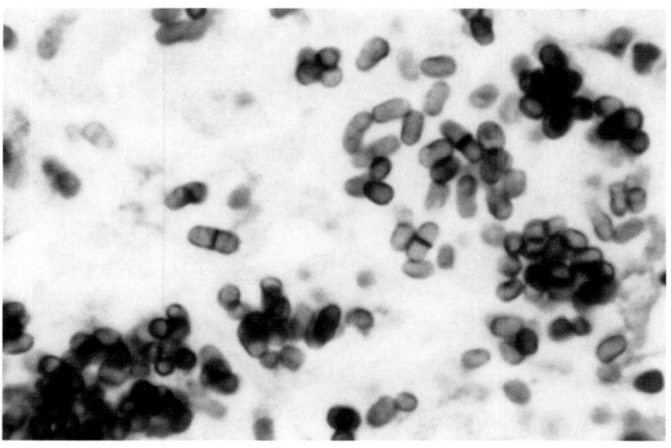

FIGURE 64-15 Gomori methenamine silver–stained yeast forms of *Talaromyces marneffei,* including forms with single, wide, transverse septa *(center).* (From Connor DH, Schwartz DA: *Pathology of infectious diseases,* Stamford, Conn, 1997, Appleton & Lange.)

Epidemiology

T. marneffei has emerged as a prominent mycotic pathogen among HIV-infected individuals in Southeast Asia (see Figure 64-2). Imported cases have been reported in Europe and the United States. Although infection has been seen in immunocompetent hosts, the vast majority of infections since 1987 have been in patients with AIDS or other immunocompromised hosts residing in, or who have visited, Southeast Asia or southern China. Talaromycosis (penicilliosis) marneffei has become an early indicator of HIV infection in that part of the world. *T. marneffei* has been isolated from bamboo rats and occasionally from soil. Laboratory-acquired infection has been reported in an immunocompromised individual exposed to the mycelial form in culture.

Clinical Syndromes

Talaromycosis marneffei is manifested when a susceptible host inhales conidia of *T. marneffei* from the environment, and disseminated infection develops. The infection may mimic tuberculosis, leishmaniasis, and other AIDS-related opportunistic infections such as histoplasmosis and cryptococcosis. Patients present with fever, cough, pulmonary infiltrates, lymphadenopathy, organomegaly, anemia, leukopenia, and thrombocytopenia. Skin lesions reflect hematogenous dissemination and appear as molluscum contagiosum–like lesions on the face and trunk.

Laboratory Diagnosis

T. marneffei is readily recovered from clinical specimens, including blood, bone marrow, bronchoalveolar lavage specimens, and tissue. In culture at 25° C to 30° C, isolation of a mold that exhibits typical *Penicillium*-like morphology and a diffusible red pigment is highly suggestive. Conversion to the yeast phase at 37° C is confirmatory. Microscopic detection of elliptic fission yeasts inside phagocytes in buffy coat preparations or smears of bone marrow, ulcerative skin lesions, or lymph nodes is diagnostic (see Figure 64-15). Serologic tests that detect antigen and antibody have been developed, although no standardized commercial tests are available. PCR and DNA sequencing methods have been applied for both direct detection from clinical samples and identification of *T. marneffei* from culture.

Treatment

A lipid formulation of amphotericin B, voriconazole, and itraconazole are often used to treat infection with *T. marneffei.* Administration of amphotericin B for 2 weeks should be followed by itraconazole for another 10 weeks. AIDS patients may require lifelong treatment with itraconazole or voriconazole to prevent relapses of the infection. Fluconazole therapy has been associated with a high rate of failure and is not recommended. The echinocandins as well as posaconazole and terbinafine may be useful, but more data are required.

Bibliography

Anstead GM, Sutton DA, Graybill JR: Adiaspiromycosis causing respiratory failure and a review of human infections due to *Emmonsia* and *Chrysosporium* spp., *J Clin Microbiol* 50:1346–1354, 2012.

Brandt ME, et al: *Histoplasma, Blastomyces, Coccidioides,* and other dimorphic fungi causing systemic mycoses. In Versalovic J, et al, editors:

Manual of clinical microbiology, ed 10, Washington, DC, 2011, American Society for Microbiology Press.

Brown J, Benedict K, Park BJ, et al: Coccidioidomycosis: epidemiology, *Clin Epidemiol* 5:185–197, 2013.

Connor DH, Schwartz DA: *Pathology of infectious diseases*, Stamford, Conn, 1997, Appleton & Lange.

Kauffman CA: Histoplasmosis: a clinical and laboratory update, *Clin Microbiol Rev* 20:115, 1997.

Kenyon C, Bonorchis K, Corcoran C, et al: A dimorphic fungus causing disseminated infection in South Africa, *N Engl J Med* 369:1416–1424, 2013.

Restrepo A, Gomez BL, Tobon A: Paracoccidioidomycosis: Latin America's own fungal disorder, *Curr Fungal Infect Rep* 6:303–311, 2012.

Roy M, Benedict K, Deak E, et al: A large community outbreak of blastomycosis in Wisconsin with geographic and ethnic clustering, *Clin Infect Dis* 57:655–662, 2013.

Smith JA, Kauffman CA: Blastomycosis, *Proc Am Thorac Soc* 7:173–180, 2010.

Vanittanakom N, Cooper CR Jr, Fisher MC, et al: *Penicillium marneffei* infection and recent advances in the epidemiology and molecular biology aspects, *Clin Microbiol Rev* 19:95, 2006.

CHAPTER

65 OPPORTUNISTIC MYCOSES

George is a 45-year-old man who underwent an allogeneic stem cell transplant as part of his treatment for acute leukemia. The transplant went well, and after engraftment George was discharged from the hospital. During the course of his transplant, George's physicians placed him on antifungal prophylaxis with voriconazole because of concerns regarding aspergillosis, which had been a problem in the hospital over the past few years. After discharge, George did well and his antifungal prophylaxis was continued; however, on a clinical visit on day 140 post transplant, he was noted to have a rash and elevated liver function studies. About 1 week later, he began having bloody diarrhea, and his physician became concerned about graft-versus-host disease (GVHD). A rectal biopsy was performed, confirming GVHD, and George's immunosuppressive regimen was increased, as was his daily dose of voriconazole. The signs and symptoms of GVHD continued, and eventually George was readmitted to the hospital, where he was found to be confused, febrile, and short of breath. A chest radiograph showed a wedge-shaped infiltrate in the right lower lung field, and imaging studies of his sinuses showed bilateral opacification.

1. What is the differential diagnosis of this process?
2. About which fungal pathogens would you be concerned in an immunosuppressed individual receiving voriconazole prophylaxis?
3. How would you go about making a diagnosis?
4. What course of therapy would you undertake?

Answers to these questions are available on StudentConsult.com.

• SUMMARIES CLINICALLY SIGNIFICANT ORGANISMS

Candidiasis

Trigger Words

Candida, pseudohyphae, endogenous, exogenous, yeast and pseudohyphae, immunocompromised, vaginal thrush, oropharyngeal

Biology, Virulence, and Disease

- Opportunistic yeasts causing infections ranging from superficial mucosal and cutaneous disease to hematogenously disseminated, often fatal, infections
- Vast majority of infections are due to five major species: *C. albicans, C. glabrata, C. parapsilosis, C. tropicalis,* and *C. krusei.*
- Morphology ranges from budding yeasts to pseudohyphae and true hyphae
- Reproduction is by formation of blastoconidia (buds)
- Most important group of opportunistic fungal pathogens
- May be community acquired (mucosal infections) or hospital associated (invasive disease)

Epidemiology

- *Candida* spp. are known colonizers of humans and other warm-blooded animals
- Primary site of colonization is gastrointestinal tract; commensals in the vagina, urethra, skin, and nails
- Most infections are endogenous, involving normally commensal host flora
- Exogenous transmission in hospitals also occurs
- *C. albicans* predominates in most types of infection
- Consequences of *Candida* bloodstream infections (BSIs) are severe; risk factors include hematologic malignancies and neutropenia, abdominal surgery, prematurity in infants, and age > 70 years

Diagnosis

- Clinical appearance, direct microscopic examination, and culture
- Hematogenously disseminated infections and candidemia difficult to diagnose on clinical grounds alone
- Laboratory diagnosis involves procurement of appropriate clinical material, followed by direct microscopic examination, culture, and (increasingly) application of molecular, antigenic, and proteomic analysis

Treatment, Prevention, and Control

- Mucosal and cutaneous infection: topical and systemically active antifungal agents include azoles (itraconazole, fluconazole, miconazole, many others), polyenes (amphotericin B and nystatin)

- Invasive candidiasis and candidemia: oral or intravenous administration depending on antifungal agent and severity of disease and/or immunosuppression; azoles (fluconazole, voriconazole, posaconazole, isavuconazole), echinocandins (anidulafungin, caspofungin, micafungin), amphotericin B formulations (deoxycholate and lipid formulations), flucytosine

Cryptococcosis

Trigger Words

Capsule, budding yeast, CNS, neurotropic, India ink, antigen, AIDS

Biology, Virulence, and Disease

- Systemic mycosis caused by the fungi *Cryptococcus neoformans* and *C. gattii*
- *C. neoformans* includes capsular serotypes A, D, and AD; var. *grubii* (serotype A) and var. *neoformans* (serotype D)
- *C. gattii* includes serotypes B and C
- Spherical to oval, encapsulated, yeastlike organisms that replicate by budding
- Both species may cause pulmonary, hematogenously disseminated, and central nervous system (CNS) disease

Epidemiology

- Usually acquired by inhaling aerosolized cells of *C. neoformans* and *C. gattii*
- Both species pathogenic for immunocompetent individuals
- *C. neoformans:* most often encountered as opportunistic pathogen; found worldwide in soil contaminated with avian excreta
- *C. gattii:* found in tropical and subtropical climates in association with eucalyptus trees; the focus in the Pacific Northwest has been associated with Douglas fir trees
- Disease is similar, although *C. gattii* infection tends to occur in immunocompetent individuals and has a lower associated mortality
- Incidence has progressively declined since early 1990s owing to widespread use of fluconazole and successful treatment of HIV infection with antiviral drugs

Diagnosis

- May present as pneumonic process or (more commonly) as CNS infection
- Diagnosis may be made by culture of blood, cerebrospinal fluid (CSF), or other clinical material
- Microscopic examination of CSF may reveal characteristic encapsulated budding yeast cells
- Cryptococcal meningitis: diagnosis by detection of polysaccharide antigen in serum or CSF

Treatment, Prevention, and Control

- Cryptococcal meningitis and other disseminated forms universally fatal if left untreated
- Antifungal therapy: amphotericin B (deoxycholate or lipid formulation) plus flucytosine followed by maintenance/consolidation therapy with fluconazole (preferred) or itraconazole
- Effective management of CNS pressure and immune reconstitution inflammatory syndrome (IRIS) crucial to successful management of cryptococcal meningitis

Aspergillosis

Trigger Words

Septate branching hyphae, hypersensitivity pneumonitis, angioinvasive, aspergilloma, conidia

Biology, Virulence, and Disease

- Broad spectrum of diseases caused by filamentous fungi (molds) of genus *Aspergillus*
- Exposure to spores in environment may cause allergic reactions in hypersensitized hosts or destructive, invasive, pulmonary, and disseminated disease in highly immunocompromised hosts
- Vast majority of infections caused by *A. fumigatus* (most common), *A. flavus, A. niger,* and *A. terreus*
- Hyaline molds that produce vast amounts of spores (conidia) that serve as infectious propagules upon inhalation by host
- Invasive aspergillosis marked by angioinvasion and tissue destruction due to infarction
- Hematogenous dissemination of infection to extrapulmonary sites (most commonly brain, heart, kidneys, GI tract, liver, spleen) common because of angioinvasive nature of fungus

Epidemiology

- *Aspergillus* spp. common worldwide; conidia ubiquitous in air, soil, decaying matter
- Within hospital environment, *Aspergillus* spp. may be found in air, showerheads, water storage tanks, potted plants
- Conidia (spores) constantly being inhaled; respiratory tract most frequent and important portal of entry
- Host reaction, associated pathologic findings, and outcome of infection depend more on host factors than virulence or pathogenesis of individual species

Diagnosis

- Serologic, culture, histopathologic, molecular, biochemical, and antigenic methods supplemented by imaging studies

Treatment, Prevention, and Control

- Treatment usually involves administration of corticosteroids coupled with pulmonary toilet
- Treatment of chronic pulmonary aspergillosis may involve steroids as well as long-term antifungal therapy, usually with an azole antifungal agent
- Prophylaxis of high-risk (neutropenic) patients usually accomplished by administration of a mold-active azole (itraconazole, posaconazole, voriconazole)
- Specific antifungal therapy of invasive aspergillosis usually involves administration of voriconazole or a lipid formulation of amphotericin B; isavuconazole has recently been cleared by the U.S. Food and Drug Administration for treatment of invasive aspergillosis
- Efforts to decrease immunosuppression and/or reconstitute host immune defenses important, as is surgical resection of infected tissue if possible
- Resection of aspergillomas only considered in instances of severe hemoptysis

The frequency of invasive mycoses caused by opportunistic fungal pathogens has increased significantly over the past 2 decades. This increase in infections is associated with excessive morbidity and mortality (see Chapter 57, Table 57-1) and is directly related to the increase in patient populations at risk for developing serious fungal infections. High-risk groups include individuals undergoing blood and marrow transplantation (BMT), solid organ transplantation, or major surgery (especially gastrointestinal [GI] surgery) and those with acquired immunodeficiency syndrome (AIDS), neoplastic disease, immunosuppressive therapy, advanced age, and premature birth (Table 65-1). The most well-known causes of opportunistic mycoses include *Candida albicans, Cryptococcus neoformans,* and *Aspergillus fumigatus* (Box 65-1). The estimated frequency of invasive mycoses caused by these pathogens is over 400,000 infections per year for *Candida,* over 1,000,000 for *C. neoformans,* and over 400,000 for *Aspergillus* (see Chapter 57, Table 57-1). In addition to these agents, of increasing importance is the growing list of "other" opportunistic fungi (see Box 65-1). New and emerging fungal pathogens include species of *Candida* and *Aspergillus* other than *C. albicans* and *A. fumigatus,* microsporidia, opportunistic yeastlike fungi (e.g., *Trichosporon, Malassezia, Rhodotorula* species, *Blastoschizomyces capitatus*), Mucormycetes, hyaline molds (e.g., *Fusarium, Sarocladium, Scedosporium, Scopulariopsis, Purpureocillium (Paecilomyces), Trichoderma* species), and a wide variety of dematiaceous fungi (see Box 65-1). Infections caused by these organisms range from catheter-related fungemia and peritonitis to more localized infections involving lung, skin, and paranasal sinuses to widespread hematogenous dissemination. Many of these fungi were previously thought to be nonpathogenic and now are recognized causes of invasive mycoses in compromised patients. Estimates of the annual incidence of the less common mycoses have been virtually nonexistent; however, data from a population-based survey conducted by the Centers for Disease Control and Prevention indicate that mucormycosis occurs at a rate of 1.7 infections per million population per year, hyalohyphomycosis (*Fusarium, Sarocladium,* etc.) at 1.2 infections per million per year, and phaeohyphomycosis (dematiaceous molds) at 1.0 infection per million per year.

Given the complexity of the patients at risk for infection and the diverse array of fungal pathogens, opportunistic mycoses pose a considerable diagnostic and therapeutic challenge. Diagnosis depends upon a heightened clinical suspicion (think **fungus**) and obtaining appropriate material for culture and histopathology. Isolation and identification of the infecting organisms is very important in properly managing infections because of the less common opportunistic fungi. Some of these organisms are inherently nonsusceptible to standard azole, echinocandin, or polyene therapy (see Chapter 61) and may require the use of alternative

Table 65-1 Predisposing Factors for Opportunistic Mycoses

Factor	Possible Role in Infection	Major Opportunistic Pathogens
Antimicrobial agents (number and duration)	Promote fungal colonization Provide intravascular access	*Candida* spp., other yeastlike fungi
Adrenal corticosteroid	Immunosuppression	*Cryptococcus neoformans, Aspergillus* spp., Mucormycetes, other molds, *Pneumocystis*
Chemotherapy	Immunosuppression	*Candida* spp., *Aspergillus* spp., *Pneumocystis*
Hematologic/solid organ malignancy	Immunosuppression	*Candida* spp., *Aspergillus* spp., Mucormycetes, other molds and yeastlike fungi, *Pneumocystis*
Previous colonization	Translocation across mucosa	*Candida* spp.
Indwelling catheter (central venous, pressure transducer, Swan-Ganz)	Direct vascular access Contaminated product	*Candida* spp., other yeastlike fungi
Total parenteral nutrition	Direct vascular access Contamination of infusate	*Candida* spp., *Malassezia* spp., other yeastlike fungi
Neutropenia (WBC < 500/mm^3)	Immunosuppression	*Aspergillus* spp., *Candida* spp., other molds and yeastlike fungi
Extensive surgery or burns	Route of infection Direct vascular access	*Candida* spp., *Fusarium* spp., Mucormycetes
Assisted ventilation	Route of infection	*Candida* spp., *Aspergillus* spp.
Hospitalization or intensive care unit stay	Exposure to pathogens Exposure to additional risk factors	*Candida* spp., other yeastlike fungi, *Aspergillus* spp.
Hemodialysis, peritoneal dialysis	Route of infection Immunosuppression	*Candida* spp., *Rhodotorula* spp., other yeastlike fungi
Malnutrition	Immunosuppression	*Pneumocystis, Candida* spp., *Cryptococcus neoformans*
HIV infection/AIDS	Immunosuppression	*Cryptococcus neoformans, Pneumocystis, Candida* spp., Microsporidia
Extremes of age	Immunosuppression Numerous comorbidities	*Candida* spp.

AIDS, Acquired immunodeficiency syndrome; *HIV,* human immunodeficiency virus; *WBC,* white blood cells.

Box 65-1 Agents of Opportunistic Mycoses*

***Candida* spp.**
C. albicans
C. glabrata
C. parapsilosis
C. tropicalis
C. krusei
C. lusitaniae
C. guilliermondii
C. dubliniensis
C. rugosa

***Cryptococcus neoformans* and Other Opportunistic Yeastlike Fungi**
C. neoformans/gattii
Malassezia spp.
Trichosporon spp.
Rhodotorula spp.
Blastoschizomyces capitatus
Microsporidia
Pneumocystis jirovecii

***Aspergillus* spp.**
A. fumigatus
A. flavus
A. niger
A. versicolor
A. terreus

Mucormycetes
Rhizopus spp.
Mucor spp.
Rhizomucor spp.
Lichtheimia corymbifera
Cunninghamella spp.

Other Hyaline Molds
Fusarium spp.
Sarocladium spp.
Scedosporium spp.
Paecilomyces spp.
Trichoderma spp.
Scopulariopsis spp.

Dematiaceous Molds
Alternaria spp.
Bipolaris spp.
Cladophialophora spp.
Curvularia spp.
Exophiala spp.
Exserohilum spp.
Wangiella spp.

*List is not all-inclusive.

antifungal agents in addition to surgical management and reversal of the underlying impairment of host defenses.

• Candidiasis

Candida spp. are clearly the most important group of opportunistic fungal pathogens. They are the third most common cause of central line–associated bloodstream infections (BSIs), exceeding that of any individual gram-negative pathogen (Table 65-2; Clinical Case 65-1). Between 1980 and the present, the frequency of *Candida* BSI has risen steadily in hospitals of all sizes and in all age groups.

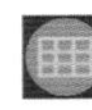

Table 65-2 Central Line–Associated Bloodstream Infections: Most Frequent Associated Pathogens—National Healthcare Safety Network

Rank	Pathogen	% of Isolates*
1	Coagulase-negative staphylococci	34.1
2	*Enterococcus* spp.	16.0
3	*Candida* spp.	11.8
4	*Staphylococcus aureus*	9.9
5	*Klebsiella pneumoniae*	4.9
6	*Enterobacter* spp.	3.9
7	*Pseudomonas aeruginosa*	3.1
8	*Escherichia coli*	2.7
9	*Acinetobacter baumannii*	2.2
10	*Klebsiella oxytoca*	0.9

Data from Hidron AI, Edwards JR, Patel J, et al: Antimicrobial-resistant pathogens associated with healthcare-associated infections: annual summary of data reported to the National Healthcare Safety Network at the Centers for Disease Control and Prevention, 2006-2007, *Infect Control Hosp Epidemiol* 29:996–1011, 2008.
*Percent of a total of 11,428 infections.

Although more than 100 species of *Candida* have been described, only a few have been implicated in clinical infections (see Box 65-1). *C. albicans* is the species most commonly isolated from clinical material and generally accounts for 90% to 100% of mucosal isolates and 40% to 70% of isolates from BSI, depending on the clinical service and the patient's underlying disease (Table 65-3). Approximately 95% of all *Candida* BSIs are accounted for by four species: *C. albicans, C. glabrata, C. parapsilosis,* and *C. tropicalis* (see Table 65-3). Among these common species, only *C. glabrata* can be said to be truly "emerging" as a cause of BSI, in part because of its intrinsic and acquired resistance to azoles and other commonly used antifungal agents. The remaining 5% of *Candida* BSI encompasses 12 to 14 different species, including *C. krusei, C. lusitaniae, C. dubliniensis,* and *C. rugosa* among others (see Box 65-1). Although these species must be considered "rare" causes of candidiasis, several have been observed to occur in nosocomial clusters and/or to exhibit innate or acquired resistance to one or more established antifungal agents.

Morphology

All *Candida* species exist as oval yeastlike forms (3 to 5 μm) that produce buds or blastoconidia. Species of *Candida* other than *C. glabrata* also produce pseudohyphae and true hyphae (Figure 65-1; also see Chapter 57, Figure 57-2A and Chapter 60, Figure 60-1). In addition, *C. albicans* forms germ tubes (Chapter 57, Figure 57-2) and terminal thick-walled chlamydoconidia (Figure 65-2). *C. glabrata,* the second most common species of *Candida* in many settings, is incapable of forming pseudohyphae, germ tubes, or true hyphae under most conditions. In histologic sections, all *Candida* spp. stain poorly with hematoxylin and eosin (H&E) and well with the periodic acid–Schiff (PAS), Gomori methenamine silver (GMS), and Gridley fungus stains.

In culture, most *Candida* spp. form smooth, white, creamy, domed colonies. *C. albicans* and other species may also undergo **phenotypic switching,** in which a single strain of *Candida* may change reversibly among several different morphotypes ranging from the typical smooth white colony composed of predominantly budding yeastlike cells to very "fuzzy" or "hairy" colonies composed primarily of pseudohyphal and hyphal forms. The frequency of the switching phenomenon is too high to result from gene mutations and too low to be attributable to mass conversion, whereby all cells in the population change their phenotype in response to signals from the environment. It is likely that switching serves as some type of master system in *C. albicans*—and other species—for rapid response at the level of individual cells to changes in the local microenvironment. It has been postulated that phenotypic switching explains the ability of *C. albicans* to survive in many different environmental microniches within the human host.

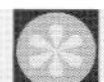

Clinical Case 65-1 Candidemia

Posteraro and associates (*J Clin Microbiol* 44:3046–3047, 2006) describe a case of recurrent fungemia in a 35-year-old woman. The patient was seen at 5 weeks' gestation after intrauterine insemination. She presented with fever, tachycardia, and hypotension. The white blood cell (WBC) count was 23,500/μl with 78% neutrophils. She experienced a spontaneous abortion. Severe chorioamnionitis was diagnosed, placental and fetal tissues were cultured, and blood cultures and vaginal swabs were obtained. The patient was treated with broad-spectrum antibacterial agents. Five days later, no clinical improvement was seen. The cultured blood and placental samples grew the yeast *Candida glabrata,* which was also isolated from the patient's vaginal cultures. On the basis of fluconazole minimal inhibitory concentrations, indicating that the organism was susceptible, the patient was placed on fluconazole. Four weeks later, she experienced complete resolution of her symptoms, with eradication of the fungus from her bloodstream. Antifungal treatment was discontinued, and the patient was sent home, where she did well. Six months later she was readmitted to the hospital with fever, chills, and fatigue. The WBC count was elevated at 21,500/μl with 73% neutrophils. Consecutive blood cultures were again positive for *C. glabrata,* which was also found in cultures of vaginal fluid. All isolates were found to be resistant to fluconazole. On the basis of these findings, the patient was treated with amphotericin B. Within 1 week, the patient's clinical condition was improved. After 1 month of amphotericin B treatment, blood cultures were sterile, and she was discharged from the hospital. Three years later, she remained free of any evidence of infection.

This is an unusual case in that the patient was not immunocompromised yet experienced recurrent candidemia with *C. glabrata.* The use of fluconazole as initial therapy, although apparently successful, induced up-regulation of drug efflux pumps in the organism and allowed later isolates to become resistant to fluconazole and other azoles.

Epidemiology

Candida spp. are known colonizers of humans and other warm-blooded animals. As such, they are found in humans and in nature worldwide. The primary site of colonization is the GI tract from mouth to rectum. They may also be found as commensals in the vagina and urethra, on the skin, and under the fingernails and toenails. *C. albicans,* the most common etiologic agent of human disease, has also been found apart from humans and animals in air, water, and soil.

It is estimated that 25% to 50% of healthy persons carry *Candida* as part of the normal flora of the mouth, with *C. albicans* accounting for 70% to 80% of isolates. Oral carriage rates are increased substantially in hospitalized patients; those with human immunodeficiency virus (HIV) infection, dentures, and diabetes; patients receiving antineoplastic chemotherapy; those receiving antibiotics; and children. Virtually all humans may carry one or more *Candida* species throughout their GI tract, and the levels of carriage may increase to that detectable in illness or other circumstances in which the host's microbial suppression mechanisms become compromised.

The predominant source of infection caused by *Candida* spp., from superficial mucosal and cutaneous disease to hematogenous dissemination, is the patient. That is, most types of candidiasis represent **endogenous** infection in which the normally commensal host flora take advantage of the "opportunity" to cause infection. To do so, there must be

Table 65-3 Species Distribution of *Candida* Bloodstream Infection Isolates by Clinical Service in the United States*

	% of Isolates by Species and Clinical Service (No. Tested)							
Species	**GMED (2554)**	**HEME (455)**	**SCT (165)**	**NICU (62)**	**SOT (292)**	**ST (629)**	**SURG (1175)**	**HIV/AIDS (82)**
C. albicans	41.3	22.0	17.6	54.8	33.2	42.1	44.5	40.2
C. glabrata	24.8	25.5	32.7	1.6	38.4	28.9	23.7	22.0
C. parapsilosis	14.5	12.3	13.9	30.6	11.3	11.6	15.4	9.8
C. tropicalis	7.7	15.4	7.9	0.0	5.5	7.6	7.1	7.3
C. krusei	2.7	16.0	19.4	0.0	2.7	2.2	1.4	3.7
Other	8.9	8.8	8.5	12.9	8.9	16.1	7.6	17.1

GMED, General medicine; *HEME,* hematologic malignancy; *HIV/AIDS,* human immunodeficiency virus/acquired immunodeficiency syndrome; *NICU,* neonatal intensive care unit; *SCT,* stem cell transplant; *SOT,* solid organ transplant; *ST,* solid tumor; *SURG,* surgical (nontransplant).

*Data compiled from Pfaller M, Neofytos D, Diekema D, et al: Epidemiology and outcomes of candidemia in 3648 patients: data from the Prospective Antifungal Therapy (PATH Alliance) registry, 2004-2008, *Diagn Microbiol Infect Dis* 74:323–331, 2012.

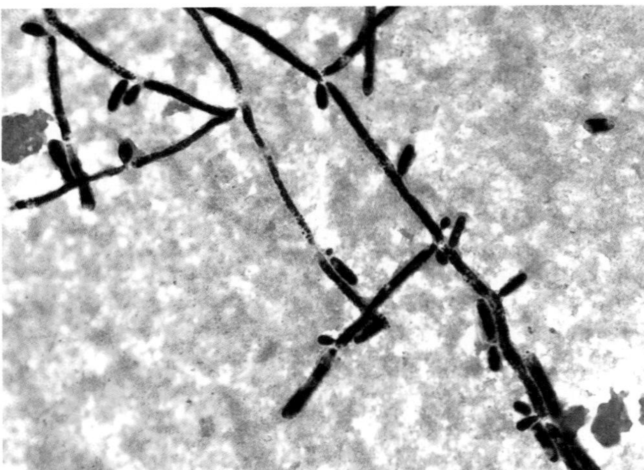

FIGURE 65-1 *Candida tropicalis* blastoconidia and pseudohyphae (Gram stain, ×1000).

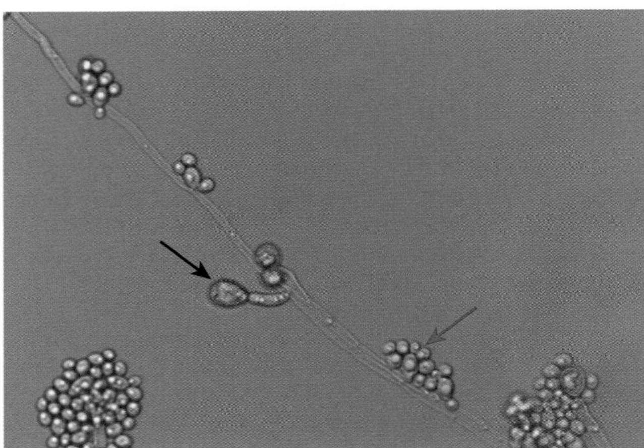

FIGURE 65-2 *Candida albicans.* Microscopic morphology in cornmeal agar showing large chlamydospores *(black arrow),* blastoconidia *(red arrow),* hyphae, and pseudohyphae.

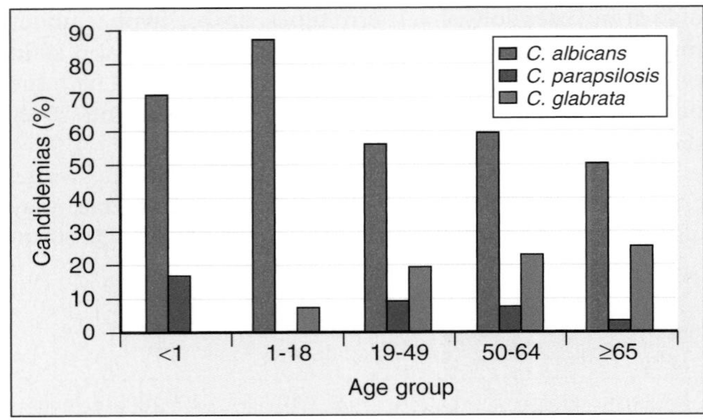

FIGURE 65-3 Percentage of all candidemias caused by selected *Candida* species in each age group. Data are from the Emerging Infections and the Epidemiology of Iowa Organisms Survey, 1998 to 2001. (Data from Pfaller MA, Diekema DJ: Epidemiology of invasive candidiasis: a persistent public health problem, *Clin Microbiol Rev* 20:133, 2007.)

a lowering of the host's anti-*Candida* barrier. In the cases of *Candida* BSI, transfer of the organism from the GI mucosa to the bloodstream requires prior overgrowth of the numbers of yeasts in their commensal habitat, coupled with a breach in the integrity of the GI mucosa.

Exogenous transmission of *Candida* may also account for a proportion of certain types of candidiasis. Examples include the use of contaminated irrigation solutions, parenteral nutrition fluids, vascular pressure transducers, cardiac valves, and corneas. Transmission of *Candida* spp. from health care workers to patients and from patient to patient has been well documented, especially in the intensive care unit environment. The hands of health care workers serve as potential reservoirs for nosocomial transmission of *Candida* spp.

Among the various species of *Candida* capable of causing human infection (see Box 65-1 and Table 65-3), *C. albicans* predominates in most types of infection. Infections of genital, cutaneous, and oral sites almost always involve *C. albicans*. A wider array of *Candida* spp. is seen causing BSI and other forms of invasive candidiasis, and although *C. albicans* usually predominates (see Table 65-3), the frequency with which this and other species of *Candida* are isolated from blood varies considerably according to the clinical service (see Table 65-3), the age of the patient (Figure 65-3), and the local, regional, or global setting (Table 65-4). Whereas *C. albicans* and *C. parapsilosis* predominate as causes of BSI among infants and children, a decrease in *C. albicans* and *C. parapsilosis* infections and a prominent increase in *C. glabrata* infections is seen among older individuals (see Figure 65-3). Likewise, although *C. glabrata* is the second most common species causing BSI in North America, it is seen at a lower frequency in Latin America, where *C. parapsilosis* and *C. tropicalis* are more common (see Table 65-4). The differences in the number and types of *Candida* spp. causing infections may be influenced by numerous factors, including patient age, increased immunosuppression, antifungal drug exposure, or differences in infection-control practices. Each one of these factors, alone or in combination, may affect the prevalence of different *Candida* spp. in each institution. For example, the use of azoles (e.g., fluconazole) for antifungal prophylaxis in hematologic malignancy patients and recipients of stem cell transplantation may increase the likelihood of infections caused by *C. glabrata* and *C. krusei,* two species with decreased susceptibility to this class of antifungals (see Table 65-3). Likewise, breaks in infection-control precautions and in the proper care of vascular catheters may lead to more infections with *C. parapsilosis,* the predominant species isolated from the hands of health care workers and a frequent cause of catheter-related fungemia.

The consequences of *Candida* BSI in the hospitalized patient are severe. Hospitalized patients with candidemia have been shown to be at a twofold greater risk of death in the hospital than those with noncandidal BSI. Among all patients with nosocomial (hospital-acquired) BSI, candidemia was found to be an independent predictor of death in hospitals. Although estimates of mortality may be confounded by the serious nature of the underlying diseases in many of these patients, matched cohort studies have confirmed that the mortality directly attributable to the fungal infection is quite

Table 65-4 Species Distribution of *Candida* Bloodstream Infection Isolates by Geographic Region

Region	No. of Isolates	% of Isolates by Species				
		CA	CG	CP	CT	CK
Asia-Pacific	366	44.8	14.2	25.4	12.0	0.8
Europe	1097	50.3	16.0	17.8	8.1	2.6
Latin America	433	43.0	8.8	24.0	17.6	1.8
North America	1211	41.5	25.3	14.3	9.0	3.3
TOTAL	**3107**	45.2	18.4	18.2	10.3	2.5

Modified from Pfaller MA, Messer SA, Woosley LN, et al: Echinocandin and triazole antifungal susceptibility profiles for clinical opportunistic yeast and mold isolates collected from 2010 to 2011: application of new CLSI clinical breakpoints and epidemiological cutoff values for characterization of geographic and temporal trends of antifungal resistance, *J Clin Microbiol* 51:2571–2581, 2013.

CA, Candida albicans; CG, C. glabrata; CK, C. krusei; CP, C. parapsilosis; CT, C. tropicalis.

Table 65-5 Excess Mortality Attributable to Nosocomial Infections with *Candida* and *Aspergillus*

Type of Mortality Rate	Percent Mortality		
	*Candida**		*Aspergillus*[†]
	1988	2001	1991
Crude mortality			
Cases	57	61	95
Controls	19	12	10
Attributable mortality	38	49	85

*Patients with candidemia. Data from Wey SB, Mori M, Pfaller MA, et al: Hospital-acquired candidemia. The attributable mortality and excess length of stay, *Arch Intern Med* 148:2642–2645, 1988; and Gudlaugsson O, Gillespie S, Lee K, et al: Attributable mortality of nosocomial candidemia, revisited, *Clin Infect Dis* 37:1172–1177, 2003.

[†]Bone marrow transplant patients with invasive pulmonary aspergillosis. Data from Pannuti CS, Gingrich RD, Pfaller MA, et al: Nosocomial pneumonia in adult patients undergoing bone marrow transplantation: a 9-year study, *J Clin Oncol* 9:77–84, 1991.

high (Table 65-5). Notably, the excess or attributable mortality resulting from candidemia has not decreased from that observed in the mid-1980s to that observed in the present day, despite the introduction of new antifungal agents with good activity against most species of *Candida*.

Clearly, more is known about the epidemiology of nosocomial candidemia than any other fungal infection. The accumulated evidence allows one to propose a general view of nosocomial candidemia (Figure 65-4). Certain hospitalized individuals are clearly at increased risk of acquiring candidemia during hospitalization because of their underlying medical condition: patients with hematologic malignancies and/or neutropenia, those undergoing GI surgery, premature infants, and patients older than 70 years (see Table 65-1 and Figure 65-4). Compared to control subjects without the specific risk factors or exposures, the likelihood of these already high-risk patients contracting candidemia

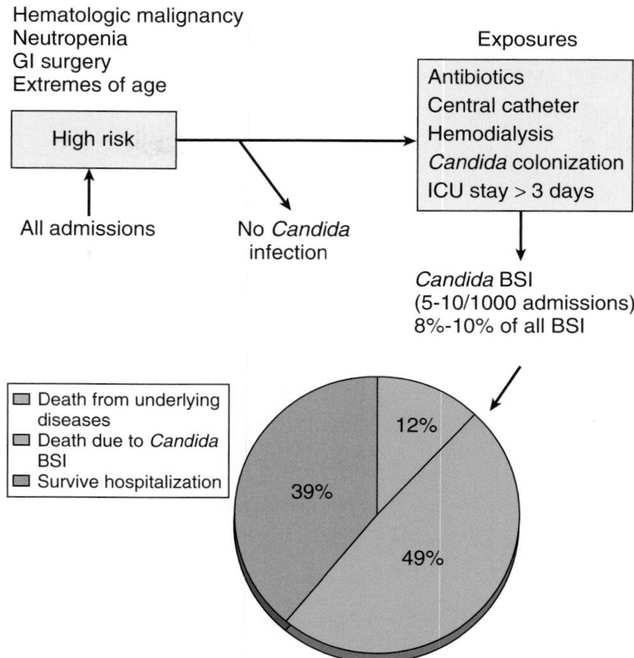

FIGURE 65-4 Global view of hospital-acquired candidemia. *BSI,* Bloodstream infections; *GI,* gastrointestinal; *ICU,* intensive care unit. (Modified from Lockhart SR et al: The epidemiology of fungal infections. In Anaissie EJ, McGinnis MR, Pfaller MA, editors: *Clinical mycology,* ed 2, New York, 2009, Churchill Livingstone.)

in the hospital is approximately 2 times greater for each class of antibiotics they receive, 7 times greater if they have a central venous catheter, 10 times greater if *Candida* has been found to be colonizing other anatomic sites, and 18 times greater if they have undergone acute hemodialysis. Hospitalization in the intensive care unit setting provides the opportunity for transmission of *Candida* among patients and has been shown to be an additional independent risk factor.

The available epidemiologic data indicates that between 20 and 40 of every 1000 high-risk patients exposed to the above risk factors will contract BSI caused by *Candida* spp. (8% to 10% of all nosocomial BSI; see Table 65-2). Approximately 49% of these patients will die as a result of their infection, 12% will die of their underlying disease, and 39% will survive hospitalization (see Figure 65-4). This picture has not changed (and may even be worse) from that seen in the mid-1980s. The outcome for almost half of those patients with candidemia could be improved by more effective means of prevention, diagnosis, and therapy. Clearly the most desirable of these is prevention, which is best approached by rigorous control of the exposures—especially limiting use of broad-spectrum antibiotics, improving catheter care, and adhering to infection-control practices.

Clinical Syndromes

Given the right setting, *Candida* spp. can cause clinically apparent infection of virtually any organ system (Table 65-6). Infections range from superficial mucosal and cutaneous candidiasis to widespread hematogenous dissemination involving target organs such as the liver, spleen, kidney, heart, and brain. In the latter situation, the mortality directly

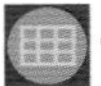

Table 65-6 Types of *Candida* Infection and Associated Predisposing Factors

Type of Disease	Predisposing Factors	Type of Disease	Predisposing Factors
Oropharyngeal infection	Age extremes	Endocarditis	Major surgery
	Denture wearers		Previous valvular disease
	Diabetes mellitus		Prosthetic valve
	Antibiotic use		Intravenous drug use
	Radiotherapy for head and neck cancer		Long-term central venous catheter
	Inhaled and systemic steroids	Pericarditis	Thoracic surgery
	Cytotoxic chemotherapy		Immunosuppression
	HIV infection	CNS infection	CNS surgery
	Hematologic malignancies		Ventriculoperitoneal shunt
	Stem cell or solid organ transplantation		Ocular surgery
Esophagitis	Systemic corticosteroids	Ocular infection	Trauma
	AIDS		Surgery
	Cancer	Bone and joint infection	Trauma
	Stem cell or solid organ transplantation		Intraarticular injections
Vulvovaginal infection	Oral contraceptives		Diabetic foot
	Pregnancy	Abdominal infection	Perforation
	Diabetes mellitus		Abdominal surgery
	Systemic corticosteroids		Anastomotic leaks
	HIV infection		Pancreatitis
	Antibiotic use		Continuous ambulatory peritoneal dialysis
Infections of the skin and nails	Local moisture and occlusion	Hematogenous infection	Solid organ transplantation
	Immersion of hands in water		Colonization
	Peripheral vascular disease		Prolonged antibiotic use
Chronic mucocutaneous candidiasis	T-lymphocyte defects		Abdominal surgery
			Intensive care support
Urinary tract infection	Indwelling urinary catheter		Total parenteral nutrition
	Urinary obstruction		Hemodialysis
	Urinary procedures		Immunosuppression
	Diabetes mellitus		Extremes of age
Pneumonia	Aspiration (rare)		Stem cell transplantation
			Vascular catheters

Modified from Dignani MC, Solomkin JS, Anaissie EJ: *Candida*. In Anaissie EJ, McGinnis MR, Pfaller MA, editors: *Clinical mycology,* ed 2, New York, 2009, Churchill Livingstone.
AIDS, Acquired immunodeficiency syndrome; *CNS,* central nervous system; *HIV,* human immunodeficiency virus.

attributable to the infectious process approaches 50% (see Table 65-5 and Figure 65-4).

Mucosal infections caused by *Candida* spp. (known as "thrush") may be limited to the oropharynx or extend to the esophagus and the entire GI tract. In women, the vaginal mucosa is also a common site of infection. These infections are generally seen in individuals with local or generalized immunosuppression or in those settings in which candidal overgrowth is favored (see Table 65-6). These infections usually present as white "cottage cheese"–like patches on the mucosal surface. Other presentations include the **pseudomembranous** type, which reveals a raw bleeding surface when scraped; the **erythematous** type—flat, red, occasionally sore areas; candidal **leukoplakia**—nonremovable white thickening of epithelium caused by *Candida* spp.; and angular **cheilitis**—sore fissures at the corners of the mouth.

Candida spp. may cause localized skin infection in areas where the skin surface is occluded and moist (e.g., groin, axillae, toe webs, breast folds). These infections present as a pruritic rash with erythematous vesiculopustular lesions.

Onychomycosis and paronychia may occur in the setting of a mixed microbial flora, including *Candida*. The species most commonly involved are *C. albicans, C. parapsilosis,* and *C. guilliermondii.*

Skin lesions may also appear during the course of hematogenous dissemination. These lesions are of major diagnostic importance; they can be directly biopsied and thus provide an etiologic diagnosis of a systemic process.

Chronic mucocutaneous candidiasis is a rare condition marked by a deficiency in T-lymphocyte responsiveness to *Candida* spp. These patients suffer from severe unremitting mucocutaneous *Candida* lesions, including extensive nail involvement and vaginitis. The lesions may become quite large with a disfiguring granulomatous appearance.

Urinary tract involvement with *Candida* spp. ranges from asymptomatic bladder colonization to renal abscesses secondary to hematogenous seeding. Bladder colonization with *Candida* spp. is essentially not seen unless a patient requires an indwelling bladder catheter, has diabetes, suffers from urinary obstruction, or has had prior urinary procedures. Benign colonization of the bladder is most common in these settings, but urethritis and/or cystitis may occur. Hematogenous seeding of the kidney may result in renal abscess, papillary necrosis, or "fungus ball" of the ureter or renal pelvis.

Candida peritonitis may be seen in the setting of chronic ambulatory peritoneal dialysis or after GI surgery, anastomotic leak, or intestinal perforation. These infections may remain localized to the abdomen, involve adjacent organs, or lead to hematogenous candidiasis.

Hematogenous candidiasis may be acute or chronic and usually results in seeding of deep tissues, including the abdominal viscera, heart, eyes, bones and joints, and brain. Chronic hepatosplenic candidiasis may occur after overt or occult fungemia and presents as an indolent process marked by fever, elevated alkaline phosphatase, and multiple lesions in the liver and spleen.

Central nervous system (CNS) candidiasis may occur secondary to hematogenous disease or be associated with neurosurgical procedures and ventriculoperitoneal shunts. This process may mimic bacterial meningitis, or the course may be indolent or chronic.

Most cardiac involvement with *Candida* spp. is the result of hematogenous seeding of a prosthetic or damaged heart valve, the myocardium, or pericardial space. Implantation of heart valves contaminated with *C. parapsilosis* has been reported. The clinical presentation resembles bacterial endocarditis, with fever and a new or changing heart murmur. The vegetations are classically large and friable, and embolic events are more common with endocarditis caused by *Candida* spp. than with bacterial endocarditis.

The eye is frequently involved in patients with hematogenous candidiasis, presenting as chorioretinitis and endophthalmitis. For this reason, all patients at risk for candidemia should receive careful and frequent ophthalmologic examinations. Traumatic keratitis may also be seen.

Bone and joint infections caused by *Candida* spp. are almost always sequelae of candidemia. Often these infections will present several months after successful treatment of candidemia. Similarly, occult or "transient" candidemia may result in seeding of a skeletal focus that becomes clinically apparent at a later time. Vertebral osteomyelitis is a frequent presentation, with local pain and low-grade fever.

Although hematogenous candidiasis is most often an endogenous infection arising from the GI or genitourinary tract, it may also result from contamination of an indwelling vascular catheter. Organisms transferred to the hub or lumen of the catheter may form a biofilm within the catheter lumen and subsequently spread into the circulation. Although such infections are no less serious than those arising from an endogenous source, they may be dealt with somewhat more successfully because removal of the catheter essentially removes the nidus of infection. Of course, if the infected catheter resulted in the seeding of distant organs, the consequences and problems in treating the infection would be the same as those arising from an endogenous source.

Laboratory Diagnosis

Laboratory diagnosis of candidiasis involves procurement of appropriate clinical material followed by direct microscopic examination and culture (see Chapter 60). Scrapings of mucosal or cutaneous lesions may be examined directly after treatment with 10% to 20% potassium hydroxide (KOH) containing calcofluor white. The budding yeastlike forms and pseudohyphae are easily detected upon examination with a fluorescence microscope (see Figure 60-1). Culture on standard mycologic medium will allow isolation of the organism for subsequent identification to species. Increasingly, such specimens are plated directly on a selective chromogenic medium such as CHROMagar Candida, which allows detection of mixed species of *Candida* within the specimen and rapid identification of *C. albicans* (green colonies) and *C. tropicalis* (blue colonies) based on their morphologic appearance (Figure 65-5).

All other types of infection require culture for diagnosis unless tissue can be obtained for histopathologic examination (see Chapter 60). Whenever possible, skin lesions should be biopsied and histologic sections stained with GMS or another fungal-specific stain. Visualization of characteristic budding yeasts and pseudohyphae is sufficient for the diagnosis of candidiasis (Figure 65-6). Cultures of blood, tissue,

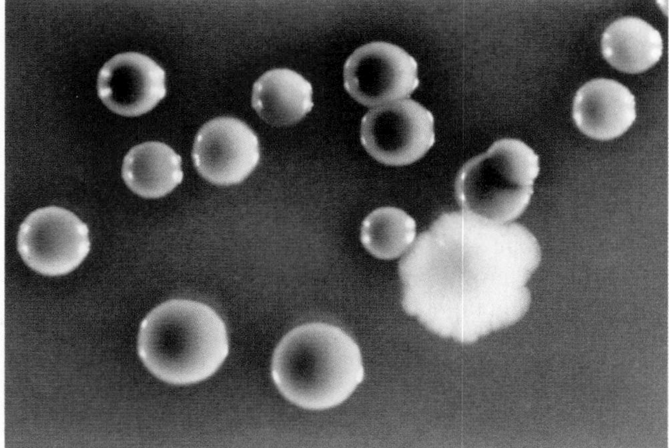

FIGURE 65-5 Differentiation of *Candida* species by isolates on CHROMagar Candida. The green colonies are *C. albicans,* the blue-gray colonies are *C. tropicalis,* and the large, rough, pale pink colony is *C. krusei.* The smooth pink or mauve colonies are another yeast species (only *C. albicans, C. tropicalis,* and *C. krusei* can be reliably recognized on this media; other species have colonies ranging from white to pink to mauve). (From Anaissie EJ, McGinnis MR, Pfaller MA, editors: *Clinical mycology,* ed 2, New York, 2009, Churchill Livingstone.)

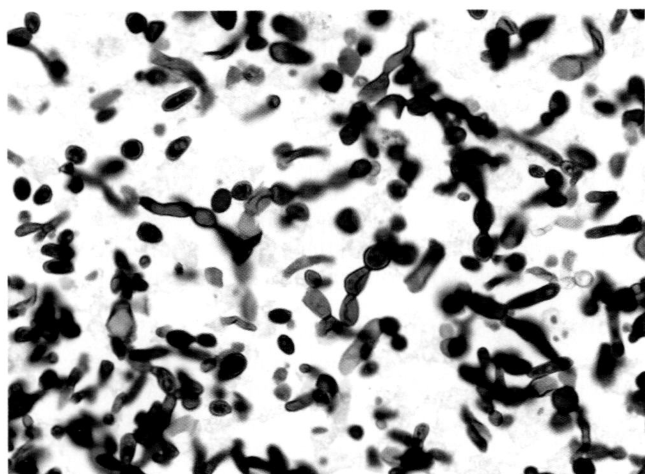

FIGURE 65-6 *Candida* stained with Gomori methenamine silver demonstrating budding yeasts and pseudohyphae (×1000).

and normally sterile body fluids should also be performed. Identification of *Candida* isolates to species level is important, given the differences in response to various antifungal agents (see Chapter 61). This can be accomplished as described in Chapter 60, using the germ-tube test (*C. albicans*), various chromogenic media/tests (see Figure 65-5), peptide nucleic acid–fluorescence in situ hybridization (PNA-FISH), and commercially available sugar assimilation panels. Alternatively, the use of proteomics provides a rapid, accurate, and cost-effective means of species identification.

Immunologic, biochemical, and molecular markers for the diagnosis of candidiasis are described in Chapter 60. Although these methods are not widely available at the present time, recent breakthroughs in direct detection technology hold great promise for the rapid diagnosis of invasive candidiasis.

Treatment, Prevention, and Control

There are a wide variety of treatment options for candidiasis (see Chapter 61). Mucosal and cutaneous infections may be treated with a number of different topical creams, lotions, ointments, and suppositories containing various azole antifungal agents (see Table 61-1). Oral systemic therapy of these infections may also be accomplished with either fluconazole or itraconazole.

Bladder colonization or cystitis may be treated with either instillation of amphotericin B directly into the bladder (bladder wash) or by oral administration of fluconazole. Both of these measures will likely be unsuccessful if the bladder catheter cannot be removed.

More deep-seated infections require systemic therapy, the choice of which depends upon the type of infection, infecting species, and overall status of the host. In many instances, oral fluconazole may be quite effective in treating candidiasis. It may be used in the treatment of peritonitis, as well as in more long-term maintenance therapy of invasive disease after an initial intravenous course of therapy. Fluconazole is efficacious when administered intravenously for the treatment of candidemia in nonneutropenic patients. Patients who become candidemic while on fluconazole prophylaxis or those with documented infection caused by *C. krusei* or fluconazole-resistant *C. glabrata* require treatment with either amphotericin B (conventional or lipid formulation) or an echinocandin (anidulafungin, caspofungin, or micafungin). In clinical settings where *C. glabrata* or *C. krusei* are plausible etiologic agents (e.g., prior fluconazole therapy/prophylaxis or an endemic situation), initial therapy with either an echinocandin or an amphotericin B formulation is advised, with a switch to fluconazole (less toxic than amphotericin B, less expensive, and orally available versus echinocandins) based upon final species identification and susceptibility test results. In every instance, care should be taken to remove the nidus of infection if possible. Thus vascular catheters should be removed or changed, abscesses should be drained, and other potentially infected implanted materials should be removed to the extent possible. Likewise, efforts should be directed toward immune reconstitution.

As in most infectious diseases, prevention is clearly preferable to treatment of an established candidal infection. Avoidance of broad-spectrum antimicrobial agents, meticulous catheter care, and rigorous adherence to infection-control precautions are musts. Decreased colonization achieved by fluconazole prophylaxis has been shown to be efficacious when employed in **specific** high-risk groups, such as BMT patients and liver transplant patients. Such prophylaxis carries with it the potential for selecting for or creating strains or species that are resistant to the agent administered. This in fact has been seen with the emergence of fluconazole-resistant *C. glabrata* and *C. krusei* in certain institutions, but the overall benefit in the high-risk patient groups outweighs the risk. Transfer of this approach to other patient groups, however, is fraught with problems and should not be undertaken without careful study and risk stratification to identify those individuals most likely to benefit from antifungal prophylaxis.

• Opportunistic Mycoses Caused by *Cryptococcus neoformans* and Other Noncandidal Yeastlike Fungi

In the same manner *Candida* species have taken advantage of immunocompromising conditions, indwelling devices, and broad-spectrum antibiotic use, so too have a number of non-*Candida* yeastlike fungi found an "opportunity" to colonize and infect immunocompromised patients. These organisms may occupy environmental niches or be found in food and water and can be normal human microbial flora. The list of these opportunistic yeasts is long, but we will limit this discussion to two major pathogens, *C. neoformans* and *Cryptococcus gattii,* and four genera that pose particular problems as opportunistic pathogens: *Malassezia* spp., *Trichosporon* spp., *Rhodotorula* spp., and *Blastoschizomyces capitatus* (teleomorph, *Dipodascus capitatus*).

Cryptococcosis

Cryptococcosis (Clinical Case 65-2) is a systemic mycosis caused by the encapsulated, basidiomycetous, yeastlike fungi *C. neoformans* and *C. gattii. C. neoformans* is worldwide in distribution and found as a ubiquitous saprophyte of soil, especially soil enriched with pigeon droppings. *C. neoformans* includes capsular serotypes A, D, and AD, and *C. gattii* includes serotypes B and C. *C. neoformans* is further divided

Clinical Case 65-2 Cryptococcosis

Pappas and colleagues (www.FrontlineFungus.org) describe a case of cryptococcosis in a heart transplant recipient. The 56-year-old patient, who underwent heart transplantation surgery 3 years earlier, presented with new-onset cellulitis of his left leg and a mild headache of 2 weeks' duration. The patient was on chronic immunosuppressive therapy with cyclosporine, azathioprine, and prednisone and was admitted for intravenous (IV) antibiotics. Despite 5 days of IV nafcillin, the patient failed to improve, and a skin biopsy of the cellulitic area was obtained for histopathologic studies and culture. Laboratory results revealed the presence of a yeast consistent with *Cryptococcus neoformans.* A lumbar puncture was also performed, and examination of the cerebrospinal fluid (CSF) disclosed cloudy fluid and an elevated opening pressure of 420 mm H_2O. Microscopic examination revealed encapsulated budding yeast forms. Cryptococcal antigen titers of CSF and blood were markedly elevated. Blood, CSF, and skin biopsy cultures grew *C. neoformans.* Systemic antifungal therapy with amphotericin B and flucytosine was initiated. Unfortunately, the patient suffered progressive mental status decline despite aggressive management of intracranial pressure and maximizing doses of antifungals. He experienced slow, progressive decline, leading to death 13 days after initiation of antifungal therapy. CSF cultures obtained 2 days before death remained positive for *C. neoformans.*

The patient in this case was highly immunocompromised and presented with cellulitis and headache. Such a presentation should arouse suspicion of an atypical pathogen such as *C. neoformans.* Given the high mortality associated with cryptococcal infection, rapid and accurate diagnosis is important. Unfortunately, despite these efforts and use of aggressive therapy, many such patients will succumb to the infection.

into two varieties, var. *grubii* (serotype A) and var. *neoformans* (serotype D).

Morphology

Microscopically, *C. neoformans* and *C. gattii* are spherical to oval, encapsulated, yeastlike organisms, 2 to 20 μm in diameter. Replication is by budding from a relatively narrow base. Single buds are usually formed, but multiple buds and chains of budding cells are sometimes present (Figure 65-7). Germ tubes, hyphae, and pseudohyphae are usually absent in clinical material.

In tissue and upon staining with India ink, the cells are variable in size, spherical, oval, or elliptic, and are surrounded by optically clear, smoothly contoured, spherical zones or "halos" that represent the extracellular polysaccharide capsule (Figure 65-8). The capsule is a distinctive marker that may have a diameter of up to five times that of the fungal cell and is readily detected with a mucin stain such as Mayer mucicarmine (Figure 65-9). The organism stains poorly with H&E but is easily detected with PAS and GMS stains. The cell wall of *C. neoformans* contains melanin, which may be demonstrated by staining with the Fontana-Masson stain.

Epidemiology

Cryptococcosis is usually acquired by inhaling aerosolized cells of *C. neoformans* and *C. gattii* from the environment (Figure 65-10). Subsequent dissemination from the lungs, usually to the CNS, produces clinical disease in susceptible individuals. Primary cutaneous cryptococcosis may occur after transcutaneous inoculation but is rare.

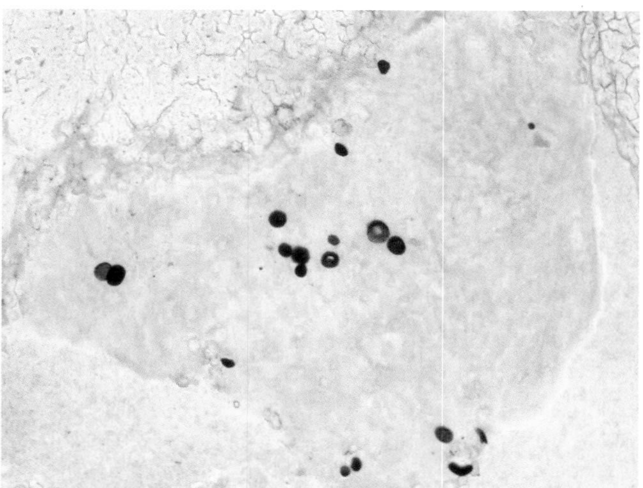

FIGURE 65-7 *Cryptococcus neoformans.* Microscopic morphology, Gomori methenamine silver stain.

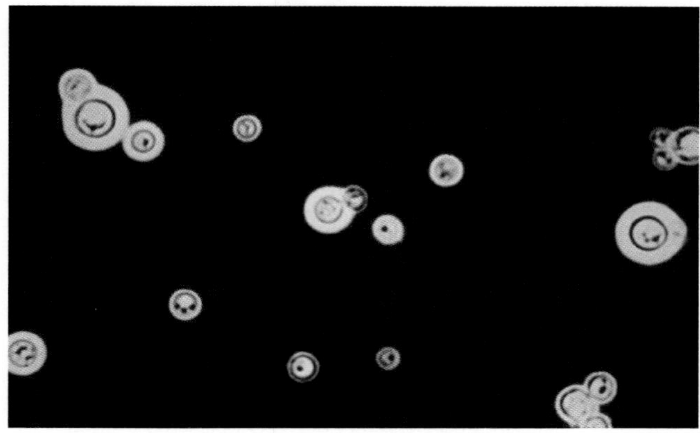

FIGURE 65-8 *Cryptococcus neoformans.* India ink preparation demonstrating the large capsule surrounding budding yeast cells (×1000).

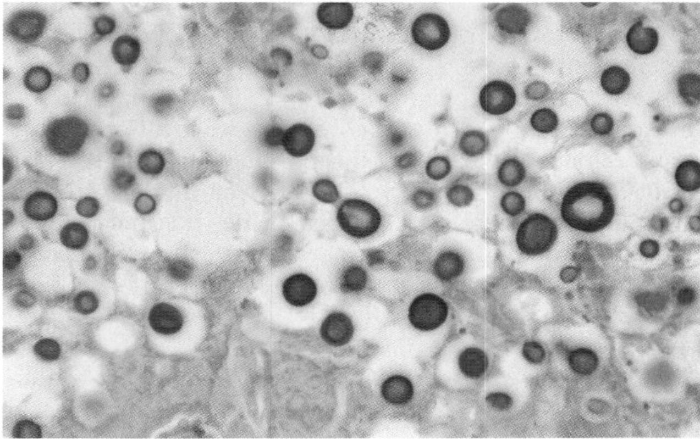

FIGURE 65-9 *Cryptococcus neoformans* stained with mucicarmine (×1000).

Although both *C. neoformans* and *C. gattii* are pathogenic for immunocompetent individuals, *C. neoformans* is most often encountered as an opportunistic pathogen. It is the most common cause of fungal meningitis and tends to occur in patients with defective cellular immunity.

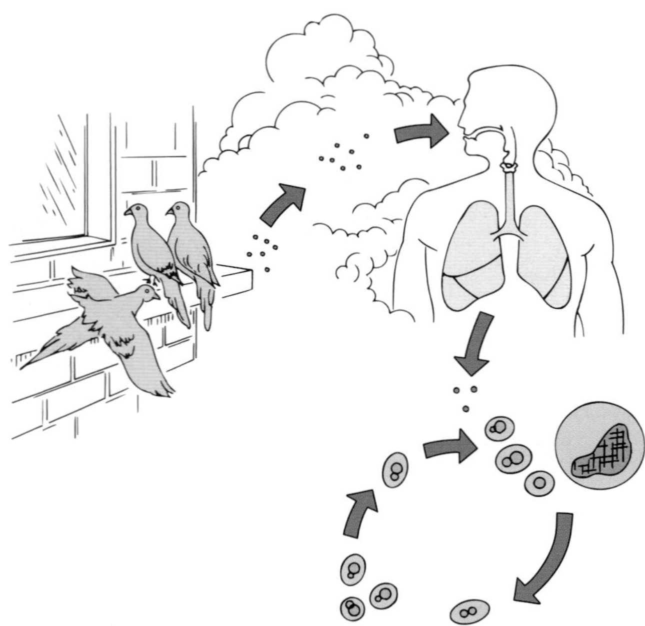

FIGURE 65-10 Natural history of saprobic and parasitic cycle of *Cryptococcus neoformans.*

Whereas *C. neoformans* var. *neoformans* and var. *grubii* are found worldwide in association with soil contaminated with avian excreta, *C. gattii* is generally found in tropical and subtropical climates in association with eucalyptus trees. An endemic focus of *C. gattii* has been identified in Vancouver Island, British Columbia, and in Oregon and Washington state, extending down into California. Sporadic cases of *C. gattii* infection have been detected in several different areas of the United States. Both *C. neoformans* (var. *neoformans* and var. *grubii*) and *C. gattii* cause a similar disease, although *C. gattii* infection tends to occur in immunocompetent individuals and has a lower associated mortality but more severe neurologic sequelae because of CNS granuloma formation.

C. neoformans is a major opportunistic pathogen of patients with AIDS. Individuals with $CD4^+$ lymphocyte counts of less than $200/mm^3$ are at high risk for CNS and disseminated cryptococcosis. The incidence of cryptococcosis seems to have peaked in the United States in the early 1990s (65.5 infections per million per year) and has progressively declined since then because of the widespread use of fluconazole and, more importantly, successful treatment of HIV infection with new antiretroviral drugs.

Clinical Syndromes

Cryptococcosis may present as a pneumonic process or more commonly as a CNS infection secondary to hematogenous and lymphatic spread from a primary pulmonary focus. Less often, a more widely disseminated infection may be seen with cutaneous, mucocutaneous, osseous, and visceral forms of the disease.

Pulmonary cryptococcosis is variable in presentation, from an asymptomatic process to a more fulminant bilateral pneumonia. Nodular infiltrates may be either unilateral or bilateral, becoming more diffuse in severe infections. Cavitation is rare.

Table 65-7 Sensitivity of Antigen Detection, India Ink Microscopy, and Culture of Cerebrospinal Fluid in the Diagnosis of Cryptococcal Meningitis

	% Sensitivity	
Test	**AIDS Patients**	**Non-AIDS Patients**
Antigen	100	86-95
India ink	82	50
Culture	100	90

Modified from Viviani MA, Tortorano AM: *Cryptococcus.* In Anaissie EJ, McGinnis MR, Pfaller MA, editors: *Clinical mycology,* ed 2, New York, 2009, Churchill Livingstone.

AIDS, Acquired immunodeficiency syndrome.

C. neoformans and *C. gattii* are highly neurotropic, and the most common form of disease is cerebromeningeal. The course of disease is variable and may be quite chronic; however, it is inevitably fatal if untreated. Both meninges and the underlying brain tissue are involved, and the clinical presentation is that of fever, headache, meningismus, visual disturbances, abnormal mental status, and seizures. The clinical picture is highly dependent upon the patient's immune status and tends to be dramatically severe in AIDS patients and other severely compromised patients treated with steroids or other immunosuppressive agents.

Parenchymal lesions (cryptococcomas) are uncommon in infections caused by *C. neoformans* but are the most common presentation of CNS cryptococcosis in immunocompetent hosts infected with *C. gattii.*

Other manifestations of disseminated cryptococcosis include skin lesions, which occur in 10% to 15% of patients and may mimic those of molluscum contagiosum; ocular infections, including chorioretinitis, vitritis, and ocular nerve invasion; osseous lesions involving the vertebrae and bony prominences; and prostatic involvement, which may be an asymptomatic reservoir of infection.

Laboratory Diagnosis

The diagnosis of infection caused by *C. neoformans* and *C. gattii* may be made by culture of blood, cerebrospinal fluid (CSF), or other clinical material (see Chapter 60). Microscopic examination of CSF may reveal the characteristic encapsulated budding yeast cells. The cells of *C. neoformans,* when present in CSF or other clinical material, may be visualized with Gram stain (see Chapter 60, Figure 60-2), India ink (see Figure 65-8), or other stains (see Figure 65-7). Culture of clinical material on routine mycologic media will produce mucoid colonies composed of round, encapsulated, budding yeast cells that are urease positive within 3 to 5 days. Species identification may be accomplished by carbohydrate assimilation testing, by growth on niger seed agar (*C. neoformans* colonies become brown to black in color), or by directly testing for phenoloxidase activity (positive).

Most commonly, however, the diagnosis of cryptococcal meningitis is made by direct detection of the capsular polysaccharide antigen in serum or CSF (Table 65-7). Detection of cryptococcal antigen is accomplished by using one of several commercially available latex agglutination or enzyme immunoassay kits. Development of a lateral flow antigen detection assay provides a potential point-of-care test for use in the field. These assays have been shown to be rapid, sensitive, and specific for the diagnosis of cryptococcal disease due to both *C. neoformans* and *C. gattii* (see Table 65-7). Whereas the β-D-glucan test is not useful for diagnosis of cryptococcosis, molecular methods such as polymerase chain reaction (PCR) show great promise.

Treatment

Cryptococcal meningitis (and other disseminated forms of cryptococcosis) is universally fatal if left untreated. In addition to prompt administration of appropriate antifungal therapy, effective management of CNS pressure and immune reconstitution inflammatory syndrome (IRIS) are crucial to successful treatment of cryptococcal meningitis. All patients should receive amphotericin B plus flucytosine acutely for 2 weeks (induction therapy), followed by 8-week consolidation with either oral fluconazole (preferred) or itraconazole. AIDS patients generally require lifelong maintenance therapy with either fluconazole or itraconazole. In non-AIDS patients, treatment may be discontinued after the consolidation therapy; however, relapse may be seen in up to 26% of these patients within 3 to 6 months after discontinuation of therapy. Thus a prolonged consolidation treatment with an azole for up to 1 year may be advisable even with patients without AIDS.

Treatment of these patients should be followed both clinically and mycologically. Mycologic follow-up requires repeat lumbar puncture to be performed (1) at the end of the 2-week induction therapy to ensure sterilization of the CSF, (2) at the end of the consolidation therapy, and (3) whenever indicated by a change in clinical status during follow-up. CSF samples collected during follow-up must be cultured. Determination of CSF protein, glucose, cell count, and cryptococcal antigen titer are helpful in assessing the response to therapy but are not highly predictive of outcome. Failure to sterilize the CSF by day 14 of therapy is indicative of a much higher probability that the consolidation therapy will fail.

Other Mycoses Caused by Yeastlike Fungi

Among the non-*Candida*, non-*Cryptococcus* yeastlike pathogens, nosocomial infections caused by *Malassezia* spp., *Trichosporon* spp., *Rhodotorula* spp., and *Blastoschizomyces capitatus* are most prominent, either because they are difficult to detect or because they may pose particular problems with respect to antifungal resistance.

Infections caused by *Malassezia* spp. (*M. furfur* and *M. pachydermatis*) are usually catheter related and tend to occur in premature infants or other patients receiving lipid infusions. Both of these organisms are budding yeasts (Figure 65-11; also see Chapter 62, Figure 62-2). *M. furfur* is a common skin colonizer and the etiologic agent of tinea (pityriasis) versicolor (see Chapter 62), whereas *M. pachydermatis* is a frequent cause of otitis in dogs, as well as a human skin commensal.

Among the *Malassezia* spp., *M. furfur* is known for its requirement for exogenous lipid for growth. This growth requirement, plus its ecologic niche on skin, explains some of the epidemiology of *M. furfur* because nosocomial infections caused by this organism are directly related to administration of intravenous lipid supplements through a central venous catheter. Although *M. pachydermatis* does not require exogenous lipids for growth, fatty acids do stimulate its growth, and infections caused by this organism have been associated with parenteral nutrition and intravenous lipid administration. Although most infections with *Malassezia* spp. are sporadic, outbreaks of fungemia have been observed among infants receiving intravenous lipid supplementation. Growth of the organism is favored by the lipid-rich infusion, and the organism gains access to the bloodstream via the catheter. One notable outbreak of *M. pachydermatis* fungemia in a pediatric intensive care unit was linked to nurses who owned dogs with *M. pachydermatis* otitis. The outbreak strain was found on the hands of the nurses and at least one of the affected dogs.

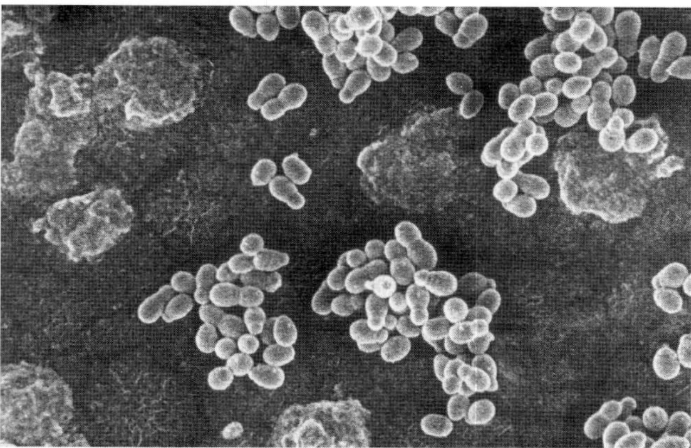

FIGURE 65-11 Scanning electron micrograph of *Malassezia furfur* adhering to the lumen of a central venous catheter. (Courtesy S.A. Messer.)

Malassezia spp. should be considered when yeasts are seen microscopically in blood culture bottles or clinical material but no organisms are recovered on routine agar medium. To isolate *Malassezia* spp. (especially *M. furfur*) on agar medium, the plates must be inoculated and then overlaid with sterile olive oil. Olive oil provides the lipid requirement, and growth should be detected in 3 to 5 days.

Treatment of fungemia caused by *Malassezia* spp. does not usually require administration of antifungal agents. The infection subsides once the lipid infusion is stopped and the intravascular lines are removed.

The genus *Trichosporon* currently consists of six species that are of clinical significance: *T. asahii* and *T. mucoides* are known to cause deep invasive infections, *T. asteroides* and *T. cutaneum* cause superficial skin infections, *T. ovoides* causes white piedra of the scalp, and *T. inkin* causes that of the pubic hair. Confusingly, most of the literature regarding deep-seated trichosporonosis refers to the older nomenclature *T. beigelii*. Morphologically, these organisms are similar and appear in clinical material as hyphae, arthroconidia, and budding yeast cells.

Trichosporon causes catheter-associated fungemia in neutropenic patients but also may gain entrance to the bloodstream via the respiratory or GI tract. Widespread hematogenous dissemination may manifest as positive blood cultures and multiple cutaneous lesions. Chronic hepatic trichosporonosis may mimic hepatic candidiasis and is seen upon recovery from neutropenia. *Trichosporon* has been reported as the most common cause of noncandidal yeast infection in patients with hematologic malignancies and carries mortality in excess of 80%. Susceptibility to amphotericin B is variable, and this agent lacks fungicidal activity against *Trichosporon*. Clinical failures with amphotericin B, fluconazole, and combinations of the two have been reported, and the outcome is generally dismal in the absence of neutrophil recovery. *Trichosporon* species are resistant to the echinocandins but appear to respond clinically to treatment with voriconazole.

Rhodotorula spp. are characterized by the production of carotenoid pigments (produce pink to red colonies) and variably encapsulated, multilateral, budding yeast cells. Species of *Rhodotorula* include *R. glutinis, R. mucilaginosa* (syn. *R. rubra*), and *R. minuta*. These yeastlike fungi are found as commensals on skin, nails, and mucous membranes, as well as in cheese and milk products and environmental sources, including air, soil, shower curtains, bathtub grout, and toothbrushes. *Rhodotorula* species are emerging as important human pathogens in immunocompromised patients and those with indwelling devices. *Rhodotorula* has been implicated as a cause of central venous catheter infection and fungemia, ocular infections, peritonitis, and meningitis. Amphotericin B has excellent activity against *Rhodotorula* and, coupled with catheter removal, is an optimal approach to infections with this organism. Flucytosine has excellent activity as well but should not be considered for monotherapy. Neither fluconazole nor the echinocandins should be used to treat infections caused by *Rhodotorula* species, and the role of the new extended-spectrum triazoles (e.g., voriconazole and posaconazole) is uncertain pending clinical data.

Among the emerging opportunistic yeastlike pathogens, *Blastoschizomyces capitatus* (teleomorph *D. capitatus*) is a rarely described fungus that produces severe systemic infection in immunocompromised patients, especially those with hematologic malignancies. This organism produces hyphae and arthroconidia, is widely distributed in nature, and may be found as part of the normal skin flora. Infection with *B. capitatus* presents similar to that with *Trichosporon* in neutropenic patients, with frequent fungemia and multiorgan (including brain) dissemination and a mortality rate of 60% to 80%. Blood cultures are usually positive. As with *Trichosporon,* a chronic disseminated form similar to chronic disseminated candidiasis may be seen upon resolution of neutropenia.

The optimal approach to therapy of infections caused by *B. capitatus* is not yet defined. Some clinicians feel that *B. capitatus* has decreased susceptibility to amphotericin B. The excellent in vitro activity of voriconazole suggests that it may be a useful agent for treatment of infections caused by this organism. Rapid removal of central venous catheters, adjuvant immunotherapy, and novel antifungal therapies (e.g., voriconazole or high-dose fluconazole plus amphotericin B) are recommended for treatment of this rare but devastating infection.

• Microsporidia

Physiology and Structure

Microsporidia are nucleated, single-celled, obligately intracellular parasites that were considered to be primitive eukaryotic organisms based on the presence of prokaryote-like ribosomes and the apparent absence of true Golgi membranes, peroxisomes, and mitochondria. The microsporidia, however, were recently reclassified with the fungi, based on observations that include the presence of chitin in the spore wall, identification of a mitochondrial *HSP70* gene, and phylogenetic analyses of genes encoding β-tubulin, large subunit RNA polymerase II, translocation elongation factors EF-1 alpha and EF-2, and glutamyl synthase. Mature organisms now appear to possess mitochondrial-derived organelles, and Golgi-like membranes have been identified in association with polar filament formation. The organisms are characterized by the structure of their spores, which have a complex tubular extrusion mechanism used for injecting the infective material (sporoplasm) into cells. Microsporidia have been detected in human tissues and implicated as participants in human disease. Fourteen microsporidian species have been identified as human pathogens: *Anncaliia* (formerly *Brachiola*) *algerae, Anncaliia* (formerly *Brachiola*) *connori, Anncaliia vesicularum, Encephalitozoon cuniculi, Encephalitozoon hellem, Encephalitozoon intestinalis* (syn. *Septata intestinalis*), *Enterocytozoon bienusi, Microsporidium ceylonensis, Microsporidium africanum, Nosema ocularum, Pleistophora ronneafiei, Trachipleistophora hominis, Trachipleistophora anthropophthera,* and *Vittaforma corneae.* Of these, *E. bieneusi* and *E. intestinalis* are the two most common causes of enteric disease, whereas most of the species incriminated in extraintestinal and disseminated disease belong to the *Encephalitozoon* genera: *E. hellem, E. cuniculi,* and *E. intestinalis.* Other species—*A. connori, V. corneae, T. anthropophthera,* and *T. hominis*—have been described in rare cases of disseminated microsporidiosis.

Pathogenesis

Infection with microsporidia is initiated by ingestion of spores. After ingestion, the spores pass into the duodenum, where the sporoplasm with its nuclear material is injected into an adjacent cell in the small intestine. Once inside a suitable host cell, the microsporidia multiply extensively, either within a **parasitophorous vacuole** or free within the cytoplasm. The intracellular multiplication includes a phase of repeated divisions by binary fission **(merogony)** and a phase culminating in spore formation **(sporogony).** The parasites spread from cell to cell, causing cell death and local inflammation. Although some species are highly selective in the cell type they invade, collectively the microsporidia are capable of infecting every organ of the body, and disseminated infections have been described in severely immunocompromised individuals. After sporogony the mature spores containing the infective sporoplasm may be excreted into the environment, thus continuing the cycle.

Epidemiology

Microsporidia are distributed worldwide and have a wide host range among invertebrate and vertebrate animals. *E. bieneusi* and *E. (S.) intestinalis* have gained increasing attention as causes of chronic diarrhea in patients with AIDS. Both *Encephalitozoon*-like and *Enterocytozoon*-like organisms have been reported in the tissues of AIDS patients with hepatitis and peritonitis. *Trachipleistophora* and *Nosema* are known to cause myositis in immunocompromised patients. *Nosema* species have caused localized keratitis, as well as disseminated infection in a child with severe combined immunodeficiency. *Microsporidium* species and *E. hellem* have caused infection of the human cornea.

Although the reservoir for human infection is unknown, transmission is likely accomplished by ingestion of spores that have been shed in the urine and feces of infected animals or individuals. As with cryptosporidial infection, individuals with AIDS and other cellular immune defects appear to be at increased risk for infection with microsporidia.

Clinical Syndromes

Clinical signs and symptoms of microsporidiosis are quite variable in the human cases reported (Clinical Case 65-3). Intestinal infection caused by *E. bieneusi* in patients with AIDS is marked by persistent and debilitating diarrhea similar to that seen in patients with cryptosporidiosis, cyclosporiasis, and cystisosporiasis. The clinical presentation of infection with other species of microsporidia depends on the organ system involved and ranges from localized ocular pain and loss of vision (*Microsporidium* and *Nosema* species) to neurologic disturbances and hepatitis (*E. cuniculi*) to a more generalized picture of dissemination with fever, vomiting, diarrhea, and malabsorption (*Nosema* species). In a report of disseminated infection with *A. connori*, the organism was observed involving the muscles of the stomach, bowel, arteries, diaphragm, and heart and the parenchymal cells of the liver, lungs, and adrenal glands.

Clinical Case 65-3 Microsporidiosis

Coyle and colleagues (*N Engl J Med* 351:42–47, 2004) described a case of fatal myositis caused by the microsporidian *Brachiola (Anncaliia) algerae*. The patient was a 57-year-old woman with rheumatoid arthritis and diabetes who presented with a 6-week history of increasing fatigue, generalized muscle and joint pain, profound weakness, and fever. She was taking immunosuppressive agents (prednisone, methotrexate, leflunomide) for rheumatoid arthritis and had no evidence of human immunodeficiency virus (HIV) infection. In the 6 months before admission, she began taking infliximab, a monoclonal antibody with high binding affinity for tumor necrosis factor (TNF)-α. The patient resided in a small town in northeastern Pennsylvania and had no recent travel history. She had no contact with animals. On admission, her serum creatine kinase was elevated, and a test for HIV was negative. A muscle biopsy from the left anterior thigh contained microorganisms that were consistent with microsporidia. The morphologic appearance suggested *Brachiola (Anncaliia)* species, and the identity was confirmed by polymerase chain reaction with the use of primers specific for *B. (A.) algerae*, a mosquito pathogen.

The muscle pain worsened, and the patient became increasingly debilitated, requiring mechanical ventilation after respiratory insufficiency developed. Despite administration of albendazole and itraconazole, a repeat muscle biopsy from the right quadriceps muscle revealed microsporidia. Four weeks after admission, the patient died from a massive cerebrovascular infarction. A postmortem muscle biopsy revealed necrosis and persistent organisms.

B. (A.) algerae is a well-known microsporidian pathogen of mosquitoes but had not been reported previously to cause myositis in humans. The present case report illustrates that insect pathogens such as *B. (A.) algerae* are capable of causing disseminated disease in humans. Anti-TNF-α therapy (infliximab) may have predisposed the patient to infection with this agent.

Laboratory Diagnosis

Diagnosis of microsporidia infection may be made by detection of the organisms in biopsy material and by light-microscopic examination of CSF and urine. Spores measuring between 1.0 and 2.0 μm may be visualized by Gram (gram-positive), acid-fast, periodic acid–Schiff, immunochemical, modified trichrome, and Giemsa staining techniques. A chromotrope-based staining technique for light-microscopic detection of *E. bieneusi* and *E. (S.) intestinalis* spores in stool and duodenal aspirates has also been described. Electron microscopy is considered the gold standard for diagnostic confirmation of microsporidiosis and for identification to genus and species level; however, its sensitivity is unknown. Additional diagnostic techniques, including PCR, culture, and serologic testing, are under investigation. These techniques are not yet considered reliable enough for routine diagnosis. Molecular methods may also be used to identify the infecting organism to genus and species.

Treatment, Prevention, and Control

Management of microsporidial infection most often includes oral treatment with the drug albendazole. Clinical studies have demonstrated the efficacy of albendazole against species of the *Encephalitazoon* genus in HIV-infected patients, for whom it is the treatment of choice for intestinal, ocular, and disseminated microsporidiosis, although it is only partially active against *E. bieneusi*. Fumagillin has been used successfully against species of the *Encephalitozoon* genus and against *V. corneae* in vitro and in humans for the treatment of *E. bieneusi* intestinal microsporidiosis. Nitazoxanide has activity against *E. intestinalis* and *V. corneae* and has been effective in treating infection caused by *E. bieneusi* in AIDS patients. As with most opportunistic infections, immune reconstitution associated with antiretroviral therapy plays a key role in eradicating microsporidia in HIV-infected patients, and effective antiretroviral therapy is likely to reduce the incidence of infections caused by microsporidia in the future.

As with *Cryptosporidium*, preventing microsporidial infection is difficult. The same methods of improved personal hygiene and sanitation used for intestinal protozoa should be maintained with this disease.

• Aspergillosis

Aspergillosis (Clinical Case 65-4) comprises a broad spectrum of diseases caused by members of the genus *Aspergillus* (Box 65-2). Exposure to *Aspergillus* in the environment may cause allergic reactions in hypersensitized hosts or destructive, invasive, pulmonary, and disseminated disease in highly immunosuppressed individuals. Although approximately 19 species of *Aspergillus* have been documented as agents of human disease, the majority of infections are caused by *A. fumigatus, A. flavus, A. niger,* and *A. terreus.* Molecular taxonomic studies have shown that all of the aforementioned species are actually species complexes that contain morphologically indistinguishable cryptic species, some of which may exhibit important antifungal resistance profiles and pathogenic features.

Clinical Case 65-4 Invasive Aspergillosis

Guha and associates (*Infect Med* 24[Suppl 8]:8–11, 2007) describe a case of invasive aspergillosis in a renal transplant recipient. The patient was a 34-year-old woman who presented with a 2-day history of weakness, dizziness, left calf pain, and black tarry stools. She denied chest pain, cough, or shortness of breath. Her past medical history was significant for diabetes leading to renal failure, for which she received a cadaveric renal transplant in 2002. Three weeks before presentation, acute graft rejection developed. She was placed on an immunosuppressive regimen of alemtuzumab, tacrolimus, sirolimus, and prednisone. On admission, she was tachycardic, hypotensive, and febrile. Physical examination revealed a tender venous cord palpable in the popliteal fossa. An initial chest radiograph showed no abnormalities. Laboratory studies showed anemia and azotemia. The white blood cell count was 4800/μl with 80% neutrophils. The patient was given four units of packed red blood cells, and empirical treatment with gatifloxacin was started. Blood cultures were positive for *Escherichia coli* susceptible to gatifloxacin. On hospital day 6, a vesicular rash developed on the buttocks and left calf, cultures of which were positive for herpes simplex virus, and she was placed on acyclovir. The patient's clinical condition stabilized except for her renal function, and intermittent hemodialysis was started on hospital day 8. On hospital day 12, the patient exhibited decreased responsiveness, became obtunded, and was intubated for respiratory distress. A chest radiograph showed diffuse bilateral lung nodules. Culture of bronchoalveolar lavage fluid was positive for *Aspergillus* species, and viral inclusion bodies suggestive of cytomegalovirus were seen. Her immunosuppression was decreased, and liposomal amphotericin B was started. The patient experienced an acute myocardial infarction and became comatose. Multiple acute infarcts in the frontal lobe and cerebellum were seen on a magnetic resonance imaging scan of the brain. The patient's condition continued to deteriorate, and multiple skin nodules developed on her arms and trunk. Biopsy specimens of the skin nodules grew *Aspergillus flavus* on culture. The patient subsequently died on hospital day 23. At autopsy, *A. flavus* was detected in multiple organs, including heart, lung, adrenal gland, thyroid, kidney, and liver.

This case serves as an extreme example of disseminated aspergillosis in an immunocompromised host.

Morphology

Aspergillus spp. grow in culture as hyaline molds. On a gross level, the colonies of *Aspergillus* may be black, brown, green, yellow, white, or other colors, depending upon the species and the growth conditions. Colonial appearance may provide an initial suggestion as to the species of *Aspergillus,* but definitive identification requires microscopic examination of the hyphae and the structure of the conidial head.

Aspergilli grow as branched septate hyphae that produce conidial heads when exposed to air in culture and tissue. A conidial head consists of a conidiophore with a terminal vesicle, on which are borne one or two layers of phialides, or sterigmata (see Chapter 57, Figure 57-3B). The elongated phialides in turn produce columns of spherical conidia, which are the infectious propagules from which the mycelial phase of the fungus develops. Identification of individual species of *Aspergillus* depends in part on the difference in their conidial heads, including the arrangement and morphology of the conidia (Figures 65-12 and 65-13). In many instances, the cryptic species within a species complex can require molecular methods for identification.

Box 65-2 Spectrum of Diseases Caused by *Aspergillus* Species

Allergic Reactions
Nasal cavity
Paranasal sinuses
Lower respiratory tract

Colonization
Obstructed paranasal sinuses
Bronchi
Preformed pulmonary cavities

Superficial Cutaneous Infections
Wounds
Catheter sites

Limited Invasive Infections
Mildly immunodeficient patients
Bronchi
Pulmonary parenchyma

Frankly Invasive Pulmonary Infection
Severely immunodeficient patients
Pulmonary vasculature and parenchyma
Systemic dissemination
Death

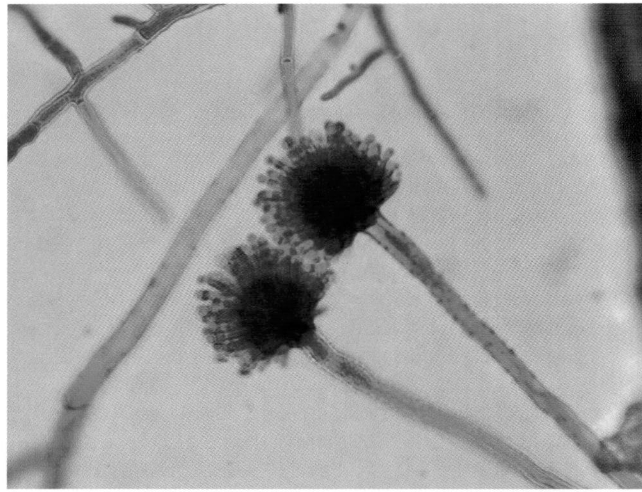

FIGURE 65-12 *Aspergillus fumigatus.* Lactophenol cotton blue preparation showing conidial heads.

In tissue, the hyphae of *Aspergillus* spp. stain poorly with H&E but are well visualized by the PAS, GMS, and Gridley fungal stains (Figure 65-14). The hyphae are homogeneous, uniform in width (3 to 6 μm), with parallel contours, regular septations, and a progressive treelike pattern of branching (see Figure 65-14). The branches are dichotomous and usually arise at acute (≈45-degree) angles. The hyphae may be seen within blood vessels (angioinvasion), causing thrombosis. The conidial heads are rarely seen in tissue but may arise within a cavity (Figure 65-15). The important species *A. terreus* can be identified in tissue by its spherical or oval aleurioconidia that develop from the lateral walls of the mycelium (Figure 65-16). Otherwise, the hyphae of pathogenic *Aspergillus* spp. are morphologically indistinguishable from one another in tissue.

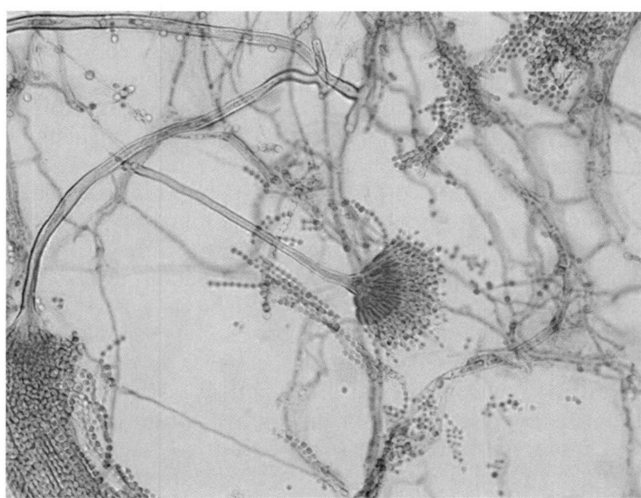

FIGURE 65-13 *Aspergillus terreus.* Lactophenol cotton blue preparation showing conidial head.

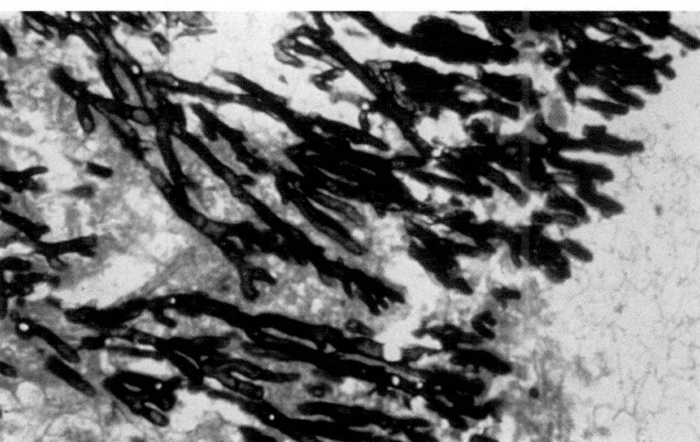

FIGURE 65-14 *Aspergillus* in tissue showing acute-angle branching, septate hyphae (Gomori methenamine silver, ×1000).

Epidemiology

Aspergillus spp. are common throughout the world. Their conidia are ubiquitous in air, soil, and decaying matter. Within the hospital environment, *Aspergillus* spp. may be found in air, showerheads, hospital water storage tanks, and potted plants. As a result, the conidia are constantly being inhaled. The type of host reaction, associated pathologic findings, and ultimate outcome of infection depend more on host factors than on the virulence or pathogenesis of the individual *Aspergillus* spp. The respiratory tract is the most frequent and most important portal of entry.

Clinical Syndromes

The allergic manifestations of aspergillosis constitute a spectrum of presentations based on the degree of hypersensitivity to *Aspergillus* antigens. In the bronchopulmonary form, asthma, pulmonary infiltrates, peripheral eosinophilia, elevated serum immunoglobulin (Ig)E, and evidence of hypersensitivity to *Aspergillus* antigens (skin test) may be seen. Allergic sinusitis shows laboratory evidence of hypersensitivity to go along with upper respiratory symptoms of nasal obstruction and discharge, headache, and facial pain.

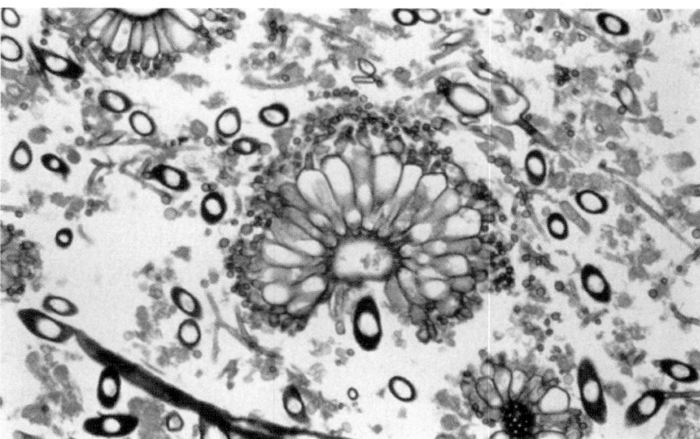

FIGURE 65-15 *Aspergillus niger* in a cavitary lung lesion showing both hyphae and conidial head (Gomori methenamine silver, ×1000).

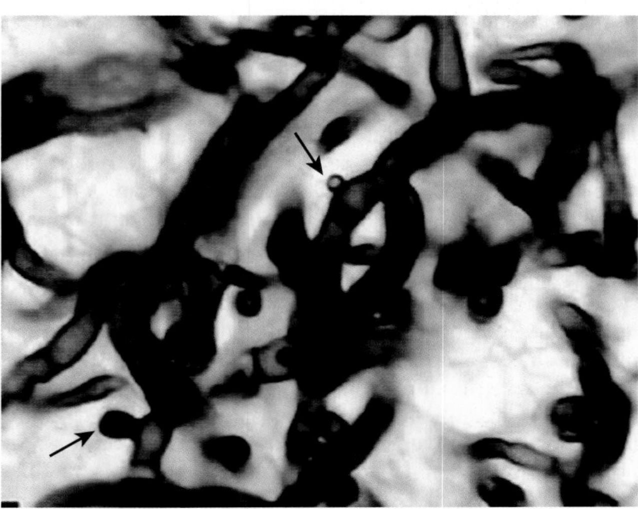

FIGURE 65-16 *Aspergillus terreus* in tissue. *Arrows* point to aleurioconidia (Gomori methenamine silver, ×1000). (From Walsh TJ, Petraitis V, Petraitiene R, et al: Experimental pulmonary aspergillosis due to *Aspergillus terreus:* pathogenesis and treatment of an emerging fungal pathogen resistant to amphotericin B, *J Infect Dis* 188:305–319, 2003.)

Both the paranasal sinuses and the lower airways may become colonized with *Aspergillus* spp., resulting in obstructive bronchial aspergillosis and true aspergilloma ("fungus ball"). Obstructive bronchial aspergillosis usually occurs in the setting of underlying pulmonary disease such as cystic fibrosis, chronic bronchitis, or bronchiectasis. The condition is marked by formation of bronchial casts or plugs composed of hyphal elements and mucinous material. Symptoms remain those of the underlying disease; no tissue injury results, and no treatment is necessary. An aspergilloma can form either in the paranasal sinuses or in a preformed pulmonary cavity secondary to old tuberculosis or other chronic cavitary lung disease. Aspergillomas may be seen on radiographic examination but usually are asymptomatic. Treatment is generally not warranted unless pulmonary hemorrhage occurs. In the event of pulmonary hemorrhage, which may be severe and life threatening, surgical excision of the cavity and fungus ball is indicated. Likewise, radical debridement of the paranasal sinuses may be necessary to alleviate any symptomatology or hemorrhage caused by a fungus ball of the sinuses.

Forms of invasive aspergillosis run the gamut from superficially invasive disease that may occur in the setting of mild immunosuppression (e.g., low-dose steroid therapy, collagen vascular disease, or diabetes) to destructive, locally invasive pulmonary or disseminated aspergillosis. The more limited forms of invasion generally include necrotizing pseudomembranous bronchial aspergillosis and chronic necrotizing pulmonary aspergillosis. Bronchial aspergillosis may cause wheezing, dyspnea, and hemoptysis. Most patients with chronic necrotizing pulmonary aspergillosis have underlying structural pulmonary disease, which may be treated with low-dose corticosteroids. This is a chronic infection that may be locally destructive, with the development of infiltrates and fungus balls seen on radiographic examination. It is not associated with vascular invasion or dissemination. Surgical resection of affected areas and administration of antifungal therapy are efficacious in treating this condition.

Invasive pulmonary aspergillosis and disseminated aspergillosis are devastating infections seen in severely neutropenic and immunodeficient patients. The major predisposing factors for this infectious complication include neutrophil count less than 500/mm^3, cytotoxic chemotherapy, and corticosteroid therapy. Patients present with fever and pulmonary infiltrates, often accompanied by pleuritic chest pain and hemoptysis. Definitive diagnosis is often delayed because sputum and blood cultures are usually negative. The mortality of this infection despite specific antifungal therapy is quite high, usually exceeding 70% (see Table 65-5). Hematogenous dissemination of infection to extrapulmonary sites is common because of the angioinvasive nature of the fungus. Sites most often involved include brain, heart, kidneys, GI tract, liver, and spleen.

Laboratory Diagnosis

As with other ubiquitous fungi, the diagnosis of aspergillosis necessitates caution when evaluating the isolation of an *Aspergillus* species from clinical specimens. Recovery from surgically removed tissue or sterile sites, accompanied by positive histopathology (moniliaceous septate, dichotomously branching hyphae), should always be considered significant; isolation from normally contaminated (e.g., respiratory) sites requires closer scrutiny.

Most etiologic agents of aspergillosis grow readily on routine mycologic media lacking cycloheximide. Species-level identification of the major human pathogens can be made by observing cultural and microscopic characteristics from growth on potato dextrose agar. Microscopic morphology (conidiophores, vesicles, metulae, phialides, conidia) is best observed with a slide culture and is necessary for species identification.

Invasive aspergillosis caused by *A. fumigatus* and most other species is rarely documented by positive blood cultures. In fact, most bloodstream isolates of *Aspergillus* species have been shown to represent pseudofungemia or terminal events at autopsy. Notably, *A. terreus,* among all species of *Aspergillus,* has been shown to cause true aspergillemia. Similar to other angioinvasive filamentous fungi (e.g., *Fusarium, Scedosporium* spp.), *A. terreus* is capable of adventitious sporulation in which yeastlike spores (aleurioconidia) are formed in tissue and are more likely to be detected in blood obtained for culture (see Figure 65-16). Recognition of these aleurioconidia on microscopic examination of tissue, fine-needle aspirates, or bronchoscopy specimens can allow a rapid presumptive identification of *A. terreus.*

Rapid diagnosis of invasive aspergillosis has been advanced by the development of immunoassays for the *Aspergillus* galactomannan antigen in serum. This test employs an enzyme immunoassay format and is available as a commercial kit or from reference laboratories. This test appears to be reasonably specific but exhibits variable sensitivity. It is best used on serial specimens from high-risk (primarily neutropenic and BMT) patients as an early indication to begin empirical or preemptive antifungal therapy and more aggressively pursue a definitive diagnosis. The β-D-glucan test has been applied to the diagnosis of invasive aspergillosis, but it suffers from a lack of specificity. In contrast, PCR-based assays have proven to be both sensitive and specific for the diagnosis of invasive aspergillosis, and efforts to standardize this method are ongoing.

Treatment and Prevention

Prevention of aspergillosis in high-risk patients is paramount. Neutropenic and other high-risk patients are generally housed in facilities where the air is filtered to minimize exposure to *Aspergillus* conidia.

Specific antifungal therapy of aspergillosis usually involves administration of voriconazole or one of the lipid formulations of amphotericin B. It is important to realize that *A. terreus* is considered resistant to amphotericin B and should be treated with an alternative agent such as voriconazole. The introduction of voriconazole provides a treatment option that is more efficacious and less toxic than amphotericin B (see Chapter 61). Recently, combination therapy with voriconazole plus anidulafungin was found to have promising activity when compared to the use of either drug alone. Concomitant efforts to decrease immunosuppression and/or reconstitute host immune defenses are important components of the treatment of aspergillosis. Likewise, surgical resection of involved areas is recommended if possible. Resistance to the mold-active triazoles (isavuconazole, itraconazole, posaconazole, voriconazole) is uncommon but has been reported from numerous locations worldwide. A potential link to the use of azole fungicides in agriculture has been reported from the Netherlands.

• Mucormycosis

Mucormycosis refers to diseases caused by fungi of the subphyla Mucoromycotina and Entomophthoromycotina. The principal human pathogens among the Mucormycetes are encompassed by two orders: Mucorales and Entomophthorales. The order Entomophthorales contains two pathogenic genera, *Conidiobolus* and *Basidiobolus.* These agents generally incite a chronic granulomatous infection of subcutaneous tissues and are discussed in Chapter 63.

In the order Mucorales, pathogenic genera include *Rhizopus, Mucor, Lichtheimia* (formerly *Absidia*), *Rhizomucor, Saksenaea, Cunninghamella, Syncephalastrum,* and *Apophysomyces.* Infections caused by Mucormycetes are rare,

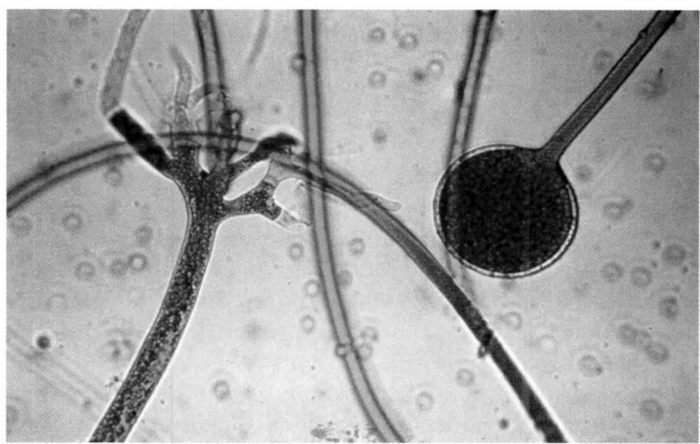

FIGURE 65-17 *Rhizopus* sp. showing sporangium and rhizoids.

occurring at an annual rate of 1.7 infections per million population in the United States. Unfortunately, when they do occur, infections caused by these agents are generally acute and rapidly progressive, with mortality rates of 70% to 100%.

Morphology

Macroscopically, the pathogenic Mucorales grow rapidly, producing gray to brown woolly colonies within 12 to 18 hours. Further identification to genus and species level is based upon microscopic morphology. Microscopically, the Mucormycetes are molds with broad hyaline, sparsely septate, coenocytic hyphae. The asexual spores of the order Mucorales are contained within a sporangium and are referred to as **sporangiospores.** The sporangia are borne at the tips of stalklike sporangiophores that terminate in a bulbous swelling called the **columella** (Figure 65-17; also see Chapter 57, Figure 57-3A). The presence of rootlike structures called **rhizoids** is helpful in identifying specific genera within the Mucorales. As with the aspergilli, identification of the Mucorales is best accomplished by molecular methods.

In tissue, Mucormycetes (order Mucorales) are seen as ribbon-like, aseptate or sparsely septate, moniliaceous (nonpigmented) hyphae (Figure 65-18). In contrast to *Aspergillus* spp. and other hyaline molds, the diameter of the hyphae often exceeds 10 μm, and the hyphae are irregularly contoured and pleomorphic, often folding and twisting back upon themselves. The pattern of hyphal branching is haphazard and nonprogressive, and branches typically arise from the parent hyphae at right angles. The walls of the hyphae are thin, stain weakly with GMS and other fungal stains, and are often more easily detected with H&E (see Figure 65-18). The Mucormycetes are typically angioinvasive.

Epidemiology

Mucormycosis is a sporadic disease that occurs worldwide. *Rhizopus arrhizus* is the most common cause of human mucormycosis; however, additional species of *Rhizopus, Rhizomucor, Lichtheimia,* and *Cunninghamella* are known to cause invasive disease in hospitalized individuals. The organisms are ubiquitous in soil and decaying vegetation, and infection may be acquired by inhalation, ingestion, or contamination of wounds with sporangiospores from the environment. As with *Aspergillus* spp., nosocomial spread of Mucormycetes may occur by way of air-conditioning systems, particularly during construction. Focal outbreaks of mucormycosis have also been associated with the use of contaminated adhesive bandages or tape in surgical wound dressings, resulting in primary cutaneous mucormycosis.

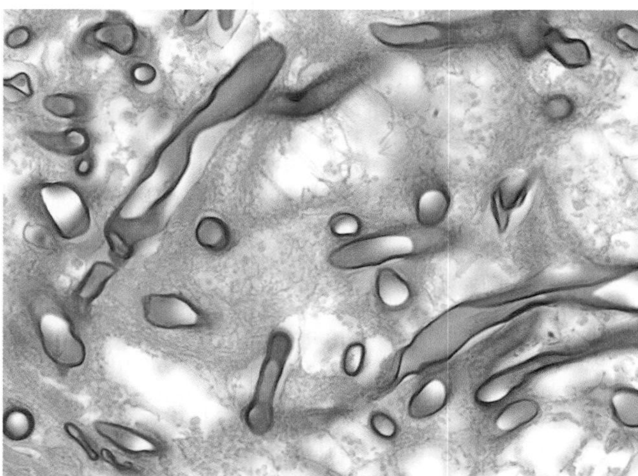

FIGURE 65-18 *Rhizopus* sp. in tissue showing broad, ribbon-like, aseptate hyphae (hematoxylin and eosin, ×1000).

Invasive mucormycosis occurs in immunocompromised patients and is similar clinically to aspergillosis. It is estimated that Mucormycetes may cause infection in 1% to 9% of solid organ transplants, especially those with underlying diabetes mellitus. Risk factors include corticosteroid and deferoxamine therapy, diabetic ketoacidosis, renal failure, hematologic malignancy, myelosuppression, and exposure to hospital construction activity. Mucormycosis has been seen after BMT in patients receiving antifungal prophylaxis with voriconazole, an agent that is not active against the Mucormycetes.

Clinical Syndromes

There are several clinical forms of mucormycosis caused by members of the order Mucorales. Rhinocerebral mucormycosis is an acute invasive infection of the nasal cavity, paranasal sinuses, and orbit that involves the facial structures and extends into the CNS, involving the meninges and brain. Most of these infections occur in patients with metabolic acidosis, particularly diabetic ketoacidosis, and those with hematologic malignancies.

Pulmonary mucormycosis occurs as a primary infection in neutropenic patients and may be misdiagnosed as invasive aspergillosis. The pulmonary lesions are infarctive as a result of hyphal invasion and subsequent thrombosis of large pulmonary vessels. Chest radiographs show a rapidly progressive bronchopneumonia, segmented or lobar consolidation, and signs of cavitation. Fungus-ball formation mimicking aspergilloma may be seen. Pulmonary hemorrhage with fatal hemoptysis may be seen as a result of vascular invasion by the fungus.

The angioinvasive nature of the mucoraceous Mucormycetes often produces disseminated infection with tissue infarction of various organs. Symptoms at presentation point to neurologic, pulmonary, or GI involvement. Involvement of the GI tract often results in massive hemorrhage or perforation.

Cutaneous mucormycosis may be a sign of hematogenous dissemination. Lesions tend to be nodular with an ecchymotic center. Primary cutaneous mucormycosis may occur after traumatic injury, in surgical dressings, or as colonization of burn wounds. The infection may be superficial or extend rapidly into the subcutaneous tissues. The aftermath of the devastating tornados of 2011 in the United States saw several cases of deeply invasive mucormycosis in non-immunocompromised individuals secondary to cutaneous inoculation by flying debris.

Laboratory Diagnosis

Because of the extremely poor prognosis of mucormycosis, every effort should be made to obtain tissue for direct microscopic examination, histologic study, and culture. The Mucormycetes are an extremely ubiquitous group of fungi, so demonstration of characteristic fungal elements in tissue merits considerably more importance than simple isolation in culture.

Appropriate specimens include scrapings of nasal mucosa, aspirates of sinus contents, bronchial alveolar lavage fluid, and biopsy of any and all necrotic infected tissue. Direct examination of material mounted in KOH with calcofluor white may reveal the broad aseptate hyphae. Histopathologic sections stained with H&E or PAS are most useful (see Figure 65-18). Broad, irregularly branched, pauciseptate, twisted hyphae can be observed.

Tissue for culture should be minced, not homogenized, and placed on standard mycologic media without cycloheximide. Negative cultures are common, occurring about 40% of the time, despite the microscopic demonstration of hyphae in tissue. The diagnosis of mucormycosis cannot be established or rejected based on culture alone. It depends on a panel of evidence gathered by both the clinician and microbiologist. Unfortunately, no widely available serologic or molecular tests specific for the Mucormycetes are available yet (see Chapter 60).

Treatment

Amphotericin B remains the first-line therapy for mucormycosis, often supplemented by surgical debridement and immune reconstitution. Most Mucormycetes appear quite susceptible to amphotericin B and are generally not susceptible to the azoles or echinocandins (see Chapter 61). Among the extended-spectrum triazoles, however, posaconazole and isavuconazole stand out in that they appear to have useful activity against many of the Mucormycetes. Both of these triazoles have documented efficacy in murine models of mucormycosis and in limited experience in the treatment of infections in humans. In contrast, voriconazole is inactive against these agents, and breakthrough mucormycosis has been reported in BMT patients receiving voriconazole prophylaxis.

• Mycoses Caused by Other Hyaline Molds

The list of hyaline molds, also known as **hyalohyphomycetes,** is quite long, and it is well beyond the scope of this chapter to discuss them all (see Box 65-1). The taxonomically diverse agents of hyalohyphomycosis (infection caused by nonpigmented molds) do share several characteristics in that many exhibit decreased susceptibility to a number of antifungal agents, and when present in tissue, they appear as hyaline (nonpigmented), septate, branching, filamentous fungi that may be indistinguishable from *Aspergillus.* Culture is necessary to identify these agents and may be critical in determining the most appropriate therapy.

Although infections caused by most of these fungi are relatively uncommon, they appear to be increasing in incidence. Most disseminated infections are thought to be acquired by inhalation of spores or by the progression of previously localized cutaneous lesions. In this chapter, the discussion of specific genera is limited to selected clinically important hyaline molds: *Fusarium* spp., *Scedosporium* spp., *Sarocladium* spp., *Paecilomyces* spp., *Purpureocillium* spp., *Trichoderma* spp., and *Scopulariopsis* spp. These organisms tend to cause infections in neutropenic patients, are often disseminated in nature, and are almost uniformly fatal in the absence of immune reconstitution. Several of these organisms are capable of adventitious conidiation (generation of spores in tissue) with concomitant hematogenous dissemination, positive blood cultures, and multiple cutaneous lesions.

Fusarium species have been recognized with increased frequency as causes of disseminated infection in immunocompromised patients. *Fusarium* is also an important cause of fungal keratitis, especially among contact lens wearers. The most common species isolated from clinical specimens include *Fusarium moniliforme, F. solani,* and *F. oxysporum.* The hallmark of disseminated fusariosis is the appearance of multiple purpuric cutaneous nodules with central necrosis (Clinical Case 65-5). Biopsy of these nodules generally reveals branching, hyaline, septate hyphae invading dermal

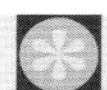

Clinical Case 65-5 Fusariosis

Badley and associates (www.FrontlineFungus.org) describe a 38-year-old man, undergoing chemotherapy for recently diagnosed acute myeloid leukemia, who developed neutropenia and fever. He was placed on broad-spectrum antibacterial agents but remained febrile after 96 hours. A left internal jugular catheter was in place. Blood and urine cultures showed no growth. To combat a potential fungal infection, voriconazole was added to the therapeutic regimen. After 1 week of treatment, the patient was still febrile and neutropenic, and his antifungal therapy was changed to caspofungin. Four days later, the patient developed a mildly painful rash. Initially the rash developed on the upper extremities and consisted of papular, erythematous, plaquelike lesions with centers that became necrotic. Blood cultures and skin biopsy specimens were sent to the laboratory for analysis. The laboratory report indicated that the blood cultures were positive for "yeast" based on the presence of budding cells and pseudohyphae. The skin biopsy showed "mold" consistent with *Aspergillus.* However, serum galactomannan testing was negative. All cultures grew *Fusarium solani.* The patient's caspofungin was discontinued, and he was switched to a lipid preparation of amphotericin B and voriconazole. Despite the antifungal therapy, the lesions increased in number over the next 2 weeks and spread throughout his extremities, trunk, and face. The neutropenia and fever persisted, and he died approximately 3 weeks after the initial diagnosis.

The combination of skin lesions and positive blood cultures is a typical finding in fusariosis. Although "yeast" was reported from the blood cultures, closer examination revealed the microconidia and hyphae of *Fusarium.* Likewise, the appearance of septate hyphae in the skin biopsy could represent a number of different hyaline molds, including *Fusarium.*

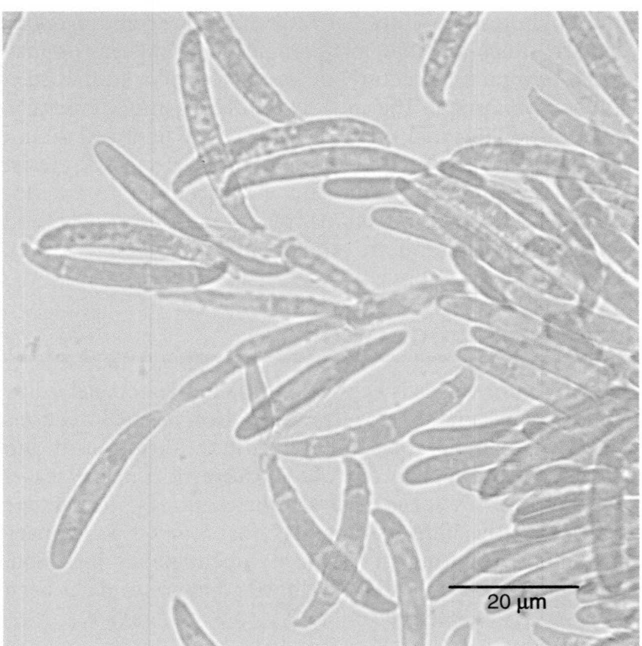

FIGURE 65-19 *Fusarium* sp. in culture showing characteristic "sickle-shaped" macroconidia. (From Long SS, Pickering LK, Prober CG: *Principles and practice of pediatric infectious diseases,* Philadelphia, 2012, Saunders, Fig. 245-2.)

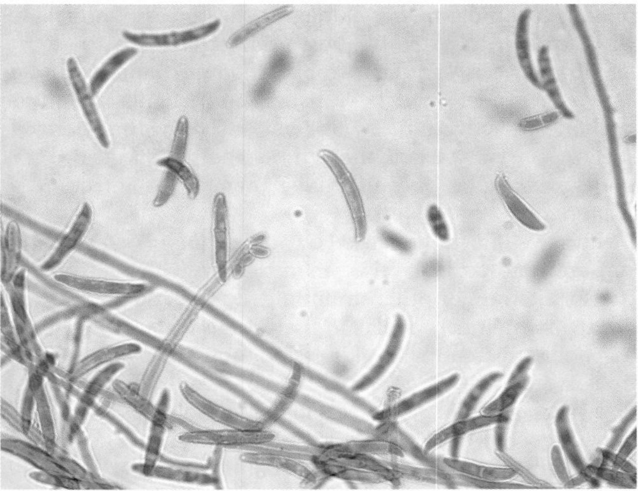

FIGURE 65-20 *Fusarium oxysporum.* Lactophenol cotton blue preparation.

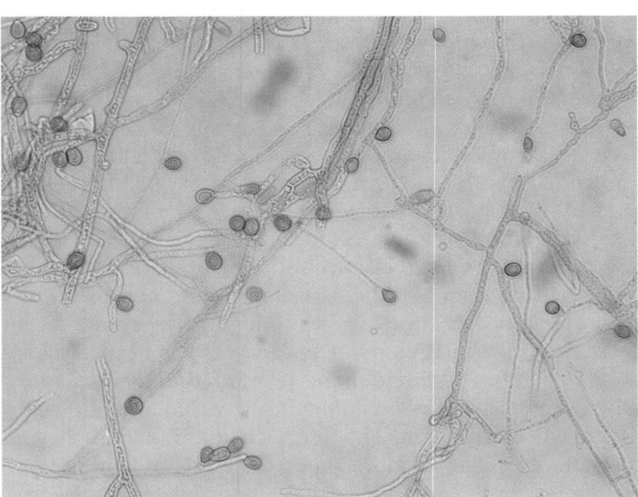

FIGURE 65-21 *Scedosporium apiospermum (Pseudallescheria apiosperma).* Lactophenol cotton blue preparation showing conidia and septate hyphae.

blood vessels (Figure 65-19). Cultures of biopsy material and blood are useful in establishing the diagnosis of *Fusarium* infection. Although blood cultures are virtually always negative in invasive infections caused by *Aspergillus* spp., approximately 75% of patients with fusariosis will have positive blood cultures. In culture, colonies of *Fusarium* spp. are rapidly growing, cottony to woolly, flat, and spreading. Colors may include blue-green, beige, salmon, lavender, red, violet, and purple. Microscopically, *Fusarium* spp. are characterized by the production of both macroconidia and microconidia. Microconidia are single or double celled, ovoid to cylindrical, and generally borne as mucous balls or short chains. Macroconidia are fusiform or sickle shaped and many celled (see Figures 65-19 and 65-20). *Fusarium* spp. often appear resistant to amphotericin B in vitro, and breakthrough infections occur frequently in patients treated with this agent. Voriconazole and posaconazole have been used successfully in some patients with amphotericin B–refractory fusariosis. Primary therapy with a lipid formulation of amphotericin B, voriconazole, or posaconazole, plus vigorous efforts at immune reconstitution, is recommended for treatment of fusariosis.

Within the genus *Scedosporium, S. apiospermum* (teleomorph *Pseudallescheria apiosperma*) and *S. prolificans* represent two important antifungal-resistant opportunistic pathogens. *S. apiospermum* may be readily isolated from soil and is an occasional cause of mycetoma worldwide; however, it is also the cause of serious disseminated and localized infection in immunocompromised patients. In addition to widespread disseminated disease, *S. apiospermum* has been reported to cause corneal ulcers, endophthalmitis, sinusitis, pneumonia, endocarditis, meningitis, arthritis, and osteomyelitis. *S. apiospermum* is indistinguishable from *Aspergillus* spp. and other agents of hyalohyphomycosis on histopathologic examination. Such distinction is important clinically because *S. apiospermum* is resistant to amphotericin B and susceptible to voriconazole and posaconazole. In culture, colonies are woolly to cottony and are initially white, becoming smoky brown to green. Microscopically, conidia are one celled, elongate, and pale brown and are borne singly or in balls on either short or long conidiophores (Figure 65-21).

S. prolificans (formerly *S. inflatum*) is a potentially virulent and highly aggressive emerging agent of hyalohyphomycosis. Although far less important than *Fusarium* or *S. apiospermum,* infections caused by *S. prolificans* are associated with soft-tissue trauma and are characterized by widespread local invasion, tissue necrosis, and osteomyelitis. *S. prolificans* resembles *S. apiospermum* in macroscopic and microscopic morphology. The formation by *S. prolificans* of annelloconidia in wet clumps at the apices of annellides with **swollen bases** is the most useful characteristic in differentiating this organism from *S. apiospermum. S. prolificans* is considered to be resistant to virtually all of the systemically active antifungal agents, including the extended-spectrum triazoles and the echinocandins. Surgical resection remains the only definitive therapy for infection by *S. prolificans.*

Invasive infections caused by *Sarocladium (Acremonium)* spp. are almost exclusively seen in patients with neutropenia, transplantation, or other immunodeficiency conditions and occur in a manner similar to that of *Fusarium,* with hematogenously disseminated skin lesions and positive blood cultures. Species of *Sarocladium* are commonly found in soil, decaying vegetation, and decaying food. Colonies are whitish gray or rose, with a velvety to cottony surface. The conidia may be single celled in chains or a conidial mass arising from short, unbranched, tapered phialides. The optimal treatment for infections caused by *Sarocladium* spp. has not been established. Resistance is seen to amphotericin B, itraconazole, and the echinocandins. A recent report of successful treatment of a pulmonary infection caused by *Sarocladium* (formerly *Acremonium) strictum* with posaconazole suggests that the new triazoles may be useful in treatment of *Sarocladium/Acremonium* infections.

Although uncommon, *Paecilomyces* spp. may cause invasive disease in organ and hematopoietic stem cell recipients, individuals with AIDS, and other immunocompromised patients. The portal of infection is often through breaks in the skin or intravascular catheters. Dissemination of the infection may be aided by adventitious conidiation that takes place within tissues. The two most common medically important species are *P. lilacinus* and *P. variotti.* In a recent taxonomic shuffle, *Paecilomyces lilacinus* has been assigned to the genus *Purpureocillium (Purpureocillium lilacinus).* Microscopically, the *Paecilomyces* spp. conidia are unicellular, ovoid to fusiform, and form chains. Phialides have a swollen base and a long, tapered neck. Susceptibility to amphotericin B is variable, with resistance seen with *P. lilacinus.* Voriconazole has been used successfully to treat both severe cutaneous infection and disseminated disease.

Trichoderma spp. are excellent examples of fungi previously labeled as nonpathogenic that have emerged as important opportunistic pathogens in immunocompromised patients and in patients undergoing peritoneal dialysis. Fatal disseminated disease caused by *T. longibrachiatum* occurs in patients with hematologic malignancies, after BMT or solid organ transplantation. Most *Trichoderma* spp. show decreased susceptibility to amphotericin B, itraconazole, fluconazole, and flucytosine. Voriconazole appears to be active against the few isolates tested.

Scopulariopsis spp. are ubiquitous soil saprobes that have been rarely implicated in invasive human disease. *S. brevicaulis* is the most frequently isolated species. Infection is usually confined to the nails; however, serious deep infection has been noted in neutropenic leukemia patients and after BMT. Both local and disseminated infections have been described, with involvement of the nasal septum, skin and soft tissues, blood, lungs, and brain. Diagnosis is made by culture and histopathology. *Scopulariopsis* spp. grow moderately to rapidly on standard mycologic media. Colonies are initially smooth, becoming granular to powdery with age. Conidiophores are simple or branched; the conidiogenous cells are annellides that form singly or in clusters or may form a broomlike structure, or scopula, similar to that seen with *Penicillium* spp. The annelloconidia are smooth initially, become rough at maturity, are shaped like light bulbs, and form basipetal chains. *Scopulariopsis* spp. are usually resistant to itraconazole and moderately susceptible to amphotericin B. Invasive infections may require surgical and medical treatment and are often fatal.

• Phaeohyphomycosis

Phaeohyphomycosis is defined as tissue infection caused by dematiaceous (pigmented) hyphae and/or yeasts. Infections caused by dematiaceous fungi constitute a significant and increasingly prevalent group of opportunistic fungal diseases and may take the form of disseminated disease or become localized to the lung, paranasal sinuses, or CNS. Primary inoculation, resulting in localized subcutaneous infection, occurs commonly in underdeveloped countries and has been discussed in Chapter 63.

The dematiaceous fungi that have been documented to cause human infection encompass a large number of different genera; however, the more common causes of human infection include *Alternaria, Bipolaris, Cladosporium, Curvularia,* and *Exserohilum* species. In addition, several of the dematiaceous fungi appear to be neurotropic: *Cladophialophora bantiana, Bipolaris (Curvularia) spicifera, Exophiala* spp., *Wangiella dermatitidis, Ramichloridium obovoideum,* and *Chaetomium atrobrunneum.* Brain abscess is the most common CNS presentation. *Bipolaris* (*Curvularia*) spp. and *Exserohilum* spp. infections may present initially as sinusitis, which then extends into the CNS. *Exserohilum rostratum* was implicated in a large iatrogenic outbreak in the United States due to contaminated methylprednisolone preparations, leading to numerous fatal cases of meningitis and CNS vasculitis in otherwise immunocompetent individuals. Notably, both PCR and the β-D-glucan test were quite useful in diagnosis and management of these patients.

In tissue, hyphae with or without yeast forms are present. Most often, the pale brown to dark melanin-like pigment within the cell wall is apparent in H&E- or Papanicolaou-stained tissue (Figure 65-22). Staining with the Fontana-Masson technique (a melanin-specific stain) may help visualize the dematiaceous elements.

Dematiaceous fungi differ considerably in the clinical spectrum of infection and response to therapy. Furthermore, the different genera are not readily distinguished on histopathologic examination. Thus an accurate microbiological diagnosis based on culture of the infected tissue is important for optimal clinical management of infections caused by these fungi.

Alternaria spp. are important causes of paranasal sinusitis in both healthy and immunocompromised individuals. Other sites of infection include skin and soft tissue, cornea, lower respiratory tract, and peritoneum. *Alternaria alternata* is the best-documented human pathogen in this genus. In culture, *Alternaria* colonies are rapidly growing, cottony, and gray to black. The conidiophores are usually solitary and simple or branched. The conidia develop in branching chains and are dematiaceous, muriform, and smooth or rough and

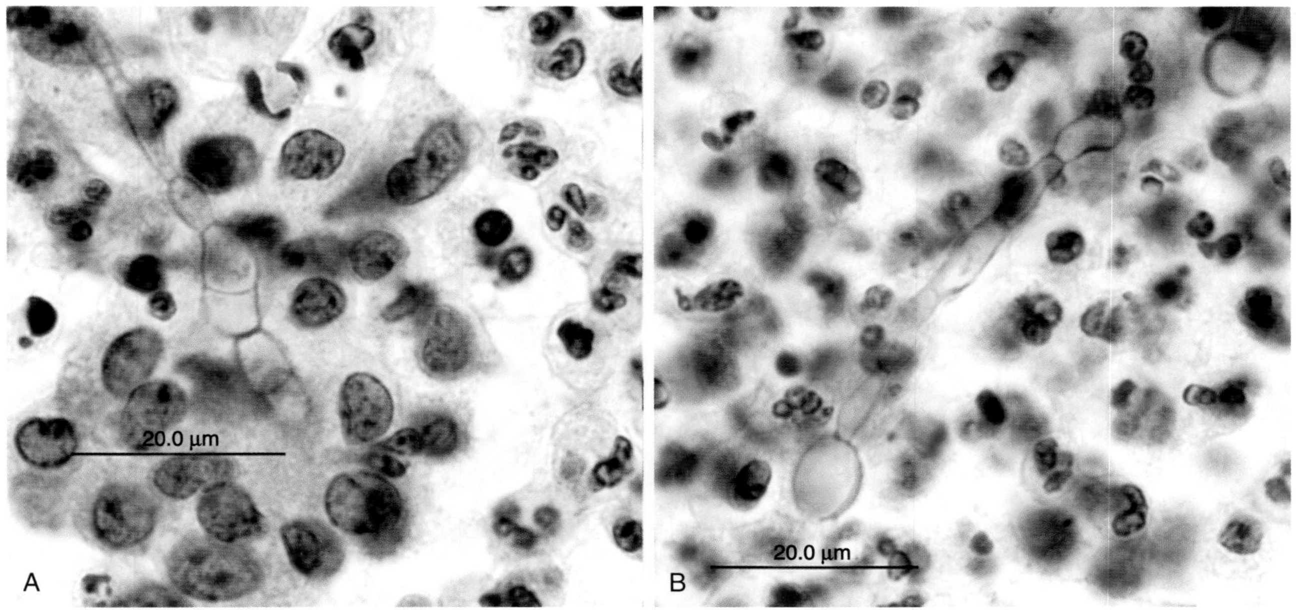

FIGURE 65-22 **A** and **B,** Fine-needle aspirate of a fluctuant mass showing the pigmented hyphae of *Phialophora verrucosa* (Papanicolaou). (From Anaissie EJ, McGinnis MR, Pfaller MA, editors: *Clinical mycology,* ed 2, New York, 2009, Churchill Livingstone.)

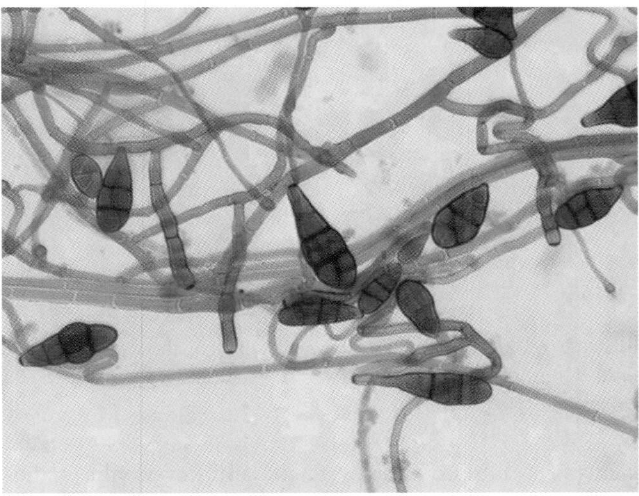

FIGURE 65-23 *Alternaria* sp. Lactophenol cotton blue preparation showing darkly pigmented chains of muriform conidia.

taper toward the distal end with a short beak at their apices (Figure 65-23).

Cladosporium spp. usually cause superficial cutaneous infections but may cause deep infections as well. These fungi are rapidly growing with a velvety olive gray to black colony. The conidiophores arise from the hyphae and are dematiaceous, tall, and branching. The conidia may be smooth or rough and single to several celled and form branching chains at the apex of the conidiophore.

Curvularia spp. are ubiquitous inhabitants of the soil and have been implicated in both disseminated and local infections. Sites of infection include endocarditis, local catheter, nasal septum and paranasal sinuses, lower respiratory tract, skin and subcutaneous tissues, bones, and cornea. In tissue, the hyphae may appear nonpigmented. Common species found to be etiologic agents of human infection include *C. geniculata, C. lunata, C. pallescens,* and *C. senegalensis.* In culture, colonies are rapidly growing, woolly, and gray to grayish black. Microscopically, the conidia are dematiaceous, solitary or in groups, septate, simple or branched, sympodial, and geniculate.

Infections caused by the genera *Bipolaris* and *Exserohilum* present similarly to those of *Aspergillus* spp., except that the disease progresses more slowly. Clinical presentations include dissemination with vascular invasion and tissue necrosis, involvement of the CNS and paranasal sinuses, and association with allergic bronchopulmonary disease. These organisms cause sinusitis in "normal" (atopic or asthmatic) hosts and more invasive disease in immunocompromised hosts. In culture, both *Bipolaris* and *Exserohilum* form rapidly growing, woolly, gray to black colonies. Microscopically, the conidiophores are sympodial and geniculate. The conidia are dematiaceous, oblong to cylindrical, and multicelled (Figure 65-24). The preponderant *Bipolaris* species in human infections are *Bipolaris australiensis, B. hawaiiensis,* and *B. spicifera.* Recently these species have been transferred to the genus *Curvularia.*

The optimal treatment of deep-seated phaeohyphomycosis has not yet been established, although it most often includes early administration of amphotericin B and aggressive surgical excision. Despite these efforts, phaeohyphomycosis does not respond well to treatment and relapses are common. Posaconazole has been used successfully to treat disseminated infection caused by *Exophiala spinifera.* In those patients with brain abscesses, complete excision of the lesion has been associated with improved survival. Long-term triazole (posaconazole or voriconazole) therapy coupled with repeated surgical excision may prevent recurrences. Treatment of the iatrogenic cases of infection due to *E. rostratum* included lipid formulations of amphotericin B and voriconazole.

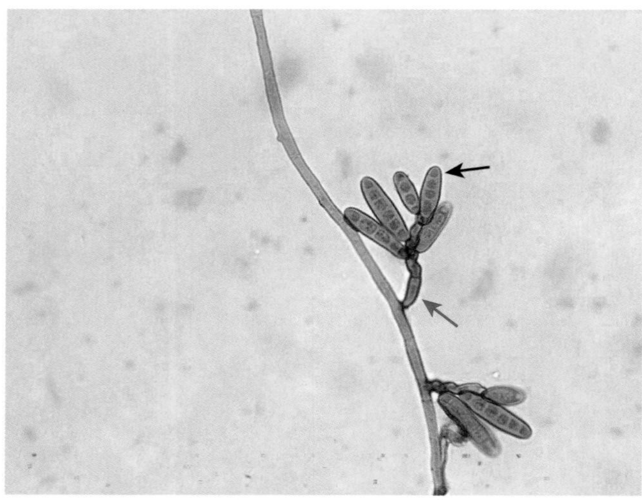

FIGURE 65-24 *Bipolaris (Curvularia)* sp. Lactophenol cotton blue preparation showing pigmented conidia *(black arrow)* borne on geniculate conidiophores *(red arrow).*

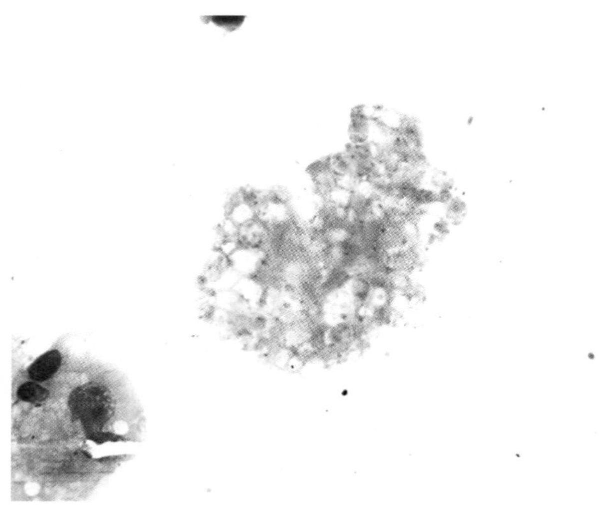

FIGURE 65-25 *Pneumocystis jirovecii* in bronchoalveolar lavage fluid. Giemsa stain shows intracystic forms (×1000).

• Pneumocystosis

Pneumocystis jirovecii (formerly *Pneumocystis carinii*) is an organism that causes infection almost exclusively in debilitated and immunosuppressed patients, especially those with HIV infection. It is the most common opportunistic infection among individuals with AIDS; however, the incidence has decreased considerably in recent years with the use of highly active antiretroviral therapy. Although it was previously considered to be a protozoan parasite, molecular and genetic evidence place it among the fungi (see Chapter 57).

The life cycle of *P. jirovecii* includes both sexual and asexual components. During the course of human infection, *P. jirovecii* may exist as free trophic forms (1.5 to 5 μm in diameter), as a uninucleate sporocyst (4 to 5 μm), or as a cyst (5 μm) containing up to eight ovoid to fusiform intracystic bodies (Figure 65-25). After rupture of the cyst, the cyst wall may be seen as an empty collapsed structure (Figure 65-26).

The reservoir for *P. jirovecii* in nature is unknown. Although airborne transmission has been documented experimentally among rodents, the rodent strains are genetically distinct from those of humans, making it unlikely that rodents serve as a zoonotic reservoir for human disease.

The respiratory tract is the main portal of entry for *P. jirovecii* in humans. Pneumonia is clearly the most common presentation of pneumocystosis, although extrapulmonary manifestations may be seen among AIDS patients. Involvement of lymph nodes, spleen, bone marrow, liver, small bowel, genitourinary tract, eyes, ears, skin, bone, and thyroid have been reported. Recent evidence suggests that both reactivation of quiescent old infection and primary infection can occur. Malnourished, debilitated, and immunosuppressed patients, especially AIDS patients with low CD4 counts (<200/μl), are at high risk of infection.

The hallmark of *P. jirovecii* infection is an interstitial pneumonitis with a mononuclear infiltrate composed predominantly of plasma cells. The onset of disease is insidious, with signs and symptoms including dyspnea, cyanosis, tachypnea, nonproductive cough, and fever. The radiographic appearance is typically one of diffuse interstitial infiltrates with a ground-glass appearance extending from the hilar region, but radiographs may appear normal or show nodules or cavitation. The mortality rate is high among untreated patients, and death is due to respiratory failure.

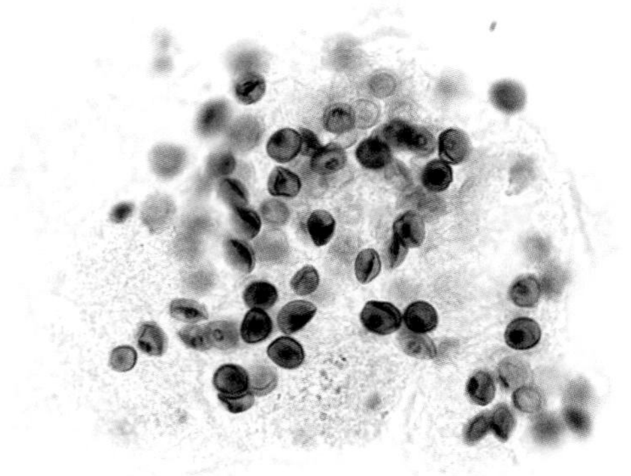

FIGURE 65-26 *Pneumocystis jirovecii* in bronchoalveolar lavage fluid. Gomori methenamine silver stain shows typical intact and collapsed cysts (×1000).

Histologically, a foamy exudate is seen within the alveolar spaces, with an intense interstitial infiltrate composed predominantly of plasma cells. Other patterns, including diffuse alveolar damage, noncaseating granulomatous inflammation, and infarct-like coagulative necrosis may also be seen.

The diagnosis of *P. jirovecii* infection is almost entirely based upon microscopic examination of clinical material, including bronchoalveolar lavage (BAL) fluid, bronchial brushing, induced sputum, and transbronchial or open-lung biopsy specimens. Examination of BAL fluid has been shown to have a sensitivity of 90% to 100% and usually precludes the need for transbronchial or open-lung biopsy. Microscopic examination of induced sputum may be useful in AIDS patients with a very high organism load; however, it has a 20% to 25% false-negative rate. A variety of histologic and cytologic stains have been used to detect *P. jirovecii:* GMS, Giemsa, PAS, toluidine blue, calcofluor white, and immunofluorescence. The Giemsa stain demonstrates the trophic forms but does not stain the cyst wall (see Figure 65-25), whereas the GMS stain is specific for the cyst wall (see Figure 65-26). Immunofluorescent techniques stain both trophic forms and the cyst wall. The β-D-glucan test has proven to be quite useful for rapid diagnosis of *Pneumocystis* pneumonia with a high degree of sensitivity and specificity. Likewise PCR is quite promising and is commercially available in Europe.

The cornerstone for both prophylaxis and treatment is trimethoprim-sulfamethoxazole. Alternative therapies have been used in AIDS patients; they include pentamidine, trimethoprim-dapsone, clindamycin-primaquine, atovaquone, and trimetrexate.

Bibliography

Anaissie EJ, McGinnis MR, Pfaller MA: *Clinical mycology*, ed 2, New York, 2009, Churchill Livingstone.

Chandler FW, Watts JC: *Pathologic diagnosis of fungal infections*, Chicago, 1987, American Society for Clinical Pathology Press.

Diekema DJ, Messer SA, Hollis RJ, et al: A global evaluation of voriconazole activity tested against recent clinical isolates of *Candida* spp, *Diagn Microbiol Infect Dis* 63:233–236, 2009.

Dignani MC, Solomkin JS, Anaissie EJ: *Candida*. In Anaissie EJ, McGinnis MR, Pfaller MA, editors: *Clinical mycology*, ed 2, New York, 2009, Churchill Livingstone.

Gudlaugsson O, Gillespie S, Lee K, et al: Attributable mortality of nosocomial candidemia, revisited, *Clin Infect Dis* 37:1172–1177, 2003.

Hidron AI, Edwards JR, Patel J, et al: Antimicrobial-resistant pathogens associated with healthcare-associated infections: annual summary of data reported to the National Healthcare Safety Network at the Centers for Disease Control and Prevention, 2006–2007, *Infect Control Hosp Epidemiol* 29:996–1011, 2008.

Lockhart SR, et al: The epidemiology of fungal infections. In Anaissie EJ, McGinnis MR, Pfaller MA, editors: *Clinical mycology*, ed 2, New York, 2009, Churchill Livingstone.

Pannuti CS, Gingrich RD, Pfaller MA, et al: Nosocomial pneumonia in adult patients undergoing bone marrow transplantation: a 9-year study, *J Clin Oncol* 9:1, 1991.

Pfaller MA, Diekema DJ: Epidemiology of invasive candidiasis: a persistent public health problem, *Clin Microbiol Rev* 20:133–163, 2007.

Pfaller MA, Diekema DJ: Epidemiology of invasive mycoses in North America, *Crit Rev Microbiol* 36:1–53, 2010.

Pfaller M, Neofytos D, Diekema D, et al: Epidemiology and outcomes of candidemia in 3648 patients: data from the Prospective Antifungal Therapy (PATH Alliance) registry, 2004-2008, *Diagn Microbiol Infect Dis* 74:323–331, 2012.

Pfaller MA, Messer SA, Woosley LN, et al: Echinocandin and triazole antifungal susceptibility profiles for clinical opportunistic yeast and mold isolates collected from 2010 to 2011: application of new CLSI clinical breakpoints and epidemiological cutoff values for characterization of geographic and temporal trends of antifungal resistance, *J Clin Microbiol* 51:2571–2581, 2013.

Viviani MA, Tortorano AM: *Cryptococcus*. In Anaissie EJ, McGinnis MR, Pfaller MA, editors: *Clinical mycology*, ed 2, New York, 2009, Churchill Livingstone.

Wey SB, Mori M, Pfaller MA, et al: Hospital-acquired candidemia: attributable mortality and excess length of stay, *Arch Intern Med* 148:2642–2645, 1988.

CHAPTER

FUNGAL AND FUNGAL-LIKE INFECTIONS OF UNUSUAL OR UNCERTAIN ETIOLOGY

Jim is a 50-year-old ex-smoker who went to his family physician for an annual physical examination. In the process, a chest radiograph revealed a nodule in the left upper lobe of his lung. Because of his age and prior smoking history, Jim underwent a thoracotomy, and the nodule was excised. Pathologic examination revealed fibrosis and several large spherical structures but no evidence of cancer.

1. What is the differential diagnosis of a solitary lung nodule?
2. Describe how one can differentiate the spherules of *Rhinosporidium seeberi* from those of *Coccidioides immitis* and *Emmonsia* spp.
3. Describe the disease process of adiaspiromycosis.
4. Which of the following agents can be identified using commercially available yeast identification systems?
   a. *Lacazia loboi*
   b. *Pythium insidiosum*
   c. *Rhinosporidium seeberi*
   d. *Prototheca wickerhamii*

Answers to these questions are available on StudentConsult.com.

• SUMMARIES CLINICALLY SIGNIFICANT ORGANISMS

Chlorellosis

Trigger Words

Chloroplasts, green lesions, water exposure, alga

Biology, Virulence, and Disease

- Infection of humans and animals caused by a unicellular green alga of genus *Chlorella*
- *Chlorella:* unicellular, ovoid, spherical or polygonal, reproduce by endosporulation
- Fresh lesions in liver, lymph nodes, cutaneous tissue are green on gross examination; smears reveal organisms that contain green refractile granules (chloroplasts)
- A single human infection reported thus far; most infections occur in sheep and cattle

Epidemiology

- A single human infection in Nebraska; resulted from exposure of a surgical wound to river water
- Infections in domestic and wild animals range from lymph node and deep organ involvement to cutaneous and subcutaneous lesions, presumably related to exposure to water containing the organism

Diagnosis

- *Chlorella* spp. infections diagnosed by culture and histopathologic examination of infected tissue
- On culture, colonies are bright green
- Wet mounts of wound exudate or touch preparations of infected tissue reveal ovoid, endosporulating cells with characteristic green cytoplasmic granules
- In tissue, cells stain with GMS and PAS but not H&E stains

Treatment, Prevention, and Control

- Repeat debridement, irrigation with Dakin solution, gauze packing and removal for drainage and granulation
- Amphotericin B therapy combined with administration of tetracycline may be useful

Lacaziosis

Trigger Words

Cutaneous trauma, soil, vegetation, water, dolphins, cutaneous nodules, tropical

Biology, Virulence, and Disease

- Chronic fungal skin infection caused by *Lacazia loboi*
- *L. loboi:* ascomycete fungus, reproduces by sequential budding, forms chains of spherical to oval cells connected by narrow tubelike bridges
- Slowly developing cutaneous nodules of varying size and shape
- Nodular keloid-like lesions most common; occur on the face, ears, arms, legs, feet
- Lesions increase in size and number over a period of 40 to 50 years
- Most patients asymptomatic; no systemic manifestations of disease

Epidemiology

- Human disease endemic in tropical regions of Central and South America
- *L. loboi* considered a saprophyte of soil and vegetation
- Mode of infection: cutaneous trauma; occurs in individuals involved in farming and jungle clearing
- Lacaziosis occurs in both marine and fresh water dolphins, suggesting an aquatic reservoir

Diagnosis

- Based on demonstrating yeast cells in lesion exudate or tissue sections
- Biopsy reveals a dispersed granulomatous infiltrate and numerous fungal forms in dermis and subcutaneous tissue

Treatment, Prevention, and Control

- Surgical excision of localized lesions
- Does not respond to antifungal therapy

Rhinosporidiosis

Trigger Words

Polypoid lesions, oropharynx, sporangium, trophocyte, endoconidia, granulomatous

Biology, Virulence, and Disease

- Granulomatous disease of humans and animals caused by *Rhinosporidium seeberi*
- Characterized by development of nasopharyngeal and ocular conjunctival polyps
- Two developmental forms seen in tissue: a large spherical form (sporangia) and a smaller trophic form

Epidemiology

- ≈90% of all known cases of rhinosporidiosis occur in India and Sri Lanka
- Natural habitat unknown
- Occurs primarily in men aged 20 to 40
- Appears to be associated with both rural and aquatic environments
- No evidence rhinosporidiosis is contagious

Diagnosis

- Histopathologic examination of affected tissues; distinctive appearance of trophocytes and sporangia in routine H&E-stained tissue is diagnostic
- *R. seeberi* has not been grown in culture

Treatment, Prevention, and Control

- Only effective form of treatment is surgical excision of lesions
- Recurrences common

Thus far we have discussed mycotic processes caused by reasonably well-characterized fungi that may serve as colonizers, opportunistic pathogens, or true pathogens. Although many of these organisms have undergone minor taxonomic reclassification over time, they all share the characteristics of the kingdom Fungi (see Chapter 57). One notable exception to this statement is *Pneumocystis jirovecii* (formerly *Pneumocystis carinii*), an organism formerly considered to be a protozoan and now classified as a fungus of the class Pneumocystidiomycetes based on molecular evidence (see Chapters 57 and 65). The fact that *P. jirovecii* cannot be grown on artificial media has complicated its characterization and assignment to the proper taxonomic category. In this chapter, we will discuss several infections that historically have been considered to represent fungal or "fungal-like" processes based on clinical and histopathologic presentation but, similar to *P. jirovecii*, have been difficult to classify because they cannot be grown on artificial media. In one instance, recent molecular evidence has suggested that an organism previously thought to be a fungus *(Rhinosporidium seeberi)* is in fact a protistan parasite. We also discuss two algal infections and two unusual infections caused by the oomycetes *Pythium insidiosum* and *Lagenidium* spp. In addition to being unusual as well as uncommon, these infections are all diagnosed based on detection of characteristic structures on histopathologic examination of tissue. A listing of the infections, etiologic agents, and typical morphology in tissue is provided in Table 66-1.

• Adiaspiromycosis

In humans, adiaspiromycosis is a rare self-limited pulmonary infection caused by inhalation of the asexual conidia of the soil saprophytes *Emmonsia crescens* and *Emmonsia parva.* Synonyms include **haplomycosis** or **adiasporosis.** Disseminated and pulmonary infections attributed to the dimorphic species *Emmonsia pasteuriana* and an *E. pasteuriana*–like species are discussed in Chapter 64.

Morphology

The fungi *E. crescens* and *E. parva* grow as molds in culture at room temperature and in nature. The hyphae are septate and branched. The small (2 to 4 µm) aleurioconidia are borne on conidiophores that arise at right angles to the vegetative hyphae. Upon incubation at 40° C in vitro, or when introduced into the lungs, the conidia transform into **adiaconidia,** which then undergo massive enlargement but show no evidence of replication (e.g., budding, endospore formation).

When mature, the adiaconidia are thick-walled spherules measuring 200 to 400 µm or more in diameter (Figure 66-1; see Table 66-1). The walls of the spherule are refractile, 20 to 70 µm thick, and when stained with hematoxylin and eosin (H&E) stain, comprise two layers: a narrow outer eosinophilic layer containing periodic fenestrations and a broad hyaline inner layer composed predominantly of chitin (see Figure 66-1). The conidial walls stain with Gomori methenamine silver (GMS), periodic acid–Schiff (PAS), and the Gridley fungus stains but not with mucicarmine (Table 66-2). In human lung tissue, the adiaconidia are usually empty but may contain small eosinophilic globules along the inner surface of the walls (see Figure 66-1).

Epidemiology

Although human adiaspiromycosis is uncommon, the infection is prevalent in rodents worldwide. Likewise, the fungus may be found in nature, predominantly in temperate zones. Human disease has been reported from France, Czechoslovakia, Russia, Honduras, Guatemala, Venezuela, and Brazil. Rodents may serve as a zoonotic reservoir for the disease. The likely mode of infection is by inhalation of fungal conidia aerosolized by contaminated soil.

Table 66-1 Morphologic Features of Fungal and Fungal-Like Infections of Unusual or Uncertain Etiology

Disease	Etiologic Agent(s)	Typical Morphology in Tissue	Usual Host Reaction
Adiaspiromycosis	*Emmonsia* spp.	Large adiaconidia, 200-400 μm diameter with thick (20-70 μm) walls; see Figure 66-1	Granulomatous fibrotic and noncaseating
Chlorellosis	*Chlorella* spp. (chlorophyllous green alga)	Unicellular, endosporulating, round organisms, 4-15 μm diameter, containing multiple cytoplasmic granules (chloroplasts); lesions are green pigmented; see Figure 66-2	Pyogranulomatous
Lacaziosis (Lobomycosis)	*Lacazia loboi (Loboa loboi)*	Spherical budding yeasts, 5-12 μm diameter, that form chains of cells connected by tubelike structures; secondary budding may be present; see Figure 66-3	Granulomatous
Protothecosis	*Prototheca wickerhamii, Prototheca zopfii* (achlorophyllous green algae)	Spherical, oval, or polyhedral spherules, 2-25 μm diameter, containing 2-20 endospores when mature; see Figure 66-5	Variable; no reaction to granulomatous
Pythiosis insidiosi Lagenidiosis	*Pythium insidiosum, Lagenidium* spp. (not true fungi; belong to the protistal kingdom Stramenopila)	Hyphae and short hyphal fragments that are hyaline, thin-walled, pauciseptate, irregularly branched, 5-7 μm *(Pythium)* to 9-18 μm *(Lagenidium)* wide with nonparallel contours; angioinvasive; see Figure 66-6	Granulomatous, necrotizing, suppurative, arteritis
Rhinosporidiosis	*Rhinosporidium seeberi* (aquatic protistan parasite of the Mesomycetozoa clade)	Large sporangia (100-350 μm diameter) with thin walls (3-5 μm) that enclose numerous endospores (6-8 μm diameter) with a zonal distribution; see Figure 66-7	Nonspecific chronic inflammatory or granulomatous

Data from Chandler FW, Watts JC: *Pathologic diagnosis of fungal infections,* Chicago, 1987, American Society for Clinical Pathology Press; and Connor DH, Chandler FW, Schwartz DA, et al: *Pathology of infectious diseases,* vol 2, Stamford, Conn, 1997, Appleton & Lange.

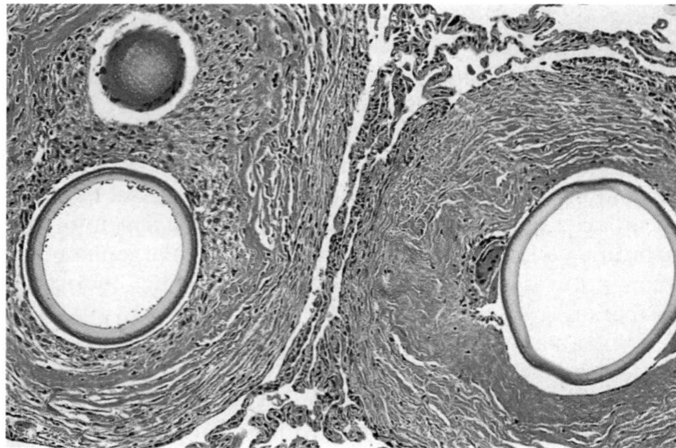

FIGURE 66-1 Pulmonary adiaspiromycosis. Hematoxylin and eosin (H&E) stain defines two layers in the wall of the adiaconidium. Each adiaconidium has evoked a fibrogranulomatous response (H&E, ×40). (From Connor DH, Chandler FW, Schwartz DA, et al: *Pathology of infectious diseases,* vol 2, Stamford, Conn, 1997, Appleton & Lange.)

Clinical Syndromes

As with many fungal infections, most cases of documented adiaspiromycosis have been asymptomatic. Pulmonary nodules may be detected radiographically or incidentally at autopsy or in surgical specimens of lung removed for another reason.

Three forms of human adiaspiromycosis have been recognized: solitary granuloma, localized granulomatous disease, and diffuse disseminated granulomatous disease. Patients with the disseminated granulomatous form of pulmonary adiaspiromycosis may experience fever, cough, and progressive dyspnea caused by compression and displacement of distal airways and alveolar parenchyma by the expanding granulomas. Fungal replication in the lungs does not occur, and dissemination to extrapulmonary sites has not been reported. Disease severity appears to be entirely commensurate with the number of conidia inhaled.

Laboratory Diagnosis

The diagnosis of adiaspiromycosis is established by histopathologic examination of affected lung and identification of the characteristic adiaconidia. Each adiaconidium is surrounded by an epithelioid and giant-cell granulomatous response, which is further encompassed by a dense capsule of fibrous tissue (see Figure 66-1). All of the granulomas are at a similar stage of development, reflecting a one-time exposure without subsequent replication within the lung.

The spherules represented by the adiaconidia should not be confused with those of *C. immitis* or *R. seeberi,* two other organisms that produce large spherules in tissue (see Table 66-2). In contrast to *C. immitis,* the adiaconidia of *Emmonsia* spp. are much larger, have a thicker wall, and do not contain endospores. The sporangia of *R. seeberi* are distinguished by the zonation of the sporangiospores and the distinctive eosinophilic globules seen within the mature sporangiospores (see Table 66-2). No other fungus of medical importance has walls as thick as those of the adiaconidia of *Emmonsia* spp. Culture of infected tissue is not useful because the adiaconidia do not represent a replicative form of the fungus.

Treatment

Human pulmonary adiaspiromycosis is a self-limited infection. Specific antifungal therapy is not necessary.

Table 66-2 Comparative Morphologic Features of Fungi and Fungal-Like Organisms That Appear as Large Spherules in Tissue

	Organisms		
Feature	***Coccidioides immitis***	***Rhinosporidium seeberi****	***Emmonsia* spp.**†
External diameter of spherule (μm)	20-200	10-350	200-400
Thickness of spherule wall (μm)	1-2	3-5	20-70
Diameter of endospores (μm)	2-5	6-10‡	None
Pigmentation	None	None	None
Hyphae or arthroconidia	Rare	None	None
Host reaction	Necrotic granulomas	Mucosal polyps with acute and chronic inflammation	Fibrotic granulomas
Growth in culture	+	–	±§
Special stain reactions			
Gomori methenamine silver	+	+	+
Periodic acid–Schiff	+	+	+
Mucicarmine	–	+	–

Modified from Chandler FW, Watts JC: *Pathologic diagnosis of fungal infections,* Chicago, 1987, American Society for Clinical Pathology Press.

*Not a fungus. Newly classified as an aquatic protistan parasite of the Mesomycetozoa clade.

†Adiaconidia.

‡Endospores arranged in characteristic zonal distribution. Mature endospores contain distinctive eosinophilic globules.

§Grows as a mold on agar medium. Organism not recoverable from tissue.

• Chlorellosis

Chlorellosis is an infection of humans and animals caused by a unicellular green alga of the genus *Chlorella.* In contrast to *Prototheca,* another alga that causes human infection, *Chlorella* contains chloroplasts that give the lesions of chlorellosis a distinct green color. Most infections with this organism occur in sheep and cattle. A single human infection has been reported thus far.

Morphology

Chlorella spp. are unicellular, ovoid, spherical, or polygonal, and 4 to 5 μm in diameter. They reproduce by endosporulation. The organisms contain numerous green chloroplasts that appear as cytoplasmic granules. The chloroplasts contain starch granules that stain intensely with GMS, PAS, and Gridley fungal stains. The cell walls may appear doubly contoured (Figure 66-2; see Table 66-1). *Chlorella* spp. reproduce asexually by internal septation and cytoplasmic cleavage, producing up to 20 daughter cells (sporangiospores) within the sporangium (parent cell). Upon maturation, the outer wall of the sporangium ruptures, releasing the sporangiospores, each of which goes on to produce sporangiospores of its own.

Epidemiology

The single human case took place in Nebraska and resulted from exposure of a surgical wound to river water. Infections in domestic (sheep and cattle) and wild animals (beaver) range from lymph node and deep organ involvement to cutaneous and subcutaneous lesions, presumably related to exposure to water containing the organism.

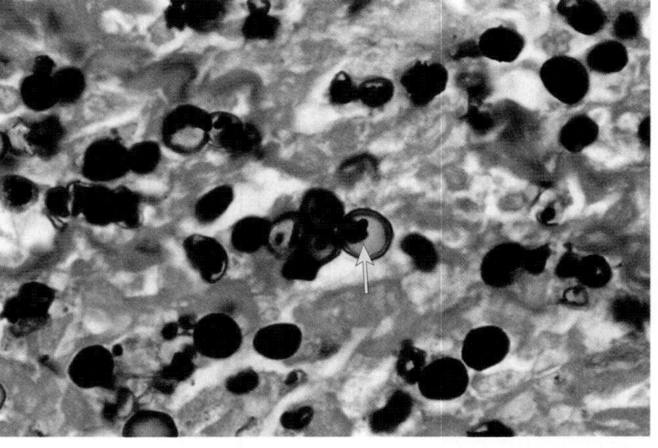

FIGURE 66-2 *Chlorella* sp. showing intracellular chloroplasts *(arrow)* and doubly contoured cell wall (Gomori methenamine silver, ×400). (From Connor DH, Chandler FW, Schwartz DA, et al: *Pathology of infectious diseases,* vol 2, Stamford, Conn, 1997, Appleton & Lange.)

Clinical Syndromes

As noted above, the human case of chlorellosis involved a healing surgical wound contaminated with river water. The wound subsequently drained a greenish yellow exudate. The infection was cured by repeated surgical debridement over a 10-month period. In animals, fresh lesions in liver, lymph nodes, and subcutaneous tissue are green on gross examination, and smears reveal organisms that contain green refractile granules (chloroplasts).

Laboratory Diagnosis

Infections caused by *Chlorella* spp. may be diagnosed by culture and by histopathologic examination of infected tissue. The organism grows well on most solid media, producing bright green colonies. Wet mounts of wound exudate or touch preparations of infected tissue reveal ovoid endosporulating cells with characteristic green cytoplasmic granules representing chloroplasts. In tissue, the cells stain well with GMS and PAS but not H&E stains. They may be distinguished histopathologically from *Prototheca* by the intracellular chloroplasts.

Treatment

Treatment in the only human case of chlorellosis consisted of repeat debridement, irrigation with Dakin solution, and gauze packing and removal for drainage and granulation. Alternatively, amphotericin B therapy combined with administration of tetracycline has proven efficacious in the treatment of protothecosis and may be useful for chlorellosis as well.

• Lacaziosis (Lobomycosis)

Lacaziosis (Clinical Case 66-1) is a chronic fungal infection of the skin caused by *Lacazia loboi* (formerly *Loboa loboi*). *L. loboi* is currently classified as an ascomycete fungus in the order Onygenales and the family Ajellomycetaceae. The disease is seen primarily in the South and Central American tropics. Natural infection occurs only in humans and dolphins, although it has been reproduced experimentally by injecting infected tissue into hamsters and armadillos. The organism has never been cultured in vitro.

Morphology

L. loboi is spherical to oval and yeastlike in appearance. The fungi are 6 to 12 μm in diameter and have a thick double-refractile cell wall. *L. loboi* reproduces by sequential budding and usually forms chains of cells connected by narrow tubelike bridges (Figure 66-3). Some of the cells may have one or two secondary buds and may be mistaken for the "pilot's wheel" form of *Paracoccidioides brasiliensis*. *L. loboi* is usually intracellular, although extracellular forms may be seen.

Epidemiology

The human disease is endemic in the tropical regions of Central and South America and has been reported in central and western Brazil, Bolivia, Colombia, Costa Rica, Ecuador, Guyana, French Guiana, Mexico, Panama, Peru, Surinam, and Venezuela. Isolated cases have been reported from Holland, and a single case has been reported in the United States in a patient with a history of travel to Venezuela.

L. loboi is believed to be a saprophyte of soil or vegetation, and lacaziosis predominates in tropical regions with thick vegetation, such as the Amazon rain forests. Cutaneous trauma is believed to be the mode of infection. A plant reservoir has not been identified.

Given that lacaziosis occurs in marine dolphins and freshwater dolphins, an aquatic habitat is likely as well. Infection among dolphins has been reported for Florida, the Texas coast, the Spanish-French coast, the South Brazilian coast,

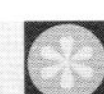

Clinical Case 66-1 **Lacaziosis**

Elsayed and associates (*Emerg Infect Dis* 10:715–718, 2004) described a case of lacaziosis (lobomycosis) in a Canadian geologist. The patient presented to her dermatologist with a slowly growing, 1.5-cm diameter, dusky red, nontender, plaquelike lesion surrounded by keloidal scar on the posterior aspect of her right upper arm. It was located at the site of a scar from a previous excision attempt of a similar lesion 2 years earlier. The original lesion was first noticed while the patient was visiting Southeast Asia in 1996, although she did not seek medical attention until returning to Canada 1 year later. At that time, coccidioidomycosis was diagnosed, based on a history of travel to an endemic region and on the presence of oval, yeastlike organisms in histologic sections. However, *Coccidioides immitis* was never cultured from the lesion, and serologic studies for this infection remained negative. She remained well until a new lesion reappeared at the site of the scar and gradually increased in size. The patient had an extensive travel history, including prolonged stays in Mexico, Costa Rica, South America, Indonesia, and the Philippines. During her travels, she generally lived in rural camps and had extensive exposure to fresh water, soil, and underground caves. Her medical history included episodes of amoebic dysentery, dengue fever, and intestinal helminthiasis but was otherwise unremarkable. Biopsied specimens of the new lesion were obtained and submitted for pathologic and microbiological examination. The hematoxylin and eosin–stained sections showed a diffuse superficial and deep granulomatous dermatitis with multinucleated giant cells. Intracellular and extracellular unstained fungal cells with thick refractile walls were seen. The fungal cells stained strongly with periodic acid–Schiff and Gomori methenamine silver stains; cells were spherical or lemon shaped, approximately 10 μm in diameter and uniform in size. They were arranged as single cells or in short budding chains joined by narrow tubelike bridges. The organisms were not cultivatable. Fungal morphology was consistent with *Lacazia (Loboa) loboi*. The lesion was completely excised, with no subsequent recurrence. This disease should be suspected in patients with single or multiple keloidal skin lesions, particularly if they have traveled to remote areas of Latin America.

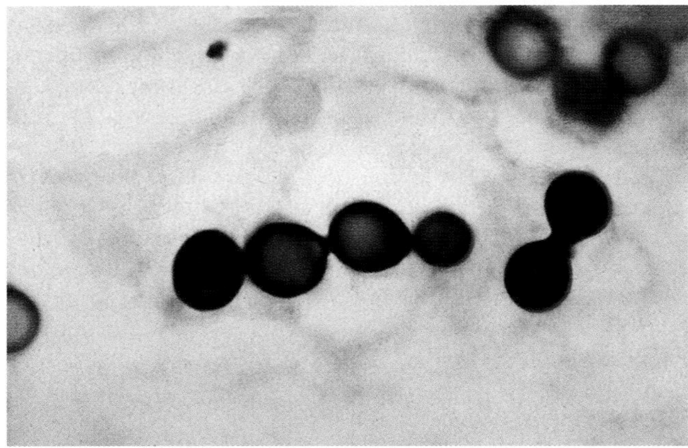

FIGURE 66-3 *Lacazia loboi*. The fungi form a single chain with individual cells joined by tubelike bridges (Gridley, ×400). (From Nikolaidis G, Rosen T: Lobomycosis. In Connor DH, Chandler FW, Schwartz DA, et al, editors: *Pathology of infectious diseases*, Norwalk, CT, 1997, Appleton & Lange.)

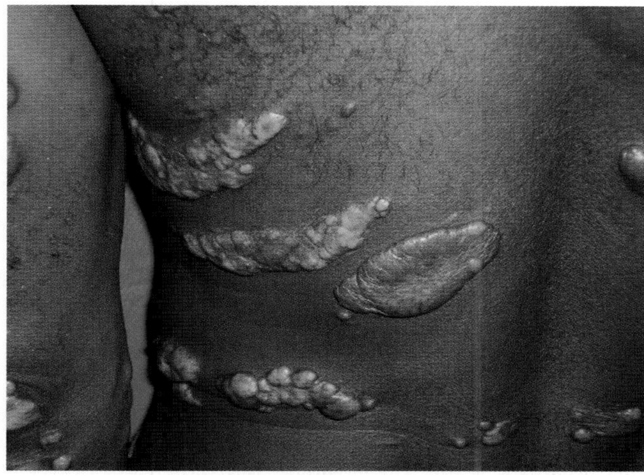

FIGURE 66-4 Multiple keloid-like lesions of lacaziosis. (From Bolognia J, Jorizzo JL, Schaffer JV: *Dermatology,* London, 2012, Saunders, Fig. 77-25B; courtesy Regina Carneiro, MD, and Caroline Brandao, MD.)

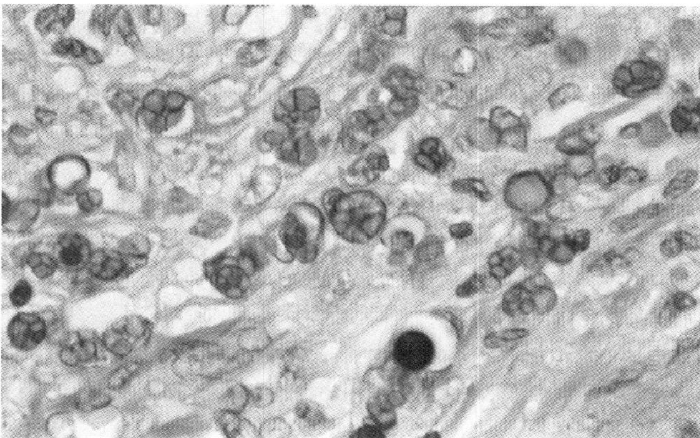

FIGURE 66-5 *Prototheca wickerhamii.* Single and endosporulating algal cells that are readily demonstrated with the periodic acid–Schiff stain. A classic "morula" form is present (×1000).

and the Surinam River estuary. One instance of dolphin-to-human transmission has been reported; however, there is no evidence of human-to-human transmission.

Lacaziosis occurs primarily in men, or in women who are involved in farming and jungle clearing. Farmers, miners, hunters, and rubber plant workers have an increased incidence of disease. There is no racial predilection, and lobomycosis affects all age groups, with the peak age of onset being 20 to 40 years.

Clinical Syndromes

Lacaziosis is characterized by slowly developing cutaneous nodules of varying size and shape (Figure 66-4). The dermal lesions are polymorphic, ranging from macules, papules, keloidal nodules, and plaques to verrucous and ulcerated lesions, all of which may be present in a single patient (see Figure 66-4). The nodular keloid-like lesion is the most common. The disease is characterized by a long dormancy period of months to years. The increase in the number and size of lesions is also a slow process, progressing over a period of 40 to 50 years. Lesions tend to arise on traumatized areas of skin, such as the face, ears, arms, legs, and feet. The disease does not involve mucous membranes or internal organs. Local cutaneous spread may occur through autoinoculation. Aside from occasional pruritus and hypesthesia or anesthesia of the affected area, patients are asymptomatic. There are no systemic manifestations of the disease.

Laboratory Diagnosis

Diagnosis is based on demonstrating the presence of the characteristic yeast cells in lesion exudate or tissue sections. Biopsy reveals a dispersed granulomatous infiltrate along with numerous fungal forms in the dermis and subcutaneous tissue. The granuloma consists primarily of giant cells, macrophages, and epithelioid cells. Both the giant cells and macrophages contain fungi that have been phagocytosed.

L. loboi stains intensely with both GMS and PAS stains. H&E stain reveals the thick, doubly contoured, hyaline cell wall and one or more hematoxylinophilic nuclei.

Although the lesions of lacaziosis resemble keloids on a gross level, microscopically, keloids have marked fibrosis, which is not the case with lacaziosis. Similarly, keloids lack granulomas and fungal elements. The morphology and pattern of budding of *L. loboi* are distinctive and should not be confused with that of *P. brasiliensis* (multiple buds, variable size), *Blastomyces dermatitidis,* and *Histoplasma capsulatum* var. *duboisii* (no chains of cells) or *Sporothrix schenckii* and *H. capsulatum* var. *capsulatum* (both smaller, 2 to 8 µm versus 5 to 12 µm). The latter fungi will also grow in culture, whereas *L. loboi* has never been cultured in vitro.

Treatment

Surgical excision of localized lesions is the optimal therapy. More widespread disease usually recurs when treated surgically and does not respond to antifungal therapy. Clofazimine has been used in these situations, but at this time medical treatment of lacaziosis is not satisfactory.

• Protothecosis

Protothecosis is an infection of humans and animals caused by achlorophyllous algae of the genus *Prototheca.* These organisms belong to the same family as the green algae of the genus *Chlorella.* Two species, *P. wickerhamii* and *P. zopfii,* are known to cause infection. Three forms of human protothecosis have been described: cutaneous, olecranon bursitis, and disseminated.

Morphology

The protothecae are unicellular oval or spherical organisms that reproduce asexually by internal septation and irregular cleavage within hyaline sporangia. Each sporangium contains between 2 and 20 sporangiospores arranged in a "morula" configuration (Figure 66-5). The sporangiospores are released after rupture of the sporangium and in turn develop into mature endosporulating forms. The cells measure 3 to 30 µm in diameter and differ from those of *Chlorella* by the lack of chloroplasts. Protothecae differ from fungi by the lack of glucosamine in their cell walls. The two species of *Prototheca* that cause human disease differ from one another in size: *P. wickerhamii* measures 3 to 15 µm in diameter, whereas *P. zopfii* measures 7 to 30 μm in diameter. Both species are readily stained with PAS, GMS, and the Gridley fungus stain (see Figure 66-5) and are gram-positive organisms.

Epidemiology

Prototheca spp. are ubiquitous environmental saprobes that have been isolated from grass, soil, water, and both wild and domestic animals. Human protothecosis has been reported on all continents with the exception of Antarctica.

Clinical Syndromes

At least half of all cases of protothecosis are simple cutaneous infections. For the most part, these infections occur in patients who are immunocompromised because of immunosuppressive therapy, acquired immunodeficiency syndrome (AIDS), malnutrition, renal or hepatic disease, cancer, or autoimmune disorders. Lesions usually arise in areas exposed to traumatic implantation and present in an indolent fashion as nodules, papules, or as an eczematoid eruption.

Individuals presenting with olecranon bursitis are usually not immunocompromised, but most report some sort of penetrating or nonpenetrating trauma to the affected elbow. Signs and symptoms of olecranon bursitis usually occur several weeks after the trauma and include mild induration of the bursa, tenderness, erythema, and production of a variable amount of serosanguineous fluid.

Disseminated protothecosis is rare but has been reported in individuals with no known immunologic deficiency. One patient with visceral protothecosis presented with abdominal pain and abnormal liver function studies that were initially considered to be the result of cholangitis. The patient had multiple peritoneal nodules that resembled metastatic cancer but were in fact manifestations of protothecosis. Another patient presented with protothecal lesions on the forehead and nose.

Laboratory Diagnosis

Prototheca spp. grow easily on a wide variety of solid media at 30° C to 37° C. Colonies are yeastlike, white, and creamy in appearance and consistency. A wet mount of the culture material may be stained with lactophenol cotton blue to reveal the characteristic sporangia and sporangiospores. The organisms are quite metabolically active and may be identified to species using one of several commercially available yeast identification panels to determine the carbohydrate assimilation profile.

On histopathologic examination of infected tissue, *Prototheca* spp. appear as sporangiospores that are wedge shaped and arranged in a radial or "morula" pattern within the sporangium (see Figure 66-5). The organisms are best visualized by stains used to demonstrate fungi in tissue: the GMS, PAS, and Gridley fungus procedures. In addition to the size differences noted above, the two species of *Prototheca* differ in that *P. wickerhamii* tends to form very symmetric morula forms, whereas these forms are rare with *P. zopfii,* which exhibits more random internal divisions. The inflammatory response in protothecosis is predominantly granulomatous.

Treatment

Treatment of olecranon bursitis usually involves bursectomy. Repeated drainage has failed; however, drainage coupled with local instillation of amphotericin B was curative in one patient. Treatment of cutaneous protothecosis with a variety of topical and systemic antibacterial, antifungal, and antiprotozoal agents has been unsuccessful. Local excision coupled with topical amphotericin B, systemic tetracycline, and systemic ketoconazole has proven useful despite ketoconazole-related hepatotoxicity. Disseminated protothecosis has been treated with systemic antifungal agents; both amphotericin B and ketoconazole have been used.

• Pythiosis Insidiosi

Pythiosis (Clinical Case 66-2) insidiosi is a "fungal-like" infection of humans and animals caused by the plant pathogen *P. insidiosum.* Although described as an "aquatic fungus," this organism is not a true fungus but rather an oomycete that belongs to the protistal kingdom Stramenopila near the green algae and some lower plants in the evolutionary tree. In humans, pythiosis causes keratitis and orbital infections as well as a cutaneous and subcutaneous vascular process marked by rapidly developing granulomatous lesions, leading to progressive arterial insufficiency, tissue infarction, aneurysms, and occasionally death. In animals (cats, dogs, horses,

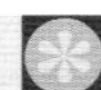

Clinical Case 66-2 Pythiosis

Bosco and associates (*Emerg Infect Dis* 11:715–718, 2005) described a case of pythiosis in a 49-year-old Brazilian man. The patient was admitted to the hospital for treatment of a skin lesion on his leg, initially diagnosed as cutaneous mucormycosis. The patient stated that a small pustule developed on his left leg 3 months earlier, 1 week after he fished in a lake with standing water. The pustule was initially diagnosed as bacterial cellulitis; it was treated with intravenous antibiotics, with no improvement. A biopsy of the lesion showed a suppurative granulomatous inflammation associated with several nonseptate hyphae (shown by Gomori methenamine silver stain), a finding that led to the diagnosis of mucormycosis. The treatment was changed to amphotericin B. After receiving 575 mg (cumulative dosage) of amphotericin B plus two surgical debridements, the patient showed only slight improvement; he was then transferred to another hospital. At admission, the physical exam showed a pretibial ulcer 15 cm in diameter, with an infiltrating and nodular proximal border. Serum chemistries showed azotemia, hypokalemia, and anemia as adverse effects of the amphotericin B treatment. His white blood cell count was 4200/mm^3 with 9% eosinophils. His blood glucose was normal and human immunodeficiency virus serology was negative. Results of a second biopsy again suggested mucormycosis. The patient received itraconazole and potassium iodide, with no significant improvement. Attempts to isolate the organism in the laboratory failed. With progression of the disease, an extensive surgical debridement was considered. A course of amphotericin B was begun, and the lesion was debrided down to and including the fascia lata. A skin graft was placed and produced an acceptable recovery. Tissue was submitted for culture and molecular testing using the generic primers for fungal internal transcribed spacer (ITS) regions of ribosomal DNA. Cultures grew colorless colonies, which on microscopic examination showed broad, branched, and sparsely septate hyphae without fruiting bodies, which were later identified as *Pythium insidiosum.* Use of the polymerase chain reaction, followed by sequencing of the ITS amplicons, gave results showing 100% identity with *P. insidiosum.* This case illustrates the clinical and diagnostic issues surrounding human pythiosis.

cattle), it is an osseous, subcutaneous, or pulmonary infection. Dogs and horses may also present with intestinal infection.

Morphology

P. insidiosum grows as white colonies with submerged vegetative hyphae and short aerial hyphae on solid culture medium. Because this organism is a plant pathogen, it requires water cultures containing the appropriate leaves to produce zoosporangia and zoospores in vitro. In nature, it produces biflagellate zoospores that attach and penetrate the leaves of various grasses and water lilies. The zoospores have a strong tropism for skin and hair, as well as water lily and grass leaves. If zoospores contact injured tissue, they encyst, form germ tubes that produce hyphae, and cause invasive disease.

In tissue, *P. insidiosum* exists as hyaline pauciseptate thin-walled hyphae or hyphal fragments that branch infrequently. The hyphal elements are 5 to 7 μm wide with nonparallel contours and superficially resemble those of Mucormyceta (Figure 66-6). Like the Mucormycetes, *P. insidiosum* is angioinvasive. In tissue the hyphal elements of *P. insidiosum* stain with GMS but not with H&E or other fungal stains.

Epidemiology

P. insidiosum grows in aquatic to wet environments in tropical to subtropical regions. Reports of pythiosis have come from Australia, Costa Rica, India, Japan, New Guinea, Thailand, and the United States.

Clinical Syndromes

Human disease caused by *P. insidiosum* has occurred in patients with thalassemia who developed pythiosis insidiosi of the lower limbs. The disease process was marked by progressive ischemia of the lower limbs, necrosis, thrombosis of major arteries caused by hyphal invasion, gangrene, aneurism formation, and ultimately fatal hemorrhage. Orbital pythiosis has been misdiagnosed as a mucormycotic fungal infection. Less serious forms of the infection include keratitis and localized cutaneous infections after injury.

In horses, pythiosis presents as localized inflammation and necrotic sores of the legs and lower abdomen with necrotic cores. Septic arthritis, osteitis, and tenosynovitis are also common.

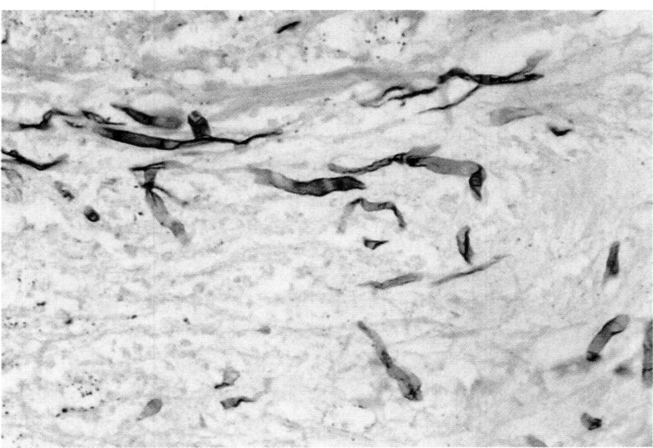

FIGURE 66-6 *Pythium insidiosum* invading an arterial wall. Infrequently septate, weakly stained hyphae and hyphal fragments resemble those of Mucormycetes (Gomori methenamine silver, ×160). (From Connor DH, Chandler FW, Schwartz DA, et al: *Pathology of infectious diseases,* vol 2, Stamford, Conn, 1997, Appleton & Lange.)

Laboratory Diagnosis

The organism may be isolated from fresh clinical material seeded onto mycologic medium such as Sabouraud glucose agar. Demonstration of biflagellate zoospores may be accomplished using water cultures with grass or lily bait incubated at 37° C for 1 hour. Serologic assays using either the enzyme-linked immunosorbent assay or Western blot technologies have been useful in the early detection of the disease in humans and animals.

Histopathologic examination of infected tissue shows a necrotizing arteritis and thrombosis. Vascular invasion by sparsely septate, irregularly branched hyphae is seen (see Figure 66-6). The acute perivascular inflammatory reaction is eventually replaced by granulomas that contain sparse hyphae and hyphal fragments. The hyphal elements of *P. insidiosum* may be surrounded by the eosinophilic Splendore-Hoeppli phenomenon. Pythiosis insidiosi in humans must be differentiated from cutaneous and subcutaneous mucormycosis, sporotrichosis, mycetoma, and neoplasms.

Treatment

Although potassium iodide has been used to treat cutaneous infections, medical treatment of pythiosis insidiosi is generally not effective. Surgical debridement and excision of infected tissue has been used with some success. There is some evidence that azole antifungal agents (e.g., fluconazole, ketoconazole, itraconazole, miconazole) exhibit in vitro activity against this organism. A case of orbital pythiosis responded well to a combination of itraconazole and terbinafine, although this combination has not been useful in other cases of pythiosis. Immunotherapy has been useful in the treatment of equine pythiosis and has a 55% cure rate in human disease.

• Lagenidiosis

Like *P. insidiosum, Lagenidium* spp. is an oomycete that causes infections in mammals, rarely in humans. Members of the genus *Lagenidium* also cause infections in lower animals including crabs, nematodes, and mosquito larvae among others. In mammals the infection presents with involvement of the skin and subsequently disseminates to blood vessels. These organisms are currently classified within the Kingdom Stramenopila, Phylum Heterokontophyta, Class Oomycota, Order Lagenidiales, and Family Lagenidiaceae.

Morphology

In contrast to other pathogens covered in this chapter, *Lagenidium* spp. grow readily on routine fungal isolation media. On agar media these organisms grow readily at 37° C as white to yellow submerged colonies without aerial mycelia. Similar to *P. insidiosum, Lagenidium* spp. produce 9- to 18-μm ribbon-like hyphae with spherical structures 20 to 45 μm in diameter. In liquid media vesicles may be seen at the tips of the undifferentiated hyphae. The presence of sexual structures (oogonia) has not yet been described. The two species mentioned in the literature thus far, *L. caninum* and *L. karlingii,* have not undergone a formal taxonomic description.

Epidemiology

At the present time, most of the cases of lagenidiosis in mammals have been reported in the United States and in the same areas as *P. insidiosum* infections: the States bordering the Gulf of Mexico, as well as Arkansas, Georgia, Illinois, Indiana, Maryland, North and South Carolina, Tennessee, and Virginia among others. *Lagenidium* completes its life cycle in aquatic environments, possibly using plants or lower animal hosts. In addition to the regions noted, a case of human keratitis caused by *Lagenidium* has been reported from Thailand, and lagenidiosis in a dog has been reported from Australia. It is thought that infection is initiated when zoospores present in a contaminated environment gain entry through open skin injuries. Lagenidiosis does not appear to be transmitted from one infected host to another, and attempts to establish infection in mice have been unsuccessful.

Clinical Syndrome

As with *P. insidiosum, Lagenidium* spp. cause infections ranging from superficial cutaneous to subcutaneous and arterial involvement. Systemic infection appears to be rare. In humans and animals the sites of infection are cornea, gastrointestinal tract, and limbs.

Laboratory Diagnosis

The diagnosis of infection with *Lagenidium* spp. may be made by direct microscopy and culture of material taken from the site of infection. On microscopic examination of cytologic specimens stained with Giemsa, *Lagenidium* spp. appear as broad branched hyphae. In culture on Sabouraud dextrose agar, white to yellowish flat glabrous colonies submerged in the agar may be seen following incubation at 37° C for 24 to 48 hours. Microscopically the hyphae are coenocytic and broad (9 to 18 μm), with large spherical structures connected by short segments of hyphae. Observation of spherical structures connected by small tubules may be used to differentiate *Lagenidium* spp. from *P. insidiosum;* however, molecular studies have often been required to make this distinction. Detection of antibodies using both enzyme-linked immunosorbent assay (ELISA) and Western blot assays have been used for both diagnosis and monitoring of response to therapy. A strong cross-reaction with *P. insidiosum* antigens has been observed with ELISA testing.

Treatment

In contrast to fungi, the oomycetes lack ergosterol in their cytoplasmic membranes, thus precluding efficacy with antifungal agents directed at this sterol pathway. Despite this feature, several antifungal agents have been employed both clinically and in vitro, with mixed results. As with pythiosis, early surgical resection is recommended as the treatment of choice.

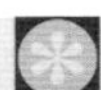 **Clinical Case 66-3 Rhinosporidiosis**

Gaines and Clay (*South Med J* 89:65–67, 1996) described three cases of rhinosporidiosis in young boys who had not traveled outside the United States. In fact, there was no history of their having traveled outside the state of Georgia. All the patients lived in rural areas in the northeast portion of the state. One had a polypoid conjunctival lesion, and the other two had nasal polyps. In each case, the lesions were excised, and histopathologic examination revealed structures morphologically typical of *Rhinosporidium seeberi.* No other treatment was given, and follow-up showed no evidence of recurrence. Despite the very rare nature of these cases, the distinctive appearance of the developmental forms of *R. seeberi* in histopathologic sections is diagnostic.

• Rhinosporidiosis

Rhinosporidiosis (Clinical Case 66-3) is a granulomatous disease of humans and animals that is characterized by the development of polyps that primarily affect the nasopharynx and the ocular conjunctiva of infected individuals. The disease is caused by *R. seeberi,* an organism with a confusing taxonomic history. This organism has been considered to be a protozoan, a fungus, and most recently has been placed in a novel clade of aquatic protistan parasites, the Mesomycetozoa. Because *R. seeberi* will not grow in synthetic media, this reclassification was based on sequence analysis of the 18S small-subunit ribosomal deoxyribonucleic acid (rDNA) of this organism. This analysis placed *R. seeberi* among the Mesomycetozoa (formerly DRIP: ***D****ermocystidium*, **R**osette agent, ***I****chthyophonus*, and ***P****sorospermium*), a clade of fish parasites that form a branch of the evolutionary tree near the animal-fungal divergence.

Morphology

Given that *R. seeberi* will not grow on artificial media, the morphologic descriptions are entirely based on the organism as it appears in infected tissue. Two developmental forms of *R. seeberi* are seen in tissue: the large spherical form (sporangia) and the smaller trophocyte. The sporangium is considered the mature form of the organism and measures 100 to 350 μm in diameter. The sporangial wall is 3 to 5 μm thick and is composed of an inner hyaline layer and thin outer eosinophilic layer. The sporangium contains numerous endoconidia arranged in a characteristic zonal formation, whereby the small, flattened, uninucleate immature endoconidia (1 to 2 μm) form a crescentic mass at the periphery of one wall of the sporangium, with the larger maturing and mature endoconidia arranged sequentially toward the center. The mature endoconidia range in size from 5 to 20 μm in diameter and contain multiple refractile cytoplasmic globules. This zonal arrangement of immature, maturing, and fully mature endoconidia is diagnostic of this pathogen and distinguishes it from other spherical endosporulating organisms in the tissue (see Table 66-2).

The trophocytes are considered to develop directly from endoconidia that have been released from the sporangium. The trophocytes range in size from 10 to 100 μm in diameter and have refractile eosinophilic walls (2 to 3 μm thick), granular cytoplasm, and a round, pale nucleus with a prominent nucleolus. Ultimately, the trophocytes enlarge and transform into mature sporangia through a process of endosporulation.

The walls of both the sporangia and endoconidia stain with both GMS and PAS fungal stains. In addition, the walls

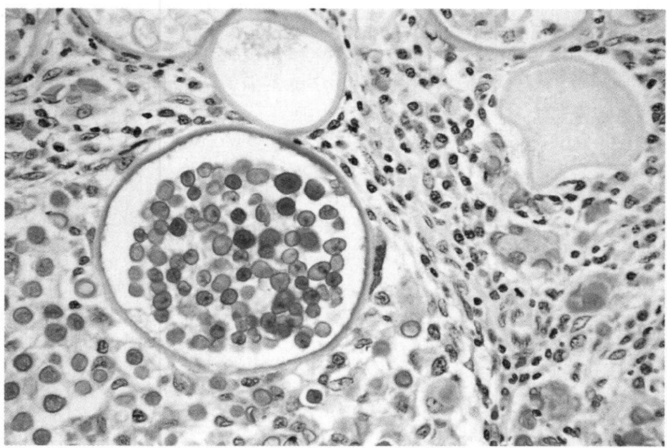

FIGURE 66-7 Mature sporangium of *Rhinosporidium seeberi.* Walls of the mature endoconidia are carminophilic (Mayer mucicarmine, ×100). (From Connor DH, Chandler FW, Schwartz DA, et al: *Pathology of infectious diseases,* vol 2, Stamford, Conn, 1997, Appleton & Lange.)

of the endoconidia and the inner wall of the sporangium stain positively with the mucin stain mucicarmine (Figure 66-7; see Table 66-2).

Epidemiology

Approximately 90% of all known cases of rhinosporidiosis occur in India and Sri Lanka. The disease also occurs in the Americas, Europe, and Africa. The natural habitat and the extent of distribution of *R. seeberi* in nature are unknown. The disease occurs primarily in young men 20 to 40 years old and appears to be associated with both rural and aquatic environments. There is no evidence that rhinosporidiosis is contagious.

Clinical Syndrome

Rhinosporidiosis manifests as slow-growing polypoid or tumor-like masses, usually of the nasal mucosa or conjunctiva. Lesions may also be seen in the paranasal sinuses, larynx, and external genitalia. Secondary spread to surrounding skin is thought to result from autoinoculation by scratching. In most patients, the disease remains localized, and symptoms are primarily nasal obstruction and bleeding resulting from polyp formation. Limited systemic dissemination has been reported but is rare.

Laboratory Diagnosis

The diagnosis of rhinosporidiosis is made by histopathologic examination of the affected tissue. The distinctive appearance of the trophocytes and sporangia in routine H&E-stained sections is diagnostic. Although other organisms that occur in tissue in the form of large spherules may be mistaken for *R. seeberi,* they are usually easily differentiated from this organism by consideration of the tissue involved and the morphologic and staining characteristics of the spherule and the endoconidia (see Table 66-2).

Treatment

The only effective form of treatment is surgical excision of the lesions. Recurrences are common, especially in mucosal sites such as the oropharynx and paranasal sinuses, where complete excision is often difficult to achieve.

Bibliography

Burns RA, Roy JS, Woods C, et al: Report of the first human case of lobomycosis in the United States, *J Clin Microbiol* 38:1283–1285, 2000.

Chandler FW, Watts JC: *Pathologic diagnosis of fungal infections*, Chicago, 1987, American Society for Clinical Pathology Press.

Connor DH, Chandler FW, Schwartz DA, et al: *Pathology of infectious diseases*, vol 2, Stamford, Conn, 1997, Appleton & Lange.

Fredericks DN, Jolley JA, Lepp PW, et al: *Rhinosporidium seeberi:* a human pathogen from a novel group of aquatic protistan parasites, *Emerg Infect Dis* 6:273–282, 2000.

Grooters AM: Pythiosis, lagenidiosis, and zygomycosis in small animals, *Vet Clin Small Anim* 33:695–720, 2003.

Herr RA, Ajello L, Taylor JW, et al: Phylogenetic analysis of *Rhinosporidium seeberi's* 18S small-subunit ribosomal DNA groups this pathogen among members of the protoctistan Mesomycetozoa clade, *J Clin Microbiol* 37:2750–2754, 1999.

Krajaejun T, Sathapatayavongs B, Pracharktam R, et al: Clinical and epidemiological analysis of human pythiosis in Thailand, *Clin Infect Dis* 43:569–576, 2006.

Lass-Florl C, Mayr A: Human protothecosis, *Clin Microbiol Rev* 20:230–242, 2007.

Mendoza L, Prasla SH, Ajello L: Orbital pythiosis: a nonfungal disease mimicking orbital mycotic infections, with a retrospective review of the literature, *Mycoses* 47:14–23, 2004.

Mendoza L, Vilela R: *Lacazia, Pythium,* and *Rhinosporidium*. In Versalovic J, et al, editors: *Manual of clinical microbiology*, ed 10, Washington, DC, 2011, American Society for Microbiology Press.

Reinprayoon U, Permpalung N, Kasetsuwan N, et al: *Lagenidium* sp. Ocular infection mimicking ocular pythiosis, *J Clin Microbiol* 51:2778–2780, 2013.

Taborda PR, Taborda VA, McGinnis MR: *Lacazia loboi* gen. nov., comb. nov., the etiologic agent of lobomycosis, *J Clin Microbiol* 37:2031–2033, 1999.

CHAPTER

67

MYCOTOXINS AND MYCOTOXICOSES

A 42-year-old man in India ate homegrown maize for several days and started developing symptoms of hepatitis. The patient was eventually rushed to the hospital, where he died of acute hepatic failure.

1. What was the most likely cause of his acute liver failure?
   a. Ochratoxin
   b. Aflatoxin
   c. Hepatitis A
   d. Citreoviridin
2. What organism was most likely responsible for this toxic illness?
   a. *Aspergillus fumigatus*
   b. *Aspergillus terreus*
   c. *Fusarium moniliforme*
   d. *Aspergillus flavus*
3. What are the long-term consequences of chronic low-level exposure to this mycotoxin?
   a. Hepatocellular carcinoma
   b. Aplastic anemia
   c. Esophageal cancer
   d. Bladder cancer

Answers to these questions are available on StudentConsult.com.

• SUMMARIES CLINICALLY SIGNIFICANT MYCOTOXINS AND MYCOTOXICOSES

Mycotoxins and Mycotoxicoses

Trigger Words

Contaminated grain, aflatoxin, carcinogen, mold, nephrotoxin, hepatotoxin, pancytopenia

Biology, Virulence, and Disease

- Mycotoxins are secondary fungal metabolites that cause diseases, known collectively as mycotoxicoses, after ingestion, inhalation or direct contact with the toxin
- Among the most important mycotoxins and their primary toxic effects are: aflatoxins (carcinogens), citrinin (nephrotoxin), ergot alkaloids (convulsive and gangrenous), fumonsins (carcinogens), ochratoxin (nephrotoxin), trichothecenes (bone marrow toxicity), stachybotryotoxins (neurotoxin)
- Mycotoxins are produced by filamentous fungi (molds), many of which may also serve as opportunistic pathogens that cause invasive disease in immunocompromised individuals
- Mycotoxicoses may manifest as acute or chronic disease, ranging from rapid death to tumor formation
- There are more than 100 toxigenic fungi and more than 300 compounds recognized as mycotoxins

Epidemiology

- The number of people affected is unknown
- The majority of mycotoxicoses result from eating contaminated foods (grains, peanuts, sugarcane, hay), most commonly caused by preharvest contamination of the material by toxigenic fungi that are plant pathogens
- Common in resource-poor countries where methods of food handling and storage are inadequate, malnutrition is prevalent and there are few regulations to protect exposed populations

Diagnosis

- Given the wide range of toxins and very diverse clinical signs and symptoms the diagnosis is usually made on epidemiologic grounds that point to an exposure to contaminated foodstuffs or exposure to domiciles or workplaces where mold has been observed (sick building syndrome)
- For many mycotoxicoses the link between the toxin and/or mold and clinical disease is quite tentative

Treatment, Prevention, and Control

- Aside from supportive therapy, there are almost no treatments for mycotoxin exposure
- In some cases of acute hepatotoxicity liver transplantation has been lifesaving
- Mycotoxicoses are not communicable from person-to-person

In addition to their role as opportunistic pathogens, filamentous fungi can produce toxins that have been implicated in a variety of illnesses and clinical syndromes in humans and animals. These mycotoxins are secondary fungal metabolites that cause diseases, known collectively as **mycotoxicoses**, after ingestion, inhalation, or direct contact with the toxin (Figure 67-1). Mycotoxicoses may manifest as acute or chronic disease ranging from rapid death to tumor formation. In this regard, mycotoxicoses are analogous to the pathologies caused by other "poisons" such as pesticides or heavy metal residues. The presenting symptoms and severity of a mycotoxicosis depend on the type of mycotoxin, amount and duration of exposure, route of exposure, and age, sex, and health of the exposed individual. In addition, a variety of other circumstances (e.g., malnutrition, alcohol abuse, infectious disease status, other toxin exposures) may act synergistically to compound the effect and severity of mycotoxin poisoning.

There are more than 100 toxigenic fungi and more than 300 compounds now recognized as mycotoxins. The number of people affected by mycotoxicoses, however, is unknown. The majority of mycotoxicoses result from eating contaminated foods. The occurrence of mycotoxins in foods is most commonly caused by preharvest contamination of the material by toxigenic fungi that are plant pathogens. In addition, stored grains may be damaged by insects or moisture, providing a portal of entry for toxigenic fungi present in the storage environment. Mycotoxicoses are more common in resource-poor countries where methods of food handling and storage are inadequate, malnutrition is prevalent, and there are few regulations designed to protect exposed populations.

Some mycotoxins are dermonecrotic, and cutaneous or mucosal contact with mold-infected substrates may result in disease. Likewise, inhalation of spore-borne toxins also constitutes an important form of exposure. Aside from supportive therapy, there are almost no treatments for mycotoxin exposure. Fortunately, mycotoxicoses are not communicable from person to person.

Among fungal plant pathogens, the elaboration of mycotoxins plays a role in causing or exacerbating the plant disease. Although mycotoxins may be poisonous to humans, and some may have potent immunosuppressive properties, there is very little evidence that mycotoxins enhance the ability of the fungus to grow and cause disease in vertebrate hosts. Fungi such as *Aspergillus fumigatus* that are both important opportunistic pathogens and capable of producing gliotoxins (inhibitors of T-cell activation and proliferation) generally do

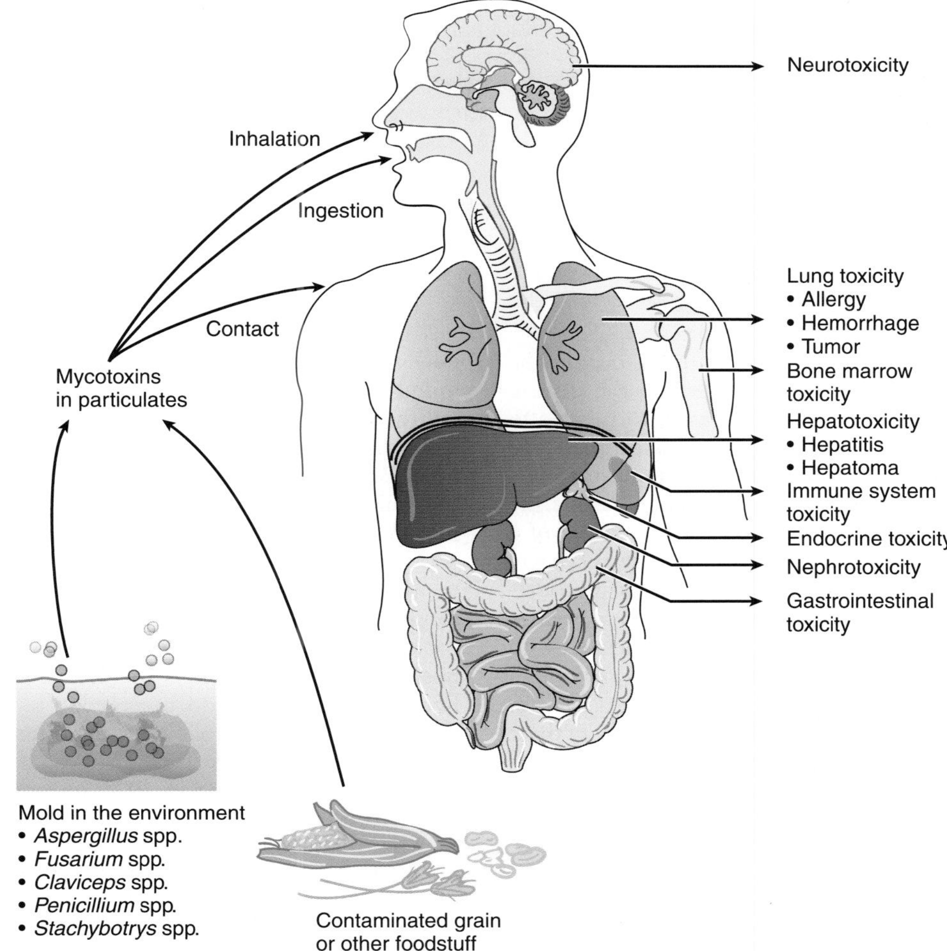

FIGURE 67-1 Various exposures and influences of mycotoxins. (Modified from Richard JL: Mycotoxins and human disease. In Anaissie EJ, McGinnis MR, Pfaller MA, editors: *Clinical mycology,* ed 2, New York, 2009, Churchill Livingstone.)

Table 67-1 Mycotoxin-Related Illnesses Postulated to Affect Humans, Based on Analytic or Epidemiologic Data

Disease	Toxin	Substrate	Fungus	Clinical Presentation
Akakabi-byo (red mold disease)	*Fusarium* metabolites	Wheat, barley, oats, rice	*Fusarium* spp.	Headaches, vomiting, diarrhea
Alimentary toxic aleukia (ATA)	Trichothecenes (T-2 toxin, diacetoxyscirpenol [DAS])	Cereal grains (toxic bread)	*Fusarium* spp.	Vomiting, diarrhea, angina, skin inflammation
Balkan endemic nephropathy (BEN)	Ochratoxin	Cereal grains	*Aspergillus* spp. *Penicillium* spp.	Chronic nephritis
Cardiac beriberi	Citreoviridin	Rice	*Penicillium* spp.	Palpitations, vomiting, mania, respiratory failure
Ergotism (gangrenous and convulsive)	Ergot alkaloids	Rye, cereal grains	*Claviceps purpurea* *Claviceps fusiformis*	Gangrenous: vasoconstriction, edema, pruritus, necrosis of extremities Convulsive: numbness, tingling, pruritus, cramps, seizures, hallucinations
Esophageal cancer	Fumonisins	Corn	*Fusarium moniliforme*	Dysphagia, pain, hemorrhage
Hepatitis and hepatic cancer	Aflatoxins	Cereal grains, peanuts	*Aspergillus flavus* *Aspergillus parasiticus*	Acute and chronic hepatitis, liver failure
Kodua poisoning	Cyclopiazonic acid	Millet	*Penicillium* spp. *Aspergillus* spp.	Somnolence, tremors, giddiness
Moldy sugarcane poisoning	3-Nitropropionic acid	Sugarcane	*Arthrinium* spp.	Dystonia, seizures, carpopedal spasms, coma
Onyalai disease	*Fusarium* metabolites	Millet	*Fusarium* spp.	Thrombocytopenia, purpura
Stachybotryotoxicosis	Trichothecenes (T-2 toxin, DAS)	Hay, cereal grains, fodder (skin contact, inhaled hay dust)	*Stachybotrys, Fusarium, Myrothecium, Trichoderma, Cephalosporium* spp.	Tremors, loss of vision, dermonecrosis, gastrointestinal bleeding (horses and cattle), nasal inflammation, dermatitis, headache, fatigue, respiratory symptoms (humans), idiopathic pulmonary hemorrhage of infants (?)
Yellow rice disease	Citrinin	Wheat, oats, barley, rice	*Penicillium* spp. *Aspergillus* spp.	Nephropathy

Data from Kuhn DM, Ghannoum MA: Indoor mold, toxigenic fungi, and *Stachybotrys chartarum:* infectious disease perspective, *Clin Microbiol Rev* 16:144–172, 2003; Smith M, McGinnis MR: Mycotoxins and their effect on humans. In Anaissie EJ, McGinnis MR, Pfaller MA, editors: *Clinical mycology,* ed 2, New York, 2009, Churchill Livingstone; and Bennett JW, Klich M: Mycotoxins, *Clin Microbiol Rev* 16:497–516, 2003.

not produce the toxin in significant amounts during the course of human disease to have an effect on the disease process. Whereas an opportunistic fungus must be able to grow at human body temperature (37° C) to cause disease, the optimum temperature for biosynthesis of most mycotoxins is much lower (20° C to 30° C). For these and other reasons, the importance of mycotoxin exposure during the course of a mycotic infection with a toxigenic fungus is largely unknown.

In the remainder of this chapter, we will discuss mycotoxins that have been implicated in human disease, as well as metabolites produced by molds that may be associated with human foods or living/working environments. Although mushroom poisoning is a form of mycotoxicosis, it will not be discussed herein. A listing of mycotoxicoses where there is considerable evidence for involvement of a specific mycotoxin is provided in Table 67-1. It should be noted that this list is meant to be representative and not all inclusive.

• Aflatoxins

The aflatoxins (Clinical Case 67-1) are produced primarily by *Aspergillus flavus* and *Aspergillus parasiticus,* but many other species of *Aspergillus* produce aflatoxins as well. *A. flavus* is the most common aflatoxin-producing species found in agriculture and may produce as much as 10^6 mg/kg. The commodities most often affected in the United States are corn, cottonseed, peanuts, and certain tree nuts. Aflatoxin B1 is the most potent natural carcinogen known and the major aflatoxin produced by toxigenic strains; however, more than a dozen other aflatoxins have been described.

Aflatoxin is associated with both toxicity and carcinogenicity in human and animal populations. Acute aflatoxicosis results in death, whereas chronic aflatoxicosis results in more prolonged pathologic changes, including cancer and immunosuppression. The liver is the primary target organ, and liver damage has been documented in rodents, poultry, and nonhuman primates following ingestion of aflatoxin B1. Acute aflatoxicosis has been manifested in humans as an acute hepatitis. In India in 1974, an outbreak of hepatitis occurred in which 100 people died following consumption of maize that was heavily contaminated with aflatoxin. Aflatoxin B1 was detected in high concentration in the livers of those individuals who died.

It has been hypothesized that both kwashiorkor, a severe malnutrition disease, and Reye syndrome, marked by encephalopathy and fatty degeneration of the viscera, represent forms of pediatric aflatoxicosis. Although aflatoxins

Clinical Case 67-1 Acute Aflatoxicosis

Nyikal and colleagues (*MMWR Morb Mortal Wkly Rep* 53:790–793, 2004) described an outbreak of aflatoxin poisoning in Kenya. During January to June 2004, the Kenya Ministry of Health (MOH) and partners identified 317 cases of acute hepatic failure in eastern Kenya; 125 cases occurred in persons who subsequently died during the illness. Seven patients had serum samples analyzed at the Kenya Medical Research Institute, and all were negative for viruses known to cause hepatic disease in Kenya. Because aflatoxicosis outbreaks had occurred previously in that geographic area, the MOH suspected that the unusually high number of patients with acute hepatic failure might have acquired aflatoxicosis from eating contaminated maize. Public health officials sampled maize from the affected area and found concentrations of aflatoxin B1 as high as 4400 parts per billion (ppb), which is 220 times greater than the 20 ppb limit for food suggested by Kenyan authorities. A case-control study found that homegrown maize kernels from case (acute hepatic failure) households had higher concentrations of aflatoxins than did kernels from control households. Aflatoxin concentrations in maize and serum and positive hepatitis B surface antigen titers were all independently associated with case status. Although aflatoxicosis outbreaks have occurred periodically in Africa and Asia, this outbreak resulted in the largest number of fatalities ever documented. To prevent future aflatoxin outbreaks, it is necessary to explore public health interventions that promote effective production, storage, and processing of homegrown and commercial maize.

have been found in the livers of children with kwashiorkor and in Reye syndrome patients, a strong cause-and-effect relationship between aflatoxin exposure and these disease states has not been established.

Chronic low-level exposure to aflatoxins in the diet is considered a risk factor for the development of **hepatocellular carcinoma.** Such exposure has been shown experimentally to produce cancer in many animal species. Hepatocellular carcinoma is one of the leading causes of cancer mortality in Asia and Africa, and several epidemiologic investigations have shown that increased aflatoxin ingestion correlates with increased risk.

The primary mode of human exposure to aflatoxins is consumption of contaminated foods such as peanuts and cereal grains. Aflatoxins can be aerosolized and have been detected in air near farm sources, as well as in dust. Aflatoxin is a pulmonary carcinogen in experimental animals; however, evidence that airborne aflatoxin exposure leads to cancer in humans is generally weak.

The mechanism of aflatoxin-induced carcinogenesis is thought to involve tumor promotion or progression. There is evidence that aflatoxin is involved in the activation of proto-oncogenes *(c-MYC, c-Ha-RAS, Ki-RAS,* and *N-RAS)* and also may cause mutations in the tumor suppressor gene *TP53*. Aflatoxin exposure and *TP53* mutations have been tightly linked in epidemiologic studies in Africa and China. Specifically, aflatoxin exposure has been linked to a *TP53* mutation whereby a G-to-T transversion at codon 249 occurs. This particular mutation has been called the first example of a **"carcinogen-specific"** biomarker that remains fixed in human tissue. This biomarker has been used in epidemiologic studies to establish the link between aflatoxins and hepatic cancer and also to show that cofactors such as infection with hepatitis B virus increase the risk of hepatocellular cancer substantially.

Significant aflatoxin exposure is uncommon among those living in developed countries where sufficient amounts of food are available and regulations exist to monitor the level of aflatoxin in those foods. Notably, liver cancer incidence rates are 2 to 10 times higher in resource-poor countries than in developed countries. In those countries where food supplies are limited and people are facing starvation or where regulations are nonexistent or not enforced, routine ingestion of aflatoxin may occur.

• Citrinin

Citrinin is produced by several species of *Penicillium* and *Aspergillus,* including strains used to produce cheese *(P. camemberti)* and sake *(A. oryzae)*. Citrinin acts as a potent nephrotoxin in all animal species tested and has been associated with **yellow rice disease** in Japan (see Table 67-1). Citrinin may act synergistically with another nephrotoxin, ochratoxin A. Citrinin is regularly associated with human foods, including wheat, oats, rye, corn, barley, and rice; however, its significance as a cause of human disease is unknown.

• Ergot Alkaloids

Ergot alkaloids constitute a family of compounds derived from a tetracyclic ergoline ring system. Lysergic acid is a structure common to all ergot alkaloids, and the hallucinogen lysergic acid diethylamide (LSD) was discovered as a result of research with these compounds.

Mixtures of these alkaloids are produced within the sclerotia, or ergots, of common grass pathogens of the genus *Claviceps.* The ergots are hardened masses of fungal tissue (sclerotia) that are formed when the fungus invades the floret and replaces the grain of wheat, barley, or rye. The ergots are ingested when the contaminated grain is used to make bread or cereals. The two forms of **ergotism,** convulsive and gangrenous (see Table 67-1), are thought to result from different modes of action of the various alkaloids produced by different species of *Claviceps.* The gangrenous form, marked by peripheral vasoconstriction and necrosis of the distal extremities, is associated primarily with ingestion of wheat and rye contaminated with *Claviceps purpurea* and containing alkaloids of the ergotamine group. In addition to tissue infarction and necrosis, the gangrenous form of ergotism is associated with edema, pruritus, and sensations varying from pricking to severe muscle pain.

Convulsive ergotism has been associated with ingestion of millet contaminated by *Claviceps fusiformis.* Neurologic, or convulsive, ergotism is marked by muscle spasms, seizures, and hallucinations. The ergot of pearl millet implicated in an outbreak of convulsive ergotism in India in 1974 contained alkaloids of the clavine group.

Apparently, different species of *Claviceps* produce different alkaloids, although the substrate likely also plays a role in the composition of the secondary metabolites. Although modern methods of grain cleaning have virtually eliminated ergotism as a human disease, it is still an important veterinary problem. Cattle, pigs, sheep, and poultry are the animals at highest risk. Clinical symptoms of ergotism among these animals include gangrene, abortion, seizures, and ataxia.

• Fumonisins

Fumonisins are produced by a number of *Fusarium* species. The major species of economic importance is *F. moniliforme (F. verticillioides),* a corn pathogen. Fumonisins, especially fumonisin B1, interfere with sphingolipid metabolism and cause **leukoencephalomalacia** (severe necrotizing brain disease) in horses, pulmonary edema and hydrothorax in pigs, and hepatotoxic and carcinogenic effects in the liver of rats. Fumonisin B1 has been associated with a higher incidence of **esophageal cancer** in people living in South Africa, China, and Italy. It may be isolated in high concentrations in cornmeal and corn grits. Although this evidence is intriguing, multiple factors, including other mycotoxins, have been implicated in the etiology of human esophageal cancer.

Acute intoxication with fumonisin B1 has been observed in India, where consumption of unleavened bread made from moldy corn caused transient abdominal pain and diarrhea. Fumonisins have also been shown to cause neural tube defects in experimental animals and may have a role in human cases. Fumonisins have been classified as group 2B carcinogens (probably carcinogenic) by the International Agency for Research on Cancer.

• Ochratoxin

Ochratoxin belongs to a group of secondary metabolites produced by *Aspergillus* and *Penicillium* species found on cereals, coffee, bread, and foods of animal origin (e.g., pork). Ochratoxin A (OA) is the most common and most toxic chemical in its class. OA is nephrotoxic, teratogenic, and carcinogenic in all animals tested. It has been implicated in porcine nephropathy, as well as urinary tract tumors, and may cause cholinergic responses such as bronchospasm, vasodilation, and smooth muscle contraction.

Ochratoxin has been linked to a disease known as **Balkan endemic nephropathy (BEN),** a chronic progressive nephritis seen in populations living in areas bordering the Danube River in parts of Romania, Bulgaria, and the former Yugoslavia. In addition, individuals with BEN also suffer from a high frequency of renal tumors. Ochratoxin contamination of food and the presence of OA in human serum have been shown to be more common in families with BEN and those with urinary tract tumors than in unaffected families. Despite this evidence, a number of other factors (e.g., genetics, heavy metals, possible occult infectious agents) may also contribute to this disease. Although much of the evidence for the cause of BEN leans toward ochratoxin, the evidence is not conclusive. Regardless, its acute nephrotoxicity, immunosuppressive action, and teratogenic effects in animals, coupled with its propensity to be carried through the food chain, merit concern and further investigation.

• Trichothecenes

The trichothecenes (Clinical Case 67-2) are all tricyclic sesquiterpenoid metabolites that are produced by a number of fungi, including *Fusarium, Myrothecium, Stachybotrys, Trichoderma,* and *Cephalosporium* spp. (see Table 67-1). There are more than 148 natural trichothecenes, of which at least 40 are mycotoxins. Trichothecenes act by inhibiting various aspects of protein synthesis in eukaryotic cells. The most potent of these mycotoxins are T-2 toxin, diacetoxyscirpenol (DAS), deoxynivalenol (DON or vomitoxin), and fusarenon-X. These mycotoxins are commonly found as food and feed contaminants, the consumption of which can result in gastrointestinal hemorrhage and vomiting; direct contact causes dermatitis.

So-called **moldy grain intoxication** of humans and animals is well documented in Japan. Such intoxications have been attributed to *Fusarium* mycotoxins. **Akakabi-byo toxicosis,** or **red mold disease,** is believed to be caused by ingestion of grain contaminated with *Fusarium graminearum* (see Table 67-1).

T-2 toxin, DAS, and DON are the most widely studied of the fusarial trichothecenes. Symptoms produced by these agents include effects on almost every system of the vertebrate body. T-2 toxin and DAS appear to be the most potent and exhibit both cytotoxic and immunosuppressive activity. They cause a wide range of gastrointestinal, dermatologic, and neurologic symptoms and also decrease host resistance

Clinical Case 67-2 *Stachybotrys* and Acute Idiopathic Pulmonary Hemorrhage

Colin and colleagues (*MMWR Morb Mortal Wkly Rep* 53:817–820, 2004) described an investigation of acute idiopathic pulmonary hemorrhage (AIPH) in infants in Massachusetts. During 1993 to 1996, investigation of cases of AIPH among infants in Cleveland, Ohio, suggested an association between AIPH and being male, exposure to molds (notably *Stachybotrys chartarum*), exposure to tobacco smoke, and lack of breastfeeding. However, reviews of that investigation by the Centers for Disease Control and Prevention (CDC) identified shortcomings in the methodology and determined that no association between AIPH and exposure to molds had been established. It was recommended that CDC collaborate with state and local public health officials to investigate future cases of AIPH, particularly when clusters are identified. During December 2002 to June 2003, four cases of AIPH among full-term infants were reported in the Boston area. In a 4-month period, three of the infants were patients at the same hospital, which typically has one case of AIPH among infants per year. The CDC, in collaboration with the Massachusetts Department of Public Health, investigated this cluster and determined that two of the infants had von Willebrand disease (vWD), an inherited bleeding disorder, and one had borderline test results for vWD. The findings suggest that the infants with AIPH might have an underlying acquired or genetic susceptibility that predisposed them to pulmonary bleeding.

All the infants in this cluster also were exposed to certain environmental factors that might have affected their lungs, including environmental tobacco smoke, particulate matter (e.g., construction dust), and mold. *Cladosporium* and *Penicillium,* the molds most commonly identified in each of the homes, typically are the most abundant fungal genera in indoor air. Total fungal spore counts in two of the homes were at concentrations that have been associated with increased risk for lower respiratory illness, and all four infants were treated presumptively for respiratory infections before their hemorrhagic episodes. Only seven spores of *S. chartarum* were found in one home, and a single spore was found in another. Although the full significance of spore counts is not known, toxic and other non–immunoglobulin (Ig)E-mediated health effects that have been hypothesized to occur with exposure to *S. chartarum* appear unlikely to have contributed to these AIPH cases.

to infection with various microbes. DON is a common contaminant of grains used in animal feed. When ingested in high doses, it causes vomiting and diarrhea; at lower doses, farm animals exhibit weight loss and food refusal.

Both T-2 toxin and DAS have been implicated in a human disease known as **alimentary toxic aleukia (ATA).** The most important outbreak of ATA occurred in Russia during World War II. Thousands of people became sick after eating overwintered grain contaminated with *Fusarium sporotrichioides* and *Fusarium poae.* The disease was characterized by several stages, with initial oral mucosal ulceration and gastroenteritis followed by pancytopenia, bleeding from the nose, mouth, and vagina, hypotension, and vertigo. The high acute mortality rate was augmented by opportunistic bacterial infections during the later neutropenic stages of the disease. Although the two species of *Fusarium* that were isolated from the moldy grain were subsequently shown to be able to produce T-2 toxin and other trichothecenes, no attempt was made to document the presence of these mycotoxins in the grain or the affected people. Almost all signs of ATA have been documented in animals given T-2 toxin; however, the association between the toxin and human disease remains merely speculative.

Stachybotryotoxicosis is a well-described disease among horses and cattle consuming moldy straw and hay contaminated with *Stachybotrys.* Equine stachybotryotoxicosis is characterized by acute neurologic signs such as tremors, incoordination, and loss of vision and more chronic manifestations such as dermonecrosis, leukopenia, and gastrointestinal bleeding. Humans handling moldy hay have exhibited contact dermatitis, as well as mucosal inflammation, fever, chest pain, and leukopenia secondary to inhalation of dust from the hay. Macrocyclic trichothecenes were isolated from the contaminated hay.

Given these findings, and because *Stachybotrys* grows well on wet building materials (e.g., ceiling tiles, wood fiber boards, dust-lined air-conditioning ducts), toxins from this fungus have become suspect in illnesses of humans living or working in *Stachybotrys*-contaminated buildings. Complaints of pulmonary irritation, headaches, fatigue, malaise, and diarrhea have been registered by residents and workers in buildings (so-called sick building syndrome [SBS]) contaminated with *Stachybotrys chartarum. Stachybotrys* has also been associated with **idiopathic pulmonary hemorrhage** of infants; however, a cause-and-effect relationship has not been proven. Critical evaluation of the available literature has failed to find supportive evidence for serious human illness caused by *Stachybotrys* exposure in the contemporary human environment.

• Other Mycotoxins and Purported Mycotoxicoses

Given the wide variety of environmental molds that have been shown to be capable of producing mycotoxins, it is not surprising that there is a vast literature describing the potential role of these agents in human and animal disease states. Unfortunately, much of this literature is quite flawed, and critical review almost always finds it to be lacking in rigorous proof of a cause-and-effect relationship between mycotoxins and human disease.

Cyclopiazonic acid is an indole tetramic acid that is a specific inhibitor of calcium-dependent ATPase and induces alterations in ion transport across cell membranes. It is produced by many species of *Penicillium* and *Aspergillus,* including *A. flavus.* Consumption of millet that was heavily contaminated with molds and contained high levels of cyclopiazonic acid produced a condition known as **Kodua poisoning,** characterized by giddiness and nausea (see Table 67-1).

Cardiac beriberi, a condition seen in Japan and other Asian countries in the early 20th century, has been associated with the yellow rice toxins citreoviridin, citrinin, and related compounds. This disease is characterized by palpitations, nausea, vomiting, respiratory distress, hypotension, and violent mania, leading to respiratory failure and death. The neurologic symptoms and respiratory failure have been reproduced in animals given citreoviridin.

Several rare and obscure diseases have been purported to be mycotoxicosis, often with minimal objective evidence. These include **Kashin-Beck disease** in Russia, **Onyalai disease** in Africa, and **moldy sugar cane disease** in China (see Table 67-1).

It is difficult to prove that a disease is a mycotoxicosis. Even known toxigenic molds may be present in foods or the environment and not produce toxin. The mere isolation of mold from cultures of a given substrate is not the same as detection of a specific mycotoxin. Likewise, even when mycotoxins are detected, it is difficult to prove conclusively that they are the cause of specific acute or chronic disease states. Regardless, valid concerns do exist with respect to the relationship between mycotoxins and human disease. Examples of certain fungus-disease associations are reasonably well documented in the literature, including ATA from *Fusarium,* liver disease from *Aspergillus,* and ergotism from *Claviceps* spp. Other than these examples, the evidence is tenuous. It is likely that mycotoxins do pose an important danger to the health of humans and animals, the extent of which can only be determined by rigorous, well-designed clinical and laboratory studies.

Bibliography

Bennett JW, Klich M: Mycotoxins, *Clin Microbial Rev* 16:497–516, 2003.

Isham NC, et al: Mycotoxins. In Versalovic J, et al, editors: *Manual of clinical microbiology,* ed 10, Washington, DC, 2011, American Society for Microbiology Press.

Kuhn DM, Ghannoum MA: Indoor mold, toxigenic fungi, and *Stachybotrys chartarum*: infectious disease perspective, *Clin Microbiol Rev* 16:144–172, 2003.

Smith M, McGinnis MR: Mycotoxins and their effect on humans. In Anaissie EJ, McGinnis MR, Pfaller MA, editors: *Clinical mycology,* ed 2, New York, 2009, Churchill Livingstone.

van der Fels-Klerx HJ, Olesen JE, Naustvoll LJ, et al: Climate change impacts on natural toxins in food production systems, exemplified by deoxynivalenol in wheat and diarrhetic shellfish toxins, *Food Addit Contam Part A Chem Anal Control Expo Risk Assess* 29:1647–1659, 2012.

Woloshuk CP, Shim WB: Aflatoxins, fumonisins, and trichothecenes: a convergence of knowledge, *FEMS Microbiol Rev* 37:94–109, 2013.

SECTION

7

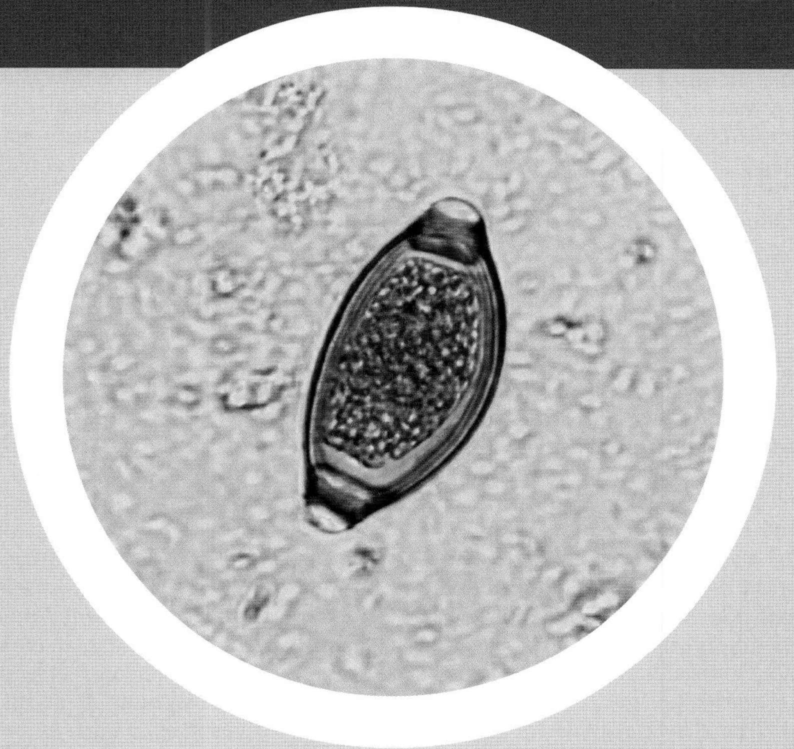

PARASITOLOGY

CHAPTER

68 PARASITIC CLASSIFICATION, STRUCTURE, AND REPLICATION

This chapter provides an introduction to parasite classification and physiology. This brief review is intended to enhance the reader's comprehension of the interrelationships among parasitic organisms, their epidemiology and transmission of disease, the specific disease processes involved, and the possibilities for prevention and control of maladies. We have deliberately attempted to simplify the taxonomy by using it to address the major divisions involved in medical parasitology: intestinal and urogenital protozoa, blood and tissue protozoa, nematodes, trematodes, cestodes, and arthropods.

• Importance of Parasites

Medical parasitology is the study of invertebrate animals capable of causing disease in humans and other animals. Although parasitic diseases are frequently considered "tropical" and thus of little importance to physicians practicing in the more temperate developed countries of the world, it is clear that the world has become a very small place and that physicians' knowledge of parasitic diseases is essential. The global impact of parasitic infections and the number of parasite-associated deaths is staggering and must be of concern to all health care workers (Table 68-1). Increasingly, tourists, missionaries, Peace Corps volunteers, and others are visiting and working for extended periods of time in exotic remote parts of the world. Thus they are at risk for parasitic and other infections that are rare in the United States and other more developed countries. Another source of infected patients is the ever-increasing number of refugees from developing countries. Finally, the profound immunosuppression problems that accompany advances in medical therapy (e.g., organ transplantation), as well as those associated with persons infected with the human immunodeficiency virus, place a growing number of individuals at risk for developing infections caused by certain parasites. Given these considerations, clinicians and laboratory workers should be aware of the possibility of parasitic disease and should be trained in ordering, performing, and interpreting the appropriate laboratory tests to aid in diagnosis and therapy.

• Classification and Structure

The parasites of humans are classified within three eukaryotic kingdoms: Protozoa, Animalia (Metazoa), and Stramenopila (formerly Chromista) (Table 68-2). Traditionally, parasite classification has taken into account the morphology of intracytoplasmic structures, such as the nucleus, type of locomotive organelles, and mode of reproduction (Table 68-3). More recently, the new taxonomic consensus has emerged based mainly on advances in our understanding of the biochemistry and molecular biology of lower organisms (e.g., Protozoa and Stramenopila). Comparisons of small subunit ribosomal ribonucleic acid (SSU rRNA) and protein sequences have made it possible to arrange organisms within groups based on evolutionary distances. Furthermore, identification of certain organelles found in eukaryotic cells, with their prokaryote origins, has made it possible to organize all living organisms within a realistic and evolutionarily sound overall taxonomic scheme. The Protozoa and Stramenopila are animals whose life functions occur in a single cell. Members of the kingdom Animalia, also known as **metazoans,** are multicellular animals in which life functions occur in cellular structures organized as tissue and organ systems.

Protozoa

Protozoa are simple microorganisms that range in size from 2 to 100 μm. Their protoplasm is enclosed by a cell membrane and contains numerous organelles, including a membrane-bound nucleus, an endoplasmic reticulum, food-storage granules, and contractile and digestive vacuoles. The nucleus contains clumped or dispersed chromatin and a central karyosome. Organs of motility vary from simple cytoplasmic extrusions or pseudopods to more complex structures such as flagella or cilia. The kingdom Protozoa comprises 13 major subgroups, or phyla, 7 of which are the concern of medical parasitology.

Flagellates: Metamonada, Parabasala, Percolozoa, and Euglenozoa

Previously grouped under the former subphylum Mastigophora, the flagellates are now distributed under four phyla: Metamonada, Parabasala, Percolozoa, and Euglenozoa. The flagellates move by lashing their whiplike flagella. The number and position of the flagella vary a great deal in different species. In addition, specialized structures associated with the flagella may produce a characteristic morphologic appearance that may be useful in species identification.

Amoebozoa

The phylum Amoebozoa, containing the amebae, is equivalent to the old subphylum Sarcodina. Locomotion of amebae is accomplished by the extrusion of pseudopodia ("false

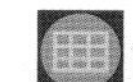

Table 68-1 Estimated Worldwide Disease Burden of Parasitic Infections

Infection	Estimated No. Infected	Deaths (Annual)*
Malaria	>500 million	2.5 million
Lymphatic filariasis	128 million	0
Leishmaniasis	2 million	59,000
Hookworm	>1 billion	—
Schistosomiasis	200 million	500,000 to 1 million
Trichuriasis	900 million	—
African trypanosomiasis	100,000 new cases per year	50,000
Ascariasis	1.3 billion	60,000
Onchocerciasis	17.7 million (270,000 blind)	0
Chagas disease	16-18 million	50,000

Modified from Edwards G, Krishna S: Pharmacokinetic and pharmacodynamic issues in the treatment of parasite infections, *Eur J Clin Microbiol Infect Dis* 23:233–242, 2004; Hoetz PJ, Molyneux DH, Fenwick A, et al: Control of neglected tropical diseases, *N Engl J Med* 357:1018–1027, 2007; and John DT, Petri WA Jr: *Markell and Voge's medical parasitology,* ed 9, St Louis, 2006, Saunders.

*Mortality data included where available.

Table 68-2 Medically Important Parasites

Kingdom	Phylum	Organisms
Protozoa	Metamonada (flagellates)	*Giardia, Chilomastix*
	Parabasala (flagellates)	*Dientamoeba, Trichomonas*
	Percolozoa (flagellates)	*Naegleria*
	Euglenozoa (flagellates)	*Leishmania, Trypanosoma*
	Amoebozoa (amebae)	*Acanthamoeba, Balamuthia, Entamoeba*
	Apicomplexa (sporozoans)	*Cryptosporidium, Cyclospora, Cystoisospora, Toxoplasma, Babesia, Plasmodium*
	Ciliophora (ciliates)	*Balantidium coli*
Stramenopila	Bigyra	*Blastocystis* spp.
Animalia	Nemathelminthes (Nematoda, roundworms)	*Trichinella, Trichuris, Ancylostoma, Necator, Ascaris, Dracunculus, Enterobius, Strongyloides*
	Platyhelminthes	Trematodes, cestodes
	Arthropoda	Crustaceans, spiders, insects, true bugs

feet"). Amebae are phagocytic and contain mitochondria with tubular cristae.

Apicomplexa

Phylum Apicomplexa organisms are often referred to as **Sporozoa** or **Coccidia.** The Apicomplexans include a large group of sexually reproducing, spore-forming protozoans with comparable life cycles and similar morphology at the electron microscopic level. These organisms have a system of organelles at their apical end that produces substances to help the organism penetrate host cells and thus become an intracellular parasite.

Ciliophora

Phylum Ciliophora consists of the ciliates, which include a variety of free-living and symbiotic species. Ciliate locomotion involves the coordinated movement of rows of hairlike structures, or cilia. Cilia are structurally similar to flagella but are usually shorter and more numerous. Some ciliates are multinucleate. The only ciliate parasite of humans, *Balantidium coli,* contains two nuclei: a large macronucleus and a small micronucleus.

Stramenopila (Formerly Chromista)

The kingdom Stramenopila was created to accommodate a number of plantlike organisms, mainly algae, that were originally chimeras between eukaryotic biflagellate hosts and symbiotic red algae that had lost their chloroplasts over evolutionary time yet still retain elements of their red algae ancestry. Although previously shuffled between the Fungi and Protozoa, *Blastocystis* spp. is now placed within the Stramenopila (phylum Bigyra, class Blastocystea) based on analysis of 18S rRNA and other molecular evidence.

Animalia (Metazoa)

The kingdom Animalia (Metazoa) includes all eukaryotic organisms that are not Protozoa, Stramenopila, or Fungi. This chapter discusses two broad groups of organisms of major importance: the helminths ("worms") and the arthropods (crabs, insects, ticks, and others).

Helminths

The helminths are complex multicellular organisms that are elongated and bilaterally symmetric. They are considerably larger than the protozoan parasites and generally are macroscopic, ranging in size from less than 1 mm to 1 m or larger. The external surface of some worms is covered with a protective cuticle, which is acellular and may be smooth or possess ridges, spines, or tubercles. The protective covering of flatworms is known as a **tegument.** Often helminths possess elaborate attachment structures such as hooks, suckers, teeth, or plates. These structures are usually located anteriorly and may be useful in classifying and identifying the organisms (see Table 68-3). Helminths typically have primitive nervous and excretory systems. Some have alimentary tracts; however, none has a circulatory system. The helminths are separated into two phyla, the Nemathelminthes and the Platyhelminthes.

Nemathelminthes

Phylum Nemathelminthes consists of the roundworms, which have cylindrical bodies. The sexes of roundworms are separate, and these organisms have a complete digestive system. The nemathelminths may be intestinal parasites or may infect the blood and tissue.

Table 68-3 Biological, Morphologic, and Physiologic Characteristics of Pathogenic Parasites

Organism Class	Morphology	Reproduction	Organelles of Locomotion	Respiration	Nutrition
Protozoa					
Ameba	Unicellular; cyst and trophocyte forms	Binary fission	Pseudopods	Facultative anaerobe	Assimilation by pinocytosis or phagocytosis
Flagellates	Unicellular; cyst and trophozoite forms; possibly intracellular	Binary fission	Flagella	Facultative anaerobe	Simple diffusion or ingestion via cytostome, pinocytosis, or phagocytosis
Ciliates	Unicellular; cysts and trophozoite	Binary fission or conjugation	Cilia	Facultative anaerobe	Ingestion via cytostome, food vacuole
Sporozoa	Unicellular, frequently intracellular; multiple forms, including trophozoites, sporozoites, cysts (oocysts), gametes	Schizogony and sporogony	None	Facultative anaerobe	Simple diffusion
Helminths					
Nematodes	Multicellular; round, smooth, spindle-shaped, tubular alimentary tract; possibility of teeth or plates for attachment	Separate sexes	No single organelle; active muscular motility	Adults: usually anaerobic; larvae: possibly aerobic	Ingestion or absorption of body fluids, tissue, or digestive contents
Trematodes	Multicellular; leaf shaped with oral and ventral suckers, blind alimentary tract	Hermaphroditic (*Schistosoma* group has separate sexes)	No single organelle; muscle-directed motility	Adults: usually anaerobic	Ingestion or absorption of body fluids, tissue, or digestive contents
Cestodes	Multicellular; head with segmented body (proglottids); lack of alimentary tract; head equipped with hooks and/or suckers for attachment	Hermaphroditic	No single organelle; usually attachment to mucosa; possible muscular motility (proglottids)	Adults: usually anaerobic	Absorption of nutrients from intestine
Arthropods					
Myriapoda	Elongated; many legs; distinctive head and trunk; poison claws on first segment	Separate sexes	Legs	Aerobic	Carnivore
Pentastomida	Wormlike; cylindrical or flattened; two distinct body regions; digestive and reproductive organs; lack of circulatory and respiratory systems	Separate sexes	Muscle-directed motility	Aerobic	Ingestion of body fluids and tissue
Crustacea	Hard external carapace; one pair of maxillae; five pairs of biramous legs	Separate sexes	Legs	Aerobic	Ingestion of body fluids and tissue, carnivorous
Chelicerata (Arachnida)	Body divided into cephalothorax and abdomen; eight legs and poisoning fangs	Separate sexes	Legs	Aerobic	Carnivore
Insecta	Body: head, thorax, and abdomen; one pair of antennae; three pairs of appendages, up to two pairs of wings	Separate sexes	Legs, wings	Aerobic	Ingestion of fluids and tissues

Platyhelminthes

Phylum Platyhelminthes consists of the flatworms, which have flattened bodies that are leaflike or resemble ribbon segments. Platyhelminthes can be further divided into trematodes and cestodes.

Trematodes, or flukes, have leaf-shaped bodies. Most are hermaphroditic, with male and female sex organs in a single body. Their digestive systems are incomplete and only have saclike tubes. Their life cycle is complex; snails serve as first intermediate hosts, and other aquatic animals or plants serve as second intermediate hosts.

Cestodes, or tapeworms, have bodies composed of ribbons of proglottids, or segments. All are hermaphroditic, and all lack digestive systems, with nutrition being absorbed through the body walls. The life cycles of some cestodes are simple and direct, whereas those of others are complex and require one or more intermediate hosts.

Arthropods

Phylum Arthropoda is the largest group of animals in the kingdom Animalia. Arthropods are complex multicellular organisms that may be involved directly in causing invasive or superficial (infestation) disease processes or indirectly as intermediate hosts and vectors of many infectious agents, including protozoan and helminthic parasites (Table 68-4). In addition, envenomation by biting and stinging arthropods can result in adverse reactions in humans that range from local allergic and hypersensitivity reactions to severe anaphylactic shock and death. There are five major categories of arthropods.

Myriapoda

The Myriapoda (formerly Chilopoda) consist of terrestrial forms such as centipedes. These organisms are of medical importance because of their venom claws, which may produce a painful "bite."

Pentastomida

The pentastomids, or tongue worms, are bloodsucking endoparasites of reptiles, birds, and mammals. Adult pentastomids are white and cylindrical or flattened parasites that possess two distinct body regions: an anterior cephalothorax and an abdomen. Humans may serve as intermediate hosts for these parasites.

Crustacea

The crustaceans include familiar aquatic forms such as crabs, crayfish, shrimp, and copepods. Several are involved as intermediate hosts in the life cycles of various intestinal or blood and tissue helminths.

Chelicerata

The Chelicerata (formerly Arachnida) consist of familiar terrestrial forms such as mites, ticks, spiders, and scorpions. Unlike insects, these animals have no wings or antennae, and adults have four pairs of legs as opposed to three pairs for insects. Of medical importance are those serving as vectors for microbial diseases (mites and ticks) or as venomous animals that bite (spiders) or sting (scorpions).

Insecta

Insecta consist of familiar aquatic and terrestrial forms such as mosquitoes, flies, midges, fleas, lice, bugs, wasps, and ants. Wings and antennae are present, and adult forms have three pairs of legs. Of medical importance are the many insects that serve as vectors for microbial diseases (mosquitoes, fleas, lice, and bugs) or as venomous animals that sting (bees, wasps, and ants).

Physiology and Replication

Protozoa

The nutritional requirements of the parasitic protozoa are generally simple and require assimilation of organic nutrients. The amebae, ameboflagellates, and certain other protozoa accomplish this assimilation by the rather primitive process of pinocytosis or phagocytosis of soluble or particulate matter (see Table 68-3). The engulfed material is enclosed in digestive vacuoles. The flagellates and ciliates generally ingest food at a definitive site or structure, the peristome or cytostome. Other unicellular parasites assimilate nutrients by simple diffusion. The ingested food material may be retained in intracytoplasmic granules or vacuoles. Undigested particles and waste may be eliminated from the cell by extrusion of the material at the cell surface. Respiration in most parasitic protozoa is accomplished by facultatively anaerobic processes.

To ensure survival under harsh or unfavorable environmental conditions, many parasitic protozoa develop into a cyst form that is less metabolically active. This cyst is surrounded by a thick external cell wall capable of protecting the organism from otherwise lethal physical and chemical insults. The cyst form is an integral part of the life cycle of many protozoan parasites and facilitates transmission of the organism from host to host in the external environment (see Table 68-4). Parasites that cannot form cysts must rely on direct transmission from host to host or require an arthropod vector to complete their life cycles (see Table 68-4).

In addition to cyst formation, many protozoan parasites have developed elaborate immunoevasive mechanisms that allow them to respond to attack by the host immune system by continuously changing their surface antigens, thus ensuring continued survival within the host. Reproduction among the protozoa is generally by simple binary fission (merogony), although the life cycle of some protozoa (e.g., sporozoans) includes cycles of multiple fission (schizogony) alternating with a period of sexual reproduction (sporogony or gametogony).

Animalia (Metazoa)

Helminths

The nutritional requirements of helminthic parasites are met by active ingestion of host tissue, fluids, or both, with resultant tissue destruction, or by more passive absorption of nutrients from the surrounding fluids and intestinal contents (see Table 68-3). The muscular motility of many helminths expends considerable energy, and the worms rapidly metabolize carbohydrates. Nutrients are stored in the form of glycogen, the content of which is high in most helminths. Similar to respiration in protozoa, respiration in helminths is primarily anaerobic, although the larval forms may require oxygen.

A significant proportion of the energy requirement of helminths is dedicated to supporting the reproductive process. Many worms are quite prolific, producing as many as 200,000 offspring each day. In general, helminthic parasites lay eggs (oviparous), although a few species may bear live young (viviparous). The resulting larvae are always morphologically distinct from the adult parasites and must undergo several developmental stages or molts before attaining adulthood.

The major protective barrier for most helminths is the tough external layer (cuticle or tegument). Worms may also secrete enzymes that destroy host cells and neutralize immunologic and cellular defense mechanisms. Similar to protozoan parasites, some helminths possess the ability to alter the antigenic properties of their external surfaces and thus evade the host immune response. This is accomplished in part by incorporating host antigens into their external cuticular layer. In this way the worm avoids immunologic recognition, and in some diseases (e.g., schistosomiasis), it allows the parasite to survive within the host for decades.

Arthropods

Arthropods have segmented bodies, paired jointed appendages, and well-developed digestive and nervous systems.

 Table 68-4 **Transmission and Distribution of Pathogenic Parasites**

Organism	Infective Form	Mechanism of Spread	Distribution
Intestinal Protozoa			
Entamoeba histolytica	Cyst/trophozoite	Indirect (fecal-oral) Direct (venereal)	Worldwide
Giardia duodenalis/intestinalis	Cyst	Fecal-oral route	Worldwide
Dientamoeba fragilis	Trophozoite ? Cyst	Fecal-oral route	Worldwide
Balantidium coli	Cyst	Fecal-oral route	Worldwide
Cystoisospora belli	Oocyst	Fecal-oral route	Worldwide
Cryptosporidium spp.	Oocyst	Fecal-oral route	Worldwide
Urogenital Protozoa			
Trichomonas vaginalis	Trophozoite	Direct (venereal) route	Worldwide
Blood and Tissue Protozoa			
Naegleria and *Acanthamoeba* spp.	Cyst/trophozoite	Direct inoculation, inhalation	Worldwide
Plasmodium spp.	Sporozoite	*Anopheles* mosquito	Tropical and subtropical areas
Babesia spp.	Pyriform body	*Ixodes* tick	North America, Europe
Toxoplasma gondii	Oocysts and tissue cysts	Fecal-oral route, carnivorism	Worldwide
Leishmania spp.	Promastigote	*Phlebotomus* sandfly	Tropical and subtropical areas
Trypanosoma cruzi	Trypomastigote	Reduviid bug	North, Central, and South America
Trypanosoma brucei	Trypomastigote	Tsetse fly	Africa
Nematodes			
Enterobius vermicularis	Egg	Fecal-oral route	Worldwide
Ascaris lumbricoides	Egg	Fecal-oral route	Areas of poor sanitation
Toxocara spp.	Egg	Fecal-oral route	Worldwide
Trichuris trichiura	Egg	Fecal-oral route	Worldwide
Ancylostoma duodenale	Filariform larva	Direct skin penetration from contaminated soil	Tropical and subtropical areas
Necator americanus	Filariform larva	Direct skin penetration, autoinfection	Tropical and subtropical areas
Strongyloides stercoralis	Filariform larva	Direct skin penetration, autoinfection	Tropical and subtropical areas
Trichinella spiralis	Encysted larva in tissue	Carnivorism	Worldwide
Wuchereria bancrofti	Third-stage larva	Mosquito	Tropical and subtropical areas
Brugia malayi	Third-stage larva	Mosquito	Tropical and subtropical areas
Loa loa	Filariform larva	*Chrysops* fly	Africa
Mansonella spp.	Third-stage larva	Biting midges or blackflies	Africa, Central and South America
Onchocerca volvulus	Third-stage larva	*Simulium* blackfly	Africa, Central and South America
Dracunculus medinensis	Third-stage larva	Ingestion of infected *Cyclops*	Africa, Asia
Dirofilaria immitis	Third-stage larva	Mosquito	Japan, Australia, United States
Trematodes			
Fasciolopsis buski	Metacercaria	Ingestion of metacercaria encysted on aquatic plants	China, Southeast Asia, India
Fasciola hepatica	Metacercaria	Metacercaria on water plants	Worldwide
Opisthorchis (Clonorchis) sinensis	Metacercaria	Metacercaria encysted in freshwater fish	China, Japan, Korea, Vietnam
Paragonimus westermani	Metacercaria	Metacercaria encysted in freshwater crustaceans	Asia, Africa, India, Latin America

Table 68-4 Transmission and Distribution of Pathogenic Parasites—cont'd

Organism	Infective Form	Mechanism of Spread	Distribution
Schistosoma spp.	Cercaria	Direct penetration of skin by free-swimming cercaria	Africa, Asia, India, Latin America
Cestodes			
Taenia solium	Cysticercus, embryonated egg or proglottid	Ingestion of infected pork; ingestion of egg (cysticercosis)	Pork-eating countries: Africa, Southeast Asia, China, Latin America
Taenia saginata	Cysticercus	Ingestion of cysticercus in meat	Worldwide
Diphyllobothrium latum	Sparganum	Ingestion of sparganum in fish	Worldwide
Echinococcus granulosus	Embryonated egg	Ingestion of eggs from infected canines	Sheep-raising countries: Europe, Asia, Africa, Australia, United States
Echinococcus multilocularis	Embryonated egg	Ingestion of eggs from infected animals, fecal-oral route	Canada, Northern United States, Central Europe
Hymenolepsis nana	Embryonated egg	Ingestion of eggs, fecal-oral route	Worldwide
Hymenolepsis diminuta	Cysticercus	Ingestion of infected beetle larvae in contaminated grain products	Worldwide
Dipylidium caninum	Cysticercoid	Ingestion of infected fleas	Worldwide

Sexes are separate. Respiration by aquatic forms is via gills and by terrestrial forms is via tubular body structures. All have a hard chitin covering as an exoskeleton.

Summary

Physician awareness of parasitic diseases is undoubtedly more critical now than at any time in the history of medical practice. Physicians today must be prepared to answer questions from patients about protection from malaria and the risks of drinking water and eating fresh fruits and vegetables in remote areas where they may be traveling. With this knowledge of parasitic diseases, the physician can also evaluate signs, symptoms, and incubation periods in returning travelers, make a diagnosis, and begin treatment for a patient with a possible parasitic disease. The risks of parasitic diseases in immunosuppressed individuals and those with acquired immunodeficiency syndrome must also be understood and taken into account.

Proper education regarding parasitic diseases in medical curricula cannot be overemphasized as a requirement for physicians whose practice includes travelers to foreign countries and refugee populations. Many of the important parasites responsible for human diseases are transmitted by arthropod vectors or are acquired by consumption of contaminated food or water. The various modes of transmission and distribution of parasitic diseases are presented in appropriate detail in the following chapters; however, the data in Table 68-4 are provided as an outline.

Bibliography

Cavalier-Smith T: A revised six-kingdom system of life, *Biol Rev* 73:203–266, 1998.

Cox FEG: History of human parasitology, *Clin Microbiol Rev* 15:595–612, 2002.

Cox FEG: Taxonomy and classification of human parasites. In Versalovic J, et al, editors: *Manual of clinical microbiology*, ed 10, Washington, DC, 2011, American Society for Microbiology Press.

Edwards G, Krishna S: Pharmacokinetic and pharmacodynamic issues in the treatment of parasite infections, *Eur J Clin Microbiol Infect Dis* 23:233–242, 2004.

Garcia LS: *Diagnostic medical parasitology*, ed 5, Washington, DC, 2006, American Society for Microbiology Press.

Hoetz PJ, Molyneux DH, Fenwick A, et al: Control of neglected tropical diseases, *N Engl J Med* 357:1018–1027, 2007.

John DT, Petri WA Jr: *Markell and Voge's medical parasitology*, ed 9, St Louis, 2006, Saunders.

Versalovic J, et al: *Manual of clinical microbiology*, ed 10, Washington, DC, 2011, American Society for Microbiology Press.

CHAPTER

69 PATHOGENESIS OF PARASITIC DISEASES

Given the wide diversity that exists among human parasites, it is not surprising that the pathogenesis of protozoan and helminthic disease is highly variable. Although the various human parasites exhibit a wide range of direct pathogenic mechanisms, in most instances, the organisms themselves are not highly virulent, are unable to replicate within the host, or have both characteristics. Thus the severity of illness caused by many parasites is related to the infecting dose and the number of organisms acquired over time. Unlike many bacterial and viral infections, parasitic infections are often chronic, lasting months to years. Repeated exposures result in an ever-increasing parasite burden. When infection with a particular organism is associated with a strong immune response, there is undoubtedly a considerable immunopathologic contribution to the disease manifestations attributed to the infection.

Important factors to consider when discussing parasite pathogenicity are listed in Box 69-1. Parasites are almost always exogenous to the human host and thus must enter the body through ingestion or direct penetration of anatomic barriers. Inoculum size and duration of exposure greatly influence the disease-causing potential of an organism. Likewise, the route of exposure is critical for most organisms. For example, pathogenic strains of *Entamoeba histolytica* are unlikely to cause disease on exposure to intact skin but may cause severe dysentery after oral ingestion. Many parasites have active self-directed means of invading the human host. Once they have invaded, parasites attach to specific host cells or organs, avoid immune detection, replicate (most protozoa and some helminths), produce toxic substances that destroy tissue, and cause disease secondary to the host's own immunologic response (see Box 69-1). In addition, some parasites physically obstruct and damage organs and tissues because of their size alone. This chapter discusses factors that are important for parasite pathogenicity and provides examples of organisms and disease processes related to each factor.

Exposure and Entry

Although many infectious diseases are caused by **endogenous** organisms that are part of the normal flora of the human host, this is not the case with most diseases caused by protozoan and helminthic parasites. These organisms are virtually always acquired from an **exogenous** source and as such have evolved numerous ways to enter the body of the human host. The most common modes of entry are oral ingestion or direct penetration through the skin or other surfaces (Table 69-1). Transmission of parasitic diseases is frequently facilitated by environmental contamination with human and animal wastes. This is most applicable to diseases transmitted by the fecal-oral route but also applies to helminthic infections such as hookworm disease and strongyloidiasis, which rely on larval penetration of the skin.

Many parasitic diseases are acquired via the bites of **arthropod** vectors. Transmission of disease in this manner is extraordinarily effective, as evidenced by the widespread distribution of diseases such as malaria, trypanosomiasis, and filariasis. Examples of parasites and their ports of entry are listed in Table 69-1. This compilation should not be considered exhaustive; rather, the list provides examples of some of the more common parasites and the means by which they enter the human body.

Additional factors that determine the outcome of the interaction between parasite and host are route of **exposure** and **inoculum** size. Most human parasites have a limited range of organs or tissues in which they can replicate or survive. For example, simple skin contact with most intestinal protozoa does not result in disease; rather, the organisms must be ingested for the disease process to be initiated. Likewise, a minimum number of organisms is required to establish infection. Although some parasitic diseases may be acquired by ingestion or inoculation of only a few organisms, a sizable inoculum is usually required. Whereas an individual may acquire malaria by a single bite of an infected female mosquito, large inocula are usually necessary to produce diseases such as amebiasis in humans.

Adherence and Replication

Most infections are initiated by the attachment of the organism to host tissues, followed by replication to establish colonization. The life cycle of a parasite is based on species and **tissue tropisms,** which determine the organs or tissues of the host in which a parasite can survive. Attachment of the parasite to host cells or tissue can be relatively nonspecific, can be mediated by mechanical or biting mouthparts, or can result from the interaction between structures on the parasite surface known as **adhesins** and specific glycoprotein or glycolipid receptors found on some cell types but not on others. Specific surface structures that facilitate parasite adhesion include surface **glycoproteins** (e.g., glycophorin A and B), complement receptors, adsorbed components of the complement cascade, fibronectin, and *N*-acetylglucosamine conjugates. Examples of some of the adherence mechanisms identified in human parasites are listed in Table 69-2.

E. histolytica is a good model for the importance of **adhesins** in virulence. The pathogenesis of invasive amebiasis requires adherence of amebae to the colonic mucosal layer, parasite attachment to and lysis of colonic epithelium and acute inflammatory cells, and resistance of the amebic trophozoites to host humoral and cell-mediated immune defense mechanisms. Amebic adherence to colonic mucins, epithelial cells, and leukocytes is mediated by a surface lectin inhibitable by galactose (gal) or *N*-acetyl-D-galactosamine (GalNAc). Binding of the galactose-inhibitable adherence lectin to carbohydrates on the host cell surface is required for *E. histolytica* trophozoites to exert their cytolytic activity. The presence of the galactose-inhibitable adherence lectin is one feature that distinguishes pathogenic from nonpathogenic strains of *E. histolytica.*

Box 69-1 Factors Associated with Parasite Pathogenicity

Infective dose and exposure
Penetration of anatomic barriers
Attachment
Replication
Cell and tissue damage
Disruption, evasion, and inactivation of host defenses

Table 69-1 Parasite Ports of Entry

Route	Examples
Ingestion	*Giardia* spp., *Entamoeba histolytica*, *Cryptosporidium* spp., cestodes, nematodes
Direct penetration	
Arthropod bite	Malaria, *Babesia* spp., filaria, *Leishmania* spp., trypanosomes
Transplacental penetration	*Toxoplasma gondii*
Organism-directed penetration	Hookworm, *Strongyloides* spp., schistosomes

Various attachment mechanisms have been associated with specific infections. For example, the **Duffy blood group antigen** acts as an attachment site for *Plasmodium vivax.* Red blood cells from most West Africans, in contrast to those from Europeans, lack the Duffy antigen. Accordingly, malaria resulting from *P. vivax* is almost unknown in West Africa. Notably, however, clinical vivax malaria has recently been reported in Duffy-negative individuals in Madagascar. The parasite and host molecules that enable this Duffy-independent invasion of human red blood cells have not yet been identified. The physical structures of parasites may act with adhesion molecules to promote attachment to host cells. *Giardia duodenalis* (formerly *intestinalis/lamblia*) is a protozoan parasite that uses a ventral disk to attach to the intestinal epithelium by a clasping or suction-like mechanism. Two recently identified adhesins, trypsin-activated *G. lamblia* lectin (taglin) and *G. lamblia* adherence molecule-1 (GLAM-1), may also be important in attachment to enterocytes. It is believed that initial contact of the parasite with the intestinal surface is facilitated by taglin, which is distributed over the surface of the parasite, and that the disk-specific GLAM-1 is responsible for avid attachment of the disk to the enterocyte surface.

After attachment to the specific cell or tissue type, the parasite may undergo replication as the next step in establishing infection. Most protozoan parasites replicate intracellularly or extracellularly in the human host, whereas replication is generally not observed with the helminths capable of establishing human infection.

Temperature may also play an important role in the ability of parasites to infect a host and cause disease. This is well illustrated by the *Leishmania* species. *Leishmania donovani* replicates well at 37° C and causes visceral leishmaniasis involving the bone marrow, liver, and spleen. In contrast, *Leishmania tropica* grows well at 25° C to 30° C but poorly at 37° C and causes an infection of the skin without involvement of deeper organs.

• Cell and Tissue Damage

Although some microorganisms may cause disease by localized multiplication and elaboration of potent microbial

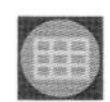

Table 69-2 Examples of Parasitic Adherence Mechanisms

Organism	Disease	Target	Mechanism of Attachment and Receptor
Plasmodium vivax	Malaria	Red blood cell	Merozoite (non–complement-mediated attachment), Duffy antigen
Plasmodium falciparum	Malaria	Red blood cell	Merozoite and glycophorin A and B
Babesia spp.	Babesiosis	Red blood cell	Complement-mediated C3b receptor
Giardia duodenalis (intestinalis/lamblia)	Diarrhea	Duodenal and jejunal epithelium	Trypsin-activated *G. lamblia* lectin and mannose-6-phosphate. *G. lamblia* adherence molecule-1 on disk
Entamoeba histolytica	Dysentery	Colonic epithelium	Lectin and *N*-acetylglucosamine conjugates
Trypanosoma cruzi	Chagas disease	Fibroblast	Penetrin, fibronectin, and fibronectin receptor
Leishmania major	Leishmaniasis	Macrophage	Adsorbed C3bi and CR3
Leishmania mexicana	Leishmaniasis	Macrophage	Surface glycoprotein (gp63) and CR2
Necator americanus *Ancylostoma duodenale*	Hookworm	Intestinal epithelium	Mechanical and biting mouth parts

toxins, most organisms initiate the disease process by invading normally sterile tissue, with subsequent replication and destruction. Parasitic protozoa and helminths are generally not known to produce toxins with potencies comparable to those of classic bacterial toxins such as anthrax toxin and botulinum toxin; however, parasitic disease can be established by elaboration of toxic products, mechanical tissue damage, and immunopathologic reactions (Table 69-3).

Numerous authors have suggested that toxic products elaborated by parasitic protozoa are responsible for at least some aspects of pathology (see Table 69-3). **Proteases** and **phospholipases** may be secreted and are released upon destruction of the parasites. These enzymes can cause host cell destruction, inflammatory responses, and gross tissue pathology. For example, the intestinal parasite *E. histolytica* produces proteinases that can degrade epithelial basement membrane and cell-anchoring proteins, disrupting epithelial cell layers. Furthermore, the amebae produce phospholipases and an ionophore-like protein that lyse the responding host neutrophils, resulting in release of neutrophil constituents that are toxic to host tissues. The expression of certain proteinases increases relative to the virulence of the strain of *E. histolytica.* In contrast to the protozoan parasites, many of the pathogenic consequences of helminthic infections are related to the size, movement, and longevity of the parasites. The host is exposed to long-term damage and immune stimulation, as well as the sheer physical consequences of being inhabited by large foreign bodies. The most obvious forms of direct damage from helminthic parasites are those resulting from mechanical blockage of internal organs or from the effects of pressure exerted by growing parasites. Large adult *Ascaris* organisms can physically block the intestine and bile ducts. Likewise, blockage of lymph flow, leading to elephantiasis, is associated with the presence of adult *Wuchereria* organisms in the lymphatic system. Some neurologic manifestations of cysticercosis are due to the pressure exerted by the slowly expanding larval cysts of *Taenia solium* on the central nervous system (CNS) and eyes. Migration of helminths (usually larval forms) through body tissues such as the skin, lungs, liver, intestines, eyes, and CNS can damage tissues directly and initiate hypersensitivity reactions.

As with many infectious agents, the manifestations of parasitic disease are due not only to the mechanical or chemical tissue damage produced by the parasite but also to host responses to the presence of the parasite. Cellular hypersensitivity is observed in protozoan and helminthic disease (Table 69-4). During a parasitic infection, host cell products such as cytokines and lymphokines are released from activated cells. These mediators influence the action of other cells and may contribute directly to the pathogenesis of parasite infections. **Immunopathologic reactions** range from acute anaphylactic reactions to cell-mediated delayed hypersensitivity reactions (see Table 69-4). The fact that many parasites are long-lived means that many inflammatory changes become irreversible, producing functional changes

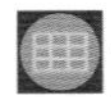
Table 69-3 Some Pathologic Mechanisms in Parasitic Diseases

Mechanism	Examples
Toxic Parasite Products	
Hydrolytic enzymes, proteinases, collagenase, elastase	Schistosomes (cercariae), *Strongyloides* spp., hookworm, *Entamoeba histolytica,* African trypanosomes, *Plasmodium falciparum*
Amebic ionophore	*Entamoeba histolytica*
Endotoxins	African trypanosomes, *Plasmodium falciparum*
Indole catabolites	Trypanosomes
Mechanical Tissue Damage	
Blockage of internal organs	*Ascaris* spp., tapeworms, schistosomes, filaria
Pressure atrophy	*Echinococcus* spp., *Cysticercus* spp.
Migration through tissue	Helminthic larvae
Immunopathology	
Hypersensitivity	See Table 69-4
Autoimmunity	See Table 69-4
Protein-losing enteropathies	Hookworm, tapeworm, *Giardia* spp., *Strongyloides* spp.
Metaplastic changes	*Opisthorchis* spp. (liver flukes), schistosomes

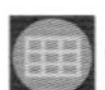
Table 69-4 Immunopathologic Reactions to Parasitic Disease

Reaction	Mechanism	Result	Example
Type 1: anaphylactic	Antigen + immunoglobulin E antibody attached to most cells: histamine release	Anaphylactic shock, bronchospasm, local inflammation	Helminth infection, African trypanosomiasis
Type 2: cytotoxic	Antibody + antigen on cell surface: complement activation or antibody-dependent cellular cytotoxicity	Lysis of cell-bearing microbial antigens	*Trypanosoma cruzi* infection
Type 3: immune complex	Antibody + extracellular antigen complex	Inflammation and tissue damage; complex deposition in glomeruli, joints, skin vessels, brain; glomerulonephritis and vasculitis	Malaria, schistosomiasis, trypanosomiasis
Type 4: cell-mediated (delayed)	Sensitized T-cell reaction with antigen, liberation of lymphokines, triggered cytotoxicity	Inflammation, mononuclear accumulation, macrophage activation Tissue damage	Leishmaniasis, schistosomiasis, trypanosomiasis

Modified from Mims C, Dimmock N, Nash A, et al: *Mims pathogenesis of infectious disease,* ed 4, London, 1995, Academic.

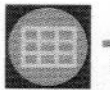 Table 69-5 Microbial Interference with or Avoidance of Immune Defenses

Type of Interference or Avoidance	Mechanism	Examples
Antigenic variation	Variation of surface antigens within the host	African trypanosomes, *Plasmodium* spp., *Babesia* spp., *Giardia* spp.
Molecular mimicry	Microbial antigens mimicking host antigens, leading to poor antibody response	*Plasmodium* spp., trypanosomes, schistosomes
Concealment of antigenic site (masking)	Acquisition of coating of host molecules	Hydatid cyst, filaria, schistosomes, trypanosomes
Intracellular location	Failure to display microbial antigen on host cell surface	*Plasmodium* spp. (red blood cells), trypanosomes, *Leishmania* spp., *Toxoplasma* spp.
	Inhibition of phagolysosomal fusion	*Toxoplasma* spp.
	Escape from phagosome into cytoplasm, with subsequent replication	*Leishmania* spp., *Trypanosoma cruzi*
Immunosuppression	Suppression of parasite-specific B- and T-cell responses	Trypanosomes, *Plasmodium* spp.
	Degradation of immunoglobulins	Schistosomes

in tissues. Examples include hyperplasia of the bile ducts secondary to the presence of liver flukes and extensive fibrosis leading to genitourinary and hepatic dysfunction in chronic schistosomiasis. Migration of larval helminths through tissues such as skin, lungs, liver, intestine, CNS, and eyes produces immune-mediated inflammatory changes in these structures. Finally, chronic inflammatory changes around parasites such as *Clonorchis (Opisthorchis) sinensis* and *Schistosoma haematobium* have been linked to the induction of carcinomatous changes in the bile ducts and bladder, respectively.

• Disruption, Evasion, and Inactivation of Host Defenses

Although the processes of cell and tissue destruction are often sufficient to initiate clinical disease, the parasite must be able to evade the host's immune defense system for the disease process to be maintained. Like other organisms, parasites elicit humoral and cell-mediated immune responses; however, parasites are particularly adept at interfering with or avoiding these defense mechanisms (Table 69-5).

Organisms can shift antigenic expression, such as that observed with the African trypanosomes. Rapid variation of expression of antigens in the glycocalyces of these organisms occurs each time the host exhibits a new humoral response. Similar changes have been observed with *Plasmodium, Babesia,* and *Giardia* species. Some organisms may produce antigens that mimic host antigens **(mimicry)** or acquire host molecules that conceal the antigenic site **(masking),** thus preventing immune recognition by the host.

Many protozoan parasites evade the immune response by assuming an intracellular location in the host. The organisms that reside in macrophages have developed a variety of mechanisms to avoid intracellular killing. These include prevention of phagolysosome fusion, resistance to killing after exposure to lysosomal enzymes, and escape of phagocytosed cells from the phagosome into the cytoplasm, with subsequent replication of the organism (see Table 69-5).

Immunosuppression of the host is often observed during the course of parasitic infections. The immunosuppression may be parasite specific or generalized, involving a response to various nonparasite and parasite antigens. Proposed mechanisms include antigen overload, antigenic competition, induction of suppressor cells, and production of lymphocyte-specific suppressor factors. Certain helminths, such as *Schistosoma mansoni,* may also produce proteinases that can degrade immunoglobulins.

Bibliography

Choi BI, Han JK, Hong ST, et al: Clonorchiasis and cholangiocarcinoma: etiologic relationship and imaging diagnosis, *Clin Microbiol Rev* 17:540–552, 2004.

Clark IA, Alleva LM, Mills AC, et al: Pathogenesis of malaria and clinically similar conditions, *Clin Microbiol Rev* 17:509–539, 2004.

Cunningham MW, Fujinami RS: *Molecular mimicry, microbes, and autoimmunity*, Washington, DC, 2000, American Society for Microbiology Press.

Espinosa-Cantellano M, Martinez-Palomo A: Pathogenesis of intestinal amebiasis: from molecules to disease, *Clin Microbiol Rev* 13:318–331, 2000.

Girones N, Cuervo H, Fresno M: *Trypanosoma cruzi*-induced molecular mimicry and Chagas disease, *Curr Top Microbiol Immunol* (vol 296), Berlin, 2005, Springer-Verlag.

Graczyk TK, Knight R, Tamang L: Mechanical transmission of human protozoan parasites by insects, *Clin Microbiol Rev* 18:128–132, 2005.

Zambrano-Villa S, Rosales-Borjas D, Carrero JC, et al: How protozoan parasites evade the immune response, *Trends Parasitol* 18:272–278, 2002.

CHAPTER

70 ROLE OF PARASITES IN DISEASE

A summary of the parasites (protozoan and helminths) most commonly associated with human disease is presented in this chapter. Although many parasites are associated with a single organ system (e.g., gastrointestinal tract) and therefore cause a disease process involving that system, some of the most dramatic manifestations of parasitic disease occur when the parasite leaves its "normal" location in the human body. Likewise, several different parasites may produce a similar disease syndrome. Management of a specific parasitic infection may differ tremendously depending on the etiologic agent, and many antiparasitic treatment regimens are quite toxic, so to guide both diagnostic and therapeutic efforts, it is useful to generate a differential diagnosis that includes the most likely parasites.

The development and prognosis of a parasitic infection often depend on factors aside from the innate virulence of the organism. In determining the possibility of a parasitic infection, the meaning of any microbiological data, and the necessity to treat and with what agent, one must take into account numerous factors, such as exposure history (e.g., travel to an endemic area), the potential infectious dose and/or organism burden, the use of prophylaxis (e.g., antimalarial prophylaxis), and the immunologic status of the host. The presentation of a given parasitic infection may be quite different in a nonimmune traveler to an endemic region versus a semiimmune resident of the same region. Likewise, treatment and prevention strategies will be different as well.

This chapter provides a very broad listing of the various parasitic agents commonly associated with infections at specific body sites and/or specific clinical manifestations (Table 70-1). This information is meant to be used in conjunction with Table 71-1 as an aid in establishing a differential diagnosis and selecting the most likely clinical specimens that will help establish a specific etiologic diagnosis. Other factors that may be important in determining the relative frequency with which specific parasites cause disease (e.g., travel and exposure history, specific clinical presentations) are covered in the individual chapters in this text or in the more comprehensive infectious disease texts cited in this and other chapters.

Table 70-1 Summary of Parasites Associated with Human Disease

System Affected and Disease	Pathogens
Blood	
Malaria	*Plasmodium falciparum, P. knowlesi, P. malariae, P. ovale, P. vivax*
Babesiosis	*Babesia* spp.
Filariasis	*Wuchereria bancrofti, Brugia malayi, Mansonella* spp., *Loa loa*
Bone Marrow	
Leishmaniasis	*Leishmania donovani, Leishmania tropica*
Central Nervous System	
Meningoencephalitis	*Naegleria fowleri, Trypanosoma brucei gambiense, T. b. rhodesiense, T. cruzi, Toxoplasma gondii*
Granulomatous encephalitis	*Acanthamoeba* spp., *Balamuthia mandrillaris*
Mass lesion Brain abscess	*T. gondii, Taenia solium, Schistosoma japonicum, Acanthamoeba* spp., *B. mandrillaris*
Eosinophilic meningitis Cerebral malaria	*Angiostrongylus cantonensis, Toxocara* spp., *Baylisascaris* (neural larva migrans), *P. falciparum*
Cerebral paragonimiasis	*Paragonimus westermani*
Eye	
Keratitis	*Acanthamoeba* spp., *Onchocerca volvulus*
Chorioretinitis Conjunctivitis	*T. gondii, O. volvulus, L. loa*
Ocular cysticercosis (mass lesion)	*T. solium*
Toxocariasis	*Toxocara* spp. (ocular larva migrans; mimics retinoblastoma)
Intestinal Tract	
Anal pruritus	*Enterobius vermicularis*
Colitis	*Entamoeba histolytica, Balantidium coli*

Table 70-1 Summary of Parasites Associated with Human Disease—cont'd

System Affected and Disease	Pathogens	System Affected and Disease	Pathogens
Diarrhea/dysentery	*E. histolytica, Giardia duodenalis (intestinalis), Cryptosporidium parvum, Cyclospora cayetanensis, Cystoisospora belli, Schistosoma mansoni, Strongyloides stercoralis, Trichuris trichiura*	**Lung**	
		Abscess	*E. histolytica, P. westermani*
		Nodule/mass	*Dirofilaria immitis, E. granulosus, E. multilocularis*
		Pneumonitis	*A. lumbricoides, S. stercoralis, Toxocara* spp., *P. westermani, T. gondii, Ancylostoma braziliense*
Toxic megacolon	*T. cruzi*		
Obstruction Perforation	*Ascaris lumbricoides, Fasciolopsis buski*	**Lymphatics**	
Rectal prolapse	*T. trichiura*	Lymphedema	*W. bancrofti, B. malayi,* other filaria
Liver, Spleen		Lymphadenopathy	*T. gondii,* trypanosomes
Abscess	*E. histolytica, Fasciola hepatica*	**Muscle**	
Hepatitis	*T. gondii*	Generalized myositis	*Trichinella spiralis, Sarcocystis lindemanni, Toxocara* spp.
Biliary obstruction	*A. lumbricoides, F. hepatica, Opisthorchis (Clonorchis) sinensis*	Myocarditis	*T. spiralis, T. cruzi, Toxocara* spp.
Cirrhosis/hepatosplenomegaly	*L. donovani, L. tropica, Toxocara canis* and *T. cati* (visceral larva migrans), *S. mansoni, S. japonicum*	**Skin and Subcutaneous Tissue**	
		Ulcerative lesion	*Leishmania* spp., *Dracunculus medinensis*
Mass lesions	*T. solium, Echinococcus granulosus, Echinococcus multilocularis*	Nodule/swellings	*O. volvulus, L. loa, T. cruzi, Acanthamoeba* spp., *Toxocara* spp.
Genitourinary		Rash/vesicles	*T. gondii, A. braziliense,* other migrating worms, schistosomes (cercarial dermatitis)
Vaginitis/urethritis	*Trichomonas vaginalis, E. vermicularis*		
Renal failure	*Plasmodium* spp., *L. donovani*	**Systemic**	
Cystitis/hematuria	*Schistosoma haematobium, P. falciparum* (blackwater fever)	General dissemination and multiple organ dysfunction	*P. falciparum, T. gondii, L. donovani, T. cruzi, Toxocara* spp., *S. stercoralis, T. spiralis*
Heart			
Myocarditis	*T. gondii, T. cruzi*	Iron deficiency, anemia	Hookworms *(Ancylostoma duodenale, Necator americanus)*
Megacardia/complete heart block	*T. cruzi*	Megaloblastic anemia (vitamin B_{12} deficiency)	*Diphyllobothrium latum*

Bibliography

Cohen J, Powderly WG: *Infectious diseases*, ed 2, St Louis, 2004, Mosby.

Connor DH, Chandler FW, Schwartz DA, et al: *Pathology of infectious diseases* (vol 2), Stamford, Conn, 1997, Appleton & Lange.

Cook G, Zumala A: *Manson's tropical diseases*, ed 21, London, 2003, Elsevier Science.

Garcia LS: *Diagnostic medical parasitology*, ed 5, Washington, DC, 2006, American Society for Microbiology Press.

John DT, Petri WA Jr: *Markell and Voge's medical parasitology*, ed 9, St Louis, 2009, Saunders.

CHAPTER

71 LABORATORY DIAGNOSIS OF PARASITIC DISEASE

The diagnosis of parasitic infections may be very difficult, particularly in the nonendemic setting. The clinical manifestations of parasitic diseases are seldom specific enough to raise the possibility of these processes in the mind of the clinician, and routine laboratory tests are seldom helpful. Although peripheral eosinophilia is widely recognized as a useful indicator of parasitic disease, this phenomenon is characteristic only of helminthic infection and even in these cases is frequently absent. Thus the physician must maintain a heightened index of suspicion and must rely on detailed travel, food intake, transfusion, and socioeconomic history to raise the possibility of parasitic disease. Proper diagnosis requires that (1) the physician consider the possibility of parasitic infection, (2) appropriate specimens be obtained and transported to the laboratory in a timely fashion, (3) the laboratory competently performs the appropriate procedures for recovery and identification of the etiologic agent, (4) the laboratory results be effectively communicated to the physician, and (5) the results be correctly interpreted by the physician and applied to the care of the patient. In addition, for most parasitic diseases, appropriate test selection and interpretation is based on an understanding of the **life cycle** of the parasite as well as the **pathogenesis** of the disease process in humans.

Numerous methods for diagnosing parasitic diseases have been described (Box 71-1). Some are useful in detecting a wide variety of parasites, and others are particularly useful for one or a few parasites. Although the mainstay of diagnostic clinical microbiology is isolation of the causative pathogen in culture, the diagnosis of parasitic diseases is accomplished almost entirely by morphologic (usually microscopic) demonstration of parasites in clinical material. Occasionally, demonstration of a specific antibody response (serodiagnosis) helps in establishing the diagnosis. The detection of parasite antigens in serum, urine, or stool now provides a rapid and sensitive means of diagnosing infection with certain organisms. Likewise, the development of nucleic acid–based assays has proven to be an excellent means of detecting and identifying a number of parasites in biological samples such as blood, stool, urine, sputum, and tissue biopsies obtained from infected patients. In general, it is better for the laboratory to offer a limited number of competently performed procedures than to offer a wide variety of infrequently and poorly performed tests.

This chapter provides a general description of the principles of specimen collection and processing necessary to diagnose most parasitic infections. Specific details of these and other procedures of general and limited usefulness may be found in several reference texts listed in the Bibliography.

• Parasite Life Cycle as an Aid in Diagnosis

Parasites may have complex life cycles involving single or multiple hosts. Understanding the life cycle of parasitic organisms is a key to understanding important features of geographic distribution, transmission, and pathogenesis of many parasitic diseases. The life cycles of parasites often suggest useful clues for diagnosis as well. For example, in the life cycle of filariae that infect humans, certain species (e.g., *Wuchereria bancrofti*) have a **"nocturnal periodicity"** in which greater numbers of microfilariae are found in peripheral blood at night. Sampling the blood of such patients during daytime hours may fail to detect the microfilariae, whereas blood specimens collected between 10 PM and 4 AM may demonstrate many microfilariae. Likewise, intestinal nematodes such as *Ascaris lumbricoides* and hookworm, which reside in the lumen of the intestine, produce large numbers of eggs that can be detected easily in the stool of an infected patient. In contrast, another intestinal nematode, *Strongyloides stercoralis,* lays its eggs in the bowel wall rather than in the intestinal lumen. As a result, the eggs are rarely seen on stool examination; to make the diagnosis, the parasitologist must be alert for the presence of larvae. Finally, parasites may cause clinical symptoms at a time when diagnostic forms are not yet present in the usual site. For example, in certain intestinal nematode infections, **migration** of larvae through the tissues may cause intense symptomatology weeks before the characteristic eggs are present in feces.

• General Diagnostic Considerations

The importance of appropriate specimen collection, the number and timing of specimens, timely transport to the laboratory, and prompt examination by an experienced microscopist cannot be overemphasized. Because the majority of parasitologic examinations and identifications are based entirely on recognizing the characteristic morphology of the organisms, any condition that may obscure or distort the morphologic appearance of the parasite may result in an erroneous identification or missed diagnosis. As noted previously and in Box 71-1, there may be alternatives to microscopy for detection and identification of certain parasites.

Box 71-1 Laboratory Methods for Diagnosing Parasitic Disease

- Macroscopic examination
- Microscopic examination
    - Wet mount
    - Permanent stains
    - Stool concentrates
- Serologic examination
    - Antibody response
    - Antigen detection
- Nucleic acid hybridization
    - Probes and amplification techniques
    - Detection
    - Identification
- Culture
- Animal inoculation
- Xenodiagnosis

These tests (e.g., antigen detection, nucleic acid amplification/detection) are becoming more widely used. They offer the promise of more rapid, sensitive, and specific diagnostic testing for parasitic diseases. These diagnostic test options may expand the testing capabilities of many laboratories, allowing laboratories with limited proficiency in parasitology to offer diagnostic testing for certain parasitic diseases. A list of common and uncommon diagnostic procedures and specimens to be collected for selected parasitic infections is provided in Table 71-1.

• Parasitic Infections of the Intestinal and Urogenital Tracts

Protozoa and helminths may colonize or infect the intestinal and urogenital tracts of humans. Most commonly, these parasites are amebae, flagellates, or nematodes (Table 71-2). However, infection with trematodes, cestodes, or ciliate or coccidian parasites may also be encountered.

In intestinal and urogenital infections, a simple wet mount or stained smear is often inadequate. Repeated specimen collection and testing are often necessary to optimize detection of organisms that are shed intermittently or in fluctuating numbers. Concentration of specimens by sedimentation or flotation techniques may be required to detect low numbers of ova (of worms) or cysts (of protozoa) in fecal specimens. Whereas routine microscopic examination of stool for ova and parasites (O&P) is useful for detecting infections caused by helminths and amebae, physicians often (inappropriately) favor this approach as a screening method for intestinal parasites and underutilize immunoassays for *Giardia* and *Cryptosporidium* despite their epidemiologic and performance superiority among patients at low risk for other parasites (e.g., helminths and *Entamoeba histolytica*).

Occasionally, specimens other than stool or urine must be examined (see Table 71-1). Optimal detection of small bowel pathogens such as *Giardia duodenalis* and *S. stercoralis* may require aspiration of duodenal contents or even small bowel biopsy. Likewise, detection of colonic parasites such as *E. histolytica* and *Schistosoma mansoni* may necessitate proctoscopic or sigmoidoscopic examination with aspiration or biopsy of mucosal lesions. Sampling of perianal skin is a useful means of recovering the eggs of *Enterobius vermicularis* (pinworm) or *Taenia* species (tapeworm).

Fecal Specimen Collection

Patients, clinicians, and laboratory personnel must be properly instructed on collection and handling of specimens. Fecal specimens should be collected in clean wide-mouthed, waterproof containers with a tight-fitting lid to ensure and maintain adequate moisture. Specimens must not be contaminated with water, soil, or urine, because water and soil may contain free-living organisms that can be mistaken for human parasites, and urine can destroy motile trophozoites and may cause helminth eggs to hatch. Stool specimens should not contain barium, bismuth, or medications containing mineral oil, antibiotics, antimalarials, or other chemical substances, because such specimens compromise the detection of intestinal parasites. Specimen collection should be delayed for 5 to 10 days to allow barium to clear and for at least 2 weeks after antibiotics such as tetracycline to allow intestinal parasites to recover from the toxic (but not curative) effects of the drugs.

Purged specimens may be collected when organisms are not detected in normally passed fecal specimens; however, only certain purgatives (sodium sulfate and buffered sodium biphosphate [phosphosoda]) are satisfactory. One series of purged specimens may be examined in place of or in addition to a series of normally passed specimens.

Unpreserved formed fecal specimens should arrive in the laboratory within 2 hours after passage. If the stool is liquid and thus more likely to contain trophozoites, it should reach the laboratory for examination within 30 minutes. Soft or loose stools should be examined within 1 hour of passage. If examination is not possible within the recommended time limits, all fresh fecal samples should be placed into preservatives such as 10% formalin, polyvinyl alcohol (PVA), merthiolate-iodine-formalin (MIF), or sodium acetate formalin (SAF). Fecal specimens may be stored at 4°C but should not be incubated or frozen.

The number of specimens required to demonstrate intestinal parasites varies depending on the quality of the specimen submitted, the accuracy of the examination performed, the severity of the infection, and the purpose for which the examination is made. If the physician is interested only in determining the presence or absence of helminths, one or two examinations may suffice, provided concentration methods are used. For a routine parasitic examination, a total of three fecal specimens is recommended. The examination of three specimens using a combination of techniques ensures detection of more than 99% of infections. In a survey conducted in the United States, examination of three specimens was required to detect 100% of infected patients (Table 71-3).

It is inappropriate for multiple specimens to be collected on the same patient on the same day. It is also not recommended for the three specimens to be submitted one each day for 3 consecutive days. The series of three specimens should be collected within no more than 10 days. Many parasites do not appear in fecal specimens in consistent numbers on a daily basis; therefore collection of specimens

Table 71-1 Body Sites, Specimen Collection, and Diagnostic Procedures for Selected Parasitic Infections

Infecting Organism	Specimen Options	Collection Methods	Diagnostic Procedure
Blood			
Plasmodium spp., *Babesia* spp., filaria, *Leishmania, Toxoplasma, Trypanosoma* spp.	Whole blood, anticoagulated	Venipuncture	Microscopic examination (Giemsa stain) or acridine orange fluorescent stain Thin film Thick film Blood concentration (filaria) Serology Antibody Antigen PCR
Bone Marrow			
Leishmania spp., *Trypanosoma cruzi*	Aspirate	Sterile	Microscopic examination (Giemsa stain) Culture
	Serum	Venipuncture	Serology (antibody) PCR
Central Nervous System			
Acanthamoeba spp., *Naegleria* spp., trypanosomes, *Toxoplasma gondii*	Spinal fluid	Sterile	Microscopic examination Wet mount Permanent stain Culture
	Serum	Venipuncture	Serology (antibody) PCR
Cutaneous Ulcers			
Leishmania spp., *Acanthamoeba* spp.	Aspirate	Sterile plus smears	Microscopic examination (Giemsa stain)
	Biopsy	Sterile, nonsterile to histology	Culture
	Serum	Venipuncture	Serology (antibody) PCR
Eye			
Acanthamoeba spp., *Loa loa*	Corneal scrapings	Sterile saline, air-dried smear	Microscopic examination Wet mount Permanent stain
	Corneal biopsy	Sterile saline	Culture
Intestinal Tract			
Entamoeba histolytica	Fresh stool	Waxed container	Microscopic examination Wet mount Permanent stains Serology Antigen (stool) Culture PCR
	Preserved stool	Formalin, PVA	
	Sigmoidoscopy material	Fresh, PVA	
		Schaudinn smears	
	Serum	Venipuncture	Serology Antibody (serum)
Giardia spp.	Fresh stool	Waxed container	Microscopic examination Wet mount Permanent stains Antigen IFA EIA Culture PCR
	Preserved stool	Formalin, PVA	
	Duodenal contents	Entero-Test or aspirate	

 **Table 71-1 Body Sites, Specimen Collection, and Diagnostic Procedures for Selected Parasitic Infections—cont'd**

Infecting Organism	Specimen Options	Collection Methods	Diagnostic Procedure
Cryptosporidium spp.	Fresh stool	Waxed container	Microscopic examination (acid-fast)
	Preserved stool	Formalin, PVA	Antigen IFA EIA
	Biopsy	Saline	PCR
Pinworm	Anal impression smear	Cellophane tape	Macroscopic examination Microscopic examination (eggs)
Helminths	Fresh stool	Waxed container	Macroscopic examination (adults)
	Preserved stool	Formalin, PVA	Microscopic examination (larvae and eggs) Culture (*Strongyloides,* fresh stool)
	Serum	Venipuncture	Serology (antibody)
Liver, Spleen			
E. histolytica, Leishmania spp.	Aspirates	Sterile, collected in four separate aliquots (liver)	Microscopic examination
	Biopsy	Sterile; nonsterile to histology	Wet mount Permanent stains Culture
	Serum	Venipuncture	Serology Antigen Antibody
Lung			
Rarely: amebae, *(E. histolytica),* trematodes *(Paragonimus westermani),* larvae *(Strongyloides stercoralis),* or cestode hooklets	Sputum	Induced, no preservative	Microscopic examination
	Lavage	No preservative	Giemsa stain Gram stain
	Transbronchial aspirate	Air-dried smears	Hematoxylin and eosin
	Brush biopsy	Air-dried smears	
	Open lung biopsy	Fresh squash preparation; nonsterile to histology	
	Serum	Venipuncture	Serology Antigen Antibody
Muscle			
Trichinella spiralis, T. cruzi	Biopsy	Nonsterile to histology	Microscopic examination (permanent stains)
	Serum	Venipuncture	Serology Antibody Antigen
Skin			
Onchocerca volvulus, Leishmania spp. Cutaneous larval migrans	Scrapings	Aseptic, smear, or vial	Microscopic examination
	Skin snip	No preservative	Wet mount Permanent stains
	Biopsy	Nonsterile to histology	
	Serum	Venipuncture	Serology (antibody) Culture (*Leishmania* spp.)
Urogenital System			
Trichomonas vaginalis	Vaginal discharge	Saline swab, culture medium	Microscopic examination
	Prostatic secretions	Saline swab, culture medium	Wet mount Permanent stains
	Urethral discharge	Saline swab, culture medium	Antigen (IFA) Culture Serology (antibody) Nucleic acid probe
Schistosoma haematobium	Urine	Single unpreserved specimen	Microscopic examination
	Biopsy	Nonsterile to histology	

EIA, Enzyme immunoassay; *IFA,* immunofluorescence assay; *PCR,* polymerase chain reaction; *PVA,* polyvinyl alcohol.

Table 71-2 Most Commonly Identified Intestinal Parasites in U.S. Laboratories

Organism	% of Total Positive Specimens (*n* = 2933)
Giardia duodenalis (lamblia)	54
Dientamoeba fragilis	25
Entamoeba histolytica/E. dispar	7
Cryptosporidium parvum	5
Ascaris lumbricoides	2
Trichuris trichiura	2
Strongyloides stercoralis	1
Enterobius vermicularis	1
Hymenolepis nana	1
Hookworm	<1
Taenia	<1
Cystoisospora spp.	<1
Cyclospora	<1
Coccidia	<1
Other helminths	<1

Data compiled from Branda JA, Lin TY, Rosenberg ES, et al: A rational approach to the stool ova and parasite examination, *Clin Infect Dis* 42:972–978, 2006; and Polage CR, Stoddard GJ, Rolfs RT, et al: Physician use of parasite tests in the United States from 1997 to 2006 and in a Utah *Cryptosporidium* outbreak in 2007, *J Clin Microbiol* 49:591–596, 2011.

Table 71-3 Number of Specimens Required to Detect Intestinal Parasites

No. of Specimens per Patient	% of Infected Patients Detected (*n* = 130)
1	71.5
2	86.9
3	100

Data compiled from Branda JA, Lin TY, Rosenberg ES, et al: A rational approach to the stool ova and parasite examination, *Clin Infect Dis* 42:972–978, 2006.

on alternate days tends to yield a higher percentage of positive findings.

It has become apparent that in the United States, submission of stool for parasitologic examination from patients with hospital-acquired diarrhea (onset > 3 days after admission) is usually inappropriate. This is because the frequency of acquisition of protozoan or helminthic parasites in a hospital is vanishingly rare. A request for stool examination for O&P in a hospitalized patient should be accompanied by a clear statement of clinical indications and only after the more common causes of hospital-acquired diarrhea (e.g., antibiotic induced) have been ruled out.

Techniques of Stool Examination

Specimens should be examined systematically by a competent microscopist for helminth eggs and larvae as well as intestinal protozoa. For optimal detection of these various infectious agents, a combination of several techniques of examination is required.

Macroscopic Examination

The fecal specimen should be examined for consistency and the presence of blood, mucus, worms, and proglottids.

Direct Wet Mount

Fresh stools should be examined under the microscope with the saline and iodine wet-mount technique to detect motile trophozoites or larvae *(Strongyloides)*. Saline and iodine wet mounts are also used to detect helminth eggs, protozoan cysts, and host cells such as leukocytes and red blood cells. This approach is also useful in examining material from sputum, urine, vaginal swabs, duodenal aspirates, sigmoidoscopy, abscesses, and tissue biopsies.

Concentration

All fecal specimens should be placed in 10% formalin to preserve parasite morphology and should be concentrated using a procedure such as formalin ethyl acetate (or formalin ether) sedimentation or zinc sulfate flotation. These methods separate protozoan cysts and helminth eggs from the bulk of fecal material and thus enhance the ability to detect small numbers of organisms usually missed by the use of only a direct smear. After concentration, the material is stained with iodine and examined microscopically.

Permanently Stained Slides

Detection and correct identification of intestinal protozoa often depend on examination of the permanently stained smear. These slides provide a permanent record of the protozoan organisms identified. The cytologic detail revealed by one of the permanent staining methods is essential for accurate identification, and most identification should be considered tentative until confirmed by the permanently stained slide. The common permanent stains used are trichrome, iron hematoxylin, and phosphotungstic acid–hematoxylin. Slides are made either by preparing smears of fresh fecal material and placing them in Schaudinn fixative solution or by fixing a small amount of fecal material in PVA fixative. It should be noted that an order for a routine microscopic examination of stool for O&P does not necessarily include special stains required to detect organisms such as *Cryptosporidium* or *Cyclospora*. If these organisms are considered in the differential diagnosis, the order for stool examination must state this explicitly so that the necessary special stains (acid-fast *[Cryptosporidium, Cyclospora]*) and procedures (immunoassay *[Cryptosporidium]* and PCR *[Cryptosporidium* and *Cyclospora]*) can be performed.

Collection and Examination of Specimens Other Than Stool

Frequently, specimens other than fecal material must be collected and examined to diagnose infections caused by intestinal pathogens. These specimens include perianal samples, sigmoidoscopic material, aspirates of duodenal contents, and liver abscess, sputum, urine, and urogenital specimens.

Perianal Specimens

Collection of perianal specimens is frequently necessary to diagnose pinworm *(E. vermicularis)* and occasionally *Taenia* (tapeworm) infections. Methods include preparation of a clear cellulose tape slide or an anal swab. Cellulose tape slide preparation is the method of choice for detection of pinworm eggs. Specimens collected by either method should be obtained in the morning before the patient bathes or goes to the bathroom. The tape method requires that the adhesive surface of the tape be pressed firmly against the right and left perianal folds and then spread onto the surface of a microscope slide. Likewise, the anal swab should be rubbed gently over the perianal area and transported to the laboratory for microscopic examination. With either collection method, the slides or swabs should be kept at 4° C if transport to the laboratory is to be delayed.

Sigmoidoscopic Material

Material from sigmoidoscopy can be helpful in the diagnosis of *E. histolytica* infection that has not been detected by routine fecal examinations. The specimens consist of scraped or aspirated material from the mucosal surface. At least six areas should be sampled. After collection, the material should be placed in a tube containing 0.85% saline and should be kept warm during transport to the laboratory. The specimens should be examined immediately for motile trophozoites.

Duodenal Aspirates

Sampling and examination of duodenal contents is a means of recovering *Strongyloides* larvae; the eggs of *Clonorchis, Opisthorchis,* and *Fasciola* species; and other small bowel parasites such as *Giardia, Cystoisospora,* and *Cryptosporidium* organisms. Specimens may be obtained by endoscopic intubation or by use of the enteric capsule or string test (Entero-Test). Endoscopic biopsy of the small intestinal mucosa may reveal *Giardia* and *Cryptosporidium* organisms as well as *Strongyloides* larvae. Specimens should be collected in saline and transported directly to the laboratory for microscopic examination.

Liver Abscess Aspirate

Suppurative lesions of the liver and subphrenic spaces may be caused by *E. histolytica* (extraintestinal amebiasis). Extraintestinal amebiasis may occur in the absence of any history of symptomatic intestinal infection. The specimen should be collected from the liver abscess margin instead of the necrotic center. The first portion removed is usually yellowish white in appearance and seldom contains amebae. Later portions, which are reddish, are more likely to contain organisms. A minimum of two separate portions of exudative material should be removed. After aspiration, collapse of the abscess and subsequent inflowing of blood often release amebae from the tissue. Subsequent aspirations may have a greater chance of revealing organisms. The aspirated material should be transported immediately to the laboratory.

Sputum

Occasionally, intestinal parasites may be detected in sputum. These organisms include the larvae of *Ascaris, Strongyloides,* and hookworm; cestode hooklets; and intestinal protozoa such as *E. histolytica* and *Cryptosporidium* species. The specimen should be a deep sputum rather than primarily saliva, and it should be delivered immediately to the laboratory. Microscopic examination should include saline wet-mount and permanently stained preparations.

Urine

Examination of urine specimens may be useful in diagnosing infections caused by *Schistosoma haematobium* (occasionally other species as well) and *Trichomonas vaginalis.* Detection of eggs in urine can be accomplished using direct detection or concentration using the sedimentation centrifugation technique. Eggs may be trapped in mucus or pus and are more frequently present in the last few drops of the specimen rather than the first portion. The production of *Schistosoma* eggs fluctuates; therefore examinations should be performed over several days. *T. vaginalis* may be found in the urinary sediment of male and female patients.

Urogenital Specimens

Urogenital specimens are collected if infection with *T. vaginalis* is suspected. Identification is based on wet-mount preparation examinations of vaginal and urethral discharges, prostatic secretions, or urine sediment. Specimens should be placed in a container with a small amount of 0.85% saline and sent immediately to the laboratory for examination. If no organisms are detected by direct wet mounts, culture may be used.

• Parasitic Infections of Blood and Tissue

Parasites localized within the blood or tissues of the host are more difficult to detect than intestinal and urogenital parasites. Microscopic examination of blood films is a direct and useful means of detecting malarial parasites, trypanosomes, and microfilariae. Unfortunately, the concentration of organisms often fluctuates, so collection of multiple specimens over several days is required. The mainstay of diagnosis is preparation of both wet mounts (microfilariae and trypanosomes) and permanently stained thick and thin blood films. Examination of sputum may reveal helminth ova (lung flukes) or larvae (*Ascaris* and *Strongyloides* species) after appropriate concentration techniques. Biopsy of skin (onchocerciasis) or muscle (trichinosis) may be required for the diagnosis of certain nematode infections (see Table 71-1).

Blood Films

The clinical diagnosis of parasitic diseases such as malaria, leishmaniasis, trypanosomiasis, and filariasis largely rests on collection of appropriately timed blood samples and expert microscopic examination of properly prepared and stained thick and thin blood films. The optimal time for obtaining blood for parasitologic examination varies with the particular parasite expected.

Because malaria is one of the few parasitic infections that can be acutely life threatening, blood collection and examination of blood films should be performed immediately if the diagnosis is suspected. Laboratories offering this service should be prepared to do so on a 24-hour basis, 7 days a week. Because the levels of parasitemia may be low or fluctuating, it is recommended that repeat blood films be obtained and examined at 6, 12, and 24 hours after the initial sample. Detection of trypanosomes in blood is occasionally possible during the early acute phase of the disease. *Trypanosoma cruzi* (Chagas disease) may also be detected during subsequent febrile periods. After several months to a year, the trypomastigotes of African trypanosomiasis (*Trypanosoma brucei rhodesiense* and *T. b. gambiense*) are better demonstrated in spinal fluid than blood. Blood samples for the detection of nocturnal microfilariae (*W. bancrofti* and *Brugia malayi*) should be obtained between 10 PM and 4 AM, whereas for the diurnal *Loa loa,* samples are obtained around noon.

Two types of blood films are prepared for the diagnosis of blood parasite infections: thin films and thick films. Although wet-mount preparations of blood films can be examined for motile parasites (microfilariae and trypanosomes), most laboratories proceed directly to preparation of thick and thin films for staining. In the thin film, blood is spread over the slide in a thin (single cell) layer and the red blood cells remain intact after fixation and staining. In the thick film, the red cells are lysed before staining and only the white blood cells, platelets, and parasites (if present) are visible. Thick films allow a larger amount of blood to be examined, which increases the possibility of detecting light infections. Unfortunately, increased distortion of the parasites makes species identification using the thick film particularly difficult. Proper use of this technique usually requires a great deal of expertise and experience.

Occasionally, other blood-concentration procedures may be used to detect light infections. Alternative concentration methods for detecting blood parasites include use of microhematocrit centrifugation, examination of buffy coat preparations, a triple centrifugation technique for detection of low numbers of trypanosomes, and a membrane filtration technique for detection of microfilariae.

Once prepared, blood films must be stained. The most dependable staining of blood parasites is obtained with Giemsa stain buffered to pH 7.0 to 7.2, although special stains may be occasionally used to identify species of microfilariae. Giemsa stain is particularly useful for the staining of protozoa (malaria and trypanosomes); however, the sheath of microfilariae may not always stain with Giemsa. In this case, hematoxylin-based stains may be used.

Specimens Other Than Blood

Examination of tissue and body fluids other than blood may be necessary, based on clinical presentation and epidemiologic considerations. Smears and concentrates of cerebrospinal fluid are necessary to detect trophozoites of *Naegleria fowleri,* trypanosomes, and larvae of the nematode *Angiostrongylus cantonensis* within the central nervous system. Cerebrospinal fluid must be promptly examined because the trophozoite forms of these parasites are very labile (trypanosomes) or tend to round up and become nonmotile *(N. fowleri).* Examination of tissue impression smears of lymph nodes, liver biopsy material, spleen, or bone marrow stained with Giemsa stain is very useful in detecting **intracellular** parasites such as *Leishmania* species and *Toxoplasma gondii.* Likewise, biopsies of various tissues are an excellent means of detecting localized or disseminated infections caused by protozoan and helminthic parasites. Saline mounts of superficial skin snips are very useful in detecting the microfilariae of *Onchocerca volvulus.* Examination of sputum (induced) is indicated when there is a question of pulmonary paragonimiasis (lung fluke) or abscess formation with *E. histolytica. Strongyloides* larvae may be detected in sputum in hyperinfection syndrome.

• Alternatives to Microscopy

In the majority of cases, the diagnosis of parasitic disease is made in the laboratory by microscopic detection and morphologic identification of the parasite in clinical specimens. In some cases, the parasite cannot be detected despite a careful search because of low or absent levels of organisms in readily available clinical material. In such cases, the clinician may need to rely on alternative methods based on the detection of parasite-derived material (antigens or nucleic acids) or by the host response to parasitic invasion (antibodies). Additional approaches used in selected infections include culture, animal inoculation, and xenodiagnosis.

Immunodiagnostics

Immunodiagnostic methods have long been used as aids in the diagnosis of parasitic diseases. The majority of these serologic tests are based on detection of specific antibody responses to the presence of the parasite. Analytical approaches include the use of classic agglutination, complement fixation, and gel diffusion methods, as well as the more modern immunofluorescence assays (IFAs), enzyme immunoassay (EIA), and Western blot assays. Antibody detection is useful and indicated in the diagnosis of many protozoan diseases (e.g., extraintestinal amebiasis, South American trypanosomiasis, leishmaniasis, transfusion-acquired malaria and babesiosis, and toxoplasmosis) and helminthic diseases (e.g., clonorchiasis, cysticercosis, hydatidosis, lymphatic filariasis, schistosomiasis, trichinellosis, and toxocariasis). There is a problem with detection of antibody as a means of diagnosis: because of the persistence of antibody for months to years after the acute infection, demonstration of antibody can rarely differentiate between acute and chronic infection.

In contrast to antibody detection, the measurement of circulating **parasite antigen** in serum, urine, or feces may provide a more appropriate marker for the presence of active infection and may also indicate parasite load. Likewise, demonstrations of specific parasite antigen in lesion fluid, such as material from an amebic abscess or fluid from a hydatid cyst, may provide a definitive diagnosis of the infecting organism. Most common antigen detection assays use an EIA format; however, immunofluorescence, radioimmunoassay, immunochromatographic, and immunoblot methods have also proved useful. Several commercial assays for the detection of parasite antigens are now available in kits. These include EIA and immunochromatographic assays for the detection of *Giardia, E. histolytica, Entamoeba dispar,* and *Cryptosporidium* species in stool, EIA for the detection of *T. vaginalis* in urogenital specimens, and IFA for the detection of *Giardia, Cryptosporidium,* and *Trichomonas* species. Several antigen detection tests are also available for detection of **blood parasites** (malaria, filariasis) in conjunction with microscopic examination of thick and thin blood smears. The reported sensitivity and specificity for most of these kits are quite good. Advantages to these approaches are labor savings and a potential increase in sensitivity. Indeed, numerous studies have shown that immunoassays are more sensitive than microscopic examination in detecting infections caused by *Giardia* and *Cryptosporidium*. Likewise, rapid diagnostic tests for detecting antigens of *Plasmodium* spp. may outperform microscopy in certain situations and are being considered for use in the field, especially because use of the more expensive artemisinin combination therapies makes a laboratory diagnosis of malaria more cost-effective than empirical therapy in the era of chloroquine resistance. Disadvantages are the loss of parasitologic expertise and the fact that in some instances the available assay tests for only a single organism, whereas conventional microscopic examination provides the opportunity to recognize many different parasites. Although antigen detection assays have been described for many other parasites, they are not widely available. The availability of a broad panel of antigen detection assays potentially would make the use of an antigen screen a viable alternative to tedious microscopic examination.

Molecular Diagnostic Approaches

In addition to immunodiagnostic methods, the diagnosis of parasitic diseases has been enhanced considerably by the application of molecular diagnostic methods based on **nucleic acid hybridization, amplification, and sequencing.** This approach takes advantage of the fact that all organisms contain nucleic acid sequences that may be used in a hybridization assay to distinguish among strains, species, and genera. Thus parasites may be simultaneously detected and identified in clinical material depending on the specificity of the molecular method employed. Another advantage of nucleic acid–based detection systems is that they are independent of the patient's immunologic status or previous infection history, thereby identifying active infection. Finally, the use of target amplification techniques (e.g., polymerase chain reaction [PCR]) provides exquisite sensitivity, allowing detection of as little as one organism in a biological sample (Table 71-4).

Nucleic acid–based methods can be used to detect parasites not only in clinical samples of blood, stool, or tissue from infected patients but also in their natural vector. The application of deoxyribonucleic acid (DNA) "fingerprinting" allows precise identification of the parasite to the subspecies or strain level and has considerable value in epidemiologic studies. Assay formats using nucleic acid probes range from dot blot and Southern hybridization methods to in situ hybridization in tissue to PCR or other target amplification methods coupled with rapid amplicon detection and characterization. The use of nonisotopic DNA labeling techniques greatly expands the potential applicability of these assays worldwide. Diagnostic kits based on these methods are not widely available; however, a commercially available direct from specimen platform that employs multiplex PCR and post-PCR melting curve analysis has recently been cleared by the U.S. Food and Drug Administration for detection of *E. histolytica, Giardia, Cyclospora,* and *Cryptosporidium* from stool (FilmArray Gastrointestinal Panel, BioFire, Salt Lake City, UT).

Irrespective of the assay format, nucleic acid probes and amplification techniques are now being used on a research basis for detection and identification of numerous species and strains, including *Plasmodium* species, *Leishmania* species, *T. cruzi, E. histolytica, Cryptosporidium,* and *T. gondii* (see Table 71-4). It must be understood that the application of nucleic acid hybridization methods to the diagnosis of parasitic diseases is still in its infancy. Widespread use of these techniques requires further development of simple procedures for sample handling and preparation and will require extensive clinical and field testing before they can be applied broadly to aid in clinical diagnosis.

Culture

Although culture is the standard for the diagnosis of most infectious diseases, it is not commonly used in the parasitology laboratory. Certain protozoan parasites (e.g., *T. vaginalis, E. histolytica, Acanthamoeba* spp., *N. fowleri, Leishmania* spp., *Plasmodium falciparum, T. cruzi, T. gondii*) can be cultured with relative ease. However, culture of other parasites has either not been successful or is too difficult or cumbersome to be of practical value in routine diagnostic efforts.

Animal Inoculation

Animal inoculation is a sensitive means of detecting infection caused by blood and tissue parasites such as *T. b. gambiense, T. b. rhodesiense, T. cruzi, Leishmania* spp., and *T. gondii*. Although useful, this approach is not practical for most diagnostic laboratories and is largely confined to research settings.

Xenodiagnosis

The technique of xenodiagnosis employs the use of laboratory-raised arthropod vectors to detect low levels of parasites in infected individuals. Classically this approach was used to diagnose Chagas disease by allowing an uninfected reduviid bug to feed on an individual suspected of

Table 71-4 Examples of Techniques for Detection of Parasitic Infections Based on PCR Analysis

Organism	Gene	Target Sensitivity (%)	Comment
Plasmodium vivax	Circumsporozoite gene	91-96	Dried blood-spotted filter paper samples are used.
Leishmania species	kDNA minicircle sequence	87-100	Results are compared to culture and microscopy of biopsy specimens.
Trypanosoma cruzi	kDNA minicircle sequence	100	Results are compared to serology and xenodiagnosis of blood samples.
Toxoplasma gondii	*B1* repetitive gene P30 major surface antigen Recombinant DNA sequences	46-99	PCR of BAL, blood, cerebrospinal fluid, and amniotic fluid show great potential for diagnosis of toxoplasmosis.
Entamoeba histolytica	P145 tandem repeat sequence SSU rRNA	96 >90	Results are compared to microscopic diagnosis of stool samples. Tests may distinguish pathogenic from nonpathogenic strains.

BAL, Bronchoalveolar lavage; *kDNA,* kinetodast deoxyribonucleic acid; *PCR,* polymerase chain reaction; *SSU rRNA,* small subunit ribosomal ribonucleic acid.

having the disease. Subsequently, the bug was dissected and examined microscopically for evidence of developmental stages of *T. cruzi.* Although this technique may be used in endemic areas, it is obviously not practical for most diagnostic laboratories.

Bibliography

Branda JA, Lin TY, Rosenberg ES, et al: A rational approach to the stool ova and parasite examination, *Clin Infect Dis* 42:972–978, 2006.

Buss SN, Leber A, Chapin K, et al: Multicenter evaluation of the BioFire FilmArray Gastrointestinal Panel for etiologic diagnosis of infectious gastroenteritis, *J Clin Microbiol* 53:915–925, 2015.

Garcia LS, Schimizu RY, Bernard CN: Detection of *Giardia lamblia, Entamoeba histolytica/Entamoeba dispar,* and *Cryptosporidium parvum* antigens in human fecal specimens using the Triage Parasite Panel enzyme immunoassay, *J Clin Microbiol* 38:3337–3340, 2000.

Garcia LS, Shimizu RY, Paltridge GP: General approaches for detection and identification of parasites. In Versalovic J, et al, editors: *Manual of clinical microbiology*, ed 10, Washington, DC, 2011, American Society for Microbiology Press.

Jones JL, Lopez A, Wahlquist SP, et al: Survey of clinical laboratory practices for parasitic diseases, *Clin Infect Dis* 38(Suppl 3):S198–S202, 2004.

McHardy IH, Wu M, Shimizu-Cohen R, et al: Detection of intestinal protozoa in the clinical laboratory, *J Clin Microbiol* 52:712–720, 2014.

Murray CK, Gasser RA Jr, Magill AJ, et al: Update on rapid diagnostic testing for malaria, *Clin Microbiol Rev* 21:97–110, 2008.

Polage CR, Stoddard GJ, Rolfs RT, et al: Physician use of parasite tests in the United States from 1997 to 2006 and in a Utah *Cryptosporidium* outbreak in 2007, *J Clin Microbiol* 49:591–596, 2011.

Rosenblatt JE: Laboratory diagnosis of infections due to blood and tissue parasites, *Clin Infect Dis* 49:1103–1108, 2009.

Shimizu R, Grimm F, Garcia LS, et al: Specimen collection, transport, and processing: parasitology. In Versalovic J, et al, editors: *Manual of clinical microbiology*, ed 10, Washington, DC, 2011, American Society for Microbiology Press.

Stensvold CR, Lebbad M, Verweij JJ: The impact of genetic diversity in protozoa on molecular diagnosis, *Trends Parasitol* 27:53–58, 2011.

Verweij JJ, Stensvold CR: Molecular testing for clinical diagnosis and epidemiological investigations of intestinal parasitic infections, *Clin Microbiol Rev* 27:371–418, 2014.

CHAPTER 72 ANTIPARASITIC AGENTS

The chemotherapeutic approach to management of infectious diseases has clearly changed the face of medicine. Unfortunately, few of the antiinfective agents that have proved so successful against bacterial pathogens have been effective against parasites. In many instances, clinicians continue to rely on antiparasitic agents from the preantibiotic era. These and some newer agents remain limited in effectiveness and are relatively toxic. Many antiparasitic agents require prolonged or parenteral administration and may be effective only in certain disease states. Fortunately, in the last 5 to 10 years, several new agents have appeared that constitute significant advances in the treatment of parasitic diseases. In each case, the previously available drugs were toxic and often ineffective.

In large part, the difficulties in treating parasitic diseases stem from the fact that parasites are **eukaryotic** organisms and thus are more similar to the human host than the more successfully treated prokaryotic bacterial pathogens. Furthermore, the chronic and prolonged course of infection, the complex life cycles, and multiple developmental stages of many parasites add to the difficulties of effective chemotherapeutic intervention. Additional complicating factors in resource-poor countries, where the majority of parasitic diseases occur, include (1) the presence of multiple infections and the high probability of reinfection, (2) the large number of persons immunocompromised by malnutrition and human immunodeficiency virus infection, and (3) the overwhelming influence of poverty and poor sanitation, which facilitate transmission of many parasitic infections. Although chemotherapeutic approaches may be used effectively to treat and prevent many parasitic infections, some agents have adverse effects or eventually meet with resistance (microbial and social). Most antiparasitic agents are too expensive for widespread use in resource-poor countries. Thus the global approach to prevention and treatment of parasitic diseases must involve several strategies, including improved hygiene and sanitation, control of the disease vector, use of **vaccinations** if available (largely unavailable for parasitic diseases), and prophylactic and therapeutic administration of safe and effective chemotherapy. Of note, large-scale chemotherapy administered one to three times per year in endemic regions has reduced transmission of (and morbidity and mortality from) certain infections, including lymphatic filariasis, onchocerciasis, schistosomiasis, and intestinal nematodes. These strategies now must also include efforts to decrease transmission of infection by the human immunodeficiency virus.

• Targets for Antiparasitic Drug Action

As eukaryotic organisms, parasites have more similarities than differences with the human host. Consequently, many antiparasitic agents act on pathways (nucleic acid synthesis, carbohydrate metabolism) or targets (neuromuscular function) shared by both the parasite and host. For this reason, developing safe and effective antiparasitic drugs based on **biochemical differences** between the parasite and host has been difficult. **Differential toxicity** is commonly achieved by preferential uptake, metabolic alteration of the drug by the parasite, or differences in susceptibility of functionally equivalent sites in the parasite and host. Fortunately, as our understanding of the basic biology and biochemistry of parasites and the mechanism of action of antimicrobial agents has improved, so has our recognition of potential parasite-specific targets for chemotherapeutic attack. Increasingly, investigators are exploiting newly completed genome projects for protozoan parasites to identify potential drug targets for high-throughput screening. Examples of the chemotherapeutic strategies that exploit the differences between parasite and host are provided in Table 72-1. These are discussed in greater detail as we deal with specific agents.

• Drug Resistance

Resistance to antimicrobial agents is an important consideration in the treatment of infections resulting from bacterial and fungal pathogens and certainly plays a role in the chemotherapy of parasitic diseases. Unfortunately, our understanding of the molecular and genetic basis for resistance to most antiparasitic agents is quite limited. Greater understanding of the epidemiology and mechanisms of drug resistance can provide valuable guidance for a better use of existing compounds and for the development of novel agents. The use of molecular markers of drug resistance has added another dimension to surveillance efforts and generated insights into the global spread of drug resistance in both protozoa and helminths. Molecular markers have been identified for *Plasmodium falciparum* resistance to chloroquine, sulfadoxine-pyramethamine, atovaquone-proguanil, and to a limited degree other antimalarials. For chloroquine and sulfadoxine-pyramethamine, these involve single nucleotide polymorphisms in genes encoding a vacuolar membrane transporter protein and enzymes involved in folate synthesis,

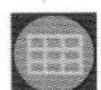

Table 72-1 **Chemotherapeutic Strategies That Exploit Differences between Parasite and Host**

Unique Site of Attack	Drug	Organism
Drug-concentrating mechanism unique to parasite	Chloroquine	*Plasmodium* spp.
Folic acid pathway (parasite unable to use exogenous folate)	Pyrimethamine or trimethoprim-sulfamethoxazole	*Plasmodium* or *Toxoplasma* spp.
Inhibitor of trypanothione-dependent mechanisms for reducing oxidized thiol groups	Arsenicals, difluoromethylornithine	Trypanosomes
Interference with neuromediators unique to parasites	Pyrantel pamoate, diethylcarbamazine	*Ascaris* spp.
Interacts with chloride channels, resulting in hyperpolarization of cells, paralysis, and death of parasites	Ivermectin	Filaria
Interaction with tubulin unique to parasites	Benzimidazoles	Many helminths
Inhibition of topoisomerase II	Pentamidine	Trypanosomes
Inhibition of pyruvate ferredoxin oxidoreductase	Nitazoxanide	*Cryptosporidium* and *Giardia*

respectively. Parasites that have developed both chloroquine and sulfadoxine-pyramethamine resistance and subsequently develop resistance to a third operational drug are termed "multidrug resistant" (MDR). Patients infected with plasmodia containing an increased copy number of *pfmdr1* (*P. falciparum* MDR 1 gene), which encodes Pfgh1, a purported transporter pump, were found to have reduced responses to mefloquine, quinine, lumefantrine, and artemisinin-based combinations containing these drugs. More recently, the *pfmrp* (MDR-associated protein) gene was associated with drug efflux in cultured parasites, and single nucleotide polymorphisms in the *pfmrp* gene were observed in recurrent infections after treatment with artemether-lumefantrine. Resistance in *P. falciparum* to the atovaquone component of atovaquone-proguanil maps to the same locus that determines atovaquone resistance in *Pneumocystis jirovecii*. These efforts have led to further studies and improved understanding of mechanisms of drug resistance in *Trichomonas* (metronidazole), *Leishmania* (pentavalent antimonials), African trypanosomes (melarsoprol, pentamidine), and schistosomes (oxamniquine). Further insights into the mechanisms of action and resistance to antiparasitic agents are necessary to optimize the effectiveness of antiparasite chemotherapy.

• Antiparasitic Agents

Although the number of effective antiparasitic agents is small relative to the vast array of antibacterial agents, the list is expanding (Table 72-2). Certainly, in many cases, the goal of antiparasitic therapy is similar to that of antibacterial therapy—to eradicate the organism rapidly and completely. In many cases, however, the agents and treatment regimens used for parasitic diseases are designed simply to decrease the parasite burden, to prevent the systemic complications of chronic infection, or both actions. Thus the goals of antiparasitic therapy, particularly as applied in endemic areas, may be quite different from those usually considered for therapy of microbial infection in the United States or other developed countries. Given the significant toxicity of many of these agents, in every case the need for treatment must be weighed against the toxicity of the drug. A decision to withhold therapy may often be correct, particularly when the drug can cause severe adverse effects.

Immunocompromised individuals pose a particular problem with respect to antiparasitic chemotherapy. On the one hand, **prophylaxis,** such as that administered for toxoplasmosis, may be effective in preventing infection. However, once infection is established, radical cure may not be possible and long-term **suppressive therapy** may be indicated. In some diseases, such as cryptosporidiosis, effective (curative) therapy is not readily available, and care must be taken to avoid unnecessary toxicity while providing supportive care for the patient.

The remainder of this chapter provides an overview of the major classes of antiprotozoal and anthelmintic agents. These and additional antiparasitic agents, their mechanisms of action, and their clinical indications are listed in Table 72-2. Treatment of specific infections is discussed in the chapters that deal with the parasites. The Bibliography lists several excellent reviews for more complete information and discussions of available antiparasitic agents.

Antiprotozoal Agents

Similar to antibacterial and antifungal agents, antiprotozoal agents are generally targeted at relatively rapidly proliferating, young, growing cells. Most commonly, these agents target nucleic acid synthesis, protein synthesis, or specific metabolic pathways (e.g., folate metabolism) unique to the protozoan parasites.

Heavy Metals

The heavy metals used for the treatment of parasitic infections include arsenical (melarsoprol) and antimonial compounds (sodium stibogluconate, meglumine antimonate). These agents are thought to oxidize sulfhydryl groups of enzymes that are essential catalysts in carbohydrate metabolism. Melarsoprol inhibits parasite pyruvate kinase, causing decreased concentrations of adenosine triphosphate (ATP), pyruvate, and phosphoenolpyruvate. Arsenicals also inhibit *sn*-glycerol-3-phosphate oxidase, which is needed for the regeneration of nicotinamide adenine dinucleotide in trypanosomes but is not found in mammalian cells. The antimonials, sodium stibogluconate and meglumine antimonate, inhibit the glycolytic enzyme phosphofructokinase and certain Krebs cycle enzymes in *Leishmania* organisms. They have also been shown to interfere with the metabolism of glutathione and trypanothione, resulting in an increased sensitivity of the organisms to oxidant stress. In each instance, the inhibition of parasite metabolism is **parasiticidal.** Unfortunately, the heavy metal compounds are toxic to the host as

Table 72-2 Mechanisms of Action and Clinical Indications for the Major Antiparasitic Agents

Drug Class	Mechanism of Action	Examples	Clinical Indications
Antiprotozoal Agents			
Heavy metals: arsenicals and antimonials	Inactivate sulfhydryl groups; disrupt glycolysis	Melarsoprol, sodium stibogluconate, meglumine antimonate	Trypanosomiasis, leishmaniasis
Aminoquinoline analogs	Accumulate in parasitized cells; interfere with DNA replication; bind to ferriprotoporphyrin IX; raise intravesicular pH; interfere with hemoglobin digestion	Chloroquine, mefloquine, quinine, primaquine, halofantrine, lumefantrine	Malaria prophylaxis and therapy Radical cure (exoerythrocytic-primaquine only)
Folic acid antagonists	Inhibit dihydropteroate synthetase and dihydrofolate reductase	Sulfonamides, pyrimethamine, trimethoprim	Toxoplasmosis, malaria, cyclosporiasis
Inhibitors of protein synthesis	Block peptide synthesis at level of ribosome	Clindamycin, spiramycin, paromomycin, tetracycline, doxycycline	Malaria, babesiosis, amebiasis, cryptosporidiosis, leishmaniasis
Diamidines	Bind DNA; interfere with uptake and function of polyamines	Pentamidine	Pneumocystosis, leishmaniasis, trypanosomiasis
Nitroimidazoles	Unclear Interact with DNA; inhibit metabolism of glucose; interfere with mitochondrial function	Metronidazole, benznidazole, tinidazole	Amebiasis, giardiasis, trichomoniasis, American trypanosomiasis (Chagas disease)
Nitrofurans	Depletion of glutathione, trypanothione, and metallothionein Oxidative stress	Nifurtimox	Chagas disease, late-stage African trypanosomiasis *(T. b. gambiense)*
Sesquiterpenes	React with heme, causing free-radical damage to parasite membranes (artemisinins); inhibit methionine aminopeptidase type 2 (fumagillin); inhibit RNA and DNA synthesis (fumagillin)	Artemisinin, artemether, artesunate Fumagillin	Malaria (artemisinins)
Ornithine analog	Inhibits ornithine decarboxylase; interferes with polyamine metabolism	Difluoromethylornithine	African trypanosomiasis
Phosphocholine analog	Disruption of cell-signaling pathways and lipid metabolism; induces apoptotic cell death	Miltefosine	Leishmaniasis
Acetanilide	Unknown	Diloxanide furoate	Intestinal amebiasis
Sulfated naphthylamine	Inhibits *sn*-glycerol-3-phosphate oxidase and glycerol-3-phosphate dehydrogenase, causing decreased ATP synthesis	Suramin	African trypanosomiasis
Thiazolides	Inhibit pyruvate-ferredoxin oxidoreductase	Nitazoxanide	Cryptosporidiosis, giardiasis
Anthelmintic Agents			
Benzimidazoles	Inhibit fumarate reductase; inhibit glucose transport; disrupt microtubular function	Mebendazole, thiabendazole, albendazole	Broad-spectrum anthelmintic: nematodes, cestodes
Tetrahydropyrimidine	Blocks neuromuscular action; inhibits fumarate reductase	Pyrantel pamoate	Ascariasis, pinworm, hookworm
Piperazines	Cause neuromuscular paralysis; stimulate phagocytic cells	Piperazine, diethylcarbamazine	Ascaris and pinworm infections
Avermectins	Block neuromuscular action; hyperpolarize nerve and muscle cells; inhibit filarial reproduction	Ivermectin	Filarial infections, strongyloidiasis, ascariasis, scabies
Pyrazinoisoquinoline	Calcium agonist Causes tetanic muscular contractions; causes tegumental disruption; provides synergy with host defenses	Praziquantel	Broad-spectrum anthelmintic: cestodes, trematodes
Phenol	Uncouples oxidative phosphorylation	Niclosamide	Intestinal tapeworm
Quinolone	Alkylates DNA; inhibits DNA, RNA, and protein synthesis	Bithionol, oxamniquine	Paragonimiasis, schistosomiasis

Continued

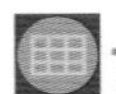

Table 72-2 **Mechanisms of Action and Clinical Indications for the Major Antiparasitic Agents—cont'd**

Drug Class	Mechanism of Action	Examples	Clinical Indications
Organophosphate	Anticholinesterase Blocks neuromuscular action	Metrifonate	Schistosomiasis
Sulfated naphthylamidine	Inhibits glycerophosphate oxidase and dehydrogenase	Suramin	Onchocerciasis

ATP, Adenosine triphosphate, *DNA,* deoxyribonucleic acid; *RNA,* ribonucleic acid.

well as the parasite. Toxicity is greatest on cells that are most metabolically active, such as neuronal, renal tubular, intestinal, and bone marrow stem cells. Their differential toxicity and therapeutic value are largely related to enhanced uptake by the parasite and its intense metabolic activity.

Melarsoprol is the drug of choice for trypanosomiasis involving the central nervous system. It can penetrate the blood-brain barrier and is effective in all stages of trypanosomiasis. The antimonial compounds are restricted to the management of leishmaniasis. Meglumine antimonate and sodium stibogluconate are important agents for the treatment of leishmaniasis and are active against all forms of the disease. Prolonged therapy is usually required for disseminated leishmaniasis, and relapses are common. Despite the use of antimonials worldwide for treatment of leishmaniasis for over 6 decades with little evidence of resistance, acquired resistance has become a clinical threat within the past 10 years. This resistance is so far unique to *Leishmania donovani,* which causes visceral leishmaniasis in the hyperendemic region of Bihar, India. The mechanism of resistance is not completely understood but likely involves activation of an efflux pump in the plasma membrane of the organism with transport of the drug out of the cells.

Quinoline Derivatives

The quinoline derivatives include the 4-aminoquinolines (chloroquine), the cinchona alkaloids (quinine, quinidine), the 8-aminoquinolines (primaquine), and the synthetic quinoline compounds (mefloquine, halofantrine, lumefantrine). These compounds all have antimalarial activity and accumulate preferentially in parasitized red blood cells. Several potential mechanisms of action have been proposed, including (1) binding to deoxyribonucleic acid (DNA) and interfering with DNA replication, (2) binding to ferriprotoporphyrin IX released from hemoglobin in infected erythrocytes, producing a toxic complex, and (3) raising the pH of the parasite's intracellular acid vesicles, thus interfering with its ability to degrade hemoglobin. Quinine, quinidine, the 4-aminoquinolines, and the synthetic quinolines rapidly destroy the erythrocytic stage of malaria and thus may be used **prophylactically** to suppress clinical illness or **therapeutically** to terminate an acute attack. The 8-aminoquinolines (e.g., primaquine) accumulate in tissue cells and destroy the extra-erythrocytic (hepatic) stages of malaria, resulting in a radical cure of the infection.

Chloroquine remains the drug of choice for prophylaxis and treatment of susceptible malaria strains. Chloroquine is active against all five *Plasmodium* species that infect humans *(P. falciparum, P. knowlesi, P. vivax, P. ovale, P. malariae)* and is well tolerated, inexpensive, and effective orally. Unfortunately, resistance of *P. falciparum* to chloroquine is widespread in Asia, Africa, and South America, greatly limiting the use of this agent. Resistance of *P. vivax* to chloroquine has also been reported from Papua New Guinea, the Solomon Islands, Indonesia, and Brazil.

Quinine and quinidine are used primarily to treat chloroquine-resistant *P. falciparum* infection. Presumably they are active against the rare chloroquine-resistant strains of *P. vivax* as well. Quinine is used orally only to treat mild attacks and by the intravenous route to treat acute attacks of MDR *P. falciparum.* Both quinine and quinidine are quite toxic and not rapidly parasiticidal; thus they should not be used alone but rather in combination with a sulfonamide or tetracycline antibiotic with antimalarial activity.

Mefloquine is a 4-quinolinemethanol antimalarial agent used for prophylaxis and treatment of falciparum malaria. It displays a high level of activity against most chloroquine-resistant parasites. Unfortunately, mefloquine-resistant strains of falciparum malaria have been reported from Southeast Asia and Africa.

Halofantrine is a synthetic phenanthrene-methanol compound with proven efficacy in the treatment of *P. vivax* and *P. falciparum* malaria. Because of its toxicity, it is not recommended for prophylaxis of malaria. Halofantrine is more active than mefloquine; however, cross-resistance between these drugs occurs. It is considered a second-line agent for the treatment of malaria because of its expense and toxicity.

Lumefantrine is also a phenanthrene-methanol compound that is available only as a fixed formulation combined with artemether. Recent studies from Cambodia have raised the possibility of declining efficacy to artemether-lumefantrine, with failure rates for the treatment of *P. falciparum* infection between 15% to 30%. Studies are ongoing to determine the contributing factors underlying this.

Folic Acid Antagonists

Similar to other organisms, protozoan parasites require folic acid for the synthesis of nucleic acids and ultimately DNA. Protozoa are unable to absorb exogenous folate and thus are susceptible to drugs that inhibit folate synthesis. The folic acid **antagonists** that are useful in treating protozoan infections include diaminopyrimidines (pyrimethamine and trimethoprim) and sulfonamides. These compounds block separate steps in the folic acid pathway. Sulfonamides inhibit the conversion of aminobenzoic acid to dihydropteroic acid. The diaminopyrimidines inhibit dihydrofolate reductase, which effectively blocks synthesis of tetrahydrofolate, a precursor necessary for the formation of purines, pyrimidines, and certain amino acids. These agents are effective at concentrations far below those needed to inhibit the mammalian enzyme, so selectivity can be attained. When a diaminopyrimidine is used with a sulfonamide, a **synergistic effect** is achieved via the blockade of two steps in the same metabolic pathway, resulting in very effective inhibition of protozoan growth.

The diaminopyrimidine trimethoprim is used with sulfamethoxazole to treat toxoplasmosis. Another diaminopyrimidine, pyrimethamine, has a high affinity for sporozoan dihydrofolate reductase and has been very effective when combined with a sulfonamide in the treatment of malaria and toxoplasmosis. Resistance to antifolates is due to specific point mutations at the active site of the parasite's dihydrofolate reductase and has been largely confined to species of plasmodia.

Inhibitors of Protein Synthesis

Several antibiotics that inhibit protein synthesis in bacteria also exhibit antiparasitic activity in vitro and in vivo. These agents include clindamycin, spiramycin, tetracycline, and doxycycline.

Clindamycin and the tetracyclines are active against *Plasmodium* species, *Babesia* species, and amebae. Doxycycline is used for chemoprophylaxis of chloroquine-resistant *P. falciparum* malaria, and tetracycline may be used with quinine for the treatment of chloroquine-resistant *P. falciparum* infection. Clindamycin may be useful in the treatment of central nervous system toxoplasmosis. Spiramycin is recommended as an alternative to the antifolates in the treatment of toxoplasmosis. Although spiramycin appears active against *Cryptosporidium* species in vitro, it has not been shown to be effective clinically for human cryptosporidiosis. Recent studies suggest that paromomycin, an older aminoglycoside, may be at least partially effective in treating cryptosporidiosis. Paromomycin, which is not systemically absorbed, is also used as a secondary drug in amebiasis and giardiasis. Recently it has been shown that treatment of the filarial parasite *Onchocerca volvulus* with doxycycline causes inhibition of worm development, blocks embryogenesis and fertility, and reduces viability. The activity of doxycycline in this organism is due to its action on the *Wolbachia* bacterial symbiont that is integral to the biology of the parasite and the disease pathogenesis.

Diamidines

Pentamidine, a diamidine, is a relatively toxic agent. Pentamidine is a polycation and may interact with DNA, or it may interfere with the uptake and function of polyamines.

Pentamidine is effective in treating the tissue forms of leishmania and the early (pre–central nervous system) forms of African trypanosomiasis. Pentamidine does not penetrate the central nervous system and therefore is not useful in the late stages of infection with *Trypanosoma brucei gambiense*. Pentamidine may also inhibit kinetoplast topoisomerase II activity and may act against trypanosomes in part by this mechanism.

Nitroimidazoles

The nitroimidazoles include the well-known antibacterial agent metronidazole, as well as benznidazole and tinidazole. The mechanism of action of these compounds is unclear. It has been suggested that they inhibit DNA and ribonucleic acid (RNA) synthesis and also inhibit the metabolism of glucose and interfere with mitochondrial function. Metronidazole binds to parasite guanine and cytosine residues, causing the loss of helical structure and breakage of DNA strands.

The nitroimidazoles have excellent penetration into body tissues and therefore are particularly effective for the treatment of disseminated amebiasis. Metronidazole is the drug of choice for trichomoniasis and is effective in the treatment of giardiasis. Benznidazole is used for the treatment of acute Chagas disease and may have benefits in chronic disease as well. Tinidazole appears to be more effective and less mutagenic than metronidazole. Tinidazole has recently been approved by the U.S. Food and Drug Administration (FDA) for the treatment of amebiasis, giardiasis, and vaginal trichomoniasis.

Sesquiterpenes

The sesquiterpenes are antimicrobial agents that are represented by the artemisinins, artemether, and artesunate. These agents react with the heme moiety, causing **free-radical damage** to parasite membranes. The artemisinins are the most active of the available antimalarial compounds and produce a fractional reduction in parasite biomass of approximately 10^4 per asexual cycle. Artemisinins have efficacy against small-ring forms as well as maturing schizonts of both *P. vivax* and *P. falciparum,* stages that are less susceptible to quinolines or quinine. The earlier-stage ring forms are immediately cleared (within 6 to 12 hours) after exposure to artemisinins. The artemisinin derivatives also have the advantage of reducing gametocyte carriage and thus transmission. These agents are highly effective when used in combination with mefloquine, halofantrine, or lumefantrine in the treatment of severe malaria, including that caused by MDR *P. falciparum.* Artemisinin-based combination treatments are now considered the best therapy for falciparum malaria, combining unrelated compounds with different molecular targets (and thus different potential mechanisms of resistance), thereby delaying the emergence of resistances. Of interest is the apparent efficacy of mefloquine-artesunate in the treatment of schistosomiasis, a helminth infection.

Atovaquone-Proguanil (Malarone)

Atovaquone is a hydroxynaphthoquinone, and proguanil is an antifolate. The combination of these two agents, Malarone, is used for the prophylaxis and treatment of malaria. Atovaquone inhibits the electron transport system in the mitochondria of parasites, thus blocking nucleic acid synthesis and inhibiting replication. Proguanil selectively inhibits plasmodial dihydrofolate reductase; however, in combination with atovaquone, it directly lowers the effective concentration at which atovaquone causes collapse of the mitochondrial membrane potential. Malarone is effective against all stages of development of *P. falciparum* and is recommended for prophylaxis and treatment of falciparum malaria. It is also active against the erythrocytic stages of *P. vivax* and *P. ovale* and shows good efficacy in the treatment of *P. malariae* infections. There are a few reports of clinical failure and resistance of *P. falciparum* isolates to Malarone associated with a single gene mutation.

Miltefosine

Miltefosine is an oral phosphocholine analog used for the treatment of visceral leishmaniasis. It is becoming increasingly important because of the growing resistance of *Leishmania* strains to the pentavalent antimonials. Miltefosine interferes with cell signaling, appears to act on key enzymes involved in the metabolism of ether lipids present on the surface of parasites, and induces apoptotic cell death, but the exact mechanisms of its parasiticidal activity are unknown. Miltefosine is active against both pentavalent antimonial-resistant and -susceptible strains of *L. donovani* and has been found to have a cure rate of 94% to 97% at 6 months in patients with visceral leishmaniasis. Resistance is due to decreased uptake of the drug. In addition to *Leishmania* spp., miltefosine has activity against *Trypanosoma cruzi, T. brucei, Entamoeba histolytica,* and *Acanthamoeba* spp. Miltefosine was approved in 2014 by the FDA for treatment of visceral, mucocutaneous, and cutaneous forms of leishmaniasis.

Nitazoxanide

Nitazoxanide is a novel 5-nitrothiazole derivative with broad-spectrum activity against numerous intestinal protozoa and helminths. Nitazoxanide inhibits pyruvate-ferredoxin oxidoreductase, an enzyme essential to anaerobic energy metabolism in protozoa, as well as anaerobic bacteria. The mechanism of action of this agent against helminths is unknown. Nitazoxanide is licensed in the United States for the treatment of cryptosporidiosis and giardiasis in immunocompetent individuals older than 12 months. It also has been shown to be effective in vitro and/or in vivo against infections caused by many enteric protozoa and helminths, including *Ascaris lumbricoides, Balantidium coli, Blastocystis, Cyclospora cayetanensis, Echinococcus* spp., *E. histolytica, Fasciola hepatica,* hookworms, *Hymenolepis nana, Cystoisospora belli, Taenia saginata, Trichomonas vaginalis,* and *Trichuris trichiura.*

Other Antiprotozoal Agents

A number of additional agents used in therapy, their mechanisms of action (if known), and clinical use are listed in Table 72-2.

Anthelmintic Agents

The strategy for the use of anthelmintic drugs is quite different from that for the use of drugs for treating most protozoal infections. Most anthelmintic drugs are targeted at **nonproliferating** adult organisms, whereas with protozoa the targets are generally younger, more rapidly proliferating cells. The helminthic life cycle is frequently quite complex, and the adaptation to survival in the human host depends strongly on (1) neuromuscular coordination for feeding movements and for maintenance of a favorable location of the worm within the host, (2) carbohydrate metabolism as the major source of energy, with glucose the primary substrate, and (3) microtubular integrity, because egg laying and hatching, larval development, glucose transport, and enzyme activity and secretion are impaired when microtubules are modified. Most anthelmintic agents are targeted at one of these biochemical functions in the adult organism.

The mechanisms of action and clinical indications for common anthelmintic agents are listed in Table 72-2.

Benzimidazoles

The benzimidazoles are broad-spectrum anthelmintic agents and include mebendazole, thiabendazole triclabendazole, and albendazole. The basic structure of these agents consists of linked imidazole and benzene rings. Three mechanisms of action have been proposed for the benzimidazoles: (1) inhibition of fumarate reductase, (2) inhibition of glucose transport, resulting in glycogen depletion, cessation of ATP formation, and paralysis or death, and (3) disruption of microtubular function. Benzimidazoles block the assembly of tubulin dimers into tubulin polymers in a process mimicked by colchicine, a powerful antimitotic and embryotoxic drug. Because tubulin is important for parasite motility, drugs such as the benzimidazoles, which bind to parasite tubulin, are thought to act against nematode parasites by reducing or eliminating their motility.

The benzimidazoles have a wide spectrum of activity, including intestinal nematodes *(Ascaris, Trichuris, Necator,* and *Ancylostoma* spp.; *Enterobius vermicularis),* as well as a number of cestodes (*Taenia, Hymenolepis,* and *Echinococcus* spp.). Triclabendazole is the agent of choice for fascioliasis and is an alternative to praziquantel for therapy of paragonimiasis and intestinal flukes. Mebendazole is active against the intestinal nematodes and the cestodes previously listed. Thiabendazole is active against a variety of nematodes, but frequent and severe side effects have limited its primary systemic use to the treatment of strongyloidiasis. Albendazole has a spectrum similar to that of mebendazole and may have greater activity against *Echinococcus* species. In addition to its broad-spectrum anthelmintic activity, albendazole also has activity against *Giardia* species. Albendazole is being increasingly used in combination with either diethylcarbamazine or ivermectin for treatment of filariasis and loiasis; it is especially useful for these infections as part of a single-dose regimen for mass chemotherapy programs.

Tetrahydropyrimidines

Pyrantel pamoate, a tetrahydropyrimidine, is a cholinergic agonist that has a powerful effect on nematode muscle cells by binding to cholinergic receptors, which results in cell depolarization and muscle contraction. This **paralytic action** on intestinal nematodes leads to expulsion of the worm from the host intestinal tract.

Pyrantel pamoate is not readily absorbed from the intestine and is active against *Ascaris* species, pinworm, and hookworm. An analog of pyrantel, oxantel, may be used with pyrantel to provide effective therapy for the three major soil-transmitted nematodes: *Ascaris* species, hookworm, and *Trichuris* species.

Piperazines

The piperazine anthelmintic used most commonly is diethylcarbamazine (DEC). DEC is predominantly a microfilaricidal agent that is thought to act by stimulating cholinergic receptors and depolarizing muscle cells, with subsequent paralysis of the worms. However, additional evidence suggests that it enhances the adherence of leukocytes to microfilariae and thus may act by altering the parasite surface membrane or by directly stimulating phagocytic cells.

DEC is active against the filariae that produce river blindness *(O. volvulus)* and lymphatic filariasis (*Wuchereria bancrofti* and *Brugia malayi*). Unfortunately, destruction of the microfilariae in the tissues may increase the pathology to the host because of the inflammatory response to the parasite antigens released on exposure to DEC. Recent information suggests that single-dose treatment with DEC may produce antiparasitic effects similar to those obtained with 14- to 21-day courses, without the severe side effects observed with the multidose regimens. In addition to its use as individual therapy for filarial infections, DEC is also used for mass community chemotherapy programs either alone or in combination with ivermectin or albendazole.

Avermectins

Ivermectin, an avermectin, acts by interacting with the chloride channel in nerve and muscle cell membranes, resulting in hyperpolarization of the affected cells and consequent paralysis and death of the parasites. The drug also inhibits the reproductive function of the adult female *O. volvulus* and alters the ability of the *O. volvulus* microfilariae to evade the host immune system.

Although ivermectin is used extensively to control gut-dwelling nematode infections in domestic and farm animals, its use in humans is limited primarily to treating ocular and lymphatic filariasis. Ivermectin is effective in the treatment of strongyloidiasis, as well as several common intestinal parasitic nematodes, including *Ascaris, Trichuris,* and *Enterobius* species. When used to treat filariasis, ivermectin has fewer side effects than DEC, and a single dose can eliminate microfilariae for up to 6 months. Ivermectin has a dramatic effect on the tissue-dwelling microfilariae of *O. volvulus* and reduces the severity of the ocular pathology seen in onchocerciasis. Because of its ability to markedly reduce the number of microfilariae in the skin of people with onchocerciasis, ivermectin has been effective in reducing the transmission of onchocerciasis in endemic areas.

Pyrazinoisoquinolines

Praziquantel, a pyrazinoisoquinoline, is an anthelmintic active against a broad spectrum of trematodes and cestodes. The drug is rapidly taken up by susceptible helminths, in which it acts as a **calcium agonist.** The entry of calcium into various cells results in elevated intracellular calcium levels, tetanic muscular contraction, and destruction of the tegument. Praziquantel appears to act with the host immune system to produce a synergistic anthelmintic effect. The drug causes disruption of the parasite surface and tegument, allowing antibodies to attack parasite antigens not normally exposed on the surface (Figure 72-1). Irreversible damage to the parasite probably occurs when complement or host leukocytes are recruited to the sites where antibody is bound.

Praziquantel has extremely broad-spectrum activity against trematodes, including *Fasciolopsis, Clonorchis, Opisthorchis, Paragonimus,* and *Schistosoma* species. It is also active against cestodes, including *Echinococcus, Taenia,* and *Dipylidium* species. Praziquantel is the drug of choice for the treatment of schistosomiasis, clonorchiasis, opisthorchiasis, and intestinal fluke infections. There is now reliable evidence that praziquantel reduces hepatosplenomegaly and portal hypertension in schistosomiasis. Most tapeworm infections respond to praziquantel. Praziquantel is also used in the treatment of neurocysticercosis and echinococcal infections, either alone or in combination with albendazole.

Phenols

Niclosamide, a phenol, is a nonabsorbable anthelmintic with selective activity against intestinal tapeworms. The drug is absorbed by gut-dwelling cestodes but not by nematodes. It acts by uncoupling oxidative phosphorylation in mitochondria, resulting in a loss of helminth ATP that ultimately immobilizes the parasite so that it is expelled with the feces. Niclosamide is effective in the treatment of intestinal tapeworms in humans and animals.

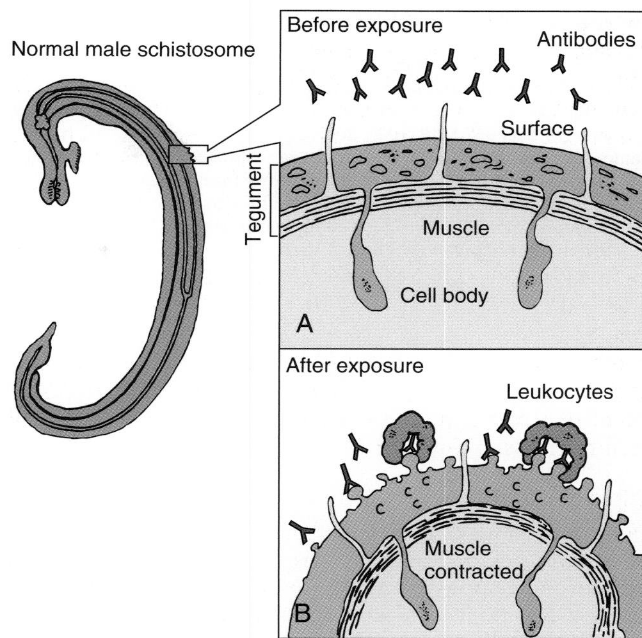

FIGURE 72-1 Before exposure to praziquantel, the schistosome is capable of avoiding the numerous antibodies directed toward surface and internally located antigens. **A,** Cross-section of the dorsal surface of a normal male schistosome. Within 1 to 2 seconds after exposure to praziquantel, the muscles of the schistosome contract because of a drug-induced influx of calcium ions into the schistosome tegument. **B,** The change in permeability of the schistosome surface toward external ions initiates the appearance of small holes and balloon-like structures, making the parasite vulnerable to antibody-mediated adherence of host leukocytes that kill the helminth. (From Wecker L, Crespo L, Dunaway G, et al: *Brody's human pharmacology: molecular to clinical,* ed 5, Philadelphia, 2010, Mosby.)

Other Anthelmintic Agents

Additional anthelmintic agents, including oxamniquine, metrifonate, and suramin, are described in Table 72-2. These agents are generally considered secondary agents for the treatment of trematode (oxamniquine and metrifonate) and filarial (suramin) infections.

Bibliography

Abubakar I, Aliyu SH, Arumugam C, et al: Treatment of cryptosporidiosis in immunocompromised individuals: systematic review and meta-analysis, *Brit J Clin Pharmacol* 63:387–393, 2007.

Baird JK: Resistance to therapies for infection by *Plasmodium vivax*, *Clin Microbiol Rev* 22:508–534, 2009.

Croft SL, Sundar S, Fairlamb AH: Drug resistance in leishmaniasis, *Clin Microbiol Rev* 19:111–126, 2006.

Edwards G, Krishna S: Pharmacokinetic and pharmacodynamic issues in the treatment of parasitic infections, *Eur J Clin Microbiol Infect Dis* 23:233–242, 2004.

Gardner TB, Hill DR: Treatment of giardiasis, *Clin Microbiol Rev* 14:114–128, 2001.

Hastings I: How artemisinin-containing combination therapies slow the spread of antimalarial drug resistance, *Trends Parasitol* 27:67–72, 2011.

Hotez PJ, Molyneux DH, Fenwick A: Control of neglected tropical diseases, *N Engl J Med* 357:1018–1027, 2007.

James CE, Hudson AL, Davey MW: Drug resistance mechanisms in helminths: is it survival of the fittest? *Trends Parasitol* 25:328–335, 2009.

Leder K, Weller PF: Antiparasitic agents. In Versalovic J, et al, editors: *Manual of clinical microbiology*, ed 10, Washington, DC, 2011, American Society for Microbiology Press.

Lin JT, Juliano JJ, Wongsrichanalai C: Drug-resistant malaria: the era of ACT, *Curr Infect Dis Rep* 12:165–173, 2010.

Secor WE, Le Bras J: Mechanisms of resistance to antiparasitic agents. In Versalovic J, et al, editors: *Manual of clinical microbiology*, ed 10, Washington, DC, 2011, American Society for Microbiology Press.

Talisuna AO, Bloland P, D'Alessandro U: History, dynamics, and public health importance of malaria parasite resistance, *Clin Microbiol Rev* 178:235–254, 2004.

Wecker L, Crespo L, Dunaway G, et al: *Brody's human pharmacology: molecular to clinical*, ed 5, Philadelphia, 2010, Mosby.

CHAPTER

INTESTINAL AND UROGENITAL PROTOZOA

A 31-year-old female veterinarian complained of diarrhea of 2 weeks' duration. She described the diarrhea as thin, watery, and non-bloody. She reported 10 to 14 diarrheal stools per day, the frequency of which was not influenced by a variety of over-the-counter antidiarrheal medications. Physical examination revealed a well-developed, well-nourished woman who appeared somewhat fatigued and mildly dehydrated. The workup included a negative human immunodeficiency virus (HIV) serologic test, a normal flexible sigmoidoscope examination, and a negative stool culture for bacterial pathogens. A microscopic examination of the stool for white blood cells was negative, as was a test for *Clostridium difficile* toxin. A stool specimen was sent for ova and parasite examination and, after appropriate concentration measures, demonstrated acid-fast oocysts.

1. Which parasite was found in the patient's stool?
2. What was the likely source of this individual's infection?
3. If this individual were HIV positive, what other intestinal pathogens would have been considered?
4. Other than conventional microscopy, what other methods could have been used to diagnose this infection?
5. Should this patient have received specific antimicrobial therapy? If so, what would have been prescribed? If not, why not?

Answers to these questions are available on StudentConsult.com.

• SUMMARIES CLINICALLY SIGNIFICANT ORGANISMS

Amebae

Trigger Words

Protozoa, amebae, trophozoite, cyst, intestinal amebiasis, extraintestinal amebiasis, hepatic amebiasis, flask-shaped ulcer, *Entamoeba*

Biology, Virulence, and Disease

- Primitive unicellular organisms with a simple two-stage life cycle
- Motility accomplished by extension of a pseudopod (false foot)
- Most amebae found in humans are commensal organisms
- Human pathogens: *Entamoeba histolytica* (most important), *E. polecki*

Epidemiology

- *E. histolytica* has worldwide distribution, with highest incidence in tropical and subtropical regions
- As many as 50% of population in some areas are infected (average prevalence, 10% to 15%); U.S. prevalence is 1% to 2%
- Many carriers asymptomatic; pass cysts in stool (reservoir)
- Main source of food and water contamination is asymptomatic carrier who passes cysts

Diagnosis

- Microscopic examination of stool allows identification of cysts and trophozoites of *E. histolytica*
- Must differentiate from nonpathogenic and commensal species of amebae
- Specific serologic tests can confirm diagnosis
- Examination of stool samples may be negative in extraintestinal amebiasis
- Newer diagnostic approaches: fecal antigen, PCR, DNA probe

Treatment, Prevention, and Control

- Acute amebiasis treated with metronidazole, followed by iodoquinol, diloxanide furoate, or paromomycin
- Carrier state may be eradicated with iodoquinol, diloxanide furoate, or paromomycin
- Elimination of cycle of infection requires introduction of adequate sanitation measures, education about routes of transmission, chlorination, and filtration of water supplies
- Travelers to developing countries should avoid consumption of water (including ice cubes), avoid unpeeled fruits and raw vegetables, boil water, and thoroughly clean fruits and vegetables before consumption

Flagellates

Trigger Words

Giardiasis, trichomoniasis, worm egg, contaminated stream, stool antigen test, flagella, wet mount, diarrhea, IgA deficiency

Biology, Virulence, and Disease

- Clinically important flagellates: *Giardia duodenalis (lamblia/intestinalis), Dientamoeba fragilis, Trichomonas vaginalis*

- *Giardia duodenalis* life cycle has both cyst and trophozoite stages; *D. fragilis* has a trophozoite stage (cyst stage in mice); *T. vaginalis* has only trophozoite stage
- Most flagellates move by lashing of flagella that pull organism through fluid environments
- Infection with *G. duodenalis* initiated by ingestion of cysts; asymptomatic carriage (50% of infected individuals); symptomatic disease ranges from mild diarrhea to a severe malabsorption syndrome
- Most infections with *D. fragilis* asymptomatic
- *T. vaginalis* causes urogenital infections
- Diseases produced by flagellates result from mechanical irritation, inflammation of gastrointestinal and genitourinary *(Trichomonas)* mucosa

Epidemiology

- *G. duodenalis* has a worldwide distribution
- Giardiasis acquired by fecal-oral route
- Risk factors for giardiasis: poor sanitary conditions, travel to known endemic areas, consumption of inadequately treated water, day-care centers, oral-anal sexual practices
- *D. fragilis* has a worldwide distribution; transmission by fecal-oral and oral-anal routes
- *T. vaginalis* has a worldwide distribution; transmission primarily by sexual intercourse

Diagnosis

- *Giardia* may be detected by microscopic examination of fecal samples or duodenal aspirates
- Detection of *Giardia* fecal antigen by enzyme immunoassay, immunofluorescent microscopy
- Infection with *D. fragilis* diagnosed by microscopic examination of fecal specimens
- Trichomoniasis: microscopic examination of vaginal or urethral discharge

Treatment, Prevention, and Control

- Drug of choice for treatment of giardiasis (both symptomatic patients and carriers): metronidazole or nitazoxanide; alternatives: furazolidone, tinidazole, paromomycin, albendazole, quinacrine
- Prevention and control of giardiasis involves avoidance of contaminated water and food
- No consensus on best approach for treating *D. fragilis* infections; infection can be avoided by adequate sanitary conditions
- Drug of choice for trichomoniasis is metronidazole; personal hygiene, avoidance of shared toilet articles and clothing, and safe sexual practices are important preventive actions

Ciliates

Trigger Words

Macronucleus, pig feces, cytostome, cilia, intestinal ulceration

Biology, Virulence, and Disease

- Protozoan organisms whose locomotion involves coordinated movement of rows of hairlike structures (cilia)
- Cilia structurally similar to flagella but usually shorter and more numerous
- *Balantidium coli:* only ciliate parasite of humans
- Disease produced by *B. coli* is similar to amebiasis; symptoms include abdominal pain, tenderness, tenesmus, nausea, anorexia, watery stools with blood and pus, ulceration of intestinal mucosa; extraintestinal infection very rare

Epidemiology

- *B. coli* distributed worldwide; swine and monkeys most important reservoirs
- Infections transmitted by fecal-oral route
- Outbreaks associated with contamination of water supplies with pig feces
- Person-to person spread has been implicated in outbreaks
- Risk factors include contact with swine and substandard hygienic conditions

Diagnosis

- Microscopic examination of feces for trophozoites and cysts

Treatment, Prevention, and Control

- Drug of choice is tetracycline; iodoquinol and metronidazole are alternatives
- Important preventive measures: personal hygiene, maintenance of sanitary conditions, careful monitoring of pig feces

Sporozoa

Trigger Words

Coccidia, oocyst, chronic diarrhea, acid-fast, fecal antigen, waterborne transmission, contaminated fruits and vegetables

Biology, Virulence, and Disease

- Sporozoa constitute a very large group of protozoa called Apicomplexa or Coccidia
- All sporozoans demonstrate typical characteristics: asexual (schizogony) and sexual (gametogony) reproduction; share alternative hosts
- Intestinal sporozoa: *Cystoisospora belli, Sarcocystis* spp., *Cryptosporidium* spp., *Cyclospora cayetanensis*
- *Cystoisospora belli:* coccidian parasite of intestinal epithelium; causes malabsorption syndrome
- *Sarcocystis* spp. can be detected in stool samples; nausea, abdominal pain, and diarrhea following ingestion of infected meat; muscular infections can occur if sporocysts ingested
- *Cryptosporidium* spp. cause intestinal disease, usually self-limited enterocolitis characterized by watery diarrhea without blood
- *Cyclospora:* illness self-limited in immunocompetent hosts, prolonged in HIV-infected individuals

Epidemiology

- *Cystoisospora* organisms distributed worldwide; disease frequent in patients with AIDS; infection reported with increasing frequency in both healthy and immuno-compromised patients
- *Sarcocystis* spp. are isolated from pigs and cattle
- *Cryptosporidium* spp. are distributed worldwide
- *C. hominis* and *C. parvum* cause most human infections; *C. ubiquitum* and *C. felis* are emerging human pathogens
- *Cyclospora:* worldwide distribution; infection acquired through contaminated water; U.S. outbreaks correlated with consumption of contaminated fruits and vegetables

Diagnosis

- *Cystoisospora belli* infection best diagnosed by careful examination of concentrated stool sediment
- *Sarcocystis* spp. sporocysts may be detected in human stool specimens
- *Cryptosporidium* spp. may be detected in unconcentrated stool specimens from immunocompromised patients with diarrhea
- Diagnosis of cyclosporiasis is based on microscopic detection of oocysts in stool
- Both *Cryptosporidium* and *Cyclospora* infections may be diagnosed by PCR

Treatment, Prevention, and Control

- *C. belli:* treatment of choice is trimethoprim-sulfamethoxazole; prevention and control effected by maintaining personal hygiene and sanitation, avoiding oral-anal sexual contact
- No known treatment for intestinal or muscular sarcocystosis in humans
- No broadly effective therapy has been developed for managing *Cryptosporidium* infections in immunocompromised patients
- Cyclosporiasis has been treated with modest success using trimethoprim-sulfamethoxazole

Protozoa may colonize and infect the oropharynx, duodenum and small bowel, colon, and urogenital tract of humans. The majority of these parasites belong to the amebae and flagellates; however, infection with ciliate and coccidian parasites may also be encountered (Table 73-1). These organisms are transmitted by the **fecal-oral route.** In the United States, transmission of intestinal protozoa is particularly problematic in day-care centers, where several outbreaks of diarrhea caused by *Giardia* or *Cryptosporidium* spp. have been documented. In other parts of the world, the spread of enteric protozoal infections may be controlled in part by improved sanitation and by chlorination and filtration of water supplies; however, this may be difficult or impossible in many developing countries.

• Amebae

Amebae are primitive **unicellular** microorganisms. Their life cycle is relatively simple and divided into two stages: the actively motile feeding stage (trophozoite) and the quiescent, resistant, infective stage (cyst). Replication is accomplished by binary fission (splitting the trophozoite) or by the development of numerous trophozoites within the mature multinucleated cyst. Motility is accomplished by extension of a **pseudopod** ("false foot"), with extrusion of the cellular ectoplasm and then drawing up of the rest of the cell in a snail-like movement to meet this pseudopod. The amebic trophozoites remain actively motile as long as the environment is favorable. The cyst form develops when the environmental temperature or moisture level drops.

Most amebae found in humans are **commensal** organisms *(Entamoeba coli, Entamoeba hartmanni, Entamoeba dispar, Entamoeba moshkovskii, Entamoeba gingivalis, Endolimax nana, Iodamoeba bütschlii).* However, *Entamoeba histolytica* is an important human pathogen. Other amebae, particularly *Entamoeba polecki,* can cause human disease but are rarely detected. The pathogenicity of *Blastocystis* spp. is still controversial. Some free-living amebae (*Naegleria fowleri, Acanthamoeba* spp.) are present in soil and in warm freshwater ponds or swimming pools and can be opportunistic human pathogens, causing meningoencephalitis or keratitis (see Chapter 74).

Table 73-1 Morphologic Identification of *Entamoeba histolytica* and *Entamoeba coli*

	*E. histolytica**	*E. coli*
Size (diameter, μm)		
Trophozoite	12-50 μm	20-30 μm
Cyst	10-20 μm	10-30 μm
Pattern of peripheral nuclear chromatin	Fine, dispersed ring	Coarse, clumped
Karyosome	Central, sharp	Eccentric, coarse
Ingested erythrocytes	Present	Absent
Cyst Structure		
No. of nuclei	1-4	1-8
Chromatoidal bars	Rounded ends	Splintered, frayed ends

**E. histolytica* is morphologically indistinguishable from the commensal species *Entamoeba dispar, Entamoeba moshkovskii,* and *Entamoeba bangladeshi.*

Entamoeba histolytica

Physiology and Structure

Cyst and trophozoite forms of *E. histolytica* are detected in fecal specimens from infected patients (Figure 73-1). Trophozoites can also be found in the crypts of the large intestine. In freshly passed stools, actively motile trophozoites can be seen, whereas in formed stools, the cysts are usually the only form recognized. For the diagnosis of amebiasis, distinguishing between the *E. histolytica* trophozoites and cysts and those of commensal amebae is important.

Pathogenesis

After ingestion, the cysts pass through the stomach, where exposure to gastric acid stimulates release of the pathogenic trophozoite in the duodenum. The trophozoites divide and produce extensive local necrosis in the large intestine. The basis for this tissue destruction is incompletely understood, although it is attributed to production of a **cytotoxin.** Attachment of *E. histolytica* trophozoites to host cells via a galactose-inhibitable adherence protein is required for cytolysis and tissue necrosis to occur. The lysis of colonic epithelial cells, human neutrophils, lymphocytes, and monocytes by trophozoites is associated with a lethal alteration of host cell membrane permeability, resulting in an irreversible increase in intracellular calcium levels. The release of toxic neutrophil constituents after the lysis of neutrophils may contribute to tissue destruction. Flask-shaped ulcerations of the intestinal mucosa are present with inflammation, hemorrhage, and secondary bacterial infection. Invasion into the deeper mucosa with extension into the peritoneal cavity may occur.

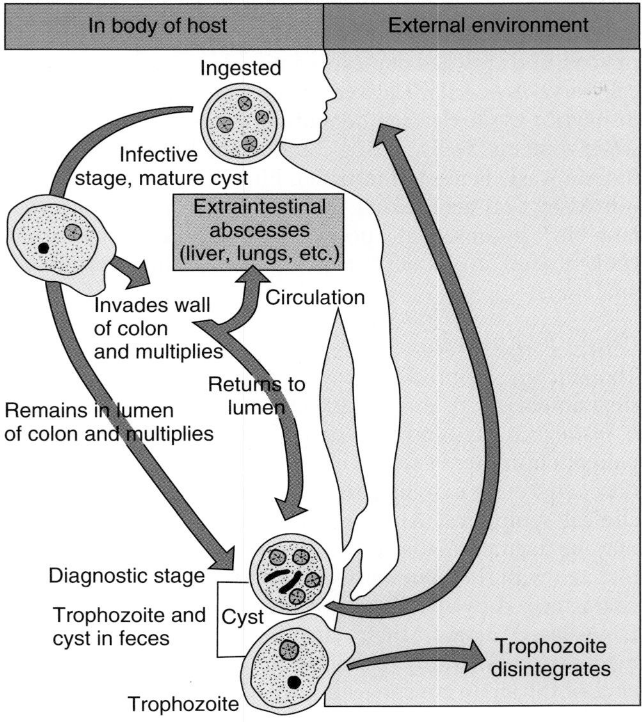

FIGURE 73-1 Life cycle of *Entamoeba histolytica.*

This can lead to secondary involvement of other organs, primarily the liver but also the lungs, brain, and heart. Extraintestinal amebiasis is associated with trophozoites. Amebae are found only in environments that have a low oxygen pressure, because the protozoa are killed by ambient oxygen concentrations.

Lectin binding, zymodeme analysis, genome deoxyribonucleic acid (DNA) analysis, and staining with specific monoclonal antibodies have been used as markers to identify invasive strains of *E. histolytica.* It is now recognized that the ameba morphologically identified as *E. histolytica* is actually four distinct species. The pathogenic species is *E. histolytica,* and the nonpathogenic species are *E. dispar, E. moshkovskii,* and *E. bangladeshi.* The zymodeme profiles and biochemical, molecular, and immunologic differences are stable and support the existence of four species. Of note, these four species are morphologically indistinguishable from one another.

Epidemiology

E. histolytica has a worldwide distribution. Although it is found in cold areas such as Alaska, Canada, and Eastern Europe, its incidence is highest in tropical and subtropical regions that have poor sanitation and contaminated water. The average prevalence of infection in these areas is 10% to 15%, with as many as 50% of the population infected in some areas. Many of the infected individuals are asymptomatic carriers who represent a reservoir for the spread of *E. histolytica* to others. The prevalence of infection in the United States is 1% to 2%.

Patients infected with *E. histolytica* pass noninfectious trophozoites and the infectious cysts in their stools. The trophozoites cannot survive in the external environment or in transport through the stomach if ingested. Therefore the main source of water and food contamination is the asymptomatic carrier who passes cysts. This is a particular problem in hospitals for the mentally ill, military and refugee camps, prisons, and crowded day-care centers. Flies and cockroaches can serve as mechanical vectors for the transmission of *E. histolytica* cysts. Sewage containing cysts can contaminate water systems, wells, springs, and agricultural areas where human waste is used as fertilizer. Finally, cysts can be transmitted by oral-anal sexual practices, with amebiasis prevalent in homosexual populations. Direct trophozoite transmission in sexual encounters can produce cutaneous amebiasis.

Clinical Syndromes

The outcome of infection may result in a carrier state, intestinal amebiasis, or extraintestinal amebiasis. If the strain of *E. histolytica* has a low virulence, the inoculum is low, or the patient's immune system is intact, the organisms may reproduce, and cysts may be passed in stool specimens, with no clinical symptoms. Although infections with *E. histolytica* may be asymptomatic, most asymptomatic individuals are infected with the noninvasive *E. dispar* or *E. moshkovskii,* as characterized by specific isoenzyme profiles (zymodemes), DNA-based assays, their susceptibility to complement-mediated lysis, and their failure to agglutinate in the presence of the lectin concanavalin A. Detection of carriers of *E. histolytica* in areas with low endemicity is important for epidemiologic purposes.

Patients with intestinal amebiasis develop clinical symptoms related to localized tissue destruction in the large intestine. These include abdominal pain, cramping, and colitis with diarrhea. More severe disease is characterized by numerous bloody stools per day. Systemic signs of infection (fever, leukocytosis, rigors) are present in patients with extraintestinal amebiasis. The liver is primarily involved because trophozoites in the blood are removed as they pass through this organ. Abscess formation is common (Clinical Case 73-1). The right lobe is most commonly involved. Pain over the liver, with hepatomegaly and elevation of the diaphragm, is observed.

Laboratory Diagnosis

Identification of *E. histolytica* trophozoites (Figure 73-2) and cysts in stools and trophozoites in tissue is diagnostic of amebic infection. Care must be taken to distinguish between these amebae and commensal amebae, as well as between these amebae and polymorphonuclear leukocytes. Microscopic examination of stool specimens is inherently insensitive because the protozoa are not usually distributed homogeneously in the specimen, and the parasites are concentrated in the intestinal ulcers and at the margins of the abscess, not in the stool or the necrotic center of the abscess. For this reason, multiple stool specimens should be collected. Extraintestinal amebiasis is sometimes diagnosed using scanning procedures for the liver and other organs. Specific serologic tests, together with microscopic

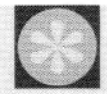

Clinical Case 73-1 **Human Immunodeficiency Virus (HIV) and Amebic Liver Abscess**

Liu and colleagues (*J Clin Gastroenterol* 33:64–68, 2001) described a 45-year-old homosexual man who developed intestinal and hepatic amebiasis. The patient initially presented with intermittent fever followed by right upper quadrant pain and diarrhea. On admission to the hospital, he was afebrile with an elevated white blood cell count and abnormal liver function tests. Stool examinations were positive for occult blood and white blood cells. He underwent colonoscopy, and multiple discrete ulcers were detected in the rectum and colon. The diagnosis of amebic colitis was confirmed by the demonstration of numerous trophozoites on histopathologic examination of colon biopsy specimens. Ultrasound examination of the abdomen revealed a large heterogeneous mass within the liver, consistent with an abscess. Percutaneous drainage of the abscess obtained chocolate-like pus, and examination of a biopsy from the margin of the abscess revealed only necrotic material without evidence of amebae. Polymerase chain reaction amplification of amebic 16S ribosomal RNA from the aspirate was positive, indicating infection with *Entamoeba histolytica.* The patient was treated with metronidazole followed by iodoquinol to eradicate the luminal amebae. Subsequent history revealed a history of travel to Thailand 2 months before the onset of the present illness. HIV serology was positive as well. The patient improved rapidly on antiamebic therapy and was discharged on antiretroviral therapy.

Although amebic cysts are frequently detected in the stools of homosexual men, previous studies in Western countries suggested that almost all isolates belonged to the nonpathogenic species *Entamoeba dispar,* and invasive amebiasis was considered rare in HIV-positive individuals. This case illustrates that invasive amebiasis, such as amebic liver abscess and colitis, can accompany HIV infection. The possible association of invasive amebiasis with HIV infection should be kept in mind for patients living in or with a history of travel to areas where *E. histolytica* is endemic.

examination of the abscess material, can confirm the diagnosis. Virtually all patients with hepatic amebiasis and most patients (>80%) with intestinal disease have positive serologic findings at the time of clinical presentation. This may be less useful in endemic areas where the prevalence of positive serologic results is higher. Examinations of stool specimens are frequently negative in extraintestinal disease. In addition to conventional microscopic and serologic tests, researchers have developed several immunologic tests for the detection of fecal antigen, as well as polymerase chain reaction (PCR) and DNA-probe assays for the detection of pathogenic strains of *E. histolytica* (versus nonpathogenic *E. dispar* and *E. moshkovskii*). These newer diagnostic approaches are promising and are now commercially available.

Treatment, Prevention, and Control

Acute fulminating amebiasis is treated with metronidazole, followed by iodoquinol, diloxanide furoate, or paromomycin. Asymptomatic carriage can be eradicated with iodoquinol, diloxanide furoate, or paromomycin. Because human infection results from ingestion of food or water contaminated with human feces or as a result of specific sexual practices, eliminating the cycle of infection requires introduction of adequate sanitation measures and education about the routes of transmission. Chlorination and filtration of water supplies may limit the spread of these and other enteric protozoal infections but are not possible in many developing countries. Physicians should alert travelers to developing countries of the risks associated with consumption of water (including ice cubes), unpeeled fruits, and raw vegetables. Water should be boiled and fruits and vegetables thoroughly cleaned before consumption.

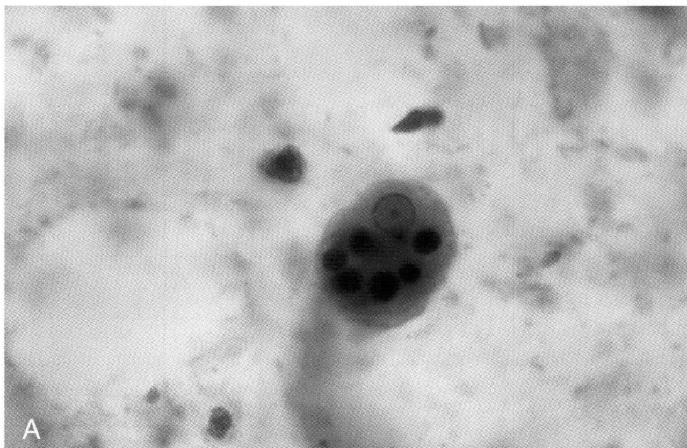

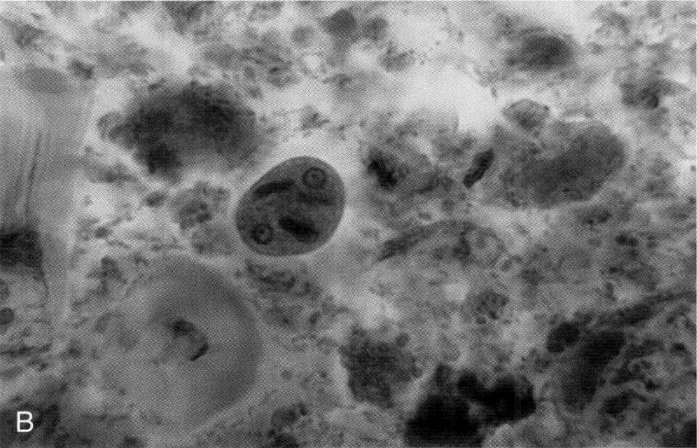

FIGURE 73-2 *Entamoeba histolytica* trophozoite (**A**) and cyst (**B**). Trophozoites are motile and vary in size from 12 to 60 μm (average, 15 to 30 μm). The single nucleus in the cell is round with a central dot (karyosome) and an even distribution of chromatin granules around the nuclear membrane. Ingested erythrocytes may be in the cytoplasm. Cysts are smaller (10 to 20 μm [average, 15 to 20 μm]) and contain one to four nuclei (usually four). Round chromatoidal bars may be in the cytoplasm. (From CDC Public Health Image Library.)

Other Intestinal Amebae

Other amebae that can parasitize the human gastrointestinal tract include *Entamoeba coli, E. hartmanni, E. polecki, E. nana, I. bütschlii,* and *Blastocystis* spp. *E. polecki,* which is primarily a parasite of pigs and monkeys, can cause human disease, a mild transient diarrhea. The diagnosis of *E. polecki* infection is confirmed by microscopic detection of cysts in stool specimens. Treatment is the same as for *E. histolytica* infections.

Blastocystis, previously regarded as a nonpathogenic yeast, is now the center of considerable controversy concerning its taxonomic position and pathogenicity. *Blastocystis* has recently been placed in the kingdom Stramenopila (formerly Chromista), based on analysis of 18S ribosomal ribonucleic acid (rRNA) and other molecular evidence. Clinically there are at least nine subtypes (genotypes) within *Blastocystis.* Recent studies have shown that no group exclusive to humans exists and that all clades have been detected in human stool. Consequently, human isolates of *Blastocystis* that in the past were referred to as *Blastocystis hominis* should be called *Blastocystis* species because there is not a single subtype specific to humans. The organism is found in stool specimens from both asymptomatic individuals and persons with persistent diarrhea. It has been suggested that the presence of large numbers of these parasites (five or more per oil-immersion microscopic field) in the absence of other intestinal pathogens indicates disease. Other investigators have concluded that "symptomatic blastocystosis" is attributable to an undetected pathogen or functional bowel problems. The organism may be detected in wet mounts or trichrome-stained smears of fecal specimens. Treatment with iodoquinol or metronidazole has been successful in eradicating the organisms from the intestine and alleviating symptoms. However, the definitive role of this organism in disease remains to be demonstrated.

The nonpathogenic intestinal amebae are important because they must be differentiated from *E. histolytica, E. polecki,* and *Blastocystis* spp. This is particularly true for *Entamoeba coli,* which is frequently detected in stool specimens collected from patients exposed to contaminated food or water. Accurate identification of intestinal amebae requires careful microscopic examination of the cyst and trophozoite forms present in stained and unstained stool specimens (see Table 73-1). Likewise, differentiation of *E. dispar* and *E. moshkovskii* from *E. histolytica* is now possible using specific immunologic reagents.

• Flagellates

The flagellates of clinical significance include *Giardia duodenalis (lamblia/intestinalis), Dientamoeba fragilis,* and

Trichomonas vaginalis. Nonpathogenic commensal flagellates, such as *Chilomastix mesnili* (enteric) and *Trichomonas tenax* (oral), may also be observed. *Giardia* organisms, similar to *E. histolytica,* have cyst and trophozoite stages in their life cycles. In contrast, no cyst stage has been observed for *Trichomonas* spp. No cyst stage of *D. fragilis* has been observed in humans, although a cyst stage has been observed in mice. Unlike the amebae, most flagellates move by the lashing of flagella that pull the organisms through fluid environments. Diseases produced by flagellates are primarily the result of mechanical irritation and inflammation. For example, *G. duodenalis (lamblia/intestinalis)* attaches to intestinal villi with an adhesive disk, resulting in localized tissue damage. Tissue invasion with extensive tissue destruction, as seen with *E. histolytica,* is rare with flagellates.

Giardia duodenalis (G. lamblia, G. intestinalis)

The literature refers to this organism as *G. duodenalis, G. lamblia,* and *G. intestinalis,* reflecting the ambiguity surrounding the classification and nomenclature of this flagellate. Further studies are necessary to determine species designations or groupings; however, *G. duodenalis* is now the accepted species designation and will be used in this chapter.

Physiology and Structure

Both cyst and trophozoite forms of *G. duodenalis* are detected in fecal specimens from infected patients (Figure 73-3).

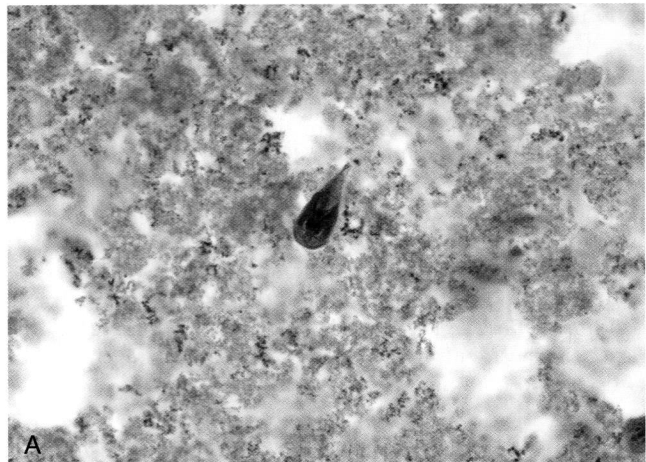

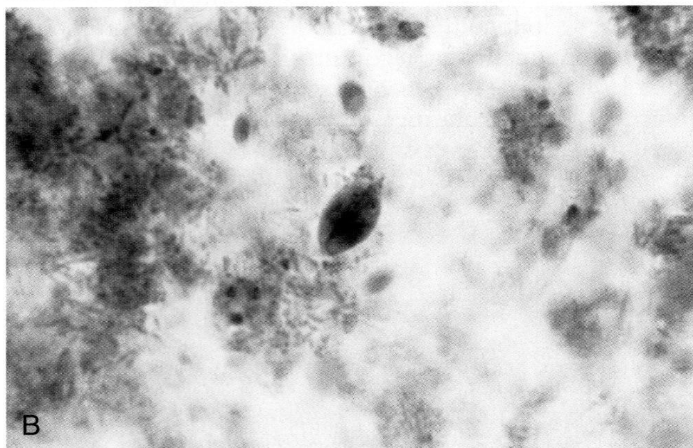

FIGURE 73-3 *Giardia duodenalis* trophozoite **(A)** and cyst **(B)**. Trophozoites are 9 to 12 µm long and 5 to 15 µm wide. Flagella are present, as are two nuclei with large central karyosomes, a large ventral sucking disk for attachment of the flagellate to the intestinal villi, and two oblong parabasal bodies below the nuclei. The morphology gives the appearance that the trophozoites are looking back at the viewer. Cysts are smaller—8 to 12 µm long and 7 to 10 µm wide. Nuclei and parabasal bodies are present. (From CDC Public Health Image Library.)

Pathogenesis

Infection with *G. duodenalis* is initiated by ingestion of cysts (Figure 73-4). The minimum infective dose for humans is estimated to be 10 to 25 cysts. Gastric acid stimulates excystation, with release of trophozoites in the duodenum and jejunum, where the organisms multiply by **binary fission.** Trophozoites can attach to intestinal villi by a prominent ventral sucking disk. Although the tips of the villi may appear flattened and inflammation of the mucosa with hyperplasia of lymphoid follicles may be observed, frank tissue necrosis does not occur. In addition, metastatic spread of disease beyond the gastrointestinal tract is very rare.

Epidemiology

Giardia has a worldwide distribution, and this flagellate has a sylvatic or "wilderness" distribution in many streams, lakes, and mountain resorts. This sylvatic distribution is maintained in reservoir animals such as beavers and muskrats. Giardiasis is acquired by consumption of inadequately treated contaminated water, ingestion of contaminated uncooked vegetables or fruits, or person-to-person spread by the fecal-oral or oral-anal route. The cyst stage is resistant to the chlorine concentrations (1 to 2 parts per million) used in most water treatment facilities. Adequate water treatment should include chemicals plus filtration.

Risk factors associated with *Giardia* infections include poor sanitary conditions, travel to known endemic areas, consumption of inadequately treated water (e.g., from contaminated mountain streams), day-care centers, and oral-anal sexual practices. Infections may occur in outbreak and endemic forms within day-care centers and other institutional settings and among family members of infected children. Scrupulous attention to hand washing and treatment of all infected individuals are important in controlling the spread of infection in these settings.

Clinical Syndromes

Giardia infection can result in either asymptomatic carriage (observed in ≈50% of infected individuals) or symptomatic disease, ranging from mild diarrhea to a severe malabsorption syndrome (Clinical Case 73-2). The incubation period before symptomatic disease develops ranges from 1 to 4 weeks (average, 10 days). The onset of disease is sudden, with foul-smelling watery diarrhea, abdominal cramps, flatulence, and steatorrhea. Blood and pus are rarely present in stool specimens, which is consistent with the absence of tissue destruction. Spontaneous recovery generally occurs after 10 to 14 days, although a more chronic disease with multiple relapses may develop. This is particularly a problem for patients with immunoglobulin (Ig)A deficiency or intestinal diverticula.

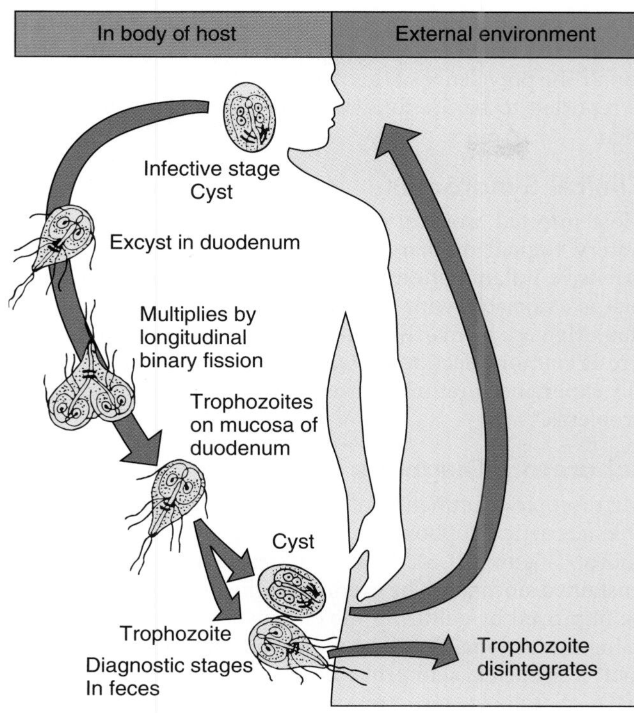

FIGURE 73-4 Life cycle of *Giardia duodenalis.*

Clinical Case 73-2 Drug-Resistant Giardiasis

Abboud and colleagues (*Clin Infect Dis* 32:1792–1794, 2001) described a case of metronidazole- and albendazole-resistant giardiasis that was successfully treated with nitazoxanide. The patient was a 32-year-old homosexual man with acquired immunodeficiency syndrome who was admitted to the hospital because of intractable diarrhea. Examination of stool revealed the presence of numerous cysts of *Giardia duodenalis (Giardia lamblia).* The patient was treated unsuccessfully five times with metronidazole and albendazole without improvement in diarrhea or cyst shedding. Although combined antiretroviral therapy was also administered, it was ineffective, and viral genotypic analysis found mutations associated with high resistance to most antiretroviral drugs. The patient was subsequently treated for giardiasis with nitazoxanide, which resulted in resolution of the diarrhea and negative results of tests for stool cyst shedding. Resistance of the infecting strain of *G. duodenalis* to both metronidazole and albendazole was confirmed by in vivo and in vitro studies. Nitazoxanide may be considered a useful alternative therapy for resistant giardiasis.

Laboratory Diagnosis

With the onset of diarrhea and abdominal discomfort, stool specimens should be examined for cysts and trophozoites (see Figure 73-3). Excretion of *Giardia* spp. may occur in "showers," with many organisms present in the stool on a given day and few or none detected the next day. For this reason, the physician should never accept the results of a single negative stool specimen as evidence that the patient is free of intestinal parasites. One stool specimen per day for 3 days should be examined. If stools remain persistently negative in a patient in whom giardiasis is highly suspected, additional specimens can be collected by duodenal aspiration, Entero-Test or string test, or biopsy of the upper small intestine. In addition to conventional microscopy, several immunologic tests for detection of **fecal antigen** are available commercially. These tests include countercurrent immunoelectrophoresis, enzyme immunoassay, an immunochromatographic assay, and indirect immunofluorescent staining. Reported sensitivities range from 88% to 98% and specificities from 87% to 100%. Numerous publications have documented the superior sensitivity of the immunoassay methods over that of routine microscopic examination of stool for detection of *Giardia.* A commercially available multiplex PCR assay for detection of *Giardia* and other enteric protozoan parasites has recently been cleared by the U.S. Food and Drug Administration (FDA) for clinical use.

Treatment, Prevention, and Control

It is important to eradicate *Giardia* spp. from asymptomatic carriers and diseased patients. The drug of choice is metronidazole or nitazoxanide, with furazolidone, tinidazole, paromomycin, albendazole, or quinacrine all acceptable alternatives. Prevention and control of giardiasis involves avoidance of contaminated water and food, especially by the traveler and outdoorsman. Protection is afforded by boiling drinking water from streams and lakes or in countries with a high incidence of endemic disease. Maintenance of properly functioning filtration systems in municipal water supplies is also required because cysts are resistant to standard chlorination procedures. Public health efforts should be made to identify the reservoir of infection to prevent spread of disease. In addition, high-risk sexual behavior should be avoided.

Dientamoeba fragilis

Physiology and Structure

D. fragilis was initially classified as an ameba; however, the internal structures of the trophozoite are typical of a flagellate. No cyst stage has been described in humans.

Epidemiology

D. fragilis has a worldwide distribution. Transmission of the delicate trophozoite is not completely understood. Some observers believe the organism can be transported from person to person inside the protective shell of worm eggs, such as those of *Enterobius vermicularis,* the pinworm. Transmission by fecal-oral and oral-anal routes does occur.

Clinical Syndromes

Most infections with *D. fragilis* are asymptomatic, with colonization of the cecum and upper colon. However, some patients may develop symptomatic disease with abdominal discomfort, flatulence, intermittent diarrhea, anorexia, and weight loss. There is no evidence of tissue invasion with this flagellate, although irritation of the intestinal mucosa occurs.

Laboratory Diagnosis

Infection is confirmed by microscopic examination of stool specimens, in which typical trophozoites can be seen. The trophozoite is small (5 to 12 μm) with one or two nuclei. The central karyosome consists of four to six discrete granules. Excretion of the parasite may fluctuate markedly from day to day, so collection of several stool samples may be necessary. Examination of a purged stool sample may also be useful.

Treatment, Prevention, and Control

Multiple differing antimicrobial agents have been used for treatment of *D. fragilis* infection, with varying success. These include doxycycline, iodoquinol, metronidazole, and secnidazole. However, there is no general consensus on the best approach for treating infections with this organism. The reservoir for this flagellate and the organism's life cycle are unknown. Thus specific recommendations for prevention and control are difficult. However, infections can be avoided by maintaining adequate sanitary conditions. Eradication of infections with *Enterobius* organisms may also reduce transmission of *Dientamoeba* infection.

Trichomonas vaginalis

Physiology and Structure

T. vaginalis is not an intestinal protozoan but rather the cause of urogenital infections. The flagellate's four flagella and short, undulating membrane are responsible for motility. *T. vaginalis* exists only as a trophozoite and is found in the urethras and vaginas of women and the urethras and prostate glands of men.

Epidemiology

This parasite has worldwide distribution, with sexual intercourse as the primary mode of transmission (Figure 73-5). Occasionally, infections have been transmitted by fomites (toilet articles, clothing), although this transmission is limited by the lability of the trophozoite form. Infants may be infected by passage through the mother's infected birth canal. The prevalence of this flagellate in developed countries is reported to be 5% to 20% in women and 2% to 10% in men.

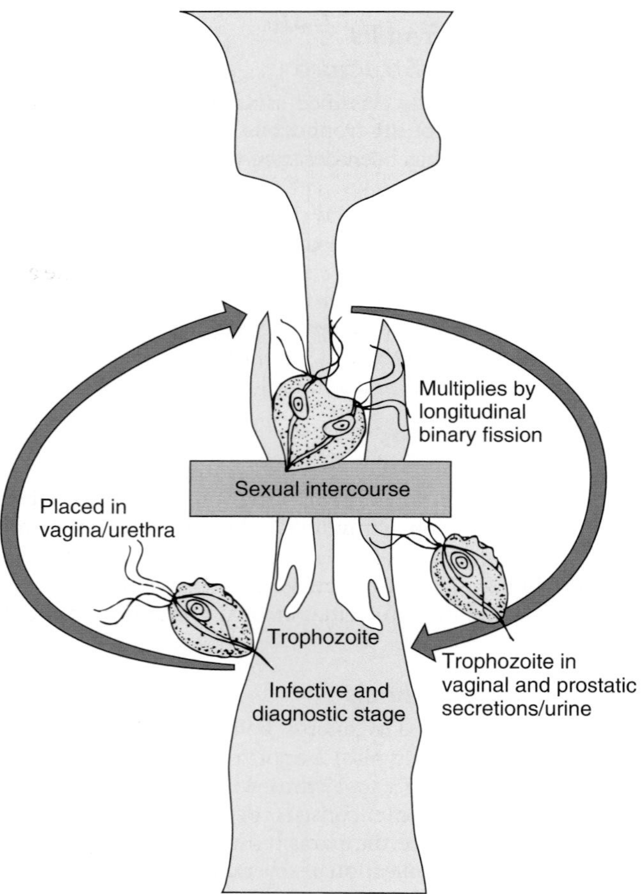

FIGURE 73-5 Life cycle of *Trichomonas vaginalis.*

Clinical Syndromes

Most infected women are asymptomatic or have a scant, watery vaginal discharge. Vaginitis may occur, with more extensive inflammation and erosion of the epithelial lining that is associated with itching, burning, and painful urination. Men are primarily asymptomatic carriers who serve as a reservoir for infections in women. However, men occasionally experience urethritis, prostatitis, and other urinary tract problems.

Laboratory Diagnosis

Microscopic examination of vaginal or urethral discharge for characteristic trophozoites is the diagnostic method of choice (Figure 73-6). Stained (Giemsa, Papanicolaou) or unstained smears can be examined. The diagnostic yield may be improved by culturing the organism (93% sensitivity) or using monoclonal fluorescent antibody staining (86% sensitivity). A nucleic acid probe assay is also available commercially. Serologic tests may be useful in epidemiologic surveillance.

Treatment, Prevention, and Control

The drug of choice is metronidazole. Both male and female sex partners must be treated to avoid reinfection. Resistance to metronidazole has been reported and may require re-treatment with higher doses. More recently, tinidazole has received FDA approval for treatment of trichomoniasis in adults and may be used as a first-line agent or for cases refractory to metronidazole. Personal hygiene, avoidance of shared toilet articles and clothing, and safe sexual practices are important preventive actions. Elimination of carriage in men is critical for eradication of disease.

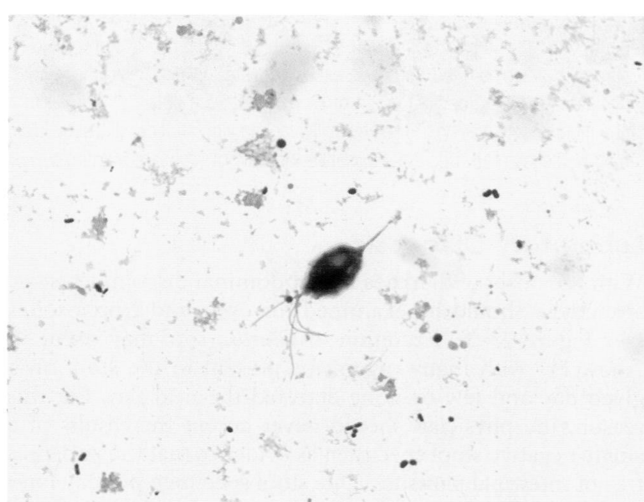

FIGURE 73-6 *Trichomonas vaginalis* trophozoite. The trophozoite is 7 to 23 μm long and 6 to 8 μm wide (average, 13 × 7 μm). The flagella and a short, undulating membrane are present at one side, and an axostyle extends through the center of the parasite.

• Ciliates

The intestinal protozoan *Balantidium coli* is the only member of the ciliate group that is pathogenic for humans. Disease produced by *B. coli* is similar to amebiasis because the organisms elaborate proteolytic and cytotoxic substances that mediate tissue invasion and intestinal ulceration.

Balantidium coli

Physiology and Structure

The life cycle of *B. coli* is simple, involving ingestion of infectious cysts, excystation, and invasion of trophozoites into the mucosal lining of the large intestine, cecum, and terminal ileum (Figure 73-7). The trophozoite is covered with rows of hairlike cilia that aid in motility. Morphologically more complex than amebae, *B. coli* has a funnel-like primitive mouth called a **cytostome,** a large and small nucleus involved in reproduction, food vacuoles, and two contractile vacuoles.

Epidemiology

B. coli is distributed worldwide. Swine and (less commonly) monkeys are the most important reservoirs. Infections are transmitted by the fecal-oral route; outbreaks are associated with contamination of water supplies with pig feces. Person-to-person spread, including through food handlers, has been implicated in outbreaks. Risk factors associated with human disease include contact with swine and substandard hygienic conditions.

Clinical Syndromes

As with other protozoan parasites, asymptomatic carriage of *B. coli* can exist. Symptomatic disease is characterized by abdominal pain and tenderness, tenesmus, nausea, anorexia, and watery stools with blood and pus. Ulceration of the intestinal mucosa, as with amebiasis, can be seen; a secondary complication caused by bacterial invasion into the eroded intestinal mucosa can occur. Extraintestinal invasion of other organs is extremely rare in balantidiasis.

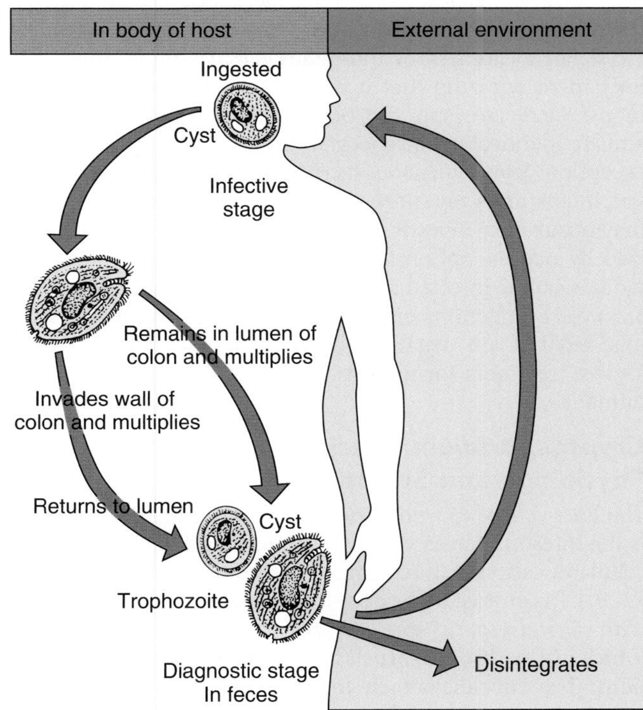

FIGURE 73-7 Life cycle of *Balantidium coli.*

Laboratory Diagnosis

Microscopic examination of feces for trophozoites and cysts is performed. The trophozoite is very large, varying in length from 50 to 200 µm and in width from 40 to 70 µm. The surface is covered with cilia, and the prominent internal structure is a **macronucleus.** A **micronucleus** is also present. Two pulsating contractile vacuoles are also seen in fresh preparations of the trophozoites. The cyst is smaller (40 to 60 µm in diameter), is surrounded by a clear refractile wall, and has a single nucleus in the cytoplasm. *B. coli* is a large organism compared with other intestinal protozoa and is readily detected in fresh, wet microscopic preparations.

Treatment, Prevention, and Control

The drug of choice is tetracycline; iodoquinol and metronidazole are alternative antimicrobials. Actions for prevention and control are similar to those for amebiasis. Appropriate personal hygiene, maintenance of sanitary conditions, and careful monitoring of pig feces are all important preventive measures.

• Sporozoa (Coccidia)

Sporozoa constitute a very large group called **Apicomplexa** or **Coccidia,** some members of which are discussed in this section with the intestinal parasites and others with the blood and tissue parasites. All sporozoans demonstrate typical characteristics, especially the existence of asexual **(schizogony)** and sexual **(gametogony)** reproduction. Most members of the group also share alternative hosts; for example, in malaria, mosquitoes harbor the sexual cycle and humans the asexual cycle. The intestinal Sporozoa discussed in this chapter are *Cystoisospora* (formerly *Isospora*), *Sarcocystis, Cryptosporidium,* and *Cyclospora* spp.

Cystoisospora (Formerly *Isospora*) *belli*

Physiology and Structure

Cystoisospora belli is a coccidian parasite of the intestinal epithelium. Both sexual and asexual reproduction in the intestinal epithelium can occur, resulting in tissue damage (Figure 73-8). The end product of gametogenesis is the oocyst, which is the diagnostic stage present in fecal specimens.

Epidemiology

Cystoisospora organisms are distributed worldwide but are infrequently detected in stool specimens. This parasite has been reported with increasing frequency in both healthy and immunocompromised patients. This is probably due to the increased awareness of disease caused by *Cystoisospora* spp. in patients with acquired immunodeficiency syndrome (AIDS). Infection with this organism follows ingestion of contaminated food or water or oral-anal sexual contact.

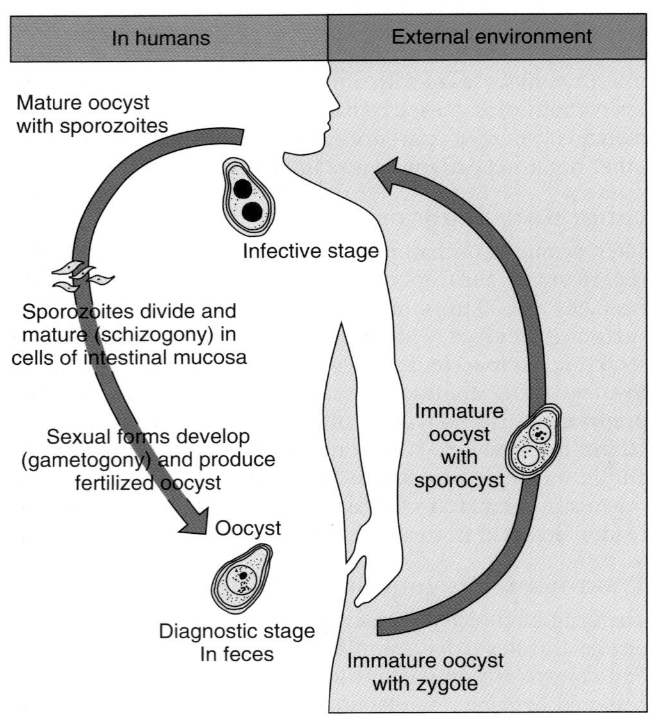

FIGURE 73-8 Life cycle of *Cystoisospora* (formerly *Isospora*) species.

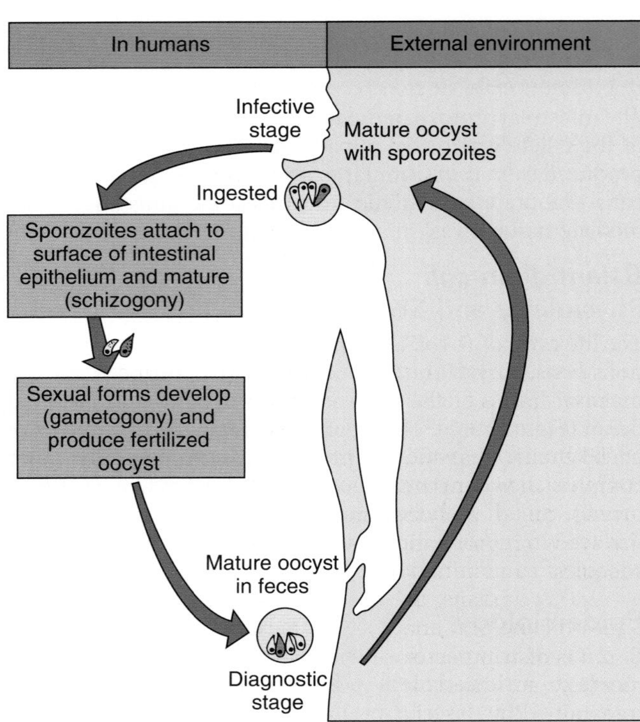

FIGURE 73-10 Life cycle of *Cryptosporidium* species.

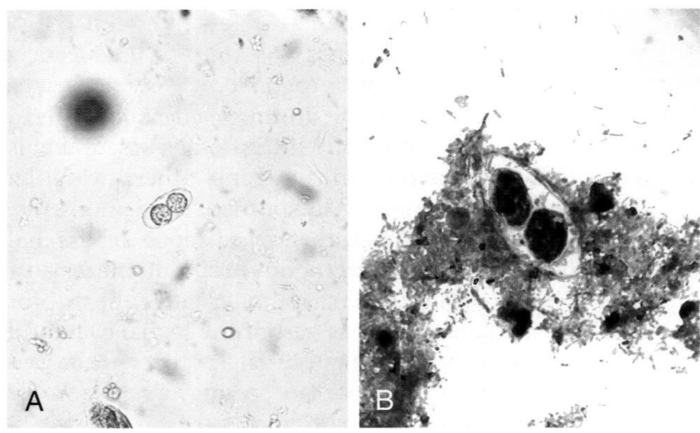

FIGURE 73-9 Oocyst of *Cystoisospora belli* containing two sporoblasts. **A,** Wet mount. **B,** Acid-fast stain. Oocysts are ovoid (≈25 µm long × 15 µm wide) with tapering ends.

Clinical Syndromes

Infected individuals may be asymptomatic carriers or suffer mild to severe gastrointestinal disease. Disease most commonly mimics giardiasis, with a malabsorption syndrome characterized by loose, foul-smelling stools. Chronic diarrhea with weight loss, anorexia, malaise, and fatigue can be seen, although it is difficult to separate this presentation from the patient's underlying disease.

Laboratory Diagnosis

Careful examination of concentrated stool sediment and special staining with iodine or a modified acid-fast procedure reveal the parasite (Figure 73-9). Small bowel biopsy has been used to establish the diagnosis when results of tests on stool specimens are negative.

Treatment, Prevention, and Control

The drug of choice is trimethoprim-sulfamethoxazole, with the combination of pyrimethamine and sulfadiazine an acceptable alternative. Prevention and control are effected by maintaining personal hygiene and highly sanitary conditions and by avoiding oral-anal sexual contact.

Sarcocystis Species

Physician awareness of the genus *Sarcocystis* is important only in recognizing that it can be detected in stool specimens. *Sarcocystis* spp. can be isolated from pigs and cattle and are identical in all aspects to *Cystoisospora* spp. with one exception: *Sarcocystis* oocysts rupture before passage in stool specimens, and only sporocysts are present. Intestinal disease may occur after ingestion of infected meat and is characterized by nausea, abdominal pain, and diarrhea. Some individuals can be infected and show no clinical signs. Muscular *Sarcocystis* infections in humans may occur if sporocysts are ingested but are usually mild or subclinical. There is no known treatment for intestinal or muscular sarcocystosis in humans.

Cryptosporidium Species

Physiology and Structure

The life cycle of *Cryptosporidium* is typical of coccidians, as is the intestinal disease, but this parasite differs in the intracellular location of the organism in the epithelial cells (Figure 73-10). In contrast to the deep intracellular invasion observed with *Cystoisospora* spp., *Cryptosporidium* organisms are found just within the brush border of the intestinal epithelium. The coccidia attach to the surface of the cells and replicate by a series of processes (merogony, gametogony, sporogony) leading to the production of new infectious oocysts. After sporogony, the mature oocysts may either excyst within the digestive tract of the host, leading to infection of new cells, or may be excreted into the environment.

Epidemiology

Cryptosporidium spp. are distributed worldwide. Infection is reported in a wide variety of animals, including mammals, reptiles, and fish. There are at least 16 different species of *Cryptosporidium;* however, *C. hominis* and *C. parvum* are the species most commonly infecting humans. *C. felis* and *C. ubiquitum* have recently been recognized as emerging pathogens. Waterborne transmission of cryptosporidiosis is now well documented as an important route of infection. The massive outbreak of cryptosporidiosis in Milwaukee in 1993 (≈300,000 individuals infected) was linked to contamination of the municipal water supply. Cryptosporidia are resistant to the usual water purification procedures (chlorination and ozone), and it is believed that runoff of local waste and surface water into municipal water supplies is an important source of contamination. Zoonotic spread from animal reservoirs to humans, as well as person-to-person spread by fecal-oral and oral-anal routes, are common means of infection. Veterinary personnel, animal handlers, and homosexuals are at particularly high risk for infection. Many outbreaks have now been described in municipal swimming pools and day-care centers, where fecal-oral transmission is common.

Clinical Syndromes (Clinical Case 73-3)

As with other protozoan infections, exposure to *Cryptosporidium* organisms may result in asymptomatic carriage. Disease in previously healthy individuals is usually a mild, self-limiting **enterocolitis** characterized by watery diarrhea without blood. Spontaneous remission after an average of 10 days is characteristic. In contrast, disease in immunocompromised patients (e.g., patients with AIDS), characterized by 50 or more stools per day and tremendous fluid loss, can be severe and last for months to years. In some patients with AIDS, disseminated *Cryptosporidium* infections have been reported.

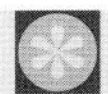

Clinical Case 73-3 Cryptosporidiosis

Quiroz and colleagues (*J Infect Dis* 181:685–700, 2000) described an outbreak of cryptosporidiosis that was linked to a food handler. In the fall of 1998, an outbreak of gastroenteritis among university students was reported to the Department of Health. Preliminary findings suggested that the illness was associated with eating at one of the campus cafeterias; four employees of this cafeteria had a similar illness. The outbreak was thought to be caused by a viral agent until *Cryptosporidium parvum* was detected in the stool specimen of several cafeteria employees. In a case-control study of 88 case patients and 67 control subjects, eating in one of two cafeterias was associated with diarrheal illness. *C. parvum* was detected in stool samples of 16 (70%) of 23 ill students and 2 of 4 ill employees. One ill food handler with laboratory-confirmed cryptosporidiosis prepared raw produce on the days surrounding the outbreak. All 25 *C. parvum* isolates submitted for DNA analysis, including three from the ill food handler, were genotype 1. This outbreak illustrates the potential for cryptosporidiosis to cause foodborne illness. Epidemiologic and molecular evidence indicate that an ill food handler was the likely outbreak source.

Laboratory Diagnosis

Cryptosporidium may be detected in large numbers in unconcentrated stool specimens obtained from immunocompromised individuals with diarrhea. Oocysts generally measure 5 to 7 microns and may be concentrated with the modified zinc sulfate centrifugal flotation technique or the Sheather sugar flotation procedure. Specimens may be stained using the modified **acid-fast** method (Figure 73-11) or by an indirect immunofluorescence assay. Both an enzyme immunoassay and an immunochromatographic assay for detecting fecal antigen are commercially available, as is a recently approved PCR panel. It should be noted that *Cryptosporidium* will not be detected on routine microscopic examination for ova and parasites (need to specify acid-fast staining) and that data now suggest that immunoassays and PCR are superior to microscopic methods for detection of this organism in fecal samples. The number of oocysts shed in stool may fluctuate; therefore a minimum of three specimens should be examined. Serologic procedures are used in epidemiologic and seroprevalence studies but are not yet widely available for diagnosing and monitoring infections.

Treatment, Prevention, and Control

Unfortunately, no broadly effective therapy has been developed for managing *Cryptosporidium* infections in immunocompromised patients. Therapeutic information is largely based on isolated reports and anecdotal information. Spiramycin may help control the diarrhea in some patients in the early stages of AIDS who have cryptosporidiosis, but it is ineffective in patients who have progressed to the later stages of AIDS. Spiramycin was no more effective than placebo in treating cryptosporidial diarrhea in infants. Nitazoxanide is approved by the FDA for treatment of cryptosporidiosis in nonimmunocompromised individuals older than 12 months, but it is not yet approved for treatment of cryptosporidiosis in immunocompromised individuals. The drugs paromomycin and azithromycin have been used to treat cryptosporidiosis in HIV-infected patients and have been shown to reduce the parasite load. There is also evidence to suggest that some antiretroviral compounds may have a direct inhibitory effect on *Cryptosporidium*. Therapy consists primarily of

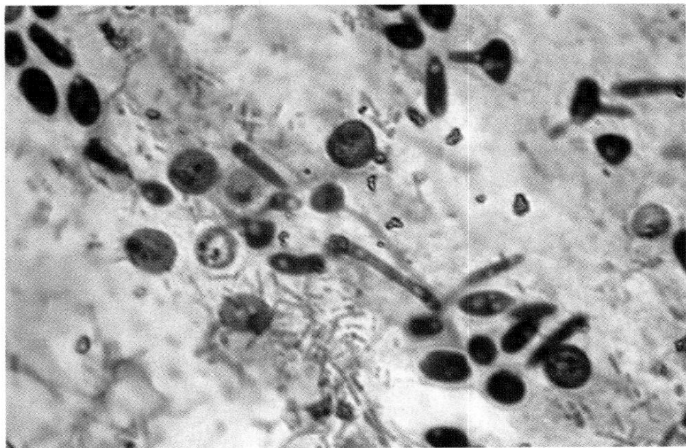

FIGURE 73-11 Acid-fast stained *Cryptosporidium* oocysts (≈5 to 7 μm in diameter). (From CDC Public Health Image Library.)

supportive measures to restore the tremendous fluid loss from the watery diarrhea.

Because of the widespread distribution of this organism in humans and other animals, preventing infection is difficult. The same methods of improved personal hygiene and sanitation used for other intestinal protozoa should be maintained for this disease. Contaminated water supplies should be treated with chlorination and filtration. In addition, avoidance of high-risk sexual activities is critical.

Cyclospora Species

Physiology and Structure

Cyclospora is a coccidian parasite that is taxonomically related to *Cystoisospora* spp., *Cryptosporidium parvum,* and *Toxoplasma gondii.* A single species infecting humans, *C. cayetanensis*, has been identified thus far.

Cyclospora organisms are similar to *Cystoisospora* in that oocysts are excreted unsporulated and require a period of time outside the host for maturation to occur. Upon ingestion, the sporulated oocyst undergoes the excystation process in the lumen of the small intestine, releasing sporozoites. Sporozoites infect cells to form type I merozoites, and these form type II merozoites. The type II merozoites differentiate within the mucosal cells into sexual stages, the microgametocytes and macrogametocytes. The macrogametocyte is fertilized by the microgametocyte and produces a zygote. Oocysts are then formed and excreted into the environment as unsporulated oocysts. The pathogenic mechanisms by which *Cyclospora* spp. cause clinical illness are unknown; however, the organism usually infects the upper small bowel and causes pronounced histopathologic changes. The organism is found within vacuoles in the cytoplasm of jejunal epithelial cells, and its presence is associated with inflammatory changes, villous atrophy, and crypt hyperplasia.

The morphologic characteristics of *Cyclospora* spp. are similar to those of *Cystoisospora* spp. and *C. parvum,* with a few exceptions. The oocysts of *Cyclospora* species are spherical and 8 to 10 µm in diameter, as opposed to the smaller oocysts of *C. parvum* (5 to 7 µm) and the much larger elliptical oocysts of *Cystoisospora* spp. (15 to 25 µm). The oocysts of *Cyclospora* spp. contain two sporocysts, each of which contain two sporozoites, which in turn contain a membrane-bound nucleus and micronemes characteristic of the sporozoans. In contrast, the *Cryptosporidium* oocyst contains four naked, or nonencysted, sporozoites, whereas the *Cystoisospora* oocyst contains two sporocysts, each containing four sporozoites.

Epidemiology

As with *Cryptosporidium, Cyclospora* is widely distributed throughout the world and infects a variety of reptiles, birds, and mammals. Although direct animal-to-human or person-to-person transmission has not been documented, there is now compelling evidence that *Cyclospora* infection is acquired through contaminated water. In areas of endemicity (e.g., Nepal), studies have documented an annual surge of cyclosporiasis that coincides with the rainy season. The prevalence of infection (symptomatic and asymptomatic) ranges from 2% to 18% in endemic areas and is estimated at 0.1% to 0.5% in developed countries. Outbreaks in the United States have occurred during the summer months and have been correlated with consumption of contaminated fruits and vegetables; transmission via contaminated water has also been suggested. Similar to *Cryptosporidium, Cyclospora* spp. are resistant to chlorination and not readily detected by methods used currently to ensure the safety of supplies of drinking water.

Clinical Syndromes

The clinical manifestations of cyclosporiasis resemble those of cryptosporidiosis: mild nausea, anorexia, abdominal cramping, and watery diarrhea. Fatigue, malaise, flatulence, and bloating have also been reported. In immunocompetent hosts, diarrhea is self-limited but may be prolonged and last for weeks. Among immunocompromised people—specifically, patients infected with HIV—clinical illness is typically prolonged and severe and is associated with a high rate of recurrence. Biliary tract infection with *Cyclospora* has been reported in two patients with AIDS.

Laboratory Diagnosis

The diagnosis of cyclosporiasis is based on microscopic detection of oocysts in stool. Oocysts may be detected by light microscopic examination of unstained fecal material (wet mount), where they appear as nonrefractile spherical to oval, slightly wrinkled bodies measuring 8 to 10 µm in diameter; they have an internal cluster of membrane-bound globules (Figure 73-12). In fresh specimens, *Cyclospora* organisms fluoresce when examined with an ultraviolet fluorescence microscope fitted with a 365-nm excitation filter.

Cyclospora oocysts may be concentrated with the modified zinc sulfate centrifugal flotation technique or the Sheather sugar flotation procedure. Organisms are acid fast and thus can be detected using one of the many acid-fast staining techniques, including the modified Ziehl-Neelsen stain or the Kinyoun acid-fast stain (Figure 73-13). A distinguishing feature of *Cyclospora* is its variable appearance on acid-fast staining, which ranges from unstained to mottled pink to deep red.

The relative sensitivity, specificity, and predictive value of the various methods for diagnosing *Cyclospora* infection are

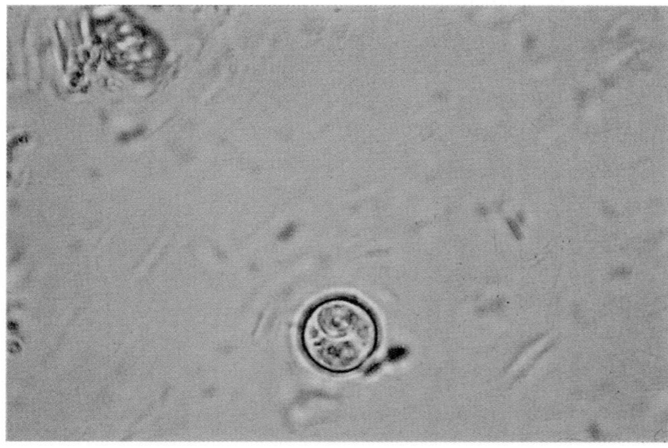

FIGURE 73-12 Sporulated oocyst of *Cyclospora cayetanensis.* The oocysts measure 8 to 10 µm in diameter and contain two sporocysts with two sporozoites (saline wet mount, ×900). (From Peters W, Pasvol G: *Color atlas of tropical medicine and parasitology*, ed 6, London, 2007, Mosby.)

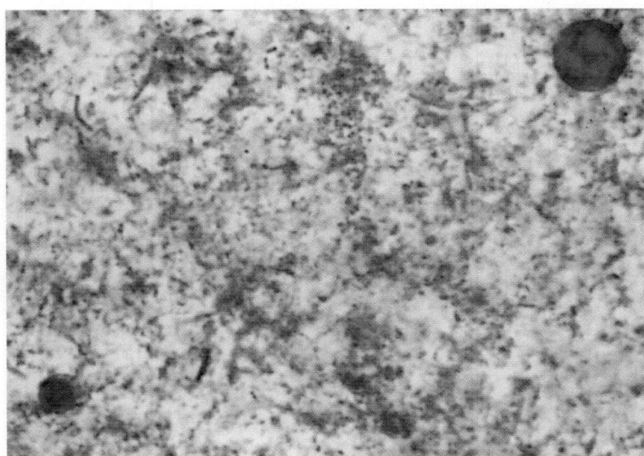

FIGURE 73-13 Oocysts of *Cryptosporidium parvum (lower left)* and *Cyclospora cayetanensis (upper right)*. Both parasites stain red with Ziehl-Neelsen stain; however, *Cyclospora* organisms typically take up variable amounts of the stain and the oocysts are larger (8 to 10 μm compared with 5 to 7 μm). (From Peters W, Pasvol G: *Color atlas of tropical medicine and parasitology*, ed 6, London, 2007, Mosby.)

not known. Currently there are no immunodiagnostic techniques to aid in the diagnosis and monitoring of these infections. The rudimentary nature of the available diagnostic techniques and the incomplete understanding of the disease process may contribute to underrecognition of *Cyclospora* infection. Notably, a multiplex PCR for detection of *Cyclospora* in stool is now commercially available.

Treatment, Prevention, and Control

The effectiveness of trimethoprim-sulfamethoxazole has been demonstrated in anecdotal reports, a large open-label study of patients infected with HIV, and a placebo-controlled trial. In HIV-infected patients, it appears that the high rate of recurrence can be attenuated with long-term suppressive therapy with trimethoprim-sulfamethoxazole. Although numerous additional agents, including metronidazole, nitazoxanide, ciprofloxacin, norfloxacin, quinacrine, nalidixic acid, tinidazole, and diloxanide furoate, have been used in various trials, the effectiveness of any one of these agents has not been proved.

As with *Cryptosporidium* spp., prevention of *Cyclospora* infection is difficult. Although *Cyclospora* organisms appear resistant to chlorination, treatment of water supplies with chlorination and filtration remains a reasonable practice. In addition, the same methods of improved personal hygiene and sanitation used for other intestinal protozoa should be used as preventive measures for this disease.

Bibliography

Abubakar I, Aliyu SH, Arumugam C, et al: Treatment of cryptosporidiosis in immunocompromised individuals: systematic review and meta-analysis, *Br J Pharmacol* 63:387–393, 2007.

Buss SN, Leber A, Chapin K, et al: Multicenter evaluation of the BioFire FilmArray Gastrointestinal Panel for etiologic diagnosis of infectious gastroenteritis, *J Clin Microbiol* 53:915–925, 2015.

Connor DH, Schwartz DA: *Pathology of infectious diseases*, Stamford, Conn, 1997, Appleton & Lange.

Espinosa-Cantellano M, Martinez-Palomo A: Pathogenesis of intestinal amebiasis: from molecules to disease, *Clin Microbiol Rev* 13:318–331, 2000.

Fayer R: *Sarcocystis* spp. in humans, *Clin Microbiol Rev* 17:894–902, 2004.

Feng Y, Xiao L: Zoonotic potential and molecular epidemiology of *Giardia* species and giardiasis, *Clin Microbiol Rev* 24:110–140, 2011.

Gardner TB, Hill DR: Treatment of giardiasis, *Clin Microbiol Rev* 14:114–128, 2001.

Leber AL, Novak-Weekly SM: Intestinal and urogenital amebae, flagellates, and ciliates. In Versalovic J, et al, editors: *Manual of clinical microbiology*, ed 10, Washington, DC, 2011, American Society for Microbiology Press.

Lindsay DS, Upton SJ, Weiss LM: *Isospora, Cyclospora,* and *Sarcocystis*. In Versalovic J, et al, editors: *Manual of clinical microbiology*, ed 10, Washington, DC, 2011, American Society for Microbiology Press.

McHardy IH, Wu M, Shmizu-Cohen R, et al: Detection of intestinal protozoa in the clinical laboratory, *J Clin Microbiol* 52:712–720, 2014.

Ortega YR, Sanchez R: Update on *Cyclospora cayetanensis,* a food-borne and waterborne parasite, *Clin Microbiol Rev* 23:218–234, 2010.

Peters W, Giles HM: *Color atlas of tropical medicine and parasitology*, ed 4, London, 1995, Mosby.

Schuster FL, Ramirez-Avila L: Current world status of *Balantidium coli*, *Clin Microbiol Rev* 21:626–638, 2008.

Stark D, Barratt JL, van Hal S, et al: Clinical significance of enteric protozoa in the immunosuppressed human population, *Clin Microbiol Rev* 22:634–650, 2009.

Tan KSW: New insights on classification, identification, and clinical relevance of *Blastocystis* spp, *Clin Microbiol Rev* 21:639–665, 2008.

Verweij JJ, Stensvold CR: Molecular testing for clinical diagnosis and epidemiological investigations of intestinal parasite infections, *Clin Microbiol Rev* 27:371–418, 2014.

CHAPTER

74 BLOOD AND TISSUE PROTOZOA

A 44-year-old heart transplant patient complained to her primary physician about headache, nausea, and vomiting approximately 1 year after transplant. She had no skin lesions. A computed tomography scan of the head demonstrated ring-enhancing lesions. A biopsy of the lesions was performed. All cultures (bacterial, fungal, viral) were negative. Special stains of the tissue revealed multiple cystlike structures of varying size.

1. What was the differential diagnosis of infectious agents in this patient? What was the most likely etiologic agent?
2. What other tests would have been done to confirm the diagnosis?
3. What aspects of the medical history might suggest a risk for infection with this agent?
4. What were the therapeutic options and the likelihood that therapy would be successful?

Answers to these questions are available on StudentConsult.com.

• SUMMARIES CLINICALLY SIGNIFICANT ORGANISMS

Plasmodium

Trigger Words

Malaria, quotidian, tertian, quartan, blackwater fever, cerebral malaria, benign tertian, malignant tertian, multiple ring forms, gametocytes, *Anopheles* mosquito, tropics and subtropics, prophylaxis

Biology, Virulence, and Disease

- Plasmodia: coccidian or sporozoan parasites of red blood cells
- Five species that infect humans share a common life cycle
- Routes of acquisition: mosquito, transfusion, needle sharing, congenital
- *P. falciparum* produces daily (quotidian) chills and fever with nausea, vomiting, diarrhea progressing to tertian (36 to 48 hours) periodicity with fulminating disease (malignant tertian); no persistent liver stage
- *P. knowlesi* produces daily (quotidian) fever, chills, headache, rigors, abdominal pain, cough (severe symptoms in 7% of cases; respiratory distress and hepatorenal failure); no persistent liver stage
- *P. vivax* causes "benign tertian malaria" with paroxysms of fever and chills every 48 hours; a spectrum of severe, life-threatening syndromes similar to that with *P. falciparum* may be seen; a liver stage may cause relapses and recrudescences
- *P. ovale* causes benign tertian malaria similar to that of *P. vivax* with both relapses and recrudescence
- *P. malariae* has a long (18 to 40 days) incubation period and causes a moderate to severe disease with a 72-hour (quartan or malarial malaria) periodicity; no persistent liver stage

Epidemiology

- Infection with *Plasmodium* spp. accounts for 1 to 5 billion febrile episodes and 1 to 3 million deaths annually, 85% of which are in Africa
- Vector—*Anopheles* mosquito—widely distributed in tropical, subtropical, and temperate regions
- *P. falciparum:* occurs almost exclusively in tropical and subtropical regions
- *P. knowlesi:* infects Old World Monkeys, and increasingly humans, in Malaysia and neighboring countries throughout Southeast Asia
- *P. vivax:* widest geographic distribution (tropics, subtropics, temperate regions); 80% of cases occur in South America and Southeast Asia
- *P. ovale:* distributed primarily in tropical Africa; also found in Asia and South America
- *P. malariae:* occurs in same tropical and subtropical areas as other malarial parasites but less prevalent

Diagnosis

- Most widely used method: detection of parasites in thick and thin blood films stained with Giemsa or Wright stain
- Antigen detection using a rapid diagnostic test (RDT); used in both the field and diagnostic laboratories as an adjunct to microscopic examination of blood films

Treatment, Prevention, and Control

- Treatment of malaria is based on history regarding travel to endemic areas, prompt clinical review and differential diagnosis, accurate and rapid laboratory work, and correct use of antimalarial drugs

- Chloroquine or parenteral quinine is drug of choice for susceptible strains of *Plasmodium;* widespread resistance to chloroquine seen with *P. falciparum* and *P. vivax*
- Chemoprophylaxis with chloroquine, doxycycline, Malarone, or mefloquine coupled with avoiding mosquito bites (netting, insect repellents, clothing) required for prevention
- Elimination of mosquito breeding places

Babesia

Trigger Words

Babesia, zoonosis, ticks, tetrad forms, splenectomy, intracellular, RBC

Biology, Virulence, and Disease

- Intracellular sporozoan parasites, morphologically resemble plasmodia
- Zoonosis infecting a variety of animals
- *Babesia microti:* usual cause of babesiosis in United States; transmitted by *Ixodes* ticks
- Incubation period of 1 to 4 weeks
- Symptoms: general malaise, fever without periodicity, headache, chills, sweating, fatigue, weakness
- Hemolytic anemia coupled with renal failure can occur
- Splenectomy or functional asplenia, immunosuppression, HIV infection, advanced age increase susceptibility to infections and more severe disease

Epidemiology

- >70 different species of *Babesia* found in Africa, Asia, Europe, North America
- *Ixodes dammini:* tick vector along U.S. northeastern seaboard
- Natural reservoir hosts: field mice, voles, other small rodents
- Disease may be severe in HIV-infected individuals
- *B. microti* increasingly transmitted by blood transfusions

Diagnosis

- Examination of blood smears is diagnostic method of choice
- Serologic tests and PCR also used to diagnose babesiosis

Treatment, Prevention, and Control

- Treatment of choice for mild to moderate illness: combination of atovaquone and azithromycin
- Treatment for severe disease: clindamycin, quinine, exchange transfusion
- Protective clothing, insect repellents can minimize tick exposure
- Prompt removal of ticks can be protective

Toxoplasma gondii

Trigger Words

Cat feces, raw meat, lymphadenitis, CNS lesion, encephalomyelitis, cat litter, congenital infection, AIDS

Biology, Virulence, and Disease

- Typical coccidian intracellular parasite found in a wide variety of animals, including birds and humans
- Essential reservoir host: common house cat and other felines
- Most *T. gondii* infections asymptomatic
- Symptoms occur when parasite moves from blood to tissues; include fever, chills, headaches, myalgia, lymphadenitis, fatigue
- Chronic disease marked by hepatitis, encephalomyelitis, and myocarditis
- Chorioretinitis may lead to blindness
- Congenital infection has serious sequelae
- Reactivation of cerebral toxoplasmosis is a major cause of encephalitis in patients with AIDS

Epidemiology

- Human infections ubiquitous
- Infection from ingestion of improperly cooked meat from intermediate-host animals or ingestion of infective oocysts from contaminated cat feces
- Transplacental infection can occur during pregnancy
- Rate of severe infection affected by patient's immune status
- Illness in immunocompromised host believed to be due to reactivation of previously latent infection rather than new exposure to organism

Diagnosis

- Increasing antibody titers documented in serially collected blood specimens
- Panel of tests—*T. gondii* serologic profile (TSP)—used to determine recent versus past acquisition of infection
- Diagnosis of *Toxoplasma* encephalitis usually involves imaging study of brain
- Microscopy, serologic and molecular techniques may be required for definitive diagnosis

Treatment, Prevention, and Control

- Treatment of choice: initial high-dose regimen of pyrimethamine plus sulfadiazine followed by lower doses of both drugs indefinitely (AIDS patients and other immunocompromised patients)
- Clindamycin or spiramycin may be used in first trimester of pregnancy
- High-risk patients may be considered for prophylaxis
- Additional preventive measures: avoid consumption and handling of raw or undercooked meat, avoid exposure to cat feces

Leishmania

Trigger Words

Kala-azar, Dumdum fever, cutaneous and mucocutaneous disease, visceral leishmaniasis, sandfly, post kala-azar dermal leishmaniasis

Biology, Virulence, and Disease

- *Leishmania:* obligate intracellular parasites transmitted from animal to human or human to human by bites from infected female sandfly
- Many different species can infect humans, producing a variety of diseases (cutaneous, diffuse cutaneous, mucocutaneous, visceral)
- Clinical syndromes depend upon species involved; most common species: cutaneous *(L. tropica),* mucocutaneous *(L. braziliensis),* visceral *(L. donovani, L. infantum),* post kala-azar dermal leishmaniasis *(L. donovani)*

Epidemiology

- Natural reservoirs: rodents, possums, anteaters, sloths, dogs, cats
- Infection may be transmitted by animal-vector-human or human-vector-human cycle, by direct contact with infected lesion, or mechanically by flies
- Mucocutaneous leishmaniasis most often occurs in Bolivia, Brazil, Peru; cutaneous leishmaniasis much more widespread throughout Middle East and in focal areas of South America
- Visceral leishmaniasis (kala-azar, Dumdum fever): ≈50,000 cases per year, 90% localized to Bangladesh, Brazil, India, Nepal, Sudan

Diagnosis

- Diagnosis of visceral, cutaneous, or mucocutaneous leishmaniasis made on clinical grounds in endemic areas
- Definitive diagnosis depends upon detecting amastigotes in clinical samples or promastigotes in culture; molecular techniques have been used for diagnosis, prognosis, and species identification

Treatment, Prevention, and Control

- Drug of choice for all forms of leishmaniasis is the pentavalent antimonial compound sodium stibogluconate (Pentostam)

- Fluconazole and miltefosine efficacious in cutaneous disease
- Stibogluconate remains drug of choice for mucocutaneous leishmaniasis
- Prevention involves prompt treatment of human infections and control of reservoir hosts, along with vector control

Trypanosomes

Trigger Words

Sleeping sickness, tsetse fly, reduvid bugs, chagoma, Romaña sign, megaesophagus, Winterbottom sign, Chagas disease

Biology, Virulence, and Disease

- Trypanosoma, a hemoflagellate, causes two distinctly different forms of disease: African trypanosomiasis and American trypanosomiasis
- African trypanosomiasis (sleeping sickness): chronic disease of several years' duration, transmitted by tsetse flies, fatal without treatment
- American trypanosomiasis (Chagas disease): asymptomatic, acute, or chronic forms, transmitted by reduvid bugs

Epidemiology

- *T. b. gambiense* limited to tropical West and Central Africa, correlating to range of tsetse fly vector
- *T. b. rhodesiense* found in East Africa, especially cattle-raising countries
- Domestic and wild game animals act as reservoir hosts for *T. b. rhodesiense*
- *T. cruzi* occurs widely in both reduvid bugs and a wide variety of reservoir animals in North, Central, South America
- Owing to chronic nature of infection, screening of solid organ and blood donors for Chagas disease has become important

Diagnosis

- Agents of sleeping sickness can be demonstrated in blood films, aspirations from lymph nodes, and concentrated spinal fluid
- *T. cruzi* can be demonstrated in blood films early in acute stage of disease

Treatment, Prevention, and Control

- Suramin: drug of choice for treating acute blood and lymphatic stages of both Gambian and Rhodesian forms of sleeping sickness; pentamidine is an alternative
- Melarsoprol: drug of choice for central nervous system disease
- Effective control measures: integrated approach to reduce human reservoir of infection, use of fly traps and insecticide
- Drugs of choice for treatment of Chagas disease: benznidazole and nifurtimox
- Vector control important: insecticide, eradication of nests, construction of homes to prevent nesting of bugs

The protozoa of blood and tissues are closely related to the intestinal protozoan parasites in practically all aspects except for their sites of infection (Box 74-1). Malaria parasites (*Plasmodium* spp.) infect both blood and tissues.

Plasmodium Species

Plasmodia are coccidian or sporozoan parasites of red blood cells, and as seen with other coccidia, they require two hosts: the mosquito for the sexual reproductive stages and humans and other animals for the asexual reproductive stages. Infection with *Plasmodium* spp. (i.e., malaria) accounts for 1 to 5 billion febrile episodes and 1 to 3 million deaths annually, 85% of which are in Africa (Clinical Case 74-1).

The five species of plasmodia that infect humans are *P. falciparum, P. knowlesi, P. vivax, P. ovale,* and *P. malariae* (Table 74-1). These species share a common life cycle, as illustrated in Figure 74-1. Human infection is initiated by the bite of an *Anopheles* mosquito, which introduces infectious plasmodia **sporozoites** via its saliva into the circulatory system. The sporozoites are carried to the parenchymal cells of the liver, where asexual reproduction **(schizogony)** occurs. This phase of growth is termed the **exoerythrocytic cycle** and lasts 8 to 25 days, depending on the plasmodial species. Some species (e.g., *P. vivax, P. ovale*) can establish a dormant hepatic phase in which the sporozoites (called **hypnozoites** or **sleeping forms**) do not divide. The presence of these viable plasmodia can lead to relapse of infections months to years after the initial clinical disease (relapsing malaria). The hepatocytes eventually rupture, liberating the plasmodia (termed **merozoites** at this stage), which in turn attach to specific receptors on the surface of erythrocytes and enter the cells, thus initiating the erythrocytic cycle.

Asexual replication progresses through a series of stages (ring, trophozoite, schizont) that culminates in rupture of the erythrocyte, releasing up to 24 merozoites, which initiates another cycle of replication by infecting other erythrocytes. Some merozoites also develop within erythrocytes into male and female **gametocytes.** If a mosquito ingests mature male and female gametocytes during a blood meal, the sexual reproductive cycle of malaria can be initiated, with eventual production of sporozoites infectious for humans. This sexual reproductive stage within the mosquito is necessary for the maintenance of malaria within a population.

Most malaria seen in the United States is acquired by visitors or residents of countries with endemic disease (imported malaria). However, the appropriate vector, the *Anopheles* mosquito, is found in several sections of the United States, and domestic transmission of disease has been

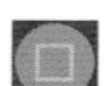
Box 74-1 Medically Important Blood and Tissue Protozoa

Plasmodium spp.
Babesia spp.
Toxoplasma spp.
Sarcocystis spp.
Acanthamoeba spp.
Balamuthia spp.
Naegleria spp.
Leishmania spp.
Trypanosoma spp.

 **Clinical Case 74-1 Malaria**

Mohin and Gupta (*Infect Dis Clin Pract* 15:209–212, 2007) described a case of severe malaria caused by *Plasmodium vivax*. The patient was a 59-year-old man who presented with a 1-day history of high-grade fever after recently returning from Guyana in South America. He did not take any medications before, during, or after the trip. He noted that his symptoms were similar to those of a malaria infection 5 years previously, also acquired in Guyana. A peripheral blood smear as part of the initial workup showed numerous red blood cells with schizonts consistent with *Plasmodium* infection, with more than 5% parasitemia. Several blood tests, including a DNA polymerase chain reaction (PCR), were sent for parasite species determination. The patient was started on quinine and doxycycline oral therapy because of concerns regarding chloroquine-resistant malaria. Subsequently, during the next 4 days, the patient developed severe thrombocytopenia and nonoliguric renal, acute respiratory, and circulatory failure despite a decrease in parasitemia to less than 0.5%. He received intravenous quinidine and an exchange transfusion to treat *Plasmodium falciparum* infection, suspected at the time because of the severity of his symptoms. The next day, however, the results of the PCR of the blood revealed the parasite to be *P. vivax* and not *P. falciparum*. The patient gradually improved and was treated with primaquine to prevent relapse.

This case shows that although unusual, severe respiratory and circulatory compromise may complicate *P. vivax* malaria. *P. vivax* should be considered if the patient's condition deteriorates despite the presence of relatively low parasite levels. As opposed to *P. falciparum, P. vivax* infections carry the additional risk of relapse, which warrants appropriate and adequate treatment. This case also emphasizes the importance of chemoprophylaxis and personal protective measures for anyone planning a trip to a malaria-infested region.

 **Table 74-1 Human Malarial Parasites**

Parasite	Disease
Plasmodium vivax	Benign tertian malaria
P. ovale	Benign tertian or ovale malaria
P. malariae	Quartan or malarial malaria
P. falciparum	Malignant tertian malaria
P. knowlesi	Simian malaria or quotidian malaria

observed (introduced malaria). In addition to transmission by mosquitos, malaria can be acquired by blood transfusions from an infected donor (transfusion malaria). This type of transmission can also occur among injection drug users who share needles and syringes ("mainline" malaria). Congenital acquisition, although rare, is also a possible mode of transmission (congenital malaria).

Plasmodium falciparum

Physiology and Structure

P. falciparum demonstrates no selectivity in host erythrocytes and invades any red blood cell (RBC) at any stage in its existence. Also, multiple merozoites can infect a single erythrocyte. Thus three or even four small rings may be seen in an infected cell (Figure 74-2). *P. falciparum* is often seen in the host cell at the very edge or periphery of the cell membrane, appearing almost as if it were "stuck" on the

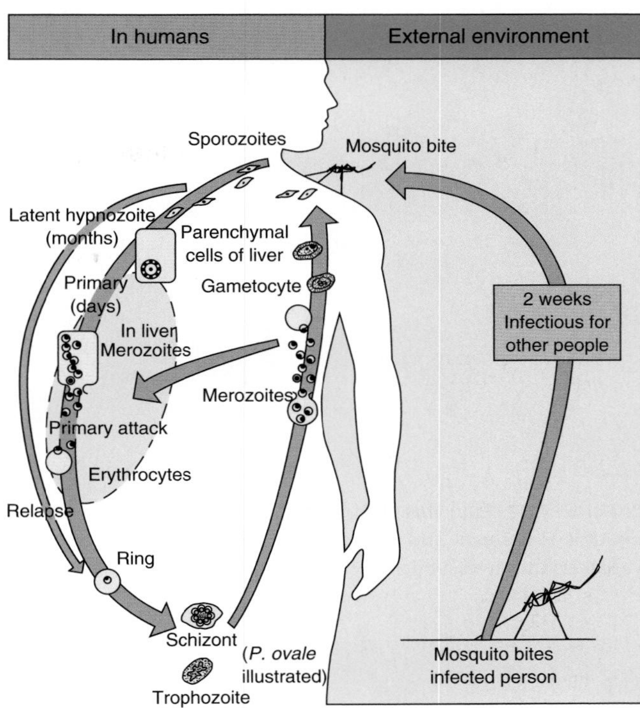

FIGURE 74-1 Life cycle of *Plasmodium* species.

outside of the cell (see Figure 74-2). This is called the **appliqué** or **accolé** position and is distinctive for this species.

Growing trophozoite stages and schizonts of *P. falciparum* are rarely seen in blood films because their forms are sequestered in the liver and spleen. Only in very heavy infections are they found in the peripheral circulation. Thus peripheral blood smears from patients with *P. falciparum* malaria characteristically contain only young ring forms and occasionally gametocytes. The typical crescentic gametocytes are diagnostic for the species (Figure 74-3). Infected RBCs do not enlarge and become distorted as they do with *P. vivax* and *P. ovale*. Occasionally, reddish granules known as **Maurer dots** are observed in *P. falciparum*.

P. falciparum, similar to *P. knowlesi* and *P. malariae,* does not produce hypnozoites in the liver. Relapses from the liver are not known to occur.

Epidemiology

P. falciparum occurs almost exclusively in tropical and subtropical regions. Co-infection with human immunodeficiency virus (HIV) is common in these regions and may pose a risk factor for severe malaria.

Clinical Syndromes

The incubation period of *P. falciparum* is the shortest of all the plasmodia, ranging from 7 to 10 days, and does not extend for months to years. After the early influenza-like symptoms, *P. falciparum* rapidly produces daily **(quotidian)** chills and fever as well as severe nausea, vomiting, and diarrhea. The periodicity of the attacks then becomes **tertian (36 to 48 hours),** and fulminating disease develops. The term **malignant tertian malaria** is appropriate for this infection. Because the symptoms of this type of malaria are similar to those of intestinal infections, the nausea, vomiting, and diar-

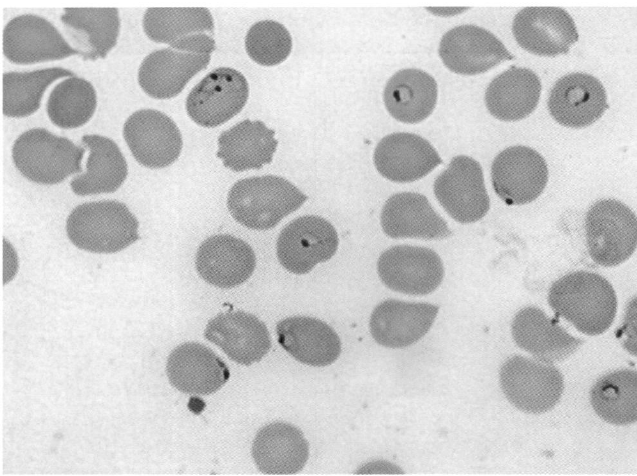

FIGURE 74-2 Ring forms of *Plasmodium falciparum.* Note the multiple ring forms and appliqué (accolé) forms within the individual erythrocytes, which is characteristic of this organism.

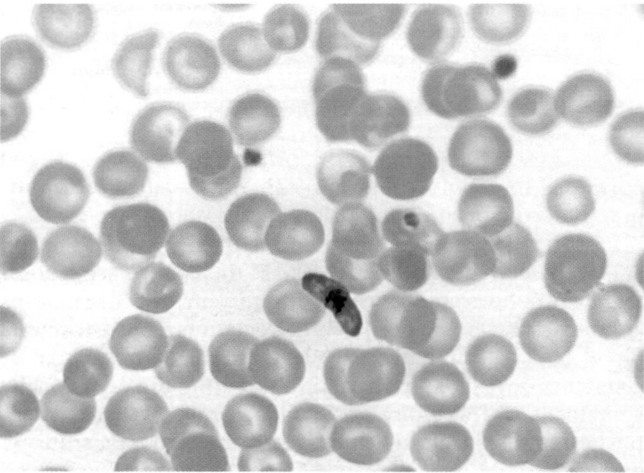

FIGURE 74-3 Mature gametocyte of *Plasmodium falciparum.* The presence of this sausage-shaped form is diagnostic of *P. falciparum* malaria.

rhea have led to the observation that malaria is "the malignant mimic."

Although any malarial infection may be fatal, *P. falciparum* is the most likely to result in death if left untreated. The increased numbers of erythrocytes infected and destroyed result in toxic cellular debris, adherence of RBCs to vascular endothelium and adjacent RBCs, and formation of capillary plugging by masses of RBCs, platelets, leukocytes, and malarial pigment.

Involvement of the brain (cerebral malaria) is most often seen in *P. falciparum* infection. Capillary plugging from an accumulation of malarial pigment and masses of cells can result in coma and death.

Kidney damage is also associated with *P. falciparum* malaria, resulting in an illness called **blackwater fever.** Intravascular hemolysis with rapid destruction of RBCs produces a marked hemoglobinuria and can result in acute renal failure, tubular necrosis, nephrotic syndrome, and death. Liver involvement is characterized by abdominal pain, vomiting of bile, severe diarrhea, and rapid dehydration.

Laboratory Diagnosis

Thick and thin blood films are searched for the characteristic rings of *P. falciparum,* which frequently occur in multiples within a single cell, as well as in the accolé position (see Figure 74-2). Also diagnostic are the distinctive crescentic gametocytes (see Figure 74-3). A high-grade parasitemia (>10% of RBCs infected) consisting only of ring forms is suggestive of *P. falciparum* infection even if no gametocytes are observed.

Laboratory personnel must perform a thorough search of the blood films because mixed infections can occur with any combination of the four species, but most often the combination is *P. falciparum* and *P. vivax.* Detection and proper reporting of a mixed infection directly affect the treatment chosen.

Increasingly, antigen detection using a **rapid diagnostic test (RDT)** is being used both in the field and in diagnostic laboratories as an adjunct to conventional microscopic diagnosis. RDTs use immunochromatographic lateral-flow strip technology and use monoclonal antibodies directed at either species-specific or pan-*Plasmodium* targets. These tests are simple, rapid (results in < 20 minutes), and inexpensive. *P. falciparum*–specific monoclonal antibodies have been developed for **histidine-rich protein 2 (HRP-2)** and *P. falciparum* lactate dehydrogenase. Targets conserved across all human malarias **(panmalarial antigens)** have been identified on ***Plasmodium*** **lactate dehydrogenase (PLDH)** and **aldolase** enzymes. Thus far, one RDT has been approved by the U.S. Food and Drug Administration (FDA): the BinaxNOW (Binax, Scarborough, Maine) Malaria test kit, based on the antigens HRP-2 and aldolase. The sensitivity and specificity of this test for detection of *P. falciparum* are 95% and 94%, respectively.

Treatment, Prevention, and Control

Treatment of malaria is based on the history regarding travel to endemic areas, prompt clinical review and differential diagnosis, accurate and rapid laboratory work, and correct use of antimalarial drugs.

Because chloroquine-resistant strains of *P. falciparum* are present in all areas of endemicity (Africa, Southeast Asia, South America), with the exception of Central America and the Caribbean, physicians must review all current protocols for proper treatment of *P. falciparum* infections, noting particularly where **chloroquine resistance** is known to occur. If the patient's history indicates that the origin is not from a chloroquine-resistant area, the drug of choice is either chloroquine or parenteral quinine. Patients infected with chloroquine-resistant *P. falciparum* (or *P. vivax*) may be treated with other agents, including mefloquine ± artesunate, artemether-lumefantrine, atovaquone-proguanil (Malarone), quinine, quinidine, pyrimethamine-sulfadoxine (Fansidar), and doxycycline. Because quinine and pyrimethamine-sulfadoxine are potentially toxic, they are used more often for treatment than prophylaxis. Amodiaquine, an analog of chloroquine, is effective against chloroquine-resistant *P. falciparum;* however, toxicity limits its use. Newer agents with excellent activity against multidrug-resistant strains of *P. falciparum* include the phenanthrene methanols, halofantrine and lumefantrine, and the artemisinins, artemether and artesunate, both sesquiterpene derivatives (see Chapter 72).

Combinations of the rapid-acting artemisinins with an existing or newly introduced antimalarial compound have been shown to be highly effective in both treatment and control of malaria caused by *P. falciparum*. The rapid reduction in parasite biomass ($\approx 10^8$-fold within 3 days) produced by the artemisinins leaves a relatively small number of organisms for the second agent (usually mefloquine or lumefantrine) to clear. This reduces considerably the exposure of the parasite population to mefloquine or lumefantrine, thus reducing the chance of an escape-resistant mutant arising from the infection. Combinations of artesunate and mefloquine and of artemether and lumefantrine have both been well tolerated and highly efficacious in the treatment of multidrug-resistant falciparum malaria in semiimmune and nonimmune individuals. Of concern are reports of prolonged parasite clearance times that have been observed in artesunate-treated patients in Western Cambodia, suggesting the possible emergence of resistance to this class of agents.

Although the rationale for red cell exchange transfusion in severe malaria is compelling, there are no prospective clinical trials comparing this therapy with others. Nonetheless, red cell exchange (or whole-blood exchange), if available, should be considered in cases of severe malaria complicated by clinical signs of cerebral malaria, acute lung injury, severe hemolysis with acidemia, shock, or a high or rising level of parasitemia despite adequate intravenous antimicrobial therapy. The use of anticonvulsants (phenobarbatone) and dexamethasone in cerebral malaria is likely to be ineffective or harmful and is not recommended.

When there is uncertainty whether the *P. falciparum* is chloroquine resistant, it is advisable to assume the strain is resistant and treat the patient accordingly. If the laboratory reports a mixed infection involving *P. falciparum* and *P. vivax*, the treatment must eradicate not only *P. falciparum* from the erythrocytes but also the liver stages of *P. vivax* to avoid relapses. Failure on the part of the laboratory to detect and report such a mixed infection can result in inappropriate treatment and unnecessary delay in accomplishing a complete cure.

Chemoprophylaxis and prompt eradication of infections are critical in breaking the mosquito-human transmission cycle. Control of mosquito breeding and protection of individuals by screening, netting, protective clothing, and insect repellents are also essential. Chloroquine resistance complicates the management of these patients but can be overcome by the physician's awareness of appropriate regimens. Immigrants from and travelers to endemic areas must be carefully screened using blood films or serologic tests to detect possible infection. The development of vaccines to protect persons living in or traveling to endemic areas is under investigation.

Plasmodium knowlesi

Physiology and Structure

Plasmodium knowlesi is a malaria parasite of **Old World monkeys** (long-tailed *[Macaca fasicularis]* and pig-tailed *[Macaca nemestrina]* macaques). *P. knowlesi* is transmitted by members of the *Anopheles leucosphyrus* group of mosquitoes that resides in the upper canopy of the forests and has infrequent contact with humans. Unlike other primate malarias, *P. knowlesi* exhibits a relaxed host specificity and is permissive in humans under natural and experimental conditions as well as in nonhuman primates. Similar to *P. falciparum,* the erythrocyte invasion by *P. knowlesi* is not restricted to young or old RBCs, which allows the development of high levels of parasitemia. It has a short life cycle of 24 hours **(quotidian),** and the development of the parasite in RBCs is not synchronous. *P. knowlesi* infection is usually misidentified as *P. falciparum* or *P. malariae* because its early trophozoites resemble the ring forms of *P. falciparum* and its later stages mimic those of *P. malariae.* In contrast to *P. falciparum, P. knowlesi* does not appear to sequester in the microvasculature, and the neurologic complications seen with *P. falciparum* infection have not been described.

RBCs infected with *P. knowlesi* exhibit a normal morphology, and all developmental stages may be seen in peripheral blood. *P. knowlesi,* similar to *P. falciparum* and *P. malariae,* does not appear to produce hypnozoites in the liver. Relapses from the liver are not known to occur.

Epidemiology

Thus far, human *P. knowlesi* infections have been described in high numbers only in Malaysia; however, because of reports of infection in the neighboring countries of Thailand, Singapore, Brunei, Indonesia, Myanmar, Vietnam, and the Philippines, it appears that *P. knowlesi* is a natural parasite of macaques throughout the Southeast Asia region.

Clinical Syndromes

The clinical and laboratory profiles of *P. knowlesi* infection are similar to those of patients infected with the other malaria parasites. Patients typically present with a nonspecific febrile illness with daily fever and chills. Other frequent symptoms include headache, rigors, malaise, abdominal pain, breathlessness, and productive cough. Tachypnea, pyrexia, and tachycardia are common clinical signs. Thrombocytopenia and mild hepatic dysfunction upon hospital admission are common.

Approximately 7% of the cases of *P. knowlesi* infection thus far have been judged as severe, using the criteria of the World Health Organization, with the most frequent complication being respiratory distress with pulmonary rather than metabolic etiology. Deaths and severe disease result from pulmonary and hepatorenal failure. Severity of infection is related to high parasitemia levels produced by its rapid and unique 24-hour erythrocyte cycle and its ability to infect all stages of RBCs. It is strongly recommended that infection with *P. knowlesi* be considered in cases in which the microscopic examination suggests *P. malariae* but in which the patient has severe disease, hyperparasitemia (>0.1%; i.e., >5000 parasites/μl), or a recent history of visiting woods or their vicinity in Southeast Asia.

Laboratory Diagnosis

Whereas the ring forms of *P. knowlesi* are morphologically similar to those of *P. falciparum,* the trophozoite, schizont, and gametocyte stages are indistinguishable from those of *P. malariae* by light microscopy. Clues to the identification of *P. knowlesi* by microscopy that are useful if present include early trophozoites with fine ring forms, double chromatin dots, and two to three parasites per RBC (resembling *P. falciparum*); trophozoites with a bird's-eye appearance and/or mature trophozoites with a band appearance resembling *P. malariae;* and mature schizonts with a higher average merozoite count (16/RBC) than in *P. malariae* (10 to 12/RBC). *P. knowlesi*–specific polymerase chain reaction (PCR) is the only reliable means of identifying this emerging species of *Plasmodium.*

At present, no commercially available RDTs are designed to specifically detect *P. knowlesi.* Performance of these mainly *P. falciparum*– and *P. vivax*–targeted RDTs in *P. knowlesi* infection has been reported in a few cases. PLDH produced by the four other *Plasmodium* species that cause human malaria is also present in *P. knowlesi.* Antibodies to the pan-malaria targets PLDH and aldolase also cross-react with those of *P. knowlesi.* At this time, the RDTs are not recommended because of the unreliable results and low sensitivity in detecting *P. knowlesi.*

Treatment, Prevention, and Control

Given the potential severity of *P. knowlesi* infection, it should be managed like *P. falciparum* malaria if the species identification is based on microscopy alone or if co-infection with *P. falciparum* cannot be excluded with certainty using PCR. *P. knowlesi* alone appears to be susceptible to numerous therapeutic alternatives, with the majority of patients responding promptly to chloroquine. As with *P. falciparum,* relapses from the liver are not known to occur.

Prevention of *P. knowlesi* infection is based on avoiding mosquito bites and taking preventive medication when indicated. Although general precautions for avoiding the bites of *Anopheles* mosquitoes probably apply, it should be recognized that current indoor control measures for malaria do not prevent zoonotic transmission of malaria by vectors that feed mainly in the forest. Zoonotic *P. knowlesi* infection is likely to pose a problem for malaria control.

Plasmodium vivax

Physiology and Structure

P. vivax (Figure 74-4) is selective in that it invades only young, immature erythrocytes. Whereas the **Duffy blood group antigen** on the RBC surface has long been considered to be the primary receptor for *P. vivax* (see Chapter 69), clinical vivax malaria has recently been reported in Duffy-negative individuals in Madagascar. The parasite and host molecules that enable this Duffy-independent *P. vivax* invasion of human RBCs are as yet unknown. In infections caused by *P. vivax,* infected RBCs are usually enlarged and contain numerous pink granules or **Schüffner dots,** the trophozoite is ring shaped but ameboid in appearance, more mature trophozoites and erythrocytic schizonts containing up to 24 merozoites are present, and the gametocytes are round. The mature schizonts often contain golden-brown **hemozoin** pigment granules **(malarial pigment).**

Epidemiology

P. vivax is the most prevalent of the human plasmodia, with the widest geographic distribution, including the tropics, subtropics, and temperate regions. The overwhelming majority (>80%) of clinical cases of vivax malaria occur in South America and Southeast Asia.

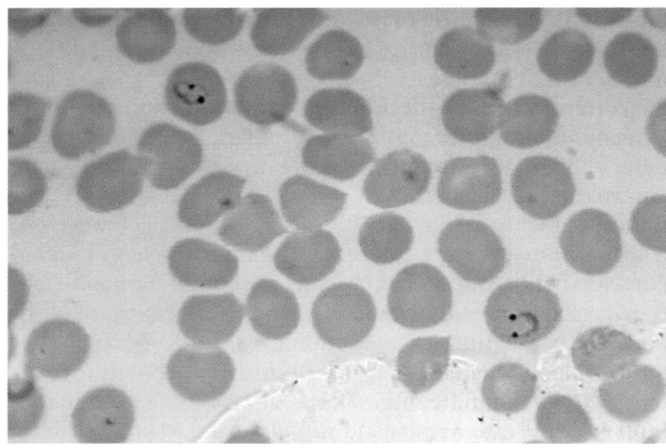

FIGURE 74-4 *Plasmodium vivax* ring forms with double chromatin dots. This feature is more reminiscent of *Plasmodium falciparum* than *P. vivax. P. vivax* rings have a large quantity of cytoplasm and a large chromatin dot as well as occasional pseudopods. The red blood cells are enlarged up to 1.5 times normal size, round, and contain fine Schüffner dots. (From CDC Public Health Image Library.)

Clinical Syndromes

After an incubation period (usually 10 to 17 days), the patient experiences vague influenza-like symptoms with headache, muscle pains, photophobia, anorexia, nausea, and vomiting.

As the infection progresses, increased numbers of rupturing erythrocytes liberate merozoites as well as toxic cellular debris and hemoglobin into the circulation. Together these produce the typical pattern of chills, fever, and malarial rigors. These **paroxysms** usually reappear periodically (generally every 48 hours) as the cycle of infection, replication, and cell lysis progresses. The paroxysms may remain relatively mild or progress to severe attacks with hours of sweating, chills, shaking, persistently high temperatures (103° F to 106° F), and exhaustion.

P. vivax causes **"benign tertian malaria,"** which refers to the cycle of paroxysms every 48 hours (in untreated patients) and the belief that most patients tolerate the attacks and can survive for years without treatment. Recent evidence, however, suggests that *P. vivax* can cause a **spectrum of severe, life-threatening syndromes** that are strikingly similar to those caused by *P. falciparum.* Reports of vivax malaria marked by delirium, seizures, renal failure, shock, hepatic dysfunction, severe anemia, lung injury, pulmonary edema, and acute respiratory distress have come from South and Southeast Asia, the Middle East, and South America. Likewise, if left untreated, chronic *P. vivax* infections can lead to brain, kidney, and liver damage as a result of the malarial pigment, cellular debris, and capillary plugging of these organs by masses of adherent erythrocytes.

Laboratory Diagnosis

Microscopic examination of thick and thin films of blood is the method of choice for confirming the clinical diagnosis of malaria and identifying the specific species responsible for disease. The thick film is a concentration method and may be used to detect the presence of organisms. With training, thick films may be used to diagnose the species as well. The thin film is most useful for establishing species identification. Blood films can be taken at any time over the course of the infection, but the best time is midway between paroxysms of chills and fever, when the greatest number of intracellular organisms is present. It may be necessary to take repeated films at intervals of 4 to 6 hours.

Serologic procedures are available, but they are used primarily for epidemiologic surveys or for screening blood donors. Serologic findings usually remain positive for approximately a year, even after complete treatment of the infection. RDTs may be used as an adjunct to microscopy in the diagnosis of malaria caused by *P. vivax;* however, the sensitivity is generally much lower than that for detection of *P. falciparum:* 69% versus 94%, respectively.

Treatment, Prevention, and Control

Treatment of *P. vivax* infection involves a combination of supportive measures and chemotherapy. Bed rest, relief of fever and headache, regulation of fluid balance, and in some cases blood transfusion are supportive therapies. The chemotherapeutic regimens are as follows:

1. Suppressive: aimed at avoiding infection and clinical symptoms (i.e., a form of prophylaxis)
2. Therapeutic: aimed at eradicating the erythrocytic cycle
3. Radical cure: aimed at eradicating the exoerythrocytic cycle in the liver
4. Gametocidal: aimed at destroying erythrocytic gametocytes to prevent mosquito transmission

Chloroquine is the drug of choice for suppression and therapeutic treatment of *P. vivax,* followed by primaquine for radical cure and elimination of gametocytes. Chloroquine-resistant forms of *P. vivax* have emerged in Indonesia, the Solomon Islands, New Guinea, and Brazil. Patients infected with chloroquine-resistant *P. vivax* may be treated with other agents, including mefloquine ± artesunate, quinine, pyrimethamine-sulfadoxine (Fansidar), and doxycycline. Primaquine is especially effective in preventing a relapse from the latent forms of *P. vivax* in the liver. Because antimalarial drugs are potentially toxic, it is imperative that physicians carefully review the recommended therapeutic regimens.

Plasmodium ovale

Physiology and Structure

P. ovale is similar to *P. vivax* in many respects, including its selectivity for young, pliable erythrocytes. As a consequence, the host cell becomes enlarged and distorted, usually in an oval form. Schüffner dots appear as pale pink granules, and the cell border is frequently fimbriated or ragged. The schizont of *P. ovale,* when mature, contains about half the number of merozoites seen in *P. vivax,* and the malarial pigment is a darker brown.

Epidemiology

P. ovale is distributed primarily in tropical Africa, where it is often more prevalent than *P. vivax.* It is also found in Asia and South America.

Clinical Syndromes

The clinical picture of tertian attacks for *P. ovale* (benign tertian or ovale malaria) infection is similar to that for *P. vivax.* Untreated infections last only about a year instead of the several years for *P. vivax.* Both relapse and recrudescence phases are similar to *P. vivax.*

Laboratory Diagnosis

As with *P. vivax,* thick and thin blood films are examined for the typical oval host cell with Schüffner dots and a ragged cell wall. Serologic tests reveal cross-reaction with *P. vivax* and other plasmodia. RDTs are not recommended for the diagnosis of *P. ovale* infection.

Treatment, Prevention, and Control

The treatment regimen, including the use of primaquine to prevent relapse from latent liver forms, is similar to that used for *P. vivax* infections. Preventing *P. ovale* infection involves the same measures as for *P. vivax* and other plasmodia.

Plasmodium malariae

Physiology and Structure

In contrast with *P. vivax* and *P. ovale, P. malariae* can infect only mature erythrocytes with relatively rigid cell membranes. As a result, the parasite's growth must conform to the size and shape of the RBC. This produces no red cell enlargement or distortion as seen in *P. vivax* and *P. ovale,* but it does result in distinctive shapes of the parasite seen in the host cell: "band and bar forms," as well as very compact dark-staining forms. The schizont of *P. malariae* shows no red cell enlargement or distortion and is usually composed of eight merozoites appearing in a rosette surrounding a dark brown central pigment granule. Occasionally, reddish granules called **Ziemann dots** appear in the host cell.

Unlike for *P. vivax* and *P. ovale,* hypnozoites for *P. malariae* are not found in the liver and relapse does not occur. Recrudescence does occur, and attacks may develop after apparent abatement of symptoms.

Epidemiology

P. malariae infection occurs primarily in the same subtropical and temperate regions as the other plasmodia but is less prevalent.

Clinical Syndromes

The incubation period for *P. malariae* is the longest of the plasmodia, usually 18 to 40 days but possibly several months to years. The early symptoms are influenza like, with fever patterns of 72 hours (quartan or malarial malaria) in periodicity. Attacks are moderate to severe and last several hours. Untreated infections may last as long as 20 years.

Laboratory Diagnosis

Observing the characteristic **bar and band forms and the rosette schizont** in thick and thin films of blood establishes the diagnosis of *P. malariae* infection. As noted, serologic tests cross react with other plasmodia. RDTs are not recommended for the diagnosis of infections with *P. malariae.*

Treatment, Prevention, and Control

Treatment is similar to that for *P. vivax* and *P. ovale* infections and must be undertaken to prevent recrudescent infections. Treatment to prevent relapse caused by latent liver forms is not required because these forms do not develop with *P. malariae.* Preventive and controlling mechanisms are as discussed for *P. vivax* and *P. ovale.*

• *Babesia* Species

Babesia spp. are intracellular sporozoan parasites that morphologically resemble plasmodia. Babesiosis is a zoonosis infecting a variety of animals such as deer, cattle, and rodents; humans are accidental hosts. Infection is transmitted by *Ixodes* ticks. *Babesia microti* is the usual cause of babesiosis in the United States.

Physiology and Structure

Human infection follows contact with an infected tick (Figure 74-5). The infectious **pyriform bodies** are introduced into the bloodstream and infect erythrocytes. The intraerythrocytic trophozoites multiply by **binary fission,** forming tetrads, and then lyse the erythrocyte, releasing the merozoites. These can reinfect other cells to maintain the infection. Infected cells can also be ingested by feeding ticks, in which additional replication can take place. Infection in the tick population can also be maintained by transovarian transmission. The infected cells in humans resemble the ring forms of *P. falciparum,* but malarial pigment or other stages of growth characteristically seen with plasmodial infections are not seen with careful examination of blood smears (Figure 74-6).

Epidemiology

More than 70 different species of *Babesia* are found in Africa, Asia, Europe, and North America, with *B. microti* responsible for disease along the northeastern seaboard of the United States (e.g., Nantucket Island, Martha's Vineyard, Shelter Island). *Ixodes dammini* is the tick vector responsible for transmitting babesiosis in this area, and the natural reservoir hosts are field mice, voles, and other small rodents. Serologic studies in endemic areas have demonstrated a high incidence of past exposure to *Babesia*. Presumably, most infections are asymptomatic or mild. *Babesia divergens,* which has been reported more frequently in Europe, causes severe, often fatal infections in people who have undergone splenectomies. Severe persistent *B. microti* parasitemia has occurred in immunosuppressed HIV-infected patients with intact spleens. Although most infections follow tick bites, *B. microti* is increasingly being transmitted by blood transfusions in the United States. A recent upsurge in transfusion-transmitted babesiosis (TTB) cases attributed to *B. microti,* coupled with at least 12 fatalities in transfusion recipients diagnosed with babesiosis, has elevated TTB to a key policy issue in transfusion medicine.

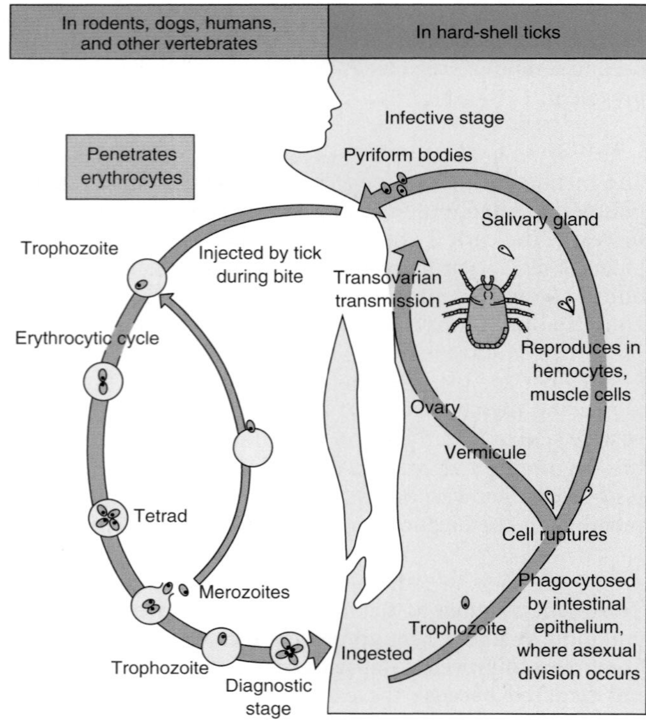

FIGURE 74-5 Life cycle of *Babesia* species.

Clinical Syndromes

After an incubation period of 1 to 4 weeks, symptomatic patients experience general malaise, fever without periodicity, headache, chills, sweating, fatigue, and weakness. As the infection progresses with increased destruction of erythrocytes, hemolytic anemia develops and the patient may experience renal failure. Hepatomegaly and splenomegaly can develop in advanced disease. Low-grade parasitemia may persist for weeks. Splenectomy or functional asplenia, immunosuppression, HIV infection, and advanced age increase a person's susceptibility to infections as well as to more severe disease.

Laboratory Diagnosis

Examination of blood smears is the diagnostic method of choice. Laboratory personnel must be experienced in differentiating *Babesia* and *Plasmodium* species. *Babesia* may mimic *P. falciparum,* with RBCs infected with multiple small ring forms (see Figure 74-6). Infected patients may have negative smears because of the low-grade parasitemia. These infections can be diagnosed by inoculating samples of blood into hamsters, which are highly susceptible to infection. Serologic tests and amplification of babesial deoxyribonucleic acid (DNA) by PCR are also available for diagnostic use.

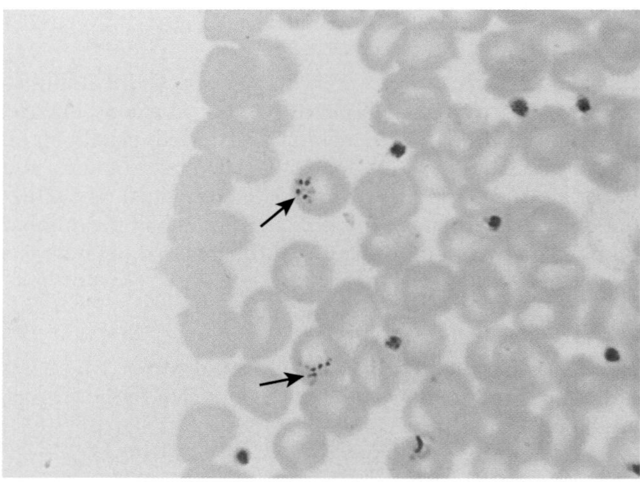

FIGURE 74-6 Ring forms of *Babesia microti.* Note the multiple ring forms *(arrows)* within the individual erythrocytes and the similarity to those of *Plasmodium falciparum* in Figure 74-3.

Treatment, Prevention, and Control

The treatment of choice for mild to moderate illness is the combination of atovaquone and azithromycin, whereas clindamycin and quinine and exchange transfusion are indicated for severe disease. Other antiprotozoal regimens, including chloroquine and pentamidine, have been used with variable results. However, most patients with mild disease recover without specific therapy. Exchange blood transfusion has also been successful in patients who have had splenectomies and who have severe infections caused by *B. microti* or *B. divergens*. The use of protective clothing and insect repellents can minimize tick exposure in endemic areas, which is critical for prevention of disease. Ticks must feed on humans for several hours before the organisms are transmitted, so prompt removal of ticks can be protective.

Toxoplasma gondii

Toxoplasma gondii is a typical coccidian parasite related to *Plasmodium*, *Cystoisospora*, and other members of the phylum Sporozoa. *T. gondii* is an intracellular parasite, and it is found in a wide variety of animals including birds and humans. Only one species exists, and there appears to be little strain-to-strain variation. The essential reservoir host of *T. gondii* is the common house cat and other felines.

Physiology and Structure

Organisms develop in the intestinal cells of the cat, as well as during an extraintestinal cycle with passage to the tissues via the bloodstream (Figure 74-7). The organisms from the intestinal cycle are passed in cat feces and mature into infective cysts within 3 to 4 days in the external environment.

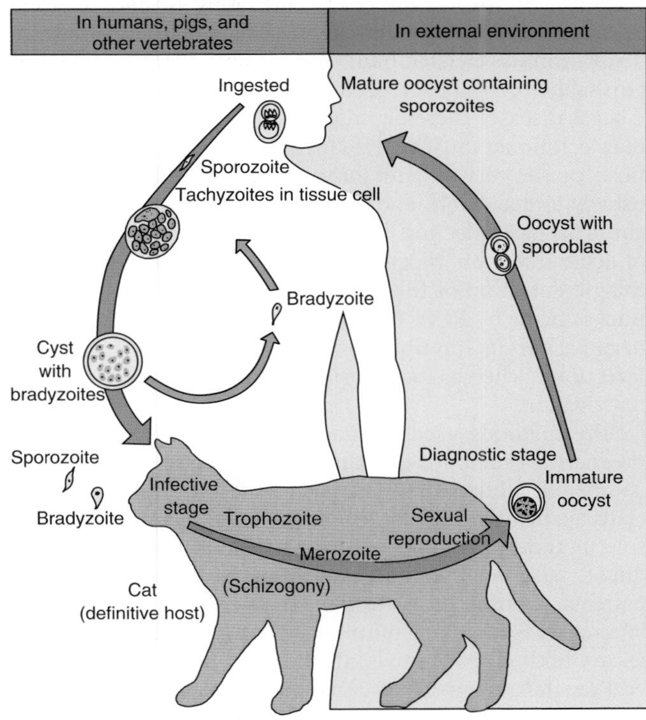

FIGURE 74-7 Life cycle of *Toxoplasma gondii*.

These oocysts are similar to those of *Cystoisospora belli*, the human intestinal protozoan parasite, and can be ingested by mice and other animals (including humans) and produce acute and chronic infection of various tissues, including brain. Infection in cats is established when the tissues of infected rodents are eaten.

Some infective forms **(trophozoites)** of the oocyst develop as slender crescentic types called **tachyzoites.** These rapidly multiplying forms are responsible for the initial infection and tissue damage. Slow-growing shorter forms called **bradyzoites** also develop and form cysts in chronic infections.

Epidemiology

Human infection with *T. gondii* is ubiquitous; however, it is increasingly apparent that certain immunocompromised individuals (patients with acquired immunodeficiency syndrome [AIDS]) are more likely to have severe manifestations. The wide variety of animals that harbor the organism—carnivores and herbivores as well as birds—accounts for the widespread transmission.

Humans become infected from two sources: (1) ingestion of improperly cooked meat from animals that serve as intermediate hosts and (2) ingestion of infective oocysts from contaminated cat feces. Serologic studies show an increased prevalence in human populations where the consumption of uncooked meat or meat juices is popular. It is noteworthy that serologic tests of human and rodent populations are negative in the few geographic areas where cats have not existed. Outbreaks of toxoplasmosis in the United States are usually traced to poorly cooked meat (e.g., hamburger) as well as contact with cat feces.

Transplacental infection can occur in pregnancy, either from infection acquired from meat and meat juices or from contact with cat feces. Transplacental infection from an infected mother has a devastating effect on the fetus. Transfusion infection via contaminated blood can occur but is not common. The sharing of needles between intravenous drug users may also facilitate transmission of *Toxoplasma.*

Although the rate of seroconversion is similar for individuals within a geographic location, the rate of severe infection is dramatically affected by the immune status of the individual. Patients with defects in cell-mediated immunity, especially those who are infected with HIV or who have had an organ transplant or immunosuppressive therapy, are most likely to have disseminated or central nervous system (CNS) disease. Illness in this setting is generally believed to be caused by reactivation of previously latent infection rather than new exposure to the organism.

Clinical Syndromes

Most *T. gondii* infections are benign and asymptomatic, with symptoms occurring as the parasite moves from the blood to tissues, where it becomes an intracellular parasite. When symptomatic disease occurs, the infection is characterized by cell destruction, reproduction of more organisms, and eventual cyst formation. Many tissues may be affected; however, the organism has a particular predilection for cells of the lung, heart, lymphoid organs, and CNS, including the eye (Clinical Case 74-2).

Symptoms of acute disease include chills, fever, headaches, myalgia, lymphadenitis, and fatigue; the symptoms

 **Clinical Case 74-2 Toxoplasmosis**

Vincent and colleagues (*Infect Med* 23:390, 2006) described a 67-year-old woman with a 3-year history of Hodgkin disease who received chemotherapy followed by autologous stem cell transplantation. Shortly afterward, she became febrile and neutropenic, and treatment with broad-spectrum antibiotics was started. The results of blood and urine cultures were negative. After resolution of neutropenia (1 month post transplantation), confusion and lethargy developed. Imaging studies of the brain revealed microinfarcts in both hemispheres and the midbrain. Findings from a lumbar puncture were unrevealing. Based on the suspicion of toxoplasmosis, pyrimethamine and sulfadiazine were added to the patient's regimen. When toxic epidermal necrolysis developed, the sulfadiazine was discontinued and clindamycin was begun. Multiorgan failure ensued, and the patient died 1 week later. At autopsy, cyst forms with bradyzoites were detected in the woman's brain and heart. Histopathologic findings and immunohistochemical staining confirmed a diagnosis of disseminated toxoplasmosis.

Disseminated toxoplasmosis is rare, especially after autologous stem cell transplantation. The likely cause of reactivation and dissemination of *Toxoplasma* in this patient was the cell-mediated immunosuppression associated with Hodgkin disease and its treatment. In addition to the brain, the heart, liver, and lungs are frequently involved in cases of disseminated toxoplasmosis.

occasionally resemble those of infectious mononucleosis. In chronic disease, the signs and symptoms include lymphadenitis, occasionally a rash, evidence of hepatitis, encephalomyelitis, and myocarditis. In some of the cases, chorioretinitis appears and may lead to blindness.

Congenital infection with *T. gondii* also occurs in infants born to mothers infected during pregnancy. If infection occurs in the first trimester, the result is spontaneous abortion, stillbirth, or severe disease. Manifestations in the infant infected after the first trimester include epilepsy, encephalitis, microcephaly, intracranial calcifications, hydrocephalus, psychomotor or mental retardation, chorioretinitis, blindness, anemia, jaundice, rash, pneumonia, diarrhea, and hypothermia. Infants may be asymptomatic at birth only to develop disease months to years later. Most often these children develop **chorioretinitis** with or without blindness or other neurologic problems, including retardation, seizures, microcephaly, and hearing loss.

In immunocompromised older patients, a different spectrum of disease is seen. Reactivation of latent toxoplasmosis is a special problem for these people. The presenting symptoms of *Toxoplasma* infection in immunocompromised patients are usually neurologic, most frequently consistent with diffuse encephalopathy, meningoencephalitis, or cerebral mass lesions. Reactivation of cerebral toxoplasmosis has emerged as a major cause of encephalitis in patients with AIDS. The disease is usually multifocal, with more than one mass lesion appearing in the brain at the same time. Symptoms are related to the location of the lesions and may include hemiparesis, seizures, visual impairment, confusion, and lethargy. Other sites of infection that have been reported include the eye, lung, and testes. Although disease is seen predominantly in patients with AIDS, it may also occur with similar manifestations in other immunocompromised patients, in particular those undergoing solid organ transplantation.

Laboratory Diagnosis

Serologic testing is required for the diagnosis of acute active infection; the diagnosis is established by the finding of increasing antibody titers documented in serially collected blood specimens. Because contact with the organism is common, assays for different isotypes of antibodies and attention to increasing titers is essential to differentiate acute active infection from previous asymptomatic or chronic infection. A panel of tests referred to as the *T. gondii* serologic profile (TSP) is used by specialized reference laboratories to determine whether the infection is consistent with acquisition recently or in the more distant past. The TSP consists of (1) the Sabin-Feldman dye test to measure immunoglobulin (Ig)G antibodies, (2) enzyme-linked immunosorbent assays (ELISAs) to measure IgM, IgA, and IgE antibodies, (3) immunosorbent agglutination assay to measure levels of IgE antibodies, and (4) differential agglutination test to measure levels of IgG antibodies.

The initial evaluation in the immunocompetent patient involves screening for IgG antibodies to *T. gondii.* Although many studies and guidelines suggest the usefulness of testing for IgM in parallel, IgM antibodies to *T. gondii* may persist for more than 12 months after an acute infection, leading to a false-positive result. If IgG titers are equivocal, serial specimens should be collected 3 weeks apart and tested in parallel. If the IgG titer is negative (<1:16), *Toxoplasma* infection is ruled out. A twofold rise in antibody titer indicates an acute infection, as does conversion from a negative to a positive result. A single high titer is not a sufficient basis for diagnosing toxoplasmosis, because IgG titers may remain elevated for many years after infection.

Toxoplasmosis in patients with malignancies, organ transplants, or AIDS is generally assumed to arise from reactivation of a chronic asymptomatic (latent) infection. The diagnosis of *Toxoplasma* encephalitis usually involves a CT or magnetic resonance imaging study of the brain. However, *Toxoplasma*-associated brain abnormalities may be indistinguishable from AIDS-related cerebral lymphoma or cerebral Chagas disease. Therefore microscopy, serologic, and molecular techniques must be used for a definitive diagnosis. Diagnosis can be very difficult for these patients; IgM antibody is usually undetectable, and the presence of IgG antibody only confirms past infection. In the absence of serologic evidence of acute infection, diagnosis can be confirmed only by histologic detection of the organism in tissues or detection of nucleic acids by PCR. Immunosuppressed patients who are negative for IgG antibodies are at risk for acute acquired infection, whereas seropositive patients are at risk of reactivation.

The methods used to diagnose acute toxoplasmosis in pregnant women are the same as those used for immunocompetent adults. The FDA has issued a warning to physicians against the use of *T. gondii* IgM commercial kits as the sole method of diagnosis during pregnancy because of frequent false-positive and false-negative results in these patients. Confirmatory testing at a *Toxoplasma* reference laboratory is highly recommended. If IgM and IgG antibodies are both absent, active infection can be excluded.

Prenatal diagnosis of congenital toxoplasmosis can be achieved by ultrasonography and amniocentesis. Amniotic fluid PCR analysis to detect *T. gondii* is the test of choice,

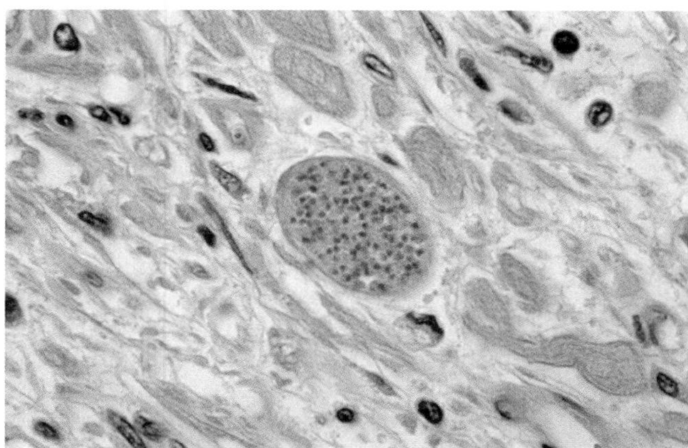

FIGURE 74-8 Cyst of *Toxoplasma gondii* in tissue. Hundreds of organisms may be present in the cyst, which may become active and initiate disease with decreased host immunity (e.g., immunosuppression in transplant patients and in diseases such as acquired immunodeficiency syndrome).

offering excellent positive and negative predictive values. Because maternal IgG antibodies are present in newborns, detection of IgA and IgM antibodies is the foundation of serodiagnosis of toxoplasmosis in the newborn.

Demonstration of these organisms as trophozoites and cysts in tissue and body fluids is the definitive method of diagnosis (Figure 74-8). Biopsy specimens from lymph nodes, brain, myocardium, or other suspected tissue, as well as body fluids, including cerebrospinal fluid (CSF), amniotic fluid, or bronchoalveolar lavage fluid, can be directly examined for the organisms. Newer monoclonal antibody–based fluorescent stains may facilitate direct detection of *T. gondii* in tissue. Culture methods for *T. gondii* are largely experimental and not usually available in clinical laboratories. The two methods available are to inoculate potentially infected material into either mouse peritoneum or tissue culture. Advances in developing PCR-based detection methods are promising and may provide rapid and sensitive approaches for detecting the organism in blood, CSF, amniotic fluid, and other clinical specimens.

Treatment, Prevention, and Control

Therapy for toxoplasmosis depends on the nature of the infectious process and the immunocompetence of the host. Most mononucleosis-like infections in normal hosts resolve spontaneously and do not require specific therapy. In contrast, disseminated or CNS infection in immunocompromised people must be treated. Before the association of *T. gondii* with HIV infection, immunocompromised patients with toxoplasmosis were treated for 4 to 6 weeks. In the setting of HIV infection, discontinuing therapy after 4 to 6 weeks is associated with a relapse rate of 25%. Such patients are currently treated with an initial high-dose regimen of pyrimethamine plus sulfadiazine and then continued on lower doses of both drugs indefinitely. Although this drug combination is the regimen of choice, toxicity (rash and bone marrow suppression) may necessitate changes to alternative agents. Clindamycin plus pyrimethamine is the best-studied alternative. Atovaquone and azithromycin (each alone or with pyrimethamine) also have some activity, although their efficacy and safety compared with those of clindamycin-pyrimethamine need to be assessed. Trimethoprim-sulfamethoxazole is another alternative to pyrimethamine-sulfadiazine for treatment of disseminated or CNS toxoplasmosis. The use of corticosteroids is indicated as part of therapy of cerebral edema and ocular infections that involve or threaten the macula.

Infections in the first trimester of pregnancy are difficult to manage because of the teratogenicity of pyrimethamine in laboratory animals. Both clindamycin and spiramycin have been substituted with apparent success. Spiramycin does not appear to be effective for the treatment of toxoplasmosis in immunocompromised patients.

As more immunocompromised patients at risk for disseminated infection are identified, greater emphasis is placed on preventive measures and specific prophylaxis. Routine serologic screening of patients before organ transplantation and early in the course of HIV infection is now being performed. Individuals with positive serologic tests are at much higher risk for the development of disease and are now being considered for prophylaxis. Trimethoprim-sulfamethoxazole, which is also used as prophylaxis to prevent *Pneumocystis jirovecii* infections, also appears to be effective at preventing infections with *T. gondii.* Additional preventive measures for pregnant women and immunocompromised hosts should include avoiding consumption and handling of raw or undercooked meat and avoiding exposure to cat feces. As is the case with other protozoa, the availability of antiretroviral therapy has led to a major reduction in AIDS-associated toxoplasmosis. In particular, cases of *Toxoplasma* encephalitis have been greatly reduced to the extent that they are now very uncommon in regions with access to antiretroviral therapy.

• *Sarcocystis lindemanni*

Sarcocystis lindemanni is a typical coccidian closely related to the intestinal forms *Sarcocystis suihominis, Sarcocystis bovihominis,* and *C. belli,* and the blood and tissue parasite *T. gondii. S. lindemanni* occurs worldwide in various animals, especially sheep, cattle, and pigs. Humans are accidentally infected only as the result of eating meat from these animals. Most infections are asymptomatic, but occasionally an infection may cause myositis, swelling of muscle, dyspnea, and eosinophilia. Infection of the myocardium has been observed but is extremely rare. There is no specific treatment for the muscle infection.

• Free-Living Amebae

Naegleria spp., *Acanthamoeba* spp., *Balamuthia* spp., *Sappinia pedata, Paravahlkampfia francinae,* and other free-living amebae are found in soil and in contaminated lakes, streams, and other water environments. Most human infections with these amebae are acquired during the warm summer months by people exposed to the amebae while swimming in contaminated water. Inhalation of cysts present in dust may account for some infections, whereas ocular infections with *Acanthamoeba* spp. are associated with the contamination of contact lenses with nonsterile cleaning solutions.

Clinical Syndromes

Naegleria, Acanthamoeba, Balamuthia, Sappinia, and *Paravahlkampfia* organisms are opportunistic pathogens. Although colonization of the nasal passages is usually asymptomatic, these amebae can invade the nasal mucosa and extend into the brain (Clinical Case 74-3). Acute primary **amebic meningoencephalitis** (PAM) is most commonly caused by *Naegleria fowleri.* Destruction of brain tissue is characterized by a fulminant, rapidly fatal meningoencephalitis. Symptoms include intense frontal headache, sore throat, fever, blocked nose with altered senses of taste and smell, stiff neck, and Kernig sign. The CSF is purulent and may contain many erythrocytes and motile amebae. Clinically, the course of the disease is rapid, with death usually occurring within 4 or 5 days. Postmortem findings show *Naegleria* trophozoites present in the brain but no evidence of cysts (Figure 74-9). Although all cases were fatal before 1970, survival has now been reported in a few cases in which the disease was rapidly diagnosed and treated.

Clinical Case 74-3 Amebic Encephalitis

Rahimian and Kleinman (*Infect Med* 22:382–385, 2005) described a 43-year-old man, originally from the Dominican Republic, who presented after a seizure. The patient had a history of diabetes and hypertension but denied any previous history of seizures. Results of a computed tomography (CT) scan without contrast were normal. Neurologic examination was unrevealing, and the patient was sent home. Approximately 2 weeks later, he was readmitted to the hospital because of a new left facial droop. A CT scan without contrast showed the new appearance of thickening and hypodensity of the right frontal gray matter. Progressive generalized weakness developed, along with paralysis of the left upper extremity. A repeat CT scan without contrast revealed an increase in the size of the right frontal hypodense area, with vasogenic edema and a new left parietal hypodense lesion. At that time, dysarthria and a bilateral occipital headache also developed. The patient was a construction worker who denied injection drug use, recent dental work, and risk factors for human immunodeficiency virus (HIV) infection. His travel history was significant only for a trip to the Dominican Republic 2 years previously. Clinical examination was remarkable for dysarthria, a left facial droop, and left upper extremity paralysis. A lumbar puncture revealed an elevated white blood cell count, a cerebrospinal fluid (CSF) protein level of 50 mg/dl, and glucose of 145 mg/dl (serum glucose was 327 mg/dl). Gram stain of the CSF was negative. A magnetic resonance imaging scan of the head showed two large ring-enhancing lesions with possible central necrosis. Results of an HIV test were negative. A brain biopsy showed lymphocytic infiltration, predominantly in the perivascular areas. A closer examination revealed trophozoites and amebic cysts consistent with a diagnosis of amebic encephalitis. Results of a polymerase chain reaction (PCR) assay were consistent with *Balamuthia mandrillaris* infection. Therapy with pentamidine was initiated, but the patient died 3 days later.

Balamuthia encephalitis has been described in both immunosuppressed and immunocompetent individuals. Many infected patients do not have a history of swimming or exposure to contaminated water. The portal of entry is believed to be the respiratory tract or skin ulceration, with dissemination to the brain. Most cases of amebic encephalitis have been diagnosed postmortem. Recently a PCR assay specific for *Balamuthia* has been used for diagnosis, as was done in this case. The majority of patients have died within weeks after the onset of neurologic symptoms, despite treatment with pentamidine.

Other small free-living amebae may rarely cause encephalitis in humans. *Sappinia diploidea* is a free-living ameba that is found in soil contaminated with the feces of elk and buffalo. *S. diploidea* was identified in an excised brain lesion from a 38-year-old immunocompetent man presenting with bifrontal headache, blurred vision, and loss of consciousness following a sinus infection. Recently a new species of the free-living ameba genus *Paravahlkampfia, P. francinae,* was isolated from the CSF of a patient with headache, sore throat, and vomiting symptoms typical of PAM. The patient recovered within a few days, suggesting that previous reports of non-fatal PAM may have been caused by this organism.

In contrast to *Naegleria, Acanthamoeba* and *Balamuthia* organisms produce granulomatous amebic encephalitis and single or multiple brain abscesses, primarily in immunocompromised individuals. The course of the disease is slower, with an incubation period of at least 10 days. The resulting disease is chronic granulomatous encephalitis with edema of the brain tissue.

Eye and skin infection caused by *Acanthamoeba* organisms may also occur. Keratitis is usually associated with eye trauma that occurred before contact with contaminated soil, dust, or water. The use of improperly cleaned contact lenses is also associated with this disease. Invasion by *Acanthamoeba* spp. produces corneal ulceration and severe ocular pain. Cases of apparent disseminated cutaneous and subcutaneous infection with *Acanthamoeba* and *Balamuthia* organisms have been described in patients with AIDS and in solid organ transplant recipients. These infections include multiple soft-tissue nodules, which on biopsy contain amebae. CNS or deep tissue involvement may also be present with this form of infection.

Laboratory Diagnosis

For the diagnosis of infections due to the free-living amebae, nasal discharge, CSF, and (in the case of eye infections) corneal scrapings should be collected. The specimens should be examined using a saline wet preparation and iodine-stained smears. Giemsa stain, Gram stain, or the fluorescent

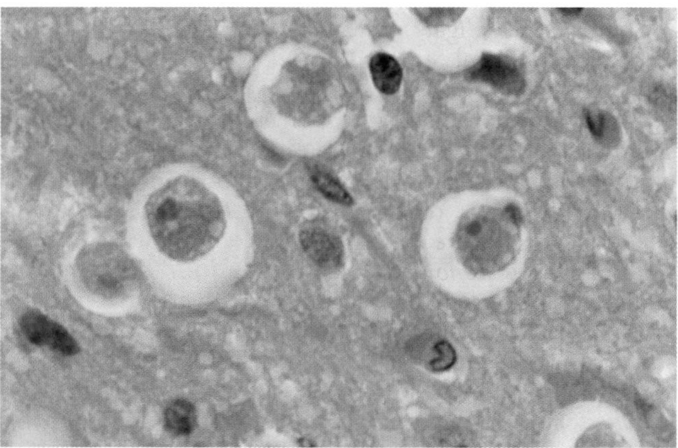

FIGURE 74-9 Numerous *Naegleria* trophozoites in brain tissue from a patient with amebic meningoencephalitis. (From CDC Public Health Image Library.)

stain calcofluor white can also be used. *Naegleria* and *Acanthamoeba* species are difficult to differentiate except by experienced microscopists. However, the observation of an ameba in a normally sterile tissue is diagnostic (see Figure 74-9). In *Naegleria* infection, only the **ameboid trophozoites** are found within the tissue, whereas with *Acanthamoeba* and *Balamuthia* infection, both trophozoites and cysts are found in tissues. Clinical specimens can be cultured on agar plates seeded with live gram-negative enteric bacilli. Amebae present in the specimens use the bacteria as a nutritional source and can be detected within 1 or 2 days by the presence of the trails that form on the agar surface as the amebae move. *Balamuthia* do not grow on agar plates used for *Naegleria* and *Acanthamoeba* but have been recovered in tissue culture using mammalian cell lines. Most cases of *Balamuthia* infection are diagnosed by immunofluorescent antibody testing. PCR has also been applied to the diagnosis of infections with all three of the free-living amebae.

Treatment, Prevention, and Control

Treatment of free-living amebic infections is largely ineffective. Amebic meningoencephalitis caused by *Naegleria, Acanthamoeba,* or *Balamuthia* is unresponsive to most antimicrobial agents. The treatment of choice for *Naegleria* infections is amphotericin B combined with miconazole and rifampin. *Acanthamoeba* infections may be treated with pentamidine, ketoconazole, and flucytosine, whereas *Balamuthia* infections have been treated with clarithromycin, fluconazole, sulfadiazine, pentamidine, and flucytosine. Amebic keratitis and cutaneous infections may respond to topical miconazole, chlorhexidine gluconate, or propamidine isethionate. Treatment of amebic keratitis may require repeated corneal transplantation or (rarely) enucleation of the eye. The wide distribution of these organisms in fresh and brackish waters makes prevention and control of infection difficult. It has been suggested that known sources of infection be off limits to bathing, diving, and water sports, although this is generally difficult to enforce. Swimming pools with cracks in the walls, allowing soil seepage, should be repaired to avoid creation of a source of infection.

Leishmania

Leishmania are obligate intracellular parasites that are transmitted from animal to human or human to human by bites from an infected female sandfly. Depending on the geographic area, many different species can infect humans, producing a variety of diseases that range from cutaneous, diffuse cutaneous, and mucocutaneous to visceral (Table 74-2). New species of *Leishmania* are being detected frequently. Whereas the older literature focused primarily on three species, *L. donovani* (visceral leishmaniasis), *L. tropica* (cutaneous leishmaniasis), and *L. braziliensis* (cutaneous leishmaniasis), the current taxonomy of leishmaniasis is in a state of flux. Species differentiation is currently based on molecular techniques rather than geographic distribution and clinical presentation.

Physiology and Structure

The life cycles of all leishmanial parasites are quite similar (Figure 74-10), whereas the associated infections differ in epidemiology, tissues affected, and clinical manifestations. The **promastigote** stage (long, slender form with a free flagellum) is present in the saliva of infected sandflies. Human infection is initiated by the bite of an infected sandfly, which injects the promastigotes into the skin, where they lose their

Table 74-2 Leishmaniasis in Humans

Parasite	Disease	Geographic Distribution
Leishmania donovani	Visceral leishmaniasis Mucocutaneous leishmaniasis Cutaneous leishmaniasis Dermal leishmanoid	Africa, Asia
L. infantum (L. chagasi)	Visceral leishmaniasis	Africa, Europe, Mediterranean area, Southwest Asia, Central and South America
L. tropica	Cutaneous leishmaniasis Visceral leishmaniasis (rare)	Afghanistan, India, Turkey, former USSR, Middle East, Africa, India
L. major	Cutaneous leishmaniasis	Middle East, Afghanistan, Africa, former USSR
L. aethiopica	Cutaneous leishmaniasis Diffuse cutaneous leishmaniasis Mucocutaneous leishmaniasis	Ethiopia, Kenya, Yemen, former USSR
L. mexicana	Cutaneous leishmaniasis Diffuse cutaneous leishmaniasis	Texas, Belize, Guatemala, Mexico
L. braziliensis	Cutaneous leishmaniasis Mucocutaneous leishmaniasis	Central and South America
L. peruviana	Cutaneous leishmaniasis	Panama, Colombia, Costa Rica
L. garnhami	Cutaneous leishmaniasis	Venezuela
L. colombiensis	Cutaneous leishmaniasis	Colombia, Panama
L. venezuelensis	Cutaneous leishmaniasis	Venezuela
L. lainsoni	Cutaneous leishmaniasis	Brazil
L. amazonensis	Cutaneous leishmaniasis Diffuse cutaneous leishmaniasis	Brazil, Venezuela
L. naiffi	Cutaneous leishmaniasis	Brazil, Caribbean Islands
L. pifanoi	Cutaneous leishmaniasis Diffuse cutaneous leishmaniasis	Brazil, Venezuela

Data from Barratt JL, Harkness J, Marriott D, et al: Importance of nonenteric protozoan infections in immunocompromised people, *Clin Microbiol Rev* 23:795–836, 2010.

USSR, Union of Soviet Socialist Republics.

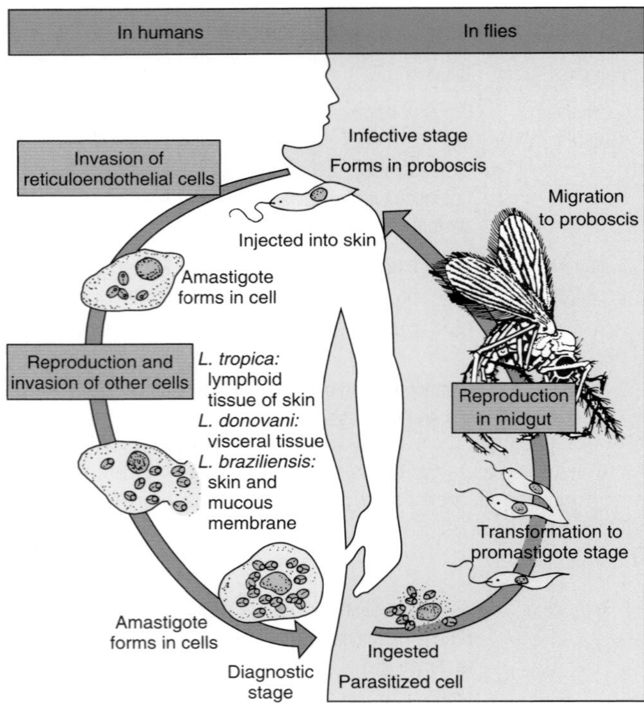

FIGURE 74-10 Life cycle of *Leishmania* species.

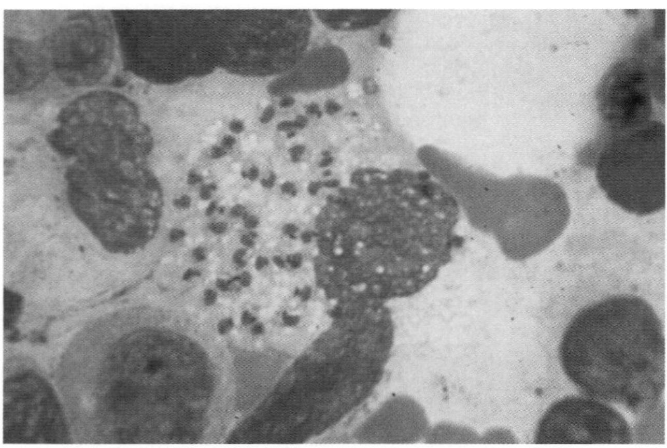

FIGURE 74-11 Giemsa-stained amastigotes (Leishman-Donovan bodies) of *Leishmania donovani* present in a touch preparation of spleen. A small, dark-staining kinetoplast can be seen next to the spherical nucleus in some parasites. (From Connor DH, Schwartz DA: *Pathology of infectious diseases,* vol 2, Stamford, Conn, 1997, Appleton & Lange.)

flagella, enter the **amastigote** stage, and invade reticuloendothelial cells. The change from promastigote to amastigote helps to avoid the host's immune response. Changes in the organism's surface molecules play an important role in macrophage attachment and evading the immune response, including manipulating the macrophage's signaling pathways. Reproduction occurs in the amastigote stage, and as cells rupture, destruction of specific tissues (e.g., cutaneous tissues, visceral organs such as liver and spleen) develops. The amastigote stage (Figure 74-11) is diagnostic for leishmaniasis as well as serving as the infectious stage for sandflies. Ingested amastigotes transform in the sandfly into the promastigote stage, which multiplies by binary fission in the fly midgut. After development, this stage migrates to the fly proboscis, where new human infection can be introduced during feeding. The life cycles of *Leishmania* organisms are similar for cutaneous, mucocutaneous, and visceral leishmaniasis, except that infected reticuloendothelial cells can be found throughout the body in visceral leishmaniasis.

Epidemiology

Leishmaniasis is a zoonosis transmitted by adult female sandflies belonging to the genera *Phlebotomus* and *Lutzomyia.* The natural reservoirs include rodents, opossums, anteaters, sloths, cats, and dogs. In areas of the world where leishmaniasis is endemic, the infection may be transmitted by a human-vector-human cycle. The infection may also be transmitted by direct contact with an infected lesion or mechanically by stable flies or dog flies.

Mucocutaneous leishmaniasis most often occurs in Bolivia, Brazil, and Peru, whereas the cutaneous form is much more widespread throughout the Middle East (Afghanistan, Algeria, Iran, Iraq, Saudi Arabia, Syria) and in focal areas in South America (Brazil, Peru). Cutaneous leishmaniasis has been diagnosed among U.S. military personnel deployed in Afghanistan, Iraq, and Kuwait.

Visceral leishmaniasis (kala-azar, Dumdum fever) occurs at a rate of approximately 500,000 new cases per year, 90% of which are localized to Bangladesh, Brazil, India, Nepal, and the Sudan. This infection may exist as an endemic, epidemic, or sporadic disease and is a zoonosis except in India, where **kala-azar** ("black fever" in Hindi) is an anthroponosis (human-vector-human). Individuals with post–kala-azar dermal leishmaniasis may be very important reservoirs for maintaining the infection in the population because of the high concentration of organisms in the skin. In contrast to cutaneous and mucocutaneous leishmaniasis, for which a large number of leishmanial species have been implicated, only *L. donovani* and *L. infantum (L. chagasi)* commonly cause visceral leishmaniasis. *L. infantum* is present in countries along the Mediterranean basin (European, Near Eastern, African) and is found in parts of China, South Africa, and the former Soviet Union, whereas *L. donovani* is concentrated in Africa and Asia. Although *L. tropica* usually causes cutaneous leishmaniasis, rare viscerotropic strains have been reported in the Middle East, Africa, and India.

Clinical Syndromes

Depending on the species of *Leishmania* involved, infection can result in a cutaneous, diffuse cutaneous, mucocutaneous, or visceral disease. With the spread of the HIV pandemic, there is increasing recognition of HIV-related visceral leishmaniasis caused by *L. donovani* in southern Asia and Africa and by *L. infantum (L. chagasi)* in South America. In these co-infected patients, leishmaniasis will manifest as an opportunistic infection, with parasites detected in atypical sites and a high associated mortality.

The first sign of **cutaneous leishmaniasis,** a red papule, appears at the site of the fly's bite between 2 weeks and 2 months after initial exposure. The lesion becomes irritated and intensely pruritic and begins to enlarge and ulcerate.

Gradually the ulcer becomes hard and crusted and exudes a thin, serous material. At this stage, secondary bacterial infection may complicate the disease. The lesion may heal without treatment in a matter of months but usually leaves a disfiguring scar. The species that is commonly associated with cutaneous leishmaniasis, *L. tropica,* may also exist in a viscerotrophic form. A disseminated nodular type of cutaneous leishmaniasis has been reported from Ethiopia, probably caused by an allergy to *L. aethiopica* antigens.

Mucocutaneous leishmaniasis is produced most often by the *L. braziliensis* complex. The incubation period and appearance of the primary cutaneous ulcers for *L. braziliensis* are similar to those found in other forms of cutaneous leishmaniasis. The essential difference in clinical disease is the involvement and destruction of mucous membranes and related tissue structures. Untreated primary lesions may develop into the mucocutaneous form in up to 80% of cases. Spread to the nasal and oral mucosa may become apparent concomitant with the primary lesion or many years after the primary lesion has healed. The mucosal lesions do not heal spontaneously, and secondary bacterial infections are common, producing severe and disfiguring facial mutilation and occasionally death.

The **visceral form of leishmaniasis** may present as fulminating rapidly fatal disease, a more chronic debilitating process, or an asymptomatic self-limiting infection. The incubation period may be from several weeks to a year, with a gradual onset of fever, diarrhea, and anemia. Chills and sweating that may resemble malaria symptoms are common early in the infection. As organisms proliferate and invade the cells of the reticuloendothelial system, marked enlargement of the liver and spleen, weight loss, and emaciation occur. Kidney damage may also occur as the cells of the glomeruli are invaded. With persistence of the disease, deeply pigmented granulomatous areas of skin, referred to as **post–kala-azar dermal leishmaniasis,** develop. In this condition, the macular or hypopigmented dermal lesions are associated with few parasites, whereas erythematous and nodular lesions are associated with abundant parasites.

Laboratory Diagnosis

Although the diagnosis of visceral, mucocutaneous, or cutaneous leishmaniasis may be made on clinical grounds in endemic areas, definitive diagnosis depends on detecting either the amastigotes in clinical specimens or the promastigotes in culture. Demonstration of the amastigotes in properly stained smears from touch preparations or ulcer biopsy specimens and cultures of ulcer tissue determines the diagnosis of cutaneous and mucocutaneous leishmaniasis. Specimens for the diagnosis of visceral leishmaniasis include splenic puncture, lymph node aspirates, liver biopsy, sternal aspirates, iliac crest bone marrow, and buffy coat preparations of venous blood. These specimens may be examined microscopically, cultured, and subjected to molecular detection methods. Molecular techniques for detection of leishmanial DNA or ribonucleic acid (RNA) have been used for diagnosis, prognosis, and species identification and are more sensitive than microscopy or culture, especially for detection of mucocutaneous leishmaniasis. Serologic tests are available but not especially useful for the diagnosis of mucocutaneous or visceral leishmaniasis. Detection of urinary antigens has been used for the diagnosis of visceral leishmaniasis.

Treatment, Prevention, and Control

At present, the drug of choice for all forms of leishmaniasis is the pentavalent antimonial compound sodium stibogluconate (Pentostam). In the past several years, ubiquitous use of this agent has been threatened by the development of drug resistance. Furthermore, drug treatment can be complicated by variation in the susceptibility of *Leishmania* spp. to drugs, variation in pharmacokinetics, and variation in drug-host immune response interaction. The toxicity of the antimonials is also considerable, and as a result, several alternative approaches to the treatment of leishmaniasis have been developed.

Standard therapy for cutaneous leishmaniasis consists of injections of antimonial compounds directly into the lesion or parenterally. Recently, both fluconazole and miltefosine have been shown to be efficacious. Other agents include amphotericin B, pentamidine, and various formulations of paromomycin. Alternatives to chemotherapy in the treatment of cutaneous leishmaniasis include cryotherapy, heat, and surgical excision.

Stibogluconate remains the drug of choice for mucocutaneous leishmaniasis, with amphotericin B as an alternative. Of note, patients clinically cured of *L. braziliensis,* which is noted for its chronicity, latency, and metastasis with mucous membrane involvement, have been found to be PCR positive up to 11 years post therapy. Follow-up with smears, cultures, and/or PCR is necessary to ensure that treatment has been effective.

The role of stibogluconate in the treatment of visceral leishmaniasis has been challenged in recent years. Although in most parts of the world, more than 95% of previously untreated patients with visceral leishmaniasis respond to pentavalent antimonials, widespread primary failure of these agents has been reported in the North Bihar region of India. The incidence of primary response was only 54%, and 8% of those initially responding to treatment relapsed. Widespread misuse of the drug is blamed for this emerging resistance. Fortunately in recent years, four new potential therapies have been introduced for visceral leishmaniasis: amphotericin B liposome formulation, oral miltefosine, a parenteral formulation of paromomycin, and oral sitamaquine (an 8-aminoquinolone). Miltefosine has shown remarkable efficacy (>95% cure rate) and tolerability. Unfortunately, preliminary data from India suggest an increasing relapse rate in patients treated with miltefosine, indicating that drug resistance could develop and strategies must be developed to prevent it.

Prevention of the various forms of leishmaniasis involves prompt treatment of human infections and control of reservoir hosts, along with insect vector control. Protection from sandflies by screening and insect repellents is also essential. Protection of forest and construction workers in endemic areas is most difficult, and disease in those places may be effectively controlled only by vaccination. Work to develop a vaccine is ongoing.

• Trypanosomes

Trypanosoma, another hemoflagellate, causes two distinctly different forms of disease (Table 74-3). One is called **African**

Table 74-3 *Trypanosoma* Species Responsible for Human Diseases

Parasite	Vector	Disease
Trypanosoma brucei gambiense and *T. b. rhodesiense*	Tsetse fly	African trypanosomiasis (sleeping sickness)
Trypanosoma cruzi	Reduviids	American trypanosomiasis (Chagas disease)

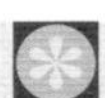

Clinical Case 74-4 Trypanosomiasis

Herwaldt and colleagues (*J Infect Dis* 181:395–399, 2000) described a case in which the mother of an 18-month-old boy in Tennessee found a triatomine bug in his crib, which she saved because it resembled a bug shown on a television program about insects that prey on mammals. An entomologist identified the bug as *Triatoma sanguisuga,* a vector of Chagas disease. The bug was found to be engorged with blood and infected with *Trypanosoma cruzi.* The child had been intermittently febrile for the preceding 2 to 3 weeks but was otherwise healthy except for pharyngeal edema and multiple insect bites of unknown type on his legs. Whole-blood specimens obtained from the child were negative by buffy coat examination and hemoculture but positive for *T. cruzi* by polymerase chain reaction and DNA hybridization, suggesting that he had low-level parasitemia. Specimens obtained after treatment with benznidazole were negative. He did not develop anti-*T. cruzi* antibody; 19 relatives and neighbors were also negative. Two of three raccoons trapped in the vicinity had positive hemocultures for *T. cruzi.* The child's case of *T. cruzi* infection—the fifth reported U.S. autochthonous case—would have been missed without his mother's attentiveness and the availability of sensitive molecular techniques. Given that infected triatomine bugs and mammalian hosts exist in the southern United States, it is not surprising that humans could become infected with *T. cruzi.* Furthermore, given the nonspecific clinical manifestations of the infection, it is likely that other cases have been overlooked.

trypanosomiasis, or sleeping sickness, and is produced by *Trypanosoma brucei gambiense* and *T. b. rhodesiense.* It is transmitted by tsetse flies. The second infection is called **American trypanosomiasis, or Chagas disease,** produced by *Trypanosoma cruzi.* It is transmitted by true bugs (triatomids, reduviids [kissing bugs]) (Clinical Case 74-4).

Trypanosoma brucei gambiense

Physiology and Structure

The life cycle of the African forms of trypanosomiasis is illustrated in Figure 74-12. The infective stage of the organism is the **trypomastigote** (Figure 74-13), which is present in the salivary glands of transmitting tsetse flies. The organism in this stage has a **free flagellum** and an **undulating membrane** running the full length of the body. The trypomastigotes enter the wound created by the fly bite and find their way into blood and lymph, eventually invading the CNS. Reproduction of the trypomastigotes in blood, lymph, and spinal fluid is by binary or longitudinal fission. These trypomastigotes in blood are then infective for biting tsetse flies, where further reproduction occurs in the midgut. The organisms then migrate to the salivary glands, where an **epimastigote** form (with a free flagellum but only a partial undulating membrane) continues reproduction to the infective trypomastigote stage. Tsetse flies become infective 4 to 6 weeks after feeding on blood from a diseased patient.

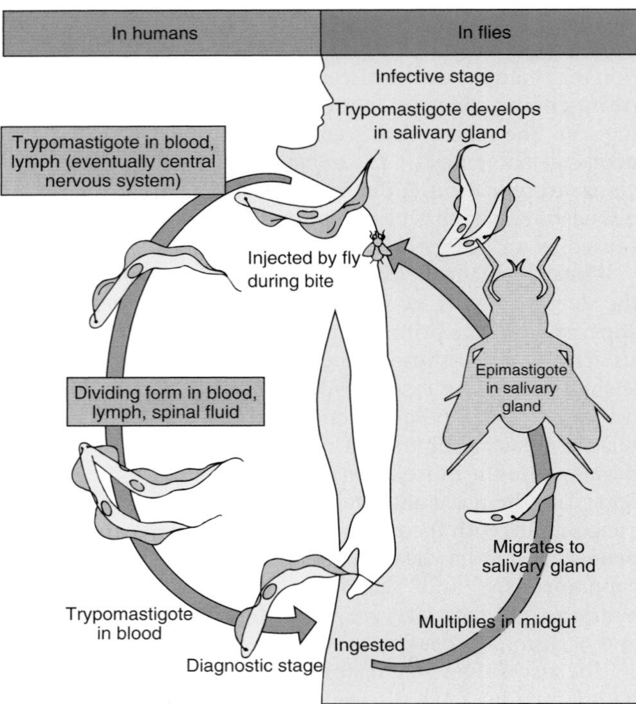

FIGURE 74-12 Life cycle of *Trypanosoma brucei.*

Epidemiology

T. b. gambiense is limited to tropical West and Central Africa, correlating to the range of the tsetse fly vector. The tsetse flies transmitting *T. b. gambiense* prefer shaded stream banks for reproduction and proximity to human dwellings. Persons who work in such areas are at greatest risk of infection. An animal reservoir has not been proved, although several species of animals have been infected experimentally.

Clinical Syndromes

The incubation period of **Gambian sleeping sickness** varies from a few days to weeks. *T. b. gambiense* produces chronic disease, often ending fatally with CNS involvement after several years' duration. One of the earliest signs of disease is an occasional **ulcer** at the site of the fly bite. As reproduction of organisms continues, the lymph nodes are invaded and fever, myalgia, arthralgia, and lymph node enlargement result. Swelling of the posterior cervical lymph nodes is characteristic of Gambian disease and is called **Winterbottom sign.** Patients in this acute phase often exhibit hyperactivity.

Chronic disease progresses to CNS involvement, with lethargy, tremors, meningoencephalitis, mental retardation, and general deterioration. In the final stages of chronic disease, convulsions, hemiplegia, and incontinence occur, and the patient becomes difficult to arouse or evoke a response, eventually progressing to a comatose state. Death is the result of CNS damage and other infections such as malaria or pneumonia.

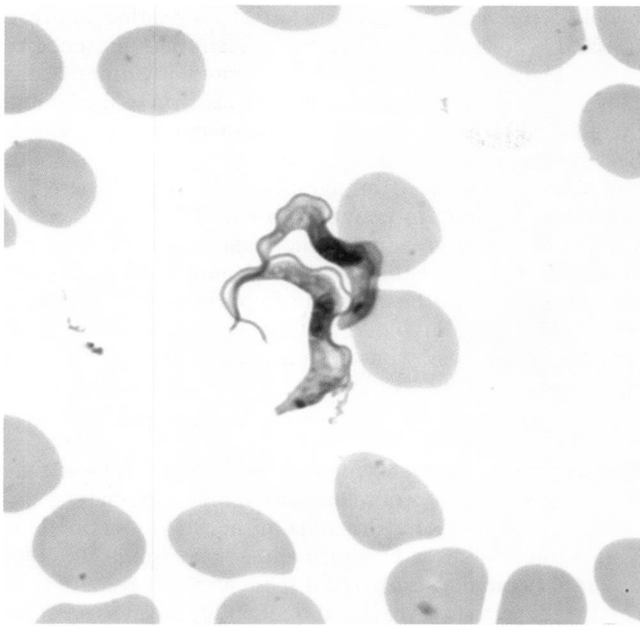

FIGURE 74-13 Trypomastigote stage of *Trypanosoma brucei gambiense* in a blood smear. (From CDC Public Health Image Library.)

Laboratory Diagnosis

Organisms can be demonstrated in thick and thin blood films, in concentrated anticoagulated blood preparations, and in aspirations from lymph nodes and concentrated spinal fluid (see Figure 74-13). Methods for concentrating parasites in blood may be helpful. Approaches include centrifugation of heparinized samples and anion-exchange chromatography. Levels of parasitemia vary widely, and several attempts to visualize the organism over a number of days may be necessary. Preparations should be fixed and stained immediately to avoid disintegration of the trypomastigotes. Serologic tests are also useful diagnostic techniques. Immunofluorescence, ELISA, precipitin, and agglutination methods have been used. Most reagents are not available commercially. Referral laboratories have used PCR to detect infections and differentiate species (*T. b. gambiense* versus *T. b. rhodesiense*), but these methods are not routinely used in the field.

Treatment, Prevention, and Control

Suramin is the drug of choice for treating the acute blood and lymphatic stages of the disease, with pentamidine as an alternative. Suramin and pentamidine do not cross the blood-brain barrier; therefore melarsoprol is the drug of choice when CNS involvement is suspected. Difluoromethylornithine (DFMO) is a cytostatic drug with activity against the acute and late (CNS) stages of the disease. The most effective control measures include an integrated approach to reduce the human reservoir of infection and the use of fly traps and insecticide; however, economic resources are limited, and effective programs have been difficult to sustain.

Trypanosoma brucei rhodesiense

Physiology and Structure

The life cycle of *T. b. rhodesiense* is similar to that of *T. b. gambiense* (see Figure 74-12), with both trypomastigote and epimastigote stages and transmission by tsetse flies.

Epidemiology

The organism is found primarily in East Africa, especially the cattle-raising countries, where tsetse flies breed in the brush rather than along stream banks. *T. b. rhodesiense* also differs from *T. b. gambiense* in that domestic animal hosts (cattle and sheep) and wild game animals act as reservoir hosts. This transmission and vector cycle makes the organism more difficult to control than *T. b. gambiense*.

Clinical Syndromes

The incubation period for *T. b. rhodesiense* is shorter than that for *T. b. gambiense*. Acute disease (fever, rigors, and myalgia) occurs more rapidly and progresses to a fulminating, rapidly fatal illness. Infected persons are usually dead within 9 to 12 months if untreated.

This more virulent organism also develops in greater numbers in the blood. Lymphadenopathy is uncommon, and CNS invasion occurs early in the infection, with lethargy, anorexia, and mental disturbance. The chronic stages described for *T. b. gambiense* are not often seen because, in addition to rapid CNS disease, the organism produces kidney damage and myocarditis, leading to death.

Laboratory Diagnosis

Examination of blood and spinal fluid is carried out as for *T. b. gambiense*. Serologic tests are available; however, the marked variability of the surface antigens of trypanosomes limits the diagnostic usefulness of this approach.

Treatment, Prevention, and Control

The same treatment protocol applies as for *T. b. gambiense*, with early treatment for the more rapid neurologic manifestations. Similar prevention and control measures are needed: tsetse fly control and use of protective clothing, screens, netting, and insect repellent. In addition, early treatment is essential to control transmission, detect infection, and determine treatment in domestic animals. Control of infection in game animals is difficult, but infection can be reduced if measures to control the tsetse fly population, specifically eradication of brush and grassland breeding sites, are applied.

Trypanosoma cruzi

Physiology and Structure

The life cycle of *T. cruzi* (Figure 74-14) differs from *T. brucei* with the development of an additional form called an **amastigote** (Figure 74-15). The amastigote is an intracellular form with no flagellum and no undulating membrane. It is smaller than the trypomastigote, oval, and found in tissues. The infective trypomastigote, which is present in the feces of a **reduviid bug ("kissing bug"),** enters the wound created by the biting, feeding bug. The bugs have been called **kissing bugs** because they frequently bite people around the mouth and in other facial sites. They are notorious for biting, feeding on blood and tissue juices, and then defecating into the wound. The organisms in the feces of the bug enter the wound; penetration is usually aided when the patient rubs or scratches the irritated site.

The trypomastigotes then migrate to other tissues (e.g., cardiac muscle, liver, brain), lose the flagellum and undulating membrane, and become the smaller, oval, intracellular amastigote form. These intracellular amastigotes multiply by

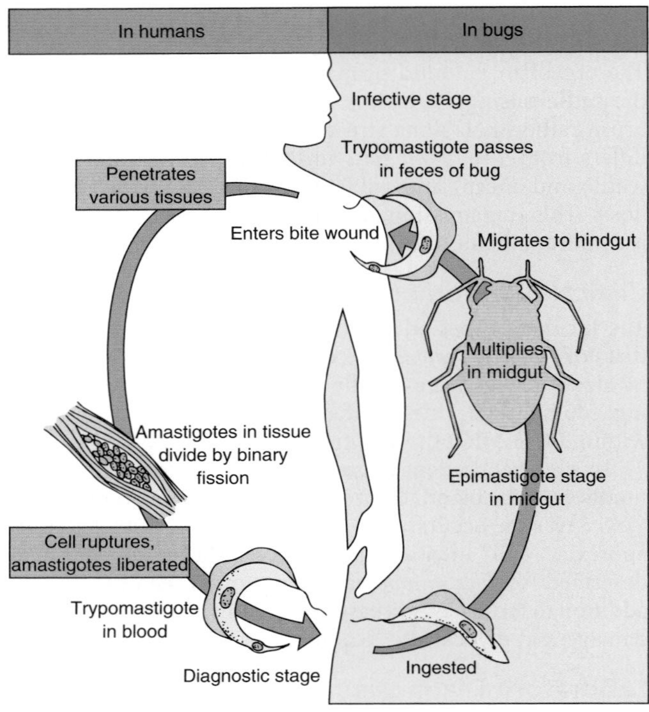

FIGURE 74-14 Life cycle of *Trypanosoma cruzi.*

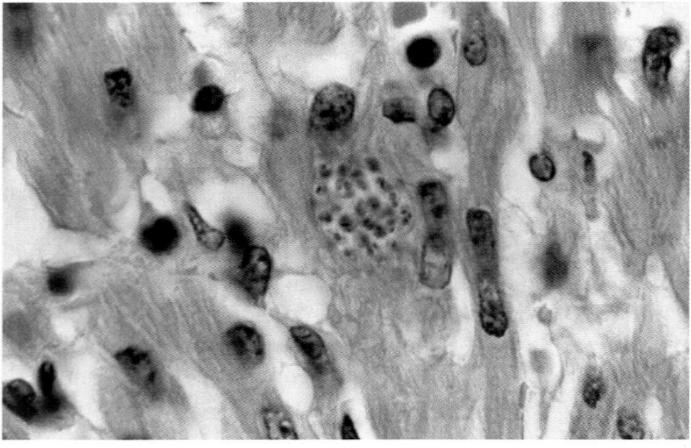

FIGURE 74-15 Amastigote stage of *Trypanosoma cruzi* in heart muscle. (From CDC Public Health Image Library.)

binary fission and eventually destroy the host cells. Then they are liberated to enter new host tissue as intracellular amastigotes or to become trypomastigotes infective for feeding reduviid bugs. Ingested trypomastigotes develop into epimastigotes in the midgut of the insect and reproduce by longitudinal binary fission. The organisms migrate to the hindgut of the bug, develop into metacyclic trypomastigotes, and then leave the bug in the feces after biting, feeding, and defecating, initiating a new human infection.

Epidemiology

T. cruzi occurs widely in both reduviid bugs and a broad spectrum of reservoir animals in North, Central, and South America. Human disease is found most often among children in South and Central America, where 16 to 18 million people are infected. There is a direct correlation between infected wild animal reservoir hosts and the presence of infected bugs whose nests are found in human homes. Naturally acquired cases of Chagas disease are rare in the United States because the bugs prefer nesting in animal burrows and because homes are not as open to nesting as those in South and Central America. Immigration from areas where the disease is endemic to countries where it is not has made Chagas disease a growing public health concern in recent years. As such, screening of solid organ and blood donors for Chagas disease has become important. In the United States, screening of blood donors with a recommended enzyme immunoassay has been implemented but is not yet mandatory.

Clinical Syndromes

Chagas disease may be asymptomatic, acute, or chronic. One of the earliest signs is development of an erythematous and indurated area called a **chagoma** at the site of the bug bite. This is often followed by a rash and edema around the eyes and face **(Romaña sign).** The disease is most severe in children younger than 5 years and frequently is seen as an acute process with CNS involvement. Acute infection is also characterized by fever, chills, malaise, myalgia, and fatigue. Parasites may be present in the blood during the acute phase; however, they are sparse in patients older than 1 year. Death may ensue a few weeks after an acute attack, the patient may recover, or the patient may enter the chronic phase as organisms proliferate and enter the heart, liver, spleen, brain, and lymph nodes.

Chronic Chagas disease is characterized by hepatosplenomegaly, myocarditis, and enlargement of the esophagus and colon as a result of the destruction of nerve cells (e.g., Auerbach plexus) and other tissues that control the growth of these organs.

Megacardia and electrocardiographic changes are commonly seen in chronic disease. Involvement of the CNS may produce granulomas in the brain, with cyst formation and a meningoencephalitis. Death from chronic Chagas disease results from tissue destruction in the many areas invaded by the organisms, and sudden death results from complete heart block and brain damage.

Laboratory Diagnosis

T. cruzi can be demonstrated in thick and thin blood films or concentrated anticoagulated blood early in the acute stage. As the infection progresses, the organisms leave the bloodstream and become difficult to find. Biopsy of lymph nodes, liver, spleen, or bone marrow may demonstrate the organisms in the amastigote stage. Culture of blood or inoculation into laboratory animals may be useful when parasitemia is low. Serologic tests are also available. In endemic areas, xenodiagnosis is widely used. Gene amplification techniques such as PCR have been used to detect the organism in the bloodstream. These approaches are not widely available and have not been adapted for use in the field.

Treatment, Prevention, and Control

Treatment of Chagas disease is limited by the lack of reliable agents. The drugs of choice are benznidazole and nifurtimox. Although both drugs have proven activity against the acute phase of disease, they are less effective against chronic

Chagas disease and have severe side effects. Alternative agents include allopurinol. Education regarding the disease, its insect transmission, and the wild animal reservoirs is critical. Bug control, eradication of nests, and construction of homes to prevent nesting of bugs are also essential. The use of dichlorodiphenyltrichloroethane (DDT) in bug-infested homes has demonstrated a drop in the transmission of malaria and Chagas disease. Screening of blood by serologic means or excluding blood donors from endemic areas prevents some infections that would otherwise be associated with transfusion therapy.

Development of a vaccine is possible because *T. cruzi* does not have the wide antigenic variation observed with the African trypanosomes.

Bibliography

Alvar J, Aparicio P, Aseffa A, et al: The relationship between leishmaniasis and AIDS: the second 10 years, *Clin Microbiol Rev* 21:334–359, 2008.

Baird JK: Resistance to therapies for infection by *Plasmodium vivax*, *Clin Microbiol Rev* 22:508–534, 2009.

Barratt JL, Harkness J, Marriott D, et al: Importance of nonenteric protozoan infections in immunocompromised people, *Clin Microbiol Rev* 23:795–836, 2010.

Bruckner DA, Labarca JA: *Leishmania* and *Trypanosoma*. In Versalovic J, et al, editors: *Manual of clinical microbiology*, ed 10, Washington, DC, 2011, American Society for Microbiology Press.

Cox-Singh J, Davis TM, Lee KS, et al: *Plasmodium knowlesi* malaria in humans is widely distributed and potentially life threatening, *Clin Infect Dis* 46:165–171, 2008.

Croft SL, Sundar S, Fairlamb AH: Drug resistance in leishmaniasis, *Clin Microbiol Rev* 19:111–126, 2006.

Kantele A, Jokiranta TS: Review of cases with the emerging fifth human malaria parasite, *Plasmodium knowlesi*, *Clin Infect Dis* 52:1356–1362, 2011.

Leiby DA: Transfusion-transmitted *Babesia* spp.: bulls-eye on *Babesia microti*, *Clin Microbiol Rev* 24:14–28, 2011.

Lin JT, Juliano JJ, Wongsrichanalai C: Drug-resistant malaria: the era of ACT, *Curr Infect Dis Rep* 12:165–173, 2010.

Menard D, Barnadas C, Bouchier C, et al: *Plasmodium vivax* clinical malaria is commonly observed in Duffy-negative Malagasy people, *Proc Natl Acad Sci U S A* 107:5967–5971, 2010.

Murray CK, Gasser RA Jr, Magill AJ, et al: Update on rapid diagnostic testing for malaria, *Clin Microbiol Rev* 21:97–110, 2008.

Rogers WO: *Plasmodium* and *Babesia*. In Versalovic J, et al, editors: *Manual of clinical microbiology*, ed 10, Washington, DC, 2011, American Society for Microbiology Press.

Visvesvara GS: Pathogenic and opportunistic free-living amebae. In Versalovic J, et al, editors: *Manual of clinical microbiology*, ed 10, Washington, DC, 2011, American Society for Microbiology Press.

CHAPTER

75 NEMATODES

A 10-year-old boy was brought in by his father for evaluation of crampy abdominal pain, nausea, and mild diarrhea that had persisted for approximately 2 weeks. On the day before evaluation, the boy reported to his parents that he passed a large worm into the toilet during a bowel movement. He flushed the worm before the parents could see it. Physical examination was completely unremarkable. The boy had no fever, cough, or rash and did not complain of anal pruritus. His travel history was unremarkable. Examination of a stool specimen revealed the diagnosis.

1. Which intestinal parasites of humans are nematodes?
2. Which nematode was likely in this case? Which organisms may be found in stool?
3. What was the most likely means of acquisition of this parasite?
4. Was this patient at risk of autoinfection?
5. Describe the life cycle of this parasite.
6. Can this parasite cause extraintestinal symptoms? Which other organs may be invaded, and what might stimulate extraintestinal invasion?

Answers to these questions are available on StudentConsult.com.

• SUMMARIES CLINICALLY SIGNIFICANT ORGANISMS

Ascaris lumbricoides

Trigger Words

Ascaris, roundworm, intestinal obstruction, pulmonary eosinophilia, decorticate, nematode

Biology, Virulence, and Disease

- Nematodes: most common helminths recognized in United States; also called roundworms
- Large (20 to 35 cm long) pink worms with moderately complex life cycle but otherwise typical of intestinal roundworm (nematode)
- Infections caused by ingestion of only a few eggs may produce no symptoms
- Even a single adult *Ascaris* worm may be dangerous: migrate to liver, penetrate intestine, cause mechanical tissue damage
- Migration of a large number of larval worms to lung may produce pneumonitis
- A tangled bolus of mature worms in intestine may lead to obstruction and perforation
- A large worm burden may result in abdominal tenderness, fever, distention, nausea

Epidemiology

- *A. lumbricoides* prevalent in areas with poor sanitation and where human feces (night soil) are used as fertilizer
- ≈1 billion people infected worldwide
- No known animal reservoir
- *Ascaris* eggs very hardy; can survive extreme temperatures, persist for months in feces and sewage

Diagnosis

- Microscopic examination of sediment of concentrated stool
- Adult worms may be visualized on abdominal radiographs; cholangiograms may reveal worms in biliary tract
- Pulmonary phase of disease may be diagnosed by finding larvae and eosinophils in sputum

Treatment, Prevention, and Control

- Treatment of symptomatic infection highly effective
- Drugs of choice: albendazole or mebendazole
- Patients with mixed infections (*Ascaris* plus other helminths, *Giardia,* or *E. histolytica)* should be treated for ascariasis first to avoid provoking worm migration
- Prevention: education, improved sanitation, avoidance of human feces as fertilizer

Onchocerca volvulus

Trigger Words

Microfilaria, macrofilaria, nodules, hanging groin, blackfly, Africa, *Wolbachia* endosymbiont, skin snip, river blindness

Biology, Virulence, and Disease

- Filariae: long, slender roundworms; parasites of blood, lymph, subcutaneous and connective tissues; transmitted by mosquitoes or biting flies
- *Onchocerca volvulus:* filarial nematode transmitted by blackfly *(Simulium damnosum)*
- Onchocerciasis affects > 18 million people worldwide; causes blindness in ≈5% of infected people

- All individual worms and all life cycle stages of *O. volvulus* contain *Wolbachia* bacterial endosymbiont
- Clinical onchocerciasis characterized by infection involving skin, subcutaneous tissue, lymph nodes, eyes
- Signs/symptoms: fever, eosinophilia, urticaria; migration of microfilariae to eyes causes severe tissue damage and blindness

Epidemiology

- *O. volvulus* endemic in many parts of Africa, especially Congo and Volta river basins; common term is "river blindness"
- Prevalence: men > women; 50% of men in endemic areas are blind before they reach age 50

Diagnosis

- Diagnosis made by demonstration of microfilariae in skin snip preparations taken from infrascapular or gluteal regions
- In patients with ocular disease, organism may be seen in anterior chamber with aid of a slit lamp

Treatment, Prevention, and Control

- Surgical removal of nodules often used to eliminate adult worms and stop production of microfilariae
- Ivermectin: single dose reduces number of microfilariae in eyes and skin
- Protection from blackfly bites, prompt diagnosis and treatment of infections to prevent transmission

The most common helminths recognized in the United States are primarily intestinal nematodes, although in other countries, nematode infections of blood and tissues can cause devastating disease. Nematodes are the most easily recognized form of intestinal parasite because of their large size and cylindrical, unsegmented bodies; hence the common name **roundworms** (Figure 75-1). These parasites live primarily as adult worms in the intestinal tract, and nematode infections are most commonly confirmed by detecting the characteristic eggs in feces. Identification of eggs should be approached in a systematic manner, taking into account the size and shape of the egg, thickness of the shell, and presence or absence of specialized structures such as polar plugs, knobs, spines, and opercula. The presence and characteristics of larvae within the eggs may also be useful. The most common nematodes of medical importance are listed in Table 75-1.

Filariae are long, slender roundworms that are parasites of blood, lymph, and subcutaneous and connective tissues. All of these nematodes are transmitted by mosquitoes or biting flies. Most produce larval worms called **microfilariae** that are demonstrated in blood specimens or subcutaneous tissues and skin snips.

• *Enterobius vermicularis*

Physiology and Structure

Enterobius vermicularis, the **pinworm,** is a small white worm that is familiar to parents who find them in the perianal folds or vagina of an infected child. Infection is initiated by ingestion of embryonated eggs (Figure 75-2). Larvae hatch in the small intestine and migrate to the large intestine, where they mature into adults in 2 to 6 weeks. Fertilization of the female by the male produces the characteristic asymmetric eggs. These eggs are laid in the perianal folds by the migrating female. As many as 20,000 eggs are deposited on the perianal skin. The eggs rapidly mature and are infectious within hours.

Epidemiology

E. vermicularis occurs worldwide but is most common in the temperate regions, where person-to-person spread is greatest in crowded conditions such as in day-care centers, schools, and mental institutions. An estimated 500 million cases of pinworm infection are reported worldwide, and this is the most common helminthic infection in North America.

Infection occurs when the eggs are ingested and the larval worm is free to develop in the intestinal mucosa. These eggs may be transmitted from hand to mouth by children scratching the perianal folds in response to the irritation caused by the migrating egg-laying female worms, or the eggs may find their way to clothing and play objects in day-care centers. They can also survive long periods in the dust that accumulates over doors, on windowsills, and under beds in rooms inhabited by infected people. Egg-laden dust can be inhaled and swallowed to produce infestation. In addition, **autoinfection ("retrofection")** can occur wherein eggs hatch in the perianal folds and larval worms migrate into the rectum and large intestine. Infected individuals who handle food can also be a source of infection. No animal reservoir for *Enterobius* is known. Physicians should be aware of the related epidemiology of *Dientamoeba fragilis;* this organism correlates well with the presence of *E. vermicularis,* with *D. fragilis* thought to be transported in the pinworm eggshell.

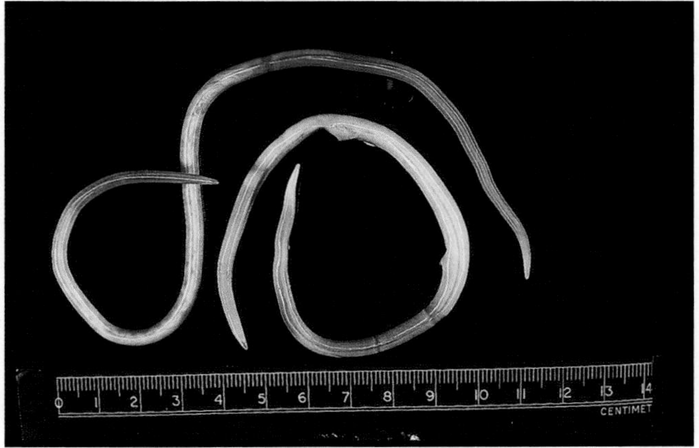

FIGURE 75-1 Adult *Ascaris lumbricoides.* (From Matthews BE, Croll NA: Comparative stereoscan electron micrographs of nematode heads, *J Nematol* 6:131–134, 1974, Figure 5.)

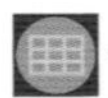 Table 75-1 **Nematodes of Medical Importance**

Parasite	Common Name	Disease
Enterobius vermicularis	Pinworm	Enterobiasis
Ascaris lumbricoides	Roundworm	Ascariasis
Toxocara canis	Dog ascaris	Visceral larva migrans
Toxocara cati	Cat ascaris	Visceral larva migrans
Baylisascaris procyonis	Raccoon ascaris	Neural larva migrans
Trichuris trichiura	Whipworm	Trichuriasis
Ancylostoma duodenale	Old World hookworm	Hookworm infection
Necator americanus	New World hookworm	Hookworm infection
Ancylostoma braziliense	Dog or cat hookworm	Cutaneous larva migrans
Strongyloides stercoralis	Threadworm	Strongyloidiasis
Trichinella spiralis	Pork worm	Trichinosis
Wuchereria bancrofti	Bancroft filaria	Filariasis
Brugia malayi	Malayan filaria	Filariasis
Loa loa	African eye worm	Loiasis
Mansonella spp.		Filariasis
Onchocerca volvulus		Onchocerciasis, river blindness
Dirofilaria immitis	Dog heartworm	Dirofilariasis
Dracunculus medinensis	Guinea worm	Dracunculosis

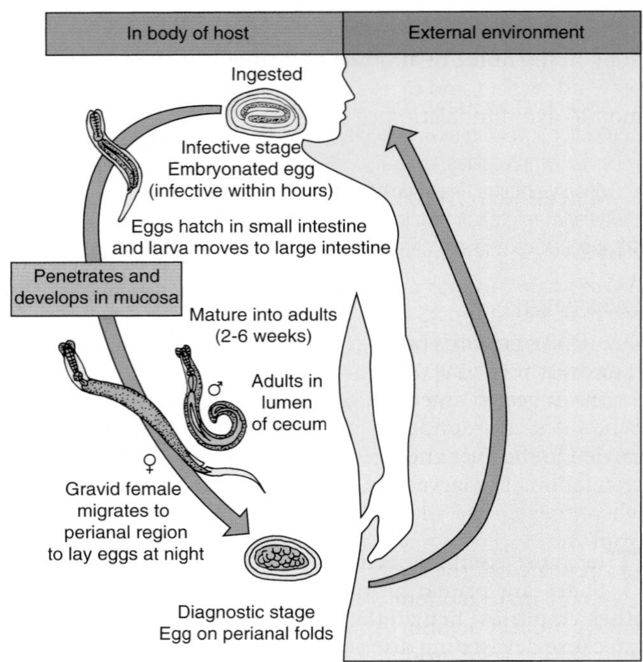

FIGURE 75-2 Life cycle of *Enterobius vermicularis.*

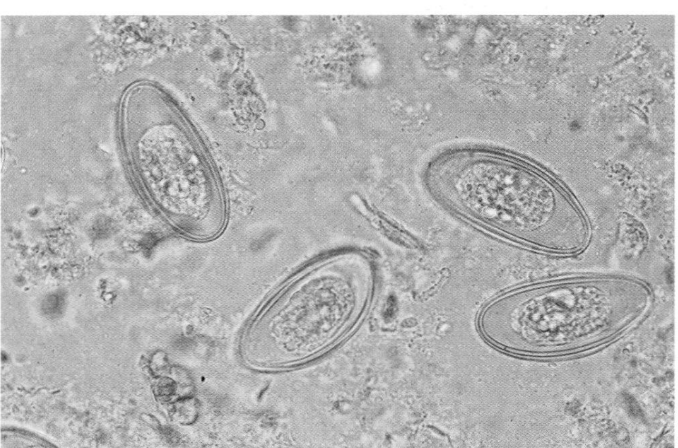

FIGURE 75-3 *Enterobius vermicularis* egg. The thin-walled eggs are 50 to 60 × 20 to 30 µm, ovoid, and flattened on one side (not because children sit on them, but this is an easy way to correlate the egg morphology with the epidemiology of the disease).

Clinical Syndromes

Many children and adults show no symptoms and serve only as carriers. Patients who are allergic to the secretions of the migrating worms experience severe pruritus, loss of sleep, and fatigue. The pruritus may cause repeated scratching of the irritated area and lead to secondary bacterial infection. Worms that migrate into the vagina may produce genitourinary problems and granulomas.

Worms attached to the bowel wall may produce inflammation and granuloma formation around the eggs. Although the adult worms may occasionally invade the appendix, there remains no proven relationship between pinworm invasion and appendicitis. Penetration through the bowel wall into the peritoneal cavity, liver, and lungs has been infrequently recorded.

Laboratory Diagnosis

The diagnosis of **enterobiasis** is usually suggested by the clinical manifestations and confirmed by detection of the characteristic eggs on the anal mucosa. Occasionally the adult worms are seen by laboratory personnel in stool specimens, but the method of choice for diagnosis involves use of an anal swab with a sticky surface that picks up the eggs (Figure 75-3) for microscopic examination. Sampling can be done with clear tape or commercially available swabs. The sample should be collected when the child arises and before bathing or defecation, to pick up eggs laid by migrating worms during the night. Parents can collect the specimen and deliver it to the physician for immediate microscopic examination. Three swabbings, 1 per day for 3 consecutive days, may be required to detect the diagnostic eggs. The eggs are rarely seen in fecal specimens. Systemic signs of infection, such as eosinophilia, are rare.

Treatment, Prevention, and Control

The drug of choice is albendazole or mebendazole. Pyrantel pamoate and piperazine are effective, but reinfection is common. To avoid reintroduction of the organism and reinfection in the family environment, it is customary to treat the entire family simultaneously. Although cure rates are high, reinfection is common. Repeat treatment after 2 weeks may be useful in preventing reinfection.

Personal hygiene, clipping of fingernails, thorough washing of bed clothes, and prompt treatment of infected individuals all contribute to control. When housecleaning is done in the home of an infected family, dusting under beds, on window sills, and over doors should be done with a damp mop to avoid inhalation of infectious eggs.

• *Ascaris lumbricoides*

Physiology and Structure

Ascaris lumbricoides are large (20 to 35 cm in length) pink worms (see Figure 75-1) that have a more complex life cycle than *E. vermicularis* but are otherwise typical of an intestinal roundworm (Figure 75-4).

The ingested infective egg releases a larval worm that penetrates the duodenal wall, enters the bloodstream, is carried to the liver and heart, and then enters the pulmonary circulation. The larvae break free in the alveoli of the lungs, where they grow and molt. In about 3 weeks, the larvae pass from the respiratory system to be coughed up, swallowed, and returned to the small intestine.

As the male and female worms mature in the small intestine (primarily jejunum), fertilization of the female by the male initiates egg production, which may amount to 200,000 eggs per day for as long as a year. Female worms can also produce unfertilized eggs in the absence of males. Eggs are found in feces 60 to 75 days after the initial infection. Fertilized eggs become infectious after approximately 2 weeks in the soil.

Epidemiology

A. lumbricoides is prevalent in areas where sanitation is poor and where human feces are used as fertilizer. Because food and water are contaminated with *Ascaris* eggs, this parasite more than any other affects the world's population. Although no animal reservoir is known for *A. lumbricoides,* an almost identical species from pigs, *Ascaris suum,* can infect humans. This species is seen in swine growers and is associated with the use of pig manure for gardening. *Ascaris* eggs are quite hardy and can survive extreme temperatures and persist for several months in feces and sewage. Ascariasis is the most common helminthic infection worldwide, with an estimated 1 billion people infected.

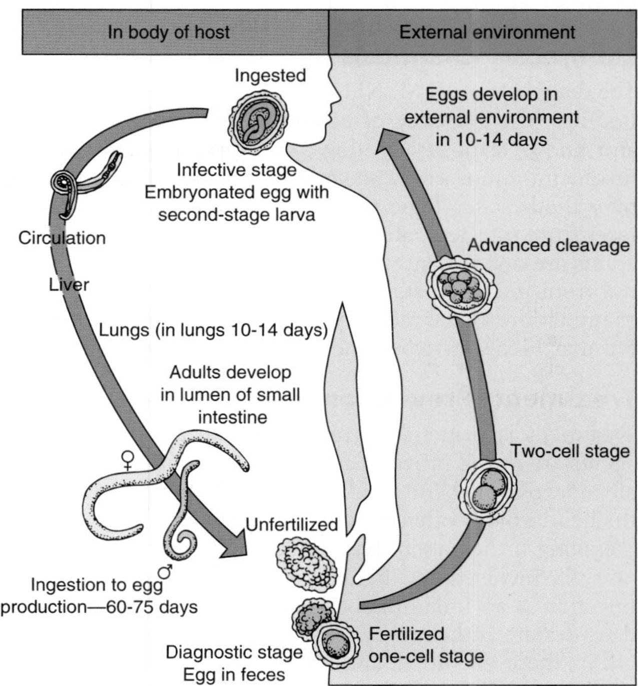

FIGURE 75-4 Life cycle of *Ascaris lumbricoides.*

Clinical Syndromes

Infections caused by ingestion of only a few eggs may produce no symptoms; however, even a single adult *Ascaris* worm may be dangerous because it can migrate into the bile duct and liver and damage tissue. Furthermore, because the worm has a tough, flexible body, it can occasionally perforate the intestine, creating peritonitis with secondary bacterial infection (Clinical Case 75-1). Adult worms do not attach to

Clinical Case 75-1 Hepatic Ascariasis

Hurtado and colleagues (*N Engl J Med* 354:1295–1303, 2006) described a case of a 36-year-old woman who presented with recurrent right upper quadrant (RUQ) abdominal pain. One year earlier, she also presented with RUQ abdominal pain, abnormal liver function tests, and positive serology for hepatitis C. An abdominal ultrasonographic examination showed biliary dilation, and endoscopic retrograde cholangiopancreatography (ERCP) showed multiple stones in the common bile duct, left hepatic duct, and left intrahepatic duct. The majority of the stones were removed. Examination of the bile-duct aspirate was negative for ova and parasites. One month before the present admission, the patient experienced recurrent RUQ pain and jaundice. Repeat ERCP again showed multiple stones in the common and left main hepatic ducts; partial removal was accomplished.

One month later, the patient was admitted with severe epigastric pain and fever. The patient was born in Vietnam and had immigrated to the United States when she was in her early 20s. She had no history of recent travel. An abdominal computed tomography scan with contrast showed abnormal perfusion of the left hepatic lobe and dilation of the left biliary radicles with multiple filling defects. ERCP showed partial obstruction of the left main hepatic duct, a few small stones, and purulent bile. Magnetic resonance imaging showed diffuse enhancement of the left lobe and left portal vein, suggestive of inflammation. Cultures of blood grew *Klebsiella pneumoniae,* and examination of a stool sample revealed a few *Strongyloides stercoralis* rhabditiform larvae. Biliary stents were placed, and the patient was treated with levofloxacin. Two weeks later, the patient was admitted to the hospital, where a partial hepatectomy was performed for treatment of recurrent pyogenic cholangitis. Gross examination of the left hepatic lobe showed ectatic bile ducts containing bile-stained calculi. Microscopic examination of the calculous material revealed collections of parasite eggs and a degenerated and fragmented nematode. *Klebsiella* spp. were identified in cultures by the microbiology laboratory. The findings were consistent with recurrent pyogenic cholangiohepatitis with infection by *Ascaris lumbricoides* and *Klebsiella* spp. In addition to antibiotics for the bacterial infection, the patient was treated with ivermectin for the *Strongyloides* infection and albendazole for the *Ascaris* organisms.

The aberrant migration of *A. lumbricoides* into the pancreatobiliary tree, with subsequent deposition of eggs followed by death and degeneration of both worm and eggs, became a nidus for calculus formation and secondary bacterial infection. Although unusual in the United States, hepatic ascariasis is estimated to contribute to more than 35% of cases of biliary and pancreatic disease in the Indian subcontinent and parts of Southeast Asia.

the intestinal mucosa but depend on constant motion to maintain their position within the bowel lumen.

After infection with many larvae, migration of worms to the lungs can produce pneumonitis resembling an asthmatic attack. Pulmonary involvement is related to the degree of hypersensitivity induced by previous infections and the intensity of the current exposure and may be accompanied by eosinophilia and oxygen desaturation. Also, a tangled bolus of mature worms in the intestine can result in obstruction, perforation, and occlusion of the appendix. As mentioned previously, migration into the bile duct, gallbladder, and liver can produce severe tissue damage. This migration can occur in response to fever, drugs other than those used to treat ascariasis, and some anesthetics. Patients with many larvae may also experience abdominal tenderness, fever, distention, and vomiting.

Laboratory Diagnosis

Examination of the sediment of concentrated stool reveals the knobby-coated, bile-stained, fertilized and unfertilized eggs. Eggs are oval, 55 to 75 μm long, and 50 μm wide. The thick-walled outer shell can be partially removed **(decorticated egg).** Occasionally adult worms pass with feces, which can be quite dramatic because of their large size (20 to 35 cm long) (see Figure 75-1). Roentgenologists may also visualize the worms in the intestine, and cholangiograms often disclose their presence in the biliary tract of the liver. The pulmonary phase of the disease may be diagnosed by the finding of larvae and eosinophils in sputum.

Treatment, Prevention, and Control

Treatment of symptomatic infection is highly effective. The drug of choice is albendazole or mebendazole; pyrantel pamoate and piperazine are alternatives. Patients with mixed parasitic infections *(A. lumbricoides,* other helminths, *Giardia duodenalis, Entamoeba histolytica)* in the stool should be treated for ascariasis first to avoid provoking worm migration and possible intestinal perforation. Education, improved sanitation, and avoidance of human feces as fertilizer are critical. A program of mass treatment in highly endemic areas has been suggested, but this may not be economically feasible. Furthermore, eggs can persist in contaminated soil for 3 years or more. Certainly, improved personal hygiene among people who handle food is an important aspect of control.

• *Toxocara* and *Baylisascaris*

Physiology and Structure

Toxocara canis, Toxocara cati, and *Baylisascaris procyonis* are ascarid worms that are naturally parasitic in the intestines of dogs, cats, and raccoons, respectively. These organisms may accidentally infect humans, producing disease states known as **visceral larva migrans (VLM), neural larva migrans (NLM),** and **ocular larva migrans (OLM).** When ingested by humans, the eggs of these worms can hatch into larval forms that cannot follow the normal developmental cycle as in the natural host. They can penetrate the human gut and reach the bloodstream and then migrate as larvae to various human tissues. *Toxocara* spp. are the most common causes of VLM and OLM, whereas *B. procyonis* is increasingly recognized as a cause of fatal NLM. Although *Toxocara* spp. do not develop beyond the migrating larval form, *B. procyonis* larvae continue to grow to a large size within the human host.

Epidemiology

Wherever infected dogs and cats are present, the eggs are a threat to humans. Likewise, contact with raccoons or their feces presents a significant risk of infection with *B. procyonis.* This is especially true for children who are exposed more readily to contaminated soil and who tend to put objects in their mouths.

Clinical Syndromes

The clinical manifestations of VLM, NLM, and OLM in humans are related to the migration of larvae through tissues. The larvae may invade any tissue of the body, where they can induce bleeding, formation of eosinophilic granulomas, and necrosis. Patients may be asymptomatic and have only eosinophilia, but they can also have serious disease directly related to the number and location of the lesions caused by the migrating larvae, as well as the degree to which the host is sensitized to the larval antigens. The organs most frequently involved are the lungs, heart, kidneys, liver, skeletal muscles, eyes, and central nervous system (CNS). NLM is a common sequela of infection with *B. procyonis* and is attributed to the extensive somatic larval migration of this species (Clinical Case 75-2). Continued growth and migration within the CNS produces extensive mechanical tissue damage. Signs and symptoms caused by the migrating larvae include cough, wheezing, fever, rash, anorexia, seizures, fatigue, and abdominal discomfort. On examination, patients may have hepatosplenomegaly and nodular pruritic skin lesions. Death may result from respiratory failure, cardiac arrhythmia, or brain damage. Ocular disease can also occur with the movement of larvae through the eye and may be mistaken for malignant retinoblastoma. Prompt diagnosis is required to avoid unnecessary enucleation.

Laboratory Diagnosis

The diagnosis of VLM, NLM, and OLM is based on clinical findings, the presence of **eosinophilia,** serologic findings, and known exposure to dogs, cats, or raccoons. Enzyme-linked immunosorbent assays are available and appear to offer the best serologic marker for disease. Examination of feces from infected patients is not useful because egg-laying adults are not present. However, examination of fecal material from infected pets often supports the diagnosis. Tissue examination for larvae may provide a definitive diagnosis but may be negative because of sampling error.

Treatment, Prevention, and Control

Treatment is primarily symptomatic because antiparasitic agents are not of proven benefit. Anthelmintic therapy with albendazole, mebendazole, diethylcarbamazine (DEC), or thiabendazole is often used. Corticosteroid therapy may be lifesaving if the patient has serious pulmonary, myocardial, or CNS involvement, because a major component of the infection is an inflammatory response to the organism. To date, despite anthelmintic treatment of cases of *B. procyonis* NLM, there are no neurologically intact survivors. These zoonoses can be greatly reduced if pet owners conscientiously eradicate worms from their animals and clean up pet

Clinical Case 75-2 Baylisascariasis

Gavin and colleagues (*Pediatr Infect Dis J* 21:971–975, 2002) described a case of a previously normal 2½-year-old boy who was admitted to hospital with fever and recent onset of encephalopathy. Past history was significant for pica and geophagia, and he was receiving ferrous sulfate for iron deficiency anemia. He was in good health until 8 days before admission, when a temperature of 38.5° C and mild cough developed. Three days before admission, he developed increasing lethargy and marked somnolence. He was irritable, confused, and ataxic. The family lived in suburban Chicago, and there were no sick contacts or pets at home. There was no travel history. On admission, he was febrile and lethargic but irritable and agitated when disturbed. Neck stiffness with generalized hypertonicity, hyperreflexia, and bilateral extensor plantar responses were present. The white blood cell (WBC) count was elevated, and eosinophilia was present. Cerebrospinal fluid (CSF) examination revealed elevated protein and WBCs, with 32% eosinophils. Gram, acid-fast, and India ink stains and bacterial and cryptococcal antigen tests were all negative. Broad-spectrum antibacterial and antiviral therapy was begun empirically; however, the patient became comatose, with opisthotonus, decerebrate posturing, hypertonicity, and tremulousness. Cranial magnetic resonance imaging demonstrated areas of increased signal involving both cerebellar hemispheres. Bacterial, fungal, mycobacterial, and viral cultures of blood and CSF were negative. Viral serologies were negative, as were tests for antibodies against *Toxocara,* cysticercosis, coccidioidomycosis, blastomycosis, and histoplasmosis. A detailed epidemiologic history revealed that 18 days before hospitalization, the family attended a picnic in a nearby suburb. Numerous raccoons were observed regularly in the vicinity, and the patient was observed playing with and eating dirt beneath the trees. CSF and serum antibodies against third-stage *Baylisascaris procyonis* were demonstrated by indirect immunofluorescence assay, with titers increasing from 1 : 4 to 1 : 1024 during a 2-week period. The patient was treated with albendazole and corticosteroids for 4 weeks but has remained severely affected with marked generalized spasticity and cortical blindness. Subsequent examination of soil and debris from the child's play site revealed thousands of infective *B. procyonis* eggs. This case underscores the devastating effects of neural larva migrans. In many regions of North America, large populations of raccoons with high rates of endemic *B. procyonis* infection (e.g., 60% to 80%) live in proximity to humans, which suggests that the risk of human infection is probably substantial.

fecal material from yards and school playgrounds. Children's play areas and sandboxes should be carefully monitored. Raccoons should not be encouraged to visit homes or yards for food, and the keeping of raccoons as pets should be strongly discouraged.

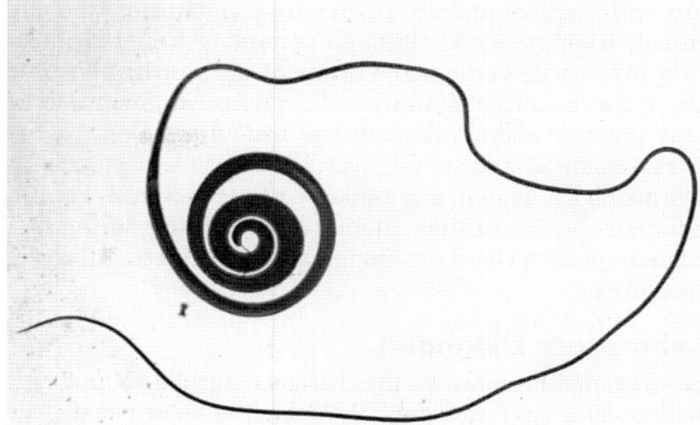

FIGURE 75-5 *Trichuris trichiura,* adult male. (From John DT, Petri WA Jr: *Markell and Voge's medical parasitology,* ed 9, Philadelphia, 2006, Elsevier.)

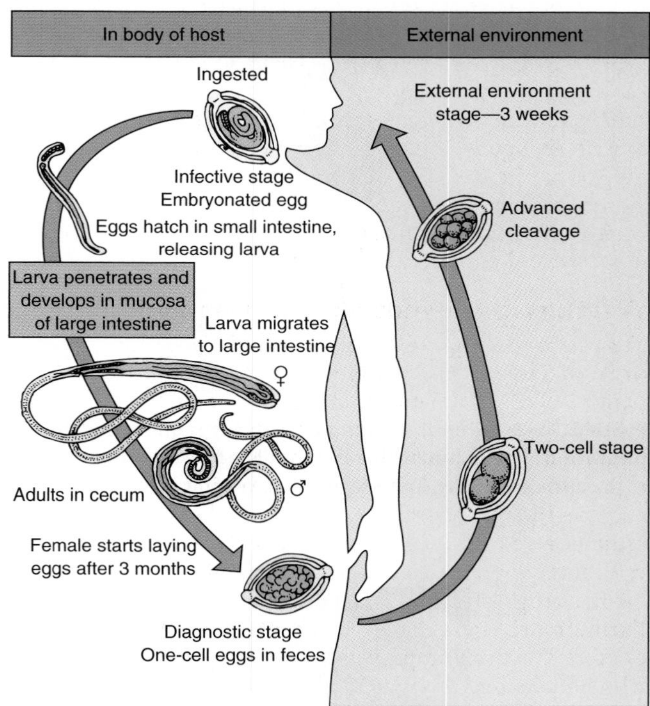

FIGURE 75-6 Life cycle of *Trichuris trichiura.*

• *Trichuris trichiura*

Physiology and Structure

Commonly called **whipworm** because it resembles the handle and lash of a whip (Figure 75-5), *Trichuris trichiura* has a simple life cycle (Figure 75-6). Ingested eggs hatch into a larval worm in the small intestine and then migrate to the cecum, where they penetrate the mucosa and mature to adults. About 3 months after the initial infection, the fertilized female worm starts laying eggs and may produce 3000 to 10,000 eggs per day. Female worms can live for as long as 8 years. Eggs passed into the soil mature and become infectious in 3 weeks. *T. trichiura* eggs are distinctive, with dark bile staining, a barrel shape, and the presence of polar plugs in the egg shell (Figure 75-7).

Epidemiology

Like *A. lumbricoides, T. trichiura* has worldwide distribution, and its prevalence is directly correlated with poor sanitation and the use of human feces as fertilizer. No animal reservoir is recognized.

Clinical Syndromes

The clinical manifestations of **trichuriasis** are generally related to the intensity of the worm burden. Most infections are with small numbers of *Trichuris* organisms and are usually asymptomatic, although secondary bacterial infection may occur because the heads of the worms penetrate deep into the intestinal mucosa. Infections with many larvae may produce abdominal pain and distention, bloody diarrhea, weakness, and weight loss. Appendicitis may occur as worms fill the lumen, and prolapse of the rectum is seen in children because of the irritation and straining during defecation. Anemia and eosinophilia are also seen in severe infections.

Laboratory Diagnosis

Stool examination reveals the characteristic bile-stained eggs with polar plugs (see Figure 75-7). Light infestations may be difficult to detect because of the paucity of eggs in stool specimens.

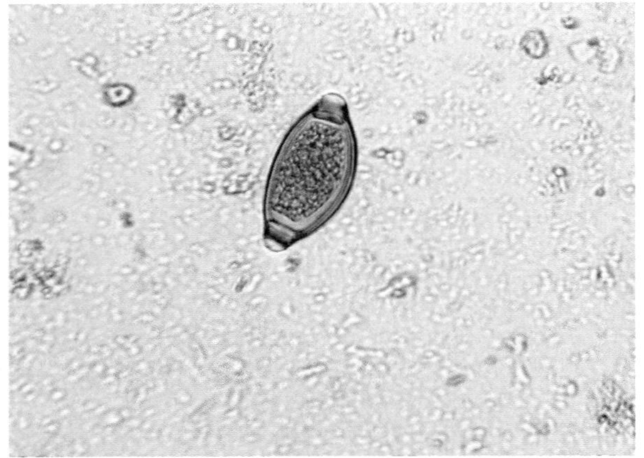

FIGURE 75-7 *Trichuris trichiura* egg. The eggs are barrel shaped, measuring 50 × 24 μm, with a thick wall and two prominent plugs at the ends. Internally, an unsegmented ovum is present.

Treatment, Prevention, and Control

The drug of choice is albendazole or mebendazole. As with *A. lumbricoides,* prevention of *T. trichiura* depends on education, good personal hygiene, adequate sanitation, and avoidance of the use of human feces as fertilizer.

• Hookworms

Ancylostoma duodenale and *Necator americanus*

Physiology and Structure

The two human hookworms are *Ancylostoma duodenale* **(Old World hookworm)** and *Necator americanus* **(New World hookworm).** Differing only in geographic distribution, structure of mouthparts (Figure 75-8), and relative size, these two species are discussed together as agents of hookworm infection. The human phase of the hookworm life cycle is initiated when a filariform (infective form) larva penetrates intact skin (Figure 75-9). The larva then enters the circulation, is carried to the lungs, and like *A. lumbricoides,* is coughed up, swallowed, and develops to adulthood in the small intestine. The adult *N. americanus* has a hooklike head that accounts for the name commonly used. Adult worms lay as many as 10,000 to 20,000 eggs per day, which are released into the feces. Egg laying is initiated 4 to 8 weeks after the initial exposure and can persist for as long as 5 years. On contact with soil, the **rhabditiform** (noninfective) larvae are released from the eggs and within 2 weeks develop into **filariform** larvae. The filariform larvae can then penetrate exposed skin (e.g., bare feet) and initiate a new cycle of human infection.

Both species have mouthparts designed for sucking blood from injured intestinal tissue. *A. duodenale* has chitinous teeth, and *N. americanus* has shearing chitinous plates (see Figure 75-8).

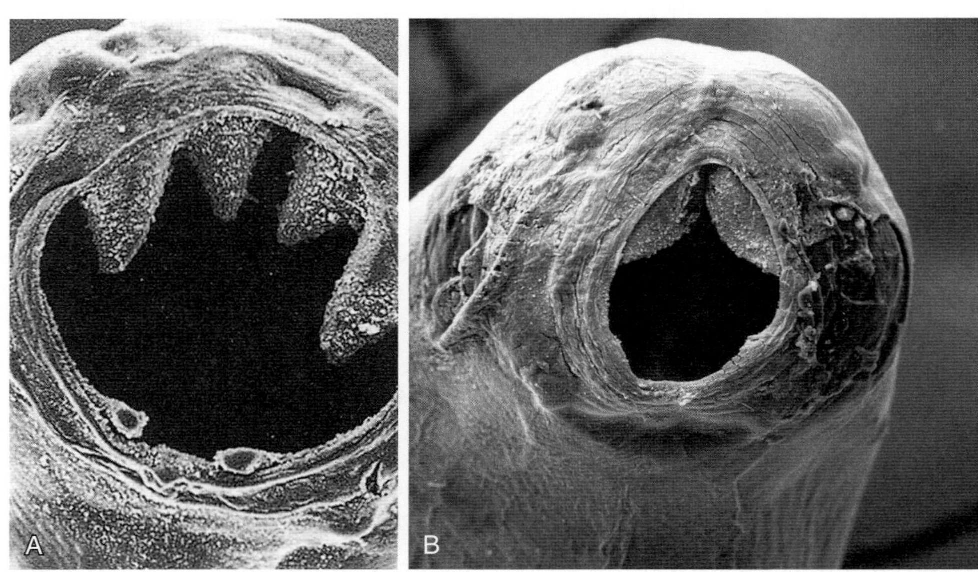

FIGURE 75-8 Scanning electron micrographs of adult hookworm mouthparts. **A,** *Ancylostoma duodenale* (×630). **B,** *Necator americanus* (×470). (From Peters W, Pasvol G: *Atlas of tropical medicine and parasitology,* ed 6, Philadelphia, 2007, Elsevier.)

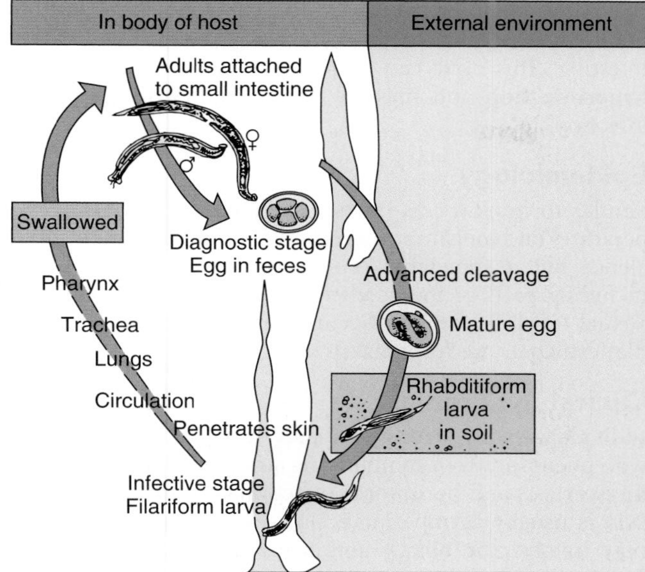

FIGURE 75-9 Life cycle of human hookworms.

Epidemiology

Transmission of hookworm infection requires the deposition of egg-containing feces on shady, well-drained soil and is favored by warm, humid (tropical) conditions. Hookworm infections are reported worldwide in places where direct contact with contaminated soil can lead to human disease, but they occur primarily in warm subtropical and tropical regions and in southern parts of the United States. It is estimated that more than 900 million individuals worldwide are infected with hookworms, including 700,000 in the United States.

Clinical Syndromes

Skin-penetrating larvae may produce an allergic reaction and rash at sites of entry, and larvae migrating in the lungs can cause pneumonitis and eosinophilia. Adult worms produce the gastrointestinal symptoms of nausea, vomiting, and diarrhea. As blood is lost due to the feeding worms, a microcytic hypochromic anemia develops. Daily blood loss is estimated at 0.15 to 0.25 ml for each adult *A. duodenale* and 0.03 ml for each adult *N. americanus.* In severe chronic infections, emaciation and mental and physical retardation may occur related to anemia from blood loss and nutritional deficiencies. Also, intestinal sites may be secondarily infected by bacteria when the worms migrate along the intestinal mucosa.

Laboratory Diagnosis

Stool examination reveals the characteristic non–bile-stained segmented eggs shown in Figure 75-10. Larvae are not found in stool specimens unless the specimen was left at ambient temperature for a day or more. The eggs of *A. duodenale* and *N. americanus* cannot be distinguished. The larvae must be examined to identify these hookworms specifically, although this is clinically unnecessary.

Treatment, Prevention, and Control

The drug of choice is albendazole or mebendazole; pyrantel pamoate is an alternative. In addition to eradication of the worms to stop blood loss, iron therapy is indicated to raise hemoglobin levels to normal. Blood transfusion may be necessary in severe cases of anemia. Education, improved sanitation, and controlled disposal of human feces are critical preventive measures. Wearing shoes in endemic areas helps reduce the prevalence of infection.

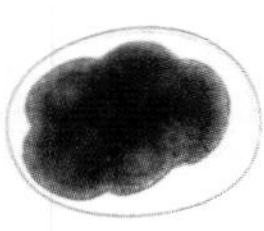

FIGURE 75-10 Human hookworm egg. Eggs are 60 to 75 μm long and 35 to 40 μm wide, are thin shelled, and enclose a developing larva.

Ancylostoma braziliense

Physiology and Structure

Ancylostoma braziliense, a species of hookworm, is naturally parasitic in the intestines of dogs and cats and accidentally infects humans. It produces a disease properly called **cutaneous larva migrans** but also called **ground itch** and **creeping eruption.** The filariform larvae of this hookworm penetrate intact skin but can develop no further in humans. The larvae remain trapped in the skin of the wrong host for weeks or months, wandering through subcutaneous tissue and creating serpentine tunnels.

Epidemiology

Similar to the situation with *Ascaris* worms, the threat of infection with *A. braziliense* is greatest among children coming into contact with soil or sandboxes contaminated with animal feces containing hookworm eggs. Infections are prevalent throughout the year on beaches in subtropical and tropical regions; in the summer, infection is reported as far north as the Canadian-U.S. border.

Clinical Syndromes

Migrating larvae may provoke a severe erythematous and vesicular reaction. Pruritus and scratching of irritated skin may lead to secondary bacterial infection. About half of patients develop transient pulmonary infiltrates with peripheral eosinophilia **(Löffler syndrome),** presumably resulting from pulmonary migration of the larvae.

Laboratory Diagnosis

Occasionally, larvae are recovered in skin biopsy or after freezing of the skin, but most diagnoses are based on the clinical appearance of the tunnels and a history of contact with dog and cat feces. The larvae are rarely found in sputum.

Treatment, Prevention, and Control

The drug of choice is albendazole; ivermectin and thiabendazole are alternatives. Antihistamines may be helpful in controlling pruritus. This zoonosis can be reduced by educating pet owners to treat their animals for worm infections and to pick up pet feces from yards, beaches, and sandboxes. In endemic areas, shoes or sandals should be worn to prevent infection.

• *Strongyloides stercoralis*

Physiology and Structure

Although the morphology of these worms and the epidemiology of their infections are similar to the hookworm, the life cycle of *Strongyloides stercoralis* (Figure 75-11) differs in three aspects: (1) eggs hatch into larvae in the intestine and before they are passed in feces, (2) larvae can mature into filariforms in the intestine and cause autoinfection, and (3) a free-living nonparasitic cycle can be established outside the human host.

In direct development, like the hookworm, a skin-penetrating *S. stercoralis* larva enters the circulation and follows the pulmonary course. It is coughed up and swallowed, and adults develop in the small intestine. Adult females burrow into the mucosa of the duodenum and reproduce parthenogenetically. Each female produces about a dozen eggs each day, which hatch within the mucosa and release **rhabditiform** larvae into the lumen of the bowel. The rhabditiform larvae are distinguished from the larvae of hookworms by their short buccal capsule and large genital primordium. The rhabditiform larvae are passed in the stool and may either continue the direct cycle by developing into infective **filariform** larvae or develop into free-living adult worms and initiate the indirect cycle.

In indirect development, the larvae in soil develop into free-living adults that produce eggs and larvae. Several generations of this nonparasitic existence may occur before new larvae become skin-penetrating parasites.

Finally, in **autoinfection,** rhabditiform larvae in the intestine do not pass with feces but become filariform larvae. These penetrate the intestinal mucosa or perianal skin and follow the course through the circulation and pulmonary structures, are coughed up, and then are swallowed; at this point, they become adults, producing more larvae in the intestine. This cycle can persist for years and can lead to **hyperinfection** and massive or disseminated, often fatal, infection.

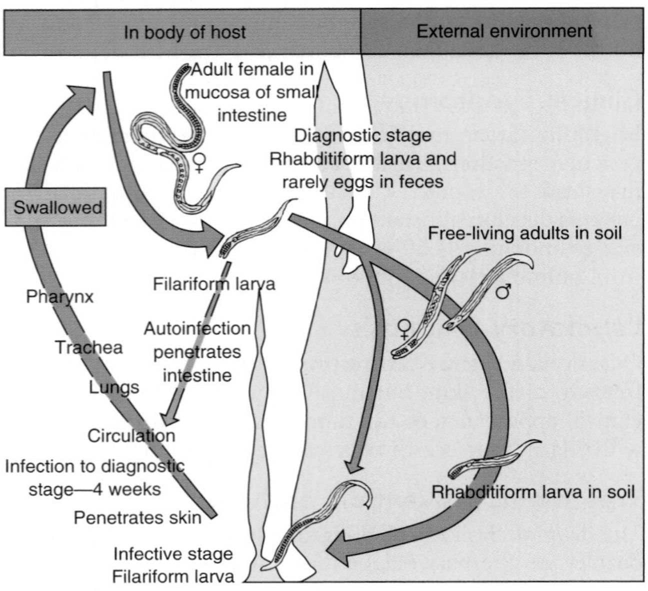

FIGURE 75-11 Life cycle of *Strongyloides stercoralis.*

Epidemiology

Similar to hookworms in its requirements for warm temperatures and moisture, *S. stercoralis* demonstrates low prevalence but a somewhat broader geographic distribution, including parts of the northern United States and Canada. Sexual transmission also occurs. Animal reservoirs such as domestic pets are recognized.

Clinical Syndromes

Individuals with **strongyloidiasis** frequently are afflicted with pneumonitis from migrating larvae, similar to that seen in ascariasis and hookworm infection. The intestinal infection is usually asymptomatic. However, heavy worm loads may involve the biliary and pancreatic ducts, the entire small bowel, and the colon, causing inflammation and ulceration leading to epigastric pain and tenderness, vomiting, diarrhea (occasionally bloody), and malabsorption. Symptoms mimicking peptic ulcer disease, coupled with peripheral eosinophilia, should strongly suggest the diagnosis of strongyloidiasis.

Autoinfection may lead to chronic strongyloidiasis that can last for years, even in nonendemic areas. Although many of these chronic infections may be asymptomatic, as many as two thirds of patients have recurring episodic symptoms referable to the involved skin, lungs, and intestinal tract. Individuals with chronic strongyloidiasis are at risk of developing severe, life-threatening hyperinfection syndrome if the host-parasite balance is disturbed by any drug or illness that compromises the host's immune status (Clinical Case 75-3). **Hyperinfection syndrome** is seen most commonly in individuals immunocompromised by malignancies (especially hematologic malignancies), corticosteroid therapy, or both. Hyperinfection syndrome has also been observed in patients who have undergone solid organ transplantation and in malnourished people. Loss of cellular immune function may be associated with the conversion of rhabditiform larvae to filariform larvae, followed by dissemination of the larvae via the circulation to virtually any organ. Most commonly, extraintestinal infection involves the lung and includes bronchospasm, diffuse infiltrates, and occasionally cavitation. Widespread dissemination that involves the abdominal lymph nodes, liver, spleen, kidneys, pancreas, thyroid, heart, brain, and meninges is common. Intestinal symptoms of hyperinfection syndrome include profound diarrhea, malabsorption, and electrolyte abnormalities. Of note, hyperinfection syndrome is associated with a mortality rate of approximately 86%. Bacterial sepsis, meningitis, peritonitis, and endocarditis secondary to larval spread from the intestine are frequent and often fatal complications of hyperinfection syndrome.

Laboratory Diagnosis

The diagnosis of strongyloidiasis may be difficult because of the intermittent passage of low numbers of first-stage larvae in stool. Examination of concentrated stool sediment reveals the larval worms (Figure 75-12), but in contrast with

Clinical Case 75-3 *Strongyloides* Hyperinfection

Gorman and colleagues (*Infect Med* 23:480, 2006) described a case of necrotizing myositis complicated by diffuse alveolar hemorrhage and sepsis after corticosteroid therapy. The patient was a 46-year-old Cambodian man with a history of Raynaud phenomenon. He presented to the rheumatology clinic with worsening symptoms of Raynaud syndrome and diffuse muscle aches. He was employed as a truck driver and had emigrated from Cambodia 30 years earlier. Pertinent laboratory studies included markedly elevated creatine kinase and aldolase levels. Pulmonary function studies showed decreased forced vital capacity, forced expiratory volume, and carbon monoxide diffusing capacity. A high-resolution computed tomography (CT) scan of the chest showed mild ground-glass changes in both lung bases and interlobular septate thickening. Muscle biopsy showed myocyte necrosis and random atrophy but no inflammatory cells. Bronchoscopy was unremarkable, and all cultures were negative. The patient was started on prednisone for presumed necrotizing myopathy secondary to undifferentiated connective tissue disease.

He was admitted to the hospital 1 month later with profound muscle weakness and dyspnea, which improved with the administration of methylprednisolone and intravenous immunoglobulin. Three weeks later, the patient was readmitted with fever, nausea, vomiting, abdominal pain, and diffuse joint pain. A CT scan of the abdomen suggested small bowel intussusception and colitis, but his symptoms improved without treatment. Another high-resolution CT scan of the chest showed early honeycombing and worsening interstitial infiltrates. The patient was scheduled for a lung biopsy; however, while awaiting the biopsy, he suffered an abrupt and fulminant deterioration, with hemoptysis and hypoxemic respiratory failure that required intubation and mechanical ventilation. A chest radiograph showed new, diffuse, bilateral infiltrates. The patient developed an acute abdomen accompanied by purpura on the lower trunk. An abdominal CT showed pancolitis. Refractory septic shock caused by *Escherichia coli* bacteremia and lactic acidosis ensued. Bronchoscopy showed diffuse alveolar hemorrhage, and numerous larvae of *Strongyloides stercoralis* were demonstrated on staining of an aspirate of endotracheal secretions. Serology was positive for anti-*Strongyloides* antibodies. Despite treatment with ivermectin, albendazole, cefepime, vancomycin, vasopressors, steroids, and dialysis, the patient died.

This case of *Strongyloides* hyperinfection syndrome emphasizes the importance of screening and treating persons at risk for latent *S. stercoralis* infection (endemic in tropical and subtropical areas) before the initiation of immunosuppressive therapy. Contact precautions should be taken in patients with hyperinfection syndrome because of the risk of infection to health care workers and visitors upon exposure to infectious larvae in the patient's stool and secretions.

hookworm infections, in *S. stercoralis* infections, eggs are generally not seen. Collecting samples from three stools, 1 per day for 3 days (as for *G. duodenalis*), is recommended because *S. stercoralis* larvae may occur in "showers," with many present one day and few or none the next. Several authors favor the **Baermann funnel gauze method** of concentrating living *S. stercoralis* larvae from fecal specimens. This method uses a funnel with a stopcock and a gauze insert. The funnel is filled with lukewarm water to a level just covering the gauze, and a specimen of stool is placed on the gauze, partially in contact with the water. The larvae in the stool migrate through the gauze into the water and then sediment into the neck of the funnel, where they may be detected by low-power microscopy. When absent from stool,

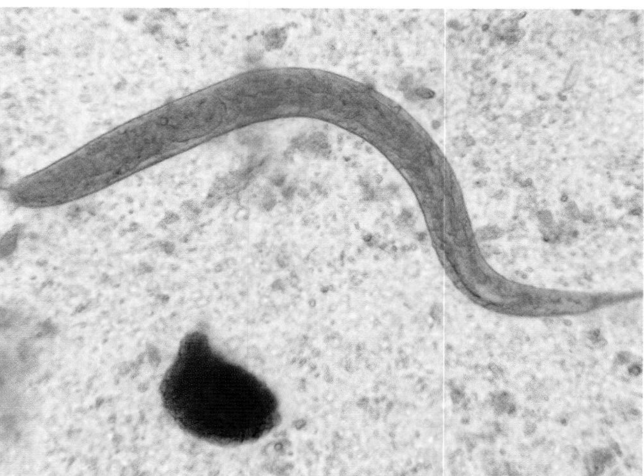

FIGURE 75-12 *Strongyloides stercoralis* larvae. The larvae are 180 to 380 μm long and 14 to 24 μm wide. They are differentiated from hookworm larvae by the length of the buccal cavity and esophagus and by the structure of the genital primordium.

larvae may be detected in duodenal aspirates or in sputum in the case of massive infection. Finally, culture of the larvae from stool using charcoal cultures or an agar plate method may be used, although these are not routine in most laboratories. Demonstration of anti-*Strongyloides* antibodies in blood may be useful as a screening test or as an adjunct for diagnosis.

Treatment, Prevention, and Control

All infected patients should be treated to prevent autoinfection and potential dissemination (hyperinfection) of the parasite. The drug of choice is ivermectin, with albendazole or mebendazole as an alternative. Patients in endemic areas who are preparing to undergo immunosuppressive therapy should have at least three stool examinations to rule out *S. stercoralis* infection and thus avoid the risks of hyperinfection syndrome. Strict infection-control measures should be enforced when clinicians care for patients with hyperinfection syndrome, because stool, saliva, vomitus, and body fluids may contain infectious filariform larvae. As with hookworm, control of *Strongyloides* spp. requires education, proper sanitation, and prompt treatment of existing infections.

Trichinella spiralis

Physiology and Structure

Trichinella spiralis is the most important cause of human disease, but other species, such as *T. pseudospiralis* and *T. britovi,* may also cause **trichinosis.** The adult form of this organism lives in the duodenal and jejunal mucosa of flesh-eating mammals worldwide. The infectious larval form is present in the striated muscles of carnivorous and omnivorous mammals. Among domestic animals, swine are most frequently involved. Figure 75-13 illustrates the simple, direct life cycle, which terminates in the musculature of humans, where the larvae eventually die and calcify.

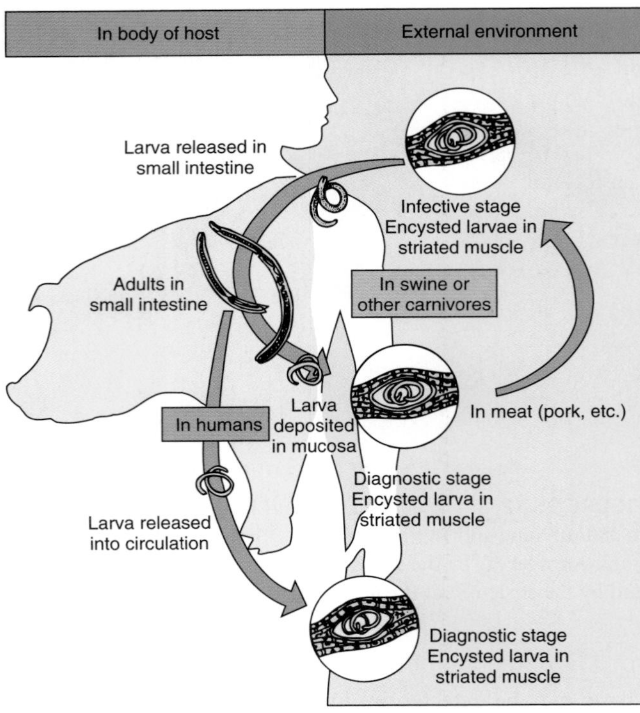

FIGURE 75-13 Life cycle of *Trichinella spiralis.*

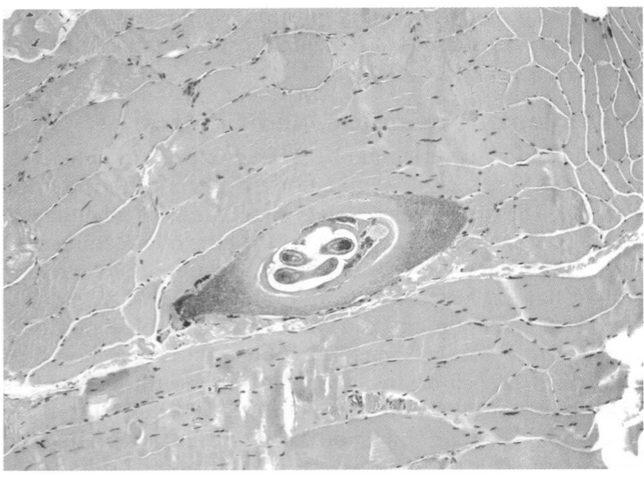

FIGURE 75-14 Encysted larva of *Trichinella spiralis* in a muscle biopsy specimen. (From CDC Public Health Image Library.)

The infection begins when meat that contains encysted larvae is digested. The larvae leave the meat in the small intestine and within 2 days develop into adult worms. A single fertilized female produces more than 1500 larvae in 1 to 3 months. These larvae move from the intestinal mucosa into the bloodstream and are carried in the circulation to various muscle sites throughout the body, where they coil in striated muscle fibers and become encysted (Figure 75-14). The muscles invaded most frequently include the extraocular muscles of the eye; the tongue; the deltoid, pectoral, and intercostal muscles; the diaphragm; and the gastrocnemius muscle. The encysted larvae remain viable for many years and are infectious if ingested by a new animal host. The muscle larvae of *T. pseudospiralis* do not induce the formation of a cyst and generate less inflammation than that of *T. spiralis*.

Epidemiology

Trichinosis occurs worldwide in humans, and its greatest prevalence is associated with the consumption of pork products. In addition to its transmission from pigs, many carnivorous and omnivorous animals harbor the organism and are potential sources of human infection. Of note, polar bears and walruses in the Arctic account for outbreaks in human populations, especially with a strain of *T. spiralis (T. natira)* that is more resistant to freezing than the *T. spiralis* strains found in the continental United States and other temperate regions. It is estimated that more than 1.5 million Americans carry live *Trichinella* cysts in their musculature and that 150,000 to 300,000 acquire new infection annually.

Clinical Syndromes

Trichinosis is one of the few tissue parasitic diseases still seen in the United States. As with other parasitic infections, most patients have minimal or no symptoms. The clinical presentation depends largely on the tissue burden of organisms and the location of the migrating larvae. Patients in whom no more than 10 larvae are deposited per gram of tissue are usually asymptomatic, those with at least 100 generally have significant disease, and those with 1000 to 5000 have a very serious course that occasionally ends in death. In mild infections with few migrating larvae, patients may experience only an influenza-like syndrome with slight fever and mild diarrhea. With more extensive larval migration, persistent fever, gastrointestinal distress, marked eosinophilia, muscle pain, and periorbital edema occur. "Splinter" hemorrhages beneath the nails, a common finding, are probably caused by vasculitis resulting from toxic secretions of the migrating larvae. In heavy infections, severe neurologic symptoms, including psychosis, meningoencephalitis, and cerebrovascular accident, may occur.

Patients who survive the migration, muscle destruction, and encystment of larvae in moderate infections experience a decline in clinical symptoms in 5 or 6 weeks. Lethal trichinosis results when myocarditis, encephalitis, and pneumonitis combine; the patient dies 4 to 6 weeks after infection. Respiratory arrest often follows heavy invasion and muscle destruction in the diaphragm.

Laboratory Diagnosis

The diagnosis is usually established with clinical observations, especially when an outbreak can be traced to consumption of improperly cooked pork or bear meat. The laboratory may confirm the diagnosis if the encysted larvae are detected in the implicated meat or in a muscle biopsy specimen from the patient. Marked **eosinophilia** is characteristically present in patients with trichinosis. Serologic procedures are also available for confirmation of the diagnosis. Significant antibody titers are usually absent before the third week of illness but then may persist for years.

Treatment, Prevention, and Control

Treatment of trichinosis is primarily symptomatic because there are no good antiparasitic agents for tissue larvae. Treatment of the adult worms in the intestine with mebendazole may halt the production of new larvae. Steroids, along with thiabendazole or mebendazole, are recommended for severe symptoms. In infections caused by *T. pseudospiralis,* albendazole may be effective. Education regarding disease transmission from pork and bear meat is essential, especially the recommendation that pork and bear meat be cooked until the interior is gray. Microwave cooking and smoking or drying meat do not kill all larvae.

Laws regulating the feeding of garbage to pigs help control transmission, as may regulations controlling the foraging of bears in garbage pits and public parks. Freezing pork, as conducted in federally inspected meat packing plants, has reduced transmission. Quick freezing of pork at −40° C effectively destroys the organisms, as does low-temperature storage at −15° C for 20 days or more.

Wuchereria bancrofti and *Brugia malayi*

Physiology and Structure

Because of their many similarities, *Wuchereria bancrofti* and *Brugia malayi* are discussed together. Human infection is initiated by the introduction of infective larvae, present in the saliva of a biting mosquito, into a bite wound (Figure 75-15). Various species of *Anopheles, Aedes,* and *Culex* mosquitoes are vectors of **Bancroft and Malayan filariasis.** The larvae migrate from the location of the bite to the lymphatic system, primarily in the arms, legs, or groin, where larval growth to adulthood occurs. From 3 to 12 months after the initial infection, the adult male worm fertilizes the female, which in turn produces the sheathed larval microfilariae that find their way into the circulation. The presence of **microfilariae** in blood is diagnostic for human disease and is infective for feeding mosquitoes. In the mosquito, the larvae move through the stomach and thoracic muscles in developmental stages and finally migrate to the proboscis. There they become infective third-stage larvae and are transmitted by the feeding mosquito. The adult form in humans can persist for as long as 10 years. These organisms harbor **bacterial endosymbionts** of the genus *Wolbachia* and depend on these endosymbionts for normal metabolic and reproductive activities. This raises the potential for the use of common antibacterial agents, such as doxycycline, to target the adult filarial worms.

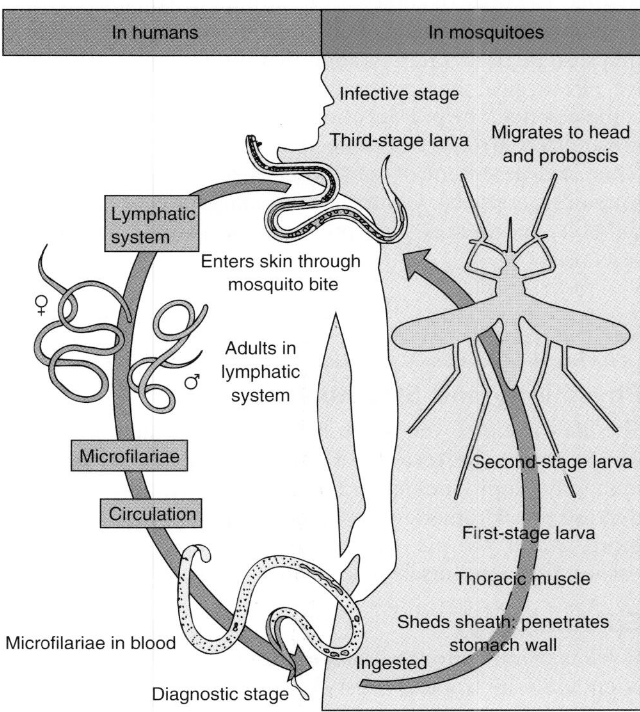

FIGURE 75-15 Life cycle of *Wuchereria bancrofti.*

Epidemiology

Infection with *W. bancrofti* occurs in tropical and subtropical areas and is endemic in central Africa, along the Mediterranean coast, and in many parts of Asia, including China, Korea, Japan, and the Philippines. It is also present in Haiti, Trinidad, Surinam, Panama, Costa Rica, and Brazil. No animal reservoir has been identified. *B. malayi* is found primarily in Malaysia, India, Thailand, Vietnam, and parts of China, Korea, Japan, and many Pacific islands. Animal reservoirs, such as cats and monkeys, are recognized.

Clinical Syndromes

In some patients, there is no sign of disease even though blood specimens may show the presence of many microfilariae. In other patients, early acute symptoms are fever, lymphangitis and lymphadenitis with chills, and recurrent febrile attacks. The acute presentation is thought to result from the inflammatory response to the presence of molting adolescent worms and dead or dying adults within the lymphatic vessels. As the infection progresses, the lymph nodes enlarge, possibly involving many parts of the body, including the extremities, scrotum, and testes, with occasional abscess formation. This results from physical obstruction of lymph in the vessels caused by the presence of adult worms and host reactivity in the lymphatic system. This process may be complicated by recurrent bacterial infections, which contribute to the tissue damage. The thickening and hypertrophy of tissues infected with the worms may lead to enlargement of tissues, especially the extremities, progressing to filarial **elephantiasis.** Filariasis of this type is thus a chronic, debilitating, and disfiguring disease requiring prompt diagnosis and treatment. Occasionally, ascites and pleural effusions secondary to rupture of the enlarged lymphatic vessels into the peritoneal or pleural cavity may be observed.

Laboratory Diagnosis

Eosinophilia is usually present during acute inflammatory episodes; however, demonstration of microfilariae in the blood is required for definitive diagnosis. As with malaria, microfilariae can be demonstrated in Giemsa-stained blood films in infections with *W. bancrofti* and *B. malayi* (Figures 75-16 and 75-17). Concentration of anticoagulated blood specimens and urine specimens are also valuable procedures. Buffy coat films concentrate the white blood cells and are useful for the detection of microfilariae. The presence of small numbers of microfilariae in blood can be detected by a membrane filtration technique in which anticoagulated blood is mixed with saline and forced through a 5-μm membrane filter. After several washes with saline or distilled water, the filter is examined microscopically for living

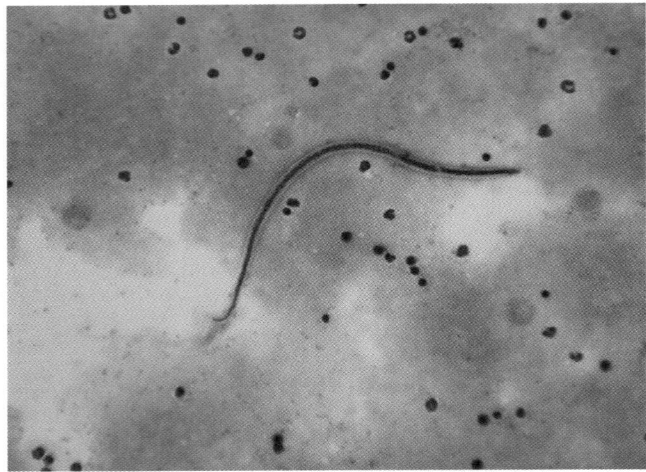

FIGURE 75-16 Giemsa stain of sheathed *Wuchereria bancrofti* microfilaria in blood smear; 245 to 295 µm long × 7 to 10 µm wide.

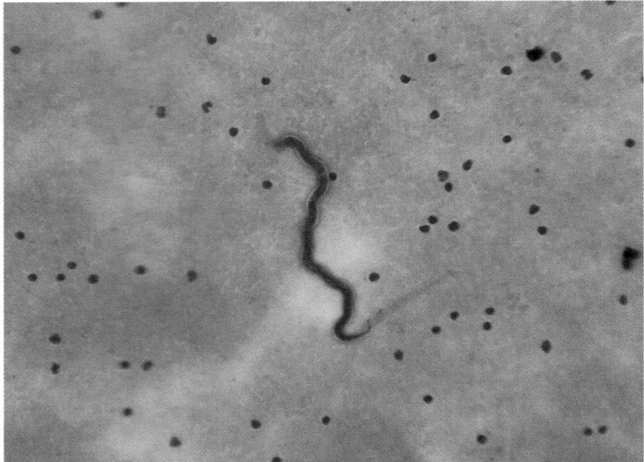

FIGURE 75-17 Giemsa stain of sheathed *Brugia malayi* microfilaria in blood smear; 180 to 230 µm long × 5 to 6 µm wide.

microfilariae, or it is dried, fixed, and stained as for a thin blood film.

W. bancrofti and *B. malayi* have both nocturnal and subperiodic periodicity in the production of microfilariae. Nocturnal periodicity results in greater numbers of microfilariae in blood at night, whereas with the subperiodic form, microfilariae are present at all times, with a peak in the afternoon.

W. bancrofti, as well as *B. malayi* and *Loa loa,* demonstrate a sheath on their microfilariae. This can be the first step in identifying the specific types of filariasis. Further identification is based on study of head and tail structures (Figure 75-18). Clinically an exact species identification is not critical, because treatment for all the filarial infections except *Onchocerca volvulus* is identical.

Serologic testing is also available through reference laboratories so that a diagnosis can be reached. Detection of circulating filarial antigens is promising but not widely available as a diagnostic test.

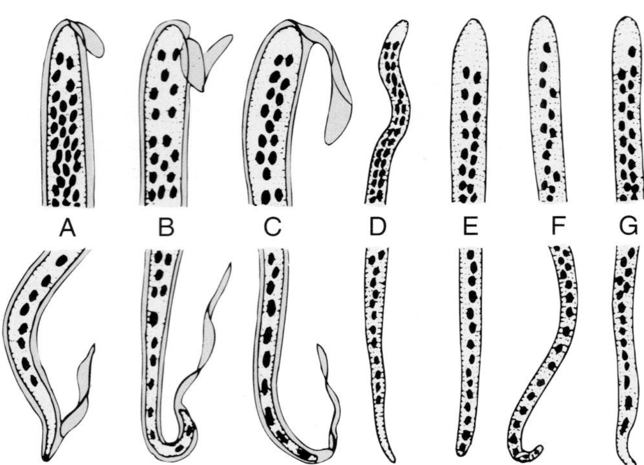

FIGURE 75-18 Differentiation of microfilariae. Identification of microfilariae is based on the presence of a sheath covering the larvae, as well as the distribution of nuclei in the tail region. **A,** *Wuchereria bancrofti.* **B,** *Brugia malayi.* **C,** *Loa loa.* **D,** *Onchocerca volvulus.* **E,** *Mansonella perstans.* **F,** *Mansonella streptocerca.* **G,** *Mansonella ozzardi.*

Treatment, Prevention, and Control

Treatment is of little benefit in most cases of chronic lymphatic filariasis because of scarring and lymphedema. At present, treatment targets the microfilarial stage. Discovery of the **bacterial endosymbiont *Wolbachia*** raises the possibility of using antibiotics such as doxycycline to treat the adult worm. This is important because (to date) there is no effective drug that targets the adult stage of these parasitic worms. The drug of choice for treatment of *W. bancrofti* and *B. malayi* microfilariae is DEC. Ivermectin and albendazole may also be used, often in combination with DEC. Supportive and surgical therapy for lymphatic obstruction may be of some cosmetic help. Education regarding filarial infections, mosquito control, use of protective clothing and insect repellents, and treatment of infections to prevent further transmission is essential. Control of *B. malayi* infections is more difficult because of the presence of disease in animal reservoirs.

• *Loa loa*

Physiology and Structure

The life cycle of *L. loa* is similar to that illustrated in Figure 75-15, except the vector is a biting fly called *Chrysops,* the mangofly. Approximately 6 months after infection, the production of microfilariae starts and can persist for 17 years or more. Adult worms can migrate through subcutaneous tissues, through muscle, and in front of the eyeball.

Epidemiology

L. loa is confined to the equatorial rain forests of Africa and is endemic in tropical West Africa, the Congo basin, and parts of Nigeria. Monkeys in these areas serve as reservoir hosts in the life cycle, with mangoflies as vectors.

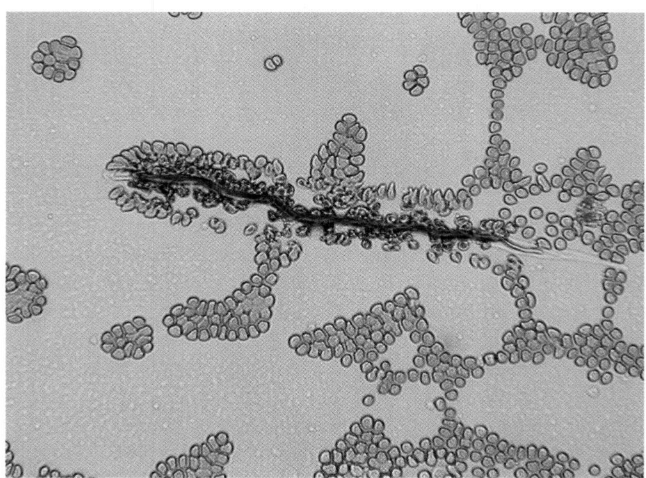

FIGURE 75-19 Giemsa stain of sheathed *Loa loa* microfilaria in blood smear; 230 to 250 μm long × 6 to 9 μm wide.

Clinical Syndromes

Symptoms usually do not appear until a year or so after the fly bite, because the worms are slow in reaching adulthood. One of the first signs of infection is the so-called **fugitive** or **Calabar swellings.** These swellings are transient and usually appear on the extremities, produced as the worms migrate through subcutaneous tissues, creating large nodular areas that are painful and pruritic. Because eosinophilia (50% to 70%) is observed, Calabar swellings are believed to result from allergic reactions to the worms or their metabolic products.

Adult *L. loa* worms can also migrate under the conjunctiva, producing irritation, painful congestion, edema of the eyelids, and impaired vision. The presence of a worm in the eye can obviously cause anxiety in the patient. The infection may be long lived and in some cases asymptomatic.

Laboratory Diagnosis

The clinical observation of Calabar swellings or migration of worms in the eye, combined with eosinophilia, should alert the physician to consider infection with *L. loa*. The microfilariae can be found in the blood (Figure 75-19). In contrast to the other filariae, *L. loa* is primarily present during the daytime. Serologic testing can also be useful for confirming the diagnosis but is not readily available.

Treatment, Prevention, and Control

DEC is effective against adults and microfilariae; however, destruction of the parasites may induce severe allergic reactions that require treatment with corticosteroids. Albendazole or ivermectin (not approved by the U.S. Food and Drug Administration) has been shown to be effective in reducing microfilarial loads. Surgical removal of worms migrating across the eye or bridge of the nose can be accomplished by immobilizing the worm with instillation of a few drops of 10% cocaine. Education regarding the infection and its vector, especially for people entering the known endemic areas, is essential. Protection from fly bites by using screening, appropriate clothing, and insect repellents, along with treatment of cases, is also critical in reducing the incidence of infection. However, the presence of disease in animal reservoirs (e.g., monkeys) limits the feasibility of controlling this disease.

Mansonella Species

Filarial infections caused by *Mansonella* spp. are less important than those previously discussed, but physicians should be aware of the names because they may encounter patients with these infections. Infections caused by these organisms are generally asymptomatic but may cause dermatitis, lymphadenitis, hydrocele, and (rarely) lymphatic obstruction resulting in elephantiasis.

All of the *Mansonella* spp. produce nonsheathed microfilariae in blood and subcutaneous tissues, and all are transmitted by biting midges (*Culicoides* spp.) or blackflies (*Simulium* spp.). Ivermectin is the treatment of choice for *M. ozzardi* and *M. streptocerca,* whereas DEC is used for *M. perstans*. Species identification, if desired, can be accomplished with blood smears, noting the structure of the microfilariae (see Figure 75-18). Serologic tests are also available.

Prevention and control require measures involving insect repellents, screening, and other precautions as for all insect-transmitted diseases.

Mansonella perstans

M. perstans occurs primarily in parts of tropical Africa and Central and South America. It may produce allergic skin reactions, edema, and Calabar swellings like those of *L. loa* infection. Reservoir hosts are chimpanzees and gorillas.

Mansonella ozzardi

M. ozzardi is found primarily in Central and South America and the West Indies. It may produce swelling of the lymph nodes and occasional hydrocele. There are no known reservoir hosts.

Mansonella streptocerca

M. streptocerca occurs primarily in Africa, especially in the Congo basin. It may produce edema in the skin and (rarely) a form of elephantiasis. Monkeys serve as reservoir hosts.

Onchocerca volvulus

Physiology and Structure

Infection occurs after the introduction of *O. volvulus* larvae through the skin during the biting and feeding of the *Simulium* (blackfly) vector (Figure 75-20). The larval worms migrate from the skin to subcutaneous tissue and develop into adult male and female worms. The adults become encased in fibrous subcutaneous nodules within which they may remain viable for as long as 15 years. The female worm, after fertilization by the male, begins producing as many as 2000 nonsheathed microfilariae each day. The microfilariae exit the capsule and migrate to the skin, eyes, and other body tissues. These nonsheathed microfilariae appearing in skin tissue are infective for feeding blackflies. Of note, all individual worms and all life-cycle stages contain the ***Wolbachia* bacterial endosymbionts.** It is now understood that

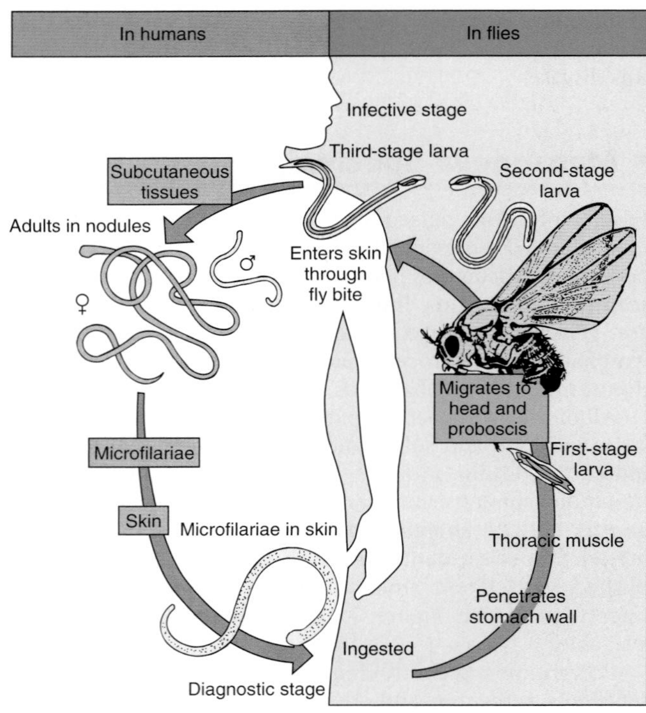

FIGURE 75-20 Life cycle of *Onchocerca volvulus.*

clearance of the endosymbionts by antibiotic treatment causes inhibition of worm development, blocks embryogenesis and fertility, and reduces worm viability. It is suggested that various biochemical pathways that are intact in *Wolbachia* but absent or incomplete in the nematode, including heme, nucleotide, and enzyme cofactor biosynthesis, may be the bacteria's contribution to nematode biology.

Epidemiology

O. volvulus is endemic in many parts of Africa, especially in the Congo and Volta river basins. In the Western Hemisphere, it occurs in many Central and South American countries. **Onchocerciasis** affects more than 18 million people worldwide and causes blindness in approximately 5% of infected people.

Several species of the blackfly genus *Simulium* serve as vectors but none so appropriately named as the principal vector, *Simulium damnosum* ("the damned blackfly"). These blackflies, or buffalo gnats, breed in fast-flowing streams, which makes control or eradication by insecticides almost impossible because the chemicals are rapidly washed away from the eggs and larvae.

There is a greater prevalence of infection in men than women in endemic areas because of their work in or near the streams where the blackflies breed. Studies in endemic areas in Africa have shown that 50% of men are totally blind before they reach 50 years of age. This accounts for the common term **river blindness,** which is applied to the disease onchocerciasis. This fear of blindness has created an additional problem in many parts of Africa because whole villages leave the area near streams and farmland that could produce food. The migrating populations then find themselves in areas where they face starvation.

Clinical Case 75-4 Onchocerciasis

Imtiaz and colleagues (*Infect Med* 22:187–189, 2005) described the case of a 21-year-old man who emigrated from Sudan to the United States 1 year before presenting with a maculopapular rash that was associated with severe pruritus. The rash and pruritus had been present for the past 3 to 4 years. In the past, the patient had undergone multiple treatments for this condition, including corticosteroids, without relief. The patient denied any systemic symptoms but did complain of blurred vision. On physical examination, his skin was somewhat thickened over different parts of the body, and he had scattered maculopapular lesions with increased pigmentation; some lesions had keloid nodules as well as wrinkling. There was no lymphadenopathy. The remainder of his evaluation was unremarkable.

Because of the presence of intense pruritus unresponsive to treatment, blurred vision, and the prevalence of onchocerciasis in his native country, skin snips were taken from the scapular area. Microfilariae of *Onchocerca volvulus* were revealed on microscopic examination. Ivermectin was prescribed, to which the patient's condition responded. Onchocerciasis, although not common in the United States, should be considered in immigrants and expatriates with suggestive symptoms if they came from areas in which the disease is endemic.

Clinical Syndromes

Clinical onchocerciasis is characterized by infection involving the skin, subcutaneous tissue, lymph nodes, and eyes (Clinical Case 75-4). The clinical manifestations of the infection are due to the acute and chronic inflammatory reaction to antigens released by the microfilariae as they migrate through the tissues. The incubation period from infectious larvae to adult worms is several months to a year. The initial signs of disease are fever, eosinophilia, and urticaria. As the worms mature, copulate, and produce microfilariae, subcutaneous nodules begin to appear on any part of the body. These nodules are most dangerous when they are present on the head and neck because the microfilariae may migrate to the eyes and cause serious tissue damage, leading to blindness. The mechanisms for development of eye disease are thought to be a combination of both direct invasion by the microfilariae and antigen-antibody complex deposition within the ocular tissues. It is now apparent that the *Wolbachia* bacterial endosymbiont plays an important role in the inflammatory pathogenesis of onchocerciasis. *Wolbachia* release after microfilarial death in the cornea causes corneal edema and opacity by inducing neutrophil and macrophage infiltration and activation in the corneal stroma. Patients progress from conjunctivitis with photophobia to punctate and sclerosing keratitis. Internal eye disease with anterior uveitis, chorioretinitis, and optic neuritis may also occur.

Within the skin, the inflammatory process results in loss of elasticity and areas of depigmentation, thickening, and atrophy. A number of skin conditions, including pruritus, hyperkeratosis, and myxedematous thickening, are related to the presence of this parasite. A form of elephantiasis called **hanging groin** also occurs when the nodules are located near the genitalia.

Laboratory Diagnosis

The diagnosis of onchocerciasis is made by the demonstration of microfilariae in skin snip preparations from the

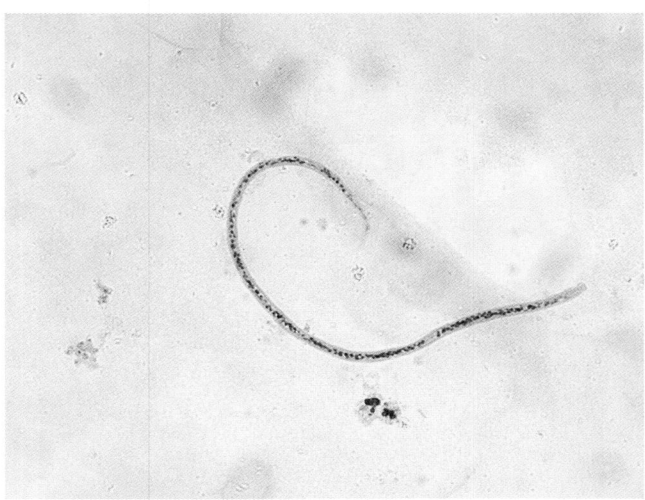

FIGURE 75-21 Giemsa-stained unsheathed *Onchocerca volvulus* microfilaria; 300 to 315 μm long × 5 to 9 μm wide.

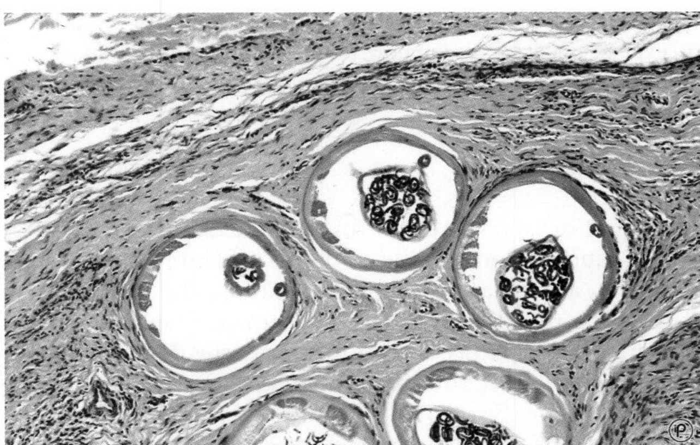

FIGURE 75-22 Cross section of an adult female *Onchocerca volvulus* in an excised nodule showing numerous microfilariae.

infrascapular or gluteal region. A sample is obtained by raising the skin with a needle and shaving the epidermal layer with a razor. The specimen is incubated in saline for several hours and is then inspected with a dissecting microscope for the presence of nonsheathed microfilariae (Figure 75-21). In patients with ocular disease, the organism may also be seen in the anterior chamber with the aid of a slit lamp. Serologic methods using recombinant antigens have been useful, as have assays using polymerase chain reaction to detect onchocercal deoxyribonucleic acid (DNA) in skin snip specimens.

Treatment, Prevention, and Control

Surgical removal of the encapsulated nodule is often performed to eliminate the adult worms and stop production of microfilariae (Figure 75-22). In addition, treatment with ivermectin is recommended. A single oral dose of ivermectin (150 mg/kg) greatly reduces the number of microfilariae in the skin and eyes, thus diminishing the likelihood of developing a disabling onchocerciasis. In endemic areas, the dose of ivermectin can be repeated every 6 to 12 months to maintain suppression of dermal and ocular microfilariae. Suppression of dermal microfilariae reduces transmission of this vector-borne disease, and thus mass chemotherapy may prove to be a successful strategy for prevention of onchocerciasis. At present, there is no firm evidence that *O. volvulus* is becoming resistant to ivermectin; however, whenever a single agent is used for disease control, with varying doses over a long period of time, it is prudent to be on guard for the possibility of resistance developing. Human field trials with antiwolbachial drugs such as doxycycline have demonstrated both sterilizing and macrofilaricidal activity. Based on these trials, doxycycline at 200 mg/day for 6 weeks is recommended for patients in whom the highest possible macrofilaricidal activity is desired and who have moved away from areas with ongoing transmission.

Education regarding the disease and its transmission is essential. Protection from blackfly bites through the use of protective clothing, screening, and insect repellents, as well as prompt diagnosis and treatment of infections to prevent further transmission, is critical.

Although control of blackfly breeding is difficult because insecticides wash away in the streams, some form of biological control of this vector may reduce fly reproduction and disease transmission.

Dirofilaria immitis

Several mosquito-transmitted filariae infect dogs, cats, raccoons, and bobcats in nature and occasionally are found in humans. *Dirofilaria immitis,* the **dog heartworm,** is notorious for forming a lethal worm bolus in the dog's heart. This nematode may also infect humans, producing a nodule called a **coin lesion** in the lung. Only very rarely have these worms been found in human hearts.

The coin lesion in the lung presents a problem for the radiologist and the surgeon because it resembles a malignancy requiring surgical removal. Unfortunately, no laboratory test can provide an accurate diagnosis of **dirofilariasis.** Peripheral eosinophilia is rare, and the radiographic features are insufficient to allow the clinician to distinguish pulmonary dirofilariasis from bronchogenic carcinoma. Serologic tests are not sufficiently sensitive or specific to preclude surgical intervention. A definitive diagnosis is made when a thoracotomy specimen is examined microscopically, revealing the typical cross sections of the parasite.

Transmission of the filarial infections can be controlled by mosquito control and prophylactic use of the drug ivermectin in dogs.

Dracunculus medinensis

The name *Dracunculus medinensis* means "little dragon of Medina." This is a very ancient worm infection thought by some scholars to be the "fiery serpent" noted by Moses with the Israelites at the Red Sea.

Physiology and Structure

D. medinensis is not a filarial worm but a tissue-invading nematode of medical importance in many parts of the world. The worms have a very simple life cycle, depending on freshwater and a microcrustacean **(copepod)** of the genus *Cyclops*

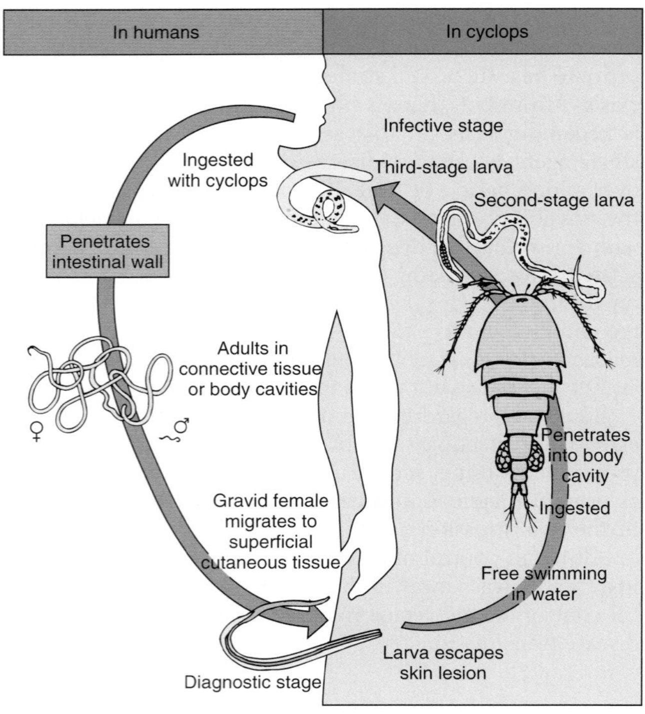

FIGURE 75-23 Life cycle of *Dracunculus medinensis.*

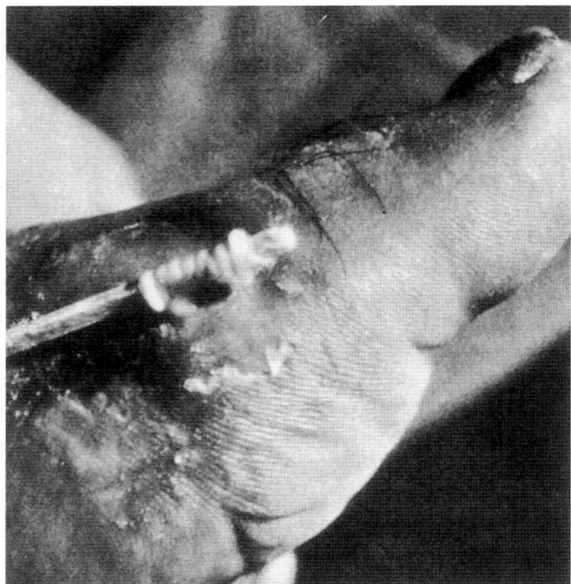

FIGURE 75-24 Removal of a *Dracunculus medinensis* adult from an exposed ulcer by winding the worm slowly around a stick. (From Binford CH, Conner DH: *Pathology of tropical and extraordinary diseases,* Washington, DC, 1976, Armed Forces Institute of Pathology.)

(Figure 75-23). When *Cyclops* spp. harboring larval *D. medinensis* are ingested in drinking water, the infection is initiated with liberation of the larvae in the stomach. These larvae penetrate the wall of the digestive tract and migrate to the retroperitoneal space, where they mature. These larvae are not microfilariae and do not appear in blood or other tissues. Male and female worms mate in the retroperitoneum, and the fertilized female then migrates to the subcutaneous tissues, usually in the extremities. When the fertilized female worm becomes gravid, a vesicle is formed in the host tissue, which will ulcerate. When the ulcer is completely formed, the worm protrudes a loop of uterus through the ulcer. On contact with water, the larval worms are released. The larvae are then ingested by the *Cyclops* spp. in freshwater, where they are then infective for humans or animals drinking the water containing the *Cyclops* spp.

Epidemiology

D. medinensis occurs in many parts of Asia and equatorial Africa, infecting an estimated 10 million people. Reservoir hosts include dogs and many fur-bearing animals that come into contact with drinking water containing infective *Cyclops* spp.

Human infections usually result from ingestion of water from so-called **step wells** where people stand or bathe in the water, at which time the gravid female worm discharges larvae from lesions on the arms, legs, feet, and ankles to infect *Cyclops* spp. in the water. Ponds and standing water are occasionally the source of infection when humans use them for drinking water.

Clinical Syndromes

Symptoms of infection usually do not appear until the gravid female creates the vesicle and the ulcer in the skin for the liberation of larval worms. This usually occurs 1 year after initial exposure. At the site of the ulcer, there are erythema and pain, as well as an allergic reaction to the worm. There is also the possibility of abscess formation and secondary bacterial infection, leading to further tissue destruction and inflammatory reaction with intense pain and sloughing of skin.

If the worm is broken in attempts to remove it, there may be toxic reactions, and if the worm dies and calcifies, there may be nodule formation and some allergic reaction. Once the gravid female worm has discharged all the larvae, it may retreat into deeper tissue, where it is gradually absorbed, or it may simply be expelled from the site.

Laboratory Diagnosis

Diagnosis is established by observing the typical ulcer and by flooding the ulcer with water to recover the larval worms when they are discharged. Occasionally, radiographic examination reveals worms in various parts of the body.

Treatment, Prevention, and Control

The ancient method of slowly wrapping the worm on a twig is still used in many endemic areas (Figure 75-24). Surgical removal is also a practical and reliable procedure for the patient. There is no evidence that any chemotherapeutic agent has a direct effect on *D. medinensis,* although various benzimidazoles may have an antiinflammatory effect and either eliminate the worm or make surgical removal easier. Treatment with mebendazole has been associated with aberrant migration of the worms, with the result that they were more likely to emerge at anatomic sites other than the lower limbs.

Education regarding the life cycle of the worm and avoidance of water contaminated with *Cyclops* spp. are critical.

Protection of drinking water by prohibiting bathing and washing of clothing in wells is essential. Persons who live in or travel to endemic areas should boil water before drinking it. The treatment of water with chemicals and the use of fish that consume *Cyclops* spp. as food also help control transmission. Prompt diagnosis and treatment of cases also limit further transmission. These preventive measures have been incorporated into an ongoing global effort to eliminate dracunculiasis with dramatic success. The annual incidence of worldwide disease has been reduced by 98%, with complete eradication in seven countries.

Bibliography

Barry M: The tail end of guinea worm—global eradication without a drug or a vaccine, *N Engl J Med* 356:2561–2564, 2007.

Despommier D: Toxocariasis: clinical aspects, epidemiology, medical ecology and molecular aspects, *Clin Microbiol Rev* 16:265–272, 2003.

Fink DL, Nutman TB: Filarial nematodes. In Versalovic J, et al, editors: *Manual of clinical microbiology*, ed 10, Washington, DC, 2011, American Society for Microbiology Press.

Garcia LS: *Diagnostic medical parasitology*, ed 5, Washington, DC, 2005, American Society for Microbiology Press.

Gavin PJ, Kazacos KR, Shulman ST: Baylisascariasis, *Clin Microbiol Rev* 18:703–718, 2005.

Gottstein B, Pozio E, Nockler K: Epidemiology, treatment, and control of trichinellosis, *Clin Microbiol Rev* 22:127–145, 2009.

Hotez PJ, Brooker S, Bethony JM, et al: Hookworm infection, *N Engl J Med* 351:799–807, 2004.

Hotez PJ, Brindley PJ, Bethony JM, et al: Helminth infections: the great neglected tropical diseases, *J Clin Invest* 118:1311–1321, 2008.

James CE, Hudson AL, Davey MW: Drug resistance mechanisms in helminths: is it survival of the fittest? *Trends Parasitol* 25:328–335, 2009.

Keiser PB, Nutman TB: *Strongyloides stercoralis* in the immunocompromised population, *Clin Microbiol Rev* 17:208–217, 2004.

Procop GW, Neafie RC: Less common helminths. In Versalovic J, et al, editors: *Manual of clinical microbiology*, ed 10, Washington, DC, 2011, American Society for Microbiology Press.

Sheorey H, Biggs BA, Traynor P: Nematodes. In Versalovic J, et al, editors: *Manual of clinical microbiology*, ed 10, Washington, DC, 2011, American Society for Microbiology Press.

Tamarozzi F, Halliday A, Gentil K, et al: Onchocerciasis: the role of *Wolbachia* bacterial endosymbionts in parasite biology, disease pathogenesis, and treatment, *Clin Microbiol Rev* 24:459–468, 2011.

CHAPTER

76 TREMATODES

A 45-year-old Egyptian man was referred for evaluation of hematuria and urinary frequency of 2 months' duration. This individual had lived in the Middle East for most of his life but for the past year lived in the United States. He denied previous renal or urologic problems. His physical examination was unremarkable. A midstream urine specimen was grossly bloody.

1. What was the differential diagnosis of hematuria in this patient?
2. What was the etiologic agent of this patient's urologic process?
3. What exposures might put an individual at risk for this infection?
4. What are the major complications of this infection?
5. How is this disease treated?

Answers to these questions are available on StudentConsult.com.

• SUMMARIES CLINICALLY SIGNIFICANT ORGANISMS

Fasciolopsis buski

Trigger Words

Aquatic vegetation, intermediate host, snail, intestinal fluke, operculum, cercariae, metacercariae, reservoir hosts

Biology, Virulence, and Disease

- Trematodes (flukes): members of Platyhelminthes; generally flat, fleshy, leaf-shaped worms
- *Fasciolopsis buski:* largest, most prevalent, most important intestinal fluke; from 1.5 to 3.0 cm long (rarely found in feces or specimens collected during surgery)
- Life cycle typical for intestinal flukes
- Symptomatology of *F. buski* infection relates directly to worm burden in small intestine; includes mucosal inflammation, ulceration and hemorrhage, abdominal discomfort and diarrhea, intestinal obstruction, eosinophilia

Epidemiology

- Distribution depends on location of appropriate snail host; most prevalent in Southeast Asia and Indian subcontinent
- Pigs, dogs, rabbits serve as reservoir hosts in endemic regions

Diagnosis

- Microscopic examination of stool reveals large, golden, bile-stained eggs with an operculum on top
- Adult worms can rarely be found in feces or specimens collected at surgery

Treatment, Prevention, and Control

- Drug of choice: praziquantel; alternative is niclosamide
- Education regarding safe consumption of infective aquatic vegetation, proper sanitation, and control of human feces reduces incidence of disease
- Snail population may be eliminated with molluscacides
- Control of reservoir hosts reduces worm transmission

Schistosomes and Schistosomiasis

Trigger Words

Snails, bladder cancer, cirrhosis, clay-pipestem fibrosis, Katayama syndrome, swimmer's itch

Biology, Virulence, and Disease

- Schistosomiasis (bilharziasis, snail fever): major parasitic infection of tropical areas, ≈200 million infections worldwide
- Three schistosomes (blood flukes) account for majority of human disease: *Schistosoma mansoni, Schistosoma haematobium, Schistosoma japonicum*
- Schistosomes differ from other flukes: male and female sexes (not hermaphroditic), oral and ventral suckers, incomplete digestive system
- Infective forms are skin-penetrating cercariae liberated from snails
- Disease results primarily from host immune response to eggs; clinical significance directly related to number and location of eggs
- Clinical manifestations of chronic infection: hepatosplenomegaly and cirrhosis, esophageal varices, bladder neck obstruction, squamous cell bladder carcinoma, transverse myelitis and other forms of CNS involvement

Epidemiology

- *S. mansoni:* most widely distributed; endemic in Africa, Saudi Arabia, Madagascar; has also become established in Western Hemisphere
- *S. japonicum* (Oriental blood fluke): found only in China, Japan, the Philippines, and on the island of Sulawesi in Indonesia

- *S. haematobium:* occurs predominantly throughout Nile Valley and many other parts of Africa
- Infection first acquired in early childhood; prevalence and intensity of infection peak at age 15-20 years; intensity declines with age
- Reservoir hosts include domestic animals, primates, rodents, marsupials
- Disease of economic progress: development of land irrigation projects in desert and tropical areas has resulted in dispersion of infected humans and snails to previously uninvolved areas

Diagnosis

- Demonstration of eggs in patient's stool or urine on microscopic examination
- Morphology of eggs specific for each species: *S. mansoni*—prominent lateral spine, *S. japonicum*—less prominent spine, *S. haematobium*—terminal spine
- Serologic tests have been developed to detect presence of specific antischistosomal antibodies; positive serology does not distinguish between current and past infection
- Ultrasound imaging useful in determining extent of disease

Treatment, Prevention, and Control

- Treatment of choice: praziquantel
- Improved sanitation, control of human fecal deposits, control of reservoir hosts are critical

Trematodes **(flukes)** are members of the Platyhelminthes and are generally flat, fleshy, leaf-shaped worms (Figure 76-1). In general, they are equipped with two muscular suckers: an oral type, which is the beginning of an incomplete digestive system, and a ventral sucker, which is simply an organ of attachment. The digestive system consists of lateral tubes that do not join to form an excretory opening. Most flukes are **hermaphroditic,** with both male and female reproductive organs in a single body. Schistosomes are the only exception; they have cylindrical bodies (like the nematodes), and separate male and female worms exist.

All flukes require intermediate hosts for the completion of their life cycles, and without exception, the first intermediate hosts are mollusks (snails and clams). In these hosts, an asexual reproductive cycle is a type of germ cell propagation. Some flukes require various second intermediate hosts before reaching the final host and developing into adult worms. This variation is discussed in the sections on individual species.

Fluke eggs are equipped with a "lid" at the top of the shell. Called an **operculum,** the lid opens to allow the larval worm to find its appropriate snail host. Schistosomes do not have an operculum; rather, the eggshell splits to liberate the larva. The medically significant trematodes are summarized in Table 76-1.

Fasciolopsis buski

A number of intestinal flukes are recognized, including *Fasciolopsis buski* (see Figure 76-1), *Heterophyes heterophyes, Metagonimus yokogawai, Echinostoma ilocanum,* and *Gastrodiscoides hominis. F. buski* is the largest, most prevalent, and most important intestinal fluke. The other flukes are similar to *F. buski* in many respects (epidemiology, clinical syndromes, treatment) and are not discussed further. It is important only that physicians recognize the relationship among these different flukes.

Physiology and Structure

This large intestinal fluke has a typical life cycle (Figure 76-2). Humans ingest the encysted larval stage **(metacercaria)** when they peel the husks from aquatic vegetation (e.g., water chestnuts) with the teeth. The metacercariae are scraped from the husk, swallowed, and develop into immature flukes in the duodenum. The fluke attaches to the mucosa of the small intestine with two muscular suckers, develops into an adult form, and undergoes self-fertilization. Egg production is initiated 3 months after the initial infection with the metacercariae. The operculated eggs pass in feces to water, where the operculum at the top of the eggshell pops open, liberating a free-swimming larval stage **(miracidium).** Glands at the pointed anterior end of the miracidium produce lytic substances that allow penetration of the soft tissues of snails. In the snail tissue, the miracidium develops through a series of stages by asexual germ cell propagation. The final stage **(cercaria)** in the snail is a free-swimming form that, after release from the snail, encysts on the aquatic vegetation, becoming the metacercariae, or infective stage.

Epidemiology

Because it depends on the distribution of its appropriate snail host, *F. buski* is found only in China, Vietnam, Thailand, parts of Indonesia, Malaysia, and India. Pigs, dogs, and rabbits serve as reservoir hosts in these endemic areas.

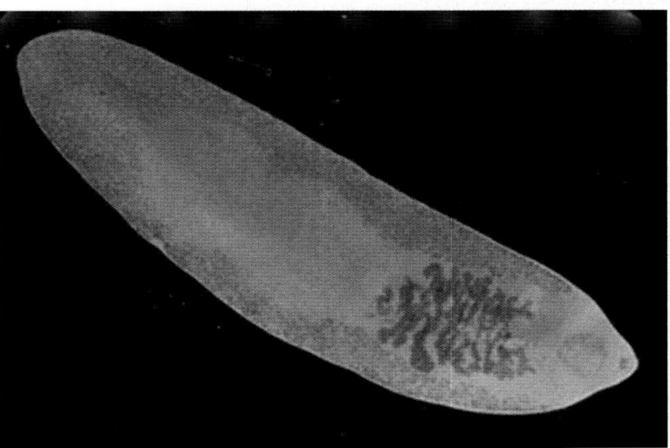

FIGURE 76-1 Adult *Fasciolopsis buski* (natural size). (From Peters W, Pasvol G: *Atlas of tropical medicine and parasitology,* ed 6, Philadelphia, 2007, Elsevier.)

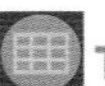 **Table 76-1 Medically Important Trematodes**

Trematode	Common Name	Intermediate Host	Biological Vector	Reservoir Host
Fasciolopsis buski	Giant intestinal fluke	Snail	Water plants (e.g., water chestnuts)	Pigs, dogs, rabbits, humans
Fasciola hepatica	Sheep liver fluke	Snail	Water plants (e.g., watercress)	Sheep, cattle, humans
Clonorchis (Opisthorchis) sinensis	Chinese liver fluke	Snail, freshwater fish	Uncooked fish	Dogs, cats, humans
Paragonimus westermani	Lung fluke	Snail, freshwater crabs, crayfish	Uncooked crabs, crayfish	Pigs, monkeys, humans
Schistosoma spp.	Blood fluke	Snail	None	Primates, rodents, domestic pets, livestock, humans

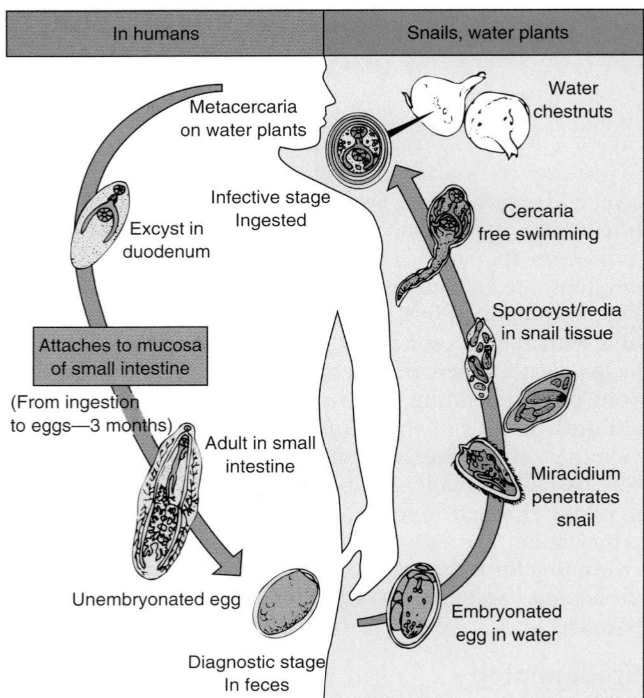

FIGURE 76-2 Life cycle of *Fasciolopsis buski* (giant intestinal fluke).

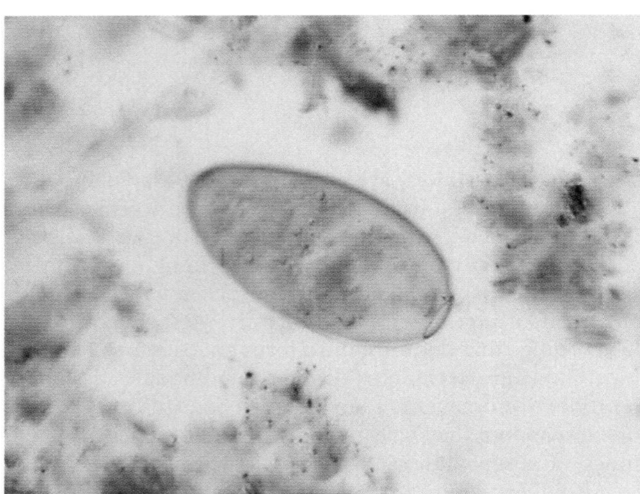

FIGURE 76-3 *Fasciolopsis buski* egg, 130 to 150 μm long × 65 to 90 μm wide, with a thin operculum at one end.

Clinical Syndromes

The symptomatology of *F. buski* infection relates directly to the worm burden in the small intestine. Attachment of the flukes in the small intestine can produce inflammation, ulceration, and hemorrhage. Severe infections produce abdominal discomfort similar to that of a duodenal ulcer, as well as diarrhea. Stools may be profuse, a malabsorption syndrome similar to giardiasis is common, and intestinal obstruction can occur. Marked eosinophilia is also present. Although death can occur, it is rare.

Laboratory Diagnosis

Stool examination reveals the large, golden, bile-stained eggs with an operculum on the top (Figure 76-3). The measurements and appearance of *F. buski* eggs are similar to those of the liver fluke *Fasciola hepatica,* and differentiation of the eggs of these species usually is not possible. Large (≈1.5 to 3.0 cm) adult flukes (see Figure 76-1) can rarely be found in feces or specimens collected at surgery.

Treatment, Prevention, and Control

The drug of choice is praziquantel, and the alternative is niclosamide. Education regarding safe consumption of infective aquatic vegetation (particularly water chestnuts), proper sanitation, and control of human feces reduces the incidence of disease. In addition, the snail population may be eliminated with molluscacides. When infection occurs, treatment should be initiated promptly to minimize its spread. Control of the reservoir hosts also reduces transmission of the worm.

• *Fasciola hepatica*

A number of liver flukes are recognized, including *F. hepatica, Clonorchis sinensis, Opisthorchis felineus,* and *Dicrocoelium dendriticum.* Only *F. hepatica* and *C. sinensis* are discussed in this chapter, although the eggs of other flukes are occasionally detected in the feces of patients in other geographic areas.

Physiology and Structure

Commonly called the **sheep liver fluke,** *F. hepatica* is a parasite of herbivores (particularly sheep and cattle) and humans. Its life cycle (Figure 76-4) is similar to that of *F. buski,* with human infection resulting from ingestion of watercress that harbors the encysted metacercariae. The larval flukes then

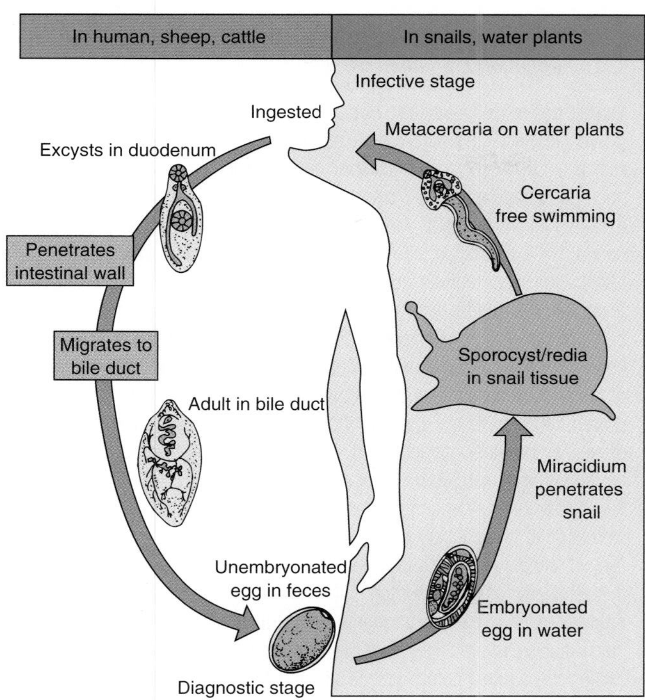

FIGURE 76-4 Life cycle of *Fasciola hepatica* (sheep liver fluke).

migrate through the duodenal wall and across the peritoneal cavity, penetrate the liver capsule, pass through the liver parenchyma, and enter the bile ducts to become adult worms. Approximately 3 to 4 months after the initial infection, the adult flukes start producing operculated eggs that are identical to those of *F. buski,* as seen in stool examination.

Epidemiology

Infections have been reported worldwide in sheep-raising areas, with the appropriate snail as an intermediate host. These areas include the former Soviet Union, Japan, Egypt, and many Latin American countries. Outbreaks are directly related to human consumption of contaminated watercress in areas where infected herbivores are present. Human infection is rare in the United States, but several well-documented cases have been reported in travelers from endemic areas.

Clinical Syndromes

Migration of the larval worm through the liver produces irritation of this tissue, tenderness, and hepatomegaly. Pain in the right upper quadrant, chills, fever, and marked eosinophilia are commonly observed. As the worms take up residence in the bile ducts, their mechanical irritation and toxic secretions produce hepatitis, hyperplasia of the epithelium, and biliary obstruction (Clinical Case 76-1). Some worms penetrate eroded areas in the ducts and invade the liver to produce necrotic foci referred to as **liver rot.** In severe infections, secondary bacterial infection can occur, and portal cirrhosis is common.

Laboratory Diagnosis

Stool examination reveals operculated eggs indistinguishable from the eggs of *F. buski* (see Figure 76-3). Exact identification is a therapeutic problem because treatment is not the same for both infections. Whereas *F. buski* responds favorably to praziquantel, *F. hepatica* does not. When exact identification is desired, examination of a sample of the patient's bile differentiates the species; if the eggs are present in bile, they are *F. hepatica,* not *F. buski,* which is limited to the small intestine. Eggs may appear in stool samples from people who have eaten infected sheep or cattle liver. The spurious nature of this finding can be confirmed by having the patient refrain from eating liver and then rechecking the stool.

Clinical Case 76-1 Fascioliasis

Echenique-Elizondo and colleagues (*JOP* 6:36–39, 2005) described a case of acute pancreatitis caused by the liver fluke *Fasciola hepatica.* The patient was a 31-year-old female who was admitted to the hospital because of a sudden onset of nausea and upper abdominal pain. She was otherwise healthy and gave a negative history of drug abuse, alcohol ingestion, gallstone disease, abdominal trauma, or surgery. On physical examination, she was markedly tender in the epigastric region and had hypoactive bowel sounds. Serum chemistries showed elevated pancreatic enzymes (amylase, lipase, pancreatic phospholipase A2, and elastase). Her white blood cell count was elevated, as were tests for alkaline phosphatase and bilirubin. Serum blood urea nitrogen, creatinine, lactate dehydrogenase, and calcium were normal. Abdominal ultrasonography and computed tomographic scan showed diffuse enlargement of the pancreas, and a cholangiogram demonstrated dilation and numerous filling defects in the common bile duct. An endoscopic sphincterotomy was performed, with extraction of numerous large flukes that were identified as *F. hepatica.* The patient was treated with a single oral dose of triclabendazole (10 mg/kg). Follow-up demonstrated normal blood chemistries and no evidence of disease 2 years postprocedure.

Treatment, Prevention, and Control

In contrast to *F. buski, F. hepatica* responds poorly to praziquantel. Treatment with bithionol or the benzimidazole compound triclabendazole has been effective. Preventive measures are similar to those for *F. buski* control; people who live in areas frequented by sheep and cattle should especially avoid ingestion of watercress and other uncooked aquatic vegetation.

• *Clonorchis sinensis*

Physiology and Structure

C. sinensis, also referred to as *Opisthorchis sinensis* in the older literature, is commonly called the **Chinese liver fluke.** Figure 76-5 illustrates its life cycle, which involves two intermediate hosts. This trematode differs from other fluke cycles in that the eggs are eaten by the snail, and then reproduction begins in the soft tissues of the snail. *C. sinensis* also requires a second intermediate host, freshwater fish, where the cercariae encyst and develop into infective metacercariae. When uncooked freshwater fish harboring metacercariae are eaten, flukes develop first in the duodenum and then migrate to the bile ducts, where they become adults. The adult fluke undergoes self-fertilization and begins producing eggs. *C. sinensis* may survive in the biliary tract for as long as 50 years, producing approximately 2000 eggs per day. These eggs pass with feces and are once again eaten by snails, reinitiating the cycle.

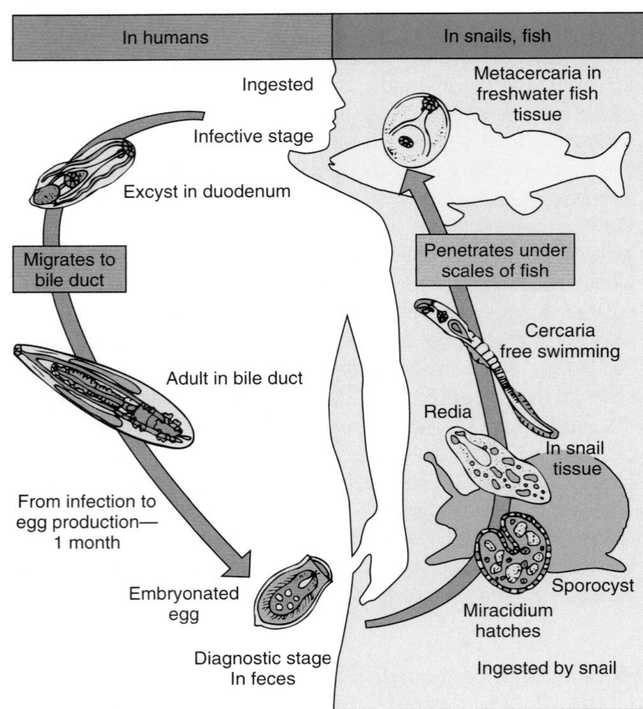

FIGURE 76-5 Life cycle of *Clonorchis sinensis* (Chinese liver fluke).

Clinical Case 76-2 Cholangitis Caused by *Clonorchis (Opisthorchis) sinensis*

Stunell and colleagues (*Eur Radiol* 16:2612–2614, 2006) described a 34-year-old Asian woman who presented to a local emergency department with a 2-day history of right upper quadrant abdominal pain, fever, and rigors. She had emigrated from Asia to Ireland 18 months earlier and gave a history of intermittent upper abdominal pain occurring over a 3-year period. On examination, she appeared acutely ill and was clammy to the touch. She was febrile, tachycardic, and had mild scleral icterus. Her abdomen was tender, with guarding in the right upper quadrant. Routine hematologic and biochemical studies revealed a marked leukocytosis and obstructive liver function tests. Contrast-enhanced computed tomography of the abdomen demonstrated evidence of multiple ovoid opacities within dilated intrahepatic bile ducts in the right lobe of the liver. The remainder of the liver parenchyma appeared normal. Upon stabilization of the patient, an endoscopic retrograde cholangiopancreatography (ERCP) was performed for biliary decompression. ERCP demonstrated intrahepatic and extrahepatic bile duct dilation, with multiple filling defects and strictures. A stool sample sent for analysis confirmed the presence of ova and adult flukes of *Clonorchis (Opisthorchis) sinensis.* The patient recovered with medical management (praziquantel) and had negative stool samples 30 days after treatment. This case, as well as Clinical Case 75-1, demonstrates the various complications of liver fluke infestation. Of note, praziquantel is the drug of choice for treating the Oriental liver fluke *(C. sinensis),* whereas triclabendazole is used to treat fascioliasis, thus emphasizing the importance of an epidemiologic history and identification of the fluke.

Epidemiology

C. sinensis is found in China, Japan, Korea, and Vietnam, where it is estimated to infect approximately 19 million people. It is one of the most frequent infections seen among Asian refugees, and it can be traced to the consumption of raw, pickled, smoked, or dried freshwater fish that harbor the viable metacercariae. Dogs, cats, and fish-eating mammals can also serve as reservoir hosts.

Clinical Syndromes (Clinical Case 76-2)

Infection in humans is usually mild and asymptomatic. Severe infections with many flukes in the bile ducts produces fever, diarrhea, epigastric pain, hepatomegaly, anorexia, and occasionally jaundice. Biliary obstruction may occur, and chronic infection can result in adenocarcinoma of the bile ducts. Invasion of the gallbladder may produce cholecystitis, cholelithiasis, and impaired liver function, as well as liver abscesses.

Laboratory Diagnosis

The diagnosis is made by recovering the distinctive eggs from stool. The eggs measure 27 to 35 μm × 12 to 19 μm and are characterized by a distinct operculum with prominent shoulders and a tiny knob at the posterior **(abopercular)** pole (Figure 76-6). In mild infections, repeated examinations of stool or duodenal aspirates may be necessary. In acute symptomatic infection, there are usually eosinophilia and an elevation of serum alkaline phosphatase levels. Radiographic imaging procedures may detect abnormalities of the biliary tract.

Treatment, Prevention, and Control

The drug of choice is praziquantel. Prevention of infection is accomplished by not eating uncooked fish and by implementing proper sanitation policies, including the disposal of human, dog, and cat feces in adequately protected sites so that they cannot contaminate water supplies where the intermediate snail and fish hosts reside.

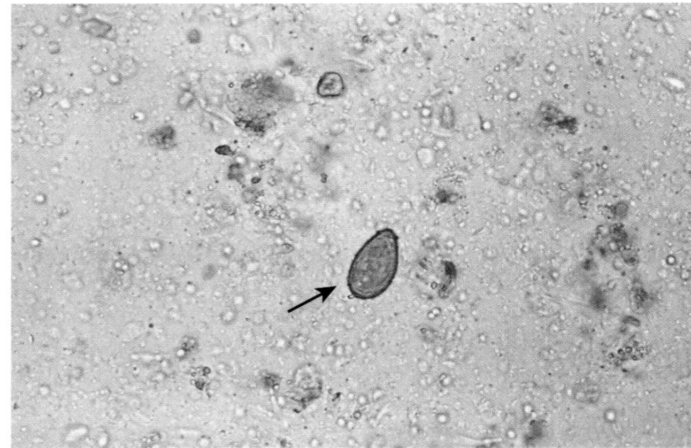

FIGURE 76-6 *Clonorchis sinensis* egg *(arrow)*. These ovoid eggs are small (27 to 35 μm long × 12 to 19 μm wide) and have a thick yellowish brown shell with a prominent operculum at one end and a small knob at the other. (From CDC Public Health Image Library.)

• *Paragonimus westermani*

Physiology and Structure

P. westermani, commonly called the **lung fluke,** is one of several species of *Paragonimus* that infect humans and many

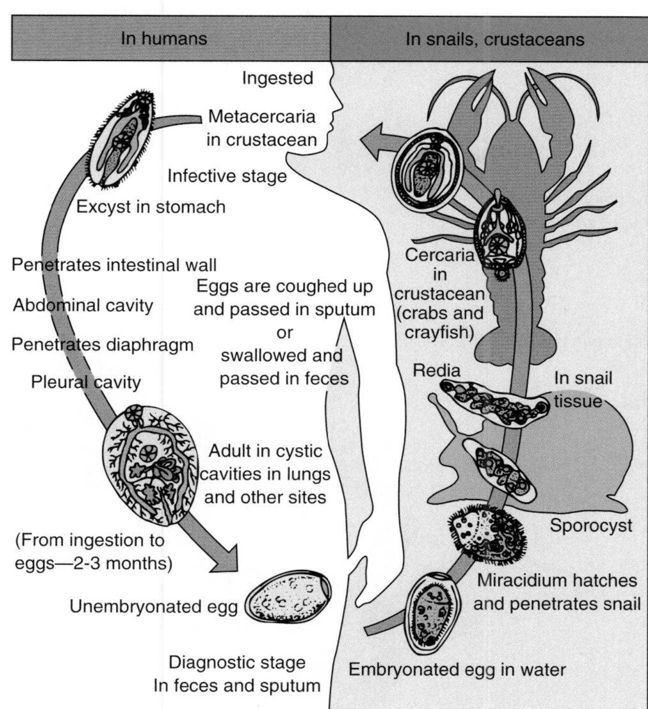

FIGURE 76-7 Life cycle of *Paragonimus westermani* (Oriental lung fluke).

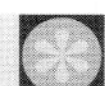

Clinical Case 76-3 Paragonimiasis

Singh and colleagues (*Indian J Med Microbiol* 23:131–134, 2005) described a case of pleuropulmonary paragonimiasis mimicking pulmonary tuberculosis. The patient was a 21-year-old man who was admitted to the hospital for progressive dyspnea, with a 1-month history of headache, fever, cough with scant hemoptysis, fatigue, pleuritic pain, anorexia, and weight loss. He had a history of antituberculous therapy for 6 months without improvement clinically. Two months before admission, after ingesting three raw crabs, he had a 3-day episode of watery diarrhea. On hospital admission, the patient was cachectic and afebrile. There were bilateral dullness to percussion and absent breath sounds in the lower two thirds of the chest. He was found to be anemic and had clubbing without lymphadenopathy, cyanosis, or jaundice. A chest radiograph showed bilateral pleural effusions that were also confirmed by computed tomography. Ultrasound-guided thoracentesis of the right lung yielded about 200 ml of yellowish fluid. The fluid was exudative and contained 2700 white blood cells/ml, 91% of which were eosinophils. Gram stain of the fluid was negative, as was culture for bacteria and fungi. Sputum smears revealed operculated yellowish eggs consistent with *Paragonimus westermani* infection. The patient was treated with a 3-day course of praziquantel and responded well. Of note, the right-sided plural effusion did not recur after the thoracentesis and praziquantel treatment. This case emphasizes the importance of making an etiologic diagnosis of a pleuropulmonary process to differentiate paragonimiasis from tuberculosis in regions where both are endemic infectious diseases.

other animals. Figure 76-7 shows a familiar fluke life cycle from egg to snail to infective metacercaria. The infective stage occurs in a second intermediate host: the muscles and gills of freshwater crabs and crayfish. In humans who ingest infected meat, the larval worm hatches in the stomach and follows an extensive migration through the intestinal wall to the abdominal cavity, then through the diaphragm, and finally to the pleural cavity. Adult worms reside in the lungs and produce eggs that are liberated from ruptured bronchioles and appear in sputum or, when swallowed, in feces.

Epidemiology

Paragonimiasis occurs in many countries in Asia, Africa, and Latin America. It can be seen in refugees from Southeast Asia. Its prevalence is directly related to consumption of uncooked freshwater crabs and crayfish. It is estimated that approximately 3 million people are infected with this lung fluke. As many as 1% of all Indochinese immigrants to the United States are infected with *P. westermani.* A wide variety of shore-feeding animals (e.g., wild boars, pigs, monkeys) serve as reservoir hosts, and some human infections result from ingestion of meat containing migrating larval worms from these reservoir hosts. Human infections endemic to the United States are usually caused by a related species, *P. kellicotti,* which is found in crabs and crayfish in eastern and midwestern waters.

Clinical Syndromes

The clinical manifestations of paragonimiasis may result from larvae migrating through tissues or from adults established in the lungs or other ectopic sites. The onset of disease coincides with larval migration and is associated with fever, chills, and high eosinophilia. The adult flukes in the lungs first produce an inflammatory reaction that results in fever, cough, and increased sputum. As the destruction of lung tissue progresses, cavitation occurs around the worms, sputum becomes blood tinged and dark with eggs (so-called rusty sputum), and patients experience severe chest pain. The resulting cavity may become secondarily infected with bacteria. Dyspnea, chronic bronchitis, bronchiectasis, and pleural effusion may be seen (Clinical Case 76-3). Chronic infections lead to fibrosis in the lung tissue. The location of larvae, adults, and eggs in ectopic sites may produce severe clinical symptoms depending on the site involved. Migration of larval worms may result in invasion of the spinal cord and brain, producing severe neurologic disease (visual problems, motor weakness, convulsive seizures) referred to as **cerebral paragonimiasis.** Migration and infection may also occur in subcutaneous sites, the abdominal cavity, and the liver.

Laboratory Diagnosis

Examination of sputum and feces reveals golden brown, operculated eggs (Figure 76-8). Pleural effusions, when present, should be examined for eggs. Chest radiographs often show infiltrates, nodular cysts, and pleural effusion. Marked eosinophilia is common. Serologic procedures are available through reference laboratories and can be helpful, particularly in cases with extrapulmonary (e.g., central nervous system) involvement.

Treatment, Prevention, and Control

The drug of choice is triclabendazole; praziquantel is an alternative. Education regarding consumption of uncooked freshwater crabs and crayfish found in endemic areas is critical. Pickling and wine soaking of crabs and crayfish do not kill the infective metacercarial stage. Proper sanitation

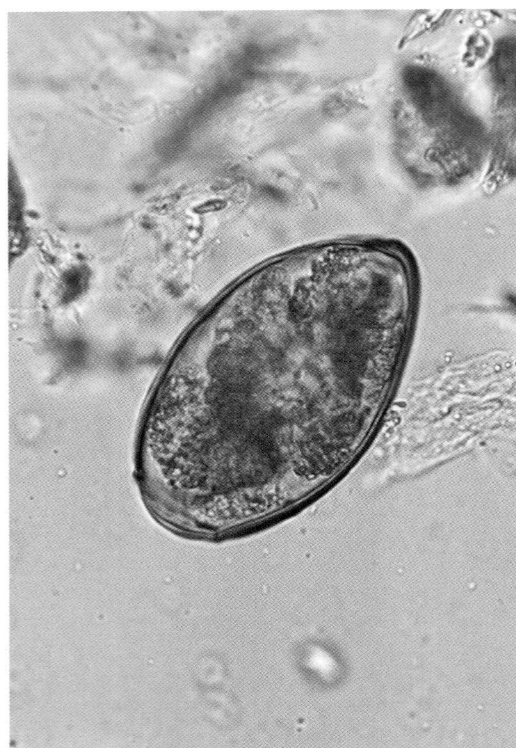

FIGURE 76-8 *Paragonimus westermani* egg. These large ovoid eggs (80 to 120 μm long × 45 to 70 μm wide) have a thick yellowish brown shell and a distinct operculum. (From CDC Public Health Image Library.)

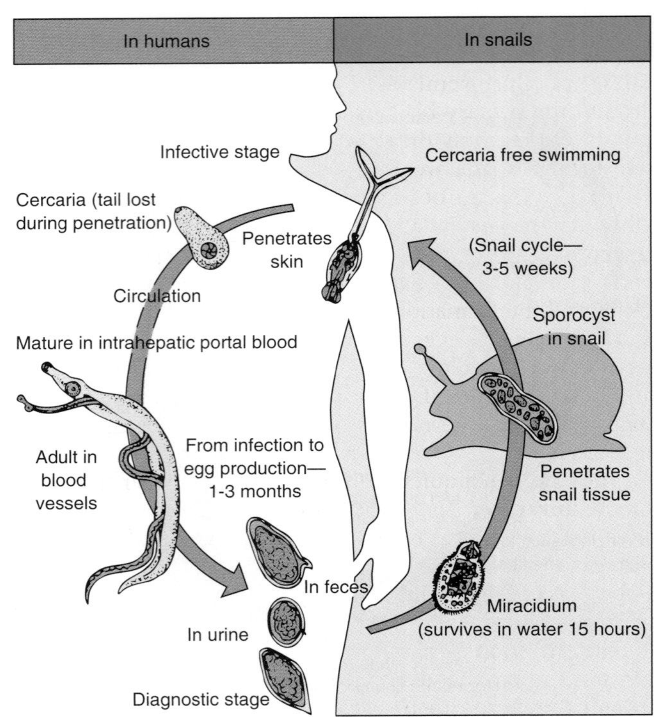

FIGURE 76-9 Life cycle of schistosomes.

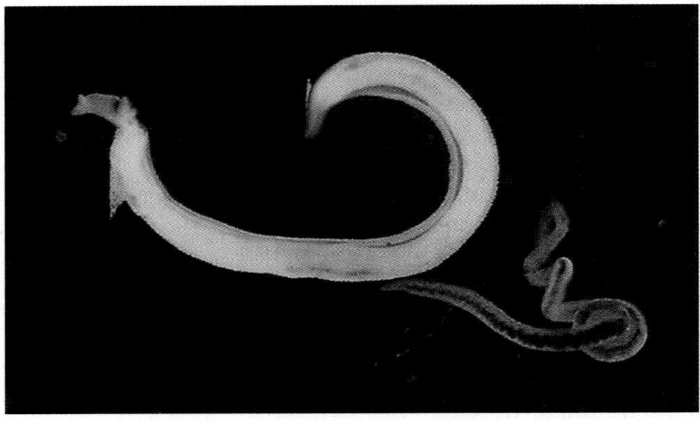

FIGURE 76-10 Living male and female *Schistosoma mansoni*. The slender female *(right)* is normally seen within the gynecophoral groove of the male *(left)* (×14). (From Peters W, Pasvol G: *Atlas of tropical medicine and parasitology,* ed 6, Philadelphia, 2007, Elsevier; courtesy Professor RE Howells.)

and control of the disposal of human feces are essential to control efforts.

• Schistosomes

Schistosomiasis is a major parasitic infection of tropical areas, with some 200 million infections worldwide. The three schistosomes most frequently associated with human disease are *Schistosoma mansoni, Schistosoma japonicum,* and *Schistosoma haematobium.* They collectively produce the disease called **schistosomiasis,** also known as **bilharziasis** or **snail fever.** As discussed earlier, the schistosomes differ from other flukes: they are male and female rather than hermaphroditic, and their eggs do not have an operculum. They also are obligate intravascular parasites and are not found in cavities, ducts, and other tissues. The infective forms are skin-penetrating **cercariae** liberated from snails, and these differ from other flukes in that they are not eaten on vegetation, in fish, or in crustaceans.

Figure 76-9 illustrates the life cycle of the different schistosomes. Infection is initiated by ciliated, free-swimming, freshwater cercariae that penetrate intact skin, enter the circulation, and develop in the intrahepatic portal circulation (*S. mansoni* and *S. japonicum*) or in the vesical, prostatic, rectal, and uterine plexuses and veins *(S. haematobium).* The female has a long, slender, cylindrical body, whereas the shorter male, which appears cylindrical, is actually flat (Figure 76-10). The cylindrical appearance derives from folding the sides of the body to produce a groove, the gynecophoral canal, in which the female resides for fertilization. Both sexes have oral and ventral suckers and an incomplete digestive system, which is typical of a fluke.

As the worms develop in the portal circulation, they elaborate a remarkable defense against host resistance. They coat themselves with substances that the host recognizes as itself; consequently, there is little host response directed against their presence in blood vessels. This protective mechanism accounts for chronic infections that may last 20 to 30 years or longer.

After developing in the portal vein, the male and female adult worms pair up and migrate to their final locations, where fertilization and egg production begin. *S. mansoni* and *S. japonicum* are found in mesenteric veins and produce intestinal schistosomiasis; *S. haematobium* occurs in veins around the urinary bladder and causes vesicular schistosomiasis. On reaching the submucosal venules of their respective locations, the worms initiate oviposition, which may continue at the rate of 300 to 3000 eggs daily for 4 to 35 years. Although the host inflammatory response to the adult worms is minimal, the eggs elicit an intense inflammatory reaction with mononuclear and polymorphonuclear cellular infiltrates and the formation of microabscesses. In addition, the larvae inside the eggs produce enzymes that aid in tissue destruction and allow the eggs to pass through the mucosa and into the lumen of the bowel and bladder, where they are passed to the external environment in feces and urine, respectively.

The eggs hatch quickly on reaching fresh water to release motile **miracidia.** The miracidia then invade the appropriate snail host, where they develop into thousands of infectious cercariae. The free-swimming cercariae are released into the water, where they are immediately infectious for humans and other mammals.

The infection is similar in all three species of human schistosomes in that disease results primarily from the host's immune response to the eggs. The very earliest signs and symptoms are due to the penetration of the cercariae through the skin. Immediate and delayed hypersensitivity to parasite antigens results in an intensely pruritic papular skin rash.

The onset of oviposition results in a symptom complex known as **Katayama syndrome,** which is marked by fever, chills, cough, urticaria, arthralgias, lymphadenopathy, splenomegaly, and abdominal pain. This syndrome is typically seen 1 to 2 months after primary exposure and may persist for 3 months or more. It is thought to result from the massive release of parasite antigens, with subsequent immune complex formation. Associated laboratory abnormalities include leukocytosis, eosinophilia, and polyclonal gammopathy.

The more chronic and significant phase of schistosomiasis is due to the presence of eggs in various tissues and the resulting formation of granulomas and fibrosis. The retained eggs induce extensive inflammation and scarring, the clinical significance of which is directly related to the location and number of eggs.

Because of differences in some aspects of disease and epidemiology, these worms are discussed as separate species.

Schistosoma mansoni

Physiology and Structure

S. mansoni usually resides in the small branches of the inferior mesenteric vein near the lower colon. The species of *Schistosoma* can be differentiated by their characteristic egg morphology (Figures 76-11 to 76-13). The eggs of *S. mansoni* are oval, possess a **sharp lateral spine,** and measure 115 to 175 μm × 45 to 70 μm (see Figure 76-11).

Epidemiology

The geographic distribution of the various species of *Schistosoma* depends on the availability of a suitable snail host. *S. mansoni* is the most widespread of the schistosomes and is endemic in Africa, Saudi Arabia, and Madagascar. It has also become well established in the Western Hemisphere, particularly in Brazil, Suriname, Venezuela, parts of the West Indies, and Puerto Rico. Cases originating in these areas may present in the United States. In all these areas, there are also reservoir hosts, specifically primates, marsupials, and rodents. Schistosomiasis may be considered a disease of economic progress; the development of massive land irrigation projects in desert and tropical areas has resulted in dispersion of infected humans and snails to previously uninvolved areas.

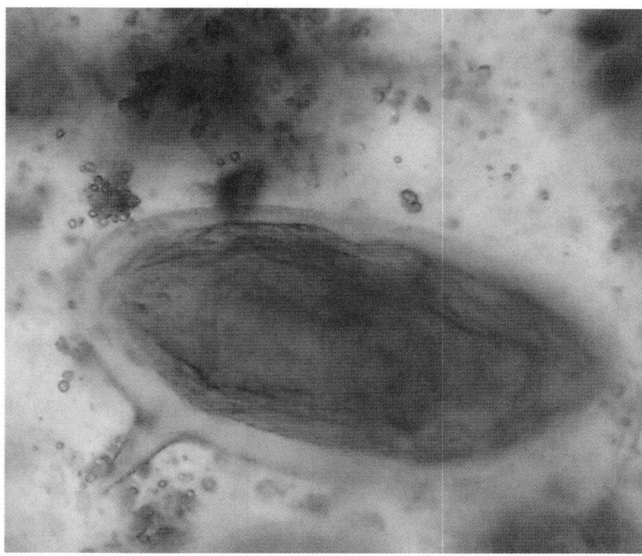

FIGURE 76-11 *Schistosoma mansoni* egg. These eggs are 115 to 175 μm long × 45 to 70 μm wide, contain a miracidium, and are enclosed in a thin shell with a prominent lateral spine.

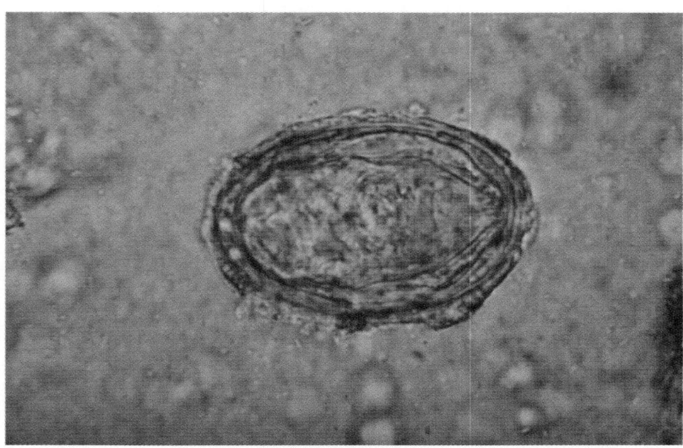

FIGURE 76-12 *Schistosoma japonicum* egg. These eggs are smaller than those of *Schistosoma mansoni* (70 to 100 μm long × 55 to 65 μm wide) and have a spine that is inconspicuous. (From CDC Public Health Image Library.)

Clinical Syndromes

Cercarial penetration of intact skin may be seen as dermatitis with allergic reactions, pruritus, and edema. Migrating worms in the lungs may produce cough; as they reach the liver, hepatitis may appear.

Infections with *S. mansoni* may produce hepatic and intestinal abnormalities. As the flukes take up residence in the mesenteric vessels and egg laying begins, fever, malaise,

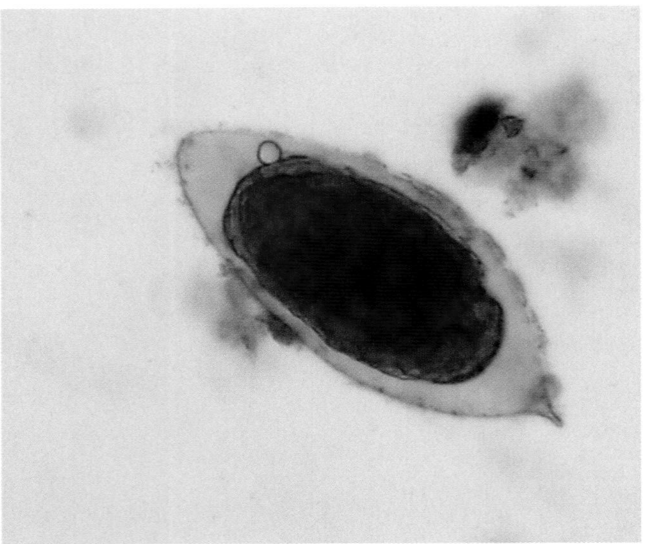

FIGURE 76-13 *Schistosoma haematobium* egg. These eggs are similar in size to those of *Schistosoma mansoni* but can be differentiated by the presence of a terminal rather than lateral spine.

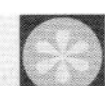

Clinical Case 76-4 Schistosomiasis

Ferrari (*Medicine [Baltimore]* 78:176–190, 1999) described a case of neuroschistosomiasis caused by *Schistosoma mansoni* in an 18-year-old Brazilian man. The patient was admitted to the hospital because of the recent onset of paraplegia. He was in good health until 33 days before admission, when he noted the onset of progressive low back pain with radiation to the lower limbs. During this period, he was evaluated three times in another institution, where radiographic films of the lower thoracic, lumbar, and sacral spine were normal. He received antiinflammatory agents, with only transient relief in his symptoms. Four weeks after the pain began, the disease progressed acutely with sexual impotence, fecal and urinary retention, and paraparesis progressing to paraplegia. At this time, the pain disappeared, replaced by a marked impairment of sensation in the lower limbs. On admission to the hospital, he gave a history of exposure to schistosomal infection. Neurologic examination revealed flaccid paraplegia, marked sensory loss, and absence of superficial and deep reflexes at and below the level T11. The cerebrospinal fluid (CSF) contained 84 white blood cells/ml (98% lymphocytes, 2% eosinophils) and 1 red blood cell, 82 mg/dl total protein, and 61 mg/dl glucose. Myelography, computed tomography–myelography, and magnetic resonance imaging showed a slight widening of the conus. The diagnosis of neuroschistosomiasis was confirmed by the demonstration of viable and dead eggs of *S. mansoni* on rectal mucosal biopsy. The concentration of CSF immunoglobulin (Ig)G against soluble egg antigen of *S. mansoni* quantitated by enzyme-linked immunosorbent assay was 1.53 μg/ml. He was treated with prednisone and praziquantel. Despite therapy, his condition remained unaltered at follow-up 7 months later. *S. mansoni* is the most frequently reported cause of schistosomal myeloradiculopathy (SMR) worldwide. SMR is among the most severe forms of schistosomiasis, and prognosis depends largely on early diagnosis and treatment.

abdominal pain, and tenderness of the liver may be observed. Deposition of eggs in the bowel mucosa results in inflammation and thickening of the bowel wall, with associated abdominal pain, diarrhea, and blood in the stool. Eggs may be carried by the portal vein to the liver, where inflammation can lead to periportal fibrosis and eventually to portal hypertension and its associated manifestations.

Chronic infection with *S. mansoni* produces a dramatic hepatosplenomegaly with large accumulations of ascitic fluid in the peritoneal cavity. On gross examination, the liver is studded with white granulomas (pseudotubercles). Although *S. mansoni* eggs are primarily deposited in the intestine, eggs may appear in the spinal cord, lungs, and other sites. A similar fibrotic process occurs at each site. Severe neurologic problems may follow when eggs are deposited in the spinal cord and brain (Clinical Case 76-4). In fatal schistosomiasis caused by *S. mansoni,* fibrous tissue, reacting to the eggs in the liver, surrounds the portal vein in a thick, grossly visible layer **("clay pipestem fibrosis").**

Laboratory Diagnosis

The diagnosis of schistosomiasis is usually established by demonstration of characteristic eggs in feces. Stool examination reveals the large golden eggs with a sharp lateral spine (see Figure 76-11). Concentration techniques may be necessary in light infections. Using rectal biopsy, the clinician can see the egg tracks laid by the worms in rectal vessels. Quantitation of egg output in stool is useful in estimating the severity of infection and in following the response to therapy. Serologic tests are also available but are largely of epidemiologic interest only. Development of newer tests using stage-specific antigens may allow the distinction of active from inactive disease and thus have greater clinical application.

Treatment, Prevention, and Control

The drug of choice is praziquantel, and the alternative is oxamniquine. Anthelmintic therapy may terminate oviposition but does not affect lesions caused by eggs already deposited in tissues. **Schistosomal dermatitis** and Katayama syndrome may be treated with administration of antihistamines and corticosteroids. Education regarding the life cycles of these worms and molluscacide control of snails are essential. Improved sanitation and control of human fecal deposits are critical. Unfortunately, treatment with praziquantel provides low cure rates in some areas, raising the specter of emerging resistance to this important therapeutic agent. The addition of artemether, an antimalarial, in combination with praziquantel has shown improved activity against *S. mansoni* and *S. haematobium.* In contrast to praziquantel, artemether acts against juvenile schistosomes in the host and may be used as a chemoprophylactic agent. Vaccine trials are in progress, but the ideal target antigen has not been identified.

Schistosoma japonicum

Physiology and Structure

S. japonicum resides in branches of the superior mesenteric vein around the small intestine and in the inferior mesenteric vessels. *S. japonicum* eggs (see Figure 76-12) are smaller, almost spherical, and possess a **tiny spine.** These eggs are produced in greater numbers than those of *S. mansoni* and *S. haematobium.* Because of the size, shape, and numbers of these eggs, they are carried to more sites in the body (liver, lungs, brain), and infection with a few *S. japonicum* adults can be more severe than infections involving similar numbers of *S. mansoni* or *S. haematobium.*

Epidemiology

This **Oriental blood fluke** is found only in China, Japan, the Philippines, and on the island of Sulawesi, Indonesia. Epidemiologic problems correlate directly with a broad range of reservoir hosts, many of which are domestic (cats, dogs, cattle, horses, pigs).

Clinical Syndromes

The initial stages of infection with *S. japonicum* are similar to those of *S. mansoni,* with dermatitis, allergic reactions, fever, and malaise, followed by abdominal discomfort and diarrhea. Katayama syndrome associated with the onset of oviposition is observed more commonly with *S. japonicum* than with *S. mansoni.* In chronic *S. japonicum* infection, hepatosplenic disease, portal hypertension, bleeding esophageal varices, and accumulation of ascitic fluid are commonly seen. Granulomas that appear as pseudotubercles in and on the liver are common, along with the clay pipestem fibrosis as described for *S. mansoni.*

S. japonicum frequently involves cerebral structures when eggs reach the brain and granulomas develop around them. Neurologic manifestations include lethargy, speech impairment, visual defects, and seizures.

Laboratory Diagnosis

Stool examination demonstrates the small golden eggs with tiny spines; usually, rectal biopsy is similarly revealing. Serologic tests are available.

Treatment, Prevention, and Control

The drug of choice is praziquantel. Prevention and control may be achieved by measures similar to those for *S. mansoni,* especially education of populations in endemic areas regarding proper water purification, sanitation, and control of human fecal deposits. Control of *S. japonicum* must also involve the broad range of reservoir hosts and consider the fact that people work in rice paddies and on irrigation projects where infected snails are present. Mass treatment may offer help, and a vaccine may be developed someday.

Schistosoma haematobium

Physiology and Structure

After development in the liver, these blood flukes migrate to the vesical, prostatic, and uterine plexuses of the venous circulation, occasionally the portal bloodstream, and only rarely other venules.

Large eggs with a **sharp terminal spine** (see Figure 76-13) are deposited in the wall of the bladder and occasionally in the uterine and prostatic tissues. Those deposited in the bladder wall can break free and are found in urine.

Epidemiology

S. haematobium occurs throughout the Nile Valley and in many other parts of Africa, including islands off the eastern coast. It also appears in Asia Minor, Cyprus, southern Portugal, and India. Reservoir hosts include monkeys, baboons, and chimpanzees.

Clinical Syndromes

Early stages of infection with *S. haematobium* are similar to those of infections involving *S. mansoni* and *S. japonicum,* with dermatitis, allergic reactions, fever, and malaise. Unlike the other two schistosomes, *S. haematobium* produces hematuria, dysuria, and urinary frequency as early symptoms. Associated with hematuria, bacteriuria is frequently a chronic condition. Egg deposition in the walls of the bladder may eventually result in scarring, with loss of bladder capacity and development of obstructive uropathy.

Patients with *S. haematobium* infections involving many flukes frequently demonstrate squamous cell carcinoma of the bladder. It is commonly stated that the leading cause of cancer of the bladder in Egypt and other parts of Africa is *S. haematobium.* The granulomas and pseudotubercles seen in the bladder may also be present in the lungs. Fibrosis of the pulmonary bed caused by egg deposition leads to dyspnea, cough, and hemoptysis.

Laboratory Diagnosis

Examination of urine specimens reveals the large, **terminally spined** eggs. Occasionally, bladder biopsy is helpful in establishing the diagnosis. *S. haematobium* eggs may appear in stool if worms have migrated to mesenteric vessels. Serologic tests are also available.

Treatment, Prevention, and Control

The drug of choice is praziquantel. At present, education, possible mass treatment, and development of a vaccine are the best approaches to control of *S. haematobium* disease. The basic problems of irrigation projects (e.g., dam building), migratory human populations, and multiple reservoir hosts make prevention and control extremely difficult. A recent report of the safety and efficacy of mefloquine-artesunate in the treatment of schistosomiasis caused by *S. hematobium* is of great interest, given the potential for the development of resistance to praziquantel among the schistosomes.

Cercarial Dermatitis

Several nonhuman schistosomes have cercariae that penetrate human skin, producing a severe dermatitis **("swimmer's itch"),** but these schistosomes cannot develop into adult worms. The natural hosts are birds and other shore-feeding animals from freshwater lakes throughout the world and a few marine beaches. The intense pruritus and urticaria from this skin penetration may lead to secondary bacterial infection from scratching the sites of infection.

Treatment consists of oral trimeprazine and topical applications of palliative agents. When indicated, sedatives may be given. Control is difficult because of bird migration and the transfer of live snails from lake to lake. Molluscacides such as copper sulfate have produced some reduction in snail populations. Immediate drying of the skin when people leave such waters offers some protection.

Bibliography

Connor DH, Schwartz DA: *Pathology of infectious diseases*, Stamford, Conn, 1997, Appleton & Lange.

Garcia LS: *Diagnostic medical parasitology*, ed 5, Washington, DC, 2006, American Society for Microbiology Press.

John DT, Petri WA Jr: *Markell and Voge's medical parasitology*, ed 9, Philadelphia, 2006, Elsevier.

Jones MK, et al: Trematodes. In Versalovic J, et al, editors: *Manual of clinical microbiology*, ed 10, Washington, DC, 2011, American Society for Microbiology Press.

Keiser J, Utzinger J: Food-borne trematodiases, *Clin Microbiol Rev* 22:466–483, 2009.

Keiser J, N'Guessan NA, Adoubryn KD, et al: Efficacy and safety of mefloquine, artesunate, mefloquine-artesunate, and praziquantel against *Schistosoma haematobium:* randomized, exploratory open-label trial, *Clin Infect Dis* 50:1205–1213, 2010.

McManus DP, Loukas A: Current status of vaccines for schistosomiasis, *Clin Microbiol Rev* 21:225–242, 2008.

Meltzer E, Artom G, Marva E, et al: Schistosomiasis among travelers: new aspects of an old disease, *Emerg Infect Dis* 12:1696–1700, 2006.

Strickland GT: *Hunter's tropical medicine and emerging infectious diseases*, Philadelphia, 2000, WB Saunders.

CHAPTER

77

CESTODES

A 30-year-old Hispanic man entered the emergency department after a focal neurologic seizure. He had recently emigrated from Mexico and was in his usual state of good health before the seizure. Neurologic examination revealed no persistent focal findings. A computed tomography (CT) scan of the head revealed multiple small cystic lesions in both cerebral hemispheres. Punctate calcification was noted in several of the lesions. A lumbar puncture revealed a glucose level of 65 mg/dl (normal) and a protein level of 38 mg/dl (normal) in cerebrospinal fluid. The white blood cell count was 20/ml (abnormal) with a differential of 5% neutrophils, 90% lymphocytes, and 5% monocytes. A purified protein derivative skin test was negative with positive controls. Serologic test for human immunodeficiency virus was negative.

1. What was the differential diagnosis of this patient's neurologic process?
2. Which parasite or parasites may have caused this condition?
3. What diagnostic tests were available for this infection?
4. What were the therapeutic options for this patient?
5. How do people become infected with this parasite?
6. What tissue sites (besides the central nervous system) may be involved? How would these additional foci of infection be documented?

Answers to these questions are available on StudentConsult.com.

• SUMMARIES CLINICALLY SIGNIFICANT ORGANISMS

Taenia solium

Trigger Words

Tapeworm, cysticercosis, proglottid, pig tapeworm, scolex, oncosphere

Biology, Virulence, and Disease

- *Taenia solium* (pork tapeworm): cestode; flat, segmented, ribbon-like body (strobila); head (scolex) equipped with four muscular cup-shaped suckers and a crown of hooklets that serve as organs of attachment
- Complex life cycle involving intermediate hosts; humans may serve as a form of intermediate host (cysticercosis) that harbors larval stages at extraintestinal sites
- Adult *T. solium* in intestine seldom causes abdominal discomfort, chronic indigestion, diarrhea
- Cysticercosis: infection of humans with larval stage of *T. solium* (cysticercus or bladder worm), which normally infects pigs

Epidemiology

- *T. solium* infection directly correlated with eating insufficiently cooked pork
- Cysticercosis found in areas where *T. solium* is prevalent; directly correlated with human fecal contamination
- *T. solium* infection and cysticercosis prevalent in Latin American countries, Africa, Asia, and Slavic countries; seen infrequently in United States

Diagnosis

- Stool examination may reveal eggs and proglottids
- Cysticercosis usually diagnosed by detection of calcified cysticerci in soft tissue roentgenograms, surgical removal of subcutaneous nodules, and visualization of cysts in the eye
- Central nervous system lesions may be detected by imaging studies
- Serologic studies may be useful in diagnosis of cysticercosis

Treatment, Prevention, and Control

- Drug of choice for *T. solium* infection: niclosamide; praziquantel, paromomycin, quinacrine effective alternatives
- Prevention of pork tapeworm infection: cook until interior of meat is gray; freeze at −20° C for at least 12 hours
- Drug of choice for cysticercosis: praziquantel or albendazole
- Surgical removal of cerebral and ocular cysts may be necessary
- Prevention and control: treatment of human cases harboring adult *T. solium,* controlled disposal of human feces

Diphyllobothrium latum

Trigger Words

Fish tapeworm, vitamin B_{12} deficiency, gefilte fish, copepod

Biology, Virulence, and Disease

- *Diphyllobothrium latum* (fish tapeworm): one of largest tapeworms infecting humans (20 to 30 feet long)
- Life cycle of *D. latum* is complex; two intermediate hosts: freshwater crustaceans, freshwater fish
- Humans infected when they eat raw or undercooked fish containing larval forms
- *D. latum* establishes infection in small bowel; may reach a length of 20 to 30 feet and produce more than 1 million eggs per day
- Most *D. latum* infections asymptomatic; symptoms include epigastric pain, abdominal cramping, nausea, weight loss

Epidemiology

- *D. latum* infection occurs worldwide, most prevalently in cool lake regions where raw or pickled fish is popular
- Insufficient cooking over campfires and tasting and seasoning "gefilte fish" account for many infections
- Dumping raw sewage into freshwater lakes contributes to propagation of this tapeworm

Diagnosis

- Microscopic examination of stool reveals bile-stained operculated egg with knob at bottom of shell
- Typical proglottids may also be detected

Treatment, Prevention, and Control

- Drug of choice is niclosamide; praziquantel and paromomycin acceptable alternatives
- Vitamin B_{12} supplementation may be necessary in people with evidence of clinical B_{12} deficiency
- Prevalence of this infection reduced by avoiding ingestion of raw or undercooked fish, controlling disposal of human waste, promptly treating infections

The bodies of cestodes, **tapeworms,** are flat and ribbon like (Figure 77-1), and the heads are equipped with organs of attachment. The head, or **scolex,** of the worm usually has four muscular cup-shaped suckers and a crown of hooklets (Figure 77-2). An exception is *Diphyllobothrium latum,* the fish tapeworm, whose scolex is equipped with a pair of long, lateral, muscular grooves and lacks hooklets.

The individual segments of tapeworms are called **proglottids** (see Figure 77-2), and the chain of proglottids is called a **strobila** (see Figure 77-1). As new proglottids develop, existing ones mature as they become more distal. The more distal proglottids are gravid, almost completely occupied by a uterus full of eggs, which are passed with the stools of the carrier, either inside completed proglottids or free after proglottid breakage. Differentiation of the various adult cestodes may be accomplished by examination of the structure of shed proglottids (length, width, number of uterine branches) or (more rarely) of the scolex (number and placement of suckers, presence or absence of hooklets).

All tapeworms are hermaphroditic, with male and female reproductive organs present in each mature proglottid. The eggs of most tapeworms are nonoperculated and contain a six-hooked **hexacanth embryo;** the one exception, *D. latum,* has an unembryonated operculated egg similar to fluke eggs. Tapeworms have no digestive system, and food is absorbed from the host intestine through the soft body wall of the worm. Most tapeworms found in the human intestine have complex life cycles involving intermediate hosts, and in some instances (cysticercosis, echinococcosis, sparganosis), humans serve as a form of intermediate host that harbors larval stages. The presence of extraintestinal larvae is at times more serious than that of adult worms in the intestine. The most common cestodes of medical importance are listed in Table 77-1.

• *Taenia solium*

Physiology and Structure

The larval stage, or **cysticercus** ("bladder worm"), of *Taenia* species consists of a scolex, which is invaginated into a fluid-filled bladder. Larval cysts develop in the tissues of the intermediate host, are 4 to 6 mm long × 7 to 11 mm wide, and have a pearl-like appearance in the tissues. After a person ingests pork muscle containing a larval worm, attachment of the scolex with its four muscular suckers and crown of hooklets (see Figure 77-2) initiates infection in the small intestine (Figure 77-3). The worm then produces proglottids until a strobila of proglottids is developed, which may be several meters in length. The sexually mature proglottids contain eggs, and as these proglottids leave the host in feces, they can contaminate water and vegetation ingested by swine. The gravid proglottids have a similar length and width (1 cm × 1 cm) and contain few (<12) lateral uterine branches (see Figure 77-2). The eggs in swine become a six-hooked larval form called an **oncosphere** that penetrates the pig's intestinal wall, migrates in the circulation to the tissues, and becomes a cysticercus to complete the cycle.

Epidemiology

T. solium infection is directly correlated with eating insufficiently cooked pork and is prevalent in Africa, India, Southeast Asia, China, Mexico, and Latin American and Slavic countries. It is seen infrequently in the United States.

Clinical Syndromes

Adult *T. solium* in the intestine seldom causes appreciable symptoms. The intestine may be irritated at sites of attachment, and abdominal discomfort, chronic indigestion, and diarrhea may occur. Most patients become aware of the infection only when they see proglottids or a strobila of proglottids in their feces.

Laboratory Diagnosis

Stool examination may reveal proglottids and eggs, and treatment may produce the entire worm for identification. The eggs are spherical, 30 to 40 μm in diameter, and possess a thick, radially striated shell containing a six-hooked hexacanth embryo (Figure 77-4). The eggs are identical to those of *Taenia saginata* **(beef tapeworm),** so eggs alone are not sufficient for species identification. Critical examination of the proglottids reveals their internal structure, which is important for the differentiation of *T. solium* and *T. saginata.* Gravid proglottids of *T. solium* are smaller than those of *T. saginata* and contain only 7 to 12 lateral uterine branches, compared with 15 to 30 for the beef tapeworm (see Figure 77-2).

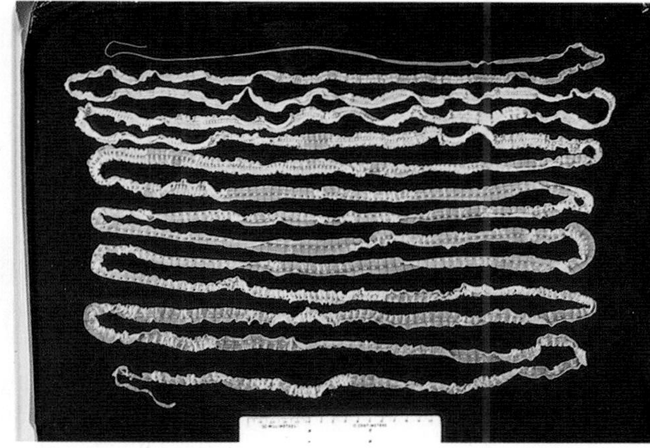

FIGURE 77-1 Intact adult *Diphyllobothrium latum.* The chain of proglottids (strobila) may reach a length of 10 meters. (From Peters W, Pasvol G: *Atlas of tropical medicine and parasitology,* ed 6, Philadelphia, 2007, Elsevier.)

Treatment, Prevention, and Control

The drug of choice is niclosamide. Praziquantel, paromomycin, or quinacrine is an effective alternative. Prevention of **pork tapeworm** infections requires that pork be either cooked until the interior of the meat is gray or frozen at −20° C for at least 12 hours. Sanitation is critical; every effort must be made to keep human feces containing *T. solium* eggs out of water and vegetation ingested by pigs.

• Cysticercosis

Physiology and Structure

Cysticercosis involves infection of people with the larval stage of *T. solium,* the cysticercus, which normally infects pigs (Figure 77-5). Human ingestion of water or vegetation contaminated with *T. solium* eggs from human feces initiates the infection. Autoinfection may occur when eggs from a person infected with the adult worm are transferred from the perianal area to the mouth on contaminated fingers. Once ingested, the eggs hatch in the stomach of the intermediate host, releasing the hexacanth embryo or oncosphere. The oncosphere penetrates the intestinal wall and migrates in the circulation to the tissues, where it develops into a cysticercus over 3 to 4 months. The cysticerci may develop in muscle, connective tissue, brain, lungs, and eyes and remain viable for as long as 5 years.

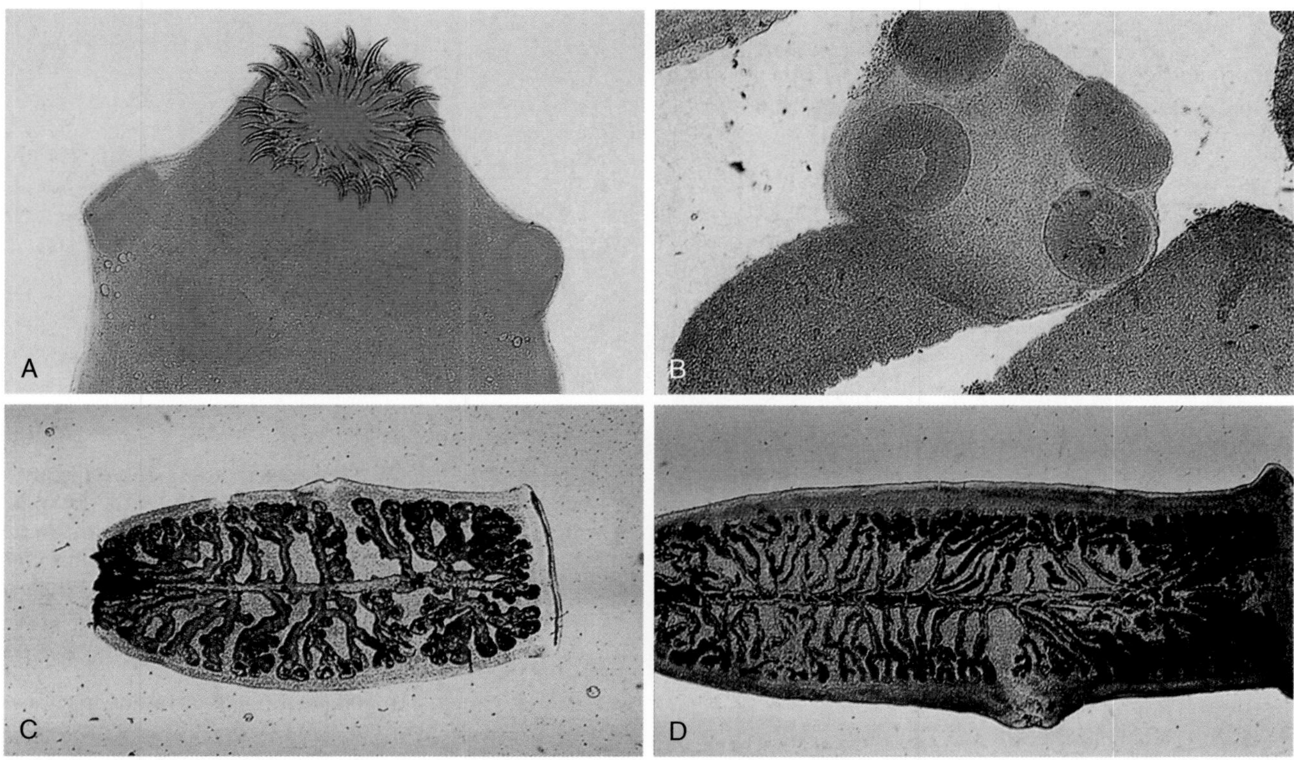

FIGURE 77-2 Scolices and proglottids of *Taenia solium* (**A** and **C**) and *Taenia saginata* (**B** and **D**). The scolex of *T. solium* (**A**) is armored with hooks in addition to four suckers. *T. saginata* has no hooks (**B**). The gravid proglottids of *T. solium* (**C**) contain a central uterus with fewer than a dozen lateral branches. The gravid segments of *T. saginata* (**D**) contain a central uterus with 15 to 20 lateral branches. (From Peters W, Pasvol G: *Atlas of tropical medicine and parasitology,* ed 6, Philadelphia, 2007, Elsevier; **C** and **D,** Courtesy Professor D. Greenwood.)

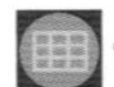

Table 77-1 Medically Important Cestodes

Cestode	Common Name	Reservoir for Larvae	Reservoir for Adults
Taenia solium	Pork tapeworm Cysticercosis	Hogs Humans	Humans —
Taenia saginata	Beef tapeworm	Cattle	Humans
Diphyllobothrium latum	Fish tapeworm	Freshwater crustaceans and fish	Humans, dogs, cats, bears
Echinococcus granulosus	Unilocular hydatid cyst	Herbivores, humans	Canines
Echinococcus multilocularis	Alveolar hydatid cyst	Herbivores, humans	Foxes, wolves, dogs, cats
Hymenolepis nana	Dwarf tapeworm	Rodents, humans	Rodents, humans
Hymenolepis diminuta	Dwarf tapeworm	Insects	Rodents, humans
Dipylidium caninum	Pumpkin seed tapeworm	Fleas	Dogs, cats

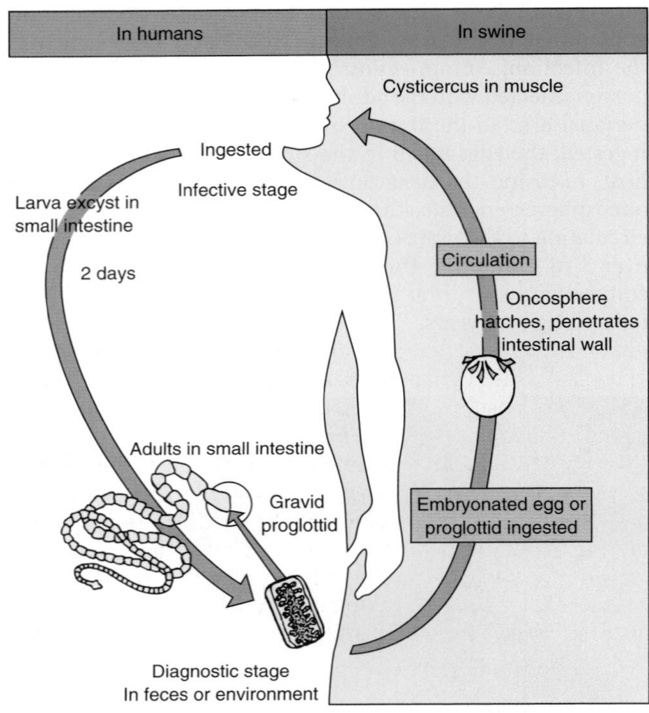

FIGURE 77-3 Life cycle of *Taenia solium* (pork tapeworm).

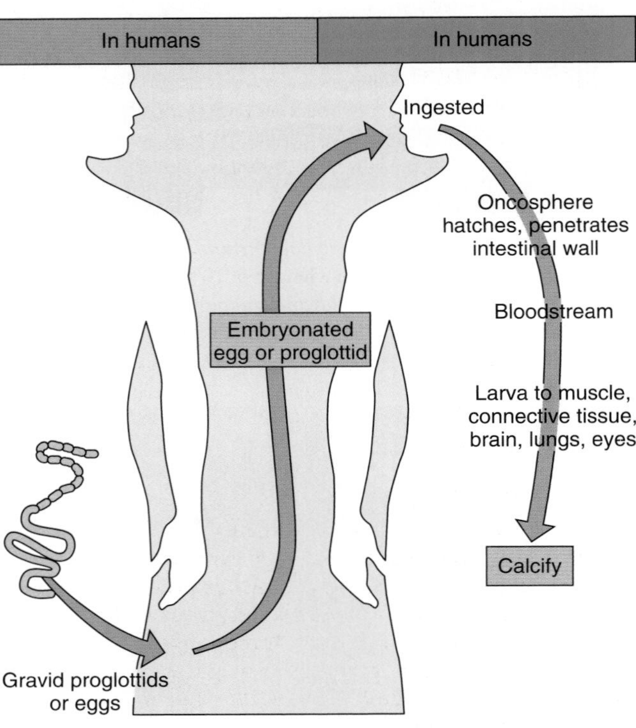

FIGURE 77-5 Development of human cysticercosis.

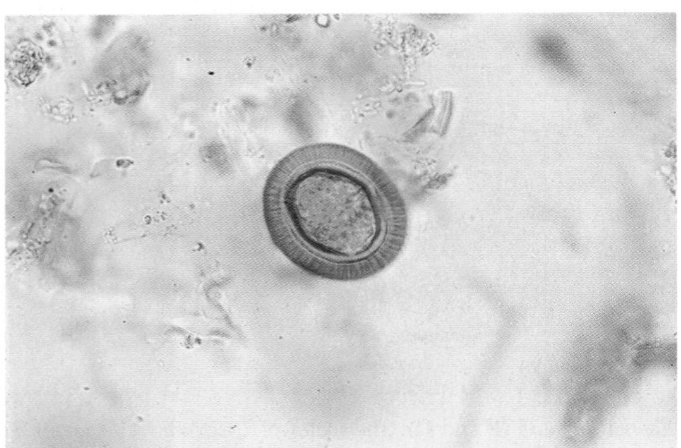

FIGURE 77-4 *Taenia* egg. The eggs are spherical, 30 to 40 μm in diameter, and contain three pairs of hooklets internally. The eggs of the different *Taenia* species cannot be differentiated.

Epidemiology

Cysticercosis is found in the areas where *T. solium* is prevalent and is directly correlated with human fecal contamination. In addition to fecal-oral transmission, autoinfection may occur when a proglottid containing eggs is regurgitated from the small intestine into the stomach, allowing the eggs to hatch and release the infectious oncosphere.

Clinical Syndromes

A few cysticerci in nonvital areas (e.g., subcutaneous tissues) may not provoke symptoms, but serious disease may follow as the cysticerci lodge in vital areas such as the brain and eyes. In the brain, they may produce hydrocephalus, meningitis, cranial nerve damage, seizures, hyperactive reflexes, and visual defects (Clinical Case 77-1). In the eye, loss of visual acuity may occur, and if the larvae lodge along the optic tract, visual field defects result. Tissue reaction to

Clinical Case 77-1 Neurocysticercosis

Chatel and colleagues (*Am J Trop Med Hyg* 60:255–256, 1999) described a case of neurocysticercosis in an Italian traveler to Latin America. The patient was a 49-year-old man with a history of a 30-day stay in Latin America (El Salvador, Colombia, Guatemala) 3 months before presentation with fever and myalgia. The clinical examination and routine laboratory test results were normal except for elevated creatine phosphokinase levels and mild eosinophilia. He received symptomatic antiinflammatory therapy, rapidly improved, and was discharged with a diagnosis of polymyositis. Two years later, he was admitted to the hospital with retroocular headache and recurrent right hemianopsia. A neurologic examination revealed a left Babinski reflex with no motor or sensory dysfunctions. Laboratory tests were unremarkable, including a negative stool examination for ova and parasites. Cerebral magnetic resonance imaging (MRI) showed the presence of several intraparenchymal, subarachnoidal, and intraventricular cysts (4 to 15 mm in diameter) with perilesional focal edema and ringlike enhancement. A specific antibody response to cysticercosis was demonstrated by enzyme-linked immunosorbent assay and immunoblotting techniques. The patient was treated with albendazole for two cycles of 8 days each. One year later, he was in good health, and cerebral MRI revealed significant reduction in the diameter of the lesions. This case provides an interesting reminder of the minimal but real risks to travelers for acquiring *Taenia solium* infections during foreign travel.

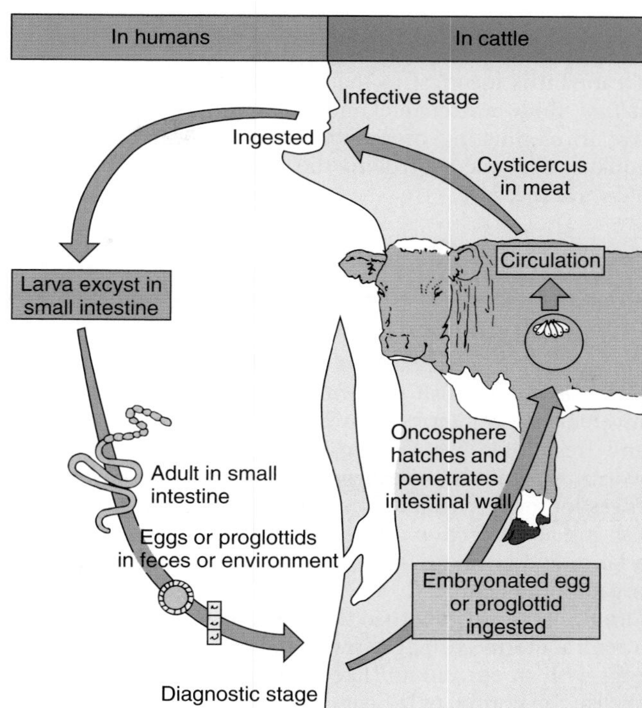

FIGURE 77-6 Life cycle of *Taenia saginata* (beef tapeworm).

viable larvae may be only moderate, thus minimizing symptoms. However, death of the larvae results in the release of antigenic material that stimulates a marked inflammatory reaction; exacerbation of symptoms can result in fever, muscle pains, and eosinophilia.

Laboratory Diagnosis

The presence of cysticerci is usually established by the appearance of calcified cysticerci in soft-tissue roentgenograms, surgical removal of subcutaneous nodules, and visualization of cysts in the eye. Central nervous system lesions may be detected by computed tomography, radioisotope scanning, or ultrasonography. Serologic studies may be useful; false-positive results may occur in people with other helminthic infections.

Treatment, Prevention, and Control

The drug of choice for cysticercosis is either praziquantel or albendazole. Concomitant steroid administration may be necessary to minimize the inflammatory response to dying larvae. Surgical removal of cerebral and ocular cysts may be necessary. Critical to prevention and control of human infection are the treatment of human cases harboring adult *T. solium* (to reduce egg transmission) and controlled disposal of human feces. These measures also reduce the likelihood of infection in pigs.

• *Taenia saginata*

Physiology and Structure

The life cycle of *T. saginata,* the beef tapeworm, is similar to that of *T. solium* (Figure 77-6), with infection resulting after cysticerci are ingested in insufficiently cooked beef. After excystment, the larvae develop into adults in the small intestine and initiate egg production in maturing proglottids. The adult worm may parasitize the jejunum and small intestine of humans for as long as 25 years, attaining a length of 10 m. In contrast with *T. solium* infections, cysticercosis produced by *T. saginata* does not occur in humans. The adult *T. saginata* worm also differs from *T. solium* in that it lacks a crown of hooklets on the scolex and has a different proglottid uterine branch structure (see Figure 77-2). The gravid proglottids are longer than they are wide (18 to 20 mm × 5 to 7 mm) and contain 15 to 30 lateral uterine branches. These facts are important in differentiating between the two tapeworms but do not affect therapy.

Epidemiology

T. saginata occurs worldwide and is one of the most frequent causes of cestode infections in the United States. Humans and cattle perpetuate the life cycle: human feces contaminate water and vegetation with eggs, which are then ingested by cattle. The cysticerci in cattle produce adult tapeworms in humans when rare or insufficiently cooked beef is eaten.

Clinical Syndromes

The syndrome that results from *T. saginata* infection is similar to intestinal infection with *T. solium.* Patients are generally asymptomatic or may complain of vague abdominal pains, chronic indigestion, and hunger pains. Proglottids may pass out of the anus directly.

Laboratory Diagnosis

The diagnosis of *T. saginata* infection is similar to that of *T. solium,* with recovery of proglottids and eggs or recovery of an entire worm whose scolex lacks hooklets. Study of the uterine branches in the proglottids differentiates *T. saginata* from *T. solium.*

Treatment, Prevention, and Control

Treatment is identical to that for the intestinal phase of *T. solium*. Both praziquantel and niclosamide are highly effective in eliminating the adult worm. Education regarding cooking beef and controlling the disposal of human feces is a critical measure.

• *Diphyllobothrium latum*

Physiology and Structure

One of the largest tapeworms (20 to 30 feet long) (see Figure 77-1), *D. latum* **(fish tapeworm)** has a complex life cycle involving two intermediate hosts: freshwater crustaceans and freshwater fish (Figure 77-7). The ribbon-like larval worm in the flesh of freshwater fish is called a **sparganum.** Ingestion of this sparganum in raw or insufficiently cooked fish initiates infection. The scolex of *D. latum* is shaped like a lance and has long lateral grooves **(bothria)** that serve as organs of attachment. The proglottids (Figure 77-8) of *D. latum* are much wider than they are long (≈8 by 4 mm), have a central uterine structure resembling a rosette, and produce eggs with an operculum (like fluke eggs) and a knob on the shell at the bottom of the egg. The adult worms may produce eggs for months or years. More than 1 million eggs per day are released into the fecal stream. On reaching fresh water, the unembryonated operculated eggs require a period of 2 to 4 weeks to develop a ciliated free-swimming larval form called a **coracidium.** The fully developed coracidium leaves the egg via the operculum and is ingested by tiny crustaceans called **copepods** (e.g., *Cyclops* and *Diaptomus* species); then the coracidium develops into a **procercoid** larval form. The crustacean harboring the larval stage is then eaten by a fish, and the infectious **plerocercoid,** or sparganum larvae, develops in the musculature of the fish. If the fish is in turn eaten by another fish, the sparganum simply migrates into the muscles of the second fish. Humans are infected when they eat raw or undercooked fish containing the larval forms.

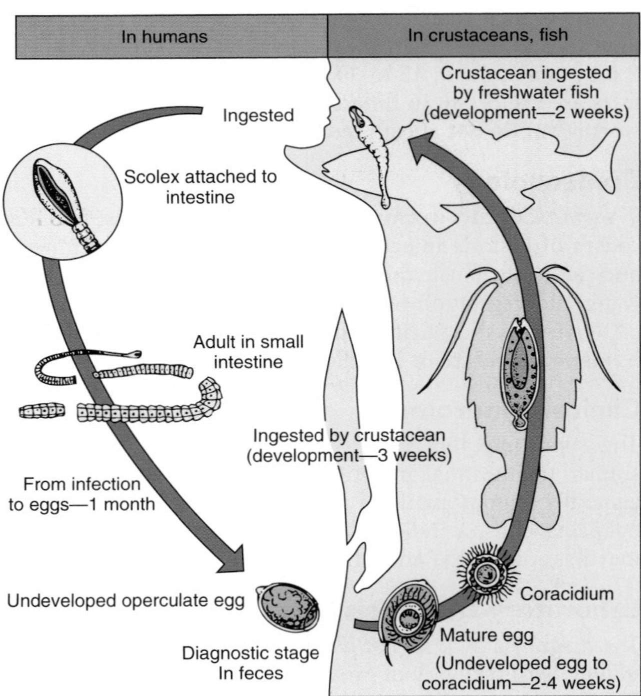

FIGURE 77-7 Life cycle of *Diphyllobothrium latum* (fish tapeworm).

Epidemiology

D. latum infection occurs worldwide, most prevalently in cool lake regions where raw or pickled fish is popular. Insufficient cooking over campfires and tasting and seasoning "gefilte fish" account for many infections. A reservoir of infected wild animals, such as bears, minks, walruses, and members of the canine and feline families that eat fish, is also a source for human infections. The practice of dumping raw sewage into freshwater lakes contributes to the propagation of this tapeworm.

Clinical Syndromes

Clinically, as is the case with most adult tapeworm infections, most *D. latum* infections are asymptomatic (Clinical Case 77-2). Occasionally, people complain of epigastric pain, abdominal cramping, nausea, vomiting, and weight loss. As many as 40% of *D. latum* carriers may have low serum levels of vitamin B_{12}, presumably because of the competition between the host and the worm for dietary vitamin B_{12}. A small percentage (0.1% to 2%) of people infected with *D. latum* develop clinical signs of vitamin B_{12} deficiency, including megaloblastic anemia and neurologic manifestations such as numbness, paresthesia, and loss of vibration sense.

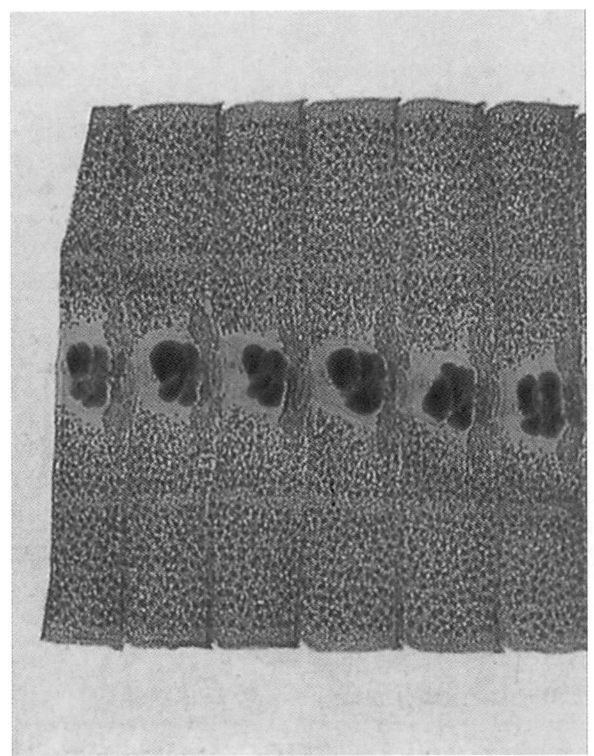

FIGURE 77-8 Proglottids of *Diphyllobothrium latum*. In contrast to those of the *Taenia*, the proglottids of *D. latum* are wider than they are long. (From Peters W, Pasvol G: *Atlas of tropical medicine and parasitology*, ed 6, Philadelphia, 2007, Elsevier.)

Clinical Case 77-2 Diphyllobothriasis

Lee and colleagues (*Korean J Parasitol* 39:319–321, 2001) reported a case of diphyllobothriasis in a young girl. A 7-year-old girl was seen in an outpatient clinic after the discharge of a chain of tapeworm proglottids measuring 42 cm in length. She had no history of eating raw fish, except once when she ate raw salmon flesh along with the rest of her family approximately 7 months earlier. The salmon was caught in a local river. She did not complain of any gastrointestinal discomfort, and all blood chemistry and hematologic studies were normal. The coprologic studies were positive for *Diphyllobothrium latum* eggs. The worm was identified as *D. latum* based on the biological characteristics of the proglottids: broad narrow external morphology, coiling of uterus, number of uterine loops, and position of the genital opening. A single dose of praziquantel 400 mg was given, but stool examination remained positive a week later. Another dose of 600 mg was given, and repeat stool examination 1 month later was negative. Among four family members who ate the raw fish, just two—the girl and her mother—were identified as being infected. Consumption of raw salmon, especially those produced by aquaculture, is a risk for human diphyllobothriasis.

FIGURE 77-9 *Diphyllobothrium latum* egg. Unlike other tapeworm eggs, *D. latum* eggs are operculated. They are 45 × 90 μm in size.

Laboratory Diagnosis

Stool examination reveals the bile-stained operculated egg with its knob at the bottom of the shell (Figure 77-9). Typical proglottids with the rosette uterine structure may also be found in stool specimens. Concentration techniques are usually not necessary, because the worms produce large numbers of ova.

Treatment, Prevention, and Control

The drug of choice is niclosamide; praziquantel and paromomycin are acceptable alternatives. Vitamin B_{12} supplementation may be necessary in people with evidence of clinical vitamin B_{12} deficiency. The prevalence of this infection is reduced by avoiding ingestion of insufficiently cooked fish, controlling the disposal of human feces (especially proper treatment of sewage before disposal in lakes), and promptly treating infections.

Sparganosis

Physiology and Structure

The larval forms of several tapeworms closely related to *D. latum* (most often *Spirometra* spp.) can produce human disease in subcutaneous sites and the eye. In these cases, humans act as the end-stage host for the larval stage, or **sparganum.** Infections are acquired primarily by drinking pond or ditch water that contains crustaceans (copepods) that carry a larval tapeworm. This larval form penetrates the intestinal wall and migrates to various sites in the body, where it develops into a sparganum. Infections may also occur if tadpoles, frogs, and snakes are ingested raw or if the flesh of these animals is applied to wounds as a poultice. The larval worm leaves the relatively cold flesh of the dead animal and migrates into the warm human flesh.

Epidemiology

Cases have been reported from various parts of the world, including the United States, but the infection is most prevalent in the East. Regardless of location, drinking contaminated water and eating raw tadpole, frog, and snake flesh lead to infection.

Clinical Syndromes

In subcutaneous sites, **sparganosis** can produce painful inflammatory tissue reactions and nodules. In the eye, the tissue reaction is intensely painful, and periorbital edema is common. Corneal ulcers may develop with ocular involvement. Ocular disease is frequently associated with the use of frog or snake flesh as a poultice over a wound near the eye.

Laboratory Diagnosis

Sections of tissue removed surgically show characteristic tapeworm features, including highly convoluted parenchyma and dark-staining calcareous corpuscles.

Treatment, Prevention, and Control

Surgical removal is the customary approach. The drug praziquantel may be used; however, no clinical data support its efficacy. Education regarding possible contamination of drinking water with crustaceans that harbor larval worms is essential, and contamination most likely occurs in pond and ditch water. Ingestion of raw frog and snake flesh or their use as poultices over wounds also should be avoided.

Echinococcus granulosus

Physiology and Structure

Infection with *Echinococcus granulosus* is another example of accidental human infection, with humans serving as dead-end intermediate hosts in a life cycle that occurs naturally in other animals. *E. granulosus* adult tapeworms are found in nature in the intestines of canines (dog, fox, wolf, coyote, jackal, dingo); the larval cyst stage is present in the viscera of herbivores (sheep, cattle, swine, deer, moose, elk) (Figure 77-10). The worm consists of a *Taenia*-like scolex with four

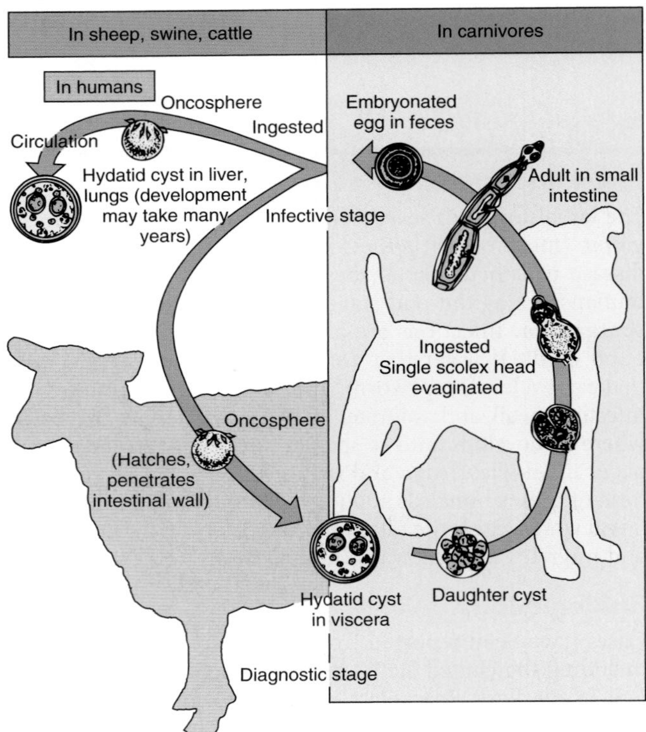

FIGURE 77-10 Life cycle of *Echinococcus granulosus.*

sucking disks and a double row of hooklets, as well as a strobila containing three proglottids: one immature, one mature, and one gravid. Adult tapeworms in the canine intestine produce infective eggs that pass in feces. The eggs are identical in appearance to those of the *Taenia* species. When these eggs are ingested by humans, a six-hooked larval stage called an **oncosphere** hatches. The oncosphere penetrates the human intestinal wall and enters the circulation to be carried to various tissue sites, primarily the liver and lungs but also the central nervous system and bone. This same cycle occurs in the viscera of herbivores. When the herbivore is killed by a canine predator or viscera is fed to canines, ingestion of cysts produces adult tapeworms in the canine intestine to complete the cycle and initiate new egg production. Adult tapeworms do not develop in the intestines of herbivores or humans.

In humans, the larvae form a unilocular **hydatid cyst,** which is a slow-growing tumor-like and space-occupying structure enclosed by a laminated germinative membrane. This membrane produces structures on its wall called **brood capsules,** where tapeworm heads (**protoscolices**) develop. Daughter cysts may develop in the original mother cyst and also produce brood capsules and protoscolices. The cysts and daughter cysts accumulate fluid as they grow. This fluid is potentially toxic; if spilled into body cavities, anaphylactic shock and death can result. Spillage and the escape of protoscolices can lead to development of cysts in other sites because the protoscolices have the germinative potential to form new cysts. Eventually the brood capsules and daughter cysts disintegrate within the mother cyst, liberating the accumulated protoscolices. These become known as **hydatid sand.** This type of echinococcal cyst is called a **unilocular cyst** to differentiate it from related cysts that grow differently. The unilocular cyst is generally about 5 cm in diameter, but some as large as 20 cm, containing almost 2 liters of cyst fluid, have been reported. The cyst may die and become calcified over long periods.

Epidemiology

Human infection with *E. granulosus* unilocular cyst is directly correlated with raising sheep in many countries in Europe, South America, Africa, Asia, Australia, and New Zealand. It occurs in Canada and in the United States, with cases reported from Alaska, Utah, New Mexico, Arizona, California, and the lower Mississippi Valley. Human infection follows ingestion of contaminated water or vegetation, as well as hand-to-mouth transmission of canine feces carrying the infective eggs.

Clinical Syndromes

Because the unilocular cyst grows slowly, 5 to 20 years may pass before any symptoms appear. In many instances, it appears that the cyst is as old as its host. The pressure of the expanding cyst in an organ is usually the first sign of infection. In the majority of cases, the cysts are located in the liver or lung. In the liver, the cyst may exert pressure on both bile ducts and blood vessels and create pain and biliary rupture. In the lungs, cysts may produce cough, dyspnea, and chest pains (Clinical Case 77-3). Rupture of the cysts may occur in 20% of cases, producing fever, urticaria, and occasionally anaphylactic shock and death, which are caused by the release of antigenic cyst contents. Cyst rupture may also lead to dissemination of infection resulting from the release of thousands of protoscolices. In bone, the cyst is responsible for erosion of the marrow cavity and the bone itself. In the brain, severe damage may occur as a result of the cyst's tumor-like growth into brain tissue.

Laboratory Diagnosis

The diagnosis of **hydatid disease** is difficult and depends primarily on clinical, radiographic, and serologic findings. Radiologic examination, scanning procedures, CT, and ultrasound techniques are all valuable and may provide the first evidence of the cyst's presence. Aspiration of cyst contents may demonstrate the presence of the protoscolices (hydatid sand); however, it is contraindicated because of the risk of anaphylaxis and dissemination of the infection. Serologic testing may be useful, but results are negative in 10% to 40% of infections.

Treatment, Prevention, and Control

Surgical resection of the cyst is the treatment of choice. In some instances, the cyst is first aspirated to remove the fluid and hydatid sand, and then it is instilled with formalin to kill and detoxify remaining fluid; finally, it is rolled into a marsupial pouch and sewn shut. If the condition is inoperable because of the cyst's location, medical therapy with high-dose albendazole, mebendazole, or praziquantel may be considered. The most important factor in preventing and controlling **echinococcosis** is education regarding transmission of infection and the role of canines in the life cycle. Proper personal hygiene and the washing of hands and cooking utensils in environments inhabited by dogs are critical. Dogs should not be allowed in the vicinity of animal

Clinical Case 77-3 Echinococcosis

Yeh and colleagues (*N Engl J Med* 357:489–494, 2007) described a 36-year-old pregnant woman at 21 weeks' gestation who presented with a 4-week history of a dry nonproductive cough. The patient denied any constitutional symptoms and had no new pets, environmental exposures, or sick contacts. It was her first pregnancy, and there were no complications. She had no medical conditions and did not smoke or drink alcohol. She was a financial consultant and enjoyed running and hiking. She had traveled to Australia, Central Asia, and sub-Saharan Africa in the past. The patient appeared well, with appropriate weight gain for the second trimester of her pregnancy. Her physical examination, including auscultation of her lungs, was normal. Her cough did not improve with use of an inhaled bronchodilator. Imaging studies were not performed because of her pregnancy. She had a normal uncomplicated vaginal delivery 4 months later. She continued to have a dry cough and presented to her physician months after delivery for a reevaluation of her cough. At that time, her physical examination and laboratory studies were unremarkable. A chest radiograph revealed a soft-tissue mass, 7 cm in diameter, adjacent to the right heart border. High-resolution computed tomography (CT) scans of the chest confirmed the presence of a homogeneous and fluid-filled structure without septa, thought to be in the mediastinum. Subsequent echocardiography also confirmed a simple cystic structure with thin walls surrounding echo-free fluid that was indenting the right atrium. On the basis of the radiographic and echocardiography findings, the clinicians caring for the patient thought that the mass was most likely a benign pericardial cyst. Because she was not experiencing dyspnea, the patient declined surgical resection. However, because of worsening cough over the next few months, she consulted a thoracic surgeon for elective resection. Intraoperative findings revealed an intraparenchymal pulmonary cyst in the right lung that was not attached to the pericardium or bronchus. The cyst was removed intact without gross spillage of the contents. Staining of the cyst wall with hematoxylin and eosin after cross-sectioning showed an acellular laminated layer. Microscopic examination of the cyst contents showed protoscolices with hooklets and suckers in a background of histiocytes and eosinophilic debris, consistent with *Echinococcus granulosus.* CT of the abdomen after removal of the thoracic cyst revealed no hepatobiliary disease. Postoperative screening for serum antibody against *Echinococcus* was positive. Praziquantel was administered for 10 days after surgery and albendazole for 1 month after surgery, with no complications. After this course of therapy, the patient had resolution of her cough and returned to her normal level of activity. There was no evidence of recurrent disease on CT follow-up 6 months after surgery.

slaughter and should never be fed the viscera of slain animals. In some areas, the killing of stray dogs has reduced the incidence of infection.

• *Echinococcus multilocularis*

Physiology and Structure

Similar to infection with *E. granulosus,* human infection with *Echinococcus multilocularis* is accidental (Figure 77-11). Adult *E. multilocularis* tapeworms are primarily found in foxes and wolves, although farm dogs and cats harbor them in some rural environments. The intermediate hosts that harbor the cyst stage are rodents (mice, voles, shrews, lemmings). Humans become infected with the cyst stage as a result of contact with fox, dog, or cat feces contaminated with eggs. Trappers and workers who handle fur pelts may become infected by inhaling fecal dust that carries eggs.

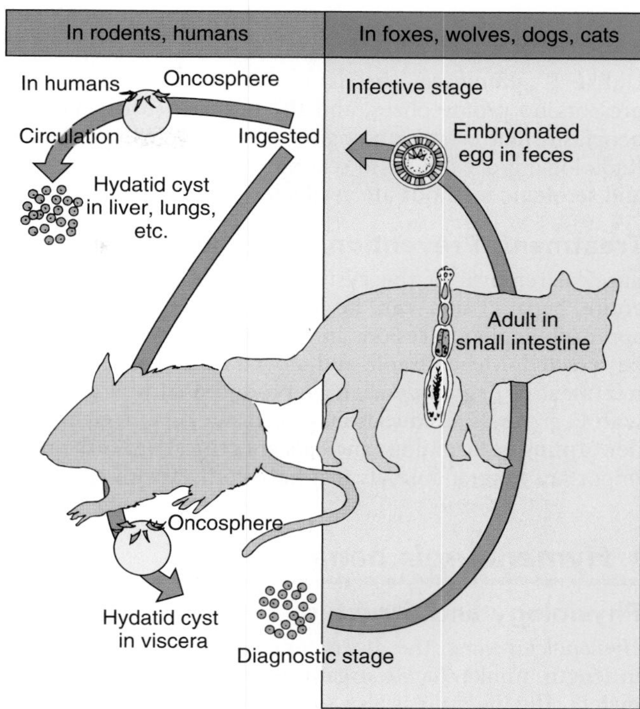

FIGURE 77-11 Life cycle of *Echinococcus multilocularis.*

Infective eggs hatch in and penetrate the intestinal tract to become oncospheres. These forms enter the circulation and take up residence primarily in the liver and lungs but also possibly in the brain.

The **alveolar hydatid cyst** develops as an alveolar or honeycombed structure that is not covered by a unilocular-limiting mother cyst–laminated membrane. The cyst grows via exogenous budding, eventually resembling a carcinoma.

Epidemiology

E. multilocularis is found primarily in northern areas such as Canada, the former Soviet Union, northern Japan, Central Europe, and Alaska, Montana, North and South Dakota, Minnesota, and Iowa in the United States. There is evidence that the life cycle may be extending to other midwestern states, where foxes and mice transmit the organism to dogs and cats and eventually to humans.

Clinical Syndromes

E. multilocularis, because of its slow growth, may be present in human tissues for many years before symptoms appear. In the liver, cysts eventually mimic a carcinoma, with liver enlargement and obstruction of biliary and portal pathways. Often the growth metastasizes to the lungs and brain. Malnutrition, ascites, and portal hypertension produced by *E. multilocularis* create the appearance of hepatic cirrhosis. Among all of the worm infections of humans, *E. multilocularis* is one of the most lethal. If the infection is left untreated, the mortality rate is approximately 70%.

Laboratory Diagnosis

Unlike *E. granulosus,* the tissue form of *E. multilocularis* presents no protoscolices, and the material so resembles a neoplasm that even pathologists mistake it for carcinoma. Radiologic procedures and scanning techniques are helpful, and serologic methods are available.

Treatment, Prevention, and Control

Surgical removal of the cyst is indicated, especially if an entire hepatic area can be resected. The same surgical approach applies to lesions in the lung, wherein a lobe can be resected. Mebendazole and albendazole, as used for the treatment of *E. granulosus,* have produced clinical cures. As with *E. granulosus,* education, proper personal hygiene, and deworming of farm dogs and cats are critical. It is extremely important to treat animals that have contact with children.

• *Hymenolepis nana*

Physiology and Structure

Hymenolepis nana, the **dwarf tapeworm,** is only 2 to 4 cm in length, unlike *Taenia* organisms, which measure several meters. The life cycle is also simple and does not require an intermediate host (Figure 77-12), although mice and beetles may be infected and enter the cycle.

Infection begins when the embryonated eggs are ingested and develop in the intestinal villi into a larval cysticercoid stage. This cysticercoid larva attaches its four muscular suckers and crown of hooklets to the small intestine, and upon maturation, the adult worm produces a strobila of egg-laden proglottids. Eggs passing in the feces are then immediately and directly infective, initiating another cycle. Infection may also be acquired by ingesting infected insect intermediate hosts.

H. nana also can cause autoinfection, with a subsequent increased worm burden. Eggs are able to hatch in the intestine, develop into a cysticercoid larva, and then grow into adult worms without leaving the host. This can lead to hyperinfection with very heavy worm burdens and severe clinical symptoms.

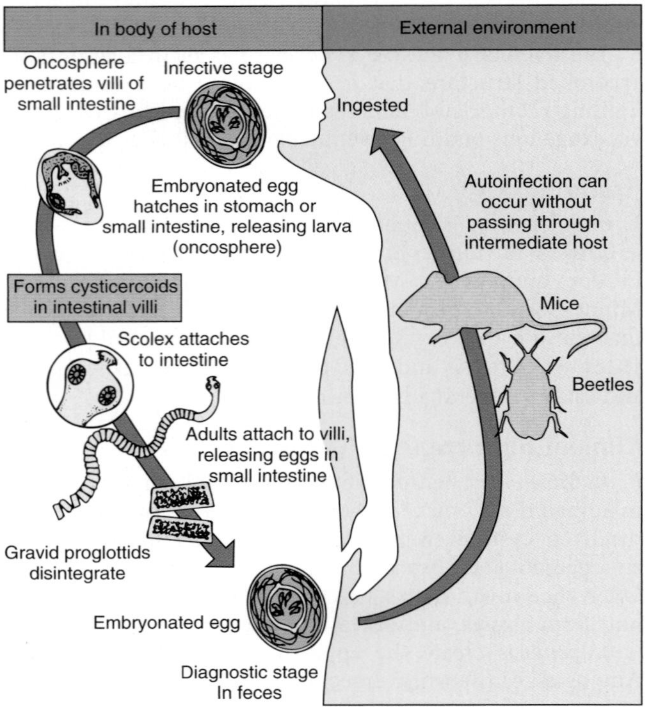

FIGURE 77-12 Life cycle of *Hymenolepis nana* (dwarf tapeworm).

Epidemiology

H. nana occurs worldwide in humans and is also a common parasite of mice. The most common tapeworm infection in North America, it occasionally develops its cysticercoid stage in beetles; humans and mice may ingest these beetles in contaminated grain and flour. Children are especially at risk of infection, and because of the simple life cycle of the parasite, families with children in day-care centers experience problems in controlling the transmission of this organism.

Clinical Syndromes

With only a few worms in the intestine, there are no symptoms. In heavy infections, especially if autoinfection and hyperinfection occur, patients experience diarrhea, abdominal pain, headache, anorexia, and other vague complaints.

Laboratory Diagnosis

Stool examination reveals the characteristic *H. nana* egg with its six-hooked embryo and polar filaments (Figure 77-13).

Treatment, Prevention, and Control

The drug of choice is praziquantel; an alternative is niclosamide. Treatment of cases, improved sanitation, and proper personal hygiene, especially in the family and institutional environments, are essential for controlling transmission of *H. nana.*

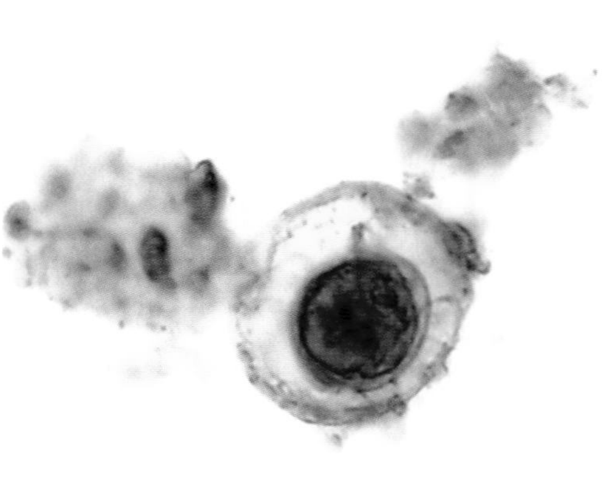

FIGURE 77-13 *Hymenolepis nana* egg. The eggs are 30 to 45 μm in diameter and have a thin shell containing a six-hooked embryo.

• Hymenolepis diminuta

Physiology and Structure

Hymenolepis diminuta, closely related to *H. nana,* is primarily a tapeworm of rats and mice, but it is also found in humans. It differs from *H. nana* in length, measuring 20 to 60 cm. The scolex lacks hooklets, and the egg is larger and bile stained and has no polar filaments (Figure 77-14). The life cycle of *H. diminuta* is more complex than that of *H. nana,* and it requires larval insects ("mealworms") to reach the infective cysticercoid stage.

Epidemiology

Infections have been found all over the world, including in the United States. Larval beetles and other larval insects become infected when they feed on rat feces that carry *H. diminuta* eggs. Humans are infected by ingesting the larval insects (mealworms) in contaminated grain products (e.g., flour, cereals).

Clinical Syndromes

Mild infections produce no symptoms, but heavier worm burdens produce nausea, abdominal discomfort, anorexia, and diarrhea.

Laboratory Diagnosis

Stool examination demonstrates the characteristic bile-stained egg that lacks polar filaments.

Treatment, Prevention, and Control

The drug of choice is niclosamide, with praziquantel as an alternative. Rodent control in areas where grain products are produced or stored is essential. Thorough inspection of uncooked grain products to detect mealworms is also important.

• Dipylidium caninum

Physiology and Structure

Dipylidium caninum, a small tapeworm averaging about 15 cm in length, is primarily a parasite of dogs and cats, but it can infect humans, especially children whose mouths are licked by infected pets. The life cycle involves development of larval worms in dog and cat fleas. These fleas, when crushed by the teeth of the infected pet, are carried on the tongue to the child's mouth when the child kisses the pet or the pet licks the child. Swallowing the infected flea leads to intestinal infection.

Because of the size and shape of the mature and terminal proglottids, *D. caninum* is often called the **pumpkin seed tapeworm.** The eggs are distinctive because they occur in packets covered with a tough clear membrane. There may be as many as 25 eggs in a packet, and a single egg free of the packet is seldom seen.

Epidemiology

D. caninum occurs worldwide, especially in children. Its distribution and transmission are directly correlated with dogs and cats infected with fleas.

Clinical Syndromes

Light infections are asymptomatic; heavier worm burdens produce abdominal discomfort, anal pruritus, and diarrhea. Anal pruritus results from active migration of the motile proglottid.

Laboratory Diagnosis

Stool examination reveals the colorless egg packets (Figure 77-15), and proglottids may be in feces brought to physicians by patients.

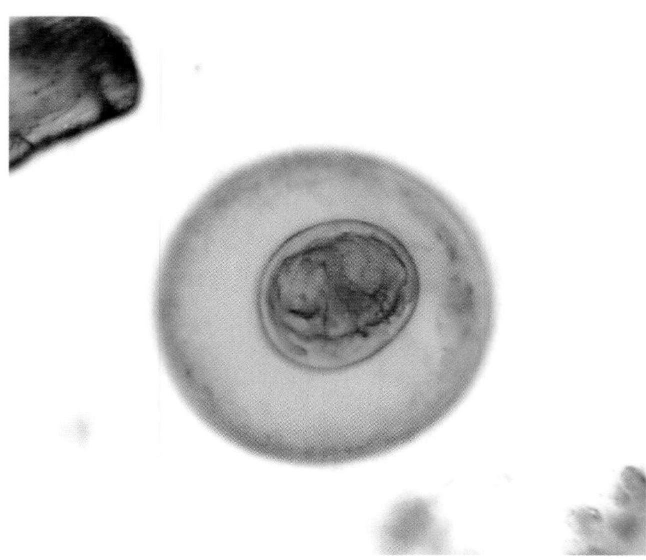

FIGURE 77-14 *Hymenolepis diminuta* egg. The eggs are large (70 to 85 µm × 60 to 80 µm) and have a six-hooked embryo surrounded by a membrane that is widely separated from the outer shell.

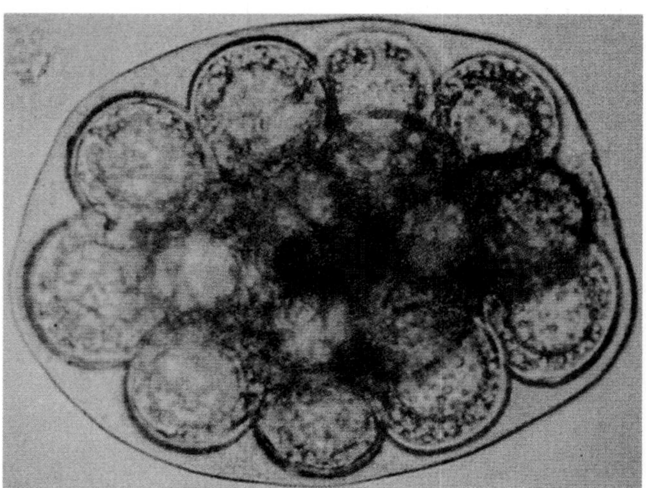

FIGURE 77-15 *Dipylidium caninum* eggs. Free eggs are rarely seen. Instead, egg packets that contain 8 to 15 six-hooked oncospheres enclosed in a thin membrane are most commonly found in fecal specimens. (From Murray PR, Baron EJ, Pfaller MA, et al: *Manual of clinical microbiology,* ed 7, Washington, DC, 1999, American Society for Microbiology Press.)

Treatment, Prevention, and Control

The drug of choice is niclosamide; praziquantel and paromomycin are alternatives. Dogs and cats should be dewormed and not be allowed to lick the mouths of children. Pets should be treated to eradicate the fleas.

Bibliography

Budke CM, Deplazes P, Torgenson PR: Global socioeconomic impact of cystic echinococcosis, *Emerg Infect Dis* 12:296–303, 2006.

Cabello FC: Salmon aquaculture and transmission of the fish tapeworm, *Emerg Infect Dis* 13:169–171, 2007.

Eckert J, Deplazes P: Biological, epidemiological, and clinical aspects of echinococcosis, a zoonosis of increasing concern, *Clin Microbiol Rev* 17:107–135, 2004.

Garcia HH, Jimenez JA, Escalante H: Cestodes. In Versalovic J, et al, editors: *Manual of clinical microbiology*, ed 10, Washington, DC, 2011, American Society for Microbiology Press.

Garcia HH, Evans CA, Nash TE, et al: Current consensus guidelines for treatment of neurocysticercosis, *Clin Microbiol Rev* 15:747–756, 2002.

Garcia LS: *Diagnostic medical parasitology*, ed 5, Washington, DC, 2006, American Society for Microbiology Press.

John DT, Petri WA Jr: *Markell and Voge's medical parasitology*, ed 9, Philadelphia, 2006, Elsevier.

Scholz T, Garcia HH, Kuchta R, et al: Update on the human broad tapeworm (genus *Diphyllobothrium*), including clinical relevance, *Clin Microbiol Rev* 22:146–160, 2009.

Sorvillo FJ, DeGiorgio C, Waterman SH: Deaths from cysticercosis, United States, *Emerg Infect Dis* 13:230–235, 2007.

CHAPTER

78 ARTHROPODS

A 4-year-old child with a complaint of itchy hands was brought in by her mother. The child stayed at a day-care center during the day while her mother worked. The girl had intense itching and a rash on her hands and arms for about 2 weeks. The itching became more severe and interfered with the child's sleep. On physical examination, the child appeared well nourished and cared for. The skin on her hands, wrists, and forearms appeared red and excoriated. Raised serpiginous "tracks" were noted on the sides of her fingers, the ventral aspects of her wrists, and in the popliteal folds. Several of the tracks were inflamed and beginning to form pustules. The mother stated that several other children at the day-care center were experiencing a similar problem.

1. What was the likely diagnosis?
2. How would this diagnosis have been confirmed?
3. How would this child have been treated, and what advice would have been given to the mother regarding prevention?
4. Did this child require antibiotic therapy? If so, why?
5. What should have been done regarding the other children at the day-care center?

Answers to these questions are available on StudentConsult.com.

• SUMMARIES CLINICALLY SIGNIFICANT ORGANISMS

Myriapoda

Trigger Words

Centipedes, maxillipeds, *Scolopendra,* Epsom salts, rubbish

Biology, Virulence, and Disease

- Myriapoda (formerly Chilopoda) consist of terrestrial forms such as centipedes
- Centipedes are elongated, multisegmented (15 to >181 segments), many-legged, tracheate arthropods
- Medically significant because of venomous claws that may produce a painful bite with localized swelling
- Bite of most centipedes harmless to humans

Epidemiology

- Most centipedes are predaceous insectivores
- Found in dark, damp environments
- Human contact almost always due to accidental exposure during outdoor activities

Diagnosis

- Gross observation of typical organism

Treatment, Prevention, and Control

- Treatment of centipede bite includes local measures (e.g., compress, Epsom salts)
- Control consists of removing rubbish near dwellings

Crustacea

Trigger Words

Crab, copepod, decapod, crayfish, intermediate host, intestinal helminth

Biology, Virulence, and Disease

- Crustaceans include familiar aquatic forms: decapods (crabs, crayfish, shrimp); copepods (water fleas)
- Several involved as intermediate hosts in life cycles of various intestinal or blood and tissue helminths

Epidemiology

- Worldwide distribution
- Helminthic diseases acquired by consuming contaminated water, ingesting uncooked flesh of intermediate host

Diagnosis

- Identification of specific helminthic parasite

Treatment, Prevention, and Control

- Depends on infecting parasite

Chelicerata (Arachnida)

Trigger Words

Spider, scorpion, mite, tick, venom, vector

Biology, Virulence, and Disease

- Chelicerata (formerly Arachnida) include familiar terrestrial forms such as mites, ticks, spiders, scorpions
- Chelicerata have no wings or antennae; adults have four pairs of legs

- Mites and ticks serve as vectors for microbial diseases; scorpions and some spiders medically significant for venomous bites

Epidemiology

- Spiders: wood and brush piles, basements
- Scorpions: southwestern United States, Mexico, Venezuela
- Mites: worldwide
- Ticks: worldwide in wooded and rural areas

Diagnosis

- Gross morphology
- Clinical and laboratory diagnosis of specific infection
- Recognition of envenomation event

Treatment, Prevention, and Control

- Symptomatic for bites
- Specific treatment for infectious disease
- Protective clothing, insect repellent, remove brush and clutter from dwellings (inside and out)

Hexapoda (Insects)

Trigger Words

Insect, mosquito, fly, flea, wasp, local reaction, vector

Biology, Virulence, and Disease

- Largest and most important of all classes of arthropods
- Accounts for ≈70% of all known species of animals; includes mosquitoes, flies, fleas, lice, roaches, bees, wasps, beetles, moths
- Body consists of head, thorax, and abdomen; one pair of antennae, three pairs of appendages, one or two pairs of wings or no wings
- Medical significance varies, related to mouthparts and feeding habits, vectors, and mechanical injury

Epidemiology

- Worldwide and extremely variable

Diagnosis

- Gross morphology
- Clinical and laboratory diagnosis of specific infection

Treatment, Prevention, and Control

- Protective clothing, insect repellent
- Insecticides, removal of habitat
- Supportive care for local reaction to bite
- Prompt removal of ticks
- Specific therapy for infection

The arthropods are the largest of the animal phyla, with more than 1 million species. The phylum Arthropoda comprises invertebrate animals with a segmented body, several pairs of jointed appendages, bilateral symmetry, and a rigid chitinous exoskeleton that is molted periodically as the animal grows. Characteristically, arthropods develop from egg to adult by a process known as **metamorphosis.** As they mature, the organisms pass through several distinct morphologic stages, including egg, larva or nymph, pupa (certain insects), and adult. Four subphyla of arthropods are of medical importance on the basis of the number or the severity of the illnesses they cause: the Myriapoda, Crustacea, Chelicerata, and Hexapoda (Insecta) (Table 78-1).

The arthropods or their larvae may affect human health in many ways. Most arthropods function indirectly in human disease; they transmit but do not produce disease. Arthropods may transmit disease mechanically, as when flies carry enteric bacterial pathogens from feces to human food. Of outstanding importance is the ability of many arthropods to act as biological **vectors and intermediate hosts** in the transmission and developmental cycle of viruses, bacteria, protozoa, and metazoa (Table 78-2). Certain arthropods may inflict direct injury by their bites or stings. Other species, such as lice, scabies mites, and tissue-invading maggots, may act as true parasites. Still other species may function as both parasites and vectors of disease.

It is not the purpose of this chapter to consider medical entomology in detail. Rather, our purpose is to provide a brief overview of several of the more important aspects of arthropods and their relationship to human disease. More detailed information on arthropods of medical importance and the therapy and control of arthropod infestations may be found in the references listed in the bibliography.

Myriapoda

Centipedes

Physiology and Structure

The centipedes are elongated, multisegmented (15 to >181 segments), many-legged, tracheate arthropods. They possess a distinct head and trunk. The body is dorsoventrally flattened, and each trunk segment bears a single pair of legs. **Maxillipeds** or venom claws are situated on the first segment and are used for capturing prey. The millipedes are sometimes classified with the centipedes; however, millipedes lack the venom claws of centipedes and have two pairs of legs per segment.

Epidemiology

Most centipedes are predaceous insectivores and commonly found in dark, damp environments, such as the areas beneath logs, among rubbish, and inside old buildings. Human bites are almost invariably the result of accidental exposure to the organism during outdoor activities.

Clinical Syndromes

Centipede bites may be extremely painful and cause swelling at the site of the bite. Reports of the effects of centipede bites on humans are conflicting. One species, *Scolopendra gigantea,* which is found in Central and South America and the Galapagos Islands, reportedly has caused several deaths.

Table 78-1 Medically Important Classes of Arthropods

Phylum	Subphylum	Organisms
Arthropoda	Myriapoda	Centipedes
	Crustacea	Copepods, decapods (crabs, crayfish), pentastomes (tongue worms)
	Chelicerata	Spiders, scorpions, mites, ticks
	Hexapoda (Insecta)	Flies, mosquitoes, lice, fleas, bugs, stinging insects

With the exception of *Scolopendra* and related tropical genera, the bite of most centipedes is harmless to humans.

Treatment, Prevention, and Control

Treatment of a centipede bite includes local measures such as the application of compresses of sodium bicarbonate or solutions of Epsom salts. Control consists of removing rubbish near dwellings.

Crustacea

Crustaceans are primarily gill-breathing arthropods of fresh and salt water. Those of medical importance are found in fresh water and serve as intermediate hosts of various worms or as endoparasites (pentastomids or tongue worms) of reptiles, birds, and mammals, including humans (see Table 78-2).

The copepods, or water fleas, are represented by the genera *Cyclops* and *Diaptomus.* The larger crustaceans, called **decapods,** include crabs and crayfish. These crustaceans also serve as the second intermediate hosts of the lung fluke *Paragonimus westermani* (see Table 78-2).

Copepods

Physiology and Structure

Copepods are small, simple aquatic organisms. They lack a carapace and have one pair of maxillae and five pairs of biramous swimming legs. Free and parasitic forms exist. The genera *Diaptomus* and *Cyclops* are medically important.

Copepods are an intermediate host in the life cycle of several human parasites, including *Dracunculus medinensis* (dracunculiasis), *Diphyllobothrium latum* (diphyllobothriasis), *Gnathostoma spinigerum* (gnathostomiasis), and *Spirometra* spp. (sparganosis). Copepods have been associated with a single case of a perirectal abscess but generally are not considered a primary cause of human infection.

Epidemiology

Copepods have a worldwide distribution and serve as intermediate hosts for helminthic diseases in the United States and Canada as well as Europe and the tropics. Human infection with these helminthic parasites results from ingesting water contaminated with copepods or from eating the raw or insufficiently cooked flesh of infected fish. Pseudooutbreaks of copepods present in human stool specimens submitted for ova and parasite examination have been reported from New York. As many as 40% of concentrated stools submitted for ova and parasite examination were found to contain copepods, presumably as a result of contamination of a hospital water supply. The single reported case of apparent human infection with copepods occurred in this hospital.

Clinical Syndromes

The clinical signs and symptoms associated with helminthic infections in which copepods serve as intermediate hosts are described in Chapters 75 and 77. The single case of apparent human infection with copepods occurred in a 22-year-old man with Crohn disease who had a perirectal abscess. Drainage of the abscess revealed purulent material that on microscopic examination contained numerous copepods surrounded by leukocytes. It was hypothesized that the copepods were introduced into preexisting perirectal lesions during sitz baths that were prepared with unfiltered tap water and may have contained copepods. Although the copepods contained within the abscess material were viable and may have been successfully feeding on body tissue, it was believed that the copepods were unlikely to have been the primary cause of the abscess.

Laboratory Diagnosis

The laboratory diagnosis of helminthic infections in which copepods serve as intermediate hosts are described in Chapters 75 and 77. In general, infection is demonstrated by detection of the infecting organism by microscopic examination of clinical material.

Treatment, Prevention, and Control

Specific treatment of copepod-associated helminthic infection is covered in Chapters 75 and 77. Prevention of these infections requires attention to standard public health measures such as chlorination and filtration of water and thorough cooking of all fish. Infected people must not be allowed to bathe in water used for drinking, and suspect water should be avoided.

Decapods

The decapods include prawns, shrimps, lobsters, crayfish, and crabs. The cephalothorax of these animals is always covered by a carapace. They have three anterior pairs of thoracic appendages that are modified into biramous maxillipeds and five posterior pairs that are developed into uniramous legs. Crabs and crayfish are medically important as the second intermediate hosts of the lung fluke *P. westermani.* The parasitic, epidemiologic, and clinical aspects of infection with *P. westermani* are described in Chapter 76. Thorough cooking of crabs and crayfish is the most effective means of preventing infection with *P. westermani.*

Pentastomida

Tongue Worms

The pentastomids, or **tongue worms,** are bloodsucking endoparasites of reptiles, birds, and mammals. Their taxonomic status is uncertain. Some scientists include pentastomids among the arthropods because their larvae superficially resemble those of mites. Others consider them annelids, and still others place them in an entirely separate phylum. For purposes of this discussion, they are considered with the arthropods. Based on molecular studies, the Pentastomida are now considered by some experts to be a subclass within the Crustacea.

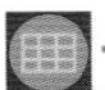 Table 78-2 **Select Human Illnesses Transmitted by Arthropods**

Primary Vector or Intermediate Host	Disease	Etiologic Agent
Chelicerata		
Mite: *Leptotrombidium* spp.	Scrub typhus (tsutsugamushi disease)	*Orientia tsutsugamushi*
Mite: *Liponyssoides sanguineus*	Rickettsial pox	*Rickettsia akari*
Tick: *Dermacentor* spp.	Tularemia	*Francisella tularensis*
Tick: *Dermacentor* spp. and other ixodid ticks	Rocky Mountain spotted fever	*Rickettsia rickettsii*
Tick: *Dermacentor, Boophilus* spp.	Q fever	*Coxiella burnetii*
Tick: *Dermacentor* spp.	Colorado tick fever	*Coltivirus*
Tick: *Ornithodoros* spp.	Relapsing fever	*Borrelia* spp.
Tick: *Ixodes* spp.	Babesiosis	*Babesia microti*
Tick: *Ixodes* spp.	Lyme disease	*Borrelia burgdorferi*
Tick: *Dermacentor variabilis, Amblyomma americanum*	Ehrlichiosis	*Ehrlichia chaffeensis*
Crustacea		
Copepod: *Cyclops* spp.	Diphyllobothriasis	*Diphyllobothrium latum*
Copepod: *Cyclops* spp.	Dracunculiasis	*Dracunculus medinensis*
Crabs, crayfish: various freshwater species	Paragonimiasis	*Paragonimus westermani*
Hexapoda (Insecta)		
Lice: *Pediculus humanus*	Epidemic typhus	*Rickettsia prowazekii*
Lice: *Pediculus humanus*	Trench fever	*Bartonella quintana*
Lice: *Pediculus humanus*	Louse-borne relapsing fever	*Borrelia recurrentis*
Flea: *Xenopsylla cheopis,* various other rodent fleas	Plague	*Yersinia pestis*
Flea: *Xenopsylla cheopis*	Murine typhus	*Rickettsia typhi*
Flea: various species	Dog tapeworm	*Dipylidium caninum*
Bug: *Triatoma, Panstrongylus* spp.	Chagas disease	*Trypanosoma cruzi*
Beetles: flour beetle	Dwarf tapeworm	*Hymenolepis nana*
Fly, gnat: *Glossina* spp. (tsetse flies)	African trypanosomiasis	*Trypanosoma brucei rhodesiense* and *T. b. gambiense*
Fly, gnat: *Simulium* spp.	Onchocerciasis	*Onchocerca volvulus*
Fly, gnat: *Chrysops* spp.	Tularemia	*Francisella tularensis*
Fly, gnat: *Phlebotomus* spp., *Lutzomyia* spp. (sandfly)	Leishmaniasis	*Leishmania* spp.
Fly, gnat: *Phlebotomus* spp.	Bartonellosis	*Bartonella bacilliformis*
Mosquito: *Anopheles* spp.	Malaria	*Plasmodium* spp.
Mosquito: *Aedes aegypti*	Yellow fever	Flavivirus
Mosquito: *Aedes* spp.	Dengue fever	Flavivirus
Mosquito: *Culiseta melanura, Coquillettidia perturbans, Aedes vexans*	Eastern equine encephalitis	Alphavirus
Mosquito: *Aedes triseriatus*	La Crosse encephalitis	Bunyavirus
Mosquito: *Culex* spp.	St. Louis encephalitis	Flavivirus
Mosquito: *Culex* spp.	Venezuelan equine encephalitis	Alphavirus
Mosquito: *Culex tarsalis*	Western equine encephalitis	Alphavirus
Mosquito: various spp.	Bancroftian filariasis	*Wuchereria bancrofti*
Mosquito: various spp.	Malayan filariasis	*Brugia* spp.
Mosquito: various spp.	Dirofilariasis	*Dirofilaria immitis*

Physiology and Structure

Tongue worms are degenerate wormlike arthropods that live primarily in the nasal and respiratory passages of reptiles, birds, and mammals. Adult pentastomids are white, cylindrical, or flattened parasites that possess two distinct body regions: an anterior head, or cephalothorax, and an abdomen. The adults are elongated and may attain a length of 1 to 10 cm. The head has a mouth and two pairs of hooks. Although the abdomen may appear annulated, it is not segmented (Figure 78-1). The pentastomids possess digestive and reproductive organs; however, they lack circulatory and respiratory systems.

The adult pentastomids are found in the lungs of reptiles *(Armillifer armillatus* and *Porocephalus crotali)* and the nasal passages of mammals *(Lingulata serrata)*. Many vertebrates, including humans, may serve as intermediate hosts. The embryonated eggs are discharged in the feces or respiratory secretions of the infected definitive host and contaminate vegetation or water, which is in turn ingested by one of several possible intermediate hosts (fish, rodents, goats, sheep, or humans). The eggs hatch in the intestine, and the primary larvae penetrate the intestinal wall and attach to the peritoneum. The larvae mature in the peritoneum and develop into infective larvae, encyst in viscera, or die and become calcified. In tissue sections, encysted larvae can be identified by acidophilic glands, a chitinous cuticle, and prominent hooks, which are present in the anterior end of the organism. Subcuticular glands and striated muscle fibers may also be observed beneath the cuticle.

Humans may also become infected by ingesting the inadequately cooked flesh of infected reptiles or other definitive hosts or by eating the infected flesh of intermediate hosts (e.g., goats, sheep) containing infective larvae. In the latter instance, the infective larvae migrate from the stomach to the nasopharyngeal tissues, where they develop into adult pentastomids and produce the symptoms of the **halzoun syndrome** (see Clinical Syndromes below). In this case, the human host is considered a temporary definitive host.

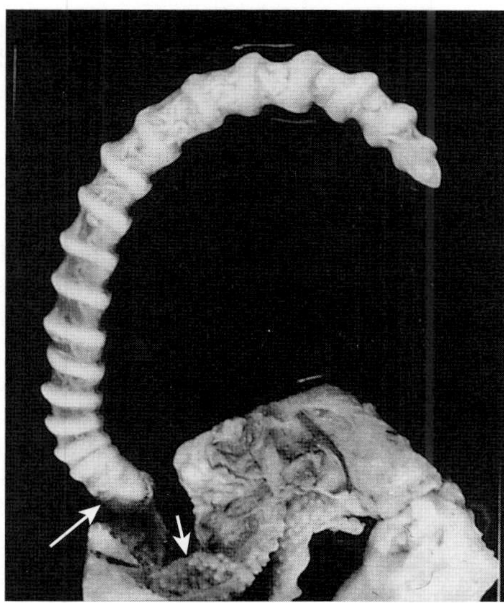

FIGURE 78-1 Adult female pentastome *(Armillifer armillatus)* attached to the respiratory surface of the lung *(short arrow)* of a rock python. Note the short cephalothorax *(long arrow)* and a long, annulated abdomen. (From Binford CH, Connor DH: *Pathology of tropical and extraordinary diseases,* vol 2, Washington, DC, 1976, Armed Forces Institute of Pathology.)

Epidemiology

Most tongue worm infections are reported in Europe, Africa, and South and Central America. The infection is common in Malaysia, where autopsy studies reveal **pentastomiasis** in up to 45% of people. As previously described, the infection is acquired by ingesting raw vegetables or water contaminated with pentastome eggs or by consuming raw or undercooked flesh of infected animals.

Clinical Syndromes

In most cases, infection is asymptomatic and is discovered accidentally during roentgenographic examination (calcified larvae), at surgery, or at autopsy. Pneumonitis, pneumothorax, peritonitis, meningitis, nephritis, and obstructive jaundice have all been ascribed to pentastomid infections; however, definitive proof of a causal relationship between disease and the presence of the parasite is frequently lacking. Localized infection of the eye has been reported, presumably secondary to direct inoculation.

Halzoun syndrome, caused by the attachment of adult pentastomes to the nasopharyngeal tissues, is characterized by pharyngeal discomfort, paroxysmal coughing, sneezing, dysphagia, and vomiting. Asphyxiation has been rarely reported.

Laboratory Diagnosis

The diagnosis is made by identifying a pentastomid in a biopsy specimen obtained at surgery or at autopsy. Occasionally, calcified larvae may be observed on radiographic films of the abdomen or chest, providing a presumptive diagnosis. There are no useful serologic tests.

Treatment, Prevention, and Control

Treatment is not usually warranted. In symptomatic patients, surgical removal of free or encysted parasites should be attempted. Preventive measures include thorough cooking of meat and vegetables and avoidance of contaminated water.

• Chelicerata (Arachnida)

Spiders

Spiders have a number of characteristic features that permit easy identification. Specifically, they possess eight legs, no antennae, a body divided into two regions (cephalothorax and abdomen), and an unsegmented abdomen with spinnerets posteriorly. All true spiders produce venom and kill their prey by biting; however, few have fangs **(chelicerae)** powerful enough to pierce human skin or venom potent enough to produce more than a transitory local skin irritation. Venomous spiders may be classified as those that cause **systemic arachnidism** and those that cause **necrotic arachnidism.** This classification is based on the type of tissue damage produced.

Systemic arachnidism is primarily caused by tarantulas and black widow spiders. Tarantulas (family Theraphosidae) are large hairy spiders of the tropics and subtropics;

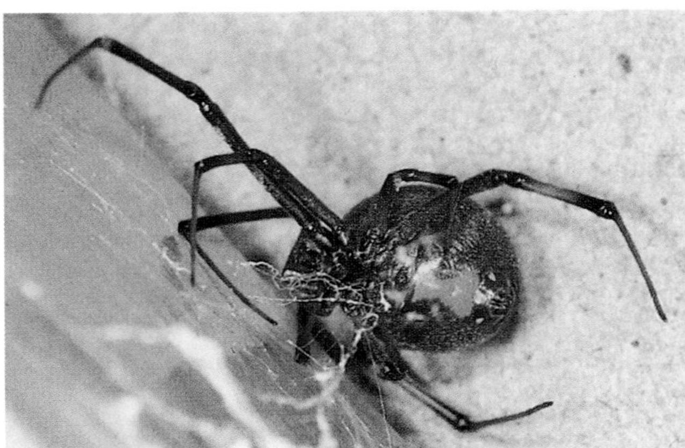

FIGURE 78-2 Female black widow spider *(Latrodectus mactans).* (From Peters W, Pasvol G: *Color atlas of tropical medicine and parasitology,* ed 6, London, 2007, Mosby.)

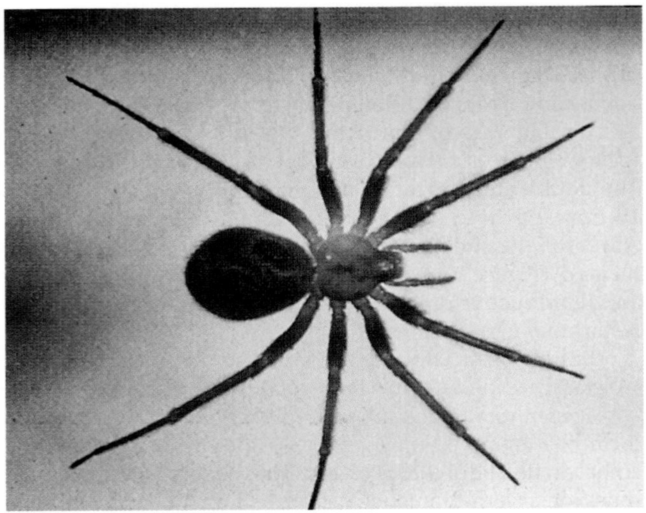

FIGURE 78-3 Female brown recluse spider *(Loxosceles laeta).* (From Peters W, Pasvol G: *Color atlas of tropical medicine and parasitology,* ed 6, London, 2007, Mosby.)

tarantulas are of little importance because they are not very aggressive and avoid human habitations. Their bite causes intense pain and a phase of agitation followed by stupor and somnolence. The black widow spider, *Latrodectus mactans,* is widespread through the southern and western United States. Related species of *Latrodectus* are found throughout temperate and tropical regions of all continents, but none is primarily domestic; thus their contact with humans is limited.

Necrotic arachnidism is produced by spiders that belong to the genus *Loxosceles.* The bites of these spiders may produce severe tissue reaction. *Loxosceles reclusa,* the brown recluse spider, is a medically important spider of this genus.

Black Widow Spiders

Physiology and Structure

The female black widow spider *(L. mactans)* is easily recognized by the presence of a globose shiny black abdomen bearing the characteristic orange or reddish hourglass marking on the ventral surface (Figure 78-2). Females vary from 5 to 13.5 mm in body length, but males are much smaller.

The venom of the black widow spider is a potent peripheral neurotoxin that is delivered by a pair of jawlike structures (chelicerae). Only the female *Latrodectus* spider is dangerous to humans; the small feeble male delivers an ineffective bite.

Epidemiology

These spiders frequent wood and brush piles, old wooden buildings, cellars, hollow logs, and privies. Given these locations, the bite is often located on the genitalia, buttocks, or extremities. Black widow spiders are common in the southern United States but are found throughout the temperate and tropical regions of both the New and Old World.

Clinical Syndromes

As is true with most cases of envenomation, the clinical picture depends on factors such as the amount of venom injected, location of the bite, and age, weight, and sensitivity of the patient. Shortly after the bite, there is a sharp pain but little or no immediate swelling. This is followed by local redness, swelling, and burning. Systemic signs and symptoms generally occur within an hour of the bite and include muscular cramps, chest pains, nausea, vomiting, diaphoresis, intestinal spasms, and visual difficulties. Abdominal tetanic cramps producing a "boardlike" abdomen are highly characteristic and may mimic an acute surgical abdomen. The acute symptoms usually subside within 48 hours; however, in severe cases, paralysis and coma may precede cardiac or respiratory failure. Mortality from the bite of the black widow spider is estimated at 4% to 5%.

Treatment, Prevention, and Control

Healthy adults usually recover, but small children or weakened people suffer considerably from these bites and may die without treatment. Muscle spasms may be severe and may require intravenous administration of calcium gluconate or other muscle relaxant agents. A specific antivenin is available and remains the treatment of choice. It is valuable if given shortly after the bite. Because it is prepared from the serum of hyperimmunized horses, patients must be tested for sensitivity to horse serum before administration. Hospitalization is advisable for the care of people with known or suspected bites.

Good housekeeping can be the simplest and most effective control for spiders in homes. This includes dusting webs and carefully removing debris from around homes and adjacent sheds. Children should be discouraged from playing on woodpiles and in woodsheds.

Brown Recluse Spiders

Physiology and Structure

Spiders producing necrotic arachnidism belong to the genus *Loxosceles.* These spiders are yellow to brown and of medium size (5 to 10 mm long) with relatively long legs (Figure 78-3). They commonly display two distinguishing characteristics: a dark fiddle- or violin-shaped marking on the dorsal side of the cephalothorax, and six eyes arranged in three pairs forming a semicircle. The venom injected by the female or male spider is a necrotoxin (that may also have hemolytic properties) and causes necrotic lesions with deep tissue damage.

Epidemiology

Four species of the genus *Loxosceles* are found in the Americas. *L. reclusa* is found in the southern and central United States, *L. arizonica* is in the western states, and *L. laeta* is in South America. *L. reclusa* is found outdoors in woodpiles and debris in warmer climates and in basements or storage areas in cooler regions. *L. laeta* is found in closets and corners of rooms. Humans are bitten only when the spider is threatened or disturbed.

Clinical Syndromes

Initially, the bite of *Loxosceles* spp. tends to be painless; however, several hours later, itching, swelling, and soreness may develop in the area of the bite. Frequently a vesicle or bleb may form at the site. General systemic symptoms are unusual but when present may include chills, headache, and nausea. Within 3 to 4 days, the bleb sloughs and may be followed by ulceration and radiating necrosis, which does not heal but continues to spread for weeks or months.

Intravascular coagulation and hemolysis may occur and be accompanied by hemoglobinuria and cardiac and renal failure. This hemolytic syndrome may be life threatening and occurs more commonly after the bite of *L. laeta*. In South America, this syndrome is known as **visceral loxoscelism.**

Diagnosis

Discrimination of a species of spider is not possible from the appearance of the lesion alone; however, a working diagnosis is commonly based on the appearance of bleb formation around puncture marks and the nature of the developing lesion. It should be noted that necrotic dermal lesions are frequently classified as loxoscelism even if the appropriate species are not known to be present in the area. The spider may be identified easily by the characteristic features previously described. An enzyme-linked immunosorbent assay has been developed to confirm the diagnosis of brown recluse spider bite but is not widely available.

Treatment, Prevention, and Control

The treatment of brown recluse spider bites is variable and based on the severity of the necrotic reaction. Most bites in the United States are inconsequential and require no specific therapy. Cleansing the bite wound and providing tetanus prophylaxis and antibiotics to prevent secondary infection may all be indicated. Healing is generally uncomplicated, and debridement or excision should not be performed for 3 to 6 weeks to allow natural healing to commence. Excision and skin grafting may be necessary for bites that have not healed in 6 to 8 weeks. Systemic therapy with corticosteroids may be useful in treating the hemolytic syndrome but are of little proven value in preventing or treating cutaneous necrosis. Although not available in the United States, an antivenin is used in South America for the treatment of visceral loxoscelism.

Preventive measures are similar to those recommended for black widow spiders. *Loxosceles* (and other) spiders may be controlled in dwellings with insecticide compounds.

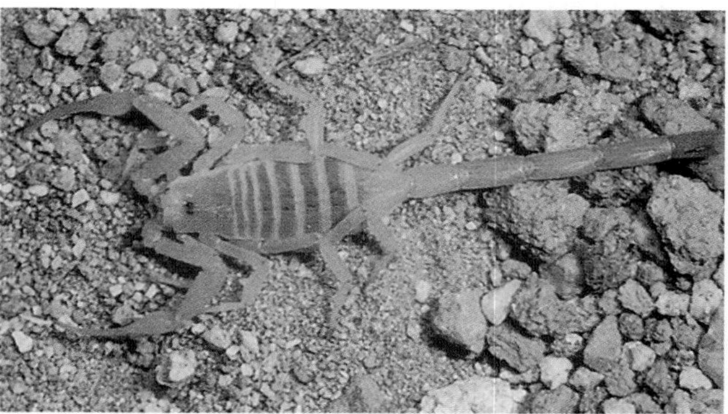

FIGURE 78-4 Scorpion (*Centruroides* spp.). (From Peters W: *A colour atlas of arthropods in clinical medicine,* London, 1992, Wolfe; courtesy Dr. J.C. Cokendolpher.)

Scorpions

Physiology and Structure

The typical scorpion is elongated with conspicuous pincer-like claws (or **pedipalps**) at the anterior end of the body, four pairs of walking legs, and a distinctly regimented abdomen that tapers to a curved, hollow, needle-like stinger (aculeus) (Figure 78-4). When the scorpion is disturbed, it uses the stinger for defense. Both male and female scorpions can sting. Venom is injected through the stinger from two venom glands in the abdomen. Most scorpions are unable to penetrate human skin or inject enough venom to cause real damage; however, a few species are capable of inflicting painful wounds that may cause death.

Epidemiology

Scorpions considered dangerous may be found in the southwestern United States, Mexico, and Venezuela. This includes several species of the genus *Centruroides,* which accounts for as many as 1000 deaths annually. Also important are several species of *Tityus* found in Trinidad, Argentina, Brazil, Guyana, and Venezuela. Children younger than 5 years are most likely to be fatally stung by scorpions.

Scorpions are nocturnal; during the day, they remain concealed under logs or rocks and in other dark moist places. At night they may invade human habitations, where they may hide in shoes, towels, clothing, and closets.

Clinical Syndromes

The effect of a scorpion sting in a patient is highly variable and depends on factors such as the species and age of the scorpion, the kind and amount of venom injected, and the age, size, and sensitivity of the person who was stung. Although the sting of many scorpions is relatively nontoxic and produces only local symptoms, other stings may be quite serious. Scorpions produce two types of venom: a neurotoxin and a hemorrhagic or hemolytic toxin. The hemolytic toxin is responsible for local reactions at the site of the sting, including radiating burning pain, swelling, discoloration, and necrosis. The neurotoxin produces minimal local reaction but rather severe systemic effects, including chills, diaphoresis, excessive salivation, difficulty speaking and swallowing, muscle spasm, tachycardia, and generalized seizures. In severe cases death may result from pulmonary edema and respiratory paralysis.

Diagnosis

Local or systemic signs and symptoms coupled with physical evidence of a single point of skin penetration are usually sufficient to establish the diagnosis. The patient may have observed the scorpion or brought it in for identification. Although scorpions are relatively easy to identify, it is important to realize that other nonpoisonous arachnids strongly resemble scorpions. An entomologist or parasitologist should be consulted if there is a taxonomic question.

Treatment, Prevention, and Control

Management of scorpion stings varies. In the absence of systemic symptoms, palliative treatment may be all that is necessary. Pain may be relieved by analgesics or local injection of Xylocaine; however, opiates appear to increase toxicity. Local cryotherapy may reduce swelling and retard systemic absorption of the toxin. Hot packs produce vasodilation and may accelerate toxin distribution systemically and are therefore contraindicated. Antivenin is available and is effective if administered soon after the sting. Antivenin is usually species specific, and without the identification of the offending agent would be administered on a presumptive basis according to the most common species in the area. Very young children with systemic symptoms should be treated as medical emergencies. Systemic symptoms and shock should be treated supportively.

Preventive measures include the use of chemical pesticides to reduce scorpion populations. Removal of debris around dwellings can reduce hiding and breeding places.

Mites

Mites are small eight-legged arthropods characterized by a saclike body and no antennae. A large number of mite species are free-living or normally associated with other vertebrates (e.g., birds, rodents) and may cause dermatitis in humans on rare occasions. The number of mites that are considered true human parasites or present real medical problems is quite small and include the housemouse mite *(Liponyssoides sanguineus),* human itch mite *(Sarcoptes scabiei),* the human follicle mite *(Demodex folliculorum),* and the chigger mite (*Leptotrombidium deliense* or *L. akamushi*). Mites affect humans in three ways: causing dermatitis, serving as vectors of infectious diseases, and acting as a source of allergens.

Itch Mites

Physiology and Structure

The itch mite *(S. scabiei)* causes an infectious skin disease variably known as **scabies, mange, or the itch.** The adult mites average 300 to 400 μm in length with an oval saclike body in which the first and second pairs of legs are widely separated from the third and fourth pairs (Figure 78-5). The body has dorsal transverse parallel ridges, spines, and hairs. The ova measure 100 to 150 μm.

Adult mites enter the skin, creating serpiginous burrows in the upper layers of the epidermis. The female mite lays her eggs in the skin burrows, and the larval and nymph stages that develop also burrow in the skin. Female mites live and deposit eggs and feces in epidermal burrows for up to 2 months. Characteristically, the preferred sites of infestation are the interdigital and popliteal folds, the wrist and inguinal regions, and the inframammary folds. The presence of the mites and their secretions cause intense itching of the involved areas. The mite is an obligate parasite and can perpetuate itself in a single host indefinitely.

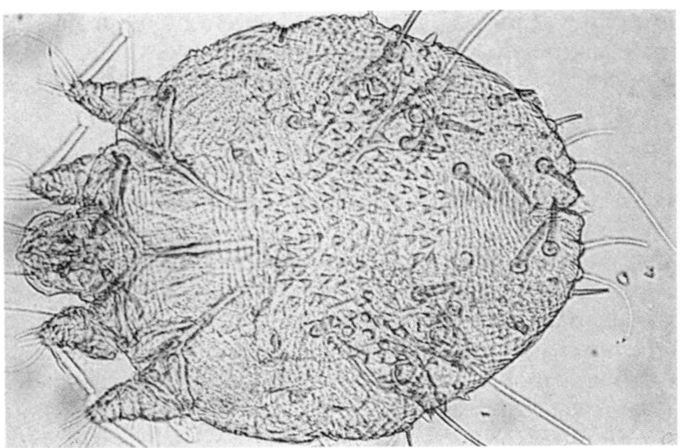

FIGURE 78-5 Scabies mite (*Sarcoptes* spp.). (From Peters W, Pasvol G: *Color atlas of tropical medicine and parasitology,* ed 6, London, 2007, Mosby.)

Epidemiology

Scabies is cosmopolitan in distribution, with an estimated global prevalence of about 300 million cases. The mite is an obligate parasite of domestic animals and humans; however, it may survive for hours to days away from the host, thus facilitating its spread. Transmission is accomplished by direct contact or contact with contaminated objects such as clothing. Sexual transmission has been well documented. Spread of the infection to other areas of the body is accomplished by scratching and manual transfer of the mite by the affected person. Scabies may occur in epidemic fashion among people in crowded conditions, such as day-care centers, nursing homes, military camps, and prisons.

Clinical Syndromes

The outstanding clinical diagnostic symptom is intense itching, usually in the interdigital folds and sides of the fingers, buttocks, external genitalia, wrists, and elbows. The uncomplicated lesions appear as short, slightly raised cutaneous burrows. At the end of the burrow, there is frequently a vesicle containing the female mite. The intense pruritus usually leads to excoriation of the skin secondary to scratching, which in turn produces crusts and secondary bacterial infection. Patients experience their first symptoms within weeks to months after exposure; however, the incubation period may be as little as 1 to 4 days in persons sensitized by prior exposure. Host hypersensitivity (delayed or type IV) probably plays an important role in determining the variable clinical manifestations of scabies.

Some immunodeficient people may develop a variant of scabies, so-called **Norwegian scabies,** characterized by generalized dermatitis with extensive scaling and crusting and the presence of thousands of mites in the epidermis. This disease is highly contagious and suggests that host immunity also plays a role in suppressing *S. scabiei.*

Diagnosis

The clinical diagnosis of scabies is based on the characteristic lesions and their distribution. The definitive diagnosis of scabies depends on the demonstration of the mite in skin scrapings. Because the adult mite is most frequently found in the terminal portions of a fresh burrow, it is best to make scrapings in these areas. The scrapings are placed on a clean microscope slide, cleared by the addition of 1 or 2 drops of a 20% solution of potassium hydroxide, covered with a coverslip, and examined under a low-power microscope. With experience, the mite and ova may be recognized. Skin biopsy may also reveal the mites and ova in tissue sections.

Treatment, Prevention, and Control

The standard, and very effective, treatment for scabies is 1% gamma benzene hexachloride (lindane) in a lotion base. One or two applications (head to toe) at weekly intervals is effective against scabies. Lindane is absorbed through the skin, and repeated applications may be toxic. For this reason its use is not advisable in treating infants, small children, or pregnant or lactating women.

Recently a 5% permethrin cream (Elimite) has replaced lindane lotions as the treatment of choice for scabies. Clinical trials have shown permethrin to be more effective and less toxic than lindane. Other preparations used to treat scabies include oral ivermectin, crotamiton sulfur (6%) preparations, benzyl benzoate, and tetraethylthiuram monosulfide. The last two preparations are not available in the United States.

Primary prevention of scabies is best achieved with good hygiene habits, personal cleanliness, and routine washing of clothing and bed linens. Secondary prevention includes identification and treatment of infected people and possibly their household and sexual contacts. In an epidemic situation, simultaneous treatment of all affected people and their contacts may be necessary. This is followed by thorough cleansing of the environment (e.g., boiling clothing and linens) and ongoing surveillance to prevent recurrence.

Human Follicle Mites

Physiology and Structure

The human follicle mites include two species of the genus *Demodex, D. folliculorum* and *D. brevis.* These mites are minute (0.1 to 0.4 mm) organisms with a wormlike body, four pairs of stubby legs, and an annulate abdomen. *D. folliculorum* parasitizes the hair follicles of the face of most adult humans, whereas *D. brevis* is found in the sebaceous glands of the head and trunk.

Epidemiology

Organisms of the *Demodex* genus are obligate parasites of the human integument and are cosmopolitan in their distribution. Infestations are uncommon in young children and increase at the time of puberty. It is estimated that 50% to 100% of adults are infested with these mites.

Clinical Syndromes

The role of *Demodex* spp. in human disease is uncertain. They have been associated with acne, blackheads, blepharitis, abnormalities of the scalp, and truncal rashes. More recently, extensive papular folliculitis resulting from *Demodex* infestation has been described in people with acquired immunodeficiency syndrome. Factors such as poor personal hygiene, increased sebum production, mite hypersensitivity, and immunosuppression may increase host susceptibility and enhance the clinical presentation of *Demodex* infestation (Clinical Case 78-1). Most people infested with these mites remain asymptomatic.

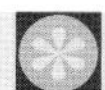
Clinical Case 78-1 *Demodex* Folliculitis

Antille and colleagues (*Arch Dermatol* 140:457–460, 2004) reported a case of *Demodex* folliculitis in a 49-year-old man. The patient had rosacea for 12 years and presented with telangiectatic and papular rosacea on the cheeks and forehead. His condition had progressively deteriorated in spite of intermittent systemic treatments with ciprofloxacin. Six months previously, the patient had stopped all treatments except antihypertensive and antiuricemic therapies. An alternating treatment with clindamycin solution and 0.03% tacrolimus ointment once daily was initially effective and well tolerated. Three weeks later, however, he experienced an acute flare with intense erythema and extensive pustulation. A pustular smear revealed an abundance of *Demodex* mites, which were also seen in a biopsy specimen that confirmed the diagnosis of rosacea. Tacrolimus treatment was discontinued, and the flare resolved rapidly with systemic ciprofloxacin therapy. Ciprofloxacin therapy was stopped 1 month later, and there was no relapse during an 11-month follow-up. This case is an example of a situation in which the immunosuppressive properties of tacrolimus facilitated the overgrowth of follicular *Demodex* mites, resulting in a pustular dermatitis.

Diagnosis

Mites may be demonstrated microscopically in material expressed from an infested follicle. They may be seen as incidental findings in histologic sections of facial skin.

Treatment

Effective treatment consists of a single application of 1% gamma benzene hexachloride.

Chigger Mites

Physiology and Structure

Chiggers are the larvae of mites of the family Trombiculidae. The adult trombiculid mites infest grass and bushes, and their larvae (i.e., chiggers) attack humans and other vertebrates, producing severe dermatitis. The larvae have three pairs of legs and are covered with characteristic branched, feather-like hairs.

The larvae appear as minute, barely visible, reddish dots attached to the skin, where they use their hooked mouth parts to ingest tissue fluids. Chiggers typically attach to the skin areas where clothing is tight or restricted (e.g., wrists, ankles, armpits, groin, waistline). After feeding, the engorged larvae fall to the ground where they molt and undergo development into nymphs and adults.

Epidemiology

Chiggers that are important in North America include the larvae of *Eutrombicula alfreddugesi* and *Eutrombicula splendens.* In Europe, the important species is the harvest mite, *Trombicula autumnalis.* Chiggers are a particular problem for outdoor enthusiasts such as campers and picnickers. In

Europe and the Americas, they are associated with intensely pruritic lesions; however, in Asia, Australia, and the western Pacific Rim, they serve as vectors of the rickettsial disease scrub typhus or tsutsugamushi fever *(Orientia tsutsugamushi)* (see Table 78-2 and Chapter 34).

Clinical Syndromes

Saliva injected into the skin at the time of mite attachment produces an intense pruritus and dermatitis. The skin lesions appear as small erythematous marks that progress to papules and may persist for weeks. Mite larvae may be visible in the center of the reddened swollen area. The irritation may be so severe that it causes fever and sleep disruption. Secondary bacterial infection of the excoriated lesions may occur.

Treatment, Prevention, and Control

Treatment for dermatitis caused by chiggers is largely symptomatic and consists of antipruritics, antihistamines, and steroids. The use of insect repellents such as *N,N*-9-diethyl-*m*-toluamide (DEET) may be of some help in prevention for persons going into chigger-infested areas.

Ticks

Physiology and Structure

Ticks are bloodsucking ectoparasites of a number of vertebrates, including humans. Ticks are opportunistic rather than host specific and tend to suck blood from a number of large and small animals. Ticks have a four-stage life cycle that includes egg, larva, nymph, and adult. Although the larva, nymph, and adult are all bloodsuckers, it is the adult tick that usually bites humans.

Ticks comprise two large families, the Ixodidae, or hard ticks, and the Argasidae, or soft ticks. Soft ticks have a leathery body that lacks a hard dorsal scutum, and the mouthparts are located ventrally and not visible from above (Figure 78-6). Hard ticks have a hard dorsal plate or scutum, and the mouthparts are clearly visible from above (Figure 78-7). Both hard and soft ticks serve as ectoparasites of humans. Soft ticks differ from hard ticks primarily in their feeding behavior. Soft ticks complete engorgement in a matter of minutes or at most a few hours; hard ticks feed slowly, taking 7 to 9 days to become engorged.

Epidemiology

Ticks are found in wooded and rural areas worldwide. In North America, the important species of hard ticks include *Dermacentor variabilis* (American dog tick), *D. andersoni* (Rocky Mountain wood tick), *Amblyomma americanum* (Lone Star tick), *Rhipicephalus sanguineus* (brown dog tick), and *Ixodes dammini* (deer tick). These ticks are found variably throughout the United States and are important vectors of several infectious diseases, including Rocky Mountain spotted fever (*Dermacentor* spp.), tularemia (*Dermacentor* spp.), Q fever (*Dermacentor* spp.), Lyme disease (*Ixodes* spp.), babesiosis (*Ixodes* spp.), and ehrlichiosis (*D. variabilis* and *A. americanum*) (see Table 78-2). Soft ticks of the genus *Ornithodoros* transmit relapsing fever spirochetes (*Borrelia* spp.) in limited areas in the West (see Table 78-2). In general, people at risk for tick exposure are involved in outdoor activities in wooded areas. Tick exposure may also occur during stays in rural cabins inhabited by small rodents, which commonly serve as hosts for ticks and other ectoparasites.

Clinical Syndromes

Tick bites are generally of minor consequence and are limited to small erythematous papules. More serious consequences of tick bite include the development of a type of paralysis resulting from substances released by ticks during feeding and transmission of a number of rickettsial, bacterial, viral, spirochetal, and protozoan diseases of humans and other animals.

Ticks may attach at any point on the body but typically favor the scalp, hairline, ears, axillae, and groin. The initial bite is usually painless, and the presence of the tick may not be detected for several hours after contact. After the tick has dropped off or has been removed manually, the area may become reddened, painful, and pruritic. The wound may

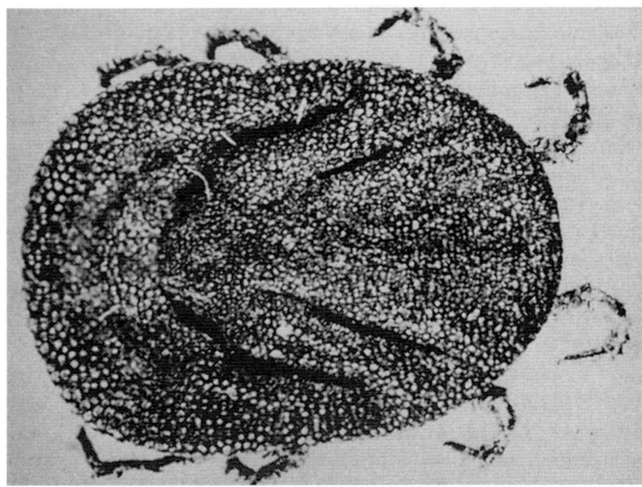

FIGURE 78-6 Soft tick (*Ornithodoros* spp.). (From Strickland GT: *Hunter's tropical medicine,* ed 7, Philadelphia, 1991, Saunders.)

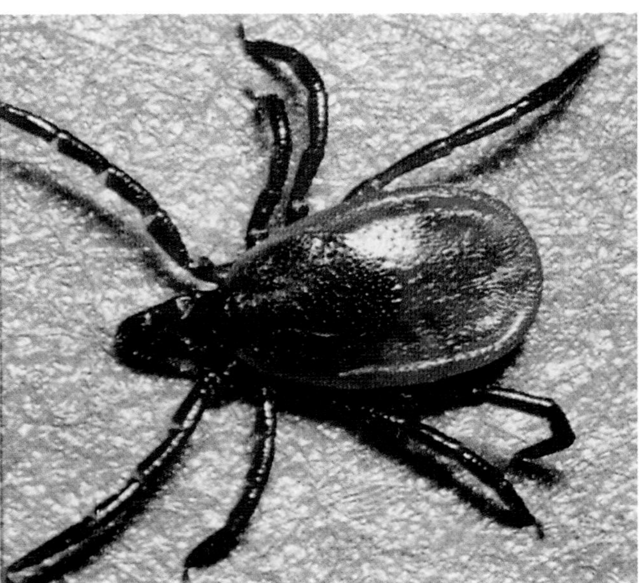

FIGURE 78-7 Hard tick *(Ixodes dammini).* (From Peters W: *A colour atlas of arthropods in clinical medicine,* London, 1992, Wolfe; courtesy Professor A. Spielman.)

 **Clinical Case 78-2 African Tick Bite Fever**

Owen and colleagues (*Arch Dermatol* 142:1312–1314, 2006) described a middle-aged woman who returned from a mission trip to Zimbabwe with an influenza-like illness and an inoculation eschar; she also had a history of travel to a game farm. Biopsy of the cutaneous lesion revealed a histopathologic pattern consistent with an infectious pathogenesis. Immunohistochemical staining confirmed the presence of rickettsial organisms. In light of the patient's history and the clinical constellation of signs and symptoms, a diagnosis of African tick bite fever was made. The patient was treated with doxycycline and had an uncomplicated course.

African tick bite fever is an illness caused by *Rickettsia africae* that has recently emerged as a significant disease among international travelers. The vector is the *Amblyomma* tick, which is endemic to sub-Saharan Africa. This is an example of just one of many rickettsial diseases transmitted by ticks.

become secondarily infected and necrotic requiring antibiotic therapy. It should be noted that upon removal of the tick, the mouthparts often remain imbedded in the skin. Removal of the mouthparts is not critical; they will either be walled off as a foreign body or be worked out in the process of scratching.

Three species of tick, *D. andersoni, D. variabilis,* and *A. americanum,* have been reported to cause **tick paralysis.** This is characterized by an ascending flaccid paralysis, fever, and general intoxication, which may lead to respiratory compromise and death. The paralysis is due to toxic substances released in the saliva of the tick and may be reversed by tick removal. Tick paralysis is observed more commonly in young children and when tick attachment is in opposition to the central nervous system (e.g., scalp, head, neck).

Ticks are also involved in the transmission of infections such as Lyme disease, Rocky Mountain spotted fever, ehrlichiosis, Colorado tick fever, relapsing fever, tularemia, Q fever, and babesiosis (Clinical Case 78-2; see also Table 78-2). The reader is referred to the appropriate sections of this book for discussion of the clinical and microbiological aspects of these infections.

Diagnosis

The diagnosis of tick bites and tick-borne diseases usually rests on the finding of a tick or a history of exposure to tick-infested areas. The identification of an organism as an adult tick is usually straightforward and based on the observations of an organism that is dorsoventrally flattened and possesses four pairs of legs and no visible segmentation (see Figures 78-6 and 78-7). An entomologist or parasitologist should be consulted if further identification is desired. The diagnosis of specific tick-borne infectious diseases is covered in the respective sections of this book.

Treatment, Prevention, and Control

Early removal of attached ticks is of primary importance and may be accomplished by steady traction on the tick body, grasped with forceps as close to the skin as possible. Care should be taken to avoid twisting or crushing the tick, which may leave the mouthparts attached to the skin or inject potentially infectious material into the wound. Steady traction is superior to noxious stimuli or occlusive techniques for the removal of ticks. After removal, the wound should be cleansed and observed for secondary infection. Because ticks may harbor highly infectious agents, the clinician should use appropriate infection-control precautions (e.g., use of gloves, hand washing, proper disposal of ticks and contaminated material) during tick removal. Tick removal is imperative in cases of tick paralysis. Unless the tick is removed, quadriplegia and respiratory paralysis may ensue; the case fatality rate without tick removal approaches 10%. Complete recovery generally is seen within 48 hours of removal.

Preventive measures used in tick-infested areas include wearing protective clothing that fits snugly about the ankles, wrists, waist, and neck so that ticks cannot gain access to the skin. Insect repellents such as DEET are generally effective. People and pets should be inspected for ticks after visits to tick-infested areas.

• Hexapoda (Insecta)

The insects, or **hexapods,** constitute the largest and most important of all the classes of arthropods, accounting for approximately 70% of all known species of animals. Insects include mosquitoes, flies, fleas, lice, roaches, bees, wasps, beetles, and moths, to name just a few. The insect body is divided into three parts—head, thorax, and abdomen—and is equipped with one pair of antennae, three pairs of appendages, and one or two pairs of wings or no wings at all. The medical significance of any insect is related to its way of life, particularly its mouthparts and feeding habits. Insects may serve as vectors for a number of bacterial, viral, protozoan, and metazoan pathogens. Certain insects may serve merely as mechanical vectors for the transmission of pathogens, whereas in other insects, the pathogens undergo multiplication or cyclic development within the insect host. The methods by which the insects transmit pathogens vary and are discussed here. Insects can also be pathogens themselves by causing mechanical injury through bites, chemical injury through the injection of toxins, and allergic reactions to materials transmitted by bites or stings. There are more than 30 orders of insects, but only those of major medical importance are discussed in this section.

Bloodsucking Diptera

Diptera is the large order of flying insects. All dipterans have a single pair of functional membranous wings and various modifications of the mouthparts, which have been adapted for piercing the skin and sucking blood or tissue juices. Their most important feature is their role as mechanical or biological vectors of a number of infectious diseases, including leishmaniasis, trypanosomiasis, malaria, filariasis, onchocerciasis, tularemia, bartonellosis, and the viral encephalitides (see Table 78-2). The bloodsucking flies include mosquitoes, sandflies, and blackflies, all of which are capable of transmitting diseases to humans. Other dipterans, such as horseflies and stableflies, are capable of inflicting painful bites but are not known to transmit human pathogens. Although the common housefly does not bite, it certainly is capable of mechanical transmission of a number of viral, bacterial, and protozoan infections to human hosts. The infectious diseases transmitted by bloodsucking flies are well covered in other chapters of this book. The following section deals only with injury resulting from the bite of these insects and the effects of salivary substances introduced into the human skin and tissues.

Mosquitoes

Physiology and Structure

Adult mosquitoes are small and have delicate legs, one pair of wings, long antennae, and greatly elongated mouthparts adapted for piercing and sucking. The two major subfamilies of mosquitoes (Culicidae family), the Anophelinae and the Culicinae, share a number of similarities in their life cycles and development. They lay eggs on or near water, are good fliers, and feed on nectar and sugars. The females of most species also feed on blood, which they require for each clutch of 100 to 200 eggs. Females may take a blood meal every 2 to 4 days. In the act of feeding, the female mosquito injects saliva that produces mechanical damage to the host but also may transmit disease and produce immediate and delayed immune reactions.

Epidemiology

Within the subfamily Anophelinae, the genus *Anopheles* contains the species responsible for transmission of human malaria. In the tropics, these mosquitoes breed continually in relation to rainfall. These species vary in their capacity for the transmission of malaria, and within each geographic area, the number of species that serve as malaria vectors is small. *Anopheles gambiae* is an important vector of malaria in sub-Saharan Africa.

Mosquitoes from *Aedes,* the largest genus of the subfamily Culicinae, are found in all habitats, ranging from the tropics to the Arctic. This species may develop overwhelming populations in marshes, tundra, pasture, or floodwater and have a severe impact on wildlife, livestock, and humans. *Aedes aegypti,* the yellow fever mosquito, usually breeds in man-made containers (flowerpots, gutters, cans) and is the primary vector of yellow fever and dengue in urban environments throughout the world.

Clinical Syndromes

Mechanical damage induced by the feeding mosquito is usually minor but may be accompanied by mild pain and irritation. The bite is usually followed within a few minutes by a small flat weal surrounded by a red flare. The delayed reaction consists of itching, swelling, and reddening of the wound region. Secondary infection may follow as a result of scratching.

Treatment, Prevention, and Control

Medical attention is usually not sought for a bite unless secondary infection occurs. Local anesthetics or antihistamines may be useful in treating reactions to mosquito bites.

Preventive measures in mosquito-infested areas include use of window screens, netting, and protective clothing. Insect repellents such as DEET are generally effective. Mosquito-control measures that involve use of insecticides have been effective in some areas.

Gnats and Biting Midges

Physiology and Structure

Ceratopogonids represent an assortment of tiny flies such as **gnats, midges,** and **punkies.** The majority of the flies that attack humans belong to the genus *Culicoides;* they are minute (0.5 to 4 mm long) and slender enough to pass through the fine mesh of ordinary window screens. The females suck blood and typically feed at dusk, when they may attack in large numbers.

Epidemiology

Biting midges may be important pests in beach and resort areas near salt marshes. Those of the genus *Culicoides* are the main vectors of filariasis in Africa and the New World tropics.

Clinical Syndromes

The mouthparts of biting midges are lancet like and produce a painful bite. Bites may produce local lesions lasting hours or days.

Treatment, Prevention, and Control

Local treatment is palliative, with lotions, anesthetics, and antiseptic measures. The treatment of breeding sites with pesticides and repellents may be useful against some of the common species of these pests.

Sandflies

Physiology and Structure

Sandflies, or mothflies, belong to a single subfamily of the Psychodidae, the Phlebotominae. They are small (1 to 3 mm), delicate, hairy, weak-flying insects that suck the blood of humans, dogs, and rodents. They transmit a number of infections, including leishmaniasis (see Table 78-2). Female flies become infected when they feed on infected people.

Epidemiology

Phlebotomine larvae develop in nonaquatic habitats such as moist soil, stone walls, and rubbish heaps. In many areas, sandflies cause problems as pests. They also serve as vectors of infectious diseases such as leishmaniasis in the Mediterranean, the Middle East, Asia, and Latin America.

Clinical Syndromes

The bite may be painful and pruritic around the local lesion. Sensitized people may have allergic reactions. **Sandfly fever** is characterized by severe frontal headaches, malaise, retro-orbital pain, anorexia, and nausea.

Treatment, Prevention, and Control

Sandflies are very sensitive to insecticides, which should be applied to breeding sites and window screens. Various insect repellents may also be useful.

Blackflies

Physiology and Structure

Members of the family Simuliidae are commonly called **blackflies** or **buffalo gnats.** They are 1 to 5 mm long, hump-backed, and have mouthparts consisting of six "blades" that are capable of tearing skin (Figure 78-8). Blackflies are bloodsucking insects and breed in fast-flowing streams and rivers. They are of major importance as vectors of onchocerciasis (see Table 78-2).

Epidemiology

Blackflies are common in Africa and South America, where they serve as vectors of onchocerciasis. In North America,

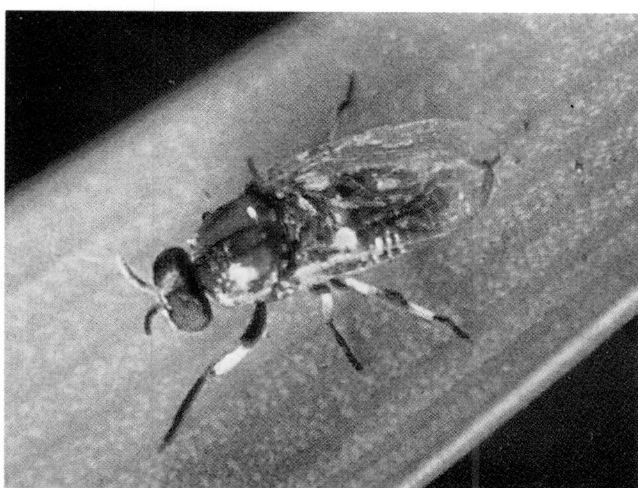

FIGURE 78-8 Blackfly (*Simulium* spp.), the vector of onchocerciasis. (From Peters W: *A colour atlas of arthropods in clinical medicine,* London, 1992, Wolfe; courtesy Dr. S. Meredith.)

they are common around the lake regions of Canada and the northern United States. They are pests to hunters and fisherman in these areas. In large numbers, they may cause significant blood loss and pose a major threat to wild and domestic animals.

Clinical Syndromes

A variety of responses have been observed in humans after the bite of blackflies. The bite of the female can tear the skin surface and induce bleeding that continues for some time after the fly has departed. There is usually a distinct hemorrhagic spot at the site of the bite. Multiple bites may result in considerable blood loss. The bite is painful and accompanied by local inflammation, itching, and swelling.

The local reaction may also be accompanied by a systemic response that varies according to the number of bites and the sensitivity of the person. This syndrome is known as **blackfly fever** and is marked by headache, fever, and adenitis. It usually subsides within 48 hours and is considered a hypersensitivity reaction to the salivary secretions of the fly.

In addition to local and systemic responses to blackfly bites, a **hemorrhagic syndrome** has been described after bites of blackflies in certain areas of Brazil. This syndrome resembles thrombocytopenic purpura and is characterized by local and disseminated cutaneous hemorrhages associated with mucosal bleeding. It is thought that this hemorrhagic syndrome may be produced by a hypersensitivity phenomenon or response to a toxin caused by multiple blackfly bites.

Diagnosis

The blackfly bite is marked characteristically by a point of dried blood and subcutaneous hemorrhage at the wound site. In people with the hemorrhagic syndrome, platelet counts are reduced; there is a prolonged bleeding time and poor clot retraction in about half of patients.

Treatment, Prevention, and Control

Treatment includes the usual palliative measures (e.g., anesthetics, antihistamines, lotions) to relieve local pruritus and swelling. Patients with the hemorrhagic syndrome have shown marked improvement with corticosteroid therapy.

Preventive measures include protective clothing. In general, insect repellents are ineffective against blackflies. Some control is achieved by pouring insecticides into rivers and streams.

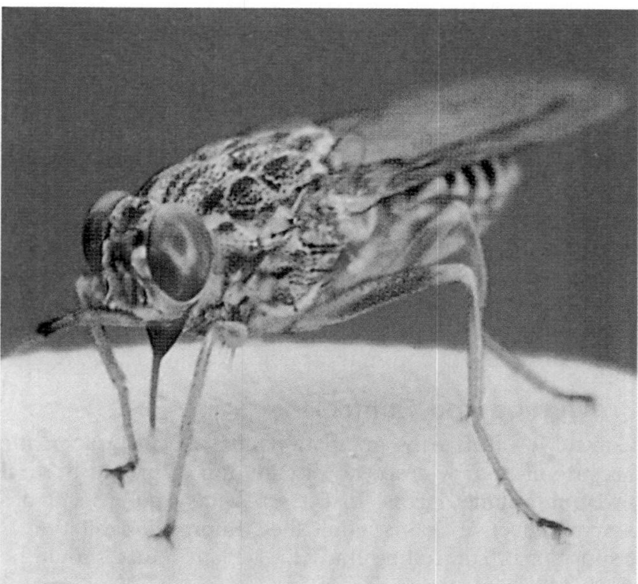

FIGURE 78-9 Tsetse fly, the vector of African trypanosomiasis. (From Peters W: *A colour atlas of arthropods in clinical medicine,* London, 1992, Wolfe; courtesy Wellcome Foundation, Berkhamsted, England.)

Horseflies and Deerflies

The family Tabanidae consists of species including horseflies, deerflies, gadflies, and mangoflies that attack mainly animals. They are large, ranging in length from 7 to 30 mm. The males feed on plant juices, the females on blood. In the act of biting, the female fly leaves a deep wound, causing blood to flow, which the fly laps up. The fly may serve as a mechanical vector of infectious diseases when the fly's mouthparts become contaminated on one host and transfer organisms to the next. These flies are not considered important vectors of infectious disease in humans.

Muscoid Flies

Physiology and Structure

The muscoid flies include three medically important insects: the housefly, *Musca domestica;* the stablefly, *Stomoxys calcitrans;* and the **tsetse flies** of the genus *Glossina.* The stablefly, often mistaken for the housefly, is a true bloodsucker capable of serving as a short-term mechanical vector of a number of bacterial, viral, and protozoal infections. The tsetse fly (Figure 78-9) is also a biting fly and serves as the biological vector and intermediate host for the agents of African trypanosomiasis, *Trypanosoma brucei rhodesiense* and *T. b. gambiense.* The common housefly represents a host of genera that are nonpiercing or contaminating flies. Because of their living and feeding habits, they mechanically transmit diverse agents to humans.

Epidemiology

The tsetse fly is found in the eastern and central regions of Africa, where it is of major medical and veterinary importance as the intermediate host and biological vector of a number of trypanosomes that infect humans and animals. The housefly and stablefly are cosmopolitan in distribution and serve as indicators of poor sanitation. The housefly, *M. domestica,* lays eggs on any matter (feces, garbage, decaying plant matter) that will serve as food for developing fly larvae (maggots). Stableflies commonly lay eggs in moist, decaying vegetable matter such as grass clippings or compost heaps found in suburban communities.

Prevention and Control

Control of tsetse fly populations has been problematic because of their widespread distribution in primarily rural and undeveloped areas. Insect repellents and insecticides may be effective against adult flies. Improved sanitation is important in controlling houseflies. Plant refuse should be protected from rain or destroyed.

Myiasis-Causing Flies

Myiasis is the term applied to the disease produced by maggots that live parasitically in human tissues. Clinically, myiasis may be classified according to the body part involved (e.g., nasal, intestinal, or urinary myiasis). The number of myiasis-producing flies and the diversity in lifestyle requirements are enormous. Only the host relations and sites of predilection of some of the more important species are covered in this section.

Specific myiasis refers to myiasis caused by flies that require a host for larval development. One important example is the human botfly, *Dermatobia hominis,* which is found in the humid regions of Mexico and Central and South America. The adult botfly attaches her eggs to the abdomen of blood-sucking flies or mosquitoes, which in turn distribute the eggs while obtaining a blood meal from an animal or human. The larvae enter the skin through the wound created by the biting insect. The larvae develop over 40 to 50 days, during which time a painful lesion known as a **warble** appears (Clinical Case 78-3). When the larvae reach maturity, they leave the host to pupate. The resulting lesion may take weeks to months to heal and may become secondarily infected. If the larva dies before leaving the skin, an abscess forms.

Semispecific myiasis is caused by flies that normally lay their eggs on decaying animal or plant matter; it develops in a host if entry is facilitated by the presence of wounds or sores. Representatives of this group include the greenbottle fly, *Phaenicia;* bluebottle flies, *Cochliomyia;* and blackbottle flies, *Phormia.* These flies are worldwide in distribution, and their presence is encouraged by poor sanitation. They occasionally lay their eggs on the open sores or wounds of animals and humans. Another group that causes myiasis in humans is the flesh flies, or sarcophagids. These flies have a worldwide distribution and normally breed in decomposing matter. They may deposit their larvae on foods that if ingested may serve as a source of infection.

Flies that produce **accidental myiasis** have no requirement for development in a host. Accidental infection may occur when eggs are deposited on oral or genitourinary openings and the resulting larvae gain entry into the intestinal or genitourinary tract. Flies that may produce accidental myiasis include *M. domestica,* the common housefly.

Sucking Lice

Physiology and Structure

Although several species of lice *(Anoplura)* infest humans as blood-feeding parasites, only the body louse is important in medicine as the vector of the rickettsia of typhus and trench fevers and the vector of the spirochetes of relapsing fever (see Table 78-2). The **body louse,** *Pediculus humanus,* and the **head louse,** *P. humanus capitis,* are elongated, wingless, flattened insects with three pairs of legs and mouthpieces adapted for piercing flesh and sucking blood (Figure 78-10). The pubic or **crab louse,** *Phthirus pubis,* has a short crablike abdomen with clawed second and third legs (Figure 78-11).

 **Clinical Case 78-3 Furuncular Myiasis**

Bakos and colleagues (*Arch Dermatol* 143:123–124, 2007) described a 54-year-old woman who was seen with a 2-week history of a painful inflammatory nodule on the inner aspect of her right leg. She vaguely remembered having been bitten in that area by a "bug." After 1 week of oral antibiotic treatment prescribed to relieve the surrounding inflammatory reaction, a poorly delimited nodule was observed, with a small pore on top from which a serosanguineous fluid exuded. Dermoscopy revealed a central opening surrounded by dilated blood vessels from which a yellowish structure with black barblike spines on the extremity extruded intermittently. This corresponded to the posterior extremity of *Dermatobia hominis* (human botfly) larva. The lesion was occluded with a double layer of plaster for 24 hours, and the immobile dead larva was removed with forceps and gentle squeezing. Furuncular myiasis caused by *D. hominis* is a common disease in tropical American countries. The diagnosis of furuncular myiasis should always be considered in every boil-like lesion not responding to ordinary treatment, especially in travelers returning from tropical countries.

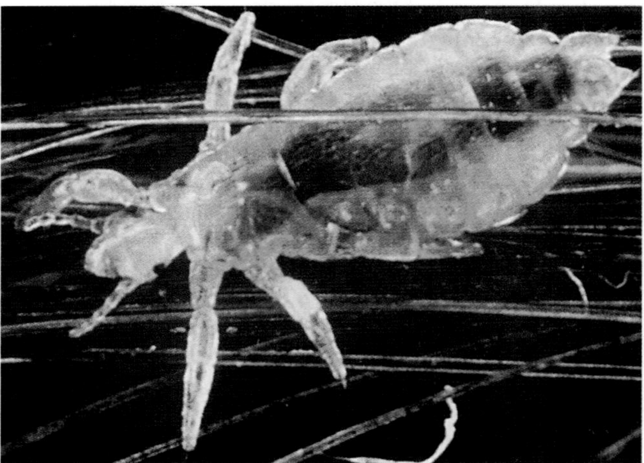

FIGURE 78-10 Body louse *(Pediculus humanus).* (From Peters W: *A colour atlas of arthropods in clinical medicine,* London, 1992, Wolfe; courtesy Oxford Scientific Films [Dr. R.J. Warren].)

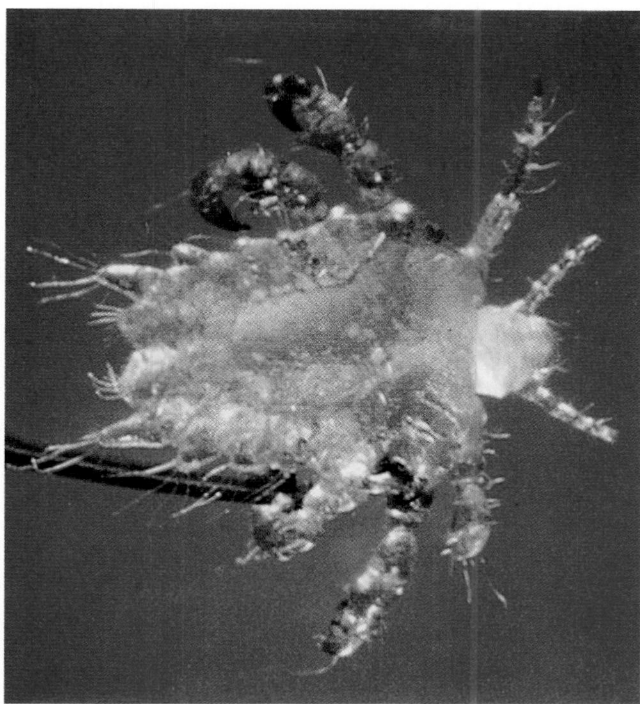

FIGURE 78-11 Crab louse *(Phthirus pubis).* (From Peters W: *A colour atlas of arthropods in clinical medicine,* London, 1992, Wolfe; courtesy Dr. R.V. Southcott.)

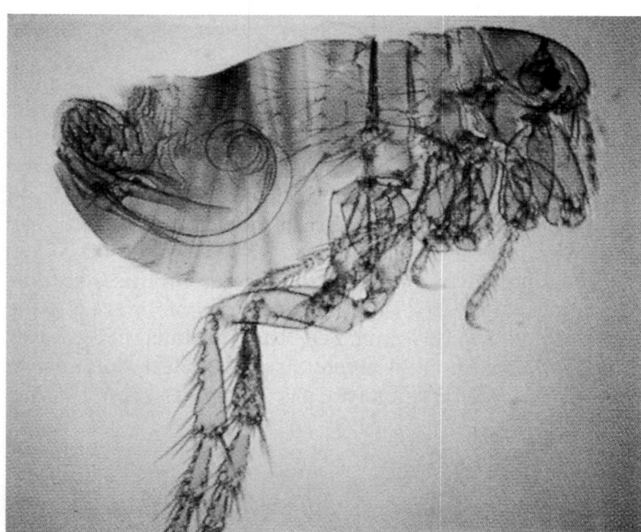

FIGURE 78-12 Flea. (From Peters W, Pasvol G: *Color atlas of tropical medicine and parasitology,* ed 6, London, 2007, Mosby.)

Epidemiology

Epidemics of head lice are reported frequently in the United States, particularly among schoolchildren. The head lice inhabit the hairs of the head and are transmitted by physical contact or sharing of hair brushes or hats. Crab lice survive on blood meals around the hairs of the pubic and perianal areas of the body. They are transmitted frequently from one person to another by sexual contact and contaminated toilet seats or clothing. Body lice are usually found on clothing. Unlike head or crab lice, they move to the body for feeding and return to the clothing after obtaining a blood meal. All of the lice inject salivary fluids into the body during the ingestion of blood, which causes varying degrees of sensitization in the human host.

Clinical Syndromes

Intense itching is the usual characteristic of infestation by lice **(pediculosis).** The patient may have pruritic red papules around the ears, face, neck, or shoulders. Secondary infection and regional adenopathy may be present.

Diagnosis

The diagnosis is made by demonstration of the lice or eggs from a patient complaining of pruritus. Frequently the patient has noticed the insects, and the diagnosis may be made over the telephone. The eggs, or **nits,** are white round objects that may be found attached to the hair shafts (head and crab lice) or on clothing (body lice).

Treatment, Prevention, and Control

Gamma benzene hexachloride (lindane) lotion applied to the entire body and left on for 24 hours is an effective treatment for lice. Shaving the hair of affected areas is a desirable adjunct. Adult lice in clothing must be destroyed by the application of lindane or dichlorodiphenyltrichloroethane (DDT) powder or by boiling. Lice may survive in the environment for up to 2 weeks; thus items such as brushes, combs, and bedding must be treated with a pediculicide or by boiling.

The best strategy for primary prevention is education and practice of good hygiene habits. Secondary prevention may be practiced by a policy of routine surveillance (e.g., scalp inspections) in schools, day-care centers, military camps, and other institutions. Repellents may be necessary for people who run a high risk of exposure in crowded conditions.

Fleas

Physiology and Structure

Fleas *(Siphonaptera)* are small wingless insects with laterally compressed bodies and long legs adapted for jumping (Figure 78-12). Their mouthparts are adapted for sucking or "siphoning" blood from the host.

Epidemiology

Fleas are cosmopolitan in distribution. Most species are adapted to a particular host; however, they can readily feed on humans, particularly when deprived of their preferred host. Fleas are important as vectors of plague and murine typhus and as intermediate hosts for dog *(Dipylidium caninum)* and rodent (*Hymenolepis* spp.) tapeworms that occasionally infect humans.

In contrast to the majority of fleas that do not invade the human integument, the **chigoe flea,** *Tunga penetrans,* may cause considerable damage by actively invading the skin. The female chigoe flea burrows into the skin, often under the toenails or between the toes, where she sucks blood and lays her eggs. The chigoe flea is found in tropical and subtropical regions of America, as well as in Africa and the Far East. It is not known to transmit human pathogens.

Clinical Syndromes

As with the bites of other bloodsucking arthropods, flea bites result in pruritic erythematous lesions of varying severity, which depends on the intensity of the infestation and the sensitivity of the bitten person. The irritation caused by the flea's saliva may produce physical findings that vary from small red welts to a diffuse red rash. Secondary infection may be a complication.

Cutaneous invasion by the chigoe flea produces an erythematous papule that is painful and pruritic. Infested tissue can become severely inflamed and ulcerated. Secondary infection is common. In severe cases, the infestation may be complicated by tetanus or gas gangrene, resulting in amputation.

Diagnosis

The diagnosis of flea infestation is inferred in a patient with annoying bites who is also a pet (dog or cat) owner. Examination of the patient and pet usually reveals the characteristic insect. Diagnosis of tungiasis is made by detecting the dark portion of the chigoe flea's abdomen as it protrudes from the skin surface in the center of an inflamed lesion.

Treatment, Prevention, and Control

Palliative treatment with antipruritics and antihistamines is indicated for most flea bites. Surgical removal of the chigoe flea is indicated.

Commercially available insecticides may control fleas at the source. Topically applied repellents can protect people against flea bites. Flea collars or powders on pets are also effective preventive measures.

Bugs

Physiology and Structure

Bugs refer specifically to two bloodsucking insects, the **bedbug** and the **triatomid bug** (Figures 78-13 and 78-14). Both bugs are characterized by a long proboscis that is folded ventrally under the body when not in use. The bedbug *(Cimex lectularius)* is a reddish brown insect approximately 4 to 5 mm long. It has short wing pads but cannot fly. The triatomid, or **"kissing" bug,** has yellow or orange markings on the body and an elongated head. Triatomid bugs have wings and are aerial.

Epidemiology

Both bedbugs and triatomid bugs are nocturnal and feed indiscriminately on most mammals. Bedbugs are cosmopolitan in distribution, whereas triatomid bugs are limited to the Americas. Bedbugs hide during the day in cracks and crevices of wooden furniture, under loose wallpaper, in the tufts of mattresses, and in box springs. Triatomid bugs live in the cracks and crevices of walls and in thatched roofs. Bedbugs do not play a role in the transmission of human disease; however, triatomid bugs are important vectors of Chagas disease (see Table 78-2 and Chapter 74).

Clinical Syndromes

The bites of bedbugs and triatomid bugs produce lesions that range from small red marks to hemorrhagic bullae. Bedbugs tend to bite in linear fashion on the trunk and arms, whereas triatomid bugs bite with higher frequency on the face. The classic periorbital edema secondary to a triatomid bite is known as the **Romaña sign.** The intensity of reaction to a bite depends on the degree of sensitization of the patient. In addition to causing local lesions, repeated exposure to bedbug bites may (rarely) lead to anaphylactic reactions or more often be associated with nervous disorders and sleeplessness in children and adults.

Diagnosis

The pattern and location of bites suggest bedbugs or triatomid bugs. The detection of tiny spots of blood on bedding or the dead insects themselves is frequently the first sign of bedbug infestation.

Treatment, Prevention, and Control

Topical palliatives are appropriate for the relief of pruritus. Antihistamines may be indicated if dermatitis is severe. Control consists of proper hygiene and environmental applications of insecticides. Control of bedbug infestations has become more challenging owing to the development of resistance to commonly used insecticides.

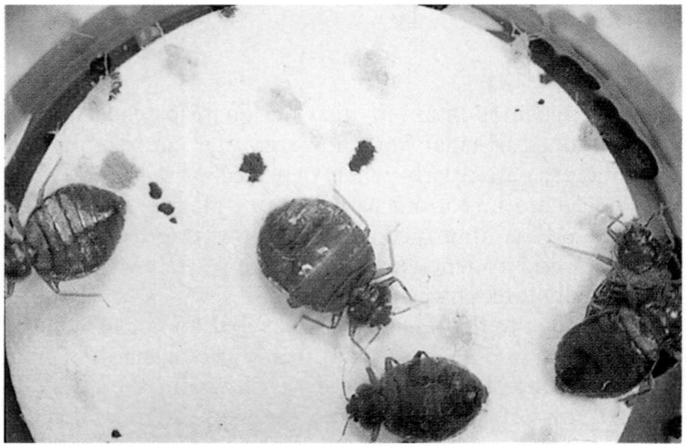

FIGURE 78-13 Bedbug *(Cimex lectularius)*. (From Peters W, Pasvol G: *Color atlas of tropical medicine and parasitology,* ed 6, London, 2007, Mosby.)

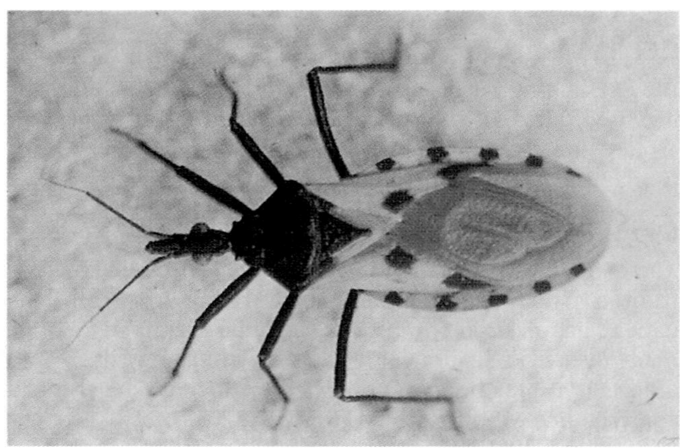

FIGURE 78-14 Triatomid bug. (From Peters W: *A colour atlas of arthropods in clinical medicine,* London, 1992, Wolfe; courtesy Dr. D. Minter.)

Stinging Insects

Physiology and Structure

The order Hymenoptera comprises bees, wasps, hornets, and ants. The modified ovipositor of the female, the apparatus for egg laying, serves as a stinging organ and is used for defense or to capture prey for food. Members of Hymenoptera are known for their complex social systems, castes, and elaborate hive or nest structures.

Epidemiology

Of the hymenopterans, the bees (Apidae) live in complex social organizations such as hives or in less structured underground nests. Only honeybees and bumblebees are of concern to humans because of their ability to sting. The Vespidae include wasps, hornets, and yellow jackets; all are aggressive insects and a major cause of stings in humans. In the act of stinging, the aroused insect inserts the sheath to open the wound. The thrust of the stylets and injection of venom immediately follow.

One group of ants of concern in the United States is the **fire ant,** *Solenopsis invicta.* Fire ants are particularly common in the southeastern states. They are well camouflaged in large hard-crusted mounds and attack when disturbed. They bite their victim with strong mandibles and then sting repeatedly.

Clinical Syndromes

An estimated 50 to 100 people die each year in the United States from reactions to stings of the hymenopterans. Severe toxic reactions, such as fever and muscle cramps, can be caused by as few as 10 stings. Allergic reactions are the most serious consequence, but others include pain, edema, pruritus, and a heat sensation at the site of the sting. Anaphylactic shock from bee stings has resulted in death in some instances.

Treatment, Prevention, and Control

No satisfactory treatment has been discovered for stings. If left in the wound, the sting apparatus should be removed immediately. Injection of epinephrine is sometimes necessary to counteract anaphylaxis (emergency kits are available by prescription for sensitive people). For relief of local discomfort, calamine lotion or a topical corticosteroid cream for more severe local lesions is helpful.

Although there are no effective repellents against these insects, their nests can be destroyed with any of several commercially available insecticidal compounds. General avoidance of areas inhabited by hymenopterans is advised for sensitive people.

Bibliography

Binford CH, Connor DH: *Pathology of tropical and extraordinary diseases*, Washington, DC, 1976, Armed Forces Institute of Pathology.

Hwang SW, Svoboda TJ, De Jong IJ, et al: Bed bug infestations in an urban environment, *Emerg Infect Dis* 11:533–537, 2005.

John DT, Petri WA Jr: *Markell and Voge's medical parasitology*, ed 9, St Louis, 2006, Saunders.

Najarian HH: *Textbook of medical parasitology*, Baltimore, 1967, Williams & Wilkins.

Peters W: *A colour atlas of arthropods in clinical medicine*, London, 1992, Wolfe.

Strickland GT: *Hunter's tropical medicine and emerging infectious diseases*, ed 8, Philadelphia, 2000, Saunders.

Swanson DL, Vetter RS: Bites of brown recluse spiders and suspected necrotic arachnidism, *N Engl J Med* 352:700–707, 2005.

Telford SR: Arthropods of medical importance. In Versalovic J, et al, editors: *Manual of clinical microbiology*, ed 10, Washington, DC, 2011, American Society for Microbiology Press.

Van Horn KG, Tatz JS, Li KI, et al: Copepods associated with a perirectal abscess and copepod pseudo-outbreaks in stools for ova and parasite examinations, *Diagn Microbiol Infect Dis* 15:561–565, 1992.

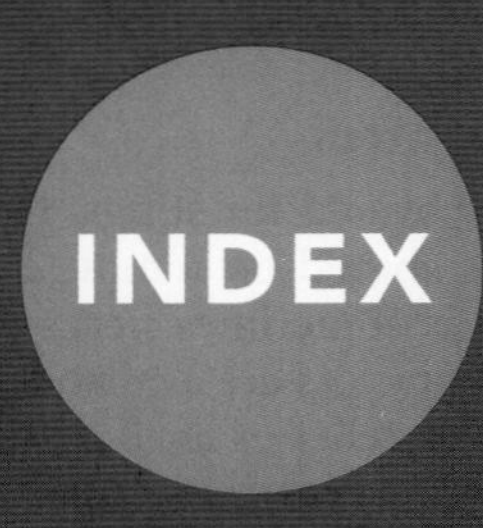

INDEX

Note: Page numbers followed by *f* indicate figures; *b*, boxes; *t*, tables.

D

E

J

K

T

U

V